GREGORY'S

Textbook Of Farriery

By
Chris Gregory
CJF, FWCF

GREGORY'S TEXTBOOK OF FARRIERY
CHRIS GREGORY, 2011

Heartland Horseshoeing School
327 SW 1st Lane
Lamar, MO. 64759 USA
heartlandhorseshoeing.com
Email: anvil@earthlink.net

First Published in the United States of America in 2011

ISBN
Library of Congress Control Number:
978-0-9833140-1-1

Editor:
Pat Tierney

Layout Design:
Christopher Nielsen

Printed by:
Walsworth Publishing Company, Inc., Marceline, Missouri, USA

Published by:
Heartland Horseshoeing School, Inc. Lamar, Missouri, USA

Printed in the USA

NOTICE:
The art and practice of farriery, in all its forms, is an ancient craft that continues to evolve. What is presented in this text has worked for the Gregory family, and the horses they have worked on, for many years. However, every horse and every situation is not only dangerous, but also variable. The author accepts no liability in the application of any of the techniques described in this work. Unfortunately, in a litigious society such as ours, a disclaimer like this has to be added. Use your head and apply good horse sense.

DEDICATION:

This work is dedicated to my soul mate,
fellow farrier, educator, and outstanding wife and mother;
Kelly Gregory, CF.

Also:
Cody Gregory, CJF, and **Jacquelyn Gregory**.
My kids are my inspiration to get out of bed every morning.

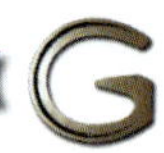

FORWARD

Years ago, there came a request for a response to a survey. The letter asked for information regarding the business or some other aspect of farriery, the exact topics I have long since forgotten, but included in the envelope was a packet of coffee and an invitation to "have a cup on me while you're responding to the questions." My first reaction was, "This guy doesn't do anything halfway." The college student who sent the survey was Chris Gregory.

Today, more than two decades later, that first impression still proves to be accurate. It will become apparent to the readers of this book that Chris does not do anything halfway.

Chris has shod horses and given clinics on at least four continents and has experienced many different shoeing disciplines while being involved with many different breeds and their hoof care needs. His extensive travels across North America and around the world have made him one of the most recognized names in the farrier industry. Chris has received many accolades from his peers; Outstanding Clinician and Educator of the Year are just a few of the many awards he has earned over the years.

Gregory's Textbook of Farriery encompasses all aspects of the art and science of farriery, even some helpful information on starting a business or developing skills as a teacher of farriery.

While the horse and its anatomy have changed very little over the centuries, our understanding of biomechanics and methods of treatment have progressed tremendously recently due to more scientific equine studies and the rapid exchange of ideas among the world's practitioners. Chris has had a major role in this new age of information through his many trade magazine articles, his onsite clinics, his school for horseshoeing, and now, this book.

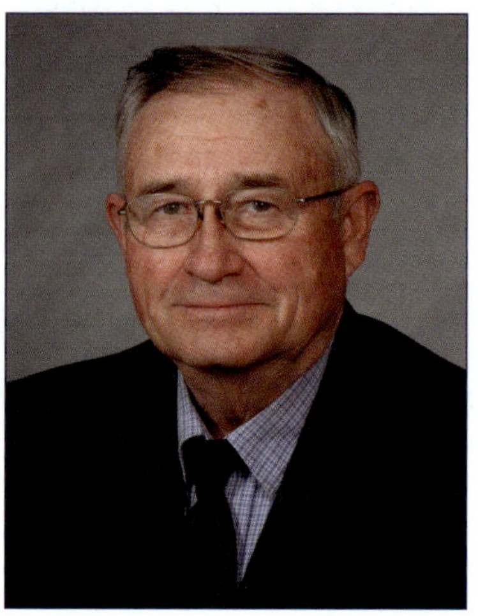

Beginning and advanced practitioner alike, as well as instructors of farriery, will find this book a great reference as will all students of the horse.

— Jim Keith, Tucumcari, NM

Jim Keith, CJF, has over 51 years experience in the farriery and blacksmithing world. He is a member of the International Horseshoeing Hall Of Fame in 1994 and was recognized as a "Farrier Industry Legend" in 2000. He is widely recognized as one of horseshoeing's top practitioners, educators and competitors. As a "self-taught" farrier, he recognizes the difficulties of "going it alone" and strongly supports all aspects of farrier education. He currently manufactures his own line of quality tools in Tucumcari, NM

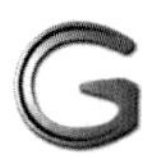

INTRODUCTION

It is hard for me to believe that this book has finally happened. This has been a long and wonderful process, and it is with joy and sorrow that I type the last of it.

I have a multitude to thank, as does any farrier who has taken this trade as far as they can. First and foremost is my wife, business partner, fellow farrier, and educator, Kelly Gregory, CF. She had the patience to allow me to forge, read, travel, write, practice, associate, and spend time with other farriers. A lot of family time was lost to the farrier trade, and I thank her for her vision of the potential. I have to thank my folks, Mike and Diana Gregory for providing my first opportunities as a farrier. There is also my son, Cody, an AFA Journeyman by the age of 15, who pushes me constantly in this craft. Cody had his DipWCF by the age of 17, and was an Associate of the Worshipful Company of Farriers by 19. It has been awe inspiring for me to watch him hone his skill and create his place in this trade. I also have an incredible daughter nemed Jacquclyn, an exceptional horsewoman, who gave feedback as I experimented with her horses. She followed a rodeo scholarship to college at McNeese State University, adn continues to train and make great horses.

For my skills, the foremost men that impacted my career are, (in chronological order), Frank Turley, CJF, Jim Poor, CJF, Ray Helmbold, CJF, Grant Moon, AWCF, Danny Ward, CJF, Kevin Hatridge, CJF, Jim Keith, CJF, Dave Showen, CJF, Bob Marshall, RSS, Ivon Bell, FWCF, Sandy Beveridge, FWCF, and Derek Gardener, AWCF. I have sat at the feet of masters, and from them I took what I was able. They make up a phenomenal group of farrier elite.

I didn't take any photos of my first 10 years of shoeing. A bad mistake because there was so much missed that would have helped some beginner avoid the mistakes that I made as a beginner. Since 1997, I have been taking pictures of any interesting foot I came across, to the tune of about 30,000 pictures. Thank you so much Melissa "Sunny" Malandrinos for categorizing them so that this book could actually happen. Sunny was a student that had to take a break from school, and asked for a project to pass the time. A request she often regretted as every surface of her home became a collage of horses' feet in photos. There are pictures in this work that have been taken by many different individuals. Some were taken by the student or customer who just happened to be standing by. Many were taken by Cody Gregory, CJF, AWCF, and a few were snapped by me.

A picture has to look like what it is depicting, so a hock is a hock is a hock, and the drawings in here are what the bones look like. In many instances, we drew from the actual bones sitting in front of us. The drawings in this book are completely orginal, and drawn either by Cody or myself, and you can easily distinguish which, as his are better than mine. However, they should all get the message across, which is the main purpose behind drawing them in the first place.

The content of this book is patially based upon the work of Dr. Doug Butler, whose book *The Principles of Horseshoeing II* I used in teaching for oer 12 years. I would like to acknowledge and thank Dr. Butler for his many contributions to the farrier industry. I have been greatly influenced by a lot of writings and books on farriery. Mainly authors like James Rooney, Colonel John Hickman and Martin Humphrey, A. W. Dollar and Albert Wheatley, Professor William Russell, Anton Lungwitz, Simon Curtis, OR Adams, Susan Harris, Jean-Marie Denoix, Hilary Clayton, Doug Butler, Klaus-Dieter Budras, W.O. Sack, Sabine Rock, and others. I did not intentionally have any direct quotes from these fine authors, and where I did, they get full credit.

The first version of this book was edited by Pat Tierney, and one of the smartest men I know named Dr. Mike Miller, MD, CJF, FWCF. Even though they spent hours agonizing over what I had written, ultimately the mistakes herein are mine and mine alone. After the first printing came out, I was amazed at the number of mispellings and small mistakes that were pointed out to me. In stepped Christine Abramo, CF. Christine is a professional of the very highest order when it comes to correcting textbooks, and she graciously went through this book. She dipped one in red ink and sent it back to me, and I have made the corrections that I could. I can never repay her immense generosity, and I would highly recommend her services if you ever write a textbook. A graduate of Heartland Horseshoeing School named Shearer Wludyka was instrumental in helping me learn how to use the software this book is laid out in, and I would like to thank her as well. Marie Leginus, CJF, from British Columbia did a lot of reading and mistake correcting. It was amazing the mistakes she found in what I thought was a final draft. She is a very smart farrier. Alice Musser, and Frank Lessiter were instrumental in getting this thing from computer to paper.

Christopher Nielsen did the outstanding layout. Although not a farrier, his creative ability is superb.

Many years ago, Frank Lessiter, of Lessiter Publications, started to publish some of my articles, and gave me a position as an Editorial Advisor. His trust in me was key to the fact that I ever wrote anything on the subject, so I owe Frank a great debt of gratitude.

Mustad Corporation, in particular Marguerite Paige and Carlos Lara, sponsored me as one of their farrier clinicians, and that trust is also one that I treasure. Through them, I have had opportunities that many farriers would not, which has allowed me a lot of learning.

The Worshipful Company of Farriers and the American Farriers Association have allowed me to rub elbows with some of the greatest farriers in the world, so I thank them as well.

My fellow farriers from around the world have freely provided knowledge, advice, and kinship. I thank the group of rugged, independent, clever, strong, and individual as they come, people who make up this trade. And of course, there is the horse. Without this noble beast, there would be no need of farriers. I have marveled at and been intrigued with this great animal for as long as I can remember, and it has been a true gift to make my living with the horse at the center of it.

Dear Reader, you have my humble thanks for buying this book. If a couple of farriers and their horses benefit from this work, it has been worth it. May you be blessed and prosper in this amazing craft, and continue to add and improve upon this effort, which is only the tip of the iceberg.

— Chris Gregory, CJF, FWCF

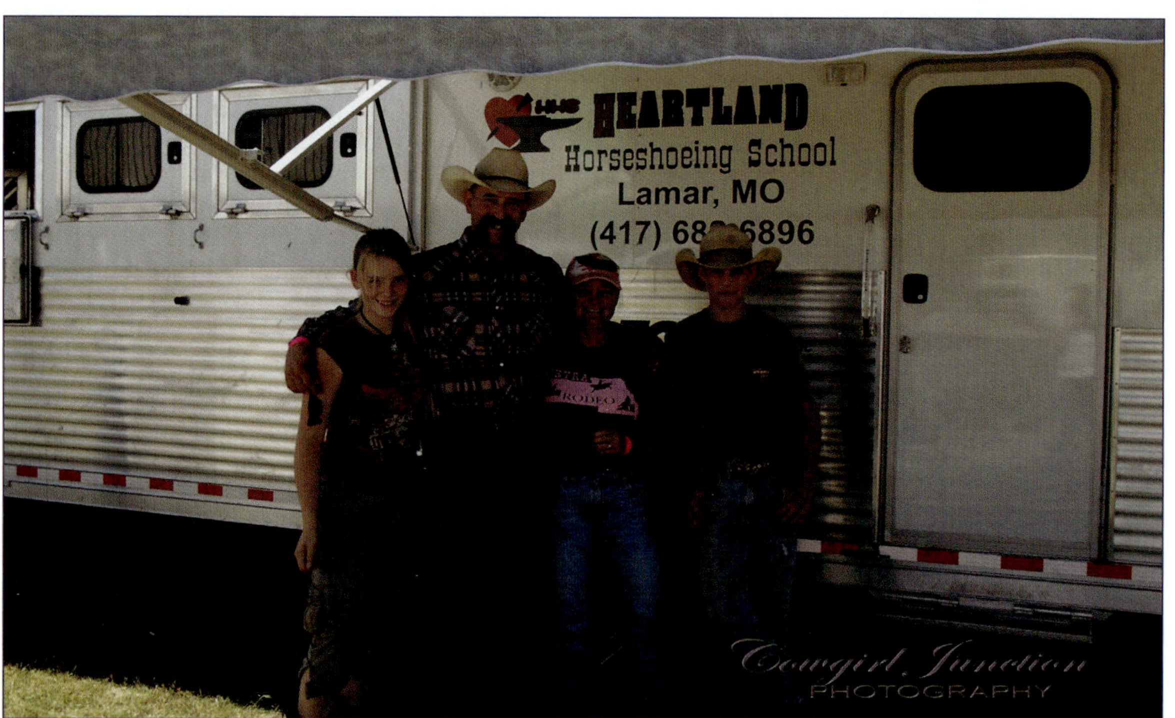

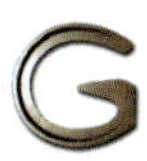

TABLE OF CONTENTS

Section 1: General Introduction and Non-Shoeing Considerations 1

Chapter 1: Welcome to the Craft 2

Chapter 2: Safety And Longevity 7

Chapter 3: Unwritten Rules and Ethics 9

Section 2: Tools and Equipment 11

Chapter 4: Farrier Tools 12

Chapter 5: Your Farrier Shop 24

Chapter 6: Your Mobile Shop 34

Section 3: Anatomy 43

Chapter 7: Anatomy Introduction 44

Chapter 8: The Foot 50

Chapter 9: Bones and Joints 65

Chapter 10: Ligaments and Tendons 98

Chapter 11: Vascular, Nerve, and Lymphatic System Basics of the Equine Leg 126

Chapter 12: Biomechanics............................134

Chapter 13: Dissection.................................151

Section 4: Conformation 157

Chapter 14: Conformation............................158

Chapter 15: Corrective Shoeing Theory........173

Section 5: Gaits 177

Chapter 16: Gaits 178

Chapter 17: Gait Faults.................................185

Section 6: Horsemanship... 197

Chapter 18: Horsemanship 198

Chapter 19: Equine Psychology 207

Section 7: General Principles of Farriery.......... 209

Chapter 20: Good Shoeing 210

Chapter 21: Trimming Considerations..........215

Chapter 22: Trimming a Hoof 218

Chapter 23: Mediolateral Balance................229

Chapter 24: Normal Shoeing on Normal Feet..233

Chapter 25: Measuring Feet for Handmades.236

Chapter 26: Shoe Selection 239

Chapter 27: Shoe Modifications....................245

Chapter 28: Clip Fitting 258

Chapter 29: Hot Fitting.................................262

Chapter 30: Nailing 266

Chapter 31: Clinching 101...........................271

Section 8: Other Shoeing...................... 279

Chapter 32: Modern Farriery........................280

Chapter 33: Bad Shoeing 294

Chapter 34: Common Sense In The Shoeing vs. Barefoot Debate 302

Chapter 35: Myths of Farriery......................306

Section 9: In the Fire.......... 311

Chapter 36: Intro to Forging.........................312

Chapter 37: Forging Basics...........................322

Chapter 38: Exercises in the Forge 336

Chapter 39: Tong Making.............................354

Chapter 40: The Basic Hind 359

Chapter 41: The Basic Front.........................371

Chapter 42: Using Concave to Make Shoes 381

Section 10: Lameness and Pathology...................... 387

Chapter 43: Lameness 389

Chapter 44: Causes of Lameness..................401

Chapter 45: Pathologies of the Horse's Foot

- **-1** Abscess 403
- **-2** Canker 413
- **-3** Club Foot 415

-4 Coffin Bone Fractures..........................418
-5 Corns 422
-6 Cracks 425
-7 Dropped Sole 435
-8 Founder and Laminitis 438
-9 Hoof Avulsion 450
-10 Keratoma 452
-11 Navicular 455
-12 Pedal Osteitis 461
-13 Quarter Cracks 463
-14 Quittor 468
-15 Sheared Heels 470
-16 Sidebone 473
-17 Soft Heel Cracks 477
-18 Sole Bruises 479
-19 Thrush 482
-20 White Line Disease 484

Chapter 46: Pathologies of the Horse's Limb

-1 Bowed Tendons 491
-2 Broken Bones......................................493
-3 Bucked Shins 495
-4 Capped Hocks and Elbows 496
-5 Carpitis 498
-6 Curb..501
-7 Osselets 503
-8 Radial Nerve Paralysis.........................505
-9 Ringbone 506
-10 Severed Tendons 511
-11 Spavin 515
-12 Splints 519
-13 Sprained Suspensory Ligament..........521
-14 Stifled and Stifle Lameness 524
-15 Stringhalt...526
-16 Thoroughpin 527
-17 Windpuffs..528

Section 11: Shoe Arsenal 531

Chapter 47: Farrier's Arsenal 532
Chapter 48: Straight Bar Shoe.......................536
Chapter 49: Egg Bar Shoe 551
Chapter 50: Heart Bar, W-Shoe and G-Bar ...561
Chapter 51: Patten Bar.................................569
Chapter 52: Z-Bar...573
Chapter 53: Aluminum Fundamentals For Farriers...578
Chapter 54: Hospital Plate............................590
Chapter 55: Extensions................................594

Section 12: Practical Application of Sound Basics....................... 601

Chapter 56: Treating Lame and Abnormal Feet

-1 Patten Bar Cases 602
-2 Z-Bar Cases...611
-3 Straight Bars 615
-4 Drastic Changes 622
-5 Heart Bar and W-Shoe 630

Section 13: Business.......... 645

Chapter 57: General Thoughts On Farriery and Standards 646
Chapter 58: Starting Your Business...............649
Chapter 59: Farrier Economics......................656
Chapter 60: Business Plan 662

Section 14: Educators Manual 665

Chapter 61: Tips on Teaching.......................666
Chapter 62: Practical Testing Strategies........669
Chapter 63: Test Questions...........................676
Chapter 64: Judging.....................................685

References 691

Index 692

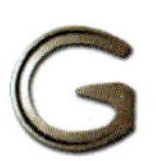

Section

1

General Introduction and Non-Shoeing Considerations

Chapter 1: Welcome to the Craft 2

Chapter 2: Safety And Longevity 7

Chapter 3: Unwritten Rules and Ethics 9

“ [8] Ask the former generation
and find out what their ancestors learned,
[9] for we were born only yesterday and know nothing,
and our days on earth are but a shadow. ”

—Job 8:8-9
—New International Version

Chapter

1 WELCOME TO THE CRAFT

If you are reading this, then you have an interest in this ancient craft of farriery. For those that are new, I would like to welcome you to this incredible world that is an art with a scientific backdrop. There is much that is still unknown, and no one of us will ever know enough about shoeing a horse. This fact keeps the trade fresh for those with a passion for horseshoeing, and perfection is an ideal that we can all strive for, yet never quite achieve. Frustrating as that sounds, it is part of what makes me get out of bed every morning happy that I have another chance to try again today.

If you do some research into the history of horseshoeing, you will find that there is not any real consensus about when and where iron shoes fixed with nails started. I have found references to Romans, Celts, Gauls, Chinese, and Greeks, and that was without looking too hard. Wherever and whoever is not important to this text, but what is important is the fact that we are still doing the same basic thing as the first farrier who ever decided that a nail could be driven into a foot. Trimming the foot as best we can, making a shoe that resembles the bottom of the foot, and attaching it to that foot with nails. The earliest reference suggests that this was first done around 400 years before the time of Christ. That makes our noble trade just over 2,400 years old. Hickman states in his book that horseshoeing extends from about 400 BC when the Gauls and the Celts first nailed a rim of iron to the hooves of their horses.

When considering the history of man and horse, it is only in recent times that the horse is no longer a necessity. Before the advent of cars, trains, tractors, planes, tanks, motorcycles, and other modern inventions, the horse was an integral part of life for the advancement of civilization. From war to colonization to agriculture to commerce, the horse was at the heart of getting things done. I often look at the countryside I live in and marvel at the idea of heading across it with my family in a wagon hitched to a team of horses. While we would think of the bravery of those pioneers, in reality, they were simply traveling with the most modern equipment for traveling available. That modern equipment just happened to be a horse.

During times of war, there is no doubt that the cavalry mounted on horses with better feet would be able to outmaneuver the cavalry with worse feet. During the American Civil War, the Confederacy was plagued by a lack of horseshoes, while the Union had plenty of ready-made keg shoes at their disposal. There were reportedly orders from the Southern Chain of Command that had the capture of horseshoes as a priority over food, ammo, clothing and weapons. It goes without saying that a cavalry of shod horses would be able to do a lot of things that a cavalry of barefoot horses could not.

The art of farriery has continued to evolve as the science of farriery makes continued advancements. Since we now understand so much more about how a foot grows, where it grows from, what it is made out of, and how shoeing affects the entire animal. We can use this knowledge to do a better job of attaching shoes to that foot. We have yet to hear a speaking horse tell us what sort of angle feels better, what kind of shoes give the best traction in all situations, how much toe length would be just right, and how they would like their feet to be held. Like a veterinarian dealing only with animals, we have to understand these things by observing the horse to see how it reacts to the changes made. That is how the horse speaks to us.

The act of trimming and shoeing a horse comes with an immense responsibility. Horses have no say in how they are shod. They are captured, led and tied up at the discretion and mercy of their owners, in front of whatever horseshoer has been selected to shoe that horse. Some horses win the horseshoe lottery and get to be shod by conscientious, caring, dedicated craftsmen who put the horse above everything else on a list of reasons why they shoe horses. Other horses are not so lucky. My challenge to you is to be one of those top farriers with the skill and knowledge to do the best shoeing that a horse can get. If you do a good job at a high standard every

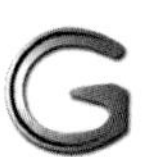

time, you will also become one of those farriers that are in demand, which leads, in turn, to prosperity.

Again, welcome to this business, craft, occupation, and trade. For me, it has gone beyond what I do to become a lifestyle and a definition of who I am. If farriery is your calling, you will spend your life in wonder that people will pay you so that you can have a good time doing what you love. And that, my friends, leads to a wonderful career.

LEARNING THE ART OF THE FARRIER

You need to know this before you start, or in the event that you have already started, you can look back on the beginning and judge me right or wrong. This art, this craft, this incredible trade is one of the hardest sets of skills to master that you will ever undertake. Because of this, there is a lot of frustration for most beginners, leading to high rates of attrition, and practitioners that are happy to achieve only average and mediocre skills. However, for a driven few, there is a chance for greatness. Push past the hard bits, relish those parts that become easy through repetition, and determine for yourself that you are going to be known for inventing horseshoeing. Lots of good times and satisfaction await those that rise to the challenge.

So, the pep talk over, how exactly should you go about learning to shoe horses? There are basically 2 main methods; apprenticeship and school. Each one has its benefits and downsides, and perhaps the best method is a combination.

I think that the single most important factor, (TSMIF, as Ivon Bell, FWCF, would say) is who teaches you. Teachers cannot teach more than he/she knows, so first, the one who is teaching should have an unrivaled skill level. Although skill as a farrier is not enough, the teacher must also have skill as a teacher. It is said that those that can't do, teach. In this industry, that just won't work. There are many gifted farriers that cannot teach anyone else how to achieve their level, but those that are not good at shoeing are also not good at teaching it. You can have the roughest bunkhouse, a shanty for a shop, and just the bare minimum when it comes to forge, anvil, and tools. You put that together with a dynamic, clever, and motivated teacher, and whether you succeed or not is up to you. The kind of teachers I am talking about will do their part, so you will have to do yours.

You should carefully look at the pros and cons for your situation, and make yourself a personal list. I am going to lay out some broad pros and cons, and you should see if any affect you. Taking this step early in your career will help you get where you want the fastest.

SCHOOL:

Pros:

- Set up for you to work on all aspects of shoeing on live horses.
- Staff will be used to dealing with beginners.
- Curriculum designed to teach farriery theory, forging, horsemanship, practical shoeing.
- You may get to work on and learn to do unruly horses.
- Fellow students may become great future contacts.

Cons:

- Some schools may not have enough live horses.
- Student:teacher ratio can be an issue.
- Many of the horses may be unruly.
- There is expense involved.
- You will have to travel away from home.

APPRENTICESHIP:

Pros:

- A lot of one-on-one education.
- May get to work on high-end horses.
- The right master can lead to you developing a high degree of skill.
- Most apprentices get to see all parts of the business from scheduling, to customer relations, to dealing with horses.

Cons:

- Can take a lot of time.
- Customers don't want the apprentice working on their animals, so oftentimes, the apprentice will pull shoes, finish, catch horses, sweep, set up the rig, grind shoes, and do everything but the actual shoeing for years.
- Many masters don't teach the theory and anatomy of farriery.
- You can end up with a bad master very easily.
- Can be treated poorly.
- Takes a lot of time.

Once you have evaluated your personal situation, the next step is to determine how to find the right school or the right apprenticeship. You should take this as seriously as you would selecting a spouse or hiring a doctor. How well you choose your school or master will have a huge impact on your future.

To pick a school, begin by gathering as much material from every school as you can. Get their flyers and brochures, look at their websites, and talk to practicing farriers about what schools are worth looking at. Make a short list of your finalists, and then take the time and effort to visit these schools while they have a class in session.

One of the most common reasons for picking one school over another is geography. Geography as it relates to horse population and weather is fine, but geography as it relates to proximity to your house is not a good reason to select a school. In the United States, many of the schools that have a colder winter will not have a lot of horses to shoe in the cold months. Most school customers are not using their horses during the winter, so that is a geographical consideration.

When you visit the school, try to spend enough time that you can visit with students in a one-on-one situation. Ask some pointed questions about what their time at the school has been like. Enough horses? How are they treated by the customers and instructors? Are they getting a lot of forge demos and classroom instruction? Are the classes being taught by the instructors, or just other students? These, and whatever other relevant questions you can think of, should be part of your interview. When you talk to the school owners, you are going to hear what they think the school is like. When you talk to students, you are going to hear what the students think the school is like. If the students are satisfied, you will probably be satisfied as well.

To find an apprenticeship, take some time to visit with local horsemen about what farriers in the area are respected. If you find one name comes up over and over, then you know that this farrier is at least doing some things right. Once you have done the legwork to make a short list of potential masters, you need to take the time to meet these farriers and find out if an apprenticeship is even a possibility.

CONTINUING EDUCATION

Once you have completed your formal education, it is imperative that you continue to learn. This is the sort of trade that you will never know enough about. One of the best ways to advance your skill set is through exposure to other good farriers. Here is some information about some of the farrier groups that you might want to gain exposure to.

FARRIER COMPANIES AND ASSOCIATIONS

Like any trade, the farrier industry has its groups that help to set standards, and offer educational opportunities. Farriery is regulated in some countries, and in these places, the groups become governing bodies and they help to set industry policy.

AMERICAN FARRIER'S ASSOCIATION

In the United States, the American Farrier's Association has been around since 1971. In 1979 they began offering testing to farriers. The AFA states that it has three levels to the certification program, these are; classification, certification, and endorsement. It is a clever system that allows farriers at almost any level to achieve a goal. Currently, you can test at the AFA Farrier level, Certified Farrier level, the Certified Tradesman Level and the Certified Journeyman Level. Above that, there is an endorsement available for Certified Journeyman Farriers called the Therapeutic Endorsement, as well as a Forging Endorsement.

Each of the exams has a theory and practical portion. The theory for all of the exams is a multiple choice, true-false type test. The practical portion for the Certified Farrier is the submission of a shoe display and shoeing 2 feet with keg shoes in an hour. For the Certified Tradesman, the candidate must shoe all 4 feet with clipped keg shoes in 1 ½ hours. The practical for the Certified Journeyman Farrier is shoeing a horse all the way around with plain stamped handmades, toe clips in front and quarter clips behind, in 2 hours. In addition, CJF candidates must make a ¾ fullered straight bar shoe to a pattern in 35 minutes.

WORSHIPFUL COMPANY OF FARRIERS

The Worshipful Company of Farriers out of the United Kingdom is the oldest and most respected organization of farriers in the world. They have a rich history that begins in 1356. The farriers of London were called together by the mayor and established as a Fellowship. Virtually all of the early work of the Company was destroyed in the great fire of London in 1666. The modern history of the Company begins with the grant of the first Charter by King Charles II on 17 January, 1674. The Charter reads:

Whereas we have been informed by ... the humble petition of our wellbeloved subjects the Brotherhood of Farryers within our Citties of London and Westminster that their art and trade is of great antiquity and of great use and benefitt to our subjects for preserving of horses and that diverse unexpert and unskilfull persons ... within the said citties ... have for want of due knowledge and skill in the right way of preserving of horses destroyed many horses in or near the same citties ... and that the said Brotherhood have not power to search and oversee such as profess the said art ... soe that the said abuses doe dayly increase ... and to invest them with power and jurisdiction for the well ordering and governing of the said Art and Trade and all such as use the same.

THE REGISTER OF FARRIERS

In January 1887, the Court appointed a Committee to consider the establishment of a register of farriers and the setting up of practical examinations in the art of making shoes for and shoeing horses. In 1889, the Court provided funds to a special Registration Account, together with the setting up of the Institute of Horse Shoeing and an organization under the auspices of the Company, of a Register, of qualified farriers not only in London but, throughout the country.

TRAINING AND EXAMINATIONS

In 1890, the Court invoked the assistance of the Lord Mayor, the Royal Agricultural Society, the Royal College of Veterinary Surgeons, and others interested in the welfare of the horse to create a scheme for training, examination and registration of farriers. Mindful of the need to improve quality, the Company introduced in 1907 further tests, which gave rise to the AFCL qualification (Associate of the Farriers Company of London), followed by an even more difficult examination in 1923 to give holders the title, Fellow of the Worshipful Company of Farriers - (FWCF).

As you can see, this is a diverse and honorable history. This track record puts the Worshipful Company of Farriers in a position where they set the highest standard of farriery in the world.

There are three levels of qualifications in the WCF. The first is a Diploma of the Worshipful Company of Farriers (DipWCF). The most common way to achieve this title is to serve a 50-month apprenticeship and then take the DipWCF exam. There is an agreement between the WCF and the AFA where an AFA Certified Journeyman Farrier with 2 years experience beyond the passing of the CJF can apply for and be granted a DipWCF. This is quite an honor bestowed upon the American farrier.

The second level is perhaps the hardest exam of farriery in the world. It is the Associateship of the Worshipful Company of Farriers (AWCF). This exam has a theory and practical portion and is actually broken down into 2 modules with 8 parts. These parts are: Exhibition of shoes; live shoeing and shoe making; modern farriery; written paper; gait analysis; live horse assessment; radiography assessment; and an oral exam. It is truly an exam that will determine one's ability to shoe horses at the highest level.

The uppermost title in the world of farriery that can be achieved is Fellowship of the Worshipful Company of Farriers. Like the other exams, there is a theory and practical aspect to this exam. As of the writing of this text, there are 35 FWCF farriers in the world still living, with the fourth American to have ever passed the exam doing so in November of 2009 at Heartland Horseshoeing School in Lamar, Missouri, U.S.A.

The exam at Heartland Horseshoeing School was a historical event, because it was the first time in the history of the WCF that its members conducted an exam on foreign soil. With a history that is as extensive as theirs, that is quite a happening. There were 10 American candidates for the AWCF, and one for the FWCF. Three of the AWCF candidates passed the entire exam, four passed either the theory or practical portion, and the FWCF candidate successfully completed the requirements for FWCF.

There are many state and regional farrier associations. Some are chapters of larger associations, and some are not. With a little bit of research, you should be able to find a local gathering of farriers. Top farriers love to help new and upcoming farriers improve their skill set. Once a farrier is at the top of his or her game, there is so much work available that helping a young farrier is not a threat or a problem. Because of this, you will have local associations that provide all sorts of learning opportunities from weekly hammer-ins to certifications and contests.

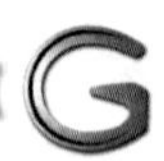

Some farriers will shoe horses for 1 year, reach a level of mediocrity, and then do that same job for 25 years in a row. They never quite learn enough to do a really nice job. Exposing yourself and your work to your peers will elevate your skills and insure that you continue to improve throughout your career.

It would be my recommendation that you determine what the best of the best are doing, and then do the same. Surrounding yourself with those that have superior skills to you will help to bring you up, while the opposite is also true. The old saying, "It is hard to soar like an eagle when you are surrounded by turkeys," is an appropriate one.

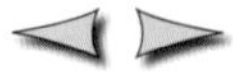

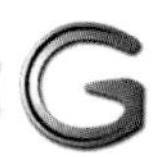

Chapter

2 SAFETY AND LONGEVITY

Farriery is not considered by most to be a long career. Not as short as that of a bull rider, but also not as long as a lot of other trades. The work is physically demanding, and there are opportunities with every horse to have a career-ending injury. The ability to handle pain is a necessity, and it helps to be a fast healer. This chapter will briefly address some of the safety concerns you should consider to lengthen your career.

Among of the most important things to protect and strengthen are your core muscles. With shoeing, there are a lot of repetitive movements that work only some muscles and not their opposing muscle groups. If you go to a gathering of older farriers, you will see that potbellies are not uncommon. Their backs are as strong as steel from the hours of bending over and holding their weight and that of the horse, but their abdominal muscles are not nearly as strong as their back muscles. This leads to imbalance, which leads to soreness, which can ultimately lead to chronic pain and problems. Staying fit with core training is essential and can add many years to your career.

If you become a "forgeaholic," you will find that the muscles in your arm will reflect your passion. At one point in my career, my right forearm measured 1 3/4 inches larger than my left forearm, and my right biceps was just over an inch larger than the left. I went to a contest in Washington and had my first arm cramps. They ended up plaguing me for many years, and I was only able to keep them at bay with nutrition and exercise designed to work muscles that were not being worked when I forged. I strongly recommend that you lift lighter weights at high repetitions as part of keeping yourself in the trade.

At the gathering of old farriers, you will also find a lot of hearing aids. The repeating clang of a hammer against a ringing anvil will do damage to your hearing, and over the years this can add up as well. I suffer from some hearing loss as a result of it, and I recommend that you use earplugs early on, instead of closing the gate once the horse is out.

Safety glasses are a must when forging. If you use safety glasses for a week, all you have to do is look at the lenses to see what your eyes have been protected from. Hot slag from the shoe can burn your eye when it sticks to it, and that leads to some discomfort. Breaking tools can send shrapnel into your eye that can permanently blind you. Losing an eye and depth perception as a farrier would not be a career-ending injury, but it would certainly make the job harder.

Your feet and toes are going to be stepped on as a farrier. Broken toes are a big nuisance, and when you break a big toe, you will be amazed at how much it affects you. I was not able to find useable protective boots to fit my feet, and I only have three toes that have not been broken. Like most things, if you can't duck it, you have to accept it. With hindsight, I should have spent the money to have some protective boots made for me. I suggest steel toes and metatarsal protectors.

Your hands are going to get burned from slag, and cut from the rasp, nails, and the edge of the hoof. In the early stages, you will get blisters from the hammer. All of this will lead to thicker skin and stronger hands, and I strongly recommend against the use of gloves. My hands do a lot of "looking" by feel where my eyes can't see; around the edge of the foot as it meets the shoe, the feel of the clip fit, the exit point of the nail, etc. The hands are trained to give a lot of information, and gloves create a barrier to that information.

Here is what I think about gloves. If you are trying to become great at any trade, you should look to those that are already great. You will see quite a few horseshoers wearing gloves, but you won't see any farriers at the World Championship Blacksmiths' Contest shoeing in gloves. Watching a certification, you are more likely to see the farriers that are going for the lower level wearing gloves than those at the top level. Now, this does not mean you cannot become a great farrier wearing gloves, but it does mean that it is not common to see the great farriers using gloves.

Depending on the type of business that you end up doing, sun protection should also be considered. I have worn a cowboy hat for years, and I find that it does not in any way hamper my ability to trim feet or forge. It also serves to protect my face and eyes from switching tails during fly season better than a ball cap ever did. I know that a lot of people don't think you can get into position with a cowboy hat on, but it has not been a problem for Cody or me. Since we are first and foremost educators, a lot of our time is spent outside under the sun. The protection we gain from wearing a cowboy hat is absolutely necessary.

Wearing your shoeing apron goes without saying, to protect you from nails that have just been driven into the foot toward your legs. Some farriers shoe in shorts, but I have never tried that. The apron should give you enough protection that you can get away with wearing shorts.

Safety, as it applies to the inanimate objects in your world, is pretty simple. Don't touch hot steel (although you are going to a few times); avoid dropping anvils on your foot — that sort of thing. Be aware of your surroundings and the potential for injury to yourself, the horse, the owner, and anything else in the area. As a professional, you should get good at predicting what may be a problem before it actually is. Stay alert and study the situations you find yourself in so that you can learn to make good decisions.

These are the basic and primary considerations for making your career a long one. I hope that you can implement these at my suggestion, and not only after you have done damage to yourself through experience. This is a great trade, and staying in it as long as you can is something that I think you will want to do.

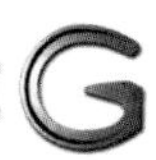

Chapter

3 UNWRITTEN RULES AND ETHICS

Of all of the trades that I know of, there are only a few that even come close to offering the kind of brotherhood and camaraderie that is shared amongst farriers. For the most part, plumbers, carpenters, painters, masons, veterinarians, etc., don't share with each other the fine points of doing their job the way farriers do. Perhaps this is due to the fact that farriers constitute a smaller group of people than other trades, or maybe because of the type of work. Most likely it is the fact that there are too few farriers to do all the work needing done. For whatever reason, this is an occupation where helping a fellow tradesman is common.

In many businesses, there is a cutthroat atmosphere in which helping the competition is seen as a bad idea. The rules for these types of trades are simple. Don't show the competition anything you know that makes the job easier. Don't help the competition when they are in a bind. Don't loan or suggest tools that make the job easier or better. And don't ever say anything nice to the customer about the competition. That seems to be the way that many people in other jobs run their business. Farriery is much different, and it is important that the newcomer understand some of this to stay out of hot water.

As a farrier, it is not good to run down other farriers. Although there is more of this in the farrier industry than I would like to see, it is not a good way to run your business. You can't look at a shoeing job with some age on it and truly know what the previous farrier had to work with. Sure, there is always something that you would have done differently, and that is how I deal with some of the terrible shoeing that I see.

When a customer asks what I think of terrible shoeing, an answer that I often use is, "It might not be how I would do it." Or "It is hard to judge what the last farrier was dealing with." With answers like this, I am not endorsing or criticizing the job, and I am able to respond without lying. I may think to myself that the last shoer should be doing something else for a living, but that is not what I say.

Many farriers get together with each other for big days. This may seem like a bad idea to the outsider, but it leads to some good friendships and makes a long day into a day of learning and fun. One of the unwritten laws of inviting a farrier friend to help you for the day is that the customer stays with the original shoer. The same goes when a young farrier is just doing a ride along.

Consider the following anecdote: Farrier John asks Farrier Sam if he can go with him for a few days. John is fresh out of school, and Sam is the top farrier in the area. At the first stop, John gets to visiting with the customer. That is breaking one of the rules. John should be there to work, and talking up the customer is not part of that work. As they visit, John and the customer find out that they have a lot in common. Their parents went to school together, they shop at the same stores, they named their kids the same names, and they have the same blood type. John and the customer are friends at first sight.

The next time the horses need shod, the customer calls John to do the shoeing. John is new, needs the money and the work, and is now in a tough spot that he may not know how to deal with. The farrier ethics of this situation require John to call Sam, tell Sam that the customer has called him, and ask Sam what he should do. By doing this, John has shown the respect to Sam that he is due as well as letting Sam know that John has decided ethics are more important than money. Sam can let John have the customer, suggest John to tell the customer no, or call the customer himself. That part of the story doesn't matter, and most of the time, Sam will gladly tell John to do the horses.

John has now put himself in a good spot with the best farrier in the area, and his success in the industry is more likely — even though he needs to spend less time visiting with Sam's customer when he is there to work.

If John takes the customer from Sam in some other way, then John is probably not going to end up doing that well as a farrier in that area. He has demonstrated a lack of character that will put him on the wrong end of the top guys. Opportunities to spend time with those guys and learn from them will be lost, and John will be seen as one of the cutthroat-type of farriers that many of the lesser skilled horse-shoers I know of are. The business will not bring him the joy that it does for the top farriers, and he is not likely to make a great living as a farrier. He just does not have the integrity that is required.

If John had met the customer in any other way, doing those horses would be fine. The fact that he met the customer as a result of being there while Sam was doing the horses is what makes it inappropriate for him to take the work without letting Sam know.

Another thing that is common in the world of the farriers is that they are always helping each other with customer service. When a horse loses a shoe and I can't get to it, I have no problem calling one of my farrier friends to see if they are going to be in the area and wouldn't mind putting the shoe on for me. I get similar calls in return. While the accountant would tell you it is not good business to do this for free, that is what happens most of the time. The other farrier will nail on a shoe for one of my customers as a favor to me, with no expectation or demand of compensation.

When I do this for other farriers, I think of it as paying it forward. Also, in this situation, it is unethical to end up with the customer's business. Simply nail on the shoe, wish the customer a good day, and go to your next stop.

There are other rules in this industry that are contrary to the normal ones of other industries. While all of these are not included here, my advice to you is to use the Golden Rule to the extreme. Anytime you are confronted with a situation, try to imagine the very best outcome if you were to be on the receiving end, and make a decision to do what is right. This will lead to lifelong friends that share a love for this great trade.

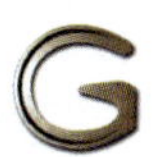

Section

2

Tools and Equipment

Chapter 4: Farrier Tools 12

Chapter 5: Your Farrier Shop 24

Chapter 6: Your Mobile Shop 34

**“ 22 Zillah also had a son, Tubal-Cain,
who forged all kinds of tools out of bronze and iron.
Tubal-Cain’s sister was Naamah. ”**

—Genesis 4:22

— New King James Version

Chapter 4 FARRIER TOOLS

If you have started pricing farrier tools, you have probably discovered that these are some pretty expensive items. Since this is such a small industry, the toolmakers that cater to farriers have to charge a premium to make up for lack of volume. That is okay, because as a farrier, you do something for a living that few can. As a result, you get to charge a premium for your skills and time. It all works out, but you need to make smart decisions when it comes to buying your equipment.

It is true that quality workmanship comes not from tools, but from the hands that wield them. Tools by themselves can do nothing, but skilled hands without tools are also at a loss. Skilled hands using quality tools is a marriage made in heaven. That is what you want to put together.

It is not always true that the more expensive something is, the better it is. But you will find that with farrier tools, this is often the case. I am going to go ahead and mention brand names for some of the tools in this textbook, but these are only my suggestions. In the case of other brands not mentioned, I may either have not had the opportunity to try them or may not have heard of them. Just because a brand is not mentioned here does not mean that I am recommending against the brand, it may just be that it does not suit me. The brands mentioned are what we currently use based on what is currently available, 10 years into the 21st century.

Here is a list of the basics that you will need to get started shoeing horses with keg shoes and some handmades. This is the minimum that I would recommend starting with. It is possible to complete a job with less than mentioned, but I would still start with the following list:

- Shoeing Box
- Shoeing Apron
- Pulloffs
- Clinch Cutter
- Clinch Block
- Clinch Gouge
- Hoof Nippers
- Crease Nail Pullers
- Clinchers
- Driving hammer
- 2 Rasps
- 2 Rasp handles
- Shoe spreaders
- Small flexible tape measure
- 2 Hoof Knives (these come in left- and right-handed models)
- Hoof testers
- Forge
- Round-horned anvil
- Anvil stand
- Vice
- 1/4," 5/16," and 3/8" Tongs
- 1.75 lb. Clipping hammer (ball peen)
- 2 lb Rounding Hammer
- Hot Fitters
- Creaser
- E-head fore punch
- Pritchels
- Butcher block brush
- Brass folding ruler
- Small wire brush
- Hoof stand
- Hoof cradle

This is not a complete and comprehensive list, but if you were to have all of this and some expendable inventory, you could shoe a lot of horses. Some items are going to wear out and have to be replaced — rasps most often. Hoof knives, nippers and wire brushes will last quite a bit longer, and a quality apron will outlast almost all of the other expendables. The rest of the gear should last for an extremely long time. Punches, pritchels and tongs will wear, but not very fast.

Following is a brief description of each of the mentioned items. The ones pictured are the types that I use, but any brand that is a quality tool will be acceptable. The final result of a good shoe on a well-prepared foot is what we are after, and if you find a brand or style of tool that suits you better, then you should use it.

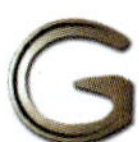

Shoeing Box. A shoeing box is basically an open toolbox that you move with you around the horse to keep all of your tools handy. I prefer an aluminum box for its weight and one with wheels, so that it is easy to move. My preferred brand is either Yoder or Raber. **(Figures 1-2)**

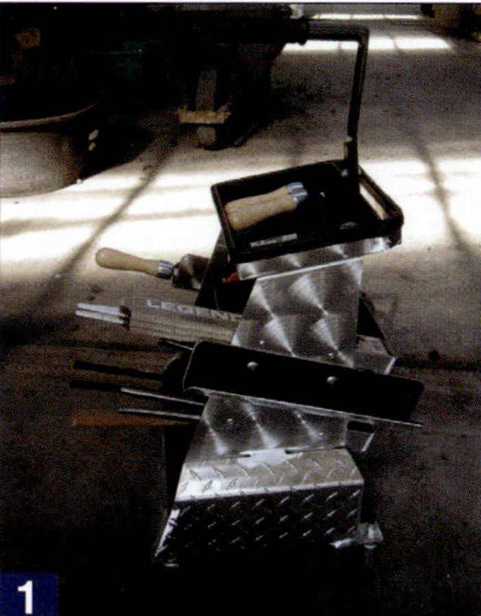

Yoder Classic shoeing box.

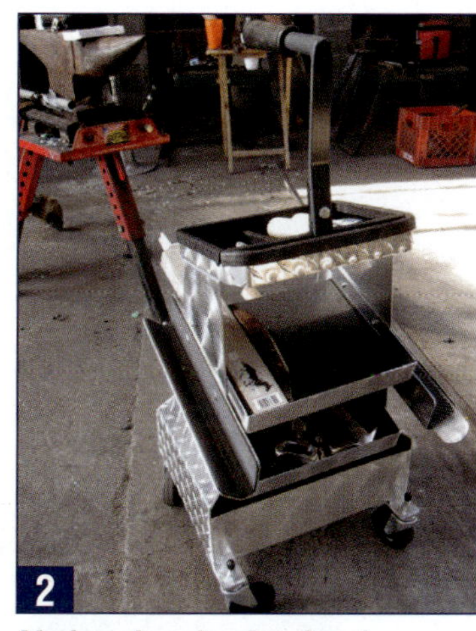

Yoder classic shoeing box.

Shoeing Apron. You will spend a long time wearing and dealing with this item. You will not really appreciate how important it is to have a good apron until you have a bad one. I have aprons made to my design. The features that make it a good apron are: It buckles in front and has an adjustable belt in back; two knife pockets; extremely durable; two leg straps; no Velcro; and the crotch area is not covered. Some farriers like break-away aprons, but they seem to break-away even when you don't want them to. **(Figures 3-4)**

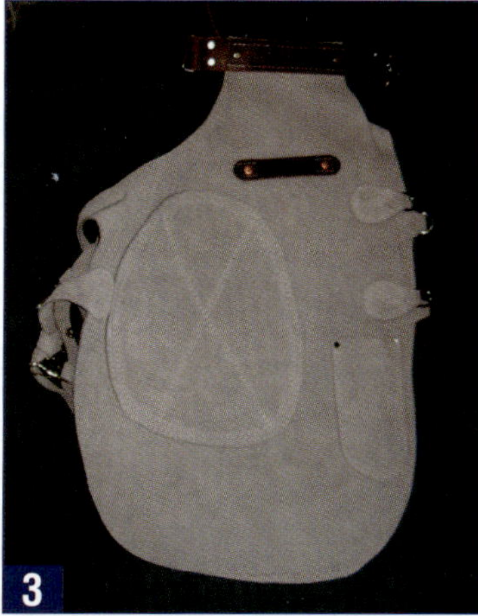

Chris Gregory Western Shoer apron without fringe.

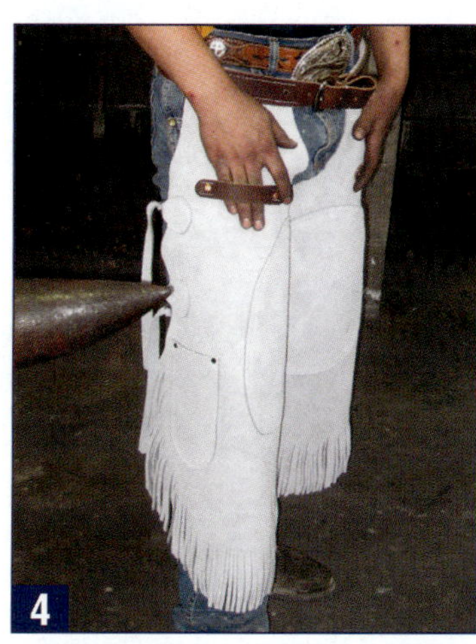

Chris Gregory Western Shoer apron with fringe.

Pulloffs. The best pulloffs that I have are from Mustad. They are sturdy, cut nails well when they need to, have a wide enough blade design to pull the shoe easily without hurting the foot, and have the ability to widen a shoe with the tooth design on the outside of the jaws. Too wide a blade can be too much pressure on the foot and be hard to use. If the blades are too narrow, they won't do enough work when you push down on them. Kelly prefers Diamond pulloffs, as they are just a little bit smaller than the Mustad. **(Figure 5)**

Clinch Cutter. This is not a tool that I use too often. As long as it stays sharp and does not take up too much room in the shoeing box, it's fine with me. **(Figure 6)**

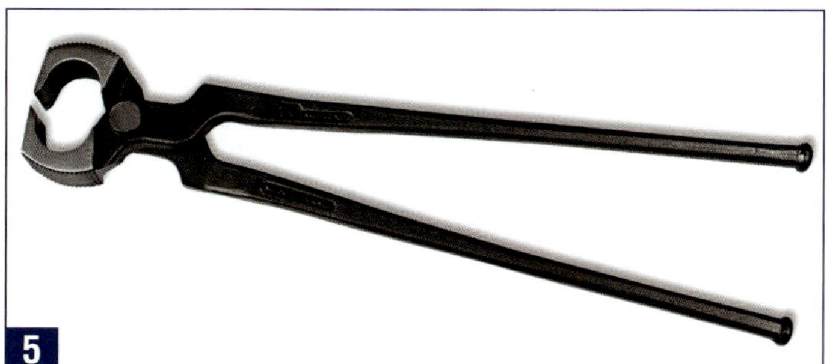

Mustad Pulloffs.

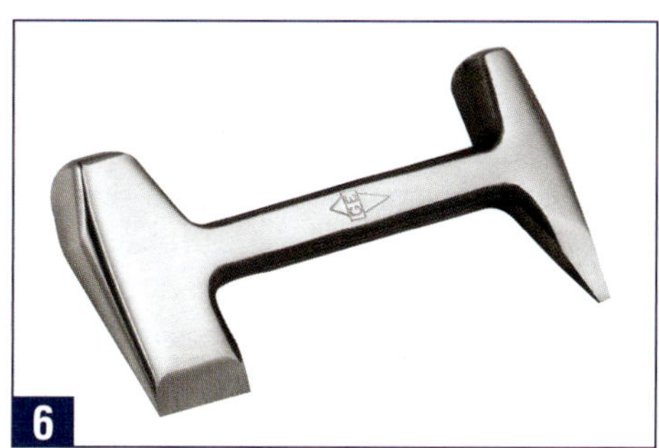

GE Clinch Cutter.

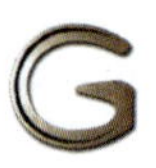

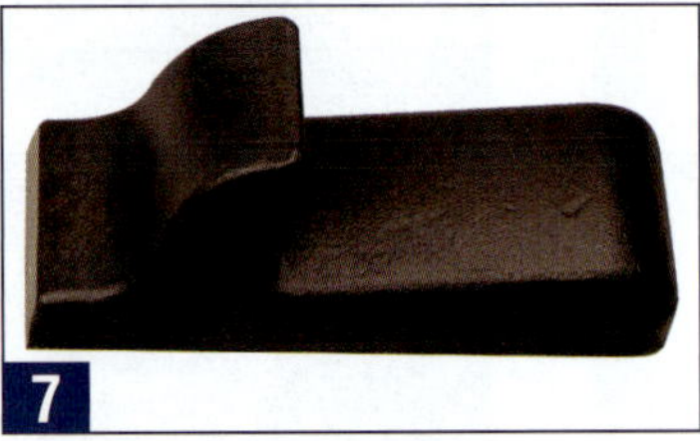

Mustad Clinch Block.

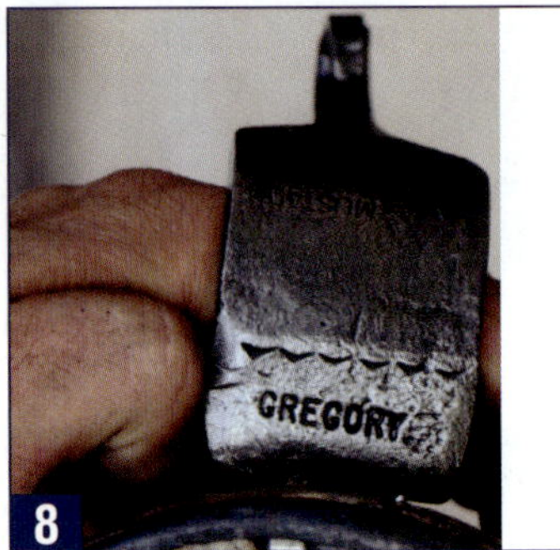

Handmade clinch block from an old rasp.

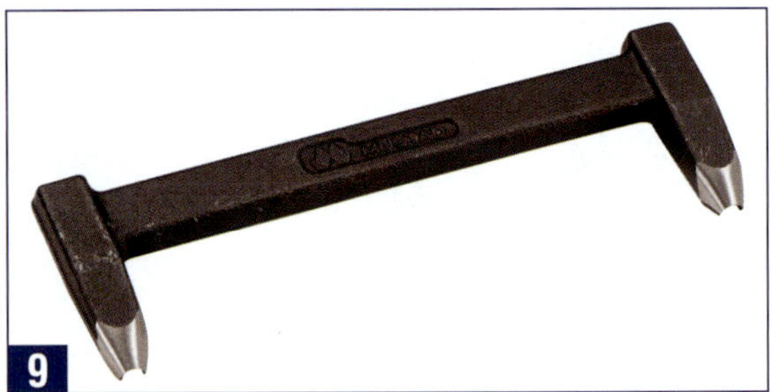

Mustad Under Clinch Gouge.

Clinch Block. I make my own clinch blocks out of old rasps. There is a description of how to make your own in the forging section of this book. A clinch block needs to be fairly heavy and easy to grab in the position that you are going to be using it. It also needs to have a solid and square working edge. Too sharp, and it will cut off the nails, too blunt, and it will not set them easily. **(Figures 7-8)**

Clinch Gouge. A clinch gouge is used to remove the little bit of hoof wall under the nail where it comes out of the foot. If done correctly, it gives the clinch a good place to seat so that it will be strong, thick and smooth. There are a couple of varieties of clinch gouges. One is called a push gouge, and I like these fine as long as they are sharp. Due to how they are used by pushing the edge against hoof and steel, they don't stay sharp, making them very difficult to use. For this reason, I like to use clinch gouges that are designed to be hammered on. **(Figure 9)**

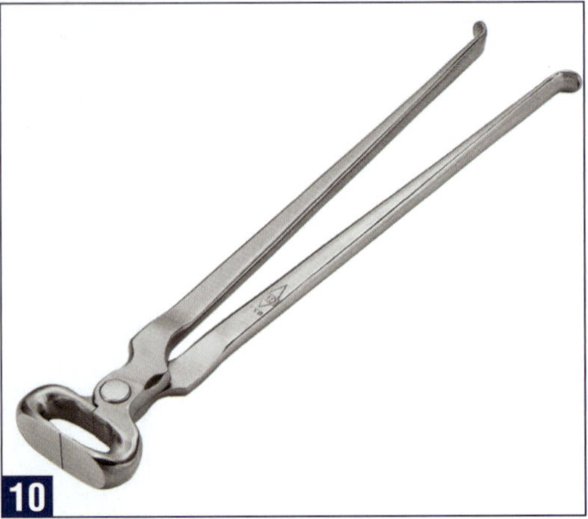

G.E. Forge & Tool hoof nippers.

Hoof Nippers. Having good quality nippers is important. This is a tool that will be used a lot, and if they are not sharp, they make the job harder. Several companies have tried, but I have yet to find a brand of nippers that beats G.E. Forge & Tool. I personally like a smaller style of nipper, like the 14" Racetrack or 12" style. However, the 15" are just as popular. While the G.E. are the most expensive, they have always been worth it. **(Figure 10)**

Crease Nail Pullers. Crease nail pullers are designed to remove horse nails from shoes once they have been driven into the foot. Since the design of a shoe is to have the nail seated deep and tight, removing that nail can be difficult. If you need to remove a nail, and you don't have a good pair of nail pullers, you will find it quite frustrating. This is a tool that will not be used too much, but one that you will be very glad to have when you need it. **(Figure 11)**

Clinchers. Clinching is basically bending over the piece of nail that comes out of the foot so that it holds the shoe on tighter. A good clinch will be thick, square and smooth against the outside of the foot. Cody likes to hammer clinch, Kelly likes to use G.E. Curved-Jaw Clinchers, and I don't mind either way. As long as you are able to bend over a consistent, square clinch every time, you should be fine with whatever brand you get. When the clinchers are brand new, they can be sharp and end up cutting nails off instead of bending them over. You may find that dulling the edges a little makes them work better. **(Figure 12)**

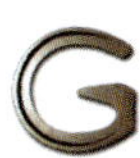

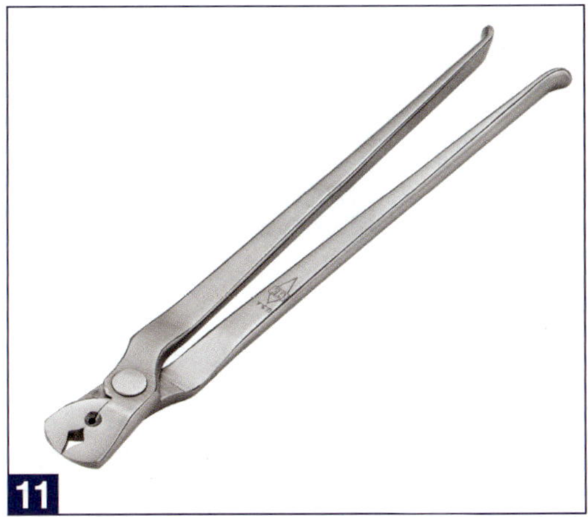

11

G.E. Forge & Tool crease nail puller.

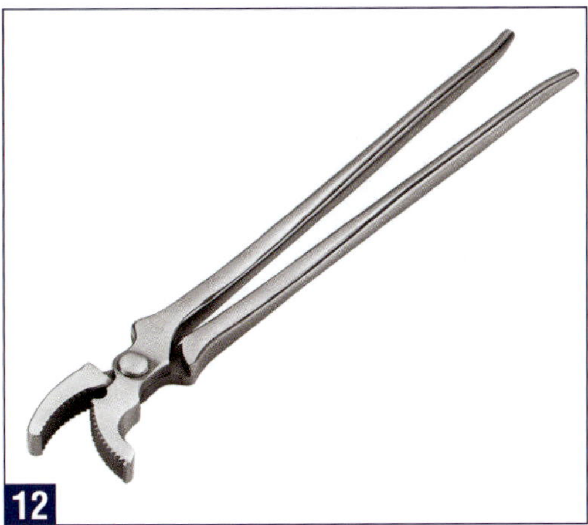

12

G.E. Forge & Tool curved jaw clinchers.

Driving Hammer. Driving hammers are designed specifically to drive horse nails into feet. Your driving hammer will be a very personal thing. I like one that is a little on the light side, and I know some very good farriers that like their driving hammers a little on the heavy side. Jim Poor at Flatland Forge in Texas makes the nicest driving hammers, and I use his 9 oz model. For hammer clinching, I like a round face on my driving hammer, so I use the light style of Mustad driving hammers. **(Figure 13-14)**

Rasps. A rasp is a file in that it is designed to remove material when it is rubbed against something. Hoof rasps are unique in that they are specifically designed to remove hoof tissue, and they have a rough side and a smooth side. I have finally found a rasp that I like best. This has been a long search because rasp quality changes often as the machines that make them have to be constantly tweaked. You think you have a great brand, and three rasps later you are ready to throw them all away. Delta Mustad Hoofcare Center has started producing a Red Tang

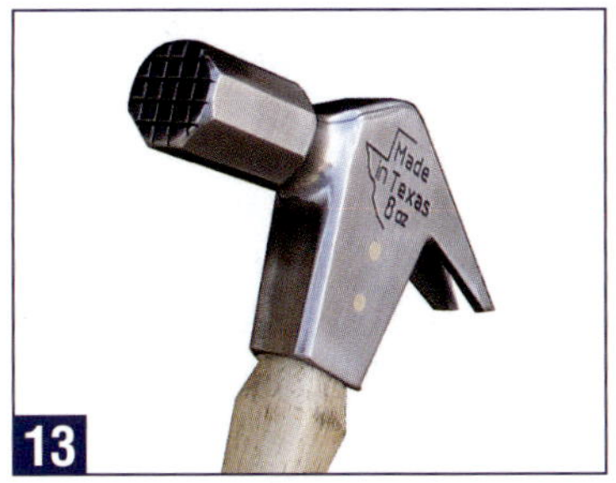

13

Flatland Forge Driving Hammer detail.

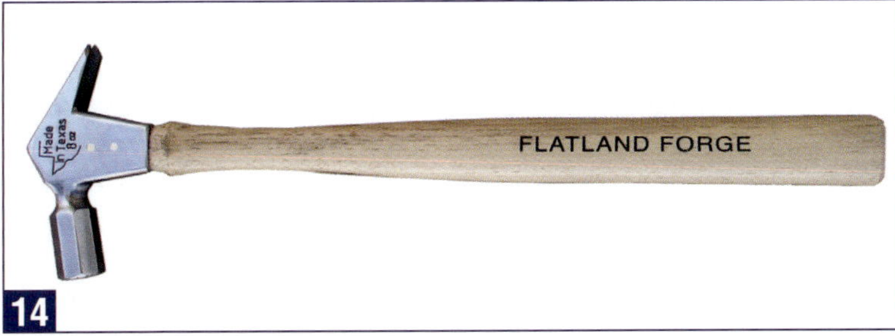

14

Flatland Forge Driving Hammer.

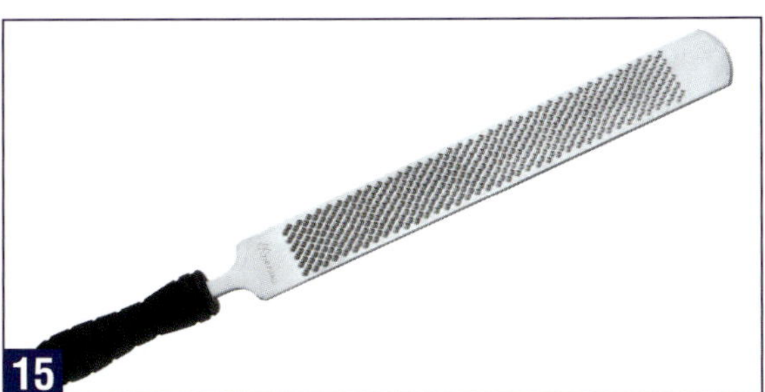

15

Mustad rasp with plastic screw-on handle.

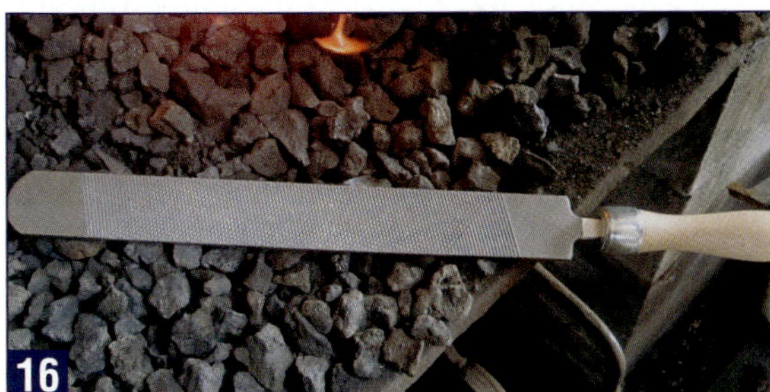

16

Heller Legend rasp, smooth side.

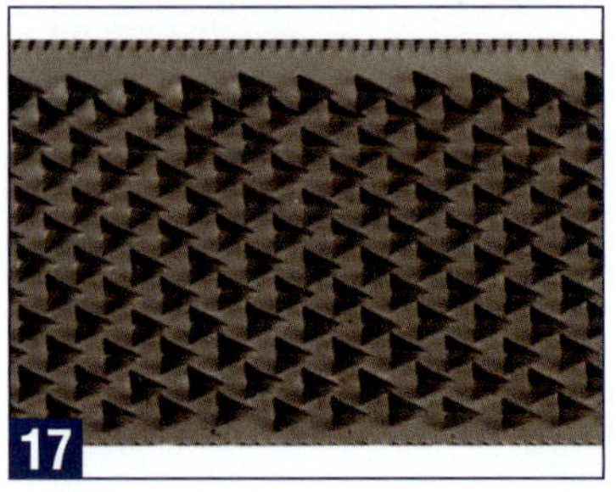
17

Close up of the rough side of a hoof rasp.

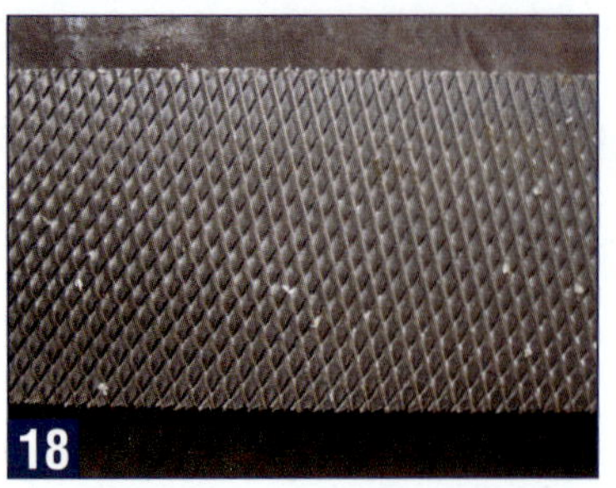
18

Detail of the smooth side of a hoof rasp.

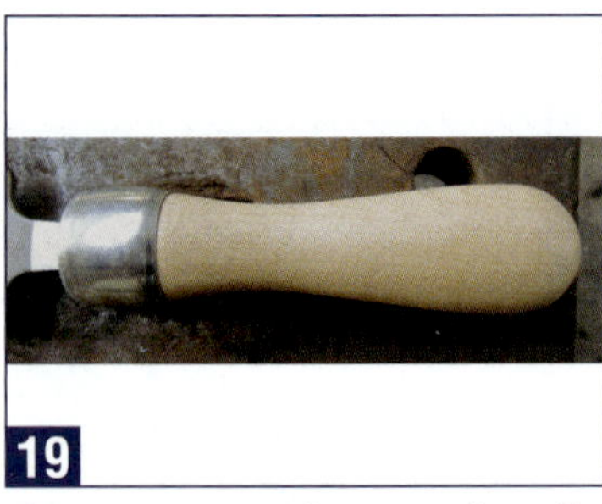
19

Screw-on wooden rasp handle.

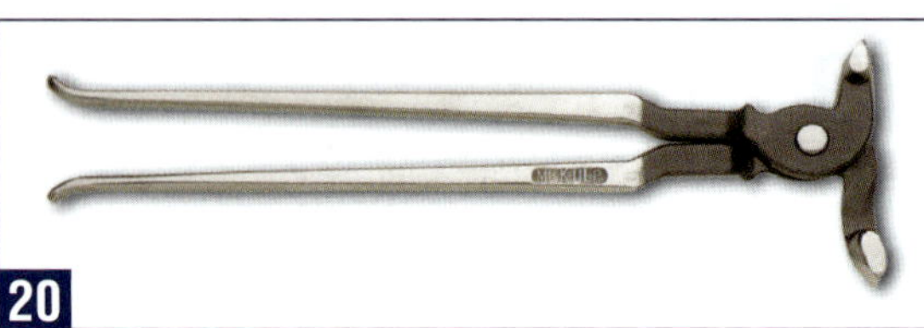
20

Kulp shoe spreaders.

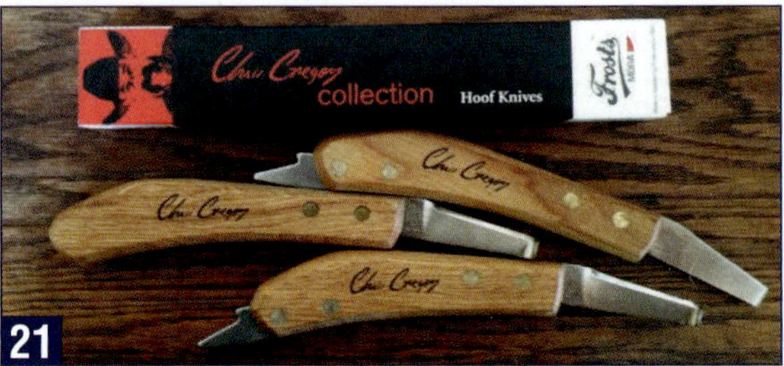

21

Photo of my knives, with and without the rooster tail.

rasp that is sharp and consistent and has a great smooth side for finishing feet, even when brand new. **(Figures 15-18)**

Finish Rasps. These are hoof rasps that have one smooth side — and the other side is smoother yet. They are not designed to take a lot of foot like a normal rasp does, but just a little bit, resulting in a smooth finish. I like the Simmons Blackmaster Finish Rasp.

Rasp Handles. Rasp handles go on the end of the rasp over the tang (the pointy bit at one end of a rasp). I like to use wooden, screw-on type handles. The ones that drive on can come off when you really need them on and some of the aluminum ones are too heavy. You should use two styles of wooden handles to differentiate between the foot rasp and the finish rasp. **(Figure 19)**

Small Flexible Tape Measure. Any brand here will do fine, but St. Croix Forge gives away a nice little model that works really well. It is also priced right.

Shoe Spreaders. We sometimes call this tool a "shoe perfecter". There will be times when you get a shoe nailed on, yet you would like to move a heel out just a tiny bit. The Kulp shoe spreaders allow you to do that without ruining the level of the shoe or smashing your fingers. There are some shoe spreaders that will slip off of the shoe and whose reins come too tightly together (experience talking here). **(Figure 20)**

Hoof Knife. Knives come in left- and right-handed models. To make a good, smooth, clean and consistent cut, I prefer a hoof knife with a pretty straight blade. When the blade has a lot of curve to it, you will make curved cuts in the sole. This leads to a sole that looks like it has scallops cut into it.

I was approached by Mora/Frost Knives of Sweden to develop a hoof knife in 2011. The result is the Chris Gregory hoof knife that you see in **Figures 21 and 22**. This knife is made to my exact specifications, and I think that it is the finest knife for the money in the farrier market. They come with or without the rooster tail, which is used as a hoof pick and for hot fitting. These knives are extraordinarily sharp, keep a good edge, and are designed for detailed and precision knife work on a horse's foot. This is an item that needs to be a perfect fit for you or you won't be able to do as good a job.

Some people like to use a loop knife for the frog. I like to use a double edged blade, or a left and a right handed knife in place of the loop knife. Loop knives are hard for me to keep as sharp as the double edged blades, or the left and right handed knives.

Figures 23 and 24 show how I use the left and right handed knives with my right hand to work on the frog.

Hoof testers. While these are not an abso-

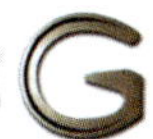

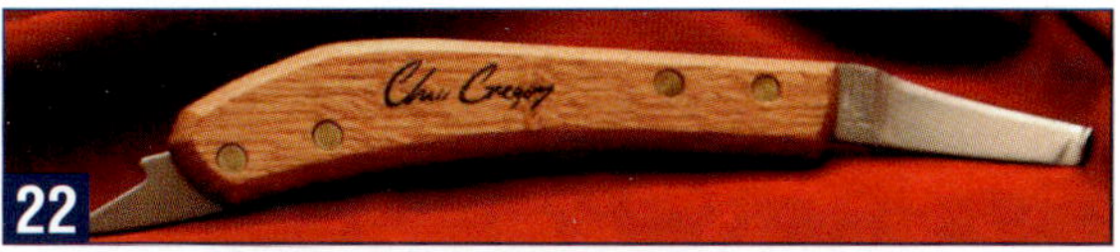

View of one of my knives with a rooster tail for cleaning the foot and hot fitting.

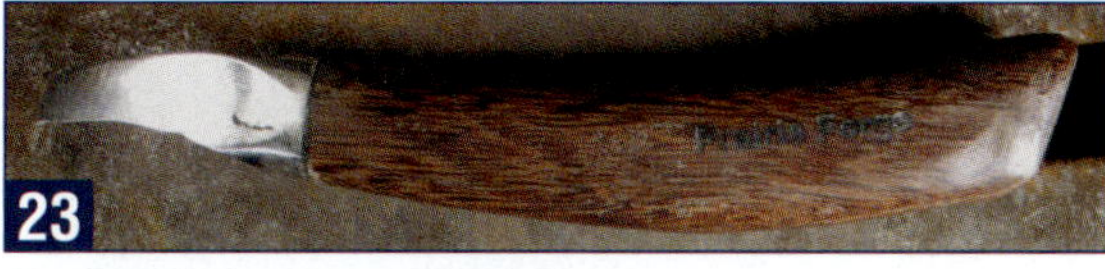

Prairie Forge Loop Knife.

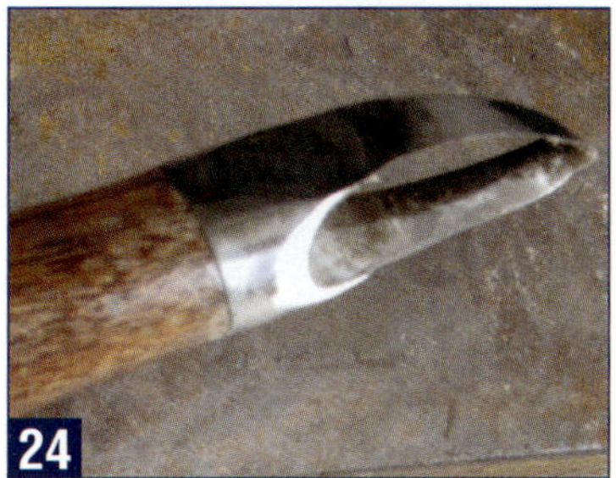

Prairie Forge Loop Knife.

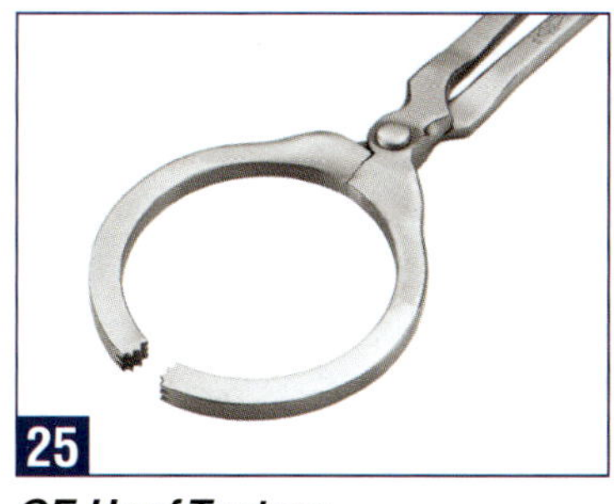

GE Hoof Testers.

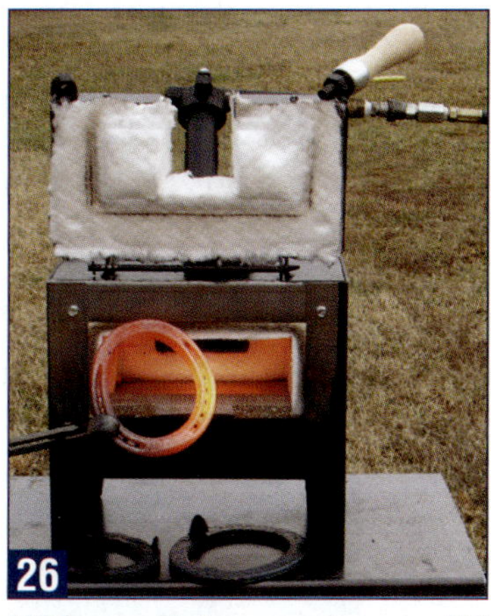

Whisper Baby, one-burner NC Forge.

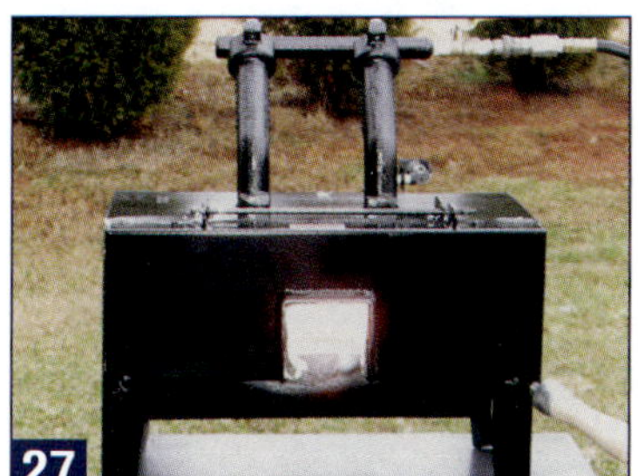

Whisper Momma, two-burner NC Forge.

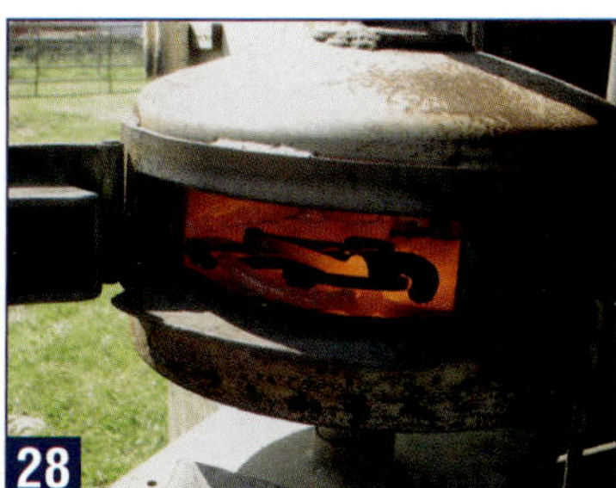

Hypona Forge.

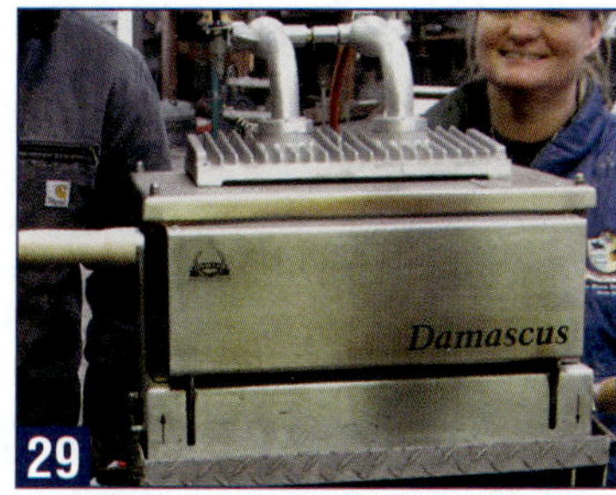

Damascus Forge from O'Dwyer in Australia.

lute necessity for the beginning farrier, I would add them to the list as soon as you are able. You have to be careful using and interpreting the results from the use of this tool, but there are many times that they are indispensable. I like large testers like the ones in **Figure 25**.

Forge. Propane forges are a clean and handy way to heat shoes and bar stock for everyday shoeing. The forge in your truck or trailer is going to take a beating from being put away hot and then bounced down the road. Because of this, you need to have one that is durable and easy to replace the liner in. For shoeing on the road, I like to use NC Tool forges. The Whisper Baby **(Figure 26)**, is fine for everyday shoeing, and if you are doing more handmades, you will like the Whisper Momma **(Figure 27)**. One of the most durable forges I ever owned was the Hypona **(Figure 28)**. In the shop, the forge is stationary and does not need to be as durable. I really like the O'Dwyer Damascus forge **(Figure 29)** and the Forgemaster Blacksmith Model.

Round-Horned Anvil. There are so many new anvils to choose from, as well as a lot of antique anvils that are still very good. As long as it has a round horn, I am happy to use it. If you are buying a new anvil for your truck, I highly recommend the Round Horn Legend, made by Anvil Brand Shoeing Supply in Illinois **(Figure 30)** or the Scott anvil, made by Scott Collier in Virginia. For your shop, it is hard to beat a Kohlswa, A1, from Sweden.

Anvil Stand. Having a good anvil stand that will secure the anvil is important. When the anvil sits loose on a block, it will be loud and bounce

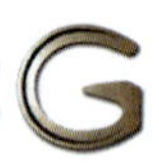

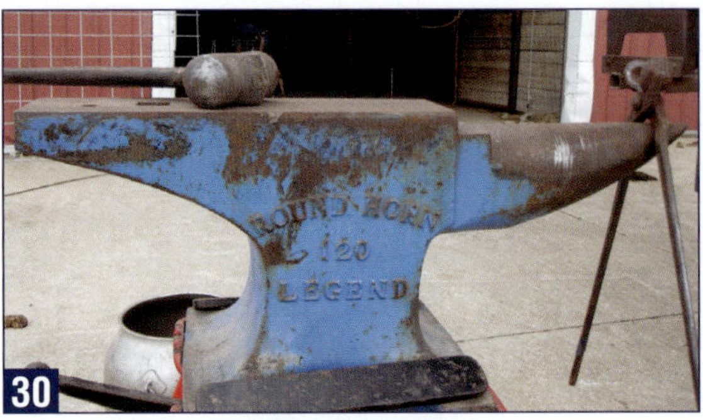

Round Horned Anvil from Anvil Brand.

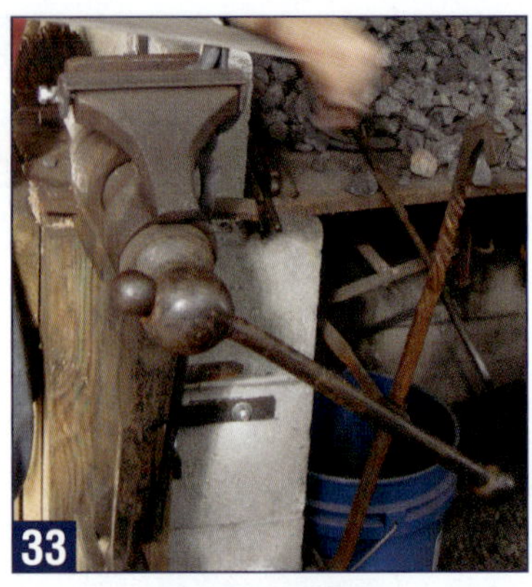

Large shop post vise.

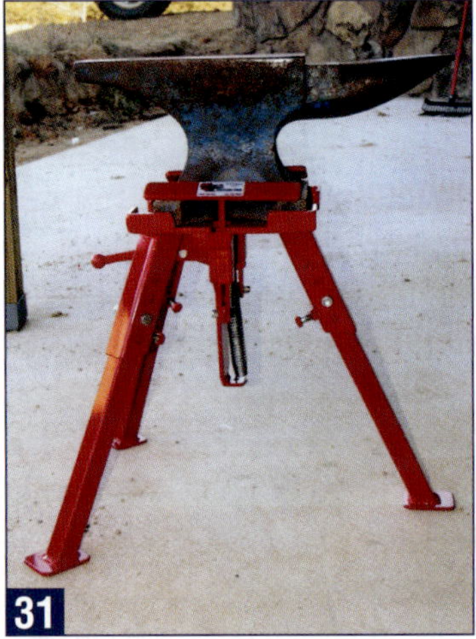

Heartland Anvil Stands from Blackwater Forge. Clamp model.

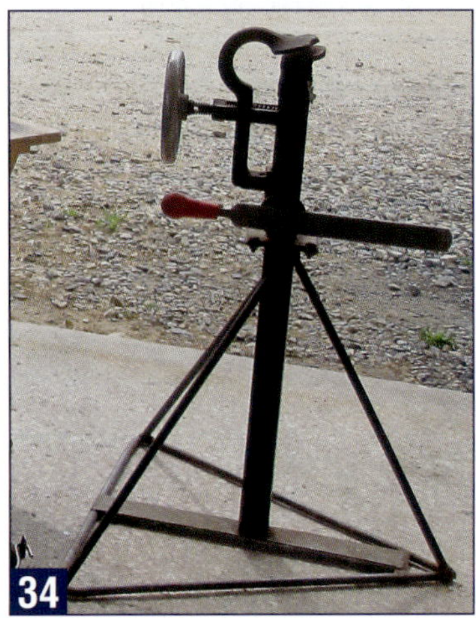

Gooseneck Vise.

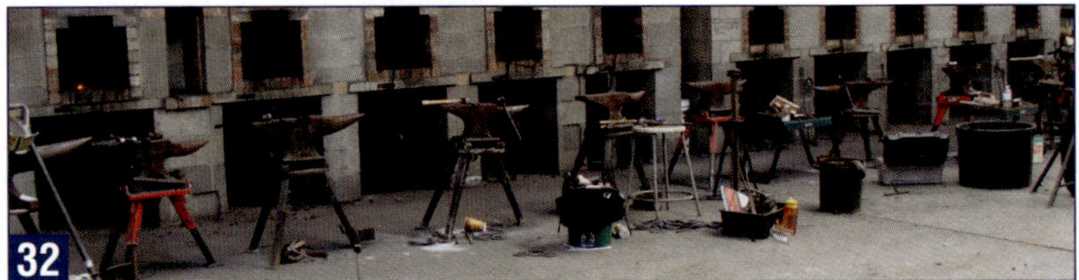

Row of shop style anvil stands in the forge at Heartland Horseshoeing School.

around when you use it. When I do clinics around the world, I am surprised at how many farriers don't have an anvil stand that works. A bouncing, ringing anvil will make you want to take a hostage, so either build or buy a good stand. Russell Colvin, CJF, from Blackwater Forge in Alabama, makes the best anvil stands that I have ever used. The style was invented - with the advice of Hall Of Fame farrier Bob Marshall - by a guy in British Columbia, Canada. At Bob's request, I later made them, but when it became too much for me, Russell took over the manufacturing. He has done an outstanding job of it, and the quality is second to none **(Figures 31-32)**.

Vise. In most blacksmith shops you will find a post vise like the one in **Figure 33**. While it is perfect for most blacksmithing applications, it is not specifically designed for a farrier. A good shoe vise will have a jaw designed for farriers and have a slant to it for easy access to the shoe. I really like the ones that are made by Billy Crothers in the UK, but the Valley Gooseneck is probably the most commonly seen one in the United States **(Figure 34)**.

Tongs: 1/4-inch, 5/16-inch, and 3/8-inch. You need to have the right-sized tongs

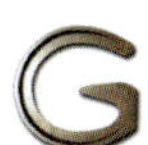

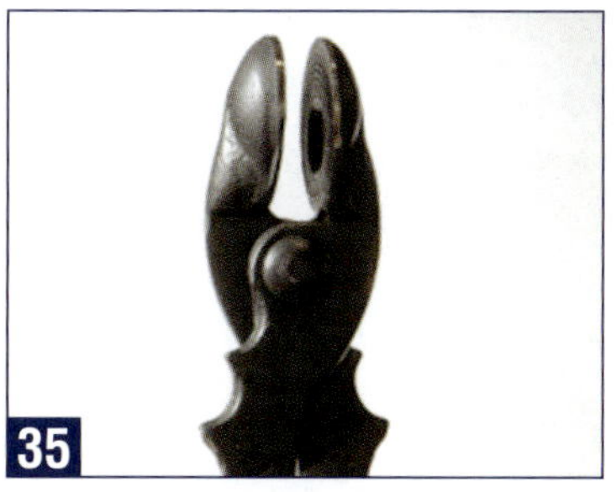
35
Jim Keith farrier tongs.

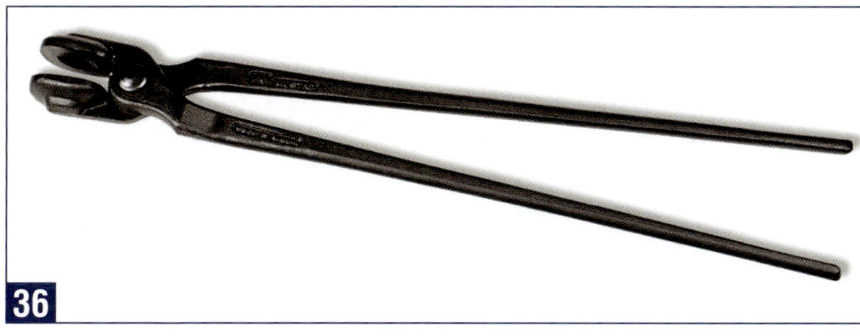
36
Mustad Farrier tongs.

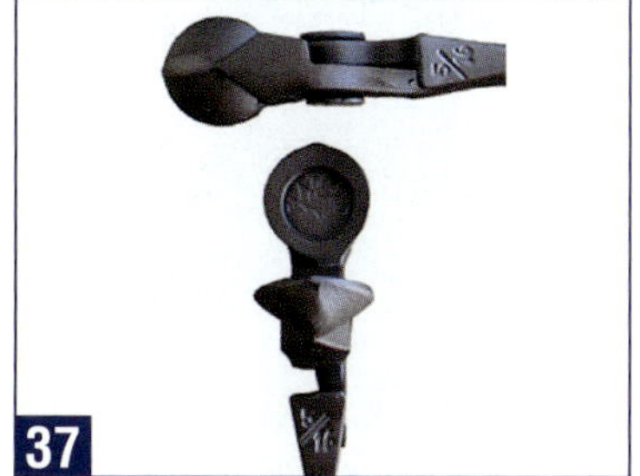
37
Flatland Forge farrier tongs detail

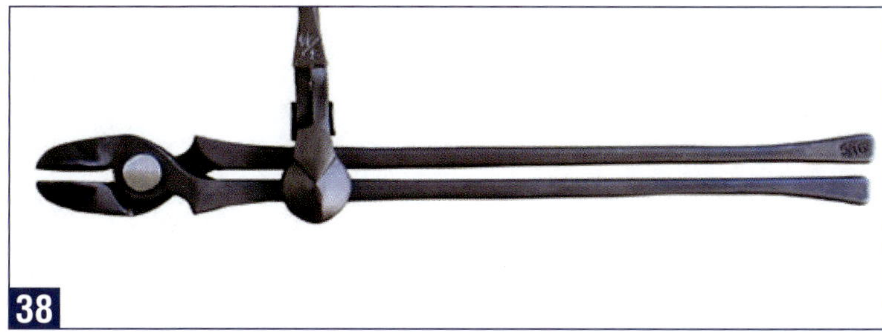
38
Flatland Forge farrier tongs.

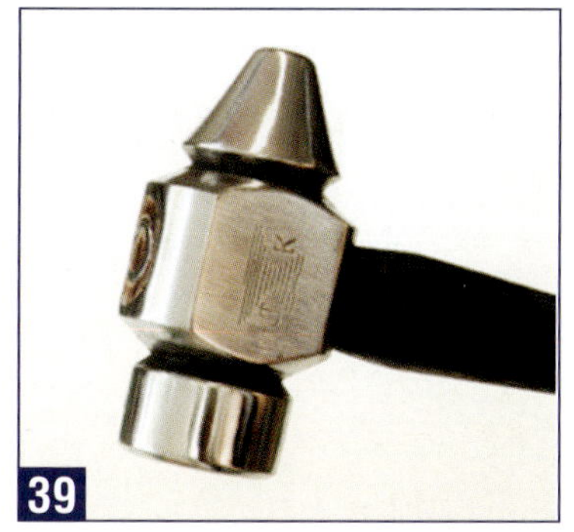
39
Kim Keith Clipping Hammer.

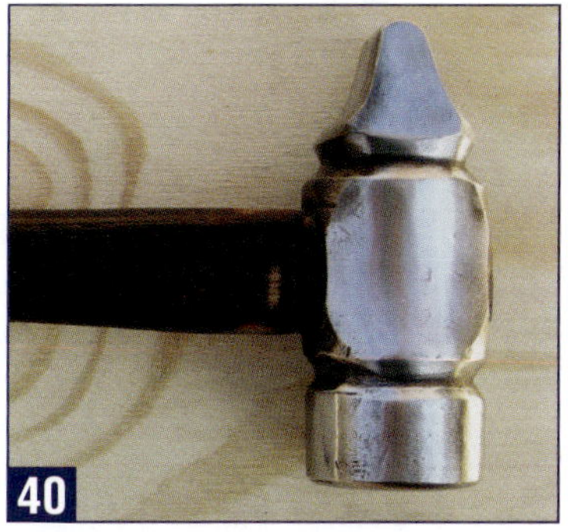
40
Bulldog Tools Clipping Hammer.

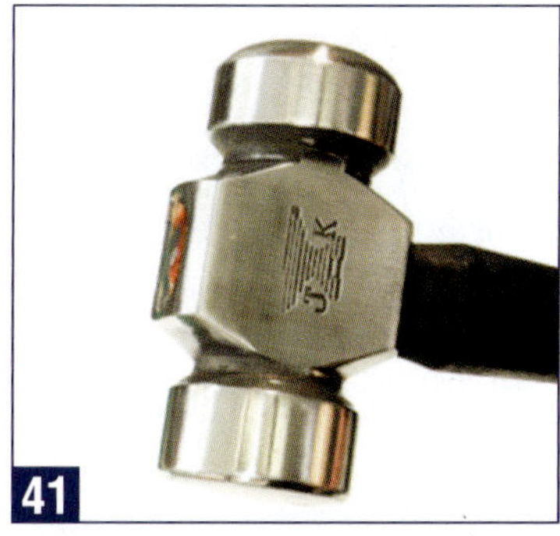
41
Jim Keith Rounding Hammer

for the stock that you are holding. They should be sturdy and strong, and hold the stock tight enough that you do not have to struggle to keep a grip. For the money, you can't beat tongs from Delta-Mustad. But Flatland Forge has come out with some tongs that are balanced extremely well and are a precision fit. They are more expensive, but if you are doing a lot of shoe making, they are worth it. Jim Keith also makes some great tongs. They are very stout, and I like to grind the jaws down when I use them. Jim Keith tongs stay to size extremely well **(Figures 35-38)**.

1.75-lb Clipping Hammer. (Ball Peen) There are a lot of ways to pull clips, but I prefer to do it with a ball-peen style hammer. Jim Keith from Jim Keith Tools in Tucumcari, NM., makes a very nice clipping hammer. The design of the peen is perfect for pulling out a great clip source, and his hammers are all durable and well balanced **(Figures 39-40)**.

2-lb Rounding Hammer. This is a hammer that has a flat face on one side, and a round face on

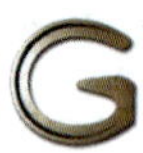

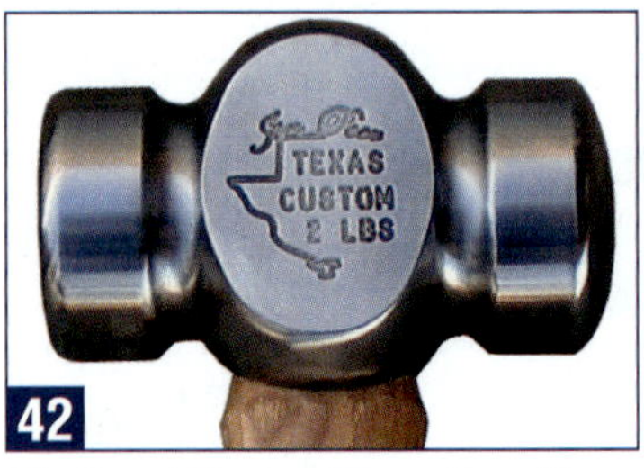

Flatland Forge Rounding Hammer detail.

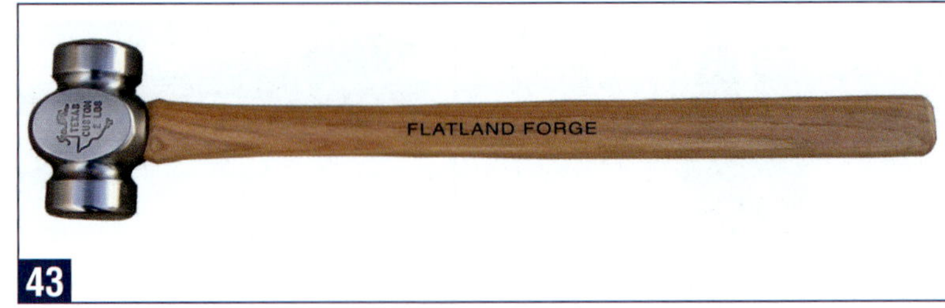

Flatland Forge Rounding Hammer.

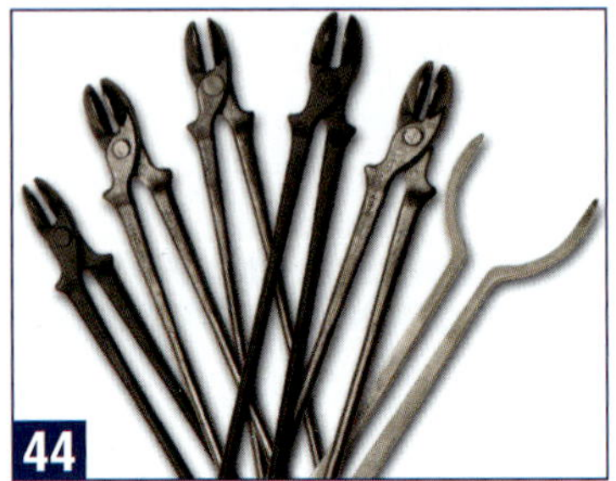

Delta tongs, Hot Fitters on the right.

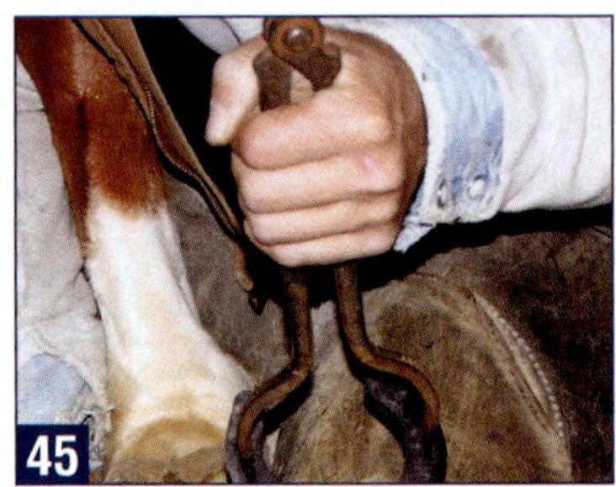

Handmade Hot Fitters in use.

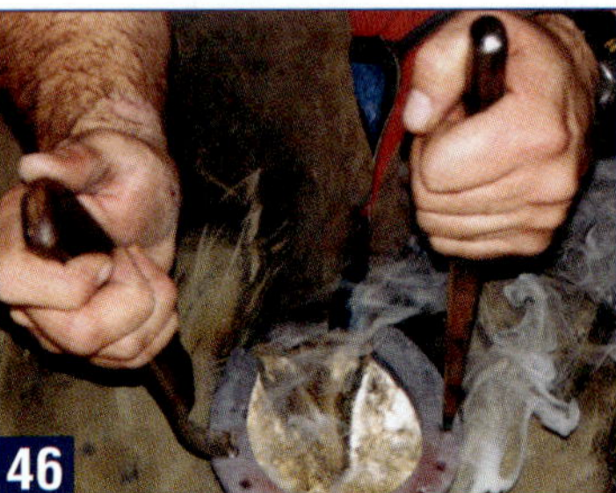

Hot fitting with a carrying pritchel.

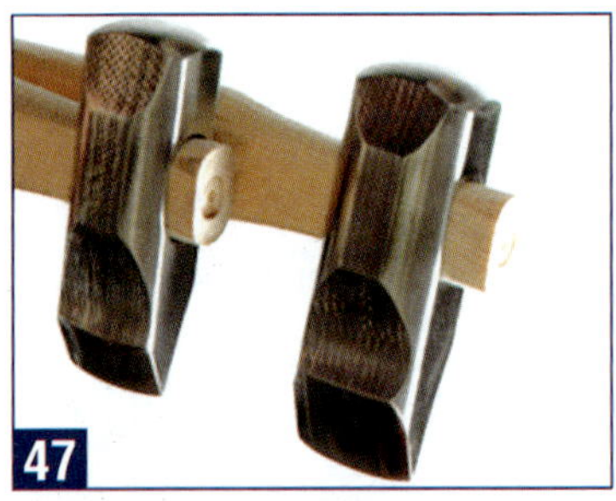

Jim Keith Creasers.

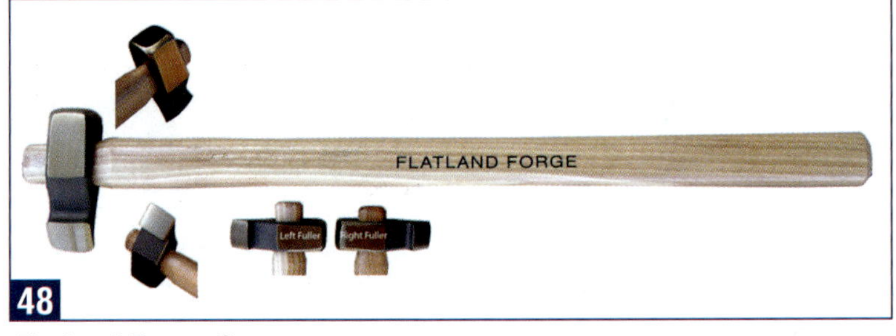

Flatland Forge Creaser.

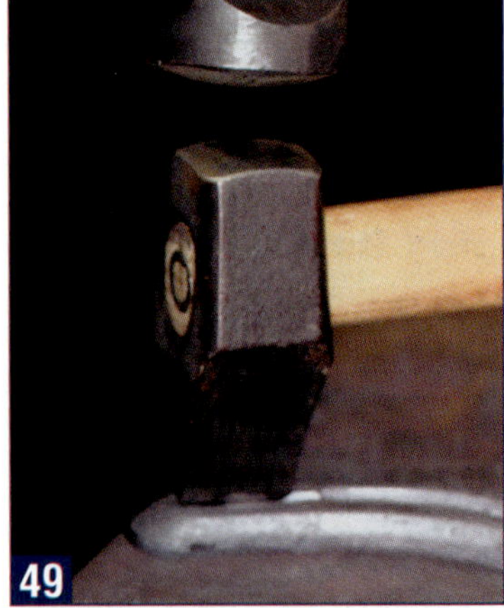

Mustad Creaser.

the other. Two pounds is the most common weight, but you need to get a weight that fits your forging style. Flatland Forge and Jim Keith Tools make really nice rounding hammers, and Delta Mustad Hoofcare Center has one of the best economy rounding hammers on the market **(Figures 41-43)**.

Hot Fitters. Hot fitters are a tool for carrying a hot shoe to a horse's foot and burning it on. You can make a pair easily out of an old pair of tongs by forging the ends of the reins out like commercially available hot fitters. You can also use a carrying pritchel for hot fitting **(Figures 44-46)**.

Creaser. A creaser, also called a fuller, is a tool that makes the cut in a horseshoe where the nails are placed. There are several designs of creasers on the

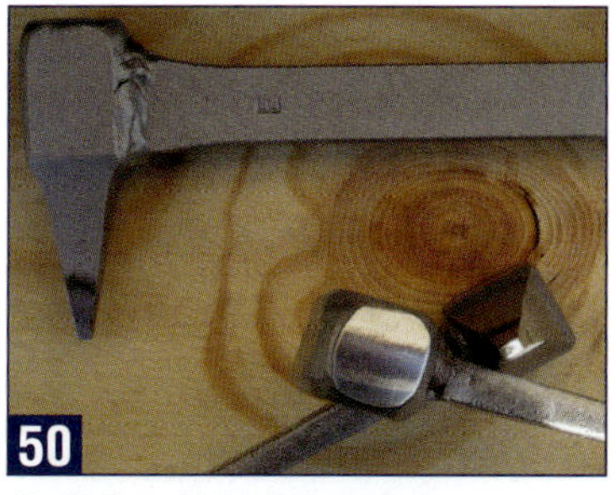

Bulldog E-head punch.

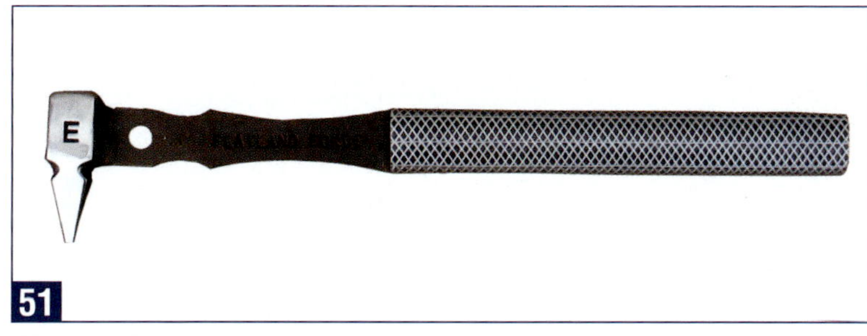

Flatland Forge E-head punch.

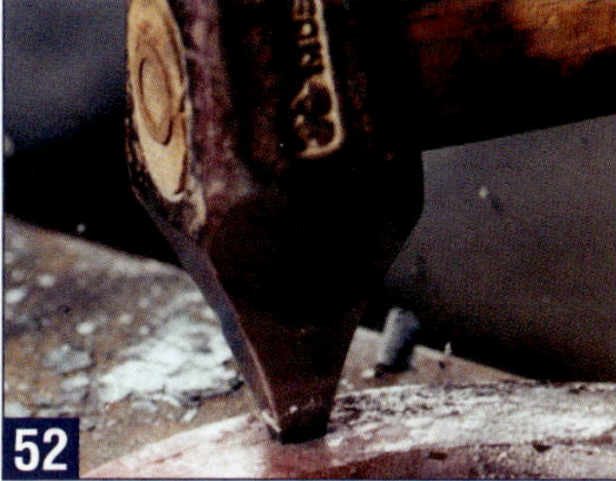

Mustad E-head punch.

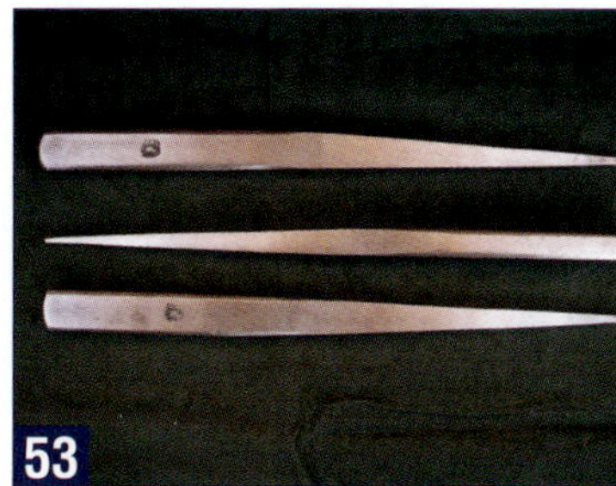

Bulldog Pritchels.

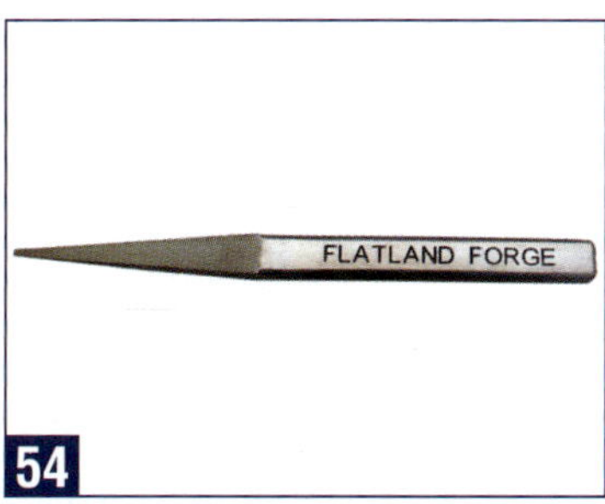

Flatland Forge Pritchel.

market, but I like the ones made by Jim Keith the best. Flatland Forge also makes a really nice creaser. They seem to penetrate really well, and they hold up good. For an economy model, it is hard to beat the Delta Mustad Hoofcare Center creasers **(Figures 47-49)**.

E-head Fore Punch. When you are making handmade shoes, the nail head shaped hole is made by a fore punch. There are 2 basic styles, an E-head, (E stands for European) and a city head. The E-head is the most accepted style for a plain stamped shoe, so that is the main punch that I would get. When you punch a shoe for E-head type nails, you only need one punch and one pritchel. If you are punching for city-head nails, you need the fore punch, a drift and a pritchel. There are a lot of good fore punches, but my preference is the Bulldog Brand made by Butch Hockaday in Virginia. Flatland Forge and Delta Mustad both make nice ones as well **(Figures 50-52)**.

Pritchels. The pritchel is a punch that removes the tiny piece of steel left at the bottom of a nail hole after the fore punch has been driven into the shoe. The important thing to look for when you buy a pritchel is that it has a long taper. I really like the ones made by both Bulldog and Flatland Forge **(Figures 53-54)**.

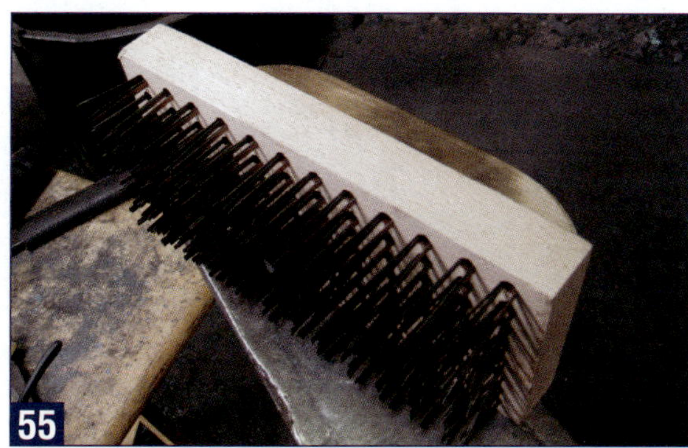

Butcher Block Brush.

Butcher Block Brush. A butcher block brush is a wire brush with stiff and heavy bristles. They are used to brush scale off of hot steel. You can get them in a small or large size, and I find the large ones to be well worth the extra expense **(Figure 55)**.

Brass Folding Ruler. This is a ruler used to measure bar stock and feet. Most will have standard measurements on one side and metric measurements on the other. You need to be able to measure steel that is longer than 12 inches, so most of these fold in the middle. Jim Keith makes one that works just fine **(Figure 56)**.

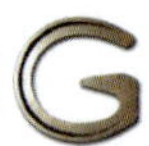

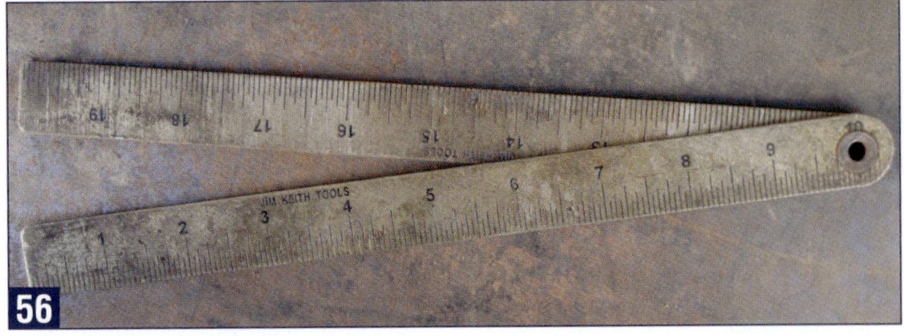

Jim Keith folding brass ruler.

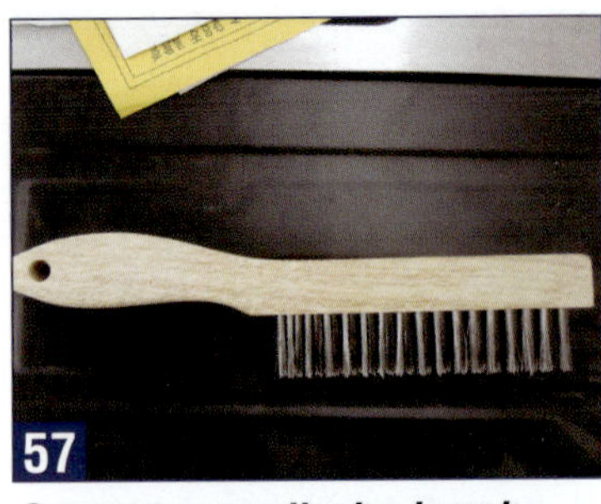

Common small wire brush.

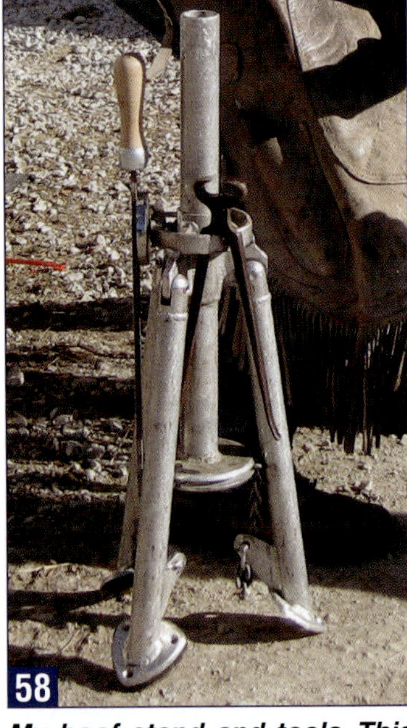

My hoof stand and tools. This stand was invented and made by Alexi Gutierrez.

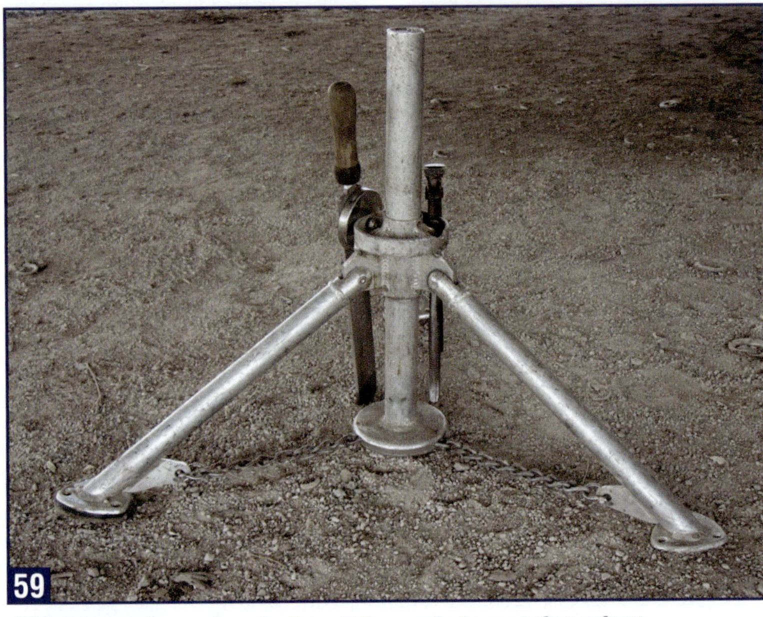

Side view of my stand when it is ready to use for a foot.

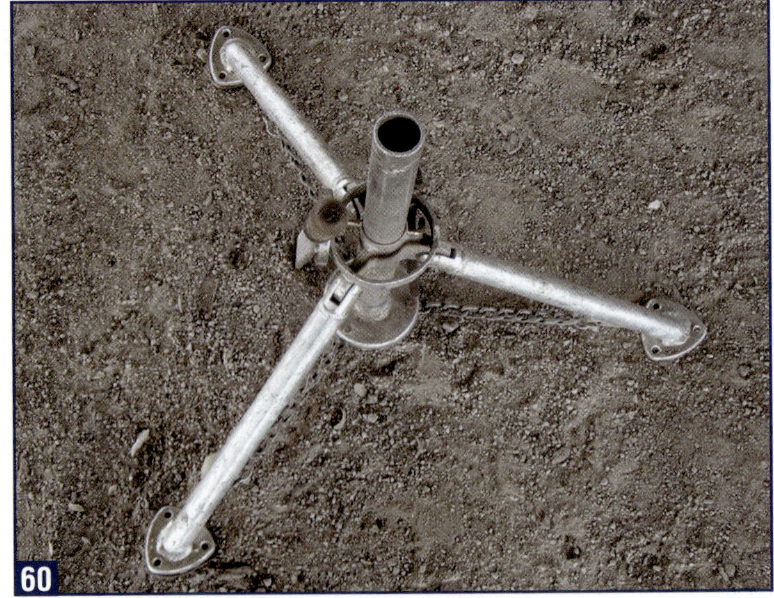

Top view of my stand when it ready to use for a foot.

Small Wire Brush. This is just an ordinary wire brush that you can get at any hardware store. It is for cleaning out the feet, and I recommend that you get one with longer wire instead of shorter. It allows deeper access into the commissures and seat of corn **(Figure 57)**.

Hoof Stand. A hoof stand is used to place the foot on when you are finishing the outside. Cody does not like to use one, but if I leave it behind, I go back for it before I do another horse.

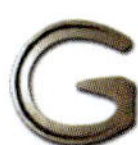

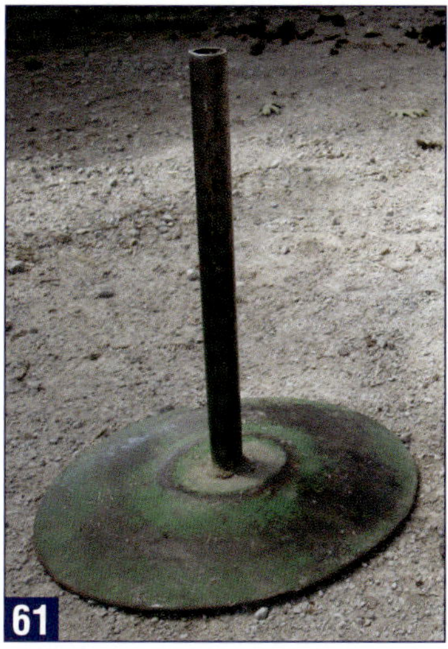

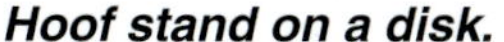
Hoof stand on a disk.

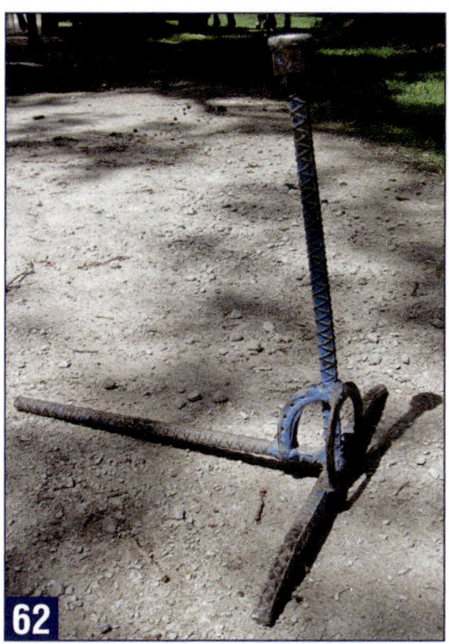

Hoof stand made from rebar.

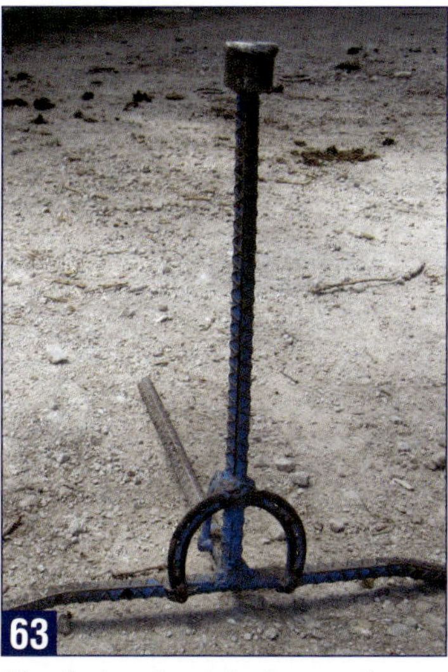

Hoof stand made from rebar.

A good friend of mine named Alexi Gutierrez has made the one that I use. It is a folding style, and I like it well. **(Figure 58-60)** I don't like the ones with a disc or round base. They do not seem sturdy to me on uneven ground, but that is a personal choice. **(Figure 61)** One of the strongest styles is pictured in **Figures 62-63**, and I would recommend making one yourself. You can make one like the one pictured for very little money.

Hoof Cradle. Hoof cradles are basically a platform to place the foot on when you are working on the bottom of it. They can be used on front feet, but I find this to be awkward.

On the hind feet, they hold the feet in a very good position, and they also make horses more comfortable. I have seen several occasions where a horse that was difficult to work on in a traditional way was quite happy to have its foot on a cradle. The one that I use is made by Hoofjack. **(Figure 64)**

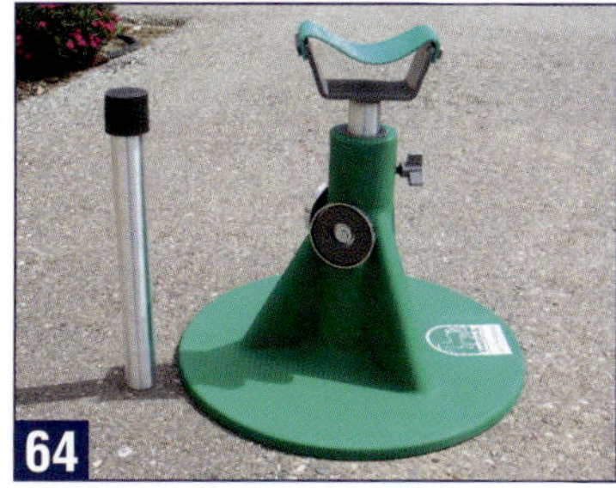

Hoofjack hoof cradle and hoof stand in one.

As stated at the beginning of this chapter, this is not a comprehensive list. You will find that there are many other items that you can add to this list. I found throughout my career that the better I got at shoeing, the less equipment I needed. The amount of things in my truck just kept diminishing until I found that I had a very Spartan rig. There is a tendency to replace skill with inventory, and I would warn against that. Go the other way, and replace inventory with skill.

Now that you have a full toolbox of shiny new toys, let's get busy learning how to use them.

Chapter 5 YOUR FARRIER SHOP

Having a nice shop to work and shoe in is the ambition of a lot of farriers. There are advantages to having customers bring horses to you. You don't have to pay for fuel, worry about being late, do more horses than scheduled, or wait for customers to show up while you wait at their homes or stables. You can also have a greater inventory that you are not hauling around with you. Of course, there are downsides too. If your shop is at your house, you can have customers coming to your house when you may not want them there. You can end up waiting for inconsiderate customers that don't show up on time, and some customers won't leave, even though the work is done. You will have to decide if having a shop to shoe out of works for you or not.

Regardless of whether you shoe out of your shop or not, you will still benefit from having an area where you can warehouse supplies and a place to forge that does not require setting up your rig every time. It takes a lot more self-discipline to come home at night and set up your rig to practice than it does to simply walk out to the shop and light a forge. So, I would suggest you plan a shop as soon as you can.

The first item of business is to create a safe and comfortable shoeing area. Whether you like cross-ties or hitching rails is up to you. I personally prefer a hitching rail, mainly due to the fact that the type of horses that I shoe are not used to cross-ties. It is different in other parts of the country, where horses are cross-tied more often.

The shoeing area should be well-lit, level, and easily accessible for both man and beast. This shoeing area at the Army School of Farriery in Melton Mowbray is one of the better set ups you will find. The horses are tied to rings in the wall, and the forges are close enough without being too close **(Figures 1 - 2)**. In **Figure 3**, you can see the shoeing area at Heartland Horseshoeing School. It is covered by a roof, but has a dirt floor, is not lit, and there are no walls on it. Horses like the openness, but it is not possible to completely eliminate having to deal with the elements in a situation like this one. Since the school is only open during the warmer months and during the day, this is fine for this situation. Very few horses stand as well as the Brazilian horses in **Figure 4**. I am not sure which one is the holder.

This shoeing area in **Figure 5** is at the Northern Melbourne Institute of TAFE (NMIT) in Australia.

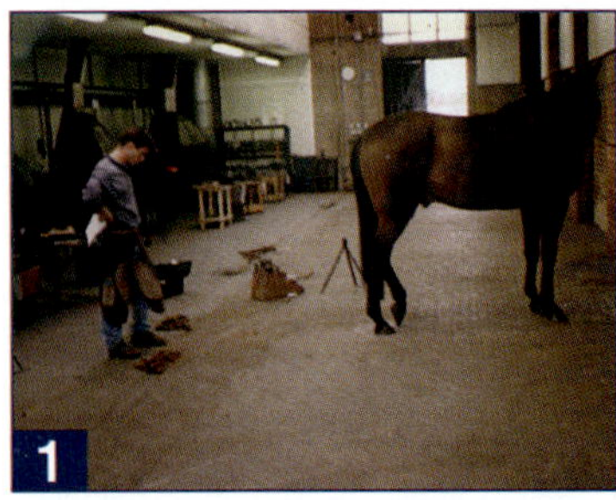

Good friend, Irish farrier, Paul Duddy, AWCF, in the Army School of Farriery at Melton Mowbray in 1997. Paul took an AWCF Prep Course with me that was taught by Sergeant Major of Farriery, Ivon Bell, FWCF (hons), and here he is contemplating the task that SGMF Bell has set for him.

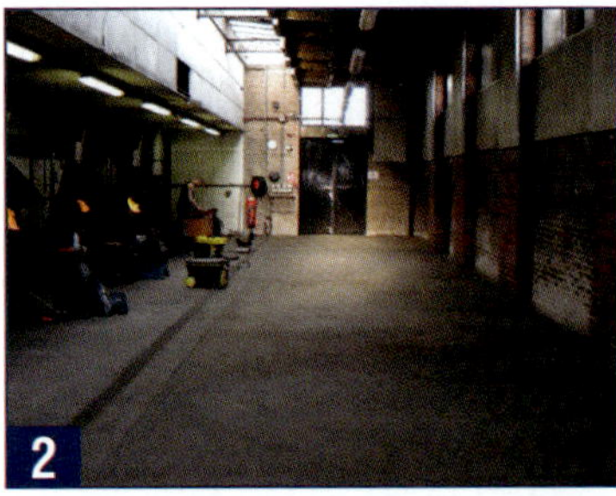

The same forge in Melton Mowbray, 2009.

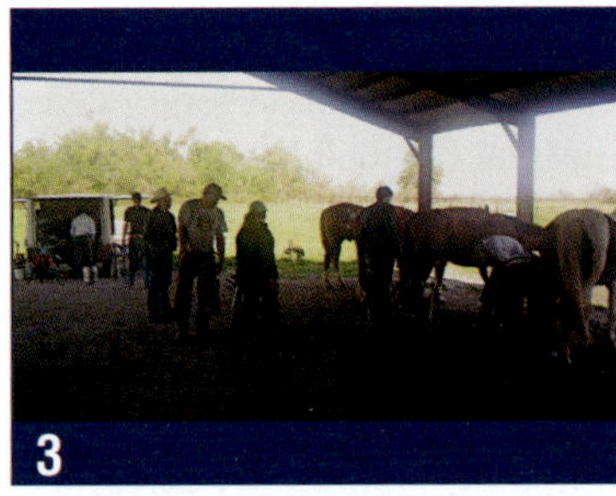

Shoeing area at Heartland Horseshoeing School.

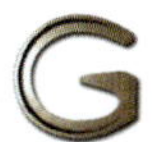

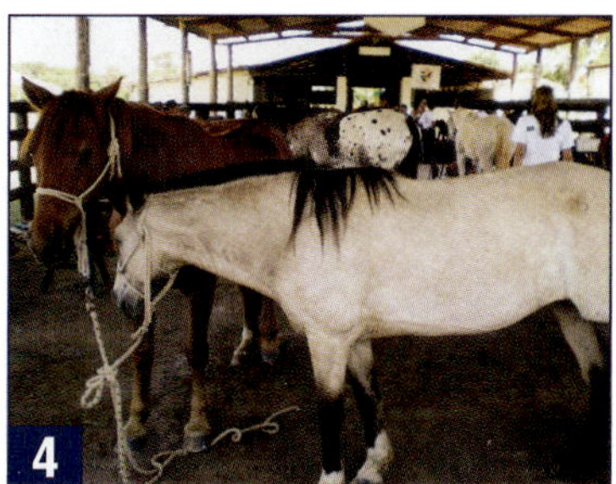

Some good Brazilian horses at a farrier exam at the Universidade do Cavalo.

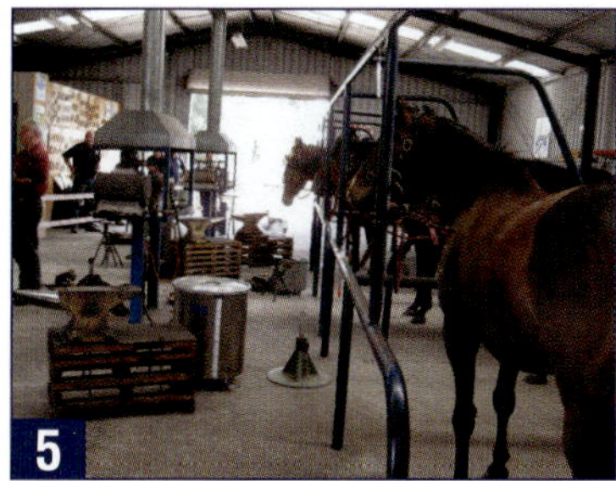

Shop at NMIT in Melbourne, Australia.

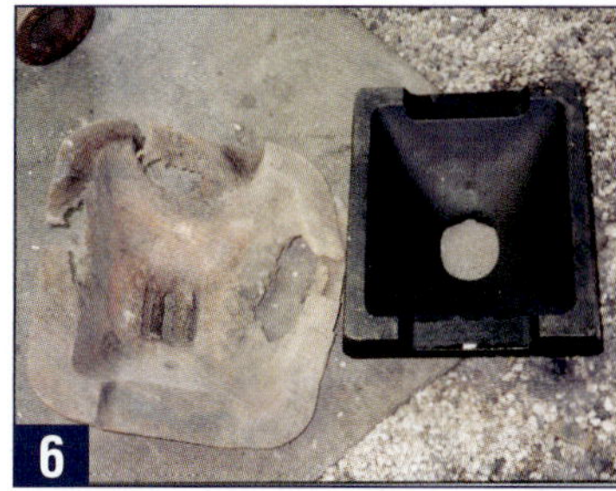

Burned up coal firepot next to a new coke firepot.

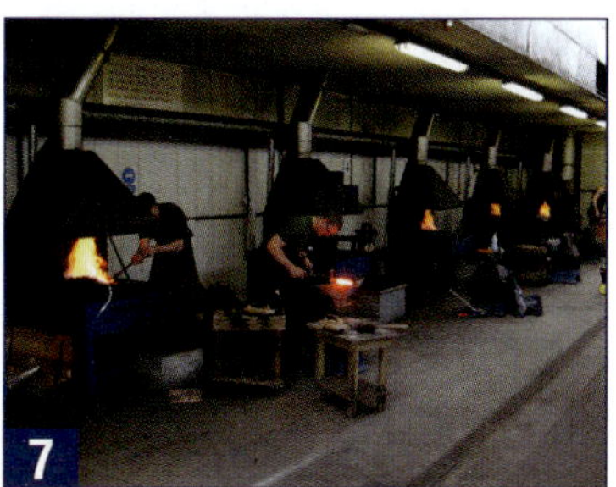

Forges in Melton Mowbray in 2009.

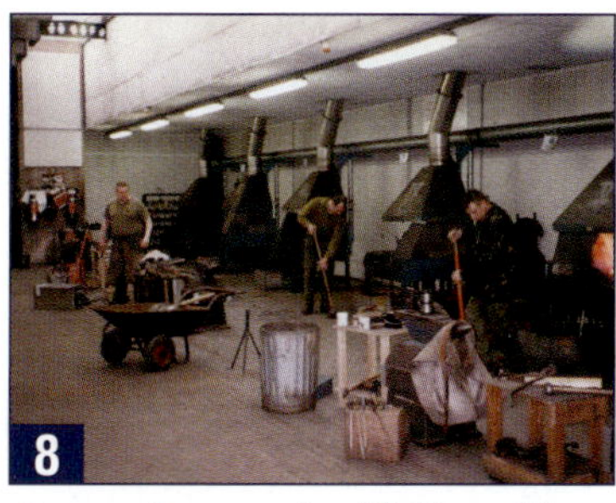

Same forges in Melton Mowbray, 1997.

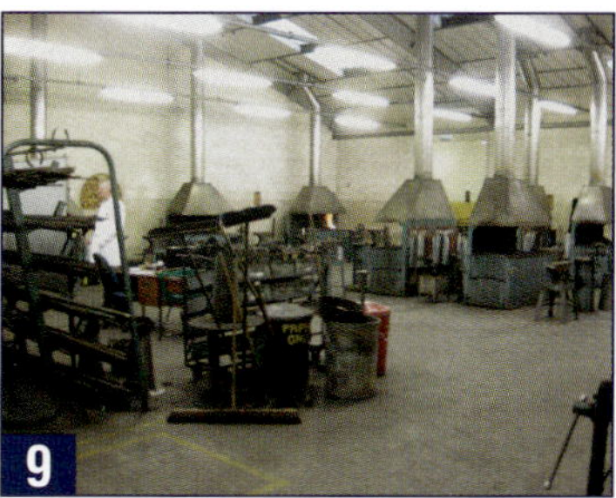

Forges at the Hereford School of Farriery and Blacksmithing.

It is well-designed and safe, as well as allowing easy access to the forges, which is an important part of a good shoeing area.

Next, you need to establish your forging area. I highly recommend a coal/coke forge. This is an old fashioned method of burning coal or coke to produce heat. These type of forges produce heat that far surpasses that of propane forges, and once you get good at the art of using one, you will wish that you had it to use on every horse.

The bottom-blast coal/coke fire is a very basic concept. There is a bowl called the firepot that has an opening in the bottom for forced air to come through. This hole is called the tuyere (pronounced tweer). Most firepots will have a clinker breaker in the opening that you can use to help break up the clinker that will form over the tuyere as the coke is consumed, but most clinker breakers only move the material around a little bit, without doing any real breaking. Note of caution, in **Figure 6**, you can see a coal fire pot that has been destroyed by burning coke in it. Coke firepots are much thicker to withstand the excessive heat from the coke fire.

There is also a side-blast coke fire that is popular in England. This is an easier model to use, but you have to have a water-cooled tuyere, and putting a side-blast forge together is more expensive to do. There is also the inherent maintenance problem with having to keep the basin of water full. As soon as the water evaporates, the tuyere will burn up. Here are some pictures **(Figures 7 - 8)** of the Army School of Farriery in Melton Mowbray, Leistershire, United Kingdom. These are side-blast fires, and they are very good. Here is the forge Hereford Blacksmith School and Hereford School of Farriery **(Figure 9)**. The air supply is in the concrete, with the blowers sitting outside. One blower supplies 10 forges. It is a fantastic facility, as you can see.

The advantages of bottom blast forges are that they are easy and inexpensive, while the advantage of the side-blasts is that you don't have to deal with clinker as often as you do when you are using a bottom blast. In my schools, we have always had bottom-blast forges, and the students have done fine with them.

We have 20 bricked-in coke fires at my school. There is one unit with two fires for Cody and me. The design was copied from Mike Miller, CJF, FWCF, who copied it from Jim Poor, CJF. It is a side-draw forge, where the chimney is placed beside

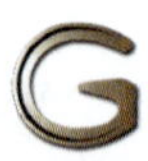

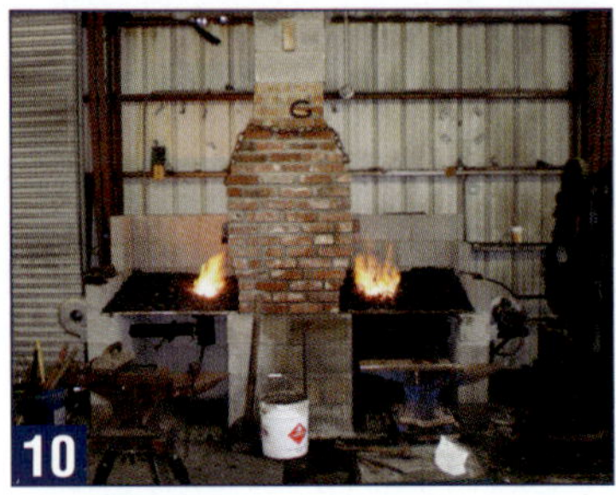

10

My forge on the left, Cody's on the right.

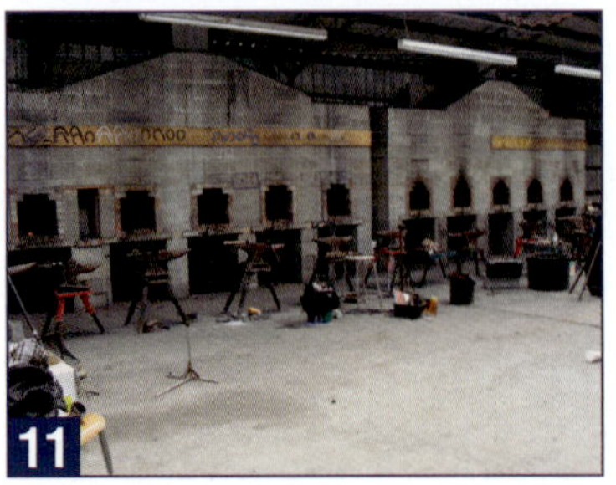

11

One bank of forges in the shop at Heartland Horseshoeing School.

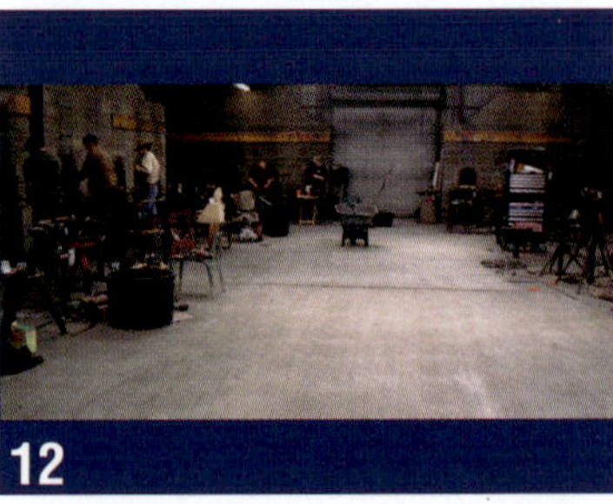

12

The rest of the forges at Heartland Horseshoeing School.

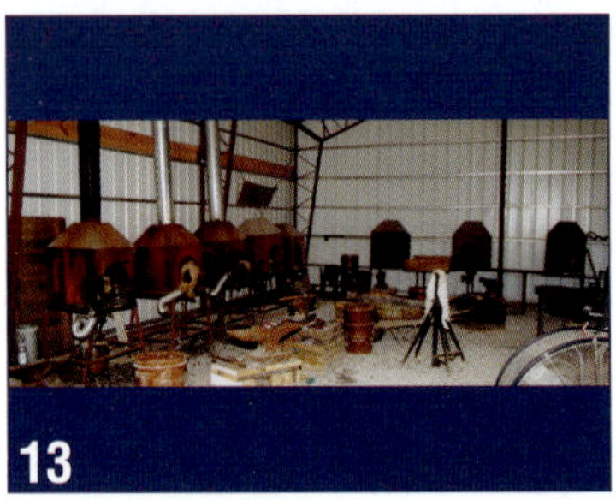

13

The early days in the forge at Heartland Horseshoeing School, probably 1997.

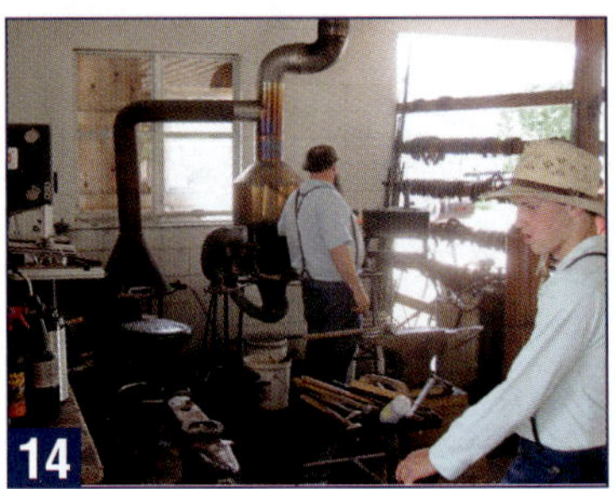

14

Abner's shop.

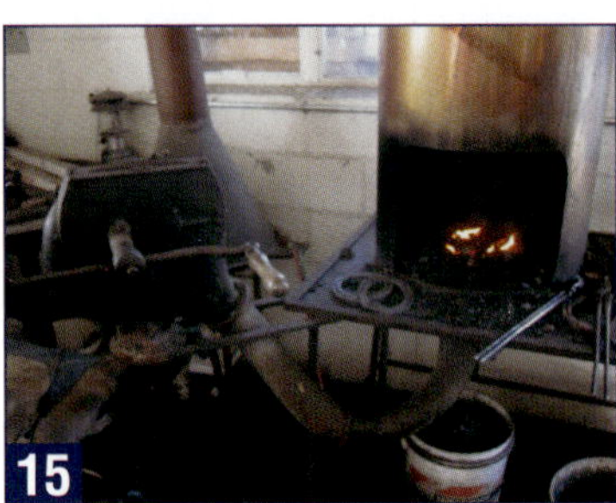

15

Abner's forge

the firepot instead of over it. This gives you more room to work in the fire **(Figure 10)**.

For the students, there are 18 forges, and the firepots are encased under the brick chimneys **(Figures 11 and 12)**. Beside every forge is a lever that controls an air gate. This air gate controls the amount of blast that each forge receives, and the amount of blast determines how hot the fire gets. More air, more heat. **Figure 13** is a shot of the inside of the shop in the early days of Heartland Horseshoeing School. Notice that the forges are all hand-cranked coal forges.

To build a good forge, all you really need to have is a solid table with a hole in it that will accept a firepot, a firepot to punt into the hole, and a good blower. The blowers that we use are called paddle-wheel blowers. Paddle-wheel blowers have more pressure than most other types and they will push the air through the system. Some blower styles, such as the squirrel-cage type, can move a large volume of air, but they don't have as much pressure. I have tried to use squirrel-cage blowers before, and they do not work well for coke forges. The system you see in **Figure 11** has 10 forges operating off of one blower. It is a blower that is used to move grain in some storage and processing operations.

When you burn coal, you make your own coke from the coal, and that is what you end up burning as your heat source. There are a lot of noxious chemicals (volatiles) that are released in that coal smoke, and this can be a problem if you have neighbors or poor ventilation. I prefer to buy a good blacksmith coke, something that does not have a lot of clinker, or produce fumes or smoke when burned.

In **Figure 14**, you can see the shop of a friend of mine in Delmarva named Abner Hershfield. He does not have electricity, so he shoes with a hand-crank coal forge **(Figures 14 and 15)**. We used hand cranks until we started using coke instead of coal. Coke requires so much more air than a coal fire that the hand crank proved inadequate. **Figure 16** is a picture of the hand-cranked coal forge that I learned to forge in at Frank Turley's Blacksmith School in 1990. I had been shoeing for over 3 years when I went to his course, and it was a real turning point in my career.

LIGHTING THE FIRE

As a young farrier and aspiring blacksmith, I wanted badly to use a coal forge. However, it was

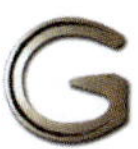

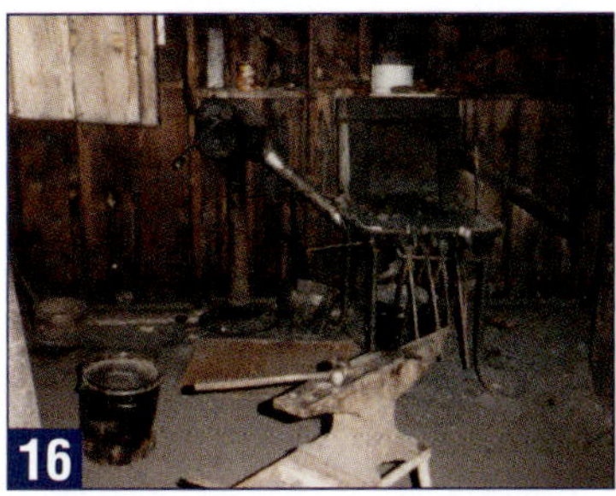

16

The first coal forge I worked on at Frank Turley's in Santa Fe, NM.

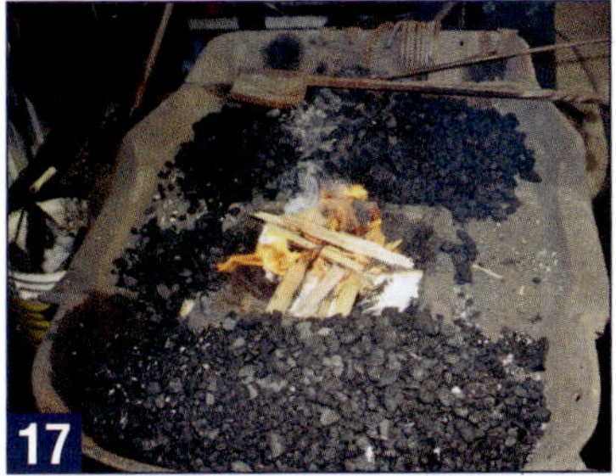

17

Wood ready to light for a coke fire.

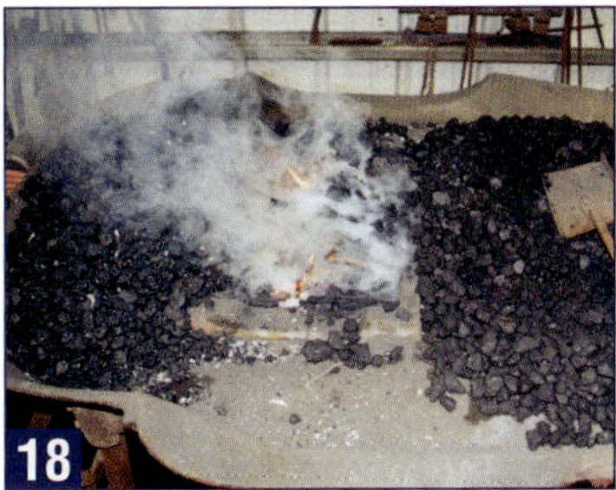

18

The wood is lit, small amount of blast, covered with coke.

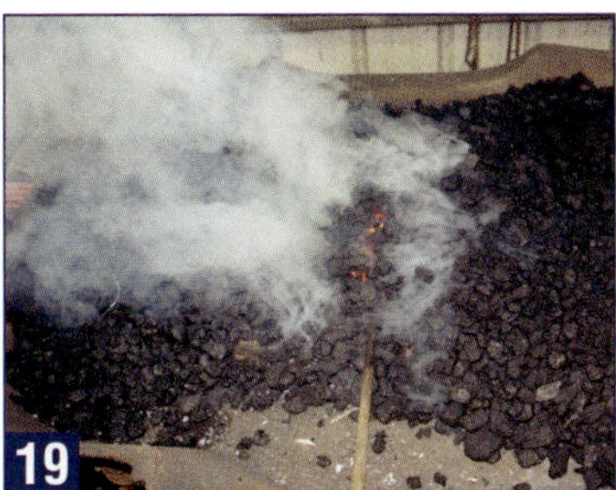

19

More coke added.

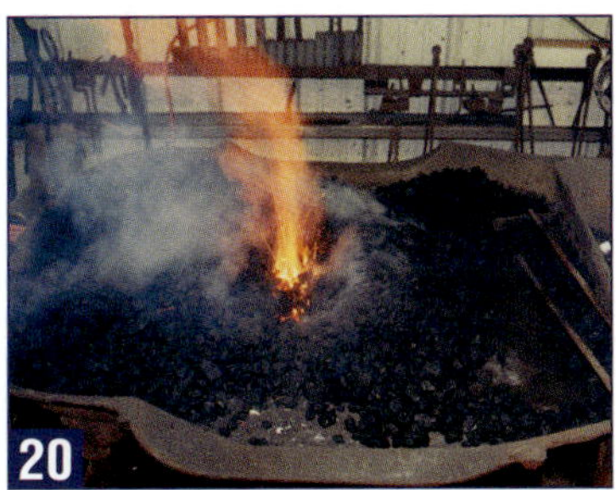

20

The fire is igniting the coke well, and the wood is about burned away.

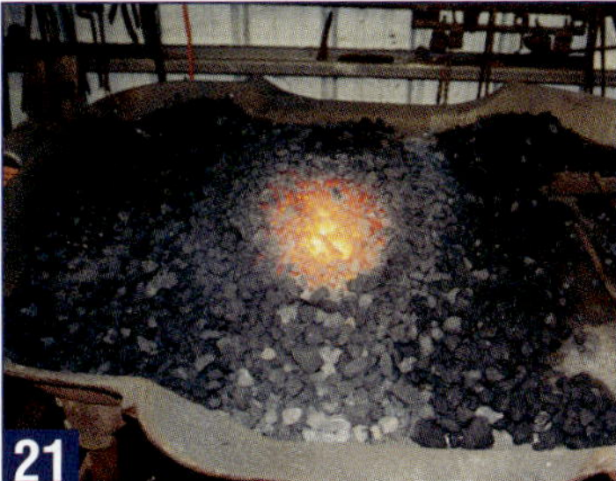

21

A well-lit fire.

about impossible to find a good book with a description of how to even light the fire. So I will take some time here to go over how to get a fire going, as well as how to use it efficiently. I have found that being good in the fire is one of the often-overlooked essential elements to being a great blacksmith. Being bad in the fire is like the great roper that is not a good horseman.

Lighting the fire will take some practice when you first start. Coal is much easier to light than coke, and it will stay lit much longer without an air blast than coke will. To light coal, you can roll up several balls of newspaper, place them in the firepot, light the paper, and put a very light blast to it from the air supply. Place some green coal, (not yet coked or burned) or better yet, some coke from the fire before, over the burning paper. Slowly increase the blast and amount of coke on the fire as it lights.

With coke, you need to use wood to start the fire. Cut up some kindling and start a small fire in the fire pot **(Figure 17)**. Tom Clark, from the Ozark School of Blacksmithing, used to soak down the wood with kerosene. As the fire gets going, give it a small blast from your blower, and slowly cover it with coke. Place more coke over the fire as more coke ignites **(Figures 18 and 19)**. Increase the blast slightly, as well. At this point in the lighting operation, there will be a lot of smoke. With good coke, the smoke is from the wood burning, not the coke.

As the coke starts to ignite, you will hear a popping sound as trapped water steams and breaks the coke apart. This is a good thing to hear, because it is an indication that you are getting your fire going. The hardest part of this is to keep yourself from raking and poking the fire as it lights. You are more apt to cause problems than help it, so I have my students get it started and then walk away for a couple minutes.

In **Figure 20**, you can see that the fire is well ignited. There is good flame coming from the center of the fire and very little smoke. You should be four to five minutes into the lighting operation by this point. **Figure 21** shows a good working fire: No smoke, hot coals, and a well-contained center.

You can make a forge lighter with a propane-fired flame-thrower. While this does work, I find that you end up with a fire that is quite high in the firepot. A high fire is one where there is unlit coke between the bottom of the firepot and the center of the fire. This makes it hard to get a good heat, and

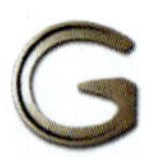

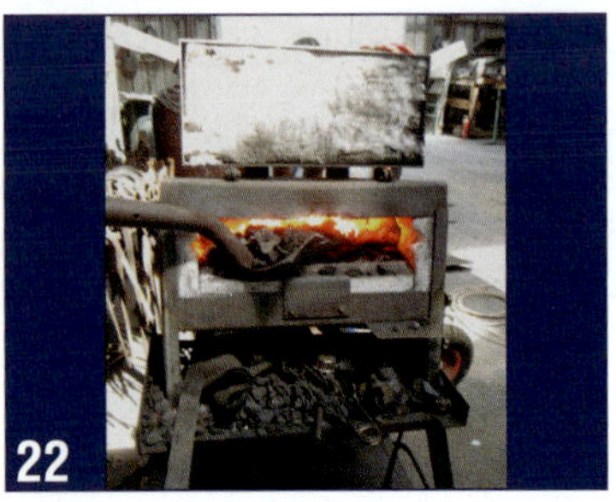
Shovel of coke being lit in a gas fire

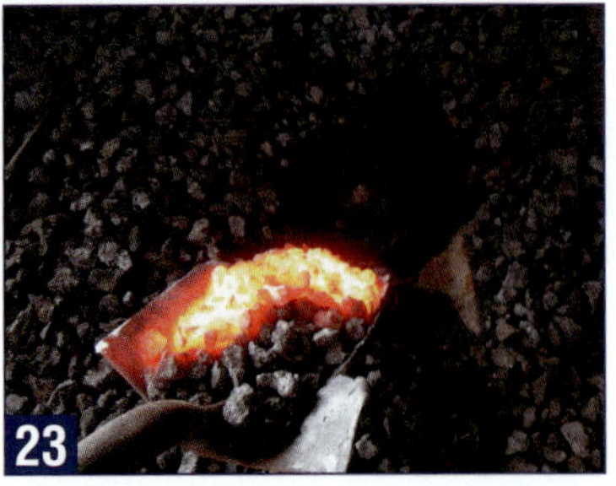
Placing the lit coals in the bottom of the firepot.

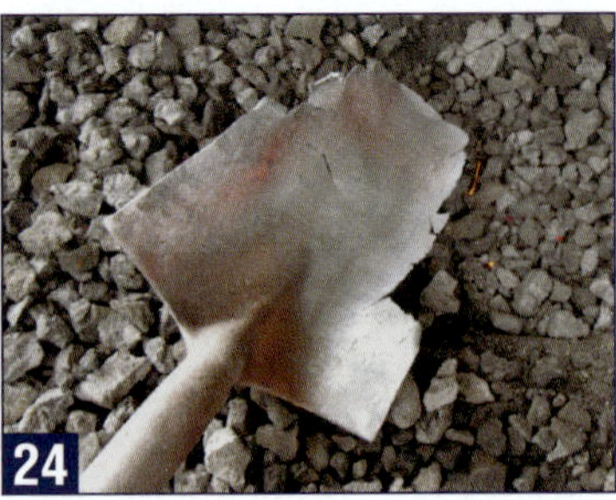
A well-used shovel.

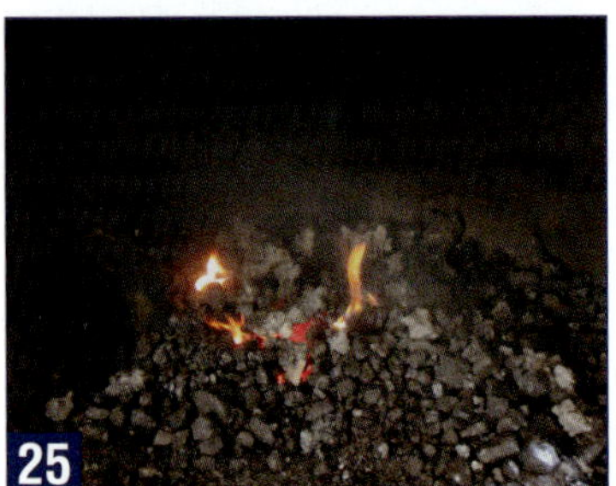
Coal fire full of freshly broken coke that had formed around it.

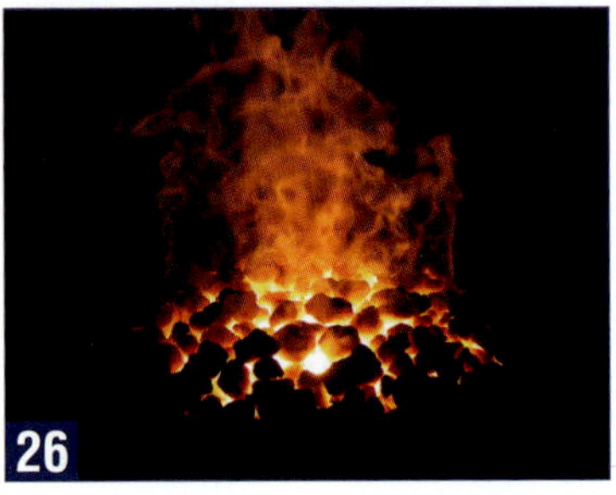
A very hot fire ready to use.

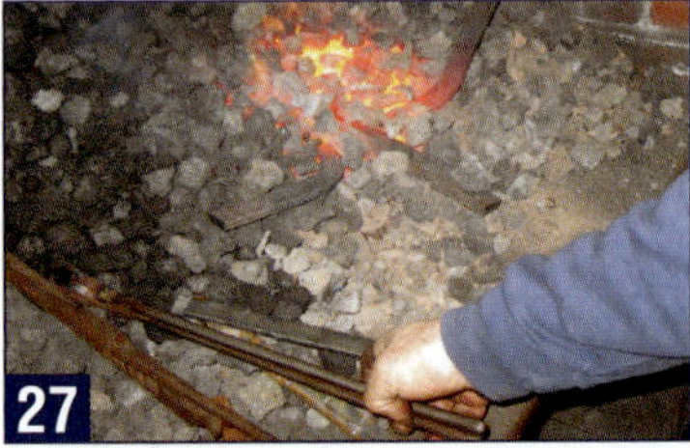
Working three pieces in a coke fire. Pieces are placed so that they won't burn, and the piece that you are wanting hot is in the center of the fire.

you spend more time trying to get your fire moved around in the firepot.

My favorite method is to light a shovelful of coke in a propane forge and throw the lighted coals into the firepot **(Figures 22 - 23)**. I give a light blast from the blower and cover over the top with unlit coke. Once one fire is going, you can shovel out a pile of lit coals to light the next fire. This is the easiest way to do it, but it is hard on shovels **(Figure 24)**.

WORKING IN COAL

When you are using coal, you are actually getting heat from burning the coke that results from burning the coal. Here is how it works. You have a blast coming through the tuyere, and this causes the coal to burn. As it burns, the volatiles are burned out of it. These go up the chimney, hopefully, in the form of a dense smoke. Ideally, you will get most of this smoke to ignite as well, but that does take a certain amount of heat that you won't have at the beginning of the lighting sequence.

The coal that is burned will stick together and form large, porous, pumice-looking coke. It will be light and soft, and you can easily break it up with your rake or poker. You can see the difference in the coke in **Figure 25** compared to the fire in **Figure 21**. The coke is going to be consumed as you work, and you will be constantly breaking it from the sides of your fire and making more coke with the coal behind it. As it burns, you will end up with a hollow area in your fire, sometimes referred to as a fire cave. Some people, mainly hobbyists, think this is a good thing to forge in, but it is not. This is just an area where you have burned away the fuel that you need to get your metal hot. This cave is an indication that you need to break away more coke off the top and sides of your fire.

A coal fire has a tendency to spread laterally across the forge. You can use a sprinkler can to water down the coal around the fire and keep it from igniting prematurely. Be careful to not use so much water that you get your cast-iron firepot wet while it is hot. If you do, you are taking a chance of cracking it.

Coal has the advantages of being easy to light, and staying lit for a long time if you need to do other things while forging. You can take a lunch break, come back to the forge and turn on the air, and generally still have a fire. When I worked exclusively in coal, it was not uncommon to still have

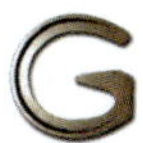

enough hot coals to light a fire the next morning by simply turning the crank on the blower.

WORKING IN COKE

You can purchase commercial coke to use in your blacksmithing. Buying a premade coke is actually more cost efficient than buying coal, but most people don't understand this. The reason coal seems cheaper is that it is cheaper by the ton. However, buying a ton of coal does not mean you will get a ton of coke out of it. In fact, you certainly will not. Commercially made coke is produced by heating coal in a recovery oven. This is like a massive pressure cooker, and it heats the volatiles out of the coal in the absence of oxygen. This prevents the burning of fixed carbon and creates a hotter and denser coke than a blacksmith can make in the normal shop situation.

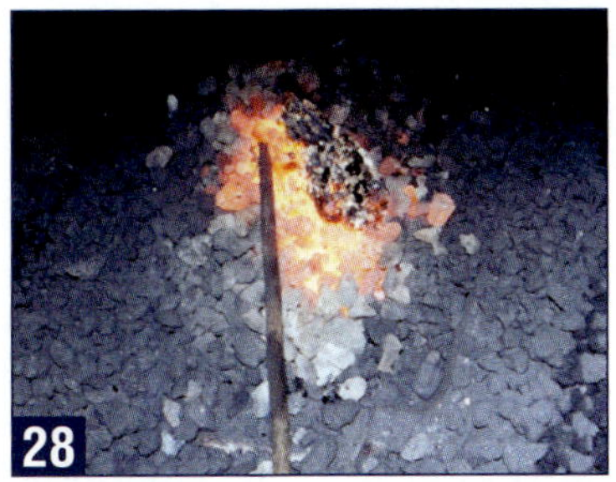

Cleaning a hot fire full of clinker.

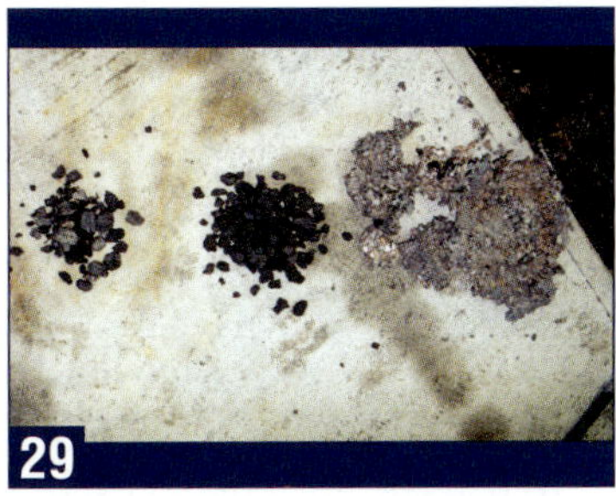

Coke on the left, coal in the center, clinker on the right.

Coke requires a lot of blast from the blower to keep it going. While not impossible, it is harder to keep a coke fire going with a hand-crank blower. As soon as the fire does not get forced air, it will start to go out. This makes it a harder medium for shoeing if you are spending time on the horse and not tending the fire. You can put a block of wood in the fire and open the ash gate to allow some air from below, but once the wood is burned away, the coke will quit burning.

On the positive side, the fire will not spread out across the forge, so you won't need to have a sprinkler can. Like the coal fire, the more air you use, the hotter the fire will get. With a coal fire, you will add fuel from the sides. With a coke fire, you will drag fuel on to the top of the fire.

Ideally, I want my coke fire to look somewhat like a low hill with an intense fire in the middle of it like the fire in **Figure 26**. The heart of my fire will be in middle of the hill, level with the top edge of the firepot. Think of your fire as the sun. Right in the middle is the hottest, and as you move away from the fire, it will be less hot.

THE FIRE

In a coal or coke fire, the heat will be coming from below the steel if you have the steel in the right place. You should try to place the material in the fire level so that it is in the heart of the fire. Try to keep from pushing cold, unlit fuel into the fire when you put the piece in the fire. If you drag cold fuel into the fire, it will cause the fire to have cold spots.

As fuel is consumed, more needs to be added. Many people don't manage their fires well, and the fire will become flat. The hill will become more like a pond of fire between two mounds. Having a fire without fuel is not efficient, so pay attention to managing your fire.

If the material you are working is rectangular, you can put it in the fire flat to make it get hotter faster. Placing the material on edge will slow down the time it takes the steel to get hot **(Figure 27)**. You should also turn off the blast when you are putting material into, or taking material out of the fire. With the blast blowing hard, you can have a lot of hot, burning coals follow the piece out of the fire and land amidst your hair, clothes, hands, and whatever else it can get on. It also conserves fuel if you are not running the fire when you don't need it.

After forging for some time, you will develop clinker in the bottom of the fire. This clinker is created by ash content in the coal or coke being melted from the heat of the fire. These clinkers become molten like lava and will settle over the tuyere. When they do, they constrict the amount of air that can reach the fire as well as allow oxygen to get through to your work without being consumed. That is why it can be harder to weld in a fire that has a lot of clinker in it.

You can clean the fire without putting it out by turning off the blast for a while and allowing the molten clinker to solidify. This will take three to five minutes, depending on how hot the fire is. Once it is a solid mass, you can fish it out with your fire poker as in **Figure 28**. In **Figure 29**, you can see from left to right, commercial coke, green coal, and clinker.

PROPERTIES OF FUEL

If you are going to have a coal or coke fire, there are some things that you need to know about the product you are burning. This information is from Ed Avolio, who is the dealer of a product called L-Brand® Coke. This is the coke that we use at the school and has been used many times at the World Champion Blacksmiths' Competition in Calgary.

When you are looking for blacksmith coal, there are some basic things to know. First you should find out what the coke button is for that coal. The coke button indicates how well that coal will coke. The coke button ranges from 1 to 9, and anything with a 7 or higher will coke. Coal with coke buttons below 7 are usually rated as steam coals.

Next, you want coal that has as fine a particle size as possible. Lump coal has to be crushed before coking, so if you get too large a size, there is the added time smashing it up before you get to use it.

It is also important to know the amount of combustible gases, known as volatiles, in the coal. The higher the amount of volatiles, the less coke will be made from that coal. When you buy coal, basing the purchase simply on BTUs (British Thermal Units), is not necessarily a good economy indicator. Knowing the volatiles is important as well, because if that coal has 35% volatiles, you will lose that 35% in weight and BTUs when it is coked. A low volatile coal, 18% to 20%, is the best to get for coke yield. The higher the volatiles, the more noxious the smoke and soot.

Ash content will remain in the coke and usually has a significant effect with high volatile coal in the 30% to 35% range. Sulfur doest not affect the coking ability, but is does make the coal smell bad when it is burned. A higher sulfur content may also cause the clinker to stick more to any metal being worked, so that is a concern for blacksmithing.

When you are buying coke, the characteristics you are looking for are a size of 1-inch to 1-1/4-inch pieces. Any larger than that and you can't get the metal into the fire. Smaller, and the blast from your air supply will blow it out of the firepot.

You want a consistent coke, which means that the fire and clinker will react in the same way all the time. The ash content should be below 9%, which is about as good as you can get in that size coke, and you want your sulfur content below 0.7%. The BTU content is a good indicator of quality, since it relates to the amount of heat available for forging. A very good number is 12,500 BTUs. You can get higher BTUs with larger sizes, but they have to be crushed for blacksmithing.

So there is a bunch of information that you can use to select a quality coal or coke to work with. I recommend that you get a sample before buying a huge quantity. If you have a terrible product, it will be more of a hassle than productive. If you use a good product, you will wonder why you ever forged in a propane forge.

GAS FORGES

I came into this trade as the atmospheric propane forge was making its debut. There were still quite a few farriers toting portable coal forges in their rigs in the late '80s. Propane was fine for shaping keg shoes, but it seemed too cold for welding and general shoe building. Someone finally figured out the process and the flux needed. Since those days, propane forges have come a long ways and become a lot more efficient and hotter.

Speaking of propane forges, you will also need one of these in your shop. They are easy to shoe out of, faster to light, and they definitely have a place in the modern shop. The main use that ours gets in the school is to light the coke fires, which is fast and easy, but perhaps not cheap. I do occasionally use it for shoeing if I have only one horse to do and it is a horse that I am not making handmades for.

One thing that I have found out is that I can get my stock a little bit hotter and actually do less damage to my liner with welding by putting coke in the gas forge. You can see the coke in the fire in **Figure 30**, where I am brazing an aluminum bar shoe. When you weld or braze in a propane forge, there will be molten flux that can get on the liner. Every time you use the forge, that material causes a little bit more of the liner to get damaged. This causes us to have to get a new liner about once a year in the rig forges, but the forges that have had coke in them seem to hold up much better. The shoes that are made or worked in the forge with coke in the bottom of it are also cleaner. I think that the coke consumes some of the oxygen that would cause oxidation to the outside of the shoe.

You can see a really clever mobile cart with a nO'Dwyer Damascus Forge and anvil on it in **Figure 31**.

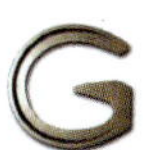

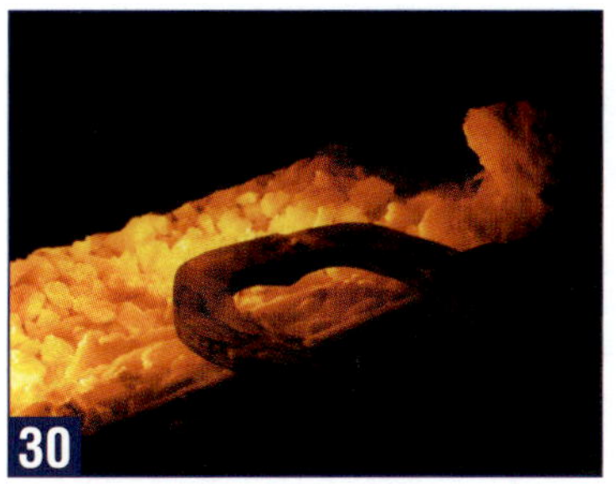

30 *Gas forge full of coke.*

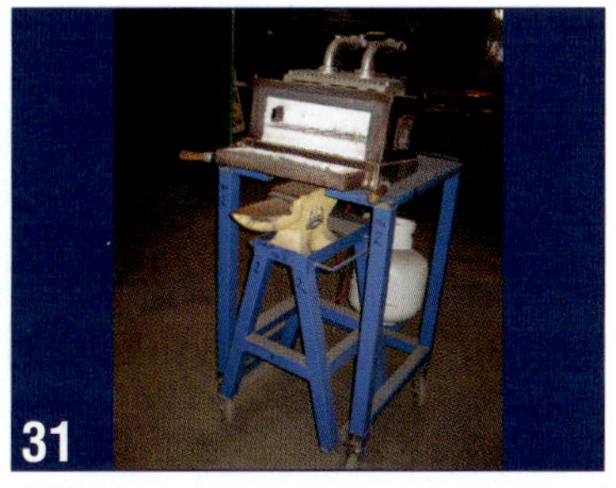

31 *O'Dwyer Damascus forge and anvil on a mobile cart.*

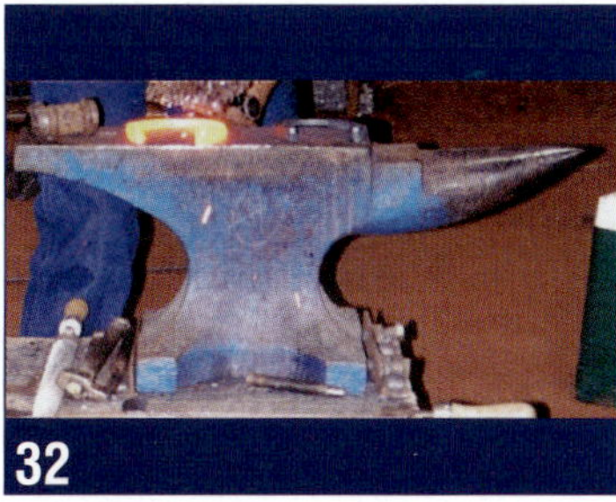

32 *Swedish-made Kohlswa A1, 200- lb anvil.*

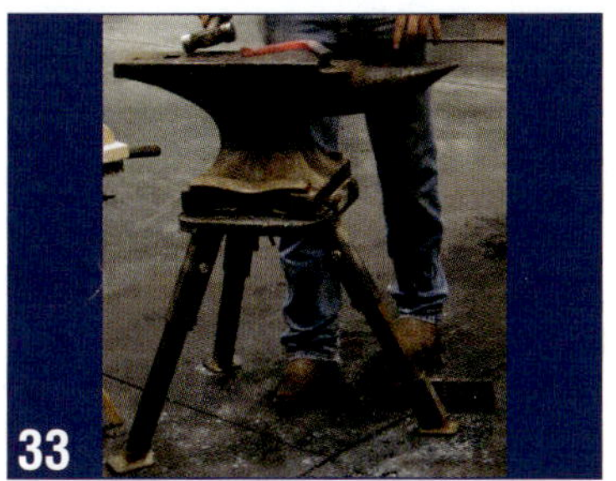

33 *Another picture of the Kohlswa on a Heartland Anvil Stand.*

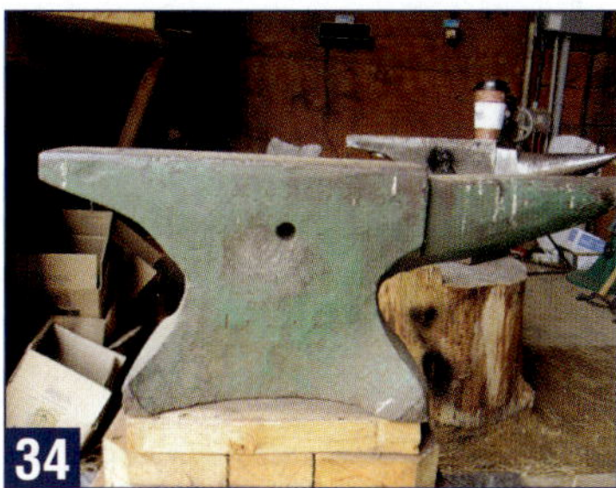

34 *Old English Mouse Hole Forge anvil with a hole in it. I don't know what the hole is for, and I never saw another one with it.*

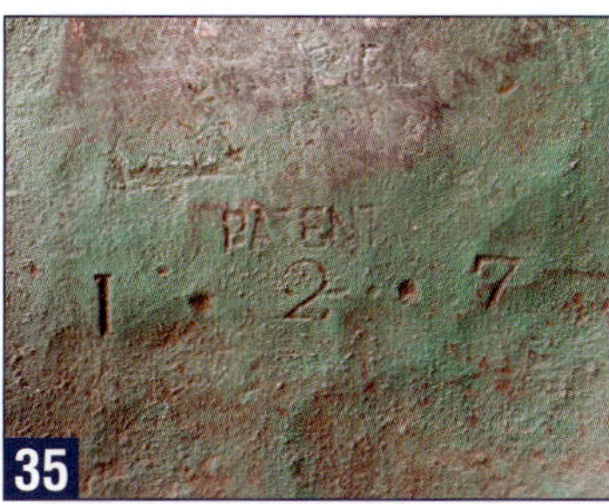

35 *Numbers on the Mouse Hole Anvil. 1 = 112 lbs. + (2 X 28) = 56 lbs. + 27 lbs. Total weight is 195 lbs.*

ANVILS

It takes extra self-discipline to come home from a long day of shoeing and set up your rig one more time to make shoes and practice. Having to set up the rig can be that little hump that makes you sit on the couch instead of picking up your hammer. So, I think it is important to set up a shop as soon as you can. This way you don't have to move your truck anvil again when it is time to work in the shop.

For a shop anvil, I recommend something in the 200-pound range. This is too heavy for your rig, but not so heavy that you can't move it around the shop when you have to or load it for a contest. The anvil in **Figures 32 - 33** is one of our 200-pound Kohlswa A1 models. It is a Swedish-made anvil, and quite popular amongst American farrier competitors.

Most American-made anvils will have the weight of the anvil on the side in pounds. Many European anvils will have the weight in kilograms. The old English anvils had a system that used hundred-weight, quarters of hundredweight, and odd pounds. With these, it takes a little math to figure the weight, but here is the formula: A hundredweight is the equivalent of 112 pounds. The first number is the number of hundredweights in that anvil. The second number is for the quarters of hundred-weight, so this number will be a 3 or lower. Once the second number would get to 4, that would be another hundredweight, so it would increase the first number. The last number is odd pounds that are less than a quarter of hundredweight. So, the last number will never be greater than 27.

So if you see one of these old English anvils, you can determine the weight with that information. Here are a couple examples:

Numbers on the side of the anvil: 1 1 7
Formula:
(1 X 112) + (1 X 28) + 7 = 147-pound anvil.

Numbers on the side of the anvil: 2 3 21
Formula:
(2 x 112) + (3 x 28) + 21
224 + 84 + 21= 329-pound anvil.

Confusing, I know, but it was their system for a long time, and knowing that now allows you to not get ripped off when buying or selling anvils by the pound. The anvil shown in **Figures 34 - 35** is owned by Mike

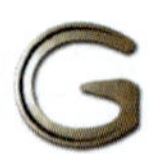

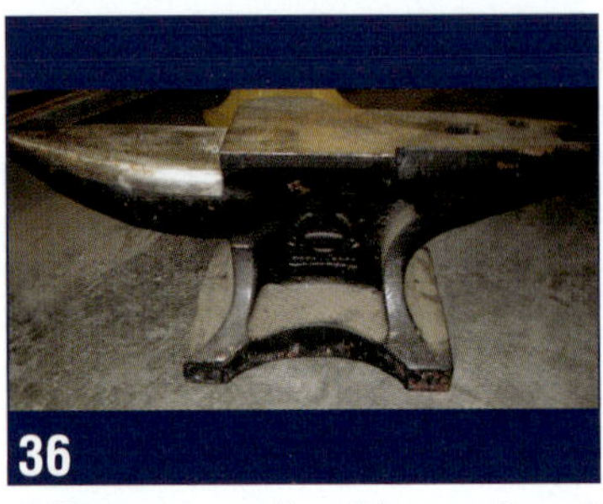
O'Dwyer anvil with a church window.

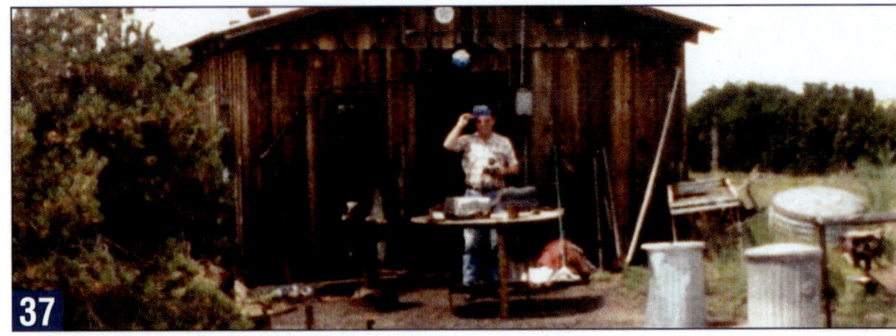
The outside of Frank Turley's shop in 1990.

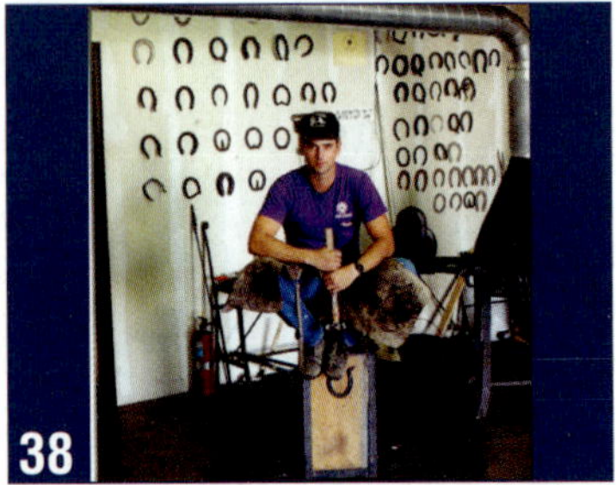
Me sitting on the anvil in the first school that I ran in Colorado in 1992.

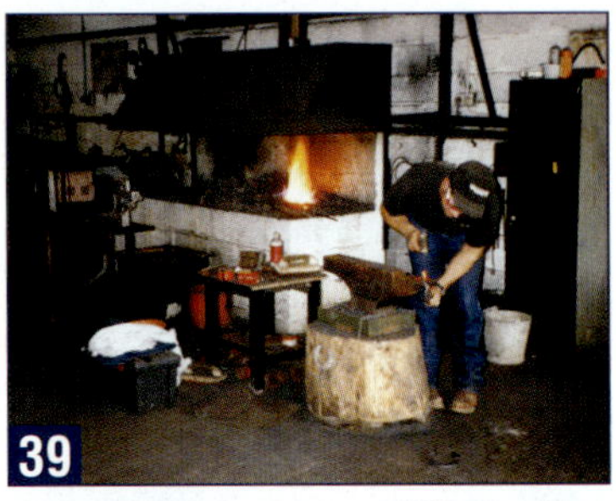
Sandy Beveridge, FWCF, shop in Scotland.

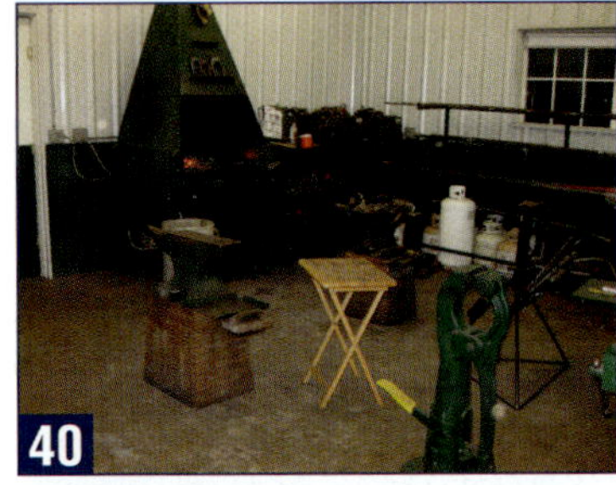
Dallas Morgan, CJF, shop in Locke, NY.

Bailey, CJF, from Delaware. It weighs 195 pounds as you can see by using the formula.

Anvils come in a variety of shapes and sizes. You can see a modern O'Dwyer with a hollowed-out area through the body in **Figure 36**. This was a tactic used in olden times to save on iron, and used here on the O'Dwyer to reduce the weight. The common name for this feature is a Church Window.

There are several features that I want in my anvils, but the most important of all is a round horn. With shoe building, a round horn gives you radiuses that you can use to predict where a shoe is going to bend or straighten. By simply pushing that steel into those radiuses, you can make a shape for a foot. The perimeter of a foot is several radiuses put together, and shaping shoes preperly requires finding those radiuses on the horn.

I also like a flat face and a few good edges. New anvils will have sharp edges, so one of the first things that needs to be done is to grind those edges down slightly. From the step, back about 3 inches on both the near and off edge of the face, I like about a 1/4-inch radius. I then put about a 1/8-inch radius down the rest of the edges till I get to the heel. At the heel, I will make the near edge a 3/8-inch radius, and the far edge I take to the a 1/4-inch radius. A sharp edge will mark and cut your work, while a softer corner will allow you to bend and clip without cutting or ruining your shoes.

Complete your shop equipment with a good vise and some odd power tools like belt sanders and a cut-off saw, and you are ready to spend some time getting great at this trade.

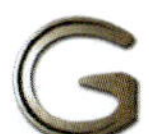

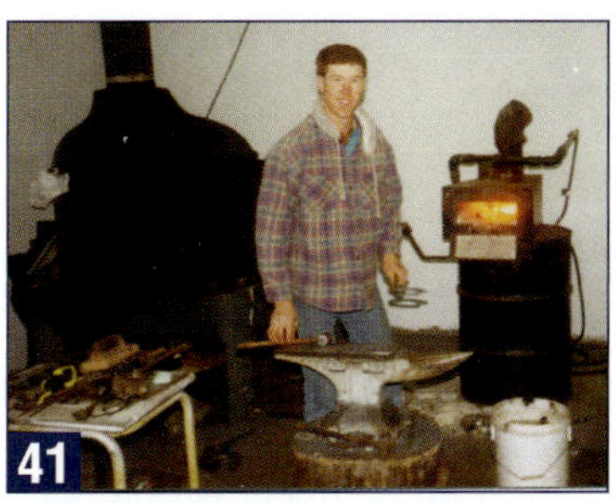

Dallas standing in Bob Marshall's shop in Mission, British Columbia, 1995.

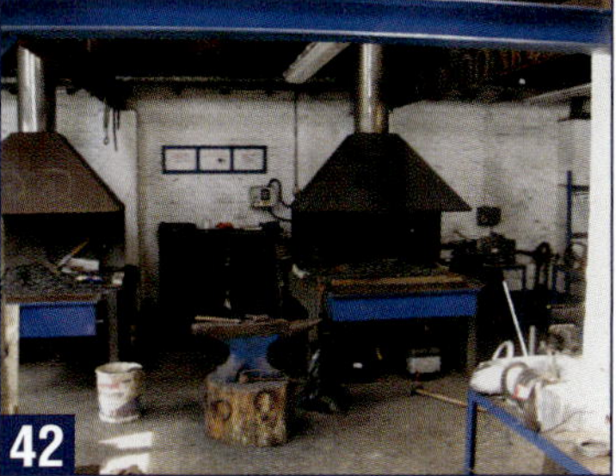

Simon Curtis, FWCF, shop in New Market, England.

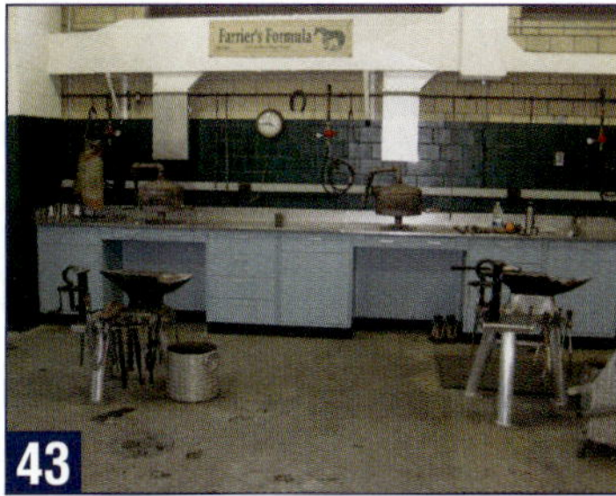

Student's shop at Cornell University. Taught by Mike Wildenstein, FWCF.

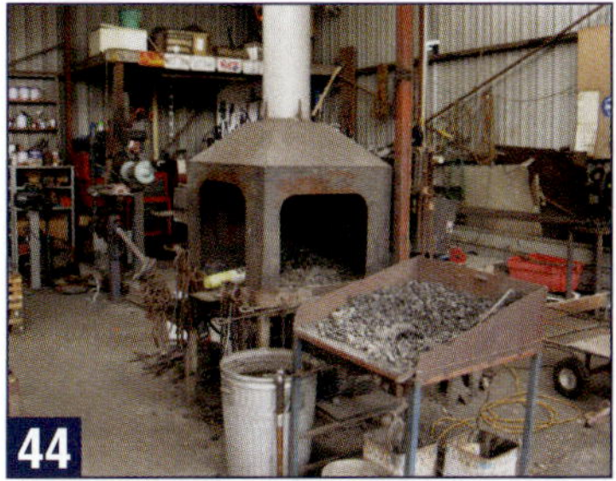

Dean Lewis, World Champion Blacksmith, shop in Australia.

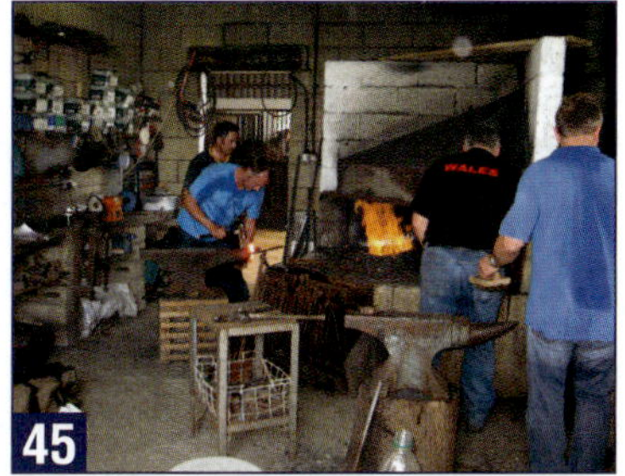

The Welsh team practicing in 2009 at Andy Martin's shop. From left to right is Andy Martin, Billy Crothers, Grant Moon and Jim Blurton.

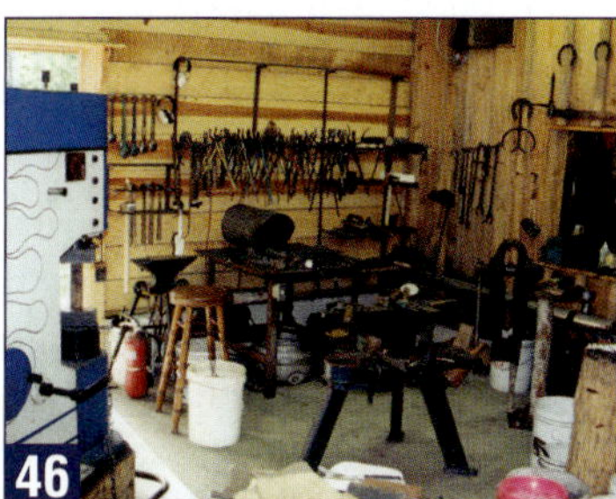

Tom Clark's shop at the Ozark School of Blacksmithing in Potosi, Missouri in 2002.

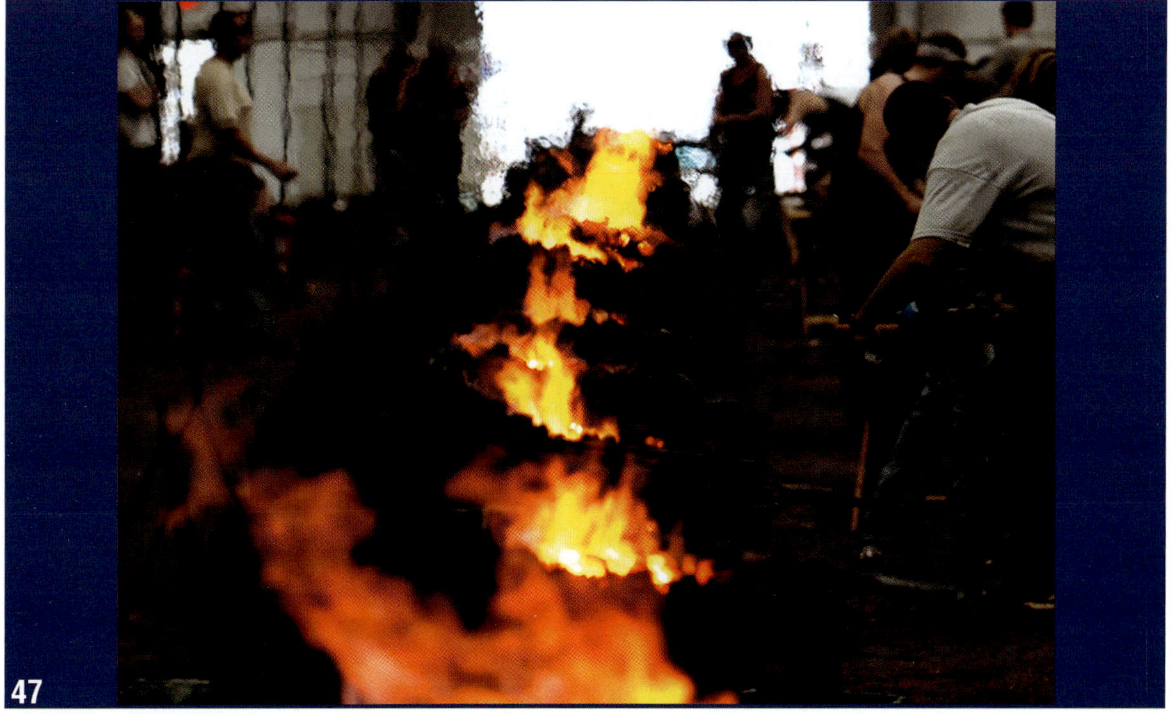

The fires in Calgary.

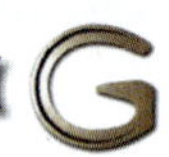

Chapter 6 YOUR MOBILE SHOP

In the modern age of farriery, it is important that you are able to take your shop to where the horses are. At one time, it was common for the horses to go to the blacksmith shop for shoeing, but now the opposite is true.

Throughout my career, I have had numerous rigs. What they all had in common was that they were inexpensive and simple. One of my first rigs was in the back of a truck that also pulled my gooseneck trailer to rodeos **(Figure 1)**. As a result, my forge had its own little box by the tailgate, and the tools and inventory went in a toolbox behind the cab. When farrier contests replaced rodeo for me, I ended up with a dedicated shoeing rig **(Figures 2-4)**. It was great, but it had way more room than I needed. That rig ended up on 3 different trucks before I sold it to another farrier **(Figure 5)**. Over many years, I ended up with several different trailers, and find that I like having a trailer for a rig better than having a truck.

There is always debate about which is best, a truck or a trailer. The answer is individual and based on your preferences, geography, driving ability, clientele served, and lifestyle. With that in mind, let's explore some of these topics and hopefully help you come to a conclusion that fits you.

First is preference. I grew up with trailers behind every truck, so hauling a trailer is not a problem. You can quickly learn how to back and turn with a trailer, especially with one that is as short as most shoeing trailers will be. I know many people who do not like the looks of a trailer, don't like having to plan where to park because they have a trailer attached, and dread having to back up with one. If you fall into that category, you should be leaning toward a truck.

Geography can be an important consideration. When I had my business in Colorado, there were several customers in the mountains that would have been difficult to serve with a trailer due to the roads and driveways you had to take to get to them. Switchback turns, steep mountainsides, and roads with no shoulder would have made using even a small trailer hard. Once the weather got bad, a trailer would have been impossible for some of those places. If you are in that sort of geographical location, you should lean toward a truck. Here in

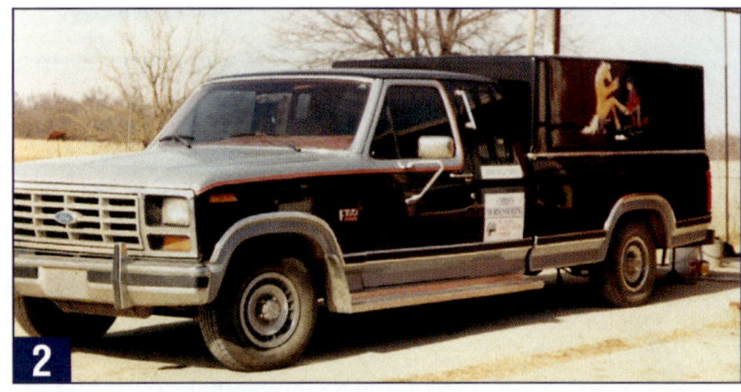
2
My third rig, 1989.

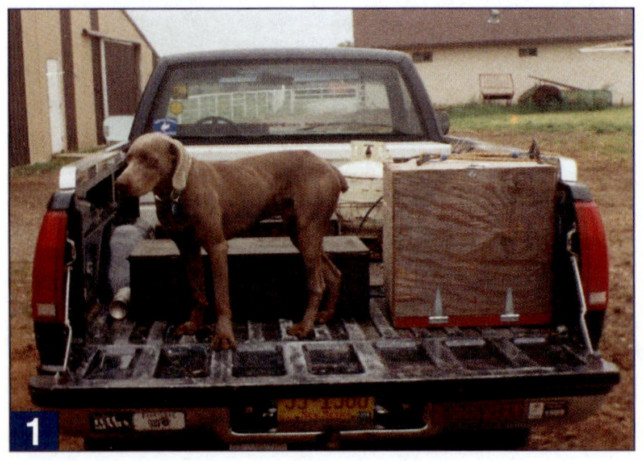
1
One of my only pictures of my second rig.

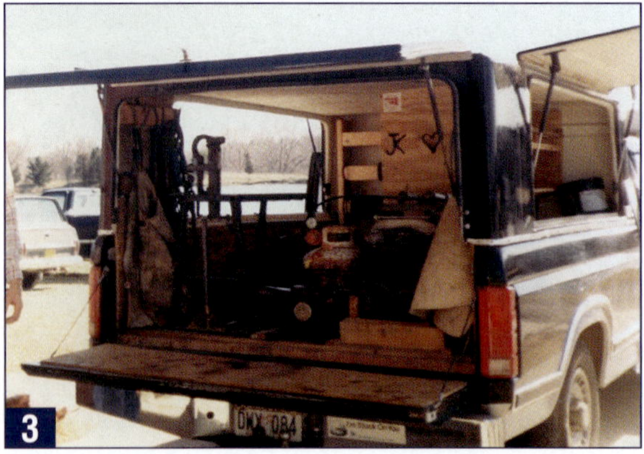
3
The inside set up.

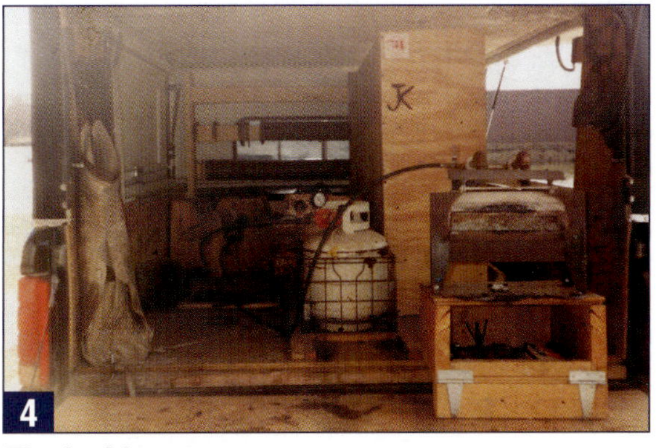

4

The inside set up.

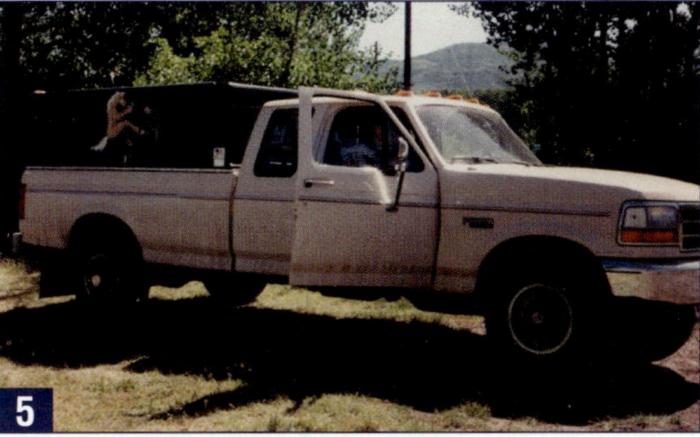

5

Same topper, different truck.

Missouri, I have been able to get everywhere I need to with a trailer, and I think that is probably true for the majority of the United States.

You have to decide for yourself if you have the driving ability to handle a trailer. As for clientele served, it will go hand in hand with geography. Take these into consideration as you decide what to put together for a rig, and perhaps even make pros vs. cons list like the ones below.

TRAILER

Pros:

1. When your truck breaks down, you don't lose your rig.
2. May be able to keep the same rig through the life of several trucks.
3. Can be unhooked to free the vehicle for other uses.
4. Has better resale value than a vehicle.
5. May be easier to park inside alleys and barns if it is small enough.

Cons:

1. May ride rougher than a vehicle, which can be hard on equipment.
2. Often dustier inside than a rig on a truck.
3. Can be hard to get in to certain spots.
4. Increases cost by decreasing gas mileage.
5. Toll roads may charge by the axle.

TRUCK MOUNTED RIG

Pros:

1. Easier to drive, park, back, and maneuver your rig to where you want it.
2. Better shock absorption for your equipment.

Cons:

1. When your truck breaks down, you are without a rig.
2. Loses value more quickly than a trailer.
3. The truck becomes dedicated to one use, requiring you to have another truck for many activities not related to shoeing.

Your lists will be different, but I would suggest making them if you are struggling choosing between a truck and trailer.

EQUIPMENT

Okay, now that the decision of how to get the equipment to the horse has been made, let's determine what equipment to take. You need to have the basics: forge, anvil, vice, tongs, propane, bar stock, shoes, nails, floor tools, forge tools, and hoof and anvil stands.

That would be the absolute minimum, but if you are like most farriers, it's just a start. If your rig is big enough, you may find that pretty soon you have about 25 varieties of shoes in 5 sizes each, 14 sizes of nails, (even though 10 of them are the same length), power equipment that you rarely need, and a lot of other power equipment that you use every time you open your rig.

It can get out of hand, so you may want to make an inventory list, check it regularly, and make sure that you aren't hauling around a bunch of stuff that you will never need.

The anvil should be light enough that you can maneuver it easily. In my youth, I used a 156-pound anvil in my rig because I was shoeing with all handmades. With age, I have found a 120-pound round-horned anvil that I like just as well **(Figure 6)**. If your rig sits high, like a 1-ton truck bed, you may want to make a swing-out on your rear bumper or truck frame to give you easy access to the anvil, like

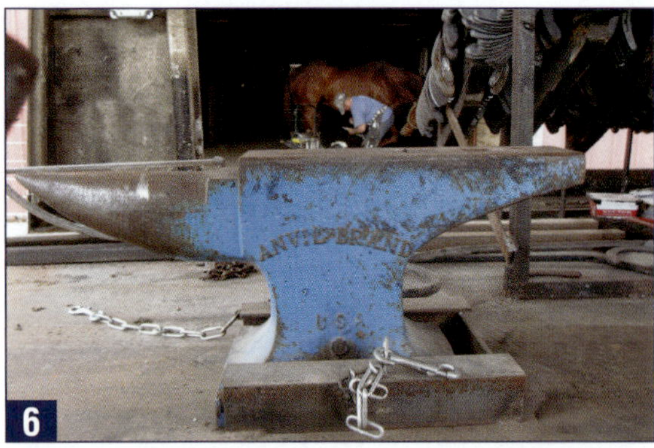

The anvil we use in our rig.

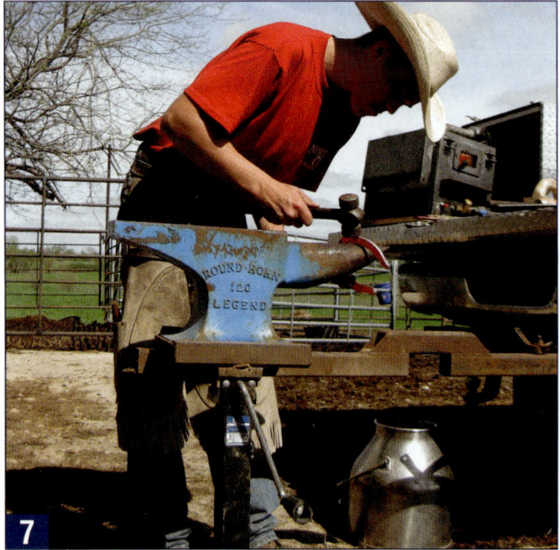

Cody's swing-out on his first rig.

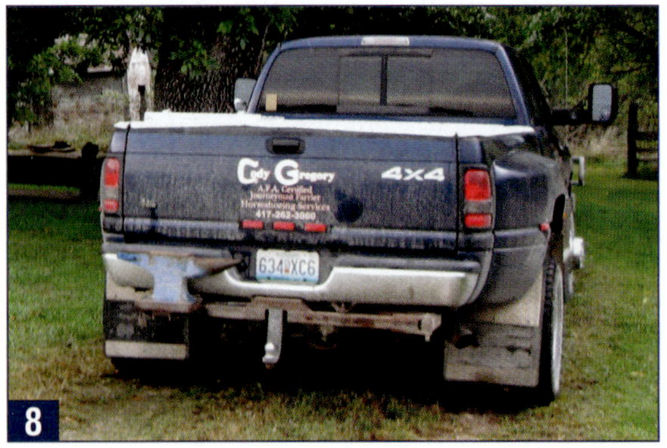

The back of Cody's first rig with the anvil swing-out.

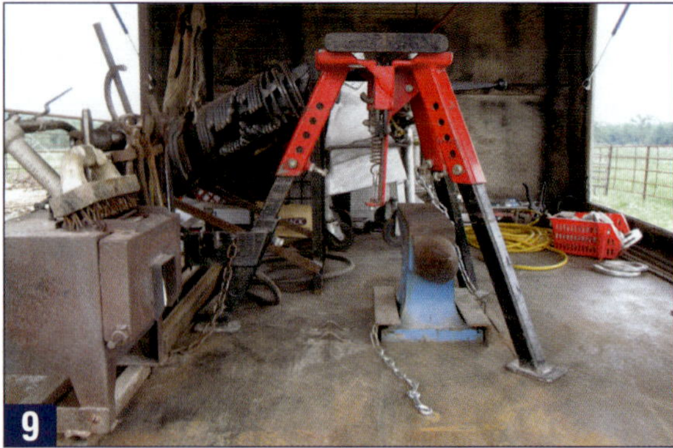

Interior of my rig

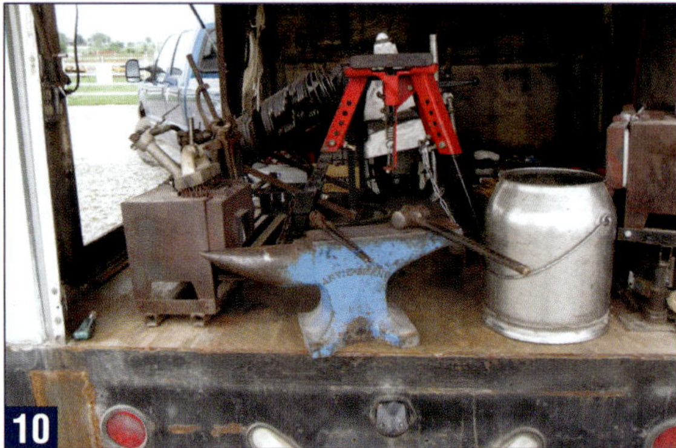

Interior of my rig

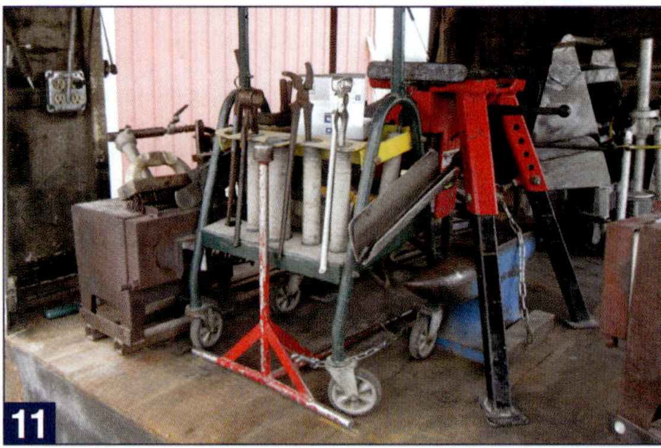

Interior of my rig

Cody had on his first rig **(Figure 7-8)**. You should organize your rig so that the anvil stand comes out of the rig ahead of the anvil and is loaded after the anvil **(Figure 9)**. In **Figure 10**, you can see that I can do quick fix-ups if I have a lost shoe without having to unload everything.

Arrange things so that you can get your shoeing box and hoof stand out without unloading anything

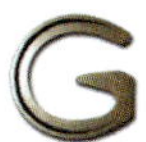

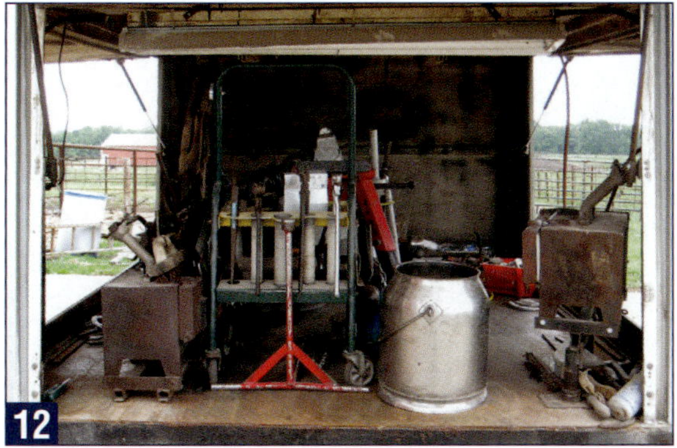

12 *Interior of my rig*

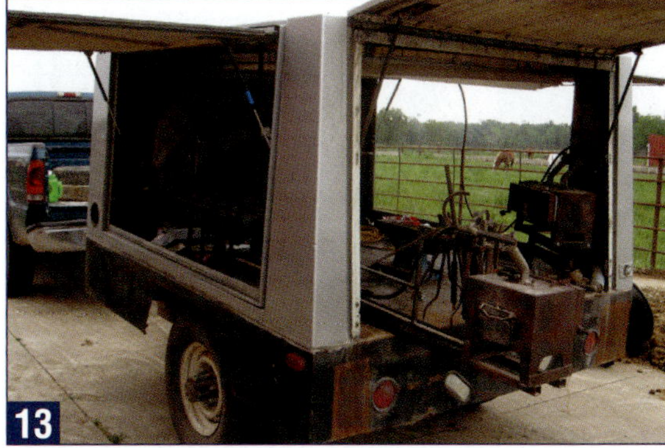

13 *Interior of my rig*

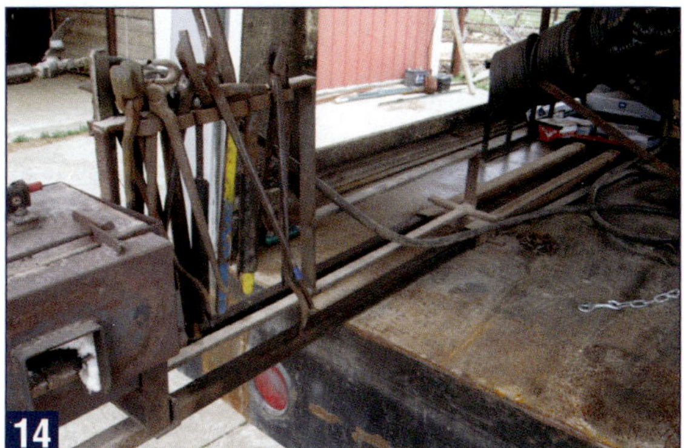

14 *Forge slide out*

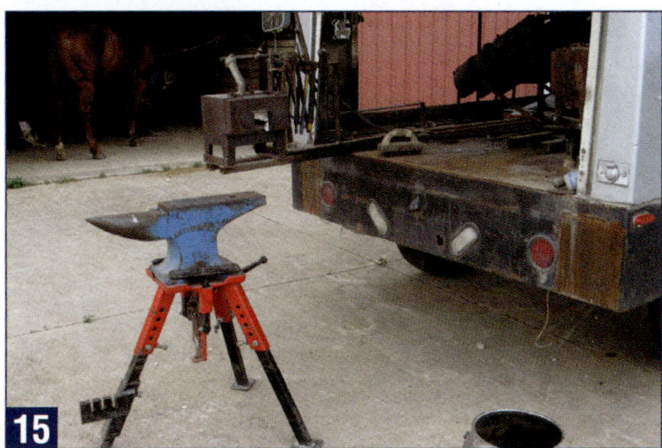

15 *Where the anvil sits in relation to the forge.*

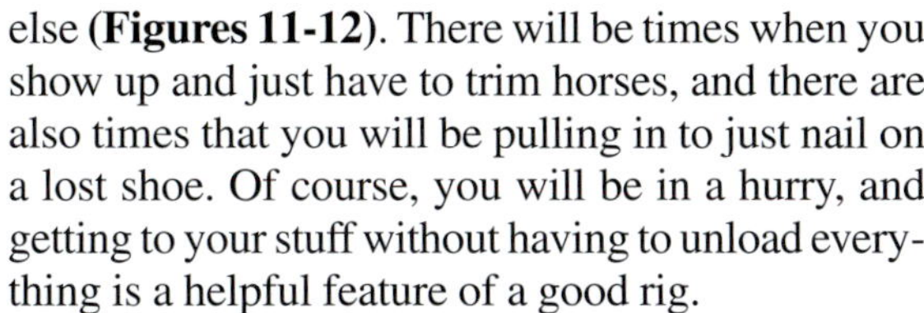

else **(Figures 11-12)**. There will be times when you show up and just have to trim horses, and there are also times that you will be pulling in to just nail on a lost shoe. Of course, you will be in a hurry, and getting to your stuff without having to unload everything is a helpful feature of a good rig.

I like my forge to swing or slide out. As you can see, there are 2 forges in the rig in **Figures 13-14**. With as many shoers as we have going together, the extra forge is very handy. There is often another anvil in this rig as well; it is the same make and size as the one pictured.

Arrange your workstation so that the anvil ends up sitting in a handy place for the forge **(Figure 15)**. The forge should have a design that allows you to heat the center of your stock for making shoes. However, since there are rear or side ports in a forge like that, be certain that you don't have it situated so that it melts taillights or burns away paint. You should also have easy access for opening, closing, and changing out propane bottles. This often gets forgotten when people set up their rigs. It becomes a hassle if a design error requires that everything be unloaded for you to get to the propane. I also like to have 2 propane bottles so that I have a backup when needed.

Finally, you should look at weight distribution of equipment and inventory so that you are not putting all of the weight to one side or the other. With a trailer, you want to be certain that there is tongue weight. I have seen some trailers that were set up so that the weight was behind the axles, which will cause the trailer to be pulling up on the hitch all the time. That can be a dangerous setup.

Design your rig so that it is easy and fast to set up. The best rigs that I have had required less than a minute to set up. That can be a big savings in time when you have a long day. Consider if you had a rig that takes 5 minutes to set up, and 3 minutes to put away. If you happen to have 4 stops in a day, that is an extra 32 minutes you put into your day, compared to the potential total of 8 total minutes with a 1-minute setup and another to load. It can add up to several hours over weeks, months, or years

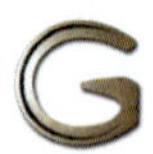

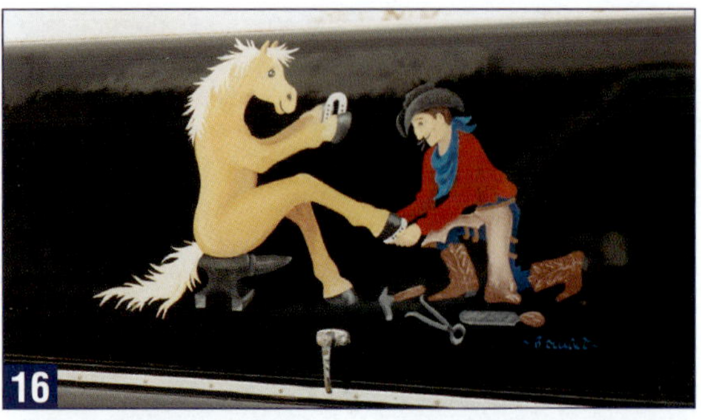
16
My first logo.

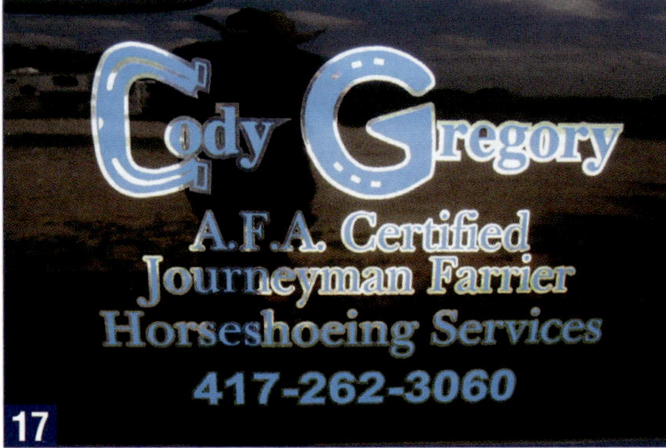

17
Cody's lettering

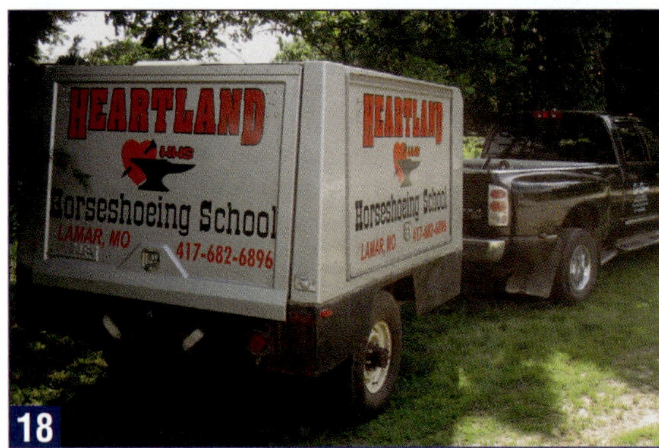

18
This is the outside of the rig that Kelly and I use personally.

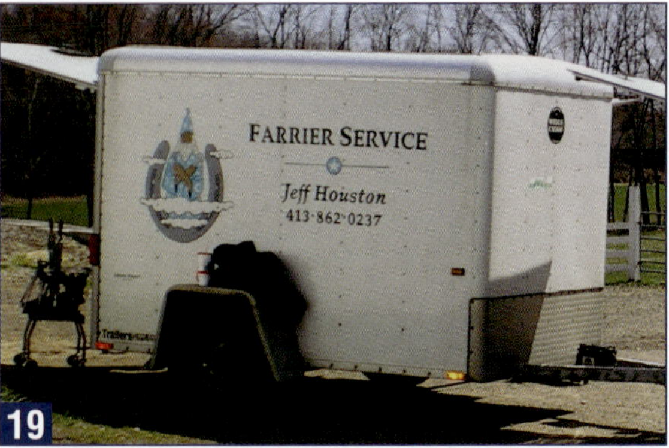

19
Jeff Houston's lettering

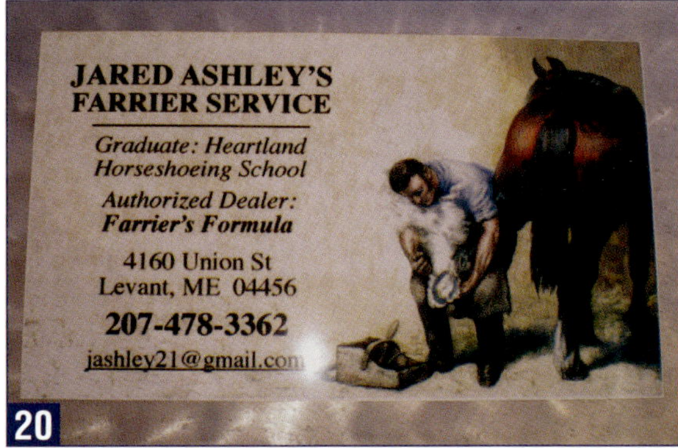

20
Jared Ashley's signage.

Finally is the issue of signage. Once you are established, you may not want to have any mobile advertising, but it is an inexpensive way for a lot of potential customers to learn about you. As with business cards, you should not cut corners when it comes to lettering and signage on your rig. One of my first rigs had the logo you see in **Figure 16**. It got a lot of comments, even from non-horse people. **Figure 17** shows Cody's rig. **Figure 18** shows our current rig. **Figure 19** shows the rig of Jeff Houston in New England. Jared Ashley, a graduate of Heartland Horseshoeing School, uses the rig in **Figure 20**.

As you can see, each of these is a little different, but they all indicate what the person hauling the trailer or driving the truck does for a living. You never know where that next big customer is going to come from, but it just may be the traffic you are sitting in.

Whether you add lettering to the outside of your rig or not is a personal business decision. Many farriers get so busy at a certain point of their career that they are trying to avoid extra calls. However, if you are that busy, you should be saying no by quoting such a high price that the customer is the one saying it. That will lead to a few that say yes to the high price, and this leads to a higher income.

For design ideas, I thought I would show a few rigs that you might be able to get some ideas from. First are some pictures of the rig belonging to my good friend Jeff Houston. In **Figures 21-24**, you can

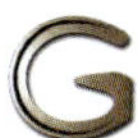

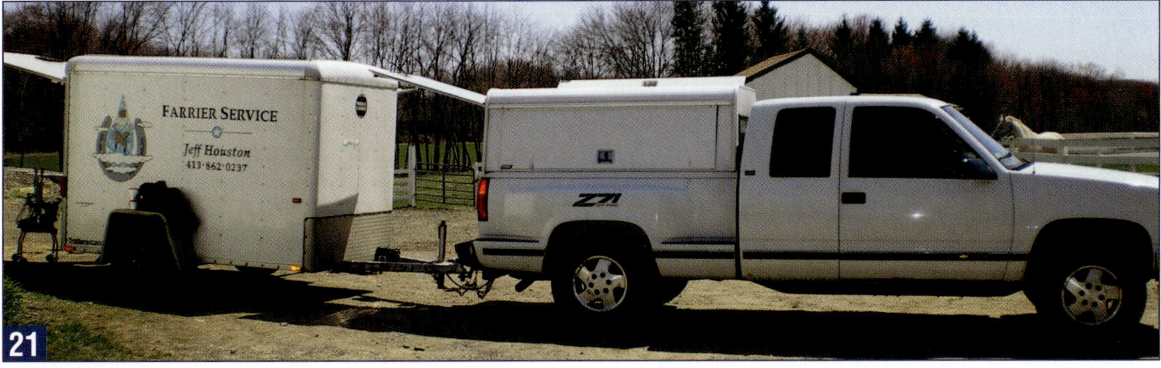

21

Jeff's set up.

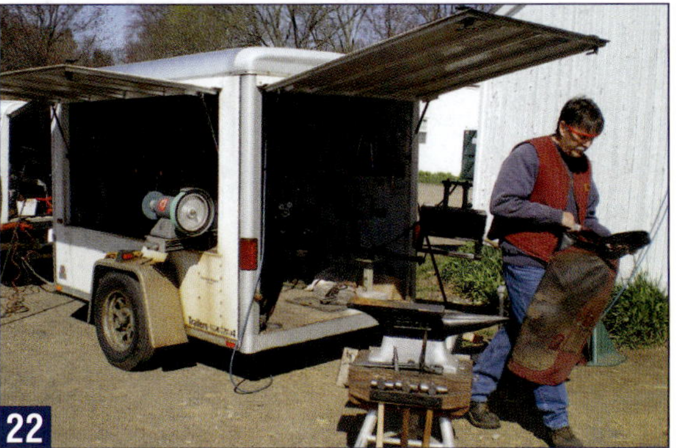

22

Jeff with his rig open, set up, and ready to work.

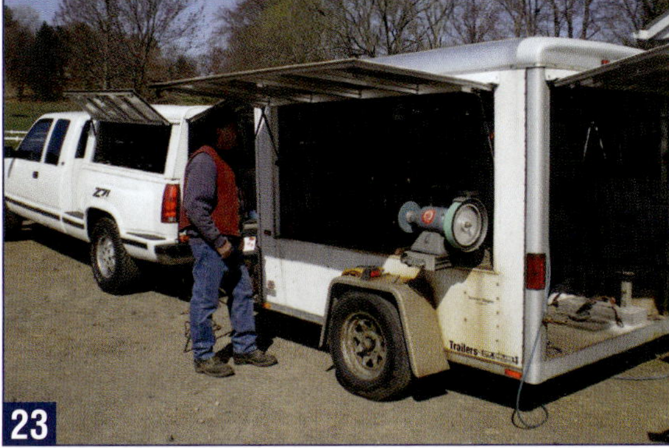

23

Vendor door side.

see some photos of his rig in action. This is a fairly inexpensive route to go, and there is a lot of room for you to add your personal preferences to the design. He has a trailer with a vendor's door. This is a big door that opens on the side to allow easier access to tools and inventory. You can see that there are drill presses, grinders, forge swing-out, and plenty of room. By having a rig created in a trailer with other uses, you may find that there is a bigger market for selling the trailer when you no longer need it as a farrier rig.

Next are some photos from Stone Well Bodies and Equipment of Genoa, N.Y. You can see that these are the top-end of farrier rigs, and that there are a lot of items designed to make your job easier. From the anvil and forge swing-outs to the drawer, shelf and rack designs, these are the ultimate in farrier rigs. I have never personally owned one, but that does not mean that I haven't wanted to. It simply means that I was able to make a living without it.

Figures 25-46 show some Stone Well creations

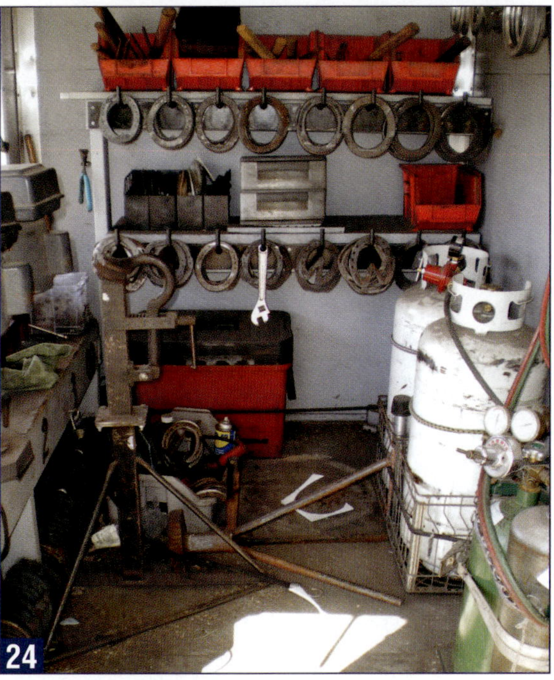

24

Interior of Jeff's rig.

to fire-up your creativity for your own design or as a goal for something you could one day own. You can see a lot of design input from the experience of many top-notch farriers. Take some time to put together a rig that makes your life easier.

In some areas and situations, a nice rig can be an important part of your image; particularly where there are more expensive horses and high-dollar shoers. In these places, the cost of a fancy rig may be justified.

Your rig is an investment. Just like a saddle for a trainer, or a lawnmower for a lawn-service business. Look carefully at what suits the situation that you find yourself working in, and then make an informed decision on what you need for a rig.

These are various designs of the top end of farrier rigs.

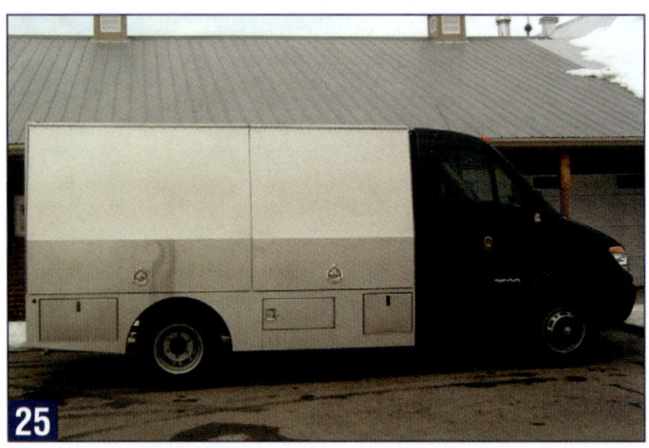

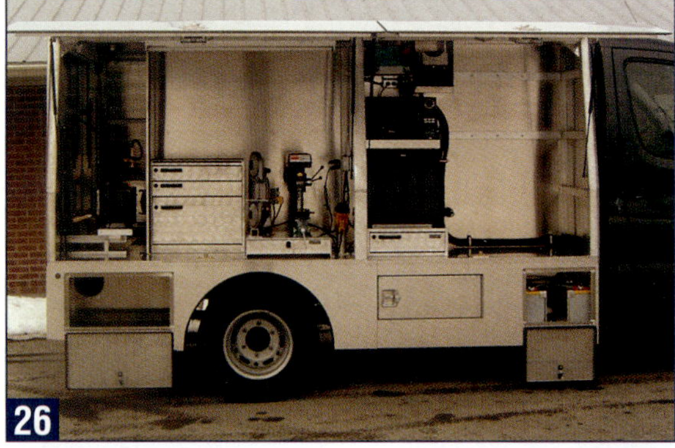

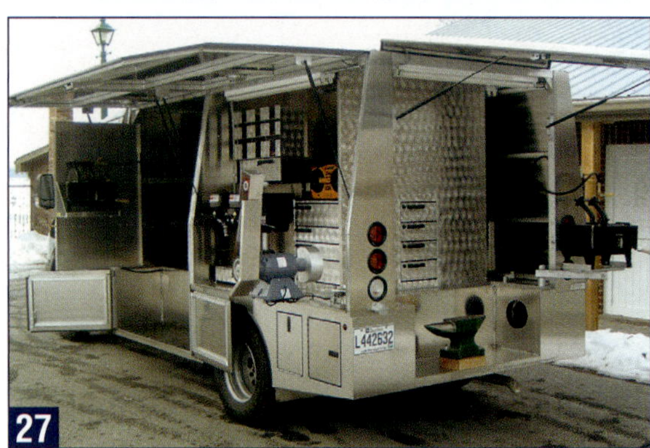

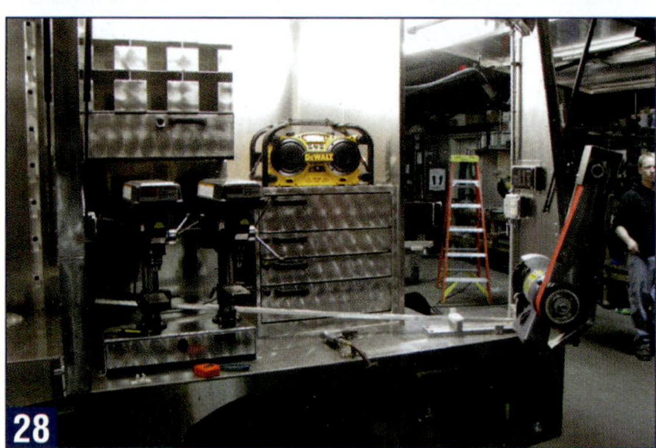

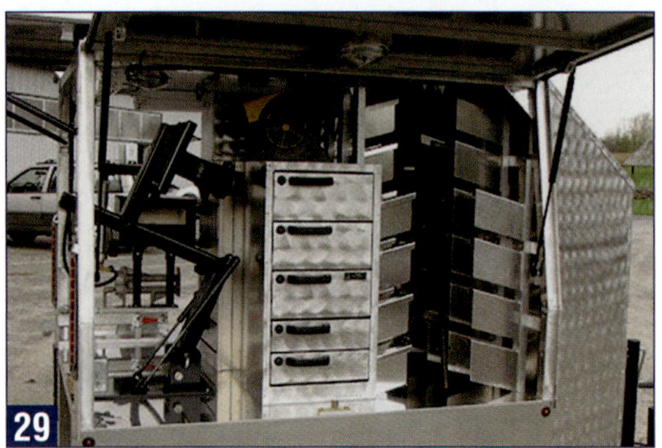

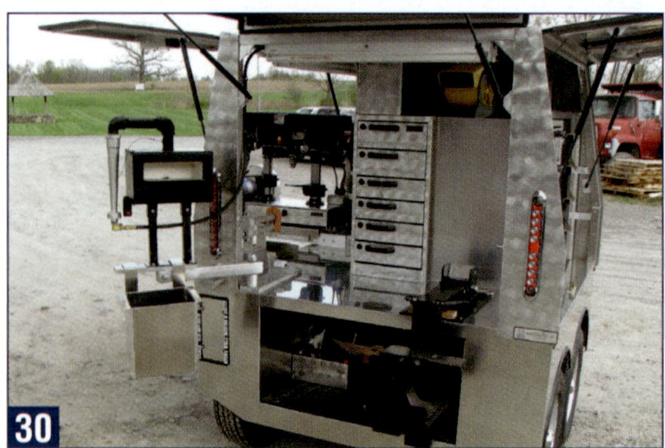

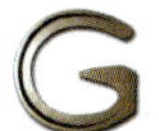

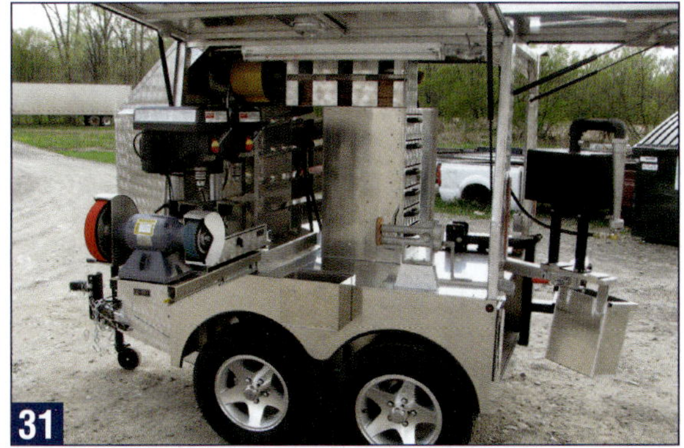

31

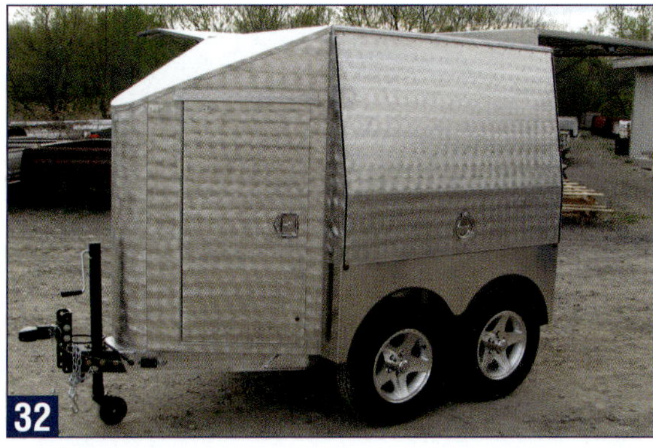

32

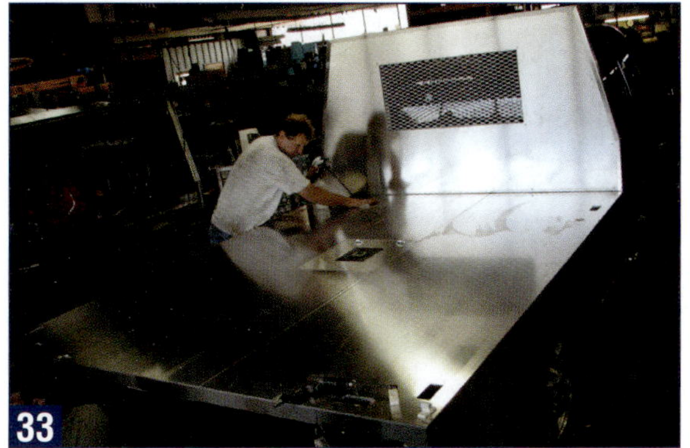

33

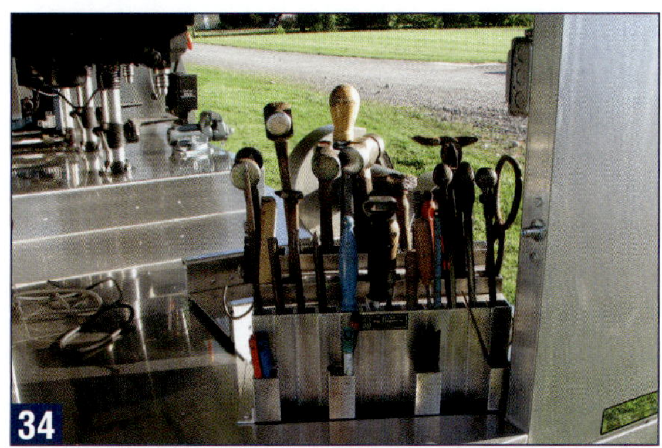

34

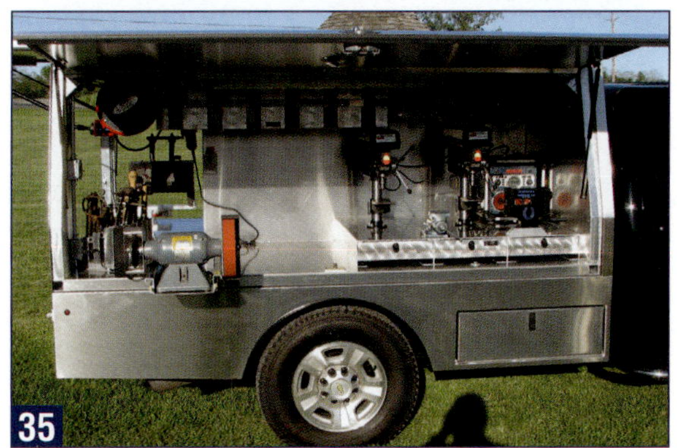

35

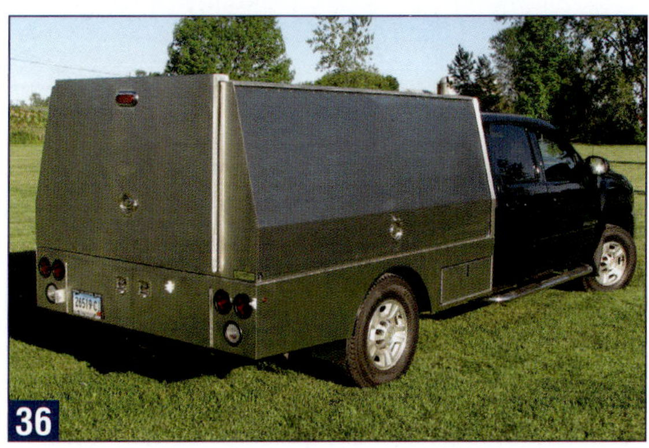

36

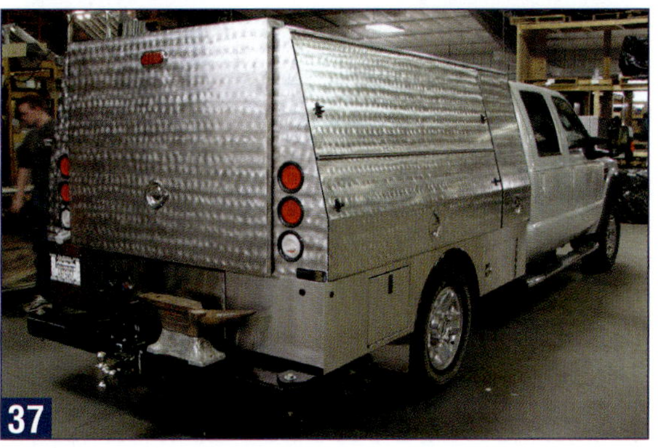

37

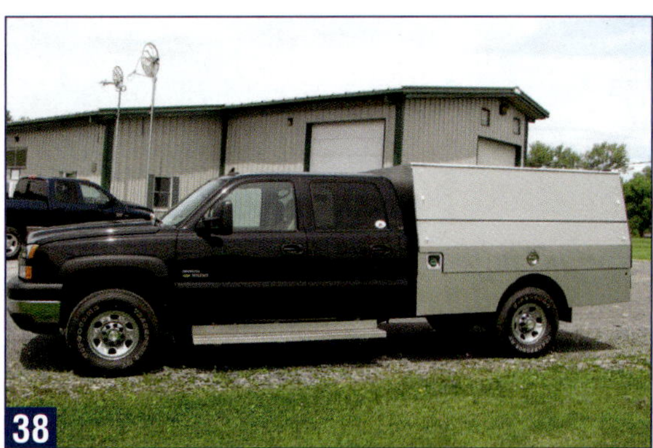

38

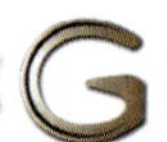

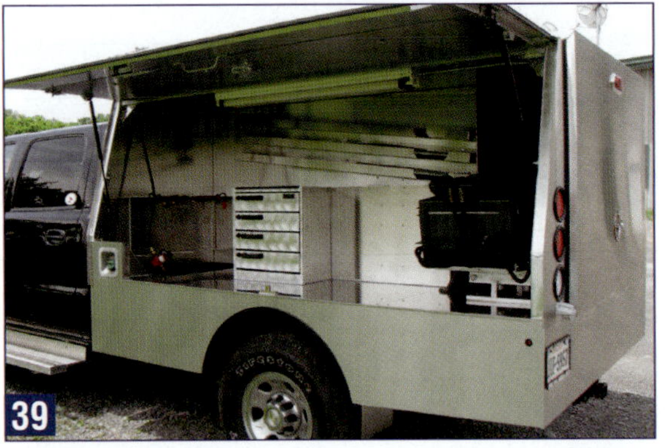
39

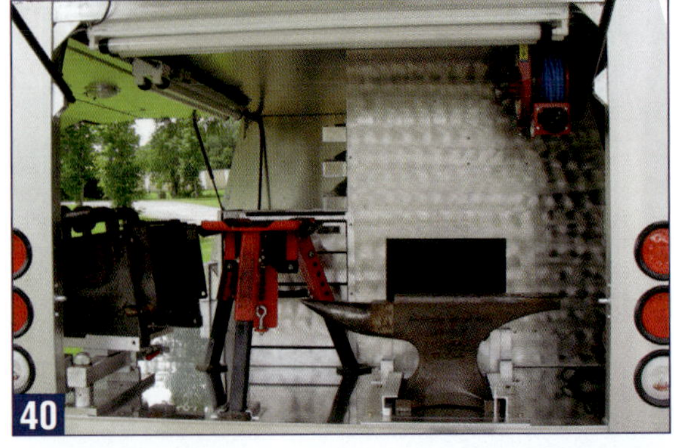
40

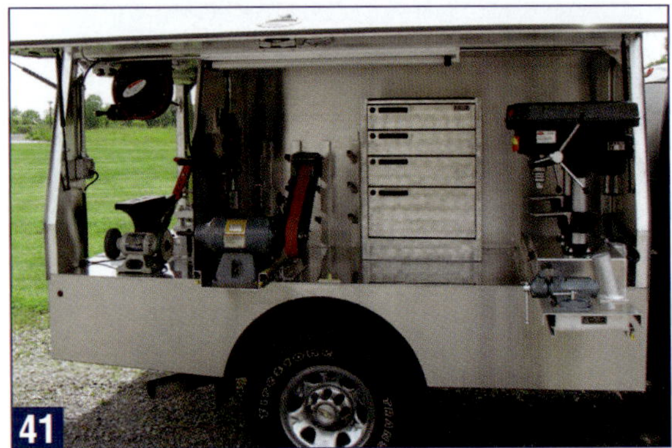
41

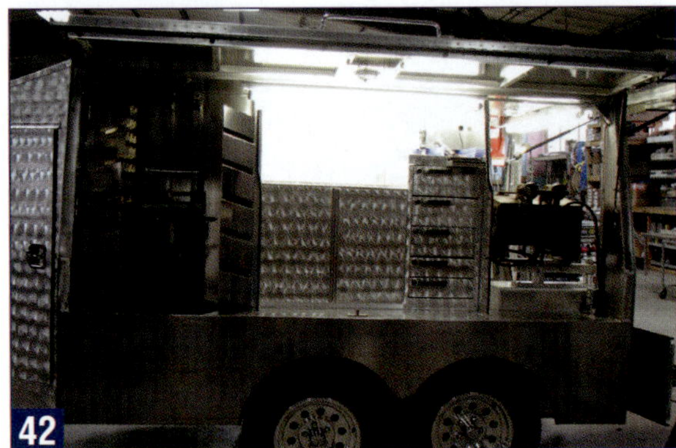
42

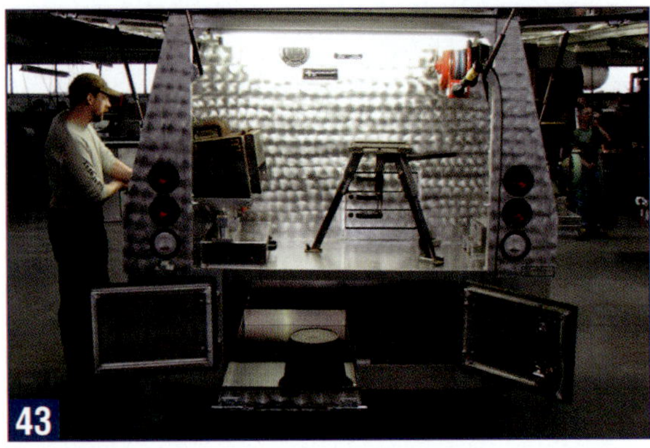
43

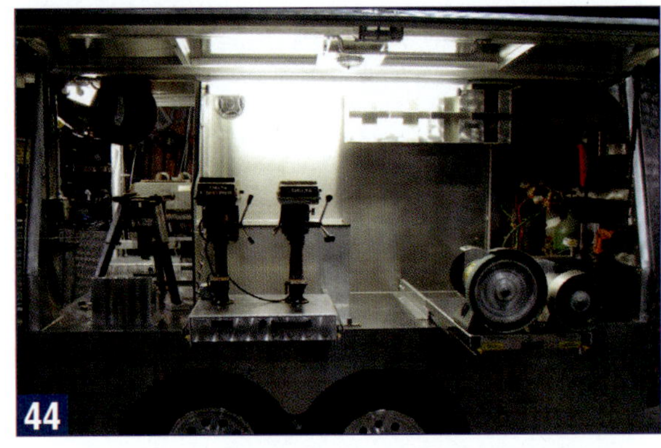
44

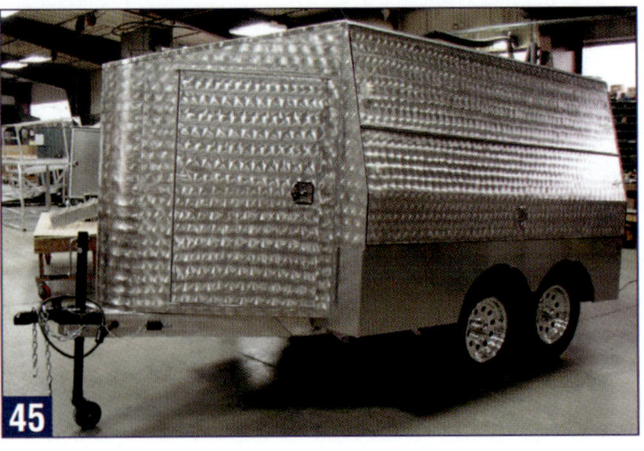
45

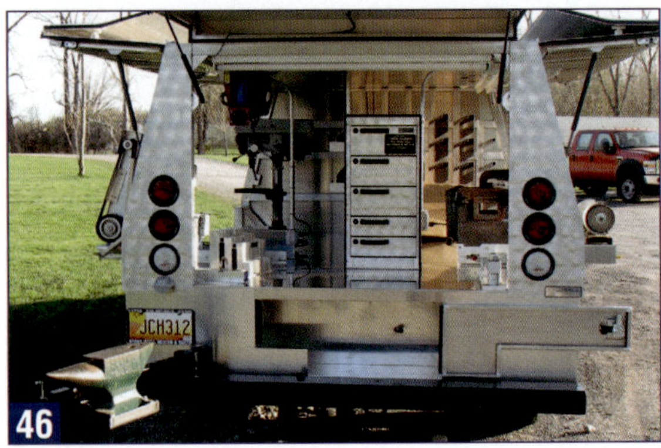
46

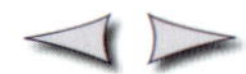

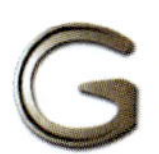

Section

3

Anatomy

Chapter 7: Anatomy Introduction 44

Chapter 8: The Foot 50

Chapter 9: Bones and Joints 65

Chapter 10: Ligaments and Tendons 98

Chapter 11: Vascular, Nerve, and Lymphatic System Basics of the Equine Leg 126

Chapter 12: Biomechanics 134

Chapter 13: Dissection 151

" 11 Clothe me with skin and flesh,
And knit me together with bones and sinews?"

—Job 10:11
—New King James Version

" 16 Lo now, his strength is in his loins,
and his force is in the navel of his belly.
17 He moveth his tail like a cedar:
the sinews of his stones are wrapped together.
18 His bones are as strong pieces of brass;
his bones are like bars of iron. "

—Job 40:16-18
—New King James Version

Chapter

7 ANATOMY INTRODUCTION

Ultimately, farriery is an art with a scientific backdrop that at its core, should be applied to a horse's foot with the aim of improving how the horse moves. So often, we as farriers become obsessed with how the foot looks when we are done, how well our shoes stay on, how much money we can make, and other parts of this craft that don't aim directly on how a horse moves. This goes for the lame horse as well, since we should be applying shoes in an attempt to decrease or eliminate that lameness, if possible.

Since the desired end result for a customer is for the horse to move as well as it can, we need to have a good foundation in basic equine anatomy. With any biomechanical system, there is a lot that is going on that we take for granted. The more that you know about these systems in the horse, the more you can determine how trimming and shoeing will affect the whole.

This section is going to be aimed primarily at the leg, which is the anatomical portion of the horse from the knee and hock down. While the leg is the main realm of the farrier, we should also have a familiarity with other systems that the leg attaches to. That is what this introduction chapter is about.

As you study anatomy, you will get the impression that everything is understood and neatly laid out in the horse's body. This is far from the truth. There are controversy and gray areas, and what looks neat and easy in a diagram can be hard to determine when actually cutting into the tissue. What is laid out in this section is the best of my understanding from research and actual dissections. I encourage you to do some dissections with a critical eye as you look for abnormal anatomy and pathology.

Having written this textbook primarily for teaching, I recommend that you read the chapters in this section in order, beginning with this one.

ANATOMY

Anatomy knowledge is one of the biggest factors that separates the average horseshoers from the great farriers. Without truly understanding how the structur come together to live, grow, move, and regenerate, a practitioner of this craft is at a big disadvantage. Often, the horseshoer without a grasp of anatomy will apply shoeing theory based only on what they are taught. This is okay for the horse if the shoer has been taught by someone with superior skills, but can be a disaster if the teacher was as ignorant as the student. Horses that possess a foot or conformation outside of normal will also suffer at the hands of an ignorant shoer who is unable to adapt technique based on sound anatomical principles.

The demand for horseshoers is currently so great, that a person does not have to be competent to make a living shoeing horses. Being available and having basic business management skills has provided many unskilled horseshoers with a way to earn a living. As a result of this demand, the industry has been able to produce and market many products and theories that do not make sense from an anatomical view. If horseshoers were more knowledgeable and skilled, many of the products, gimmicks, and trimming theories that I have seen in my career would never have made it past the first trial. We have unfortunately replaced a lot of skills with inventory and product.

Because you do not want to be one of the practitioners applying foolish theory, you must become so educated about anatomy that vets are asking you questions. Anatomy can be learned by anyone. It requires memorization, and if you have the desire and drive, you can become great at understanding anatomy.

Having taught this craft to people from all walks of life since 1992, I have found a few things that can help you learn. The anatomy section is designed to help you make your anatomy study easier. First, you need to get some index cards and colored pencils. You are going to make a set of anatomy flashcards. The process of making them will teach you quite a lot, and by using flash cards, you will study the items you don't know well. After making the flash-

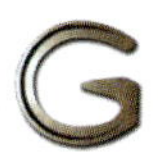

cards, you will place the ones you know well in one pile, and those you don't know well in another. As you continue your study, the pile of what you know will grow, and the pile of what you don't know will shrink.

Another thing you need to know is the terminology that is used for anatomical discussion. When you hear a vet or doctor string a bunch of anatomical terms together, it may sound quite confusing to the layman. However, the use of proper terminology makes it possible to be very specific. When I listen to someone speak Portuguese, I am lost. But, if I spoke Portuguese, there would be no problem. Anatomical terminology is the same way. Once you are able to think in the proper terms, it is easy to understand everything you hear and read.

Most of the shoeing textbooks that I know of begin the anatomy section with bones, and move from there to ligaments and tendons, leaving the hoof for later. Since the intent of this book is to be used by actual students and farrier educators, I am going to start with some terminology, and then continue with the foot. You will be dealing with feet quite early in most schools, so you need to know about them first.

Take the time to get this right. What you are about to learn will become the foundation of all your future learning and decisions when it comes to shoeing a horse. Those who skip the process of learning anatomy do so at their own peril and to the detriment of the horse.

ANATOMICAL TERMINOLOGY:

Here are some of the necessary terms:

Limb: Appendage from the trunk of the horse that includes the leg.

Leg: Portion of the limb from the knee or hock down.

Digit: Portion of the leg from the fetlock down.

Dorsal: The front aspect of the legs.

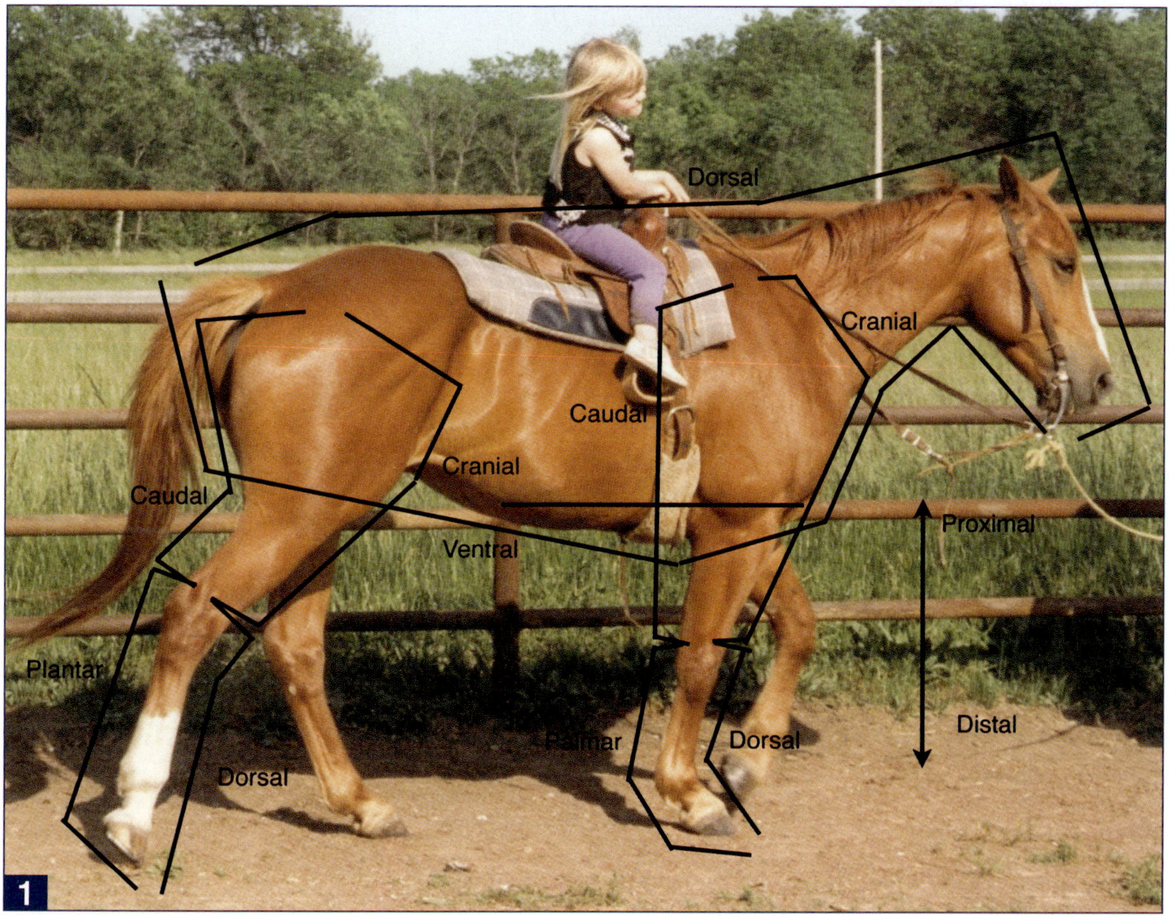

1

Location of terms

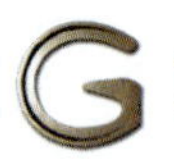

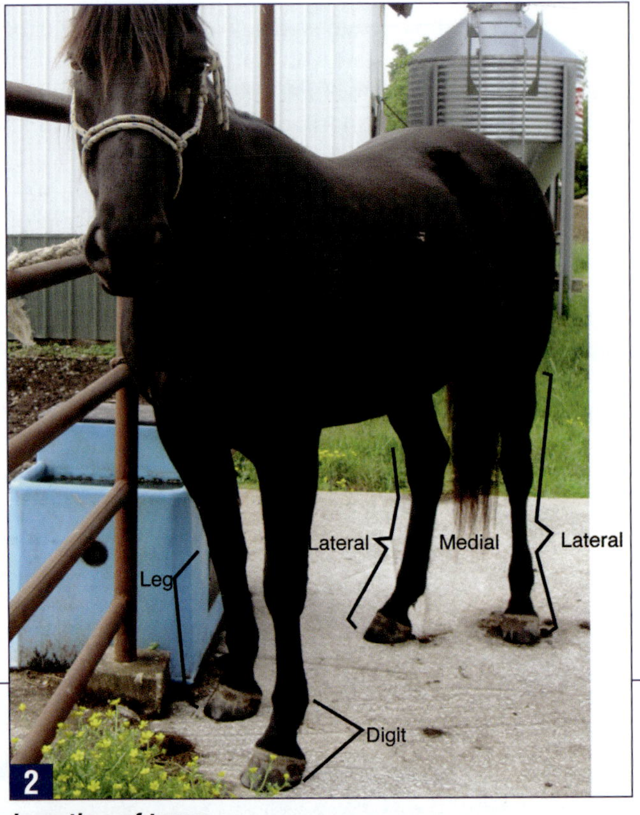

2 *Location of terms*

Palmar: The back surface of the front legs.

Plantar: The back surface of the hind legs.

Solar: Referring to the palmar and plantar aspect of the coffin bone, as well as the ground surface of the foot.

Cranial: The front surface of the upper limbs.

Caudal: The back surface of the upper limbs.

Proximal: Closest to the center of mass.

Distal: Furthest from the center of mass.

Medial: To the inside of the limb.

Lateral: To the outside of the limb.

Hoof: Horny covering on the outside of the bottom of the leg. Made of six regions.

Corium: Sensitive structure that creates and nourishes a horny structure.

Flex: Decrease the degree of, or angle

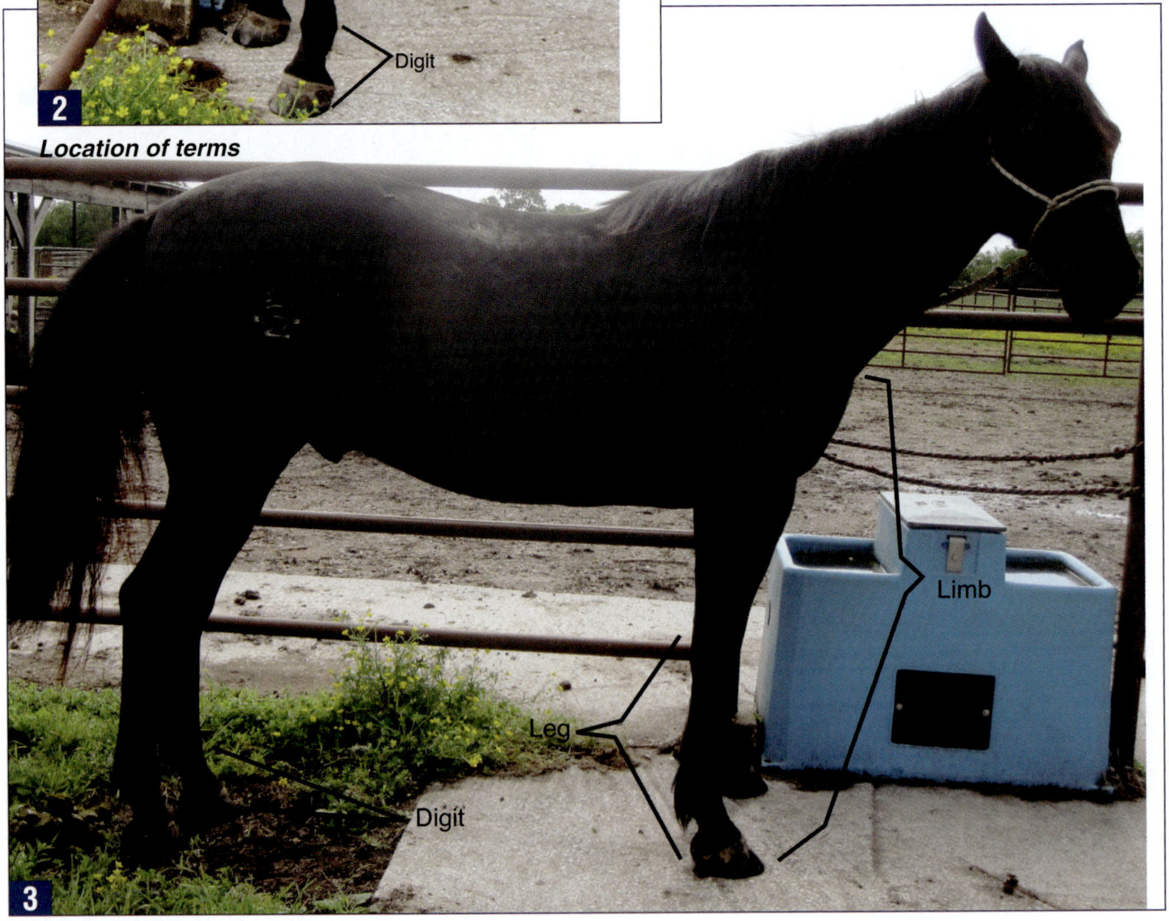

3 *Location of terms*

of a joint.

Extend: Increase the degree of, or angle of a joint.

Near: Always the left side of the horse, regardless of where you are standing in relation to the horse. Compare to port of a ship; like port, the word near has four letters as does the word left.

Off: Always the right side of the horse, regardless of your position. Opposite of near.

You will notice that the words anterior and posterior are not mentioned. The reason for this is that those terms should only be used in reference to the eye if you are talking about a quadruped. When someone says A-P (Anterior-Posterior) Balance, which is hoof pastern axis, it should be D-P (dorsal-palmar) Balance. The knowledge of the exact definition of these simple terms should give you an advantage when it comes to reading and discussing equine anatomy.

If you look at **Figures 1-3**, you will see several of the terms that we just defined as identified on a horse. In **Figure 4**, the horse has both front legs flexed and is about to extend them. In **Figure 5**, both front legs are extended and in front of the horse, and in **Figure 6**, the near front leg is extended, while the off front is flexed and just about to extend.

The parts of the horse that concern the farrier the most are as below, with a general description and definition of some of these structures. They are all covered in greater detail in later chapters.

Bones: The framework and the levers of the body. There are approximately 205 bones in the horse's skeleton. There is what is known as the axial skeleton that includes the ribs, breastbone, skull and spine, and the appendicular skeleton is made up of the pelvis and limbs. Long bones are primarily levers, while short bones absorb concussion. Flat bones like the ribs and bones found in the skull, protect vital organs and provide a large area of attachment for muscle.

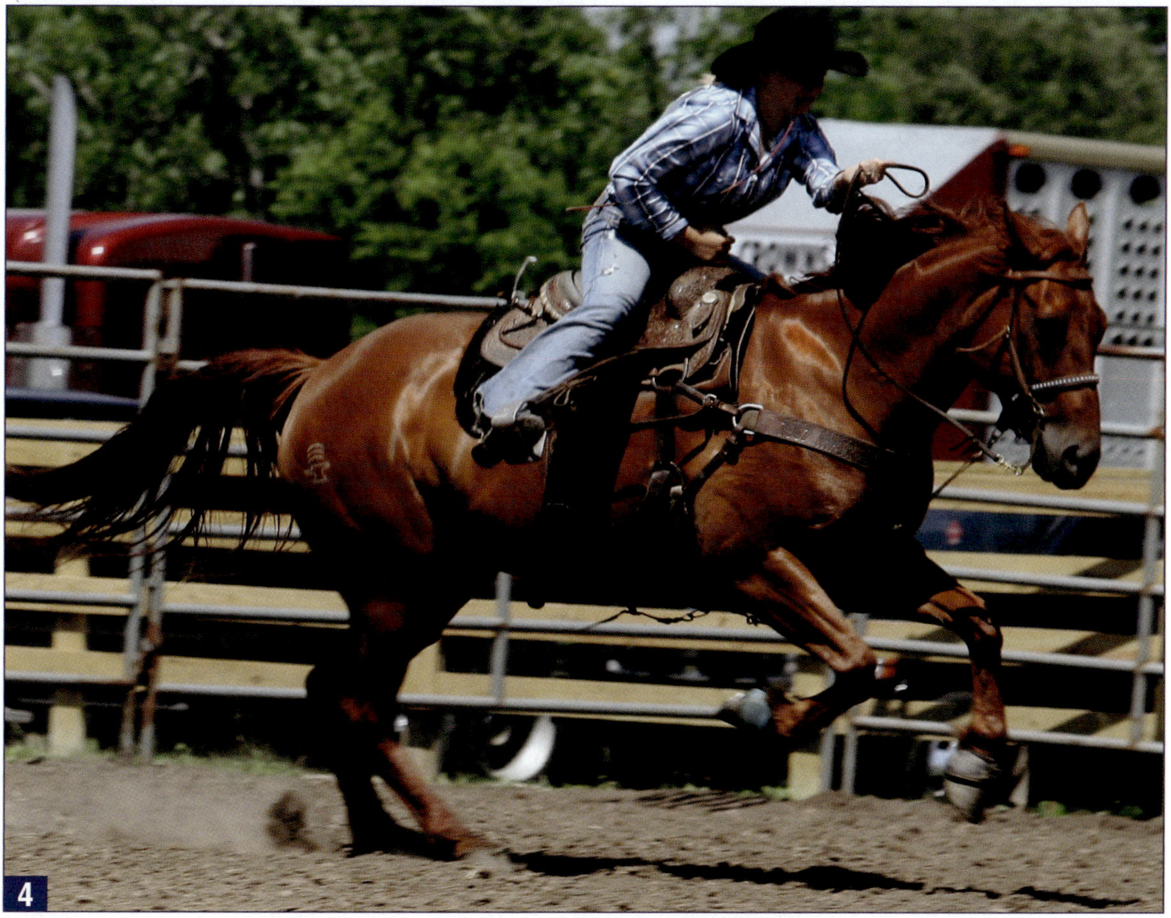

4

Both front legs are flexed at the knee, just about to extend completely.

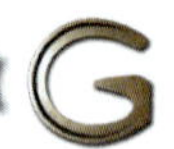

Joints: Any area where two bones come together is a joint. There are ligamentous joints, with only ligament between them, such as where the splint bones meet the cannon bone. There are cartilaginous joints, such as those between the vertebrae of the spinal column, and then there are synovial joints. These are joints that are surrounded by a capsular ligament that is filled with synovial fluid. The bones of these joints have a covering of articular cartilage where they meet to create a slick surface as well as absorb shock. In the limb, there are 3 categories of synovial joints: First is the hinge joint, known anatomically as a ginglymus joint. The fetlock is a good example. Next is the ball-and-socket joint, known anatomically as an enarthrodial joint. The shoulder and the hip joints are good examples. Finally is the plane joint, anatomically called an arthrodial joint. The carpometacarpal is a good example.

Tendons: Tissue that attach the muscles to the bones. Tendons are highly inelastic, and they glide in lubricated sheaths that are called synovial sheaths. Tendons are tough, fibrous, and are used for movement.

Muscles: Fibrous tissue that has the ability to contract. Attached to bones via tendons, muscles contract to move the skeleton. Muscles can only pull, not push, so one group of muscles on one side of a bony system will contract to pull on that system, and then relax as the opposing muscles on the other side contract to pull the system in the opposite direction.

Ligaments: Strong connective tissue that binds bones together. Most ligaments connect bone to

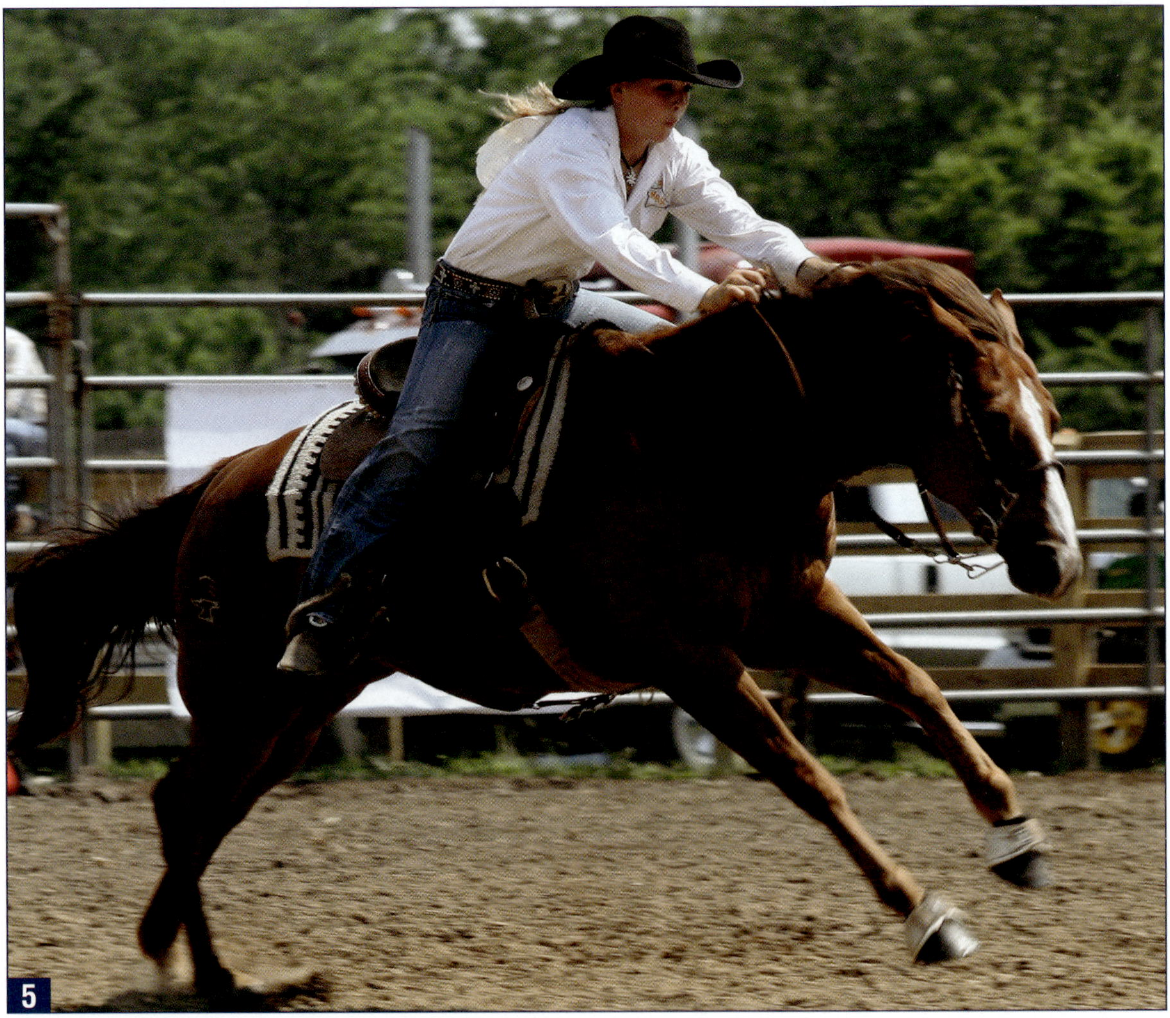

5

Both front legs are extended in front of the horse.

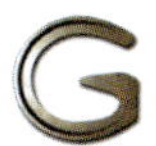

bone, but there are some notable exceptions. Most ligament tissue is also elastic, but again, there are exceptions to that rule as well. The primary function of ligaments is to support the skeleton.

Fascia: Layers of fibrous tissue found throughout the body. Fascia surrounds muscles, nerves, bones, organs, and blood vessels and interpenetrates most of the horse's body.

Arteries: Thick-walled, muscular vessels that resemble small hoses. Arteries transport bright red, oxygenated blood from the heart to the rest of the body.

Veins: Veins are collapsible, thin-walled vessels that return the blood from the extremities to the heart. Veins run next to arteries in the limbs, but the dark red, deoxygenated blood is traveling the opposite direction.

Nerves: Nerves are cable-like bundles of axons that convey information to the brain. They provide a common pathway for the elcrochemical nerve impulses that let's the brain know what the extremity is feeling. In the leg, there are primarily sensory nerves, which feel pressure, heat, cold, pain, etc. Going to the muscles are motor nerves, and these tell the muscles when to contract.

This chapter covers some very basic anatomical information that you need to posses to go forward into the realm of specific anatomy. With the terminology learned and some general definitions of different types of structures, you are ready to go into the next phase of learning equine anatomy as needed by a farrier.

Once you have a firm grasp on the anatomy of the leg, you will possess a confidence with shoeing that not all farriers have. You will be able to shoe the better horses, work in the nicer barns, demand more for your work, and be the farrier in your area that is considered the best. Anatomy knowledge is only one more of the many skills that is required of the great farrier.

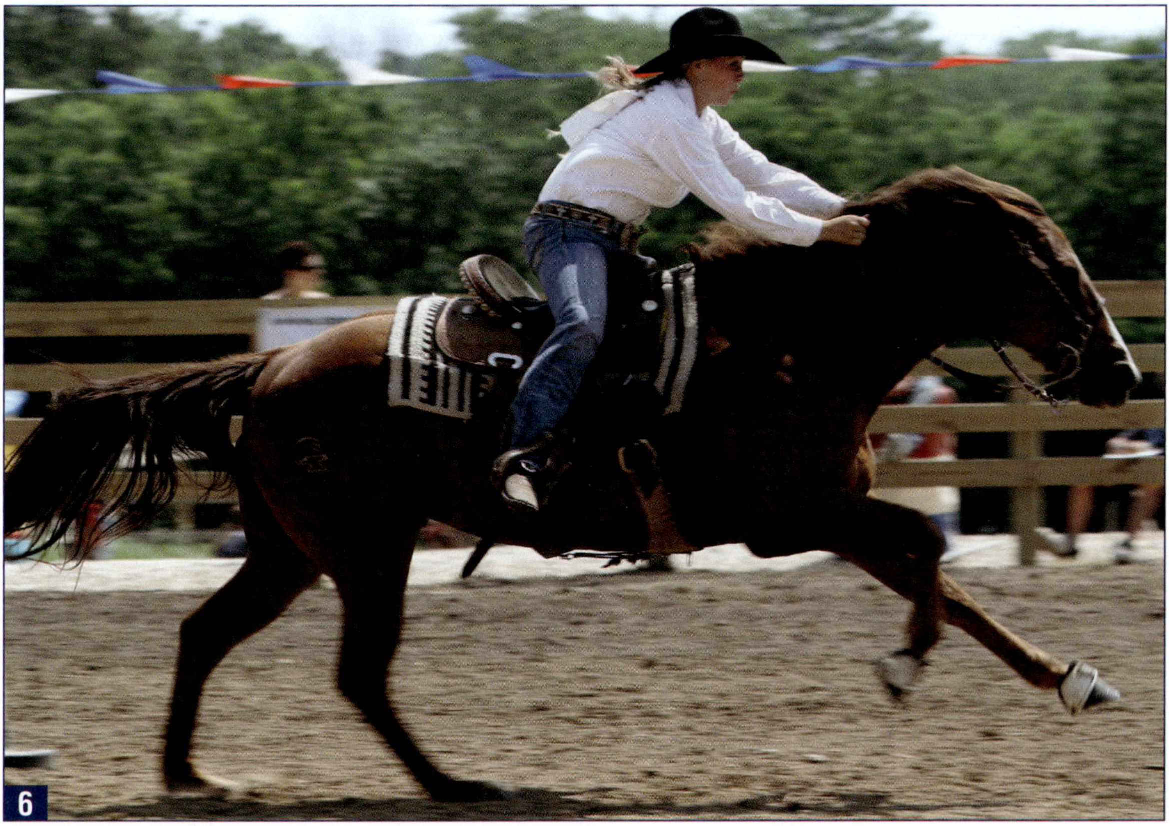

6

Near front extended, and off front flexed in the knee.

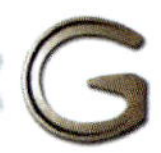

Chapter

8 THE FOOT

The foot is the hoof and everything inside of it, if you were to cut it off at the coronary band. When talking about the hoof alone, it consits of six regions of horny (insensitive) tissue on the distal end of the horse's leg.

The hoof is technically known as ungula (ungulae if plural), and it is an incredibly intelligently designed structure and system. It provides protection, traction, shock absorption and force redirection, and also constantly replenishes itself for the life of the horse. The more I study the hoof, the more I am awed by its complexity and its simplicity. There are no man-made inventions that can do the job of a hoof. I hope that your study of the foot will bring you some amazement as well.

The surface anatomy of the hoof is depicted in **Figure 1**. Just above the hoof, you can see there is an area that is slightly distended. This is known as the hoof head. Just below that is where the periople attaches the hoof wall to the skin. The white, powdery tissue below that is the remnant of the periople that remains attached to the hoof wall as it grows downward from the coronary band. The bulk of what can be seen from the outside is the hoof wall itself.

The bottom (solar surface) of the foot can be divided into several areas. From the drawing of **Figure 2**, you can see the toe, toe quarter, quarter, heel quarter, buttress, bars, commissures, seat of corn, white line, sole, frog, cleft of frog, and bulbs. These areas are the part of the foot that concern the farrier more than any other portion of equine anatomy. This is where we do most of our work, and it is imperative to the soundness of the horse that we understand how to sculpt and maintain what we are looking at.

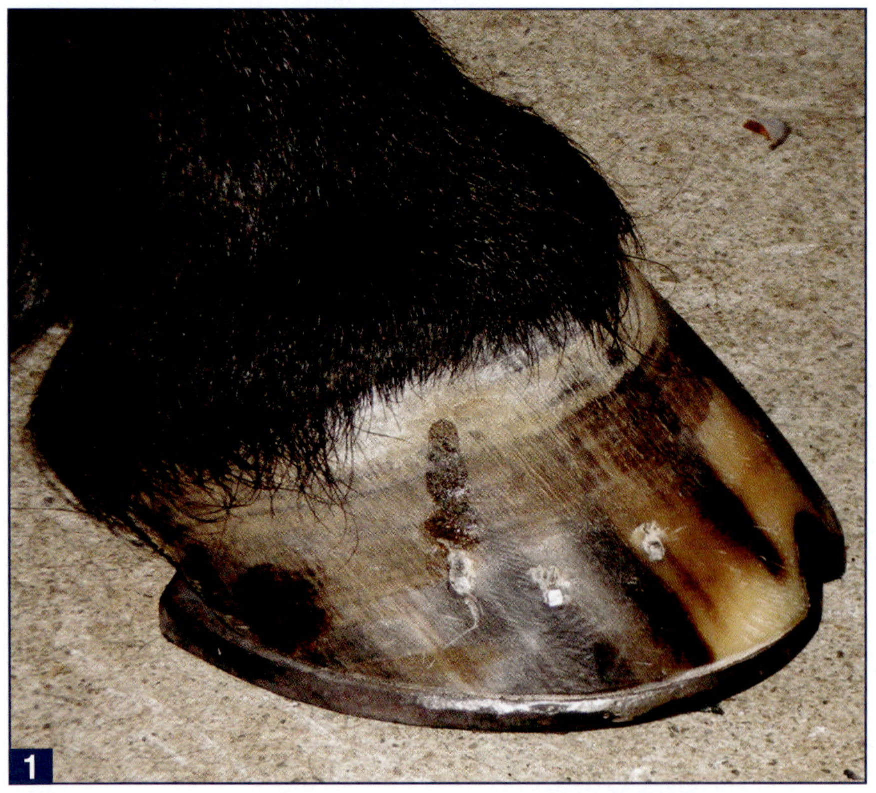

1

External structures of the foot. How most people know a hoof.

The hoof itself is completely insensitive. Another way of saying insensitive is to call that structure horny or epidermal. There are six external structures that are identified in **Figure 2**. Each of these structures is produced by a corium in much the same way as skin is created.

You will remember from the definitions that a corium is a sensitive structure that produces and nourishes a horny structure. These coriums are also known as dermal.

Part of our job as farriers is to nip, knife, rasp, sand, and sculpt these horny structures in

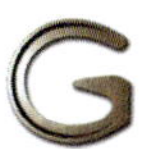

an effort to improve them. If your efforts do not result in improvement, you need to re-examine what you are doing, and why. For example, if the sole is being knifed only so that it can appear cleaner, yet it is getting thin enough to present potential harm, you should knife less. However, if there is excess sole that is in need of removal, your knifing is improving that foot toward an ideal. **Figures 3-5** are photos of a normal hind foot that has been neglected and has grown excessive length. One half of the foot has been trimmed to show the contrast.

All of the coriums for the hoof are covered with papillae, which is plural for papilla. Papillae are small, nipple-shaped protuberance that are found

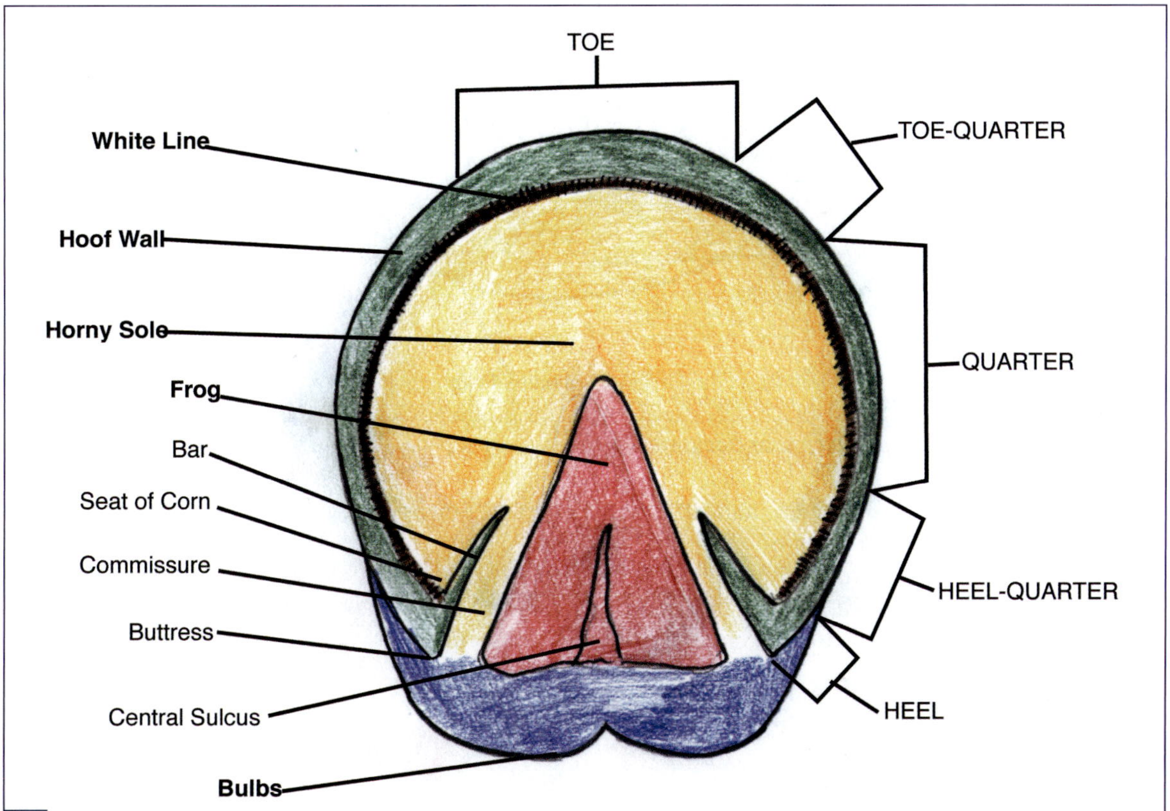

Drawing of the solar surface.

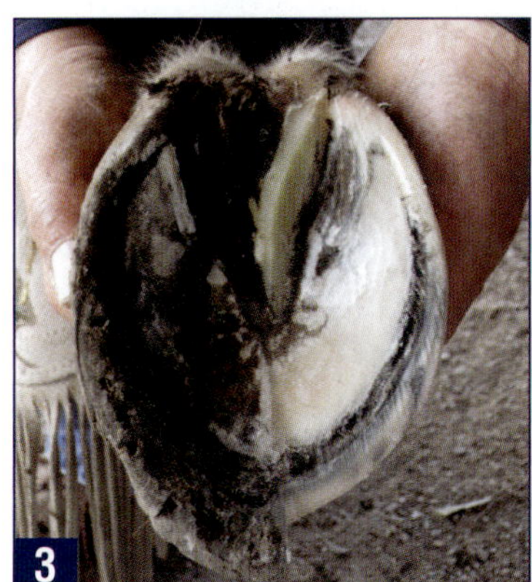

Partially trimmed foot.

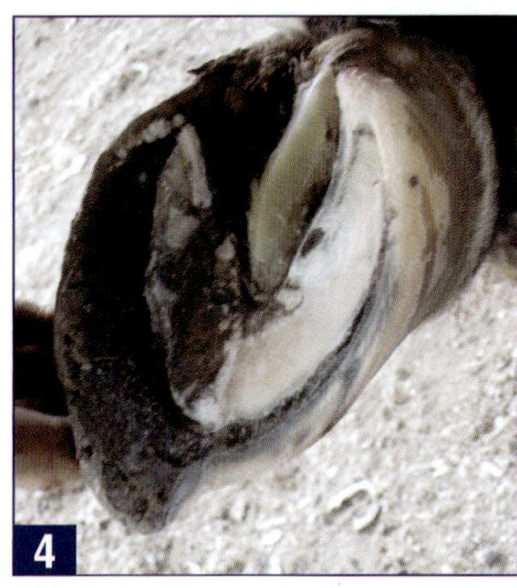

Angled view of the partially trimmed foot.

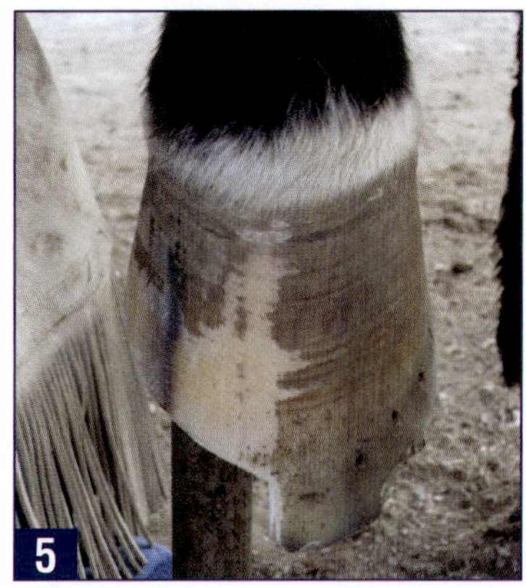

Dorsal view of half trimmed foot.

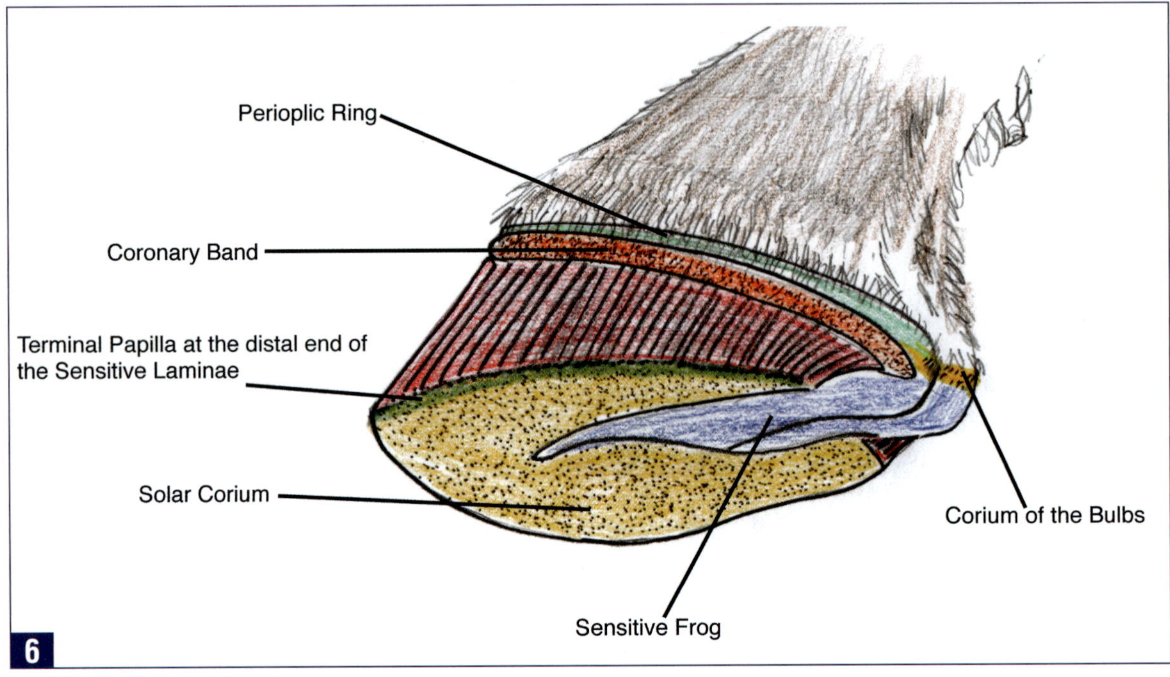

Drawing of the dermal structures, or coriums.

at the base of teeth, hair, feathers, and different horny growths such as the parts of a hoof. This stubble-like conformation multiplies the surface area of tissue many times. The drawing in **Figure 6** represent the coriums of the foot, while **Figure 9** depicts how the horny structure of the hoof would fit with the coriums. **Figures 7-8** show a dissected foot to compare to **Figure 6**, and **Figures 10-11** are pictures of a dissected foot, and can be compared to **Figure 9**.

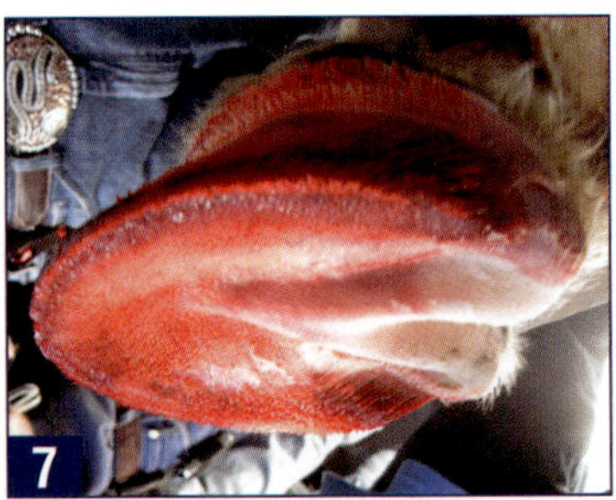

Picture of a dissected model.

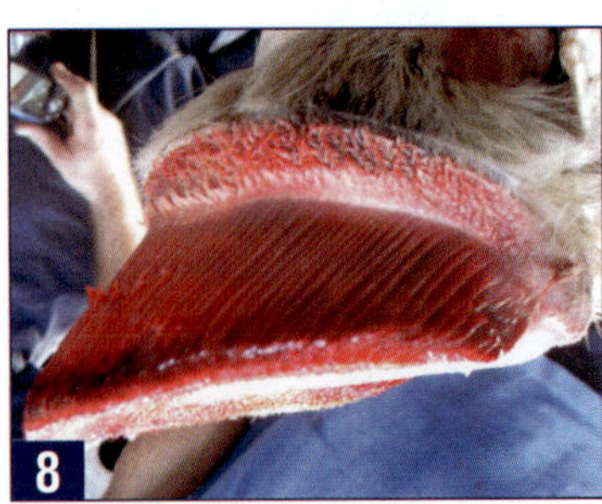

Same model, different angle.

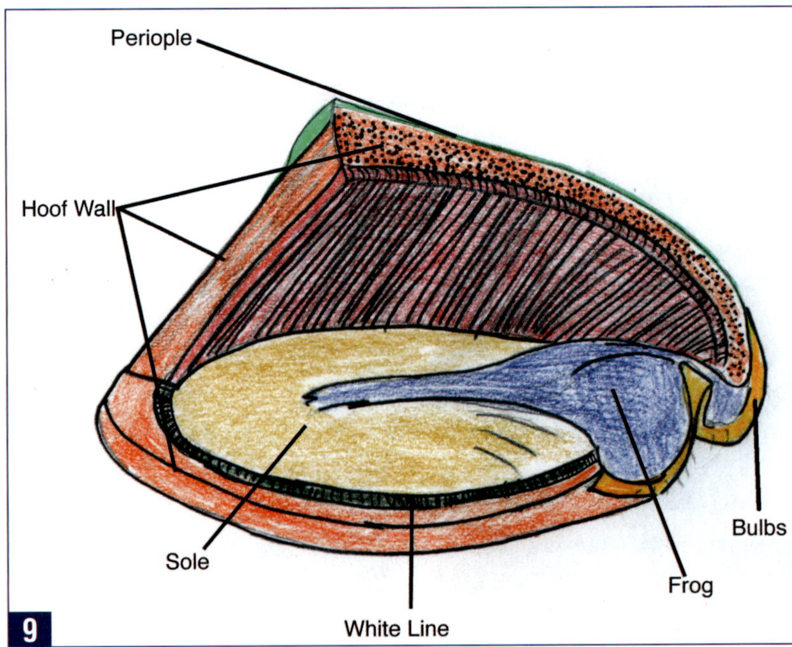

Drawing of the epidermal structures, or horny regions.

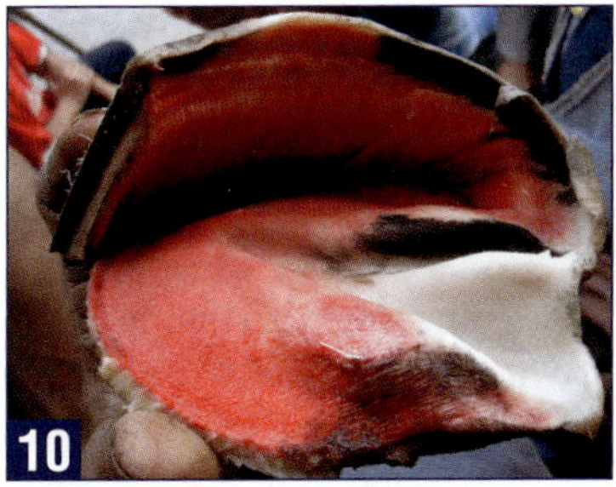

Picture of a dissected model.

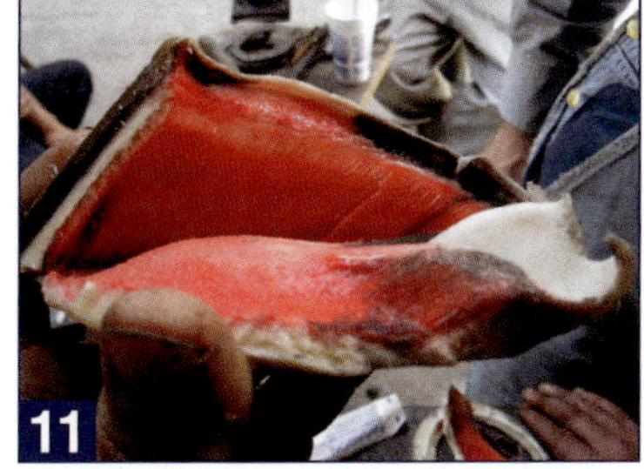

Same model, different angle.

Between all of the dermal (sensitive) and epidermal (horny) tissues is something that is called the basement membrane. This is where the foot is grown from. It is a tough tissue that completely surrounds the sensitive foot.

The hoof is divided into six regions: periople (*limbus ungulae*), wall (*paries ungulae*), white line (*zona alba*), sole (*solae ungulae*), frog (*cuneus ungulae*), and bulbs (*torus ungulae*). [10] The term ungula (or ungulae if plural) is the technical name for the hoof itself

PERIOPLE (limbus ungulae)

Figures 12-13

The proximal edge of the hoof wall is attached to the skin by a tissue called the periople. The periople is produced by the perioplic corium, also sometimes called the perioplic ring. The papillae

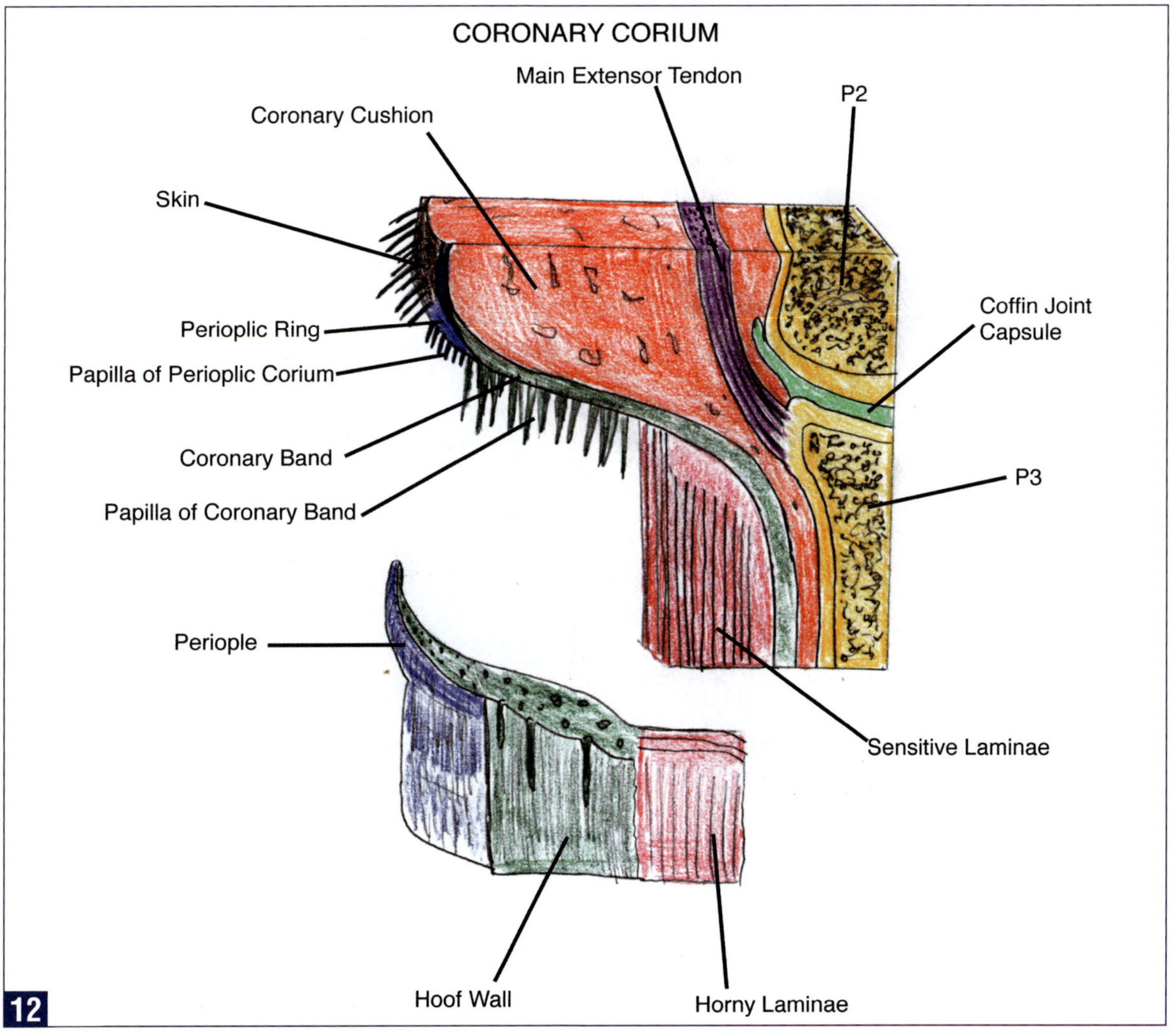

CORONARY CORIUM

Main Extensor Tendon

P2

Coronary Cushion

Skin

Coffin Joint Capsule

Perioplic Ring

Papilla of Perioplic Corium

Coronary Band

P3

Papilla of Coronary Band

Periople

Sensitive Laminae

Hoof Wall

Horny Laminae

12

Drawing of the coronary area.

of the perioplic ring originate just proximal to the coronary band. For comparison, the periople is much like our cuticle that connects our skin to our nail.

The periople performs the duty of connecting two dissimilar structures, hard hoof wall and supple skin. It allows for protection to the underlying coronary band, and allows for the inherent movement of the hoof and skin as the horse moves.

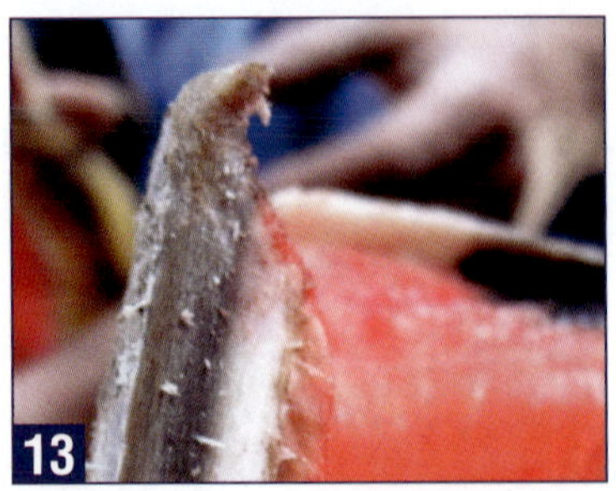

13 ***Picture that corresponds with the horny portion of the drawing in figure 12.***

As the hoof grows downward, the periople will often stay attached to the stratum externum for an inch or so from the coronary band. There is a thin layer of cells as well that are known as the stratum tectorium (stratum externum), and this is actually between the periople and the stratum medium. Many of the old time farriers were very against removing or damaging this periople with the thought that it was essential to proper hoof moisture. In fact, once it is no longer protecting sensitive structures, it has done its job. I am not suggesting that it be removed; just letting you know that it is not necessarily detrimental to do so.

In some horses, the periople may become engorged with moisture when they are in a wet environment. I have had customers become concerned when their horse comes in on a dewy morning with a thick, white, skin like tissue on the outside of the foot, extending an inch below the coronary band. This is only a natural reaction to the moisture, and not a concern. You could compare it to the skin on your fingers if you stay in the bath too long.

HOOF WALL (paries ungulae)

Figures 14-18

The hoof wall is the hardest of the horny hoof structures. It is also the largest, and the most visible when the horse is standing. It has been often stated

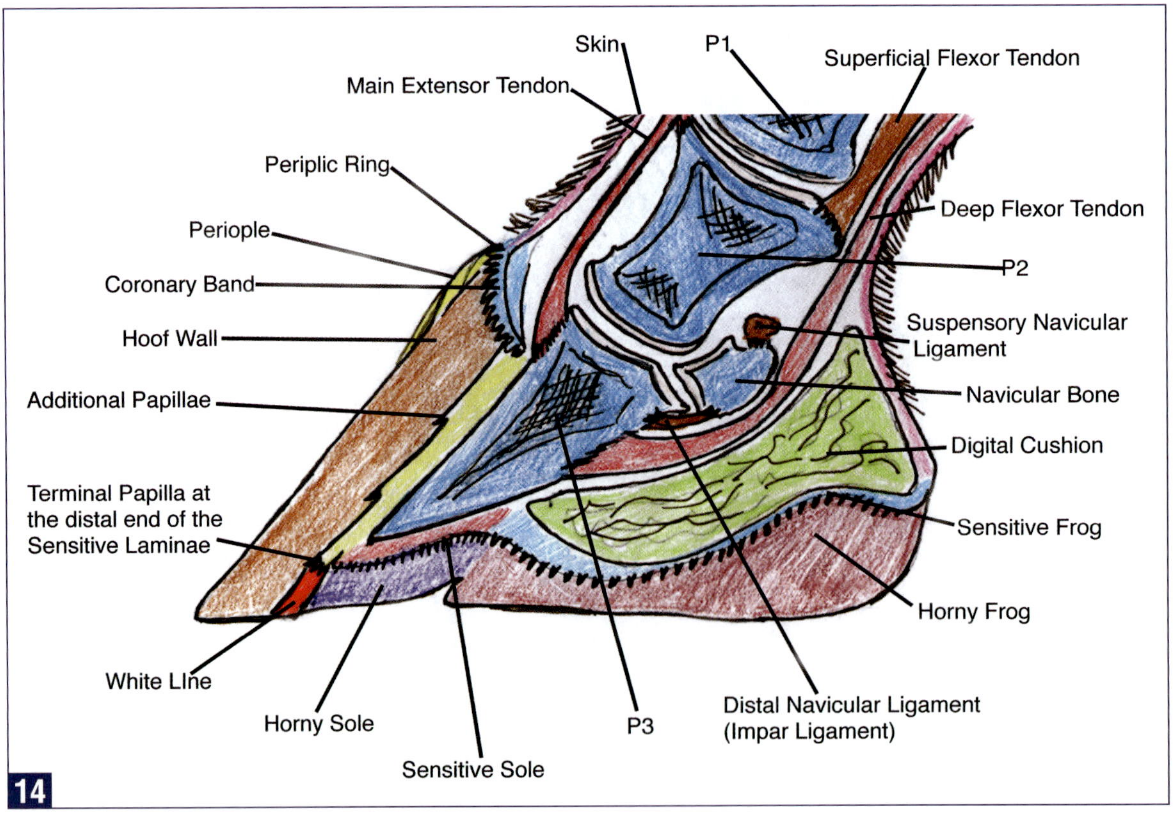

Skin
P1
Superficial Flexor Tendon
Main Extensor Tendon
Periplic Ring
Deep Flexor Tendon
Periople
Coronary Band
P2
Hoof Wall
Suspensory Navicular Ligament
Additional Papillae
Navicular Bone
Digital Cushion
Terminal Papilla at the distal end of the Sensitive Laminae
Sensitive Frog
Horny Frog
White LIne
Horny Sole
P3
Distal Navicular Ligament (Impar Ligament)
Sensitive Sole

14 ***Drawing of a sagital section of a horses' foot.***

that the average moisture content of the hoof wall is around 25%, but the environment the horse lives in will heavily impact the amount.

The hoof wall grows primarily from the coronary band, (coronet, coronary corium, or corona ungulae). The coronary band lies in an indentation at the proximal edge of the hoof wall, just distal to the perioplic ring. There are also some horn-producing papillae that exist in the sensitive laminae. You can see these depicted and labeled in **Figure 14**. These add to the hoof wall as it grows downward from the coronary band, so it is correct to state that there is some hoof wall added from an area other than the coronary band. You need to be aware that this is not commonly known, so if you are taking an older farriery exam, you actually might be expected to give the "old" answer — that the entire hoof wall

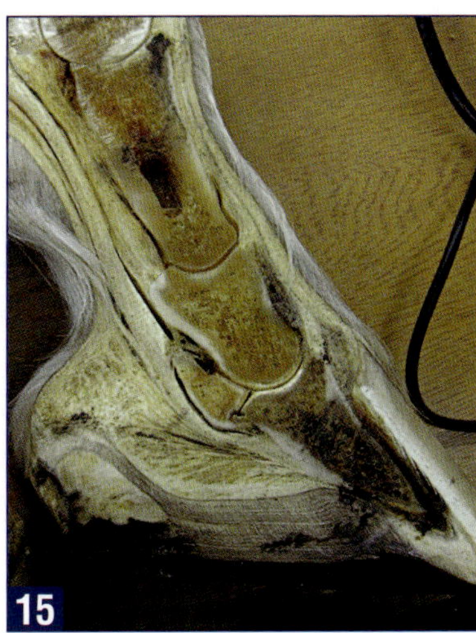

15

Picture of a freeze-dried model of the sagital section.

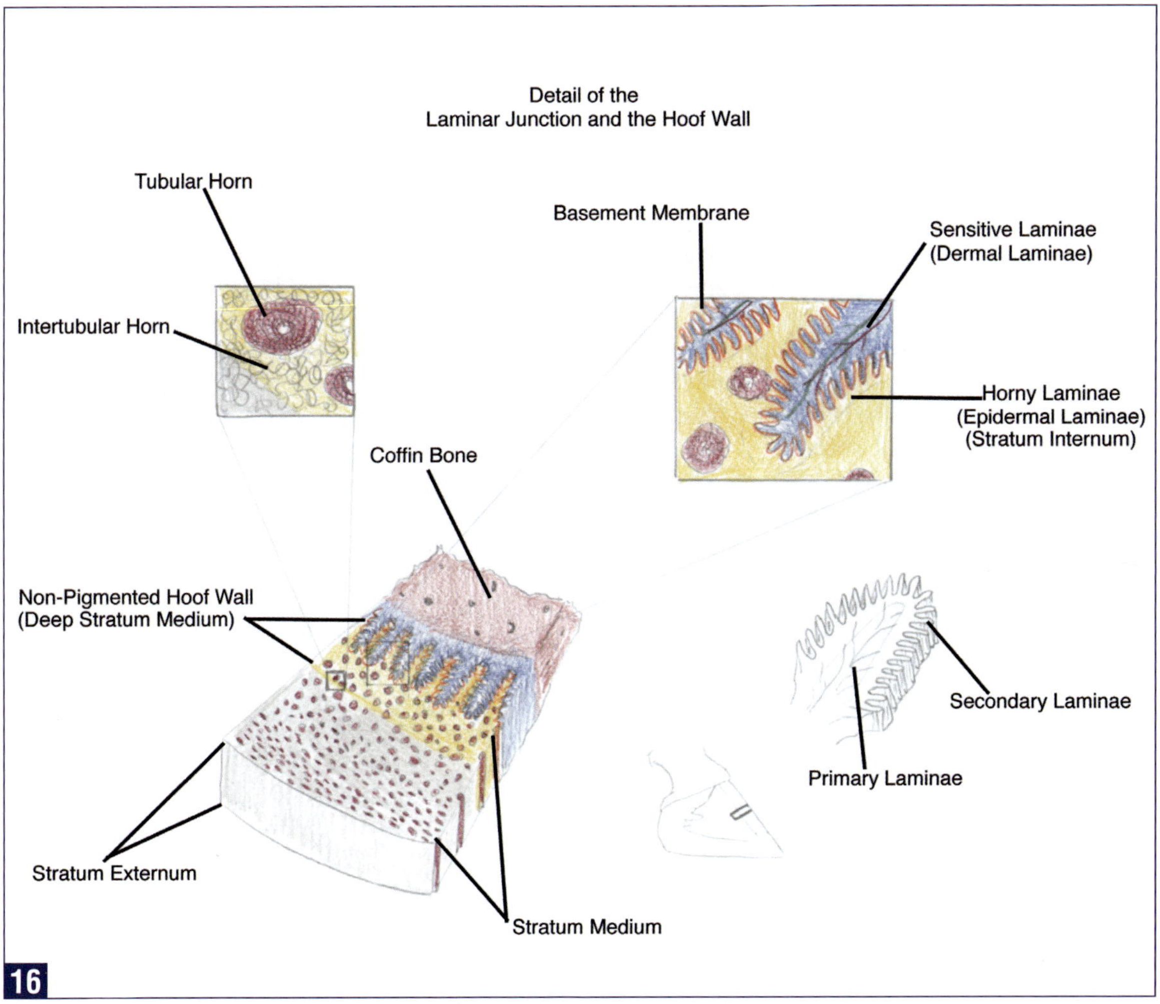

16

Drawing that depicts the hoof wall and the laminar interface.

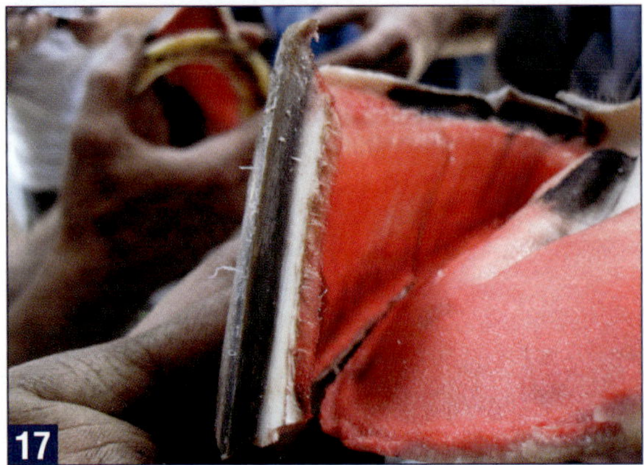

Picture of sagital section of hoof wall.

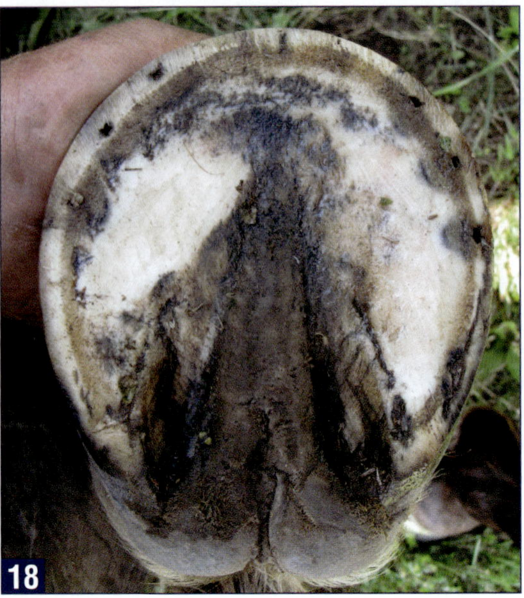

Bottom of the foot showing the bars.

is created from the coronary band. **Figure 15** is a photograph of a freeze-dried model.

There are two types of tissue produced by these papillae as seen in **Figure 16**. These are tubular horn, produced by the outside of each papilla, and intertubular horn, produced between the papilla.

Tubular horn is like a multi-layered straw (tubule). These tubules are held together by the intertubular horn. Intertubular horn is a tough bonding material that exists between the tubules. Tubular horn by itself would be like a bundle of straw. Intertubular horn by itself would be like dirt clod made of clay. Together, they become incredibly strong, like an adobe brick. I have seen some texts refer to a tissue known as intratubular horn, and it is said that it is inside each tubule. From the best sources that I have, intratubular horn does not exist.

There are three different layered regions to the hoof wall, each one having a name beginning with the term stratum. The word stratum is defined as: Any of the layers of differentiated tissue forming an anatomical structure (**Figure 17**).

The outermost is called the stratum externum or stratum tectorium. There are no tubules in this layer. It is simply a thin layer of cells that is known as the hoof varnish. It is located under the periople proximally and is exposed once the periople has detached from the growing foot. The stratum externum extends only a short way down the hoof before it is worn away.

I have found in different literature that the term stratum tectorium is often used when talking about the stratum externum. In fact, stratum tectorium is just a different term for the same thing. According to Dr. David Hood, the word tectorium is Latin for overlying structure or roof. This has led to some confusion about the number of layers of the hoof wall. There are three layers, not four.

The middle layer of the hoof wall is called the stratum medium, and it is the thickest portion of the hoof wall. The outside of the stratum medium has a flatter and denser tubular structure. It gets less dense as you go from superficial to deep. This dense tubule type of composition aids in protecting the underlying structures from environmental hazards. A dense, flat tubule makes the foot much tougher to permeate, and having a hoof wall that has tubules of different strength and structure adds to the overall strength.

In this area, the tubules are somewhat less dense, and the hoof wall is slightly softer than in the stratum externum. There is often pigment in the stratum medium until you get to the inner area. This inner area is a non pigmented layer of hoof wall that lies just outside the white line as you look at the bottom of the foot. I have heard this white area of the hoof wall referred to as the water line, and to the novice, it can easily be mistaken for the actual "white line."

The deepest layer on the inside of the hoof wall is the stratum internum. This layer is in an ornately folded and refolded pattern as it composes the horny laminae. It stops at the basement membrane, and is also non-pigmented tissue like the innermost layer

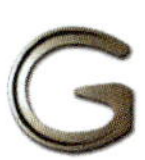

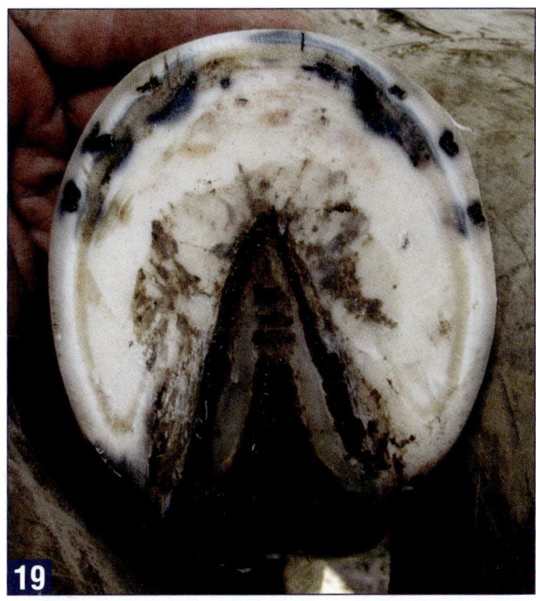

19 *White line, clean at the toe, coloring from the nails where the nail pattern is located.*

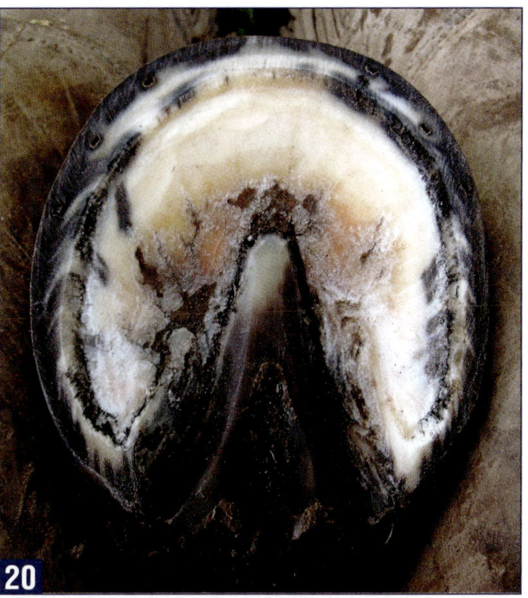

20 *Dark hooves make it easier to see the white area of the "water line" just outside the white line.*

of the stratum medium.

If you consider the shape of the proximal hoof wall as drawn in **Figure 14**, you will see that there is a depression along the border that is referred to as the coronary groove. This covers the coronary band or coronet. The bulk of the hoof wall grows from the papillae of the coronary band. The papillae does not stick out at 90 degrees to the coronary band. They lie down like combed hair, pointing distally. Since the coronary band is at this changing angle in the coronary groove, the proximal papillae are actually flatter and denser. These just happen to be the ones that make the part of the hoof wall with the denser and flatter tubules. As you continue to examine the papillae in the different areas of the coronary band, the reason for the shape of the tubules becomes evident. Superficially, the papilla are flat and dense (like the tubules); and deep, the papillae are more widely spaced (like the tubules).

On the bottom of the foot, there is hoof-wall tissue that angles dorsal from the heels along the sides of the frog. This hoof wall is called the bars, and is created by the coronary band. When the coronary band gets to the heels of the foot, it angles forward along the sides of the frog. The periople continues around the foot to attach the skin to the back of the foot and cover the bulbs. You can see from **Figure 18** where the bars come forward along the sides of the frog.

THE WHITE LINE (zona alba)

Figures 19-25

Immediately inside the hoof wall on the bottom of the foot is an area known as the zona alba, or white line. This is the junction of the sole and the hoof wall, and is actually yellowish in color with striations present in the normal hoof as in the toe area of **Figure 19**. When a foot has been shod, there will be some staining from the corrosion of the nails that can make black marks in the wall, sole, and white line, and these are also visible on **Figure 19**. On dark feet, there is a whiter area just outside (abaxial to) the white line that is indicative of the innermost later of the stratum medium. This can be seen in the toe area of **Figure 20**.

This white area is called the water line by some and is not the actual white line that we are discussing here. However, there is debate about what the term szona alba and white line are referring to.

The NAV (Nirvanna Anatomica Veterinaria) defines the white line as described above, so that is the definition we are going with. The job of the white line is to join the sole to the hoof wall, so it is basically connecting two dissimilar structures.

A lot of farriers do not understand the true location and size of the white line. I have had many explain to me that they believed the white line went all the way to the coronary band. Some of this is

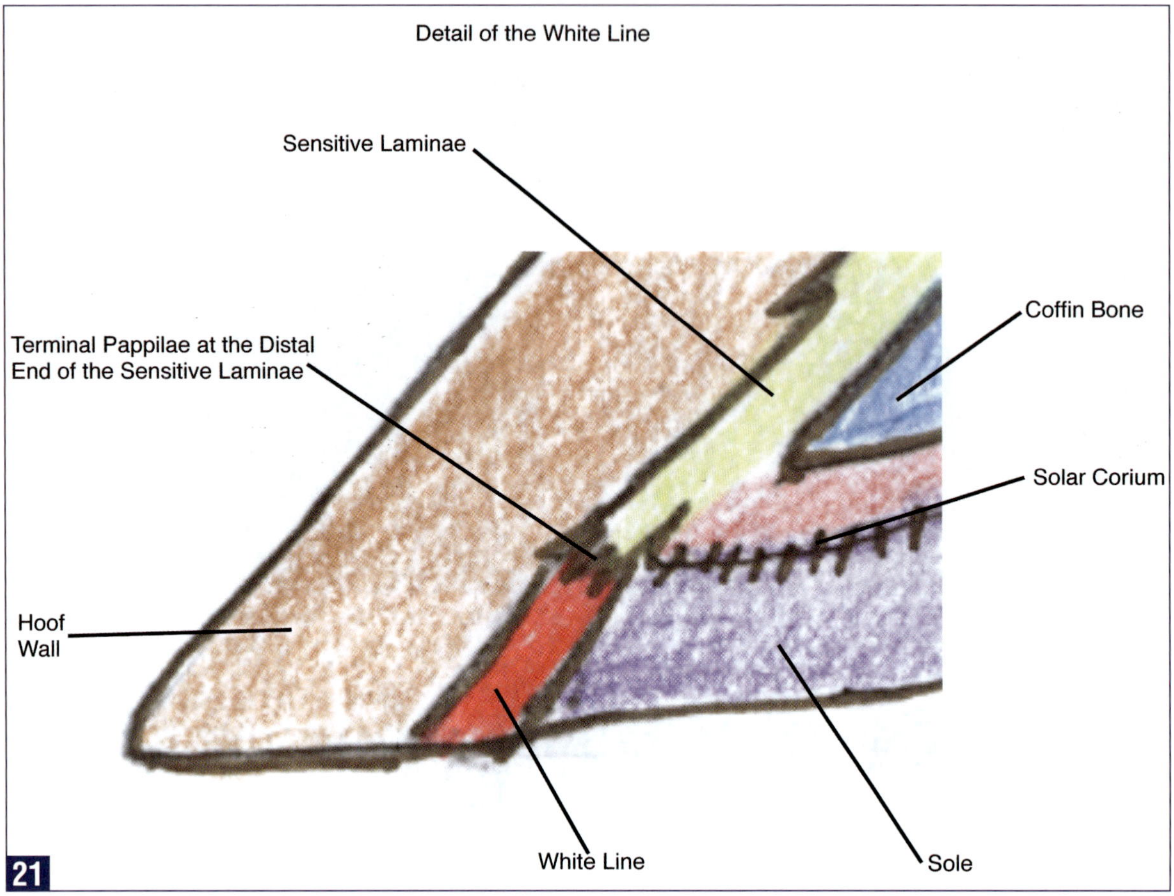

Detail of the White Line

Sensitive Laminae
Coffin Bone
Terminal Pappilae at the Distal End of the Sensitive Laminae
Solar Corium
Hoof Wall
White Line
Sole

21

Drawing of the white line.

from misinformation in textbooks, and some of it is due to white line disease, which I believe should be called white line/stratum internum disease.

The white line is produced by the terminal papillae at the distal end of the sensitive laminae (**Figures 21-22**). These papillae produce a new

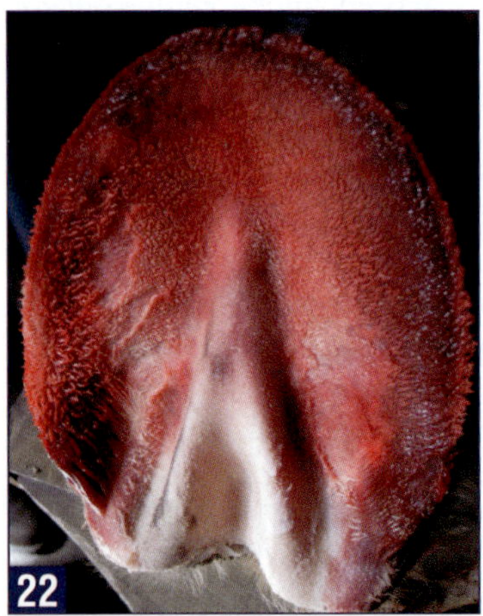

Corium of the white line around the outside perimeter of the coffin bone.

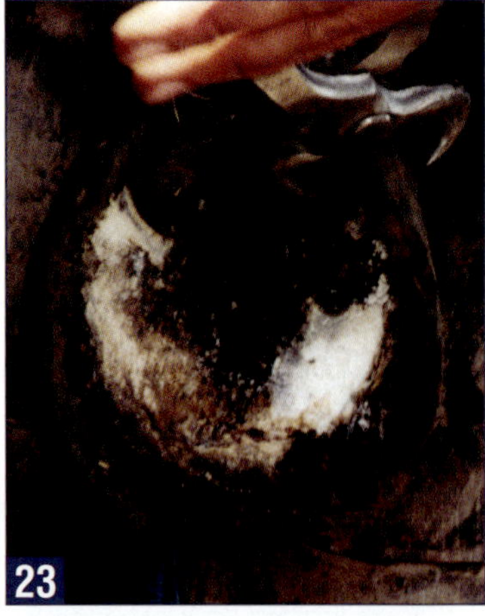

Untrimmed foundered foot.

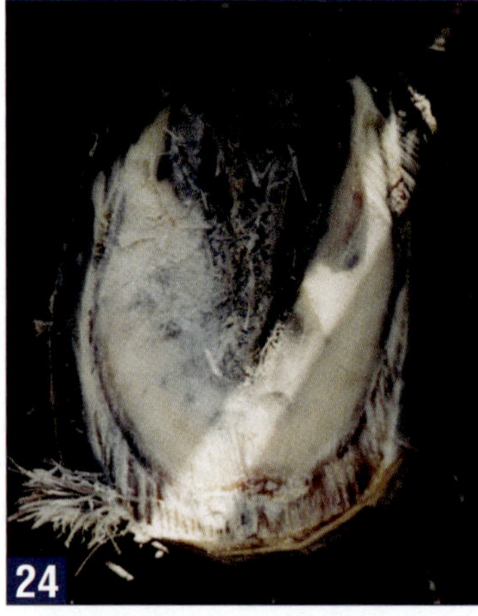

In the trimming process. Notice the width and appearance of the white line.

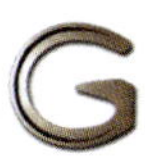

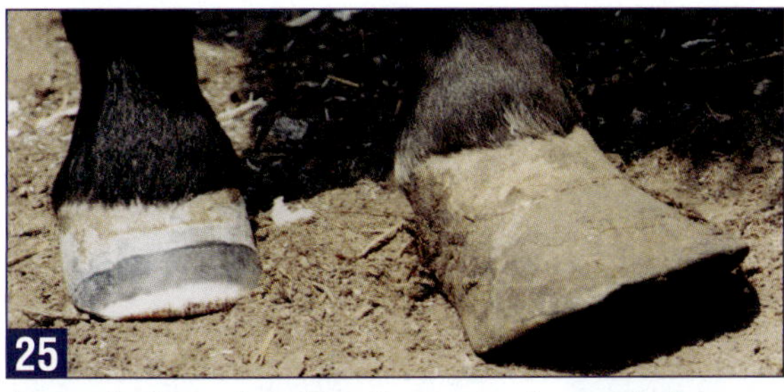

Dorsal view showing the non pigmented innermost stratum medium.

tissue that combines with the horny laminae on the inside of the stratum internum. This new tissue bonds the sole and hoof wall together. Once you are proximal to the distal border of the coffin bone, the white line does not exist, only horny and sensitive laminae.

The horny laminae, or stratum internum, continue to move past the sensitive laminae as hoof wall is produced at the coronary band. This horny laminae is going to make up part of the white line, and that is why the white line has the striations you see from the solar surface of the foot. In fact, if you look at the bottom of some chronically foundered feet, the white line will look like the underside of a mushroom cap. **Figures 23-25** are of a foundered foot being trimmed, and we can see a lot of what we have been discussing in these photos. **Figure 23** is the untrimmed foot. In **Figure 24**, you can see how the stretched white line looks, as well as the non-pigmented area of the stratum medium. **Figure 25** shows this the best. There is a white strip across the front of the foot showing that the black outer area of the stratum medium has been dressed through to show the "water line."

While the white line can be distorted, it is a pretty good indicator of the true shape of the coffin bone, and it is also a guide for the placement of nails. A well-made shoe will have the exit depth of the nails coincide with the white line. Nails driven outside of the white line will often break up the hoof, and those driven inside will often enter sensitive structures. The photos that show nail holes outside of the area of the white line are indicative of feet that have had old shoes removed and the foot trimmed.

EPIDERMAL SOLE (solae ungulae)

Figures 26-29

The epidermal, or horny, sole is produced by the sensitive sole, also called the solar corium. The sensitive sole is covered with papillae. When you do a dissection, they will look like red beard stubble (**Figure 26**). The horny sole makes up the area inside the white line, and is attached solidly to the base of the horny frog (**Figure 27**). It is also said to have moisture content of 33%.

The horny sole is a major component in the protection of the coffin bone and the sensitive structures inside the foot. It also has some flexibility that allows it to change shape to a certain degree and flatten as the foot bears weight. Ideally, it will be concave, which adds to its strength.

During normal use, the horse will slough the older horny sole tissue as new sole is produced from the solar corium. However, once shoes are added to protect the foot, the normal sloughing will not occur. As a result, part of the farriers' responsi-

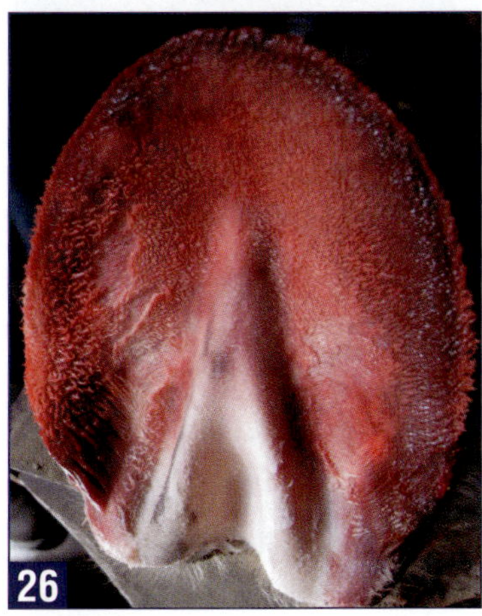

Solar corium.

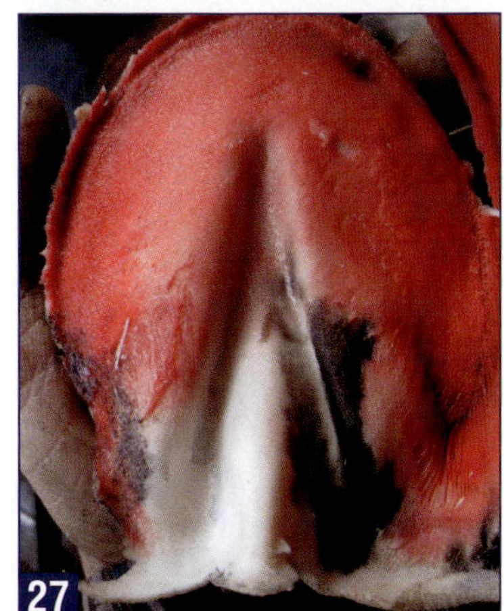

Horny sole and frog.

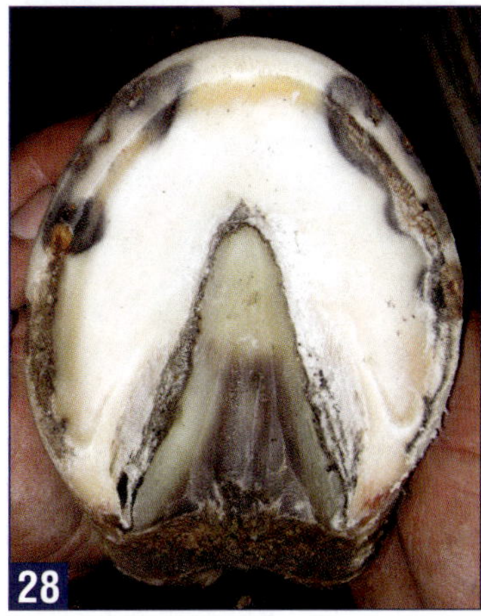

Clean, shiny sole.

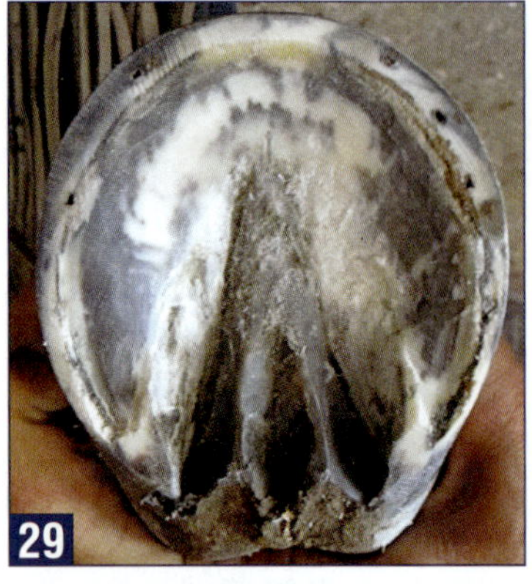

Pigmented sole.

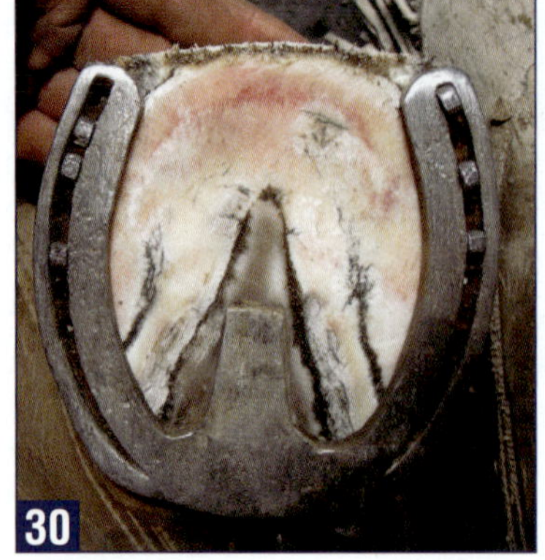

Bruised sole.

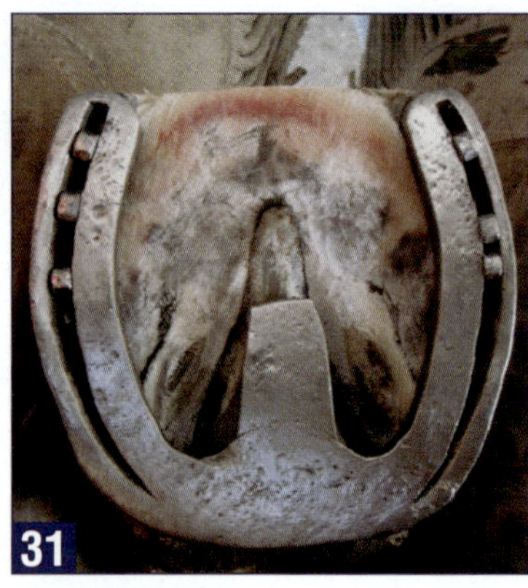

Bruised sole.

bility it to remove that excess sole when the foot is trimmed. Knowing how much sole to remove and where from comes with experience and guidance. As a general rule, you want to knife until the sole has a smooth and shiny consistency (**Figure 28**).

The oldest sole will be chalky and will come out easily most of the time. As you get past that to the newer sole, it is almost like carving a very soft wood. It is not uncommon to find pigment in the sole. This does not play a role in strength or thickness (**Figure 29**). Bruising is also quite common in the horny sole, as seen in the foundered feet seen in **Figures 30-31**.

Some older textbooks recommend trimming the

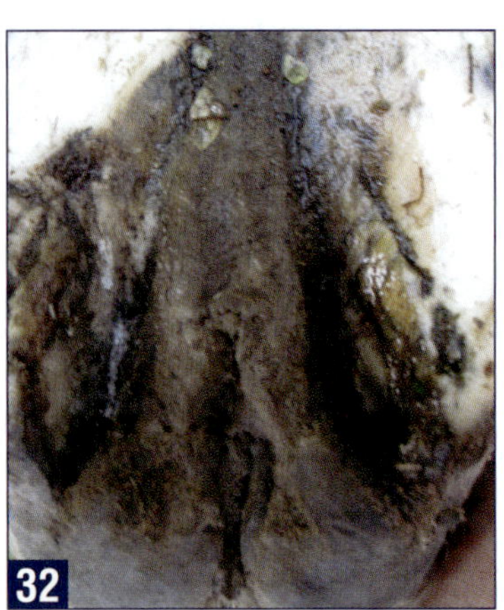

Untrimmed frog.

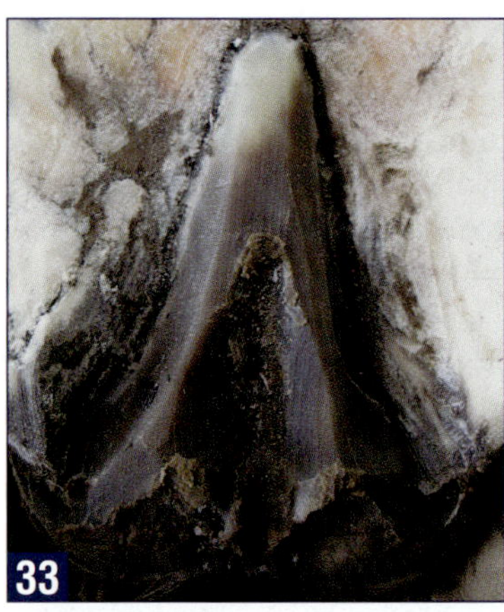

Trimmed frog

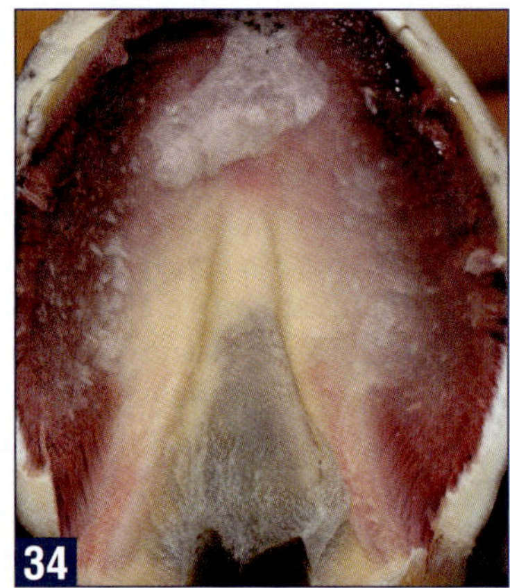

Dermal frog, (sensitive)

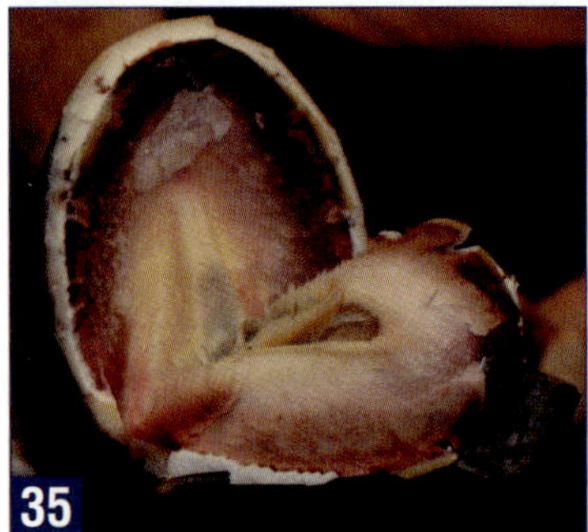

The horny frog and sole pull off as one during dissections.

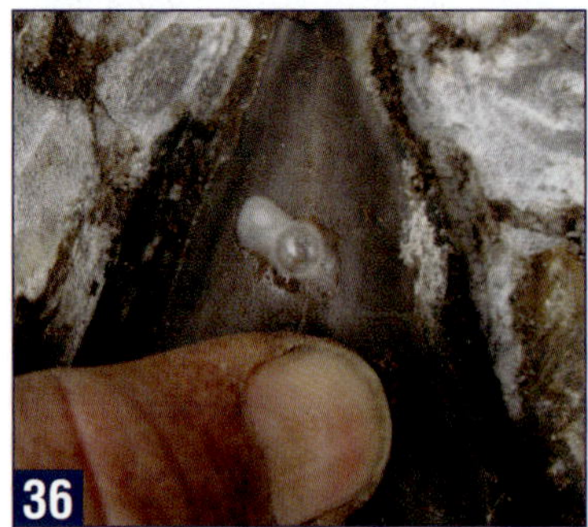

Fat deposit from the merocrine gland.

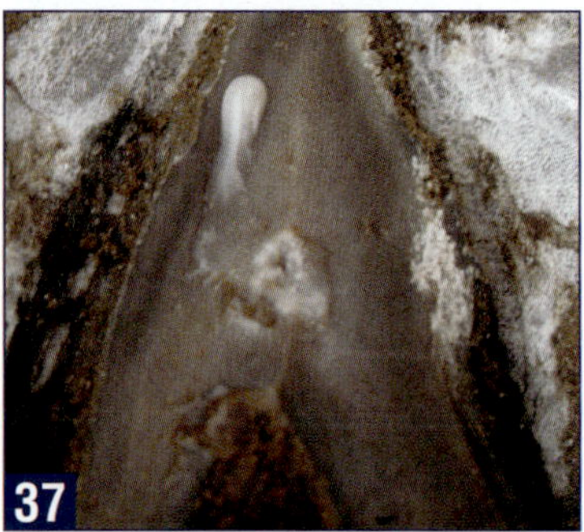

The hole where the fat deposit was located.

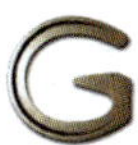

sole until it gives to thumb pressure. This is rarely a good idea. I would compare it to removing the callous from your hand. Removing a little would be fine, but creating a pink finger could be painful.

EPIDERMAL FROG (cuneus ungulae)

Figures 32-38

The epidermal, or horny, frog is a long, triangular piece of rubber-like tissue that is found in the solar-center-rear of the horse's foot. **Figure 32** shows an untrimmed frog, while **Figure 33** shows one that has been trimmed to remove excess growth. The **Figure 32** frog does not need to be trimmed, in my opinion. The frog has been blamed and credited for innumerable things throughout history, and it is a pretty amazing piece of the foot puzzle. It was thought to act as a pump to get blood back up the leg, but this has been proven false. The frog is created and nourished by the sensitive frog as seen in **Figure 34**. I believe that the frog plays a part in helping the foot to expand when the frog has ground contact. It also can provide traction and stopping power due to its shape and consistency; kind of like a gum-sole boot compared to a boot with a leather sole. The frog also provides a great deal of shock absorption as well.

In temperate climates, the frog is said to have moisture content of 50%. However, in really dry climates, it can get so dry and hard that cutting it is like chipping stone.

The two halves to the frog are divided by the central sulcus, or frog cleft, which is a separation through the middle of the frog. On both sides, there are some grooves that are known as commissures. These are sometimes called sulci, or more correctly, peracuneal sulci. At the deepest level of these collateral grooves, the frog and sole are tightly joined to the horny sole. You will find that both the horny frog and sole pull out as one unit when doing a dissection (**Figure 35**). This strong connection is one of the reasons that ground contact may not be as critical as some barefoot trimmers claim.

Occasionally, you will hit a pocket of milky, greasy fluid when you trim the frog. This is a deposit of a fatty liquid that is produced by the merocrine gland in the plantar cushion (**Figures 36-37**). The first time that this happens to young farriers, it can make them nervous. But don't worry; it is a normal and harmless thing and is part of what makes the moisture content of the frog so high. In **Figure 38**, you can see where the frog has grown so long that it has covered the outside of the heel. There are striations in the hoof wall and the frog that can easily be seen.

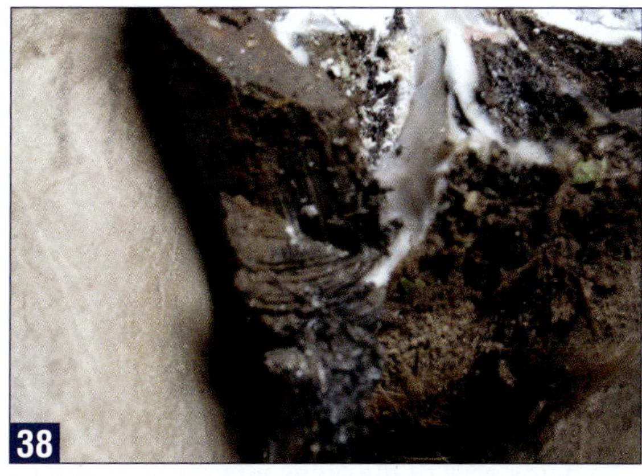

Striations in the hoof wall at the heel and the frog where the frog had grown over the heel.

In the American Midwest, the frog will often shed every spring and every fall. I have heard reports of a frog shedding its outer layer up to six times a year, although I have not seen this personally. When the frog is first shed, the frog underneath can be sensitive, and horses can become sore until it hardens. Again, it can be like us losing a callous.

BULBS (torus ungulae)

Figures 39-40

The bulbs are two rounded and hairless structures found at the most palmar or plantar portion of the foot (**Figure 39**). They are rarely discussed in farrier textbooks, other than to describe them as continua-

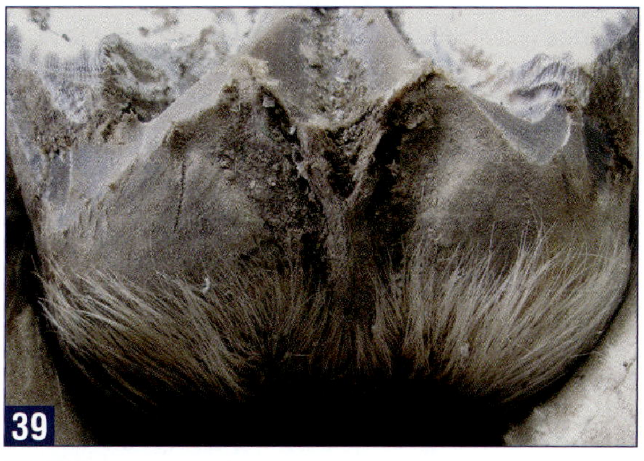

Bulbs.

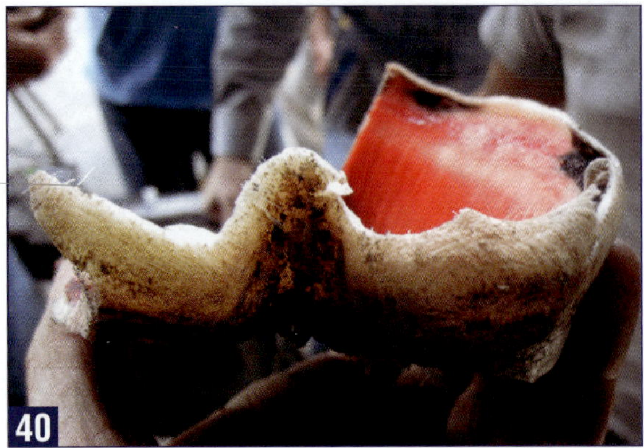

The horny area of the bulbs after being removed during dissection.

tion of the periople, with which they blend (**Figure 40**). However, they are their own structures.

The bulbs grow downward from the corium of the bulbs that is in line with the coronet, and they attach the skin to the heel region of the foot and frog in a thicker and tougher attachment than the periople alone provides. Since the heels of the hoof have a sharp angle and more movement than the rest of the hoof wall, having a stronger attachment to the skin is critical. The thickness of the attachment also allows for the sharpness of the heel to be covered by the roundness of the bulbs.

HOOF GROWTH

Hoof growth involves two basic procedures: Proliferation, which is the reproduction of cells, and cornification, which is the subsequent hardening of those cells.

These processes begin with the coriums or dermal portions of the foot. They create the horny structures, which are also known as epidermal structures, like our skin. Surrounding the dermal regions is a structure that is known as the basement membrane. This is a thin, permanent layer that acts as a filter between the dermal and epidermal layers and allows blood and nutrients to pass through from the dermal to epidermal cells as needed.

The basal epidermal cells are located just outside the basement membrane, and these cells constantly reproduce new cells to create the hoof. As these cells reproduce, the new cells push the older ones away, and hoof growth is occurring. As these cells are continually being displaced, they go through a process that is known as cornification.

Cornification describes the process whereby a cell goes from being a basal epidermal cell to becoming a hard, resilient horny dermal cell.

As a cell begins the process of cornification, it differentiates. This is a process where the cell changes dramatically in shape, size, and physical properties. As it continues to move away, it becomes what is known as a transitional cell, and finally ends up as a more fully cornified dermal cell.

Cornification will create an epidermal cell that is extremely hard, as in hoof wall, or softer, as in the frog. Proper nutrition is essential for the production of a quality hoof.

As the hoof wall grows from the coronary band, it is pushed away from the coronary band, one cell at a time. The stratum internum, which is the horny laminae, is pushed past the sensitive laminae as the wall continues to grow. The sensitive lamina are a permanent structure on the coffin bone, and the horny laminae are an insensitive structure that are continually being replaced at the coronary band. When the horny laminae reaches the end of the coffin bone, and thus the end of the sensitive laminae, the terminal papillae of the sensitive laminae form a new tissue to create the white line.

LAMINAR ATTACHMENT

Figure 41

As you know, the hoof wall is attached to the coffin bone by the laminae. There are sensitive (dermal) laminae and horny (epidermal) laminae. The basement membrane between attaches them to each other. When you pull the hoof wall off of the coffin bone in a dissection, you will see a series of ridges or folds between the hoof wall and coffin bone. These are the laminae. The large folds on the coffin bone are the primary sensitive laminae, and the large folds on the inside of the hoof wall are the primary horny laminae.

These interdigitate with each other. This means that there are folds in the sensitive laminae that are matched by the horny laminae, and they fit together with each other, much like the teeth of a zipper.

On each of the large primary folds, there are extremely small secondary folds. The secondary laminae on each primary lamina multiply the attachment area between the hoof wall and coffin bone. In fact, secondary laminae give the hoof as much as 600% more attachment area than would the primary laminae alone.

The number of primary lamina leaves will

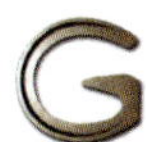

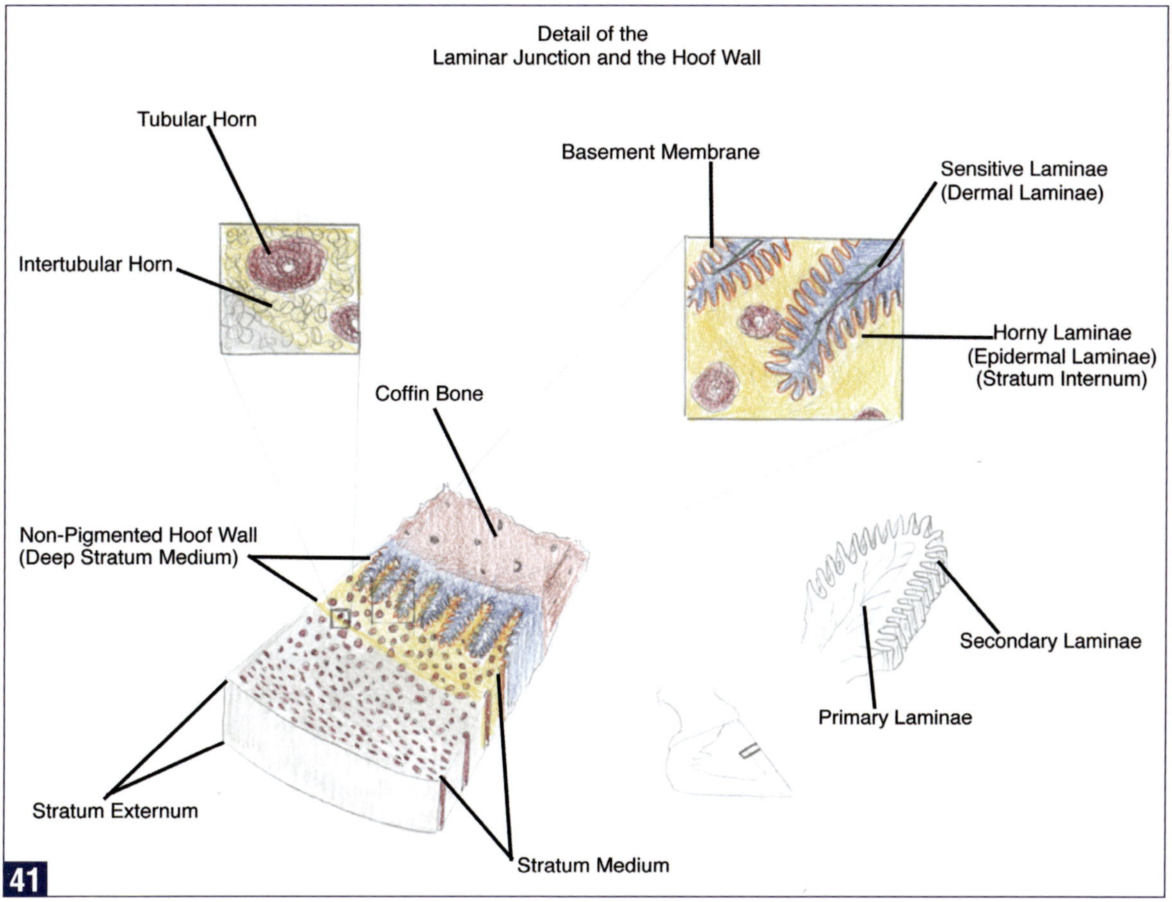

Detail of the
Laminar Junction and the Hoof Wall

Tubular Horn
Intertubular Horn
Basement Membrane
Sensitive Laminae
(Dermal Laminae)
Horny Laminae
(Epidermal Laminae)
(Stratum Internum)
Coffin Bone
Non-Pigmented Hoof Wall
(Deep Stratum Medium)
Secondary Laminae
Primary Laminae
Stratum Externum
Stratum Medium

41

Laminar interface.

vary, depending on the size of the foot as well as other genetic factors. Most horses will have between 500 and 700 primary horny laminae and a matching number of primary sensitive laminae leaves. Although it has generally been taught that there are 100 secondary laminae for each primary lamina, that number will also vary from horse to horse. It is an incredible design that allows the dispersion and absorption of concussion as well as allowing the foot to continue to grow downward.

FRONTS AND HINDS

Figures 42-43

There is a difference between the shape of a common hind foot and that of a common front foot. I believe that this difference in design serves a very important function. A front foot that has the same radius from the widest point on either side allows the horse to break over in any direction when travelling, making steering easier. The sharper toe on

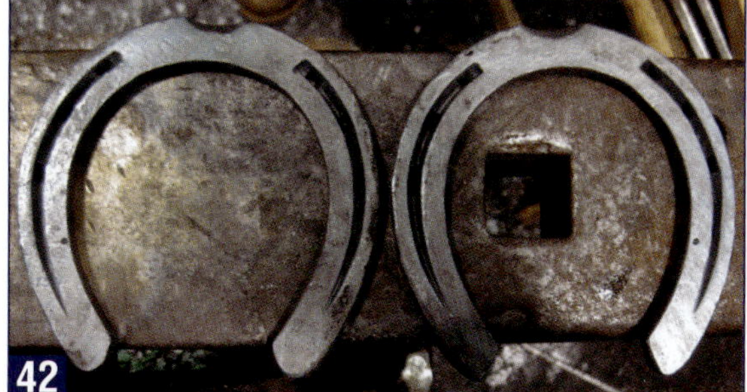

42

Front shoes.

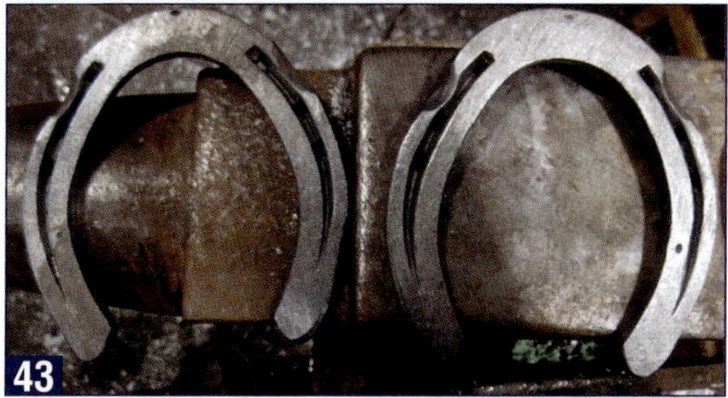

43

Hind shoes.

the hind foot allows the horse to have more traction for driving itself forward. These shapes are also reflected in the transverse section of the cannon bones of the front and hind legs.

While there are normal shapes for front and hind feet, they can also come in a variety of other shapes. The foot is shaped by many factors, such as limb conformation, genetics, injury, nutrition, environment, age, wear, and trimming, as well as others. It is the job of the farrier to make the foot as close to the ideal as possible and set it up for continued normal growth. When you trim a foot, it is possible to make it take on abnormal growth and wear patterns by applying some of the controversial trimming theories. When you see this happen from trimming cycle to trimming cycle, you need to evaluate why it is happening and what you are trying to accomplish.

HOOF MOISTURE CONTENT

The larger horny parts of the foot all have different moisture contents based on their job, location and composition. The percentages mentioned here would be what are considered ideal, but the environment is a huge factor. Since a horse stands on its feet on the ground, the wetter the environment, the wetter the feet, and vice versa.

The water content of the foot comes from the blood and the environment. A certain amount of evaporation will occur, which the body will replace as needed. When you trim a horse that is standing on a rubber mat or clean concrete, you will see it leave a wet footprint (**Figure 44**). This is hoof moisture that is left on the floor from the cut foot. When you hot-fit that foot, you will see that there is only wetness left on the floor inside the rim of the hot-fit shoe. In essence, hot-fitting the shoe has cauterized the tubules that you just nipped and rasped. This is another argument in favor of hot-fitting.

I am generally against the use of hoof dressing. Most hoof dressings will create a varnish on the outside of the foot, making a barrier to water and taking the environment out of the equation. The natural evaporation of internal moisture and intake of external moisture is stopped. A hoof dressing also seals any bacteria on the hoof against it and this can potentially be a bad thing.

Constant use of a hoof dressing can make a foot dependent on it and put the horse in a bad situation if the dressing is not available. Like the lips of a

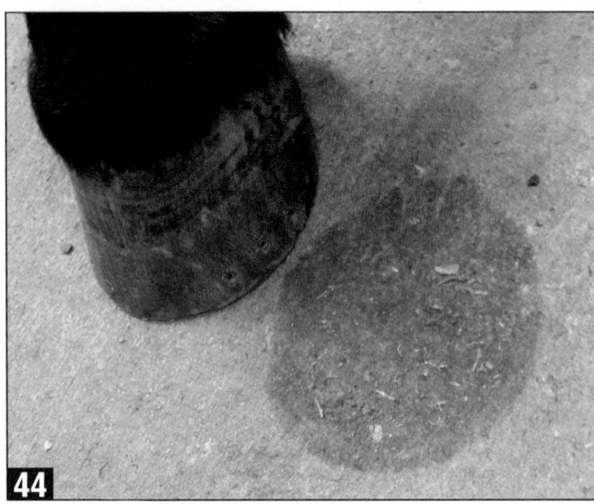

Wet hoof print from a newly trimmed foot.

person addicted to lip balm or the nose of a person addicted to nasal spray.

There are a couple of instances where I find hoof dressing to be a good thing. First, right after dressing the outer hoof wall, a hoof dressing can replace the stratum tectorium for a few days. Applied immediately after dressing the foot, once every 6 weeks or so, may be beneficial to help protect the tubules that have just been cut through. This means that a foot will receive hoof dressing around 8 times a year.

I would also recommend hoof dressing if you are going to move a horse from one harsh environment to another, for instance, from the swamps of Florida to the deserts of Nevada, or vice versa. You can start using a hoof dressing every few days for the month leading up to the move. Once you get to where you are going, continue using hoof dressing, but use less and less until the foot becomes acclimated.

If a horse were to be walked from Nevada to Florida, the amount of time that it would take would allow the foot enough time to acclimate on its own. Going by truck and trailer would not allow enough time for the natural acclimation to the moisture difference.

CONCLUSION

As you can see, there is a lot to learn and know about the hoof. Since this is the main thing that you are going to be working on, you can't learn enough about it.

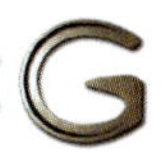

Chapter

9 BONES AND JOINTS

Bones are a remarkable part of anatomy. The long bones are formed during development through a process known as endochondral ossification. (Endo means center and chondro is the root word for cartilage.) The bone starts as a cartilage model at around 30 days of development, and it will grow in length from continuous cell division. **Figure 1** shows the bones at different stages of development in the uterus.

A thick skin of periosteum develops at about 50 days around the shaft of the bone, or diaphysis, and as the bone grows, the periosteum becomes thinner. Most long bones grow from 3 ossification centers. One in the diaphysis, and one each in the epiphysis at the ends of the bone, which are easily identified at 180 days. Cartilage between the diaphysis and the epiphysis is known as the physis or epiphyseal growth plate, and the long bones grow in length from these areas. Bones such as the navicular bone, carpal bones, tarsal bones, and coffin bone only have one ossification center, so these bones do not have a physis.

Bones can be classified into 5 categories:

- **Long Bones:** These act as levers, store minerals, aid in locomotion, and are found in the limbs.
- **Short Bones:** Primarily absorb concussion. Found in the carpus and tarsus.
- **Flat Bones:** Create cavities to protect vital organs. Found in the skull.
- **Irregular bones:** Protect the spinal cord, so these are the vertebrae.
- **Sesamoid bones:** Bones that act as a fulcrum for a tendon. The navicular bone in the foot, the sesamoid bones at the back of the fetlock, and the accessory carpal bone behind the knee are some primary examples.

Bones are dynamic and constantly change and remodel to accommodate the loads that are exerted on them. The oldest bone cell in a horse's body will be somewhere around 5 years old, which means that the oldest bone is no older than 5 years of age. As the body breaks down old bone on a cellular level, new bone cells are constantly being added to make the bone stronger with consideration to how it is

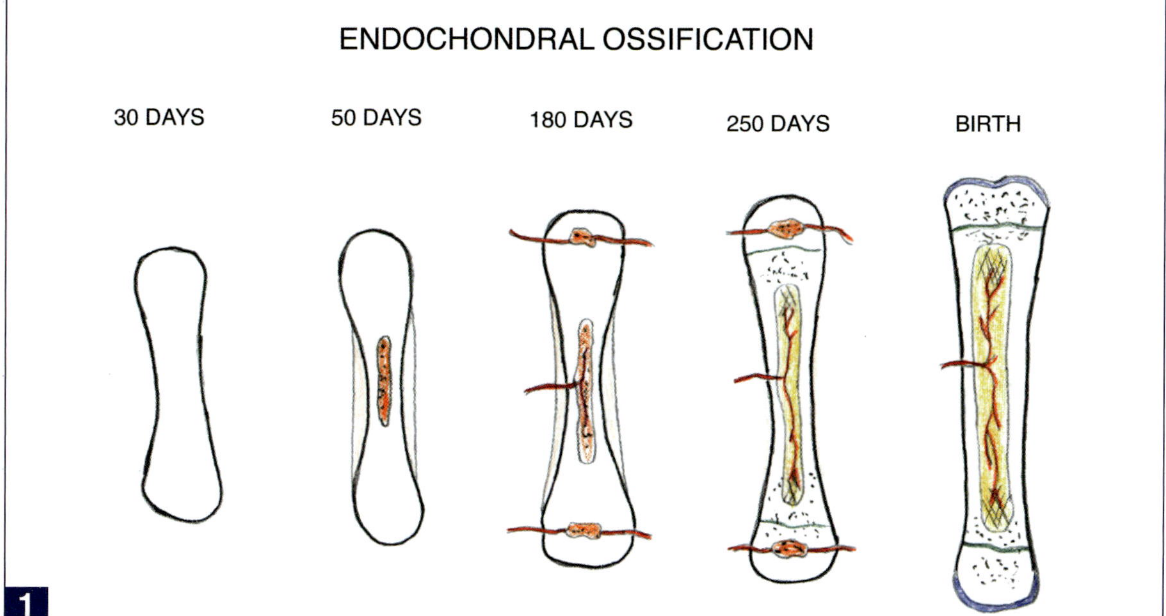

Drawing of the development of the long bones in utero

currently being stressed.

For my students, I make them learn to draw the cross section of a bone so that they can identify some basic parts **(Figures 2 - 3).** It is really handy to make drawings and then use colored pencils to make the drawing stick in your memory better. The parts of the bones are listed and described below:

- **Articular cartilage:** the tissue found on the ends of bones that are involved in synovial joints.

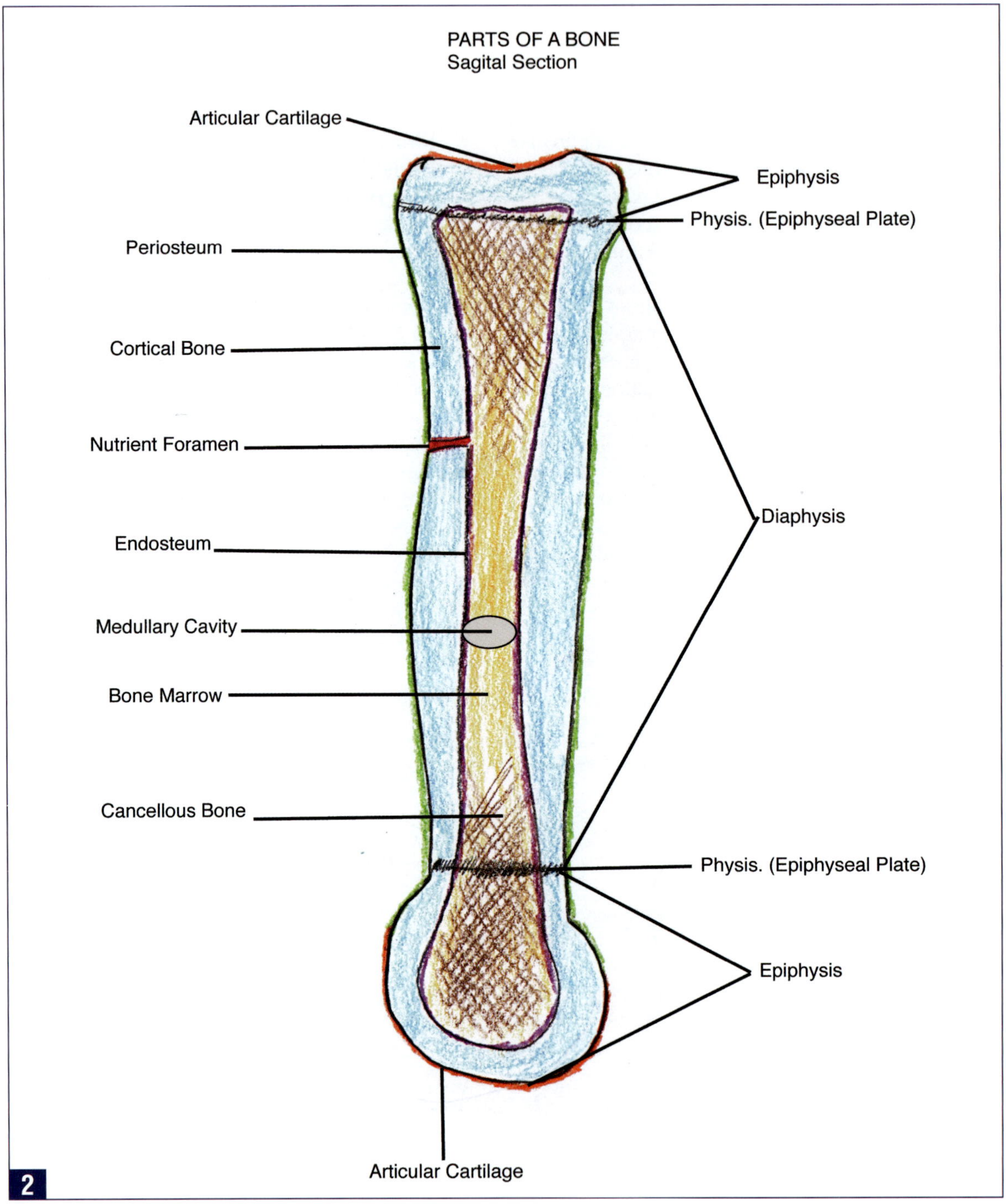

2

Sagital section of the cannon bone.

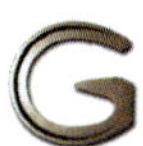

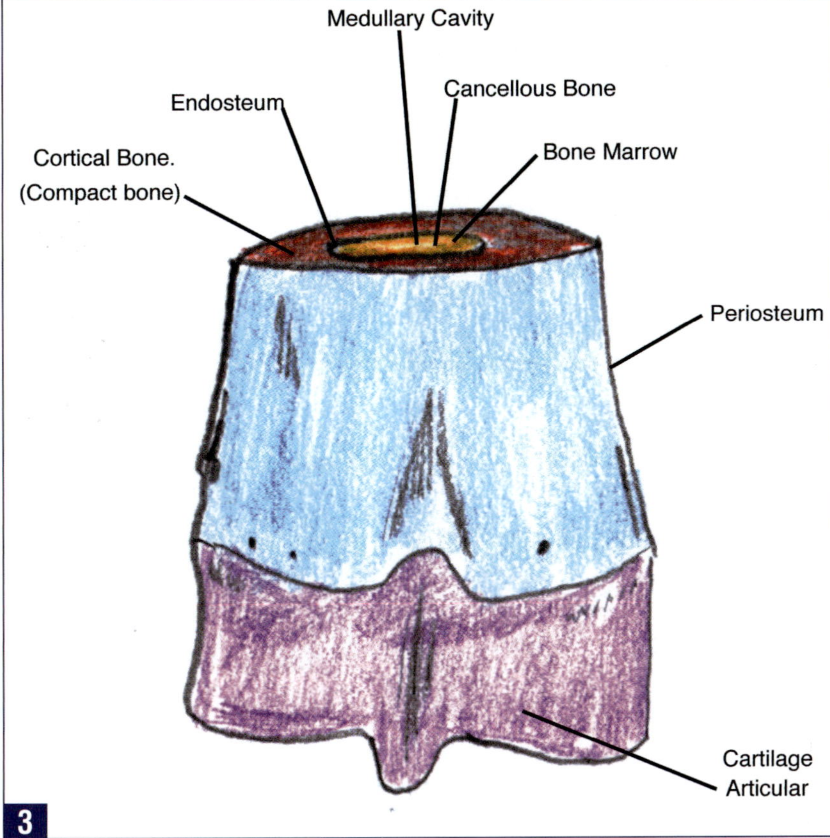

Transverse section of the cannon bone.

- **Periosteum:** Fibrous membrane that covers the outside of bones.
- **Cortical Bone:** Also called compact bone, this is the hard, thick, outer shell (cortex) of a bone.
- **Endosteum:** Fibrous membrane that lines the inside of the cortical bone, or medullary cavity.
- **Medullary Cavity:** The inside area of the long bones that is lined by the endosteum, filled with bone marrow, and has cancellous bone towards either end.
- **Nutrient Foramen:** A hole in a bone that allows nutrients to pass into the medullary cavity.
- **Bone Marrow:** A soft material that fills the medullary cavity and the spaces in the matrix of the cancellous bone.
- **Cancellous Bone:** Porous bone tissue that is found inside the medullary cavity. It is densest at the ends of the bone and may be absent in the center.
- **Physis:** Also known as an epiphyseal plate, this is an area of the long bones between the epiphysis and diaphysis where long bones grow quickly in length from.
- **Diaphysis:** The shaft area of the bone found between the growth areas on the end.
- **Epiphysis:** The ends of long bones outside the diaphysis.

In the long bones, there is a physis that allows for accelerated growth. There are actually two of these toward the end of the long bones, and they become inactive at different times. If you were to boil the bones of a newborn foal, you would find that there are a lot more parts when you get done than you thought there would be; these are the epiphysis and diaphysis separating at the physis. Looking at the photo of a freeze-dried sagital model in **Figure 4**, you can see the white lines going across the proximal and distal portion of P1. The proximal one is more evident because it closes at a later time than the distal one. This particular model is of a newborn that still has not lost the rubbery covering on the bottom of the foot that it is born with. This covering is called eponychium. Many horsemen will refer to these as golden slippers, and they help protect the mare from the hard edges of a horny hoof.

In **Figures 5 - 6**, the physis on the long bones is easily evident. While the closure time of the growth plates can be influenced by many factors such as heredity, pressure, diet, injury, environment, etc, the more distal the bone, the earlier the plate closure time. The following chart can serve as a broad approximation of closure times:

Proximal P2	3 to 6 months
Proximal P1	4 to 6 months
Distal Cannon Bone	6 to 9 months
Distal Tibia	18 to 24 months
Distal Radius	24 to 30 months

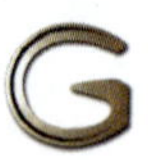

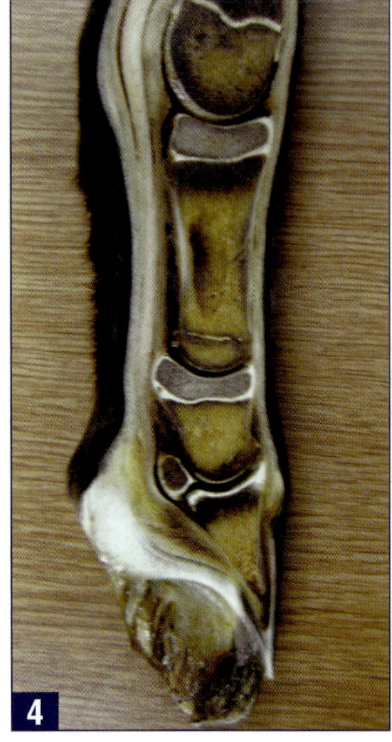

Sagittal section of a cadaver leg from a newborn foal.

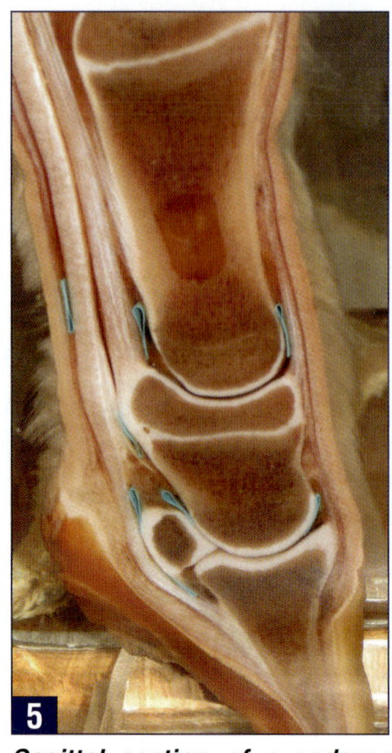

Sagittal section of a cadaver leg from a foal.

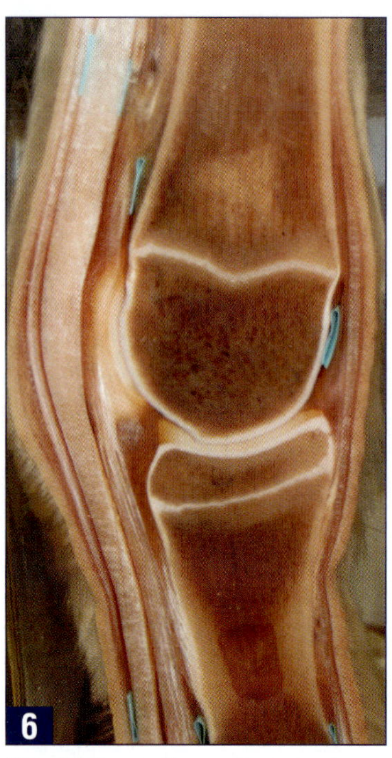

Sagittal section of a cadaver leg from a foal, fetlock joint.

Other bones, such as those in the skull, are formed through a process that is called intramembranous ossification. This process does not rely on the ossification centers like a long bone does, instead, it involves a matrix of connective tissue fibers. When the bones are completely formed, they do have similar composition, they are just created with a different process.

Bone constantly remodels to withstand the forces that are exerted upon it. Throughout the life of the horse, bone tissue is being broken down and replaced as the body thickens the area of the bone that is being worked the hardest. The practical application of this knowledge can prevent you from causing problems by radically trimming a horse that has a balance problem. Consider a 15-year old roping horse that has a toed-in stance that he has had his entire life. His foot conformation is high medial, low lateral, and the foot is situated to the inside of the bony column. The lateral side of the bones in the leg have taken the brunt of the workload, and the cortex of the lateral side is thick, while the medial cortex is comparably thinner. If you were to trim the foot to correct the stance, you might very well cause the medial side of the bones to fail from forces that they are not accustomed to.

Considering the way that individual bones are put together indicates how they are stressed in everyday life. With a composition of hard tissue like that in the compact bone, combined with cancellous bone found inside the medullary cavity, there is hardness mixed with tensile strength. Both properties are valuable when considering what a bone goes through, and together, they create a skeleton that is able to withstand the demands of being a horse.

APPENDICULAR SKELETON, (LIMBS)

The bones from the trunk to the ground are known as the limb, or appendicular skeleton. The limbs contain the leg and digit as well. The front limb **(Figure 7)** is known as the thoracic limb. The hind limb **(Figure 11)** is called the pelvic limb. You can see the scapula in **Figure 8**, the humerus in **Figure 9,** and the ulna and radius that are fused together in **Figure 10**. To help you remember these bones, think of the acronym SHUR. It stands for scapula, humerus, ulna, radius.

The pelvic limb, **(Figure 11)** is attached to the backbone by the sacroiliac joint, so the force of propulsion is directly transferred to the skeleton. You can see the pelvis in **Figure 12**, **Figures 13 -14**

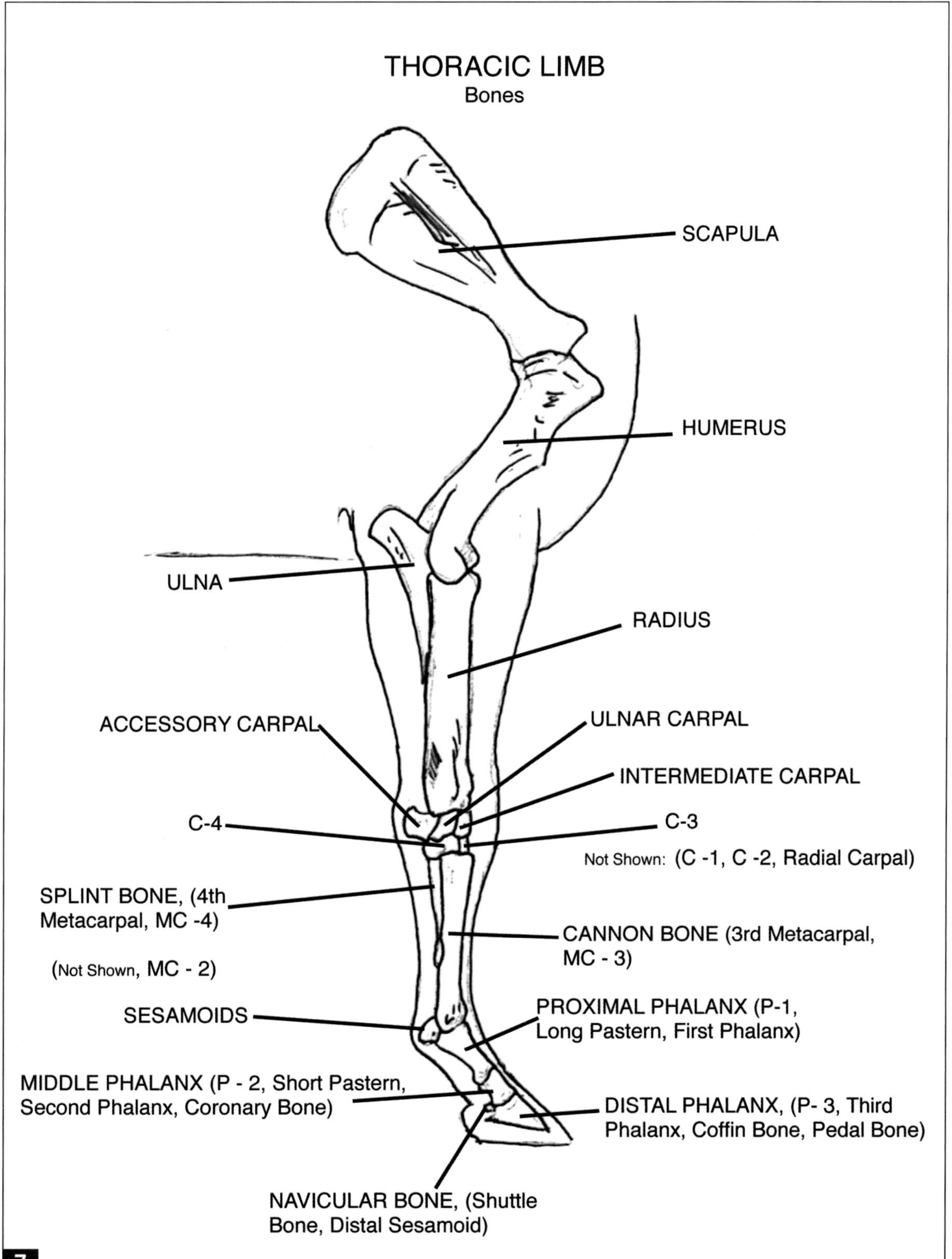

THORACIC LIMB
Bones

SCAPULA

HUMERUS

ULNA

RADIUS

ACCESSORY CARPAL

ULNAR CARPAL

INTERMEDIATE CARPAL

C-4

C-3

Not Shown: (C -1, C -2, Radial Carpal)

SPLINT BONE, (4th Metacarpal, MC -4)

(Not Shown, MC - 2)

CANNON BONE (3rd Metacarpal, MC - 3)

SESAMOIDS

PROXIMAL PHALANX (P-1, Long Pastern, First Phalanx)

MIDDLE PHALANX (P - 2, Short Pastern, Second Phalanx, Coronary Bone)

DISTAL PHALANX, (P- 3, Third Phalanx, Coffin Bone, Pedal Bone)

NAVICULAR BONE, (Shuttle Bone, Distal Sesamoid)

7

Drawing of the thoracic limb.

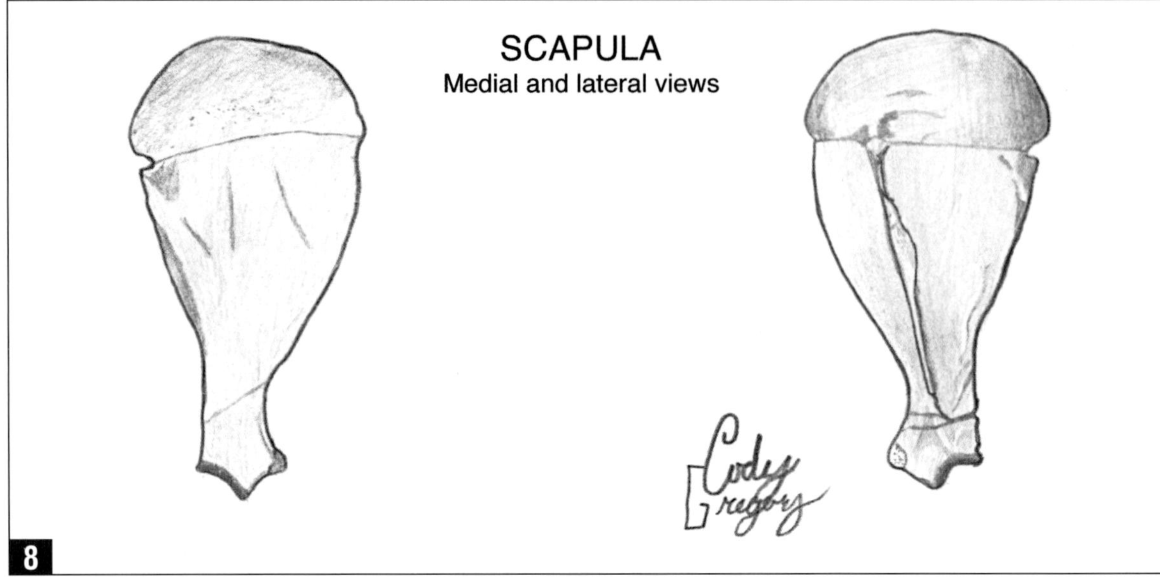

Scapula.

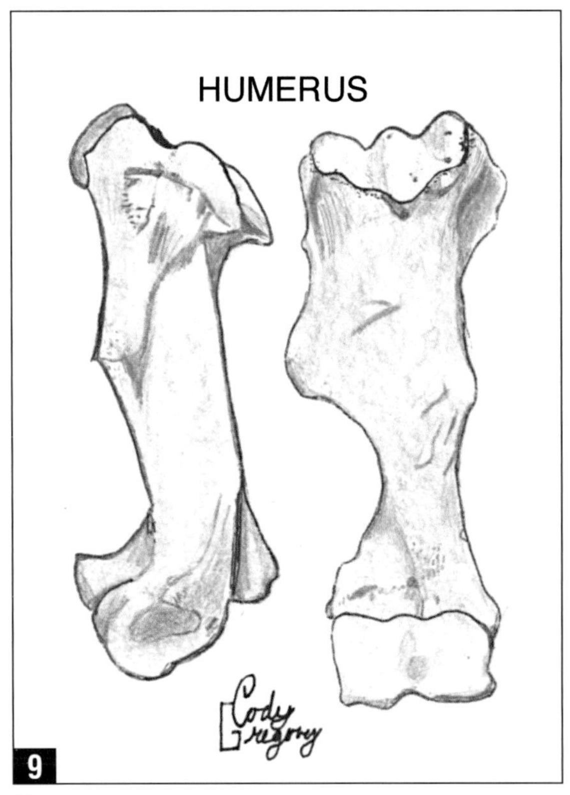

Humerus.

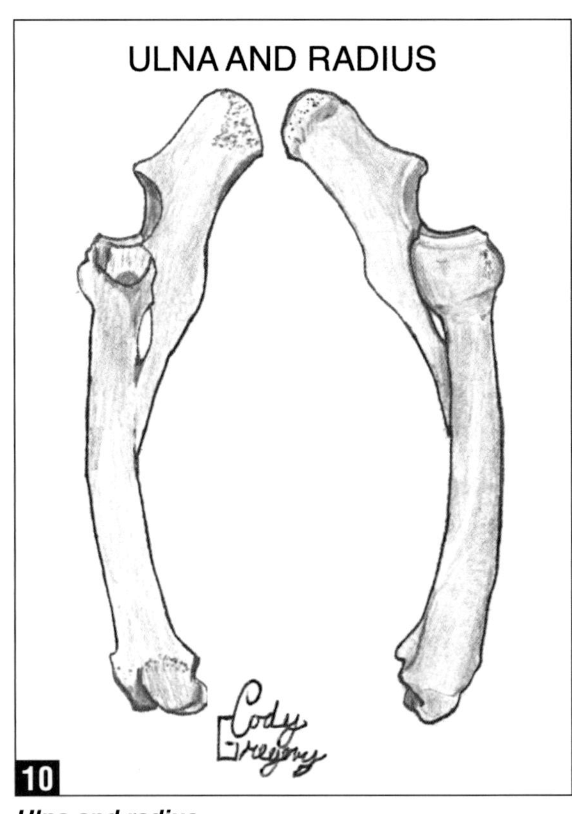

Ulna and radius.

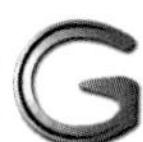

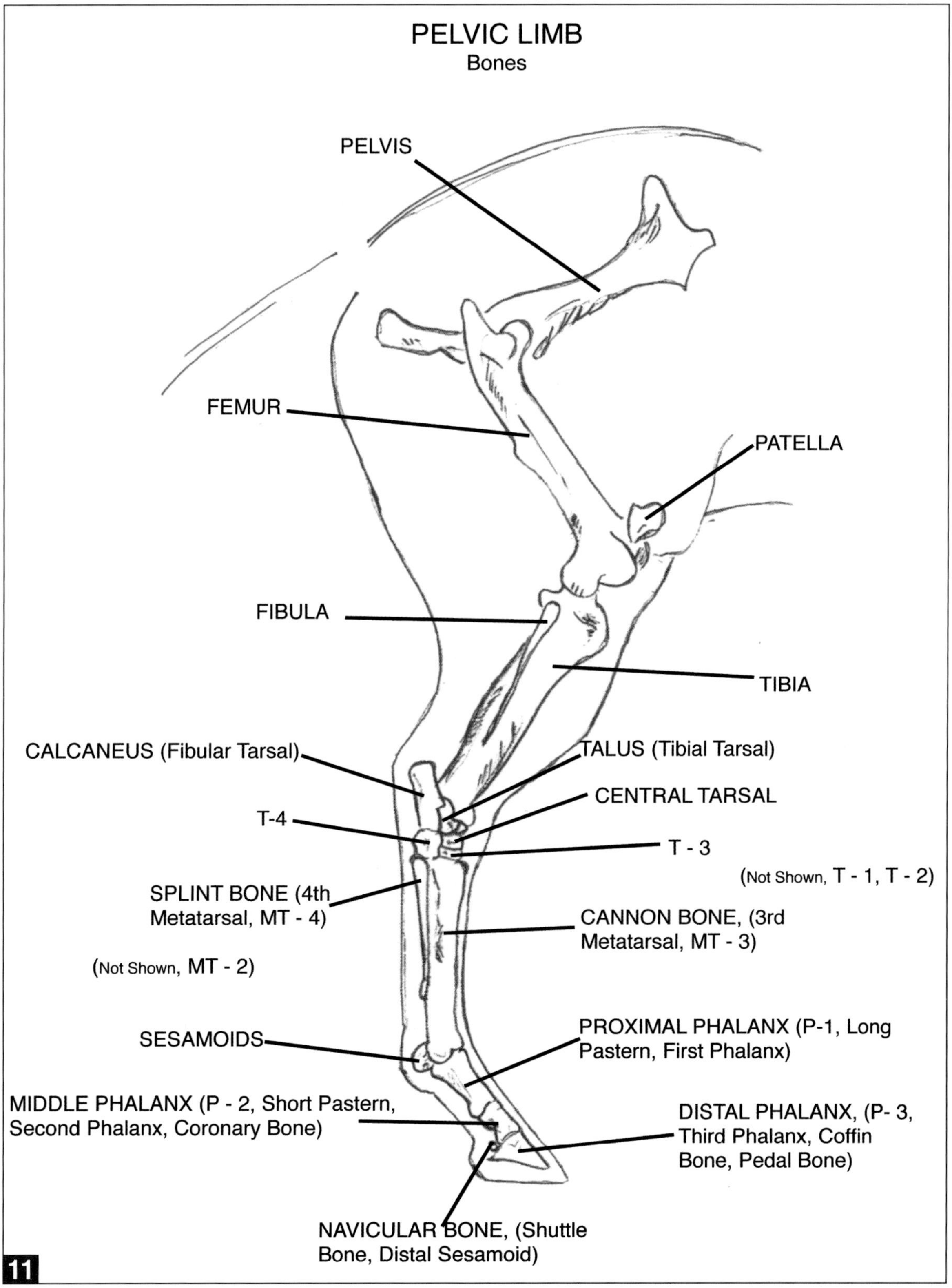

PELVIC LIMB

Bones

PELVIS

FEMUR

PATELLA

FIBULA

TIBIA

CALCANEUS (Fibular Tarsal)

TALUS (Tibial Tarsal)

CENTRAL TARSAL

T-4

T - 3

(Not Shown, T - 1, T - 2)

SPLINT BONE (4th Metatarsal, MT - 4)

CANNON BONE, (3rd Metatarsal, MT - 3)

(Not Shown, MT - 2)

SESAMOIDS

PROXIMAL PHALANX (P-1, Long Pastern, First Phalanx)

MIDDLE PHALANX (P - 2, Short Pastern, Second Phalanx, Coronary Bone)

DISTAL PHALANX, (P- 3, Third Phalanx, Coffin Bone, Pedal Bone)

NAVICULAR BONE, (Shuttle Bone, Distal Sesamoid)

11

Drawing of the pelvic limb.

PELVIS

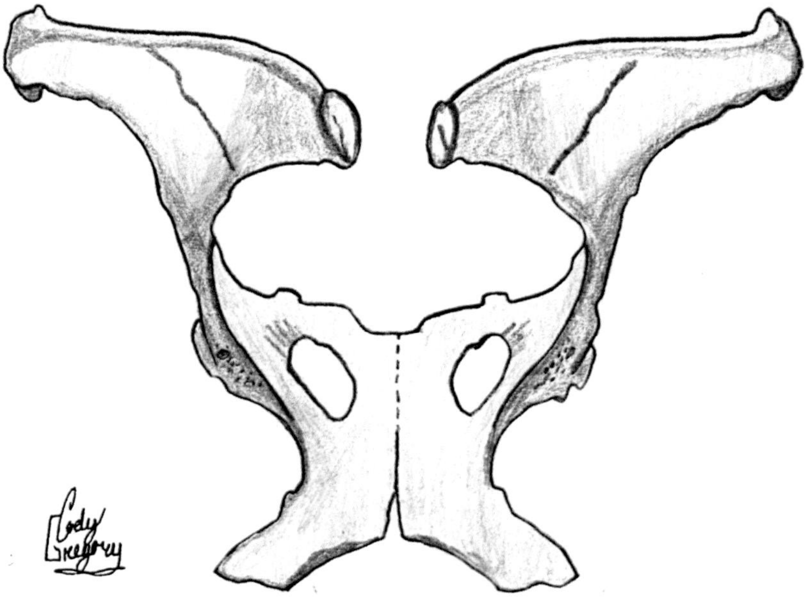

Cody Gregory

12

Pelvis.

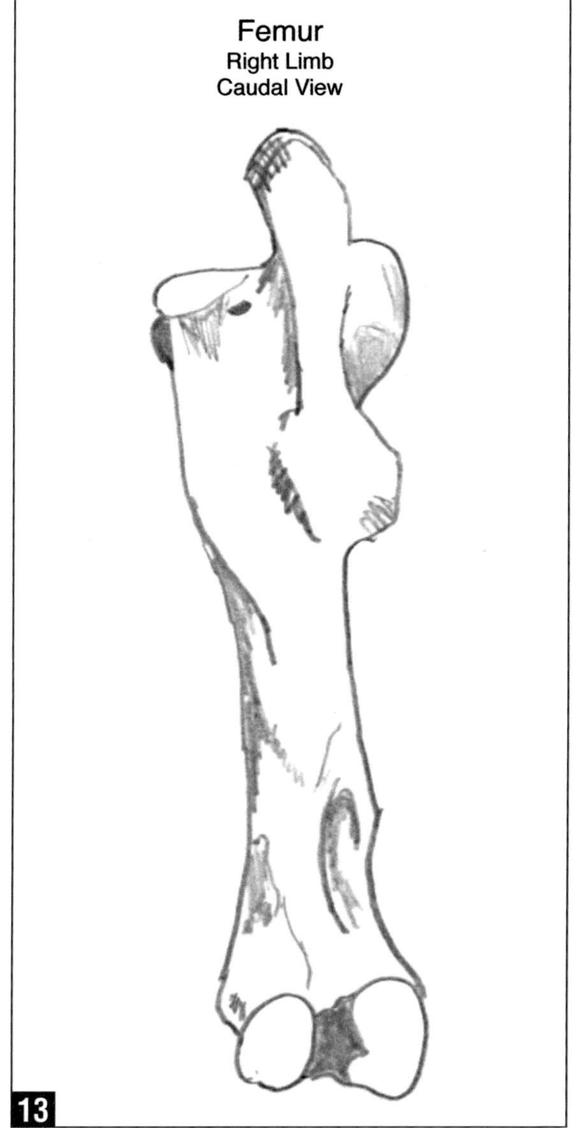

Femur.

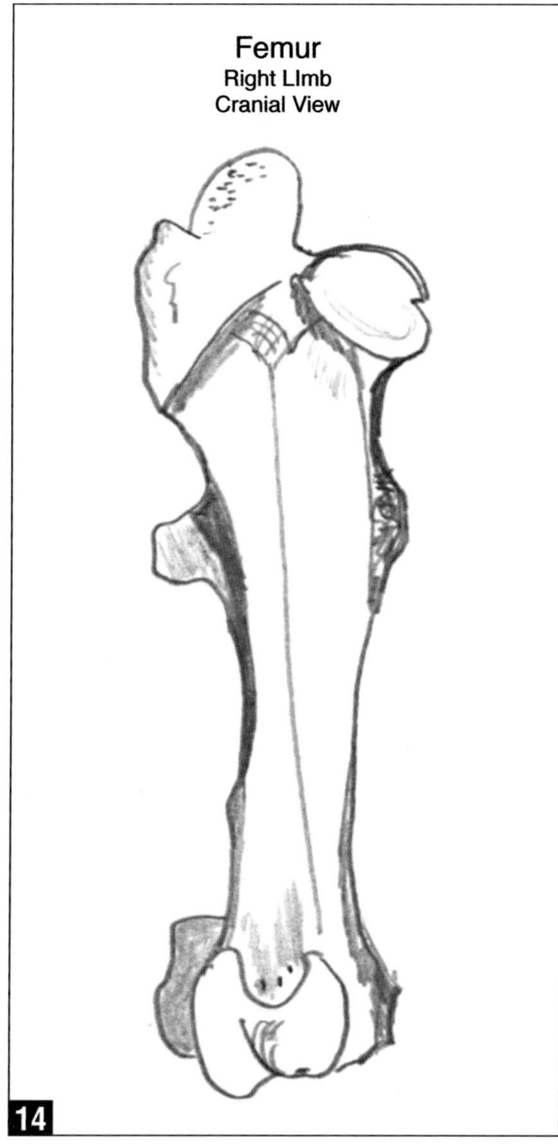

Femur.

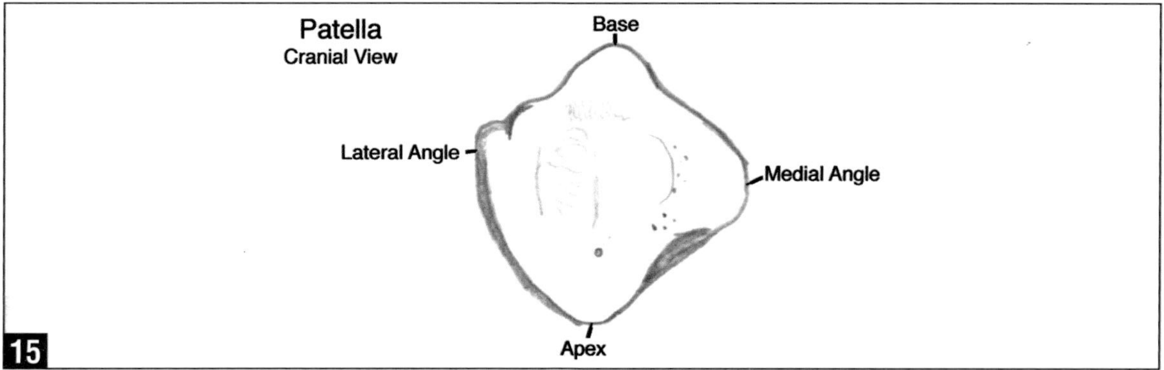

Patella.

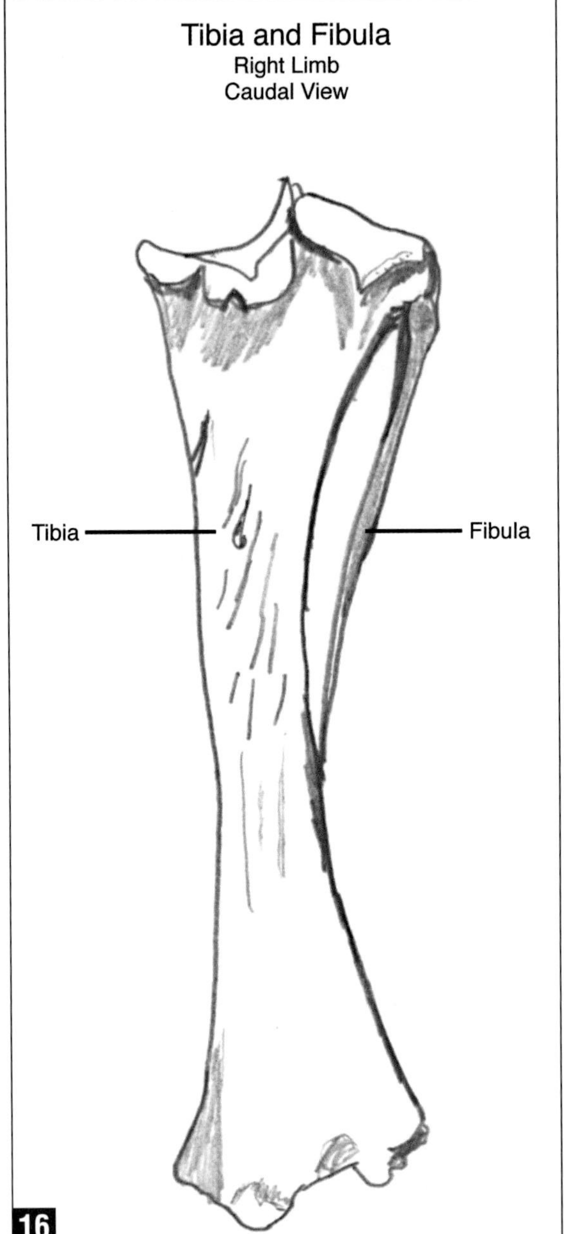

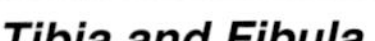
Tibia and Fibula.

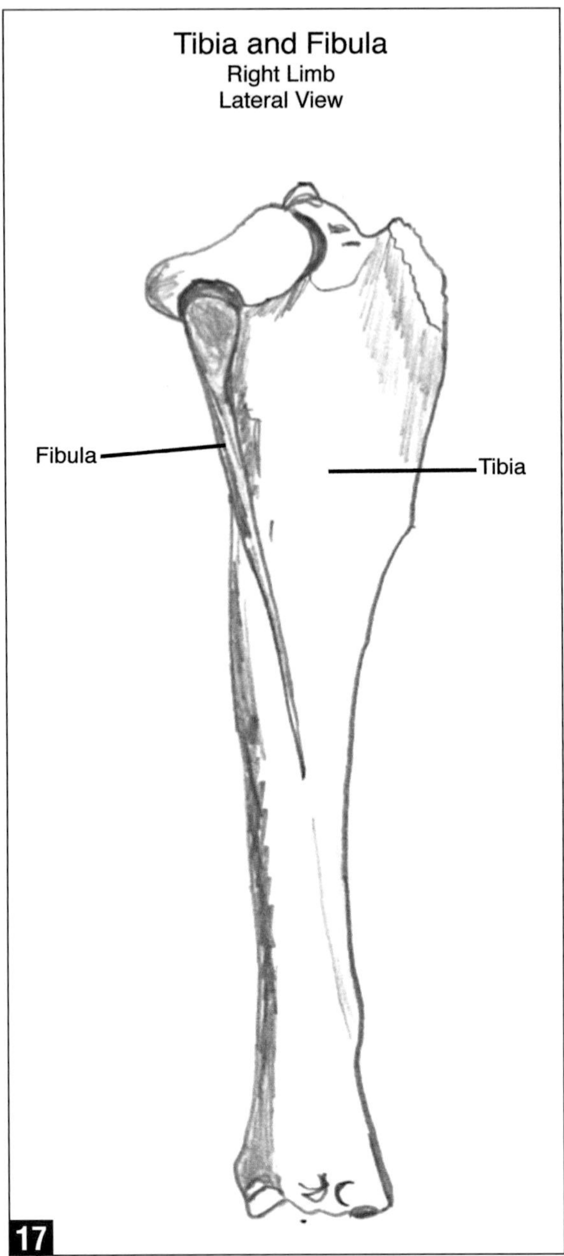

Tibia and Fibula.

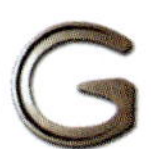

are drawings of the femur, **Figure 15** is the patella, and **Figures 16 - 17** are of the tibia and fibula. The first letters of each bone would be PFPFT, which unfortunately does not make a word. In the horse, both the ulna in the front limb, and the fibula in the hind limb, are small enough that they do not go all the way to the carpus or tarsus as they do in humans. This is one of the reasons that the horse does not have the flexibility in the carpus or tarsus that we do.

The thoracic limb is attached to the trunk by muscle, tendon, ligament, and fascia but does not have a joint in the normal sense of the word. The hind limb is attached to the pelvis by the hip joint, and the pelvis is attached to the spine through the sacroiliac joint, so there are joints in the attachments of the hind limb to the body.

It is great for a farrier to know all of the musculature, ligaments and tendons in the upper limb, but it is not an absolute necessity. For my students, they must learn the bones as seen in **Figures 7 - 11**, be able to draw them all at the right angles, and know where the muscles of the extensor and flexor tendons originate. The rest of the muscle and connective tissue is beyond the scope of this book.

LEG

The leg of the equine officially begins at the distal end of the radius in the thoracic limb, and the distal end of the tibia in the pelvic limb. This means that the carpus and tarsus are included in the leg.

CARPUS (Figures 18-23)

The drawings here are of the left carpus. **Figure 18** is a lateral view, **Figure 19** is the medial view, **Figure 20** is the dorsal view, and **Figure 21** is the palmar view. Additionally, **Figure 22** is a drawing of the proximal aspects of the proximal row of carpal bones, and **Figure 23** is the proximal aspect of the distal row.

The carpus is the anatomical equivalent to the human wrist, even though it is called the knee in a

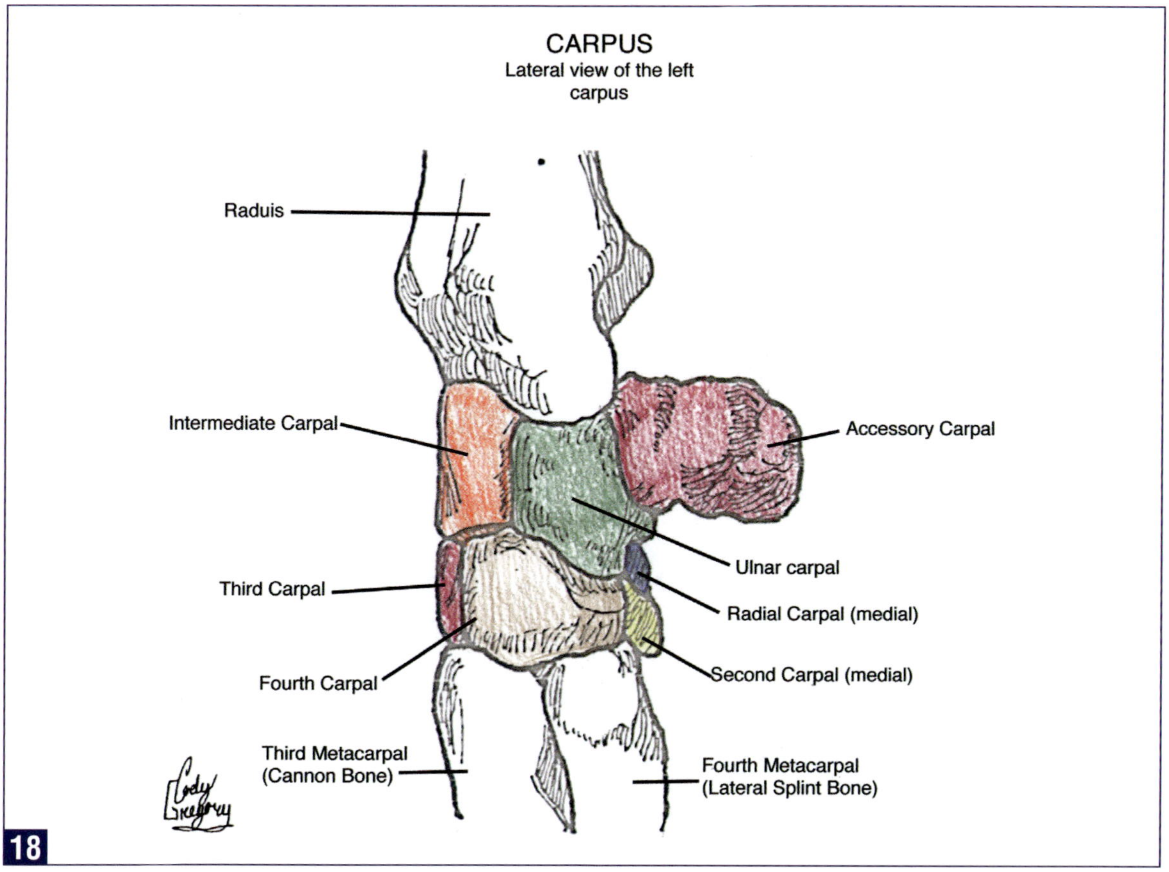

CARPUS
Lateral view of the left carpus

Raduis
Intermediate Carpal
Accessory Carpal
Ulnar carpal
Third Carpal
Radial Carpal (medial)
Fourth Carpal
Second Carpal (medial)
Third Metacarpal (Cannon Bone)
Fourth Metacarpal (Lateral Splint Bone)

18

Lateral view of the left carpus.

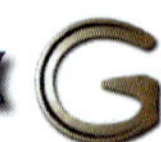

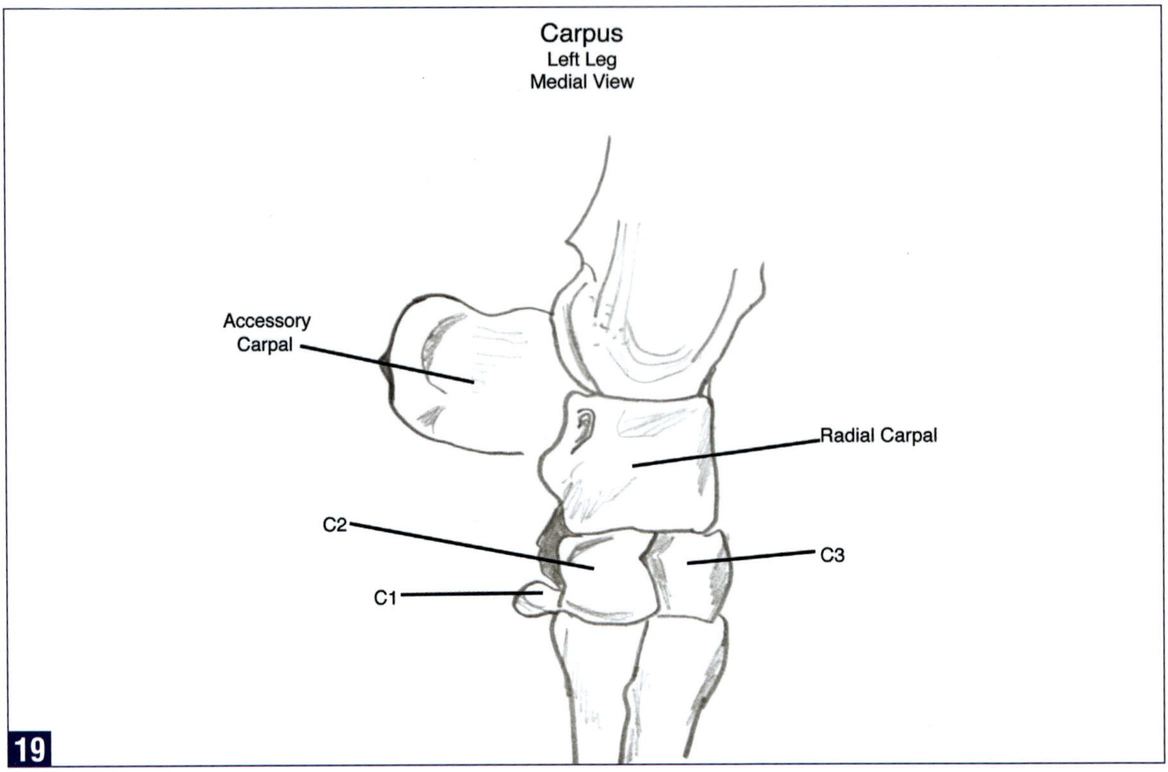

Carpus
Left Leg
Medial View

Accessory Carpal
Radial Carpal
C2
C3
C1

19

Medial View of the left carpus.

CARPUS
Dorsal View of the left Carpus

Radius
Intermediate Carpal
Radial Carpal
Ulnar Carpal
Fourth Carpal
Third Carpal
Fourth Metacarpal (Lateral Splint Bone)
Second Metarcarpal (Medial Splint Bone)
Third Metacarpal (Cannon Bone)

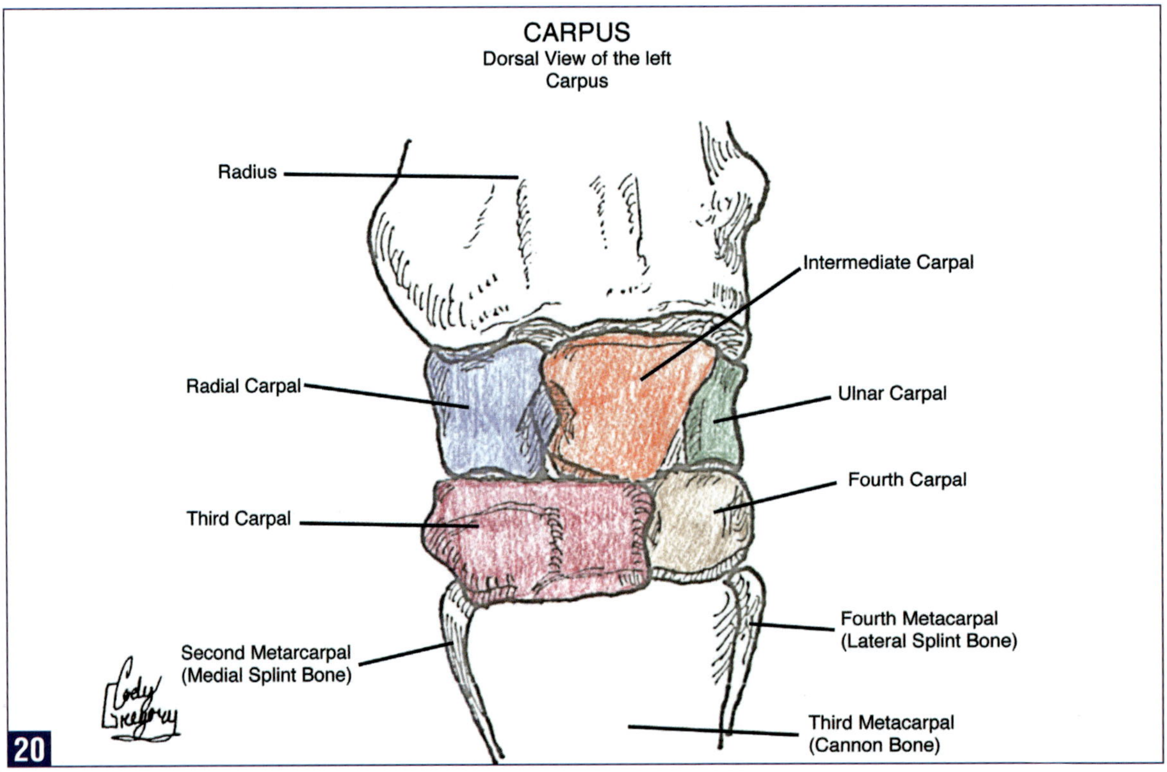

20

Dorsal view of the left carpus.

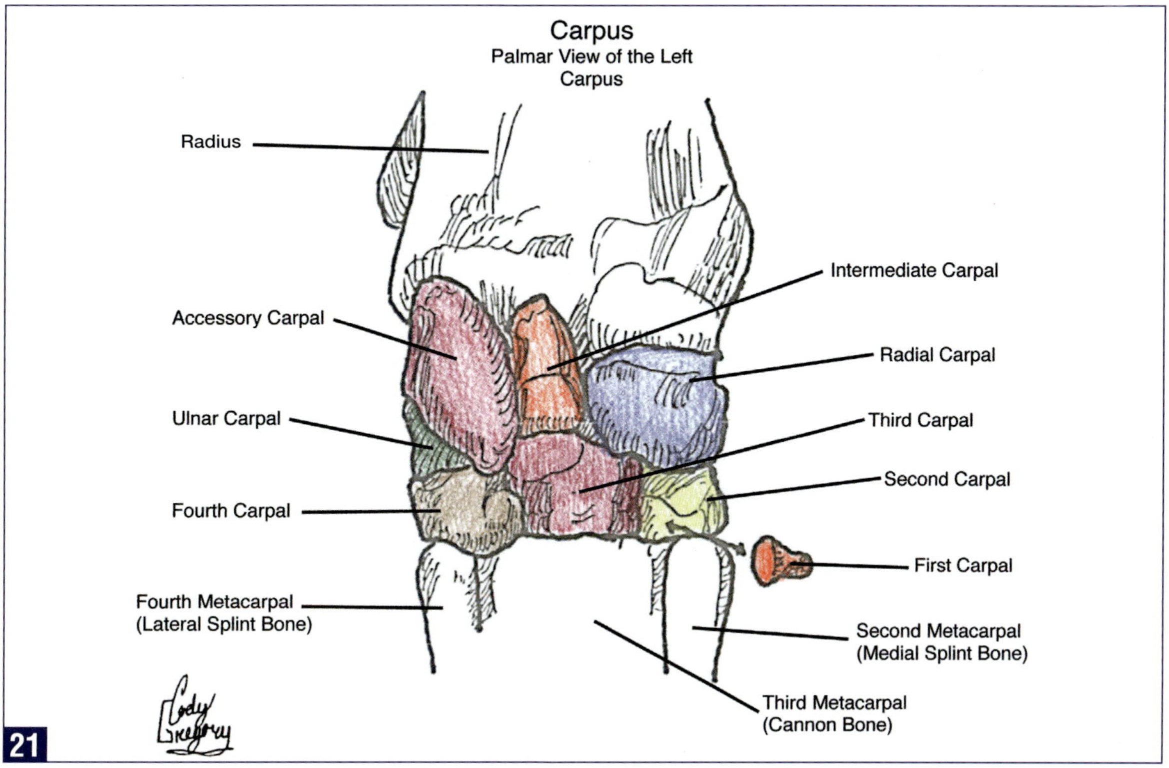

Carpus
Palmar View of the Left
Carpus

Radius
Accessory Carpal
Ulnar Carpal
Fourth Carpal
Fourth Metacarpal
(Lateral Splint Bone)
Intermediate Carpal
Radial Carpal
Third Carpal
Second Carpal
First Carpal
Second Metacarpal
(Medial Splint Bone)
Third Metacarpal
(Cannon Bone)

21

Palmar view of the left carpus.

Carpus
Left Leg
Proximal Row of Carpal Bones
Proximal View

Intermediate Carpal
Radial Carpal
Ulnar Carpal
Intercarpal Joints
Accessory Carpal

22

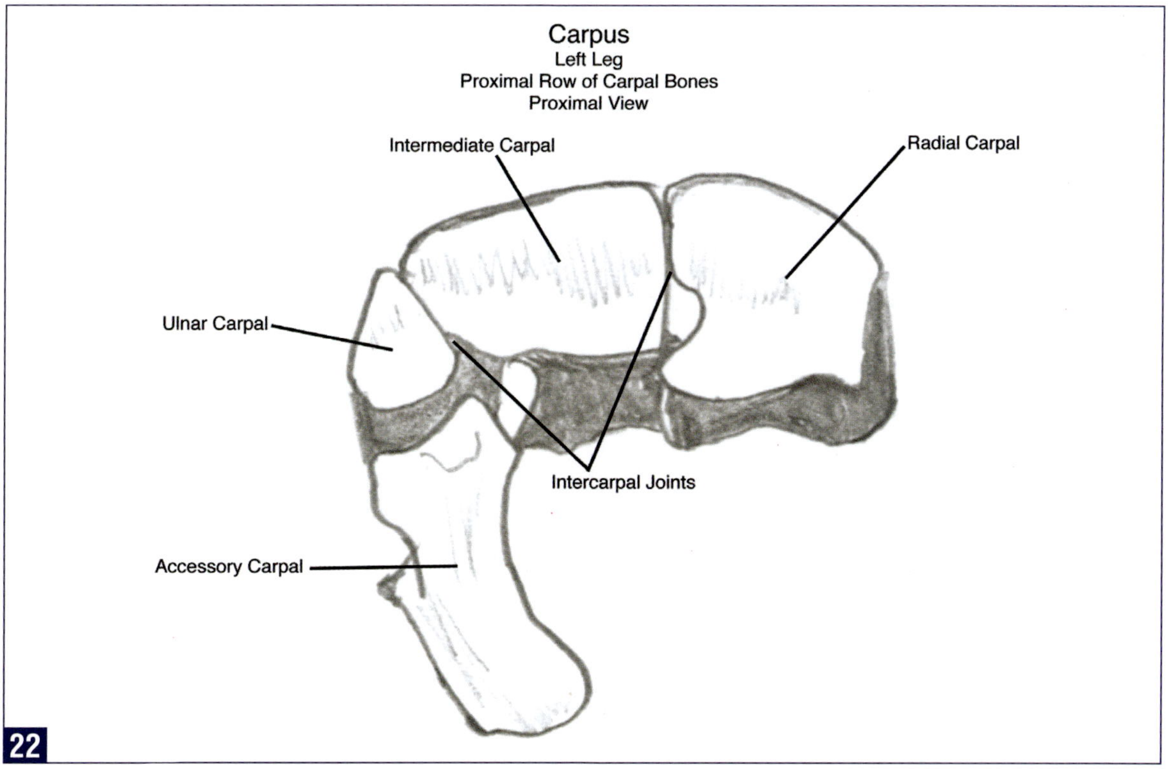

Proximal view, proximal row of carpal bones.

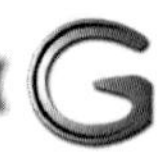

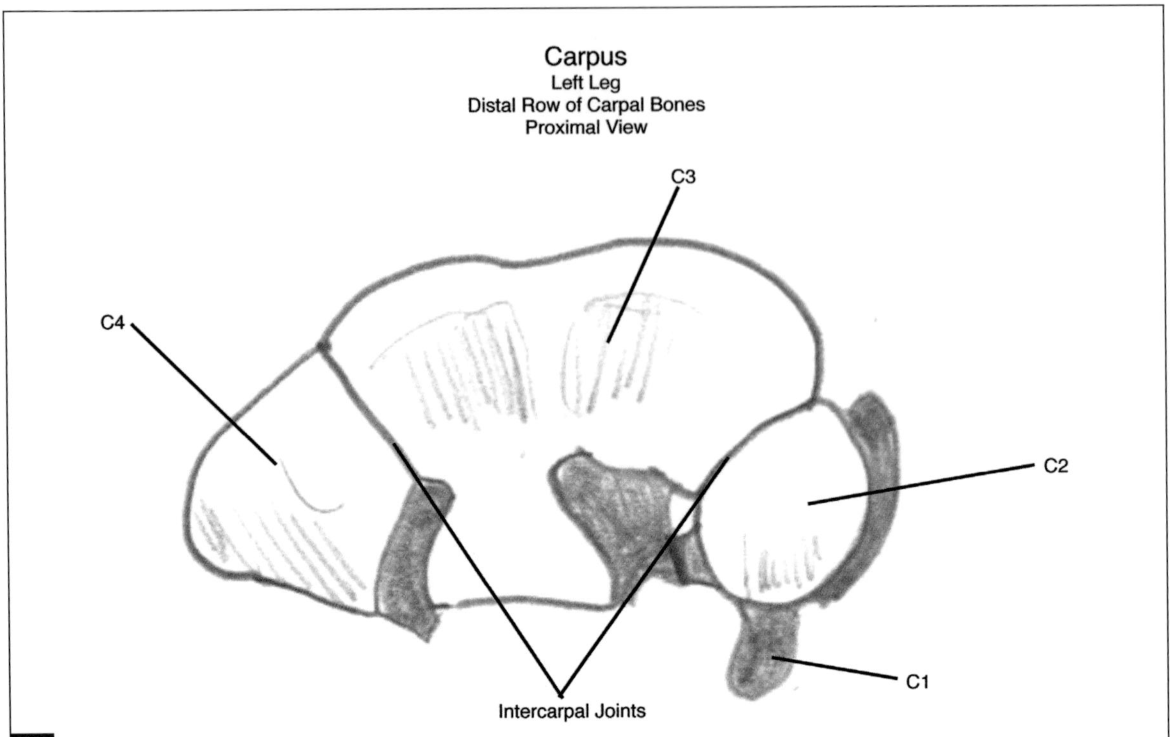

Carpus
Left Leg
Distal Row of Carpal Bones
Proximal View

C3
C4
C2
C1
Intercarpal Joints

23

Proximal view, distal row of carpal bones.

horse. It is composed of 7 more or less cube-shaped bones. In some instances there is an additional carpal bone, known as C1. If present, C1 is about the size of a pencil eraser and is located on the distal medial aspect of the carpus, detailed in **Figures 19-21, and 23**.

The bones of the carpus are arranged in two rows. The proximal row contains four bones that are named. The bottom row generally has three bones that are numbered, and occasionally has four bones. From a skyline view, the proximal row, from medial to lateral contain; the radial carpal, intermediate carpal, ulnar carpal, and accessory carpal. The accessory carpal is located lateral palmar and does not bear as much weight as the other carpal bones since it is located behind the knee. It does provide for the attachment of the flexor carpi ulnaris and ulnaris lateralis tendons, and it is considered to be a sesamoid bone.

The distal row of carpals contains three bones

most of the time, and occasionally an additional vestigial bone. From a skyline view, moving medial to lateral, there is C2 (distal to the radial carpal), C3 (distal to the intermediate carpal), and C4 (distal to the ulnar carpal).

TARSUS
(Figures 24-27)

The drawings of the tarsus are from the right leg. **Figure 24** is the lateral view, **Figure 25** is the medial view, **Figure 26** is a dorsal view, and **Figure 27** is a plantar view.

The tarsus is the anatomical equivalent to the human ankle and is commonly referred to as the hock. There are seven bones of various shapes in the hock, although T1 and T2 fuse together, making only six pieces when dissecting the tarsus.

Three of the bones in the tarsus are named, while four are numbered. Proximal plantar is the calcaneus, (fibular tarsal). This is the largest bone in the hock, and provides for the proximal attachment of the superficial flexor tendon. Dorsal medial to the calcaneus is the talus (tibial tarsal). Immediately distal to the talus and calcaneus is the central tarsal bone. This is a disc-shaped bone. Lateral to the central tarsal and T3, and distal to the calcaneus,

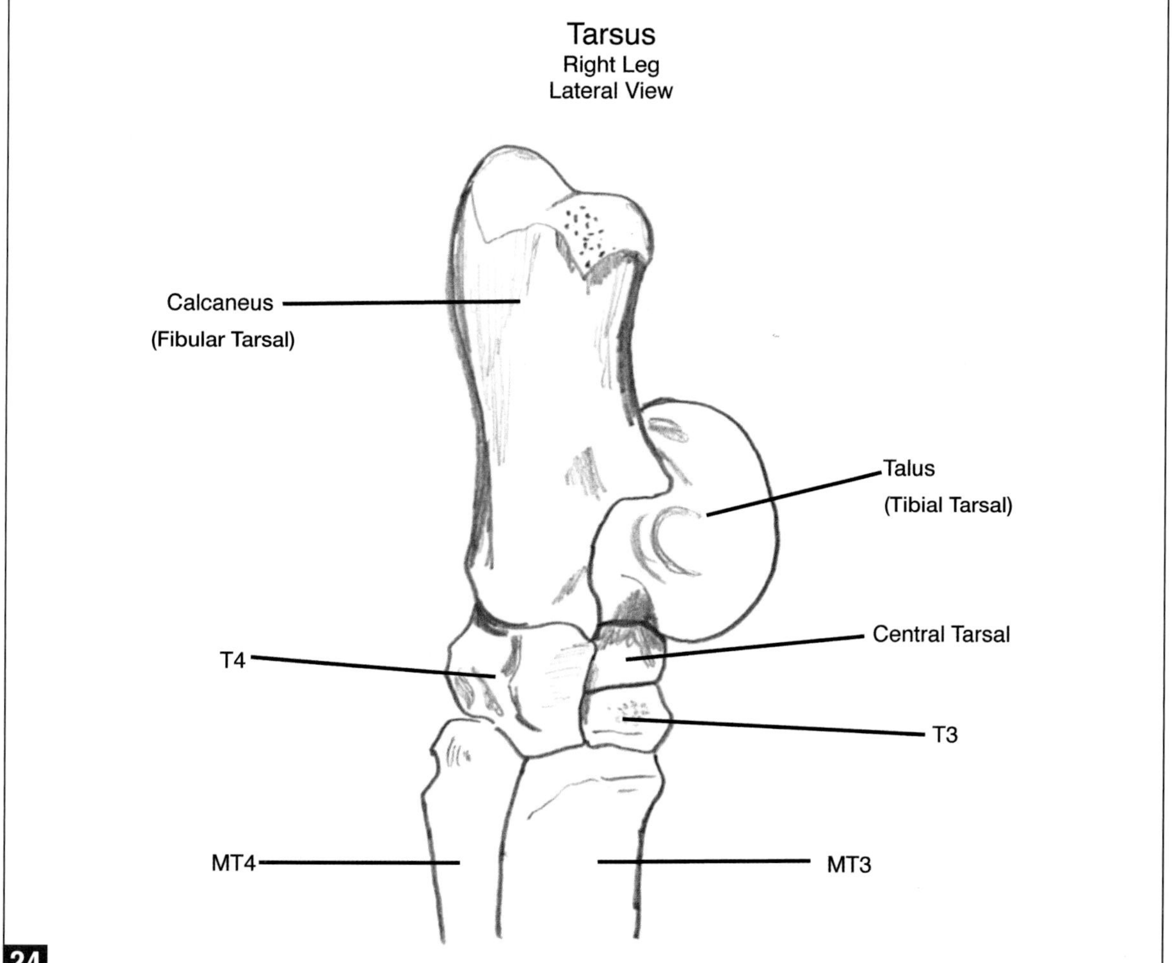

Tarsus
Right Leg
Lateral View

Calcaneus
(Fibular Tarsal)
Talus
(Tibial Tarsal)
Central Tarsal
T4
T3
MT4
MT3

24

Lateral view of right tarsus.

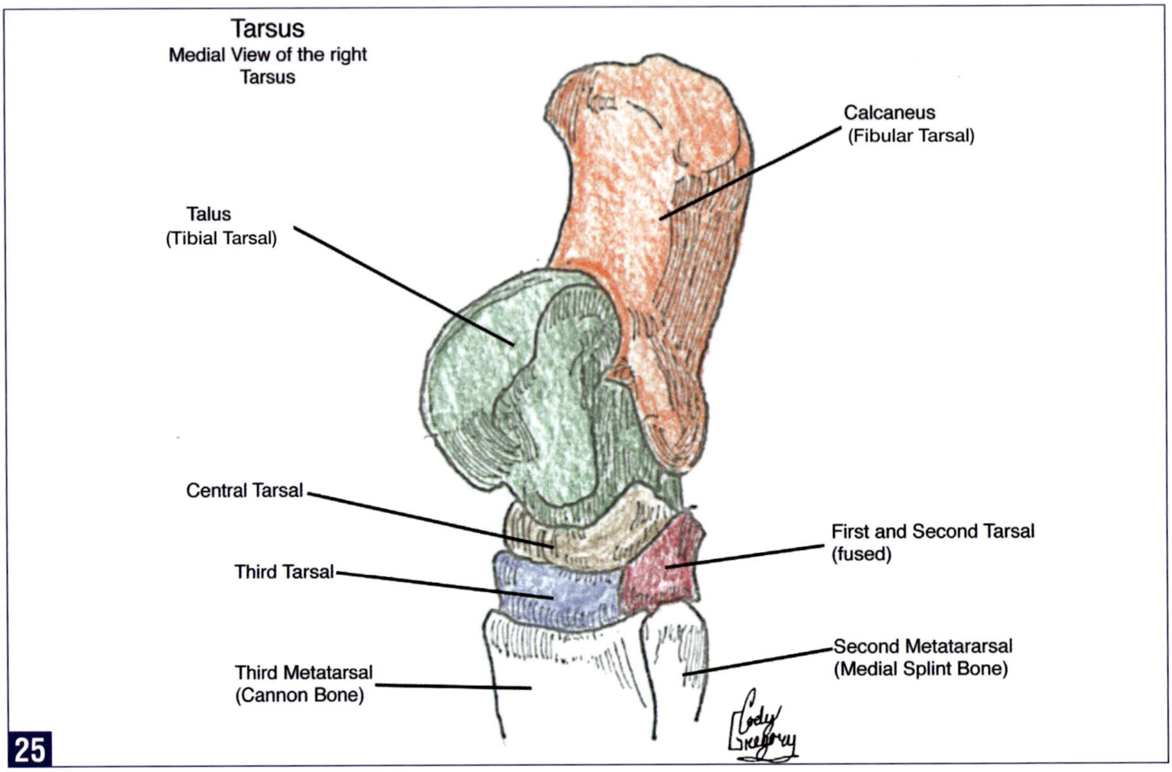

Tarsus
Medial View of the right
Tarsus

Calcaneus
(Fibular Tarsal)

Talus
(Tibial Tarsal)

Central Tarsal

First and Second Tarsal
(fused)

Third Tarsal

Second Metatararsal
(Medial Splint Bone)

Third Metatarsal
(Cannon Bone)

Cody Gregory

25

Medial view of the right tarsus.

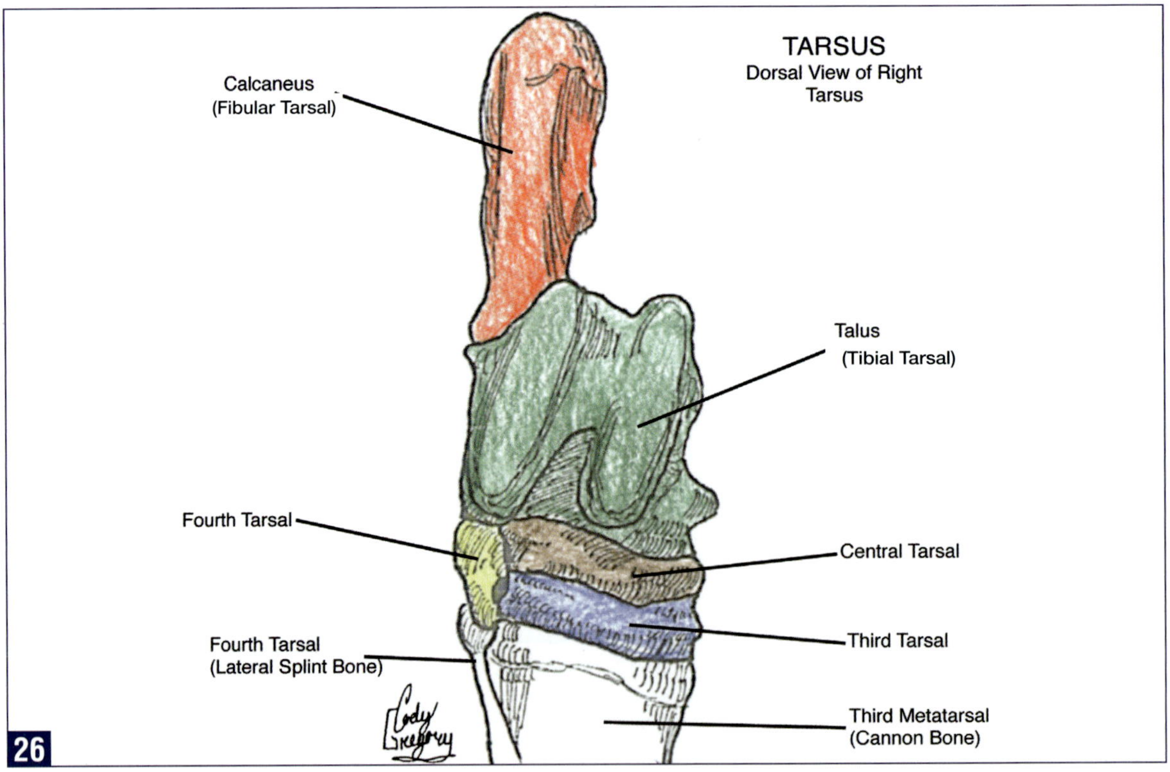

TARSUS
Dorsal View of Right
Tarsus

Calcaneus
(Fibular Tarsal)

Talus
(Tibial Tarsal)

Fourth Tarsal

Central Tarsal

Third Tarsal

Fourth Tarsal
(Lateral Splint Bone)

Third Metatarsal
(Cannon Bone)

Cody Gregory

26

Dorsal view of right tarsus.

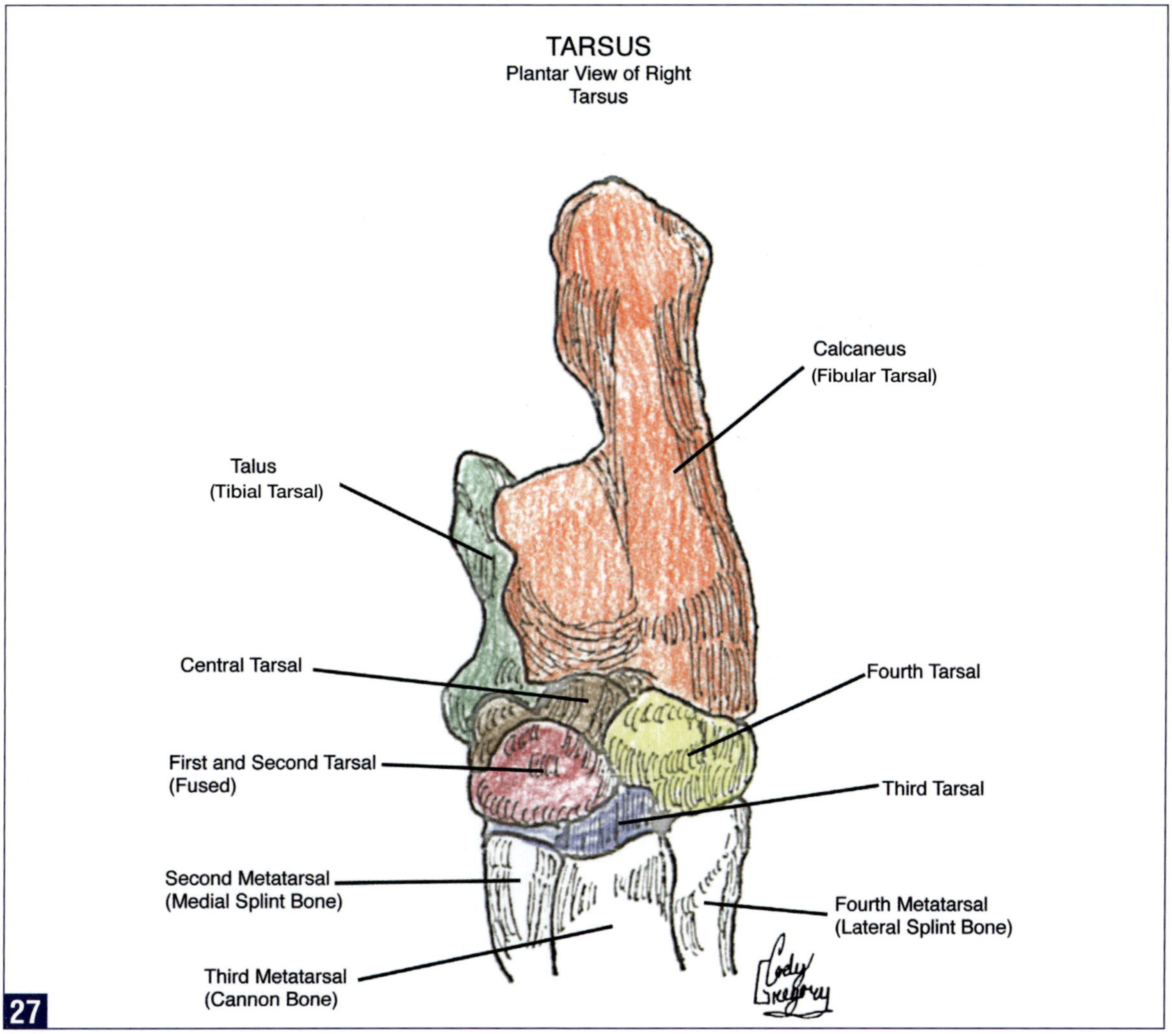

TARSUS
Plantar View of Right
Tarsus

Calcaneus
(Fibular Tarsal)

Talus
(Tibial Tarsal)

Central Tarsal

Fourth Tarsal

First and Second Tarsal
(Fused)

Third Tarsal

Second Metatarsal
(Medial Splint Bone)

Fourth Metatarsal
(Lateral Splint Bone)

Third Metatarsal
(Cannon Bone)

27

Plantar view of the right tarsus.

is T4. Distal to the central tarsal is the disc-shaped T3, and T1 –T2 is located distally to the central tarsal,and medial/plantar to T3. I know all of this description is confusing, so take some time to carefully study it while looking at the diagrams.

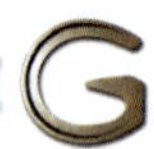

SPLINT BONES (Figures 28-29)

The splint bones in the front leg are known as the second and fourth metacarpals, and in the hind leg, as the second and fourth metatarsals. They join the cannon bone by the attachment of ligaments known as interosseus ligaments, **(Figure 28)**, which I compare to Velcro. This ligamentous attachment allows the cannon and splint bones to grow independently of each other, as well as provide some concussion absorption. If you look carefully at the splint bone on the right side of **Figure 29**, you can see that it has a bone growth, (osteophyte) on it.

Common teaching indicates that the interosseus ligaments ossify when the horse has reached physical maturity around the age of 6. At this point, they should be solidly attached to the cannon bone. However, through the experience of many dissections, I find this to be false. The interosseus ligaments seem to ossify less often on the front legs than the hinds, and I have dissected the limbs of a 36-year-old horse that did not have any of the splints attached solidly to the cannon bones. I think it is normal for the splint bones to become attached to the cannon bone through the ossification of the interosseus ligaments, but it is also normal for it not to happen.

Proximally, the second metacarpal articulates with the second and third carpal bones, so there are 2 facets on the articular surface. The fourth metacarpal articulates with the fourth carpal, so there is only one facet on that bone, making it easy to determine medial from lateral splint bones. On the pelvic limb, the fourth metatarsal is the largest of all the splint bones. It articulates with T4 proximal to it. The second metatarsal articulates with T1 and T2 above it, which are fused together.

When anatomy is numbered in the limb, the smaller numbers are generally medial and the larger numbers are lateral. Thus, MC2 is the medial splint

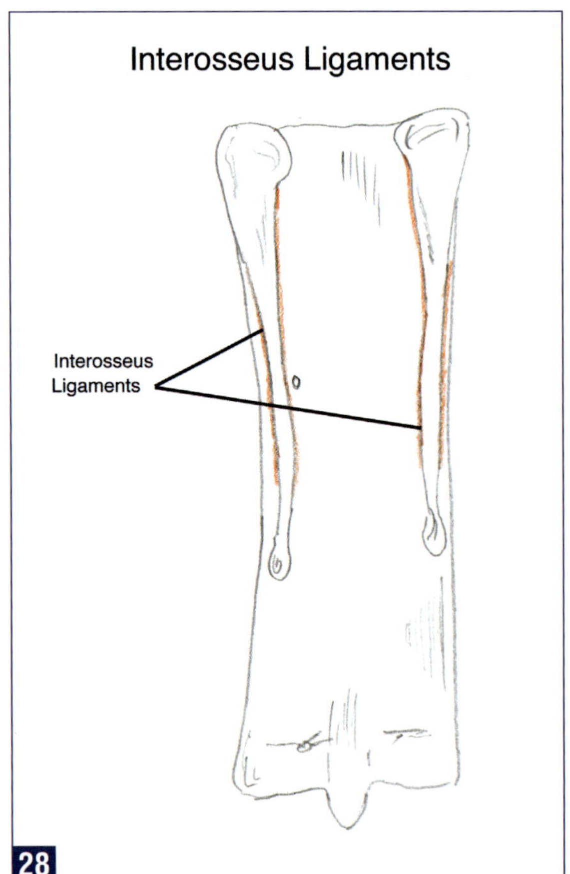

The cannon bone with the splint bones and interosseus ligaments.

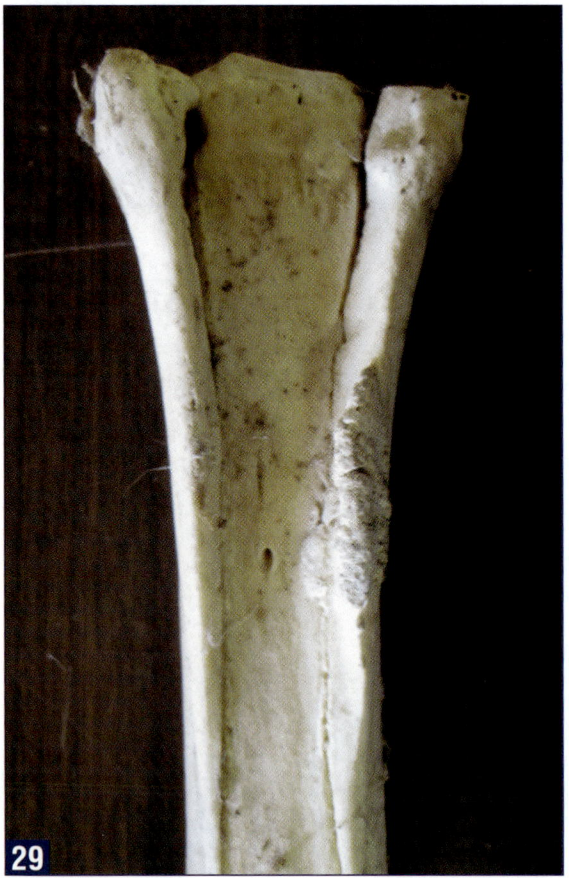

Cannon and splint bones.

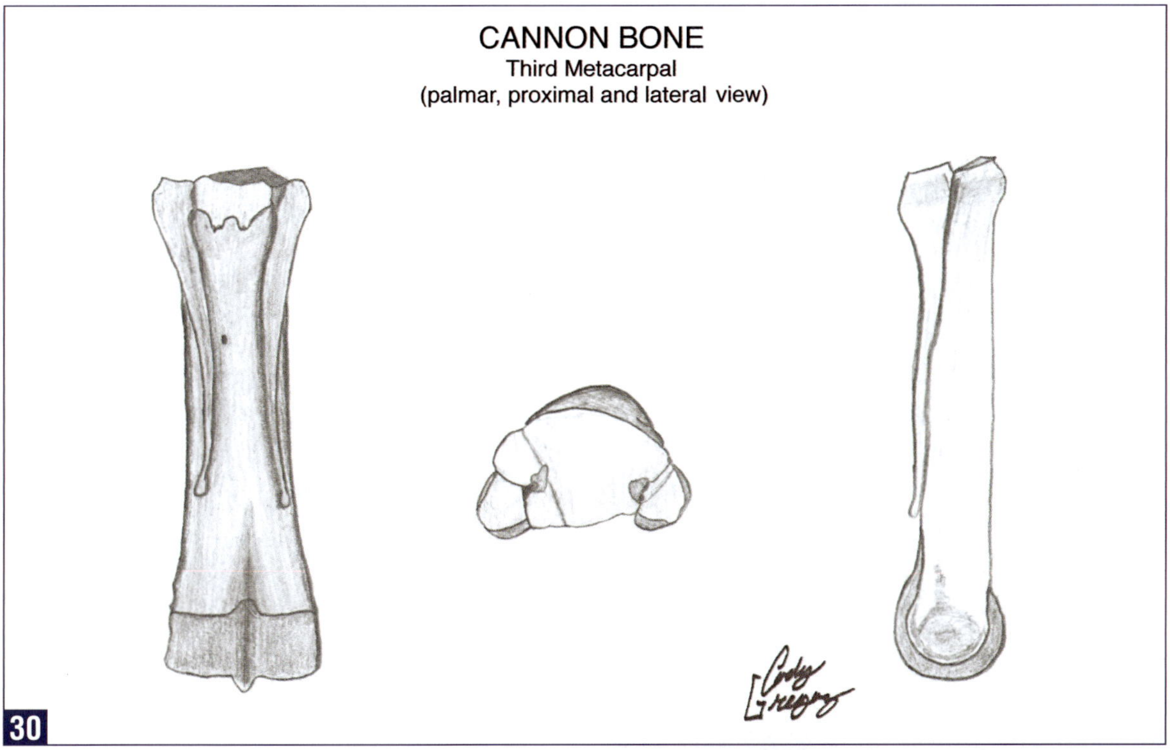

CANNON BONE
Third Metacarpal
(palmar, proximal and lateral view)

30

Front cannon bone.

bone, and MC4 is the lateral one.

CANNON BONE (Figures 30-34)

The cannon bone (**Figure 30**) is also known as the third metacarpal in the front leg and the third metatarsal in the hind leg. It is the longest bone in the leg, remembering that the leg begins at distal radius and distal tibia. **Figure 31** is of a front cannon bone lying next to the hind cannon bone from the same sized horses. You can easily see the length difference.

On the front leg, the cannon bone has a transverse section that is similar in shape to a front foot. The hind cannon bone will have a shap similar to that of a hind foot. You can see this in the cut cross section of the cannon bones in **Figure 32**. Looking at **Figure 33**, you can see the proximal end of the cannon bone really reflects the shape of the foot. The front cannon bone is also about 15% shorter on average than the hind cannon bone on the same horse. The hind leg is more involved with leverage, while the front is more involved with steering and weight support.

There is a sagittal ridge at the distal end of the

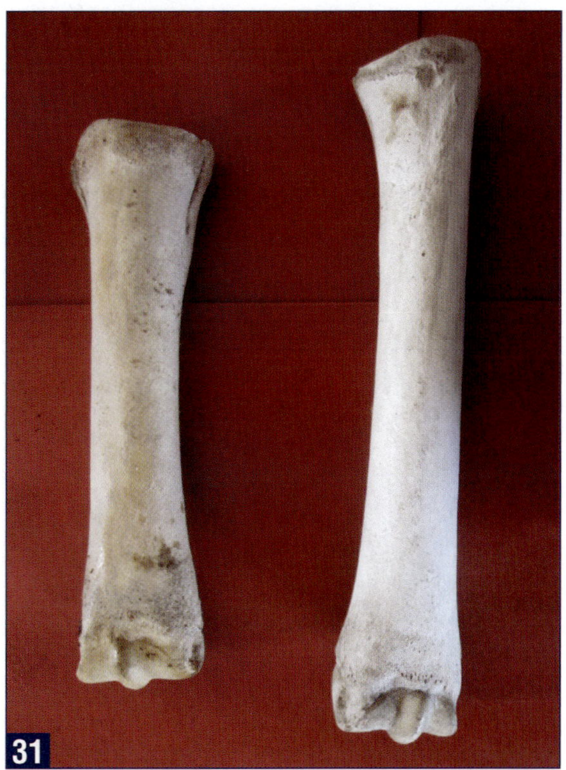

31

Front cannon bone on the left, and a hind cannon bone on the right from the similar size horses.

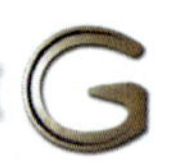

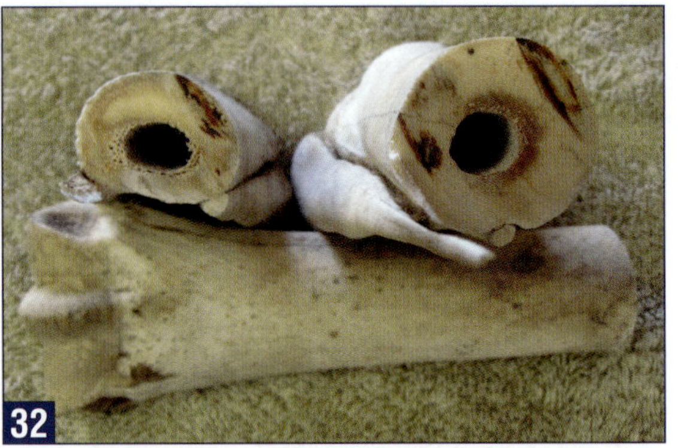

32

Transverse section of the cannon bones. Front on the left side, hind on the right.

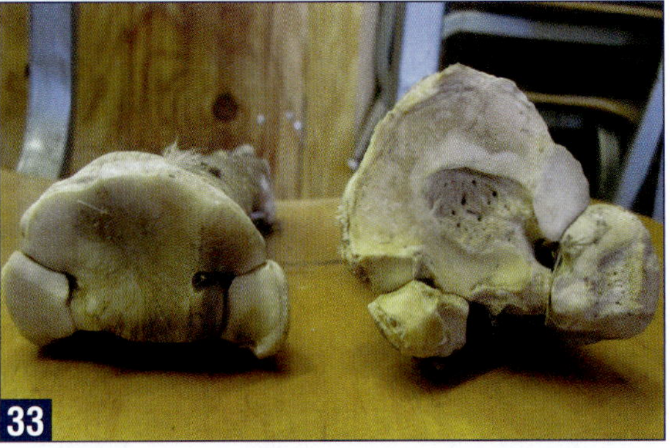

33

Proximal aspect of the cannon bones. Front on left, hind on right.

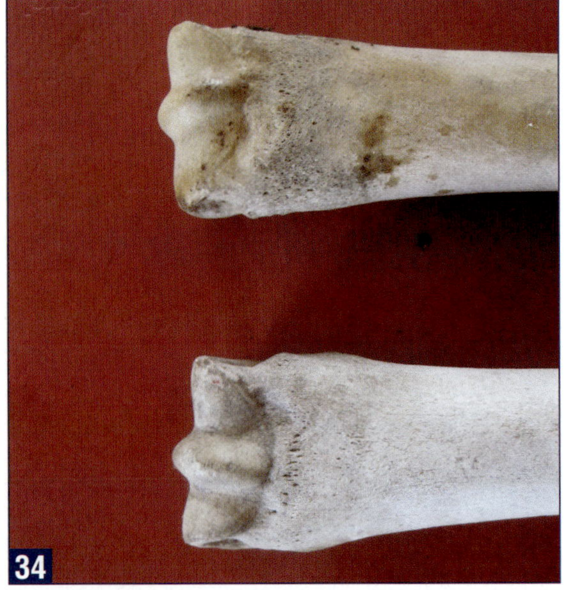

34

Distal sagittal ridges on the cannon bones.

cannon bone **(Figure 34)** that matches a groove in proximal P1 to make the fetlock joint. Proximally, the cannon bone on the front leg interacts with the second, third, and fourth carpal bones to make up the distal portion of the carpometacarpal joint. On the hind leg, the proximal third metatarsal articulates with the first, second, third, and fourth tarsals.

SESAMOIDS (Figures 35-37)

The sesamoid bones are pyramidal in shape with rounded edges instead of sharp ones. In **Figure 35,** you can see the palmar aspect of the sesamoid bones, and **Figure 36** shows the dorsal aspect, which is almost entirely covered with articular cartilage where the sesamoids contact the cannon bone.

There are two sesamoid bones located palmar/plantar to the fetlock joint. From a lateral view, they will be positioned just proximal to the palmar/plantar proximal edge of P1, articulating in the fetlock joint with the distal palmar/plantar aspect of the cannon bone **(figure 37).**

The function of the sesamoid bones is to change the direction of pull exerted on the bones when the muscles pull on the tendons. Since the tendons

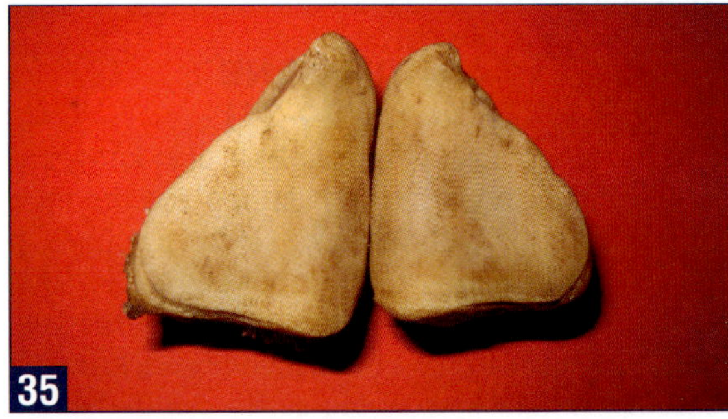

35

Dorsal view of sesamoid bones.

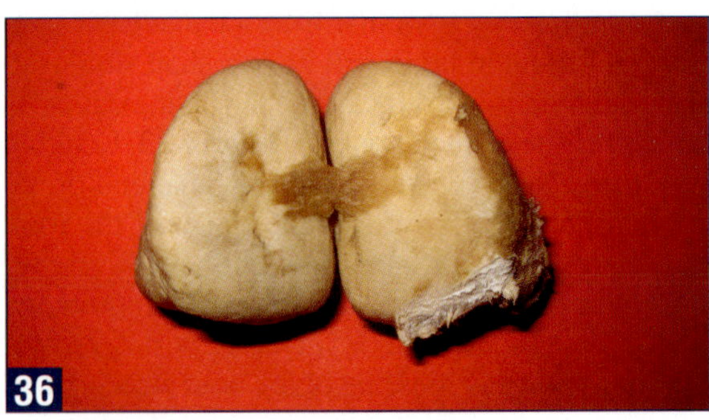

36

Palmar view of sesamoid bones

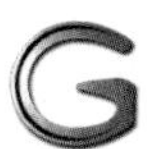

pass over the sesamoids, the direction that force is exerted on the bones is such that the foot and digit are pulled around in a palmar direction instead of more proximally. Imagine if the tendons were against the fetlock joint without the sesamoids. In this situation, when the tendons were pulled, the foot would have to overcome the weight of the horse without as much leverage. The sesamoids function like a fulcrum, giving the tendons a mechanical advantage.

Additionally, the sesamoids provide for a larger surface area for the fetlock joint. When you examine the dorsal aspect of the sesamoids, it is covered with articular cartilage where it contacts the palmar/plantar distal cannon bone.

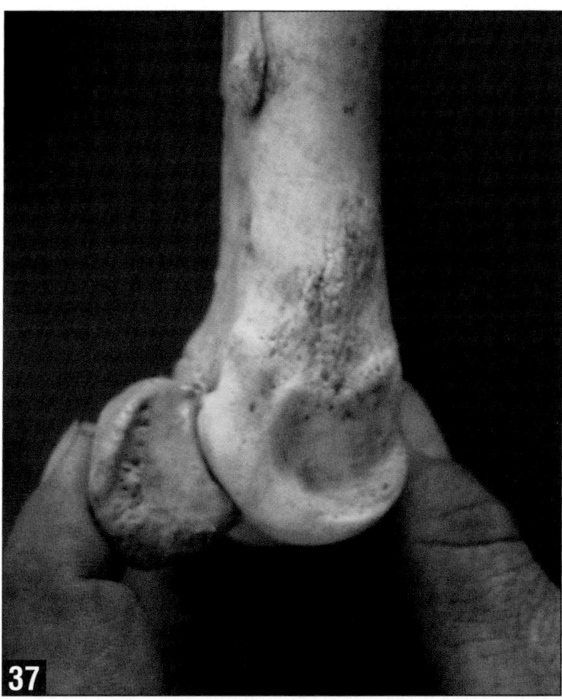

Lateral view of distal cannon bone with a sesamoid bone in position.

THE DIGIT (Figures 38-39)

The digit begins at the fetlock joint and is composed of the first, second, and third phalanx as well as the navicular bone. **Figure 38** is a dorsal view of the bones that compose the digit. **Figure 39** is a palmar view of the same bones.

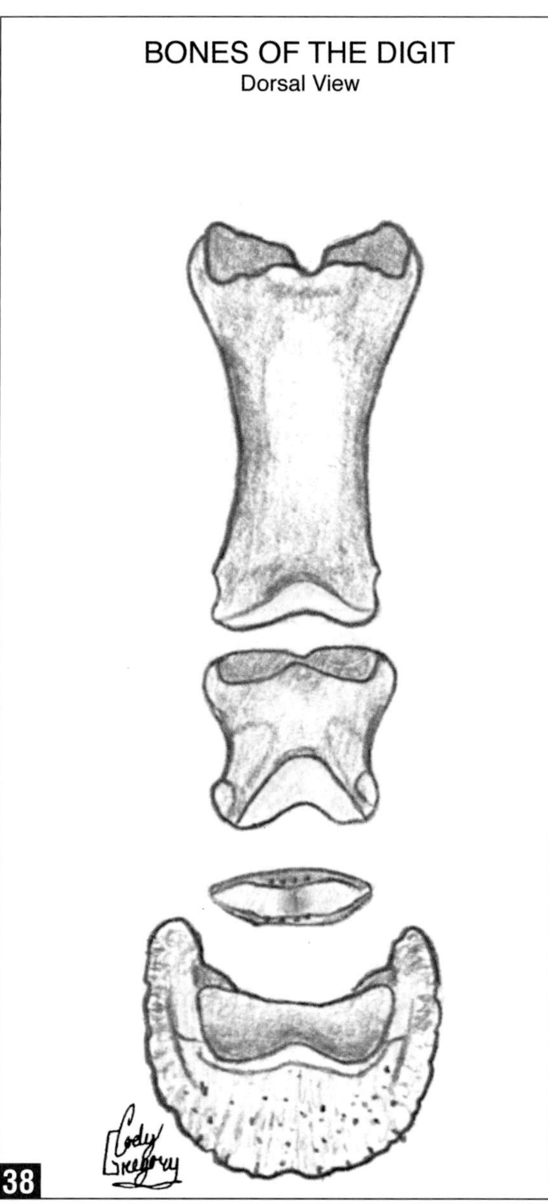

Drawing of the dorsal aspect of the bones in the digit.

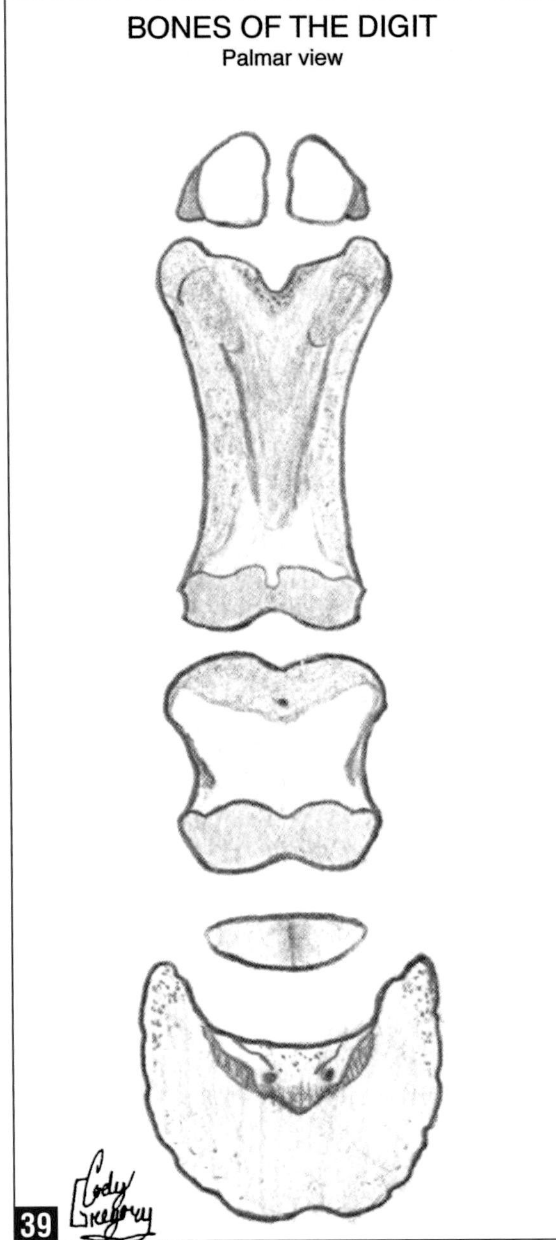

Palmar aspect of the bones in the digit.

FIRST PHALANX (Figures 40-42)

In **Figure 40**, you can see the palmar aspect of P1, **Figure 41** is the dorsal view, and **Figure 42** is a lateral view.

The first phalanx is also known as the proximal phalanx, long pastern, and P1. It is the most proximal bone in the digit. It is larger proximal, tapering towards the distal end. At the distal end, it makes up the proximal portion of the pastern joint. Proximally, it makes up the distal portion of the fetlock joint. P1 takes a tremendous amount of stress under normal conditions.

SECOND PHALANX (Figures 43-45)

Figure 43 is the palmar view of P2, **Figure 44** the dorsal, and **Figure 45** is the lateral aspect.

The second phalanx is also known as the middle phalanx, short pastern, P2, and coronary bone. From a dorsal view it appears to be as long as it is wide, but from the lateral view it is not as thick as it is wide or long. P2 is a strong bone due to its shape, and it provides area for the attachment of quite a bit of ligament and tendon compared to its size. The distal end of P2 forms the proximal portion of the coffin joint, while the proximal end of P2 forms the distal portion of the pastern joint.

NAVICULAR BONE (Figure 46-50)

Figure 46 is the dorsal view that is covered in articular cartilage where the navicular bone articulates with distal P2 in the coffin joint. **Figure 47** is the palmar view of the navicular bone where the deep flexor passes over it. **Figure 48** is the proximal end of the navicular bone, **Figure 49** is the distal edge, and **Figure 50** is the distal edge of a navicular bone with enlarged channels for blood supply (nutrient foramen).

Also known as the distal sesamoid and shuttle bone, named as a comparison to a weavers shuttle, the navicular bone is located palmar/plantar to the coffin bone, and articulates in the coffin joint. From and external lateral view of the foot, the general location of the navicular bone is at the widest part of the foot, half an inch below the coronary band. There is articular cartilage on the dorsal surface that moves with the distal palmar/plantar aspect of distal P2. **Figure 46** On the opposite side of the navicular bone, the deep flexor tendon passes over on its way to the semilunar crest of the coffin bone. **Figure 47** This aspect of the navicular bone is covered with fibrocartilage to provide a smooth surface for the deep flexor tendon.

The synovial sheath on the dorsal deep flexor tendon ends before the deep flexor tendon reaches the navicular bone. Because the tendon has to pass

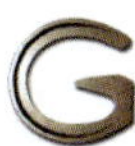

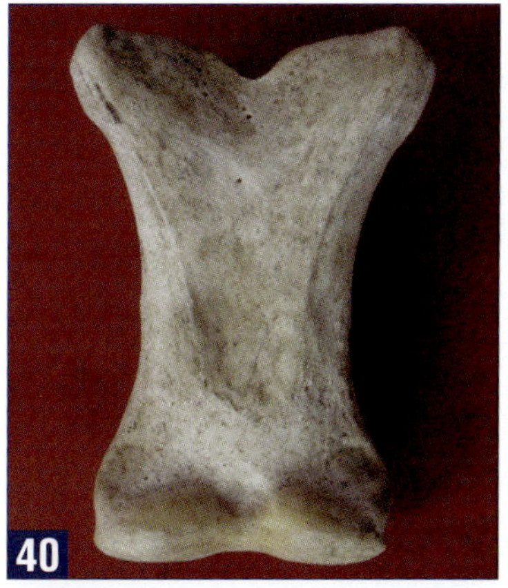

Palmar P1.

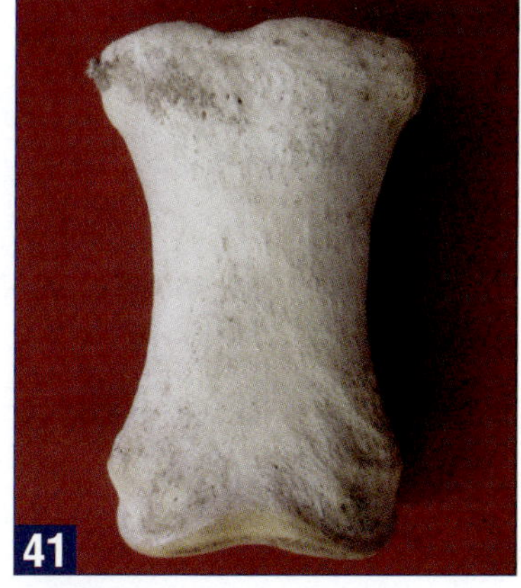

Dorsal P1.

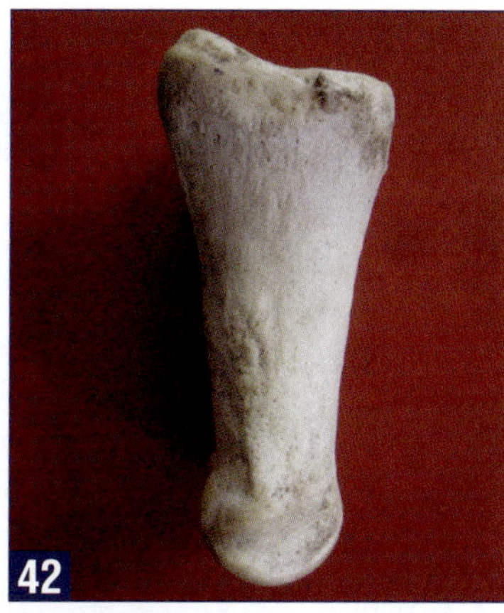

Lateral P1.

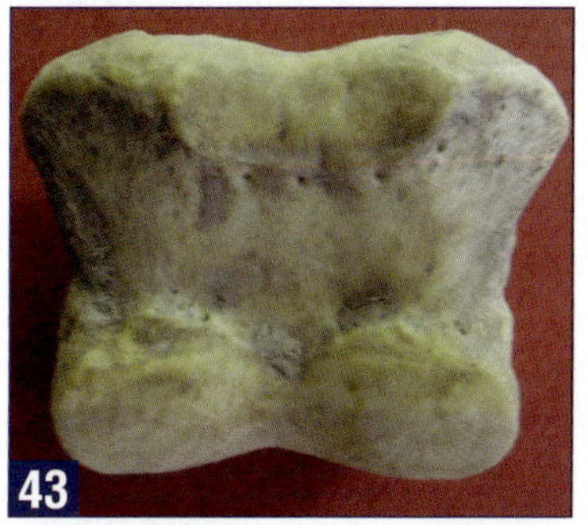

Palmar P2.

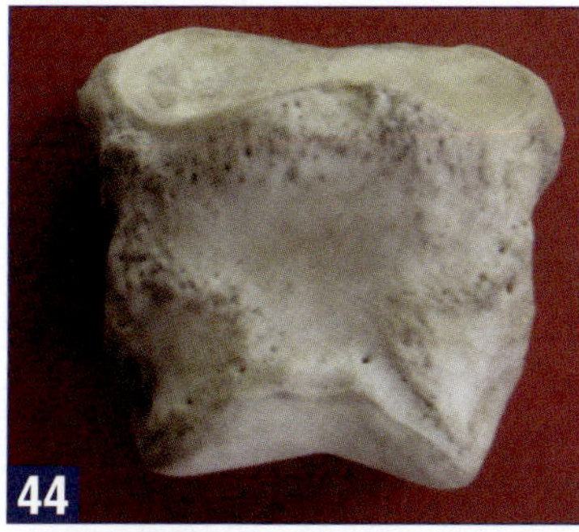

Dorsal P2.

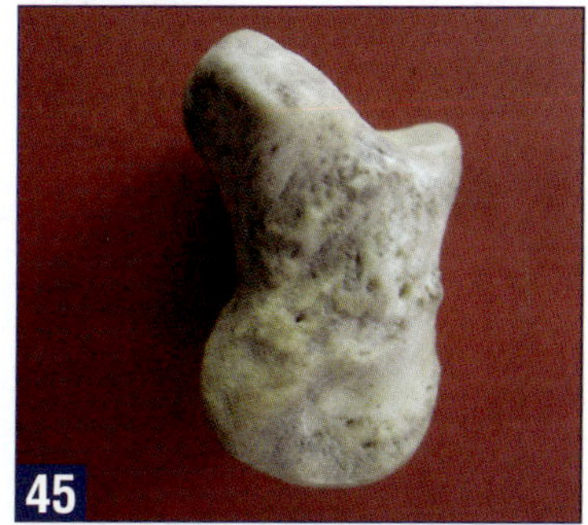

Lateral P2.

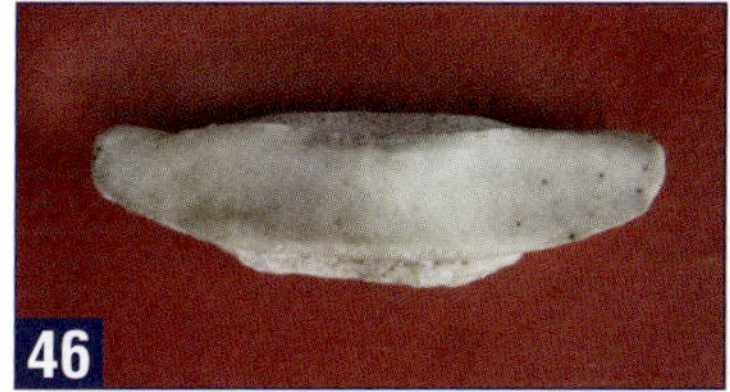

Dorsal navicular bone.

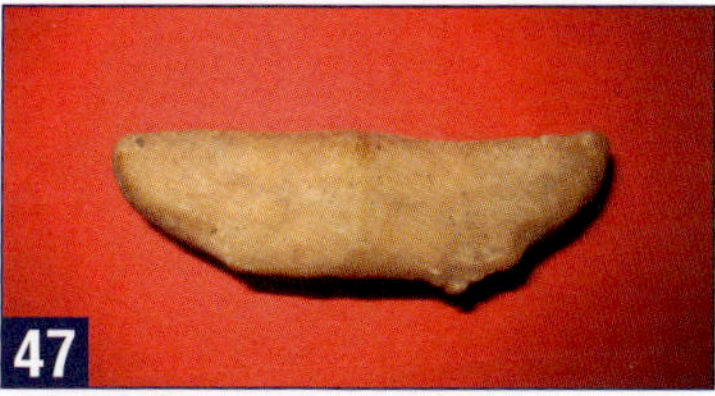

Palmar navicular bone.

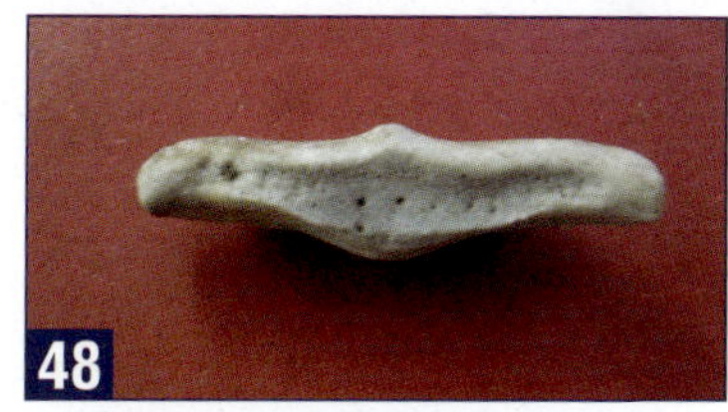

Proximal navicular bone.

over the bone without a synovial sheath, there is a bursa sack located here. Commonly known as the navicular bursa, the anatomical name is the bursa podotrochlearis.

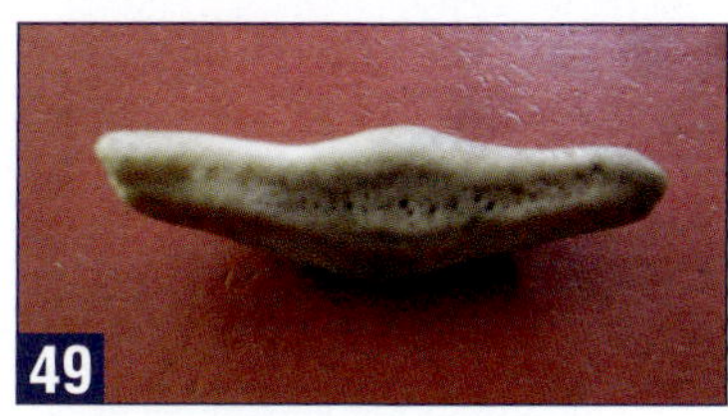

Distal navicular bone.

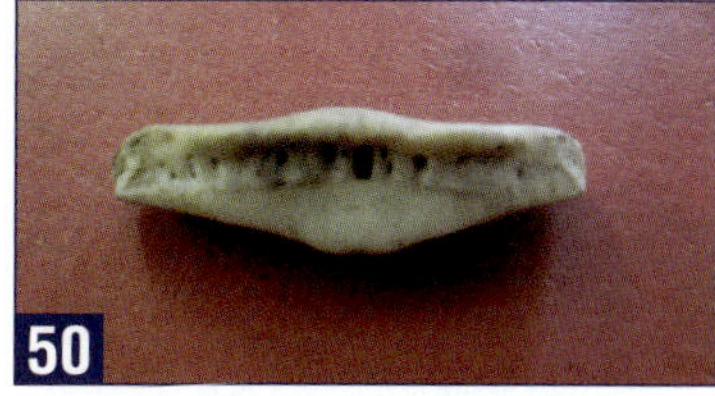

Distal navicular bone with enlarged vascular channels.

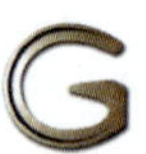

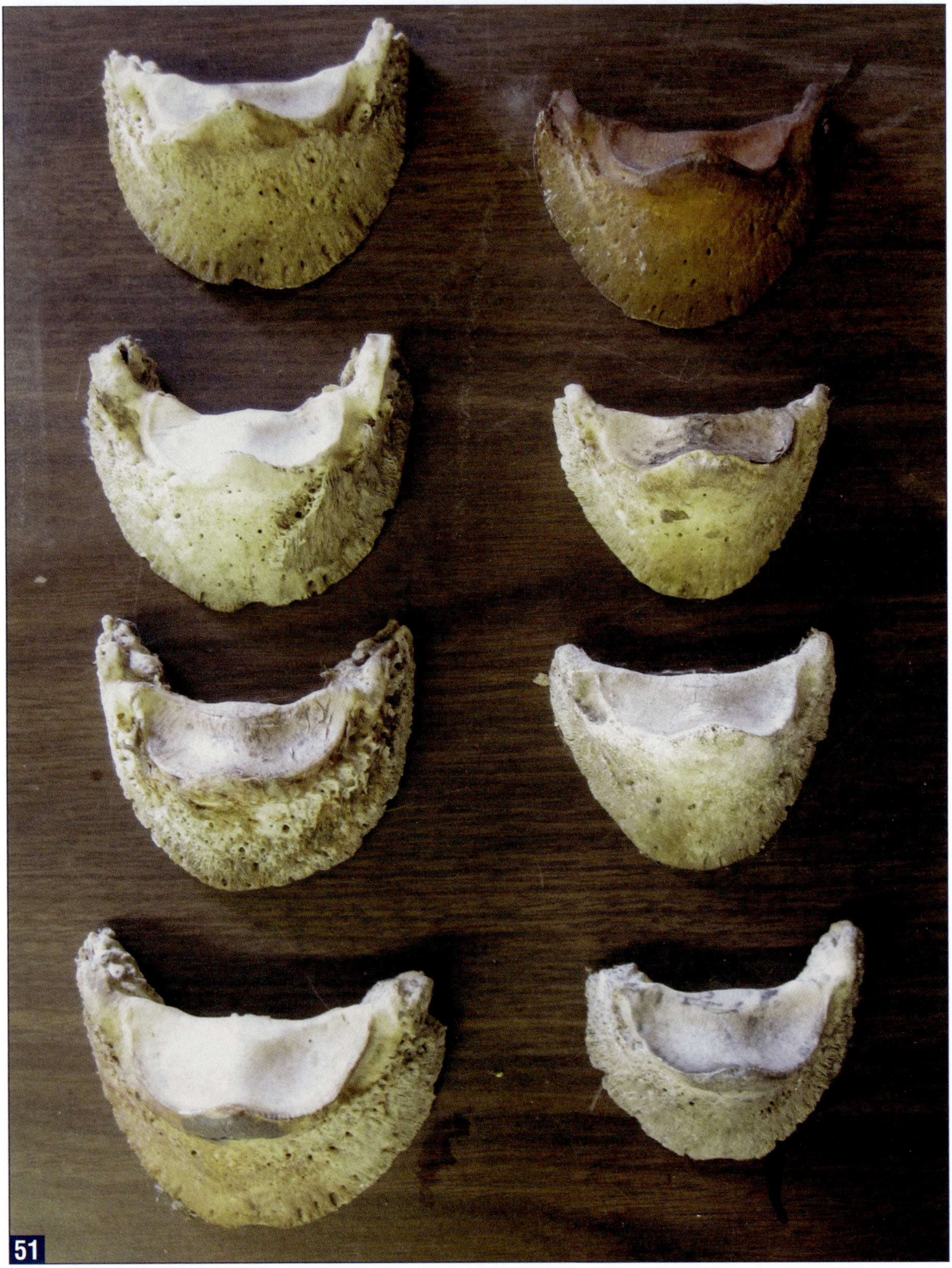

51

Rows of coffin bones, fronts on left, hinds on right.

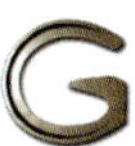

COFFIN BONE (Figures 51-57)

The coffin bone has several names. It is called the third phalanx, distal phalanx, P3, and pedal bone. It has a shape that is represented by the hoof capsule, and a front coffin bone is easily distinguished from a hind coffin bone. The row of coffin bones on the left in **Figure 51** are front coffin bones, and those on the right are hind coffin bones. On the distal dorsal border of the coffin bone there is often a notch that is known as the crenna of the coffin bone. **(Figures 52-53)** It has been suggested as a toe-stay that would work like a key in a motor shaft, however I doubt that this is the purpose of the crenna. With the strength and abundance of laminae, a toe-stay working as a key is not needed. All of the bones in the digit have a crest, groove, ridge, or anatomically significant point in the middle of the bone, and the crenna is that point on the distal aspect of the coffin bone.

It is amazing that this bone has such a sharp edge around the distal border, yet this is the area closest to the ground. Because the hoof capsule itself serves as an exoskeleton of sorts, the coffin bone is well protected. From a lateral view, the coffin bone should have a straight dorsal border with a sharp distal edge, as you can see from the coffin bone in **Figure 54**. With certain lameness issues, such as founder and pedal osteitis, you can end up with a coffin bone that looks like the one in **Figure 55**.

When you compare the tissue of the coffin bone to other bones, you will see that it is quite porous. All of these holes in the surface of the bone are there for blood supply to the coriums. The coffin bone does not weigh as much as other bones of similar size due to the porous nature of the bone.

The coffin bone serves as the last insertion point for both the deep flexor tendon and the main extensor tendon. The proximal surface of the coffin bone articulates with the distal surface of the second phalanx.

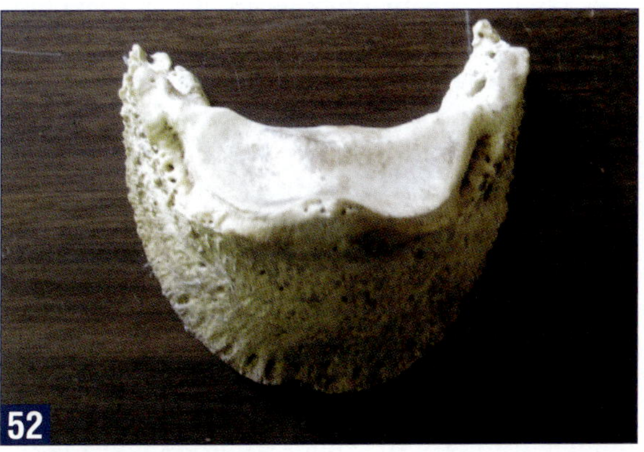

Proximal view of P3.

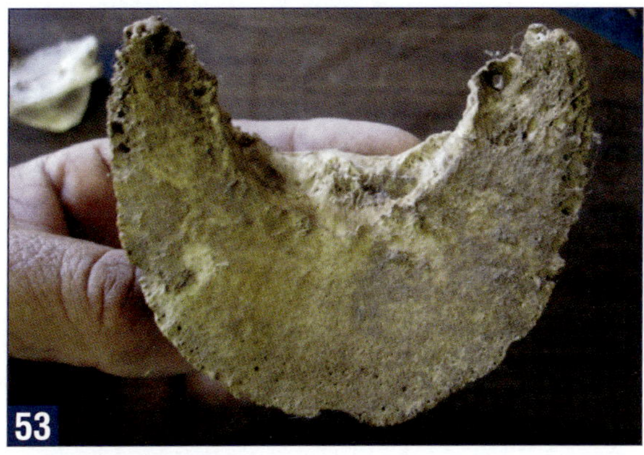

Solar view of P3.

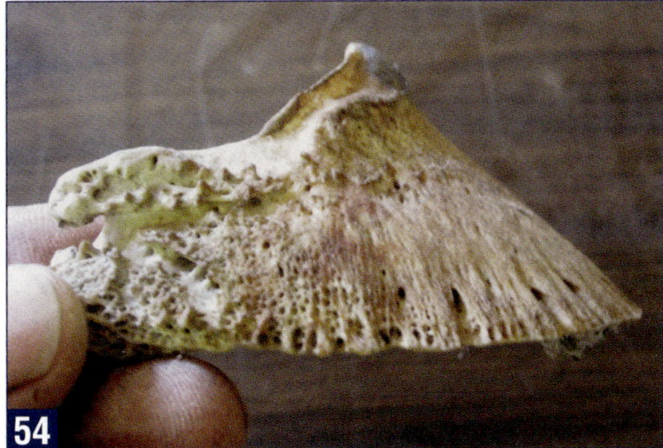

Lateral view of normal P3.

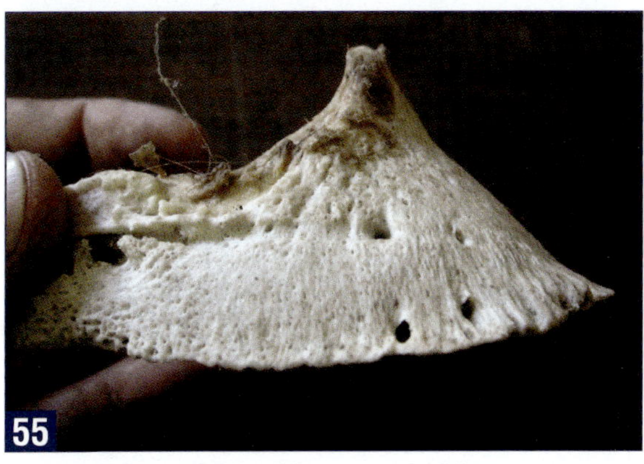

Lateral view of P3 with some problems.

COLLATERAL CARTILAGES

The collateral cartilages, (lateral cartilages or hoof cartilages) extend off of the wings of the coffin bone, and they may be considered extensions of P3 made from hyaline cartilage. Hyaline cartilage does not have nerve supply, so damage to the cartilage directly does not cause pain.

In many horses, these collateral cartilages will ossify (turn into bone) from the type of work they do, conformation, injury, etc. When this happens, the foot may take on a much different shape, and there is always a danger of them fracturing. **Figures 56 and 57** are of a coffin bone with one of the collateral cartilages having ossified. When only one does, this is known as unilateral sidebone. It is called bilateral sidebone when both collateral cartilages are involved.

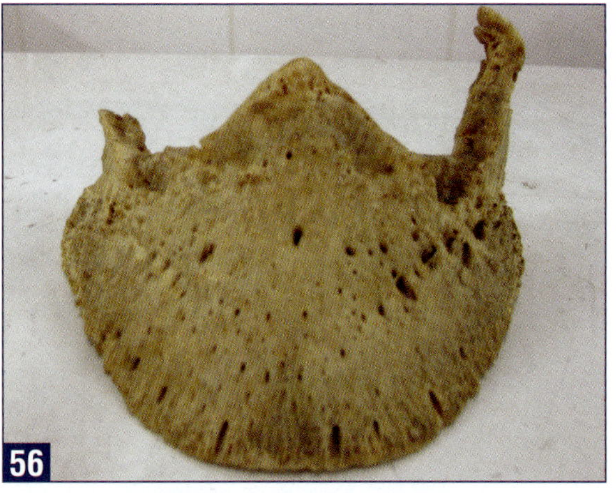

P3 with a sidebone.

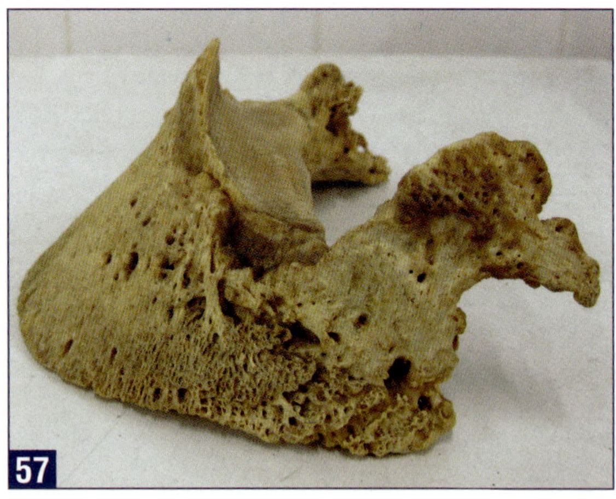

P3 with a sidebone.

JOINTS:

A joint occurs at any place that two bones meet.

There are three primary categories of joints. One is cartilaginous joints, like those found between the vertebrae. Next is ligamentous joints, like those found between the splint bones and cannon bone where only ligaments are found, and there is little movement. The joints that we as farriers are most interested in are the synovial joints. These are surrounded by a joint capsule, include articular cartilage, and contain synovial fluid.

In the category of synovial joints, there are three types. These are:

hinge joints	(ginglymus)
plane joints	(arthrodial)
ball and socket joints	(enarthrodial)

Joints allow for movement of the bones involved,as well as dissipation of shock and force. Articular cartilage does not have nerve supply, so the compression of the cartilage in a joint under load does not cause pain. Only when the cartilage fails does the bone feel pain associated with that failure.

An interesting thing for you to experiment with is the way that the joints go together when you are examining bone models. I suggest that you get several bone models, both front and hind, and look at how well all of the different bones from different horses still go together. I am always amazed at how well the cannon bone off the hind leg of a 25-year-old quarter horse fits with P1 from the hind leg of a 2-year-old quarter horse.

Figure 58 shows all of the joints in the thoracic limb, and **Figure 59** shows all of the joints in the pelvic limb.

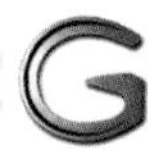

THORACIC LIMB
Joints

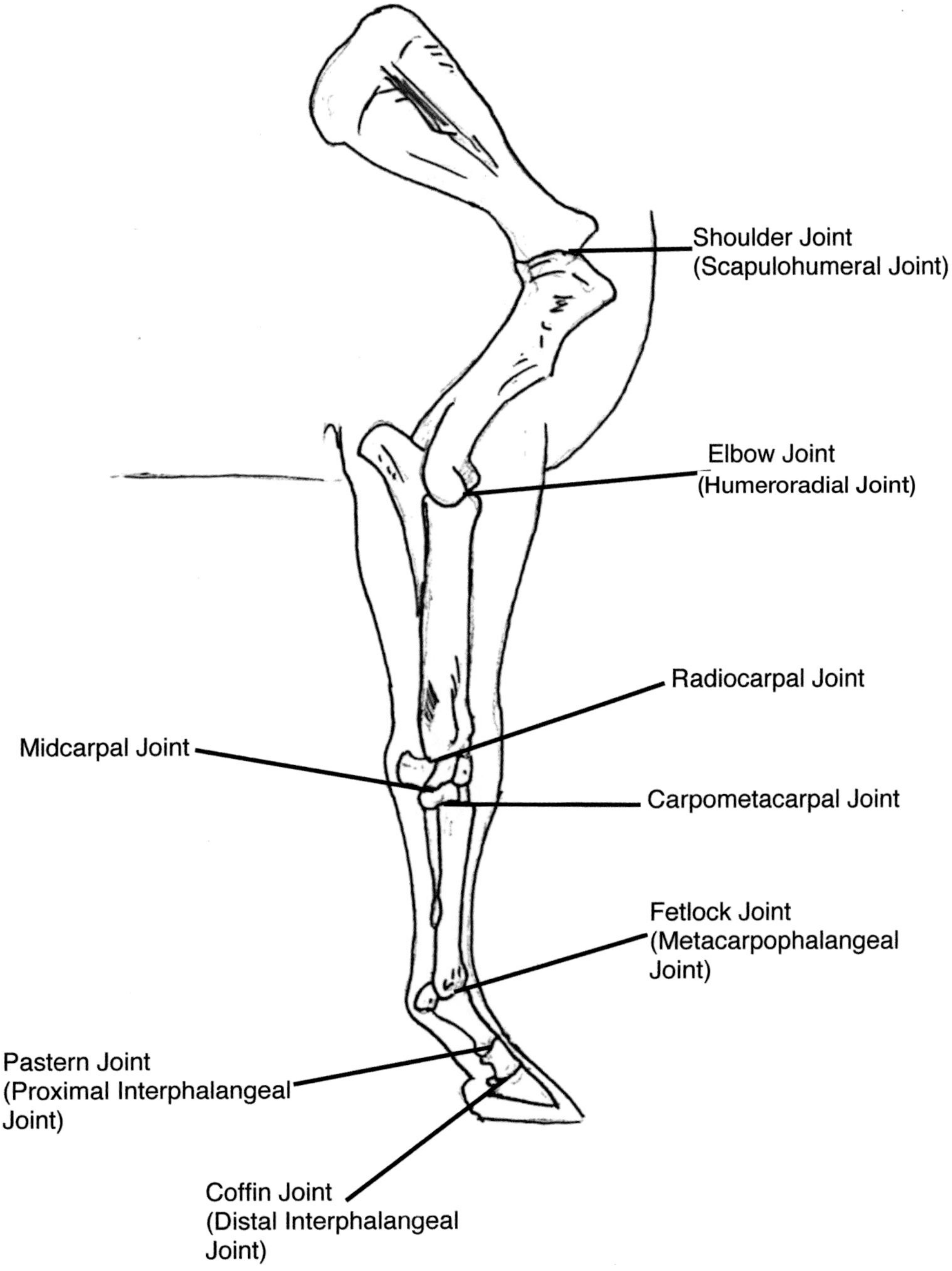

Shoulder Joint
(Scapulohumeral Joint)

Elbow Joint
(Humeroradial Joint)

Radiocarpal Joint

Midcarpal Joint

Carpometacarpal Joint

Fetlock Joint
(Metacarpophalangeal Joint)

Pastern Joint
(Proximal Interphalangeal Joint)

Coffin Joint
(Distal Interphalangeal Joint)

58

Joints in the thoracic limb

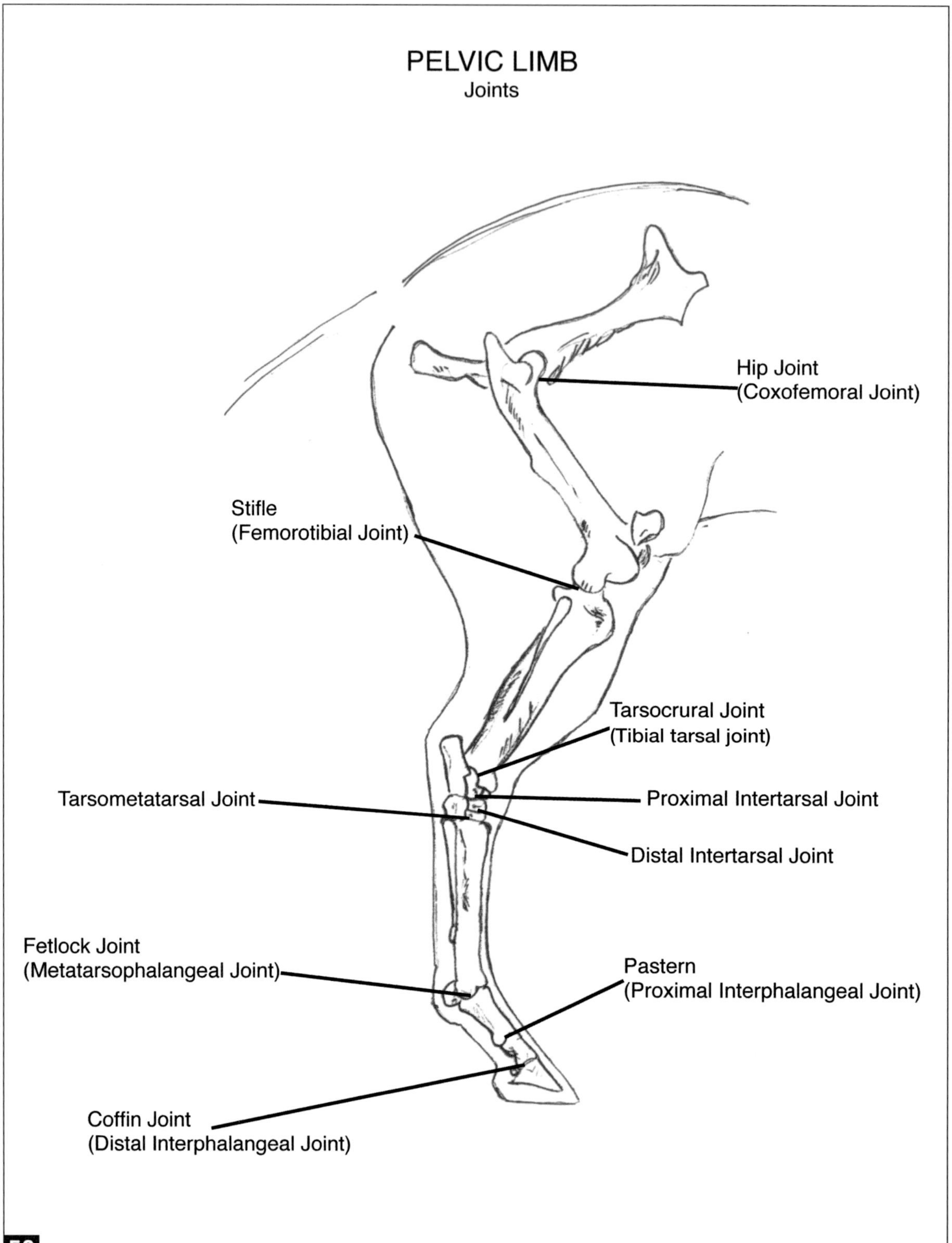

PELVIC LIMB
Joints

59

Joints in the pelvic limb

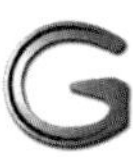

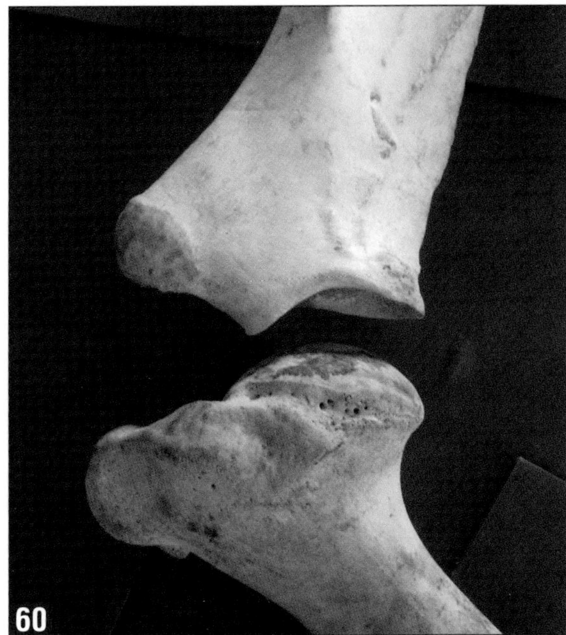

Detail of the shoulder joint.

BALL AND SOCKET JOINTS

There are two primary ball and socket joints in the limb. The shoulder joint, which is the joint between the scapula and the humerus, and the hip joint, which is the joint between the pelvis and the femur. When I first envisioned a ball and socket joint, I had it in my head that it was like the ball on a pickup and the hitch that goes over it. With the experience of dissection, I was astonished to find that the ball and socket joint is more of a bulge and depression joint. Obviously, the more enclosed the ball in a tighter socket, the less movement possible. However, there is so little encapsulation by the ball that I was surprised it could stay together. **Figure 60** is of the shoulder joint where the scapula meets the humerus.

PLANE JOINTS

A plane joint mainly allows sliding lateral movement. These types of joints play a large role in absorbing and redirecting concussion as well as allowing the horse more freedom to travel on uneven terrain. The best examples in the leg are the carpometacarpal joint and the tarsometatarsal joint. These joints do not open to any large degree when the legs are flexed or extended. Also, the vertical areas between individual carpal and tarsal bones can mostly be considered plane joints as well.

HINGE JOINTS

Hinge joints allow for a large range of movement in only two directions. For the most part, this movement is in the sagittal plane. One of the properties of a hinge joint is that it is extremely resistant to lateral movement. In fact, lateral movement to any great degree will cause catastrophic failure of that joint.

One of the best examples of a hinge joint is the fetlock joint where the cannon bone meets P1. There is a sagittal ridge on the end of the cannon bone that matches the sagittal groove on proximal P1. This allows the fetlock to fold and extend, but not accept lateral movement.

COMBINATIONS

There are several joints that act as a hinge joint, yet they allow for lateral movement like plane joints. The coffin joint is a good example, as it allows the foot to flex and extend, yet also negotiate uneven terrain. If it did not allow for that lateral movement, the horse would be much more susceptible to ligament injuries in the coffin joint.

CARPAL JOINTS (Figure 61)

Figure 61 is the dorsal view of the carpus. There are three joints in the carpus; radiocarpal joing, midcarpal joint, and carpometacarpal joint.

The radiocarpal joint (antebrachiocarpal joint), is where the radius meets the top row of carpals. Between the two rows there is the midcarpal (middle carpal) joint. This joint is often called the intercarpal joint, but the vertical joints that exist between the individual carpal bones are also known as intercarpal joints. This can cause some confusion when working with a vet, so be aware of it and make sure that you are both on the same page. Between the distal row of carpals and the metacarpus is the carpometacarpal joint. When the knee is flexed, the radiocarpal joint and the midcarpal joint open, acting as hinge joints. The radiocarpal joint opens about twice as far as the midcarpal joint. The carpometacarpal joint does not open, so it is a plane joint.

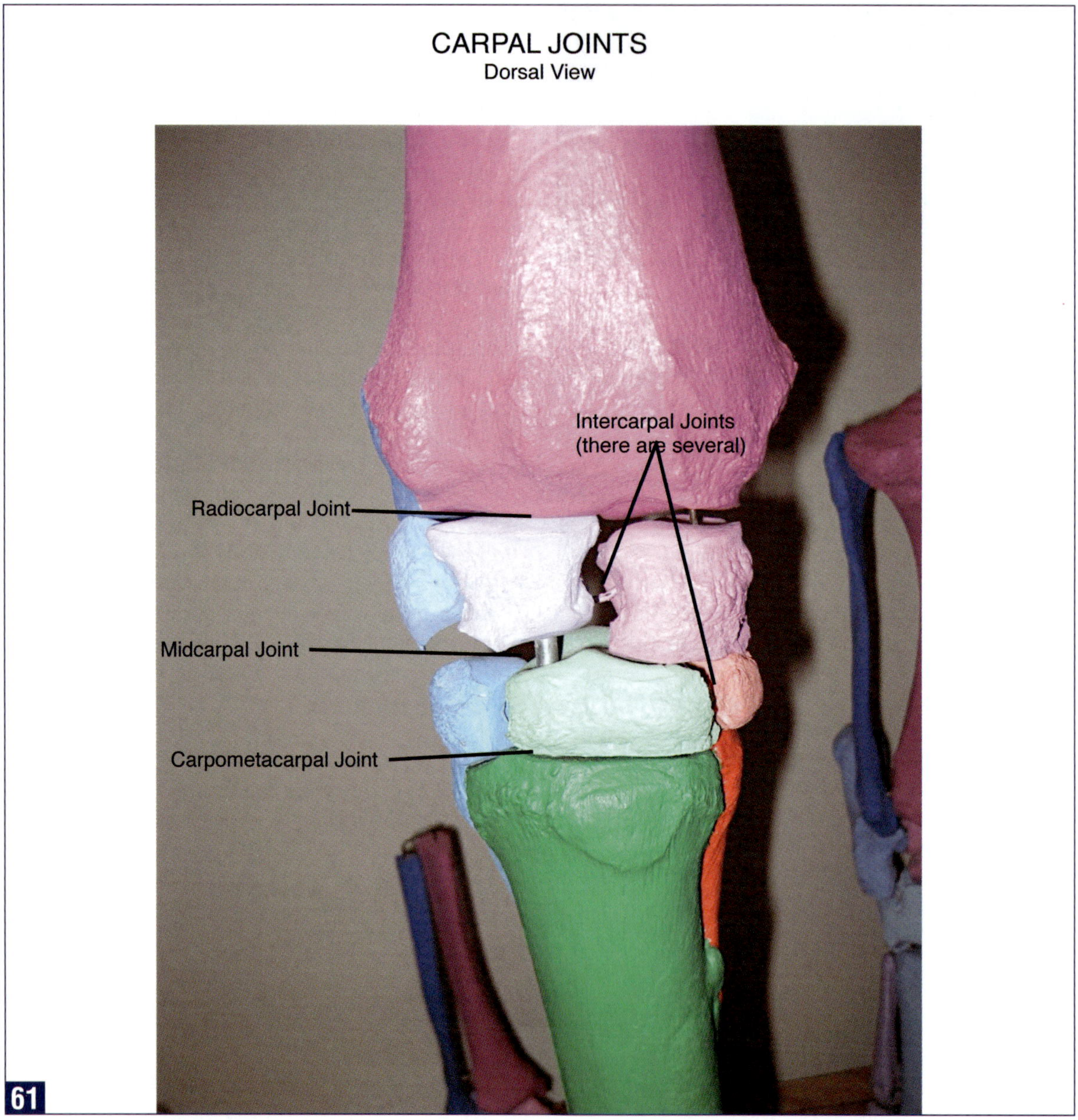

CARPAL JOINTS
Dorsal View

Intercarpal Joints
(there are several)
Radiocarpal Joint
Midcarpal Joint
Carpometacarpal Joint

61

Dorsal view of the carpus.

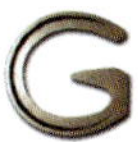

TARSAL JOINTS (Figure 62)

Figure 62 is the dorsal view of the tarsus.

There are 4 joints in the tarsus. Where the tibia meets the trochlea of the talus there is a joint known as the tibiotarsal joint. It is also referred to as the tarsocrural joint. Between the distal talus, distal calcaneus, and proximal central tarsal and proximal T4 is the proximal intertarsal joint. The distal intertarsal joint is located where the central tarsal meets T3 as well as part of T1 and T2. Between the distal row of tarsals and the metatarsus is located the tarsometatarsal joint. The primary movement in the hock is the tarsocrural joint, which is a hinge joint.

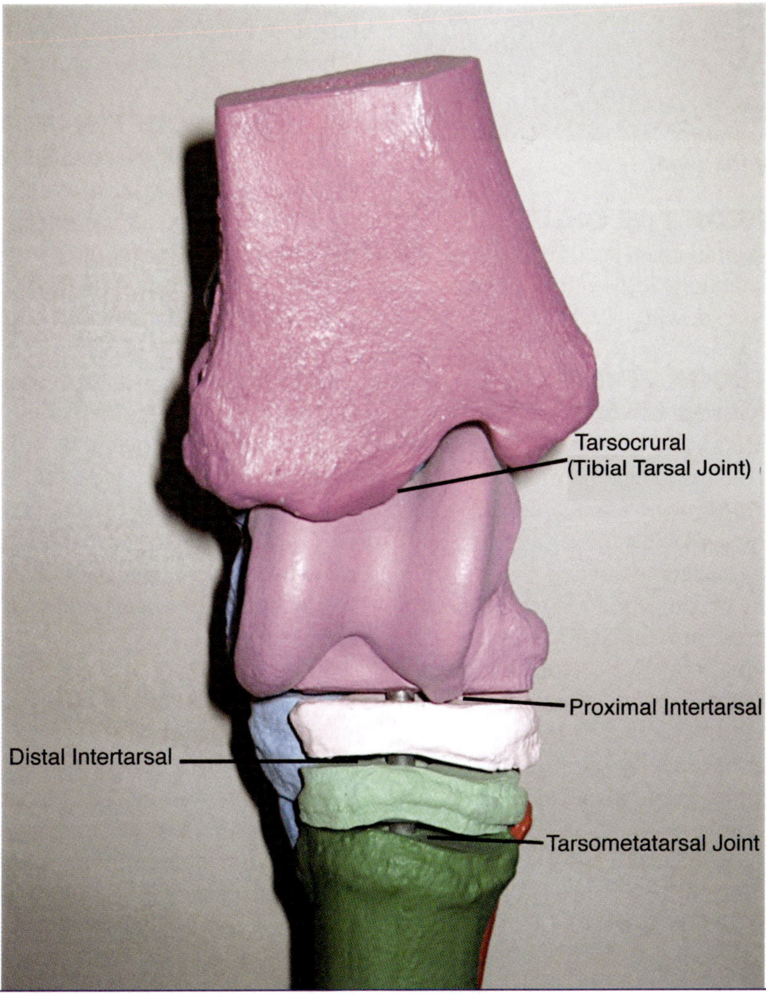

Dorsal view of the tarsus.

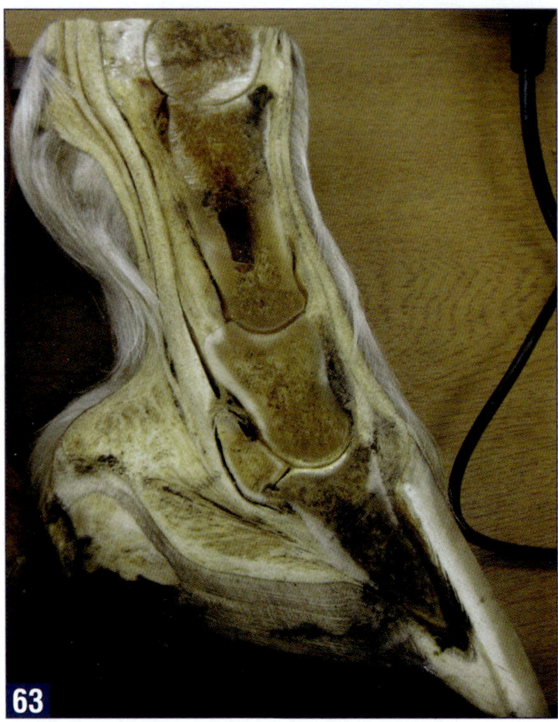

Sagittal section of the digit.

JOINTS OF THE DIGIT

Figure 63 is a sagittal cross section of the digit, and you can see inside the middle of the joints from the distal cannon bone down.

FETLOCK JOINT (Figures 64-65)

This joint is anatomically known as metacarpophalangeal joint in the front leg, and metatarsophalangeal, in the hind. **Figure 64** is the fetlock joint from the palmar view without the sesamoids, and **figure 65** is with the sesamoids added.

The fetlock joint is composed of the distal end of the cannon bone, the proximal end of P1, and the sesamoid bones. This joint allows for free movement on the sagittal plane but no lateral movement. The condyle, or sagittal ridge, on the distal end of the cannon bone fits exactly into the groove on proximal P1. Proximal P1 is also larger than the distal end of the cannon bone, just as proximal P2 is larger where it meets distal P1.

PASTERN JOINT (Figures 66-67)

Anatomically known as the proximal interphalangeal joint, **figure 66** is a palmar view, and **figure 67** is the dorsal view with the bones separated.

This joint is formed between distal P1 and proximal P2. The pastern joint is a hinge joint that has plane joint characteristics. P1 tapers down from proximal to distal, and the distal area that meets with P2 is smaller than the area of P2. This is an interesting thing in equine anatomy and suggests that concussion and load have been well dissipated by the time that they reach distal P1.

P1 and P2 can be considered a long rod that has very little movement in the pastern joint. The pastern joint is strongly held by the collateral ligaments, the pastern ligaments, the straight sesamoidian ligament, as well as the insertion of the superficial flexor tendon. Over all of that, you will find fascia, the digital annular ligaments, the extensor branches of the suspensory ligament, and the main extensor tendon. In effect, the pastern joint allows for the length of the pastern and gives it tensile strength. In other words, it is strong enough to bend.

COFFIN JOINT (Figures 68-71)

Anatomically known as the distal interphalangeal joint, **Figure 68** is a dorsal view, **Figure 69** is the plantar view without the navicular, **Figure 70** has the navicular bone added, and **Figure 71** is a solar view with the navicular bone in place.

The coffin joint is composed of distal P2, proximal P3, and the dorsal aspect of the navicular bone. It is the most distal joint in the horse and allows for quite a range of movement. It is primarily a hinge joint but does allow for a lot of lateral flexibility. You can pick up a foot and move the hoof capsule from side to side to see just how much movement is allowed by the coffin joint. This property is essential as horses have to navigate through all types of terrain.

SYNOVIAL FLUID

Synovial fluid is also known as joint oil. It is comprised of a mucopolysaccharide known as hyaluronic acid, and also contains substances called lubricin, proteinases and collagenases. It is secreted by the synovial membrane found on the inside of a joint capsule as well as the synovial sheaths found around tendons, and bursa sacs where tendon or muscle passes over bone prominence without the advantage of a synovial sheath.

Synovial fluid has non-newtonian flow charac-

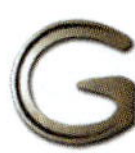

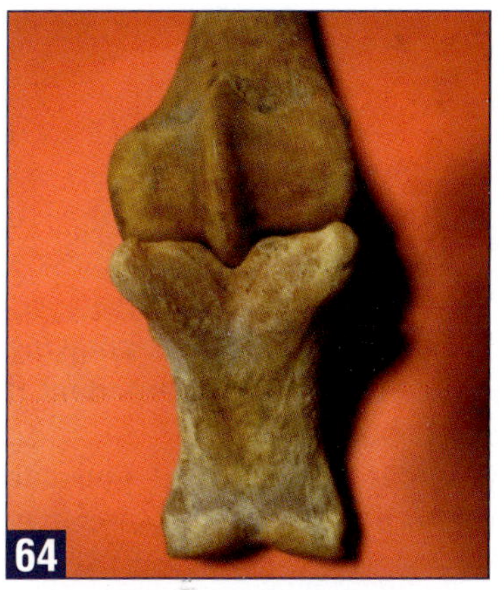
Palmar view of the fetlock joint without the sesamoids.

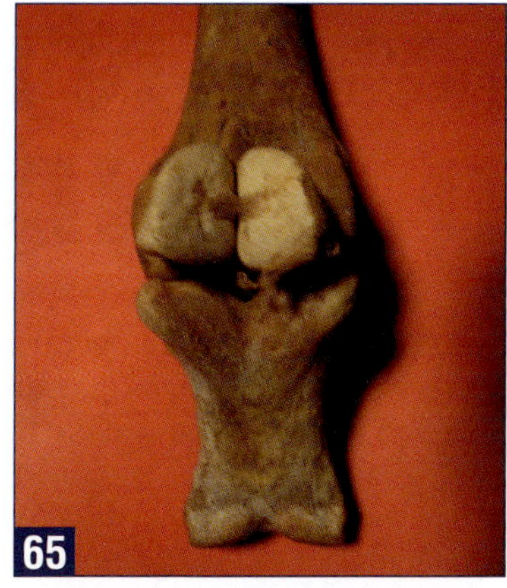
Palmar view of the fetlock joint with the sesamoids.

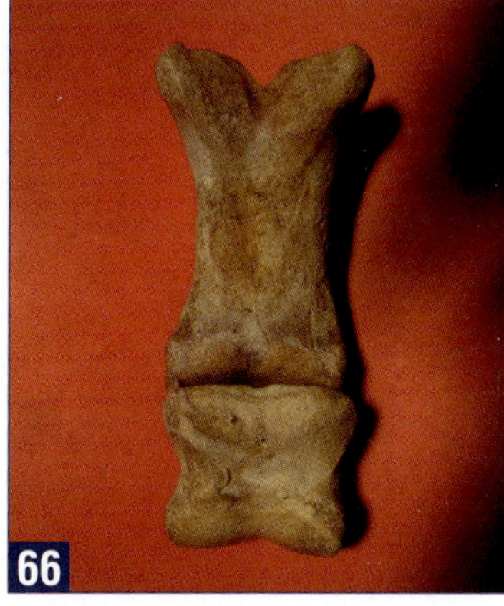
Palmar view of the pastern joint.

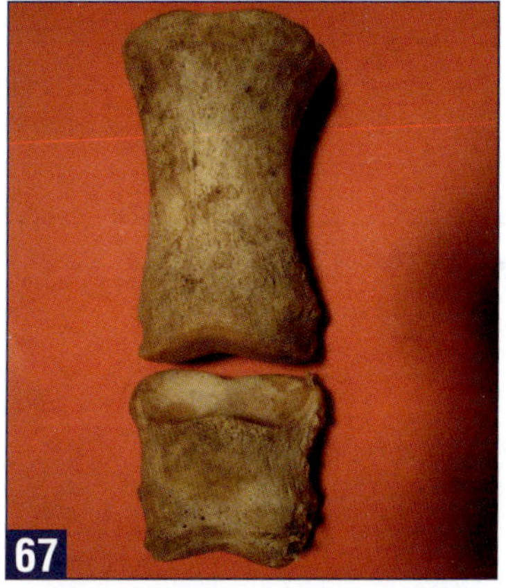
Dorsal view of the pastern joint.

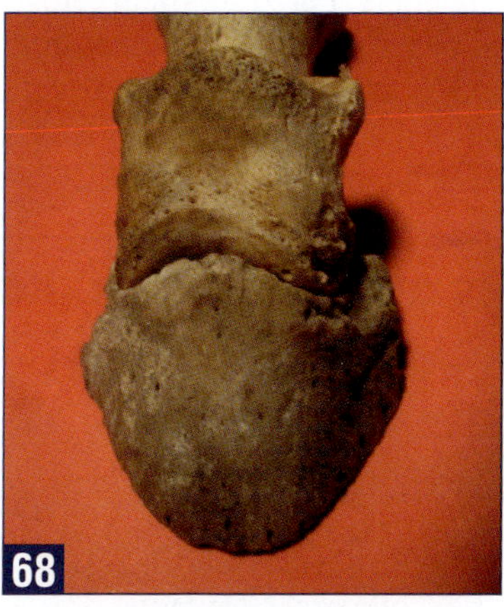
Dorsal view of the coffin joint.

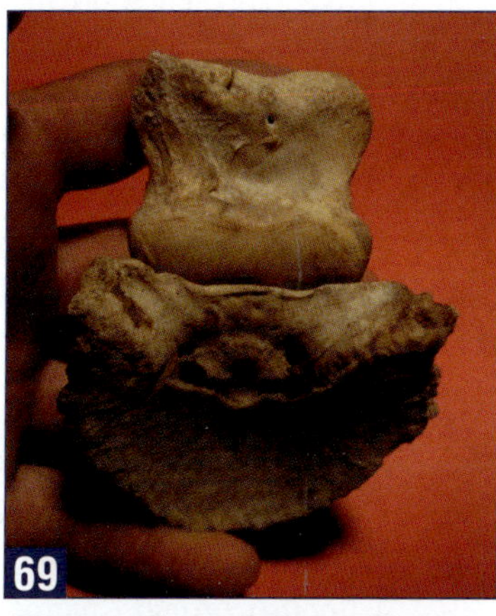
Plantar view of the coffin joint without the navicular bone.

teristics, which means that it does not have a constant viscosity. It covers all surfaces of the articular cartilage, and when the joint bears weight, the synovial fluid is squeezed out from between the bones mechanically, leaving a thin layer of fluid on the surface of the cartilage. This process is known as weeping lubrication.

When you are doing a dissection, you can manipulate the articular surfaces of the bones against each other to feel how little friction there is in a joint.

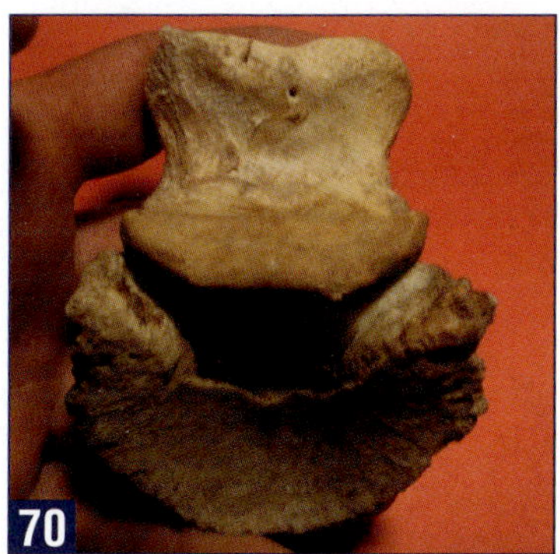
Plantar view of the coffin joint with the navicular bone.

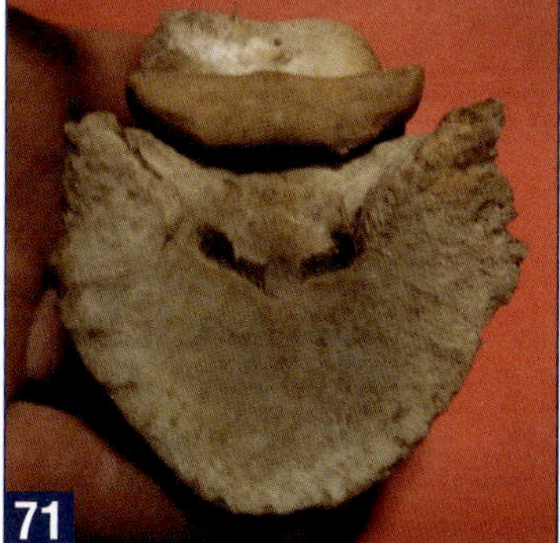
Solar view of the coffin bone and navicular bone.

Understanding how the bones are shaped, where they are located, how they connect and interact, as well as what they are made of, allows you to better understand how what you do to the foot can impact the whole horse. This is critical knowledge if you intend to be a leader in the farrier industry.

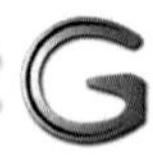

Chapter 10 LIGAMENTS AND TENDONS

The primary function of ligaments is to support the skeleton of the horse. Some of them serve to bear weight, while some serve to hold things together and increase rigidity. Ligaments are connective tissue that mostly connect bone to bone and are mostly elastic. There are 27 individual ligaments that I insist on my students knowing. Although we may identify some as only one ligament in the text, they may represent more than one ligament. For instance, the collateral sesamoidian ligaments count as one when writing them out, but there are actually two collateral sesamoidian ligaments on each leg.

The following ligaments are large basic ligamentous structures that exist in the leg, and knowing where they are and how they work is important if you want to be great at shoeing horses.

Like most things that you learn, if you can break this material into bite-size pieces, it can be easier to learn the whole. For this reason, we put the ligaments into categories. You can begin the process of learning your ligaments by first learning a small category, adding another small category, and continue in that manner again and again until you have learned them all.

The table below lists of the ligaments in their respective categories.

CATEGORY 1. EXCEPTIONS OF THE BONE-TO-BONE RULE

1. Suspensory Ligament
2. Ligament of the Ergot
3. Radial (Superior) Check Ligament
4. Subcarpal (Inferior) Check Ligament
5. Subtarsal Check Ligament
6. Chondrocompedal Ligament of the Collateral Cartilages.
7. Chondrocoronal Ligament of the Collateral Cartilages.
8. Chondrotendinous Ligament of the Collateral Cartilages
9. Chondroungular Ligament of the Collateral Cartilages
10. Transverse Lamina (T) Ligament

Name:	Origin:	Insertion:	Function:
Suspensory Ligament	Palmar/plantar proximal cannon, distal row of carpals/tarsals	Sesamoids, main extensor tendon	Support fetlock, energy return, weight bearing
Ligament of the ergot	Ergot	Distal digital annular ligament	Vestigial
Radial Check Ligament (superior)	Radius	Superficial flexor tendon	Prevent overstress of superficial flexor tendon
Subcarpal check ligament (inferior)	Distal row of carpals	Deep flexor tendon	Prevent overstress of deep flexor tendon
Subtarsal check ligament	Distal row of tarsals	Deep flexor tendon	Vestigial
Chondrocompedal	Distal P1	Collateral cartilages	Support collateral cartilages

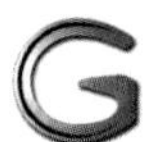

Chondrocoronal	Collateral cartilages	P2	Support collateral cartilages
Chondrotendinous	Collateral cartilages	Main extensor tendon	Support collateral cartilages
Chondroungular	Collateral Cartilages	P3	Support collateral cartilages
Transverse Lamina (T) Ligament	Deep flexor tendon	P2	Separate synovial sheath from navicular bursa

CATEGORY 2. SESAMOIDIAN LIGAMENTS

1. Superficial (Y or Straight) Sesamoidian Ligament
2. Middle (V or Oblique) Sesamoidian Ligament
3. Deep (X or Cruciate) Sesamoidian Ligament
4. Short Sesamoidian Ligament
5. Intersesamoidian Ligament
6. Collateral Sesamoidian Ligament

Name:	Origin:	Insertion:	Function:
Superficial Sesamoidian ligament (Y or Straight)	Sesamoids	P2	Rigidity of the fetlock
Middle sesamoidian ligament (V or Oblique)	Sesamoids	Distal P1	Rigidity of the fetlock
Deep sesamoidian ligament (X or Cruciate)	Sesamoids	Proximal P1	Hold sesamoids in position
Short sesamoidian ligaments	Sesamoids	Proximal P1	Hold sesamoids in position
Intersesamoidian ligament	Sesamoid	Sesamoid	Forms groove for flexor tendons
Collateral sesamoidian ligaments	Sesamoids	Collaterally on distal cannon bone and proximal P1	Hold sesamoids forward in position

CATEGORY 3. ANNULAR LIGAMENTS

1. Palmar/Plantar Annular Ligament
2. Proximal Digital Annular Ligament
3. Distal Digital Annular Ligament

Name:	Origin:	Insertion:	Function:
Palmar/plantar annular ligament	Distal cannon	Distal cannon	Holds tendons against the joint when flexed
Proximal digital annular ligament	P1 and P2	P1 and P2	Holds tendons against the joint when flexed
Distal digital annular ligament	P1 and P2	P1 and P2	Holds tendon against the joint when flexed

CATEGORY 4. NAVICULAR LIGAMENTS

1. Suspensory Navicular Ligament
2. Distal (Impar) Navicular Ligament

Name:	Origin:	Insertion:	Function:
Suspensory navicular ligament	Collateral distal P1	Proximal edge of the navicular bone	Support navicular bone
Distal navicular ligament, (Impar)	Dorsal navicular bone	Palmar/plantar P3	Support navicular bone

CATEGORY 5. PASTERN LIGAMENTS

1. Axial Pastern Ligaments
2. Abaxial Pastern Ligaments

Name:	Origin:	Insertion:	Function:
Axial Pastern ligaments	Distal palmar/plantar P1	Proximal palmar/plantar P2	Strengthen pastern joint
Abaxial Pastern ligaments	Distal palmar/plantar P1	Proximal palmar/plantar P2	Strengthen pastern joint

CATEGORY 6. LIGAMENTS THAT DO NOT FIT INTO A CATEGORY

1. Interosseus Ligaments
2. Plantar Ligament
3. Capsular Ligament
4. Collateral Ligament

Name:	Origin:	Insertion:	Function:
Interosseus ligaments	Cannon bone	Splint bones	Hold splint bones in position
Plantar ligament	Calcaneus	4th tarsal and MT4	Rigidity of the hock and energy return
Capsular ligaments	All synovial joints	All synovial joints	Compose capsule to hold synovial fluid
Collateral ligaments	Collaterally on proximal bone in synovial joints	Collaterally on distal bone in synovial joints	Strengthen joints and support of lateral movement

The total count of these 5 categories adds up to 27 ligaments. Learn them bit by bit, and make them part of your permanent memory. Now, let's go into each one individually to see where they are and what they do.

When we talk about ligaments, we often start by giving their origin and insertion. In anatomy, the origin is generally proximal to the insertion, and the point that a muscle, tendon or ligament attaches to a bone is called the enthesis (entheses plural).

With the exception of a few ligaments that run horizontally, we begin by stating the origin, then the course of the ligament, then the insertions and finally the function. For instance, to give this information for the plantar ligament, you would say, "The plantar ligament is found only on the hind limb, originating in the calcaneus, just distal to the calcanean process. The plantar ligament courses distad and inserts into the 4th tarsal and 4th metatarsal. The plantar ligament gives rigidity to the hock, and aids in strengthening the position of the calcaneus bone as well as an energy return that helps the horse when moving." When you first read that it is a mouthful. As such, you need to reread it, draw it, talk about it, ask your instructor about it, and spend some time getting to know it.

When you see the suffix "ad", and in distad, it indicates moving in a direction from a given point. The suffix "ally" indicates something is positioned at a point. For instance, a ligament may course distad from origin to insertion, and a bone may be located distally to another bone.

For some students, it is easier for them to lay things out in a different format. That is why I laid out all of the ligaments in a list format. As long as you don't leave out important stuff like origins, insertions and functions, that is fine.

Beyond that, you can make flash cards with all the pertinent information as well as a drawing. The act of making it will help, and being able to study just what you don't know is a big help as well.

CATEGORY 1. LIGAMENTS THAT ARE AN EXCEPTION OF THE BONE-TO-BONE RULE

1. Suspensory Ligament: (Figures 1-2)

The suspensory ligament is the largest ligament in the leg (from knee or hock down) and is often referred to as the interosseus muscle or interosseus tendon. These names are used because it is located between the splint bones, and there is microscopic evidence of both muscle and tendon fiber in the suspensory ligament.

It originates at the proximal palmar/plantar cannon bone, with attachments to the distal row of carpals and tarsals as well, and courses distad between the splint bones. At the distal end of the splint bones where the nodules are located, the suspensory ligament divides into two pieces (bifurcates). Each portion then inserts into the proximal collateral portions of the proximal sesamoids. From each branch, another

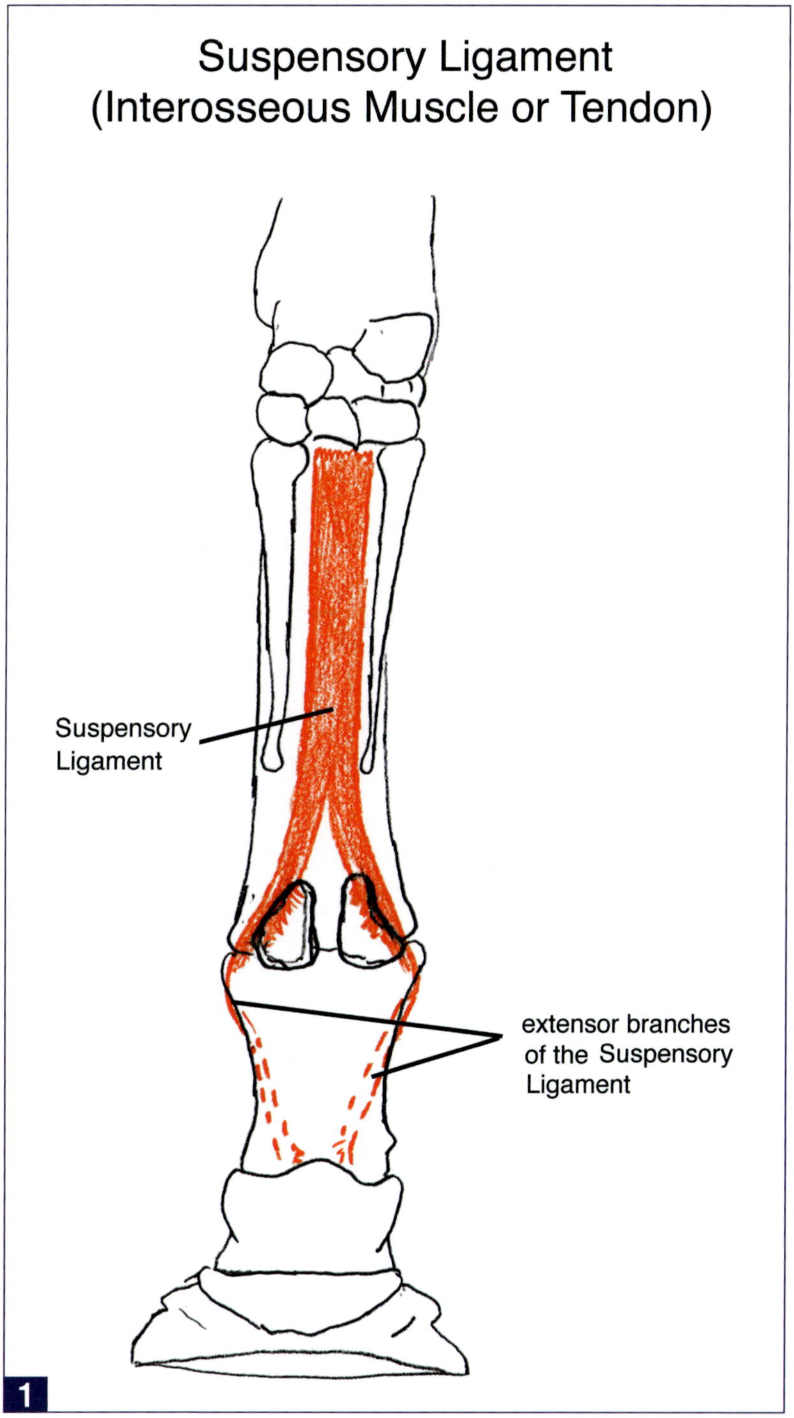

Suspensory Ligament (Interosseous Muscle or Tendon)

Suspensory Ligament

extensor branches of the Suspensory Ligament

1

smaller branch arises, and it courses dorso-distad and inserts into the main extensor tendon. This insertion is at the level of the pastern joint and is in large part responsible for making the main extensor tendon so wide from this point down. This final insertion is what puts the suspensory ligament into this category. These two branches that insert into the main extensor tendon are referred to as the extensor branches of the suspensory ligament, and they can often be easily seen and identified on live horses.

The functions of the suspensory ligament are to bear a substantial amount of weight, provide energy return as the horse moves, support the fetlock joint during load, and aid in widening the main extensor

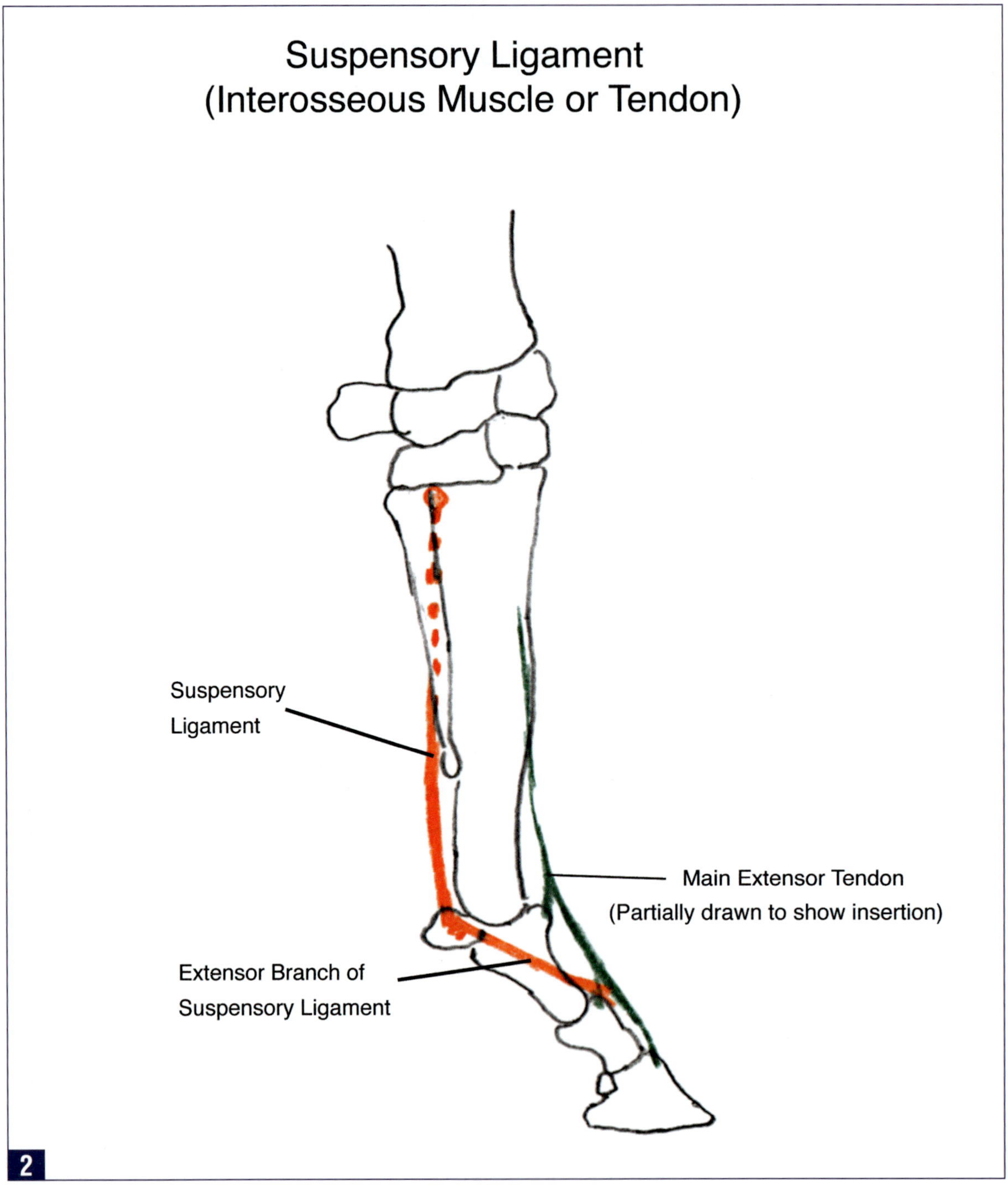

2

tendon. It is a very important ligament in the leg.

2. Ligament of the Ergot (Figure 3)

The ligament of the ergot is a small and insignificant ligament. It originates at the ergot, which is a thickened area of the skin at the back of the fetlock. In some animals, primarily drafts and ponies, the ergot may grow a piece of horn. This horn is similar to the chestnuts that grow out from the inside of the knee and hock, although not as thick. The ligament of the ergot courses dorso-distad and generally inserts into the distal digital annular ligament. It is considered vestigial, which is an anatomical term that means not needed.

It can be difficult to distinguish the ligament of the ergot from nerves when doing a dissection. The ligament of the ergot appears as a thin, white, strong tissue that resembles a nerve, but on careful inspection of the cross section, you will see a difference between the two tissues. To help you identify it, be careful when you remove the skin at the back of the fetlock. The ligament of the ergot will be imbedded in fascia and attached to the skin. If you have been diligent enough, you can follow its course to the distal digital annular ligament.

Ligament of the Ergot

Ergot

Ligament of the Ergot

Distal Digital Annular Ligament

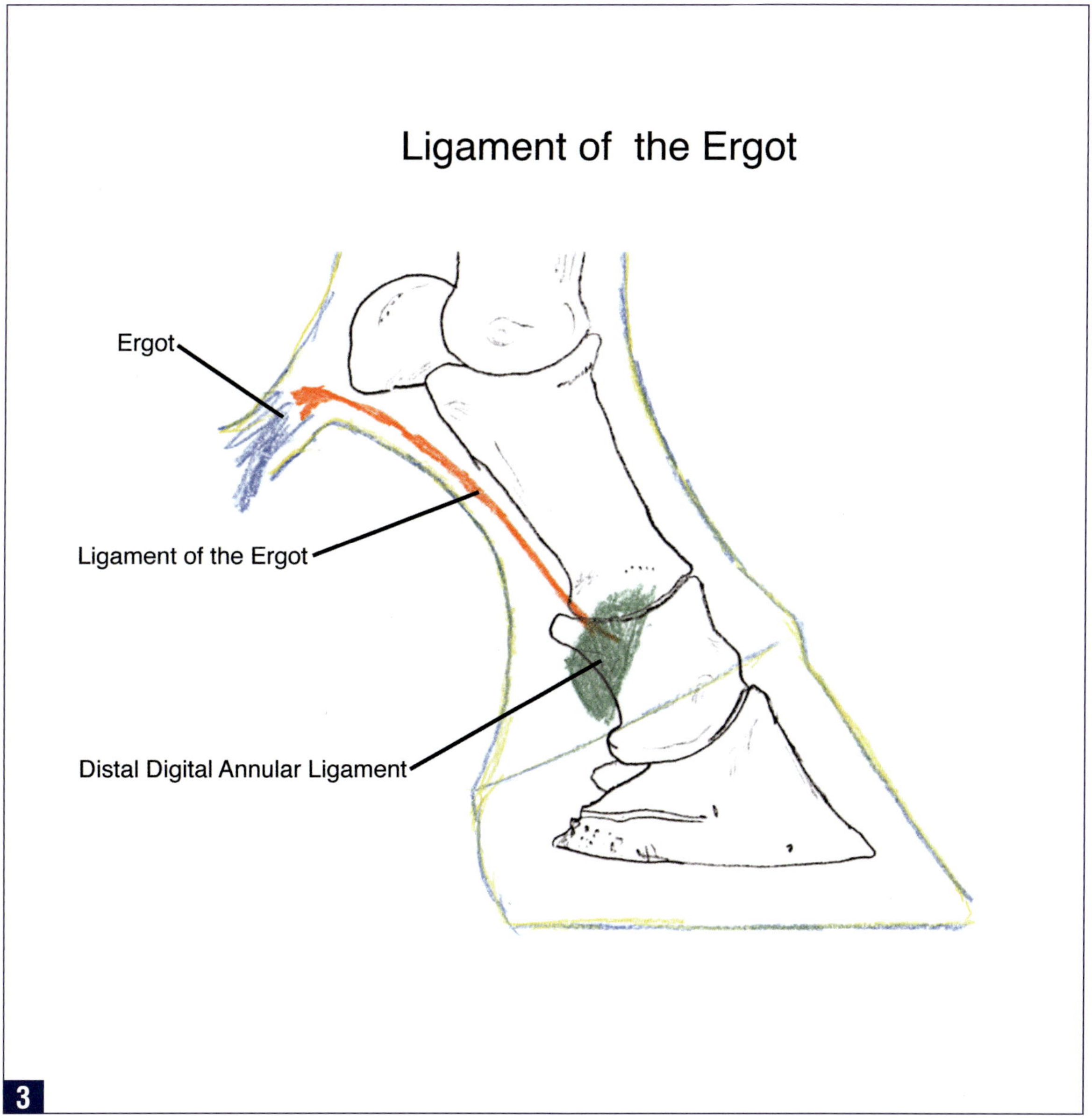

3

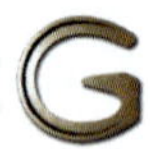

3. Radial (Superior) Check Ligament (Figure 4)

The radial check ligament is on the thoracic limb. It is called superior due to its proximal location when compared to the inferior check ligament, although the inferior check ligament is thicker and stronger. The radial check ligament originates at the radius, about one third of the way from the distal end of the bone. It courses distad inserting into the superficial flexor tendon.

Check Ligaments
Thoracic Limb

Superficial Flexor Tendon

Radial (Superior) Check Ligament

Subcarpal (Inferior) Check Ligament

Deep Flexor Tendon

4

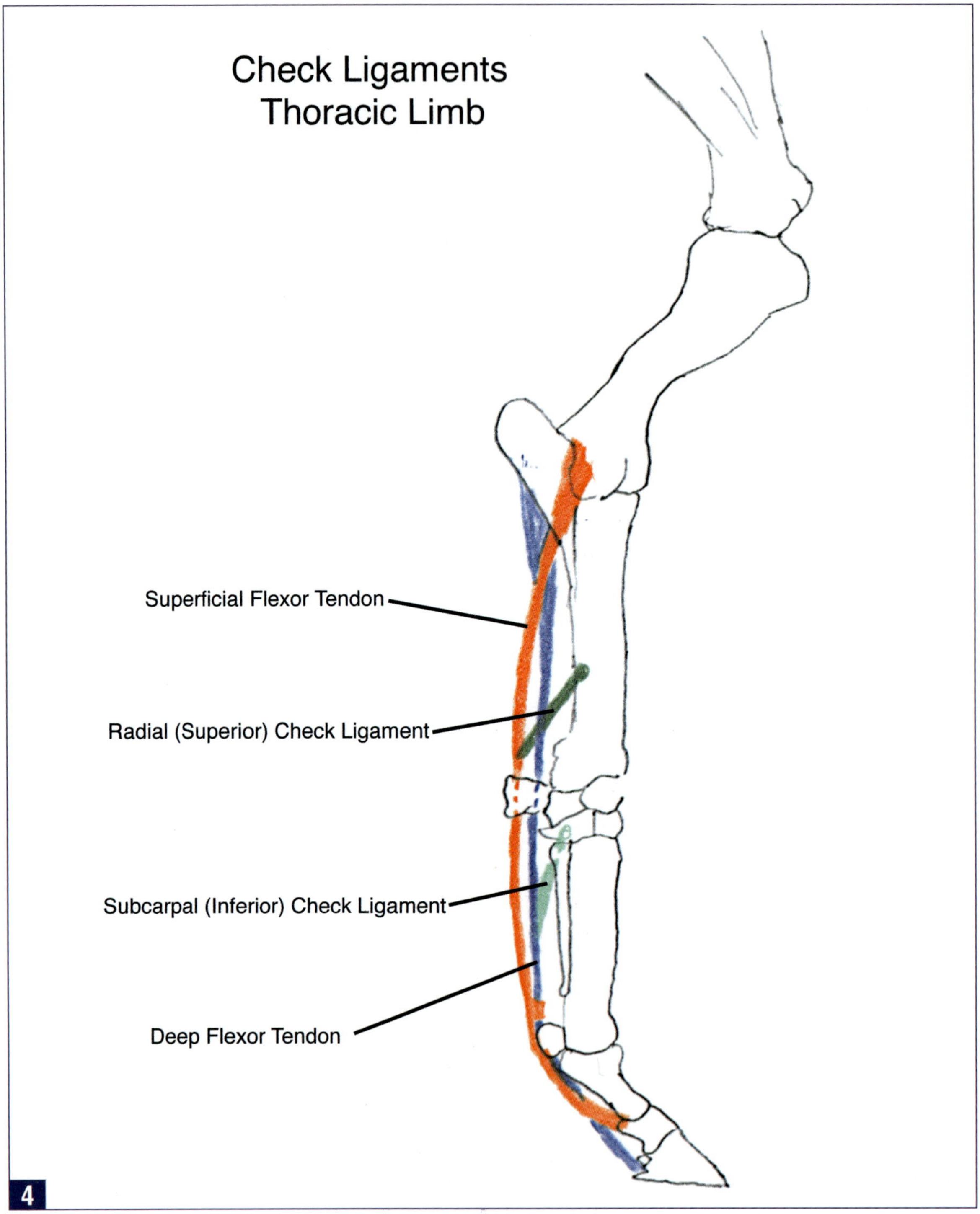

4. Subcarpal (Inferior) Check Ligament (Figure 4)

Found only on the thoracic limb, the subcarpal check ligament originates at the palmar distal row of carpal bones, courses distad, and inserts into the deep flexor tendon. It is called the inferior check ligament because it is located distally to the radial check ligament. This ligament is thick, strong, and is the largest of the check ligaments. When you do a dissection, you can cut across the subcarpal check ligament and the deep flexor tendon to see the difference in the consistency and appearance of the different types of tissue.

5. Subtarsal Check Ligament (Figure 5)

The subtarsal check ligament is found on the pelvic limb. It originates at the plantar distal tarsus, courses distad, and inserts into the deep flexor tendon. The subtarsal check ligament is as thin as a piece of spaghetti and is considered by most to be vestigial. It is sometimes absent in horses and, generally absent in mules.

Check ligaments prevent overstrain on the tendons to which they are attached. Since a ligament does have more elasticity than a tendon, the check ligaments can prevent excessive forces from being applied to the tendons by essentially dampening the blow as the horse bears weight. There is not a check ligament on the superficial flexor tendon of the pelvic limb since it inserts at the calcanean process. Additional support would be redundant.

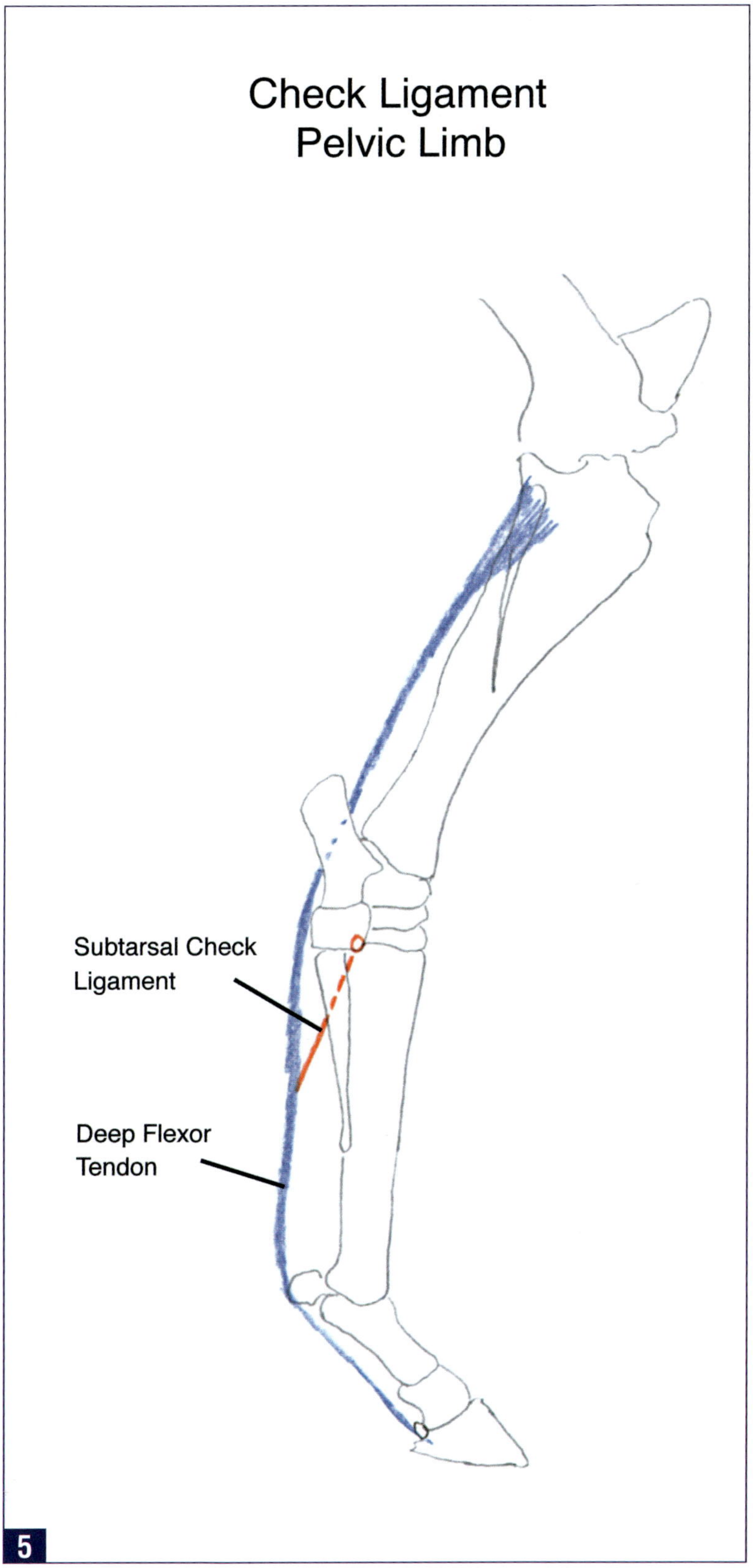

Check Ligament
Pelvic Limb

Subtarsal Check Ligament

Deep Flexor Tendon

5

6. Chondrocompedal Ligament of the Collateral Cartilages (Figure 6)

The chondrocompedal ligament is the most proximal of the ligaments of the collateral cartilages. Originating at distal P1, this ligament courses distad and inserts into the palmar/plantar proximal aspect of the collateral cartilages.

7. Chondrocoronal Ligament of the Collateral Cartilages (Figure 6)

The chondrocoronal ligament originates at the collateral sides of P2, runs diagonally palmar/plantar distad and inserts into the collateral cartilages. This is such a short ligament in an area with a lot of other tissues that it may be difficult to distinguish.

8. Chondrotendinous Ligament of the Collateral Cartilages (Figure 6)

The previous 2 chondro ligaments have connected bone to cartilage. The chondrotendinous ligament horizontally connects the collateral cartilages to the main extensor tendon.

9. Chondroungular Ligament of the Collateral Cartilages (Figure 6)

The chondroungular ligament is the most distal of the ligaments of the collateral cartilages. It attaches the distal border of the collateral cartilages to the coffin bone.

All of the ligaments of the collateral cartilages have a similar function in that they attach to the collateral cartilages to help hold them in position.

Ligaments of the Collateral Cartilages

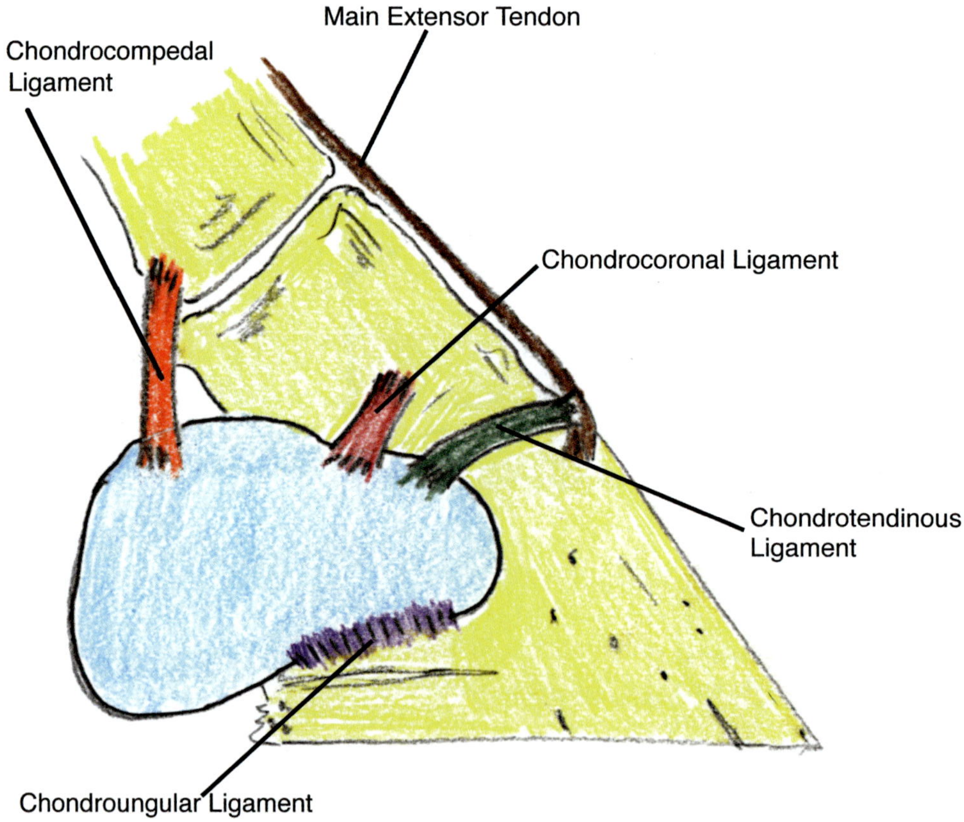

6

10. Transverse Lamina (T Ligament) (Figure 7)

I debated about whether or not to include this structure in this textbook, but decided to go ahead as it is hard to find information about this equine anatomical part. The synovial sheath on the dorsal aspect of the deep flexor tendon extends further than the synovial sheath on the palmar/plantar aspect of the deep flexor tendon. Where the sheath stops, there is the so-called T ligament, which is a band of fibrous tissue that separates the synovial sheath of the deep flexor tendon from the joint capsule of the coffin joint and the navicular (podotrochlear) bursa sac. With this being the case, the T ligament connects tendon-sheath- bone. It is the bit of red tissue that extends from the deep flexor tendon to P2 in diagram 7.

This ligament is referred to as the transverse lamina in anatomical terminology. It is very thin, and appears almost translucent. The deep flexor tendon at this point in the leg has become wide and flat, changing shape dramatically from the mostly round cross section that it has at the proximal cannon bone. From the lateral view of the diagram, it is hard to imagine just how wide it is, but the T ligament is as wide as the deep flexor tendon is in this area.

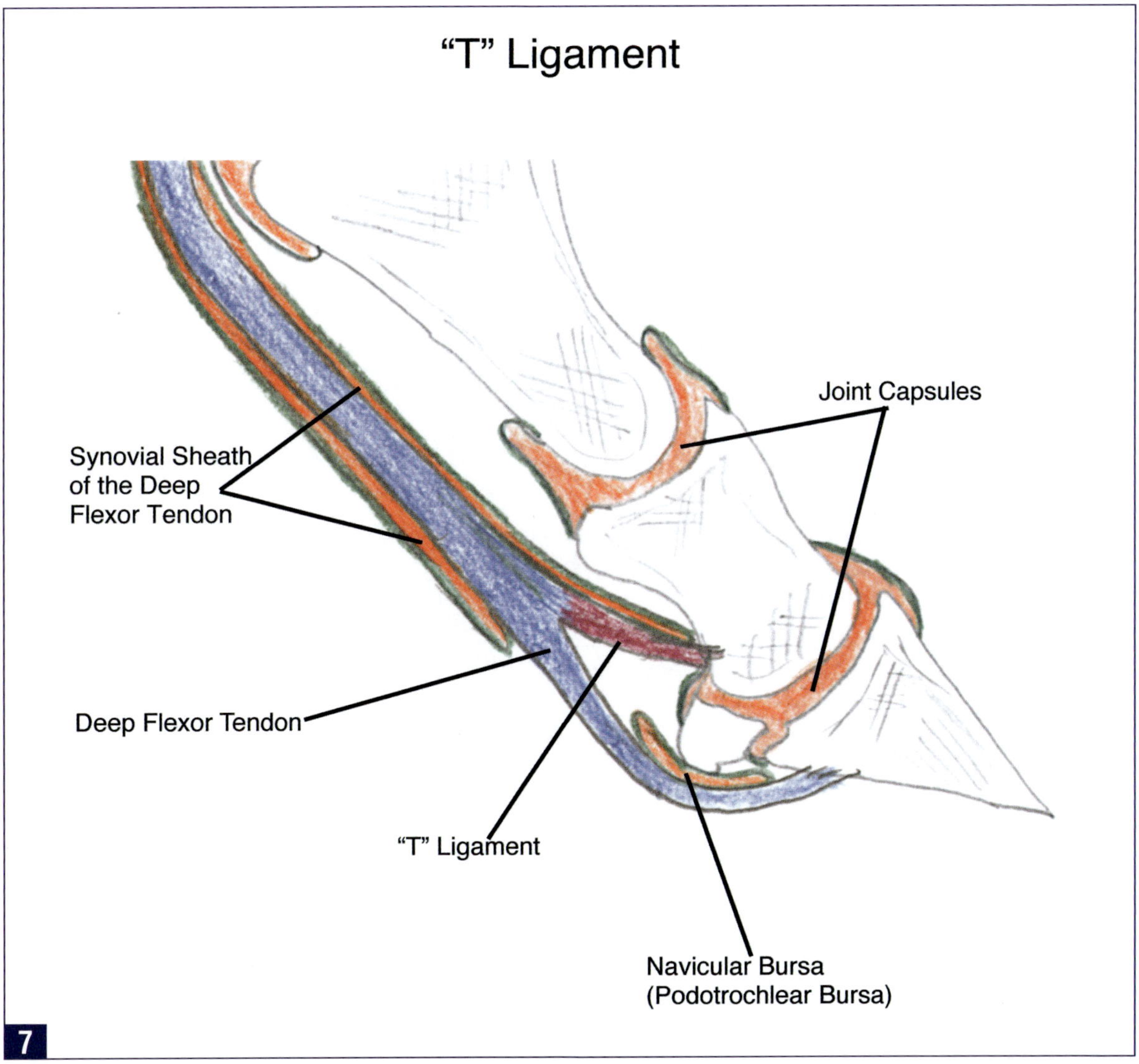

CATEGORY 2. SESAMOIDIAN LIGAMENTS:

1. Superficial (Y or Straight) Sesamoidian Ligament (Figures 8 and 14)

The superficial sesamoidian ligament originates on the distal end of the proximal sesamoids, courses distad and inserts into P2. At the proximal end, you can find fibers that cross each other in such a manner that they resemble a Y. This ligament is mostly covered by the flexor tendons and the proximal digital annular ligament, but it is the most superficial of the sesamoidian ligaments below the fetlock.

The pastern is at an angle to the ground, so there is tremendous pressure on the fetlock joint when the leg bears weight. You can look at the angle of the fetlock joint on the front leg of a standing horse, but when you pick up the leg, it is so strong that you will have difficulty extending it past 180 degrees. The superficial sesamoidian ligament is an important structure that helps to make the angle of the fetlock and position of the pastern so strong. Inserting into the proximal P2, it also makes the pastern joint more rigid and strong and opposes the pull of the suspensory ligament above the fetlock. Beyond that, the superficial sesamoidian ligament provides a good deal of energy return when a horse is moving, and a lot of concussion redirection and absorption.

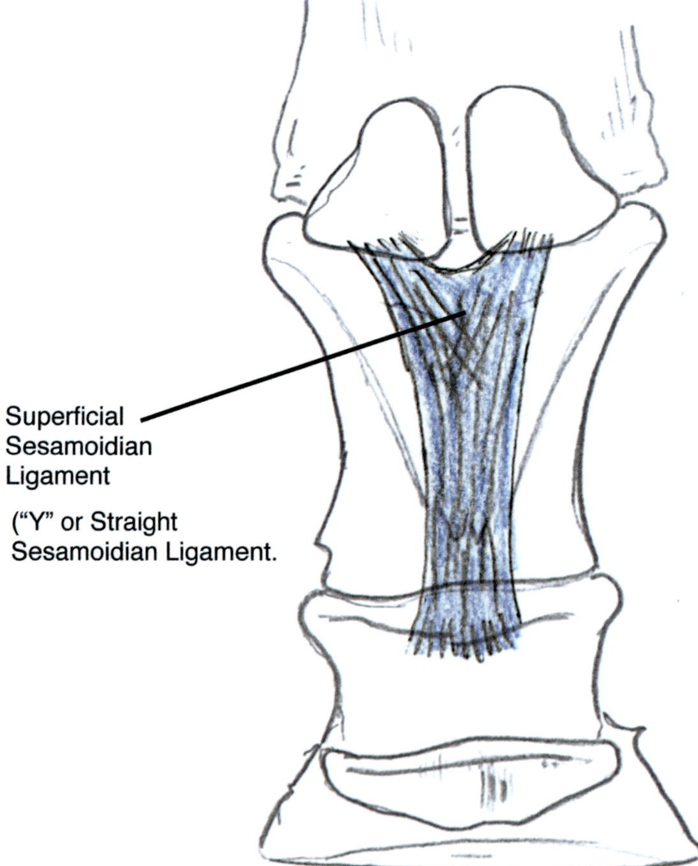

2. Middle (V or Oblique) Sesamoidian Ligament (Figures 9 and 14)

This is a V-shaped sesamoidian ligament that originates at the distal end of the proximal sesamoids, courses distad, and inserts into distal P1. If you look at the palmar/plantar surface of most long pastern bones, you will find that there is a V-shaped ridge. This is the path of the middle sesamoidian ligament, and the rougher the ridge on P1, the greater the amount of adhesions and strain from this ligament.

The middle sesamoidian ligament has a similar role to that of the superficial sesamoidian ligament in that it gives rigidity to the fetlock, provides energy return, redirects and absorbs concussion, and is a major part of allowing the pastern to have the angle that it does. Since it does not descend as far as P2, it does not play a role in the strength of the pastern joint.

Proximally, the sesamoids have the insertion of each branch of the suspensory ligament. I believe that the middle sesamoidian ligament being inserted into each bone the way that it is provides a good opposing ligament pull to that of the suspensory ligament. This is important for the fetlock to be able to deal with uneven terrain and sharp turns when a horse is moving.

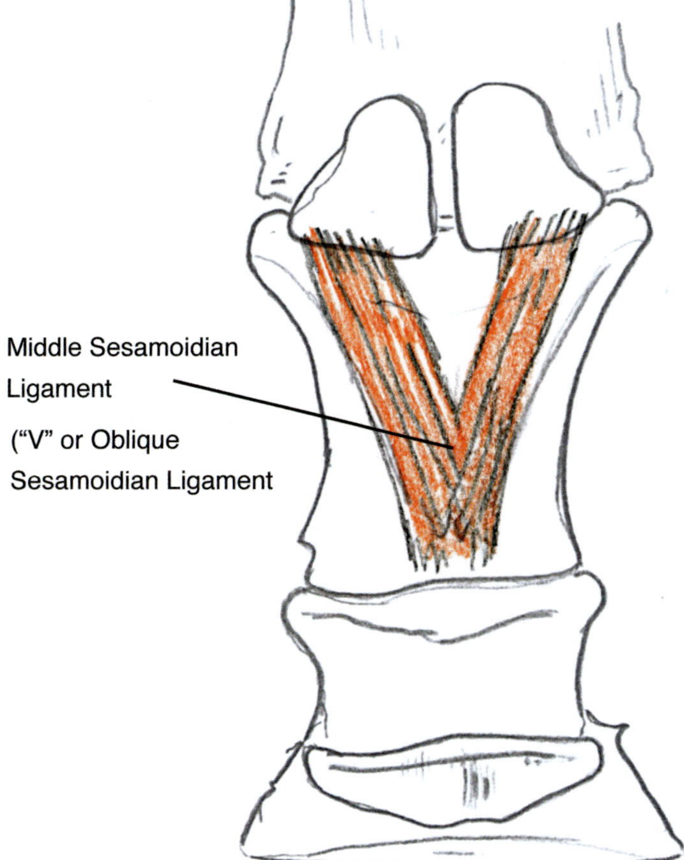

9

3. Deep (X or Cruciate) Sesamoidian Ligament (Figures 10 and 14)

The deep sesamoidian ligament is located below the sesamoids and obliquely joins the distal dorsal border of the sesamoids to proximal P1. These ligaments cross each other, forming the appearance of an X.

The deep sesamoidian ligament can be difficult to find in a dissection. I prefer to cut the collateral sesamoidian ligaments, reflect the sesamoids back by pulling on the suspensory ligament, and find it at the base of the sesamoids in the fetlock joint.

When you look at the deep sesamoidian ligament from that view, you can see that it not only holds the sesamoids dorsal in their position, but also pulls diagonally across the sesamoid bone from the inside corners, and across towards the lateral distal outside corners of the bones. Much like tying down a load on a trailer, if you have the chains pulling straight down from the load to the bed they are not nearly as stable as if they are pulling across the load from corner to corner.

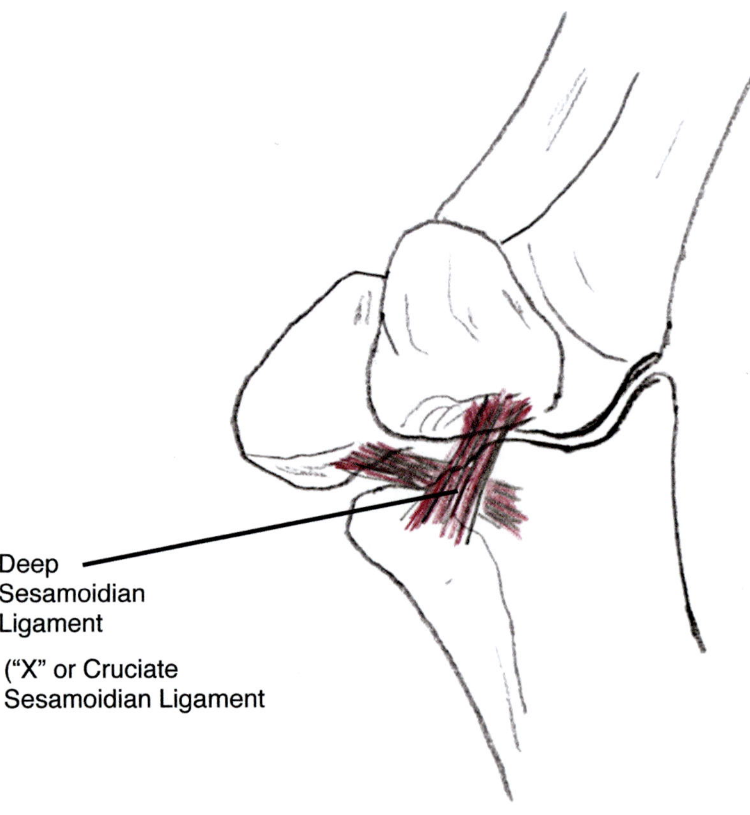

10

4. Short Sesamoidian Ligaments
(Figures 11 and 14)

There are actually two separate of these sesamoidian ligaments, one for each sesamoid bone. They lie to the sides of the deep sesamoidian ligament and connect the distal dorsal border of the sesamoids to proximal P1. When you look at the angle of the deep sesamoidian ligament, it opposes the angle of the short sesamoidian ligaments, which does pull the sesamoids from two different directions. These make the opposing chains for tying down the load as mentioned in the discussion on the deep sesamoidian ligament.

Like the deep sesamoidian ligament, I find it easiest to locate these ligaments by cutting into the fetlock joint and reflecting the sesamoid bones back. Take a rag or paper towel to wipe away the synovial fluid, thrn carefully cut into the bottom of the joint while you pull on the suspensory ligament attached to the sesamoids. You will see the tissue of both the deep sesamoidian ligament and short sesamoidian ligament as you do thid.

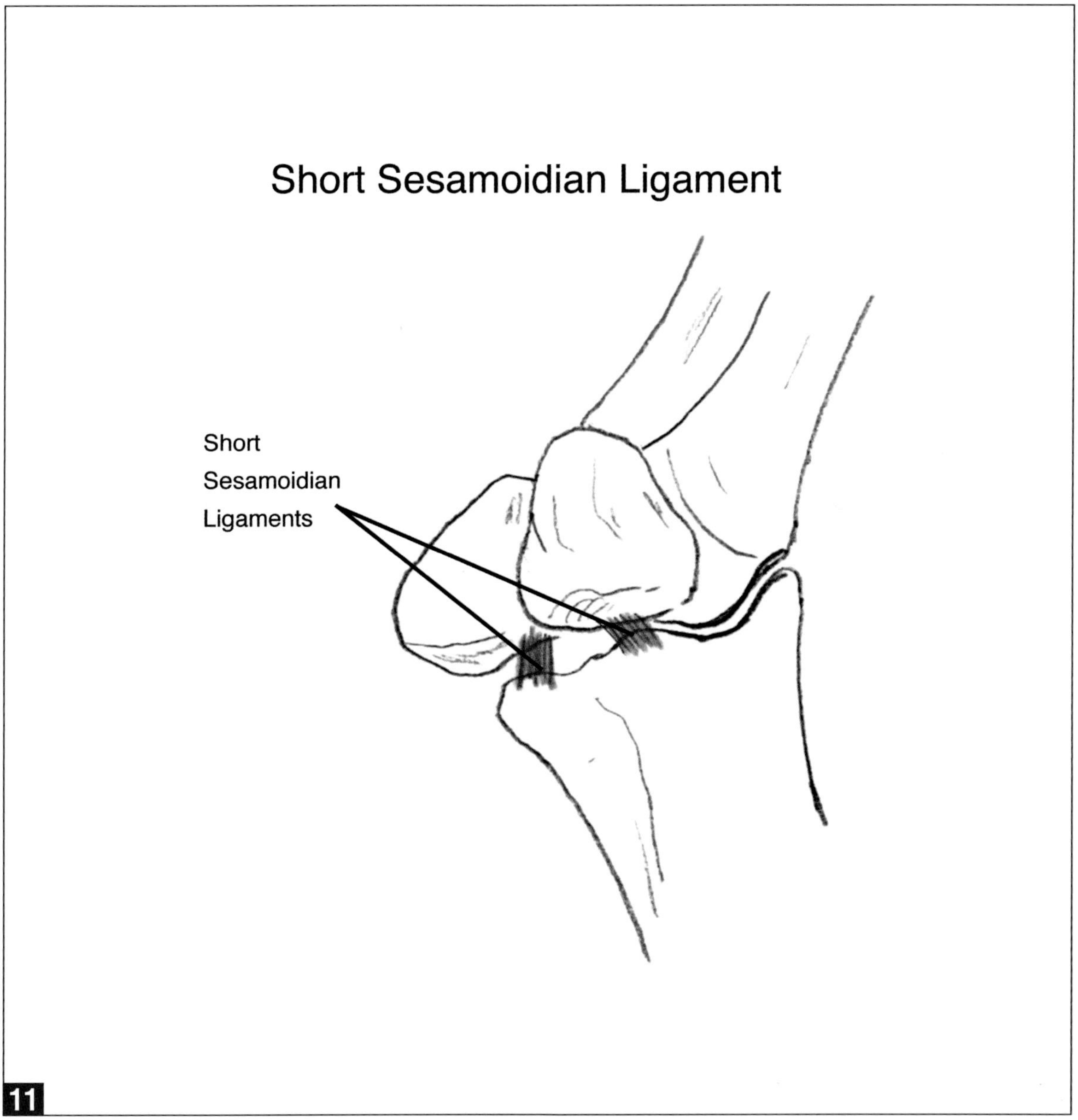

11

5. Intersesamoidian Ligament
(Figures 12 and 14)

The intersesamoidain ligament horizontally attaches the two sesamoid bones at their palmar/ plantar aspect. This ligament forms the groove that the flexor tendons glide over. It is a tough, fibrous ligament. The synovial sheath that surrounds the flexor tendons provides lubrication for the movement over the intersesamoidian ligament.

This is one of those ligaments that does not have a proximal origin and a distal insertion, which makes it difficult to add to the table found at the beginning of this chapter. When you have a ligament that runs horizontally, use terms like attaches, connects or joins.

6. Collateral Sesamoidian Ligaments
(Figures 13 and 14)

Like all collateral ligaments, the collateral sesamoidian ligament is short and attaches to the sides of joint areas. There are two collateral sesamoidian ligaments, one lateral and one medial. They connect the sesamoids to the collateral ligaments of the fetlock and may be considered a part of those ligaments as you can see from the drawing.

The sesamoidian ligaments share in the job of holding the sesamoids in place, giving rigidity to the fetlock, and helping to absorb and dampen concussion when a horse is in motion.

Intersesamoidian Ligament

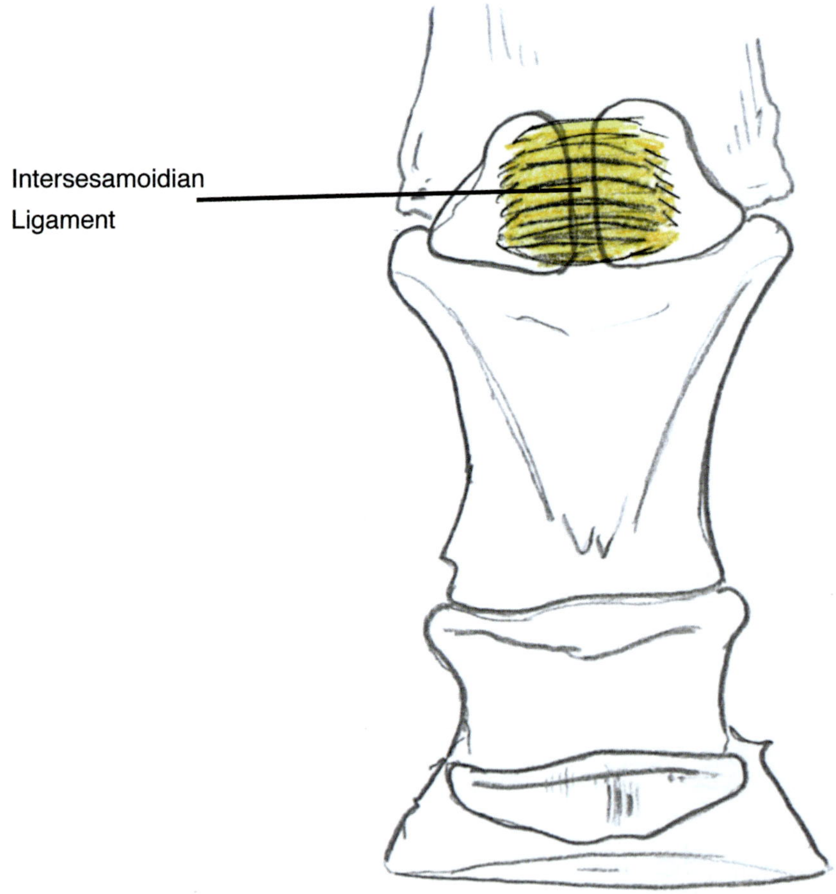

12

Collateral Sesamoidian Ligament

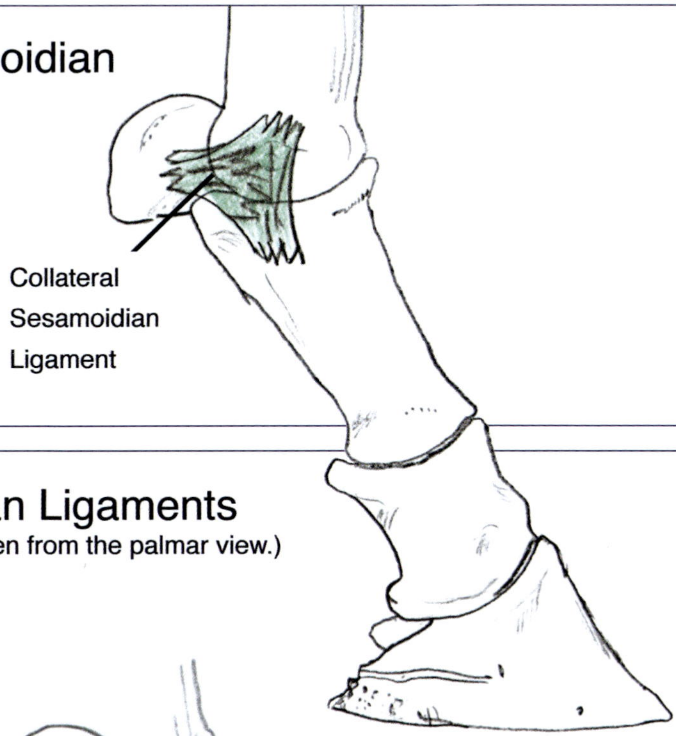

13

Sesamoidian Ligaments

(Those that can be seen from the palmar view.)

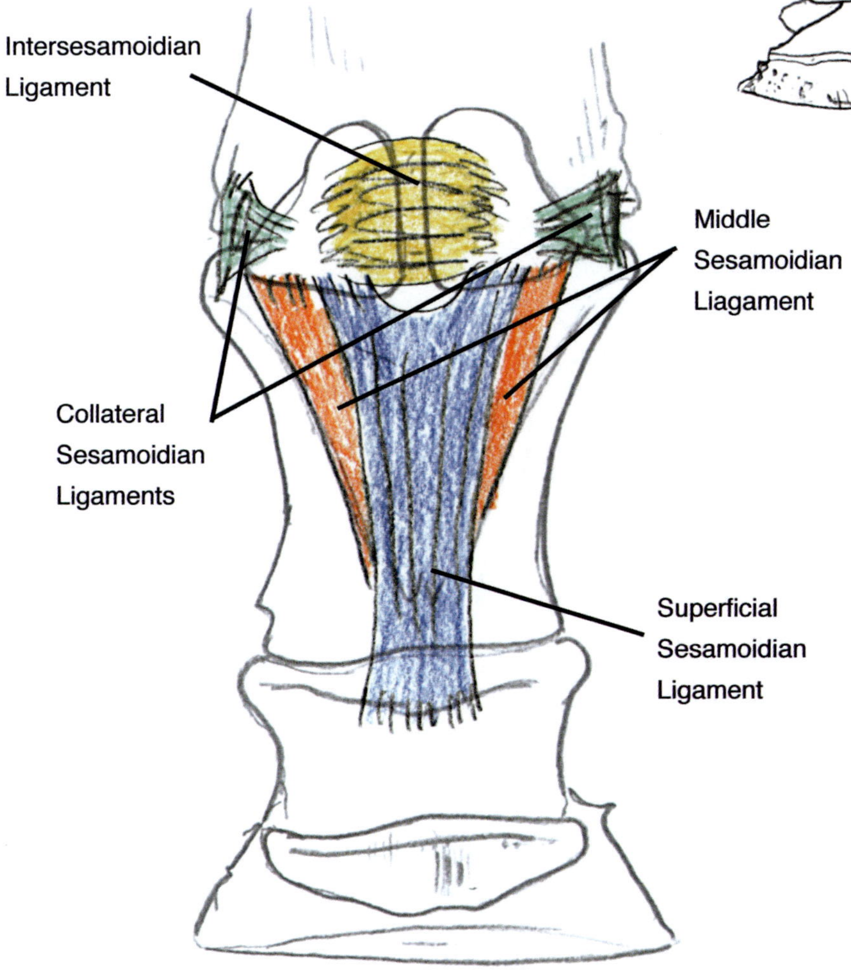

14

CATEGORY 3. ANNULAR LIGAMENTS

1. Palmar/Plantar Annular Ligament (Figure 15)

Being called palmar or plantar, depending on the limb, this annular ligament is located at the distal end of the cannon bone, and covers the sesamoids as well. It is attached to the collateral aspect of the distal cannon bone and wraps around the tendons on the palmar/plantar side of the fetlock joint.

2. Proximal Digital Annular Ligament: (Figure 15)

This used to give me some trouble, having an annular ligament with the word proximal in the name, yet being located beneath another annular ligament. The primary thing to recognize is the word digital. This proximal digital annular ligament is located on the palmar/plantar aspect of P1, and is the most proximal of the annular ligaments in the digit. It resembles the shape of an animal skin, with attachments on the collateral sides of P1 and P2.

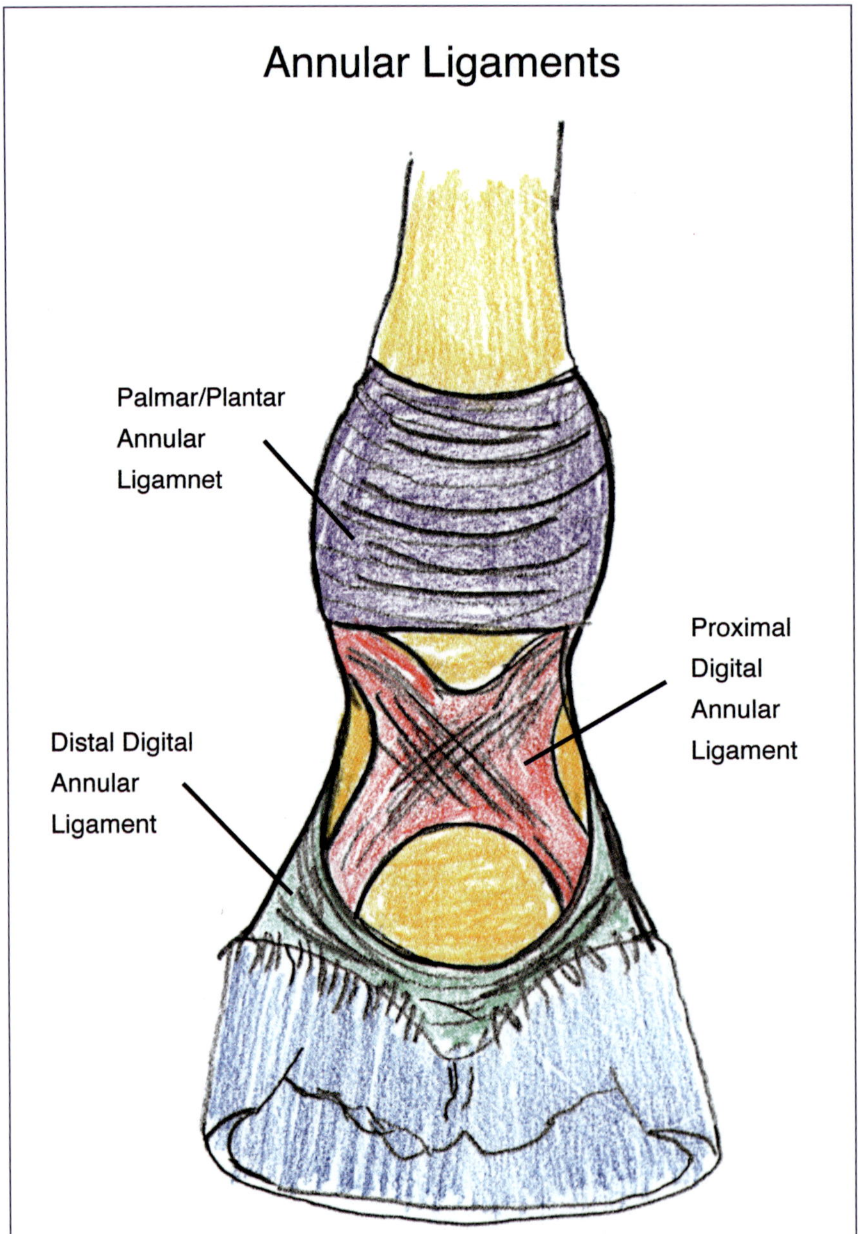

3. Distal Digital Annular Ligament (Figure 15)

Lying distal to the proximal digital annular ligament, the distal digital annular ligament is located around the back of P2. It is attached to the collateral aspect of P2 and P1, and also covers some of the distal portion of the proximal digital annular ligament.

All of the annular ligaments are thin sheets of extremely tough ligament tissue that share in the job of holding the tendons against the bones when the joints are flexed. Try thinking of them as the cable holders that are attached to the frame of a bicycle that hold the cables against the frame when you engage the brakes. This will give you an idea of how these ligaments work. They are also much less elastic than normal ligament tissue. Thinking about their function, it is obvious that if they were elastic, the horse would possess less strength.

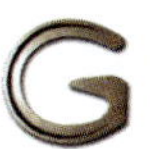

CATEGORY 4. NAVICULAR LIGAMENTS

1. Suspensory Navicular Ligament (Figures 16 – 18)

The suspensory navicular ligament originates collaterally at distal P1, courses distad down both sides of P2, and inserts into the proximal edge of the navicular bone. I often tell my students to think of this particular apparatus as a swing set, with the suspensory navicular ligament acting as the chains,and the navicular bone acting as the seat. You could make the case that P2 is sitting on the swing.

2. Distal (Impar) Navicular Ligament (Figures 16 – 18)

The impar ligament attaches the dorsal distal border of the navicular bone to the coffin bone. The attachment on the coffin bone lies just palmar/plantar to the semilunar crest of P3. This ligament runs pretty much the length of the navicular bone from side to side, but is quite short, as the navicular bone lies right against the coffin bone in this area.

The navicular bone lies in an area at the back of the coffin joint where there is not a lot of room for movement. The navicular ligaments hold the

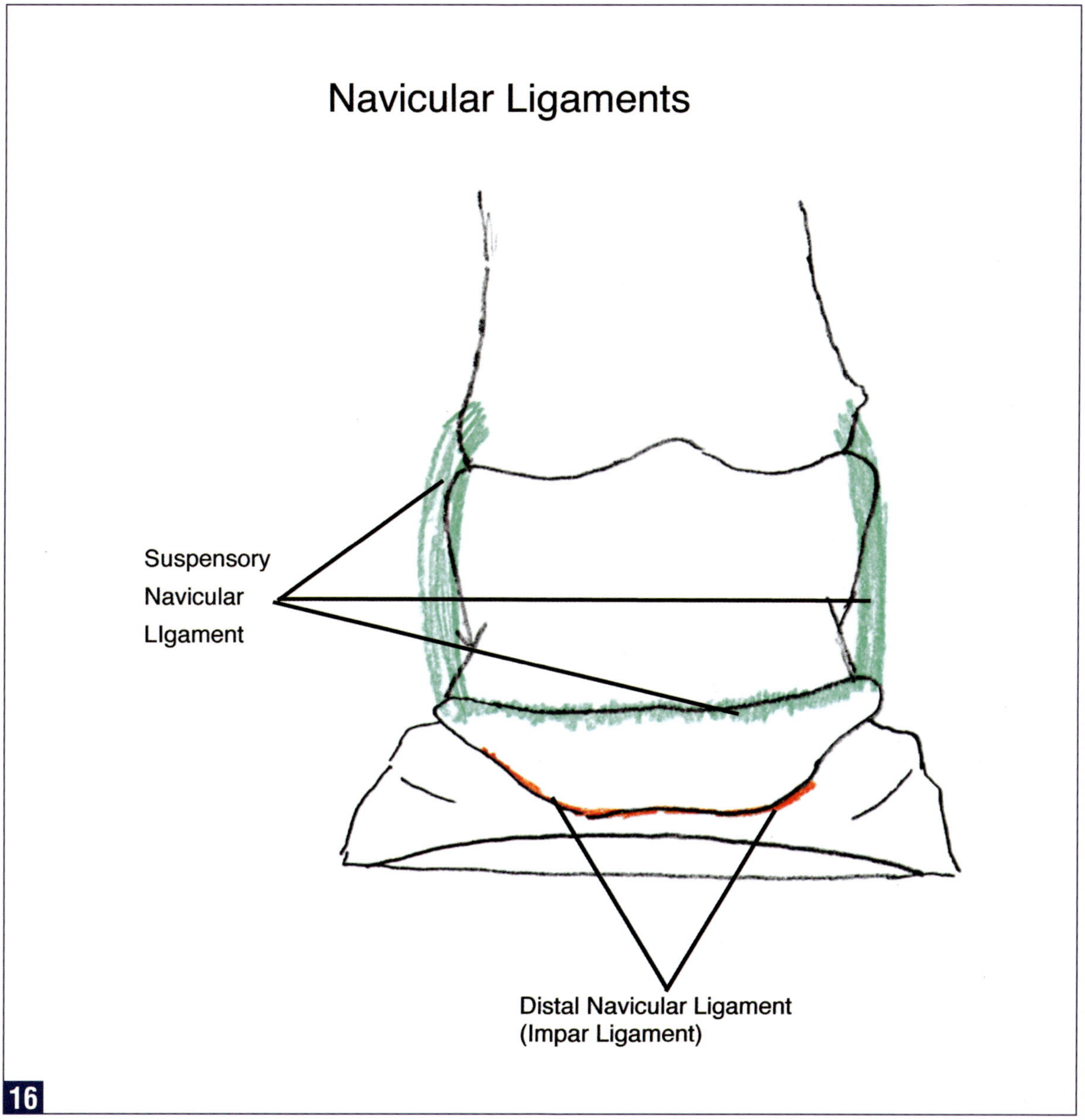

Navicular Ligaments

Suspensory Navicular LIgament

Distal Navicular Ligament (Impar Ligament)

16

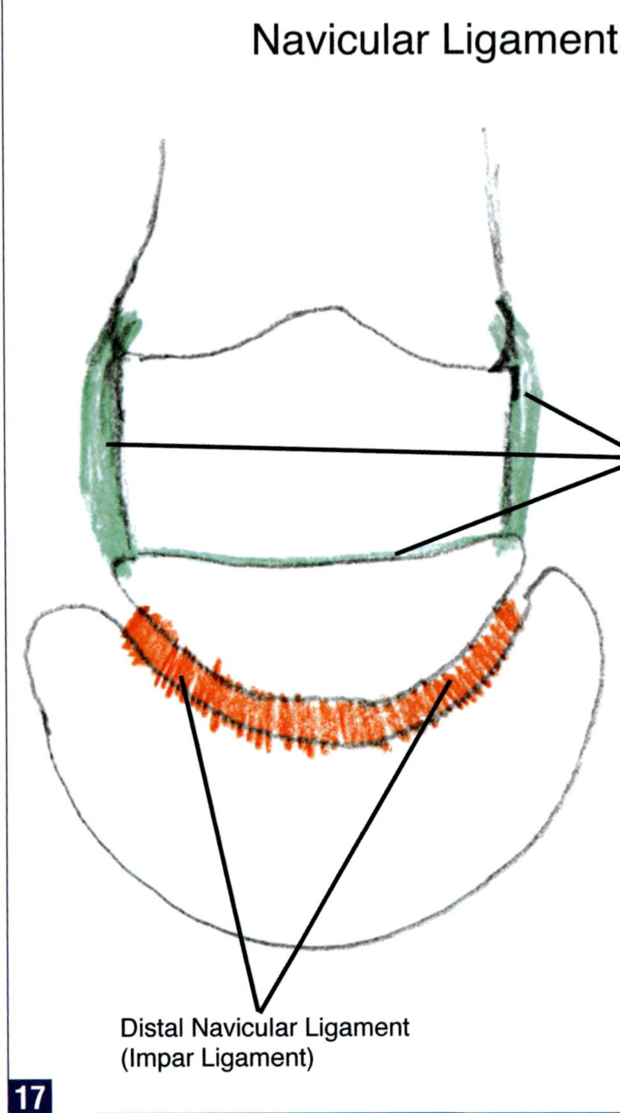

17

navicular bone in this position, and their elasticity helps to dampen the shock that the navicular bone suffers. The suspensory navicular ligament aids in absorbing the downward concussion from the boney column above, and the impar ligament aids in absorbing the strain as the fetlock descends and the horse moves over the foot into the end of the stance phase of the stride.

Navicular Ligaments

Suspensory
Navicular
Ligament

Distal Navicular Ligament
(Impar Ligament)

18

CATEGORY 5. PASTERN LIGAMENTS

1. Axial Pastern Ligaments (Figure 19)

The axial pastern ligaments originate at palmar/plantar distal P1, and insert into palmar/plantar proximal P2. There are two of these short ligaments, and they are located closer to the middle of the pastern than the abaxial pastern ligaments. That is why they are known as axial pastern ligaments.

2. Abaxial Pastern Ligaments (Figure 19)

Much like the axial pastern ligaments, the abaxial pastern ligaments originate at the palmar/plantar aspect of P1, and insert at palmar/plantar P2. Being further from the middle of the pastern is why they are known as abaxial.

The pastern joint has to be extremely strong to withstand the pressures and shock of normal use. The pastern ligaments are just part of the overall system that aids in making the pastern joint so strong and durable. They help to absorb shock when the leg is loaded and are essential in keeping the palmar/plantar portion of the pastern joint strong.

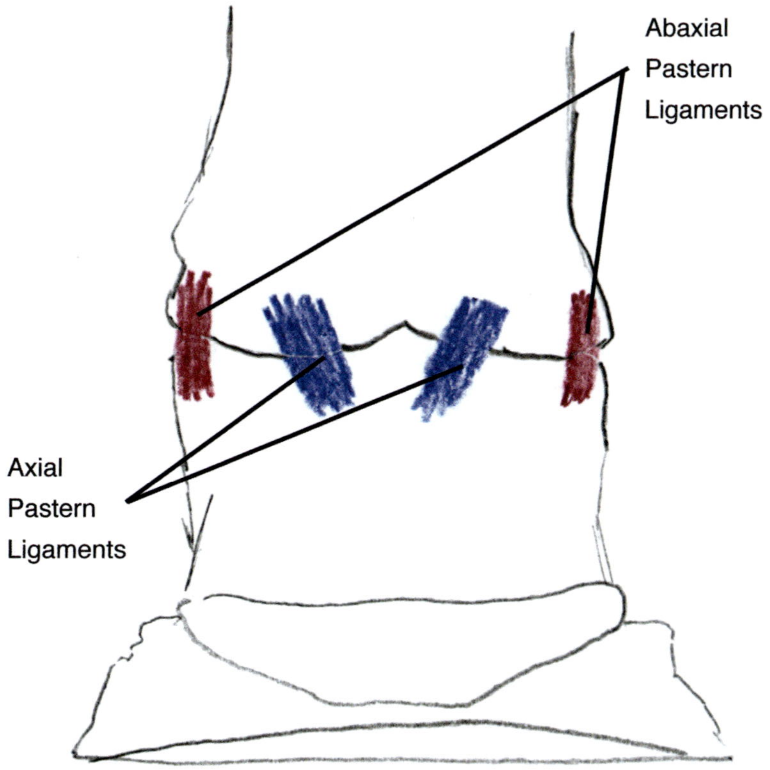

19

CATEGORY 6. LIGAMENTS THAT DON'T FIT INTO A CATEGORY

1. Interosseus Ligaments of the Splint Bones (Figure 20)

Where the splint bones lie against the cannon bone, there is a layer of ligament tissue known as the interosseus ligaments. This can be considered a ligamentous joint since there are two bones coming together, but there is not articular cartilage, synovial fluid or movement. I had often been told that these ligaments would ossify (turn to bone) when a horse was around 6 years old, but I have found many instances where even an older horse still had the splint bones separate from the cannon bone when the legs were dissected and the bones boiled. Their function is to allow for independent growth of all three metacarpal/metatarsal bones as well as aid in shock absorption as the splint bones bear some weight from the carpal and tarsal bones above.

Interosseus Ligaments

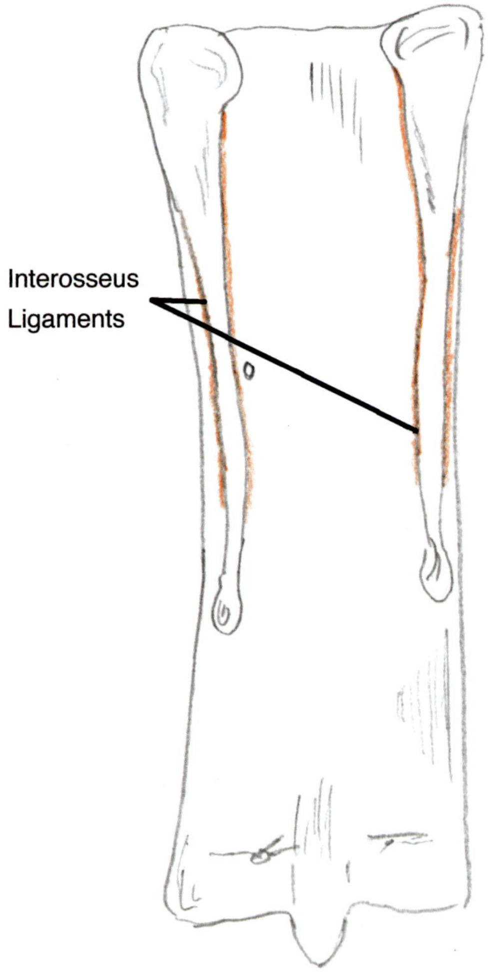

20

2. Plantar Ligament (Figure 21)

As the name would indicate, the plantar ligament is found only on the hind limb. It originates at the calcaneus, just below the calcanean process where the superficial flexor tendon inserts. Coursing distad, the plantar ligament inserts into the fourth tarsal and the fourth metatarsal. If you study the plantar aspect of the calcaneus, you can see a ridge that indicates where the plantar ligament is positioned. The primary function of the plantar ligament is to aid in the rigidity of the hock. It also provides energy return as the horse moves forward and extends the pelvic limb.

When you examine the calcaneus bone of a bone model, you will see that the entire course of the plantar ligament is rough. This roughened area is an indication of tissue attachment to a bone, so the plantar ligament is going to have small attachments where it is in contact with the calcaneus. In some cases you will find a lot of roughness, indicating excessive strain on the plantar ligament.

Horses that are sickle hocked are prone to sprain this ligament, causing a condition known as curb. The plantar ligament will swell about 4 inches below the point of the hock, and it will end up being a blemish when it heals.

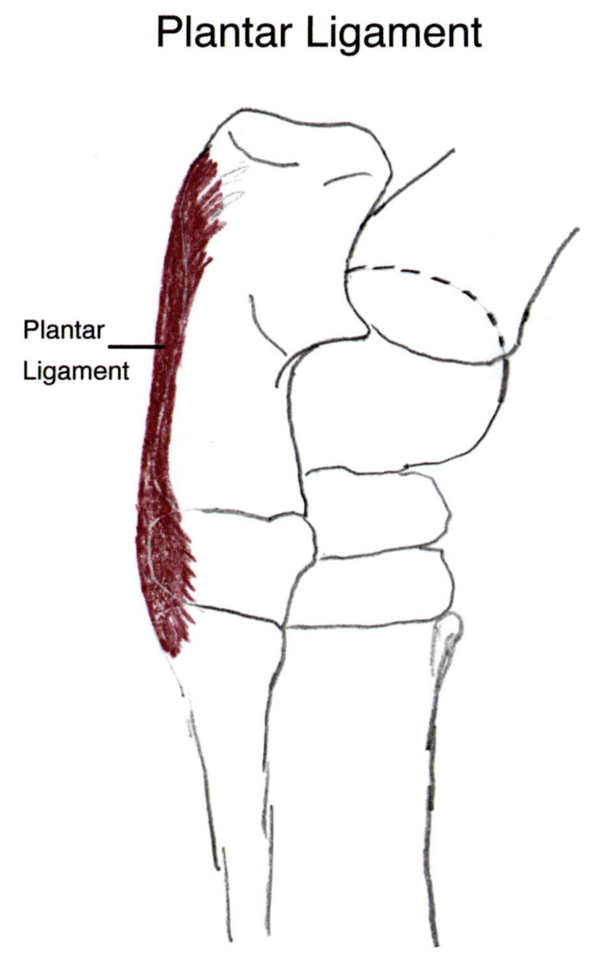

Plantar Ligament

Plantar Ligament

21

3. Capsular Ligaments (Figure 22)

Capsular ligaments are often mistakenly referred to as joint capsules. However, the capsular ligaments are just the thickened portions of the fibrous membrane surrounding a synovial joint. They have a tough, fibrous structure that surrounds synovial joints, but there is more to the joint capsule than just the ligamentous portion. There is an inner membrane known as the synovial membrane, and it produces synovial fluid.

Synovial fluid can be considered a joint oil or lubricant. It has a yolk-like consistency and has a primary function of reducing friction in the articular joints during movement. Synovial fluid is composed of hylauronic acid, lubricin, proteinases, and colleganases. It fills all empty space within the joint capsule and does not flow like normal fluid.

It is important to understand that Figure 22 is a sagital cross-section of the bones. You are seeing the middle of the bones as they would appear if they had been cut with a band saw. The joint capsule is easily defined when looking at this view.

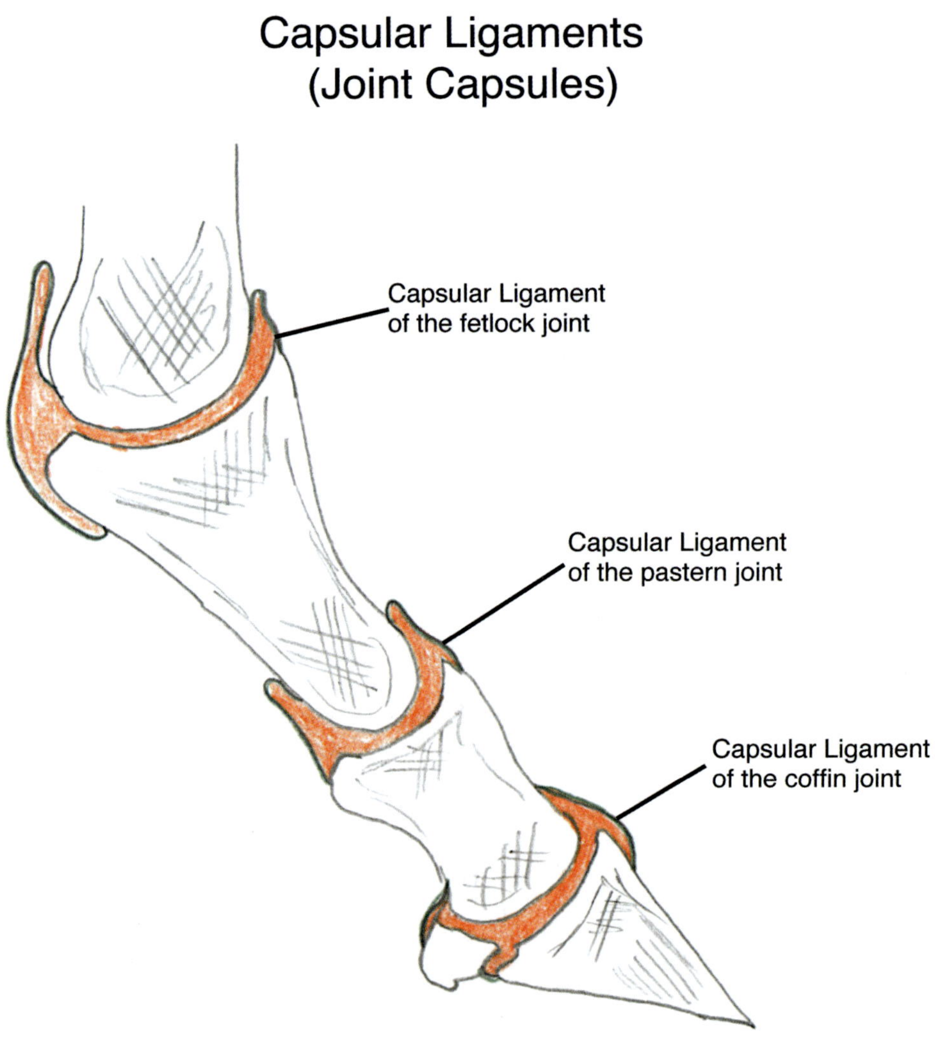

22

4. Collateral Ligaments (Figure 23)

Collateral ligaments are short ligaments that are found on the sides of many synovial joints. They do have connections to the capsular ligaments. We have already identified a couple (collateral sesamoidian ligaments), but there are several others that can be individually identified. For instance, there are the medial collateral ligaments of the coffin, pastern and fetlock joints, and the lateral collateral ligaments of the coffin, pastern, and fetlock joints. These ligaments are short, strong, cordlike tissue that helps to hold the joints together.

They are called collateral because they are found on both sides of the joints. These ligaments are crucial in allowing a horse to negotiate uneven terrain. Every time a foot lands on a slope from medial to lateral, one side of the leg is going to experience different forces than the other. When this happens, the strength and elasticity of the collateral ligaments allow the horse to continue without injury. These ligaments are also positioned in such a manner that they are more perpendicular to the ground than parallel to the bones of the pastern.

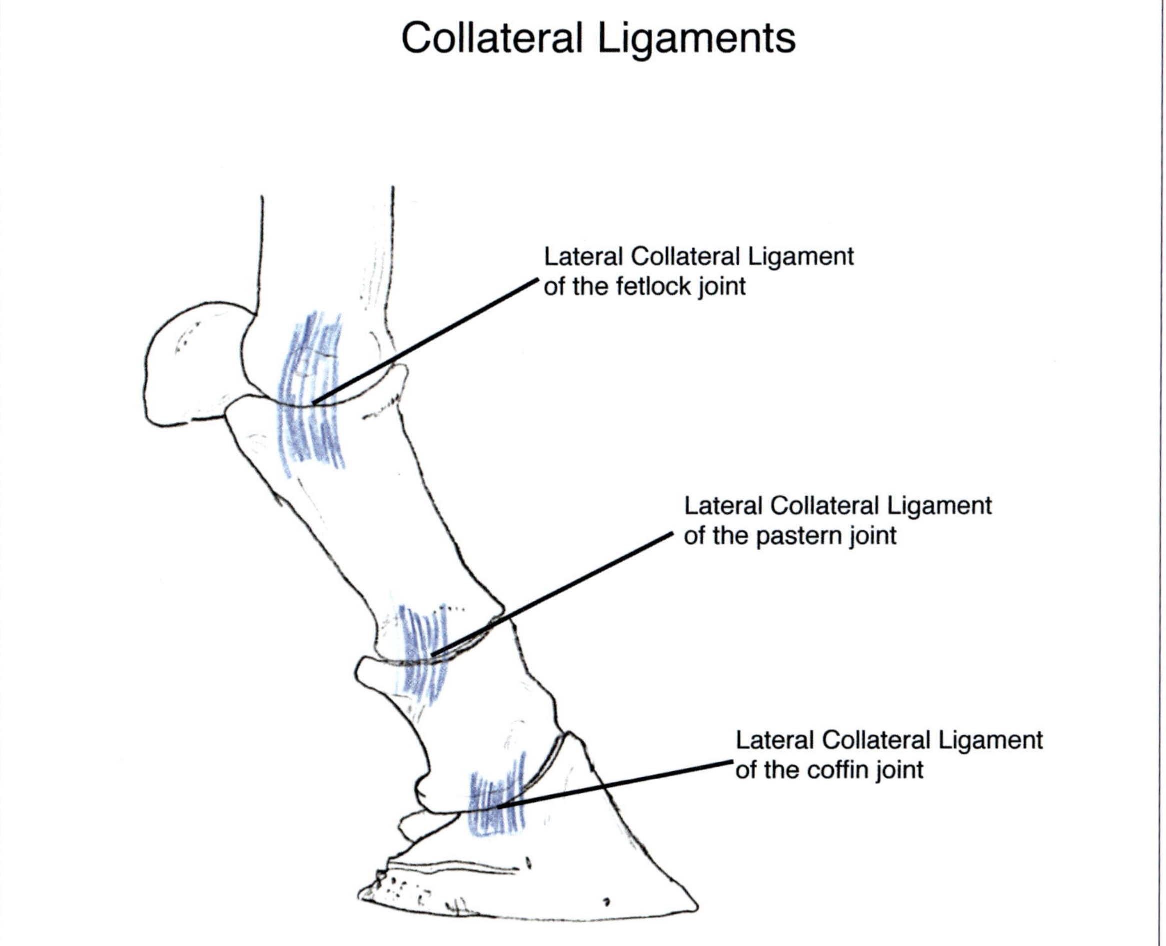

Collateral Ligaments

Lateral Collateral Ligament
of the fetlock joint

Lateral Collateral Ligament
of the pastern joint

Lateral Collateral Ligament
of the coffin joint

23

TENDONS OF THE LOWER LIMBS

The leg can be compared to a puppet when trying to describe to a customer how the anatomy works to move a horse. The bones are the main parts of the puppet, the ligaments hold the parts together, the tendons are the puppet strings, and the muscles are the puppet-master. As a muscle contracts, it pulls on a tendon, which exerts force on the bones, and this results in movement. The ligaments are there to support during load and hold together during motion.

I know that this an oversimplified view since there is a lot going on, but it is a description that can be used when explaining to folks that don't have an extensive anatomical background. You will hear that there are no muscles below the knee or hock, and as stated earlier, that is not quite the truth. There are muscular walled arteries as well as muscle tissue in the suspensory ligament, (interosseus tendon, interosseus muscle) however, the bulk of the muscle for movement is above the actual leg.

The tendons that insert into the digit are all named after the muscles that they originate from. The muscles themselves are attached to bones in the upper limb, and the tendons originate from the bottom of these muscles to insert below the fetlock. We are primarily concerned with four of these tendons. There are two on the dorsal aspect of the leg that are known as extensor tendons. Their job is to extend the leg, and these are not part of the weight-bearing structures. On the palmar/plantar aspect of the leg, are the flexor tendons. These tendons exert pull on the legs to cause propulsion, and they also are a major part of the weight-bearing system.

The properties of tendons are that they are designed to move the body, they are highly inelastic, (not totally inelastic), they glide in lubricated sheaths called synovial sheaths, and for the most part, they connect muscle to bone.

Let us cover each tendon in turn to understand where it originates and inserts, and how it works to move the horse. As I have endeavored to learn anatomy, I have often wanted to find a source that was simple and straightforward with the primary information that I was after. This part of the book is a result of my inability to find what I was after. As such, there are origins, adhesions, and attachments that are described and defined in detail that are beyond the scope of this work. What is presented here is the main information that I want my students to have when they are headed out to shoe horses for a living.

THORACIC LIMB (Figure 24)

Lateral Extensor Tendon The lateral extensor muscle originates primarily from the lateral side of the proximal radius, with some attachment to the collateral ligament of the elbow joint and the body of the ulna. The lateral extensor tendon is a pretty small and thin tendon that originates from the lateral extensor muscle, courses distad to the lateral side of the main extensor tendon, and inserts into the lateral, proximal aspect of P1. This tendon aids in extending the leg when the horse wants to bring the leg forward.

Main Extensor Tendon The main extensor tendon is the largest of the extensor tendons and is often called the common extensor tendon on the thoracic limb. The main extensor muscle has its primary origin from the lateral epicondyle of the humerus. The main extensor tendon originates from the main extensor muscle, courses distad on the lateral side of the limb and ends up at the dorsal aspect of the lower leg where it inserts into proximal P1, proximal P2, and the extensor process on the dorsal proximal area of P3. Like the name would indicate, the main extensor tendon is primarily involved with extending the leg.

Superficial Flexor Tendon: There are two primary flexor tendons that descend into the digit, so you will often see the word digital added to the superficial flexor and deep flexor tendon, i.e. Superficial digital flexor tendon. The superficial flexor muscle originates from the distal end of the humerus. The superficial flexor tendon originates from the superficial flexor muscle, courses distad, palmar to the deep flexor tendon, forms a ring around the deep flexor just proximal to the sesamoids, and bifurcates below the fetlock. At this point, the two branches that arise from the bifurcation will pass around both sides of the deep flexor tendon and insert into collateral distal P1 and collateral proximal P2. The insertions at distal P1 are such that the superficial flexor tendon and the tissue from the proximal digital annular ligament cannot be distinguished from each other. However, even if the tissue from the superficial flexor tendon were to merge with the tissue of the proximal digital annular ligament, it is still ending up attached to collateral distal P1. Because of this, I maintain that the traditional teachings of the P1 insertions are accurate.

I know this sounds confusing at first, but with

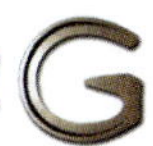

Tendons of the Thoracic Limb

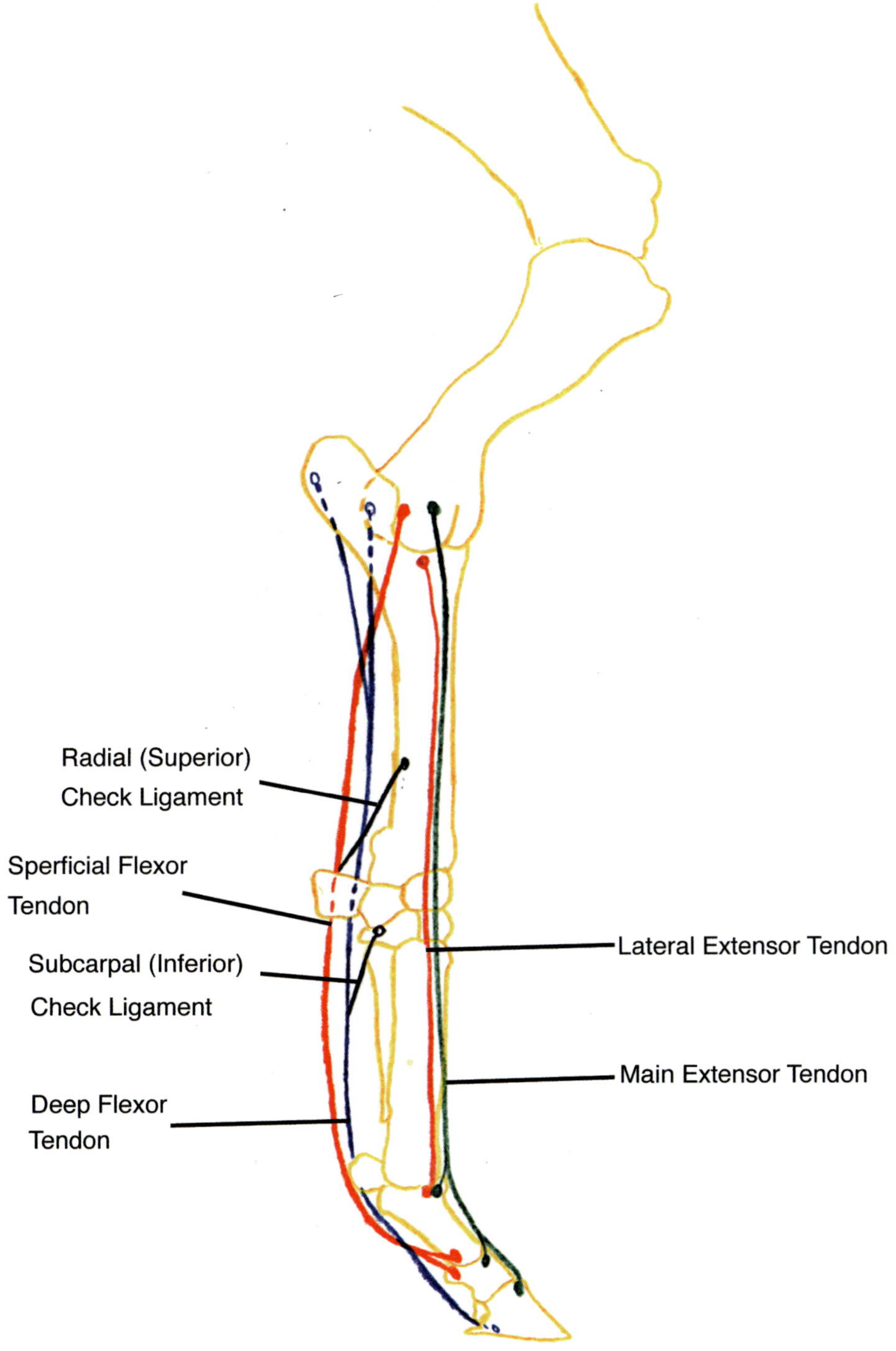

24

study it will seem pretty simple. The superficial flexor tendon actually has four insertions at the pastern joint, but many think there are only two from looking at a two dimensional drawing. Remember, the medial side will look the same.

The superficial flexor tendon flexes the leg to help propel the horse, and it is called superficial due being so close to the skin. It is also a major part of the stay apparatus, energy storage and return, and weight bearing system of the thoracic limb.

Deep Flexor Tendon: The deep flexor muscle on the thoracic limb originates from the medial epicondyle of the humerus and the ulna. The deep flexor tendon originates from the deep flexor muscle, courses distad around the sesamoids and navicular bone, and inserts into the semilunar crest on the solar surface of P3. The semilunar crest is so named because it has the shape of a partial moon. The deep flexor lies under (deep) the superficial flexor tendon until the bifurcation below the fetlock where the deep flexor becomes quite close to the skin. Like the superficial flexor tendon, the deep flexor is primarily involved in the stay apparatus, weight bearing, energy storage and return, and flexing the leg to propel the horse.

PELVIC LIMB (Figure 25)

Lateral Extensor Tendon: On the pelvic limb, there is a substantial difference between the insertion points for the lateral extensor tendon. The lateral extensor muscle primarily originates from the proximal lateral tibia, with the lateral extensor tendon inserting into the main extensor tendon (long extensor tendon) about one third of the way down the cannon bone.

One of the characteristics of a tendon is that it connects muscle to bone. This tendon is an exception to that rule. I have had the experience of a few hind leg dissections where the lateral extensor tendon appears to descend all the way to proximal P1, but even in these instances, it contacts the main extensor tendon where it normally inserts, and runs directly against it all the way down. The lateral extensor tendon aids in extending the hind foot, but actually aids in flexing the hock. This does cause some confusion due to the name of the tendon (extensor), but the leg is extending forward as the hock flexes.

Main Extensor Tendon In the hind limb, the main extensor tendon is often referred to as the long extensor tendon. The name main extensor can be applied to both the front and hind, while the names common extensor for the front and long extensor for the hind is a way to designate the difference. The main extensor muscle originates from the extensor fossa at the distal end of the femur. The main extensor tendon originates from the main extensor muscle, courses distad and inserts into proximal P1, proximal P2, and the extensor process of P3. This is similar to the insertion points on the thoracic limb. The main extensor tendon aids in extending the stifle and foot, as well as flexing the hock.

Superficial Flexor Tendon With the pelvic limb being such a big motor for propulsion, the flexor muscles are quite large and strong. The superficial flexor muscle originates on the supracondyloid fossa of the femur. The superficial flexor tendon originates at the superficial flexor muscle, courses distad and has its first insertion at the calcanean process. This is an area at the plantar, proximal aspect of the calcaneus (fibular tarsal), also known as the point of the hock. From here down, it is similar to what you have already learned about on the front limb. The superficial flexor tendon forms a ring around the deep flexor proximal to the fetlock, bifurcates below the fetlock, and inserts collaterally on distal P1, and collaterally on proximal P2. The superficial flexor tendon flexes the digit and extends the hock.

Deep Flexor Tendon When you study the deep flexor of the pelvic limb, there are several muscles that are part of the system that the deep flexor tendon arises from. To keep it simple, we will say that the deep flexor muscle originates from the proximal tibia and fibula. The deep flexor tendon originates from the deep flexor muscle, courses distad and inserts in the semilunar crest of P3. In the hock, the deep flexor passes to the dorsal medial aspect of the calcaneus, but it is similar to the deep flexor in the thoracic limb when talking about insertion points. Like the superficial flexor tendon, it flexes the foot while extending the hock. Both flexor tendons on the hind limb play a major part in bearing weight and energy storage and return.

While this is not a complete anatomy lesson, the information presented here will help you understand more fully what exactly you are doing to a horse when you trim and shoe it. It will also build a foundation to understand movement, conformation, and pathology when we get to there. Learn this well so that you can add your name to the list of great farriers before you.

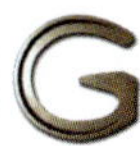

Tendons of the Pelvic Limb

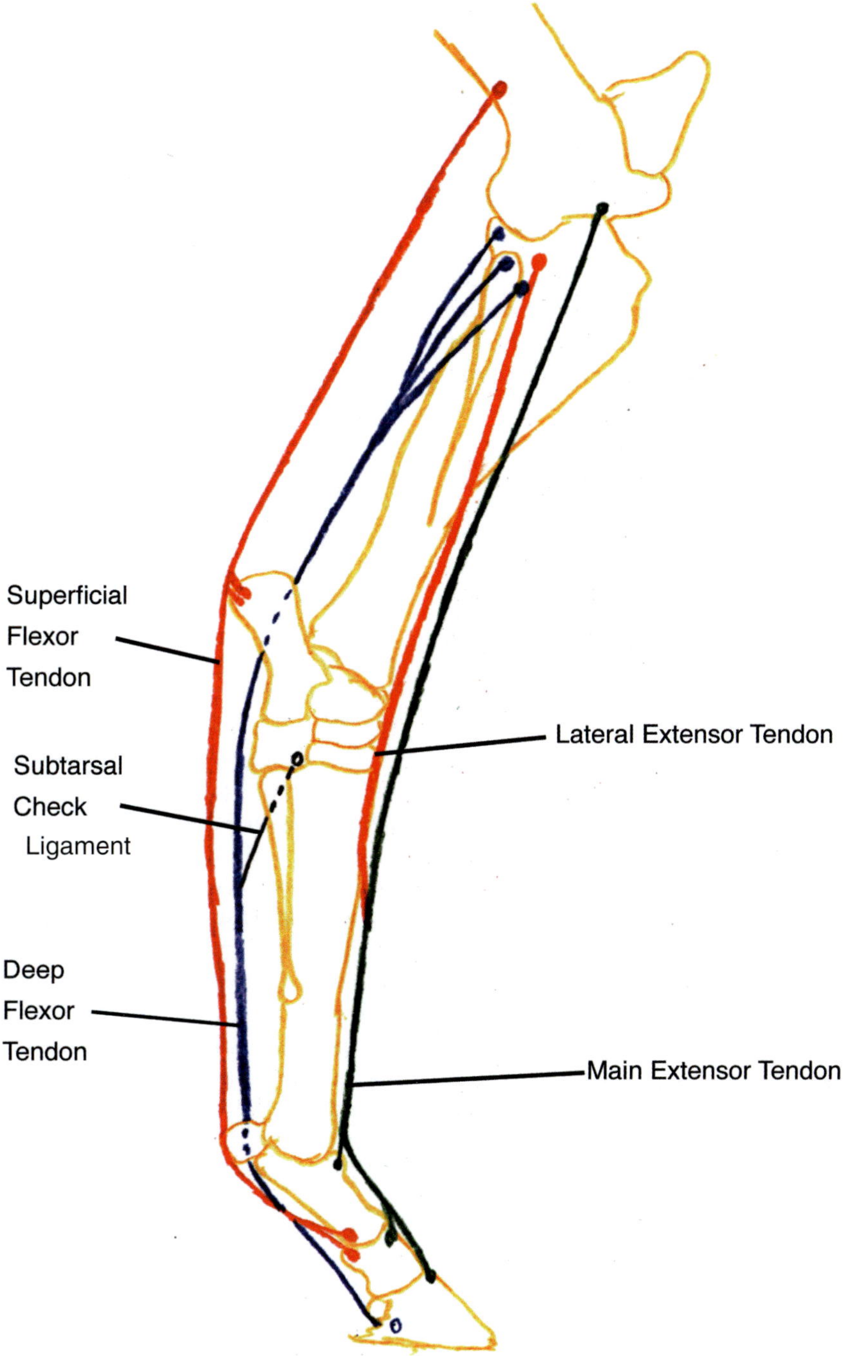

25

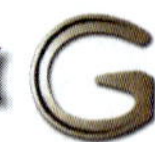

Chapter

11 VASCULAR, NERVE, AND LYMPHATIC SYSTEM BASICS OF THE EQUINE LEG

The term vascular basically means "of fluid-carrying vessels." For our purposes, we are talking mainly about the blood supply, but the lymph fluid system is also important and will also be covered.

THE ARTERIES (Figure 1-3)

The heart is basically a pump that sends blood through the body. Bright red, oxygenated blood is sent from the heart to the extremities through arteries. Arteries are thick-walled, muscular vessels. When you do a dissection, you can cut through an artery, and it will look like the cross-section of a hose. In **Figure 1**, you can see a vein, artery, and nerve on a cadaver specimen that is being dissected. The vein is on the left, the artery in the middle, and the nerve on the right. The blood enters the foot through the digital arteries. These arteries are named for where they terminate. This makes the anatomical names pretty simple. Nerves are named the same way.

Blood is supplied to the distal front leg through the median and ulnar arteries on the palmar aspect of the leg **(Figure 2)** and the transverse cubital artery on the dorsal aspect. In the hind limb, the arterial supply comes off of the femoral artery, which continues as the popliteal artery. Below the fetlock, both the front and the hind are similar. We will use the terms palmar for this chapter, even though plantar would be more appropriate if talking about the hind leg.

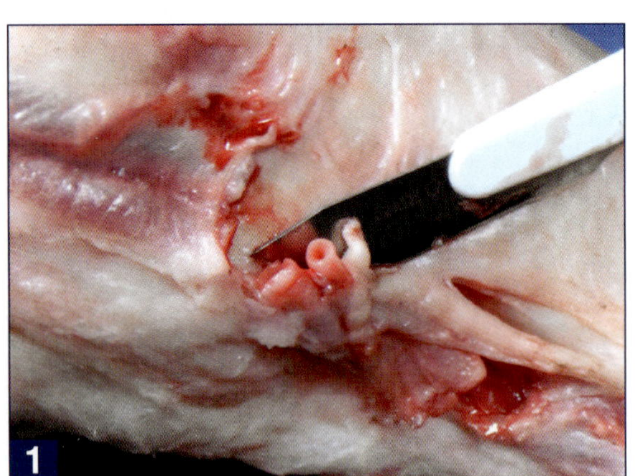
1

The majority of the blood supply to the digit comes down the palmar aspect of the leg. There are two arteries that course down the back of the leg. The lateral palmar artery is small, and the medial palmar artery (common digital artery) is the larger vessel. It bifurcates at the sesamoids to become the medial and lateral digital arteries.

It is in this area that you can easily find a pulse, as the arteries pass close to the skin and over the sesamoid bones. These branches supply blood to the entire digit. Both the lateral and medial arteries run with an associated nerve and vein in what is known as the neurovascular bundle **(Figure 3)**.

There are branches that come off of the digital arteries to supply different parts of the digit. The palmar branch of P1 joins contralateral branches and provides blood to the sesamoidian ligaments on the palmar aspect of P1. Near its origin, the palmar branch gives off a dorsal branch that joins the contralateral branch and supplies the extensor tendon.

The bulbar artery is the most palmar branch, and it supplies the skin, digital cushion, frog, and heels.

The coronal circumflex artery supplies the coronary band and heels.

On the distal palmar aspect of the coffin bone, there are two holes that are the entrance points for the terminal arch. The arteries enter each side and join each other to make a loop. There are numerous branches that come off of these arteries and pass

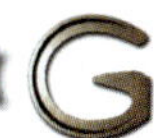

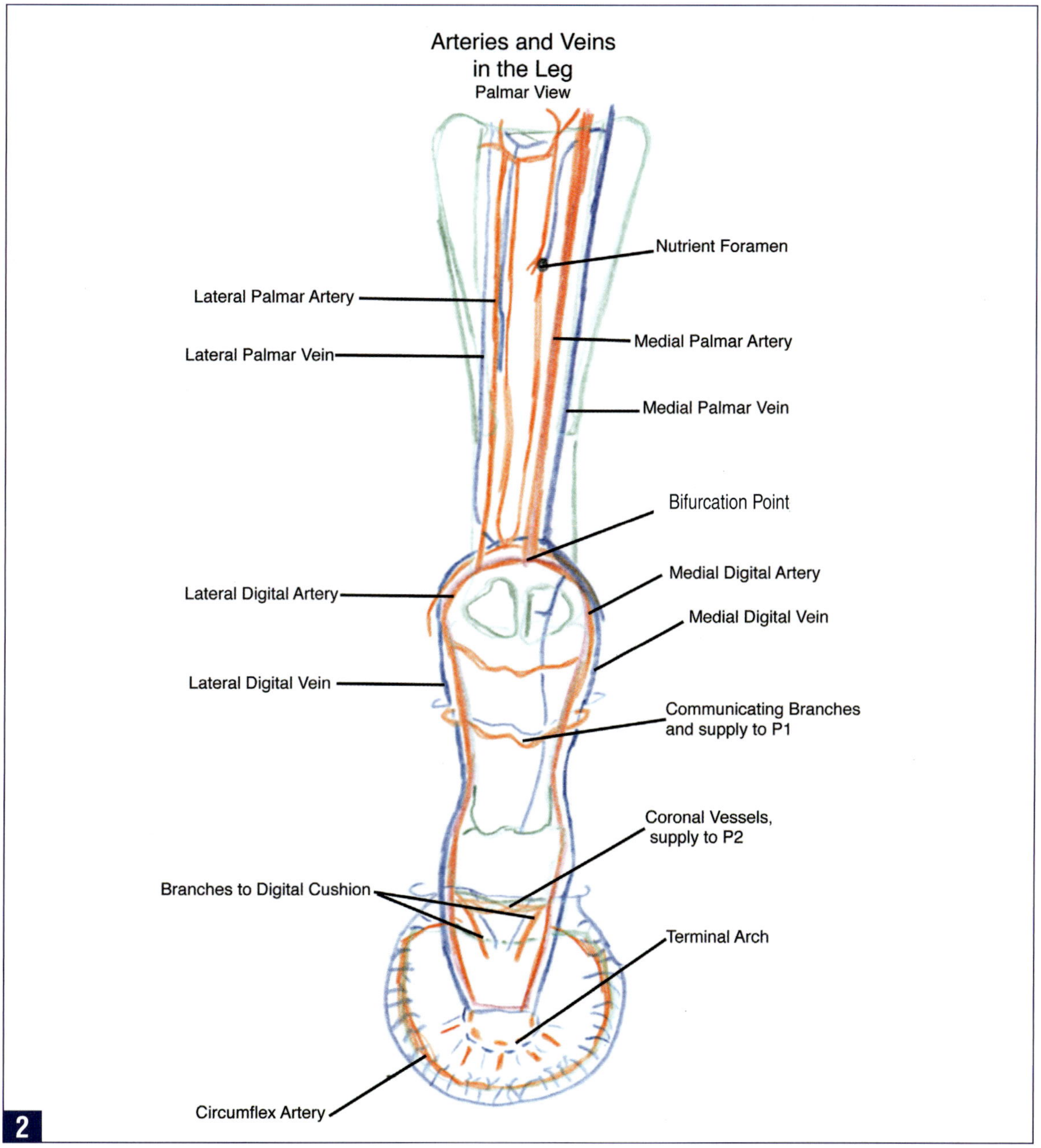

Arteries and Veins
in the Leg
Palmar View

Nutrient Foramen
Lateral Palmar Artery
Lateral Palmar Vein
Medial Palmar Artery
Medial Palmar Vein
Bifurcation Point
Medial Digital Artery
Lateral Digital Artery
Medial Digital Vein
Lateral Digital Vein
Communicating Branches and supply to P1
Coronal Vessels, supply to P2
Branches to Digital Cushion
Terminal Arch
Circumflex Artery

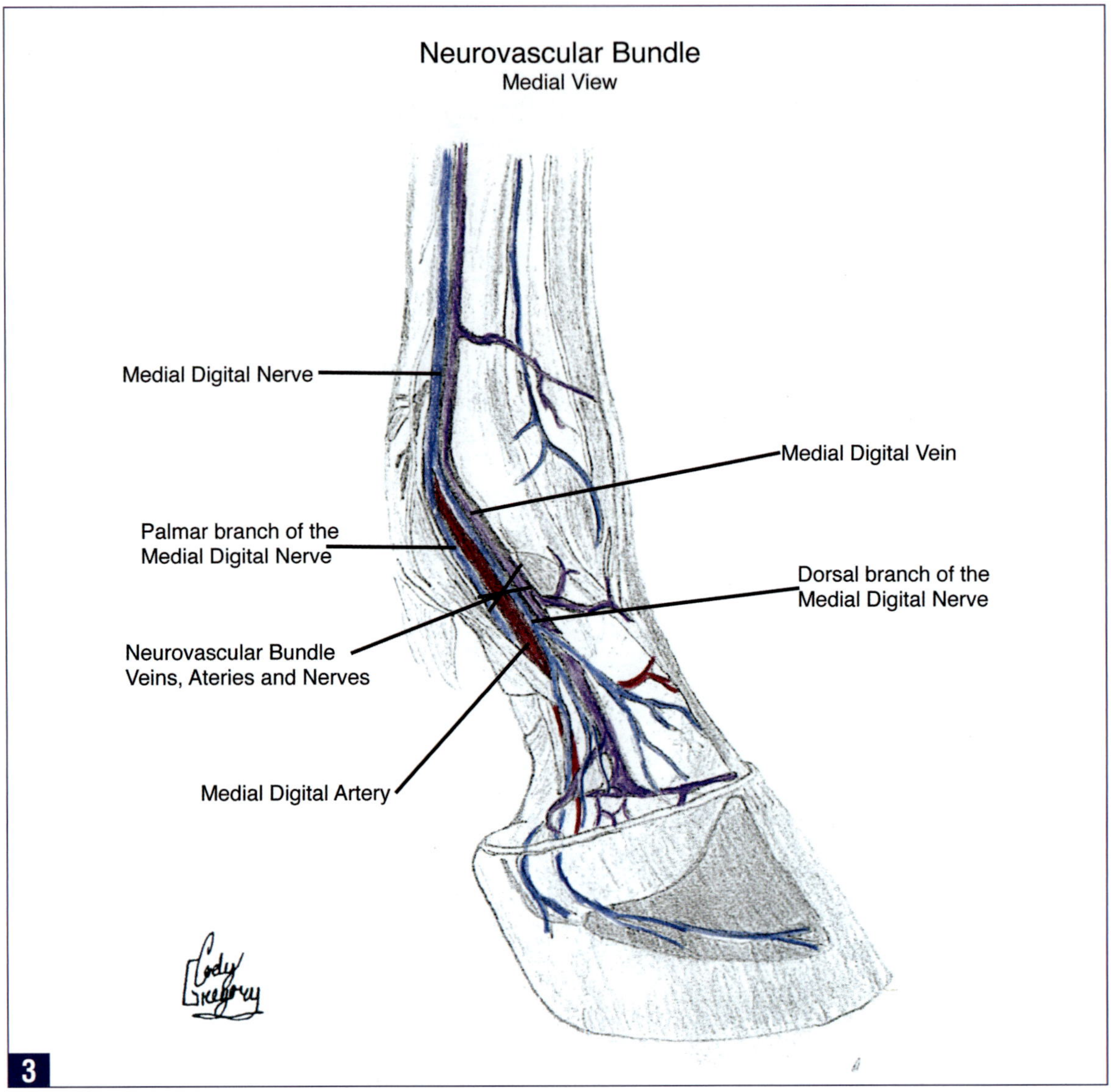

Neurovascular Bundle
Medial View

Medial Digital Nerve
Medial Digital Vein
Palmar branch of the Medial Digital Nerve
Dorsal branch of the Medial Digital Nerve
Neurovascular Bundle Veins, Ateries and Nerves
Medial Digital Artery
Cody Gregory

3

through the parietal surface of the coffin bone to nourish and supply the sensitive laminae.

Around the distal border of the coffin bone is the circumflex artery. It feeds the sensitive sole as well as the distal sensitive laminae and the corium for the white line.

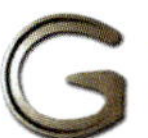

RETURN TO THE HEART (Figures 4-7)

There are three primary venous plexuses in the foot, which are an intricate network of tiny capillaries. These **(Figure 4)** are:

1. The coronary venous plexus located around the top of the hoof near the coronet.
2. The dorsal venous plexus that is located around the parietal surface of the coffin bone.
3. The solar venous plexus that is located along the solar aspect of the coffin bone.

It has been suggested that the venous plexuses also act as concussion reduction devices. This will be discussed in the chapter on biomechanics.

In **Figures 5 and 6** you can see a plastic cast of the venous plexuses. To make this, the digital artery

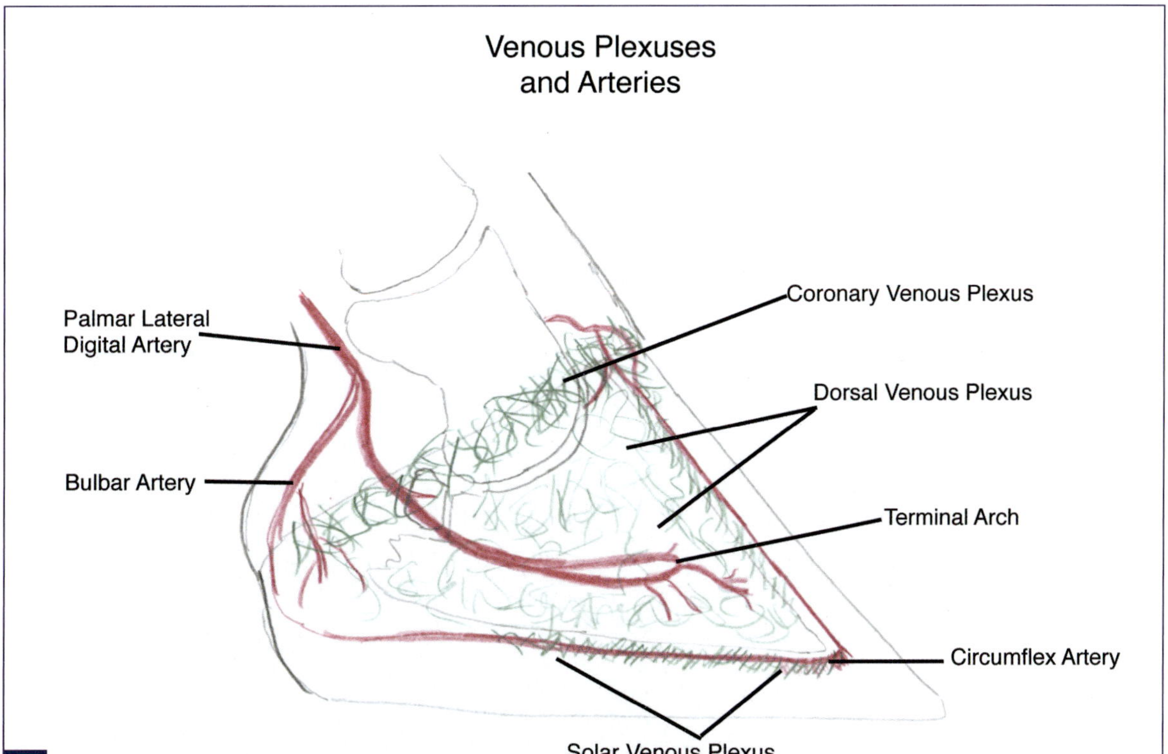

Venous Plexuses and Arteries

Palmar Lateral Digital Artery

Bulbar Artery

Coronary Venous Plexus

Dorsal Venous Plexus

Terminal Arch

Circumflex Artery

Solar Venous Plexus

4

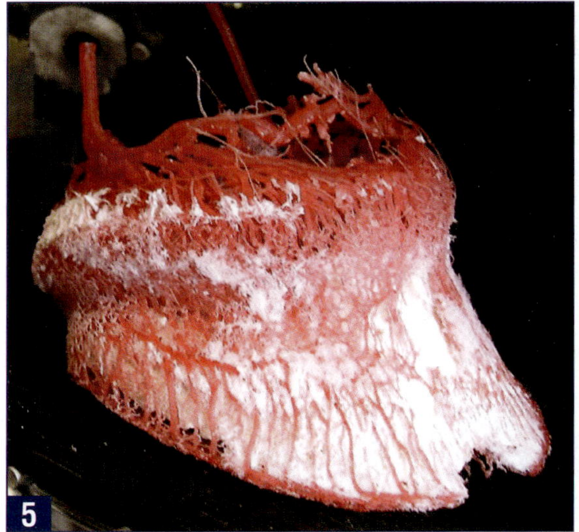

5

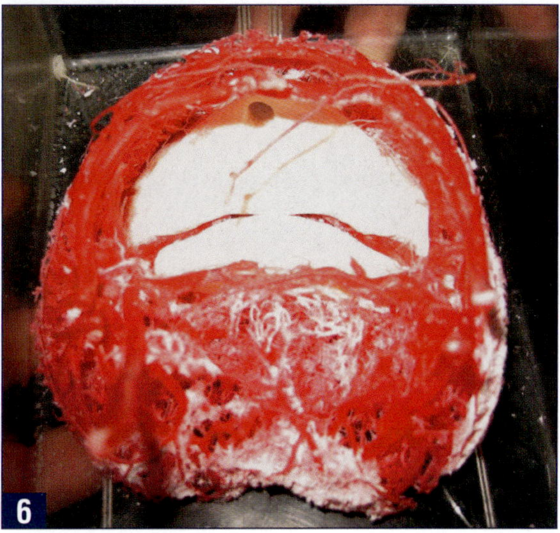

6

of a fresh cadaver leg is injected with latex so that it will leave a cast of the blood supply behind.

Figure 7 shows a venogram. The vascular system is infused with a radiopaque contrast medium. This will show up on radiographs so that the circulation of a foot can be studied.

After the blood has transferred the nutrients and oxygen to the extremities, the dark red deoxygenated blood is returned to the heart though thin-walled collapsible vessels called veins. There are reportedly check valves in the veins to prevent gravity from exerting force on the returning blood.

When the blood reaches the heart, it is infused with oxygen from the lungs and sent back through the system to resupply the tissues that make up the horse.

In addition to the arteries, capillaries, and veins, there are shunts called arteriovenous anastamoses (AVAs). AVAs connect arteries directly to veins without branching off to deliver nutrients to the extremities. These AVAs will sometimes open and, in effect, steal nutrient-rich blood from the artery, shunting it to the vein before the nutrients have been distributed. These AVAs have been strongly implicated in the cause of founder.

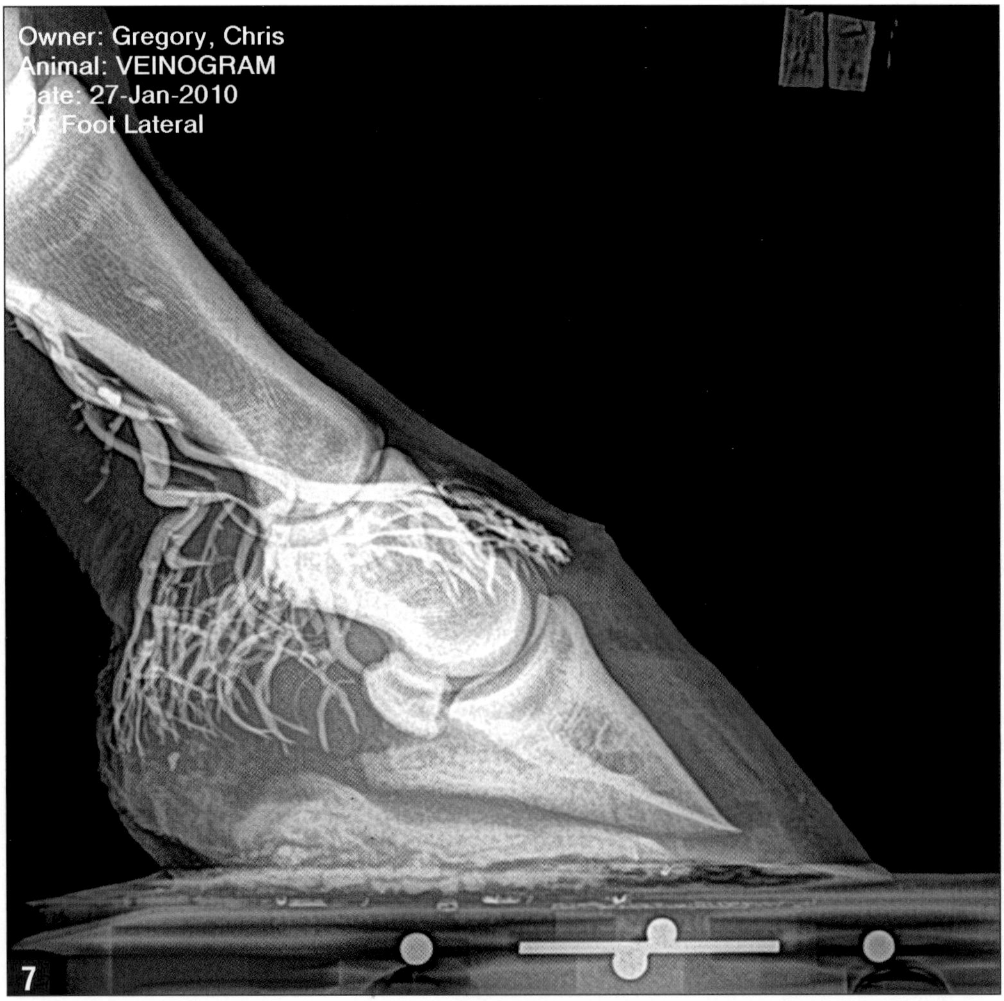

Owner: Gregory, Chris
Animal: VEINOGRAM
Date: 27-Jan-2010
RF Foot Lateral

7

NERVE SUPPLY (Figures 8-9)

The nerves that supply the leg run next to the veins and arteries that supply the leg. Remember that this is referred to as a neurovascular bundle.

There is a medial and lateral palmar/plantar nerve that runs down both sides of the suspensory ligament. It is in a space between that ligament and the deep flexor tendon, along with the veins and arteries in the neurovascular bundle.

There are numerous small branches that supply sensation to the metacarpus/metatarsus. The nerves then divide into a dorsal branch and a palmar/plantar branch at the fetlock, becoming the palmar/plantar medial and lateral digital nerves and the dorsal medial and lateral digital nerves. There are also communicating branches between the medial and lateral nerves.

After the bifurcation at the sesamoids, the palmar/plantar branch courses distad just palmar to the artery in that foot. The neurovascular bundle lies just dorsal and to both sides of the deep flexor tendon in the digit.

The plamar/plantar branch supplies the palmar/

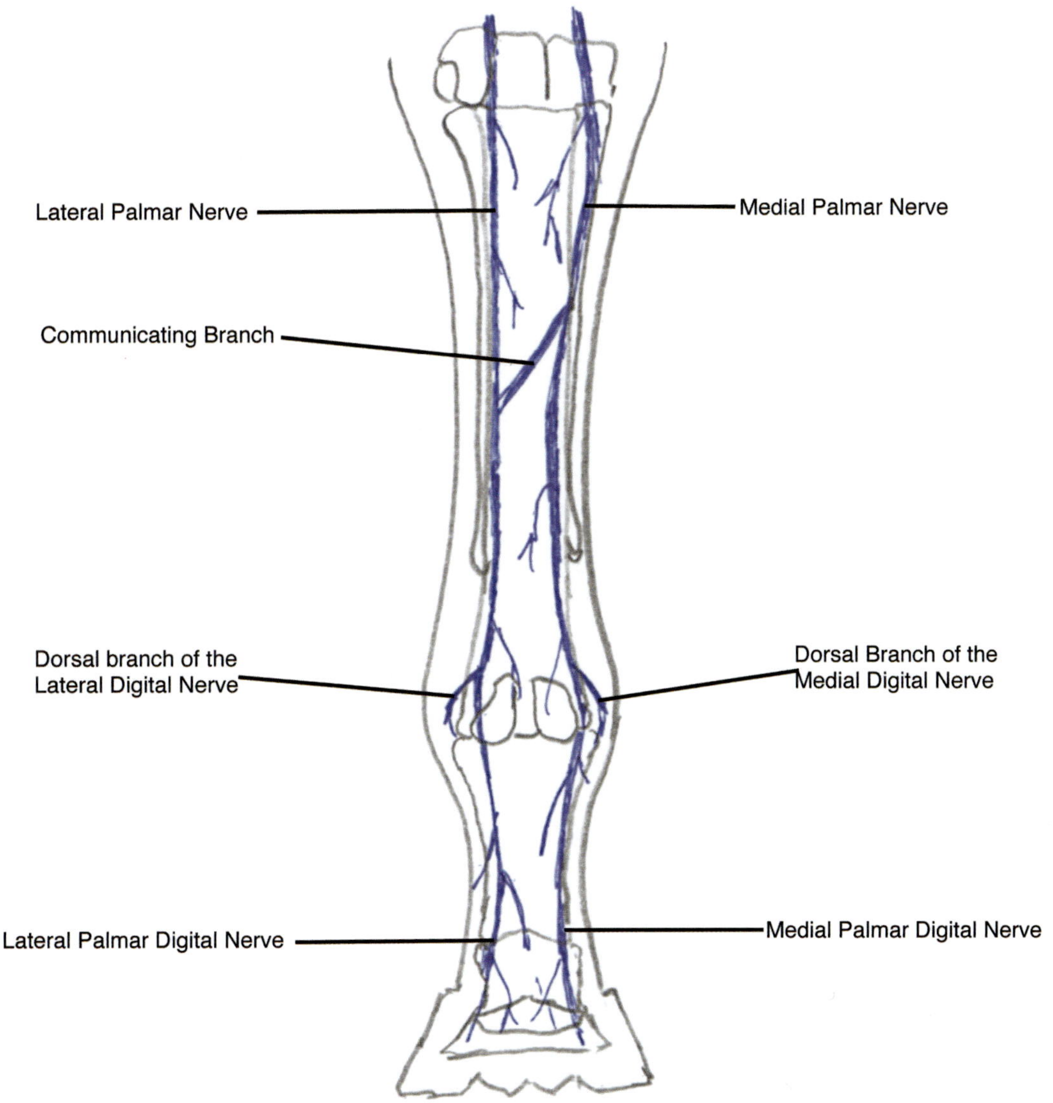

8

plantar aspect of the digit, including the skin, the deep flexor tendon, the sesamoidian ligaments, superficial flexor tendon, and hoof.

In the foot, this nerve provides sensation to the navicular region, the bulbs, heels and the digital cushion, as well as the corium of the frog, sole, and white line.

The dorsal branch supplies the dorsal aspect of the pastern, including the skin, main extensor tendon, and dorsal aspect of the coffin and pastern joints, as well as the perioplic ring and coronary band.

Nerves are perfect electrical conductors, and they convey information to the brain as an electrical impulse. There are no motor nerves below the knee or hock, only sensory nerves. The difference is that a motor nerve supplies a muscle, and sensory nerves inundate other tissue to provide information to the brain about the environment that the body is in. When a horse feels pain, heat, cold, pressure, etc., in the leg, it is conveyed to the brain. The brain interprets the information and sends a message back through the motor nerves to a muscle if the muscle needs to contract to remove the extremity from whatever it is feeling.

Take this example. You drive a nail into the quick. That causes pain in the foot, and the sensory nerves that supply that area send a message up the limb to the brain that indicates pain has been experienced by the foot. When that is received, the brain sends a message to the muscles on that limb, telling them to contract to get the foot out of danger. When they do, the horse jerks his leg to free it from the area where it is in pain. The amount of time that it takes for this to happen is called reaction time.

The sensory nerves are also important when a horse is moving. A horse cannot see its feet, so it has to rely on what it saw when it was approaching an obstacle and the experience it has from hitting objects in the past when it was forming its motor nerve wiring and learning to move. As a horse passes over an obstacle — a log, for example — it has to raise each leg at the right place in order to get over the log without tripping. It has to do that without looking at its feet. When it was young and learning to walk over obstacles, the sensory nerves would tell the brain that a collision had occurred if it hit an obstacle. The horse would learn from the information. The better that the horse got at navigating obstacles, the more surefooted it became.

For this reason, having a horse nerved with a high-nerve neurectomy is considered unethical. In the United States, almost all neurectomies are performed on the palmar branches of the digital nerve so the horse is still able to experience some sensation in the toe area.

In a high nerving, the nerve would be severed above the bifurcation at the fetlock. That would take away all sensation in the digit, and the horse would be dangerous to ride as well as a danger to itself.

There is a high incidence of hoof avulsion when a high nerving is done. Horses without sensation in their feet will pull until their leg is free when they get stuck, and this can cause the horse to pull his hoof off of the end of the leg.

THE LYMPHATIC SYSTEM

The lymphatic system is a fluid system that consists of small vessels containing lymph fluid. Lymphatic fluid itself is a relatively colorless fluid that is composed of blood plasma and white blood cells. These are called lymphocytes, and they produce antibodies to defend the body against infections. The lymph nodes are also part of this system, which works hand in hand with the circulatory system. The primary difference between the lymphatic system and the cardiovascular system is that the lymphatic system does not have a central pump, which is what the heart is for the cardiovascular system. The lymph vessels are also thinner, and do not have the muscular walls to aid in fluid movement.

Lymph fluid is moved through the body by the movement of the horse as muscles are flexed and relaxed. Tendon and ligament movement, contraction of muscles, and respiratory, circulatory, and digestive movements all contribute to the movement of the lymphatic fluid. Movement of the body pushes on the lymphatic vessels, which are squeezed by the movement, and lymphatic fluid is pushed through the system. Every time a horse inhales and exhales, the expansion and contraction of the thoracic cavity aids in moving lymphatic fluid. As the fluid moves, it carries toxins and waste away from the tissues.

A horse is approximately 70% water. Some of this is in the blood, but much more of it is in and around the cells that make up the tissues that make the horse. The lymphatic system is a big part of keeping the fluid balance in the body correct, which is of vital importance when talking about any creature with such high water content.

Any part of the body that receives circulation

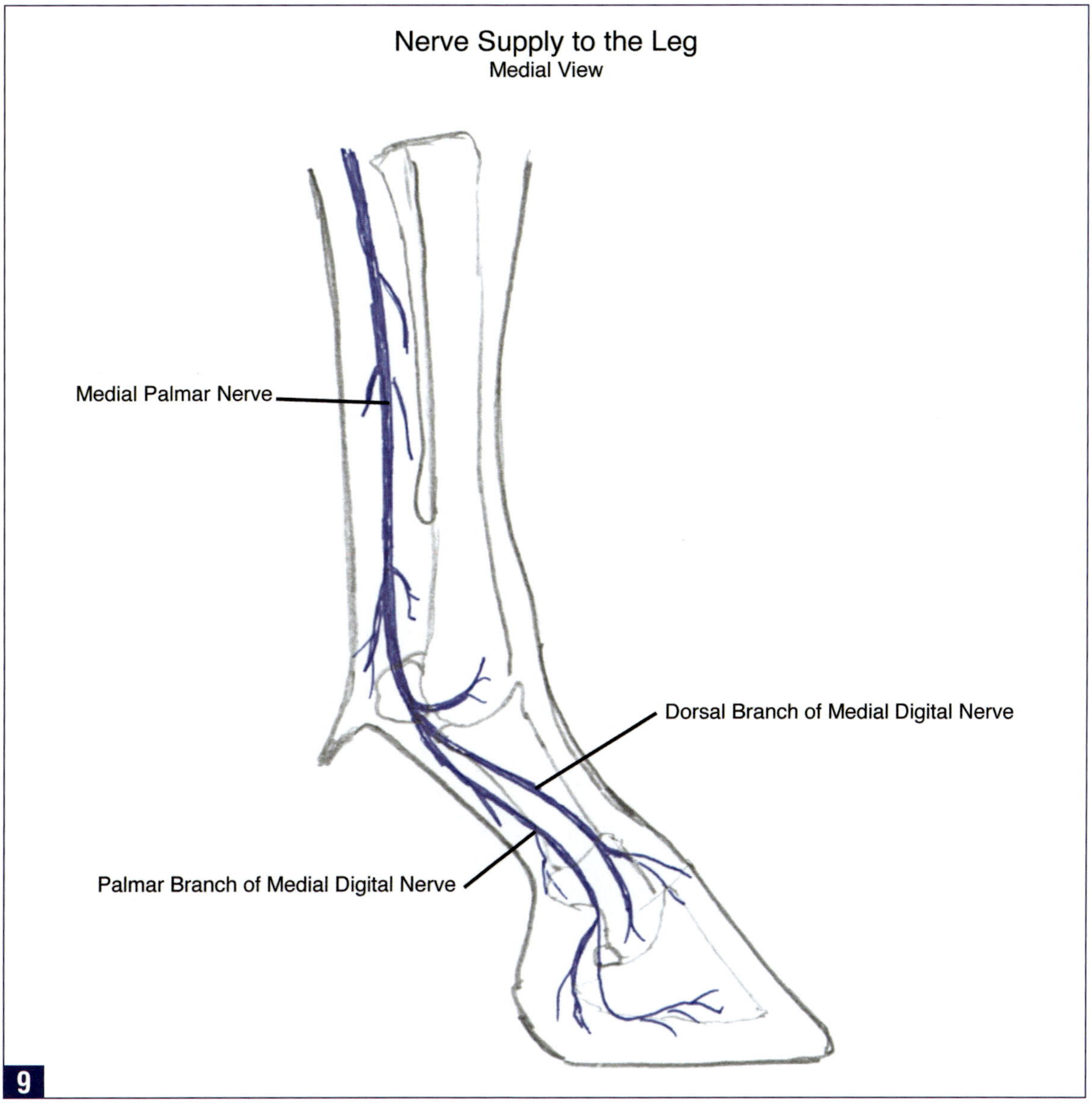

Nerve Supply to the Leg
Medial View

Medial Palmar Nerve

Dorsal Branch of Medial Digital Nerve

Palmar Branch of Medial Digital Nerve

9

is nourished by the nutrients carried on protein molecules dissolved in fluid and released by the blood into the tissue. Most waste products such as protein molecules, harmful toxins, lactic acids, and salts are removed by the lymphatic system. When the lymphatic system fails, swelling known as edema develops. This is what is known as a horse "stocking up" or being "stall stocked." This type of swelling in the legs can be identified by the lack of heat, and the way that the swollen leg will dent when palpated. With an inflammatory swelling, pushing on the leg is similar to pushing on a water balloon. As soon as you remove the pressure from your fingers, the water balloon returns to its original shape. With edema, it is similar to pressing on a gel filled sack. The indentation from pressure remains for some time, returning to its original shape slowly.

The lymphatic system is very important to the wellbeing of any mammal, and knowing the basics of how it works is just one more part of becoming a great farrier.

This chapter covers some of the basic information you need to understand about how the leg, digit,s and foot are supplied with blood and innervated. You will find this information handy as you continue to study the anatomy and movement of this incredible animal.

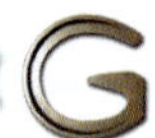

Chapter 12

BIOMECHANICS

Biomechanics refers to the application of mechanical principles from the realm of physics to living creatures. This is a huge subject, but the focus of this chapter is much smaller. In this chapter I want to discuss some very specific anatomical principles of the horse that include the stay apparatus, reciprocal apparatus, and concussion absorption and redirection, as well as the effects of changes to the hoof-pastern axis. These are the areas of static biomechanics that I feel are the essentials for a farrier, but I encourage you to delve deeper. Get some books that explore kinesiology and dynamics in the horse if you want more thorough information.

STAY APPARATUS, PASSIVE STAY APPARATUS, AND RECIPROCAL APPARATUS

The term stay apparatus is used to describe how a horse is able to stand with little effort. There is not any one component of the stay apparatus that

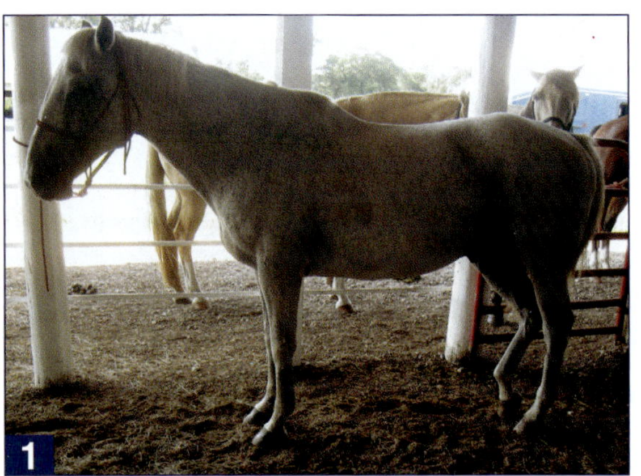

Lateral view of a horse at rest.

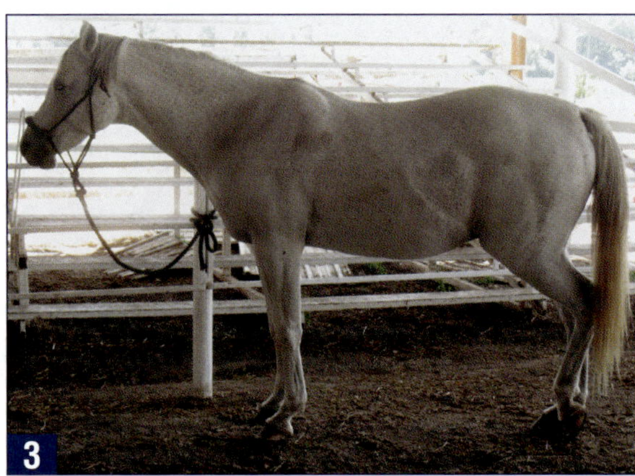

Lateral view of a horse at rest.

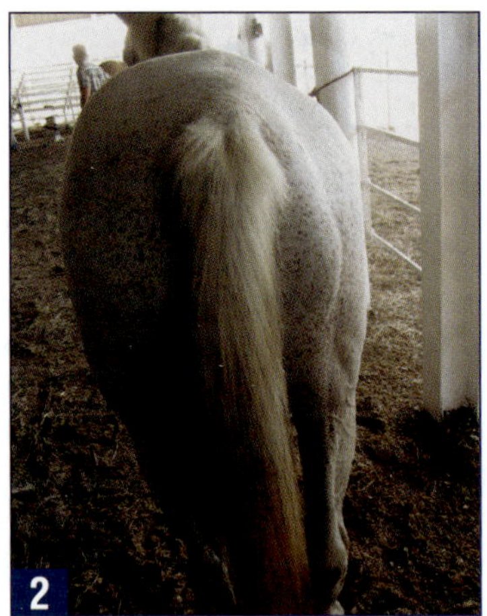

Rear vies of a horse at rest.

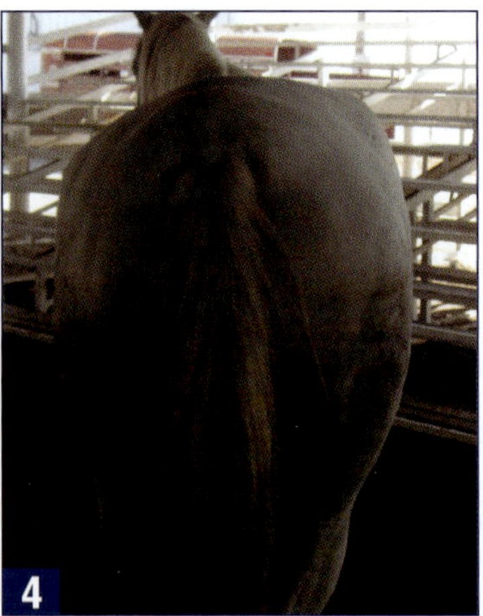

Rear view of the pelvis tilt that is common when the passive stay apparatus is engaged.

you can define, rather, it is a combination of many components. The removal of or injury to any of these components can destroy the stay apparatus.

Horses take many standing naps during the course of a day, and the average horse only requires around 2.5 hours of sleep per day. Unlike humans, the combination of several naps serves the purpose of resting the horse. The standing naps are not a deep sleep, but rather a state of rest that allows a horse to enter and recover quickly, yet still get some rest. To get into deep sleep, a horse has to lie down, and they will sleep on their sides at least once every few days if allowed to. When horses are in situations where they cannot sleep lying down for days on end, they may enter deep sleep while standing and end up falling down. This means that there is a component to the stay apparatus that requires at least some muscular control and effort. The horses in **Figures 1-4** are all in that resting state. Notice how one hind limb is resting and the pelvis is tilted.

STAY APPARATUS OF THE THORACIC LIMB

Major components of the stay apparatus in the thoracic limb are the tendons and ligaments, which do not tire like muscles. Being non-tiring tissue, they prevent the flexion of the joints in the carpus, or knee. They also help prevent the overextension of the fetlock and pastern joints that are already extended.

Since the forelimb is attached to the trunk by only muscle, tendon, ligament, and fascia (this fleshy attachment is called the synsacosis), it in itself is not a part of the stay apparatus. However, the serratus ventralis that is the main weight-bearing connection to the trunk has a lot of tendinous tissue in it. The serratus ventralis does create a sling that prevents the trunk of the horse from falling to the ground, and pulls the front limbs against the trunk since it is situated between them **(Figure 5)**.

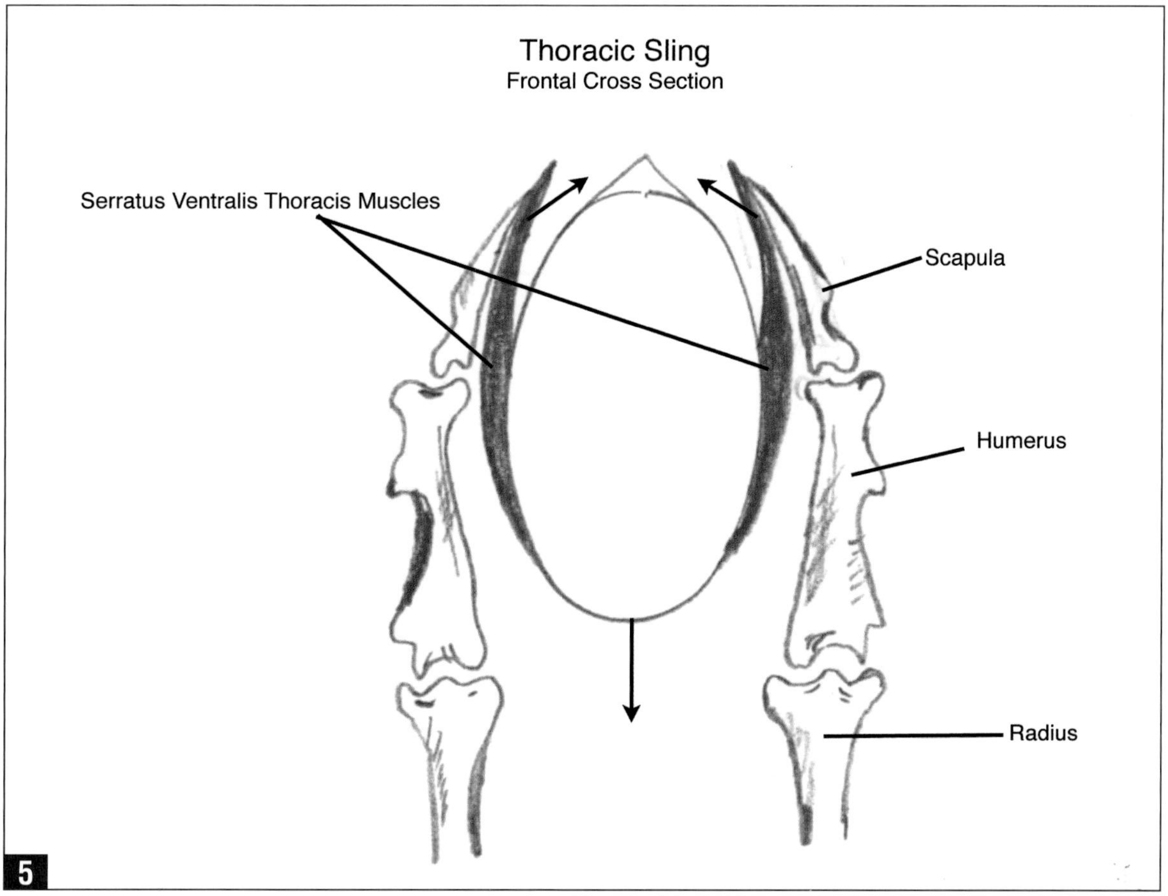

5

Thoracic sling.

Figures 6 and 7 are two drawings of the thoracic limb, each showing some of the components that make up the stay apparatus. I didn't include everything on just one drawing so that you could see these structures better.

The shoulder joint is primarily stabilized by pressure on the cranial aspect of the joint by the biceps tendon. The way that this tendon passes over the proximal humerus suggests a locking mechanism. The elbow joint is the origin for several carpal and digital flexors and extensors. This, along with the collateral ligaments of the elbow joint and the insertion of the biceps, stabilizes the joint **(Figures 6 and 7)**.

The carpus is stabilized by many anatomical structures. Cranially, the extensor carpi radialis

Components of Stay Apparatus

Biceps

Lacertus Fibrosis

Flexor Carpi Ulnaris

Ulnaris Lateralis

Extensor Carpi Radialis

Suspensory Ligament

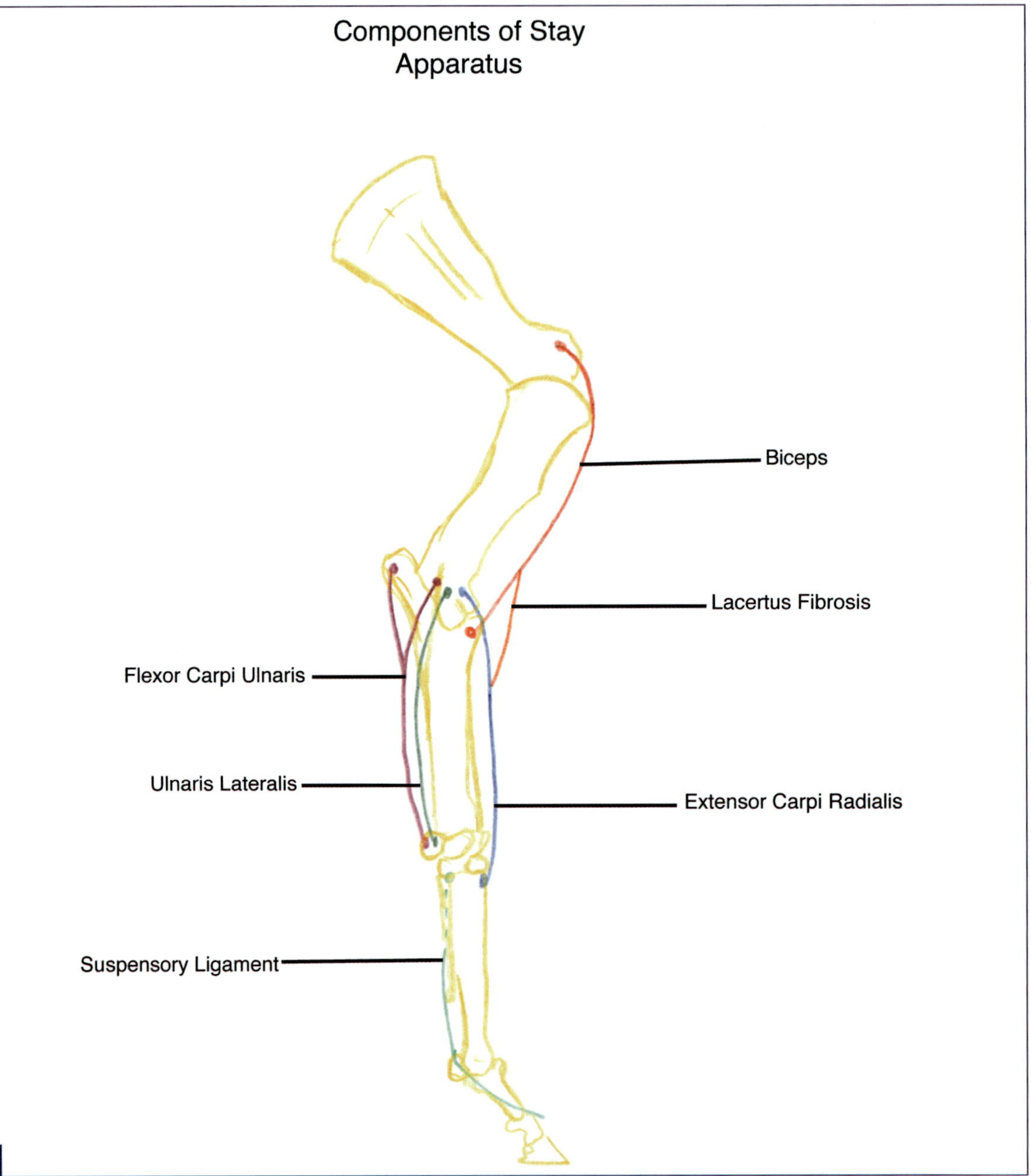

6

Front limb with some of the components of the stay apparatus.

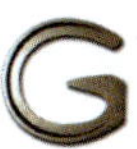

exerts pressure to keep the carpus extended. On the caudal aspect, the ulnaris lateralis and flexor carpi ulnaris insert at the accessory carpal bone, and they are kept taut by the weight of the horse, which pulls on the proximal flexor surface of the joint to keep it extended. The check ligaments of the superficial and deep flexor tendons exert pull on the joint distally, and there is the suspensory ligament that originates from the distal row of carpals and the proximal cannon bone to stabilize the joint further. Inside the carpus there are numerous non-tiring ligaments that hold the carpus together from all directions.

The fetlock joint is prevented from sinking further by the suspensory ligament, the superficial and deep flexor tendons, and the sesamoids and the

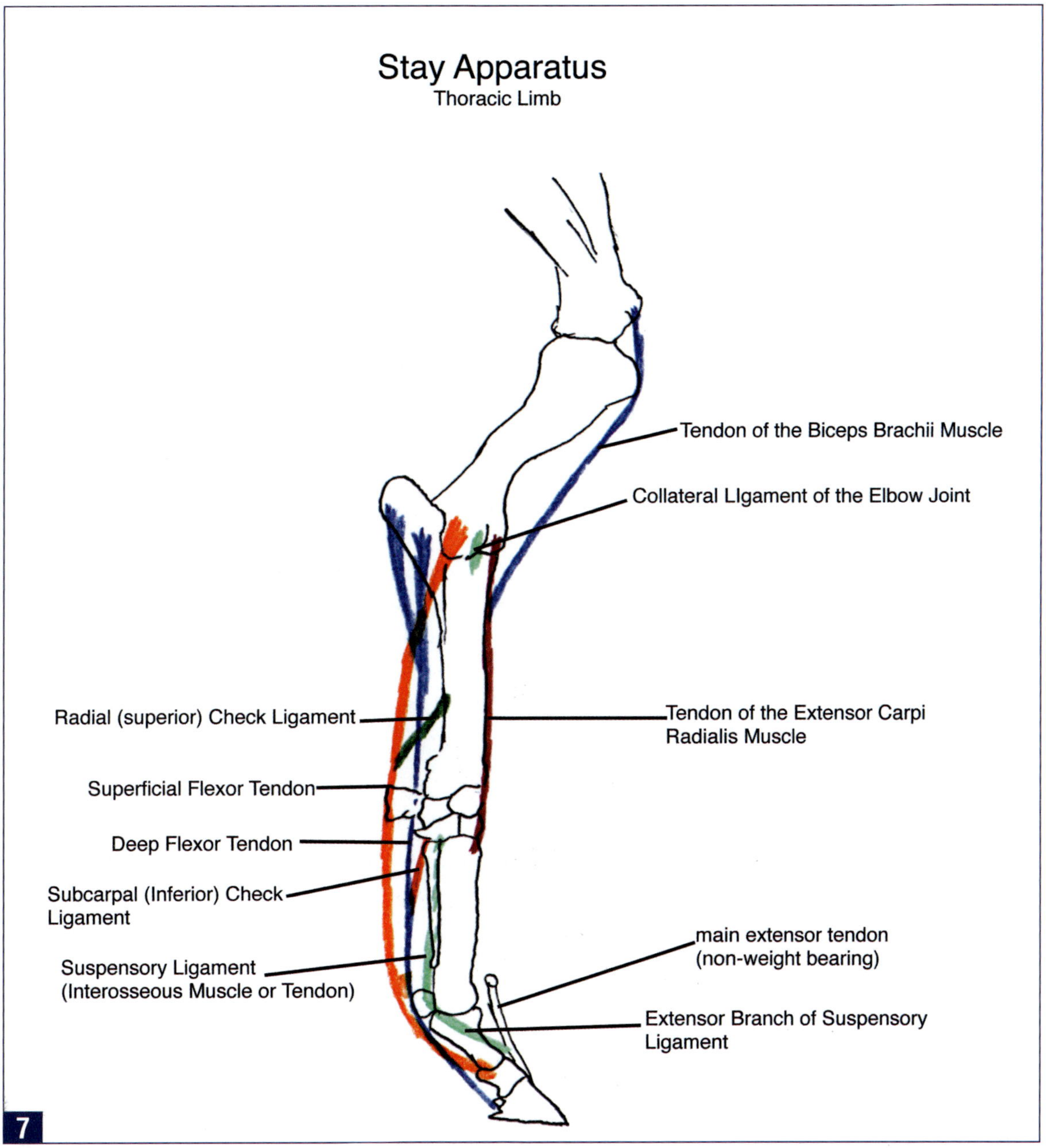

Another drawing of the front limb with additional components of the stay apparatus.

sesamoidian ligaments. It is further stabilized from lateral movement by the hinge design of the joint surfaces as well as the collateral ligaments. There is a lot of ligamentous and tendinous tissue around the fetlock joint.

The pastern joint is stabilized by the collateral ligaments, the pastern ligaments (axial and abaxial), the insertion of the superficial sesamoidian ligament, and the superficial flexor tendon.

PASSIVE STAY APPARATUS OF THE PELVIC LIMB

In the pelvic limb, the ability to stand with minimal effort is referred to as the passive stay apparatus. It is common to see a horse resting one limb, the pelvis tilted, and the weight of the hindquarters being born by one limb **(Figures 1-4)**. The horse achieves this by locking its stifle joint, which basically converts the hind limb into a pillar. When the horse stands with both limbs square in the hind limb, the patella is positioned at the proximal end of the trochlea at the distal cranial aspect of the

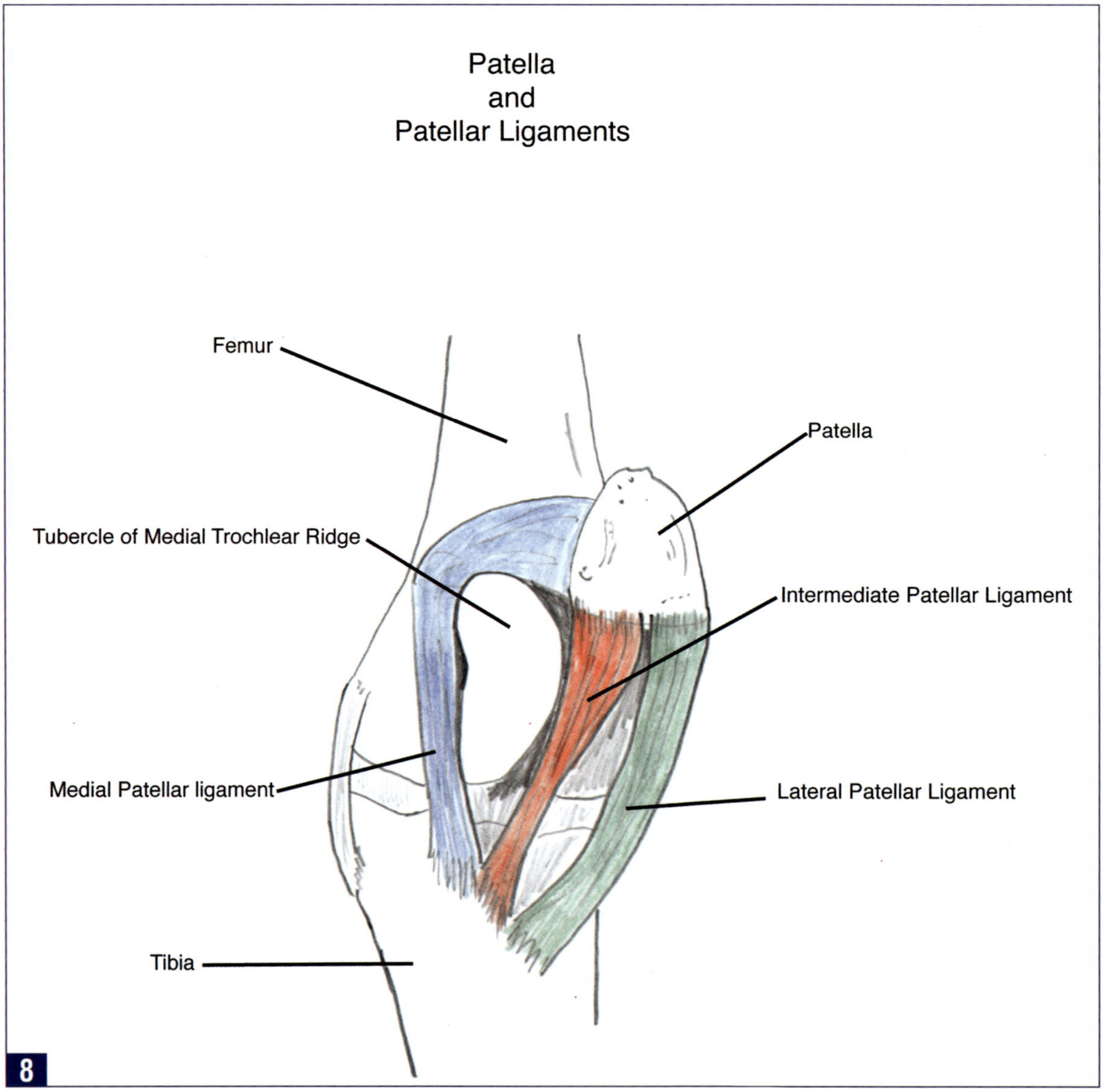

Detail of the stifle joint and the patellar ligaments.

femur (**Figure 8**). When it shifts the weight to one limb, the patella rotates medially about 15 degrees, and the fibrocartilage and medial patellar ligament slide caudally on the tubercle, fully locking the stifle joint.

The reciprocal apparatus (reciprocal mechanism) is a major component of the pelvic limb stay apparatus. The reciprocal apparatus refers to the fact that when one joint flexes in the hind limb, they all flex, and when one joint extends, they all extend. This mechanism is primarily the result of two tendinous structures **(Figure 9)**. On the caudal aspect, the superficial flexor tendon connects the caudal distal femur to the calcaneus process, continuing distad to insert collaterally on distal P1 and proximal P2. Cranially, the peroneus tertius originates from the lateral condyle of the femur and inserts into the fourth tarsal and proximal cannon bone. The peroneus tertius is tendon tissue. These two structures oppose each other, creating the reciprocal apparatus function.

To help understand this, imagine that there was a cable that started in your armpit, was bolted to your elbow, and attached to the palm of your hand. Whenever you bent your elbow, there would be pull

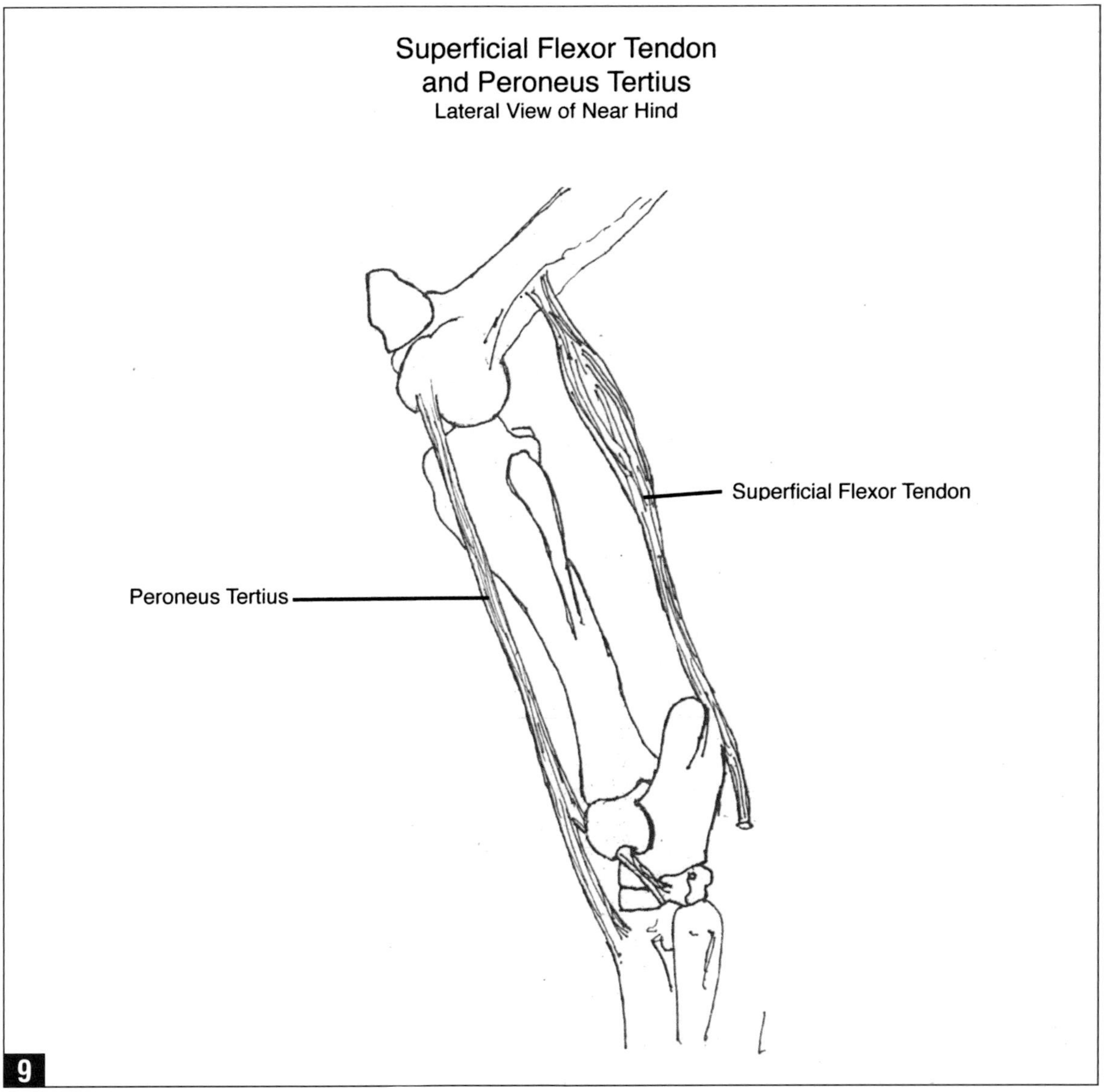

Superficial Flexor Tendon
and Peroneus Tertius
Lateral View of Near Hind

Superficial Flexor Tendon

Peroneus Tertius

9

Detail of the superficial flexor tendon and the peroneus tertius.

on the palm of your hand, which would cause your wrist to bend as well. This is how the superficial flexor tendon on the pelvic limb acts as part of the reciprocal apparatus. An opposing cable on the other side of your arm would be the peroneus tertius.

Since the stifle joint is locked when the passive stay apparatus is engaged and there is a reciprocal apparatus in the hind limbs, the horse is able to stand with almost no effort.

There are, of course, other structures involved in the stay apparatus of the hind limb, primarily the deep flexor tendon and the suspensory ligament **(Figure 10)** as well as the lower structures mentioned on the thoracic limb.

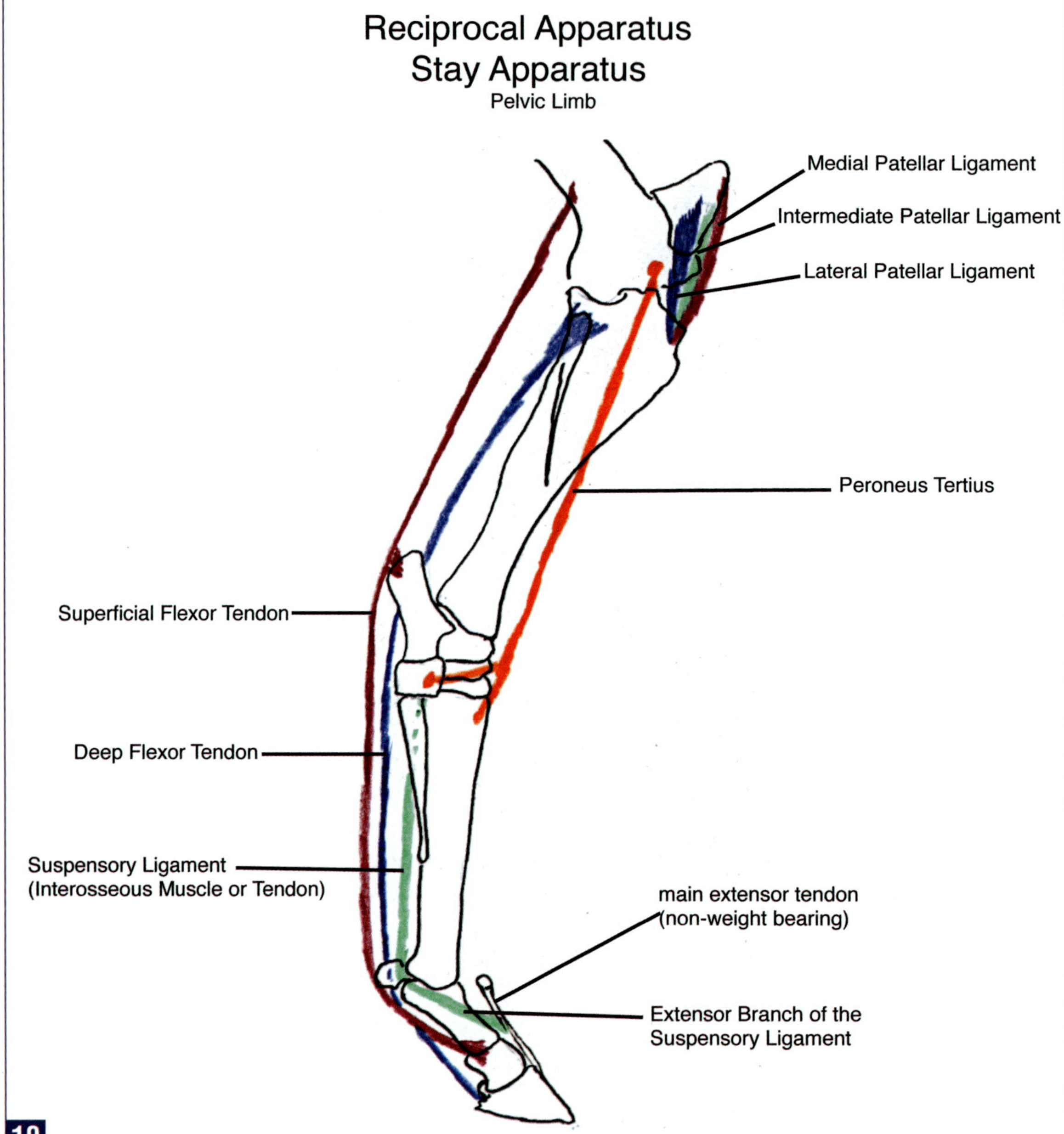

Pelvic limb and components of the passive stay apparatus and the reciprocal apparatus.

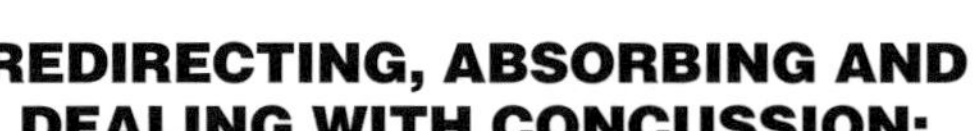

REDIRECTING, ABSORBING AND DEALING WITH CONCUSSION:

There are several angled joints in the limbs that create a system whereby the forces that are experienced by the horse are absorbed and redirected so that the body does not have to take the full brunt of the impact. Study the limb drawings in **Figures 11 and 12** to see these angles. Additionally, when a horse is moving, the angles of the joints cause the tendons and ligaments to store energy much like a

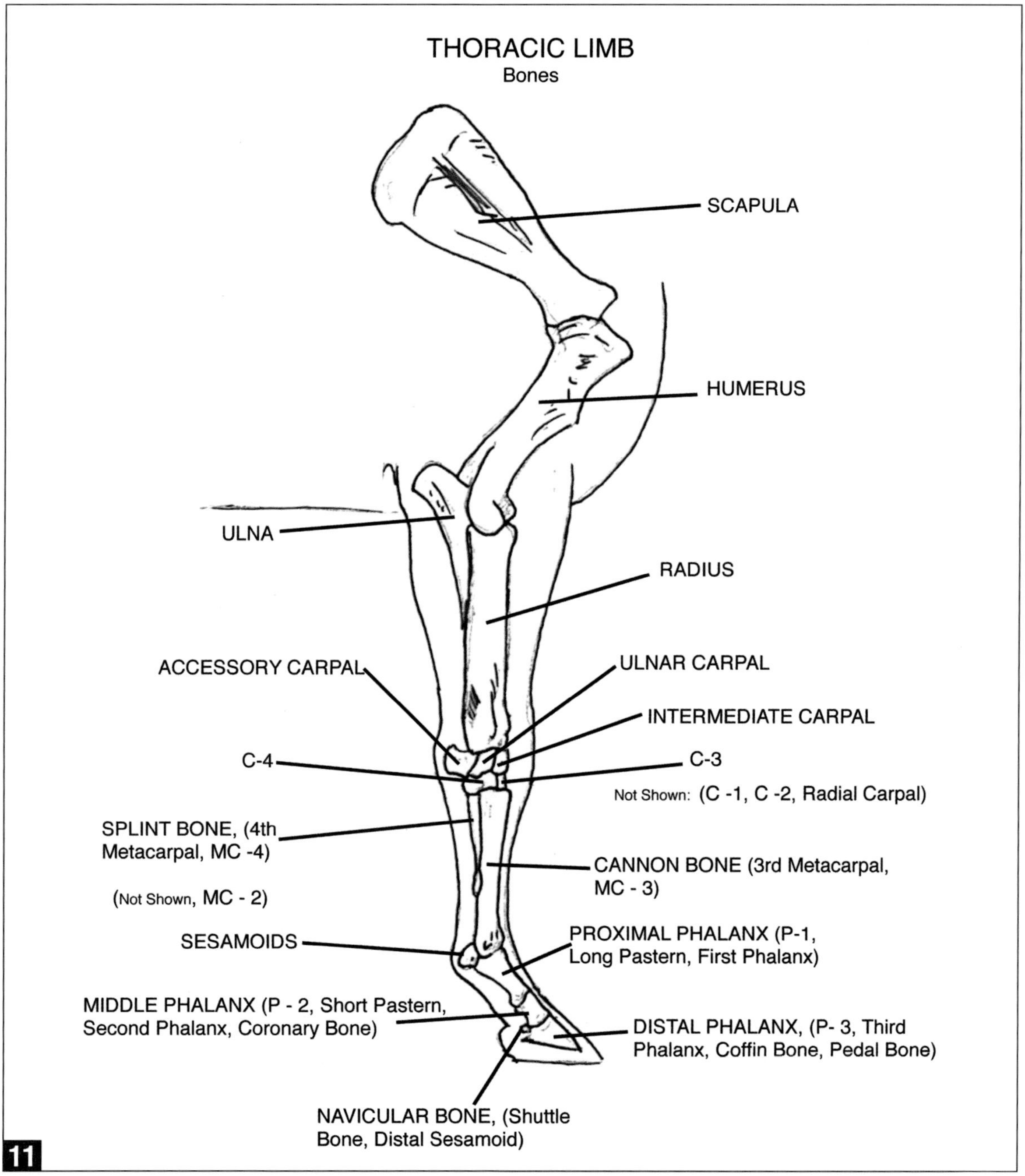

THORACIC LIMB
Bones

SCAPULA
HUMERUS
ULNA
RADIUS
ACCESSORY CARPAL
ULNAR CARPAL
INTERMEDIATE CARPAL
C-4
C-3
Not Shown: (C -1, C -2, Radial Carpal)
SPLINT BONE, (4th Metacarpal, MC -4)
(Not Shown, MC - 2)
CANNON BONE (3rd Metacarpal, MC - 3)
SESAMOIDS
PROXIMAL PHALANX (P-1, Long Pastern, First Phalanx)
MIDDLE PHALANX (P - 2, Short Pastern, Second Phalanx, Coronary Bone)
DISTAL PHALANX, (P- 3, Third Phalanx, Coffin Bone, Pedal Bone)
NAVICULAR BONE, (Shuttle Bone, Distal Sesamoid)

11

Thoracic limb.

rubber band, and this helps to propel a horse to the next step through that energy return. Without that, an animal the size of a horse would need much more muscle mass than it has to keep it going as fast and as far as it does. The muscles quickly tire, while the tendons and ligaments are non-tiring tissue. Energy return is a critical component of movement for most large animals.

If the limbs were completely straight like a pillar, every time the horse landed, there would be tremendous forces directly transferred to the body. So, the angles of the joints of the fetlock, elbow, shoulder, hock, stifle and hip are important factors. Think of these as biomechanical shock absorbers.

The distal ends of the long bones are covered with articular cartilage that is surrounded by synovial fluid. This cartilage does not have innervations like the bones do, so it is well adapted to bearing weight.

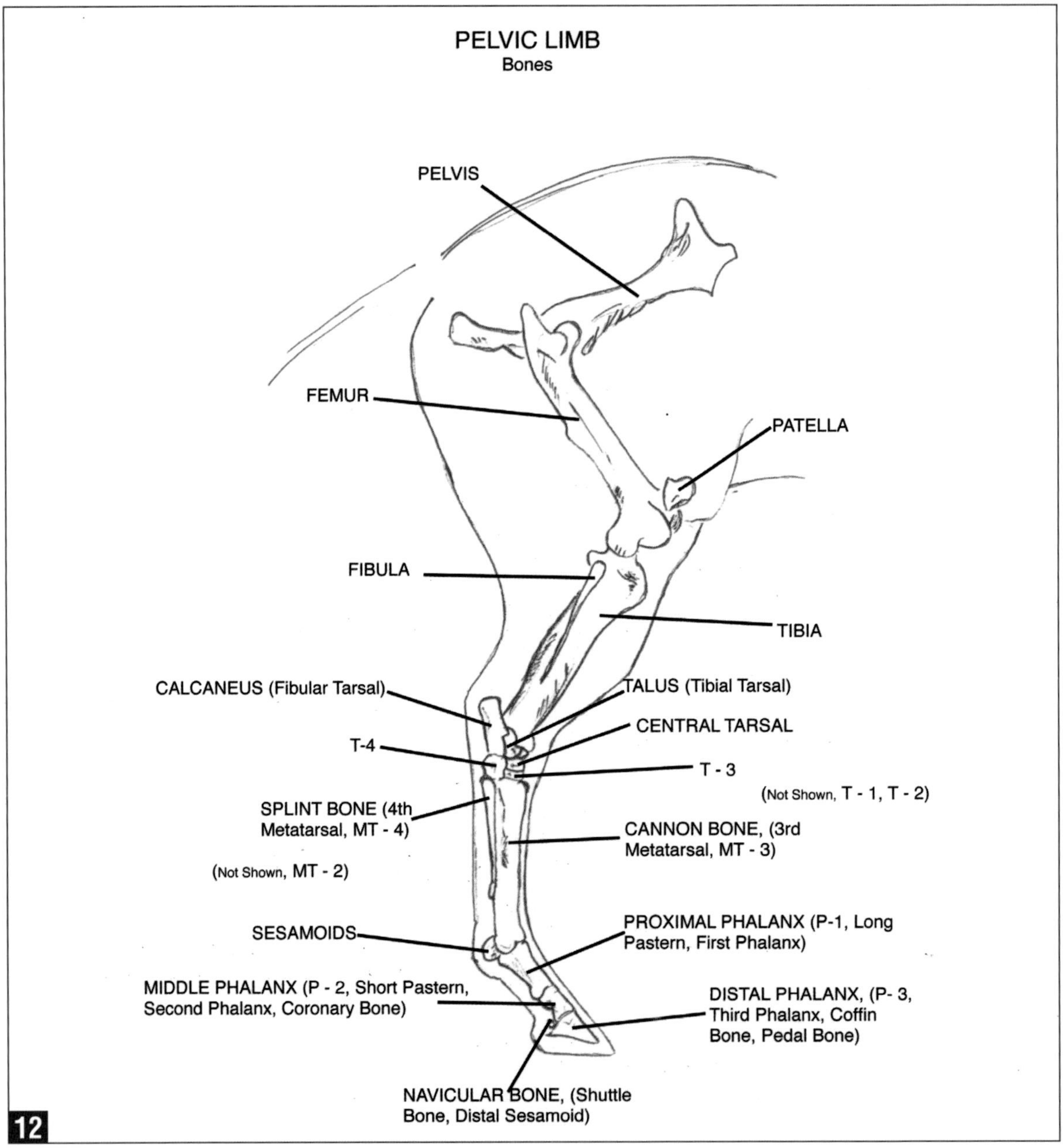

PELVIC LIMB
Bones

PELVIS
FEMUR
PATELLA
FIBULA
TIBIA
CALCANEUS (Fibular Tarsal)
TALUS (Tibial Tarsal)
CENTRAL TARSAL
T-4
T - 3
(Not Shown, T - 1, T - 2)
SPLINT BONE (4th Metatarsal, MT - 4)
CANNON BONE, (3rd Metatarsal, MT - 3)
(Not Shown, MT - 2)
SESAMOIDS
PROXIMAL PHALANX (P-1, Long Pastern, First Phalanx)
MIDDLE PHALANX (P - 2, Short Pastern, Second Phalanx, Coronary Bone)
DISTAL PHALANX, (P- 3, Third Phalanx, Coffin Bone, Pedal Bone)
NAVICULAR BONE, (Shuttle Bone, Distal Sesamoid)

12

Pelvic limb.

It also has the ability to absorb concussion, and the synovial fluid that infuses the cartilage is also a component of shock absorption.

Arrangement and shape of bones in the carpus and tarsus allow these bones to move laterally to a small degree, which is also a component of weight bearing and reducing the effects of impact on the body.

Now we get to the foot. When you consider the shape of the foot, it has the shape that you would give to a pedestal to create a large base of support for the item above. It has a larger area distally than proximally and is not connected all the way around, having the heels open. There is still a lot of debate about what exactly happens when a foot bears weight, so all I can put here is what I think is happening.

Based on the design and shape of the foot, as well as judging the wear pattern on the hoof surface of thousands of shoes, combined with research and discussion amongst some of the top farriers in the world, I think the following happens when a normal foot bears weight. The term normal is crucial to this discussion, because a diseased foot or lame animal will move differently.

At impact with the ground, the heels hit an instant before the rest of the foot. As the foot is loaded, the heels expand, the frog descends toward-sthe ground, and the sole flattens as it descends as well. The dorsal aspect of the coronet moves palmar/plantar as does the dorsal proximal hoof wall. **Figures 13 and 14** are drawings of feet with minimal load, and next to that, the same foot loaded. In **Figure 13**, the foot on the left is a standing horse, and the green line represents the position of the sole. The drawing on the right is that foot loaded with the angle changes that occur to the hoof compared to the red outline, and the descending of the sole being depicted in green. **Figure 14** is the bottom of a foot. On the left is the solar surface of a standing horse. On the right, the same foot loaded and the original position of the foot depicted in red.

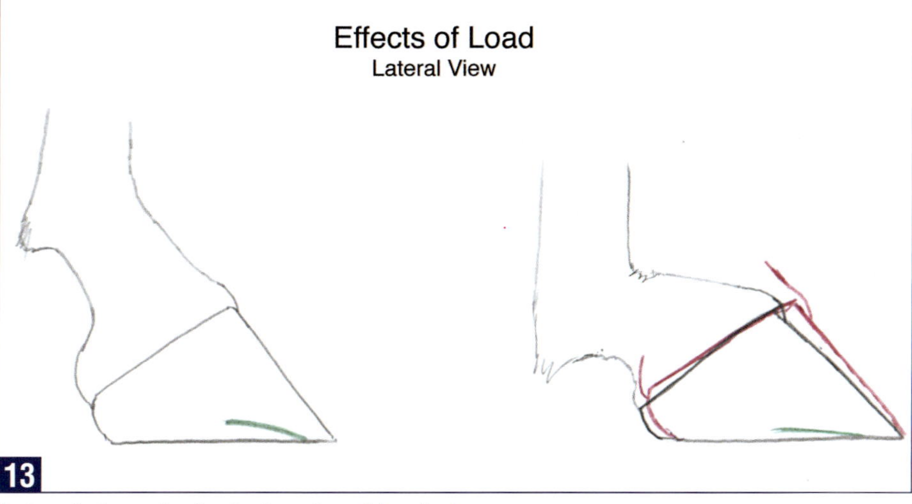

Lateral view of a foot at rest and loaded.

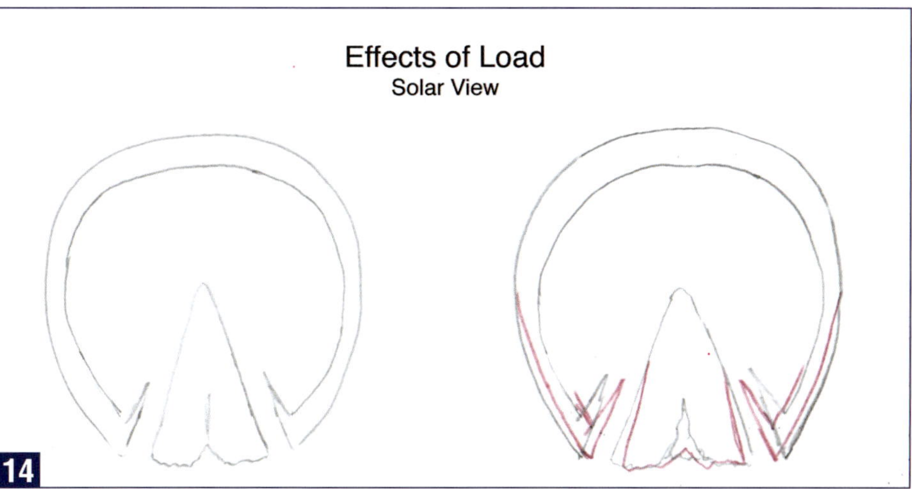

Solar view of a foot at rest and loaded.

With the widening of the heels, the top of the hoof wall at the coronet above the heels and quarters either stays the same or possibly moves inward slightly. This would help to explain the trapping of the blood in the venous plexuses during maximum load and the hydraulic cushion effect. Since the fetlock is descending, the force and angle change generated when P2 descends may prevent the top of the coronet from contracting. However, P2 could also be acting as a cork in a bottle, descending under load and trapping the blood in the hoof capsule. It can definitely put pressure on the proximal collateral cartilages.

Proximal to the frog, there is a cartilaginous tissue that is known as the digital cushion **(Figure 15)**. This fibrofatty insensitive tissue is situated distal and palmar to the coffin bone and fills the space between the frog and deep flexor tendon and the collateral cartilages. The digital cushion is compressed during loading and pushes downward on the frog, protects the deep flexor tendon, and pushes outward on the collateral cartilages. This helps to create some of the expansion at the distal heels of the hoof.

CIRCULATION AND CONCUSSION MECHANISM:

During movement, the foot loads and the heels expand. The bony column sinks into the hoof capsule, the sole descends, the frog is smashed, and the fetlock moves toward the ground. The coronary band and top of the foot are pulled palmar during loading, and this causes the blood that is in the foot to become momentarily trapped. Because it has filled the venous plexuses, these plexuses form the function of a hydraulic cushion. **Figure 16** is a drawing of the venous plexuses. There are 3 main venous plexuses; the coronary venous plexus, the dorsal venous plexus, and the solar venous plexus.

As the foot leaves the ground, the contraction of the heels, the ascension of the sole and frog, and the release of pressure at the top of the foot and coronet all aid in returning the dark-red, deoxygenated blood to the heart. What is really neat about this cycle is that it is perfectly tuned to the job the horse is doing. When a horse is moving fast and hard, there is a lot of concussion from the extra downward force causing more descent in the sole, frog, fetlock and coronet. At this time, a horse needs the more

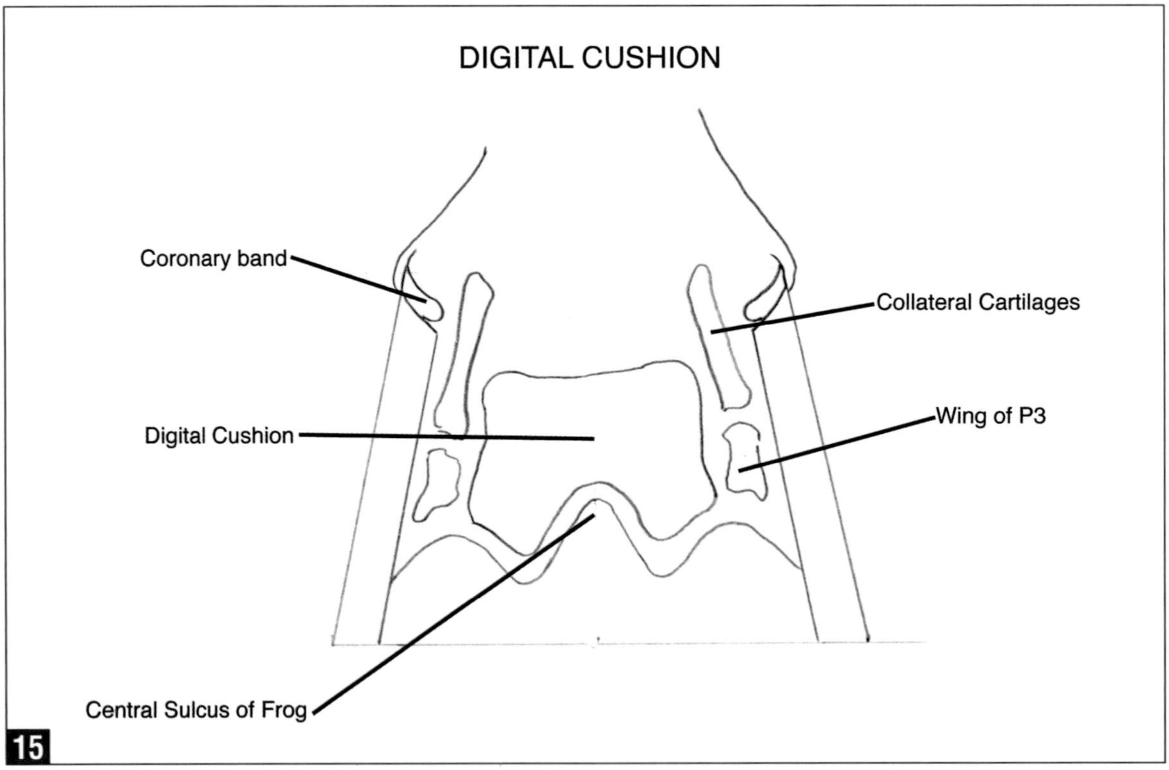

Cross section of a foot showing the digital cushion.

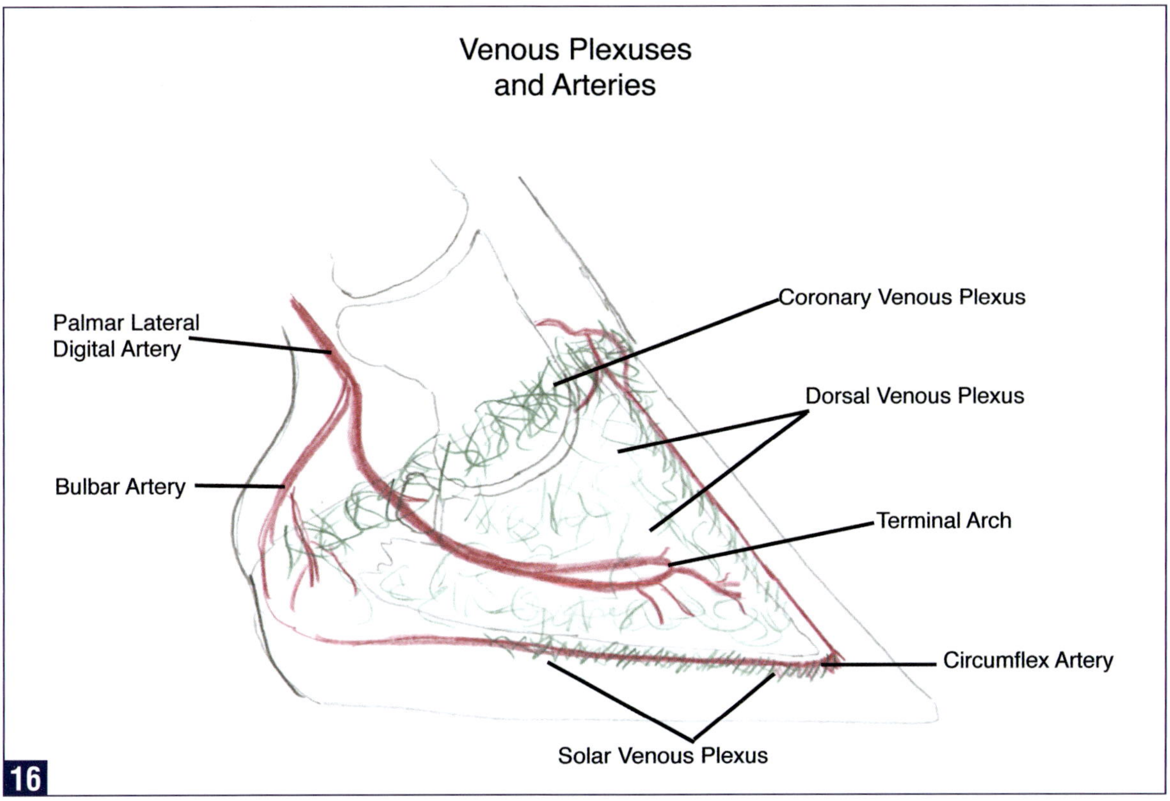

Venous plexuses.

bright-red, oxygenated blood in its extremities.

Horses that are standing still will push blood through their foot by arterial pulse. This biomechanical process of blood supply to the foot matches perfectly with the horse's activity. A horse at a walk will be using the process at a lesser percentage than a horse at a trot. The trotting horse will use it less than the horse at a lope, etc.

HOOF PASTERN AXIS AND ANGLE CHANGE: PROPER ANGLES ON FRONT FEET

When you trim the ground surface of the hoof capsule, you influence how that foot sits on the ground and accepts the load from the horse above. What you do to the angle of that foot will have an immediate impact on how the angle of the coffin bone relates to the angle of the pastern bones.

There is a concept in farriery known as "natural angle." Due to the improper commercial use of the word natural for naming a trim and shoe, the word now carries a bad connotation among many of the top farriers in the world. The use of natural in the phrase "natural angle" is meant to indicate the angle that is appropriate for that individual horse, and has no relevance to anything commercial. However, it is a label that is commonly used in the farrier industry, and one that you must be familiar with.

This angle is determined by looking at a horse from a lateral view, with the horse standing with all four feet on level ground. Lifting any one foot will give you a false reading of the natural angle by loading the other legs more than normal. This goes for taking radiographs as well. The horse should be standing as square as possible, with the front legs in the same lateral plane under the trunk. The hinds should also be in the same lateral plane.

Once you have the horse standing correctly, carefully look at the angle of the pastern as it relates to the angle of the dorsal hoof wall. Be aware that the long pastern bone is elliptical in shape and not a uniform size from top to bottom. This means that there is not any precise way to determine the exact angle of that bone with the naked eye. However, you can learn to see enough to determine if the axis of the pastern is parallel to the dorsal wall. Having these lines parallel is what is known as a proper natural angle.

Every horse has an angle that is appropriate for that horse. Some texts will dictate one angle for every horse, but that makes as little sense as dictating one shoe size for every human. The ability to accept the individual challenges that each horse will present is part of what separates the great farriers from the average horseshoers. **Figure 17** is a drawing that represents a range of angles. Any of these angles are correct for the horse pictured because the dorsal wall is straight with the axis of the pastern. Problems occur when we begin to change the angles incorrectly. You can end up with feet and pasterns like those in **Figure 18**. Notice that the angle of the pastern is not lined up with the angle

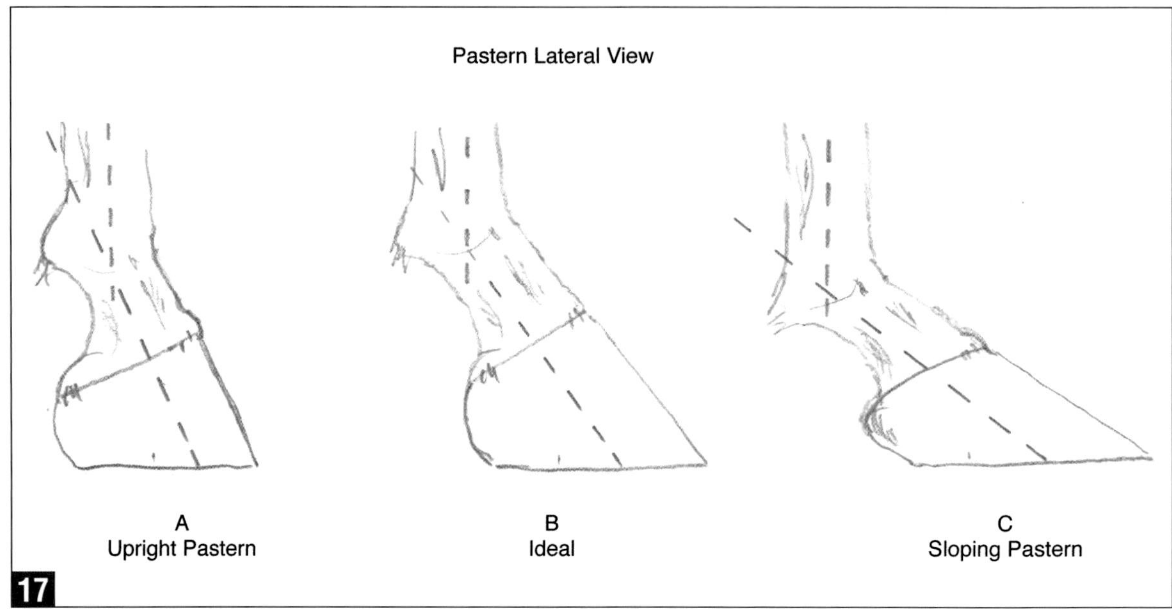

Proper natural angles.

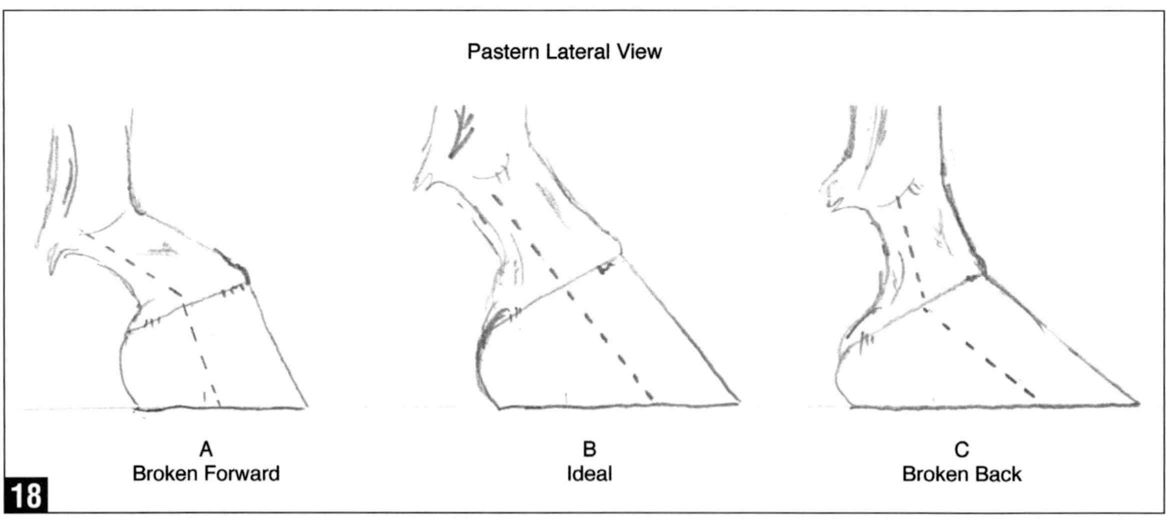

Pastern and hoof angles that are not in alignment.

of the hoof on two of the drawings.

Figure 19 is a radiograph of a horse with a very good natural angle. As you can see, a straight line will bisect the bones of the pastern and remain parallel to the dorsal wall. **Figure 20** is another horse that is at a good natural angle, but we are evaluating the angle without radiographs. Your rasp is a handy straight line to lay along the pastern and compare with the toe.

Now consider the insertion of the superficial flexor tendon (SFT) in relation to the deep flexor tendon (DFT). The SFT inserts into both

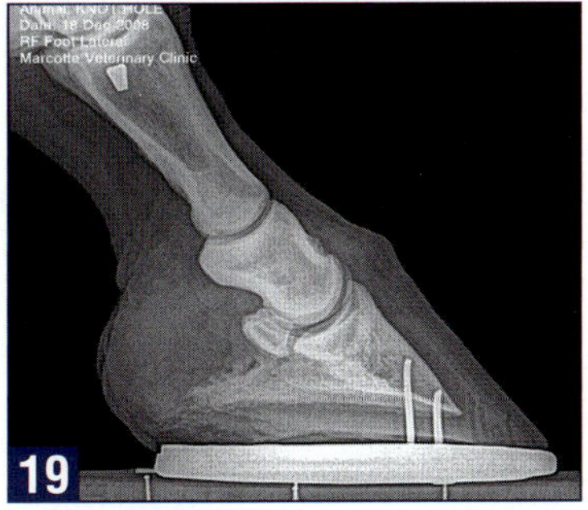

19

Radiographs of a horse with a good natural angle.

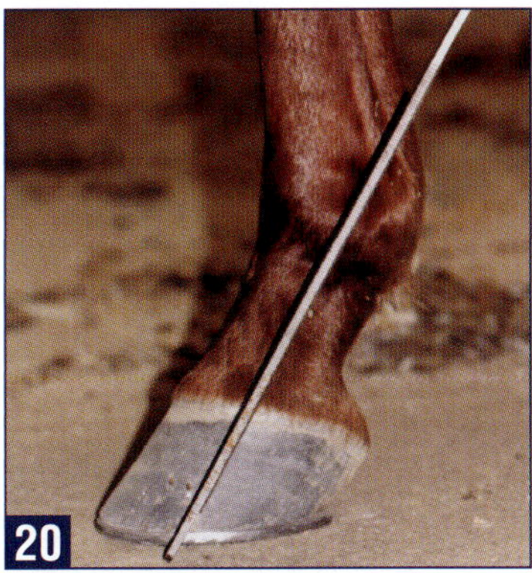

20

Evaluating the natural angle using a rasp.

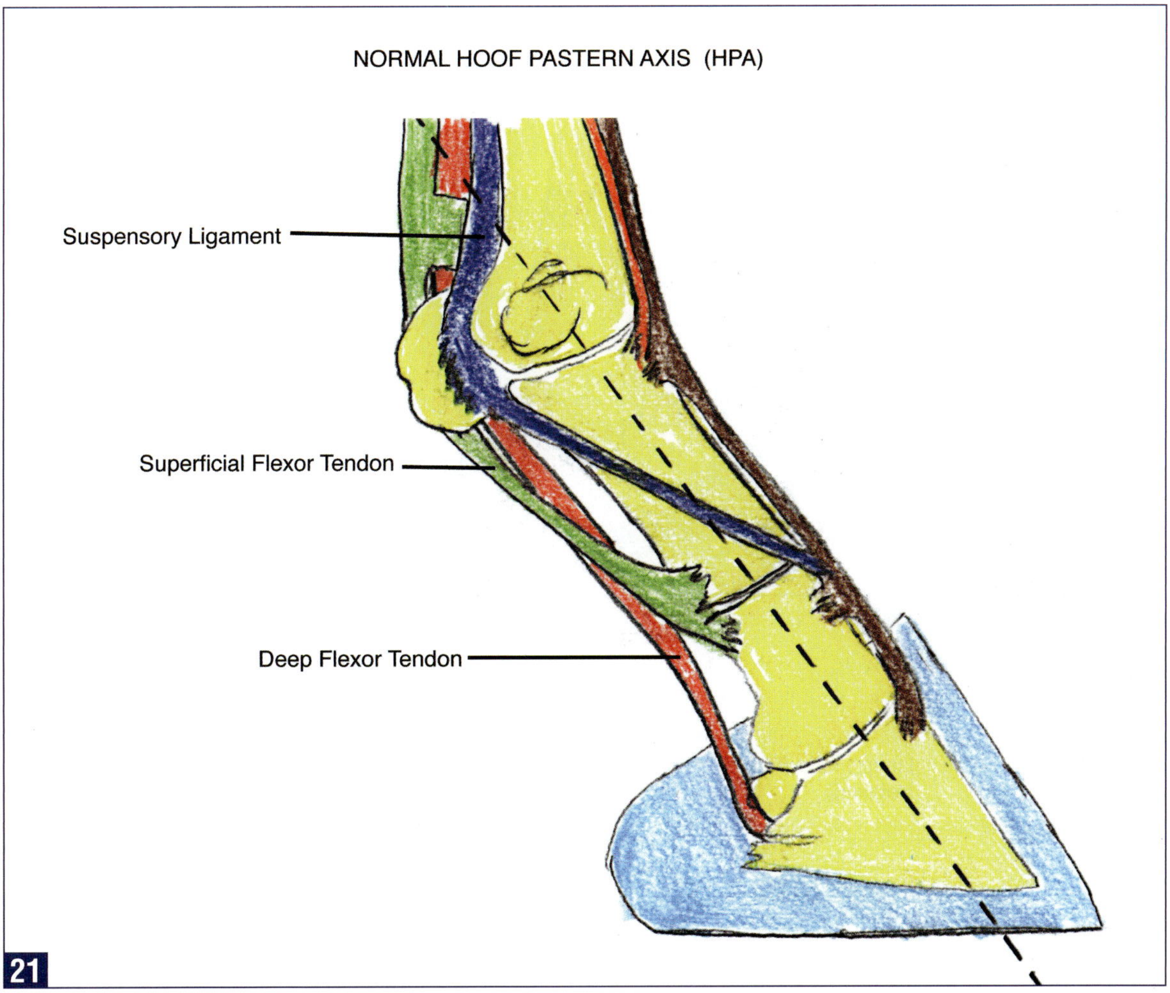

NORMAL HOOF PASTERN AXIS (HPA)

Suspensory Ligament

Superficial Flexor Tendon

Deep Flexor Tendon

21

A drawing of the lower leg that depicts a good natural angle, including the main tendons and ligaments affected.

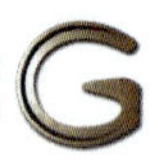

sides of the pastern joint (collaterally on distal P1 and proximal P2). The DFT inserts into the semlunar crest on the solar surface of the coffin bone. The coffin joint is located between these two insertion points. This joint allows for quite a bit of movement, and it is important to remember the way that this joint moves when trying to understand the stress applied from tendons as they react to hoof angle. It is also important to remember that the extensor tendons are not weightbearing structures. I have often had students get confused about this, so I thought that I should stress that point.

If a foot is trimmed to what is the correct angle for that horse, the tension on the flexor tendons and suspensory ligament is correct for that horse **(Figure 21)**. After a change is made to make the angle of the foot either higher or lower (steeper or shallower), the coffin bone's orientation is going to become either steeper or shallower as well. This will cause a different pull on the deep flexor tendon in relation to the superficial flexor tendon and the suspensory ligament. Here is how it works:

Increasing the angle of the foot **(Figure 22)** — raising the heel relative to the toe — brings the semilunar crest of P3 closer to the origin of the DFT at the distal end of the deep flexor muscle.

With the origin and insertion of the DFT closer to each other (increased hoof angle), there will be less stress on the DFT. With less stress, the DFT will not bear as much weight, and this will allow the fetlock to descend slightly. After this happens, the angle of the pastern is changed as the fetlock descends, causing there to be more stress on SFT.

The converse is true as well. Decreasing the

STEEP FOOT, SHALLOW PASTERN
Suspensory LIgament
(stressed)
Superficial Flexor Tendon
(stressed)
Deep Flexor Tendon
(relaxed)
22

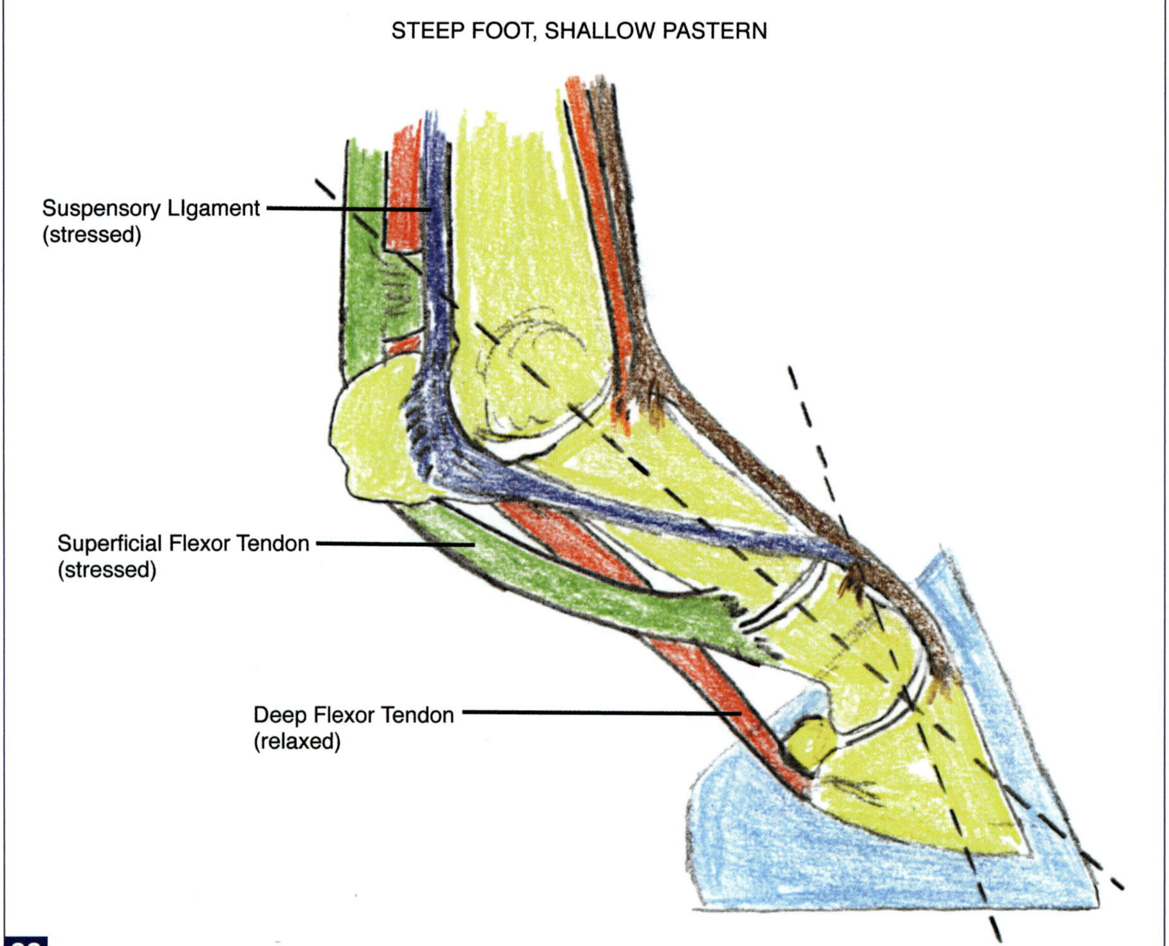

Drawing of the anatomical changes to the natural angle that can happen from trimming a foot too steep.

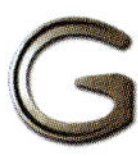

hoof angle **(Figure 23)** — lowering the heel relative to the toe — places more stress on the DFT as the origin and insertion move farther apart. As this happens, the fetlock is pushed forward and upward slightly. This new position of the fetlock makes the angle of the pastern different, which in turn decreases stress on the SFT.

One way to think about this is that after you depart from the natural angle, the foot and that pastern will go in opposite directions. Steeper foot = shallower pastern: shallower foot = steeper pastern.

Consider also that whatever happens to the SFT will also happen to the suspensory ligament. Relax the SFT, and the suspensory ligament relaxes. Stressing the SFT stresses the suspensory ligament.

Another thing to know is that the horse will be able to adjust its stance to accommodate the trim. In the front end, if the hoof angle it too steep, the horse will stand under. It will stand camped in front if the foot angle is too shallow. On the pelvic limb, the reciprocal apparatus places the foot automatically, and you will find that changing angles on hind feet does not affect the pastern as much as it does the placement of the foot on the ground in relation to the trunk.

All of these principles of angle on the front feet are extremely important if you are to understand how trimming the foot impacts the rest of the horse. When dealing with any sort of flexor tendon or suspensory ligament problem, you can make things better or worse based on how you trim the foot. Knowing how the trim affects the tendons can be the difference between a sound horse and a crippled horse.

SHALLOW FOOT, STEEP PASTERN
Suspensory Ligament (relaxed)
Superficial Flexor Tendon (relaxed)
Deep Flexor Tendon (stressed)
23

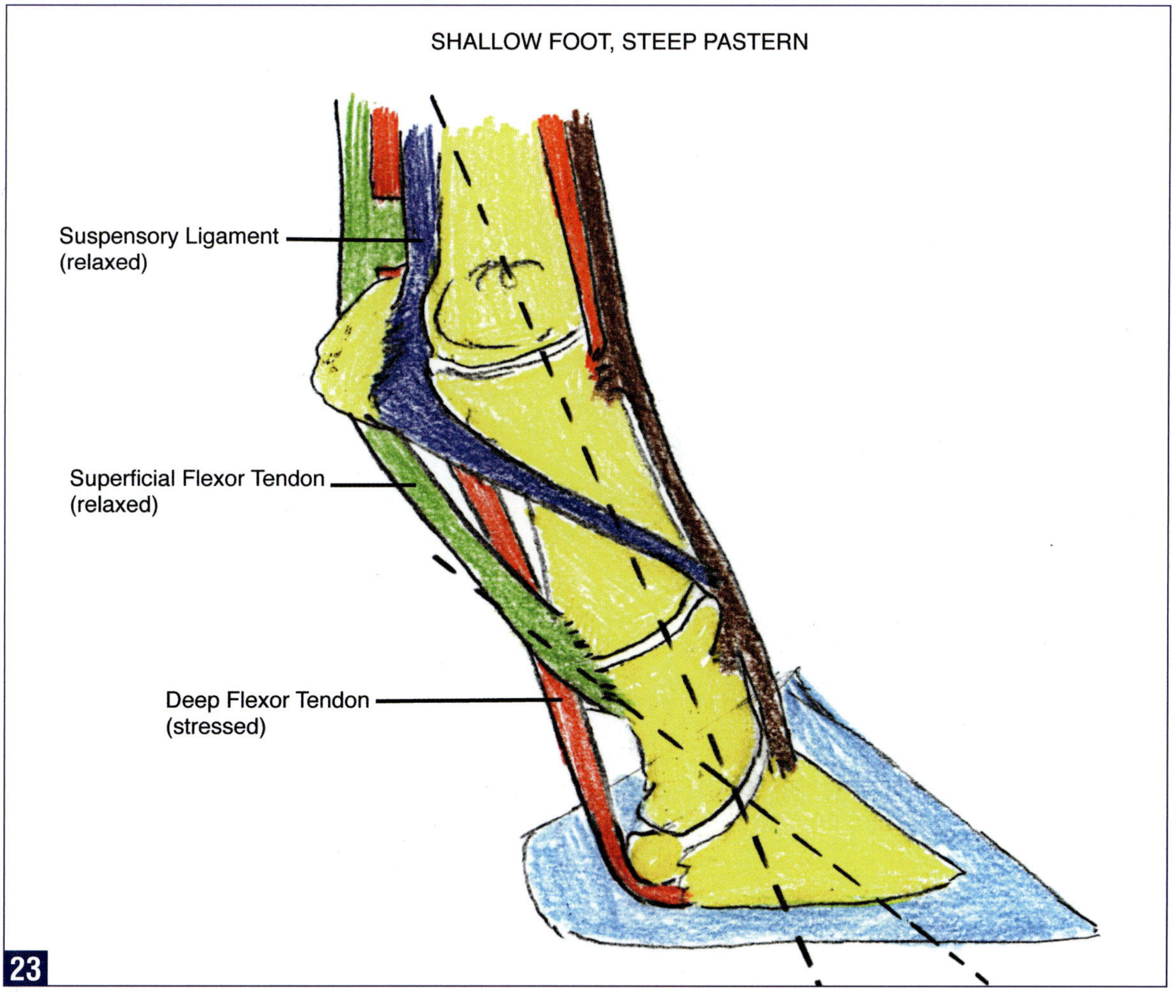

Drawing of the anatomical changes to the natural angle that can happen from trimming a foot too shallow.

Likewise, dealing with gait problems such as overreaching can be greatly influenced by the angle of the trim. Trimming a front foot steep can cause a horse to overreach when it had not done so before because the horse will stand under to accommodate the steep trim. This information can make you the hero when you correct the work of a farrier with less knowledge and skill.

Understanding how the trim on the foot impacts the entire horse is the basis of good farriery. If you don't have a firm grasp on this chapter, read it again until you do.

There is still a lot that we don't know about what exactly happens when a horse is in motion. Many researchers are developing ways to see with science and technology what we can't see with our eyes. They are studying the biomechanics of the equine, and I am excited to find out what the results of their efforts will yield. As of now, the principles outlined in this chapter are what I believe is happening to a horse.

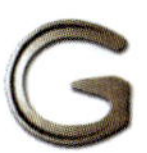

Chapter

13 DISSECTION

Your quest to become great at this trade can be greatly assisted by doing dissections. Doing a whole horse dissection can teach you a lot about this animal **(Figures 1 and 2)**, but I would start with the legs. After you have mastered the anatomy of the leg, continue learning from there and never stop.

The goal of this dissection is to see where the extensor and flexor tendons traverse down the leg. Identify and explore the course and position of the suspensory ligament, check ligaments, sesamoidian ligaments, annular ligaments, and collateral ligaments. Identify and remove the horny portions of the hoof from their respective coriums, and ultimately remove the navicular bone from the coffin joint. You will see and learn about the digital cushion, lateral cartilages, sensitive frog, sole, laminae, and coronary band.

There are few things that can teach you as much as dissecting a horse's leg. I prefer to have the leg cut off at the distal end of the radius or the distal end of the tibia. I will remove the leg with a saw. This allows me to have the entire carpus and tarsus to go with the dissection.

Begin the dissection by removing the skin. The first cut I make will be up the dorsal aspect of the cannon bone to the where the skin ends. When you remove the skin, try to avoid cutting into the tendons, ligaments, arteries, veins and nerves. The white connective tissue that you will be seperating is called fascia. Place the hoof in a vise and pull on the skin as you cut through the fascia. When you get to the top of the hoof capsule, you can decide how much skin you wish to leave at the top of the foot. Generally, a half inch is enough to see what is under the skin, yet still get the benefit of seeing the periople **(Figure 3)**.

The first thing that I like to do is to reflect back the tendons to a spot distal to the carpus or tarsus. You can cut them off if you prefer, but I like to have the extra piece to hold on to. If you are on good terms with your local vet, you can get clamps and tweezers to hold onto this slippery biological tissue. If not, needle-nosed vise grips will serve you well.

Numerous ligaments hold the carpus and tarsus together. You can decide whether or not you want to separate each bone from the others. This is time consuming but rewarding as you get to see the exact position and shape of each carpal and tarsal bone. A quick note on time; if the dissection is going to take more time than you have, you can always put it back in the freezer. Depending on your situation,

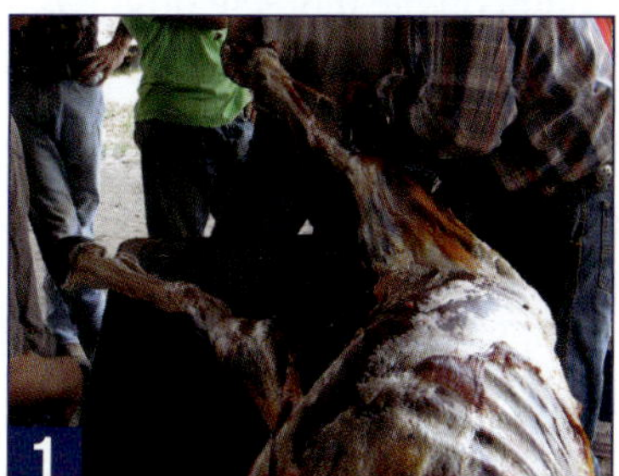

Whole horse dissection.

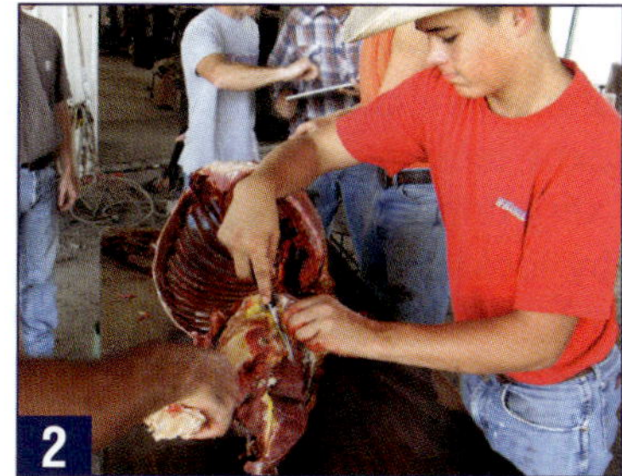

Cody working on the carcass of a pony.

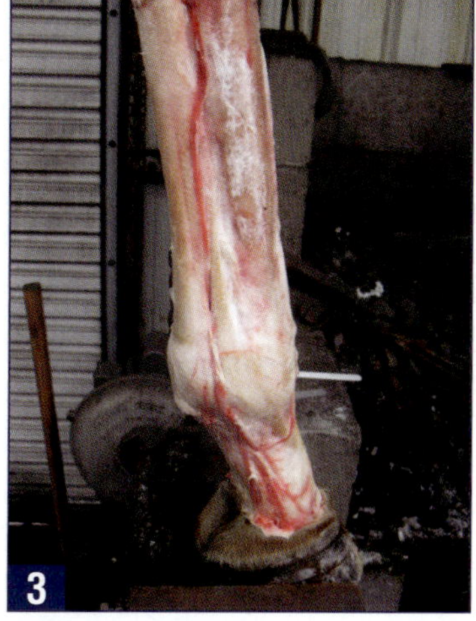

Skinned leg in vise.

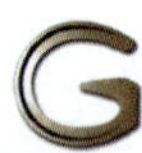

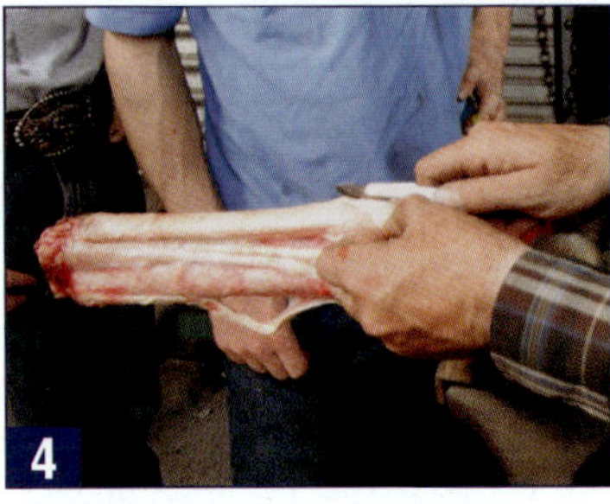
Cutting through the palmar annular ligament.

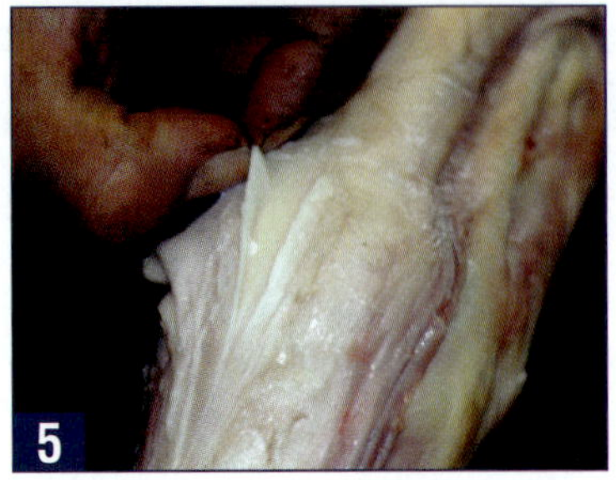
Palmar annular ligament

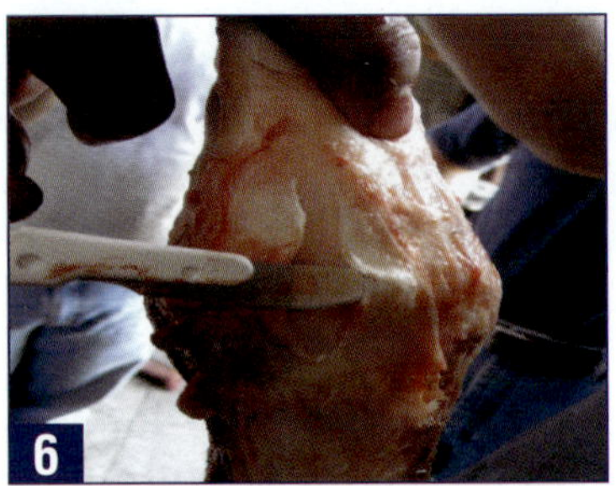

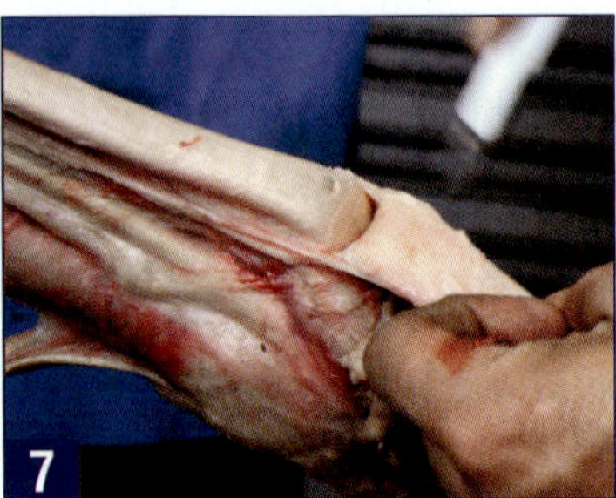
Reflecting back the superficial flexor tendon.

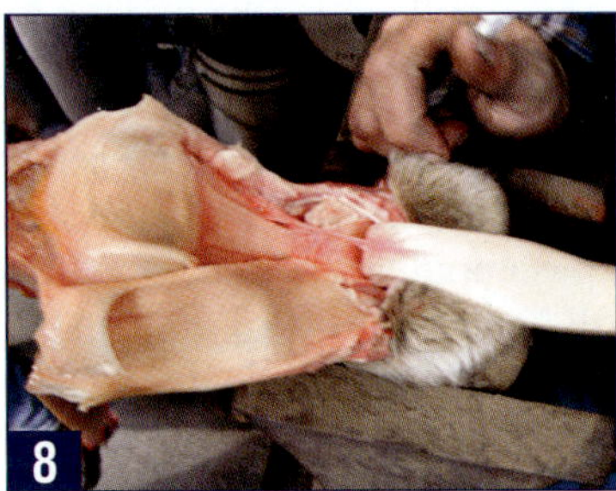
Reflecting back the deep flexor tendon.

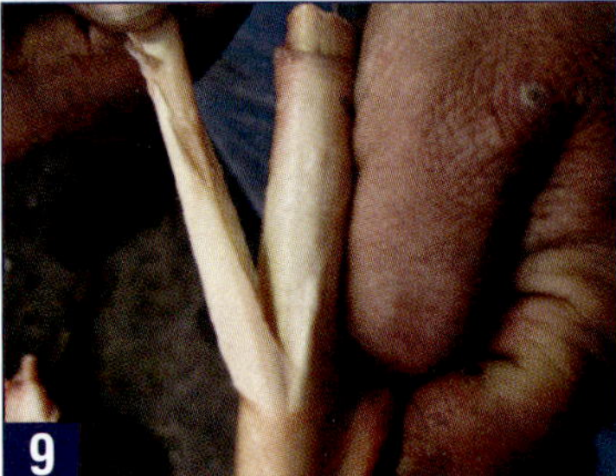
Detail of the subcarpal check ligament where it joins the deep flexor tendon.

you may need to disguise it in the freezer to keep your spouse happy.

Begin by reflecting the extensor tendons back from the cannon bone. You will notice that they are quite thin compared to the flexor tendons. Their job is to pull the leg forward against minimal resistance, while the flexor tendons have to have superior strength to push the weight of the horse forward.

With the hoof held in the vise, you can identify the tendons as you reflect them back from the leg. In **Figure 4**, I am cutting through the palmar annular ligament to allow me to pull the flexor tendons back. The palmar annular ligament is very thin and inelastic. You can see just how thin by looking at **Figures 5 and 6**. The palmar annular ligament is the piece that I am holding between my thumb and finger in **Figure 5**. The most external tendon is the superficial flexor tendon. You can see that I have reflected it away from the deep flexor tendon to the point where the superficial flexor makes a ring around the deep flexor tendon in **Figure 7**.

I like to cut through one side of the superficial flexor so that I can reflect it back and free the deep flexor tendon as it makes its way around the navicular bone to insert into the semilunar crest of P3. Run your fingers up and down the deep flexor, and you can feel how the dimensions change from round proximally to flat and wide as it passes over the back of the pastern. In **Figure 8**, I have reflected back the lower portion of the superficial flexor tendon and removed the top portion of it all together. In the picture, the deep flexor tendon is being pulled away to expose the sesamoidian ligaments underneath.

he deep flexor tendon on the thoracic limb has a check ligament on it called the subcarpal (inferior) check ligament. It is quite a thick and strong check ligament, and in **Figure 9** you can see where it attaches to the deep flexor tendon. This is the largest and strongest of the three check ligaments.

At this point in the process, I generally go back to the palmar aspect of the cannon bone and remove the suspensory ligament. This is the largest ligament in the leg (bear in mind that the leg is technically from the knee or hock down). It originates at the palmar proximal cannon bone with adhesions to the carpals or tarsals, courses distad, and bifurcates at the distal nodules of the splint bones. If you look at **Figure 10**, you will see that the striations of this ligament at the bifurcation area are very pronounced in this horse. They are not always as

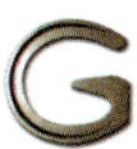

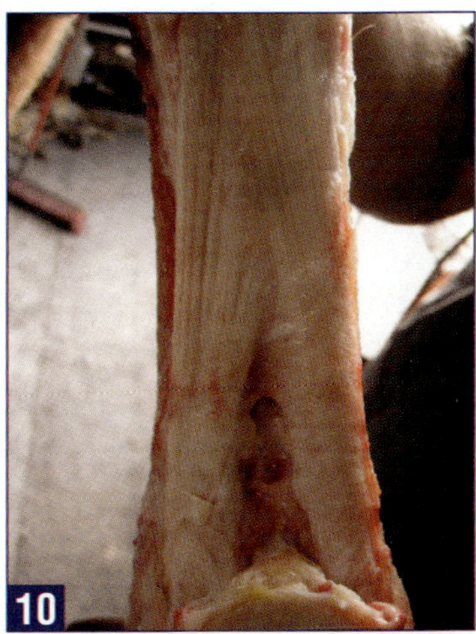

Striations in the suspensory ligament (interosseous muscle, interosseous tendon) at its' bifurcation point.

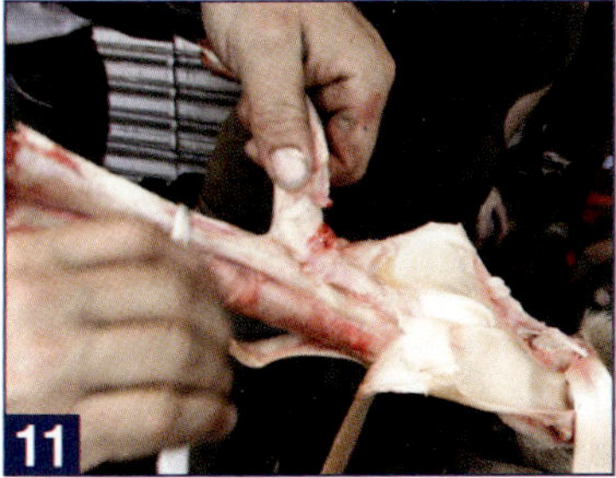

Freeing the suspensory ligament from the cannon bone,

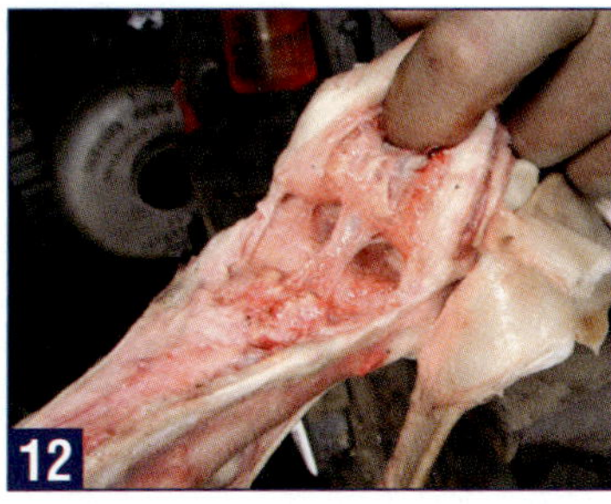

Pulling the suspensory ligament back at the sesamoids.

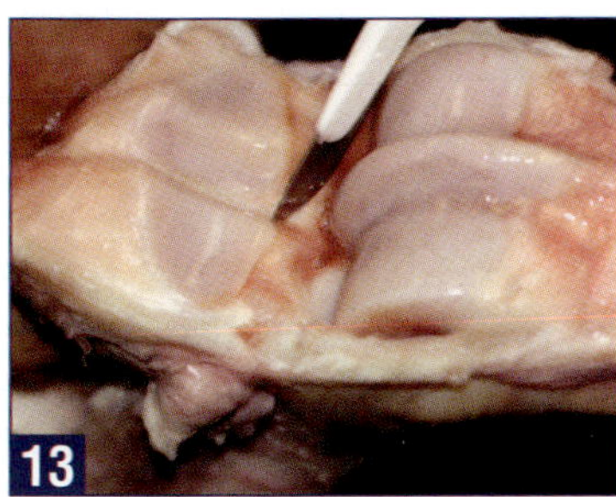

Fetlock joint with the cannon bone still in the joint.

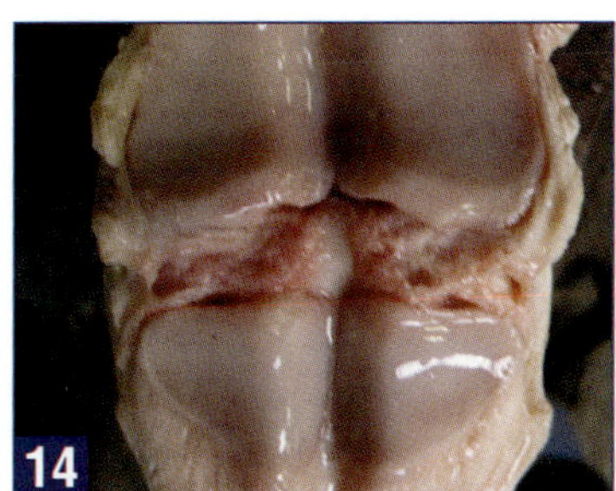

Fetlock joint with the cannon bone removed. Detail of the deep and short sesamoidian ligaments.

defined. The distal nodules are easy to find at this stage by running your fingers down the splint bones. Follow the suspensory ligament to its insertion on the sesamoids and then dorsodistad to the main extensor tendon.

Pull back on the suspensory ligament as you cut along both sides of it to reveal the proximal sesamoid bones **(Figures 11 and 12)**. The sesamoid bones make up a large portion of the fetlock joint (metacarpophalangeal joint), so when you cut through the collateral sesamoidian ligament that holds them in place, you should get into the synovial fluid of the fetlock joint.

Having found the fetlock joint, I cut around the joint to free the cannon bone from the pastern. It is amazing to feel how slick this joint surface is, and you can move the cannon boner around on top of P1 to feel the lack of friction.

There are six ligaments that are known as sesamoidian ligaments, and this is a good time to identify these. We have already cut through the bulk of the collateral sesamoidian ligament on the sides of the fetlock joint. By pulling on the suspensory ligament to reflect the sesamoidian bones away from the fetlock joint, you may be able to see the deep (X) sesamoidian ligaments and the short sesamoidian ligaments. **Figure 13** depicts the dorsal aspect of the sesamoids being pulled back and the cannon bone still attached to the proximal and dorsal aspects of P1. In **Figure 14**, the cannon bone has been removed, and the deep sesamoidian ligament is the X-shaped tissue in the middle of the picture, and the short sesamoidian ligament is the tissue on either side of the deep sesamoidian ligament. Both of these connect the distal, dorsal aspect of the sesamoid bones to proximal P1. Use a towel to wipe away the synovial fluid to see it more clearly. They can also be found from a palmar route to resemble the drawings of these ligaments in Chapter 10, Ligaments and Tendons.

Place the sesamoids back in position, and you can now see the palmar aspect of the sesamoidian ligaments and pastern. In **Figure 15**, the scalpel is touching the intersesamoidian ligament. To the right of the photo is a flap of tissue. This is part of the palmar annular ligament that was shown in **Figures**

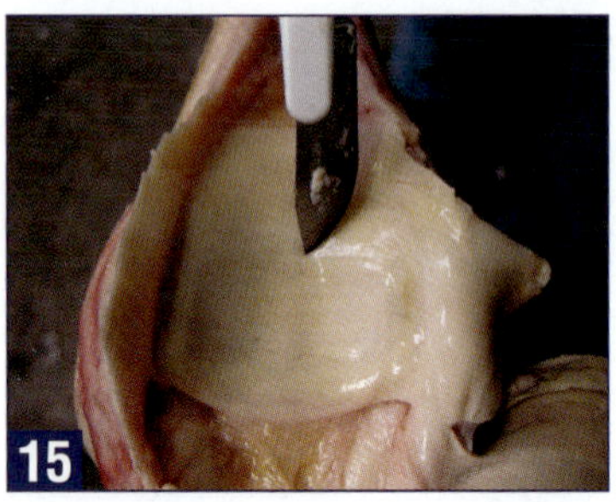

15 ***Intersesamoidian ligament with some of the palmar annular ligament attached.***

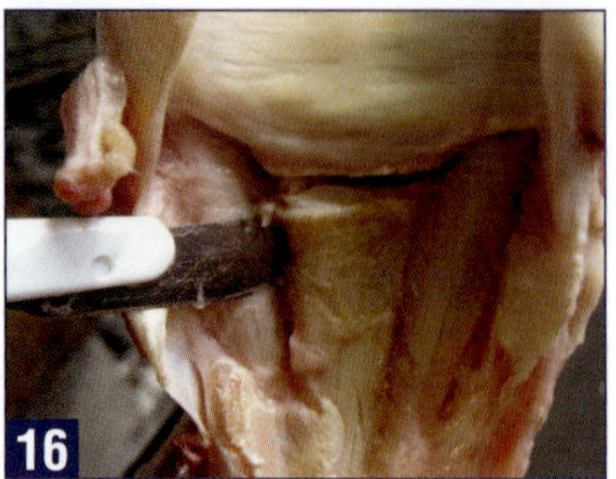

16 ***Superficial sesamoidian ligament (Y or straight sesamoidian ligament).***

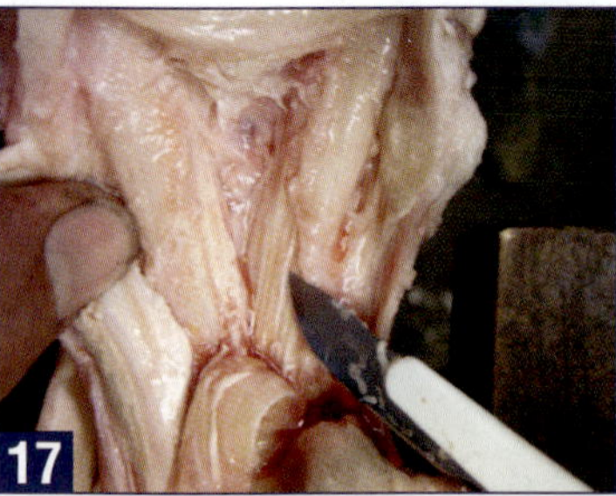

17 ***Middle sesamoidian ligament (V or oblique sesamoidian ligament).***

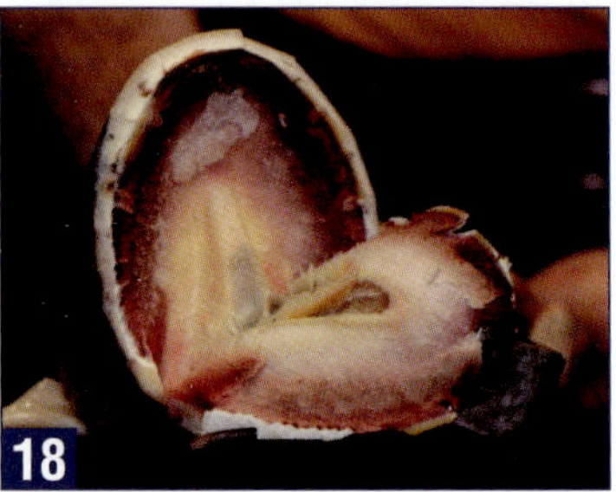

18 ***Pulling the sole off prior to removing the hoof wall.***

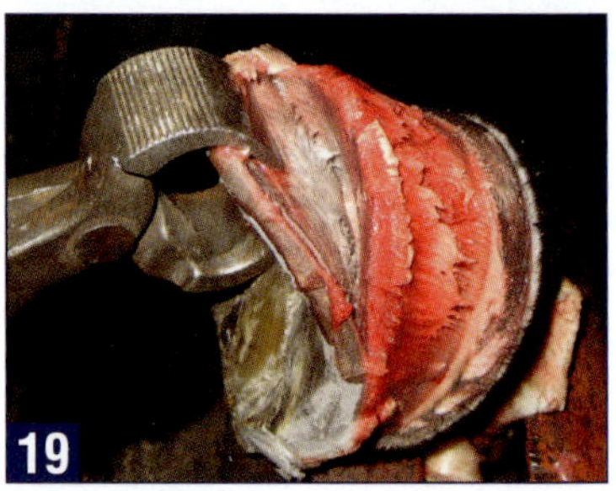

19 **20** ***Removing the sole after the hoof wall has been removed.***

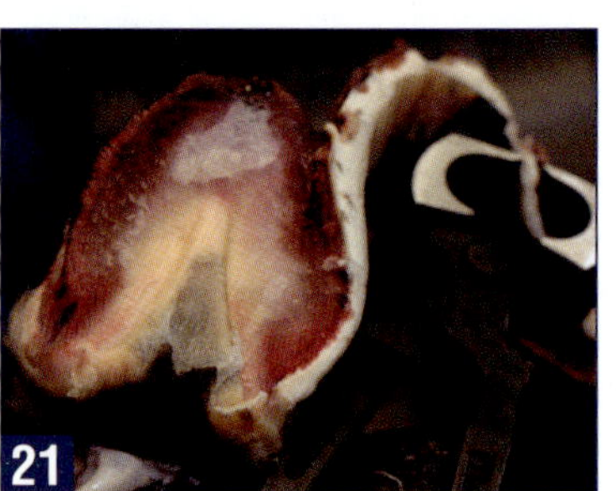

21 **22** ***Pulling the hoof wall off of the coffin bone.***

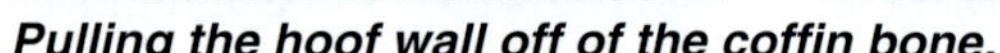

5 and 6. There are a lot of adhesions between the palmar annular ligament and the intersesamoidian ligament.

Below the intersesamoidian ligament, the straighter of the ligaments on the back of the pastern is the superficial (Y) sesamoidian ligament **(Figure 16)**. Cut this away, and you can see the middle (V) sesamoidian ligament that originates on the sesamoids and inserts into distal P1 **(Figure 17)**. If you cut it away as well and carefully cut under the sesamoid bones, you can find the deep and short sesamoidian ligaments from the palmar view.

Take the foot out of the vise and put P1 in its place. The hoof is now ready to be dissected. You can see the solar view, and this is a good time to identify all the parts. Nip from heel to heel at an angle, going right to the white line if possible. As you nip, be certain to point out to any onlookers that nipping like this is only done when working on dead feet. Depending on what you want to do, you can pull the sole off now, as in **Figure 18**, or do it after the wall is pulled away as in **Figures 19 and 20**.

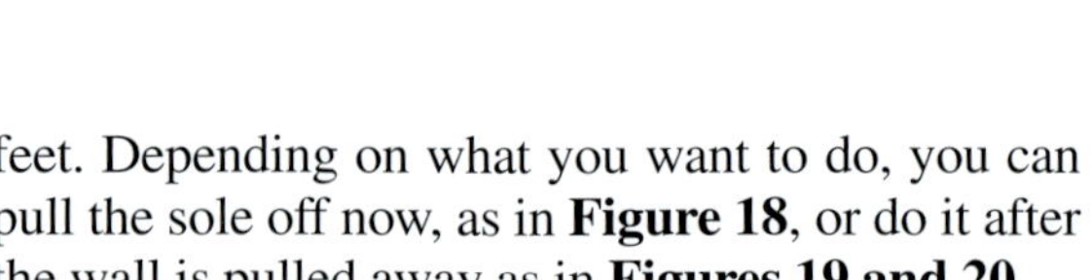

To pull the wall away, grab the wall at one heel with the pulloffs. Move the reins of the pulloffs toward the toe, tearing apart the bond between the horny and sensitive laminae **(Figures 21-22)**. You will be exposing the coffin bone covered with sensitive laminae as you pull the hoof wall off. This is such a strong connection, that you may be surprised at just how difficult it is to get the hoof wall off of the coffin bone. With the wall and sole removed,

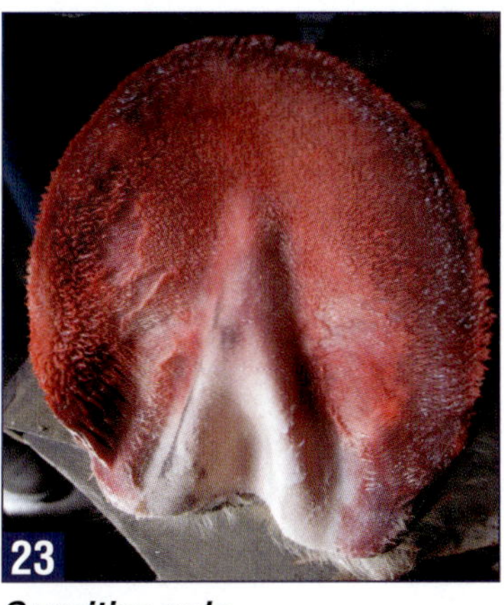

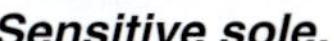

Sensitive sole.

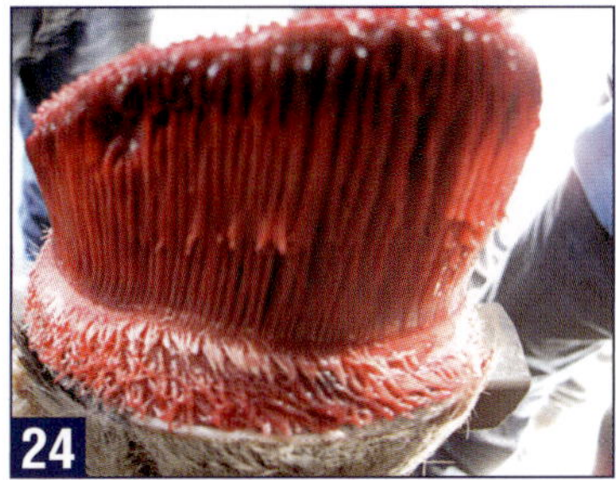

Sensitive laminae

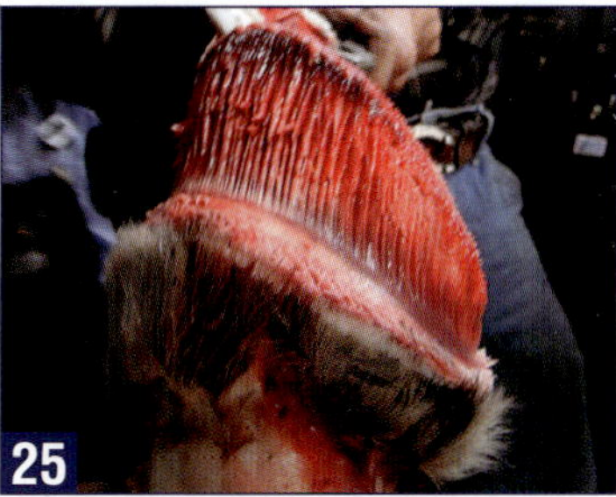

Coriums of the foot exposed.

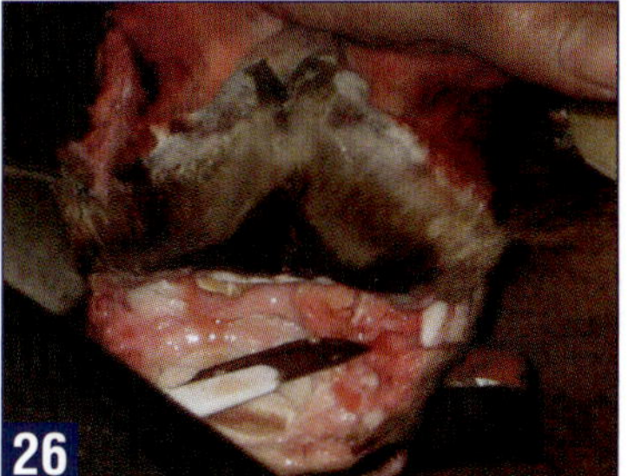

Pushing back on the toe of the foot to cut into the coffin joint.

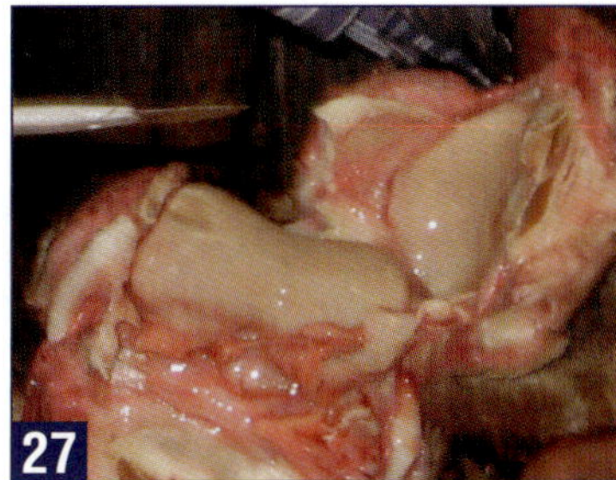

Access to the coffin joint and navicular bone with one of the collateral ligaments of the coffin joint still intact.

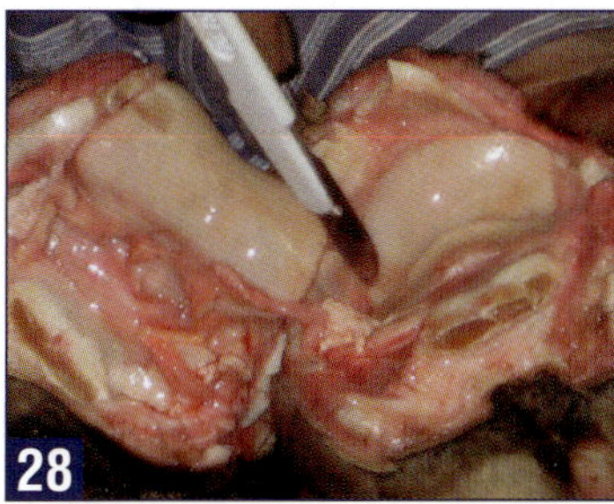

Cutting around the navicular bone.

you should be looking at the coriums of the hoof **(Figures 23-25)**.

Many basic dissections will stop at this point, but I like to cut into the coffin joint and remove the navicular bone. You can do this carefully or roughly, depending on what structures you are still trying to identify. To identify the collateral cartilages and their ligaments takes a lot of patience and careful cutting.

To remove the navicular bone in a rough manner, push back on the toe of the coffin bone as you cut into the deep flexor tendon, collateral cartilages, and eventually into the coffin joint **(Figure 26)**. I like to cut through one of the collateral ligaments of the coffin joint but leave the other complete to hold the coffin bone for me **(Figure 27)**. Cut around the navicular bone with your scalpel as you attempt to release it from its position **(Figure 28)**.

You have now exposed, touched, and defined many of the major structures of the horse's leg. The more dissections you do, the more you will learn. From time to time, you may even find unusual and abnormal anatomy, but you will always find more knowledge.

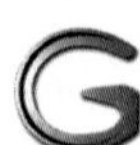

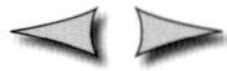

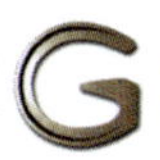

Section

4

Conformation

Chapter 14: Conformation.. 158

Chapter 15: Corrective Shoeing Theory................ 173

" 25 And God made the beast of the earth after his kind, and cattle after their kind, and every thing that creepeth upon the earth after his kind: and God saw that it was good. "

—Genesis 1:25
—King James Version

" 10 Mordecai wrote in the name of King Xerxes, sealed the dispatches with the king's signet ring, and sent them by mounted couriers, who rode fast horses especially bred for the king. "

—Esther 8:10
—New International Version

Chapter

14 CONFORMATION

Conformation means the structural arrangement, or — more specifically for horses — the proportions of a horse's body parts in relation to one another. How the horse is built will directly relate to how that horse moves. Most points of conformation are functional, not just aesthetic. When looking at a horse from a farrier's perspective, knowing how certain conformations affect certain movements is critical. The more you study equine conformation, the better your understanding can equate to success as a farrier.

In a wild environment without the interference of humans, horses will breed based on the principles of natural selection. The strong survive and reproduce while predators consume the weak. Domestic horses are bred based on the desires of their owners, and often the selection process is based on the wrong criteria. Breeding for color for instance, without considering conformation or disposition, has led to some poorly bred stock. Add to this the fact that many mares that are not sound for locomotion are still sound for breeding and can pass on the least desirable traits. As a farrier, you have to learn to deal with those undesirable traits to create as sound a horse as possible.

All the parts of a horse should be in proportion to one another. If a horse has any unusual characteristics, you should learn to see them at a glance. Horses with long legs and short backs are prone to overreach. Short-legged horses cannot move as fluidly as long-legged horses. If a horse is heavily built in the shoulders and lightly built in hindquarters, it will be heavy on the forehand, etc.

To describe weight distribution of the ideal horse, the front limb is perpendicular to the ground, and the horse will bear approximately 60% of its body weight on the front limbs. The hind cannon bones are perpendicular to the ground, and the horse will bear 40% of its body weight on the hind limb.

You can begin by looking at the head and neck, although there is nothing that you are going to be able to fix with shoeing. The horse uses its head and neck as a balancer, or counterweight, to help with movement. A long neck with an overly large head makes this more difficult than a smaller head. Generally speaking, the longer the neck, the longer the stride, as the muscles of the neck help to draw the front legs forward in movement.

The angle of the scapula determines the range of motion for the thoracic limb. This angle is often overlooked, but it is of the utmost importance. A sloping scapula rotates further back in movement, and this allows the foreleg to reach further up and forward. An upright shoulder restricts the range of motion upward and forward but does predisposes to a higher knee action.

The angle of the shoulder is often compared to the angle of the pastern, and there is a correlation, although it can be difficult to determine for several reasons. First, the scapula is an elliptically shaped bone, wider at the top than at the bottom. This means that there is a cranial angle, a caudal angle, and the axis of the bone. Next, the scapula is covered with muscle, tendon, ligament, fascia, skin and hair, making any true measurement of any angles quite difficult. Finally, there are not any really good ways to accurately compare the angle that you see at the scapula with the angle of the pastern. You have to rely solely on your eye. I'm a proponent of relying on the eye in most aspects of shoeing, but I take exception with the angle of the scapula. Generally speaking, if the shoulder is shallow, the pastern angle will be shallower, and vice versa. The shallower the angle of shoulder and pastern, the more shock absorbent the ride, but the better the chance of suspensory-related problems. The more upright the angles of the shoulder and pastern, the more concussion transferred to the horse's trunk, and the rougher the ride. These horses are prone to concussion-related lameness issues.

To begin with, it is important that you are able to determine what the ideal conformation of any part of the horse is. The ideal does not truly exist in nature, but it is something that you can judge the horses you are looking at against. With the ideal picture formed in your mind's eye, the deviations

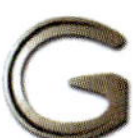

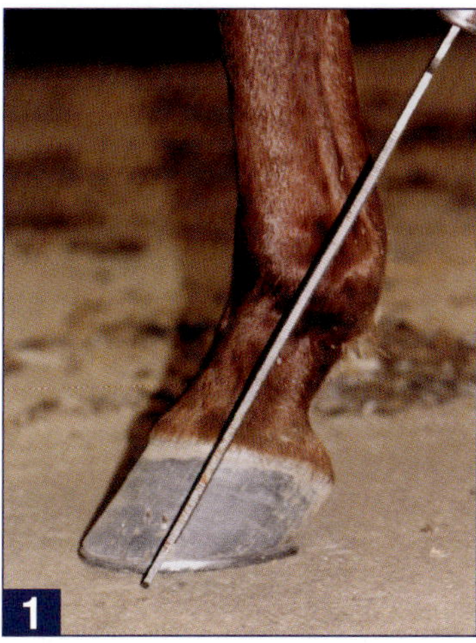

Good natural angle.

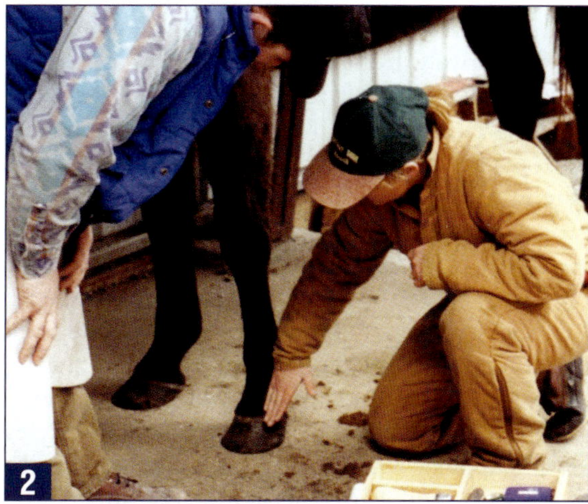

Kelly showing a student what to look for in the natural angle.

that each horse presents are more readily seen.

Deviations in the limbs can happen at any age, but most of the time, they will happen during the growth of the animal. These are commonly known as developmental orthopedic disorders (DODs).

DODs of the limbs generally fall into one of three categories. These are:

- Angular Limb Deformities (ALDs), which are a deviation in a joint that causes a horse to have a crooked limb. Most valgus and varus deviations are ALDs.
- Rotational or spiral deviations. Sometimes called vertical axis rotation, this refers to the twisting of a portion of the limb that can cause the horse to have a crooked leg. Rotational deviations can often be confused with ALDs and require careful examination.
- Flexural deformities, which are evident from a lateral view, and fall into the categories of contracture or laxity. Contracture refers to when the musculotendon structure is too short, causing the joints to flex, and laxity is when the musculotendon structure is too long, allowing the joints to dorsiflex. A club foot would be contracture, and flaccid tendons would be an example of laxity.

THORACIC LIMB

We will begin this discussion by looking at the digit. From the fetlock down is right in our realm,and is the part of the horse that we look at and understand the most.

The bones in the digit are the long pastern (P1), short pastern (P2), navicular bone, and coffin bone (P3). When a foot is trimmed, there is an immediate impact on the way that P3 will sit on the ground and load. Leaving too much foot in one area, or taking too much in another, will result in changes that can lead to long-term problems.

From a lateral view, I like to see the axis of the pastern parallel to the dorsal hoof wall as in **Figure 1**. This is an important thing that a young farrier needs to recognize, as Kelly is pointing out in **Figure 2**. Anatomically, P1 is larger proximally than distally and this can lead to an argument about what exactly is the axis and angle of the pastern. It has to be judged from the side on level ground to determine if the angle is appropriate for that horse.

There are three basic normal conformations for the pastern and hoof from the lateral view, with varying degrees of each. These are the upright pastern, the normal pastern, and the sloping pastern as seen in **A, B, and C of Figure 3**. As long as the foot and pastern have achieved a natural angle without the limb being too far out of perpendicular, then the horse is standing where that horse needs to be standing. There is nothing to fix, just conformation to accept. Young farriers often try to change the angles of the foot toward the ideal foot, even though this can be a bad idea if that horse was already at its natural angle. I find this to be especially true of horses that are ordinarily shallow. These types of feet are just shallow and sloping, and you have to accept that as part of that horse's conformation.

You can also have horses that are broken back or broken forward from a lateral view. In the normal situation, the fetlock will change angle opposite to the foot. For instance, if you increase the angle of the foot past its natural angle, the deep flexor tendon is relaxed and the fetlock can descend to make the broken forward problem even worse than it would have been without the change in the pastern. The opposite is true, where dropping the heels on a foot that is at its natural angle will cause the deep flexor tendon to tighten, pushing the fetlock up and forward, making the pastern steeper. Refer to the angle section in Chapter #12 where it discusses what happens when you relax the deep flexor tendon by increasing the angle; the superficial flexor tendon and suspensory ligament have to take up the slack. When you stress the deep flexor by lowering the angle of the foot, you relieve stress on the superficial flexor tendon and suspensory ligament. **Figure 4** shows this.

Ideal proportions of the thoracic limb would be a long scapula, a short humerus, a long radius, a short cannon bone, and a medium length pastern. These proportions result in a longer, freer stride with a greater range of motion.

From a lateral view, the bony column should be perpendicular to the ground, the cannon bone should be in line and under the radius, the knee should be straight, or bowed ever so slightly forward, and the foot and pastern should result in a natural angle.

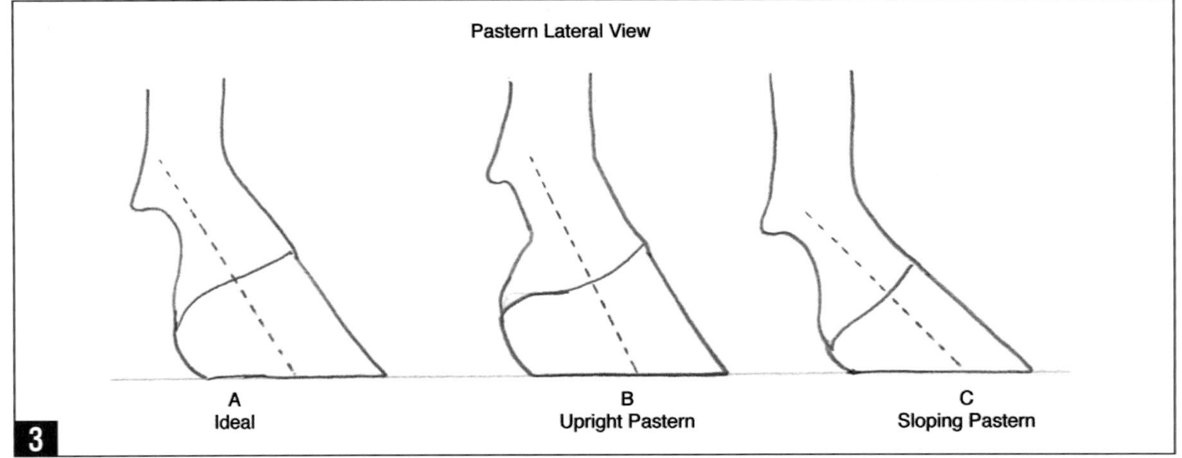

Drawing showing an upright foot, an ideal foot, and a sloping pastern and foot. All of them are at the appropriate natural angle for that particular horse.

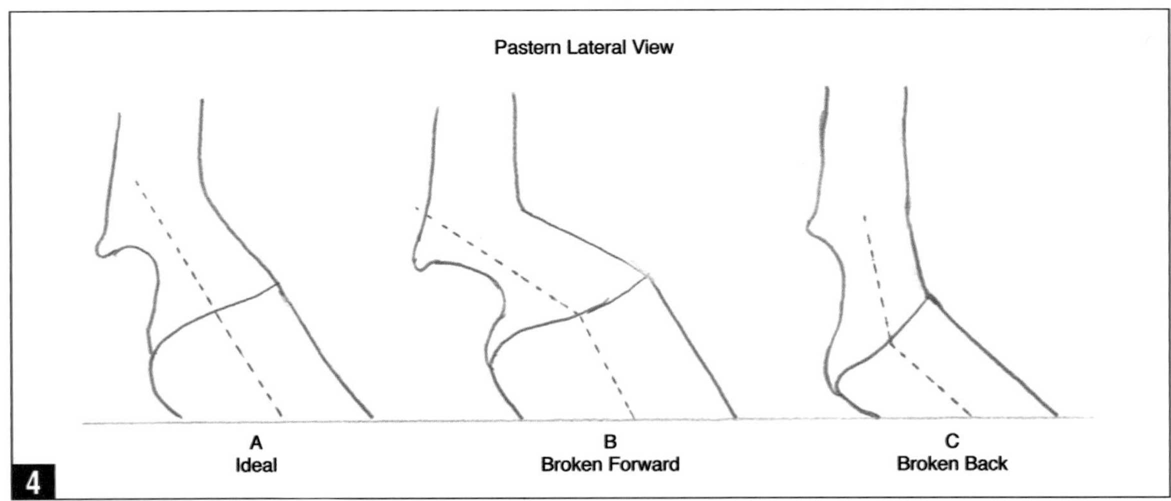

Drawing of a horse that has a broken forward hoof pastern axis (HPA), an ideal HPA, and a broken-back HPA.

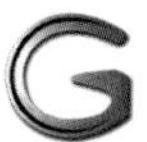

This is depicted in drawing A in **Figure 5**.

Due to my exposure to the American Quarter Horse and the use of this horse as a rodeo and cutting competitor, I don't mind if a horse is standing under slightly in the front limb, as long as it does not overreach. My rule of thumb is that the horse can stand under to the point that a line dropped from the point of the shoulder will fall in the back third of that horse's foot (B in **Figure 5**). Standing under further than this is not an acceptable stance, (C

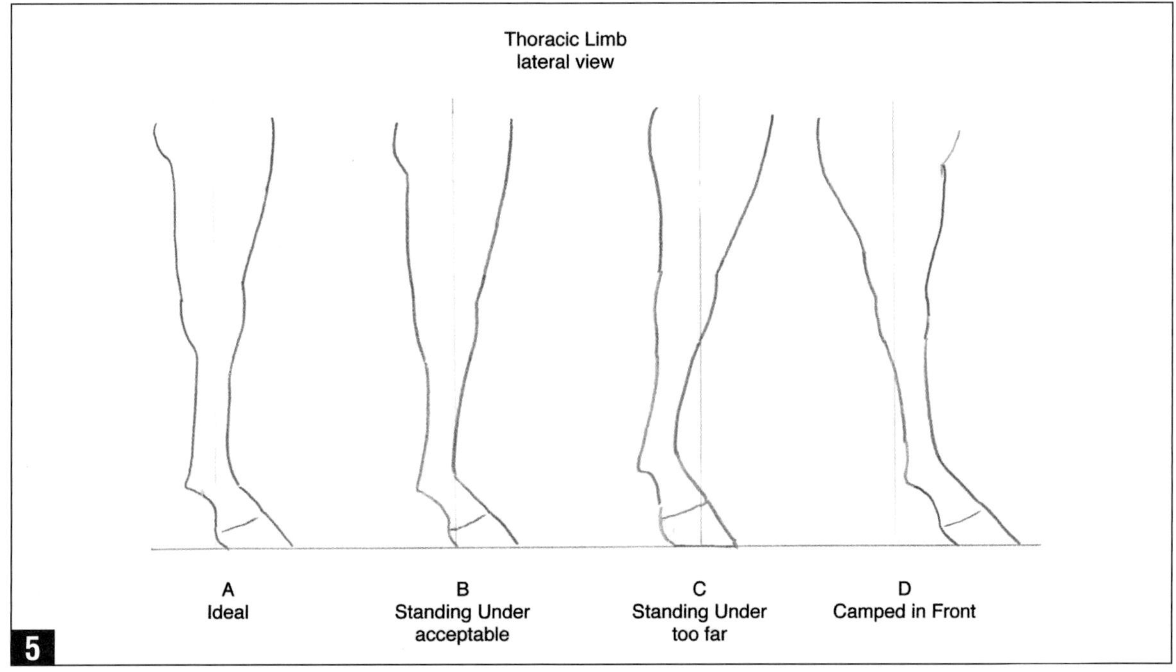

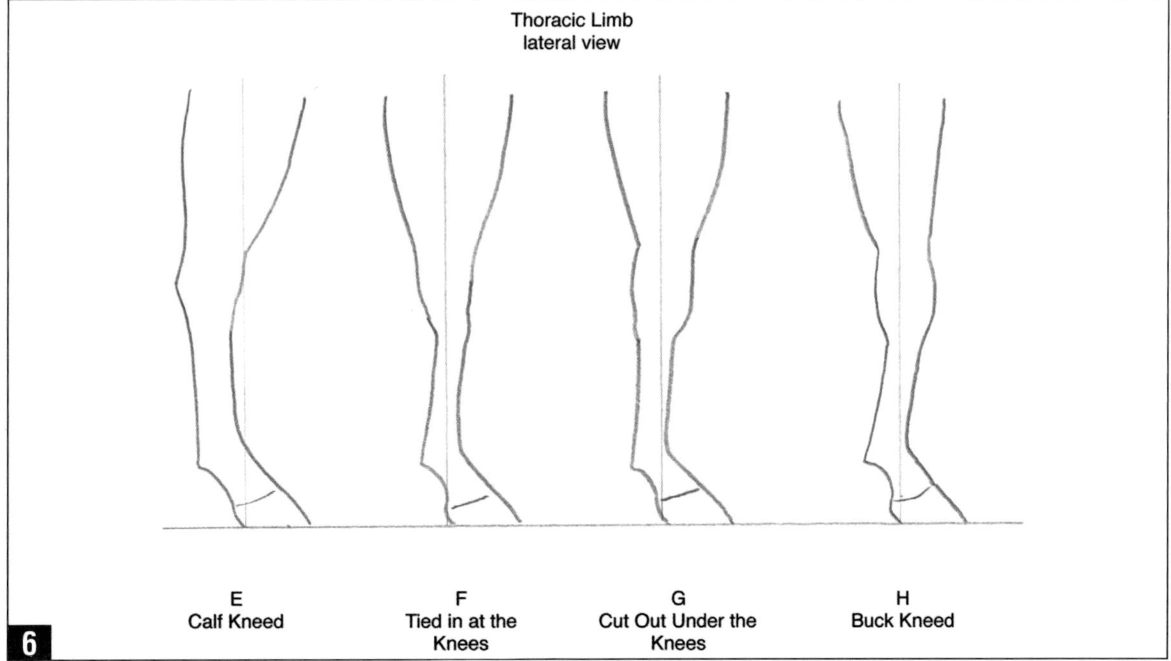

Lateral view of front limb conformation.

in **Figure 5)** and standing under even just a little will place more weight on the front limbs. If you have ever seen one of those foldable anvil stands collapse, you can imagine how moving the front limb back even a little bit can result in a problem. Think of the anvil sitting on the stand as the horse's head and neck, and the folding legs as the horse's limbs. Often, lowering the heels will cause the foot to move forward in relation to the trunk as the horse accommodates the angle of the trim, and this is referred to as camped in front (D in **Figure 5**).

There are several different conformational defects that can occur in the knee. With the arrangement of seven or eight bones, and three joints in the carpus, there is a lot of potential for the knee to have problems with how it is put together.

***Calf knees, sheep kneed, back at knees, or rearward deviation of the carpus* (E in Figure 6)**

This is perhaps one of the worst conformations that you can find in the carpus. Every time the knee bears weight, it is stressed in a manner that it was not designed for. The dorsal carpal bones are being compressed by this conformation as well as placing undue strain on the check ligaments. A horse with this conformation is prone to arthritis and chip fractures and rarely stays sound when put to work. If you have a horse like this on your books, politely tell the customer about the potential problems. By doing so, they can make an informed decision about how to use this horse. Also, when the horse does break down, you can be regarded as an intelligent farrier that forecast the problem, instead of an ignorant farrier that caused the problem. If the horse is a stud, cut it. If it is a mare, don't expose it.

***Tied in at the knees* (F in Figure 6)**

Tied in at the knees describes a conformation where the cannon bone appears to be positioned dorsally to the carpus and radius. Palmar to the distal carpus, it appears as if there is not enough mass to the tendons. This conformation is blamed for poor movement, and there is nothing that shoeing can do to change the conformation.

***Cut out under the knees* (G in Figure 6)**

Cut out under the knees refers to the cannon bone being positioned more palmarally to the carpus and radius. When you first see this conformation, it may appear as if the horse is calf kneed, but you can distinguish the difference by looking at the angle of the cannon bone to the ground. If the cannon bone is perpendicular, then it is cut out under the knees. If it is angled forward, it is calf kneed.

Like calf knees, this conformation predisposes a horse to problems, and it should be considered a poor conformation trait. To shoe this horse, you may want a rocker toe, or similar strategy, although you are not going to be able to fix the problem.

***Buck knees, goat knees, sprung knees, over in the knees, or forward deviation of the carpus* (H in Figure 6)**

This is a favorable conformation to calf knees, although if you had your choice, you would just as soon the knee was straight. This conformation can place extra strain on the sesamoid bones, superficial flexor tendon, and suspensory ligament. Most foals will appear to be buck kneed, but this disappears by about 3 months of age. In some cases, the horse will be so buck-kneed that it cannot bear weight on one leg alone without it buckling. From a shoeing standpoint, you can try to lower the angle of the foot slightly to relieve some of the stress on the superficial flexor and suspensory ligament, but this will not be a lasting fix. You may also find that slight toe extensions allow the horse to control its stance without buckling as much, but it will not enhance the horse's movement.

Open knees

This is referring to an irregular profile of the carpus, often seen in horses suffering epiphysitis (physitis) as well as in horses younger than 3 years of age. Generally, the appearance of the joints will improve with age. While this may appear as a problem, radiographically these knees have acceptable conformation.

Dorsal view

From the front, the ideal limb will be straight and perpendicular under the horse, with a line from the point of the shoulder passing through the center of the limb, knee, cannon, pastern and foot (A in **Figure 7**). Due to the biomechanics of where a foot is placed in relation to the horse's trunk, it is widely accepted that a foot will bear more weight on the inside. I have to say that I don't think that it is as much of a difference from the medial to the lateral side as I have heard some farriers say.

Many of my peers see a big difference between medial and lateral sides of feet, but I tend to try and achieve symmetry as much as a foot will allow, based on what I have seen in hundreds of coffin bones. Since this has never caused the horses that I have shod any problems, I feel that a foot can deal better when symmetrical than it can when shod and trimmed asymmetrically. After a horse has been shod several times with a symmetrically trimmed foot and symmetrically shaped shoe, the foot often becomes more symmetrical.

In common terminology, varus would be bow-legged, and valgus would be knock-kneed (B and C in **Figure 7**). If you do some research on the meaning of the words, it can be quite confusing, and it seems that the meaning of the words have changed through the years. I would recommend using the terms bow legged and knock kneed if possible, but you need to be aware of the Latin terms as they are widely used around the world as well. There are a couple ways to help you remember the differences. Valgus has a G in is, G stands for gum, and gum would make the knees stick together. Varus is pronounced as v air-us. Since it is a deviation away from center, there would be a lot of air between them.

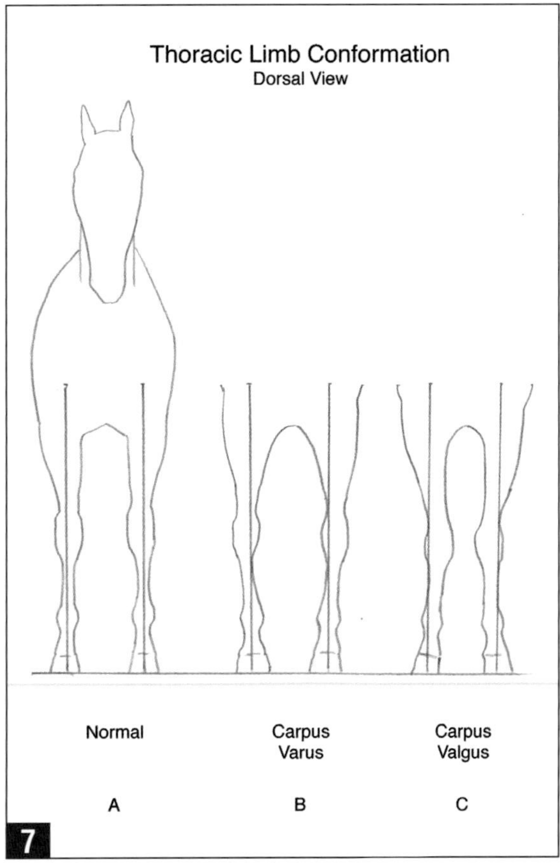

Cranial view of front limb conformation.

Varus and valgus deviations in the knee are often caused by hypoplasia of some of the carpal bones. Hypoplasia refers to a part of the body failing to develop to a proper size, thus it is too small. Hypoplasia of a carpal bone will cause that area of the carpus to be shorter than the opposite side, and that can lead to all sorts of deviations, with carpus valgus and carpus varus foremost amongst these.

A bow-legged horse is going to wear the lateral side of the foot, and a knock-kneed horse is going to wear the medial side of the foot. To correct these conformations, you might use an extension on the foot to protect and build up the side that is being worn, and if enough foot is present on the opposite side, you can trim that lower. Trim the medial side lower on the bow-legged horse, and the lateral side lower on the knock-kneed horse.

Narrow in front (D in **Figure 8**), is a straight conformation on a horse that is lightly muscled and thin. Some breeds tend to have a leaner conformation, and these horses will often be seen as narrow.

The next figure is base-wide (**E in Figure 8**). The limbs themselves seem to have a straight structure; they are just angled out from the shoulder. With a base wide conformation, the foot is on the ground in a position that is wider than the area where the limb comes out of the shoulder. This is also a common conformation in lightly built horses. Due to the position of the foot in relation to the body, this horse will put more stress on the medial side of his foot and leg, and you might trim more from the lateral side in an attempt to fix it, or place a medial extension on the foot. This conformation is often found in foals that later grow into straight horses, so I don't get too excited about doing much for base-wide youngsters unless there is excessive and rapid wear of the medial side.

Next, we have the base-narrow horse (F in **Figure 8**). This is just the opposite of the base-wide horse, with the feet being placed closer together than where the limbs come out of the shoulder. You will be more likely to see this conformation on horses that are heavily built, like an American Quarter Horse. Base-narrow horses put more stress on the lateral side of the foot and leg, wearing the lateral side and flaring the medial side. The correction would be the exact opposite than the one for the base-wide horse, so trim the foot lower on the medial side to correct the problem.

Many times a horse will have another defect in conjunction with the base-wide or base-narrow conformation. This happens because the foot is trying to place itself under the center of pressure for that bony column, so the base-wide horse may have a toed-in deviation occurring at the fetlock, and the base-narrow horse may have a toed-out deviation occurring at the fetlock. Sometimes it is an angular limb deformity, and sometimes it is vertical axis rotation.

With toed-in and toed-out horses, the deviation is occurring in the fetlock joint (G and H in **Figure 8**). This would be considered a true angular limb deformity. If you were to dissect this horse, you would find that the cannon bone is not square on the distal end. The epicondyles are in different planes and this causes the joint to be angled. This will make a horse have the toed-out or toed-in deformity. A toed-out horse may be referred to as fetlock valgus, and a toed-in horse as fetlock varus. Trim more from the side that the foot is pointing toward; the lateral side for a toed-out horse, and the medial side for a toed-in horse.

Offset knees, or bench knees (I in **Figure 8**), are a defect where the cannon bone is positioned laterally to the radius and carpus. This is a very common defect, and once you start looking for it, you will be astonished at how many horses actually have offset knees. There is nothing that a farrier can do about this, other than support the medial side of the leg if the condition is severe. This will help the limb bear weight, but it will not do anything to fix the problem.

When dealing with vertical axis rotation, a horse may appear toed in or toed out, but the fetlock will actually be square. The bony column above the fetlock may have a twist or spiral in it that makes it look as if there is an angular limb deformity. I identify this problem by carefully studying the knee. There is a normal flat spot in the knee that is rotated just a degree or two off center to the lateral side in the model horse. If you look for that flat spot and compare its position to the foot, you can determine if the horse has vertical axis rotation or not. It is easier to determine if the problem is ALD or rotational if you take radiographs of the joint, especially the fetlock.

To illustrate vertical axis rotation, stand in front of a full-length mirror with your feet pointed straight ahead. This would be our model. Now, if you leave your heels in their location, but move your toes out, you will appear to have become toed out. In fact, your ankle conformation has not changed; rather you twisted your limb to create the appearance of toed out. Now your kneecap is pointing in a slightly outward position, and this turn created the

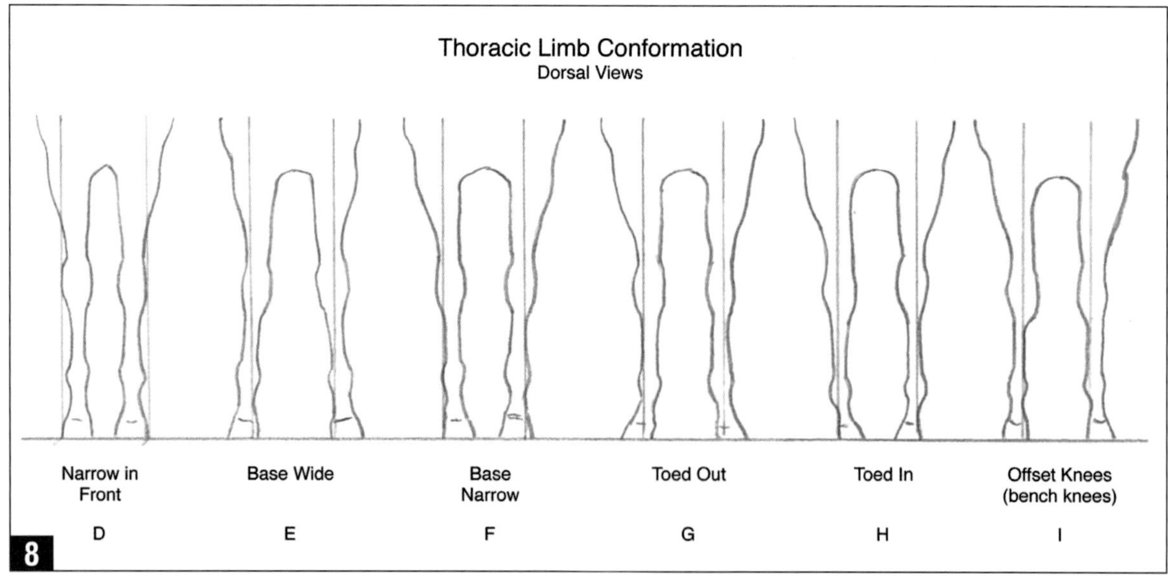

Cranial view of front limb conformation.

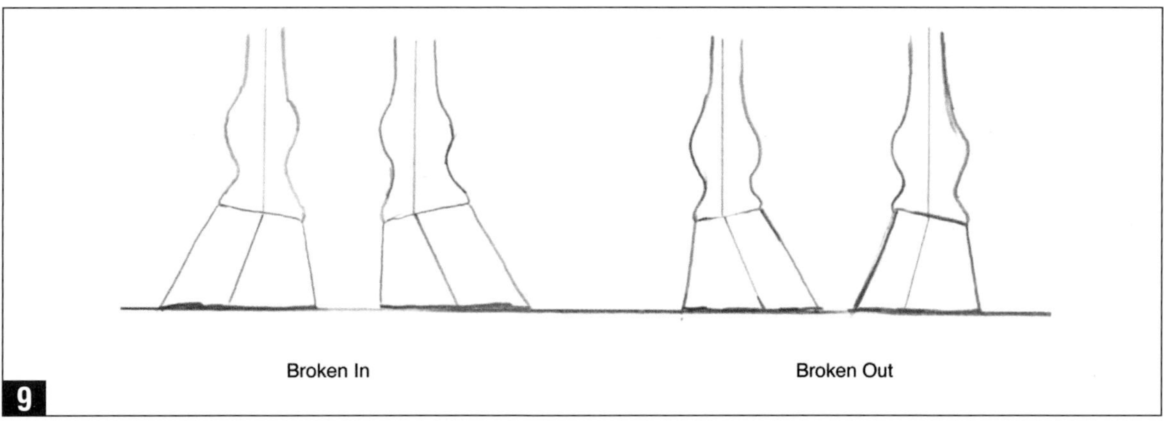

Broken in, broken out.

look. Fundamentally, this is vertical axis rotation.

Digit

If the limb is straight to the top of the foot and there is a deviation in the hoof capsule itself, the condition that you are seeing will be referred to as broken in or broken out. As in the case of toed in and toed out, if this is not taken care of by the farrier, it is more likely to become worse instead of better. The reason that it gets worse is that the lower portion of the foot will bear the most weight. As it bears more weight, it wears away more. This places even more weight on that lower portion of the foot, and the higher side will flare more. While this is happening, the foot will become even further out of balance.

The good part about these problems is that they are generally able to be improved by the farrier. If you can't trim it into a good level, you can create a shoe or apparatus that will allow you to achieve a good level. Options include using medial/lateral wedges and extensions. The drawing on the left of **Figure 9** is a broken-in stance and could be corrected by trimming the lateral side of the foot. The right drawing of **Figure 9** is a broken-out stance and could be corrected by trimming the medial side. If you notice, these look a lot like the toed-in and toed-out pictures, just remember that the deviation occurs in the foot alone. Also, it can be confusing because broken in looks toed out and vice versa.

PELVIC LIMB

The hindquarters of the horse are the engine that drives that horse. If you consider the muscle mass of the hindquarters the engine, the limbs are a system of levers that provide propulsion. The physics involved in levers and leverage indicates that some ratios are better than others. A longer line from hip to hock with a shorter cannon and a medium length pastern is the ideal for engaging the hind quarters and exerting the most power. Long cannons will predispose a horse to more action but will not be as strong as the shorter cannon.

Lateral View

The angles of the joints in the pelvic limb determine the placement of that limb. The ideal hind limb from the lateral could be described as one in which the cannon bones are perpendicular to the ground, with a line dropped from the point of the buttock running down the back of the hock and cannon (A in **Figure 10**). The center of the cannon bone lines up over the buttress of the foot. All of the joints are at appropriate angles.

Post-legged or straight behind (B in **Figure 10**) are those that do not have as much angle in them as the ideal. This conformation is good for speed, as there is not much flexion. Post-legged horses are prone to spavin and other concussion-related problems, and they do transfer more shock to their bodies.

Sickle hocks are hocks that have more bend than normal (C in **Figure 10**). The cannon bones are angled dorsally, and the feet are placed further under the horse. This conformation is good for collected gaits but not for speed. Sickle-hocked horses are predisposed to strain in the hock, such as curb. They are also more likely to overreach, since the hind feet are already closer to the fronts.

Hind limbs that are placed behind the point of the buttocks are referred to as camped behind (D in **Figure 10).** This type of conformation does not allow the horse to engage the hindquarters as effectively, so this is a weaker conformation.

Camped in front (E in **Figure 10)** looks a lot like sickle hocks, but the difference is that the legs are fairly normal when it comes to the angle of the hock, just the entire limb is angled forward. These horses will be prone to overreach.

Caudal View

I have seen the ideal caudal view of the hind limb described as being perfectly straight, with a

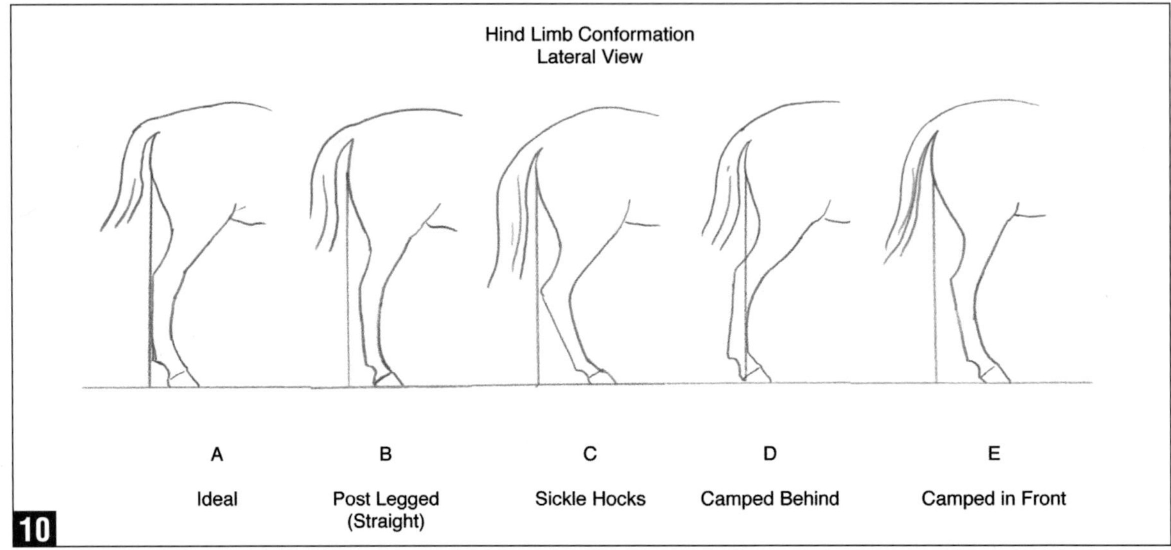

Lateral view of hind limb conformation.

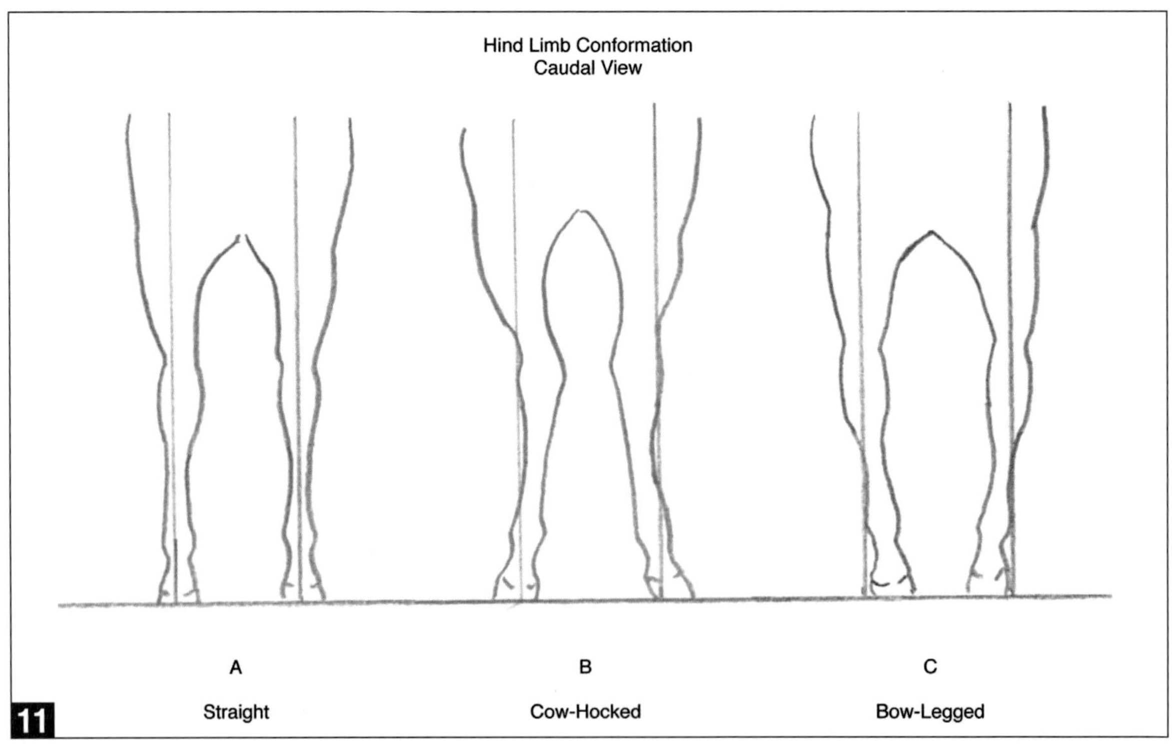

Caudal view of hind limb conformation.

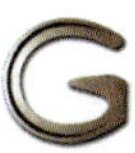

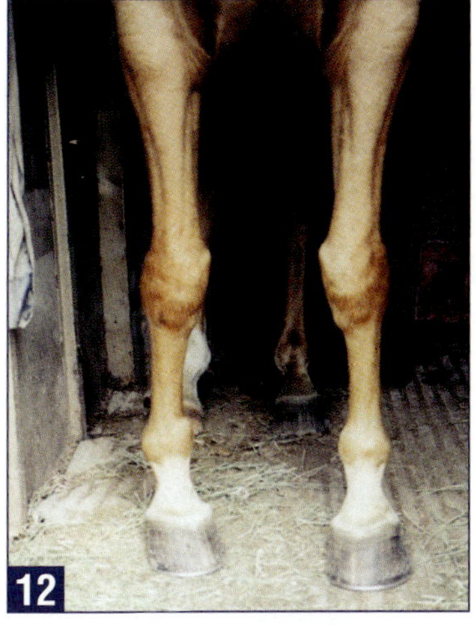

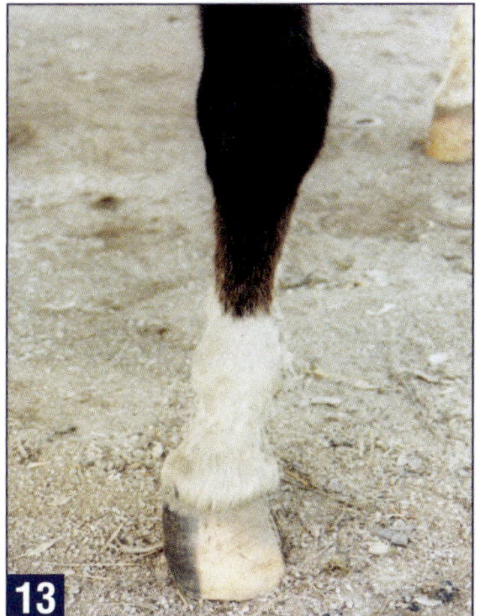

Offset knees and fetlock varus.

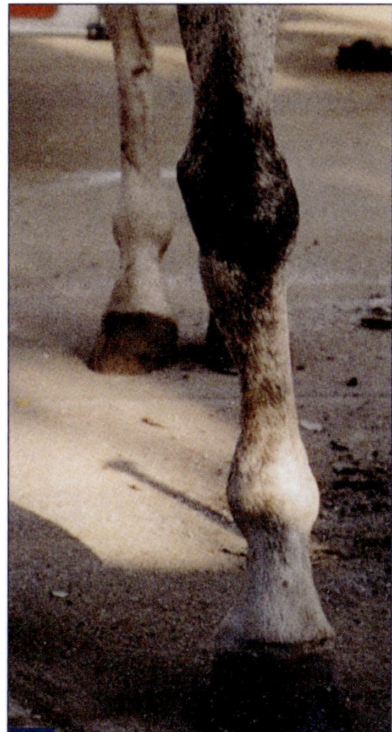

Offset knee with deformation of the splint bone and cannon bone below it.

line dropped from the point of the buttocks passing through the center of the cannon bone, pastern, and foot (A in **Figure 11**). I do not find this to be ideal because a horse with this conformation is likely to overreach, and its stifle will interfere with its trunk when it really moves out. For this reason, I label this as straight, instead of ideal as most would.

For me, the ideal would be more in line with the cow-hocked horse (B in **Figure 11**). Cow hocks are hocks that are close together, with the cannon bones angling outward. When this happens, the lateral heel and medial toe take the brunt of the stress. If you were standing just outside the shoulder in front of the horse to view the limb, the foot would line up straight under the cannon bone. If you look at the way that the tibia comes into the talus and the angle of the trochlea on the talus, it would indicate to me that the foot should be slightly turned out behind.

Horses that are bow-legged behind are the opposite of cow-hocked horses **(C in Figure 11)**. The hocks are further apart, and the cannon bones are angling inward. This is not as common as cow-hocked horses, and when you do see it, these horses will struggle to perform as well as expected.

Base-wide and base-narrow stances will be similar to what we have described in the thoracic limbs. The feet are either wider or closer than the point of the hip. The stress on the foot and hock would be similar to that described for the foot and knee on the thoracic limb.

Now that we have gone over a lot of conformation basics, I want to show some examples of horses that suffer from different conformation issues. **Figure 12** shows a horse that has some badly offset knees. The cannon bone is positioned well to the lateral side of the carpus. Looking carefully at the off front leg, you can also see a varus deviation in the fetlock so that the foot ends up being under the axis of that bony column more than it would be if it were directly under the cannon bone. This is common as the horse tries to place the platform for the limb under the center of that limb as well as it can.

Figure 13 has a knock-kneed (carpus valgus) deviation that has caused a fetlock problem that has led to a hoof distortion.

The next horse **(Figure 14)** has a badly offset knee on his near front. Over time, the proximal medial cannon bone and medial splint bone have become enlarged with bony growth. This happens as the leg responds to the uneven weight bearing. I did not take before photos, but the horse has just been shod with a medial extension so that I could place the platform closer to the axis of the bony column **(Figure 15)**.

Oftentimes in young foals, there will be deviations that make it look like a foal is at the end of

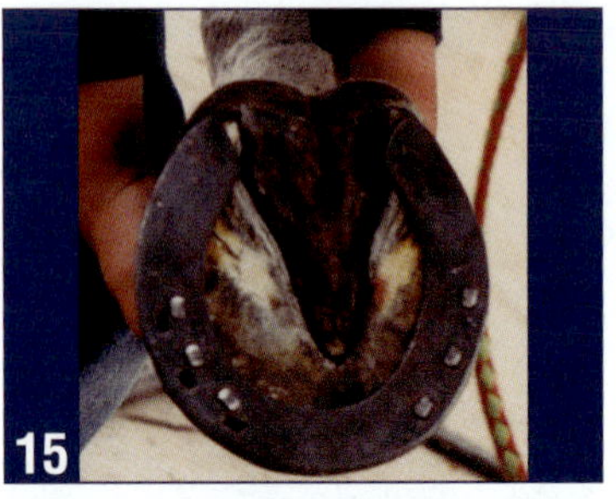

The shoe applied to the horse in Figure 14 to allow for some medial extension.

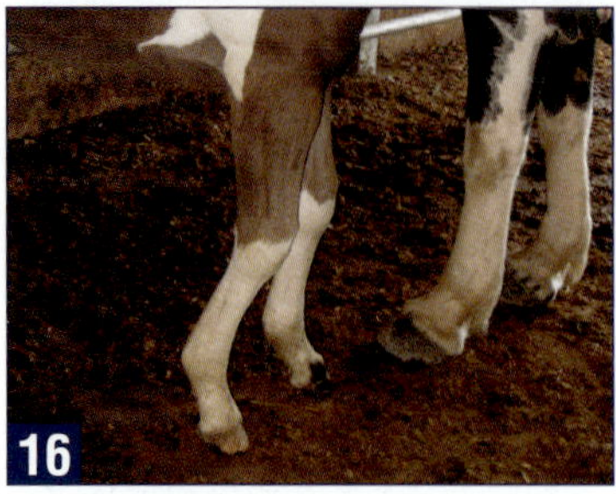

Buck-kneed foal.

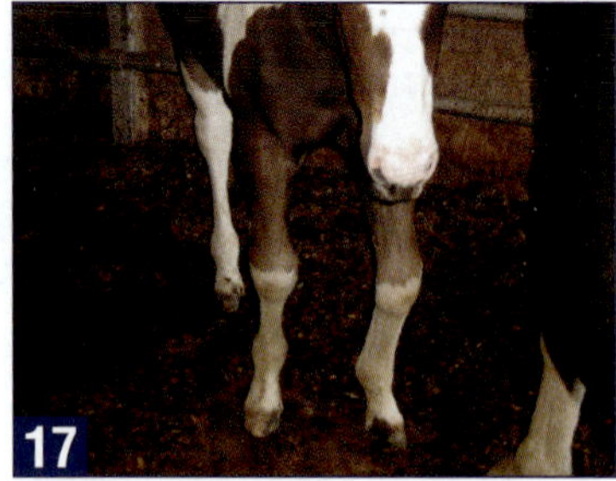

Same foal from a cranial view showing a carpus varus appearance from the severe buck-knee conformation.

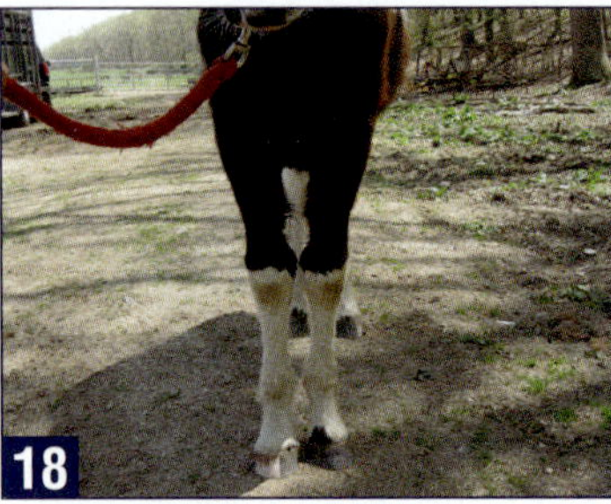

Same foal months later after corrective trimming.

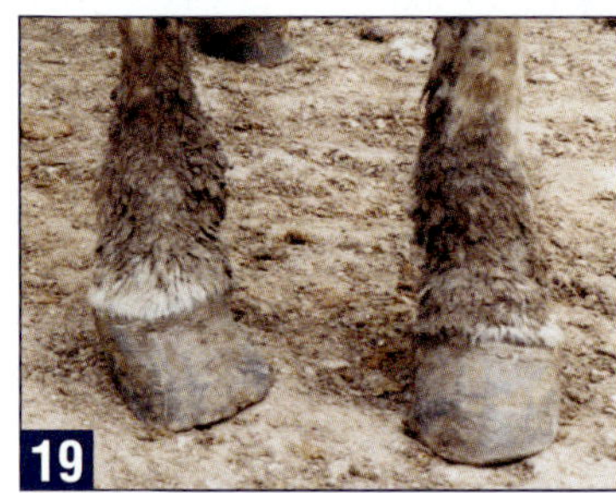

Broken-out deviation

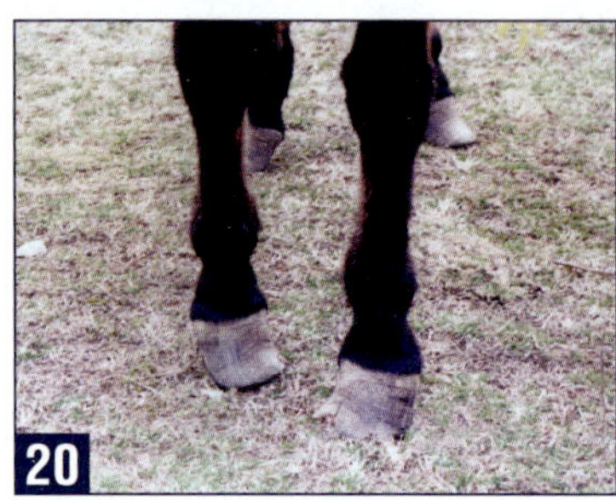

Broken-out deviation

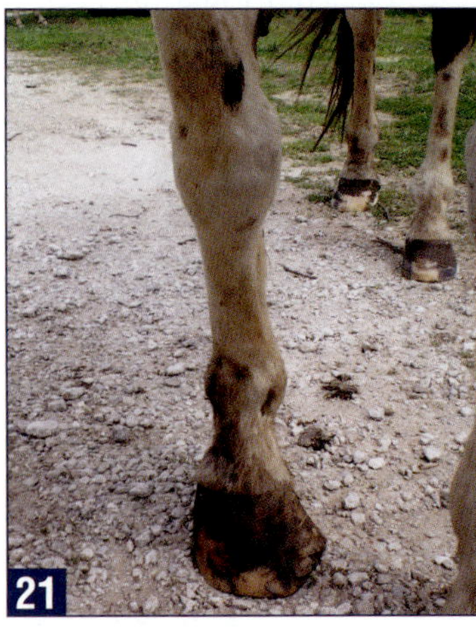

Broken-out foot on a leg that has some rotation problems.

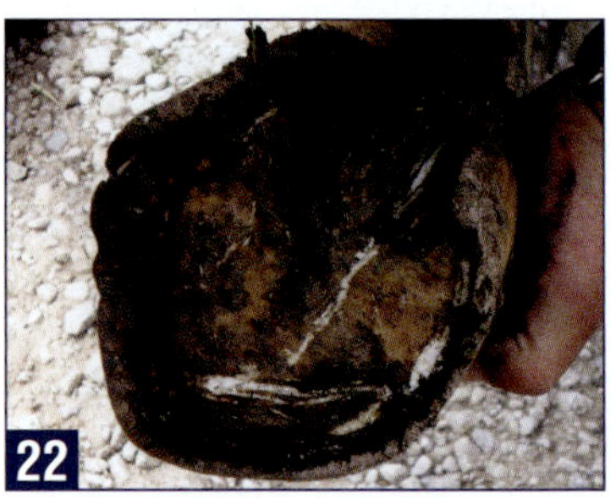

Bottom of the foot in Figure 21.

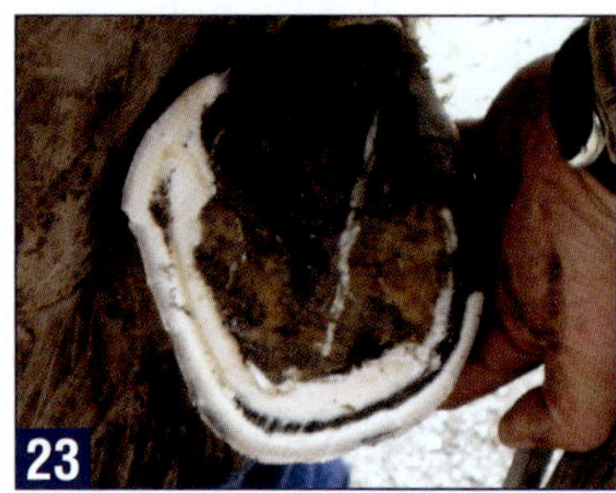

Preliminary trim.

the line. If these are flexural deformities, they will recover more often than not. The foal in **Figures 16 and 17** was about 3 weeks old when these photos were taken. Not only is there a buck-kneed condition present, the bending of the knee makes it appear there is a bow-legged (carpus varus) problem as well. With a problem like this, I will trim the feet as close to balanced as I can on a regular schedule, and take a wait-and-see approach. If the problem is still present at 35 days of age or so, I will apply an extension. This foal ended up doing fine without intervention beyond regular and correct trimming as can be seen from **Figure 18**. He is quite narrow in front, but that is a minor problem compared to what he started with.

Broken out is the most common type of deviation I see in the hoof capsule on the front feet of American Quarter Horses. This comes from the wide, heavily muscled chest and the tendency toward offset knees.

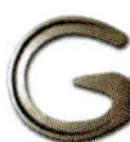

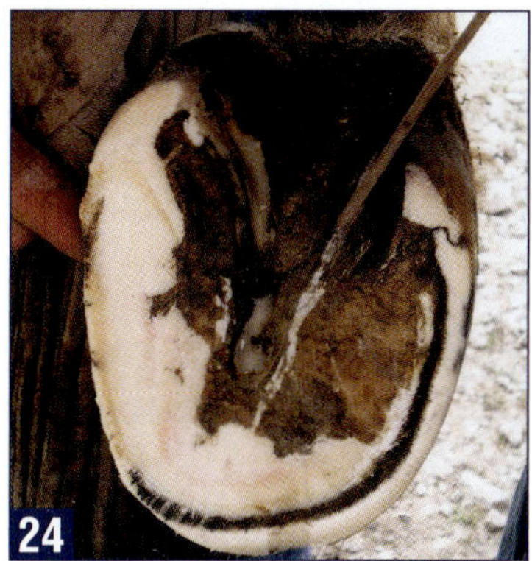
24
Finished finding the foot from the bottom.

The foot is attempting to place itself under the bony column, and with a little time, the lateral side will wear and the medial side will flare, making the problem worse than it was to start with. **Figures 19 and 20** clearly show this has happened to these horses. In **Figures 21-24**, the rotational deviation in the leg has caused the expected distortion in the foot. The length is trimmed off the bottom of the foot, and the flare is dressed.

For the horse that is going to be shod, I will often make a shoe that has a lateral wedge for horses like these last three. In **Figure 25**, a horse is presented with this common deviation. **Figure 26** is the same after being shod. The near front foot, which was the worst, has a shoe with a lateral wedge as well as a lateral extension. This has placed the foot in a more appropriate place under the bony column as well as demonstrated the need for the farrier to be able to make shoes. When this horse walks, there is marked difference between how the knee comes forward. It is fairly straight on the off front, which was the straighter foot, and swings lateral on the near front, which was the worse of the feet (**Figures 27-28**). Sometimes a trim can do

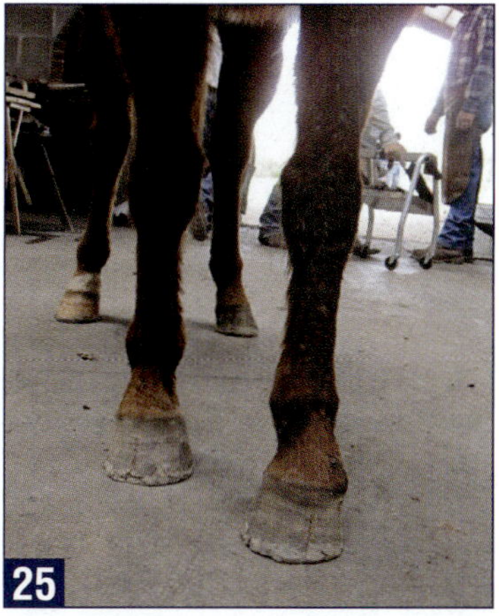
25
Crooked horse before shoeing.

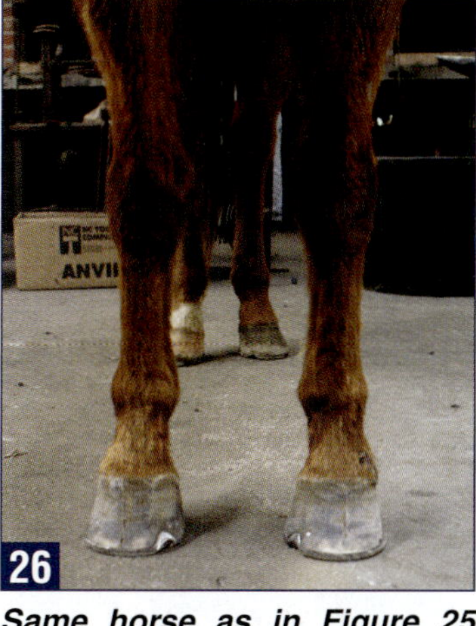

26
Same horse as in Figure 25 after shoeing with a lateral extension and wedge.

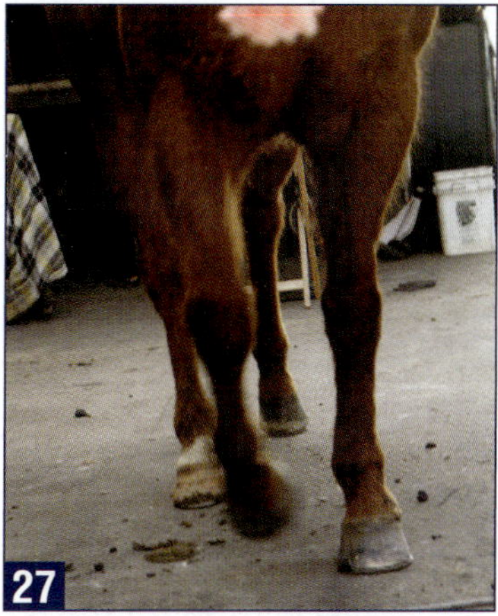
27
Picture of how the off front moves through the air.

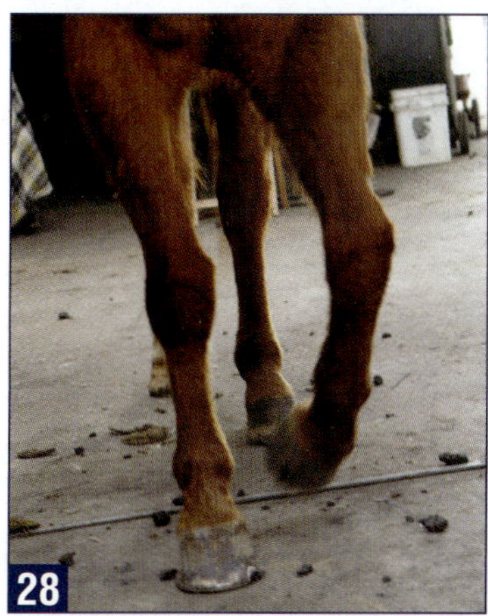
28
Picture of the how the near front moves through the air.

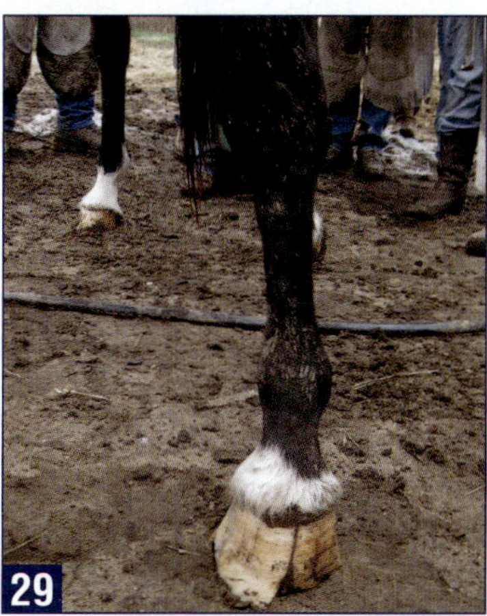
29
Crooked leg before trimming.

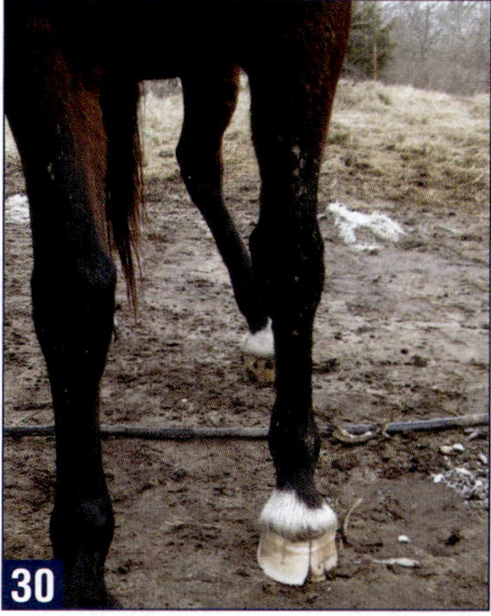
30
Crooked leg after trimming.

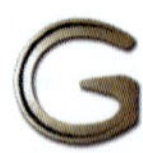

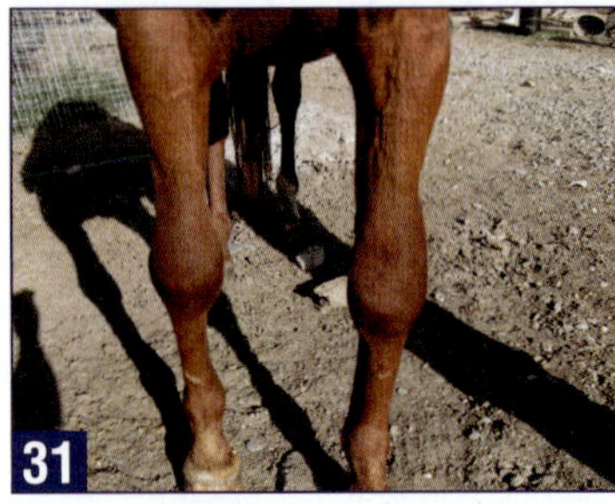

Carpus varus.

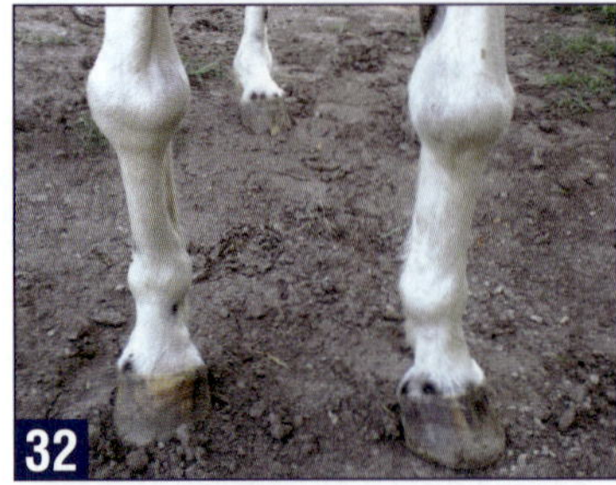

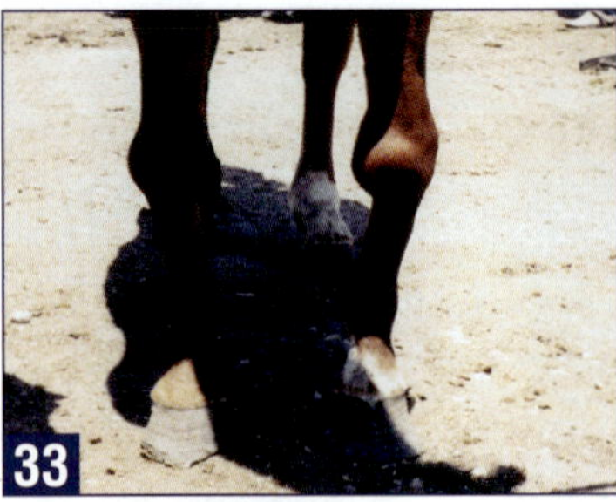

Carpus varus with arthritis of the knee, (carpitis).

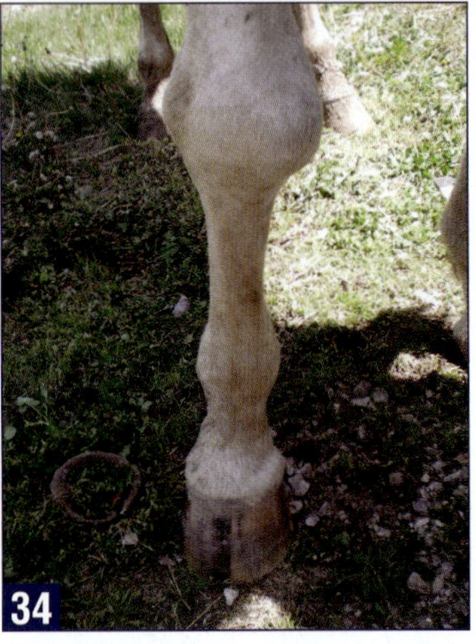

Carpitis.

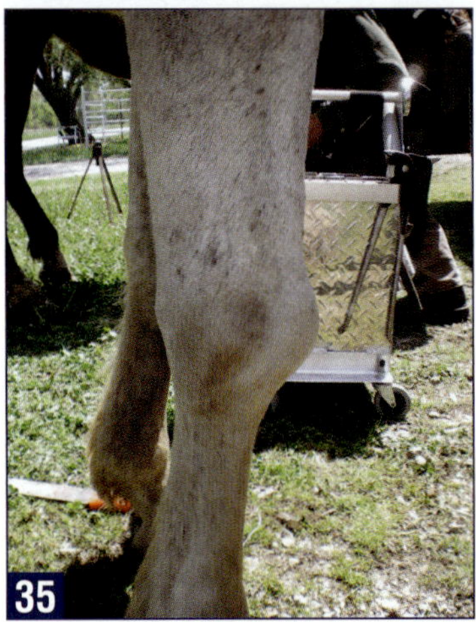

Lateral view of the carpitis making the leg also buck kneed.

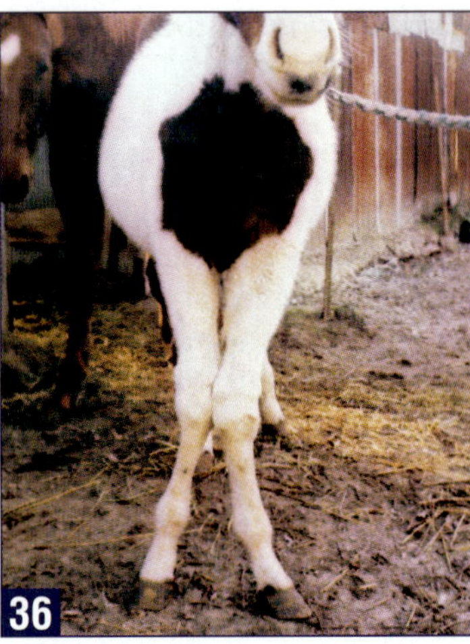

Carpus valgus.

all that is needed **(Figures 29 and 30)**, but it is imperative for the customer to keep on schedule if the changes are to become permanent.

Offset knees and carpus varus can lead to some devastating arthritis of the knee (carpitis) over time. The horse in **Figure 31** is still sound enough to use, but the horses in **Figures 32-35** have lost most of the flexion in the knee and are not sound to use. When shoeing or trimming these horses, it is good to catch them lying down so that you don't have to bend the knee to work on them. The priority is to prevent uneven wear, which is the most common foot problem that these horses will face. It may mean nailing on a shoe, but that is a horse-by-horse case, and the benefits have to be weighed against the pain caused in the process. Eventually, the knee may become fused. When this happens, the horse will not be suffering from the pain in the knee any longer, but the quality of life is questionable.

The horse featured in **Figure 36** is suffering from a valgus deformity, most likely from hypoplasia of the lateral carpal bones. This horse should be trimmed lower on the lateral side of the foot and definitely needs an extension. The next horse **(Figure 37)** is so deformed that it had to be destroyed. This is an important thing for a farrier to be able to advise a customer about. No one wants to kill a youngster, but there are conditions that are beyond the scope of current technologies to fix, and knowing that early can prevent a lot of needless suffering. In some cases where there was a desire to fix the horse at all costs, there has been some pretty severe pain for the horse that had to eventually be destroyed anyway.

When it comes to the hind leg, the horse in **Figure 38** is bow legged (tarsus varus). This is not a common thing for me to see in the horses I work on, and I am glad of that. It is a conformation that can lead to a lot of problems, and horses that are bow legged behind are not fast or athletic.

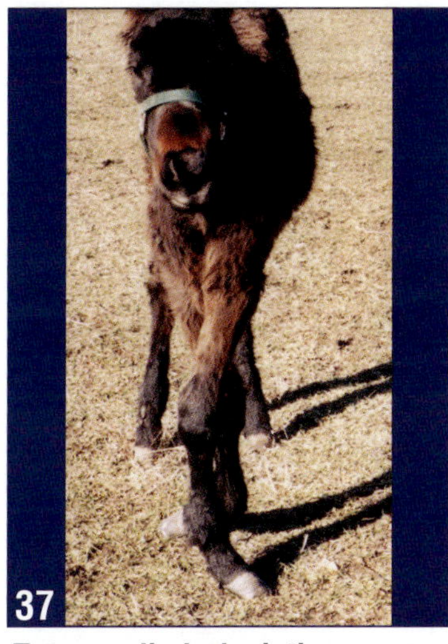

Extreme limb deviations.

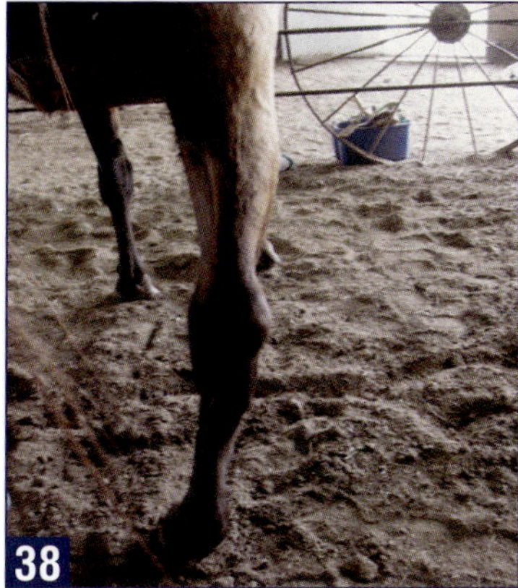

Bow-legged hind limb.

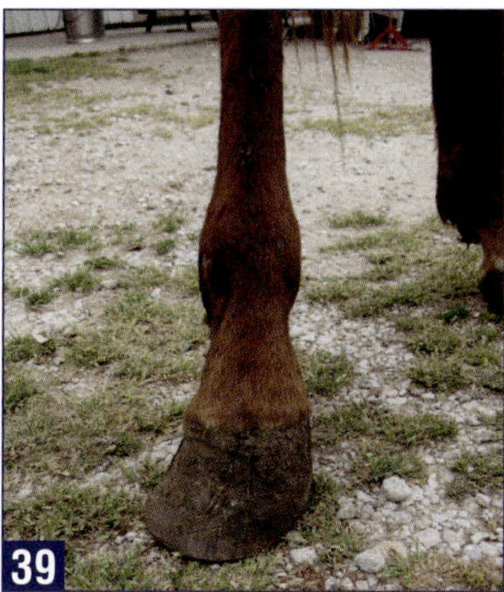

Lateral flare on a hind foot, broken in.

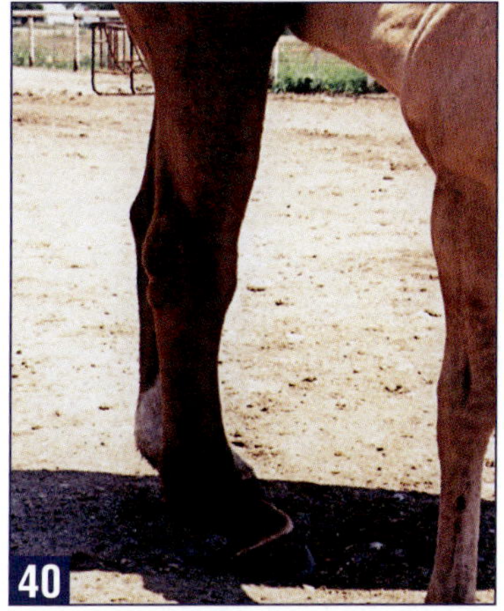

Post legged, (straight behind).

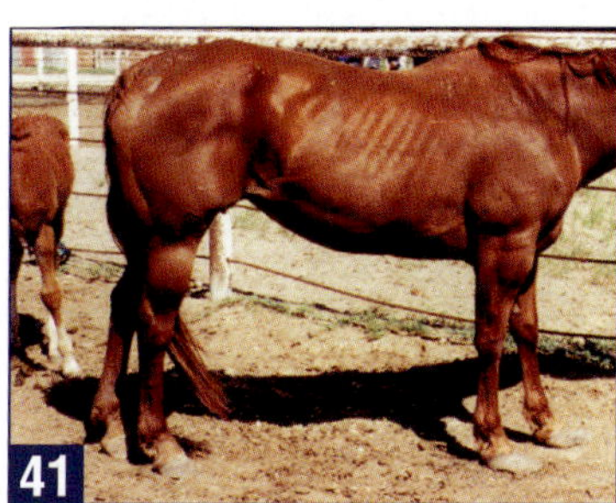

Post legged

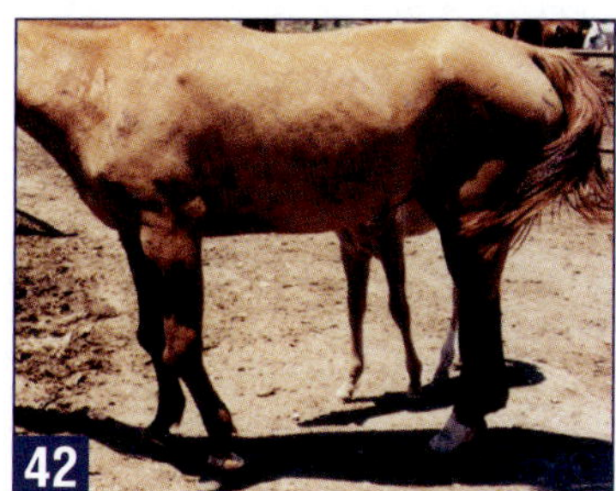

Post legged as well as carpitis.

One of the most common things to see in the hind foot is broken in **(Figure 39)**. A horse with the hind foot placed outside the bony column will have its legs spread when it tries to stop, (splatter), and there is a lot of stress placed on the joints of the digit. One of the big reasons this happens in shod horses is that shoers are judging balance for the hind foot in the air in a non-weight bearing position for the hind foot. Balance on hind feet should be judged on the ground as discussed in the chapter on trimming. To fix this problem is simple, just trim and dress more on the lateral side of the foot.

Post-legged, or straight-behind horses can be fairly common in some American Quarter Horse lines **(Figures 40-42)**. This type of conformation does lend itself to speed, but too straight can lead to all sorts of concussion related issues, such as spavin and ringbone. The horses here are all brood mares at the same Quarter Horse breeding farm, and you can see that the horse in **Figure 42** has some serious knee problems as well. Perhaps breeding horses that aren't sound enough to work isn't a very good idea. Who knew?

The youngster in **Figures 43 and 44** has a flexural deformity of the hind limbs. This makes it look like a classic case of sickle hocks, but there is more going on to cause that look. Notice the fetlocks and the angle of the pastern, and this tells you that there is more going on here then just the bony conformation.

The shoe on the horse in **Figure 45** is a lateral

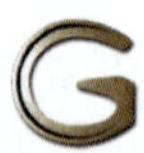

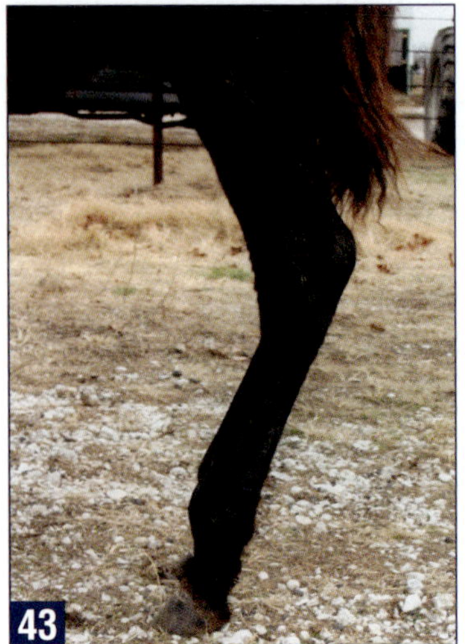

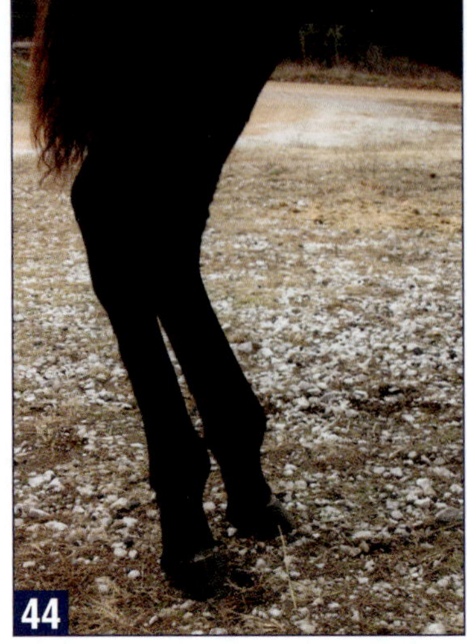

Sickle hocked with a flexural deviation.

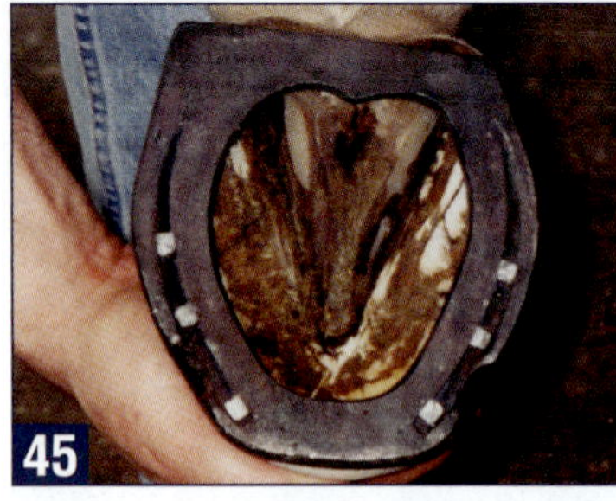

Lateral heel extension straight bar shoe for a cow-hocked horse.

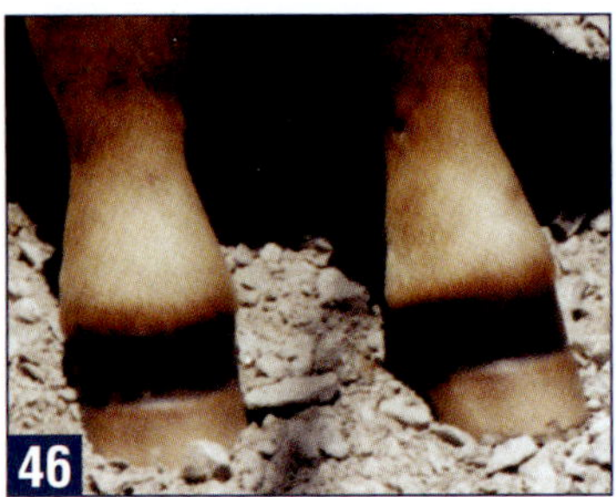

Foal's feet changing color.

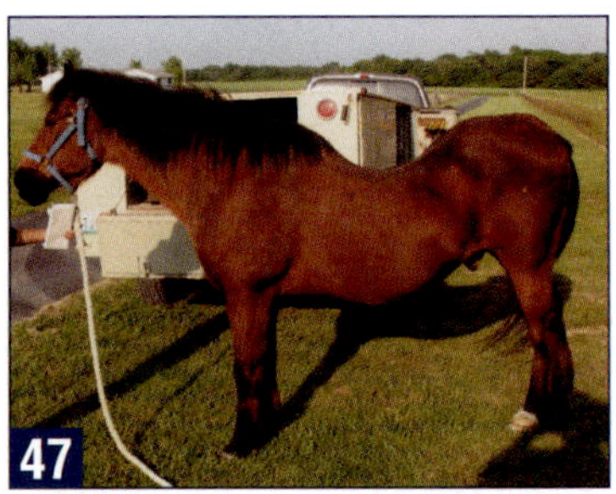

Severe sway backed horse, (lordosis).

heel extension straight bar. This is a good shoe to use on cow-hocked horses. Being cow hocked is more in line with a rotation problem then with an angular deformity, so taking the entire lateral side of the foot is not called for. The lateral toe can be lowered, but if the lateral heel is also lowered, the foot can rotate the limb right around into a cow-hocked position. As such, a shoe that extends past the lateral heel will support that side of the leg and hock and allow the horse to stand a bit straighter.

I close this chapter with a couple of unusual photos. **Figure 46** shows the feet of a foal that have changed from white to black. There is a marked line of change where the pigment started to become a part of the hoof capsule.

Figure 47 shows an old cutting horse with a severe sway back. Sway back is known as lordosis. In young horses, this is caused by hypoplastic articulations on the top of some of the vertebrae. This causes the spine to sink until it gains stability, causing a sway back. This horse always had a sway back to some degree, but here it is in its 30s, and the condition has become quite extreme.

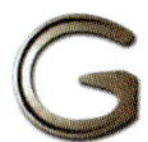

Chapter

15 CORRECTIVE SHOEING THEORY

Corrective shoeing is a term that is used quite often in the world of farriery. In fact, if you are removing tissue from a foot in any manner, it should be corrective in nature; otherwise, you should not be removing it. With that concept in mind, the term corrective shoeing should apply to every foot that you trim as you take that foot toward the ideal. However, the term is more often thought of as referring to correcting the stance of horses with less than ideal conformation. In this chapter we will look into the principles of changing stance.

As you read this chapter, refer to some of the drawings and pictures in Chapter #14, Limb Conformation.

When you are tasked to fix some of the problems seen in Chapter #14, the first thing you need to determine is whether or not the benefits outweigh the disadvantages. For me, if the horse is not interfering and there is not a compelling reason to fix a horse, I will only balance the foot and not apply a correction beyond that, especially when I am working on any horse that is over 2 years old. In an older horse, the physis has closed and any change that I try to make can potentially put a lot of pressure on the bony column and joints.

On young horses, you can fix the stance, and the horse will learn to walk in a straight manner with a good straight stance. On aged horses, if you try and fix the stance, you often mess up the gait. Since the gait is more important than the stance in most situations, I don't mind if a sound but crooked horse remains crooked. You just have to explain to the customer that pretty is as pretty does, and that making a horse sore to meet a human sense of aesthetics is not a good idea. I will also inform the customer of potential problems that result from different conformations so that they can be on the lookout for early signs of any problems.

On the horses that you decide should have a corrective procedure, there is a general rule that you lower the side that the foot is pointing toward when it is on the ground. This would be the lateral side on a knock-kneed, base-wide, broken-in, or toed-out horse. For the bow-legged, base-narrow, broken-out, or toed-in horses, that would be the medial side. Most of the correction will be toward the toe if the correction is truly an angular limb deformity without any rotation of the bony column.

When you are viewing a crooked leg, the portion of that limb that is closest to the axis for that limb will be under the most stress. For instance, the horse

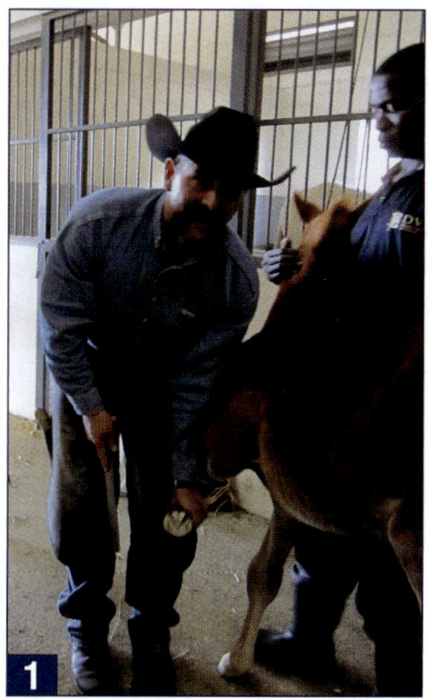

1

Trimming a racehorse foal in Africa.

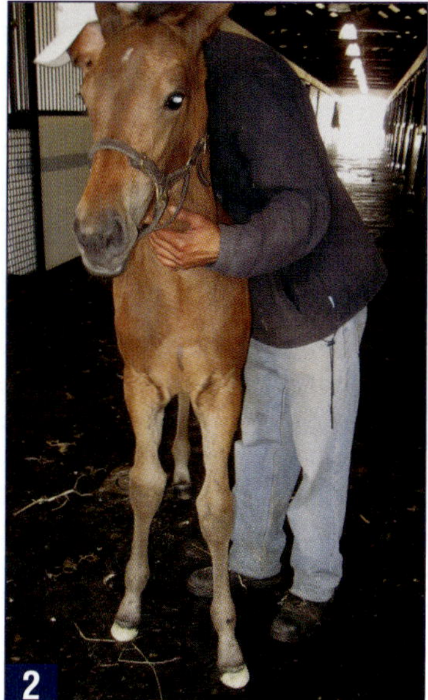

2

Lateral toe extensions on a foal with carpus valgus (knock kneed).

that is bow legged will have stress on the lateral side of the foot but on the medial side of the knee. While there may be exceptions to this rule, if you draw an imaginary line from the point of the shoulder to the ground, whatever is abnormally closest to that line will be under the most stress.

Another item that I want you to keep in mind is that the further from the foot that the deviation occurs, the harder it is to fix with shoeing. One of the great things about a horse's leg is the fact that it can absorb a lot of what it encounters on uneven terrain. This is essential to soundness, but it is also a trait that causes our attempts to fix the proximal deviations to be taken up by the joints below. The coffin joint will take a lot of the changes instantly, and the knee often gets whatever is left. I do not think it is a good idea to get radical in an attempt to affect the shoulder, rather just accept that it is generally out of the farrier's realm.

When you are dealing with horses that have vertical axis rotation you may find that you will have to go after diagonals. With angular limb deformities, the entire foot is placed toward either the medial or lateral axis of the bony column. With rotational problems, when the toe is rotating laterally, the medial toe is closest to the axis, while the lateral heel is closest to the axis in the rear of the foot.

For instance, you have a horse that has a vertical axis rotation toward the lateral side. From the front, this horse will appear to be toed out, even though the fetlock does not have an angular deformity. As the toe rotates away from the midline, the lateral heel will rotate toward the midline. As such, the medial heel and lateral toe may be long, and the foot may exhibit a perimeter where that diagonal measures longer than the opposite diagonal. Taking the entire lateral side — including the heel — would not be the right call on this horse.

If you are struggling to understand this, consider a cow-hocked horse. The toes are pointing laterally, but the lateral heels are often crushed and worn on these horses. When you pick up the foot, the lack of lateral heel is obvious, and you can easily see that the lateral toe should be trimmed. In fact, you may find that you need to make a shoe that has a trailer or lateral extension for that lateral heel. But, if you take that lateral heel in an effort to improve stance, the foot will rotate more, and the horse will look even more cow-hocked. This is a good example of the vertical axis of rotation, and you can apply the principles to the front leg as well.

LIMB

Base wide and base narrow are both conformational defects where the feet are in a different place on the perpendicular plane than where the limb comes out of the shoulder. As such, the deviation actually occurs a long way from the foot. The side opposite of the direction that the limb is pointing takes the most weight, so a horse can have other conformation defects arise out of being base wide or base narrow.

The classic correction would be to lower the lateral side of the foot on the base-wide horse and the medial side of the foot on the base-narrow horse. However, since the foot is so far from the shoulder, you will find that the lower joints negate your corrective trimming efforts. Trimming the foot to good medial/lateral balance on the long axis, and then shoeing with an extension to support the limb is a better way to go. The extension will be slight, and it will extend medially for the base-wide horse and laterally for the base-narrow horse.

If you have other conformational defects with the base-wide and base-narrow horse, try to trim so that you place the bottom of the foot under the axis of the bony column. The column may be crooked, but it will still have a point located at the bottom that is the center of pressure for weight bearing. Think about some of those abstract sculptures that have the pedestal, or foundation, placed to support their odd shape. The foot is the pedestal, and the shoe is the base of that pedestal.

KNEE

First is the bow-legged horse. With this conformation, the strategy for helping this horse is to trim the medial side of the foot. You can liken the corrective procedures to the horse that is base narrow. The big difference is that the knee is close enough to the foot that there is a better chance of improving this deviation with trimming.

The horse with knoc knees is just the opposite. Trim laterally, or shoe with a medial extension. This strategy is the same as that for the horse that is base wide.

Offset-knees are a conformation defect that cannot be fixed by shoeing. Since the cannon bone is not directly under the radius, it would require taking the carpus apart and relocating the cannon bone to fix it. So, we have to accept that the horse has offset knees and let it go at that. If there is a problem from the offset knees, you may find that shoeing with a slight medial extension can place the shoe in the center of the axis for the limb, but that does not fix the offset knees, it just makes the bony column stronger. You are supporting a bad conformation, but not changing it. The correction works if the foot is under the axis of the cannon bone. Sometimes, the fetlock will become varus from the offset knees, and you have to apply the extension to the lateral side of the foot. Look at the whole limb to determine what you need to put on the foot.

From the lateral view, we can change the placement of the front foot on the ground in relation to the shoulder by changing the angle of the foot. A horse can accommodate a trim that is not at its natural angle by moving the foot to make the stress on the tendons appropriate. If the foot is too steep, the horse may stand under to accommodate it. If the foot is too shallow, the horse may stand camped in front to accommodate it. Either way, the horse is placing the foot based on how it was trimmed. We can use this principle when dealing with overreaching, but I don't recommend that you change natural angle until you have exhausted the other potential remedies.

With calf-kneed horses, I would recommend a rocker toe to place as little stress on the leverage arm for breakover as possible. This is just a bad conformation that you aren't going to fix, but you may make the horse more comfortable with the rocker toe. Do the same if the horse is tied in at the knees or cut out under the knees. With the buck-kneed horse, shoe normally. The initials we use for shoeing normally are TLB, which stands for Trim, Level, and Balance.

HOCKS

As with the knee, there isn't a tremendous amount that can be done to make a big change in the hocks. There are some minor changes that can be made in the limb, but in general, the front limbs are more likely to react to changes than the hind. This is true for a couple of reasons. First, the scapula is not solidly attached to the trunk as the femur is to the pelvis. Second, the front limb does not have a reciprocal apparatus like the pelvic limb does. Following are some conformation defects, and suggested trimming and shoeing strategies for each.

Post-legged horses are just going to be straight from a lateral view, and there is nothing in the realm of shoeing that is going to change that.

You may help sickle hocks by increasing the angle of the hind foot and/or extending the heels on the horseshoe. By doing this, the foot may end up being placed further toward plantar, causing the hock to straighten.

With the camped-behind horse, you may have results by lowering the angle slightly, but I have not found it to be as effective as some textbook authors have. It is worth a try, and if you are shoeing that horse, don't extend the heels excessively.

Base-wide behind will also stress the medial side of the foot, causing it to wear faster. You may have good results by lowering the lateral side of the foot. For the base-narrow horse, lower the medial side of the foot.

With a cow-hocked horse, you can trim the lateral toe but stay off of the lateral heel. This is similar to the vertical axis rotation described earlier, and the lateral heel will be already worn or crushed. I have used lateral heel extension bar shoes quite successfully on this type of horse.

The bow-legged behind horse poses some additional challenges. This conformation makes it much harder for the horse to engage the hindquarters because the stifle interferes with the belly. The shoeing strategy should be to trim the medial toe and lateral heel. You may end up with an extended heel on the medial heel of the shoe, but a trailer on the medial side is not an option. A medial trailer is likely to interfere with the opposite leg and cause more problems than you had to start with.

Throughout my career, I have found that adhering to a method of shoeing that called for good, solid and traditional basics has brought about the best results. There are a lot of things that we can try to fix to please our sense of what is pretty, but these things rarely serve the horse. The horse is only of value to man if it is sound and able to do the job intended. Even if the conformation is not attractive, if the horse is sound, it is probably going to be fine to shoe the way it stands. If it ain't broke, don't fix it.

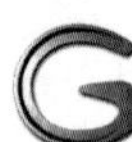

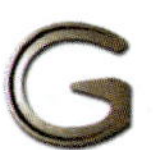

Section 5

Gaits

Chapter 16: Gaits 178

Chapter 17: Gait Faults 185

> “ 29 There are three things which are majestic in pace,
> Yes, four which are stately in walk. ”
>
> —Proverbs 30:29
>
> —New King James Version

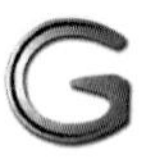

Chapter

16 GAITS

Foals are on their feet within minutes of being born. In the wild, abilities like that are common among prey animals, as birthing is a dangerous time when a predator can catch and eat mom and baby. You will find that predators need a lot of care as infants, while prey animals have instinctive abilities that are pretty amazing.

As the foal moves, its brain receives information about the obstacles that the foal is navigating. It is not possible for a horse to physically see where it steps as it places each foot, so the foal learns to move using proprioception. Proprioception is the sense of the relative position of one's own body parts. This is what allows you to touch your fingers behind your back where you can't see either hand.

For a horse, as it hits an obstacle with a foot, the body develops a sense of when it needs to lift a foot higher, or even how and when to jump certain obstacles. The better that a horse is at going through rough terrain, the more sure-footed we consider that horse. During this learning phase for the foal, the neural pathways of the brain are developing that individual horse's particular way of moving. What it ends up with are its gaits.

A gait is the pattern of a horse's steps as that horse moves. It begins with the horse deciding to go, and is accomplished stride by stride in a number of different speeds and sequences. These differences are what distinguish one gait from another.

A stride is the complete cycle of all four legs, and a step is the complete cycle of only one leg. Thus, a stride is the compilation of four steps, one from each limb. There is a lot of terminology out there to explain what happens in each step, but here is what I teach my students.

There are two basic phases for the step. These are the swing phase, which can be broken down into a dorsal and palmar stage on the front limbs,

Phases of Step
Thoracic Limb

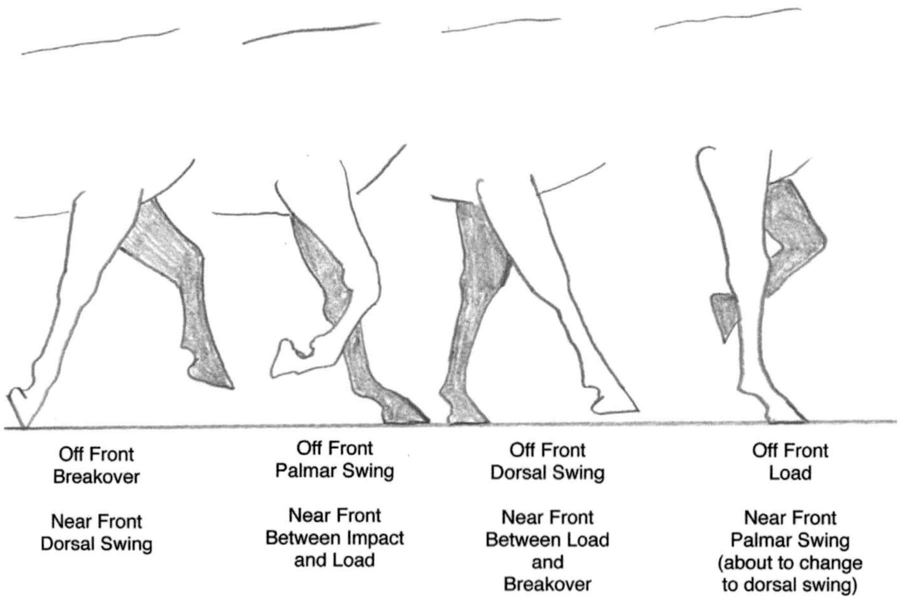

Off Front
Breakover

Near Front
Dorsal Swing

Off Front
Palmar Swing

Near Front
Between Impact
and Load

Off Front
Dorsal Swing

Near Front
Between Load
and
Breakover

Off Front
Load

Near Front
Palmar Swing
(about to change
to dorsal swing)

1

and a dorsal and plantar on the hind limbs. **Figures 1 - 2** are the front and hind limbs in different phases of their individual steps. The captions below each of the drawings explain the portion of what phase each limb is in.

The second phase of a step is the stance phase. This is anytime that the foot is on the ground, and the stance phase can be broken into the impact stage, load stage, propulsion stage, and breakover stage. Let us examine all of these more closely.

As soon as the foot leaves the ground, it enters what is knows as the swing stage. As long as that foot is behind the opposite leg, it is in the palmar (thoracic) or plantar (pelvic) stage of the swing phase. This allows you to view the swing phase in two separate segments. You will find this useful when examining lame horses. Often, you will find laymen will notice that a horse is lame because they are moving with what is called a "short stride." This is actually a misnomer. The horse is exhibiting a shorter dorsal phase on one limb (usually the sound limb), and a shorter palmar/plantar phase on the other limb. In fact, the steps are equal in distance if the horse is moving in a straight line, but the untrained eye will see it differently.

Ask a person that insists on the horse having a short stride to define the exact length of each step. For instance, the horse has an injury to the near front, and is taking a shorter palmar/longer dorsal stage with the injured near front and a longer palmar/shorter dorsal stage with the off front. So, the person answers that the near front is traveling at 6 feet per step (long stride), and the off front is only travelling 4 feet (short stride). Next, ask them to do the math on a horse that travels 10 strides, each foot having made 10 steps. In that case, the near front with the long stride will have traveled 60 feet and the off front with a short stride will have traveled 40 feet. Obviously, this is a physical impossibility since the horse can't come apart to make this statement work any more than it can to make the overreaching statement of speeding up the fronts and slowing down the hinds work.

What has happened is the horse went the same distance with each foot at each step. It just appeared to be different because the dorsal stage for the sound leg was shorter than the dorsal stage of the lame leg.

During the stance phase, the first instant where the foot hits the ground is known as the impact stage. From a textbook model point of view, we would like the foot to land flat. Feet rarely land completely flat; rather most will impact on the lateral heel region first and more so in the hind end

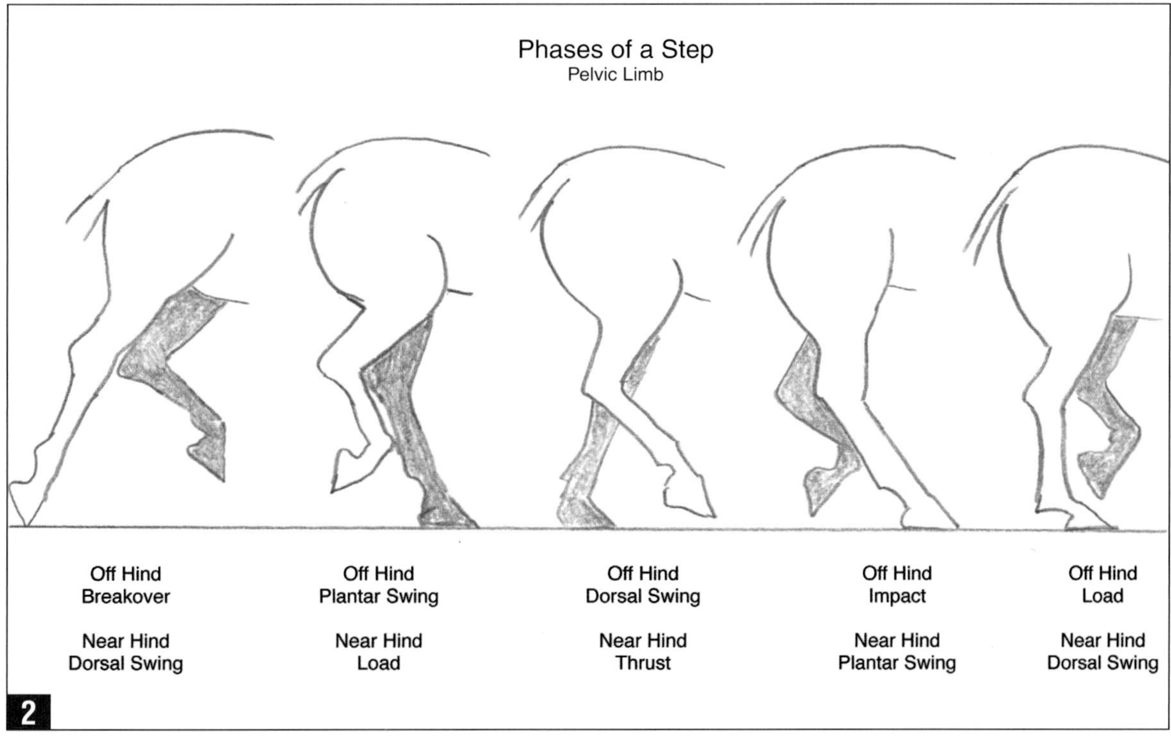

than the front. With close observation, you may be able to determine how the foot impacts at the beginning of the stance phase. However there has been a lot of research using advanced technology that can see more exactly what happens than we can with our naked eye.

The next part of the stance phase is the load stage. As the body moves over the foot on the ground, that foot will become increasingly stressed by a greater amount of the horse's body weight. Once the limb becomes vertical and the body begins to pass over the leg, the foot will enter the propulsion stage of the stance phase. This is where the limb begins to add thrust to the body to propel the horse to the next step.

The very last instant that the toe of the foot is on the ground is known as breakover. While there is debate within the farrier industry over a good definition or understanding of breakover, I define it for students like this: it is the last instant that the toe of the foot is on the ground. Throughout your career, you will hear about speeding up breakover and easing breakover. I think that it can be eased, but referring to the speed of breakover does not make much sense. It is the last instant of contact, whether that is from a rocker toe, square toe, or toe extension; the last instant is the last instant.

Once each limb has made its way through a step and arrived at the beginning of the cycle again, the horse is considered to have completed a stride at that gait. Even though it may appear that a horse begins from a standstill on the front legs, it actually begins from behind. Although the front legs have to get up and out of the way of the hind, the horse is an animal that is rear drive. The horse does not just pull itself forward with the front end, rather it pushes itself forward with the hind limbs. This is why the stride cycle of movement is described by starting with the hind foot. If you remember from the anatomy section, the pelvic limb is solidly attached to the backbone, and this allows all of the thrust to be transferred to the body to push the horse forward.

The fact that the horse is rear drive does not mean that the front end does nothing to move the horse. With the size and strength of the front muscles and the leverage allowed by the bones and their position, there is no doubt that the front limbs actively pull as the horse moves. There is also the added propulsion that is achieved by the energy storage in the tendons and ligaments of the front legs that is translated into thrust with each step. However, with the front limb being attached by a fleshy attachment (called syncosis), the horse is unable to transfer as much thrust to the body as it can with the hind limbs.

Gaits are broken into several categories. The main ones that you should know as a general farrier are:

- Lateral Gait: Cycle of movement where both legs on one side work together. The pace, walk, and the gallop are lateral gaits.
- Diagonal Gait: Cycle of movement where opposite diagonal legs work together. The trot and canter are diagonal gaits.
- Two-Beat Gait: Two feet hit the ground in unison, and then the other two feet hit the ground in unison. There are only two hoof-beat sounds to be heard The pace and the trot are two-beat gaits.
- Three-Beat Gait: Two feet hit together, and each of the other feet hit on their own. There are three hoof-beat sounds to be heard The canter is a three-beat gait.
- Four-Beat Gait: Each foot has its own, independent strike on the ground. There are four hoof-beat sounds in the stride cycle The walk and the gallop are four-beat gaits.

As you study the stride of a horse, you can determine the sequence of the feet in each different stride. You should begin the description of the sequence with the hind foot, since movement starts on the hind foot. Beyond stride, you will also have several gaits in which the horse will, at times, have no contact with the ground with any feet. This is known as suspension, so gaits with this characteristic should be noted when described.

Each step can also be analyzed by:

- **Height**, which is the highest point that the foot reaches as it moves through the swing phase. This is best seen from the side as the horse moves past the observer.
- **Trueness**, which is the amount that a foot moves from side to side as it goes through the swing phase. This is best seen from in front of, or behind a horse as it is moving.
- The **speed** of the foot as it is in the swing phase, which is obviously related to the gait that the horse is in, and the foot will go slower in the walk than in the trot, and so on.
- The **length** of the stride can be determined by measuring hoof prints. To do this, you should

measure from the same point on a hoof print to the same point on the other hoof print; for example, from the center of the toe print to the center of the toe print on the next hoof print.

The natural gaits of the horse are the walk, trot ,and gallop. These are also found in other members of the equine family such as donkeys and zebras. Some horses have been bred to have a tendency toward one type of gait or another, such as the pace, running walk, and Paso gait. Some gaits are refined by training horses to enhance their natural gaits, such as the rack, canter, and stepping pace.

As a farrier, you should make yourself familiar with the gaits of the type of horses that you are shoeing the most. If you find that you are shoeing primarily Tennessee Walking Horses, you need to become fluent in the language unique to that breed,and understand what the trainers, riders, and owners are expecting from their horses.

This textbook will define some of the basic gaits, but you may need to expand beyond this work to get more specific information about other breeds.

Remember that throughout this text, the term "near" is used to describe the left side, and the term "off" is used to describe the right side. This is common terminology among many horsemen, so we use it to make students familiar with it. Most people come to school knowing the difference between left and right, and using the terms near and off only increases their knowledge.

THE WALK (FIGURE 3)

This is a lateral, four -beat gait, so you will hear four distinctive hoof-beat sounds. Two or three feet are always on the ground, making the walk one of the most stable gaits for the horse to move at. Since there is always contact with the ground, there is no suspension to this gait.

The sequence of the feet at a walk is:

1. Near hind
2. Near fore
3. Off hind
4. Off fore

Although it may appear that one foreleg moves

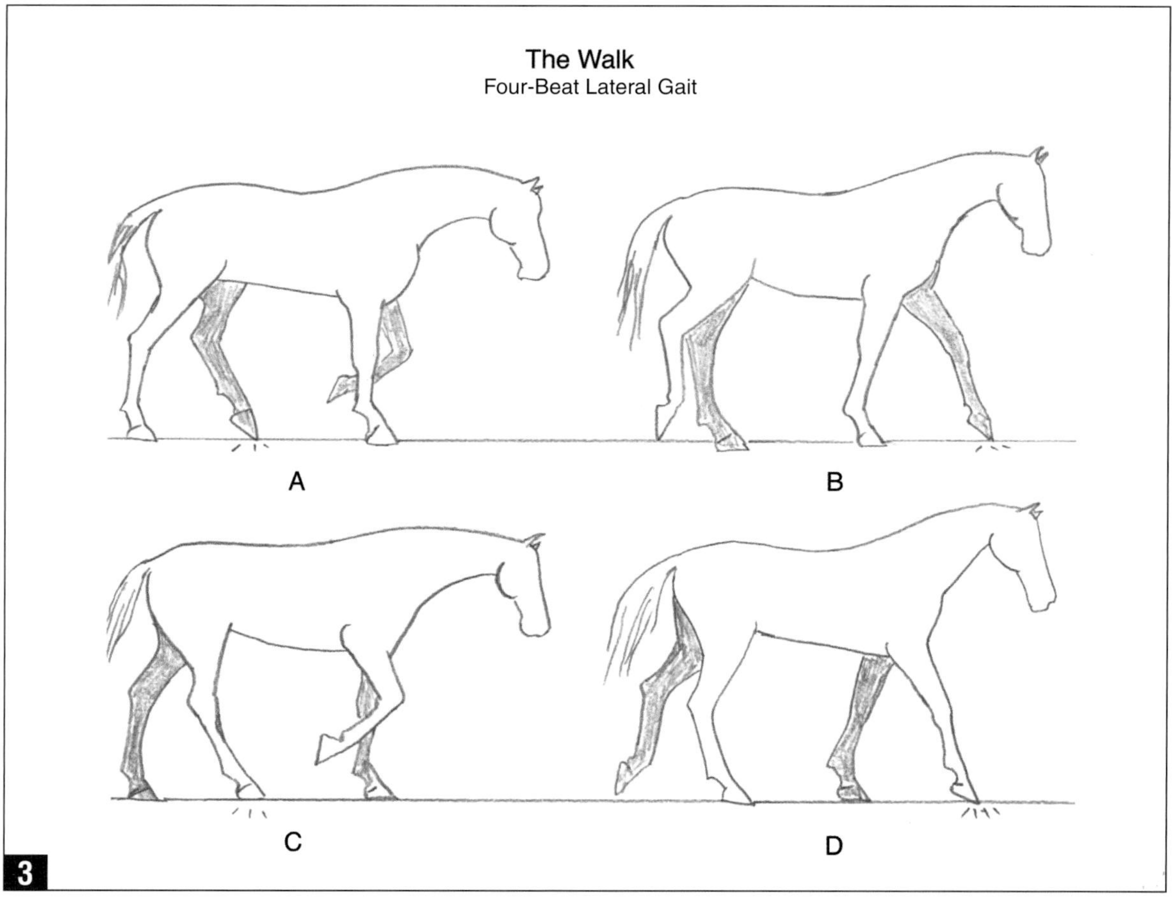

The Walk
Four-Beat Lateral Gait

A

B

C

D

3

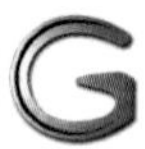

first, the walk sequence is said to start from the rear because that is where the power comes from. Each beat should be clear and distinct without shuffling, quickening or altering the rhythm. The average horse will move at about 4 miles per hour at the walk.

THE TROT (FIGURE 4)

The trot is a diagonal, 2-beat gait, so you will only hear two sounds as the horse moves at this gait. I often compare the trot to how people move when walking at a normal pace. They will swing their right arm forward as their left leg goes forward, and then the left arm swings forward as the right foot swings forward. This is a comfortable and easy way for us to move, and the trot is a comfortable and easy way for most horses to move.

To describe the sequence, you would say:

1. Off hind, near fore, suspension
2. Near hind, off fore, suspension. That instant of suspension is what makes the trot springy or bouncy.

The feet should move and land in unison, and there should only be one sound. If not, there is a good chance that the horse has a problem. The average horse will be moving around 7 or 8 miles per hour at a normal trot.

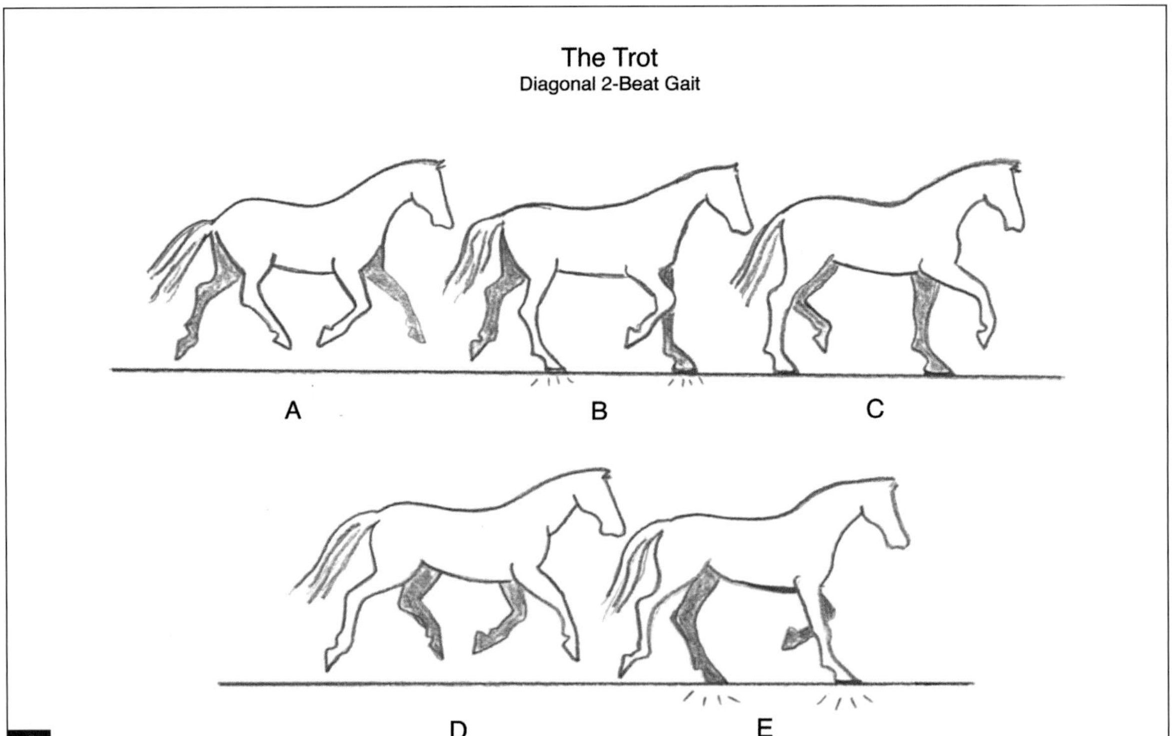

The Trot
Diagonal 2-Beat Gait

A B C

D E

4

THE CANTER (FIGURE 5)

This is a three-beat, diagonal gait with suspension. The sequence of feet would be:

1. Off hind
2. Near hind, off fore, (diagonal)
3. Near front, suspension.

This is the sequence of a horse that is in the left lead and should be turning to the left if it is being turned. The lead leg is actually the last one to land in the stride sequence, but it is also the one that is the furthest forward at the end of the sequence, just before suspension. If a horse is turned to the right while in the left lead, it is called a wrong or false lead and referred to as counter canter. This is uncomfortable to ride and clumsy for the horse to do. The sequence of feet for the right lead would be:

1. Near hind
2. Off hind, near fore
3. Off front, suspension.

The canter has a gentle motion, and is one of the most comfortable gaits for the rider. It can range in speed from 10 to 17 miles per hour.

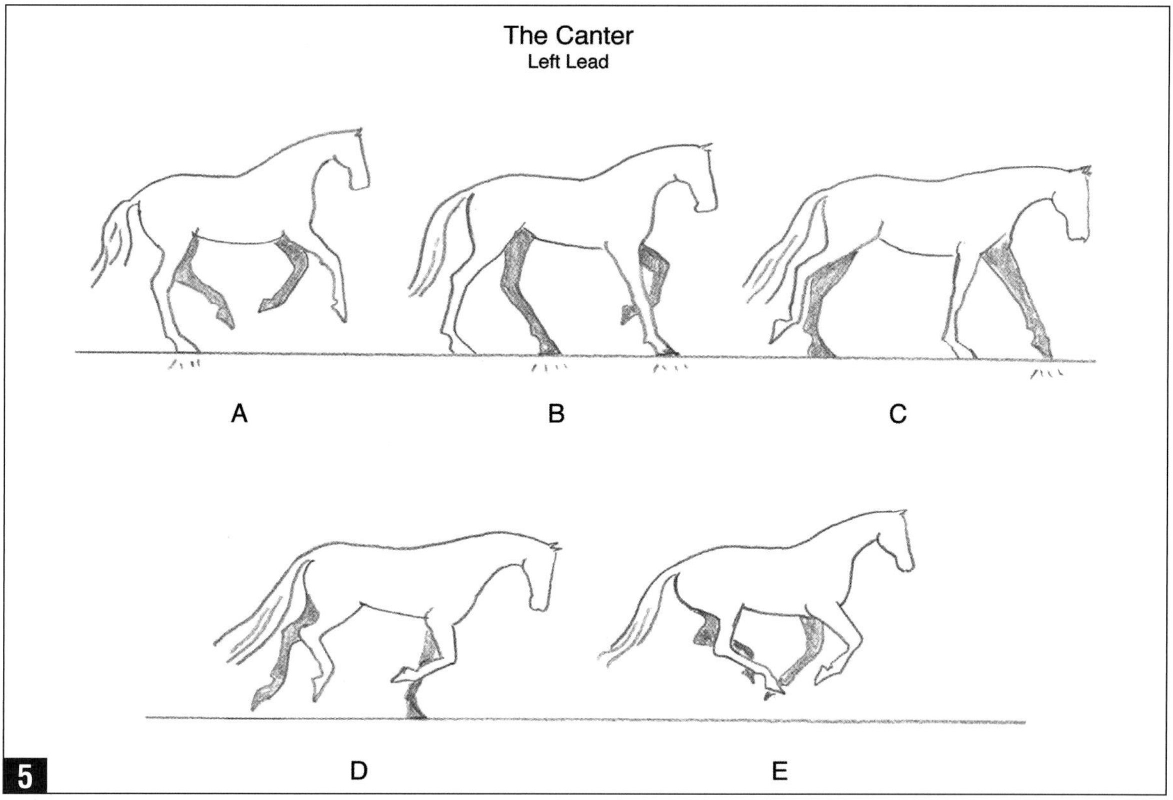

The Canter
Left Lead

A B C

D E

5

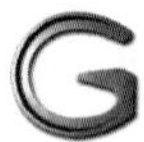

THE GALLOP (FIGURE 6)

The gallop is a fast, four-beat speed gait for the horse. There is a good amount of suspension in the gallop due to the speed that the horse is moving. The gallop is the fastest gait of the horse, averaging between 25 and 30 miles per hour, with speeds of up to 55 miles per hour being achieved by the American Quarter Horse in a sprint.

The sequence of the feet in the gallop in the left lead would be:

1. Off hind
2. Near hind
3. Off fore
4. Near fore, suspension.

This is an extended gait with a lot of engagement from the hinds.

THE PACE

This is a two-beat, lateral gait with suspension. It is very similar to the trot, with the difference being that the sides are working together instead of the diagonals. You can imagine the difference by comparing the normal person walking to the way that some foreign soldiers march with the arm and leg on the same side of the body coming forward at the same time.

To sequence the pace, you would say:

1. Near hind, near fore, suspension
2. Off hind, off fore, suspension.

The pace is difficult to ride but is flashy to watch. If a horse has the gait fault known as crossfiring, it will occur at this gait.

THE BACK

This is not a natural thing for the horse to do in the wild. If they do back, it is for a very short length before spinning and getting away in a forward movement. The back can be considered a diagonal, four-beat gait.

There are a multitude of other gaits, and some gaits that are the same, but called by different names due to the different discipline of riding. The ones in this section will get you off to a good start, but you should delve deeper into this subject if you are shoeing a horse of a particular discipline that has specialized movement.

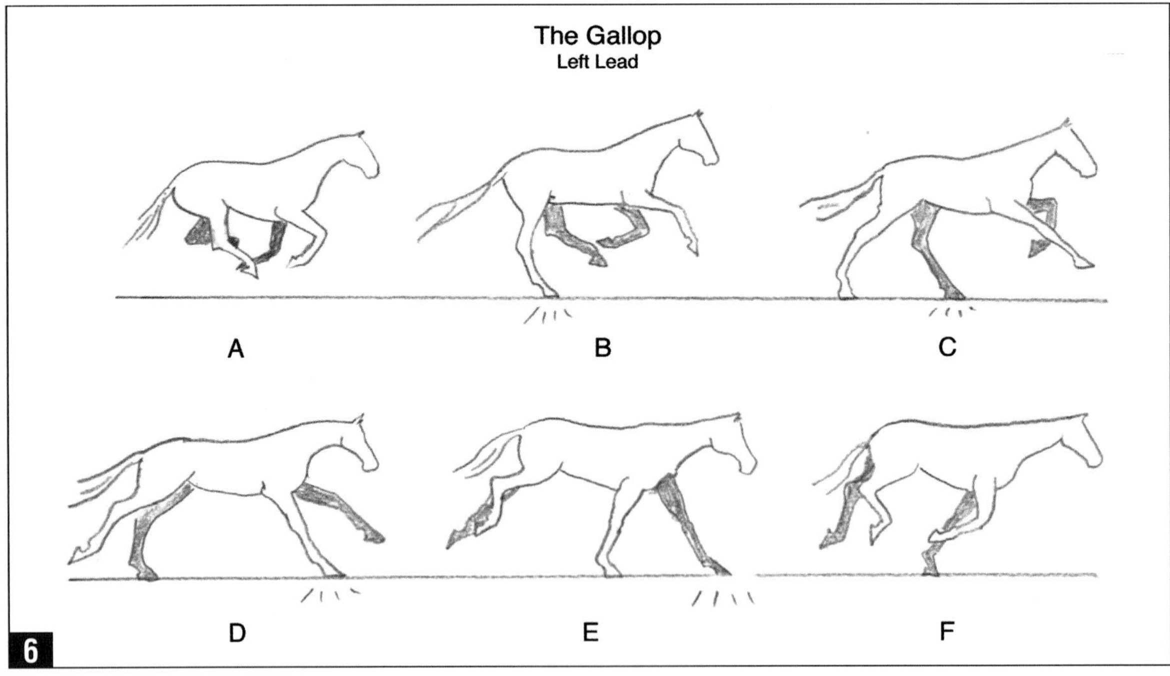

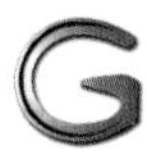

Chapter 17 GAIT FAULTS

A gait fault is when a horse does something that it should not at the desired gait. Some are annoying, such as forging at a walk, while some are damaging and dangerous, such as overreaching. For the farrier, it is important that you are able to distinguish these gait faults as well as learn to shoe in a manner to correct them.

Many gait faults are in the way that the horse is built. Bad conformation will lead to bad movement, so there is a limit to what shoeing can accomplish. However, a horse that has learned to walk with a certain conformation may develop problems if you try and change that conformation to suit aesthetic goals. You can correct the stance of a foal at a young age and the horse will develop a gait based on better conformation due to your efforts. But when the horse has learned to deal with its conformation defects without your corrections, you may have to learn to live with that conformation on the aged horse.

You will also find that many of the corrections that you can create through shoeing will vanish once the shoes are off. This should be explained to customers so that they are prepared for the changes that you are about to create, as well as how those changes can deteriorate over the course of a shoeing cycle.

The gait faults that concern the farrier the most are those in which a horse is actually hitting itself. These types of problems have potential to injure the horse, and possibly the rider if the horse happens to fall. For this reason, I don't mind getting aggressive in order to fix this sort of problem. With any gait fault that results in feet hitting other legs or feet, protective equipment is a must. Overreach boots, splint boots, scalpers, leg wraps, or whatever else the customer can come up with are important. The horse will not continue to perform if it is afraid of hurting itself.

There are instances where a horse is going to take a misstep and hit itself with another leg. After all, there are holes and unseen objects that we stumble and trip over. The same is true for a horse, which has the added disadvantage of having four legs to worry about and no way to see those legs. The horse also has to deal with a load that it didn't pack sitting on it, and that load may or may not have any business being up there.

Poorly made and ill-fitting tack can cause a lot of gait faults. Since we don't feel what a horse feels when it is saddled, we really cannot sympathize with what it's like to have a saddle that is completely wrong for that horse cinched down, then have a moving human sit in the middle of it. The shape of the saddle tree compared to the shape of a horse's withers is an important consideration when you are dealing with gait faults. Another potential problem with tack is a heavily made breast collar. In my experience of shoeing horses that are used for roping events, I have seen quite a few breast collars that did not fit the horse properly. Many of them were too wide and sat too low, and these interfere with the front legs trying to come forward. I am not surprised when a horse with one of those breast collars has a stumbling or overreaching problem.

The primary gait faults that we will discuss in this textbook are: stumbling, interfering, overreaching, forging, scalping, crossfiring, speedy cutting, elbow hitting, and toe dragging.

STUMBLING (FIGURE 1)

The definition of stumbling is interference between the toe of a foot and the ground during the swing phase of a stride. This is a problem that can be deadly to the rider and is very dangerous to the horse.

You will find that a horse may stumble on occasion in deep ground or rough terrain with a lot of obstacles, but this is not the sort of stumbling that we are concerned with. We are concerned with the chronic stumbling that happens in the absence of bad footing.

This is rarely a shoeing issue, which means that it can rarely be fixed by shoeing alone. The traditional suggestions of rocker toes or heavier shoes have not seemed to work that well in my experi-

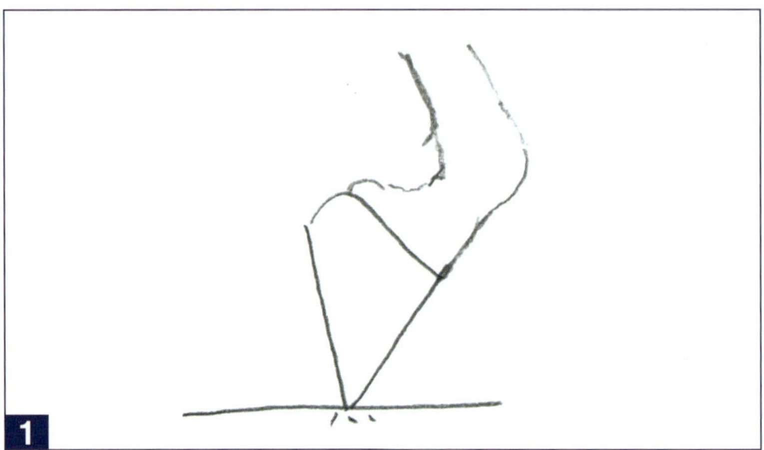

Stumbling.

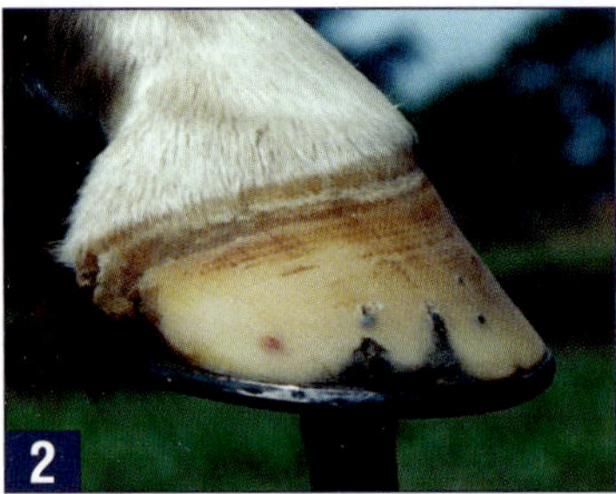

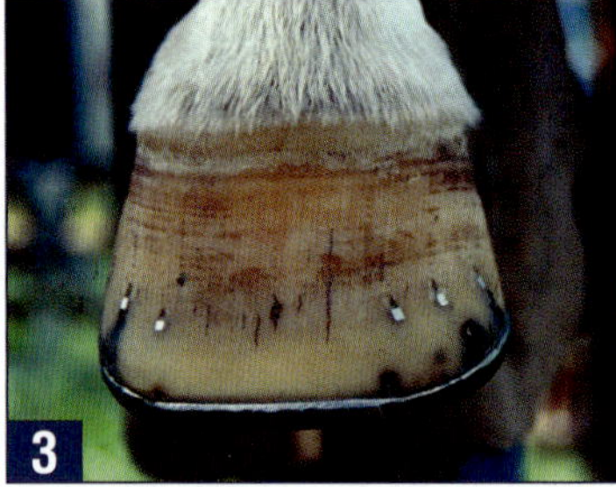

Rocker toe on foot.

ence. If a rocker toe did work, I think that it did so only because it decreased the length of the toe, and this gave the horse less material to interfere with. Changing the breakover was not the main advantage that helped the horse to avoid stumbling. However, since less length of toe will mean less length to hit the ground, a rocker toe is often the first thing I try on a stumbling horse **(Figures 2 and 3)**.

Stumbling can be caused by a number of things. The first concern is an untrained rider on a lazy horse. This is a tough one for the farrier, because it takes a lot of tact to give advice to customers about their riding skills without offending them. For the horse that only stumbles when ridden by a certain person, you will have to find a way to suggest changes in the riding style.

The next concern is the amount of work that a person is demanding from a horse. If a horse is too young or too weak for what it is being asked to do, then it is likely to stumble. Those of you who have been in the service are sure to remember some of those really tough road marches where everyone was stumbling by the end. The same thing can happen to a horse that is asked to carry too much too far. Fixing the problem is easy; simply decrease the workload.

Stumbling is a result of pain in the back or shoulders. This is a long way from the foot, and you should involve a good vet to help diagnose and treat whatever may be ailing the horse. We once had a customer with a stumbling horse that gave up on whatever we tried and started shoeing that horse himself. He tried everything he could think of. I saw the horse at the saddle club once with angles on the front feet that had to be approaching 75 degrees. Yet, the horse continued to stumble. Finally, a chiropractor adjusted the horse and it quit stumbling. There was enough pain in the withers that the horse was unable to bring its front limbs forward correctly. When you have this sort of problem, you have to be an advisor, because shoeing is not going to change anything.

Another cause of stumbling is lameness. Heel lameness if the primary culprit, but any lameness can cause a horse to have problems bringing the feet forward. If the horse is stumbling with the lame foot, I suspect heel lameness because the horse is trying to protect that heel and has its toe pointed to avoid heel impact. Horses that stumble with the sound leg are doing so because they are trying to get that leg down fast and relieve the lame leg. In either case, treat that lameness successfully, and the stumbling should go away.

As you can see, there is not an easy answer for stumbling. I suggest that you hand your customer this book and have him or her read this section, and perhaps together you can come up with a solution for this horse.

INTERFERING (FIGURE 4)

Interfering is the basic term used to describe the inside of one foot hitting the inside of the opposite leg. It can happen in the front or hind legs but is more common in the hinds.

There have been a lot of anecdotal fixes for interfering, but I have found it is easier to cause than to fix. Eddie Watson used to say that a lot of good horseshoeing is simply undoing the work that was already done to the horse. The traditional conformation that is blamed for a horse that interferes in front would be a toed-out stance. This type of conformation will encourage the foot to swing toward the inside in the swing phase of the step, and this can cause a collision. It is said that a toed-out horse will break over the medial toe, but it is rare to find a shoe that is worn at the medial toe more than the lateral toe, so I don't think this happens quite like the older textbooks on the subject indicate. I believe that some horses are just prone to swing their feet to the inside of true, while some horses are prone to wing out. But in the front feet, most horses will wear the lateral toe more than the medial.

The first thing that should be used for this horse is protective boots. The interference can happen anywhere from the knee to the foot. You can find the exact spot and how the foot is hitting by chalking the leg wraps with colored chalk. There are many types of protective wraps and boots. **Figure 5** shows a protective splint boot on the inside of the front leg. Be aware that these splints should be as thin as possible while still providing protection to the horse. The thicker they are, the greater chance of the foot hitting the excess material.

Farriers who get the balance wrong on horses that have a tendency to interfere can easily make one that is close become one that is hitting. Taking too much off of the medial side, especially towards the toe on one of these horses can be enough to cause it to hit. Fitting full, or using heavy shoes can also be a cause.

Knowing this, you can work backward to deter-

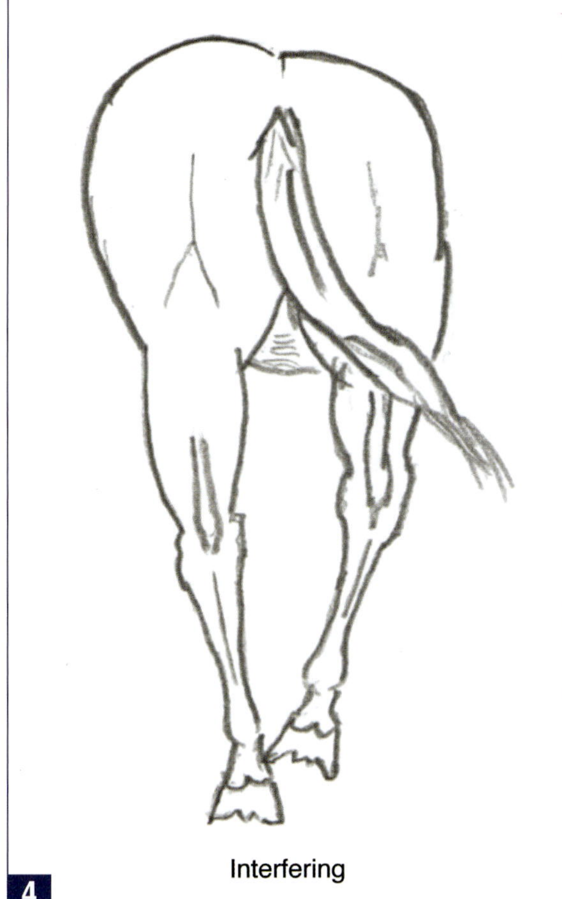

Interfering.

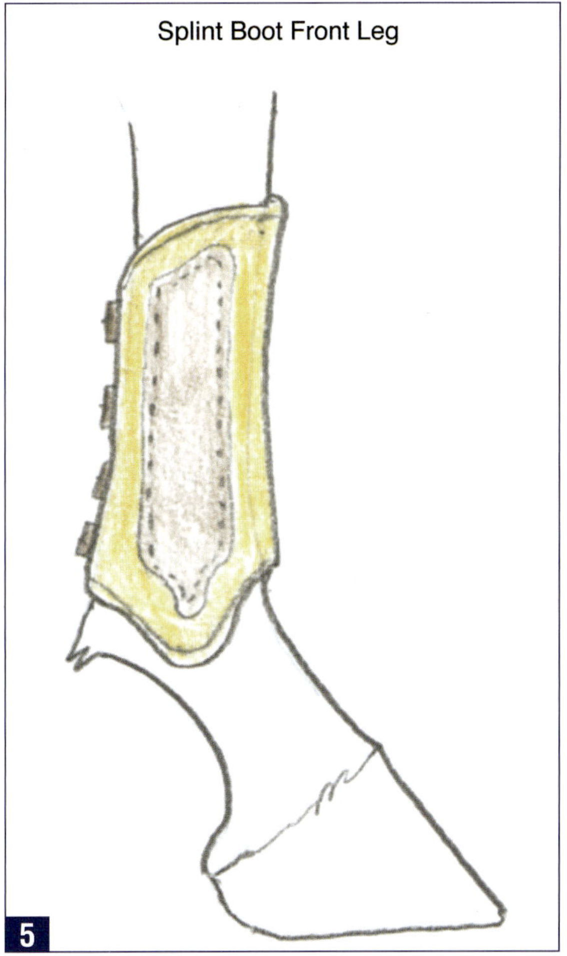

Splint boot.

mine a method of correcting the problem. You can lower the lateral side of the foot to make the horse stand, and hopefully move, straighter. You can use a lighter shoe that is fit tight on the medial side. Scott Simpson, CJF, suggests trying a side weight on some of these horses. However, if you try with weight on the outside and that doesn't work, you may need the weight on the inside. Each horse responds to side-weighted shoes differently.

Try any of these suggestions and even some combinations, but it is essential that you impress upon the rider the importance of this horse always having protective boots when being used. Adding splint boots can prevent some serious problems.

Interference on the hind legs is a different problem. This is generally found on horses that are base-narrow behind. Since the feet are starting out closer to the centerline of the body, they are more apt to hit each other as they move forward. The legs are especially likely to interfere if the horse is doing a turn where one foot has to move closer to the other leg. On the bright side, these horses will generally move with their feet further apart when they pick up speed. At least this lessens the chance of the interference being worse due to speed. As with the front feet, you should apply protective wraps and boots to these horses. **Figure 6** shows a common type of protective boot for the hind legs.

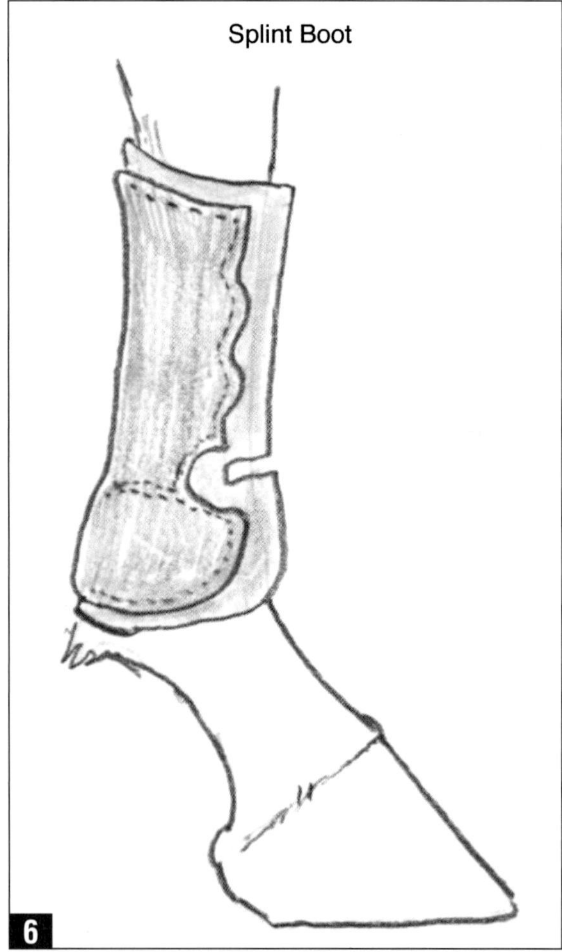

Splint boot.

If the horse has a base-narrow conformation behind, you can trim lower on the medial side to move the feet further apart. Couple this with a lateral extension on the lateral heel, and the feet should assume a stance that is further apart than the conformation would dictate.

Cow-hocked horses that interfere behind should be shod with a square-toed hind shoe with a trailer. The trailer will support the lateral heels that are trying to roll under as well as pull these heels out a little. You can trim lower on the lateral toe, but the effects of the square-toed shoe should direct breakover toward the middle of the foot.

Finally, you can try placing traction on the lateral side of the shoe. Much like the crossfiring shoe that we are about to cover, a shoe that has more traction on the lateral side and less on the medial will cause the foot to twist slightly at landing, and hopefully line it up so that it will break over straighter.

Be certain to shoe any horse with interference in a safe manner. Do not let too much steel hang out the medial side of the foot and be certain to soften the edges of the shoe with boxing and safing.

OVERREACHING, FORGING (FIGURES 7-8)

These are some of the more common problems that I have had to deal with in my career of shoeing rodeo, cutting, and the Western horse. Both of these problems relate to a timing problem where the front foot and the hind foot on the same side strike each other. Conformation can be a big part of the problem when you are dealing with horses that have a short back and long legs. These horses are built to have collisions between the front and hind feet. Tack should also be considered when dealing with this problem.

Due to the fact that the front feet have to break trail for the hind feet, deep ground, tall grass, water, mud, snow, and other rough going can also cause any horse to overreach. As such, these are exceptional reasons and not really a consideration in this discussion of the problem.

I have seen in some very popular textbooks that the way to correct overreaching and forging is to speed up the fronts and slow down the hinds. As a young farrier educator, I used to actually stand in front of my students and spout that out like I knew what I was talking about. Of course this is an impossible thing to do, and I have never had any farrier ever tell me how it should be accomplished. If you think about it, if a horse were made to go faster in the front — let's say 10 mph — and slower behind — let's say 9 mph — it would be a very short trip until the horse was torn in two. The inconvenience of a spine prevents this theory from working, but it does not hinder uninformed shoers from recommending it. See the section on shoeing myths for more on this.

Each of these problems has a specific definition. Overreaching refers to the toe of a hind foot hitting the heel region or bulbs of a front foot on the same side **(Figure 7)**. This can happen before the front foot leaves the ground, or once it is in the air. Overreaching can lead to bad cuts in the bulbs, as well as pulled shoes and horses falling because the front foot is kept from moving forward.

Forging occurs at a walk or trot, and happens when the toe of a hind foot hits the bottom of the front foot on the same side in midair **(Figure 8)**. If shod, there will be a loud clack as the shoes collide. While this is not necessarily a dangerous thing, it can be very annoying. Some horsemen say that it is a habit that a horse develops, much like people dragging their feet as they walk.

For both of these, the correction is basically the same. The theory is that you need to change the position of the hind feet in relation to the front feet. We have already established that the front of the horse is going the same speed as the rear. The step lengths are also the same. If the near front is going 6 feet, so is the off, unless the horse is moving in a circle. This goes for the hinds as well. You will have horseshoers tell you that you can speed up a step by easing breakover or even change the length of that step. You can only do this by changing the momentum of the horse. The faster it goes, the longer the stride length is going to be, and all legs are going to be affected. This means that a rocker toe placed on the fronts to get them to move out of the way faster does not really work.

So, with some of those myths debunked, consider how a horse ends up hitting itself. It is a timing problem in which the hinds are coming up before the fronts have had a chance to get out of the way.

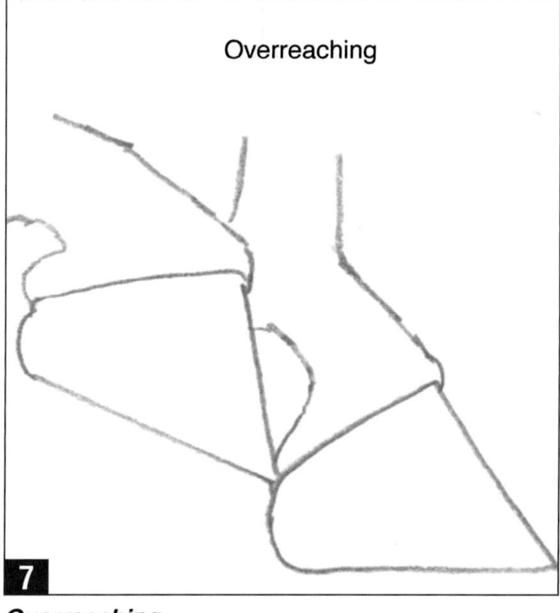

Overreaching.

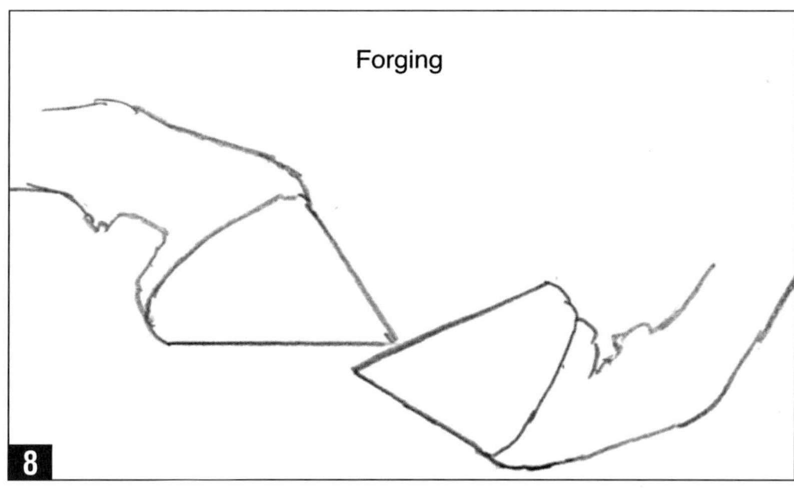

Forging.

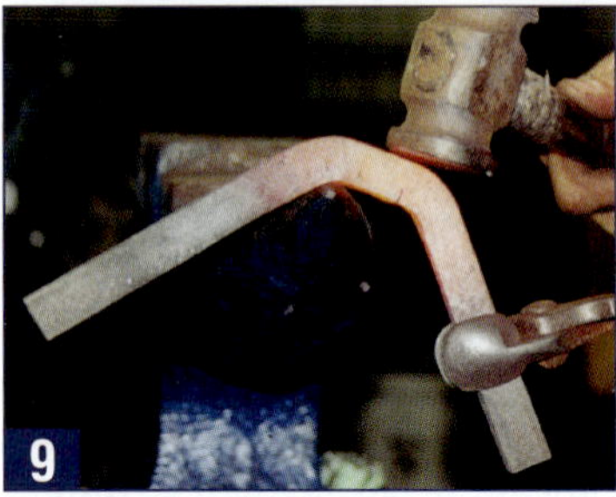

Making a square toe.

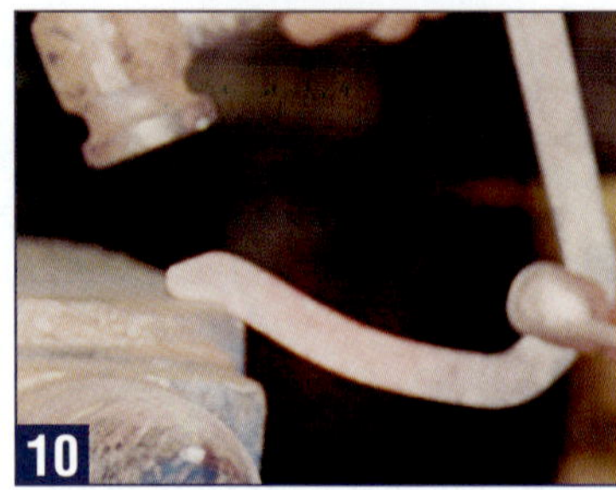

Making a trailer.

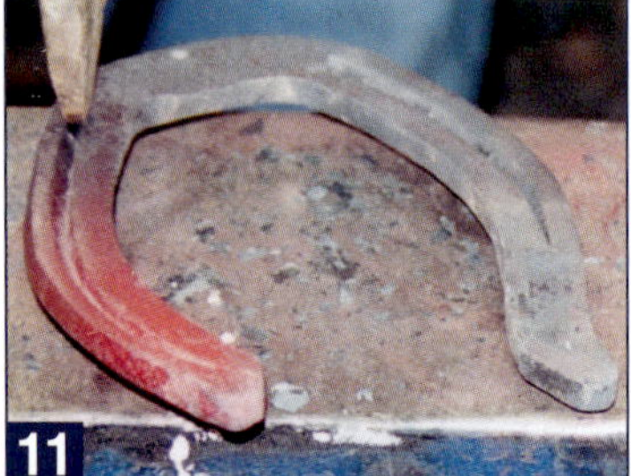

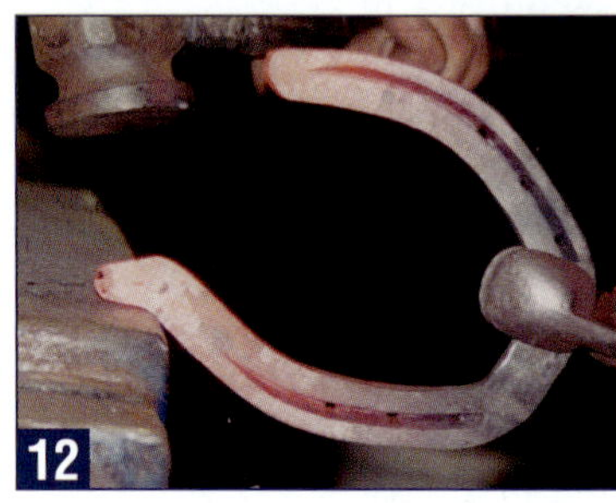

Completing the shoe.

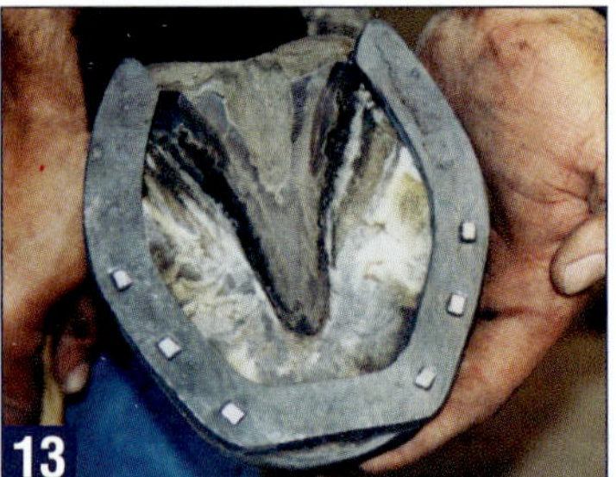

Square toe on foot.

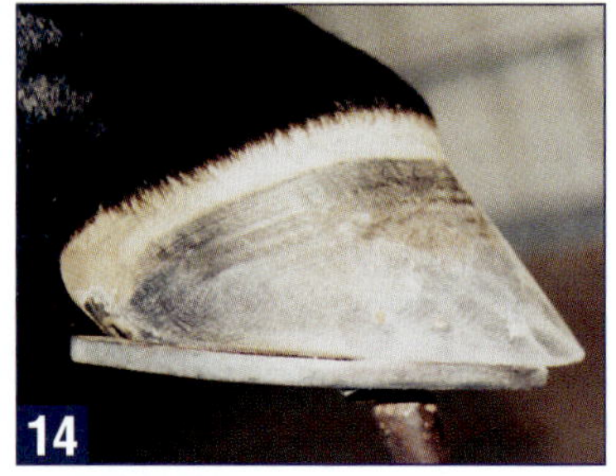

Lateral view of the square toe on the foot.

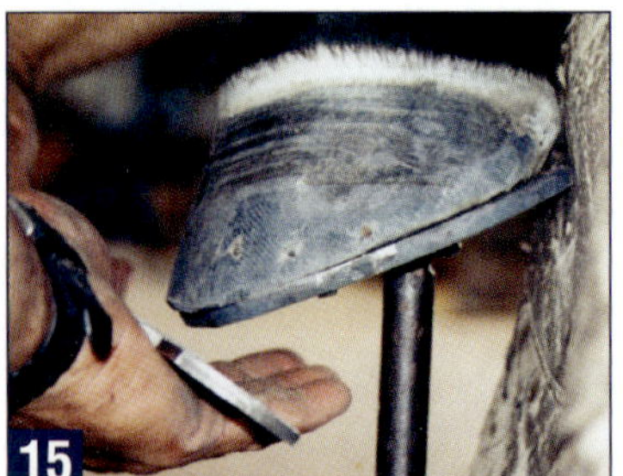

Beveling off the toe of the foot with a square toed shoe on it.

If we were able to place the hinds on the ground just a fraction further away from the fronts, the problem would be solved. So, this is how I begin my approach to fixing overreaching and forging.

The first thing that I do is trim all four feet to their natural angles. The fronts will be shod normally, no rocker toes, wedges, or special breakover patterns. I may fit the horse tighter than normal until I am certain that the problem is corrected.

On the hinds, I will use a square-toed shoe with either extended heels or a trailer **(Figures 9-12)**. The way that this shoe works is that the trailer or extended heels impact the ground when the foot is behind where it would impact the ground without the extended heels. You can say that the foot would hit the ground earlier than before, but remember that the speed of the foot and the length of the step have not changed, but simply the placement of the foot in relation to the body. Since the length and speed of the step are the same, if I get the placement of the impact for the hinds to become further from the fronts, any potential collision is averted.

The square toe results in the shoe being set back from the toe about 1/2 inch. You can make it as severe as you want to, but I will rarely set one back as far as the width of the web **(Figure 13)**. There will be hoof wall that extends past the toe of the shoe **(Figure 14)**. This material is rounded off with the rasp **(Figure 15)** and now the horse has less length to hit its front feet with. If it does hit, it will be with hoof wall that is rounded up instead of with the edge of a horseshoe. This gives the square toe two advantages over a perimeter fit.

If the horse continues to overreach or forge, I will add heel caulks to the extended heels or trailer. With the shoe extended behind the buttress of the foot, the foot will impact sooner. Since the extensions alone were not enough, if I project something downward like a heel caulk, it will impact the ground even earlier. This opens up the distance between the front and hind feet even more. I will say that I only have to do this on about one in 20 horses that overreach.

To this point, all of the correction has been on the shoe selection for the hind feet. Nothing has changed on the front feet except the addition of bell boots (**Figure 16**). If the shoes on the hind feet are still not working, I will start to change the angle that the feet are trimmed at. Trimming at angles that are not correct for the horse is the last resort to fix this problem. However, I have only had to do this on a handful of horses. The previously mentioned corrections work 99 out of 100 times, so don't change the angles away from the natural angle unless you absolutely have to.

The front feet can be trimmed at a lower angle, and the hinds can be trimmed at a steeper angle. The theory behind this trimming scheme is that the front foot will move forward on the ground as it attempts to achieve natural angle and still accept the trim. The hind foot will move backward in stance since the reciprocal apparatus on the hind limb places the foot on the ground where it is most comfortable with the natural angle of the hind foot.

I have had some farriers tell me that this was the opposite way to trim, because they were wanting to speed up the fronts and slow down the hinds. To their way of thinking, making the fronts steep would speed them up because breakover would be easier for the fronts. Trimming the hinds shallow would slow the feet down because the horse had to break over these shallow feet. As you are aware, you can't speed up the fronts and slow down the hinds. Also, that sort of trimming scheme will only move the feet toward each other when the horse is standing, and this will set the horse up to overreach.

When you are dealing with overreaching and forging, a miss by 1/2 inch is as good as a mile. There will be some horses that really challenge you when it comes to overreaching. You may find that you have to come up with other solutions like changing the breakover pattern for the front feet or applying weighted shoes to change the action of the feet. Try what I have mentioned first, but don't be afraid to think outside of the box. Anytime a horse is hitting itself with other feet it is a dangerous enough situation that it needs your help.

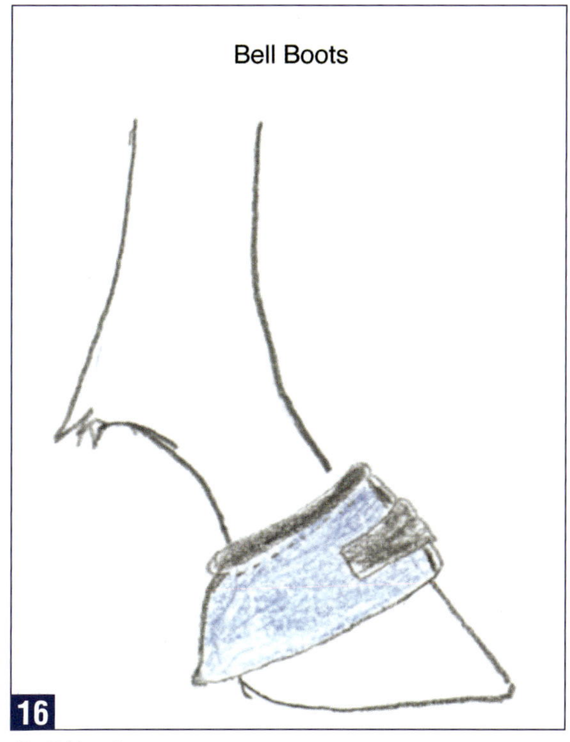

Bell Boots.

SCALPING (FIGURE 17)

Scalping occurs when the toe of the front foot hits the dorsal wall or coronary region of the hind foot. Scalping mainly occurs at an extended trot, and as such, is not the sort of thing that rodeo horses have happen too often. Standardbred trotters are known for having problems with scalping, and I have seen it happen with Amish buggy horses, which are often Standardbred racehorses that are no longer racing. Since most of the Amish buggy horses have Borium on their shoes, scalping can cause even more damage to them than on a horse shod with normal shoes.

The suggested shoeing to prevent or reduce scalping is to trim the front feet as short as you can. Many trainers will not want to do this, but a horse that is hitting itself needs to have that problem fixed. You can try using either half-round shoes or rocker toes in the front to decrease some of the length that the horse has to hit itself with as well. Add to that some small heel caulks on the hind feet to open the horse up a little bit in his stance. As with the over-reaching problem just discussed, the heel caulks will cause the hind feet to hit the ground earlier in

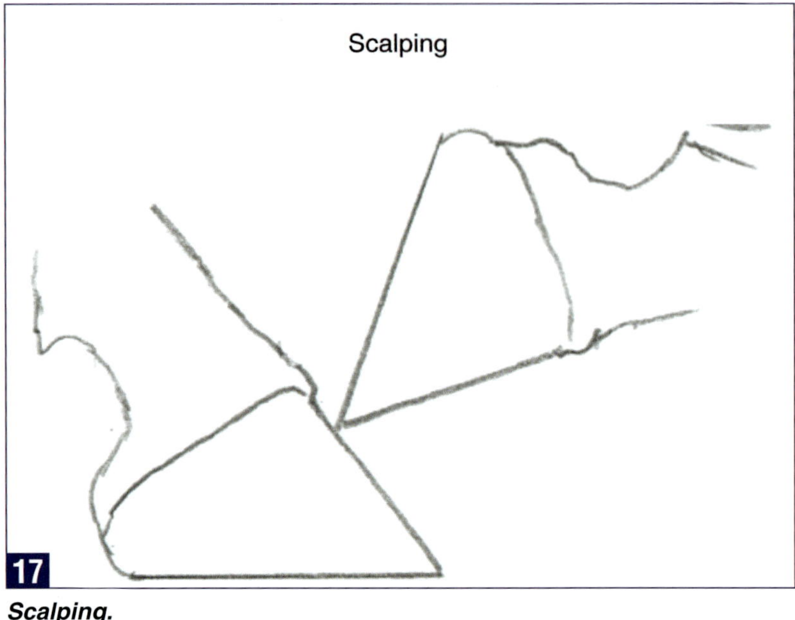

Scalping.

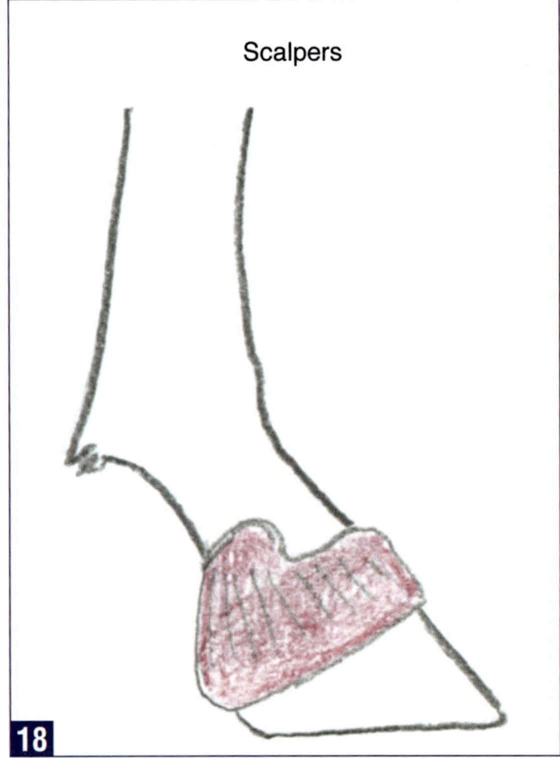

Protective boot called a scalper.

the stride, moving these feet away from the front feet.

As with the other gait faults mentioned, make sure to advise the owner to protect the legs from potential injury with boots. In this case, there are boots known as scalpers that protect the dorsal portion of the hind foot and coronary band **(Figure 18)**.

CROSSFIRING (FIGURE 19)

Crossfiring only occurs at a pace, so it is not the sort of thing that you will see with a Western type of horse. This is a collision between the medial toe of a hind foot and the medial hoof or leg of the diagonal limb. The near hind hits the off fore, or the off hind hits the near fore, while all the feet are in the air.

The two-beat gaits for a horse are the trot and pace. With a trot, the diagonals come forward together, so they stay apart from each other all the time. The pace is a lateral gait, so the hind comes forward toward the diagonal front. This is where the interference takes place.

The strategy for correcting crossfiring should be to open up the stance of the fronts or hinds or both. You can do this by trimming the fronts slightly lower on the lateral side. On the hinds, I prefer opening the stance by using a trailer or even a slight lateral extension.

The traditional crossfiring shoe is a half-round, half-swedged shoe with a trailer. If you don't have

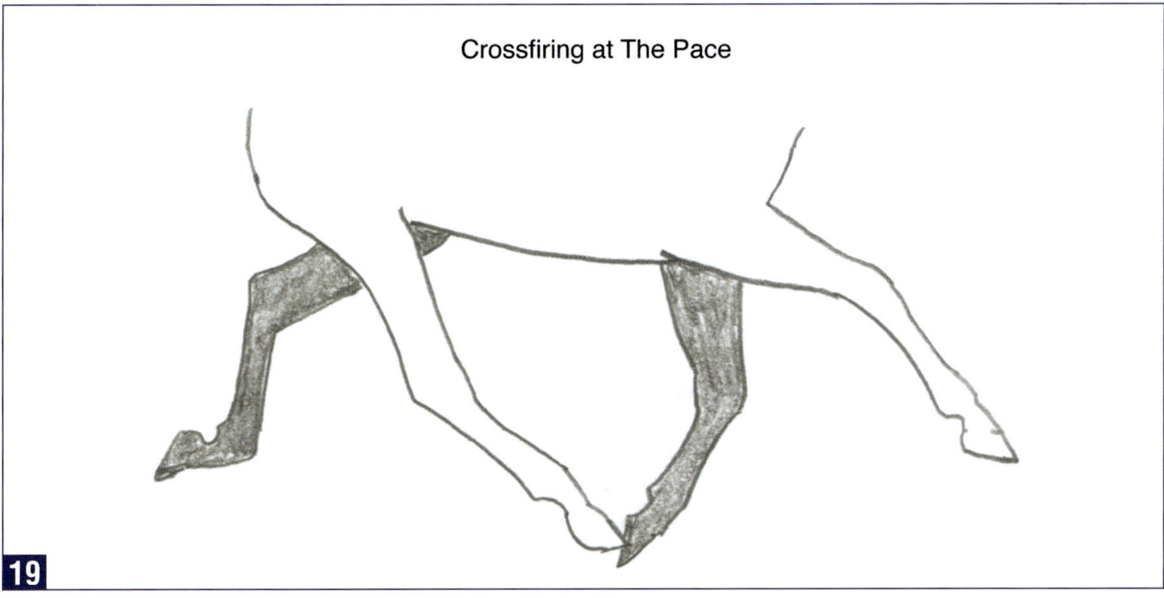

Crossfiring.

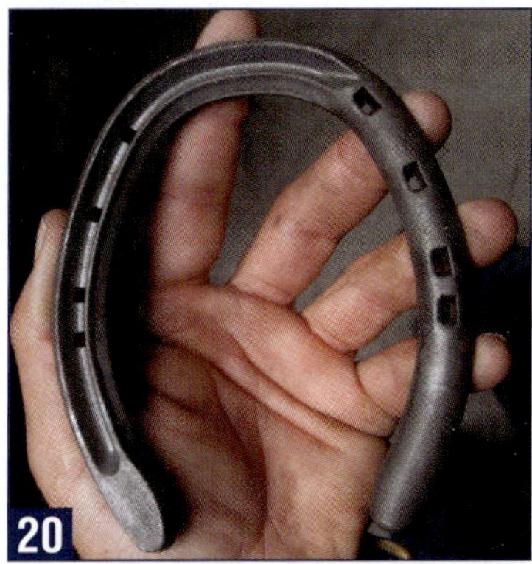

Half-round, half-swedged keg shoe that can be modified for a crossfiring horse.

a swedge block, you can make this shoe out of light concave by collapsing the concave on the medial side. You can also modify a keg shoe **(Figure 20)** like the one pictured. If the trailer by itself is not enough, try adding a heel caulk to it.

Again, you need to suggest protective boots to the owner.

SPEEDY CUTTING (FIGURE 21)

Speedy cutting refers to when a horse hits the inside of a back leg with a front foot on the same side. This happens on racing trotters as well as racehorses. In the world of trotters, they give names to this type of interference based on where the injury on the hind leg occurs. Close to and including the foot is scalping. Injuries from the coronary band to the fetlock are caused by speedy cutting. From the fetlock to the hock is known as shin hitting, and in the hock it is called hock hitting. The faster the horse is trotting, the higher the feet will hit. With racehorses, everything from the fetlock up is called speedy cutting.

Regardless of the name it is a collision between hoof and leg that has to be corrected. The principle strategy is to widen the flight of the hind legs if possible, but this can be hard to do. I recommend a half-round, half-swedged shoe, with a caulk and trailer on the hind (as you would for a crossfiring horse). On the front, use a shoe with the toe fit under the border of the wall to keep the horse from hitting itself with the shoe.

There are shin boots with a speedy cutting connection, or you can add a speedy cutting boot **(Figure 22)** to the shin boots on the hind leg. I also read about a pretty neat trick in Scott Simpson's book, *The Contemporary Horseshoer*. He recommends using pieces of chap leather and sale-barn tag glue. That stuff is pretty sticky, as you know if you have ever bought horses or cattle through the auction. Your leather patch will remain for several days. Don't put it directly on open wounds, but it will give the leg a little protection if you don't have a boot that will work.

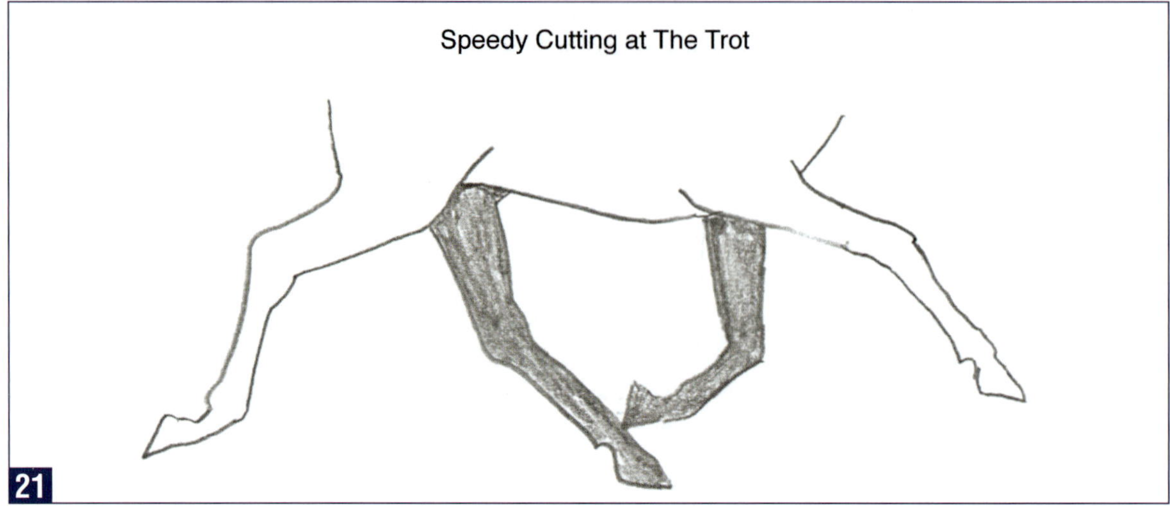

Speedy cutting.

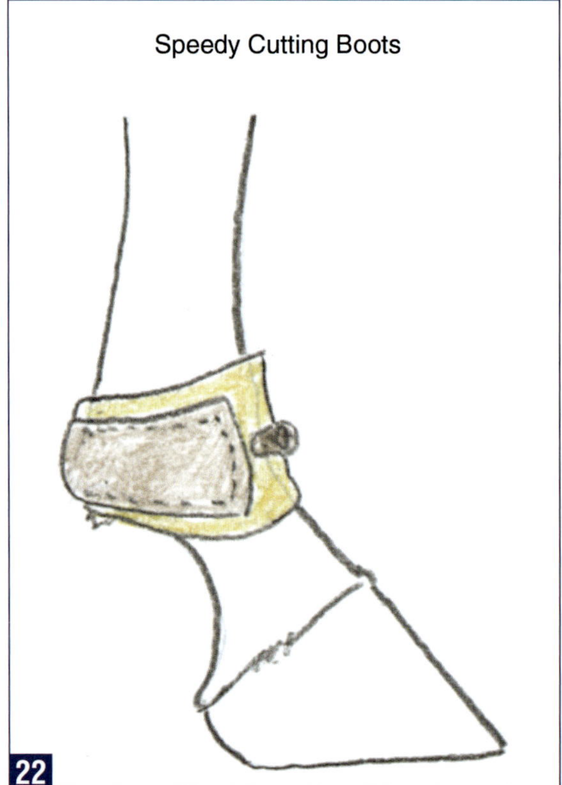

A protective boot that can be added to the splint boots and bell boots for speedy cutting.

ELBOW HITTING (FIGURE 23)

Elbow hitting occurs when a horse has enough action that the foot strikes the elbow on the same limb. This is blamed for causing what is called a shoe boil or capped elbow, (see Capped Elbow in Chapter #46-4). If the foot is hitting the elbow, you should shoe to try and keep it from happening.

The first thing to try is to use heel-weighted shoes or apply heel weight to the package that the horse already has on. If that does not work, try increasing the angle of the front feet a bit, or using more wedge pads, since the type of horses that are prone to elbow hitting are commonly shod with pads anyway. There is a protective apparatus made with straps that go over the top of the neck and cover the point of the elbows, but these are hard to keep in place as a horse moves out. The sale-barn tag cement with leather is probably a better solution.

Horses that hit in this manner will develop a condition referred to as a capped elbow or shoe boil. This is a large, soft swelling from the impact of the shoe. Horses can also get a capped elbow from lying down, rolling, and getting up on hard ground. I shoe a horse that hits its elbow when stomping because of flies. It has been suggested that a horse will hit its elbow with the shoe on the opposite leg when it is lying down, and there is even a beveled shoe used to prevent this from happening. However, I have yet to perssonally see this happen.

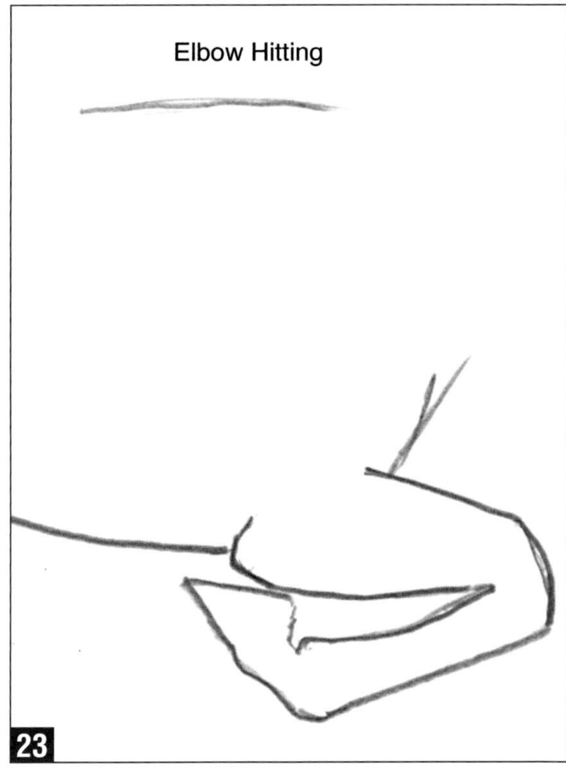

23

Elbow hitting.

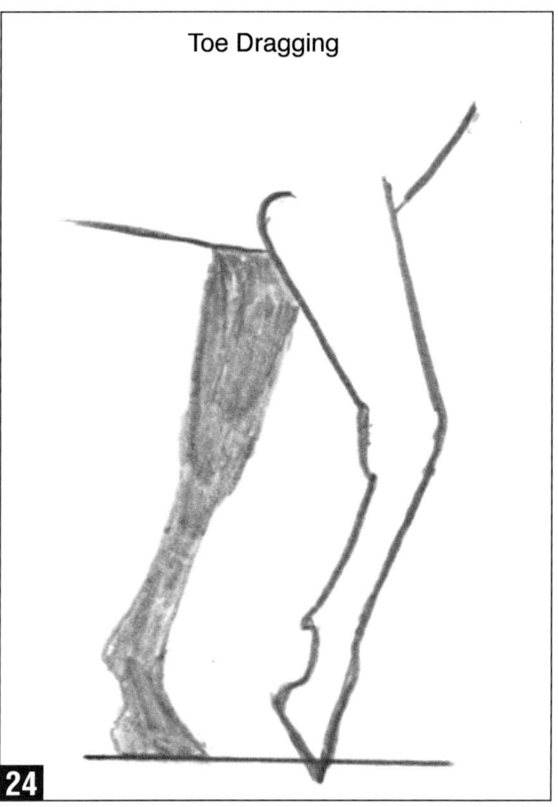

24

Toe dragging.

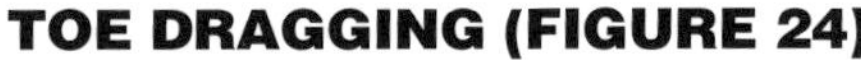

TOE DRAGGING (FIGURE 24)

This can be a really tough gait fault to correct. It happens for several reasons. First, a horse that is injured may drag the toe of one foot due to the pain of lifting that leg. Some horses have a very low arc to their step and may drag their toes anytime they are in dirt, sand, or similar terrain. Also, some horses have a lazy way of going that is similar to people who drag their feet. Once motivated to move, horses (or people) will often start to lift their feet higher.

For the injured horse, treat the lameness successfully and you will generally have corrected the problem. Some things, such as radial nerve paralysis, will be beyond the scope of the farrier, so you can only protect the toe of the foot from excessive wear from being dragged. To do this, make a shoe out of thicker stock and fit the perimeter of the toe. You may have to add borium or hard surface material to the thickness of the shoe at the toe in severe cases.

For the horse with a lower stride arc, try using a heavier shoe. While this may seem counterintuitive, most of the time the addition of weight will cause the horse to get the foot into the air higher.

An active and competent rider that keeps the horse moving can help horses that have the habit of dragging their toes. While this does nothing for the horse in pasture, it will help while the horse is being used. However, this is outside the realm of the farrier.

Gait faults come in varying degrees of severity, and it is important that the farrier be actively involved in coming up with a solution. Those mentioned in this chapter are only some of many ways that have been used to prevent horses from hitting themselves. Keep an open mind about potential solutions. Good solid basics applied with skill will often fix a lot of problems that are created by well-meaning, ignorant, and incompetent shoers who are applying a product in a way that they don't understand. Just use the simplest and least aggressive technique that will achieve the desired results.

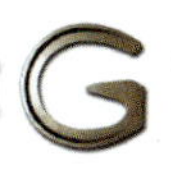

Section

6

Horsemanship

Chapter 18: Horsemanship 198

Chapter 19: Equine Psychology............................ 207

" 19 Hast thou given the horse strength?
Hast thou clothed his neck with thunder?
20 Canst thou make him afraid as a grasshopper?
The glory of his nostrils is terrible.
21 He paweth in the valley, and rejoiceth in his strength:
he goeth on to meet the armed men.
22 He mocketh at fear, and is not affrighted;
neither turneth he back from the sword.
23 The quiver rattleth against him,
the glittering spear and the shield.
24 He swalloweth the ground with fierceness and rage:
neither believeth he that it is the sound of the trumpet.
25 He saith among the trumpets, Ha, ha;
and he smelleth the battle afar off,
the thunder of the captains, and the shouting. "

—Job 39:19-25
—King James Version

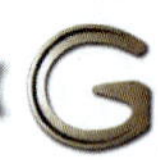

Chapter 18

HORSEMANSHIP

No one was born knowing how to handle horses. Yes, some are more adept naturally than others, but this does not mean that you cannot develop the skills to become enough of a horseman to be a great farrier. This does not entail having the ability to start a colt and make a finished heading horse. It simply means that you are able to predict what a horse is going to do and what it is thinking. You are able to make a horse more comfortable instead of more anxious. You are able to read a horse **(Figure 1)**.

My daughter, Jacquelyn, can walk into a barn full of nervous horses, and you can watch them visibly relax. They have a look on their faces that seems to say, "Oh, it's alright now. Jacquelyn is here. Everything is going to be fine." That comes from exposure to horses from youth that not everyone gets.

If you don't have that advantage, you need to learn how to become a horseman by conscious effort and study. You will have to learn how to hold still when you want to run and be quiet when you want to yell. That is okay. You can learn that.

Nothing in this chapter should be done or attempted by anyone who is not a seasoned and knowledgeable professional. It is being added here for educational purposes, not as a step-by-step guide or recommendation. Now, with the disclaimer out of the way, let's continue with this chapter.

A horse has to read you based on a lot of things that can be hard to control. A horse reads your body language (stance, posture, expression, eyes, movements, attitude) without understanding the words you say. The actual words you use do not make as big a difference to how the horse interprets the situation as the tone that you use. It could be all cuss words as far as the horse is concerned, but the tone and the way you deliver the words will make a big difference.

When you are around a horse, stay calm, confident, quiet, and move slowly, but still with a purpose. You have to let the horse know where he is compared to you on the pecking order. This is done by how you approach and handle that horse. Approach a horse like you would a beloved younger brother; full of respect, yet still in charge.

Here is something you can apply to more than just horsemanship. If you believe in yourself and your ability, that belief will be transferred to the horse, and the horse will also believe in your confidence. If you believe that you are going to have trouble, you are probably right about that as well,

It is not the best idea, but it is entirely possible to manhandle a horse. They can be roped, tied up, thrown down, and generally beaten into submission. Have I done that? Of course I have. If you run a shoeing school for very long, you run into situations that have to be handled this way. I don't like to do that, but when there is a job to, you have to get to it. In **Figure 2**, I am in a pen of horses getting ready to rope a horse to shoe. As you can see, catching the horse may be the easiest part of the job.

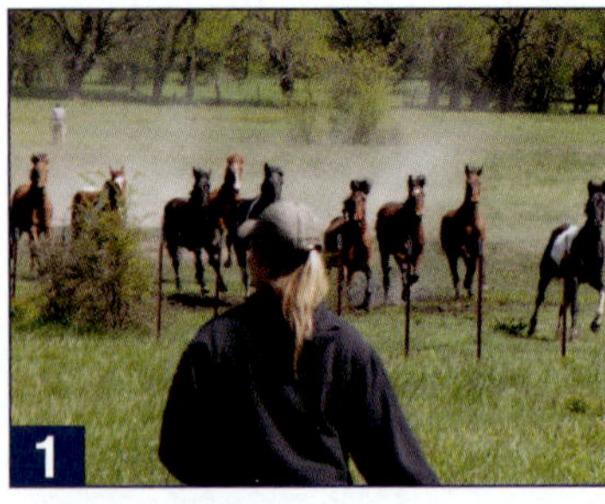

1 *Kelly headed out to catch some horses for the students to shoe.*

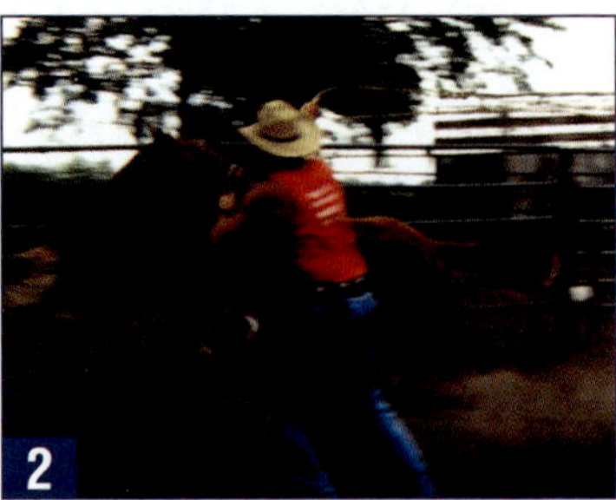

2 *Roping a horse.*

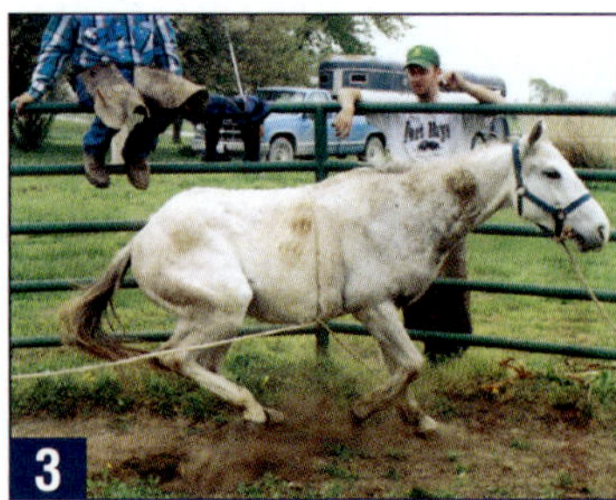

3 *Front foot tied up.*

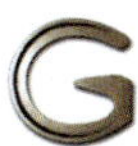

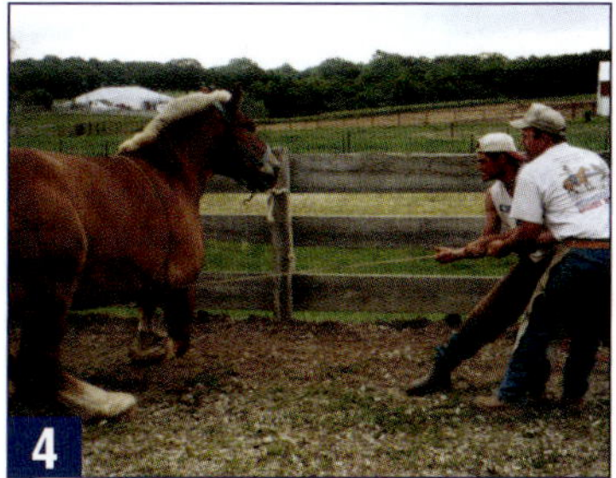

Pulling the front leg up.

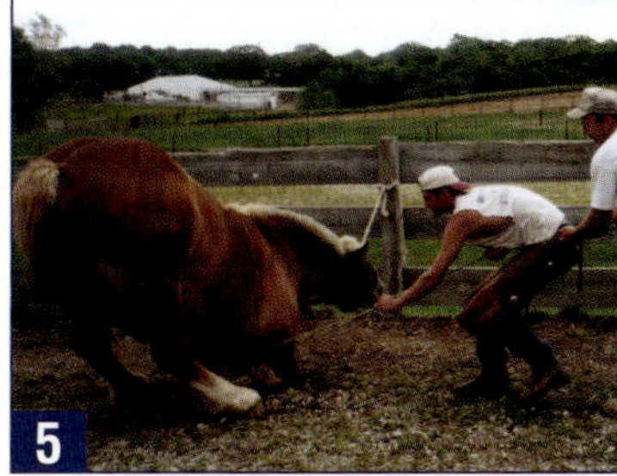

The horse bows.

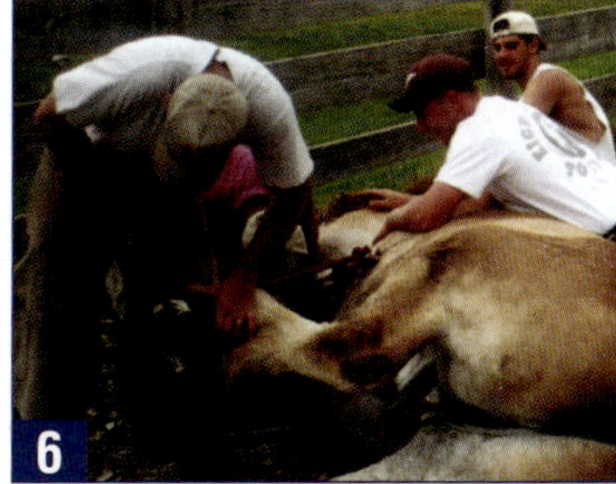

Once it lies down, get on it.

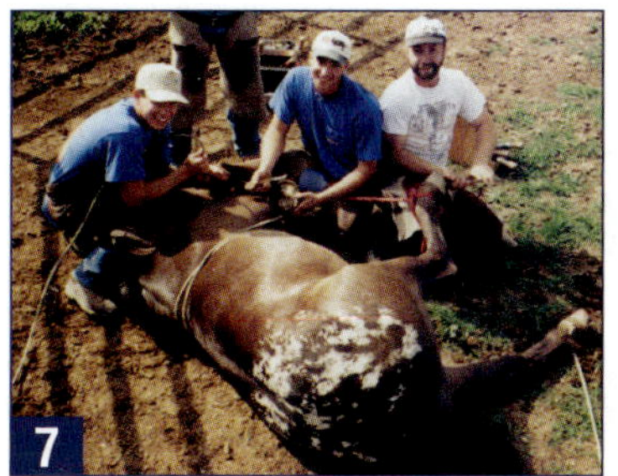

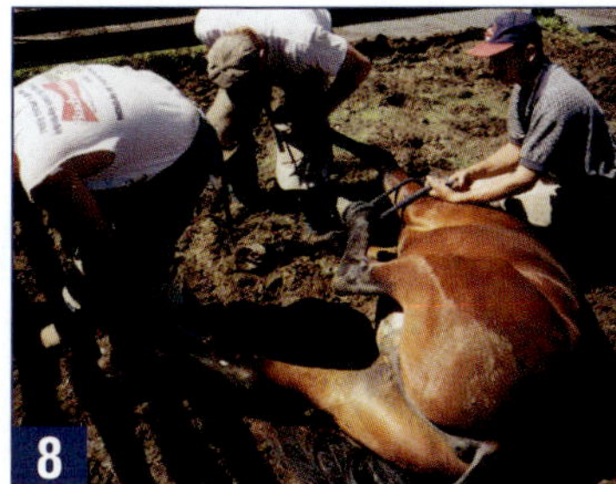

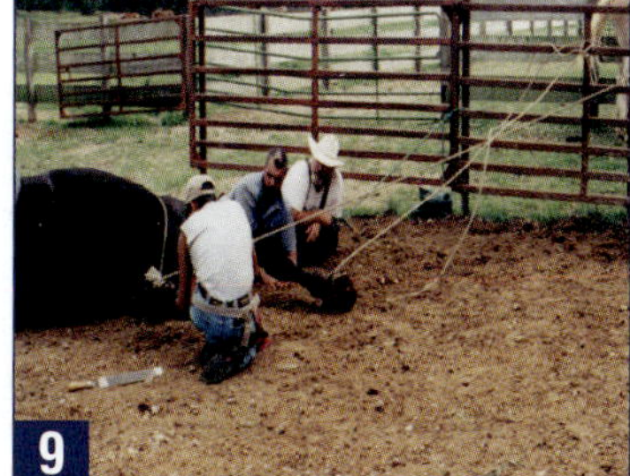

Tie the legs to posts and fences.

Bear in mind that a horse is not a car. A horse brings a personality and mentality to the situation that may put you in a position where force is the only option. Just try to get through it without hurting the horse or yourself.

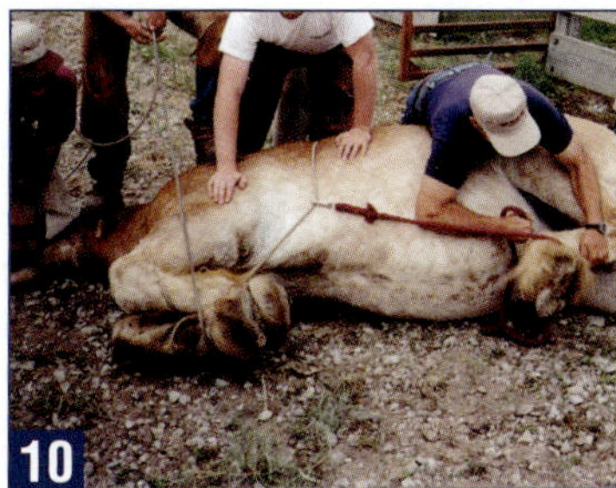

Tying the top hind leg forward.

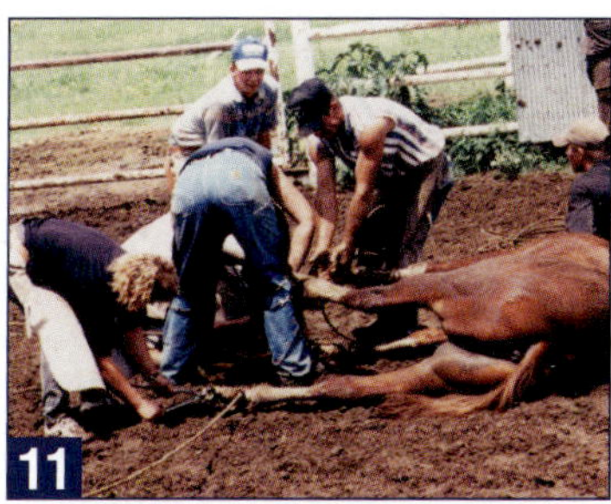

A dangerous situation with the legs not tied to anything.

I recommend getting several people involved when it comes to working on a bad horse. The school had an account with a lot of draft horses that were not much different than cattle, and the use of drugs was not an option. To trim these horses, we had to throw many of them on their side. Here are some pictures of this at a place we called the blood farm.

Begin by tying the horse long and low to a sturdy fence. Rope the front leg and pass the rope over the back and under the girth, bringing it in front of the rope that is around the foot. In **Figure 3**, you can see a horse that is ready to be thrown. When you pull, the foot with the rope on it is going to be lifted off the ground, and you will have the power to hold it since you are dallied around the horses' middle.

As the horse fights and you pull, the horse will tire and if all goes well, he will end up lying down **(Figures 4-5)**. Once the horse is down, you need your bravest soul on the head **(Figure 6)**. The other legs can be tied to other fences. You do not have to stretch the horse out here, you just need to tie the legs back far enough that it is safe. In fact, if you do stretch the horse out too much, it is more likely to fight **(Figures 7-9)**. In **Figure 10**, you can see that I am tying the top hind leg forward toward the belly. This is perhaps the most dangerous leg on a thrown horse, as it can sometimes hit the headman, and it can certainly get the trimmers. In **Figure 11**,

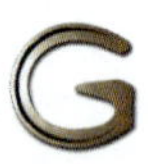

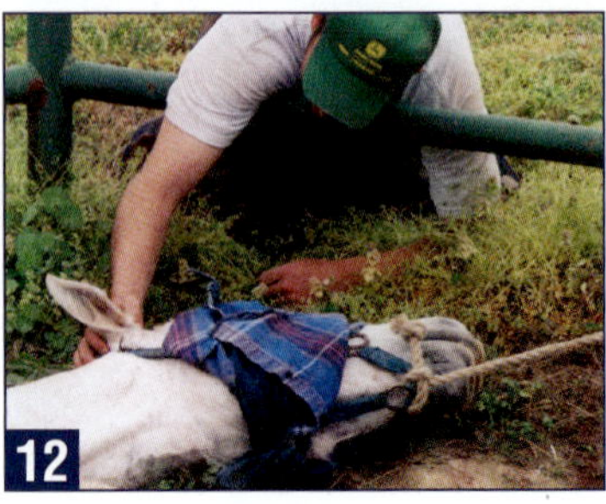
Covering the eyes.

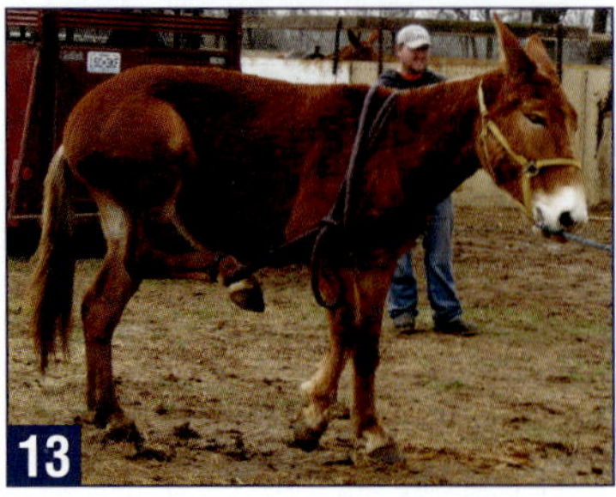
A mule in a tight scotch-hobble.

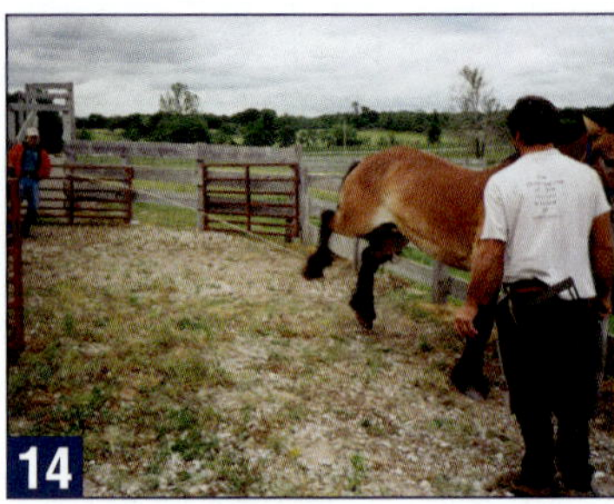
Tying a leg back.

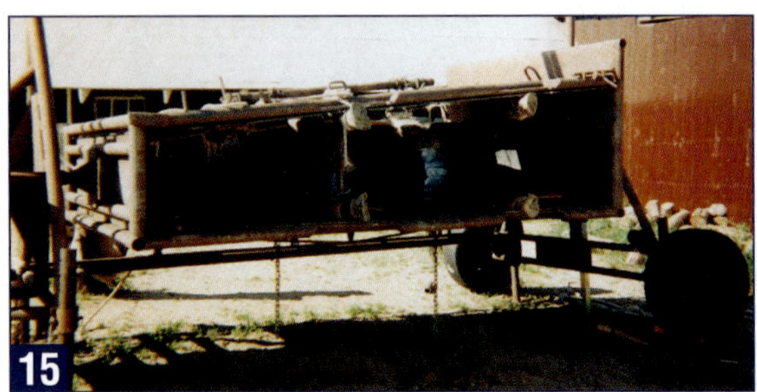

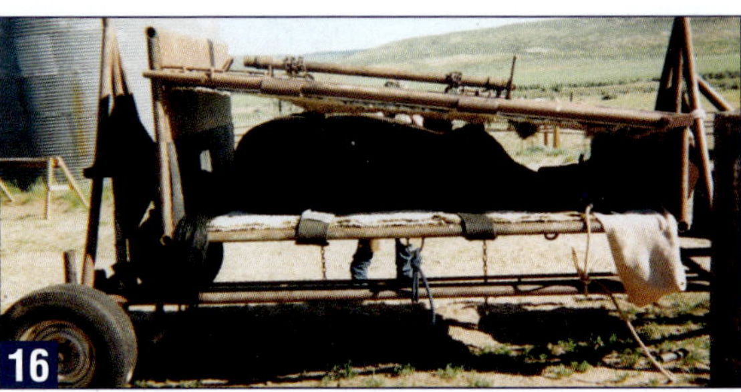
Horseshoeing turning stocks.

the top leg is not tied forward, and there are several people in harm's way. This is only done when the horse has completely quit fighting, and you are still risking bodily harm. Strike that, this should not be done at all — but we were young.

I also like to cover the horse's eyes, since this will sometimes make the horse calmer **(Figure 12)**. It is also safer for the horse's eye, and if we don't have a shirt or jacket, I will get the headman to put the edge of his shoeing apron over the eye.

Once the feet are trimmed, you can let the horse up. Try to remove as many ropes from the feet as you safely can before letting the horse up. You will find that a lot of horses hit the ground with a bad attitude but get up with a whole new lease on life. About 7 in 10 will be happy to stand still and let you work on their feet after they get up. This is a good thing, because it is all but impossible to do a good job on a horse that is tied down on its side. Finish the trim on the standing horse.

If you want to work on the horse standing but still restrained, there is a humble-hobble for the front feet and a scotch-hobble for the hind feet. Both of these can make it difficult to do a great job on a horse, but they definitely increase your safety.

To put on a humble-hobble, you can tie the front foot up as described for throwing a horse. There is also a commercially available humble-hobble that has buckles and rings in the correct spot for tying up a leg. The scotch-hobble can be made from about any rope, but I recommend cotton if you are going around the pastern.

Begin by making a loop around the neck. Pass the rope around the hind foot just above the pastern, and take the end of the rope back through the loop at the neck. Pull on the tail of the rope until the foot is just touching the ground. In **Figure 13**, you can see a mule that is trussed up in a scotch hobble. It is a little short for working on the foot, but I would rather too short than too long. Tying a leg back like the one in **Figure 14** has never worked that well for me, but I do know some farriers who swear by it.

Another option is to get a table like the one pictured. Here are some pictures a friend named Jim Rennie gave me of an operation that does a lot of horses on their side in a chute that can be spun. The horse is led in and secured, and the chute is twisted so that the horse's feet are safely exposed for shoeing. This is about as humane a way to do bad horses without drugs or training as you can get. When you come across some of these untrained animals, you may decide to build one of

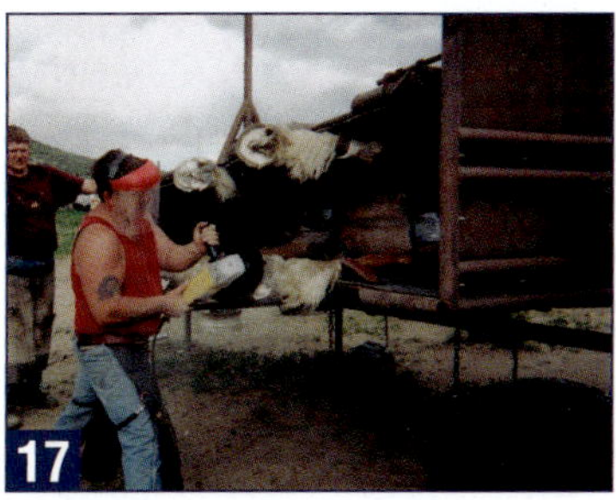

Trimming feet with a 7-inch grinder.

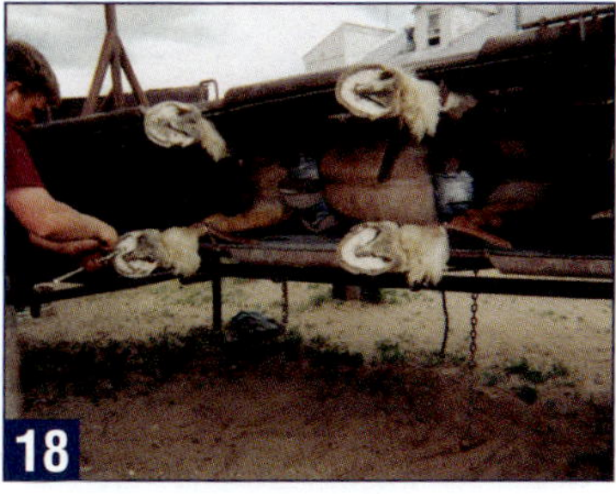

Working on the feet of a horse in the turning stocks.

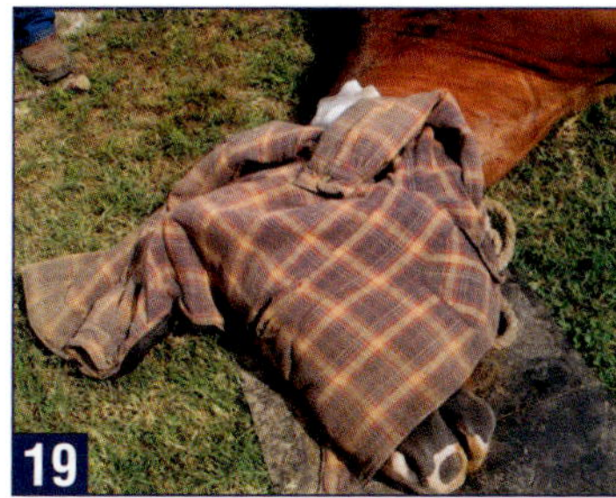

A horse that has been sedated.

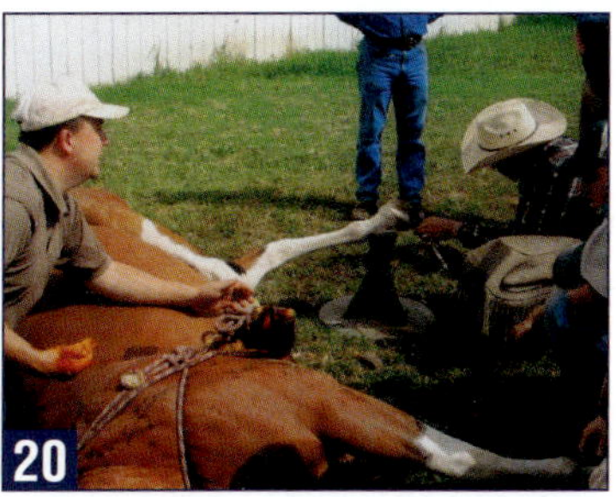

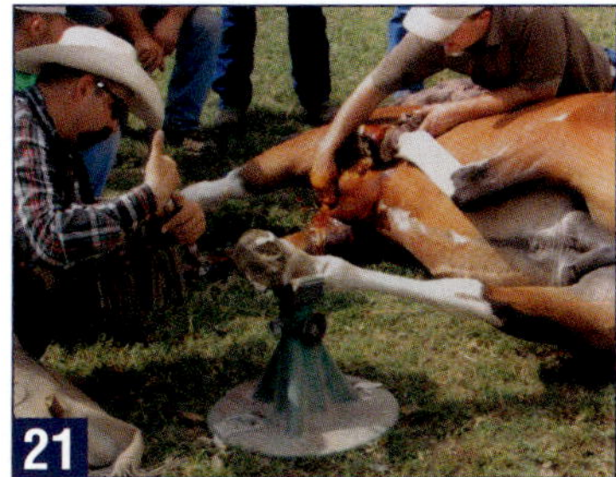

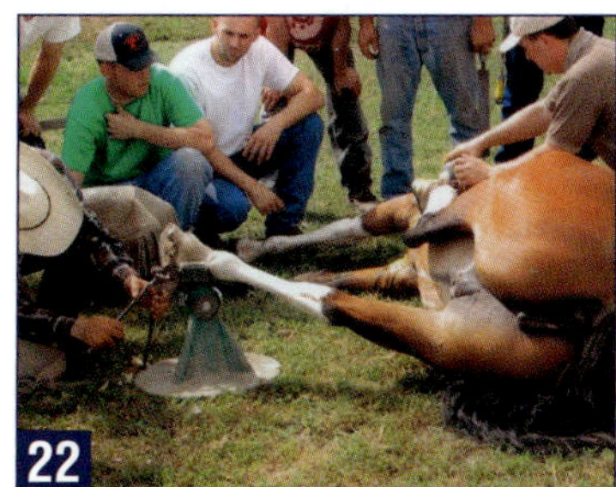

Working with a veterinarian on a sedated horse.

these chutes for yourself (**Figures 15-18**).

The next method is to use drugs. We call this "chemical training." In the old days (I can't believe that I have been around long enough to say that), the drugs that we had to use were pretty unpredictable. There were some problems with these where a horse could fire a kick at you out of the blue, and they also made a horse really heavy to work on. Another thing to worry about was the potential for a problem called penile paralysis in geldings where the penis will stay extended and not retract into the sheath. When that happens, a horse has to be put down.

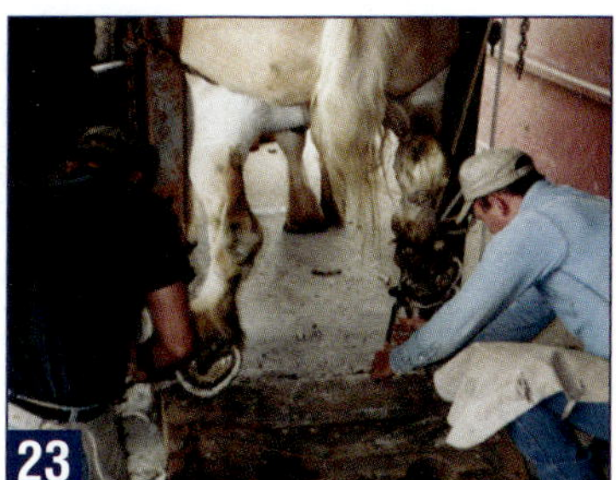

Both feet are up, both feet get trimmed.

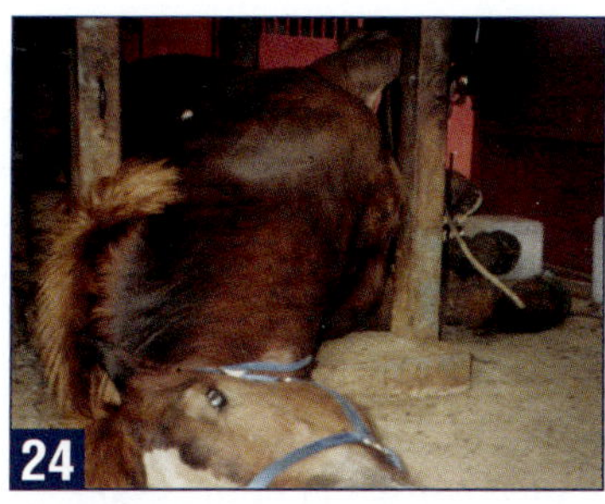

A horse on its side in the stocks.

Along came some new drugs. The horses were steadier and lighter to work on, and you had a good 45 minutes most of the time. If a horse is in pain, have the veterinarian add some pain medication to the tranquilizer, and you have a great cocktail. The main problem is the cost, but you will find that to be a problem if you get a broken leg as well.

With certain horses, it is best to have a vet come out and lay the horse down for you. In **Figures 19-22**, the work that had to be done to the feet was so extensive that the horse had to be sedated before it could be worked on. This is the safest way to work on any horse.

Finally, there are stocks that you can put a horse in. Like working on a thrown horse, it can be very difficult to do a great job in stocks. Also, you need to be certain that the stocks are well designed to prevent injury to yourself or the horse. In **Figure 23**, you can see a draft that has lifted both legs as he sat on the chain on the back of the stocks. **Figure 24** shows a draft that went down in the stocks. Unfortunately, with this pair of stocks and the

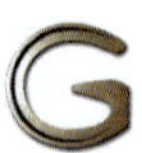

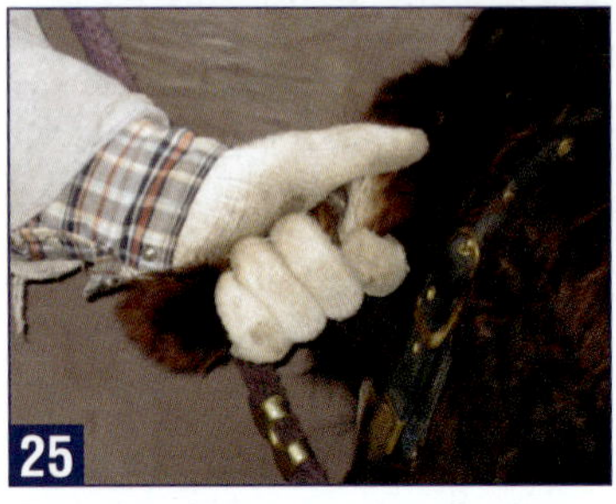
Twisting the ear on a donkey.

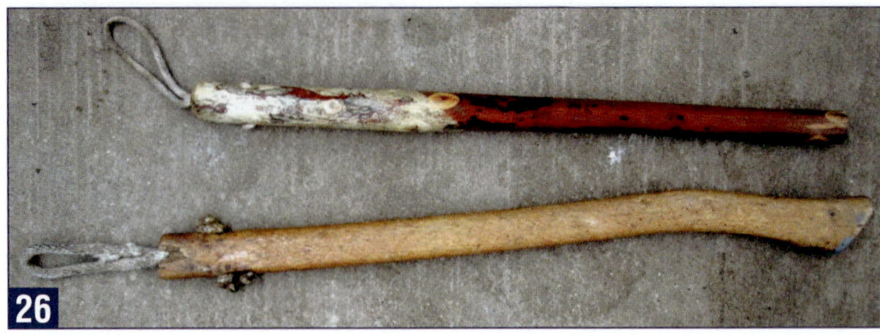
Twitches.

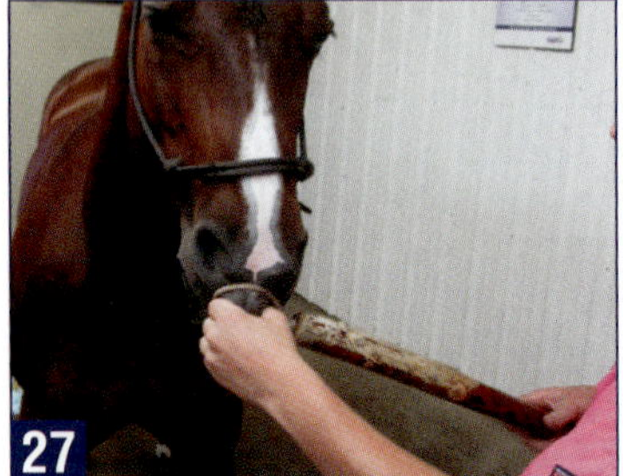
Putting a twitch on the nose.

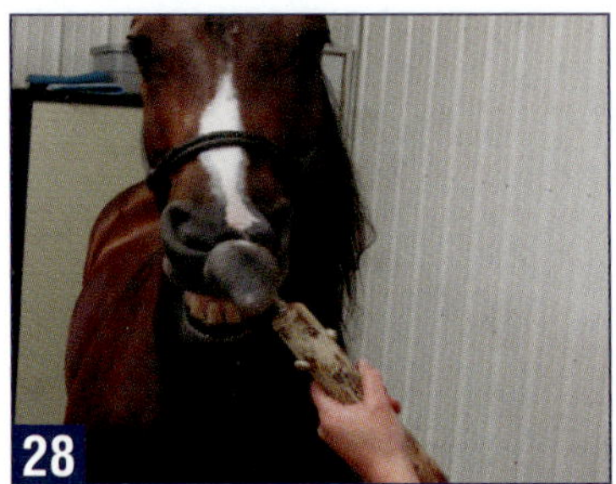
Twisting the twitch.

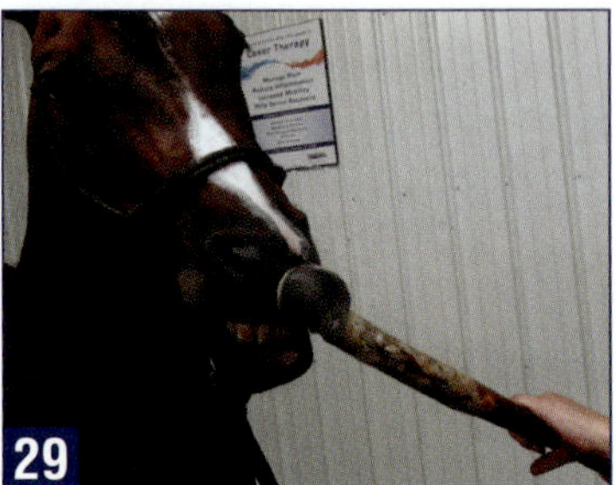
The twitch applied.

animals we had to do in them, about 1 in 5 would throw itself on its side. Stocks are my least favorite method to use for shoeing a bad horse.

There are a variety of twitches and similar items that can be applied to the ears and nose. I prefer to twist the ear by hand when necessary **(Figure 25)** and tongs can be used as a universal twitch on the upper lip. The most common twitch is made from a piece of wood with strong, thin rope at the end. The upper lip is placed in the rope, and the wooden handle is turned, causing the rope to tighten on the lip. You can see a couple of twitches in **Figure 26**, and how they are used in **Figures 27-29**.

There will be times in your career where a good barn full of nice horses comes with one or two bad horses. Perhaps you will come across one with a brand on its neck like the horse in **Figure 30**. If the freeze branded number has a US in front of it, it is a captured Mustang. Yeah, you shouldn't have to do bad horses and all that, but let's be honest. It is a part of surviving in this business, and you will be better off learning how to deal with a crazy horse than spending all your time avoiding them.

So here are the basics of working on a bad horse without using drugs or restraint techniques.

Begin on the hind feet. Tie the horse short and approach the horse slowly and confidently. To get the horse tied short, you might want to pass the lead rope back through the halter. This allows you to use the leverage of a pulley system to shorten the lead rope **(Figure 31)**. Touch the horse on the shoulder **(Figure 32)** and move to the middle of the ribcage, placing your inside hand over the horse's back. Stay close to the horse, and place some of your weight on your inside arm **(Figure 33)**. This is your safety spot. The horse can't bite you from the front or kick you from the hind.

With your outside hand, move slowly down the rump towards the hock. If the horse gets nervous or violent, try to stay close, and move your hand back up the limb to the last point that the horse was comfortable. You will continue to push the limits of what this horse will allow. Each time the horse gets nervous, simply try to go back to the last spot that the horse was comfortable. We refer to this method as "advance and retreat."

You can see that the young horse in this series is quite nervous and does not appreciate me trying to get its leg up **(Figure 34)**. As I try to get the hind foot up, the horse is squatting and turning towards

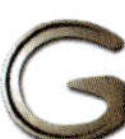

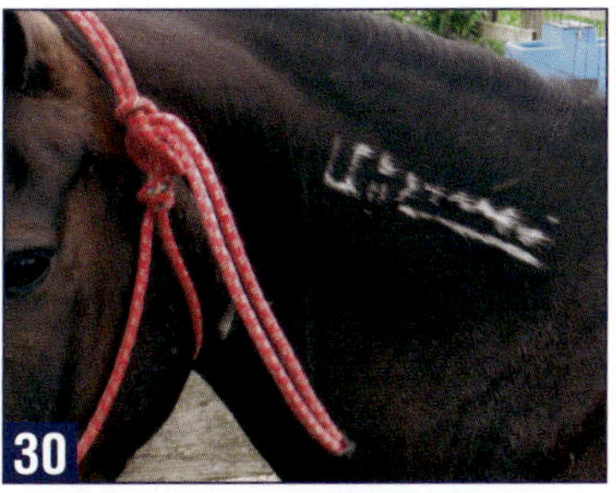
30
Freeze brand starting in US on the neck of a Mustang.

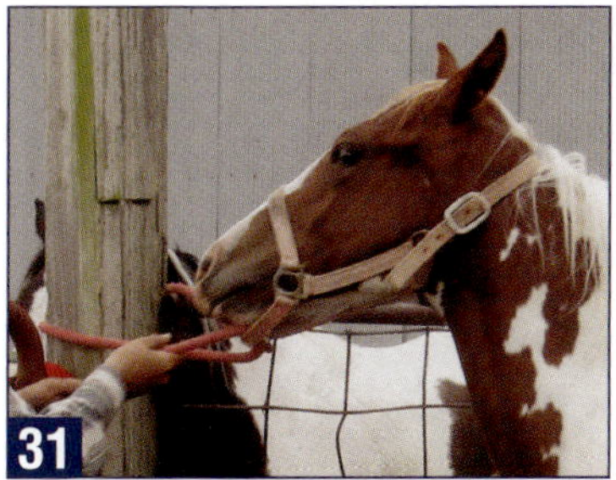
31
Tying the head short.

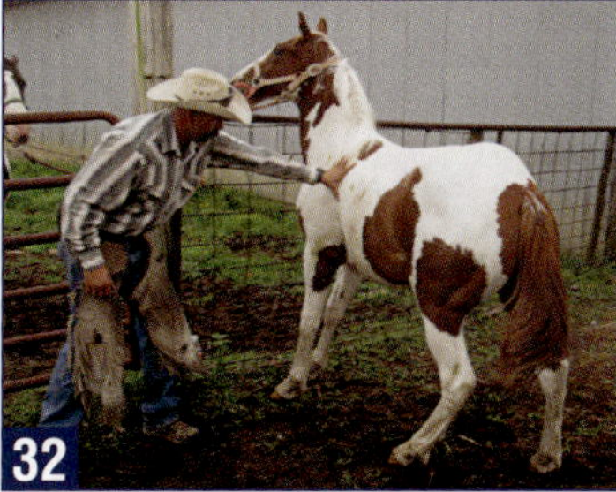
32
Approaching the shoulder of a nervous horse.

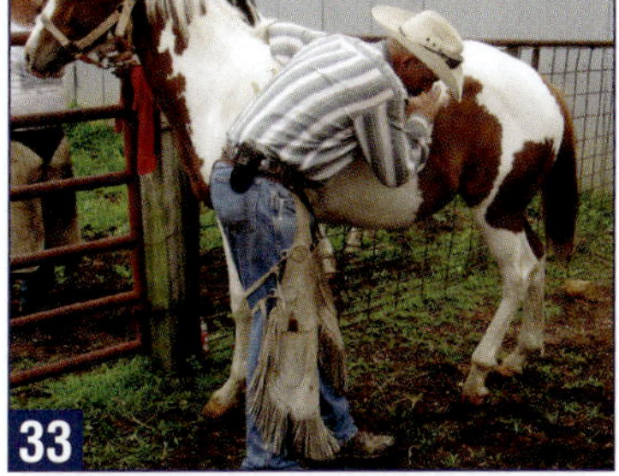
33
Safe position on the side of the horse.

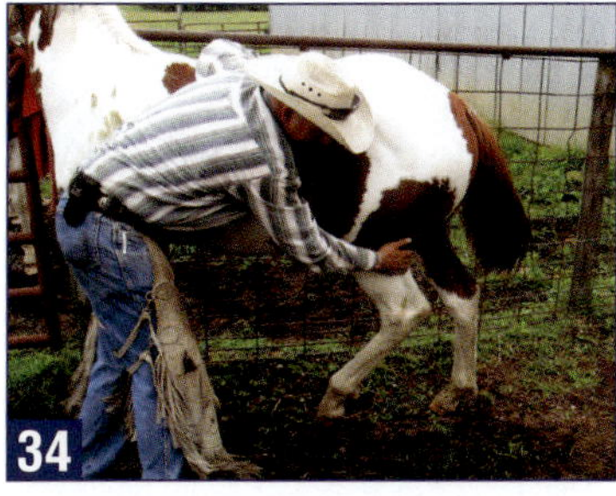
34
Reaching for the cannon bone.

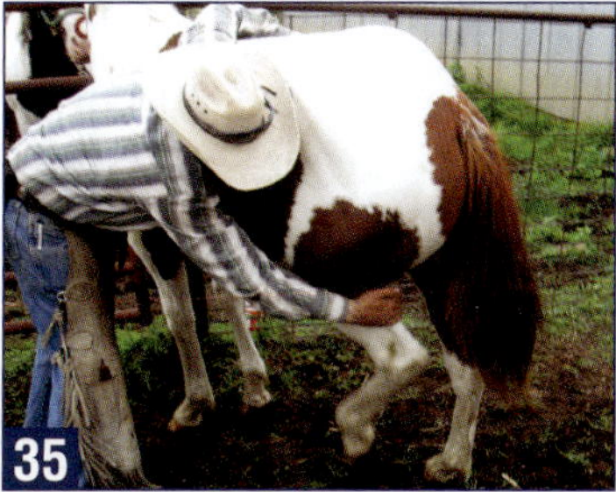
35
Horse squatting and leaning towards me.

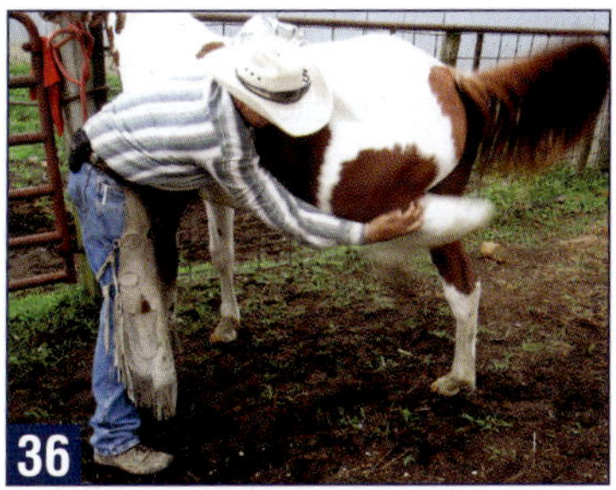
36
Cocking the leg to kick.

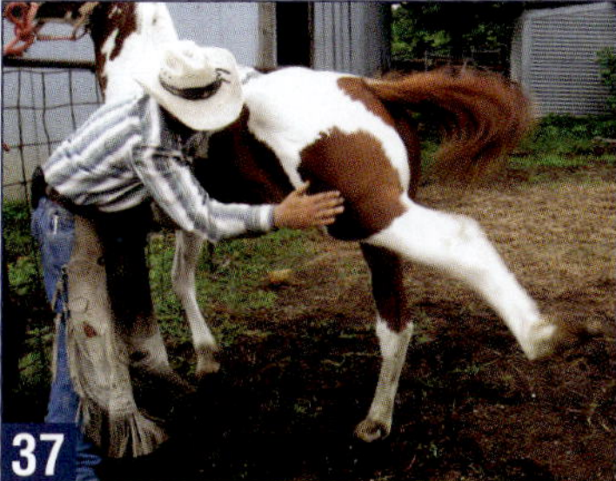
37
Sending a kick my way, I am safe.

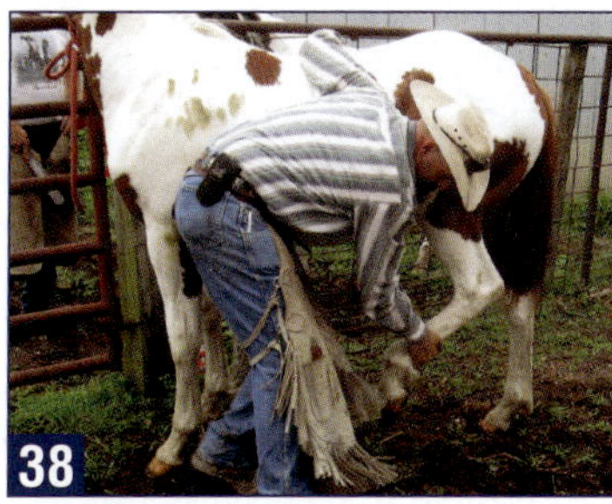
38
Getting the cannon bone.

me **(Figure 35)**, a sure sign that it will kick when the opportunity is available **(Figure 36-37)**.

If you get to where you can place your hand below the hock, try to pull gently on the cannon bone as you move the leg toward the horse's belly **(Figure 38)**. When the horse relaxes, move your inside arm down to grab the toe as in **Figure 39**. Allow the horse to settle and balance, and then grab the toe with your outside hand and reach around the hock for the foot with your inside hand **(Figure 40)**. Place your leg against the fetlock and move the foot back to work on **(Figure 41)**.

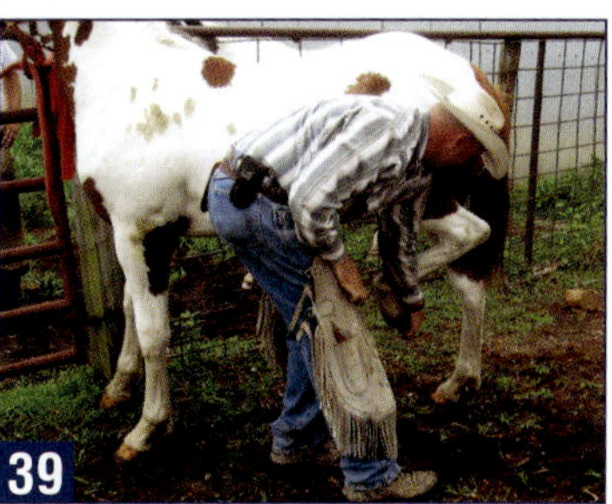
39
Grabbing the toe with my inside hand.

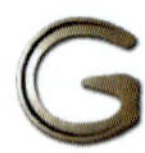

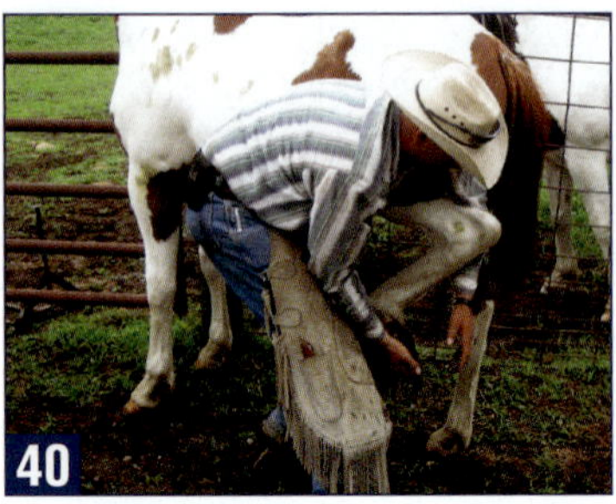

Changing hands while I reach around the hock.

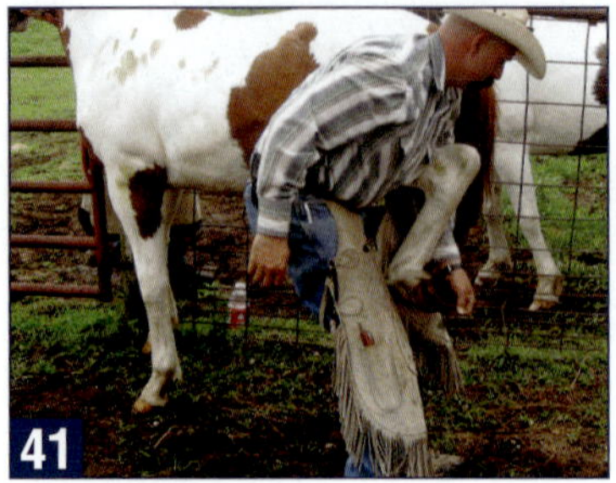

Pulling the foot back.

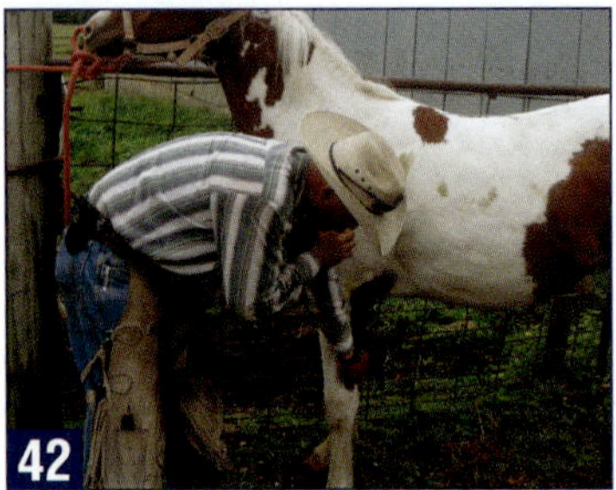

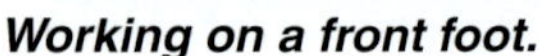

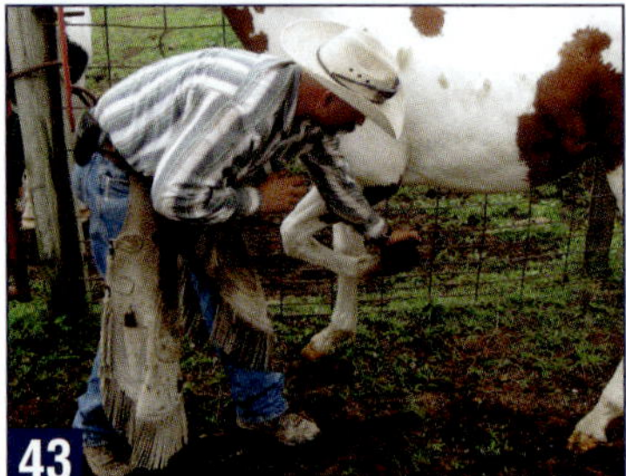

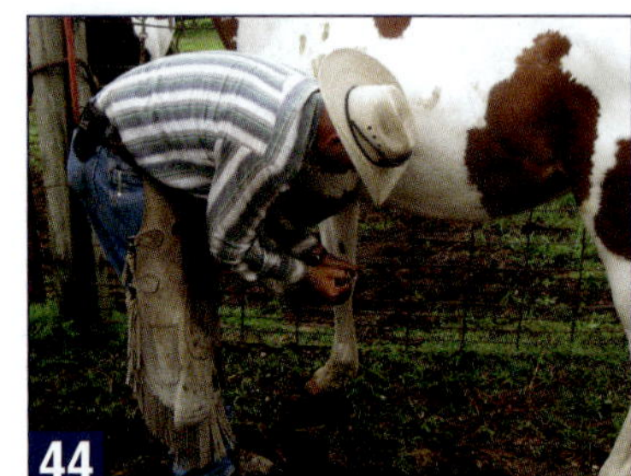

Working on a front foot.

It is easier to win the battle on the hind feet than it is on the fronts. That is why we always try to do the hind feet first on a bad horse. You can see in **Figure 42-44** that the horse has a little different view of things as I work on the front feet after conquering the hinds.

Keep working with the horse. It is important to maintain your composure. Do not lose your temper. I know this is a hard one, and every one of us has our moments when it is just too much, and we get mad at the horse. Try and remember that you should never get mad at a horse for being a horse. That is how God made them, and if you are going to work on and with them, you will have to accept it. Getting mad is apt to get you or the horse hurt, and later on you may regret it, either way.

If you are unable to get the leg up after working patiently with the horse, it is time to use a method that is one of the best horse-handling tools I have ever used.

Now this is about to sound like a commercial, and I guess it kind of is, but this is a tool that absolutely changed how we did things in about 2002.

This fellow named Rick Wheat patented an iron halter that he called the Noavel Headstall. It is like a Bosal made with a steel nosepiece. You can see Rick using it on a 3-year-old stud horse at a clinic in **Figure 45**. Like most things made to train horses, if abused, it can be way too much. However, if handled correctly, this device will make even some of the worst horses agreeable. For those of you that have no horse experience, you should get some videos or go to some clinics about the Noavel. If you use one without any training, try to remember that less is more when you bump the horse.

The Noavel works on the principle of instant pressure, instant release. Anytime you are around a horse, you are training it, for better or worse. If a horse pulls slightly when you pick up the leg and is then rewarded by getting the leg back, you have just trained the horse to get away from you by pulling on its leg. However, if the horse is punished for that action in a humane and just manner, that horse will learn that pulling on the leg creates a negative reaction instead of a positive reaction. This is the basic premise for most horse training, and the Noavel Headstall can be used to make it quick, easy and humane.

Begin by putting the Noavel on the horse. The noseband has an intentional wave in it, and it is

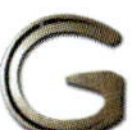

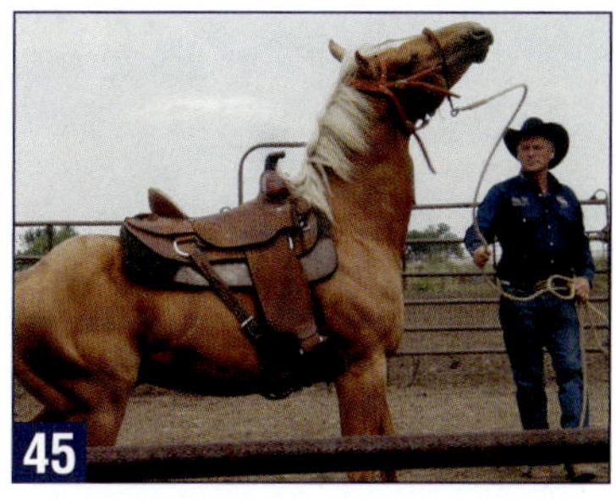
45
Rick Wheat, inventor and patent holder of the Noavel Headstall.

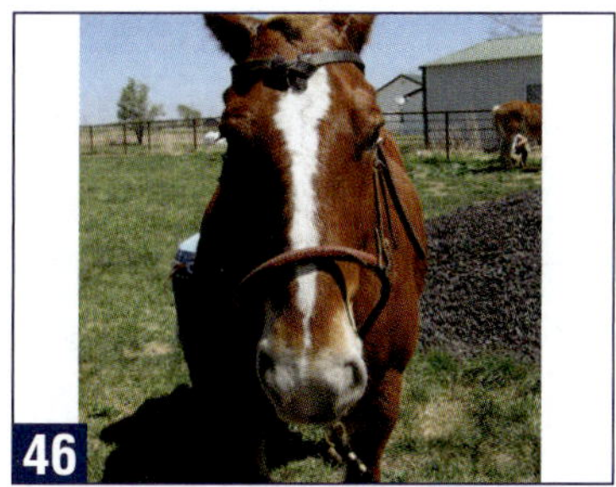
46
Front view of a Noavel on a horse.

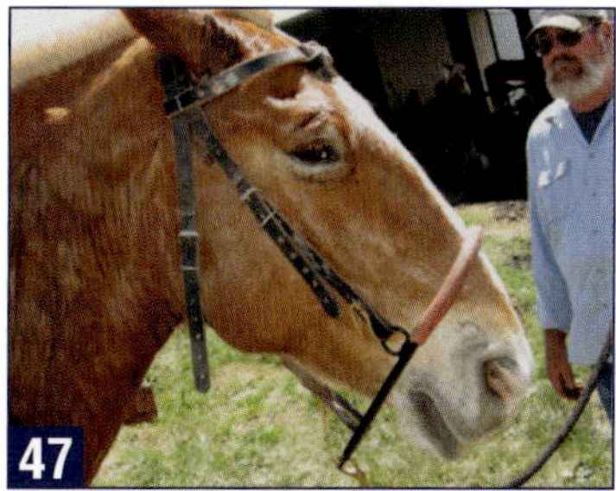
47
Side view of the Noavel on a horse.

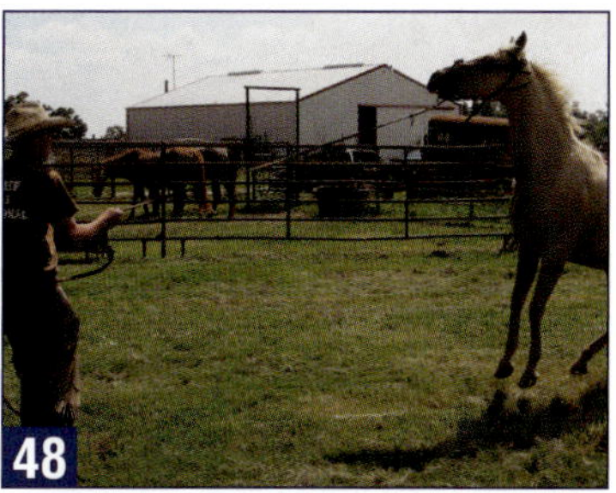
48
Cody working with a young horse.

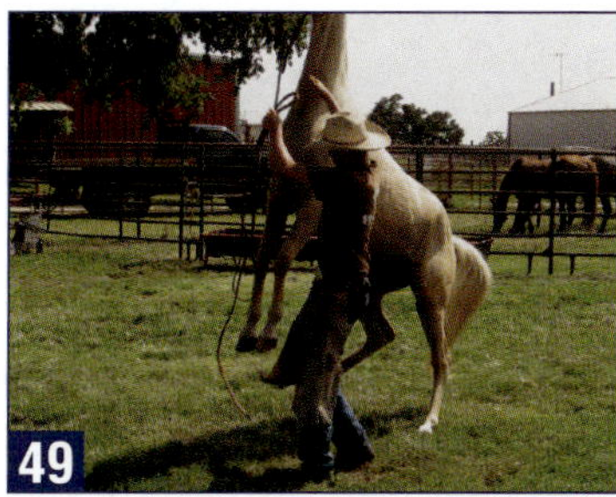
49
The horse reared to fight.

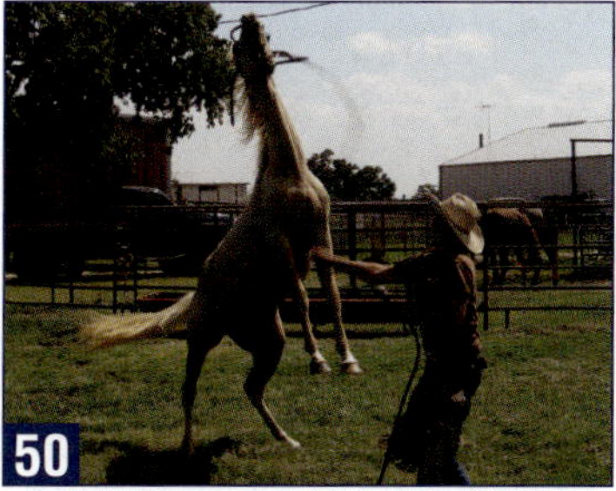
50
Cody was able to bump the horse while it was in the air.

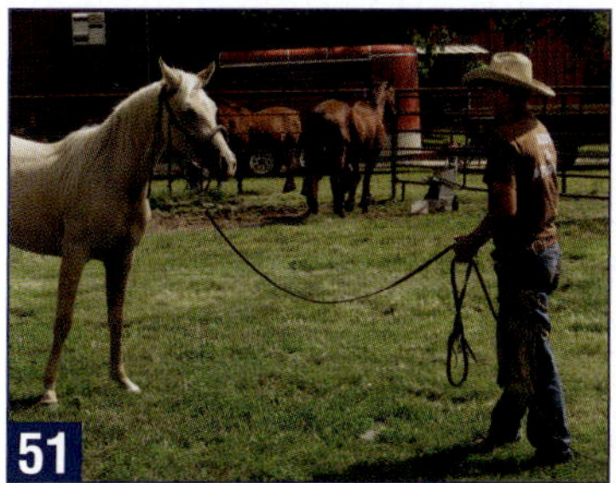
51
Bringing the horse around.

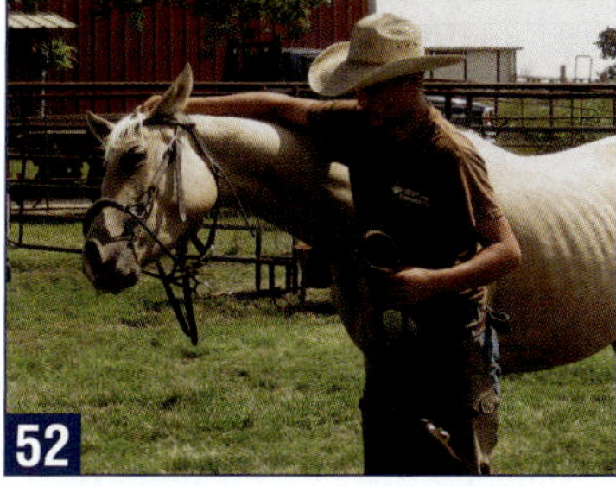
52
Working behind the left ear.

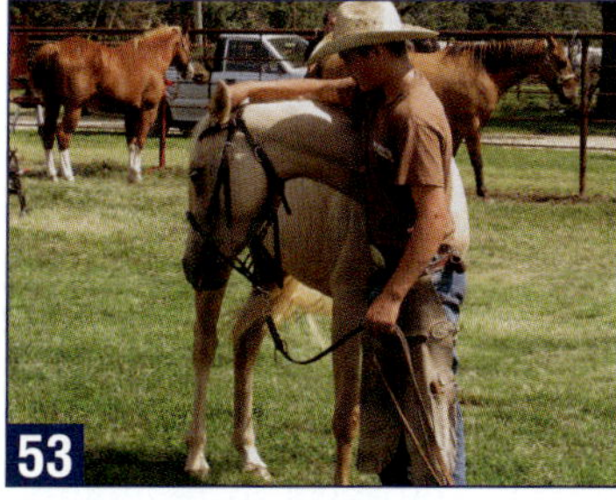
53
Staying with the ear.

designed to fit a little bit low and loose. The bar on the bottom of the noseband should contact the bone behind the soft part of the chin when it is pulled on. I try to put it so that the band is even with the first molars. This can be determined by feeling the ridges that are on the side of a horse's head **(Figure 46-47)**.

Teach the horse something simple first. Backing up is a good choice. Bump the horse lightly as you ask for a back. Get slightly more aggressive as you continue to ask for the back. The instant that one foot moves just a little bit rearward, quit bumping. The next time the horse should back with less effort on your part. Soon, the horse will be backing simply because you rattled the clip attached to the lead rope.

In **Figure 48-56**, you can see a series with Cody working with a young horse that he is holding for students to shoe. The horse is unruly and wants to fight. You can see that he is able to punish the horse while it is in the air fighting him, and finally he gets the horse to lower its head. With the head down and the horse relaxed, the horse can be shod without injury to itself, the holder, or the farrier.

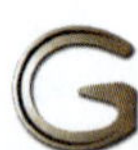

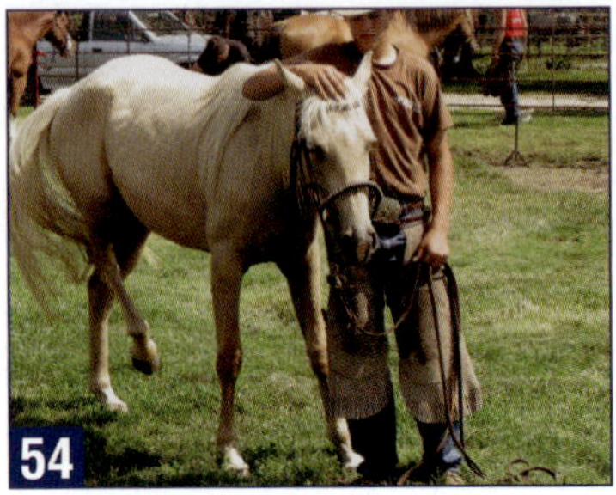

Waiting for the head to drop.

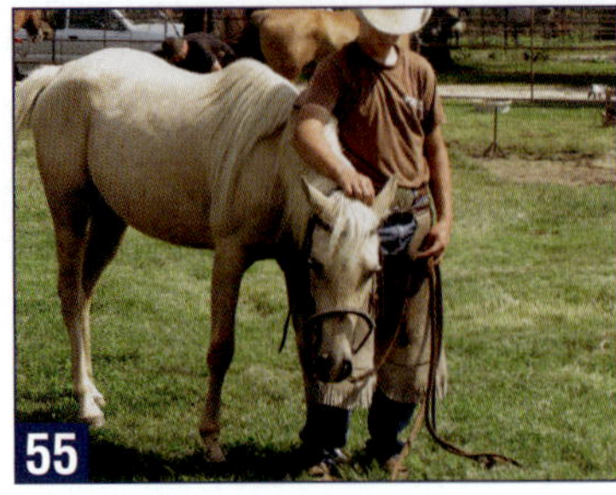

Head goes down.

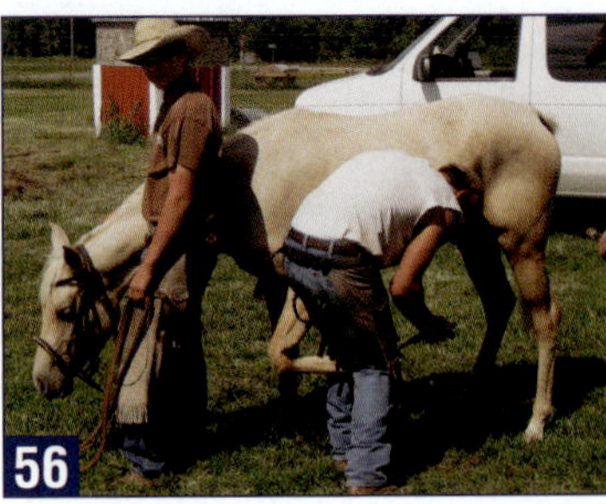

Calm and quite horse being shod by students.

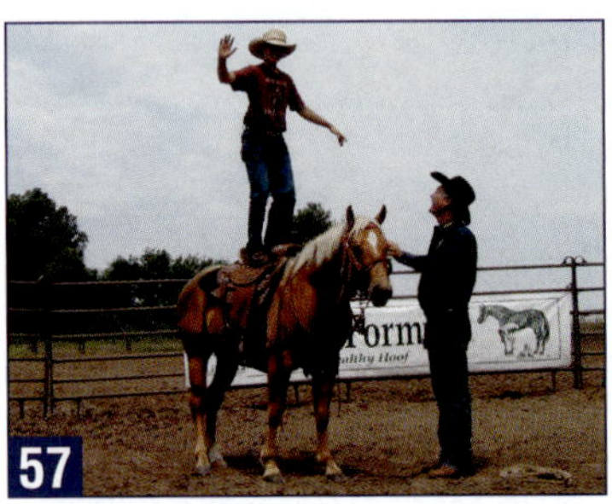

Cody standing on the young horse that Rick Wheat worked on.

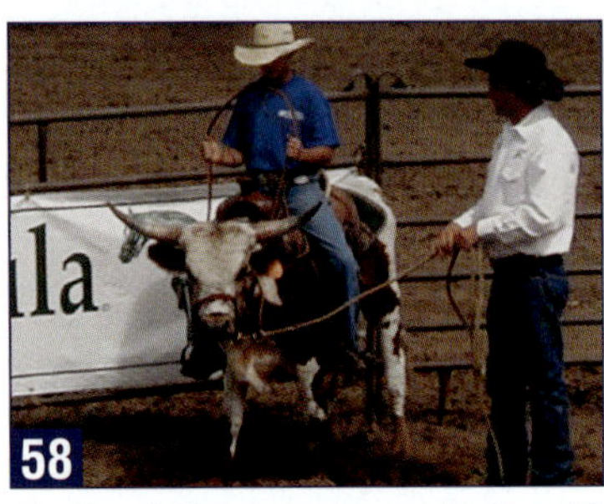

Cody riding a young bull with the Noavel Headstall.

The Noavel actually brings a horse down. Twitches, lip-chains, beatings, and other methods that work along those lines elevate a horse. They seem to make the horse nervous, angry, and ready for a fight. With the Noavel, a horse will lower its head and become accepting of what you are trying to get done. If I were guessing, I would say it does this because the horse feels comfortable knowing what it will and will not get in trouble for. This means you have to be competent at asking for the right thing in the right way at the right time. Learning this comes primarily from competent instruction and experience. In **Figure 57**, you can see that young stud that Rick started at the clinic. Cody is standing on him within a matter of minutes of Rick working with him. In **Figure 58**, Cody is riding a young bucking bull with the Noavel.

Having a good holder is essential when you are shoeing unruly animals. The holder actually has to have as much, if not more, horsemanship than the farrier. As a general rule (and there are not that many of these) the holder should stay on the same side of the horse that the shoer is working on. The reason is this: If the horse decides to charge forward, the horse will go around the holder on the side that he is being held from. If the shoer is on the opposite side, the horse will be pushed into the farrier and potentially run the farrier over.

When I am holding a Noavel on a bad horse, there is one basic rule that I make the horse understand as soon as I can. That rule is: The horse cannot move its feet for any reason without being asked. It's a pretty simple and straightforward rule. If you don't let the horse move its feet, it can't be too bad.

There are several other restraint/training methods that are common and useful. The ones mentioned are the ones I have used and like, so I will limit this text to those. Like most things with shoeing horses, there is more than one approach to getting the job done. As long as the final result is a sound horse, a sound holder, a sound farrier, and the barn not looking like a biker bar after a brawl, you can't argue with it too much.

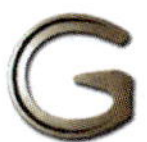

Chapter

19 EQUINE PSYCHOLOGY

It is important for the farrier to have an idea about the way that horses think and respond. Since farriers will have to handle and deal with many different horses in many different situations over the course of a day, the better they are able to read the horse, the safer everyone will stay.

One of the first considerations is that a horse is a prey animal that eats vegetation. Some of the features that have helped the horse survive and prosper are common to prey animals. Several of these traits are:

- The ability to sleep standing, requiring about 2.5 hours of sleep out of 24 hours, and attaining sleep in short naps. A horse needs to lie down to enter deep sleep and will do so if able every few days.
- Long nose allows the animal to graze with nose on the ground, but eyes above the grass.
- Lives in herds. Horses are highly social creatures that live in a linear dominance society.
- Young are able to stand and run almost immediately after birth.
- Wide and broad range of vision, except for directly behind. Monocular.
- Flight instinct, but able to bite, paw, kick, and run over predators when needed.
- Able to cover a lot of ground quickly.
- Very attentive to the surroundings.
- Curious about non-threatening objects.
- Well-adapted instinct to read the body language of humans.

Many of these traits are in sharp contrast to meat-eating predators, which humans just happen to be. We can live with or without large groups of people. Predators don't sleep standing. They also have good depth perception but a relatively small range of vision compared to the horse. However, two eyes that can focus on the same object all the time is handy for hunting.

The newborn of predators require a lot of care,

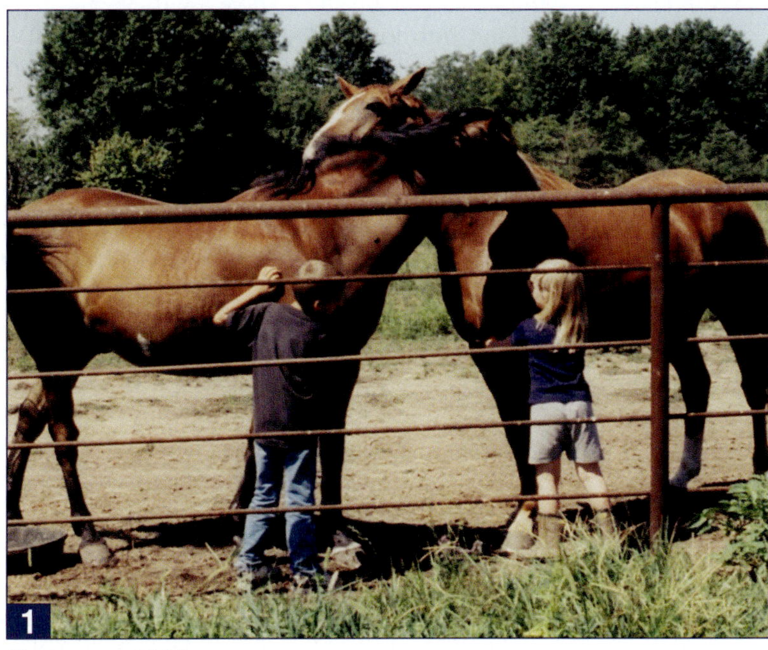

1

Horses and kids.

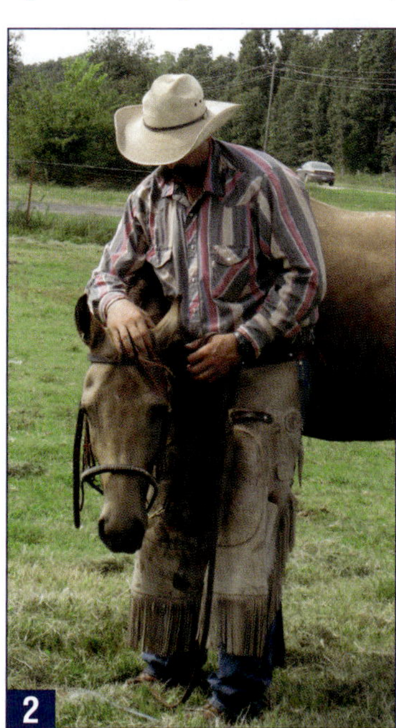

2

A horse lowering its head as it understands its place in the pecking order.

attention, and safety to reach maturity. Predators are less likely to flee as a first response, and most prey animals have pretty good speed compared to predators.

Horses are on the human menu, but we are not on theirs. On top of that, we do not naturally read body language of other species nearly as well as a horse does. All of this puts us in natural opposition to the horse, so we have to be able to adapt, understand, react, and convey appropriate signals when dealing with horses.

Since the horse is an animal that wants to flee when there is danger, you can imagine what it must be like for one to have a halter on, be tied to a post, and be surrounded by predators. The fact that the horse has become such a good friend of humans is quite remarkable. Horses can read your intentions quite well, even when you are trying to put up a front to block them from knowing. Just take the lead rope of an aggressive horse from a competent handler and hand it to someone who is afraid of horses. You can watch the change come over the horse immediately. That is something that you will see hundreds of times in your career with customers that are in over their heads, and it is up to you to control that situation.

In the wild, feral and wild horses live in groups that have a distinct pecking order. This is a matriarchal society with a boss or lead mare, several other mares, young horses, and a stallion. The boss mare is actually the one in charge and leads the herd wherever they go. She will eat the best grass as well as be the first to take a drink. To pass her on the trail would be unthinkable for a young horse that is not ready to fight for her job. With that in mind, you should never let a horse pass you when you are trying to lead it. Doing so firmly establishes in that horse's mind that you are below it in the pecking order.

The lead stallion remains on the outside of the herd to defend against predators as well as prevent any incoming young stallion that would like to challenge for the right to be the herd stallion. Although he is the top male in the herd, he still falls under the boss mare in the hierarchy.

Horses naturally form these herds, and this is where horses are comfortable; knowing exactly where they stand in the pecking order as well as where everyone else stands. When they are separated from other horses or placed in frightening situations, they are under stress and may end up being dangerous if the handler does not know how to act in the situation.

Another thing that happens in the wild is that horses will use body language to threaten another horse and follow up with violence to enforce that threat. What this means is that a horse may bare its teeth and pull its ears back at another horse to get its way. If the other horse does as the threatening horse wishes, then there is no confrontation. In the case that the threatened horse decides to put up a fight, then there is a battle that will include pawing, biting, pushing, and kicking. At the end of the battle, the hierarchy is more defined as the victor ends up one rank over the loser.

In a human–horse situation, if the horse acts threatening to the human and the human runs in fright, that horse will feel that it is above that human in the pecking order. For a farrier, that is a dangerous thing to have happen. Every time you approach that horse when it does not want you to, there is a good potential that it will try to run you off. You can end up badly hurt in such a situation.

We use a patented iron halter called the Noavel Headstall. You can read all about it in Chapter #18 on horsemanship. No matter what your method of gaining a higher spot on the pecking order, make certain that you are able to do so.

Handling horses does not require brutality, cruelty, or violence. You can look at a horse and see if it is scared, mad, hurt, tired, curious, mean, or in any other state, and then act to make the horse comfortable, all the while maintaining your spot in the pecking order. Horses will learn to trust you if you are consistent in your actions. This means that you correct a horse only when it is needed, and you refrain from correcting a horse that is doing well. Every time that you handle a horse, you are training that horse. For good or bad is up to you.

Horse psychology is really all about horse sense. No one is born knowing how to handle and act around horses. It is a learned behavior, and like shoeing, you can learn it, too. Try to spend time with a knowledgeable horseman that does not have to use violence for everything that he does with a horse. Violence is a tool, but as such, it has a specific use. Kindness, consistency, body language, and demeanor are also tools that can be used to effectively work around horses and those are the ones that your customers will appreciate.

Section

7

General Principles of Farriery

Chapter 20: Good Shoeing 210

Chapter 21: Trimming Considerations.................... 215

Chapter 22: Trimming a Hoof.................................. 218

Chapter 23: Mediolateral Balance.......................... 229

Chapter 24: Normal Shoeing on Normal Feet 233

Chapter 25: Measuring Feet for Handmades 236

Chapter 26: Shoe Selection 239

Chapter 27: Shoe Modifications 245

Chapter 28: Clip Fitting 258

Chapter 29: Hot Fitting 262

Chapter 30: Nailing... 266

Chapter 31: Clinching 101 271

"7 Some trust in chariots and some in horses,
but we trust in the name of the LORD our God."

—Psalm 20:7

—New International Version

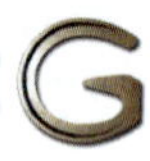

Chapter
20 GOOD SHOEING

Good, sound shoeing is something that I believe just about everyone who has ever done the job wants to achieve. A lot of incompetent shoeing occurs, but I don't think anyone gets up in the morning and says to themselves, "I wonder just how bad I can be today?" Some folks lack the work ethic to get to the highest level, and a lot of people are led astray by a lack of knowledge and the availability of gimmicks and product. To me, the best shoeing that can be done is simple, straightforward, traditional shoeing that honors some time-tested principles of straight tubular horn and symmetry. There will always be exceptions, and if you're experienced and are reading this, you've probably had many of them just pass through your memory, but the sound, normal horse should be shod with common sense and a straightforward approach.

There are very few absolutes in farriery — a fact that makes it hard to teach and harder to learn. With some trades, there are enough absolutes that a person can learn to be competent through pure memorization. But farriers must develop the skills to see what the foot should look like, compare it to what they have to work with, apply a shoe that will last till the next shoeing, and set the foot up so that it is in good shape at the next shoeing. That is a lot to know about, and the only way to get there is time and perserverance. In this chapter, I want to show some pictures of good shoeing done on sound feet by experienced craftsmen. The closer you can get your work to look like the photos in this chapter, the better farrier you will become.

Anytime that you are presenting work to farriers, draw or arrange the picture so that the toe of the horseshoe is up and the heels are down. This is the position that the horseshoer is most accustomed to seeing a foot from. When doing a presentation for horse owners, draw and arrange the pictures so that the heels are up and the toe is down.

This is just a picture chapter that is going to have the work of many farriers around the world. Some is Cody's, some are from Calgary, some from students, some from me, and some from certifications around the world. I am not going to label any of it, just put it in here for your study and enjoyment. This is good, basic, solid, and traditional work. There is shoeing in here for you to emulate. As you study these photos, you will see that none of them is perfect. There will be minor imperfections in every job you will ever do or see. However, there is some very good work here to give you a visual goal of what would constitute good horseshoeing.

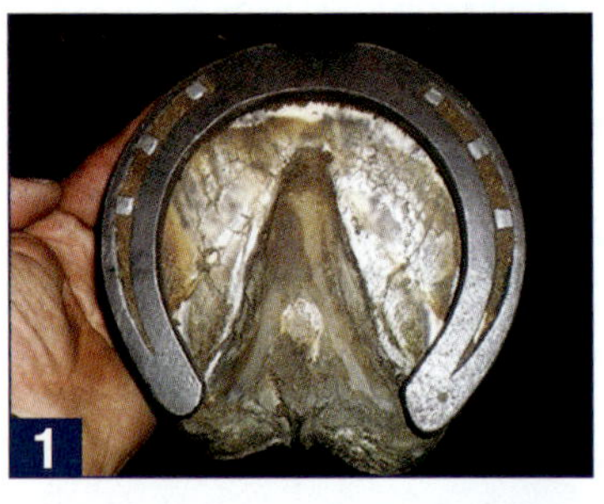

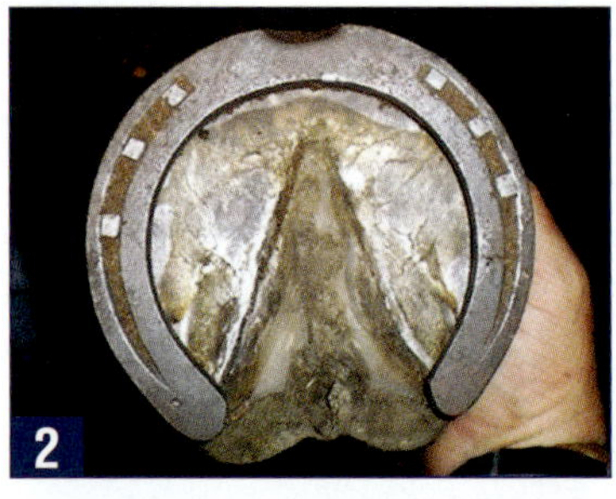

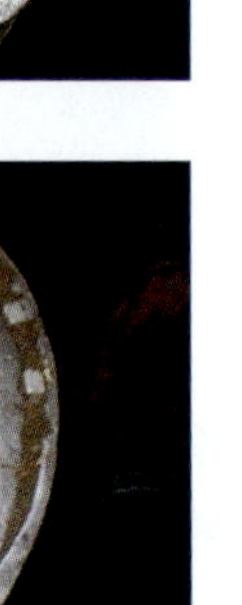

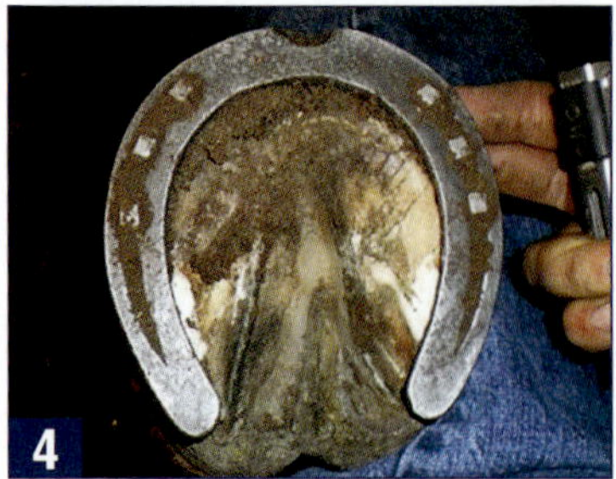

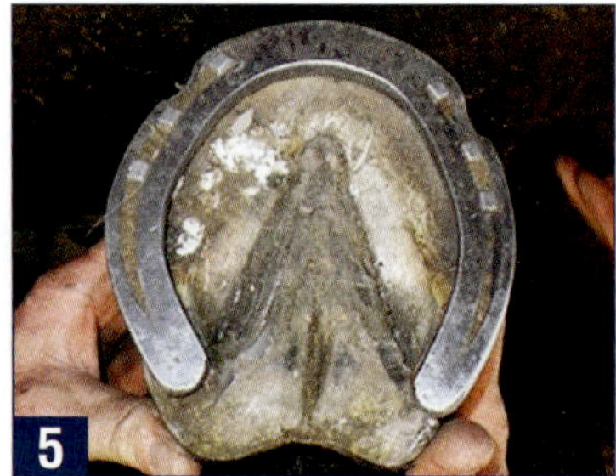

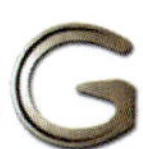

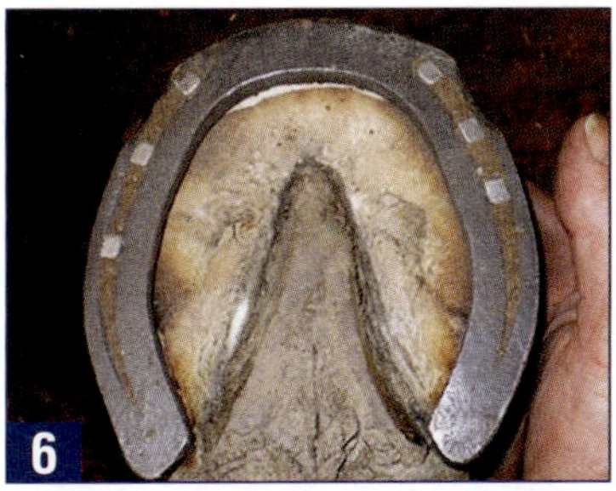

6

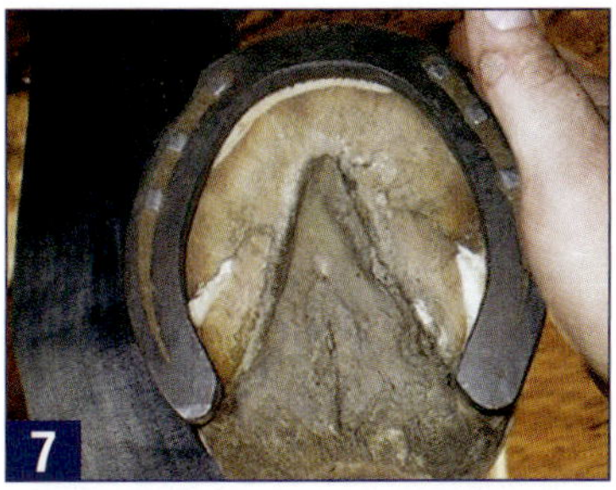

7

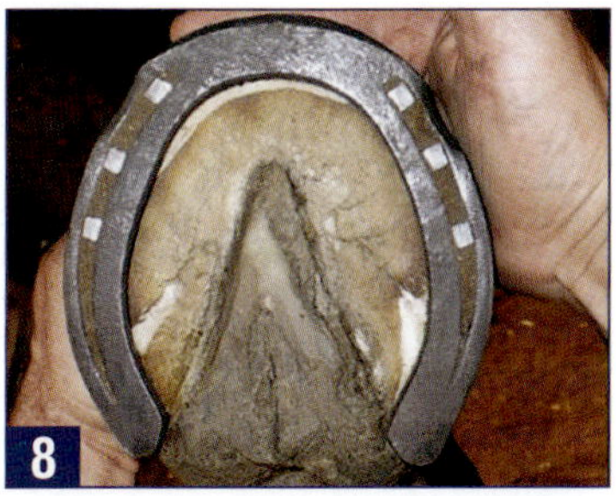

8

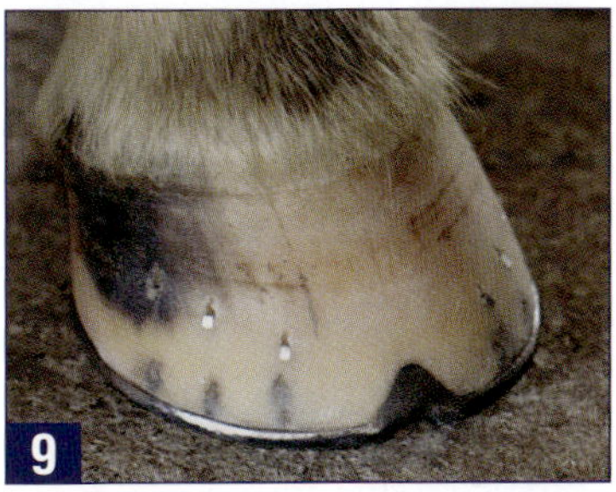

9

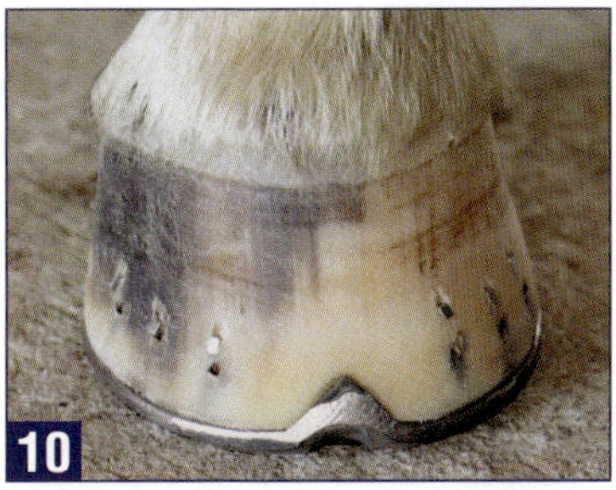

10

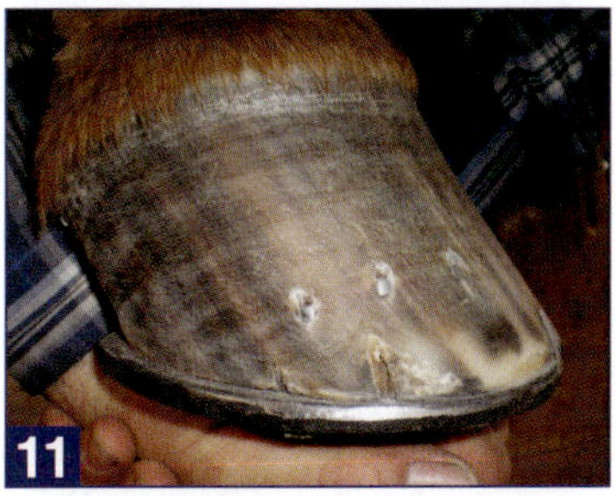

11

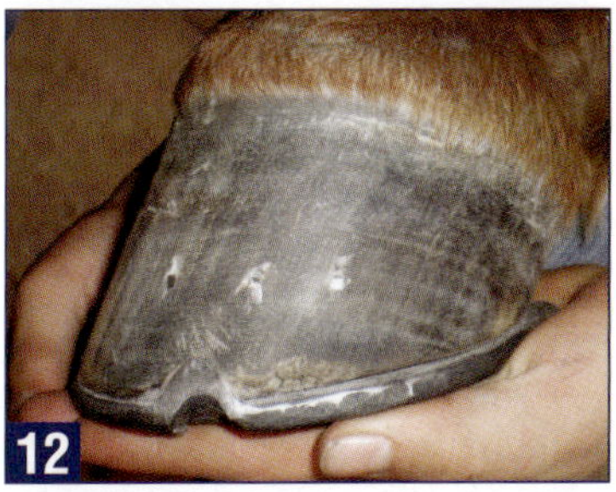

12

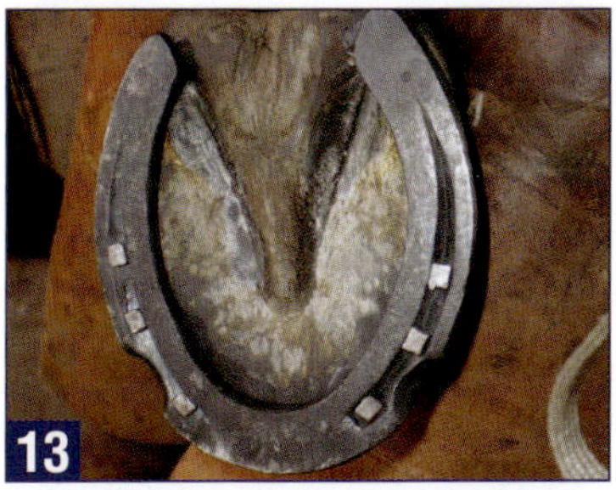

13

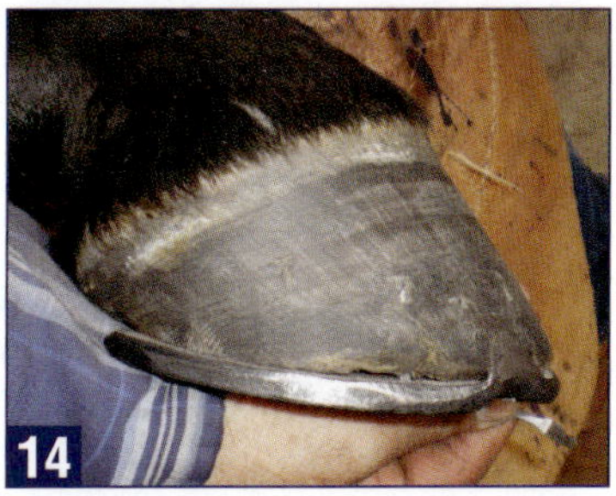

14

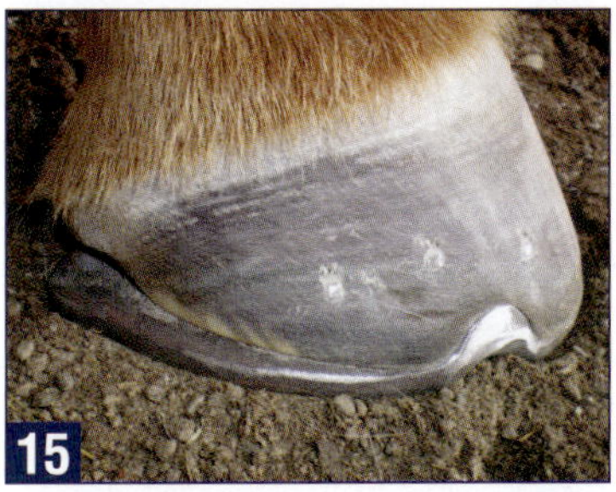

15

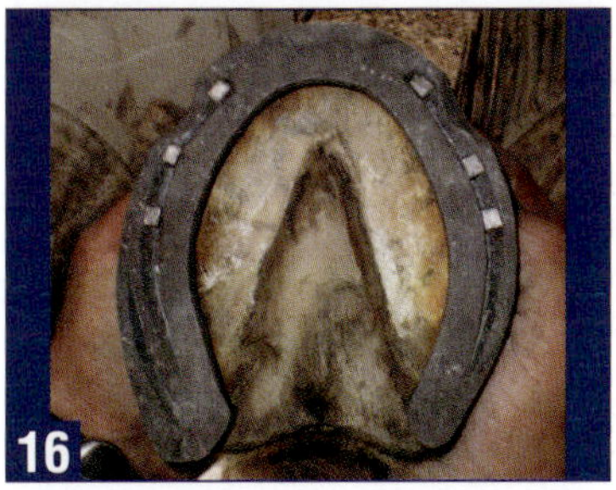

16

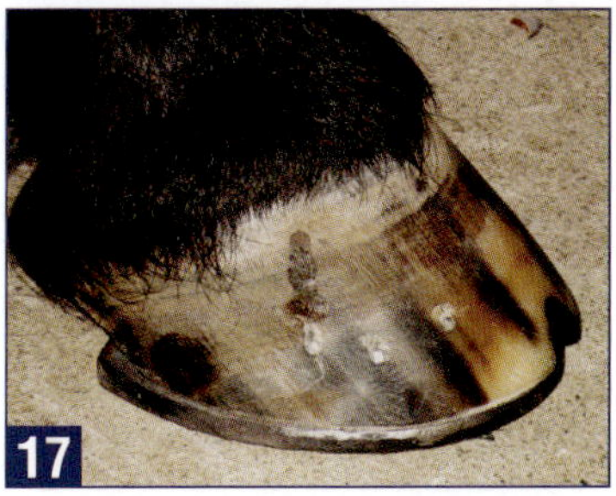

17

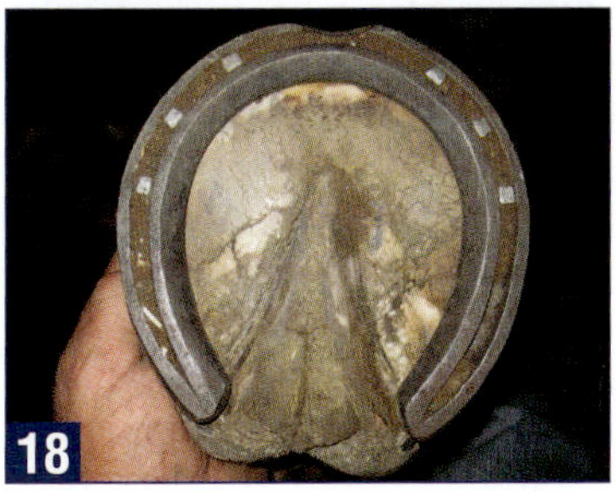

18

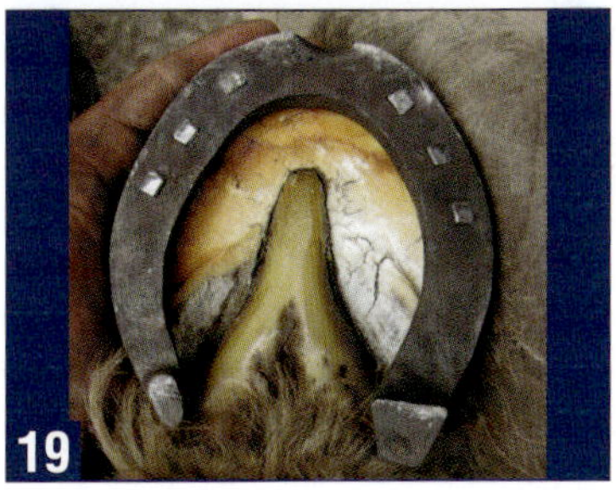

19

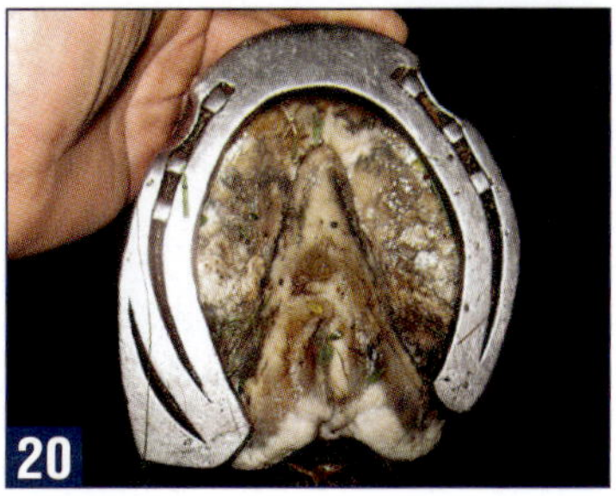

20

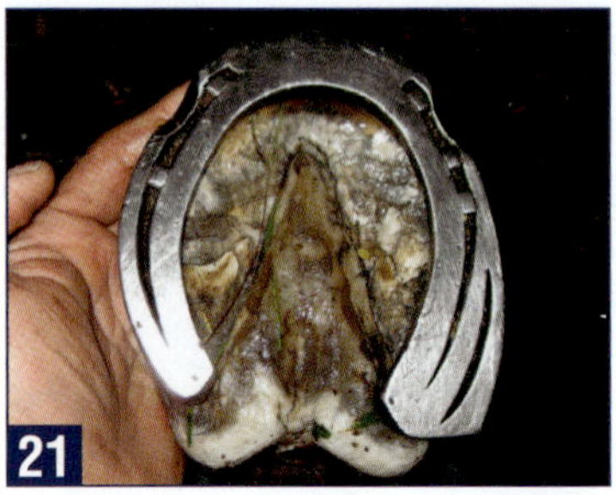

21 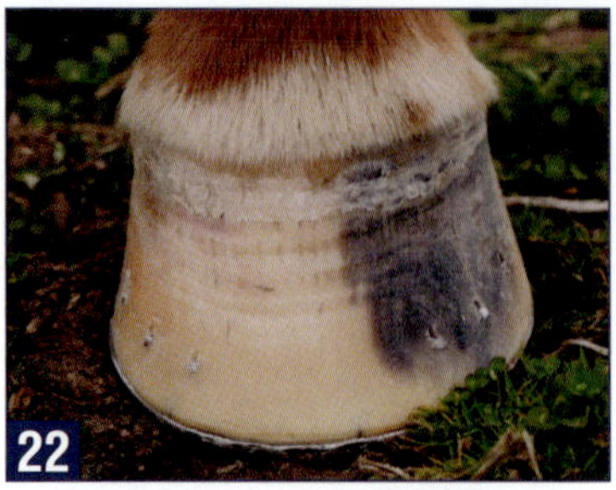 22 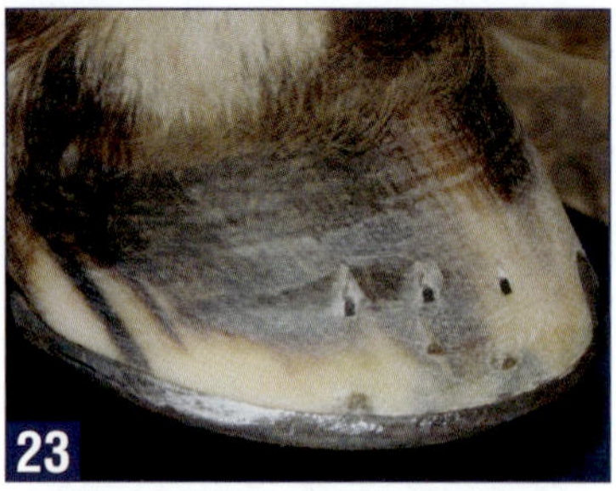 23

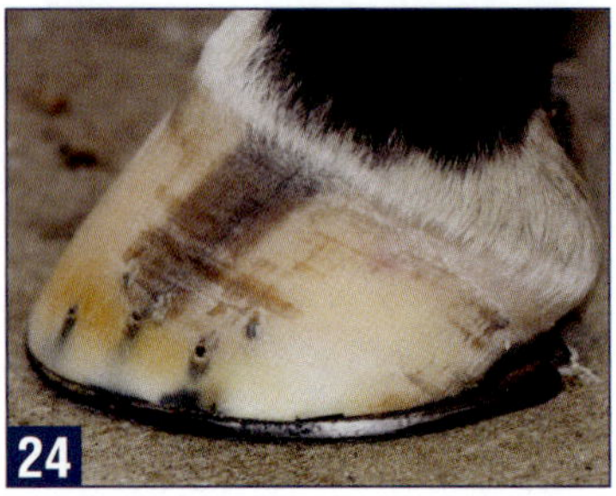

24 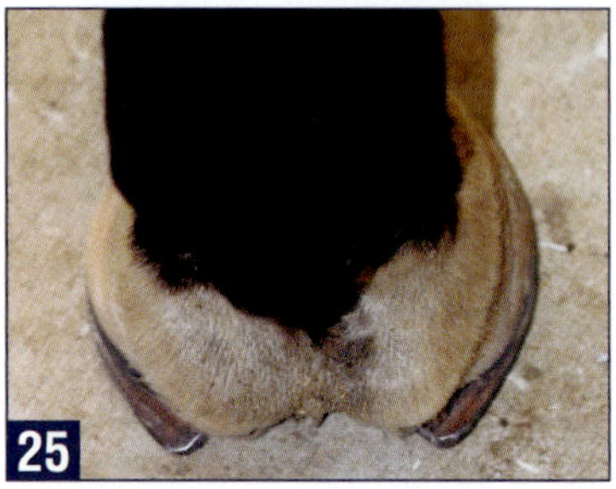 25 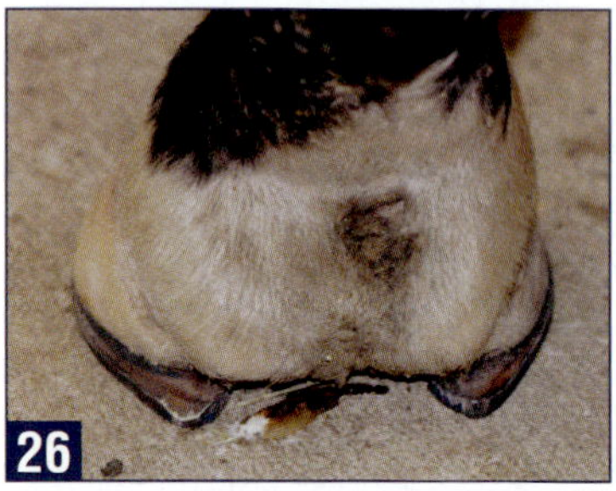 26

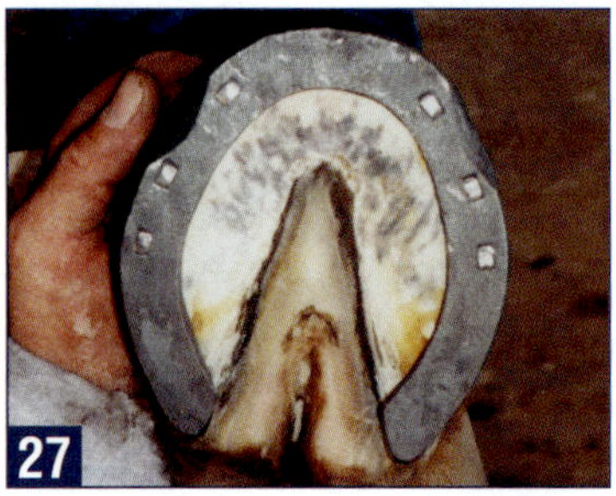

27 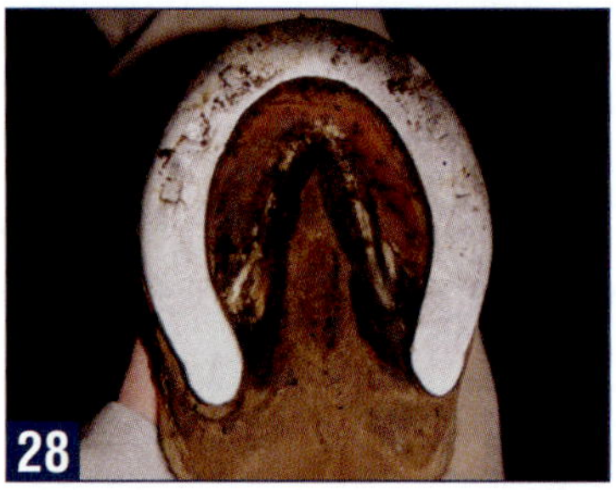 28 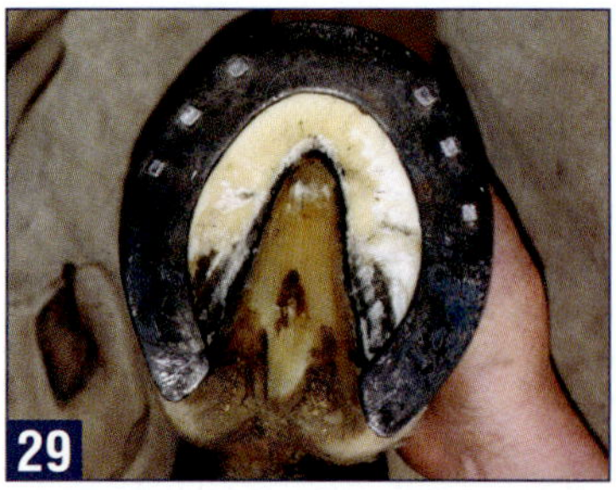 29

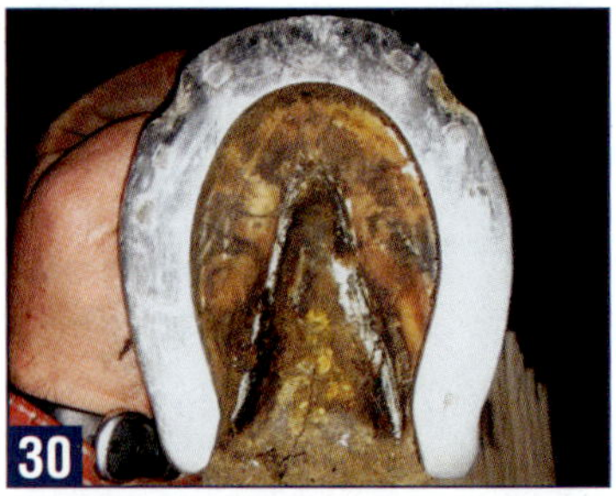

30 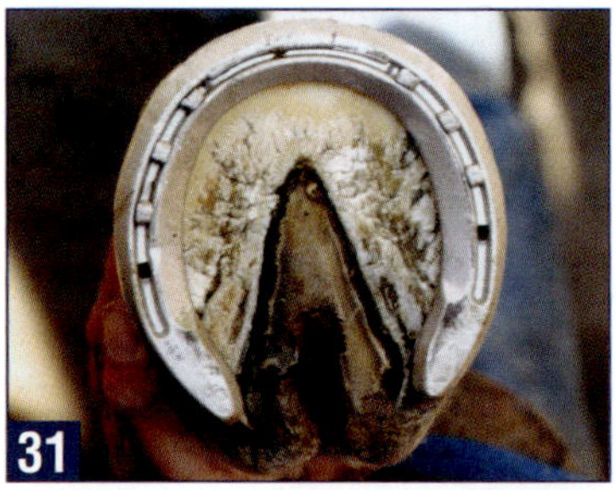 31 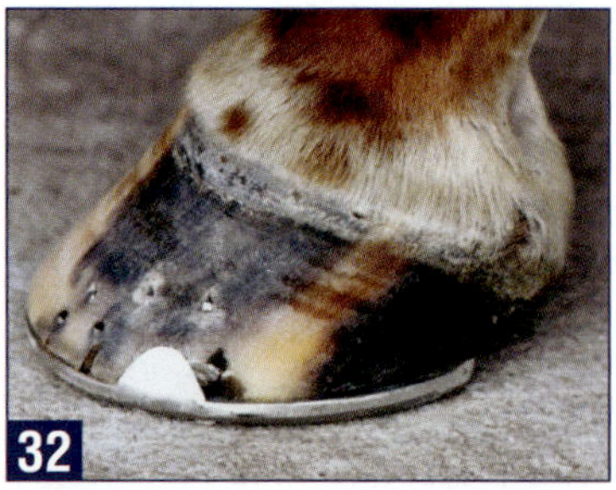 32

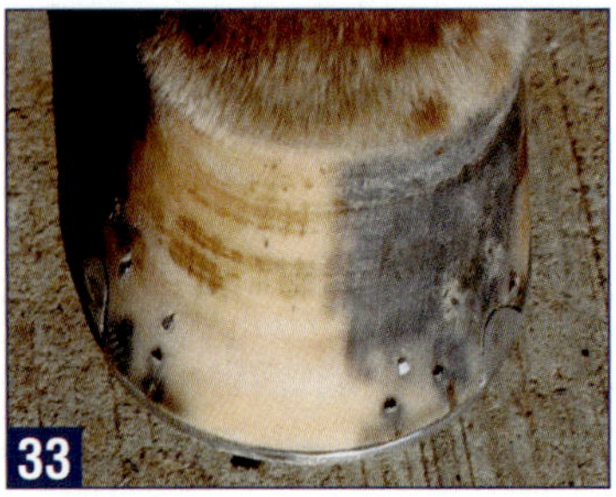

33 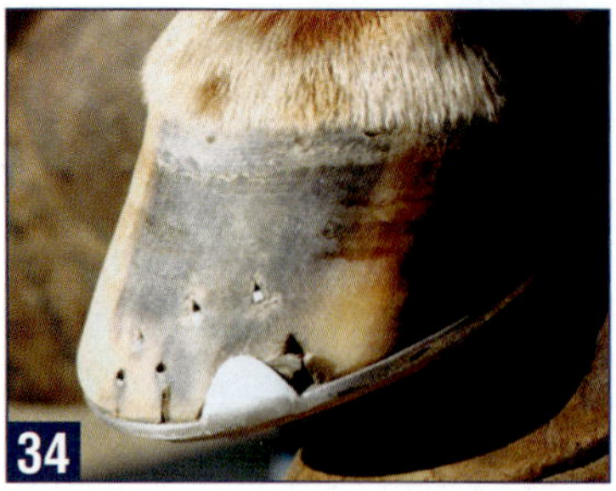 34 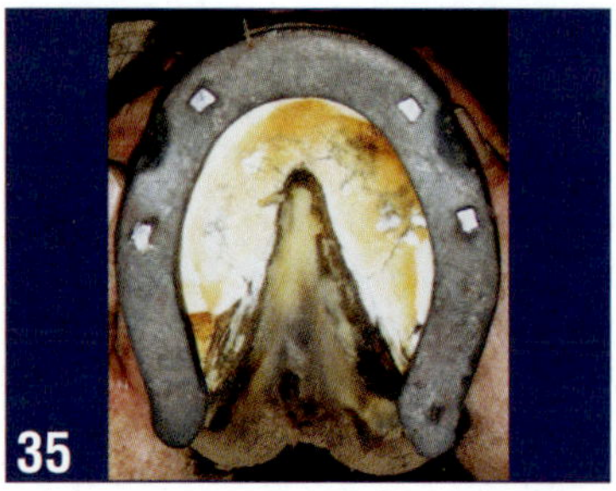 35

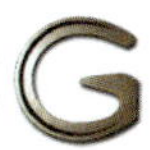

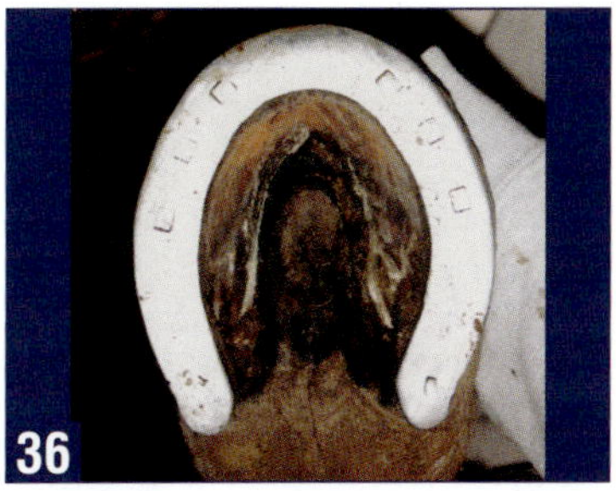

36

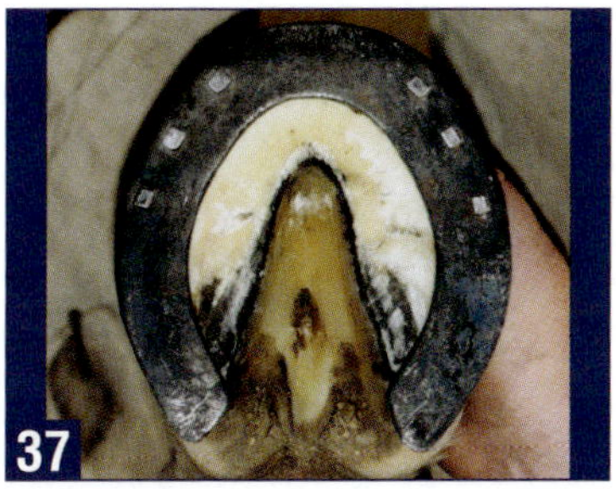

37

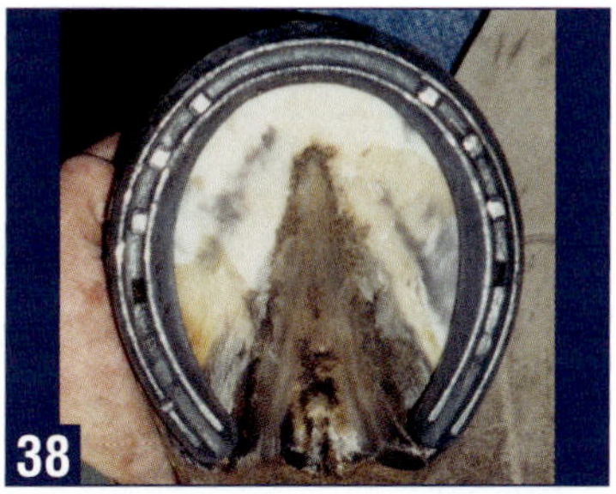

38

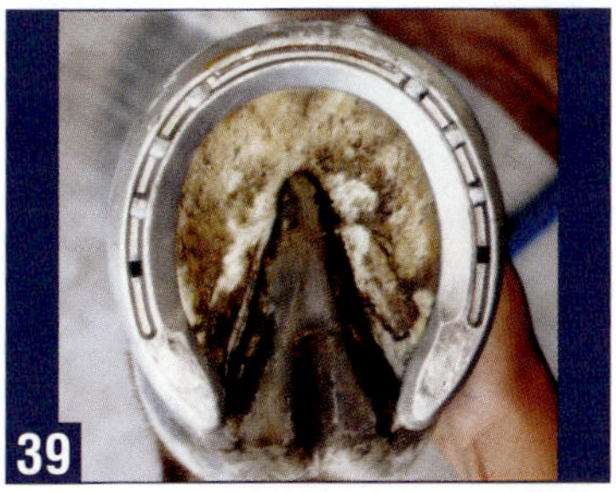

39

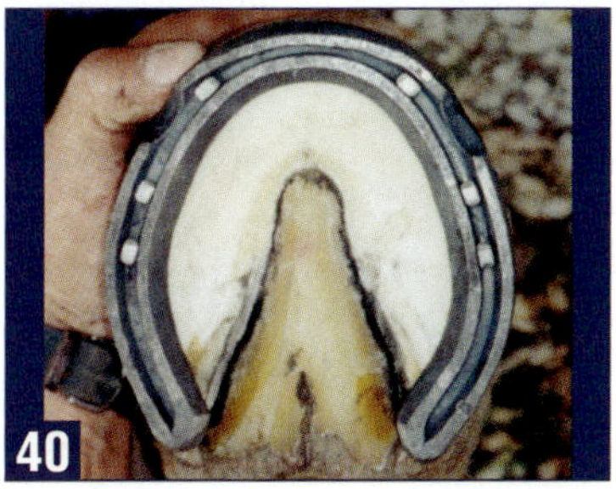

40

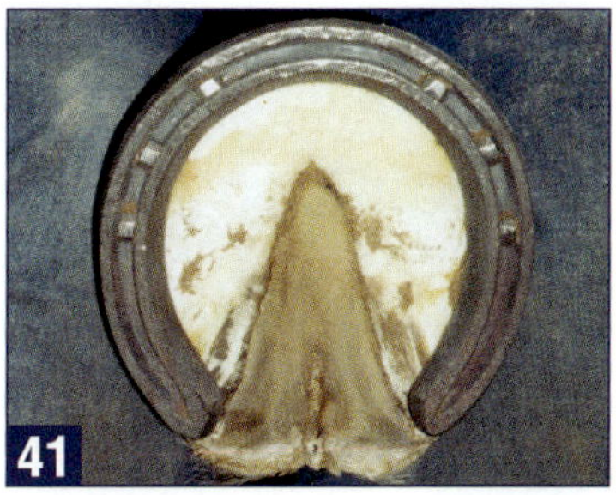

41

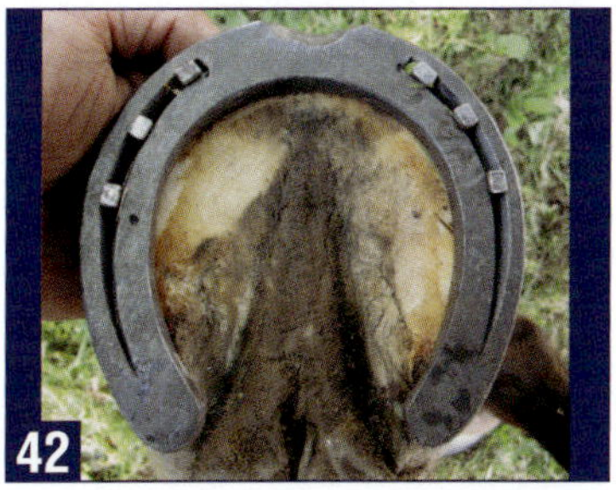

42

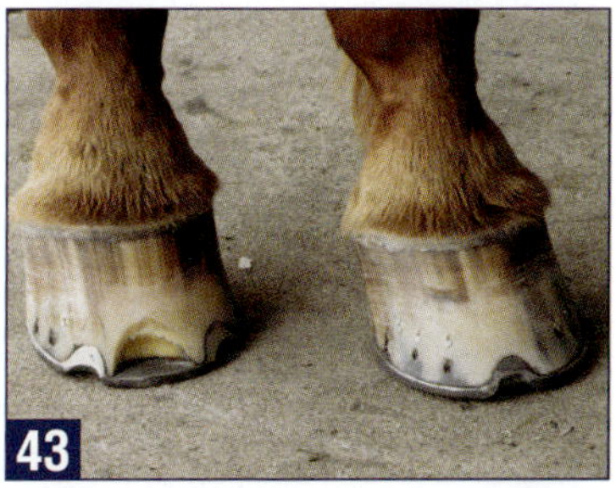

43

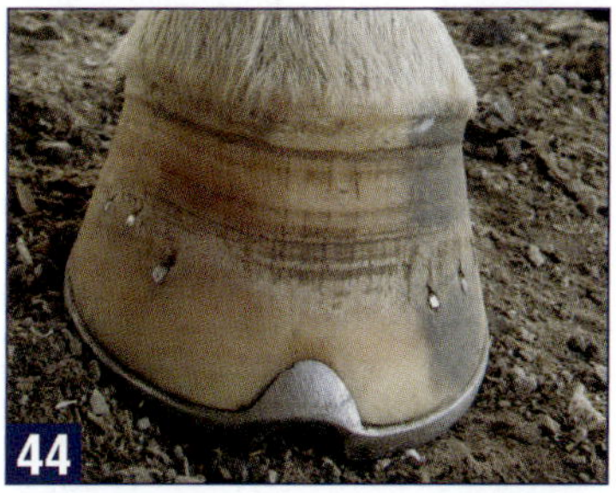

44

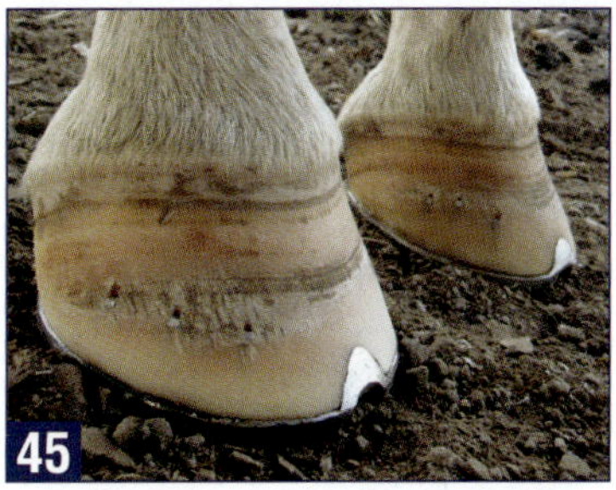

45

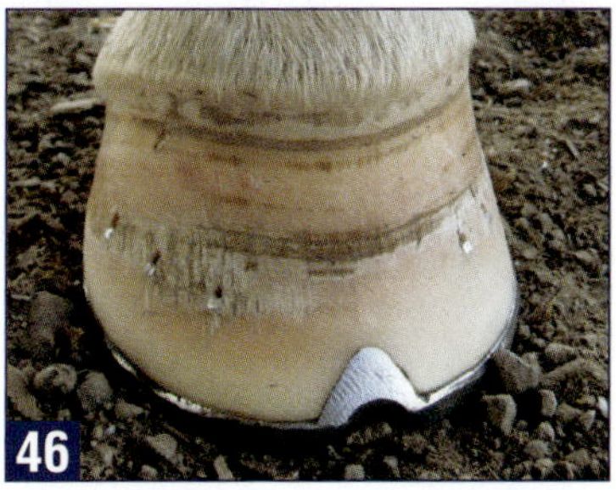

46

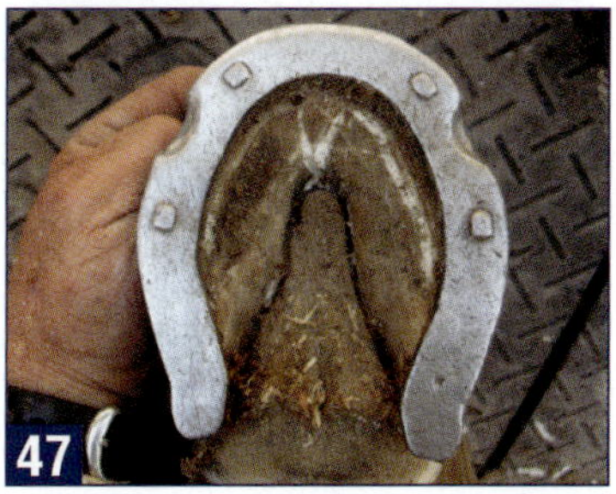

47

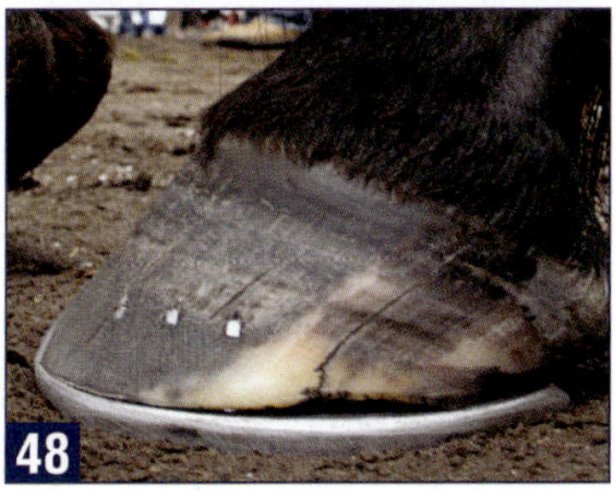

48

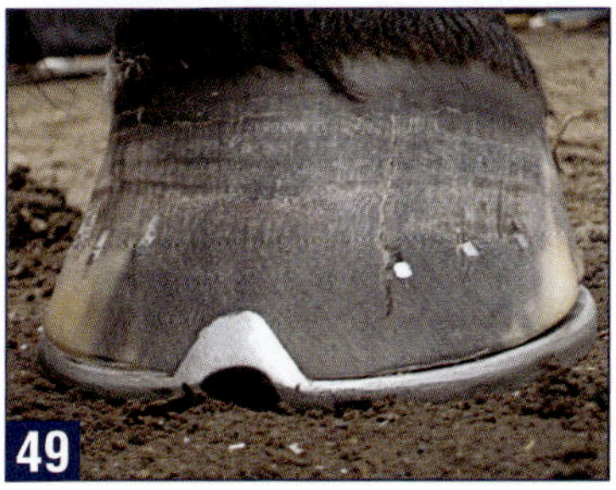

49

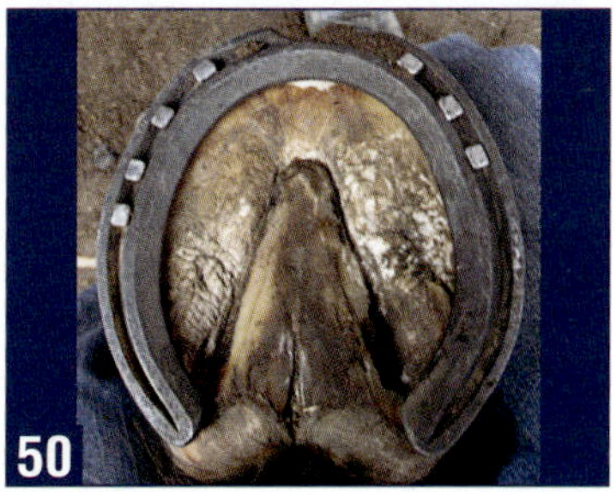

50

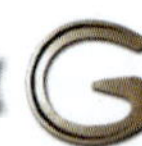

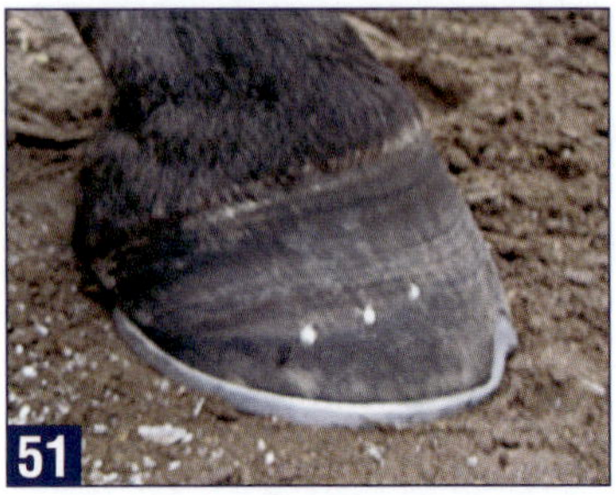

51 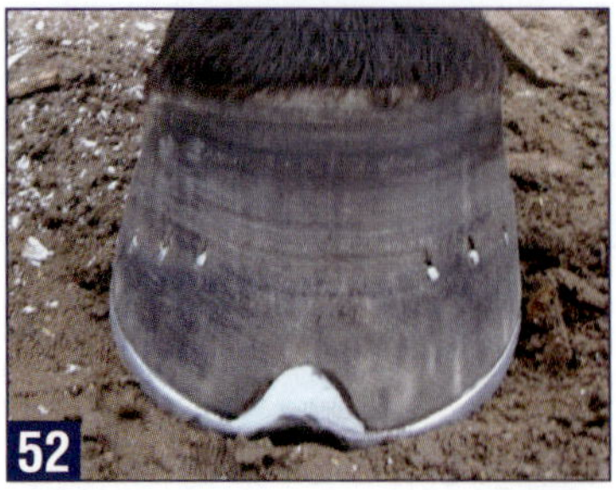 52 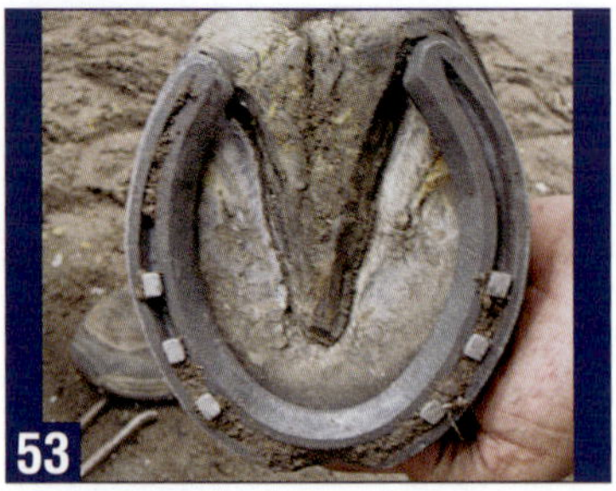 53

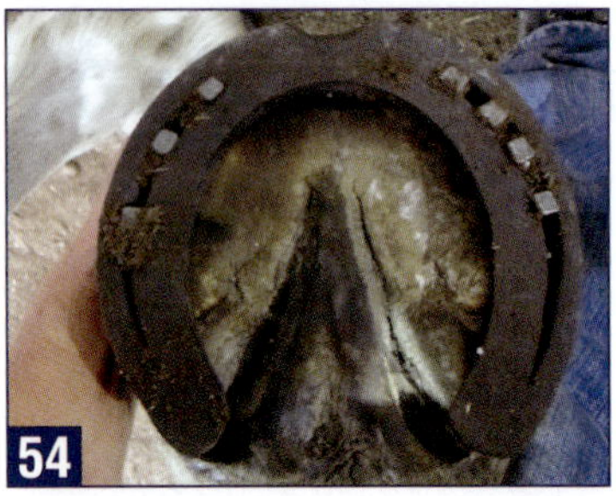

54 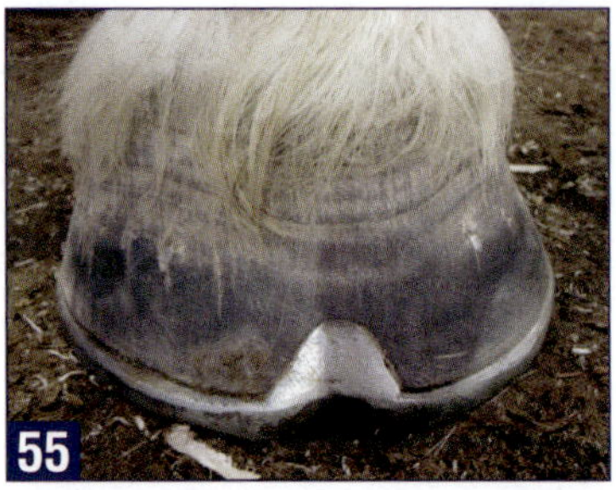 55 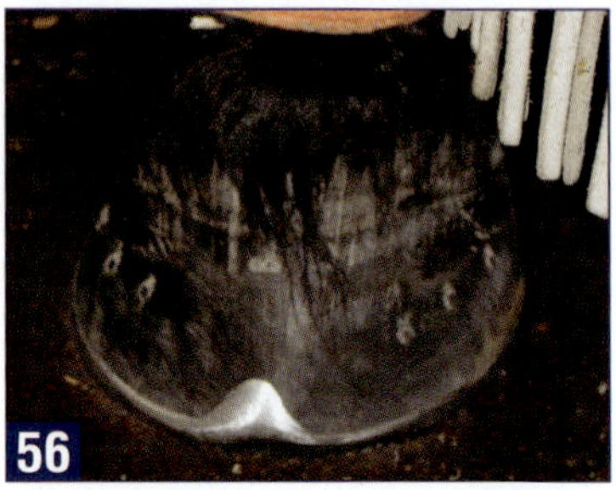 56

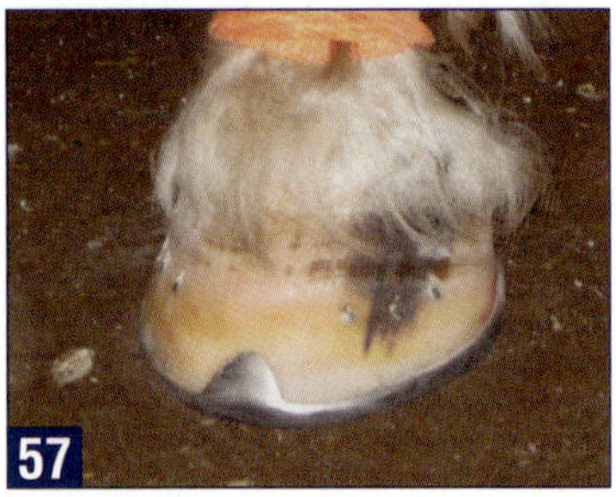

57 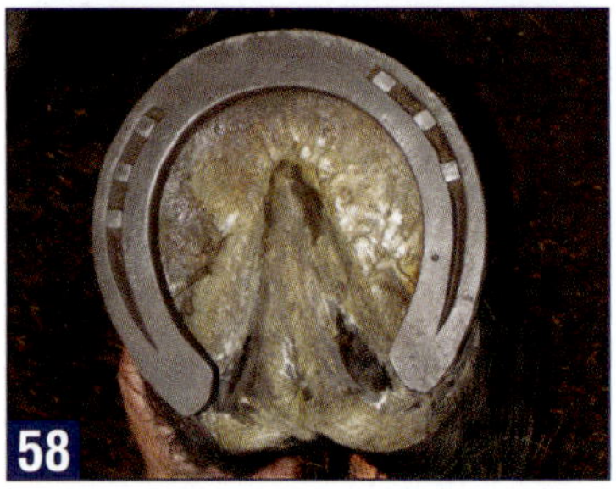 58 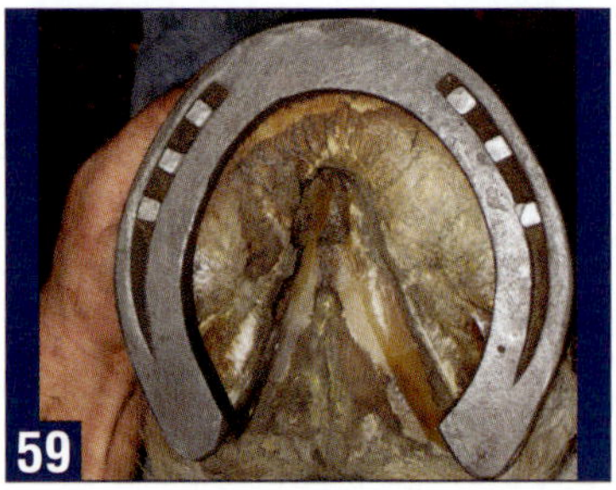 59

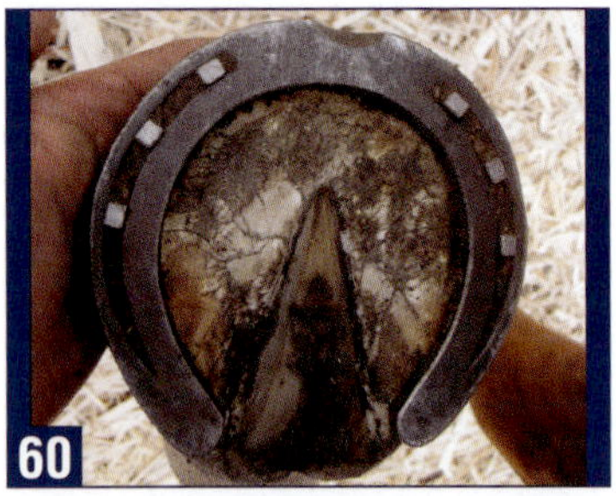

60 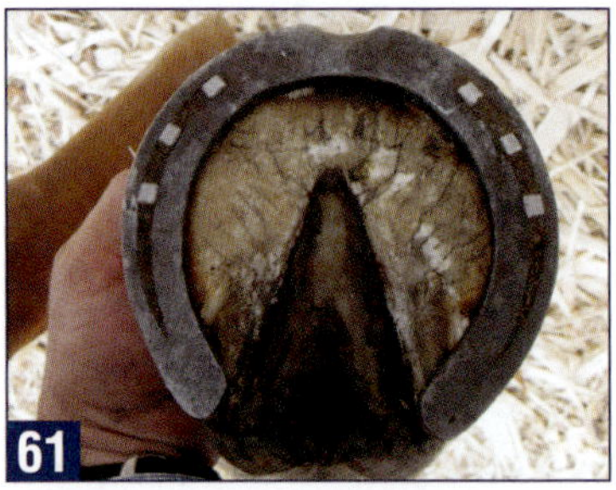 61 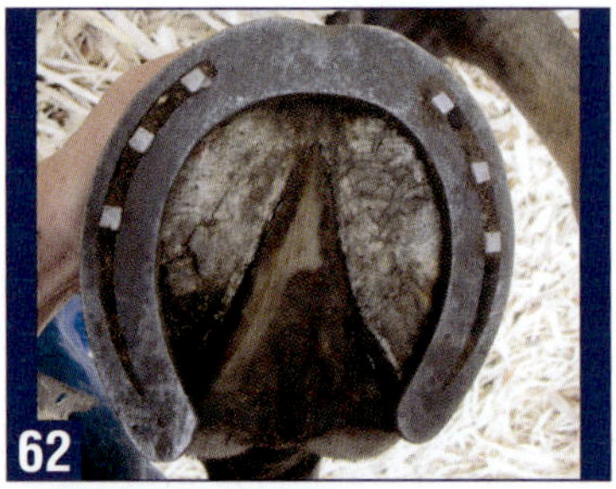 62

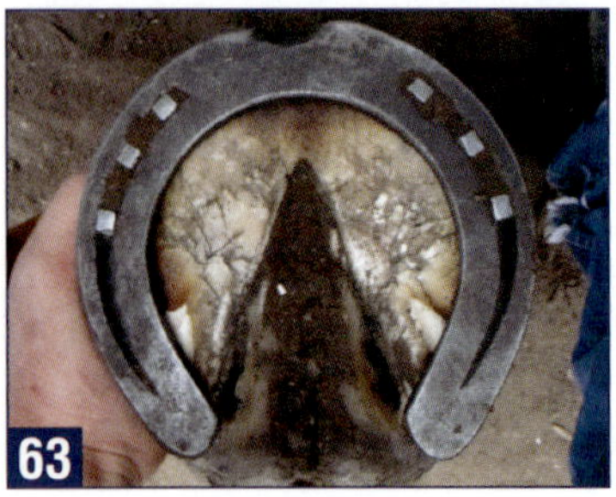

63 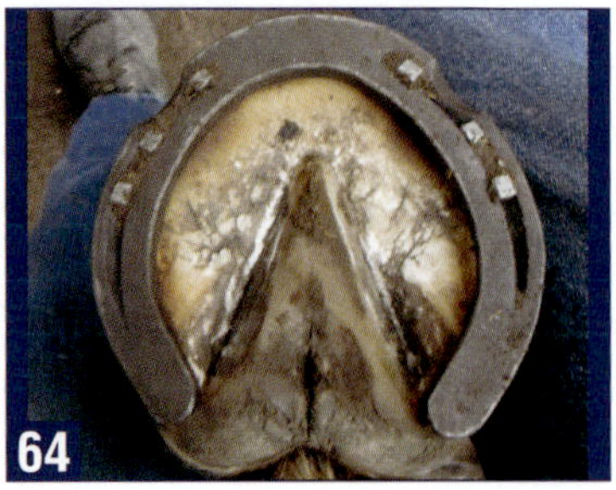 64 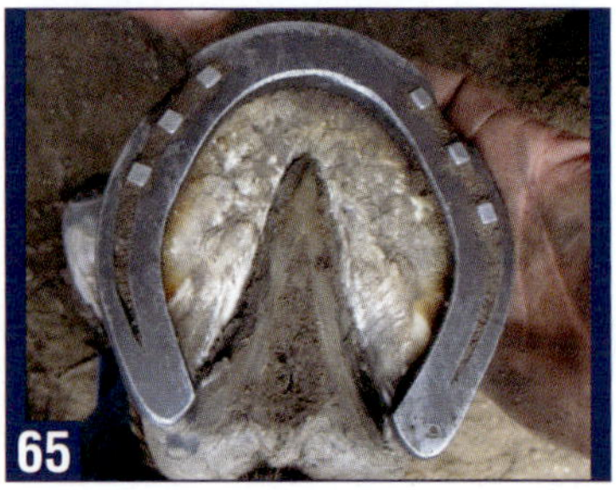 65

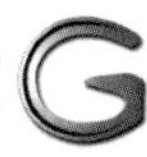

Chapter 21 TRIMMING CONSIDERATIONS

The hoof is a marvel of engineering and an object that most farriers come to respect and revere through the course of their careers. As a farrier, you are basically an artist who is modeling and carving a living medium that changes for many reasons. It changes because it is in a constant state of renewal, because of the environment, because of genetics, because of use, and because of what the farrier does or does not do to it. This requires YOU to have an unequaled knowledge of this living medium that you are about to sculpt.

There are few things that can take the stress that a horse's foot takes. It is designed to bear weight, provide traction, resist wear, adapt its growth cycles at appropriate times, provide protection to the skeleton, and become a weapon in a fight. It is hard where it needs to be hard, and softer where it needs to be softer.

For horses in the wild living without the intervention of a farrier, there is a perfect balance between growth and wear. The natural horse will eat enough to keep the hoof growing and travel enough to provide suitable wear. If these things fall out of harmony, the horse is in a situation where hoof care is needed. Horses in the wild do not live as long as domestic horses, and their lives are much harsher. One of my favorite quotes comes from a farrier friend of mine in California by the name of Bill Adams. Whenever one of his customers said that they would like for their horse to be more "natural", Bill responded, "Well, you better buy him a lion." In nature, there is no such thing as mercy or a kind death. The natural world is cruel and unforgiving. Watch a cat with a mouse or a spider with trapped fly. Life in nature is harsh and brutal. Perhaps that is why the term "natural" was used to promote that sort of trimming.

Most domestic horses are fed more than their wild cousins, and their feet are used less. When they are used, they are used in areas where they might not go of their own accord, and the added weight of human and tack lead to excessive wear. This is why farriers and horseshoes are needed.

In recent years, there has been a lot said and written about natural hoof care and the evil of horseshoes. This has created an environment in which natural hoof-care specialists do not shoe with traditional shoes and nails. Instead, they only trim the feet, reasoning that this would be more natural for this creature that was born, bred, trained, cultivated, and kept by man in captivity. This continues until the time that the foot wears more than it grows. Since they are against shoeing, they either glue something to the foot or provide a slip-on, strap-on, or Velcro-on shoe of some design or another. They are still shoeing the foot!

Part of this movement comes from the fact that it is hard to learn to do everything that a farrier needs to know how to do. If you only have to learn trimming, the number of skills needed are only a fraction of what a farrier needs to know to shoe in the traditional sense. Another cause of this movement is that incompetent traditional shoeing done by ignorant horseshoers can be very damaging. For this reason, if you are going to shoe, you must become as competent as you possibly can. The responsibility that you are undertaking when you decide to cut into a foot and drive nails into it is immense and should never be taken lightly.

As discussed in the anatomy introduction, those that are ignorant in this industry easily fall prey to people who would market products or gimmicks that do not make sense. During the last several years, there have been large numbers of people who have devised a trimming tactic based on their observations, and some of these have caused quite a bit of harm. Matt Gillis, CJF, is a good friend of mine. While editor for *Today's Pro Farrier*, his sentiments in the following paragraphs are mine exactly, but they are stated much more eloquently than I am capable of. Here is an editorial that he wrote, and has allowed me to use here. I asked Matt **(Figure 1)** to read this editorial at a clinic I did in Indiana for Marvin Schwartz.

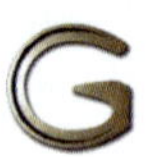

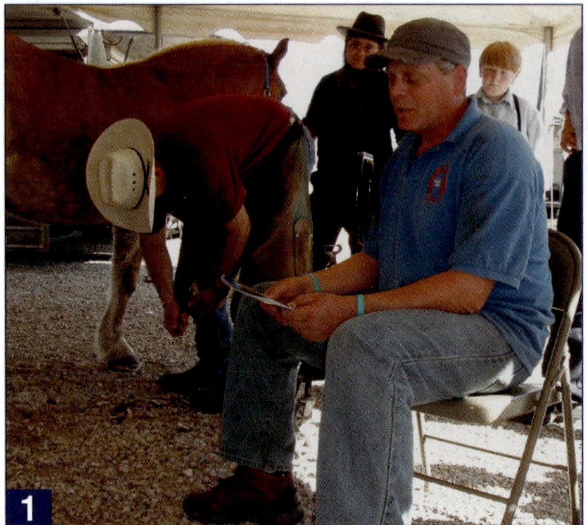

Matt Gillis shares his thoughts on "trims with a name" at an Indiana clinic.

DANGERS OF A NAMED TRIM

"What's in a name? A trim with a name is a dangerous thing. A name can provide validity when there is no merit in the method. A name can give its inventor the appearance of having been born enlightened; discovering a truth that everyone else just missed. A trim with a name is an opportunity for the incompetent to appear credible, and opportunity for liars and fools to profit.

"The Natural Barefoot Trim is a trim with a name that elicits good feelings, and a theory whose result is senseless cruelty to horses and disillusioned, confused, horse owners. The natural trim is a franchise in stupidity, and its proprietors are arrogant and presumptuous. There is no shortage of credible educational material available for students of the equine digit, and no shortage of world-class farriers with the experience to know the truth and the ability to pass it on; any claims to the contrary are disingenuous, irresponsible, and idiotic.

"The world has gone green. Raised environmental consciousness is evident throughout the world. The natural barefoot trim exploits this by using the word natural. The beauty and freedom that the American feral horse has come to symbolize are also exploited, painting a picture of an idyllic environment and life on the open range that does not exist! Nature is cruel and devoid compassion. Natural is a breeding program that is managed by hungry predators and the prospect of starvation. Natural is an otherwise insignificant injury that will become infected and result in death. Natural is a horse without a worming program, or vaccinations. Natural is no blanket, no fly mask, no shelter. Nature does not tolerate the propagation of crooked-legged and deformed foals because they are from a "good blood line." Nature will not break the ice in a horse's bucket so that it can drink water today. Nature will send vultures to watch a horse die and to feed on its carcass while it rots in the sun.

"Nature is a harsh manager that eliminates weakness at the source. Horseshoes do not prevent the domestic horse from being natural; domestication prevents the horse from being natural. Every year horses are injured and maimed and even killed by fencing, poorly constructed stalls, and ill-fitting tack. Every year fat, spoiled, horses are fed to death by well-meaning, ignorant owners, and yet the barefoot crowd would have us believe that people can achieve a more symbiotic relationship with the horse by depriving it of steel shoes. The desired end result for the barefoot trimmer is that the horse live in its 'natural barefoot state.' The desired end result of every ethical horseshoer is the soundness and usability of the horse.

"Barefooters ignore the great benefits that horseshoes have provided horses throughout history. I know that I am not alone in saying that I am a horseshoer! And I have chosen my career because of admiration for the horse; my faith has increased as I marvel at the engineering genius present in the design of the hoof. My stewardship as a caregiver is taken with the utmost seriousness, and I take great offense to the notion that I, or any other competent farrier, have done harm to horses by the proper application of steel shoes. I have managed to keep many horses sound, and many horses happy for over twenty years with nothing but a trim, but some horses need shoes and I am proud to have helped them.

"Remember Benjamin Franklin's famous quote? 'For the want of a nail, the shoe was lost; for the want of a shoe, the horse was lost; for the want of a horse, the rider was lost; being overtaken and slain by the enemy, all for the want of care about a horseshoe nail.' Today my enemy, the enemy of the rider, the enemy of the horse, is a trim with a name!"

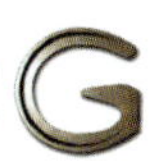

There has been a lot of anecdotal evidence against many of these 'trims with a name,' but there has only been one conclusive study that gives definite and unbiased proof about what happens to horses that are subjected to some of these trimming theories. While satisfying the thesis requirements of becoming a Fellow of the Worshipful Company of Farriers, Dr. Mike Miller, MD, CJF, FWCF, did a study on the effects of a 4-point trim compared to a conventional unnamed trim. Kelly, Cody and I were lucky enough to play a part in this study, and we helped Doc with the trimming. Dr. Miller has published this study in a book called, *The Mirage of the Natural Foot. Science and Snake Oil in the Barefoot Trimming Debate.* More information, as well as photos of this study, appear in Chapter 34, Common Sense In The Shoeing vs. Barefoot Debate.

One thing this study certainly did bring to light is the fact that the horse is an unbelievably forgiving creature. Their feet can accept a lot, and this allows people to do ignorant things to the feet, yet the horse stays sound. If the horses and their feet were less tolerant, there would be less snake oil and more people would have to shoe their horses, more farriers would have to comply with proper anatomical principles, and more horses would be lame from stupidity.

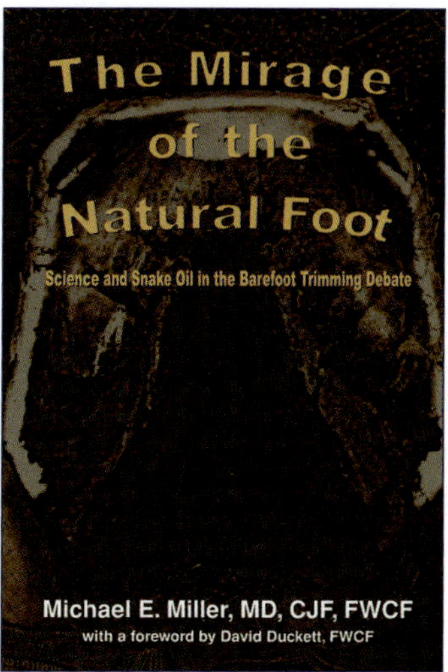

It is said elsewhere in this book, but it can't be said enough. If you plan on becoming the best farrier you can be, you need to listen to, be exposed to, learn from, and observe those that are already the best. Gaining wisdom from an idiot cannot be done, so you should not even try. Those vocal, unskilled people who lead the unsuspecting novice down the wrong road should be stopped. The best way to stop them is to become knowledgeable enough that you don't follow them. Find and learn from those in this trade that have the ability to teach and the knowledge to teach the right thing.

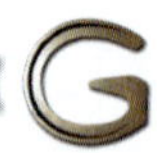

Chapter

22 TRIMMING A HOOF

There is a lot that has been written and said about trimming feet, but at the end of the day, trimming a foot is as simple as taking off horn that should not be there. That being said, sometimes what the farrier leaves is more important that what is removed. We have talked at length about anatomy and the importance of knowing everything you can about a foot. Now, it is time to get the tools out of the packages and get your hands dirty. Following are the essentials of trimming a horse.

TRIMMING

As you approach a horse, you need to begin with a mental checklist of what you see. Where is the foot in relation to the leg? How does the fetlock and knee look above that foot? Where is the bony column and foot in relation to the trunk? How does it look from the side and from the front? Go through a systematic check every time, and it will soon become an automatic thing that happens in an instant. Many seasoned farriers can know more about a horse's conformation in a matter of minutes than the owner will know in years. Become one of those farriers by starting slow.

Once you have made your assessment, it is time to start work.

There is an analogy that was once told to me by Frank Turley concerning blacksmithing. I modified it to relate to hoof prep, and for most of my teaching career, I have applied this analogy to trimming. Here it is in all of its blessed simplicity.

Trimming feet is like carving a wooden Indian. You begin with a piece of wood **(Figures 1 - 2)**. Everything that does not look like a wooden Indian, you remove. When you are done, you have a wooden Indian **(Figure 3)**.

Sounds straightforward. In fact, it is pretty simple. The important thing is that you learn what a good wooden Indian should look like. Some of what you personally perceive as a correct foot will have to do with the type of horses that you shoe and the discipline of riding that they are used for. What looks good to an Arabian show horse farrier will not look good to someone who shoes mainly rodeo and cutting horses. This I know for a fact.

Begin your quest by borrowing from the experience of someone who is seasoned and respected. In other words, spend some time with a good farrier so that you can learn what a good foot is supposed to look like. Make the decision of who this farrier is very carefully. A bad farrier is like a bad carpenter, or a bad mason, or a bad cook, etc. Bad farriers can only teach what they know, so pick someone that has a proven ability. I would suggest an AFA

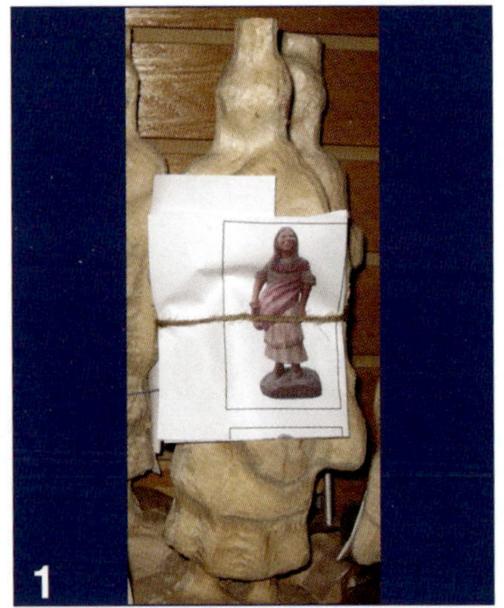

1 *Rough wooden Indian blanks.*

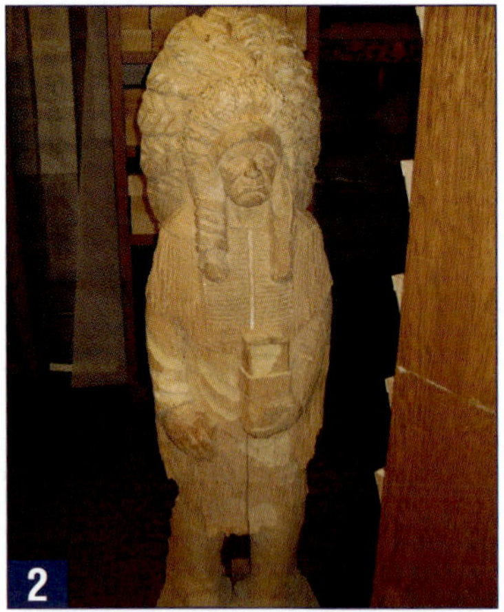

2 *Wooden Indian blank.*

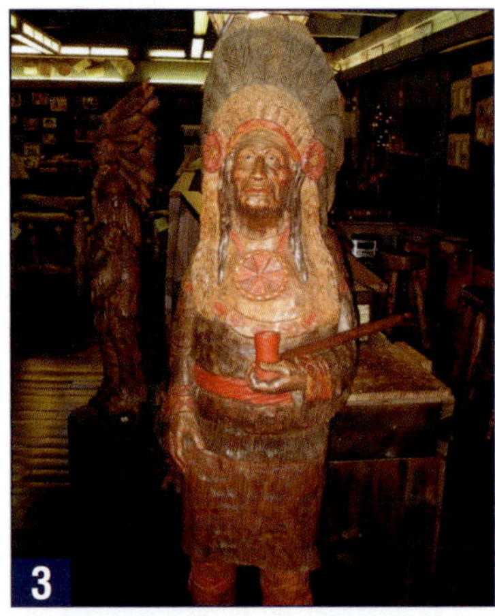

3 *Finished wooden Indian.*

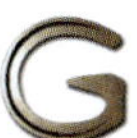

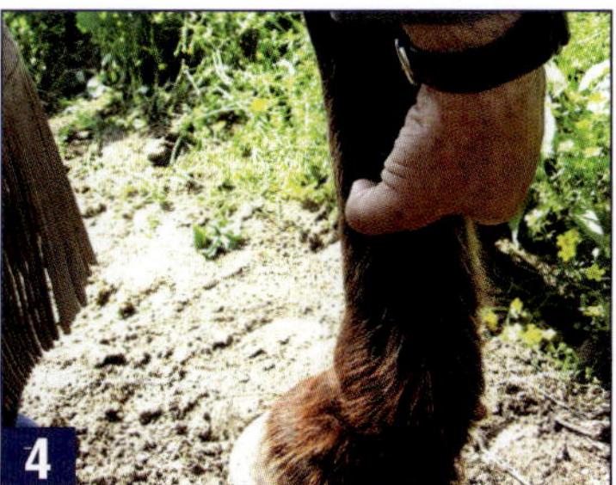

Squeezing the pick-up button on a front foot.

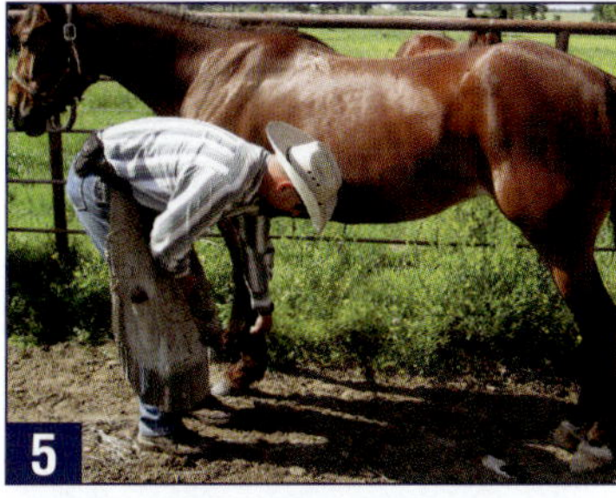

Notice how I am in a safe position as I pick up a front foot.

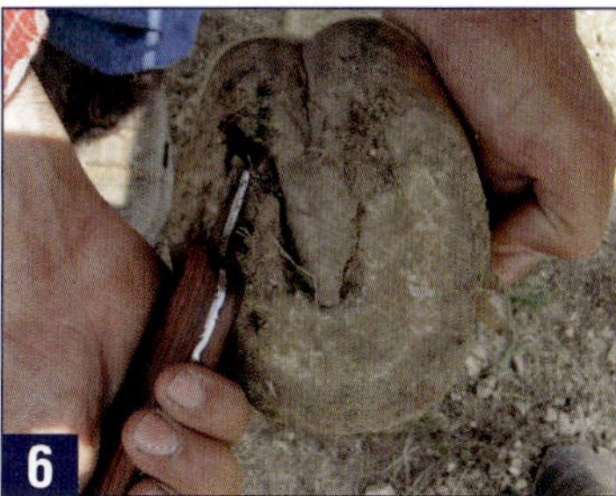

Using the pick on my knife to clean the foot.

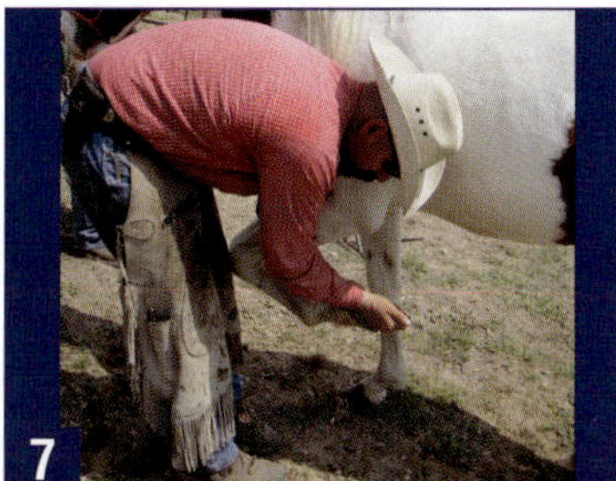

My position to clean the foot one-handed.

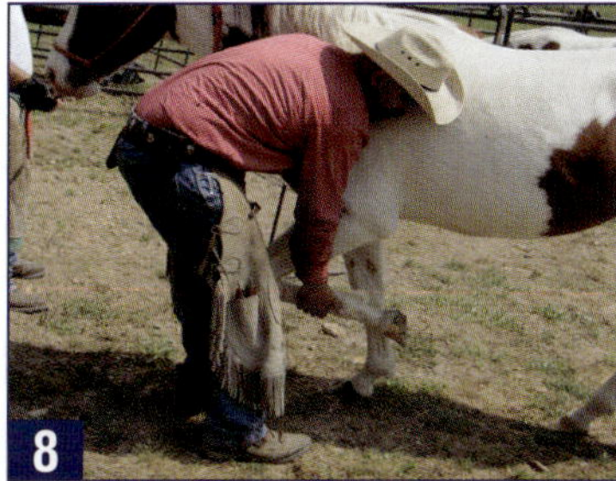

Sighting a front foot. Keep your head close to the body, and the horse's head and neck straight.

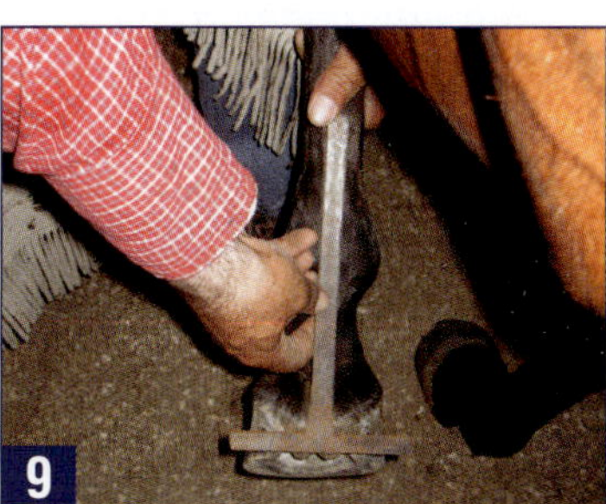

Using a T-square.

Certified Journeyman Farrier at the very least, but I would really look for a farrier who is an Associate of the Worshipful Company of Farriers if possible. They are scarce as hen's teeth but worth looking for. To become the best, you need to know what the best do.

All right, now we pick up what appears to be the longest hoof. If the horse has lost a shoe, I will generally start with the front foot that has not lost a shoe. If the horse is not shod, or has both shoes on, I will start with the one that looks the longest. You will be amazed how well you are able to determine the longest foot within just a short time of training your eye to see it. Horses that have one white sock, or a white and black hoof, or even a wide vs. narrow hoof will pose a slight optical illusion. In time, you will be able to compensate for that as well.

I begin trimming most horses on the front feet; however, it is a handy trick to begin a youngster on the hinds. You can see more about that in the chapter on dealing with behaviorally challenged horses. One thing to make a habit is to pick up feet the same way every time, and then move to the position you need to be in to work on the foot. Even if I am going to dress the front foot, I will still pick it up from the position depicted in **Figure 5**, then turn so that I bring the foot forward.

To pick up the foot, you can squeeze the area where the cannon bone and the splint bones come together on both sides of the cannon bone **(Figures 4 - 5)**. Pick an area about half way down the length of the splint bone, and you may have to use your fingernail to apply pressure. We refer to this spot as the "pick-up button."

On a barefoot horse, pick up the foot and clean it before placing it between your knees. I like to do this so that I can sight the foot prior to getting under the horse. Cleaning the foot is a one-handed job, so doing it prior to getting in trimming position will save one step **(Figure 6)**. If the hoof has a shoe on it, I will go ahead and put it between my legs so that I can pull the shoe and clean the foot prior to sighting it.

Once the foot is cleaned, I will hold the cannon bone with my outside hand and sight down the plane of the bottom of the hoof **(Figure 8)**. I am imagining that plane in comparison to the axis of the bony column from the knee down. There is a short axis, which is from the fetlock down, and there is a long axis, from the knee down. On the ideal horse,

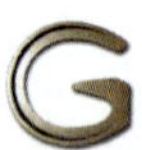

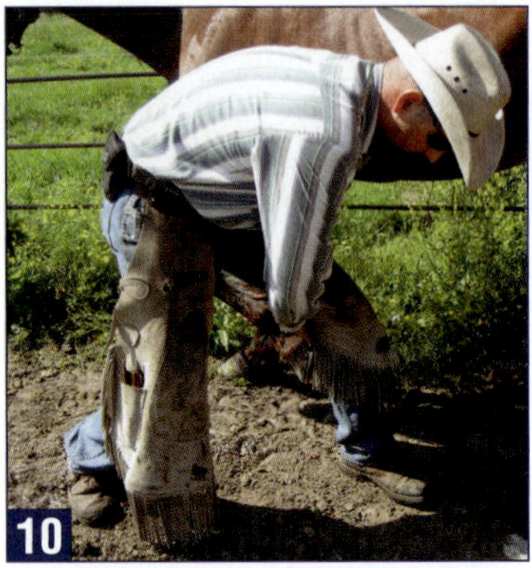
10 *Moving into position to hold a front foot.*

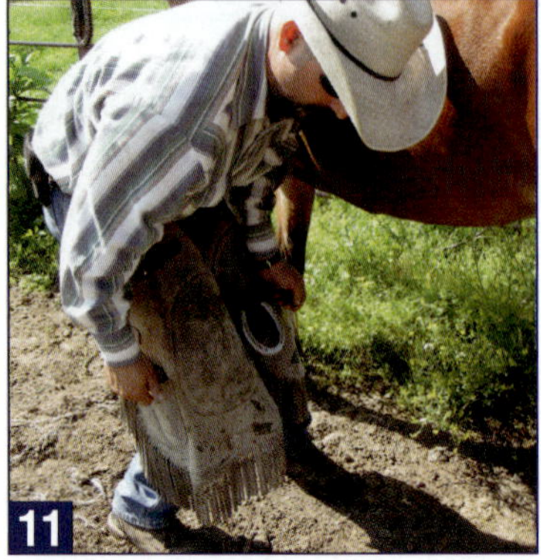
11 *Working position for a front foot.*

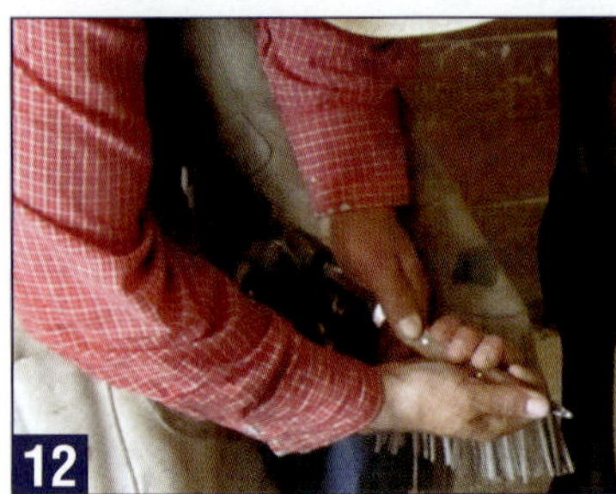
12 *Starting position for knifing.*

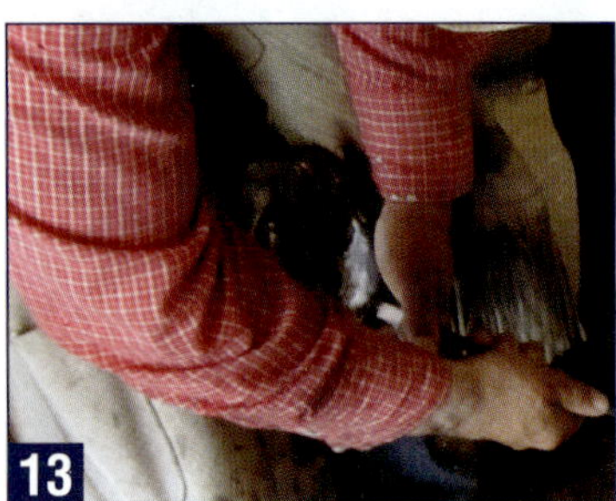
13

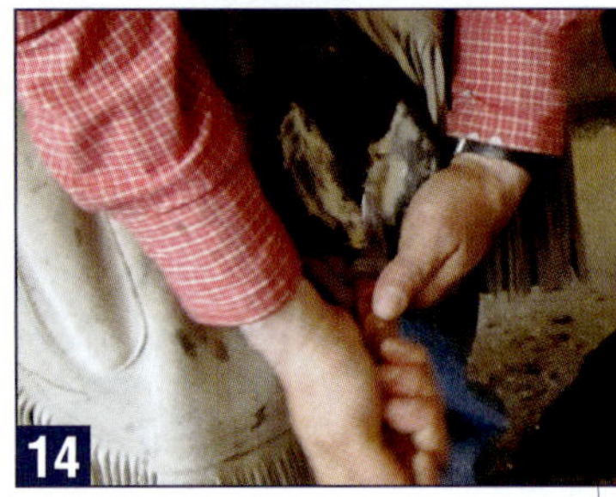
14

Moving around the foot with the hoof knife.

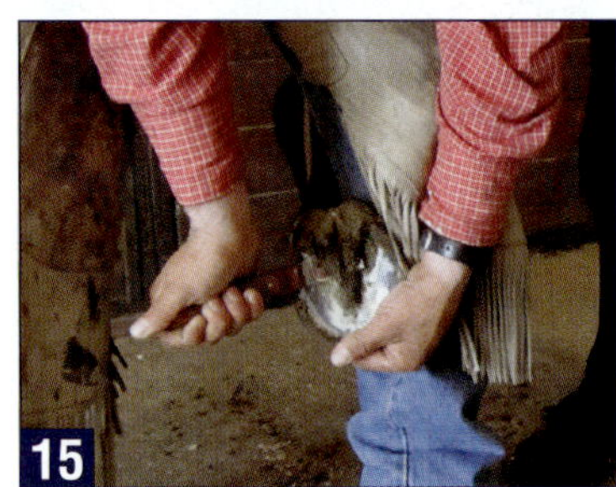
15 *Pulling up through the sole on my hammer-hand side.*

we are trying to achieve a 90-degree angle between the bottom of the foot and the long axis. A T-square can help you train your eye to see this **(Figure 9)**, although I don't personally use one.

Once I have made my determination of where to trim, I get under the horse and place the foot between my knees. To do this, step forward slightly with your inside leg **(Figure 10)**. Place your outside hand between your knees and grab the hoof. Pull slightly as you move your inside leg back toward the horse's head. Turn your toes toward each other and bend your knees. This will cause your knees to come together and squeeze the pastern, effectively holding the foot steady so that you can work on it **(Figure 11)**.

Take out your knife and begin by knifing on your tong-hand side **(Figure 12)**. Start up at the heel in the seat of corn and move around the foot, making shallow, smooth cuts **(Figures 13 and 14)**. We often tell students to cut potato chips. (Crisps if you are from England). In **Figure 15**, I am coming up on my hammer hand side. To do this, I grab the toe of the foot with my tong hand and pull the knife towards me. Be careful that you don't slip out of the foot and cut either yourself or the horse when using this move.

The knife is being used to only take away excess sole. In many instances you will find that you do not need to knife at all. Often, doing a good trim is as much about what you leave as what you take. Horses that have had shoes or live in soft terrain do not exfoliate as much sole as they should, so the hoof knife allows the farrier to do that for the horse.

Hoof-knife technique is important. When you are young and strong, you can get away with bad technique (you will pay for that someday). However, if you learn good technique that will allow you to do a lot of work with less effort, you can become an old farrier. If you are already old, good technique is a must. The knifing technique that I like the best is to anchor my tong hand on the foot with my middle, ring and pinky finger. I place the base of the knife handle against the base of my index finger and my

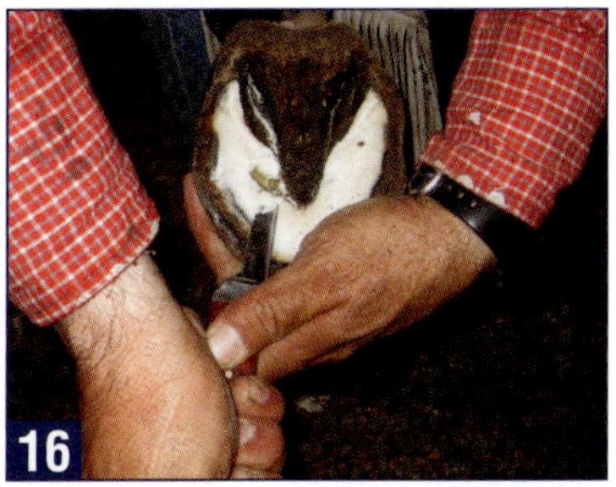

Close up of how the knife is used.

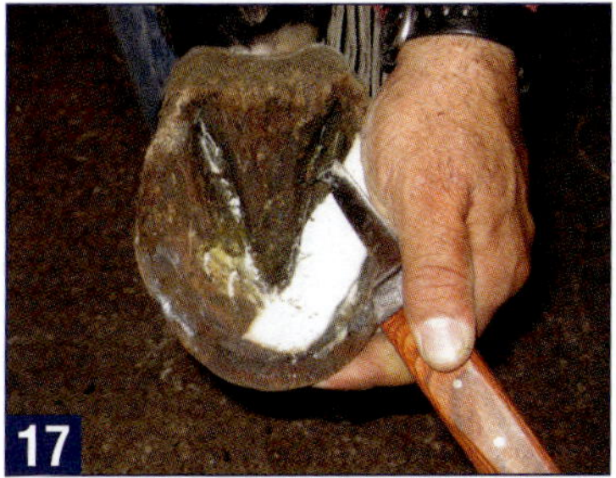

Fulcrum point for the knife at starting point of cut.

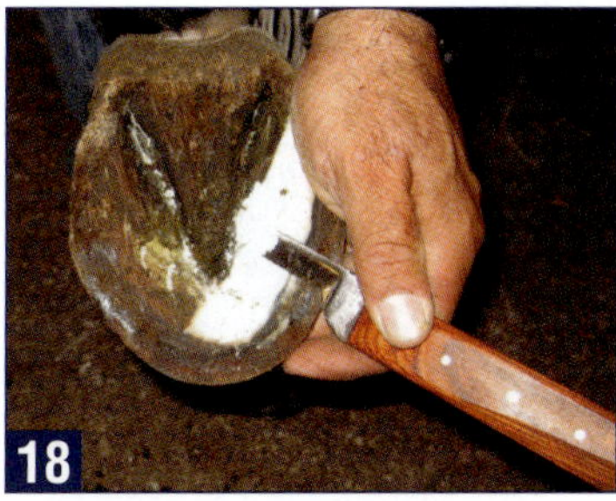

Moving through the cut.

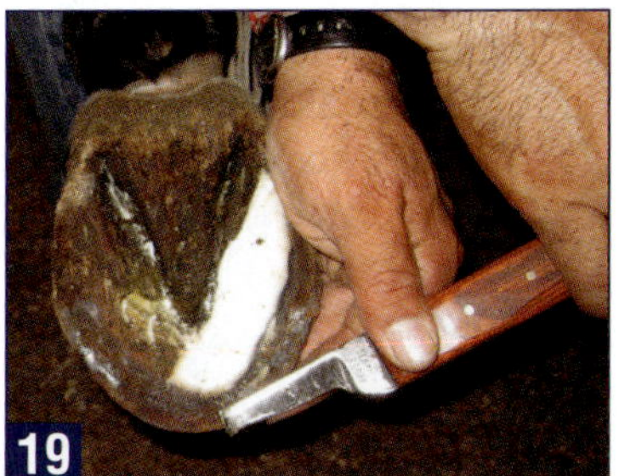

Finishing the cut.

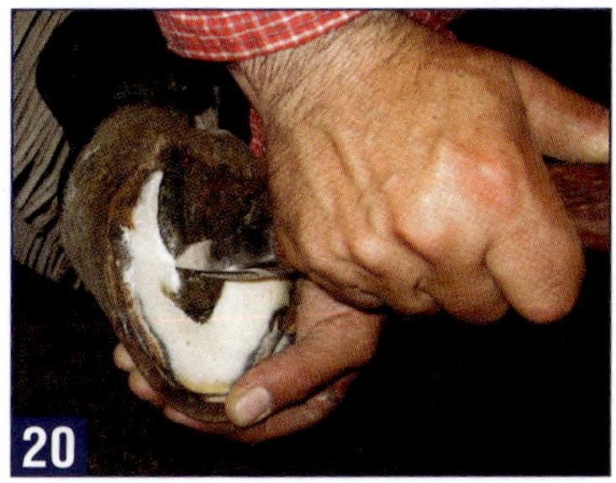

Start at the tip of the frog with your loop knife

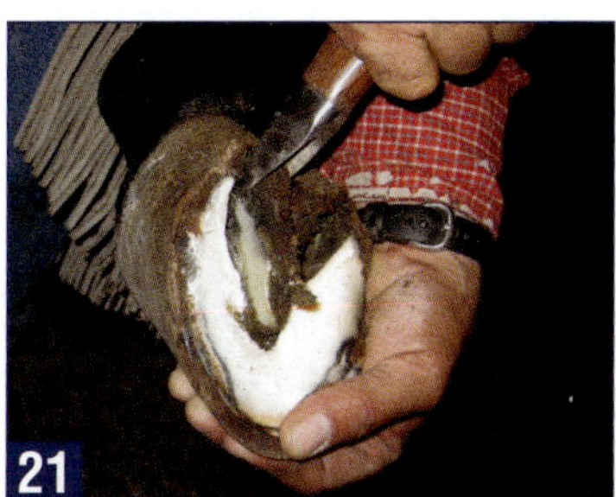

Pull upward to make a clean and smooth cut.

thumb, and push the shaft of the knife handle toward my tong hand **(Figure 16)**. Since my tong hand is acting as a fulcrum, the blade of the knife is moving toward my hammer hand. **Figures 17-19** show the movement of the knife and the placement of my tong hand as a fulcrum. I am using leverage to cut, and that makes for a great improvement in power with the knife, and a lot less effort. If you get good at this technique and couple it with a sharp knife, you will be amazed at the results.

As you knife, you are feeling the consistency of the sole, and you are looking at the texture of the dead sole. If it is chalky and cracked, this is an indication that it should be removed. Continue knifing until you reach a shiny, clean sole. You do not want the sole to give to thumb pressure as many people were taught at some of the shoeing schools in years gone by. If you are able to push on the sole and have it flex to your strength, imagine how much it will flex when the weight of the horse comes down on it. You do want it to be clean, thick and strong.

Next we will knife the frog. One of the most common questions from beginners is: How much frog can I take? There is not a textbook answer that can be given to this question. Like the trimming of the overall hoof, the frog can be looked at like a little wooden Indian of its own (perhaps a papoose). It needs to be trimmed so that it looks appropriate for that particular horse, and you will only know what that is with experience and guidance.

I personally like to use a loop-knife for this. A loop-knife is a knife that can be used as either a left- or right-hand hoof knife. Start at the dorsal tip of the frog on your hammer hand side and pull toward the heels with a smooth, even cut **(Figures 20-21)**. If you stop or saw with the knife, you will leave a little line in the frog. It won't matter to the horse, but it is an indication of skill, or lack thereof. When you get to the top, turn the knife in your hand to finish the cut and use the back of the blade to clean the inside of the bar on that side **(Figure 22)**. Repeat the steps on the opposite side of the frog **(Figures 23 - 24)**. If you look closely at **Figure 25**, you can see that I have changed my hand position a little bit to allow me to push the blade. You can use this technique instead of pulling the blade if it seems to work well for you.

On prominent frogs, the top may need to be cut off **(Figure 26)**. I like to do this after I have trimmed the sides of the frog. The central sulcus of the frog

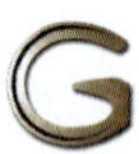

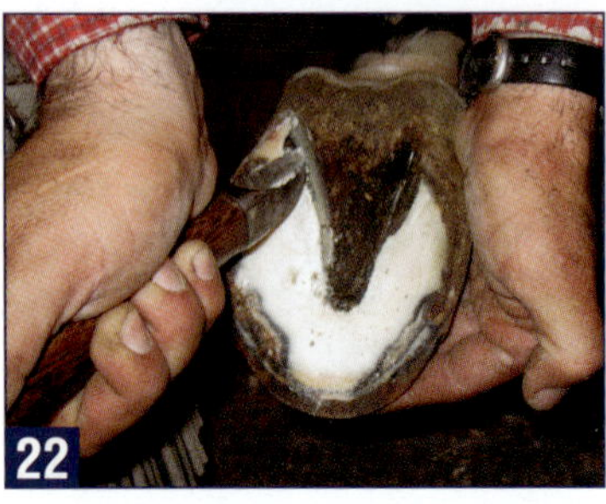

Clean the bar with the back of your loop knife blade.

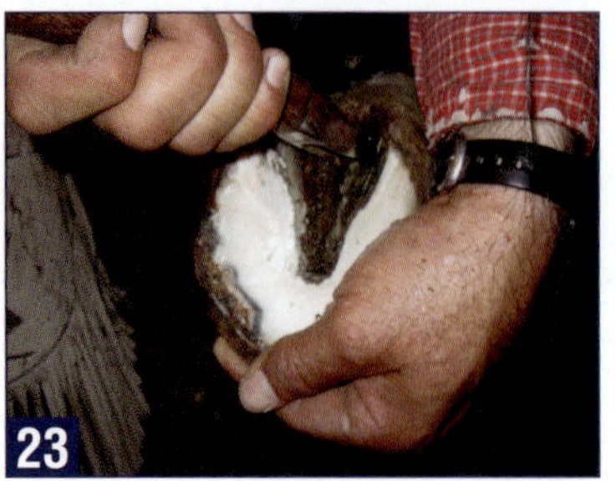

Pull up the other side of the frog.

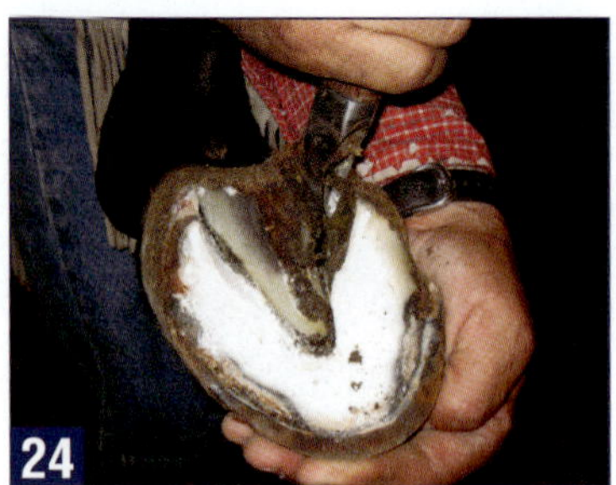

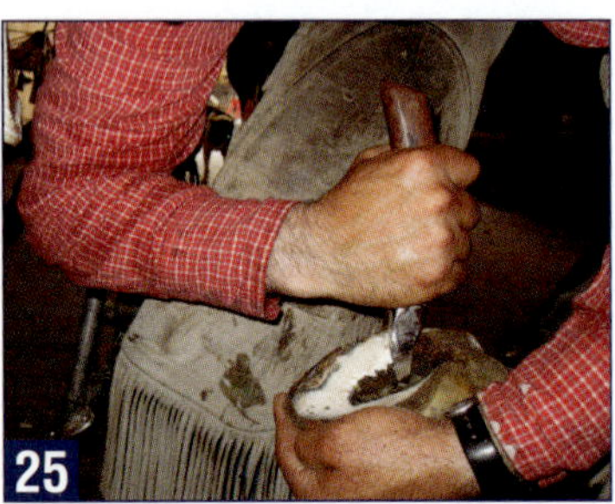

You may find it easier to push the blade up on your tong-hand side.

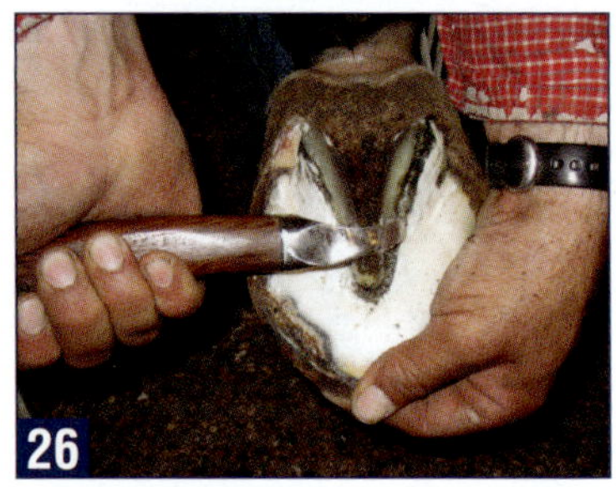

Cut off the top of the frog if needed.

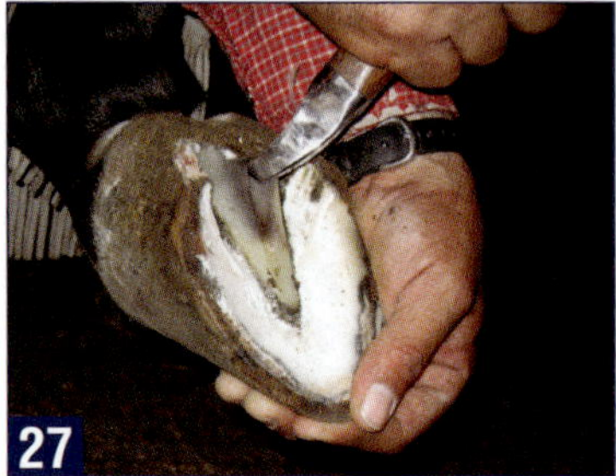

Clean up the central sulcus.

should also be trimmed if needed. Again, mimic what the sensitive frog underneath the horny frog looks like. I also like to use my loop-knife for this task (**Figure 27**).

The angle of the loop-knife is important. By and large, most farriers will lay the knife down at too shallow an angle. If you can remember what the sensitive frog looked like when you did your dissection, try to achieve that angle. Trimming the frog like this allows the commissure (paracuneal sulci) to clean easier. Less stuff stuck in there means less chance of thrush or other hygiene problems.

On the sides of the commissures, there is a continuation of the hoof wall known as the bars. These should be trimmed to the level of the sole in strong feet, and perhaps left a little bit longer in weaker, shallower feet. However, you do not want them to be so long that they collapse. When they do, there is a good chance of soreness from the pressure from that piece of horn. The inside of the bars should not be knifed on, however I do use the back edge of my loop-knife to clean the bars.

With the majority of the knife work is done, it is time to begin nipping. Some of the general rules to remember about nipping are:

A. Take small bites.
B. Hold your nippers at 90 degrees to the bottom of the foot.
C. Go slowly to learn good technique before you worry about speed.
D. Hoof can be taken but not put back.

I personally like to start at the heel on my tong-hand side. To begin, I will make certain that my nipper is flat, and I will make a nip that includes the buttress of the heel if there is enough foot to warrant it. Going slowly, I will move about half the width of the nipper blade with each cut. **Figures 28-32** show the movement of my nippers around a foot.

One problem that a lot of beginners will struggle with is taking the full amount that they want at the heel, but avoiding dipping the quarters. This problem happens because the bars can make it hard to determine where to nip in the heel. Just find your plane, and stick with it. When you get to the quarters, be careful to not follow the sole as it descends in the quarter. This is hard because you are often nipping with nothing touching the flat part of the inside nipper blade. If you become reliant on having a rest for that inside blade, you will dip a lot of quarters. Learn to nip straight.

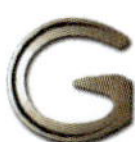

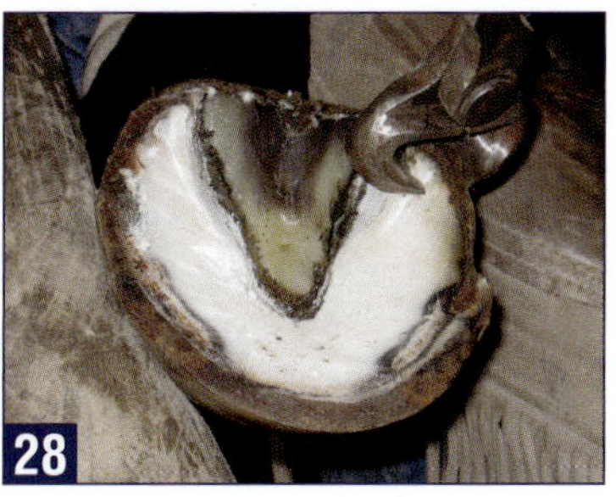

Begin nip at the heel of your tong-hand side.

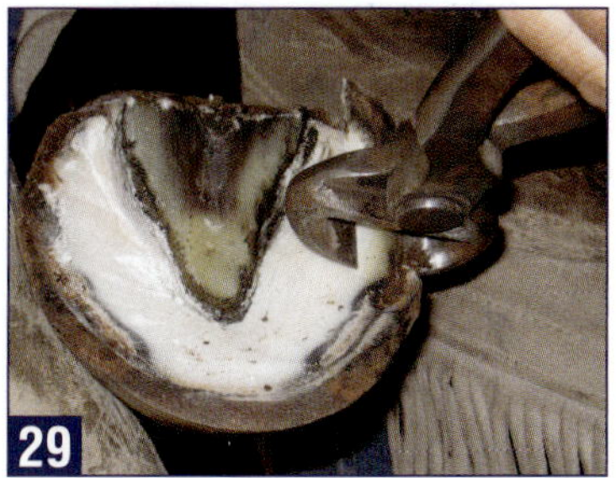

Nip towards the toe.

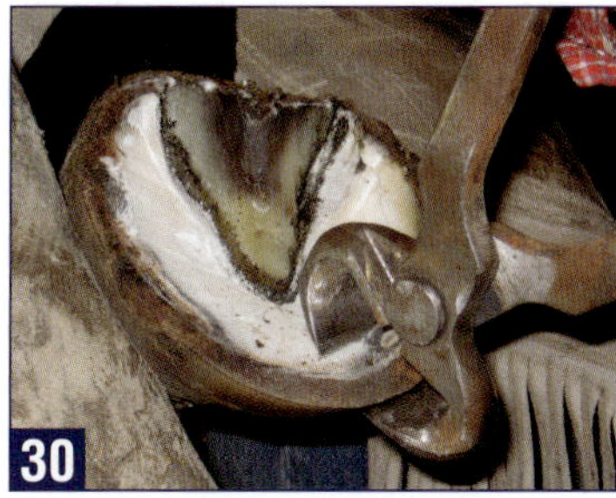

Open the nippers and twist to move into the next cut.

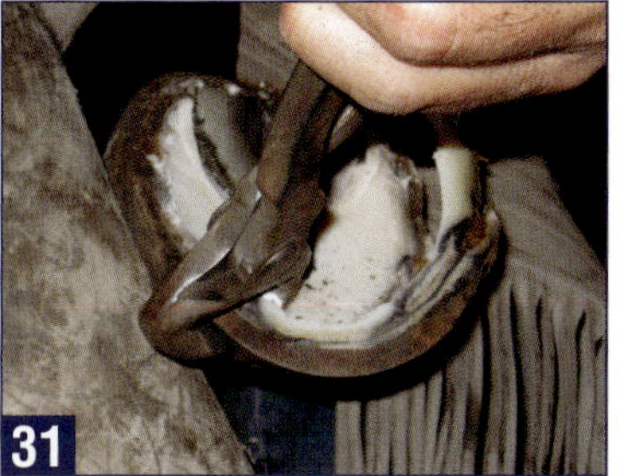

Move towards the heel on the hammer hand side

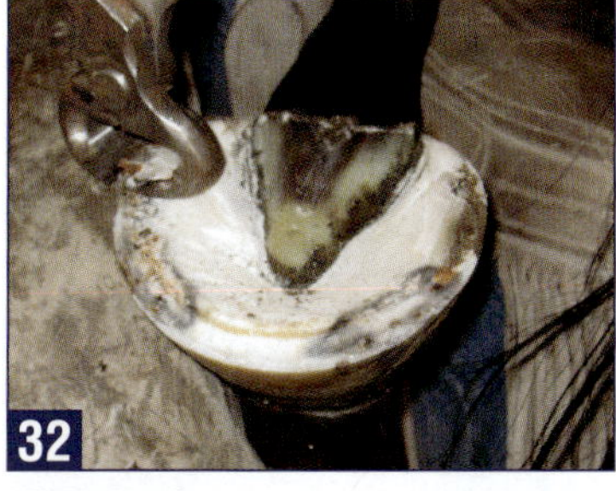

Finish nip.

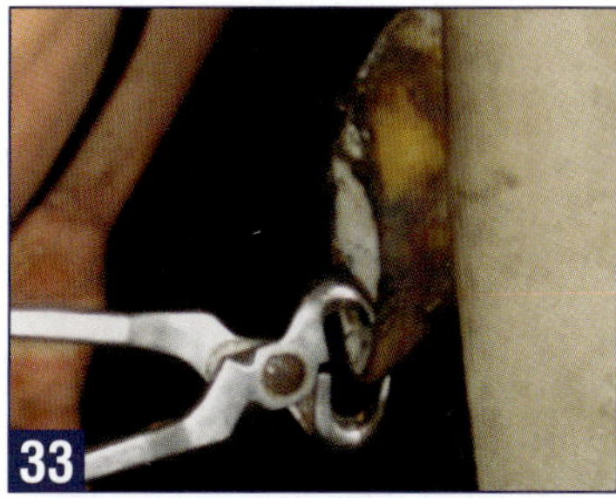

Cody likes to start at the toe.

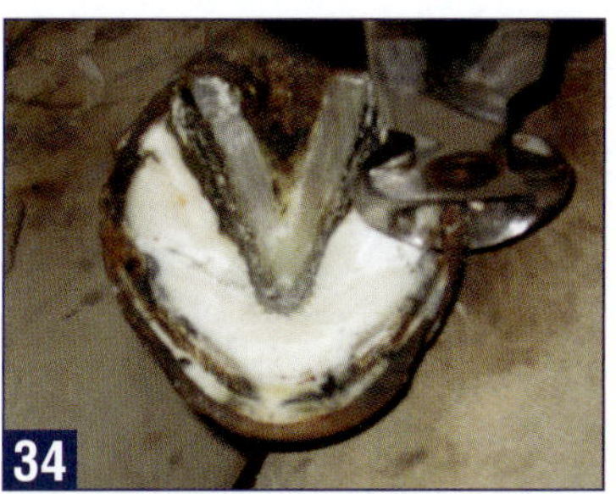

Nip toward one heel.

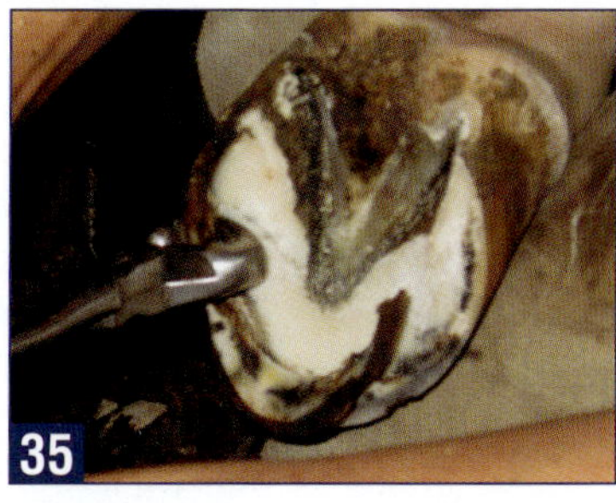

Nip from the toe to the opposite heel.

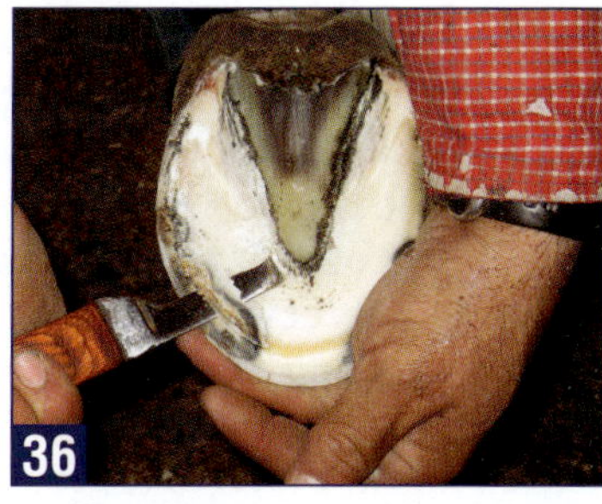

Knife off the little ridge of sole.

Try this technique to stay in a flat plane. Close the nippers to make a cut. Open them just wide enough to accept the next bite, and twist the handles slightly. This will allow the nippers to "walk" into the next area to be nipped. Close the nippers and repeat.

A lot of really good farriers (Cody included) like to start at the toe **(Figures 33-35)**. To do this, cut into the toe at a depth you deem as the appropriate amount of wall to remove, and nip toward the heels. Once you get to one heel, you will just go back to the original cut at the toe and nip back to the opposite heel. This method works just as well as the one I prefer.

After nipping, there will generally be an area of sole that protrudes beyond the plane of the just-trimmed hoof wall. Knife this down so that it is lower than the hoof wall **(Figure 36)**.

The next step is to rasp. Your rasp is one of the most dangerous tools in your shoeing box. With a sharp rasp, you will remove a tremendous amount of horn. It is extremely important that you learn to use this tool correctly. I like to start by reducing the heels to the desired plane of the foot **(Figures 37 -**

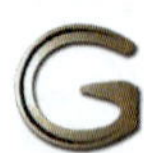

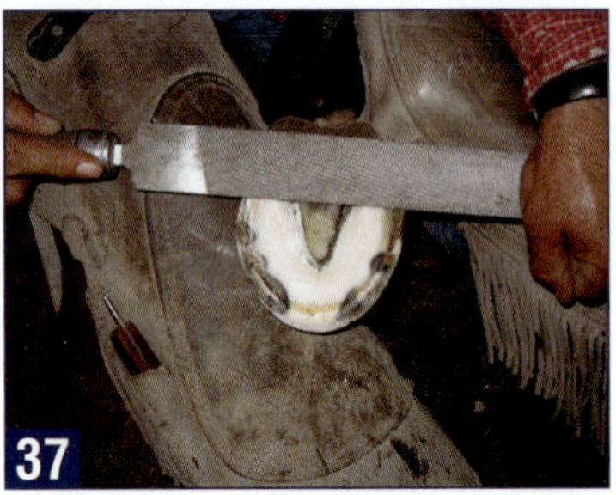

Move across heels with the rasp.

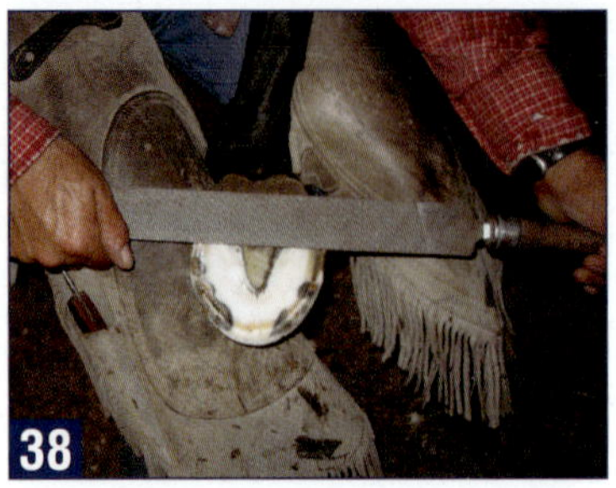

Turn the rasp around and go across the opposite heel. Try to hit the heel furthest from the handle, but barely brush the heel closest to the handle.

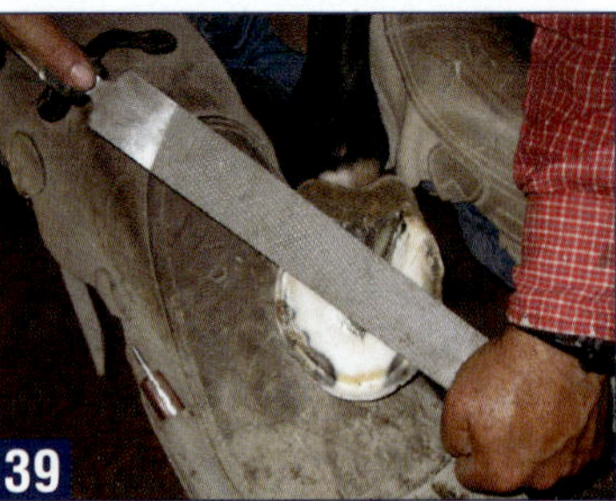

Using the heels as a guide, rasp toward the toe.

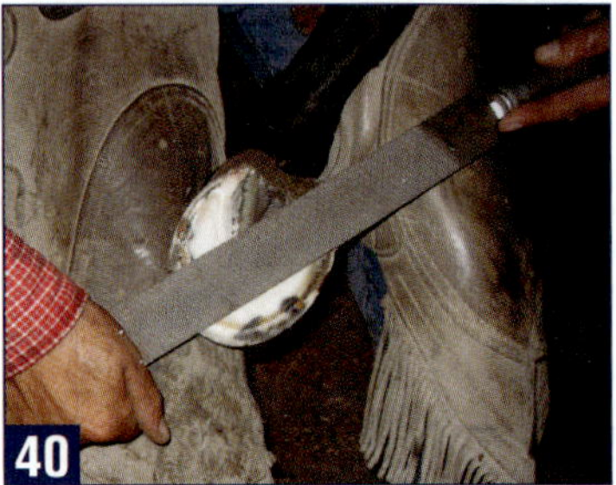

You can switch hands to rasp toward the toe.

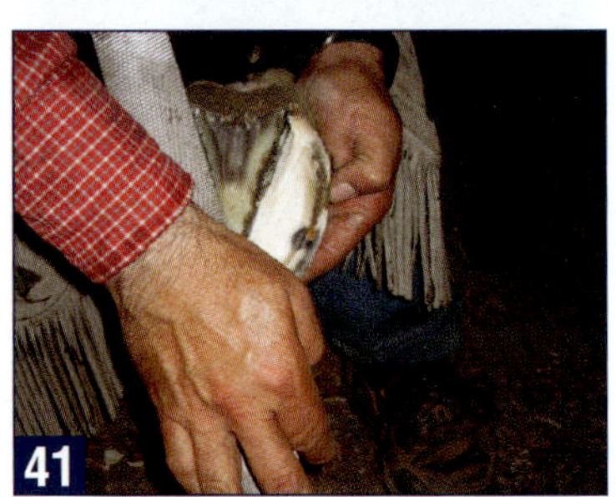

With big frogs, you may have to pull up on the rasp to hit the heels.

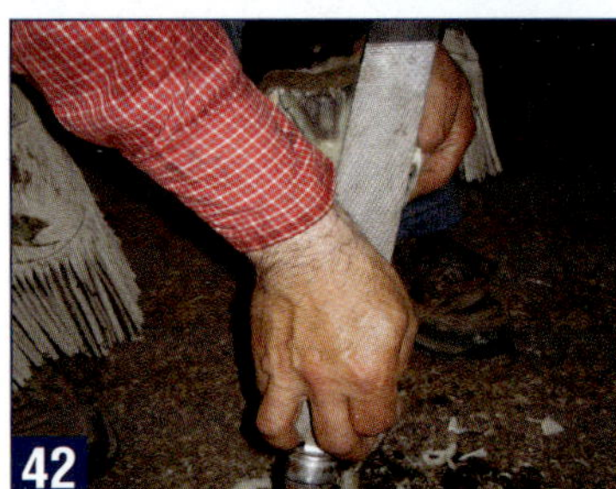

Coming up the opposite heel. Notice my hand position.

38). To do this, move the rasp toward the heel that is being removed. Be careful to prevent the handle from lifting away from the foot as you come across. If you let it lift, you will make a bevel with the outside edge of the wall lower than the inside edge.

Once one heel is done, turn the rasp around and cut across the opposite heel. The goal is to have both heels at exactly the same plane, and level with the desired finished level of the foot.

Using your heels as a guide, rasp downward toward the toe **(Figures 39 - 40)**. As you push the rasp with your hand on the handle, use your opposite hand as a guide to move the rasp across the foot. This means that the rasp is moving toward the toe as well as across the foot. On feet that have a large frog that sticks out past the bottom of the foot, you have to change your technique to get around the frog. On these feet, I pull my rasp upward towards the heel more than pushing it toward the toe **(Figures 41 - 42)**.

One of the rules we make students follow is that they cannot rasp on the sole. As soon as you see the first tooth mark on the sole, you need to do a little bit more knife work. With a hoof knife, you can feel the consistency and texture of the sole easier than with a rasp. Some of the worst sole quicks that I have seen occurred from rasping the sole because the student did not know how far they were going or how much material was being taken.

Another rule for rasping the bottom of the foot is that you should only use the rough side unless you are in a contest or certification situation. The reason for this has to do with rasp longevity, and not really about trimming the foot. A lot of rasps get discarded because the smooth side is worn out, but there is still a lot of life left in the rough side. I like to conserve my smooth side for finishing the outside of the hoof wall, so I do not use it on the bottom very often. You will find that many farriers will take 6 or 7 swipes on the bottom of the foot with the smooth side, when 1 or 2 with the rough side would suffice. When you get competent with your rasp, you will understand what I am talking about.

Once the foot is rasped to what you think is level, get out from under the horse and sight the foot once more. Here you are looking for level and flat. Remember, level is the plane on the bottom of the foot in comparison to the axis of the leg. Flat means

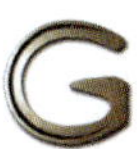

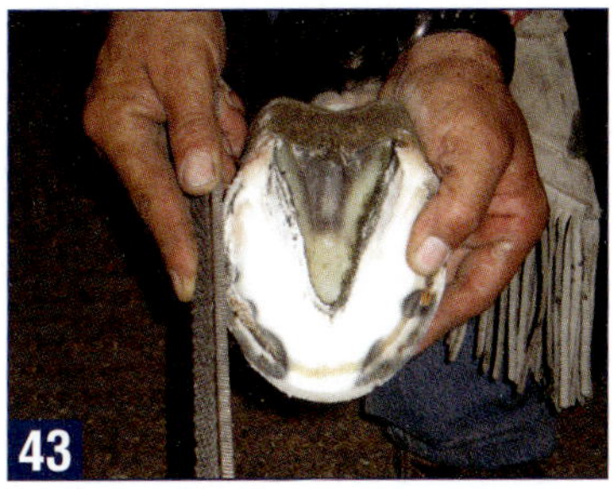

Find a good perimeter for the foot.

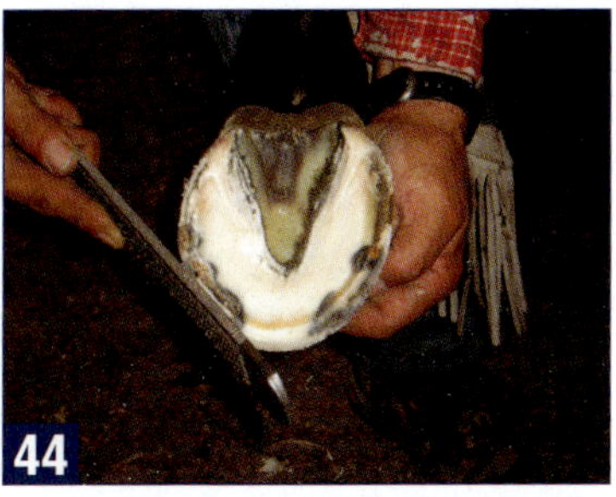

I use the smooth side of the rasp for this most of the time.

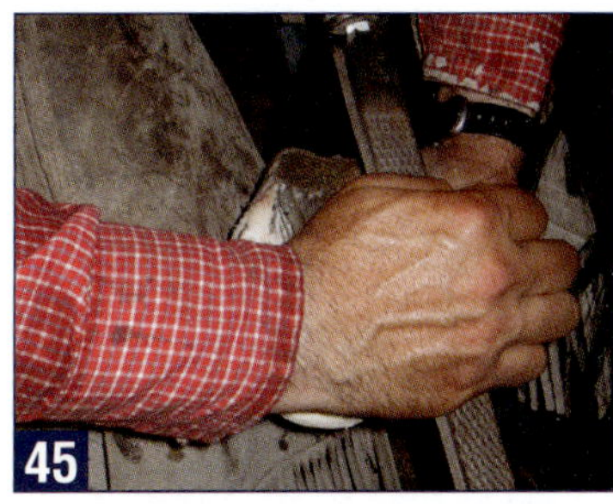

Come right around the foot.

that whatever plane you happen to have achieved on the bottom of the foot is smooth and even. You can have a flat foot that is not level.

After sighting the foot, if everything is what you wanted, get back under the horse and make a symmetrical perimeter. This is one of the most important elements of trimming that gets overlooked by a lot of people. Doing this correctly will set the horse up for the next shoeing as well as make the foot stronger now. We call this "finding the wooden Indian."

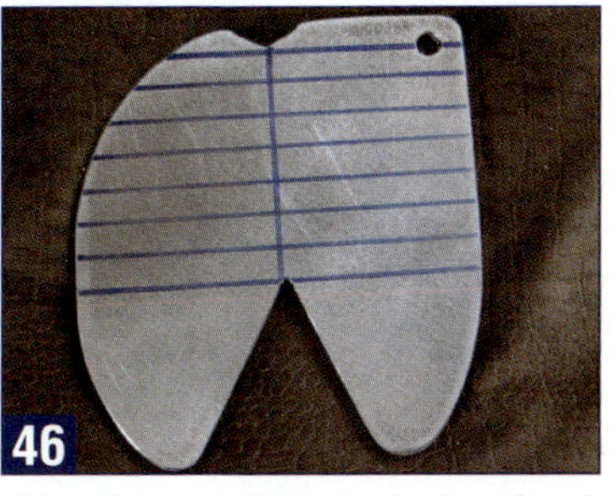

Aluminum plate to help check level on feet and shoes.

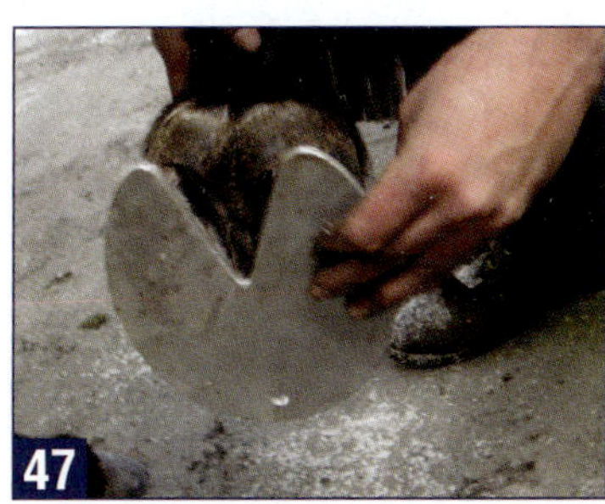

Cody using his aluminum plate to check the foot.

Begin at one heel, and rasp the perimeter with the smooth side of the rasp **(Figure 43)**. Move around the foot until you have the desired shape **(Figures 44 - 45)**. Make sure that you go through the heels all the way to the buttress. I would estimate that at least 80% of the horses I see at contests and certifications around the world are not properly finished through the heels. So many farriers will dress a foot from quarter to quarter, leaving tags, flares, and even dirt behind the widest part of the foot. If I am judging, that competitor, candidate, or student is going to have a bad day.

I heard it once said: "When you trim feet you need to be building shoes." This means you are making a shape in the foot that is easy to make or shape a shoe to. Having sharp corners makes it difficult to shape, so you should be thinking about having a smooth, even flow around the entire perimeter. To go with this saying, when you make shoes, you should be trimming feet. In a perfect situation, you trim a foot, go to the anvil and build the perfect shoe for that foot. One trip to the foot for a hot fit, quench the shoe, and done. That does not always happen, but it is what we try to achieve on a daily basis. Trimming that foot correctly is the starting point.

When I am deciding on the perimeter for a certain foot, I look at the white line, the position of the frog, the thickness of the wall, and the location of the buttress at the heels. All of these are landmarks that together, give me an indication of where I am and where I want to go with a foot. I do not like rules that state things like, "All feet must always be trimmed to the widest part of the frog," or "The white line is always the true shape of the foot." These are general suggestions that may or may not work on the horse you are working on. If they work, that is great. If not, you need to have enough knowledge to think outside of the box that rules like that put you in.

You can use a flat piece of aluminum plate to check the flatness of your foot. In **Figure 46**, you can see how this plate is cut out with a triangular area to clear any large frog. Cody is using a plate on the foot in **Figure 47**. With the solar surface of the foot trimmed, you should be looking at feet that look like **Figure 48** for a front foot or **Figure 49** for a hind.

The last part of the job is to dress the foot on the

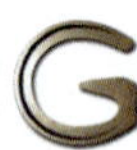

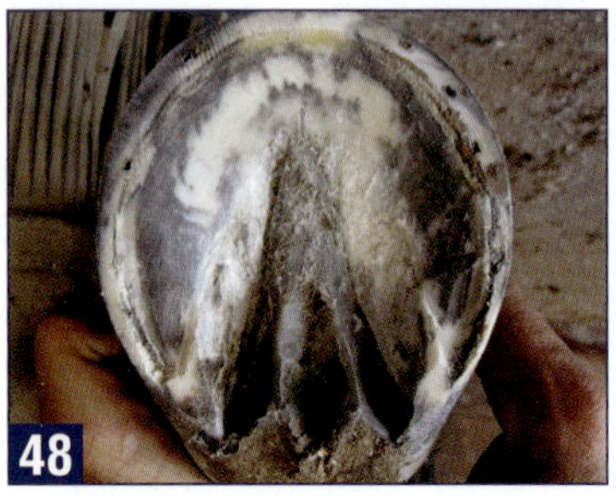
Trimmed front.

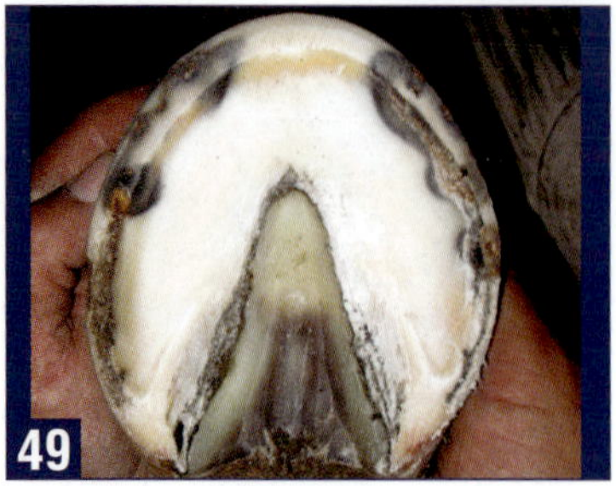
Trimmed hind.

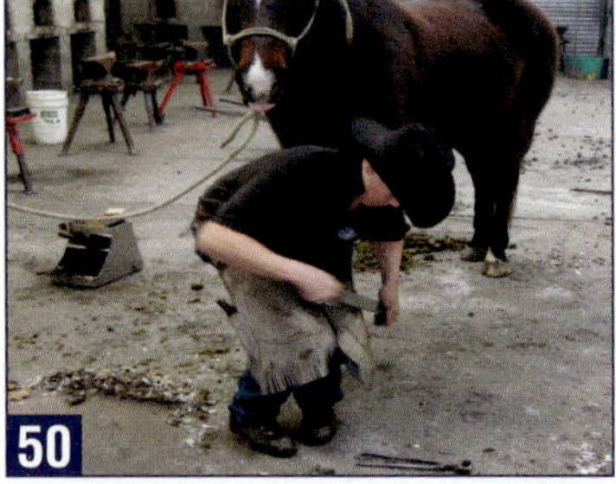

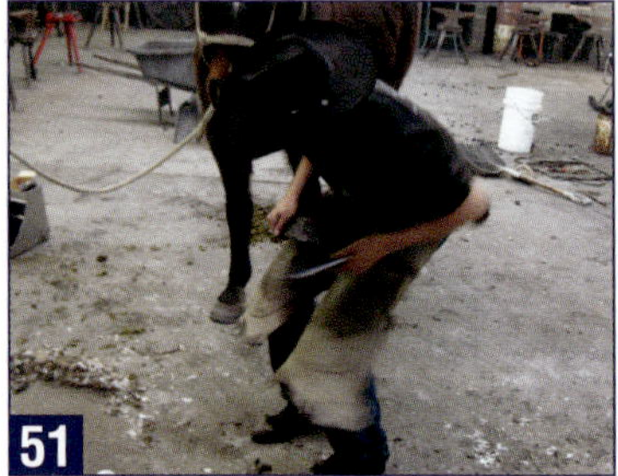
Positions Cody uses to dress a front foot.

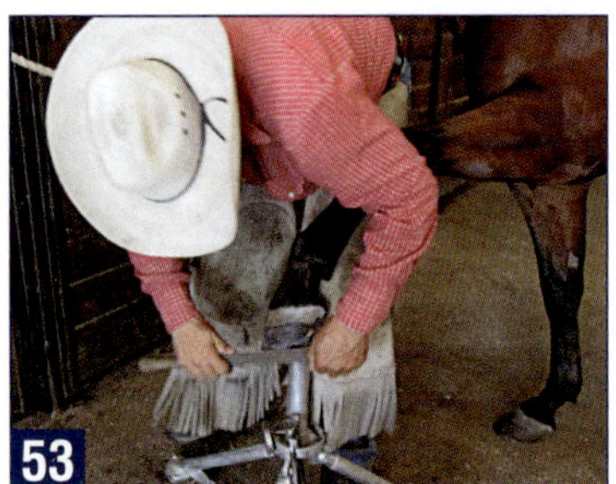
In front of the horse finishing the foot.

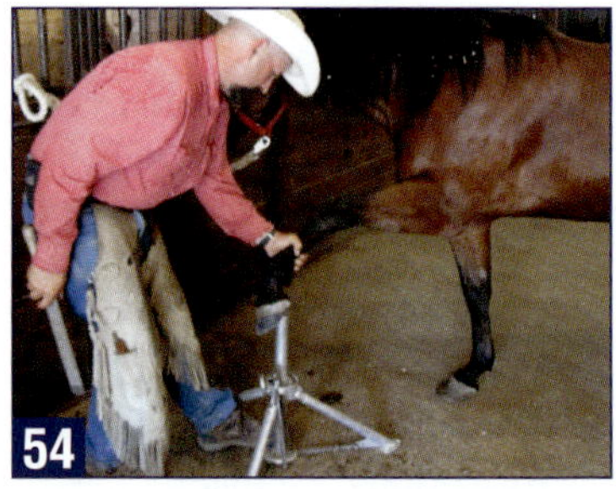
When I move around a foot on a hoof stand, I try to keep a hand on the leg.

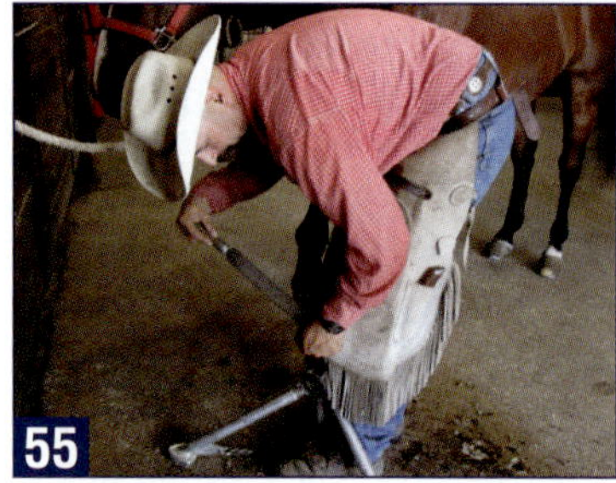
Opposite side for finishing.

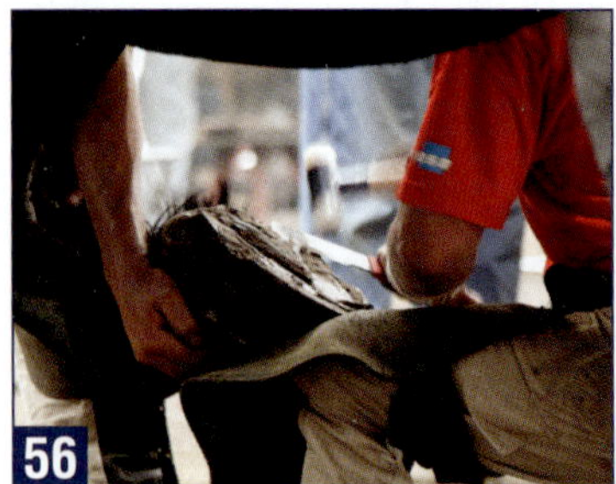
Swiss team trimming a foot at Calgary.

stand. Cody likes to use his knee **(Figures 50-52)**, but I will drive home for my hoof stand if I forget it. When I dress the foot, I know exactly where I am going because I found the perimeter for the foot while I was working on the bottom of the foot. If you have not taken the time to find the foot from the bottom, you can be easily misled when you are dressing the outside. Dress the foot with long, even strokes. Use the rough side if you have a lot of flare to come off, and then clean it up and make it smooth with the fine side of your rasp. I like to dress toward the heels with diagonal strokes. I will stand on one side while I dress the opposite side of the hoof **(Figure 53)** and then move around the horse **(Figure 54)** to finish the

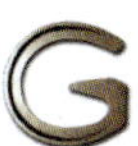

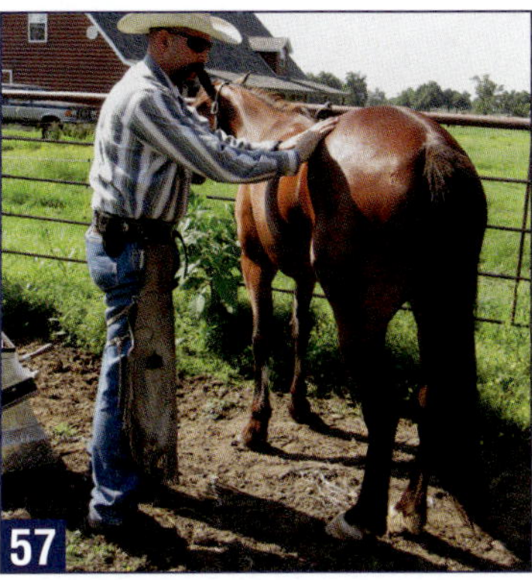

Position to begin picking up a hind foot.

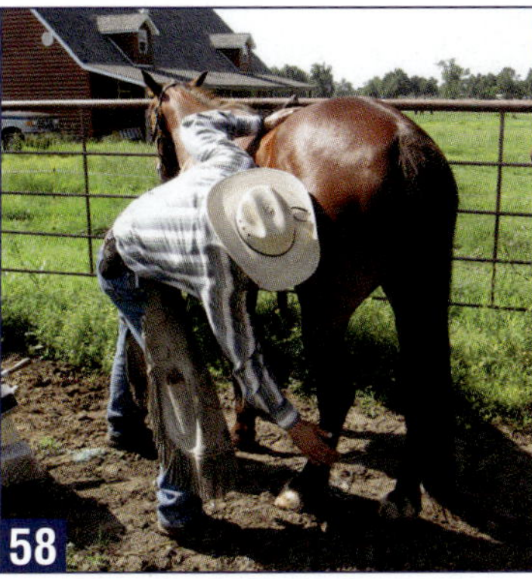

Hand on cannon bone.

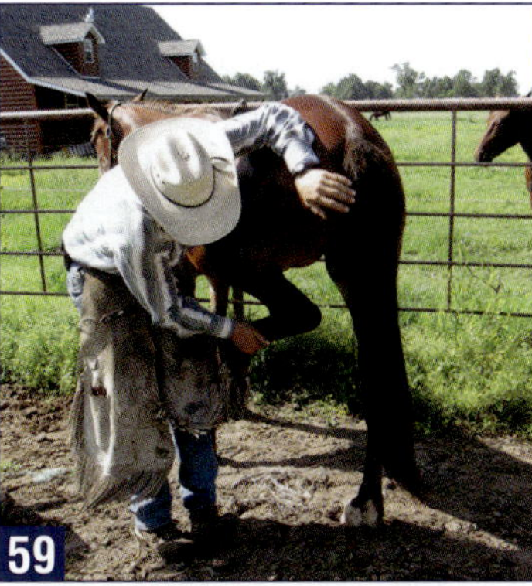

Lifting foot toward belly, and crossing over with inside hand to grab the toe.

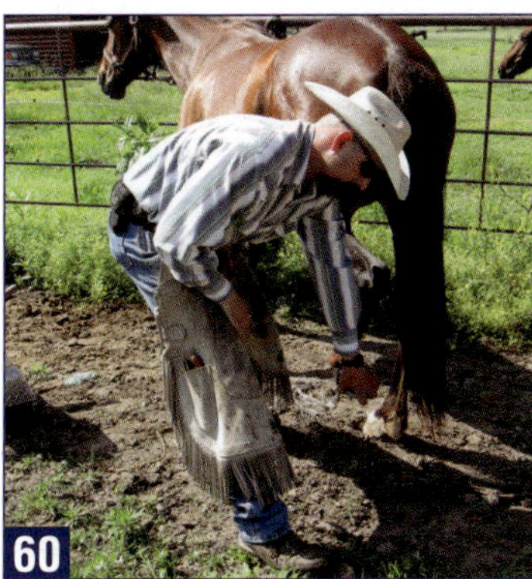

Holding the toe to allow the horse to balance.

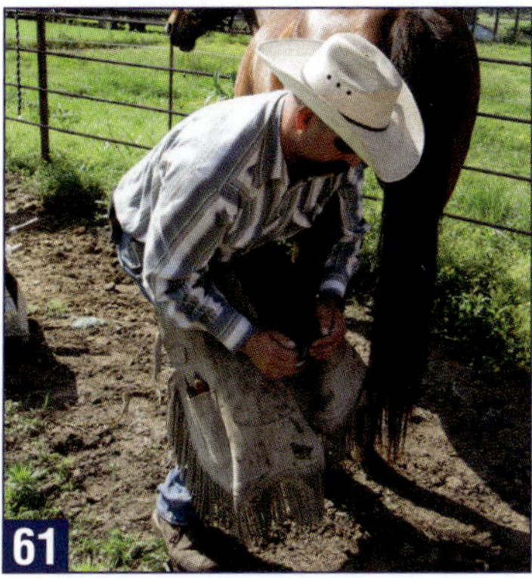

Moving into position.

other side of the foot **(Figure 55)**.

If the horse is to be shod, I will put a small bevel on the outside of the foot. For horses that are to be left barefoot, the bevel should be about three times as large as the bevel you put on a foot that is going to be shod. The bevel will keep the foot from breaking away as easily as a sharp edge would.

There are other trimming methods used around the world. In **Figure 56**, you can see some Swiss competitors at the World Championship Blacksmiths' Contest in Calgary. They trim with the customers holding the feet. This farrier is driving a toeing knife through the foot with a mallet while his partner holds the foot.

To pick up and trim hind feet, face the horse and place both hands on the hip **(Figure 57)**. Run your rearmost hand down the back of the leg to the cannon bone **(Figure 58)**. Pull forward on the cannon bone, lifting the foot toward the horse's belly **(Figure 59)**. Turn toward the rear of the horse and cross over your arm with your inside arm. Grab the toe of the foot and release the hand you had on the cannon bone **(Figure 60)**. Stay still for a couple of seconds to allow the horse to gain its balance.

I have a lot of people complain about how horses lean on them while they work on the hind feet. A horse only leans if it is allowed to. Give the horse the option of falling down or standing balanced, and it will stand balanced most of the time. If you hold the horse's weight, the horse will put it on you. The short pause after grabbing the toe of the hind foot is critical to making a horse balance on its own.

Once the horse has decided to stand, place the knee of your inside leg against the horse's fetlock. Slowly take the foot back, without jerking it or pulling it too far outside the line of the body **(Figure 61)**. Stay as low as you can, put your knees together, and rest the foot over the lap of your inside leg

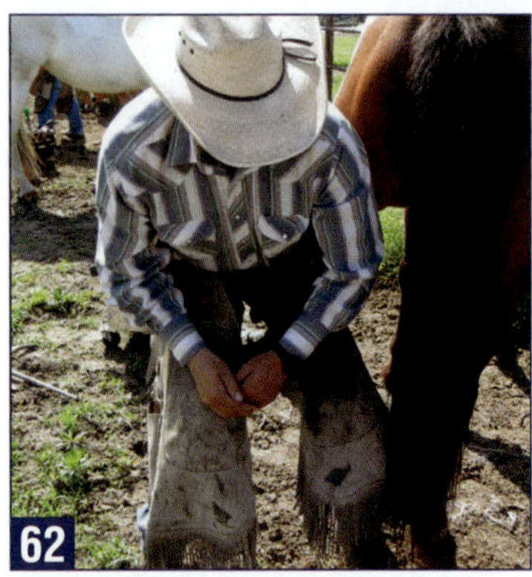

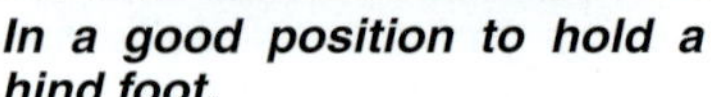
In a good position to hold a hind foot.

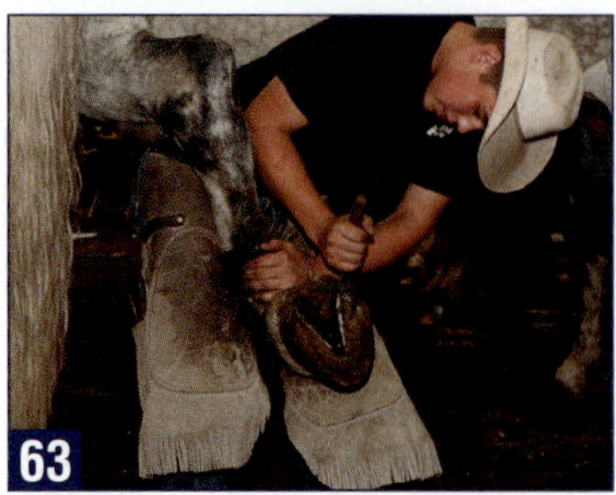

Cody holding the hind of a draft horse.

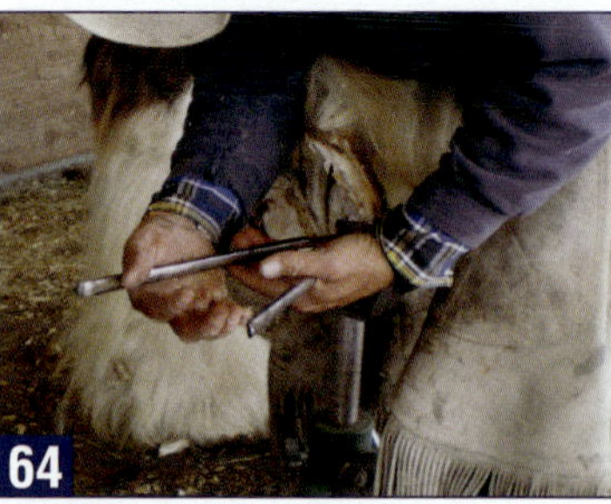

Working on a cradle.

(Figures 62 - 63). There is quite a bit of pressure from the hock on my ribcage, and this helps to hold the foot against my inside leg. If at first this feels pretty uncomfortable, you know that you are doing it correctly. With time and practice, you will find that it is not too tough a position.

A lot of farriers use a cradle for the hind feet **(Figure 64)**. I have tried to get used to a cradle but without too much success. I can knife and nip with a cradle, but I don't like to rasp or nail with one. Had I learned from the beginning, it would be a normal part of shoeing.

Trimming feet correctly is about vision and your ability to see the finished product inside the foot you are presented with, exactly like the wooden Indian carver does. Take the time to get the training needed to see what that good foot should look like, and you will become a prosperous farrier who is in demand.

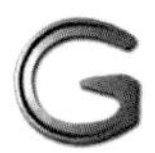

Chapter 23 MEDIOLATERAL BALANCE

Like many things in the world of farriery, balance can be controversial. I believe that most of this controversy comes from a lack of anatomical understanding and knowledge. Unfortunately, there are some vocal horseshoers that have deeply seated beliefs about what to do with feet yet who do not know enough about anatomy to have a defensible position. This does not prevent them from voicing their opinion, and we have a lot of the blind leading the blind in this industry. When everyone working on a horse is on the same page regarding anatomy, there is a common ground for discussion of balance and other items that are typically the cause of disagreement.

To evaluate mediolateral balance, the foot should be viewed in the air and on flat ground. Since there is not a reciprocal apparatus on the front limb, it is possible to see the front foot in a weight-bearing position. On the hind end, it is impossible to see the foot in the air in a weight-bearing situation. This is due to the reciprocal apparatus. Since the flexing of one joint also flexes the other joints in the hind limb, the simple act of picking up the hind foot folds the fetlock and changes how the plane on the bottom of the hoof relates to the axis of the leg.

FRONT FOOT

Begin by looking at the foot on flat ground with the horse standing square. Evaluate the conformation of the leg and limb. You will be making judgments about where the foot is placed on the ground under the limb. Any defect such as carpus valgus, toed-in, base wide, etc. will play a part in where the foot is and where it should be.

For the purpose of this discussion, we are going to discuss the straight horse. Ideally, the foot is under the axis of the radius, carpus, cannon bone, and pastern. A straight line would bisect the limb and go through the middle of the foot.

We should also distinguish between the terms "level" and "flat." When speaking about level on the bottom of the foot, we are referring to the plane of the bottom of the foot as it relates to the axis of the leg. We are usually looking for a plane that is perpendicular to the axis of the leg. When speaking of flat, we are just talking about the nature of the surface on the bottom of the foot. So, you can have a foot that is flat but not level, or level but not flat. These are important distinctions, and when you work with other farriers, you should make sure that you are both talking about the same things.

Pick up the foot and hold the cannon bone with your outside hand **(Figure 1)**. Holding with your inside hand is likely to cause you to pull the foot out too far out from under the horse. You are trying to keep the foot as close to under the body as you can. With the foot hanging loosely at the end of the leg, place you head against the horse's body and determine how the plane on the bottom of the foot relates to the axis of the leg. It is also important that you hold just the cannon bone. There is a lot of movement in the coffin joint, so if you hold the pastern or foot itself, you are likely to get a false reading of level. Next time you have a foot up, wiggle it around by just the foot. You will be surprised how much movement there is.

You will hear the terms long axis and short axis when farriers talk about mediolateral balance. Long axis refers to the axis of the cannon bone and pastern bones. Short axis is referring to the pastern alone. Horses that have faults that occur in the fetlock joint can be difficult to balance.

While you are evaluating the foot, you should be aware of how the horse is standing. The head and neck should be straight. It is amazing how much the level on the bottom of the foot changes when you allow the head to move. The foot will appear higher on the side that the head is turned towards. You can use this knowledge when competing or taking exams. If you have a holder that understands this anatomical principle, they can make a foot appear a certain way by how they hold the foot. This is valuable information if you are at a contest or certification.

There is a device called a T-square that you can use to determine whether the foot is flat in relation

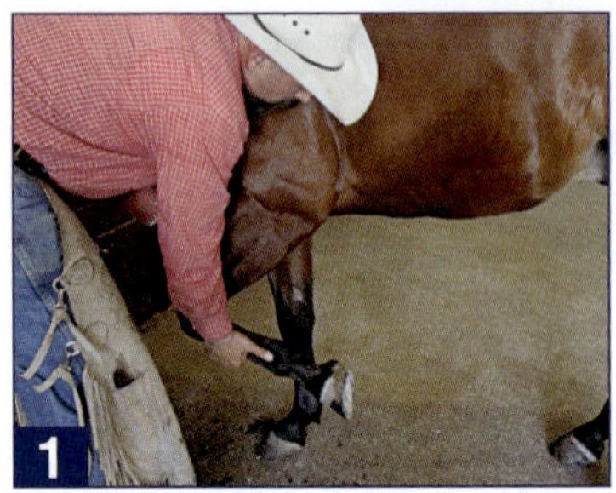

Holding a front leg to evaluate the mediolateral balance.

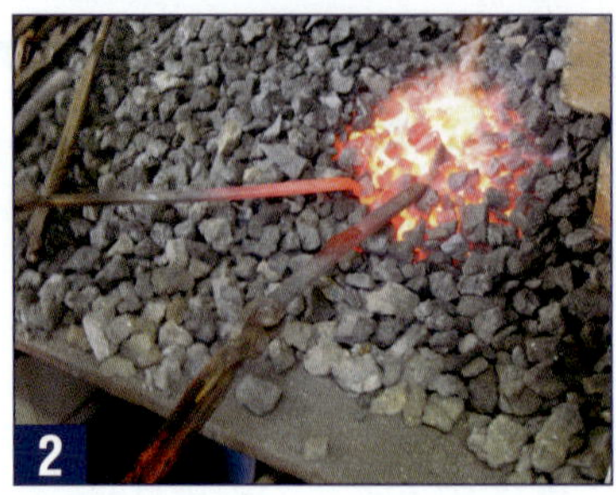

Metal ready to be welded into a T-square.

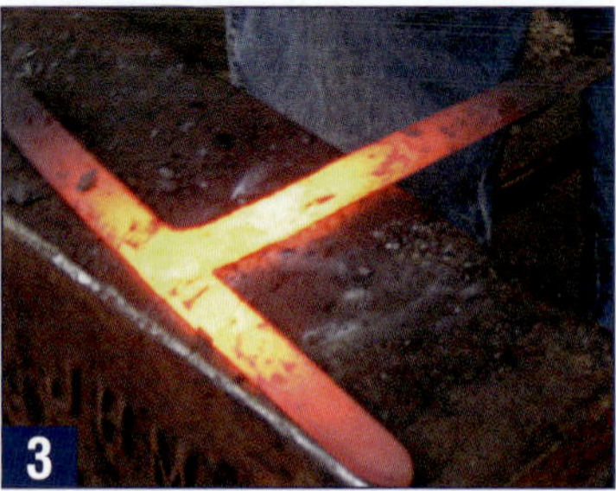

Welding the T-square.

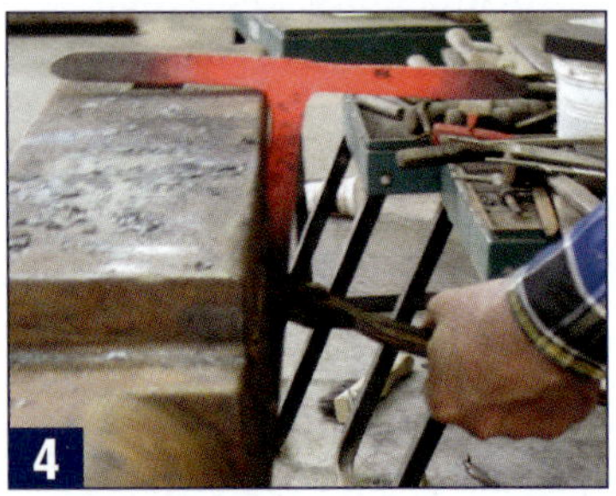

Forging to crisp up the edges of the tool.

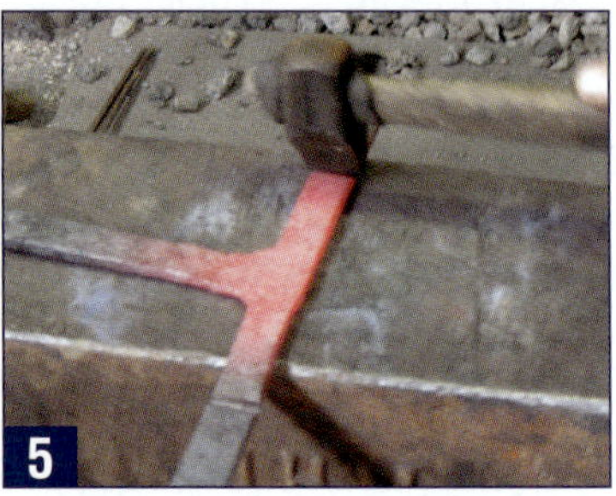

Cutting off the ends to make it as wide as a normal foot.

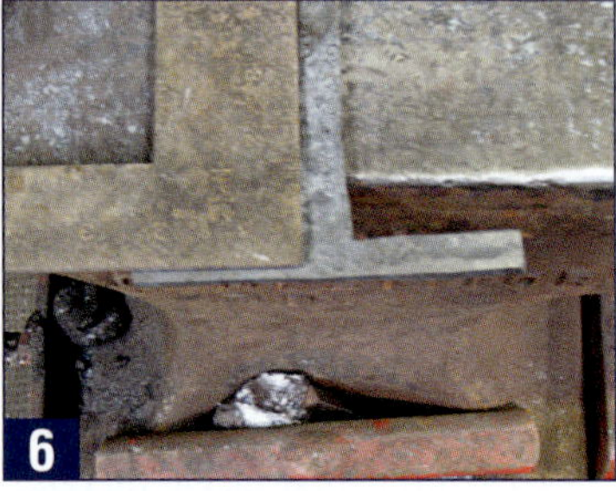

Finished T-square being compared to a square.

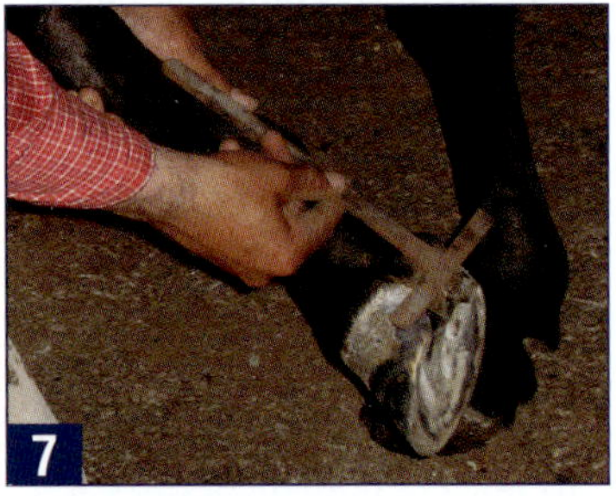

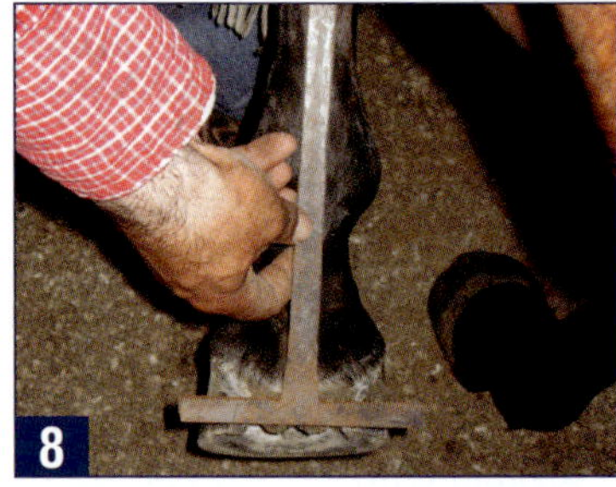

Using a T-square.

to the axis of the leg. This is an easy item to make, so here are a few pictures of making one (**Figures 2-6**).

To use this item, hold the leg as described, and lay the T-square on the palmar aspect of the leg, with the long piece on the axis of the leg. Compare the bottom of the foot to the flat end of the T-square. If you look carefully at **Figure 7**, you will see that I am holding the foot with my inside hand, but I am reaching around the medial side of the limb to hold the cannon bone from the medial side instead of the lateral side. **Figure 8** shows the T-square on the leg.

HIND FOOT

One of the most common ways of evaluating a hind foot for balance is incorrect. I was taught — as were many farriers — to let the cannon bone hang across your leg, place your head over the hock to view down the back of the leg, and then compare the bottom of the foot to what you imagine to be the axis of the cannon. I am doing this in **Figures 9 and 10**. With your knowledge of anatomy, I am certain that you can see the potential problems with this. The first is the fact that you are looking down the cannon bone in such a way that you cannot see the axis of the cannon bone, or how it would relate to the body of the horse. What you can see is whether the foot is flat or not, so this is a good method for seeing flat. Remember, there is a difference between flat and level.

The next problem is that when a hind foot is lifted, the reciprocal apparatus is engaged. Since this happens, it is not possible to see the bottom of the hind foot in a weight-bearing position. Because of this, it is more important to evaluate a hind foot on the ground than in the air. Be aware that what you see in the air may make you want to trim in a plane that contradicts what you see on the ground. What you see on the ground should win this battle. Look at **Figure 11**. This is a drawing of a dorsal view of the lower leg, showing the fetlock joint. This one is straight, and if the hind limb were lifted, the foot should fold up straight. With this kind of perfect conformation, you could evaluate the foot in the air as in **Figures 9 and 10**.

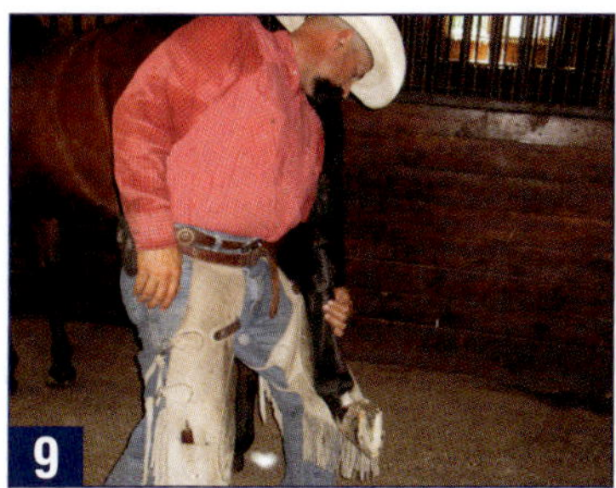

Holding a hind leg to look at the flatness of the bottom of the foot. This is an old way of evaluating mediolateral balance on the hind leg.

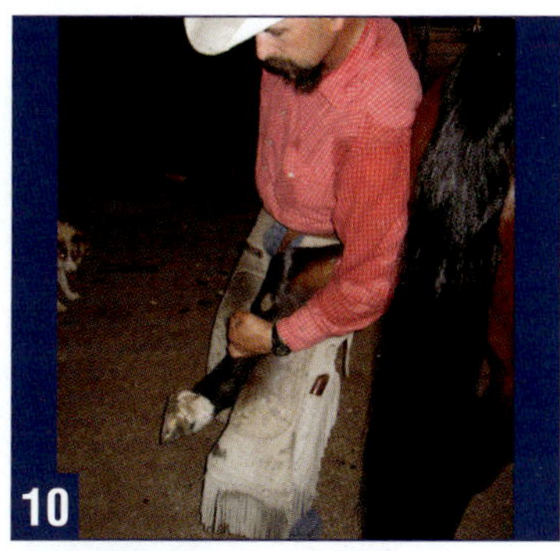

Another view of Figure 9.

However, there are very few fetlock joints that are straight. Most look like the drawing in **Figure 12**. This means that when the fetlock is bent, the foot comes up at an angle. This gives you a false view of what the bottom of the foot should be in comparison to the leg. Go back to the chapter on bones and look at the distal end of the cannon bones pictured there. You will see that the distal end is not perpendicular to the axis of the cannon bone.

Here is what happens: The foot is lifted off the ground and the fetlock bends. If the distal end of the cannon bone is not perfectly square, the foot and pastern are bent around a joint that is at an angle. This will end up making the bottom of the foot look like it is not square with the leg. When the foot is

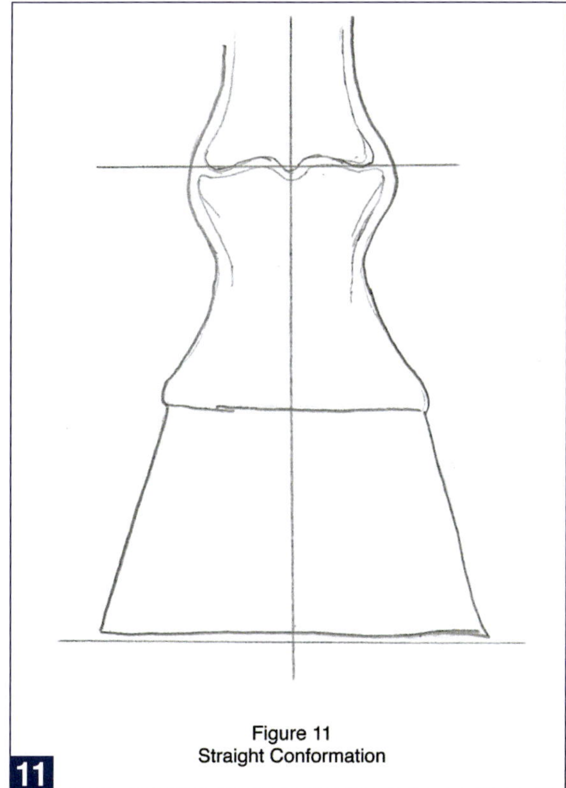

Drawing of a straight fetlock joint and foot.

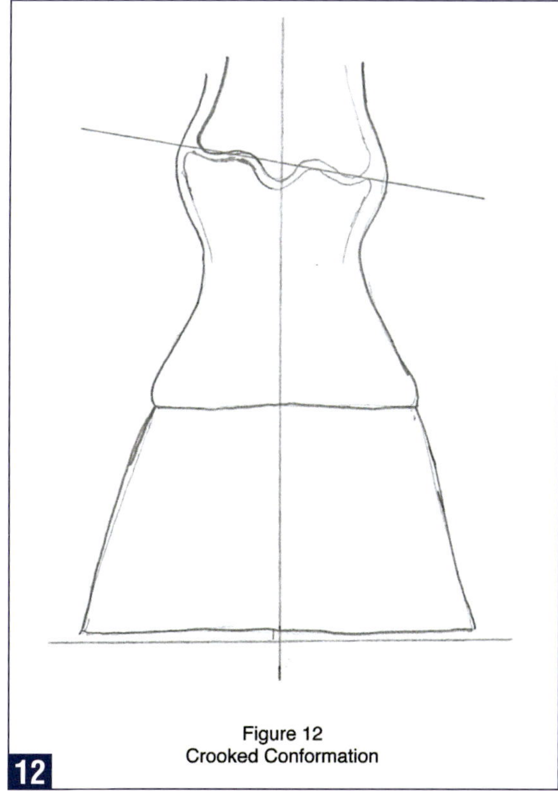

Drawing of a crooked fetlock joint straight foot.

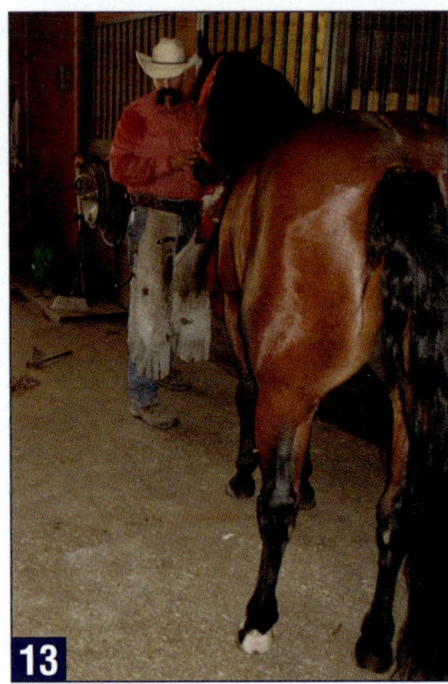
Evaluating the hind foot in a weight-bearing position.

on the ground, it is in a weight-bearing position because it is weight bearing. Any inconsistency in the fetlock will not matter to the level of the foot if it is placed under the bony column.

It does not matter at all what a foot looks like in the air. What really matters is how it is loaded when the horse is moving.

To evaluate the mediolateral balance, have the horse stand squared up on flat ground. Move to the head of the horse and stand just to the outside of the shoulder. Look at the leg and foot, determining if the foot is under the leg or not. This is what I am trying to determine for the horse in **Figure 13**.

If there is a discrepancy, the most common thing to see will be the foot on the ground to the lateral side of the leg. If that is the case, it is an indication that the foot is high lateral. On a lot of horses, when you pick up this foot that is placed on the ground to the outside of the bony column, the foot will appear to be level in the air. To correct it, the foot should be trimmed so that it looks like it is high medially when you have it in the air.

Because it looks level in the air, it is common for shoers who do not understand conformation, anatomy and the reciprocal apparatus to leave the foot there. They are not willing to do what the foot on the ground is telling them has to be done. How the foot bears weight is the most important consideration when determining how to balance a foot.

I hope that by the time you have reached this point in this textbook, you are looking at feet a little bit differently. There are a lot of things in the world of farriery that have been done by tradition for years, even though they don't make anatomical sense. Evaluating hind feet in the air is one of those things.

The end result we all want is a horse that is sound and able to do the job demanded of it. We also want this horse to last as long as possible and have a comfortable life. Knowing how to balance a foot correctly is paramount in this quest, so please be certain that you understand this chapter.

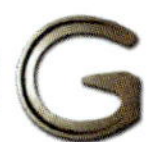

Chapter

24 NORMAL SHOEING ON NORMAL FEET

The majority of shoeing done by most farriers is ordinary shoeing on sound, normal horses. It still takes a lot of skill and practice to become good at the basic shoeing job. I have taught farriery for most of my life, and it is amazing how often I hear from prospective students that they just want to get good enough to do their own horse. If you want to be good enough to just do your own horses, you really need to be good enough to do any horse. In fact, I would like my own horses to be done as well as possible. That requires a higher level of expertise than just average standards and average skills.

For us, normal shoeing is a simple, open-heeled shoe, generally with six nails, and most of the time the shoe will be clipped. The following is the way that I shoe a horse when I am working on my own.

Tie the horse in a comfortable spot that is not too far from the forge and anvil. Twenty feet would be fine. I would like to have level ground to work on, and I don't mind if it is concrete or rubber mats. However, I have done more than my share of horses while exposed to the elements (**Figure 1**). Good lighting is also a requirement, more so now than in my youth.

Begin by giving the feet a quick look to determine which is the longest of the front feet. If they appear the same, I generally start with the near front. Why? I don't know, but it is the way I have done it for so long, it seems like there should be a reason.

I pick up that foot, put it between my knees, and pull the shoe. I will then either just clean the foot, or better yet, do my preliminary knife work on the sole and frog. At this point, I will get out from under the horse and sight the foot. For horses that do not have a shoe on, I like to clean the foot out one-handed before I get under the foot for the first time. I then sight the foot prior to getting under it. Once I sight the foot, I will know where I am going to nip (**Figures 2 and 3**).

Once the knife work is done, I nip the foot. I like to nip from the left heel through the opposite heel. Cody likes to nip from the toe back through each heel (**Figure 4**), and Kelly does it like I do. After nipping, I will take the little edge of sole off with my knife and rasp the foot flat. Next, I rasp around the perimeter of the foot, making sure to go through the heels, and create as good a shape as that foot will allow (see the section on hoof prep and the wooden Indian). Without putting the foot down, I will grab the leg with my outside hand, turn my body toward the horse, and bring the foot forward to the stand (**Figure 5**). I rasp the foot to match the perimeter that I created, and that foot is trimmed and ready to be fit.

This exact sequence will then be repeated for the

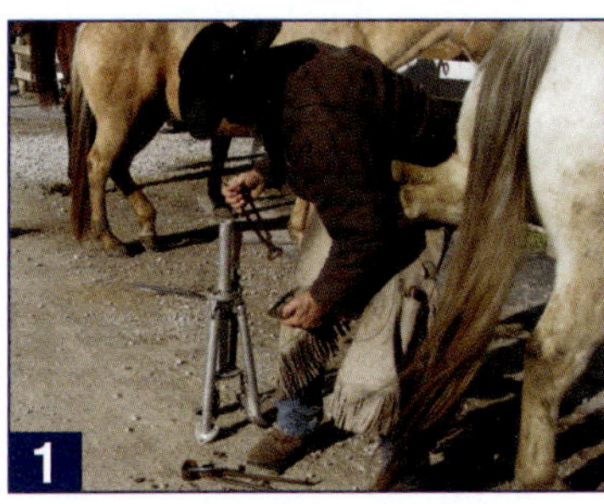

Working outside in the winter.

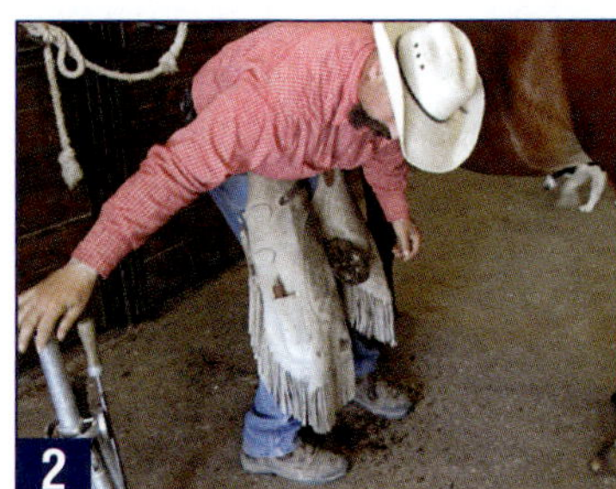

Beginning to trim.

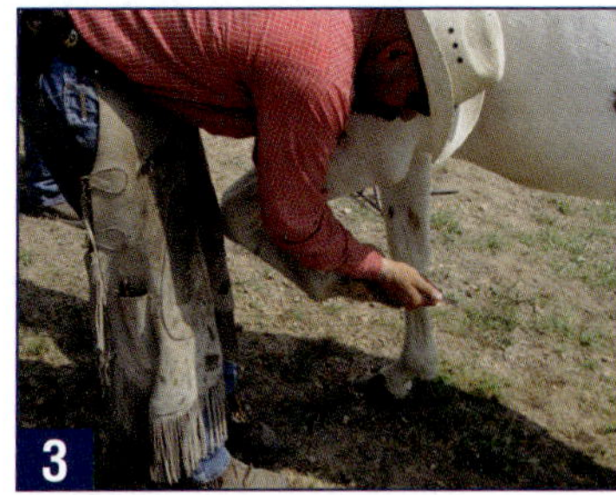

Cleaning out the foot from the outside.

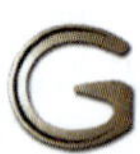

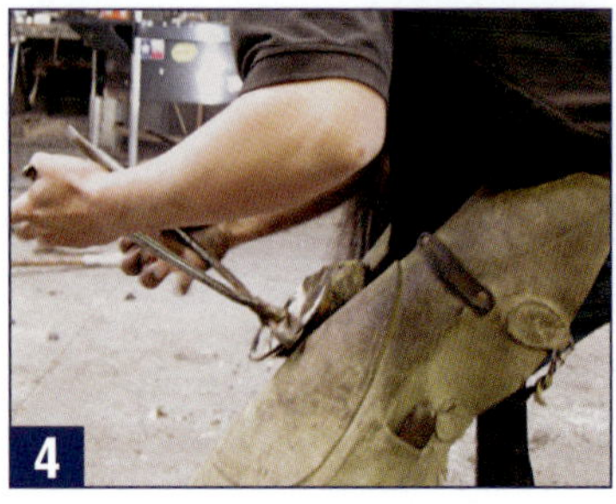
Cody nipping from the toe back.

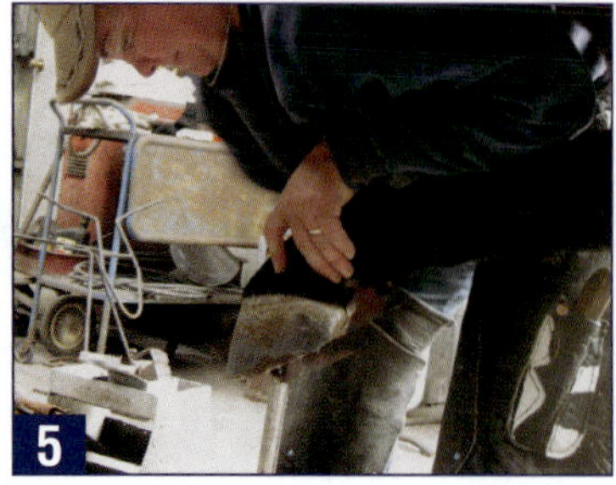
Kelly working on a hoof stand.

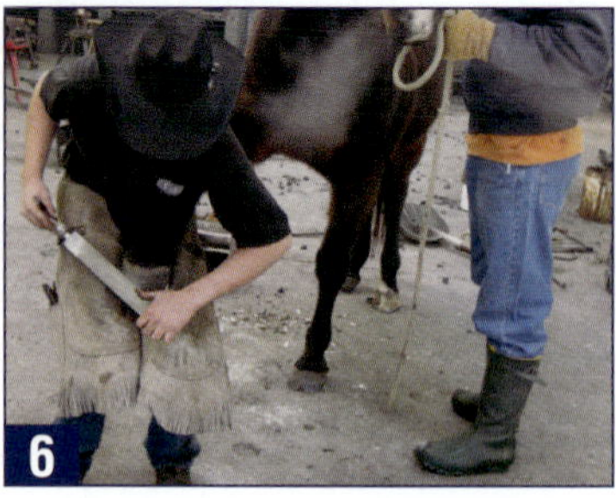
Cody dressing on high knee.

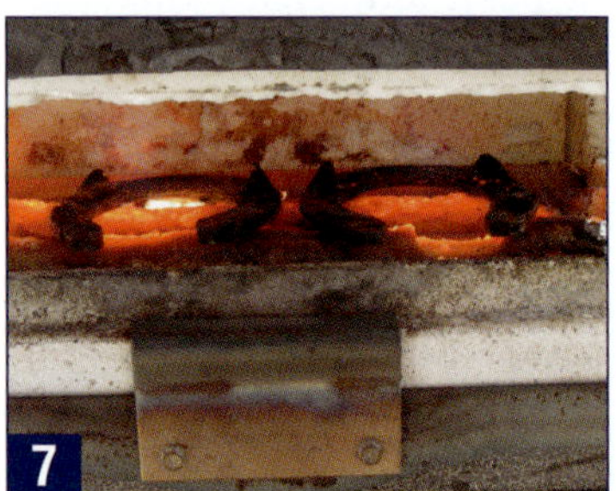
Resets in the fire.

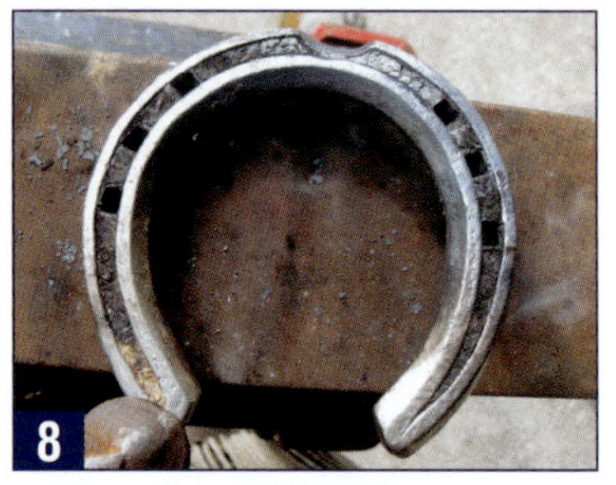
Concave shoe needing cleaning.

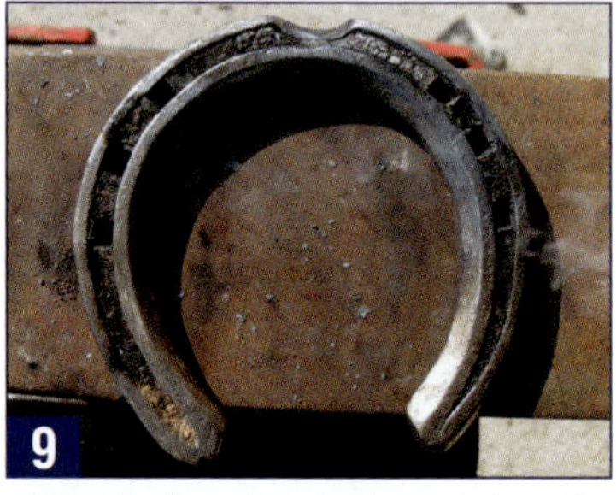
After being heated and the dirt dried out.

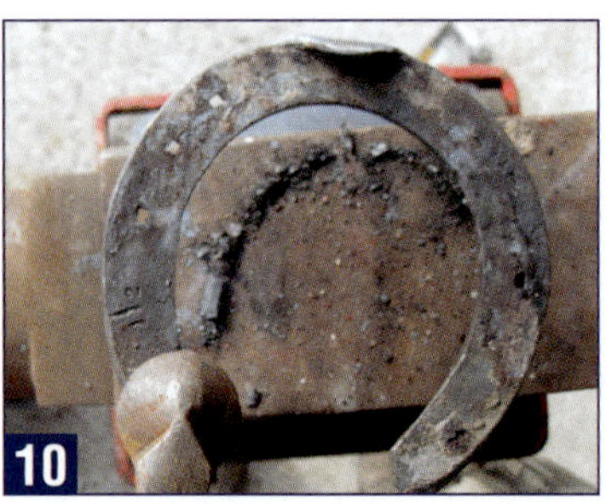
Tapping the shoe against the anvil.

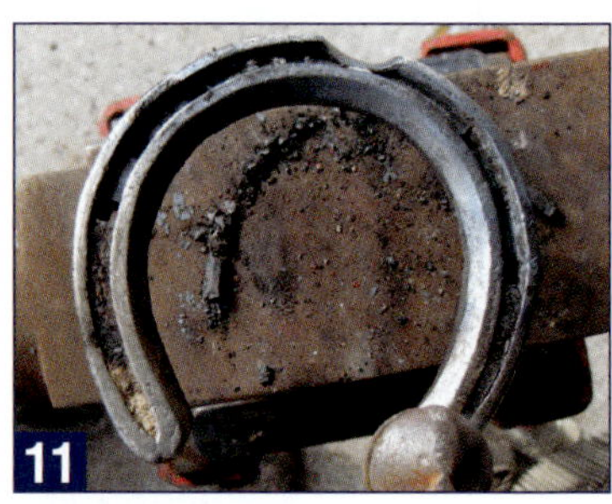
The dirt cleaned out of the groove.

next front foot. Then I move to the hind foot on the same side as the second front foot, generally the off hind. I repeat the process, with the exception that I don't put the hind foot between my legs. Also, I will grab the leg with my inside hand to move the foot to the stand. I will put that foot on my knee, and walk it forward to the stand. Cody does not like a hoof stand (youth), so he will just walk the leg forward and leave it on his knee **(Figure 6)**.

Now I get to the last foot. I will pull the shoe and knife the foot. Once that is accomplished, I will put the two front shoes in the fire **(Figure 7)**. If the horse is a reset, I will hang out at the forge for about 1 minute to heat the shoes up enough to tap and brush the mud out of the crease. I then go back to the horse and trim the final foot. The shoes will be hot and ready to shape, clip, or if resets, level. When I come back from trimming the last foot, I place the two hind shoes in the fire and fit my front shoes.

Just a quick note on resetting shoes hot. You can see in **Figure 8** that we have a concave shoe that has been pulled from the foot and still has dirt in the crease. I place the shoe in the forge for about 30 seconds, just long enough to dry out the dirt in the crease **(Figure 9)**. Be certain that you don't leave the shoe in the fire too long. Any sand in the crease will turn to glass and only clog the nail holes further. With the dirt completely dry, tap the shoe on the face of the anvil with the ground surface down **(Figure 10)**. This will cause most of the dirt to come out of the crease **(Figure 11)**. Brush the hoof surface, and the shoe is ready to heat, level **(Figure 12),** and hot fit.

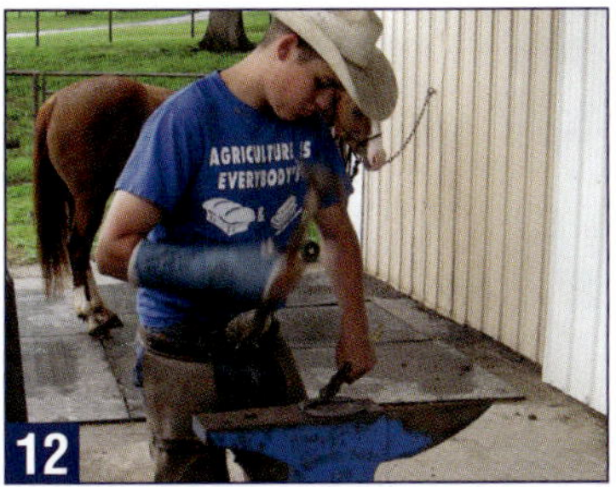

12 *Cody leveling a shoe.*

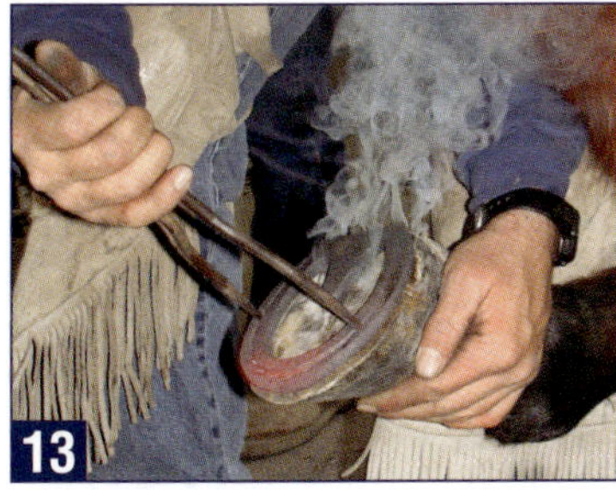

13 *Hot fitting.*

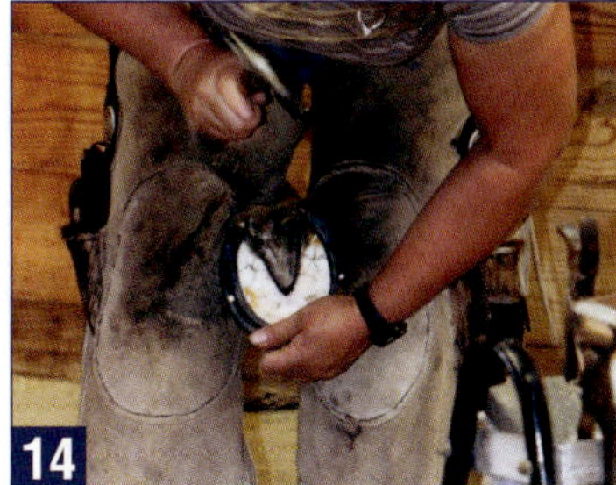

14 *Kelly nailing.*

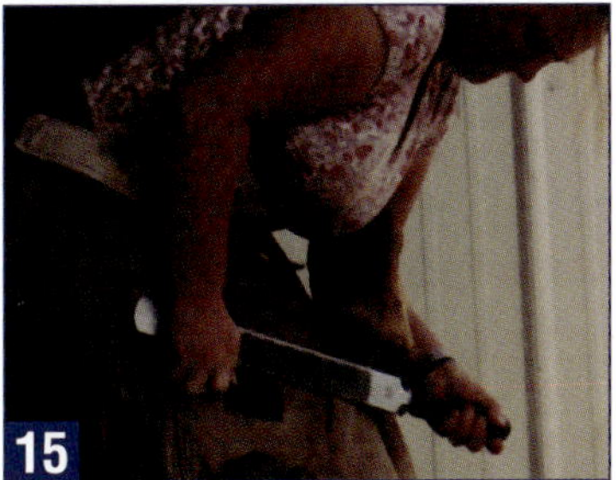

15 *Kelly finishing on her knee.*

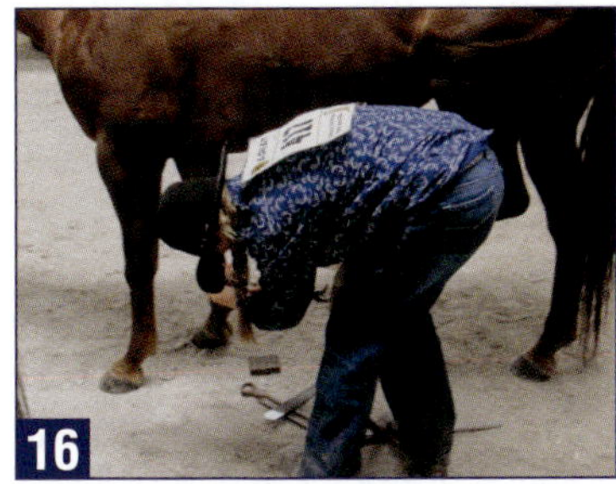

16

17 ***Jacquelyn clinching for us at a rodeo.***

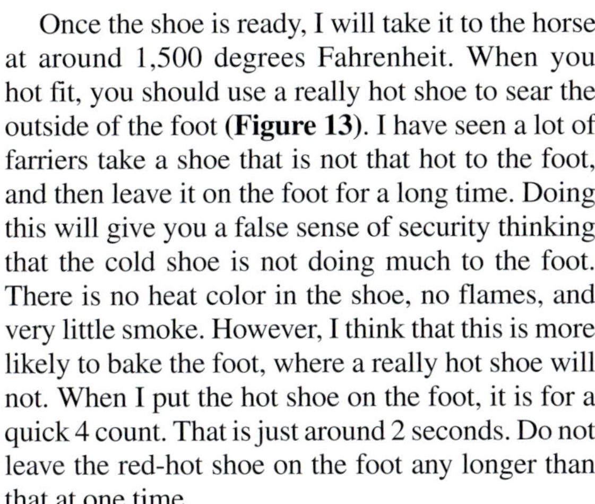

Once the shoe is ready, I will take it to the horse at around 1,500 degrees Fahrenheit. When you hot fit, you should use a really hot shoe to sear the outside of the foot **(Figure 13)**. I have seen a lot of farriers take a shoe that is not that hot to the foot, and then leave it on the foot for a long time. Doing this will give you a false sense of security thinking that the cold shoe is not doing much to the foot. There is no heat color in the shoe, no flames, and very little smoke. However, I think that this is more likely to bake the foot, where a really hot shoe will not. When I put the hot shoe on the foot, it is for a quick 4 count. That is just around 2 seconds. Do not leave the red-hot shoe on the foot any longer than that at one time.

When the shoe has clips, I will mark where the clip is with the hot clip, cut out the area for the clip, and then hot fit the shoe. In the perfect world, there will be one trip to the foot with the shoe, the shoe will fit, and I will cool it down. Since the world is not always perfect, I will go back to the anvil and do whatever minor corrections are needed to the shoe as soon as I am done with the first hot fit. I'll then quench the shoe and repeat the process with the other front shoe.

By the time the front shoes are fit, the hinds are ready to work with. I will continue with them as with the fronts. With all four shoes fit and cooled off in the quench bucket, I will take all of them to the horse to nail.

I like to nail all four shoes on **(Figure 14)** and then clinch all four feet **(Figure 15-17)**. The main reason that I don't clinch each foot right after nailing is that I have my clinching tools with the hoof stand, and I can nail without having to have all that extra equipment with me while I do it.

Regardless of the sequence you end up following, the more you can make it a routine, the more likely you are to do a consistently good job. Try to think about what you can do in your everyday work to make the job more efficient. For instance, a lot of students like to pull all the shoes before they do any trimming. Or perhaps they will even trim the bottom of each foot and then go back and dress each foot. That is not an efficient way to shoe. (I realize that is how I do the nailing and clinching, but there is a good reason for that.)

Most beginners wonder when they will finally pick up some speed at shoeing. Following a good sequence will help you get to where you are averaging a horse every 45 minutes to an hour. That is a good pace for a one-man operation. If you handle everything correctly, you can end up working an easy 6-hour day everyday and still making a good living.

Chapter 25

MEASURING FEET FOR HANDMADES

Measuring feet for handmade shoes is a complicated and controversial subject. Everyone has an opinion, formula, or a best guess.

What is the magic formula that will make the shoe right every time? This section of the book will help you find your way to the measurement formula that fits you. I don't intend to give you an exact recipe (no one can), but I do intend to teach you something about how you can control the finished result of your handmades.

Every farrier has struggled with this area of shoe building. I certainly did. I researched the subject heavily, yet my shoes did not always fit the formulas. At some point it finally fell together, but the formula was individual to me. Your formula will be individual to you, and it will take some practice to get it worked out 100%.

If you endeavor to become an American Farrier's Association Certified Journeyman Farrier, take any of the Worshipful Company of Farriers exams, or achieve the higher levels in the Farrier International Testing System (FITS) exams, your ability to make the exact size shoe needed will often be the difference between success and failure. Unfortunately, many farriers will second-guess themselves out of the right length of stock once they get to the contest or exam. The reason for this is that they don't trust their system. If this is you, it is time to get a measurement system down that works.

One of the things that I don't like about many formulas is the guesswork portion. For instance, there is a formula that has you measure the width of the foot, plus the length from the center of the toe to the longest buttress, and add 1 1/2 inches if the hoof is normal. If it is "really long" from toe to heel, you add 1/4 inch more. If it is "really wide," you reduce what you add by 1/4 inch. This type of formula leaves you hanging when it really matters. When you are under the gun, your mind will play tricks on you as you decide the difference between normal, really long, and really wide. That being said, I know a lot of talented farriers that use this formula. The big difference is that their talent allows them to make the stock work for the foot even if it is not the perfect length. This takes a LOT of practice, and by the time you get to that stage, you should have gotten past any of the measurement problems we are trying to fix now.

Since I was not able to make that sort of formula work for me when I was starting out, I decided to find a method that measured any foot without guesswork. Using the circumference method worked well. This involved measuring the foot from one heel, around the toe to the other heel; or better yet, from where I wanted the shoe to fit, around the toe to where I wanted the shoe to fit the other side. This led to a formula that took into account all of the metal required for the shoe without regard to the abnormalities that the individual hoof presented by being really wide or really long.

Here is the way to the magic formula: Cut 6 pieces of stock the same length. Mark all of them exactly the same and make 6 shoes that are the same. Once the pile is complete, measure all of the shoes from heel to heel and write down the measurements. Where you are in developing your shoe-building skills will make a big difference as to how close in size these shoes will be. Add all the measurements together and divide by 6 (finding the average). This should tell you how much the stock grew from your forging, which will in turn tell you what length you need to cut for a foot that you are using that particular stock width on.

If you used 12 inches of 5/16-by-3/4-inch stock, your math may look like this:

14 1/8" + 14" + 14" + 13 7/8" + 14 1/8" + 13 7/8" = 84"

84 divided by 6 = 14 (the average).

This means that your average piece of 5/16-by 3/4-inch stock will grow 2 inches in your shoe-making process for you. (Your formulas and measurements may be different. This is just an example.)

Now cut 6 pieces of stock that are 1/8 inch wider than the first ones. Repeat all the previous steps, and you will now have a formula for how you forge the added width. You can continue with wider or thinner stock to increase your knowledge of your personal formula. You should grow in length by twice what you gained in width. Stating it another way: If you used 12 inches of 5/16-by-3 /4-inch stock to cover a hoof that measured 14 inches from heel to heel, you would need 11 3 /4 inches if you were to use 5/16-by7/8-inch, or 11 1/2 inches if it were 5/16-by-1 inch. Your forging style may make it slightly different, but you won't know until you try.

The best part about this method is that it will be individual for you and your style of forging. The late Ivon Bell, FWCF, who ran the British Army School of Farriery, told me that the steel manufacturers have never made the right cross section of bar stock for a horse's hoof. He said that the farrier makes the right section by forging. Someone who forges the stock heavily in order to change the cross section will use a lot shorter piece than someone that mainly bends without a lot of forging.

You can use this method to find the length needed for any shoe you have to make. If you are using the method for bar shoes, you will have to add the amount of steel needed for your bar. However, with practice, you can get this measurement down pat as well. The described practice session is very helpful for preparing for the Journeyman practical and bar shoe. You will need to do a different practice session to find out how creasing affects your length. Some people will grow 1/4 inch per branch from creasing. I seem to grow about half that.

Here is a step-by-step method for making your own foot measuring tape. Refer to the checklist to make your own tape measure **(Figures 1-8)**.

1. Obtain a cloth tape measure, white cloth tape, scissors, and a clothes marker **(Figure 1)**.
2. Cut and assemble as shown **(Figure 2)**.
3. Make your specimen shoes of the desired widths and the same known length. Here I am going to make some shoes out of 12 inches of stock, measuring 3/4 inch, 7/8 inch and 1 inch" in width **(Figure 3)**.
4. These are pictures of the finished blanks **(Figures 4 and 5)**.
5. Measure the shoes so that the 12 ends at the heel of each **(Figure 6)**.
6. Mark the tape to coincide with each stock width **(Figure 7)**.
7. Here is the finished tape measure, marked for three different stock sizes. **(Figure 8)**.

Using the tape to measure feet is shown in

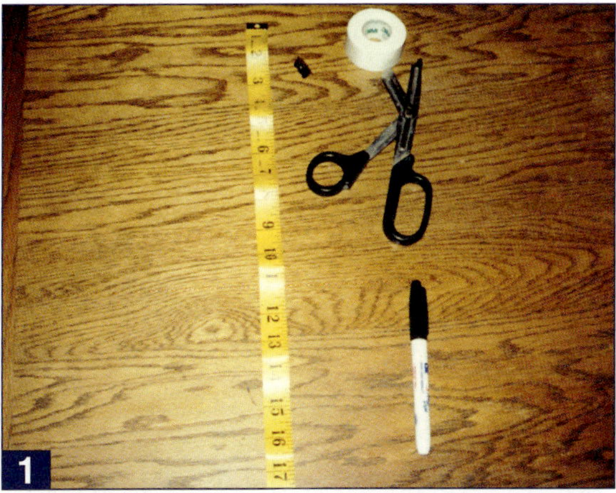
1

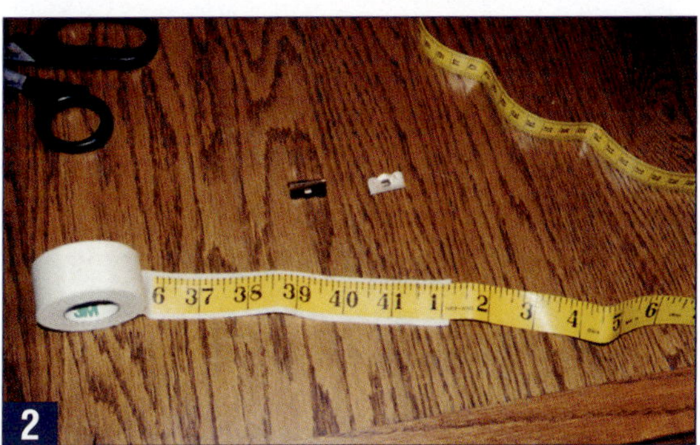
2

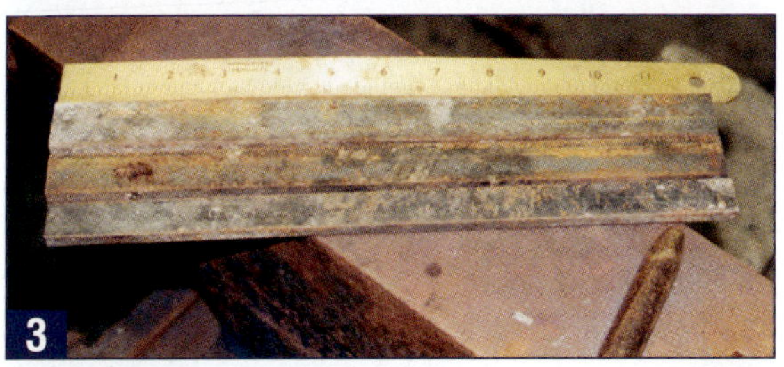
3

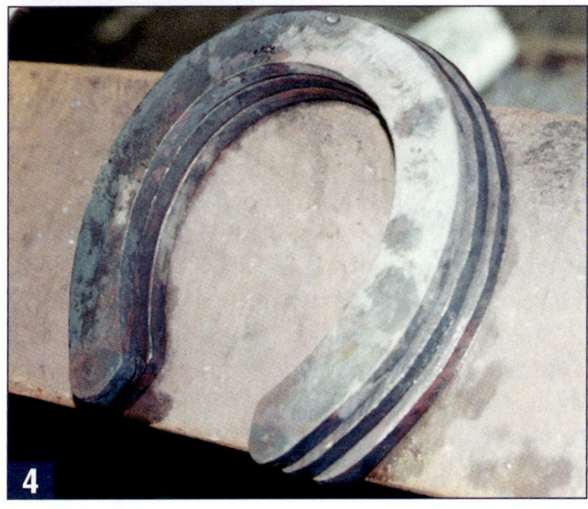
4

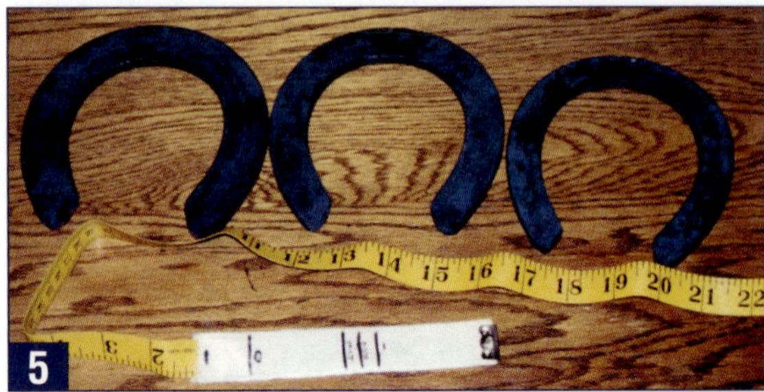

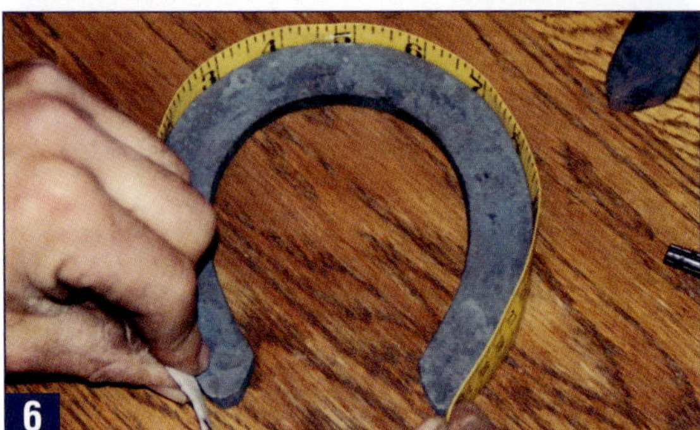

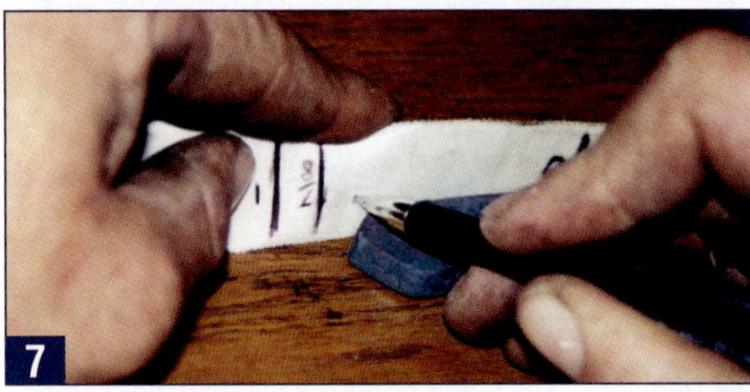

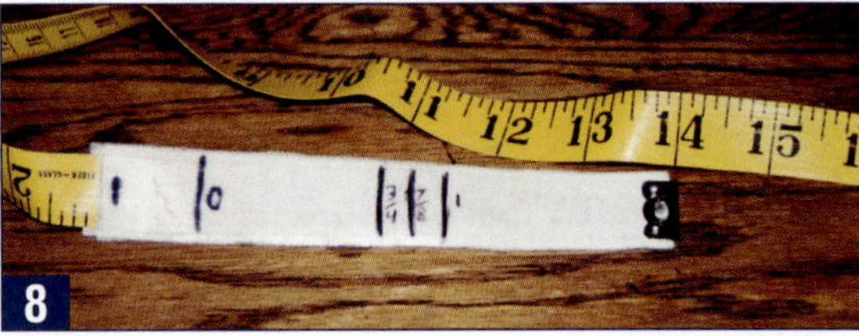

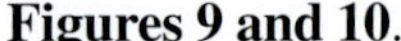

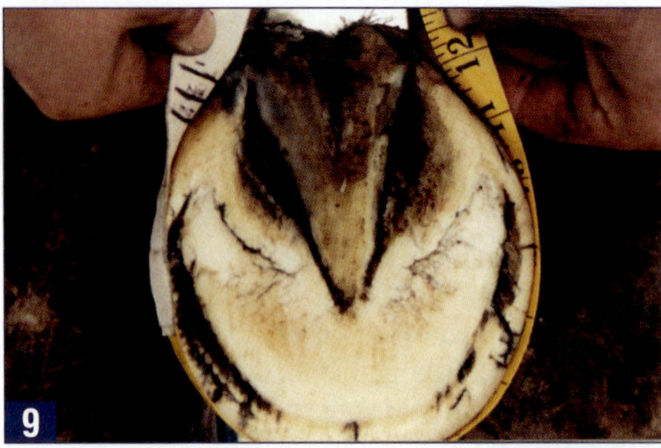

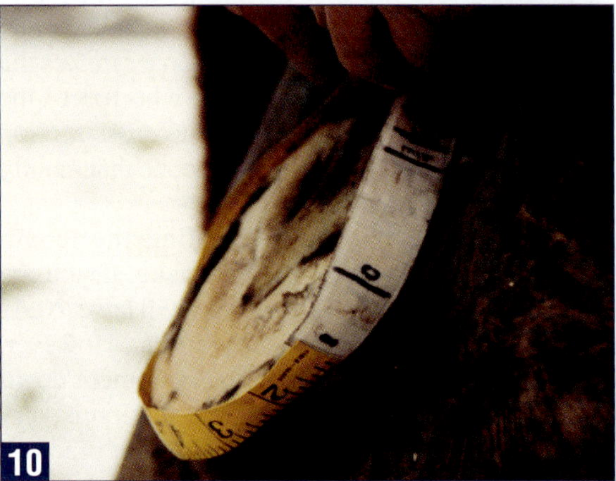

Figures 9 and 10.

Figure 9, Place the mark for your desired bar stock at one heel and measure around the foot.

Figure 10, The resulting measurement is the length of stock you need to cut for that particular hoof.

You may want to make a few of these tapes. Make one for concave stock, and one for creased or fullered shoes. The same tape can be marked with different colored ink to designate different types of shoes.

You will find that nailing on your own handmades is perhaps the best practice for shoe building there is. As you continue to raise your skill level, you will find that measuring feet is really easy, and you will be able to make any number of formulas work. At some point you may even decide that measuring is not that necessary. I call it instinctive shoeing, and I worked to get to where I did not have to measure feet to get the right shoe on. I did this to help me pass the AWCF exam where there are a lot of different types of shoes, and having a formula for all of them would be quite difficult. You should be able to make any piece of reasonable bar stock fit any reasonable foot. Measuring carefully now will help you get to the point that you don't have to measure the foot, and with practice, you won't have to measure the stock either.

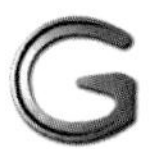

Chapter

26 SHOE SELECTION

Once you have established yourself as a farrier, you will find that most of your customers expect you to know which shoes they should use. There will be some that will insist on a certain style (often out of incorrect perceptions about that particular type of shoe), but there will also be many who will have you decide. This is an important decision. If you consider the effects of different shoes you wear, you can see why. It would be hard to play a game of football in cowboy boots, and just as hard to steer wrestle in a pair of cleats. Horses face the same challenges if they are not shod for the job they are doing.

This chapter is about selecting shoes for sound horses that are doing particular jobs. The section on pathology and pathological shoes will detail what shoes to use for different types of problems. Here we are concerned with the everyday lifestyle that the horse lives, and the jobs it does when ridden.

NORMAL KEG SHOE

Figure 1 shows a common keg shoe made by St. Croix Forge. The shape is generic, meaning that it is not a front or a hind. This is the basic type of shoe that was available before the early 1990s, when many types of pre-shaped shoes came on the market. Now, it is common to find most farriers using pre-shaped front **(Figure 2)** and pre-shaped hinds **(Figure 3)**. A quick note on business here: If you can buy the generic shoe for less, and then apply your skill to make it the shape needed, you will make more money per horse than the shoer that has to rely on the manufacturer's skill at shaping shoes.

The width of the stock that is used to make a shoe is called its web. You can see that **Figures 2 and 3** show a wide-webbed shoe, while **Figure 1** would be considered a standard width for the size of the shoe. Web width is an important consideration when selecting a shoe, as we will explain.

TRACTION

Traction, or grip, is one of the big factors you need to understand and consider when picking a shoe for a particular job. In essence, traction is a basic formula based on the amount of ground contact and the weight applied to that contact. Here is a simple example (an easy one to use with customers): If a horseshoe were made from material that ended up giving the foot 10 square inches of contact with the ground, and the horse put all 1,000 pounds of its weight on that shoe, you would have 100 pounds per square inch. Doubling the amount of shoe by widening the material would give you 20 square inches on the ground. Now, the 1,000 pounds would only be able to generate 50 pounds per square inch. This is basically what makes sliding plates work on the back of a reining horse, and rim shoes work on a barrel racer.

If you look back through the historical record of horseshoe patents, it is amazing how many of the patents were based on achieving more traction. **Figure 4** shows the drawings for a common type of patent that was being filed in the late 1800s. You can also see several old shoes that hang on the wall at The

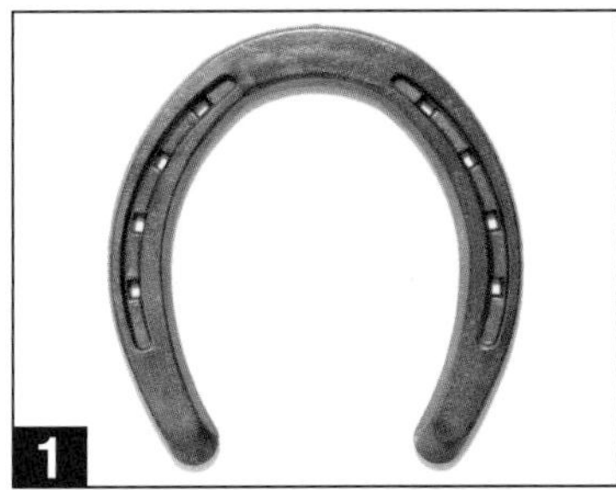

1 *Plain, generic keg shoe.*

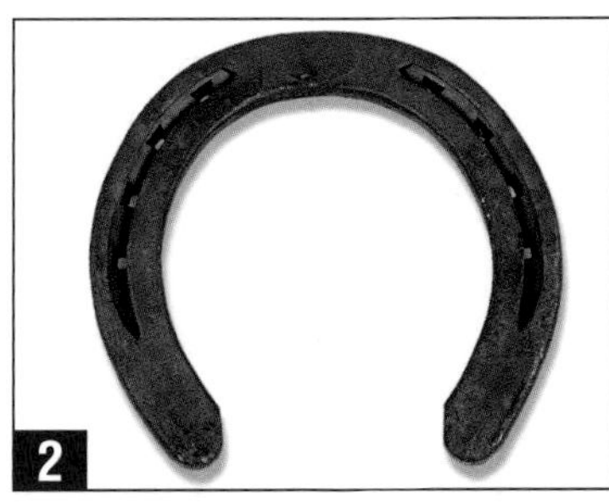

2 *Wide-webbed, front-shaped shoe.*

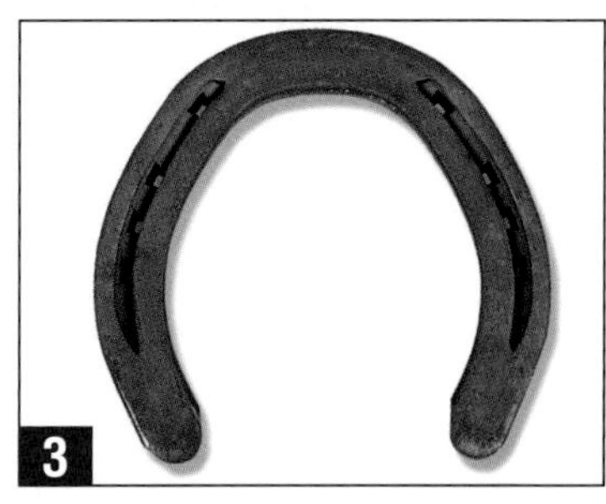

3 *Wide-webbed, hind-shaped shoe.*

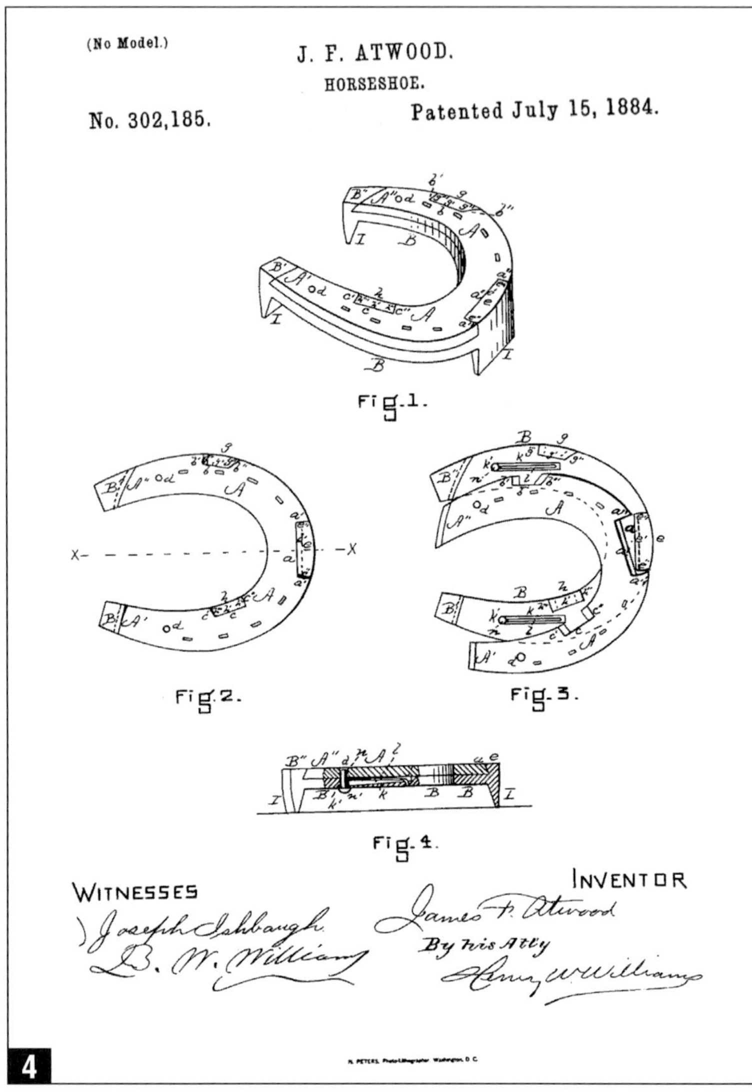

Patent drawing from the late 1800s.

Army School of Farriery in England in **Figures 5-8**. Some pretty severe traction was being applied to feet at one time. **Figure 9** shows a shoe that had tarred rope put into the groove once the shoe was nailed on the foot. It was another attempt at traction.

The next thing to consider is the terrain that the horse will be living and working in. Knowing how a horse lives normally is very important, because even a horse that is used hard will spend more time without a rider than with one. If the shoes are not compatible with its lifestyle, then you need to determine how to accomplish the owner's goals for that horse. Just look at some of the packages that are used on gaited horses. Those horses cannot be let out on their own with those shoes, so having to wear them makes constant confinement necessary. Putting sliding plates on a horse that lives in a large grass pasture surrounded by barbed wire and filled with other horses is a sure way to get a horse hurt. You are in a position to inform the owner about some of those dangers so that they don't have to learn the hard way.

My background is pretty much straight out of the world of rodeo horses, cutting horses, and trail horses. These are primarily American Quarter Horses, but there is quite a variety in the trail-horse world.

With the rodeo horse, you can get along pretty well with the normal plain shoe seen in **Figure 1** in a lot of situations. However, for serious competitors, changing the style of shoe slightly can have a big impact. For speed events that don't require a hard stop (such as steer wrestling, barrel racing, and pole bending), using concave stock **(Figure 10)**, light rims **(Figures 11 - 12),** or St. Croix Eventers **(Figures 13 - 14)** make a pretty good choice. These shoes not only have a smaller amount of steel on the ground (their primary benefit), but the crease around the shoe will pack with dirt, which can add traction. In some instances, mainly barrel racing, aluminum Eventers are a good choice **(Figure 15)**. Aluminum shoes are light, but won't withstand wear as well as steel shoes. For a bit more traction on a plain shoe, creasing through the toe **(Figure 16)** is a good idea.

On roping horses, I don't like too much traction on the hind feet due to the amount of torque that the hocks have to absorb. Many of the roping horses I shoe are done just like a cutting horse, with concave or rim shoes in front, and a light plain or a plain-stamped handmade behind. If I think the hocks can take the stress, I will use a keg shoe like the St.

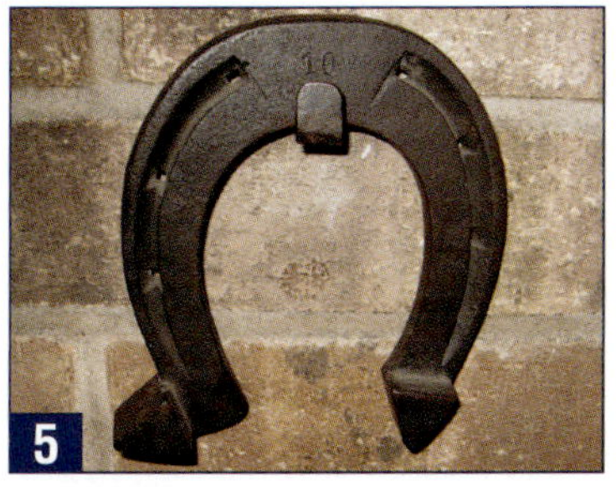

Strange shoe with large caulks.

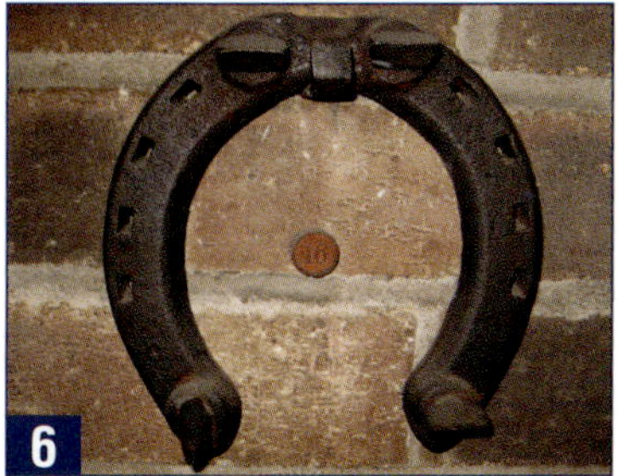

Ice shoe.

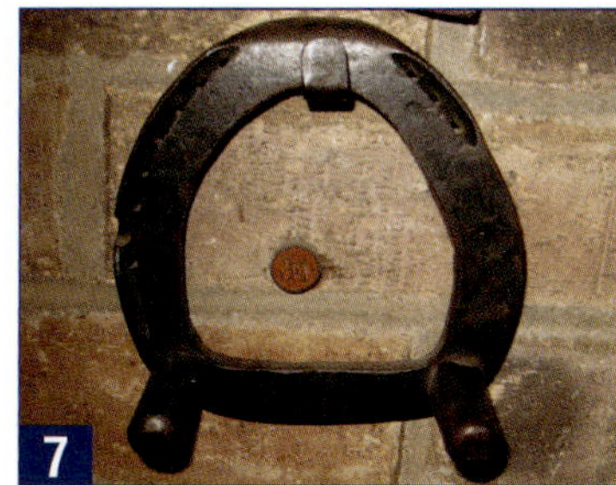

Bar shoe with long, round caulks.

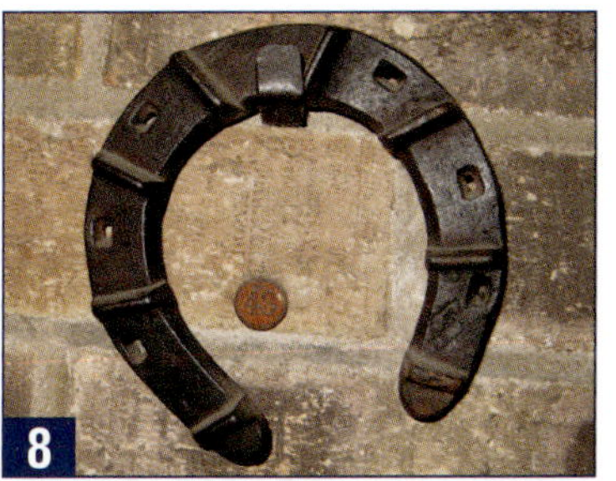

Old shoe with several bars across it.

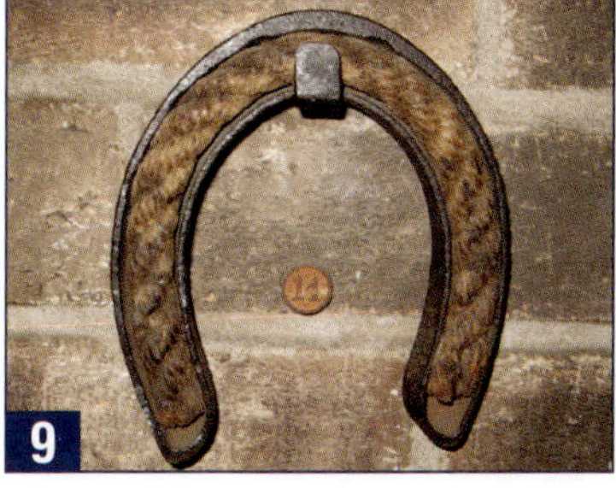

Rope shoe.

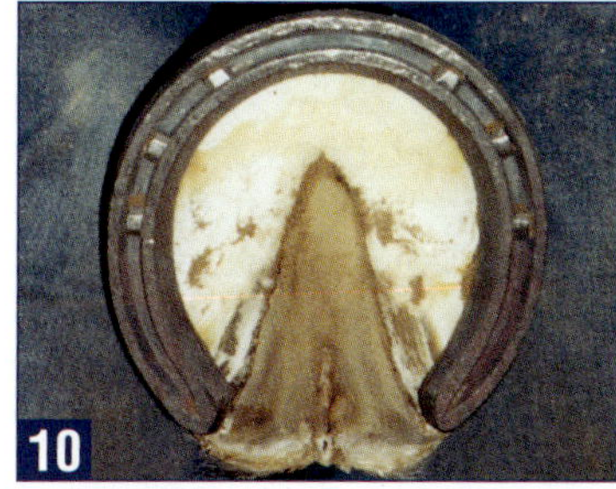

Concave front on foot.

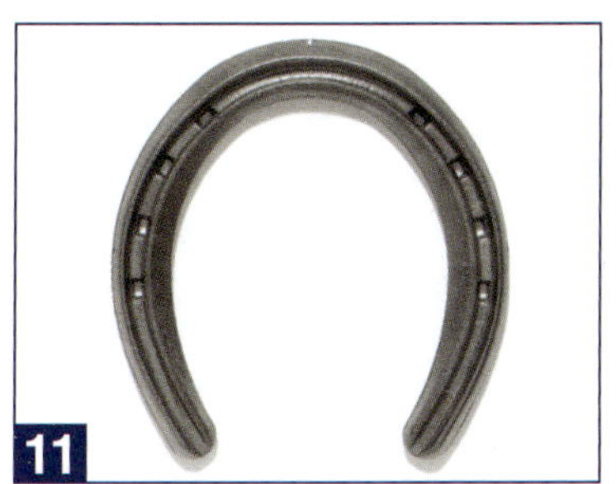

Generic rim shoe.

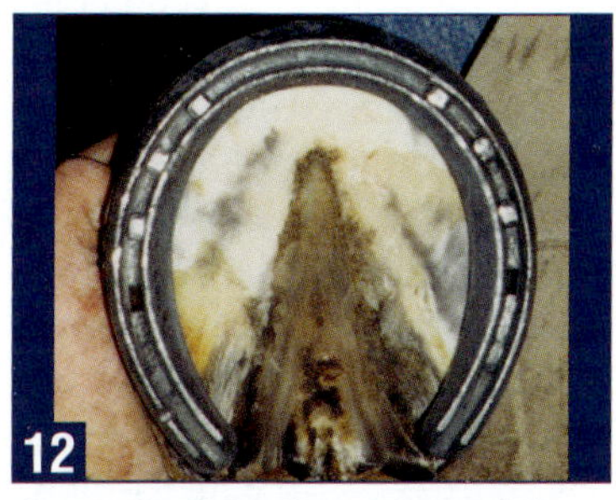

Generic rim shoe shaped for a front, and nailed to a foot.

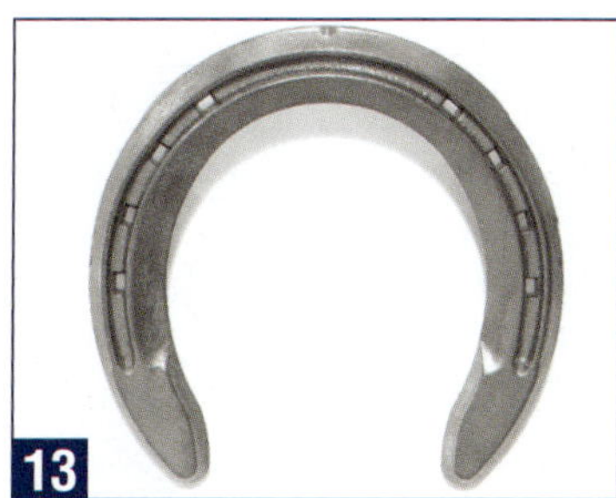

Front Eventer.

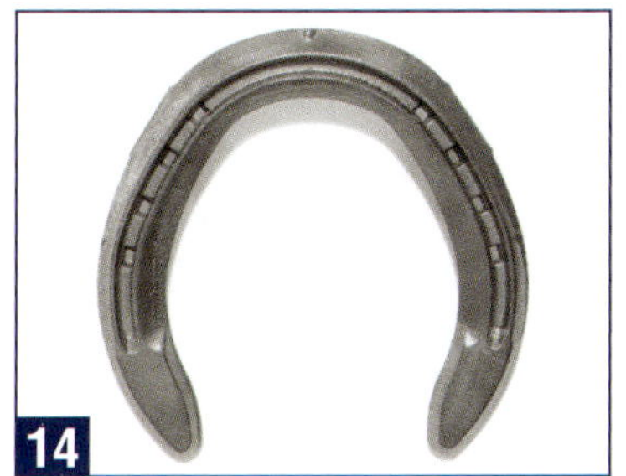

Hind Eventer

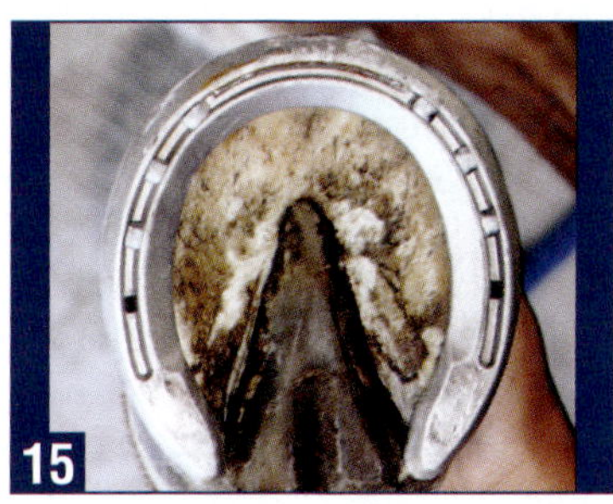

Aluminum Eventer on a foot.

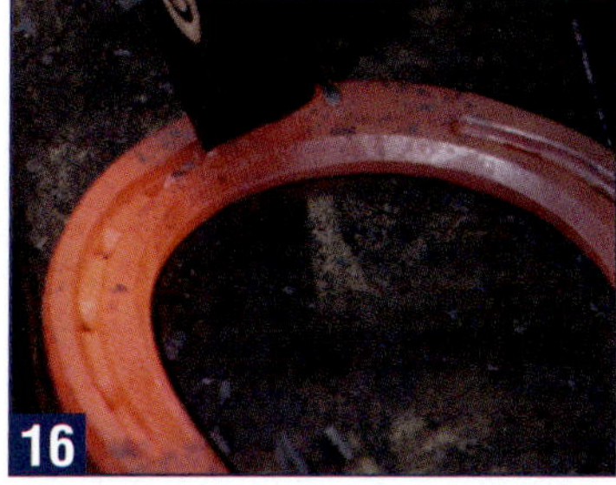

Fullering through the toe of a keg shoe.

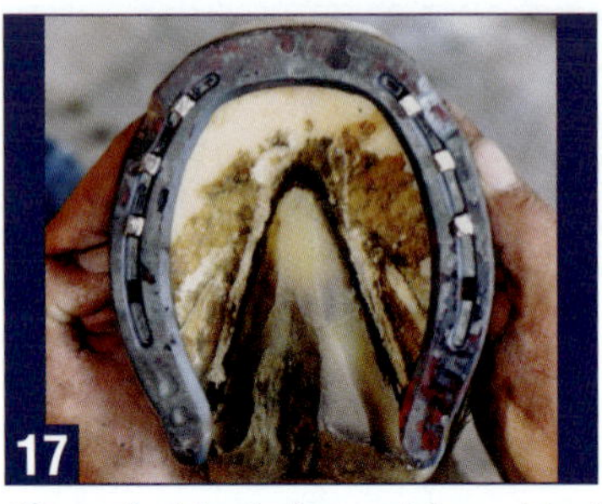

Generic hind shaped for a hind with minor extended heels.

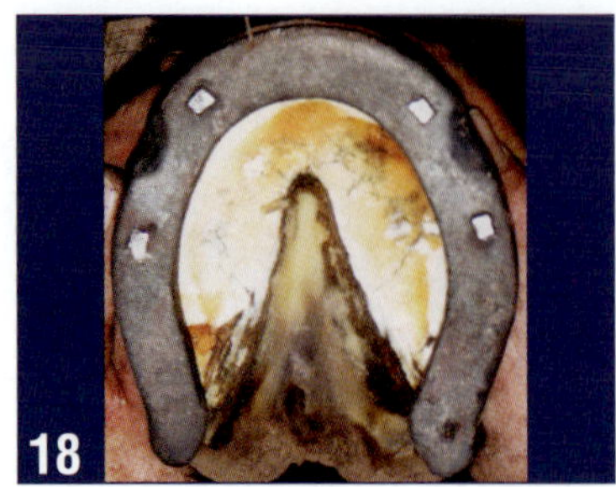

Plain stamped handmade hind.

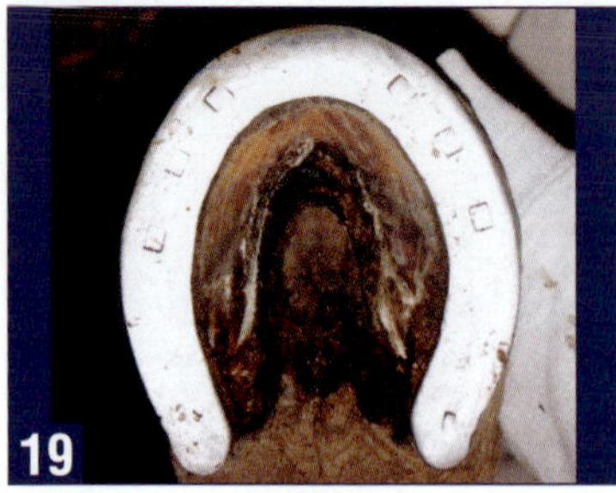

Plain stamped handmade hind with some wear on it.

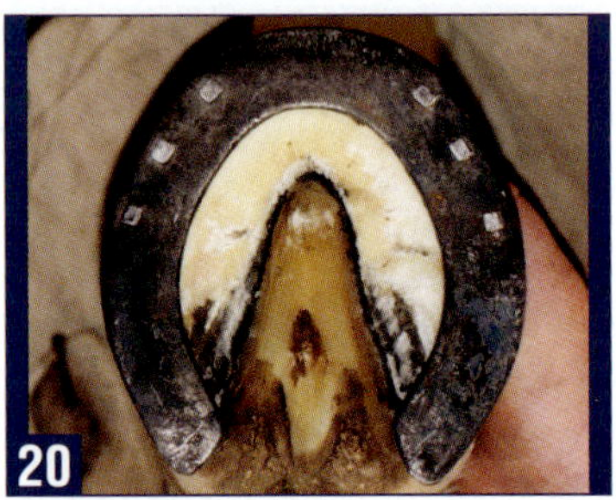

Plain stamped handmade hind from 7/8-inch stock.

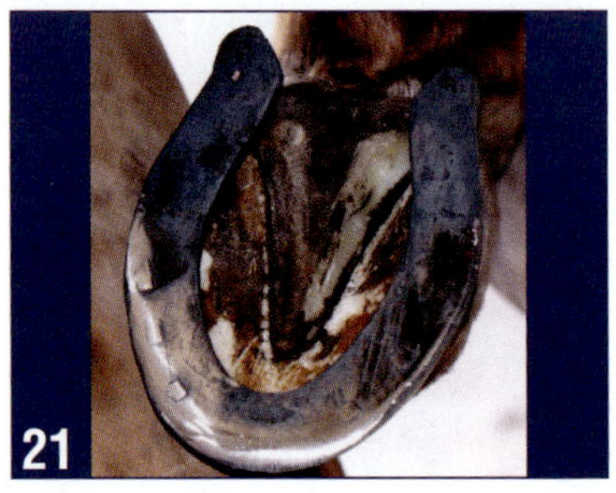

Slider plate with the nails ground off.

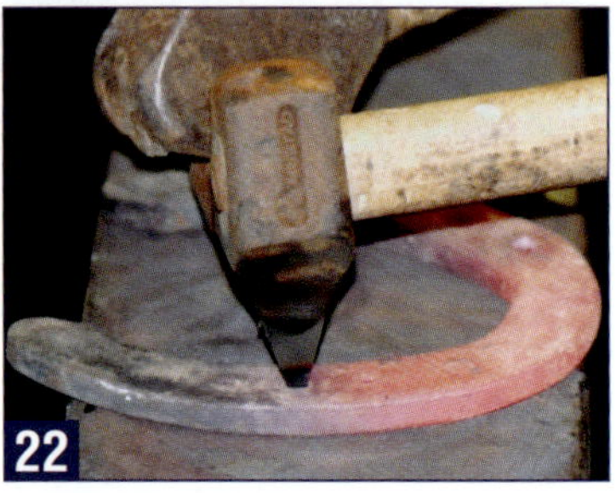

Punching plain stamped nails from the hoof surface of a keg shoe.

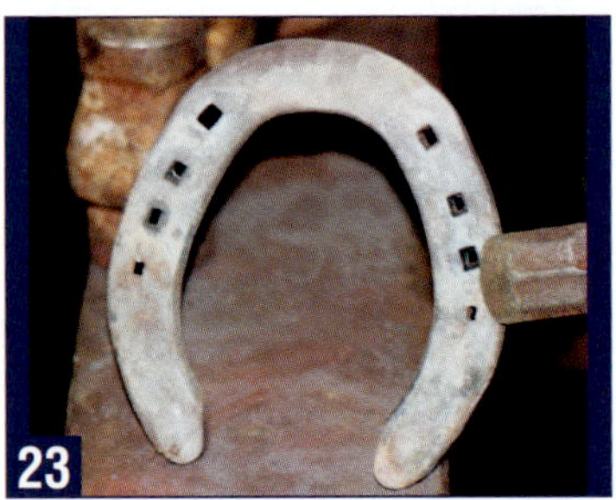

The keg shoe punched from the back to decrease traction.

Croix Lite Plain behind (**Figure 17**). To get a little less traction, I use something like a St. Croix Euro, which is just a wider keg shoe. For still less traction, I will use a plain stamped handmade and regulate the amount of traction with the width of the stock. **Figure 18** shows a plain stamped handmade with four nail holes that has just been reset. You can see in **Figure 19** how a shoe like this will wear smooth. Most commonly it will be 3/4 inch in width, but there are some that do better with 7/8 inch, like the shoe shown in **Figure 20**, or even 1 inch like the slider plate in **Figure 21**.

While I don't recommend this as a regular thing, you can plain stamp the nail holes from the back of a wide-webbed keg shoe to get the effects of a plain stamped shoe. In **Figure 22**, I am driving a fore punch from the hoof surface of a Mustad Basic, and in **Figure 23**, you can see the resulting shoe. When you do this, it does hourglass the nail holes, which, in turn, can shear the nails off more easily. The same thing goes for back-punching nail holes with a pritchel.

In many parts of the United States, you will find owners who want to have toed-and-heeled shoes on their horses. These shoes give the horse a lot of traction, but I won't use them unless I absolutely have to. Their design is handy for some very particular uses, such as on asphalt and rocky trails, but they provide too much traction for the everyday life of most horses. Trying to talk an "old timer" out of using them may be difficult, so I require customers that want toed-and-heeled shoes to supply them for their own horses. This does make them more willing to use the shoes that I have in stock, but be aware that a policy like that may cost you a customer or two. You may want to experiment with jar caulks as in **Figure 24**. You can braze on whatever sized piece

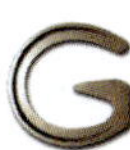

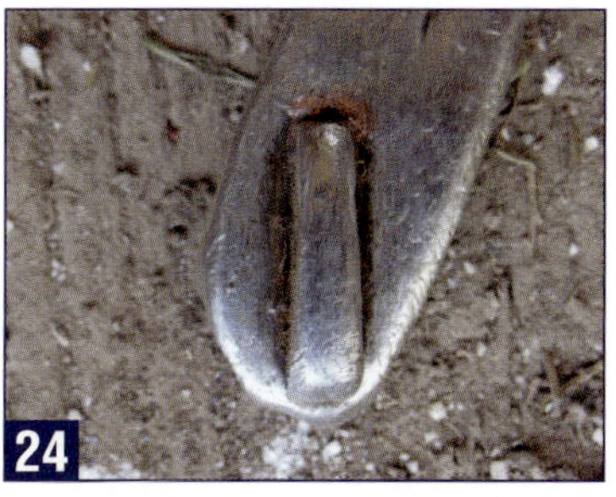

Jar caulk brazed on in the line of flight.

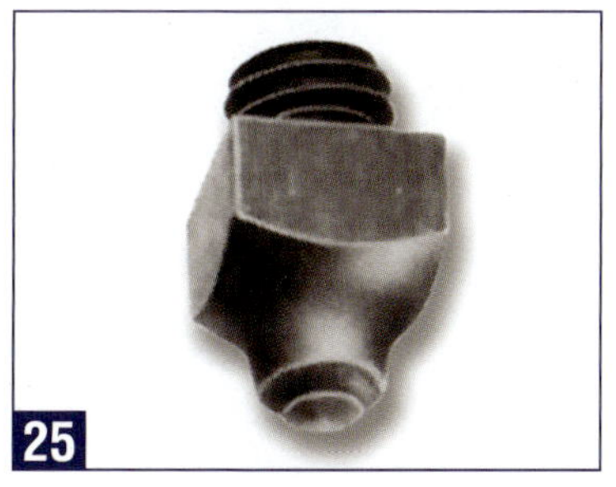

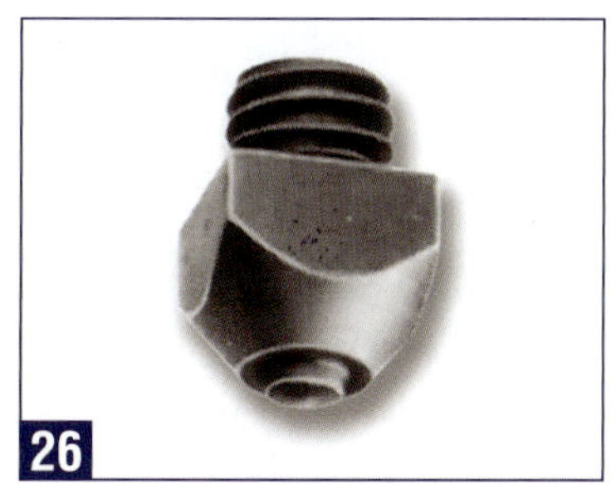

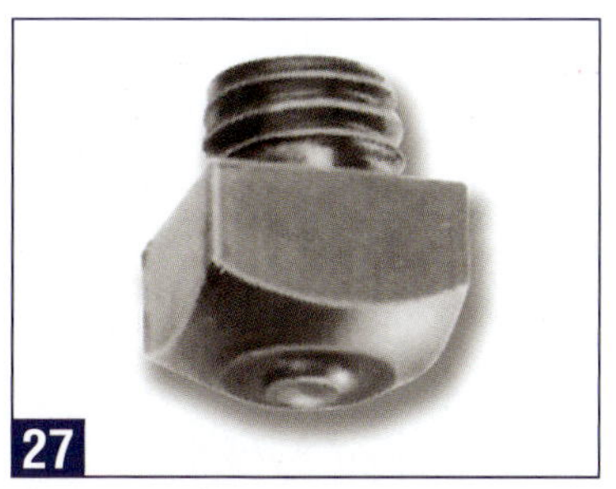

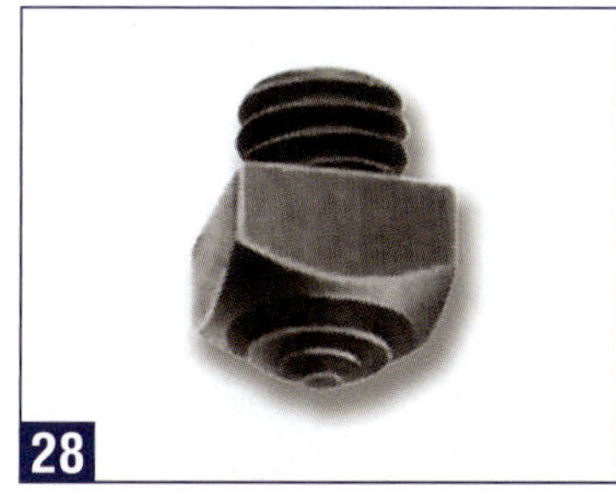

Screw-in stud.

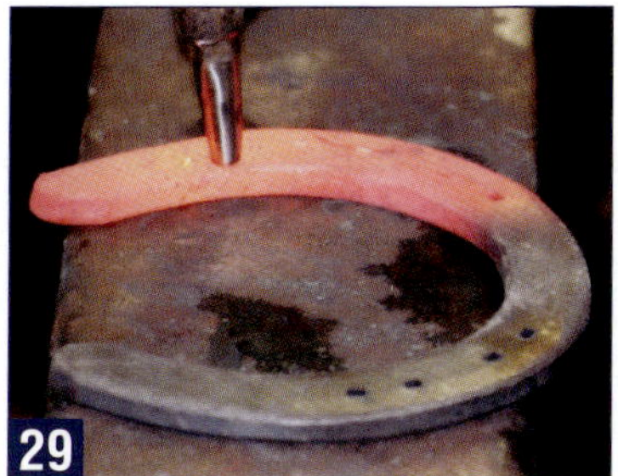

Punching a stud hole from the hoof surface of the shoe.

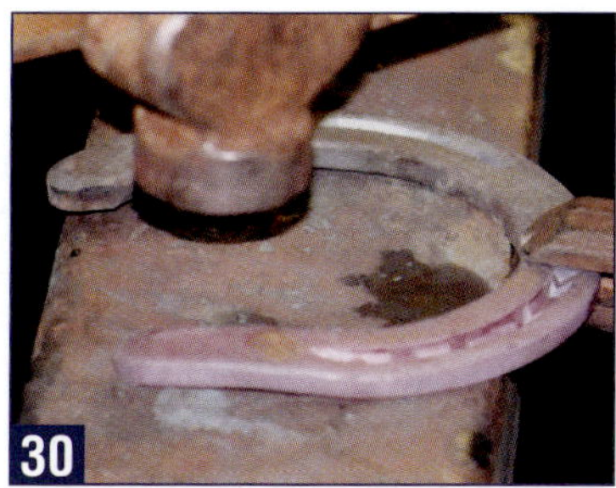

Hammering flat from the ground surface.

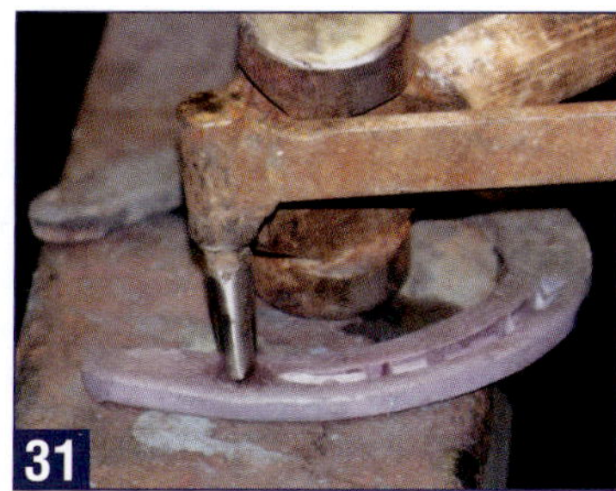

Positioning the stud punch on the ground surface.

of steel you want at whatever angle.

A concave or rim shoe is also an ideal shoe for a trail horse. I think that the amount of traction generated by a rim shoe is petty close to what a bare foot will have, even though there is a difference from the rigidity of the shoe and the fact that the traction is the same all the way around the shoe. It is hard to go wrong on the basic horse with a good set of handmade concave shoes.

Some riding disciplines require different traction from one place to another. Jumping horses are a good example. When you shoe a horse that requires the traction to change to match the footing, you can put stud holes in the shoe so that the owner can use studs of differing heights and design. **Figures 25-28** are some examples of studs that are made by Mustad. A stud hole is simply a hole that is punched or drilled in the horseshoe, and then tapped. Most are tapped for a 3/8-inch coarse thread screw, but there are other sizes of studs out there.

The process is fairly simple. Begin by punching from the hoof surface of the shoe **(Figure 29)**. Turn the shoe over and hammer on the ground surface as you would before pritcheling a nail hole **(Figure 30)**. Place the punch in the center of the shiny spot **(Figure 31)** and then move to the pritchel hole on the anvil to punch out the round slug as I am doing in **Figure 32**. You should have a perfectly round hole like the one in **Figure 33**.

Place the shoe in a vise and apply some cutting

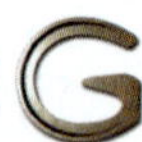

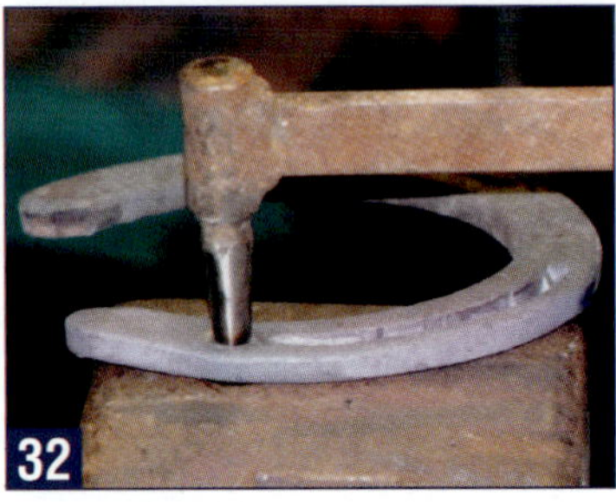

Punching out the slug.

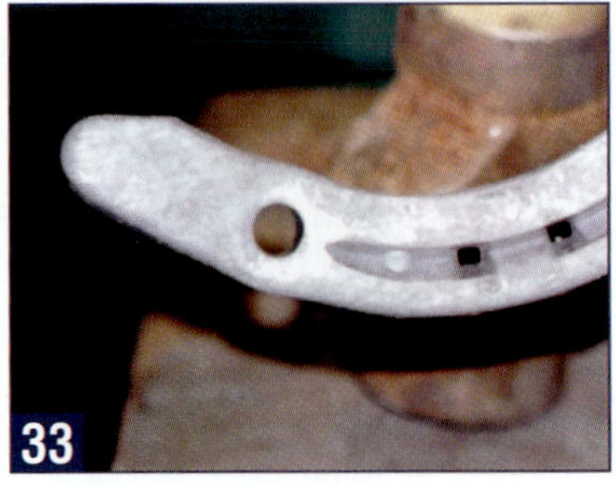

Stud hole punched.

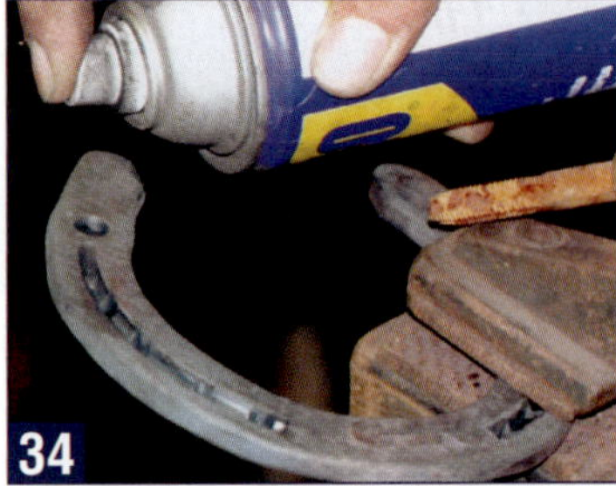

Shoe in the vise and applying cutting oil.

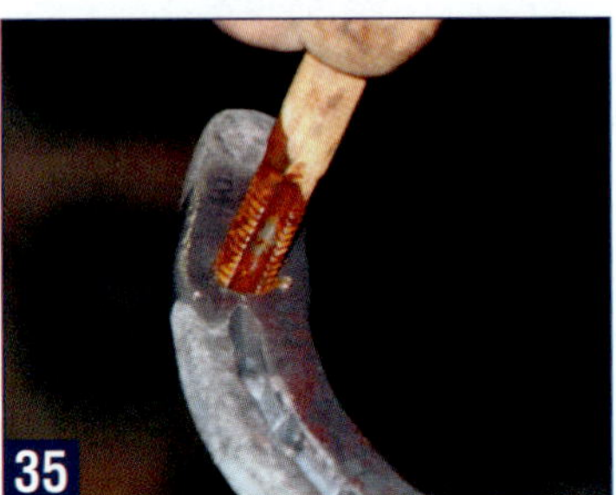

Tapping the hole.

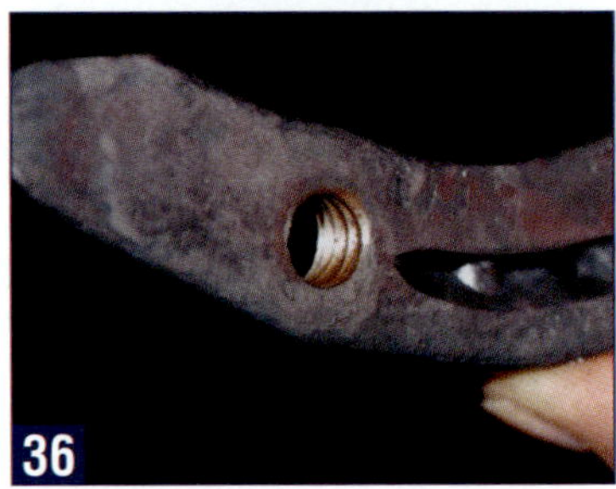

Finished hole.

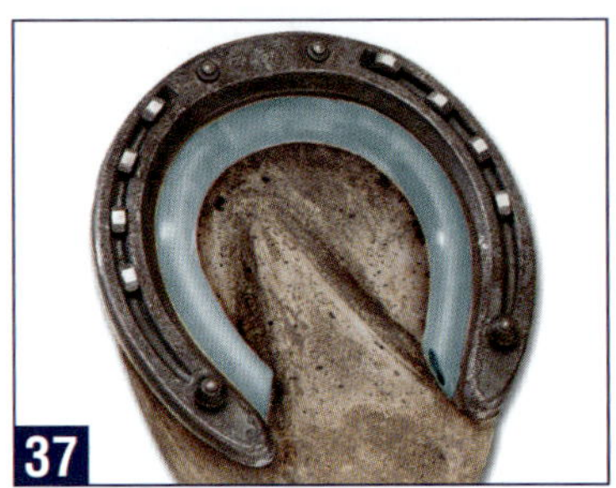

Snow-shoe set up.

oil **(Figure 34)**. Put the tap in straight, and tap from the ground surface **(Figure 35)**. When you are done, you will have a hole like the one shown in **Figure 36**. The customer can then change the traction of the shoe to accommodate the ground that they find themselves competing in.

Studs have not yet become too popular among the rodeo crowd, but there are certainly areas where they would be perfect. We have used them on barrel horses and pole horses with good success.

The position of a stud hole can differ from farrier to farrier, but I personally like to have one in the lateral heel, as close to the buttress of the foot as possible. Going forward on the branch can put a lot of stress and concussion in the quarter of the hoof, and lead to problems like quarter cracks. I don't like to have a stud on the medial side, but many people do. Place a medial stud close to the buttress as well, and be certain that you have a talk with the customer about not putting too tall or sharp a stud in that hole. There is always an inherent risk that the horse will step on its opposite foot, causing great damage with that medial stud. If you put them in the toe, try to get them as wide as possible.

When you have customers who use studs, there are a few points that you should make clear to them. Studs should only be put into the shoes for the time that the horse is working, and then be removed as soon as the event is done. They should never haul or turn out a horse with studs in its shoes, and oftentimes what they think is the right stud is too much. You may also have to teach them to properly hold the horse's feet to change the stud.

You will need to know about shoeing for snow and ice if you live in an area with drastic seasonal changes. I like to use a St. Croix Euro or a Mustad Basic for this type of shoeing. Shape and fit the shoe just as normal, and then drill out 4 holes in the shoe for drive-in studs. You should also use a snow pad. **Figure 37** is a good example of a snowshoe package.

Experience, exposure, and experimentation will be an important part of the first few years of shoeing in whatever discipline you find yourself, so be observant. Ask questions of the farriers who are shoeing in that field as well as the customers who ride those horses. Attend events featuring the type of horses you shoe, and perhaps get involved in riding them as well. With diligent practice and study, you will soon find yourself a farrier in demand amongst your chosen specialty.

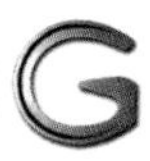

Chapter 27 SHOE MODIFICATIONS

I have been shoeing hot exclusively since 1990. Prior to that time, I did a couple years of cold work, followed by another year doing mainly cold with the occasional ceremonial forge lighting. There were many horses I shod in the early years to a standard that would embarrass me if photos existed, and I am certain that there will be a number of horses waiting in heaven for me so they can settle the score. Since you are reading this, I would assume that you are in the process of trying to improve your skills. For this, I commend you. I would also encourage you to learn the ins and outs of hot shoeing and incorporate it in your everyday work. It will not only set you apart from the rest of the shoers in your area, but it will also improve the fate of the horses in your care. It will help to shorten the line of horses in heaven waiting for you.

Oftentimes, the foot requires special handmade shoes or modifications to keg shoes that just cannot be done as well or as easily cold. From the work that we see come into the forge from around the country, there is a marked difference between the work done hot and that done cold. Since the advent of pre-shaped keg shoes, it is possible for cold shoeing to be done with well-shaped shoes. However, this is generally when the horse is helpful enough to have feet shaped like the shoe manufacturer determined was appropriate. Once the horseshoer with insufficient skills comes across that horse with a foot that does not fit the pattern, the horse suffers. You should determine that you are not going to be that horseshoer with insufficient skills.

At the end of a long day of shoeing, the last thing that a lot of cold shoers want to do is take the time and effort to put a good broad toe on a generic keg shoe, especially when the shoe out of the box could be nailed on without immediate damage. There is a difference between "okay" and "correct." As a hot shoer, it is just as easy to shape the shoe correctly as to not. In my mind, this is only one of the many arguments in favor of hot shoeing. Remember that your standard will drop to the lowest standard that you allow.

For the craftsman who wishes to be the best shoer around, a forge is a necessary piece of equipment. There is a financial argument in favor of developing the skills needed to make good, useable handmade shoes as well. If you are able to make any shoe that you might need, stocking the rig is easy and inexpensive. I have several sets of different sized keg shoes and a few lengths of bar stock. The only manufactured bar shoes in the rig are aluminum. The better you get at shoeing, the less equipment it will take. You will notice this when you clean your rig and come across an item that you haven't seen or used for 5 years. Keep it simple.

One of the hardest things for a beginner to learn is shaping shoes to the feet that they have just trimmed. Trimming is not hard to learn by itself, and neither is shaping a shoe. However, to put the two together can be difficult. I like to take a mental picture of the foot with the intended shoe already on it, and then I make that shoe I have already imagined when I go to the anvil.

Following is a description and picture essay of shaping shoes for normal fronts or hinds. It is a difficult subject to put to pen, but if you will study the photos carefully, I am certain that you can get it. We will start with the front shoe.

Begin with the toe. Find the radius of the horn that matches the foot you are fitting. Roll the shoe around the horn while you hammer lightly on the toe of the shoe **(Figures 1 and 2)**. Continue in that radius until you get to the widest part of the shoe **(Figure 3)**. At this point, twist the shoe to create a longer radius in the shoe from the widest part back through the heel **(Figure 4)**. Notice the tong position as I move the shoe around the horn, trying to keep the tongs from interfering with the inside perimeter of the shoe. Your shoe should look like the one in **Figure 5** at this point.

Turn the shoe around and repeat exactly the same moves from the toe nail on the side you are holding, right through the heel **(Figures 6-10)**. By doing the same moves from one side of the shoe to the other, the result will be a symmetrical front-shaped shoe **(Figure 10)**.

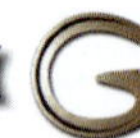

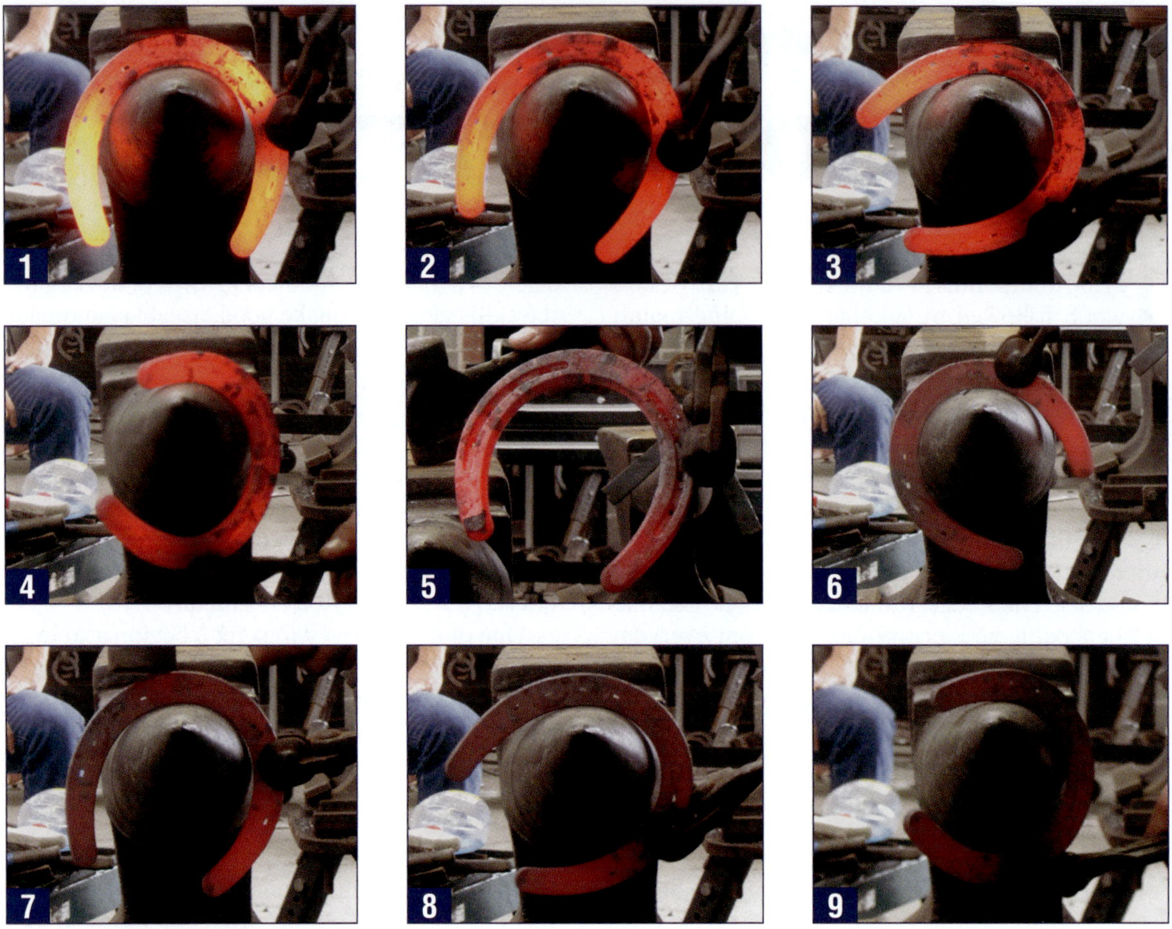

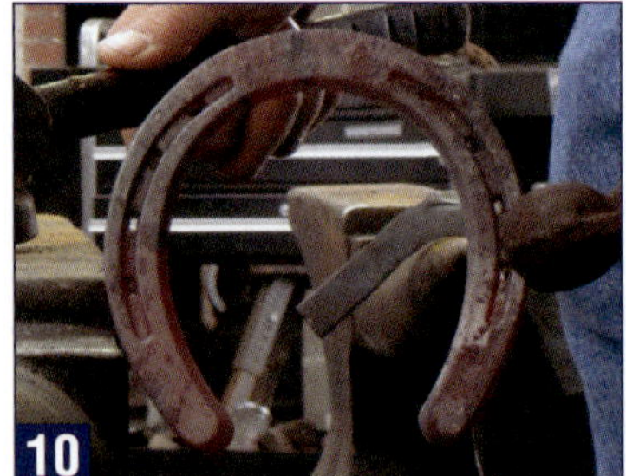

Figures 1 through 10. Steps in shaping a front shoe.

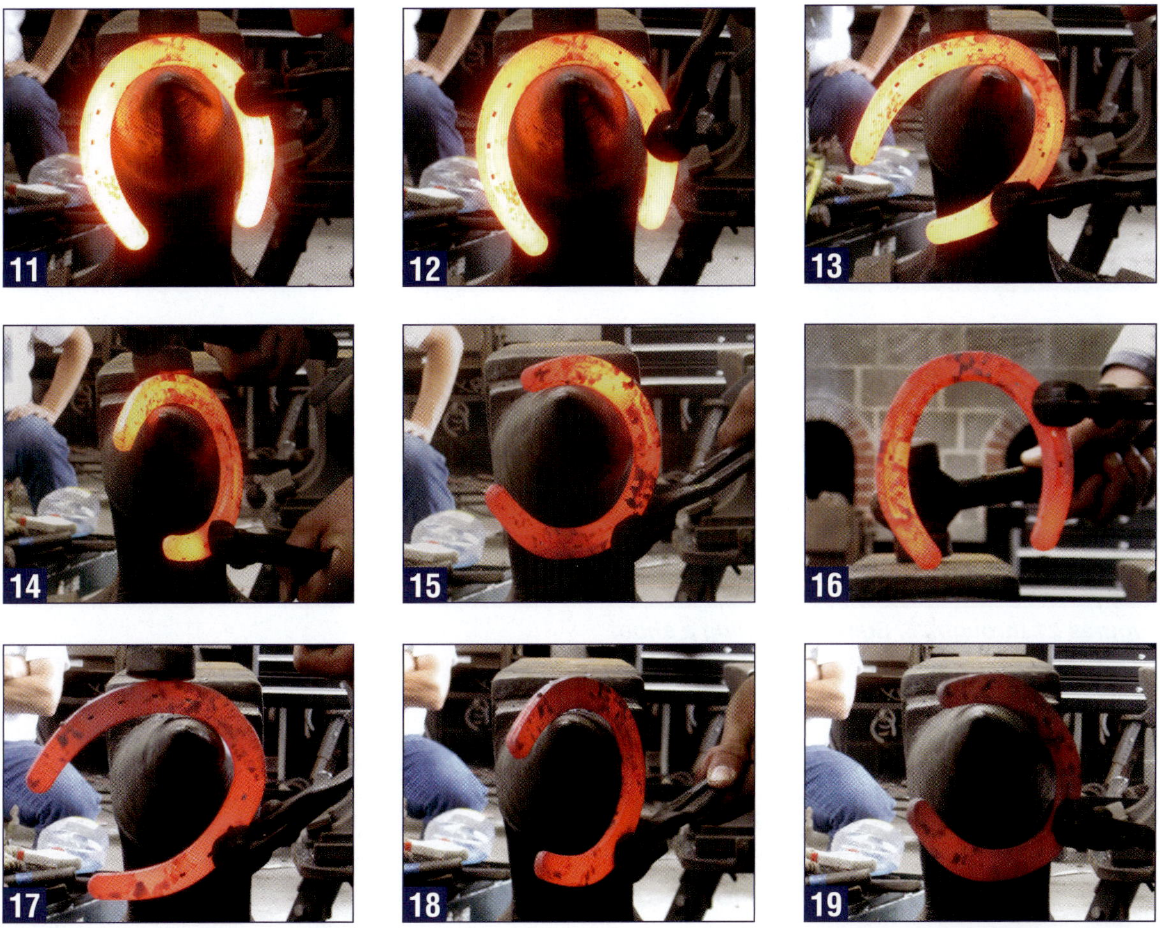

Figures 11 through 20. Steps in shaping a hind shoe.

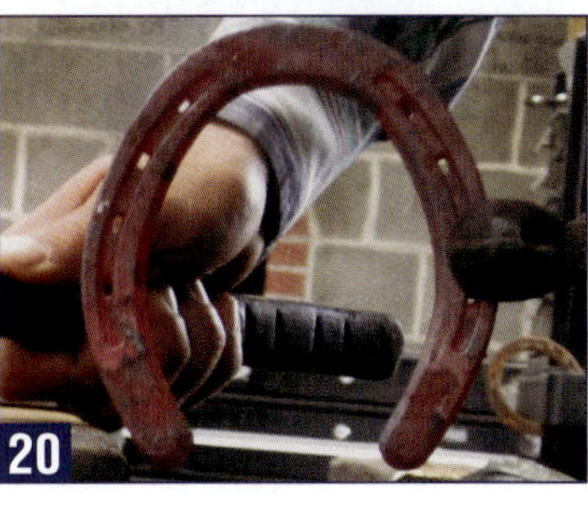

To shape a hind shoe, begin with the center of the toe as in **Figure 11**. If you study the difference between **Figures 11 and 12**, you will see that I raised my tong hand in **Figure 12**, but the shoe is in the same place as in **Figure 11**. Now, straighten your tong hand arm and set the toe by hitting lightly just past the point of contact on the horn **(Figure 13)** From this point, twist the shoe to find the long radius of the branch. Hammer lightly into the near side of the horn to straighten the branch **(Figure 14)** and move to the quarter to make that bend **(Figure 15)**. One side of the shoe is now shaped **(Figure 16)**. Turn the shoe around and repeat the process on the other branch **(Figures 17-19)** and you will have a good hind-shaped shoe **(Figure 20)**.

The method for leveling a shoe is as follows. Hold onto the heel on your tong hand side with the ground surface up **(Figure 21)**. Hammer from that side of the toe around the shoe to the opposite heel, hitting the outside of the web **(Figures 22-23)**. Grab the opposite heel with your tongs, and hammer around the shoe to the first heel you were holding **(Figure 24)** also hitting the outside of the shoe. Turn the shoe over and hold the center of the toe **(Figure 25)**. Hammer around the shoe, hitting the inside of the web **(Figure 26)**. When you get to the last inch or so of the heels, try to hit the shoe flat instead of

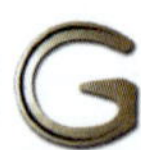

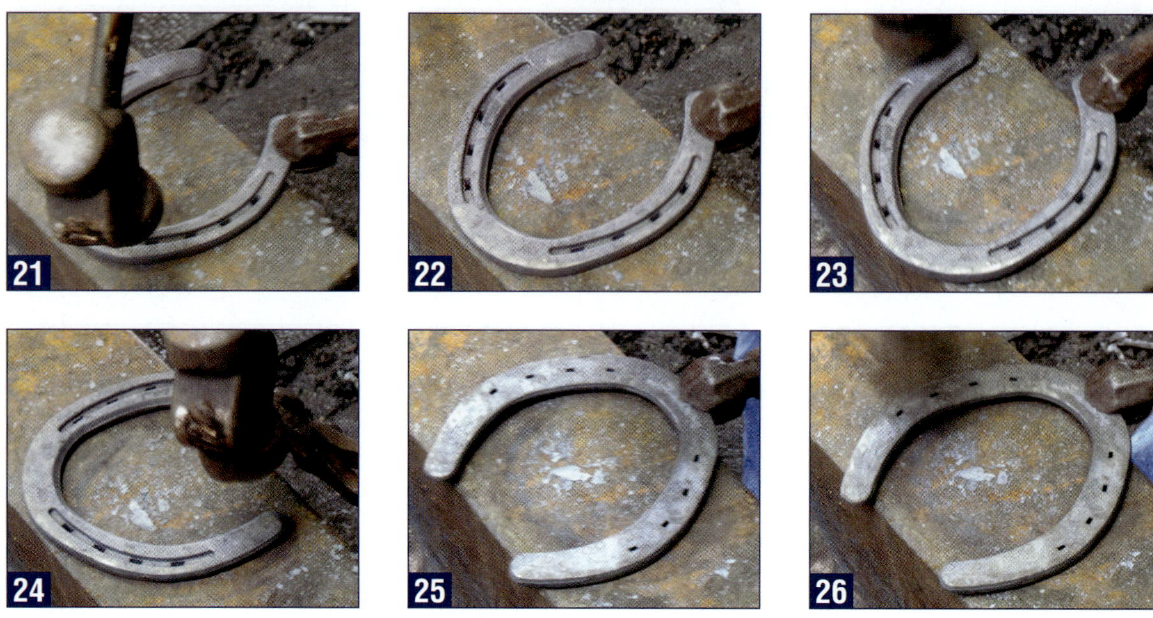

Figures 21 through 26. Steps in leveling a shoe.

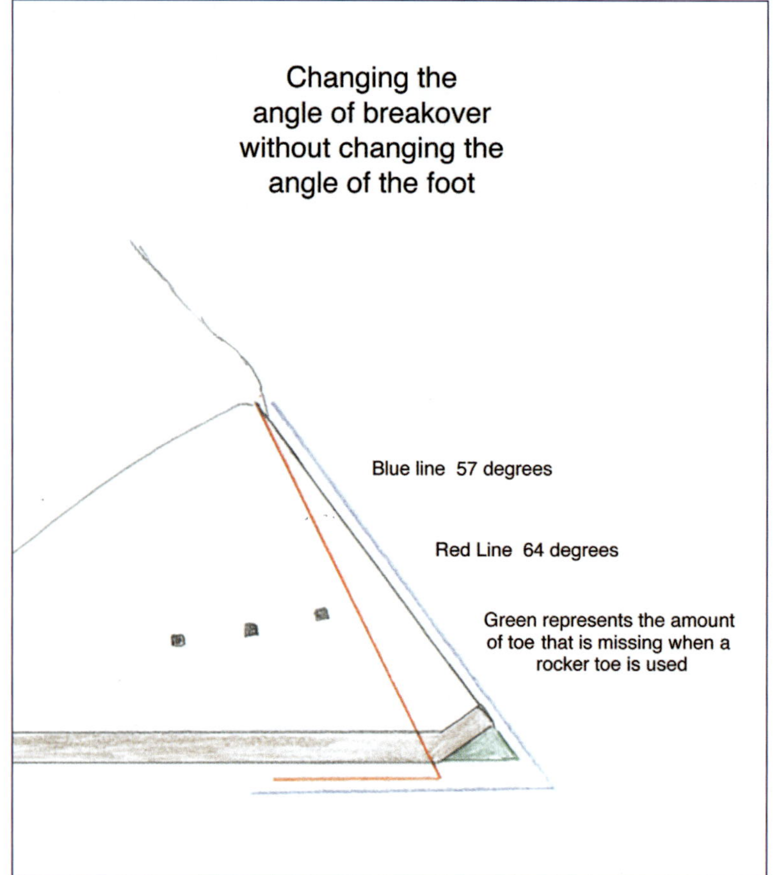

the inside of the web. This will help you avoid sprung heels.

That explains the basics of shaping. You should spend a lot of time shaping shoes from fronts to hinds and back again. This will teach you how the shoe moves when hot, and allow you to make the needed modifications for the horse.

Some of the most common modifications are the ones that are called for as part of the American Farriers' Association Certified Farrier Shoe Display. Those that have not been covered in other parts of this text can be found in this chapter.

ROCKER TOE

A rocker toe is used to change the breakover of the hoof, although there is debate about exactly how and how much. By using a rocker toe, we can change the angle of breakover without affecting the angle of the coffin bone inside the hoof capsule (drawing). This

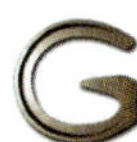

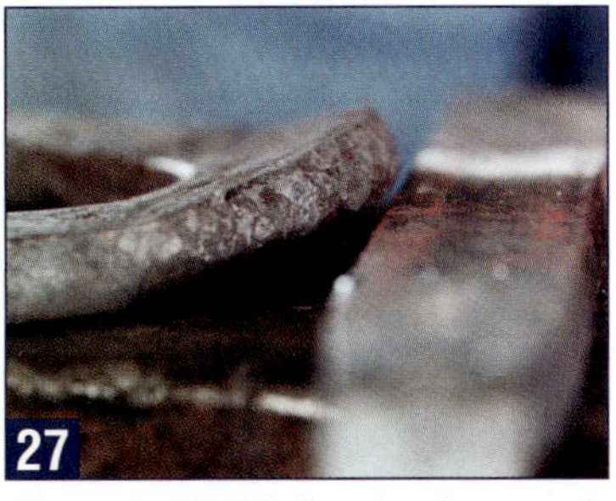

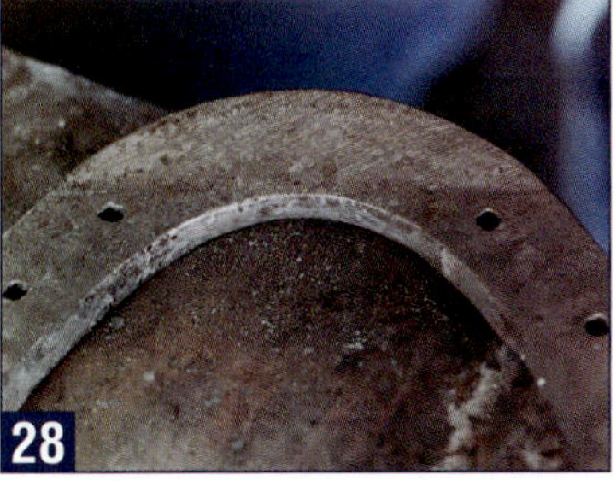

Figures 27-28. Look of a good rocker toe.

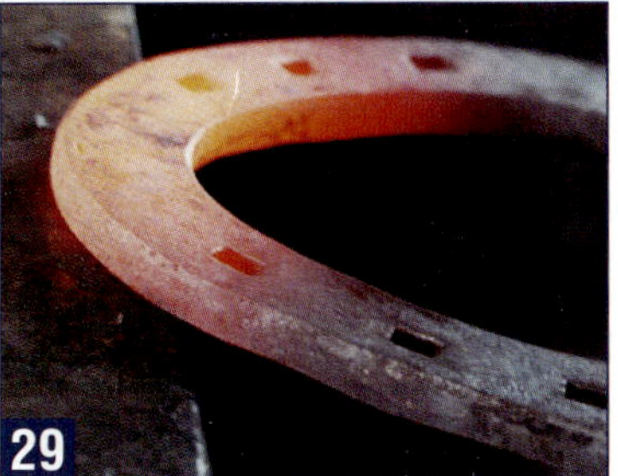

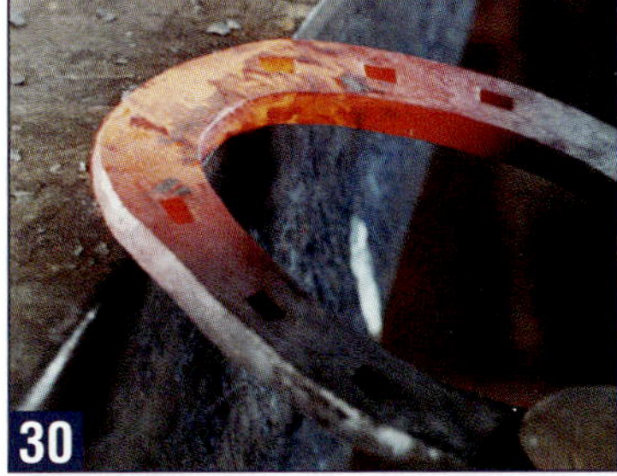

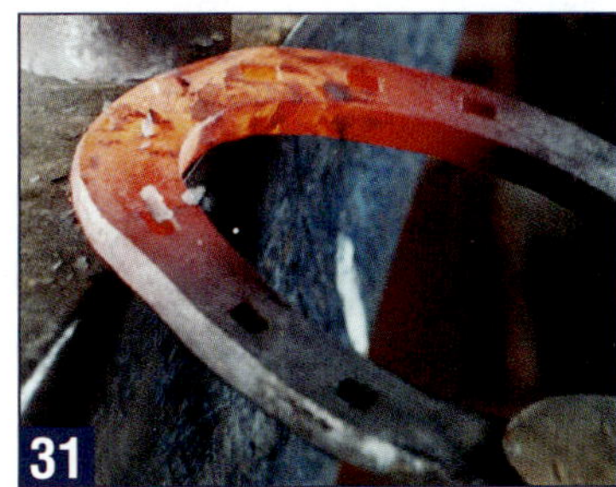

Figures 29 through 31. Making a rocker toe.

modification differs from a rolled toe and a square toe in that it breaks the plane of the foot and shoe. A rocker toe greatly increases the wearability of the shoe by moving the area of the most wear (toe) into a position where it will have less abrasion in a shoeing cycle.

I would define a rocker toe by stating that a proper rocker toe is bent to such a degree that the ground surface of the shoe at the toe is at the same level as the hoof surface of the shoe behind the rocker toe. In other words, the tip of the toe would be bent enough that there would be a 5/16-inch gap at the toe of a shoe made from 5/16-inch-thick stock when the shoe is laid on a flat surface and viewed from the side **(Figure 27)**. The thicker the stock, the more that the toe would be bent. This works out well if the stock is appropriate for the size of the hoof being shod. As for depth of the rocker toe on the stock, it should be between three-quarters and the full width of the stock **(Figure 28)**.

To apply a rocker toe to a shoe, begin by shaping or building the shoe to fit the foot. The rocker can be forged on either the near side of the anvil or over the far edge. If quarter clips are called for, pull the clips first, and use the near edge of the anvil to make the rocker toe.

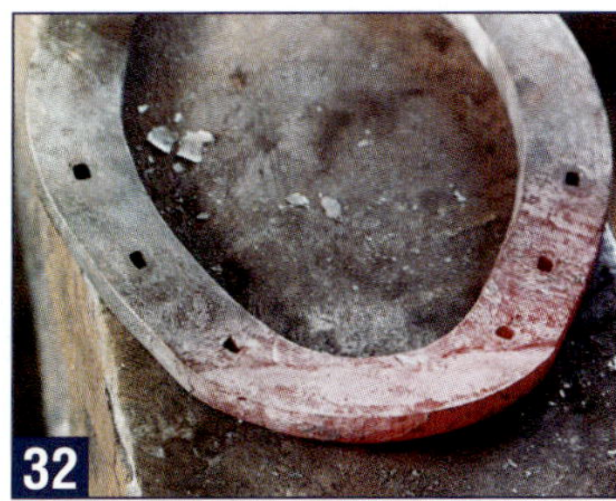

Depth of the rocker toe.

Begin by placing the desired amount of stock past the edge of the anvil **(Figure 29)**. Hold one heel of the shoe and strike the toe on the same side that you are holding **(Figure 30)**. You can either hold the opposite heel for the other side of the toe,or continue holding it as you are. By changing tong position, there is less chance of warping the level of the shoe; however, leveling the shoe is not hard to do.

After striking the second side of the toe, hammer with overlapping hammer blows from one side of the toe to the other **(Figure 31)**. It is important that the shoe does not move while this is being done, since this will cause a bunch of lines on the hoof surface of the shoe. These lines will make the

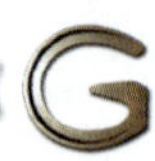

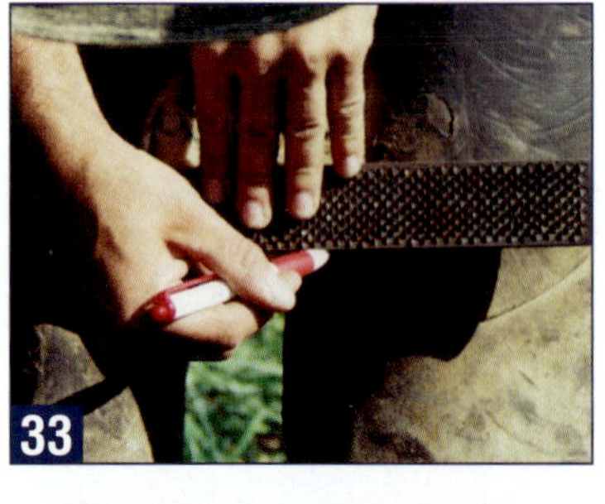

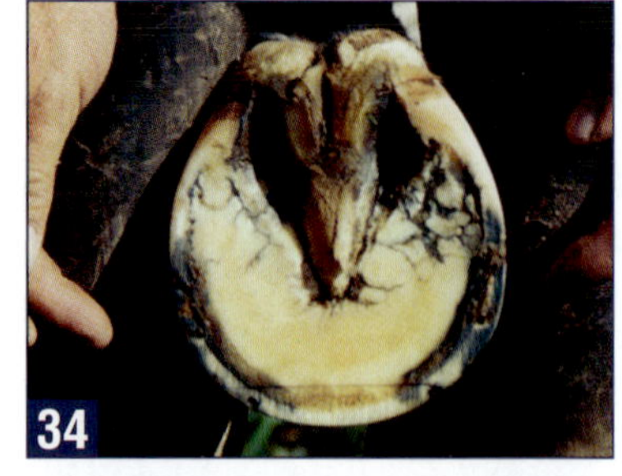

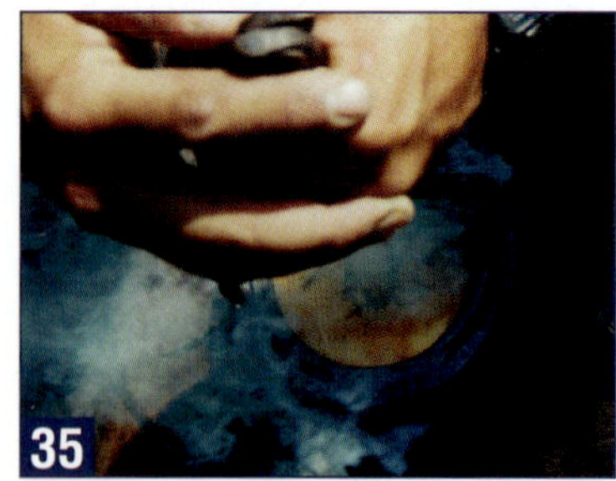

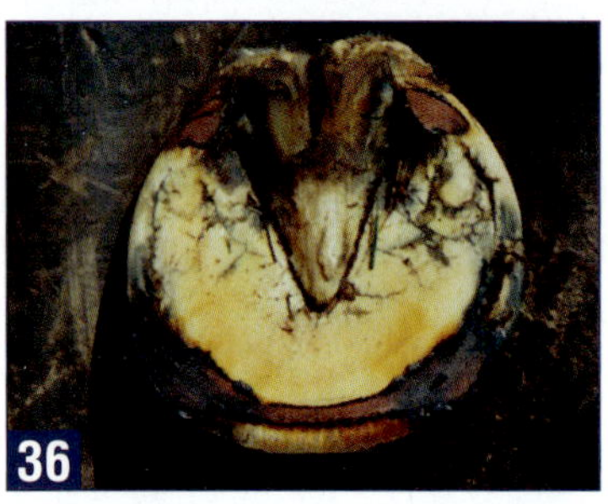

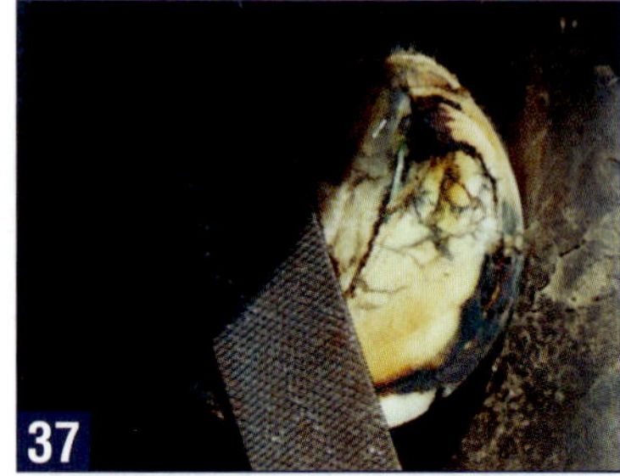

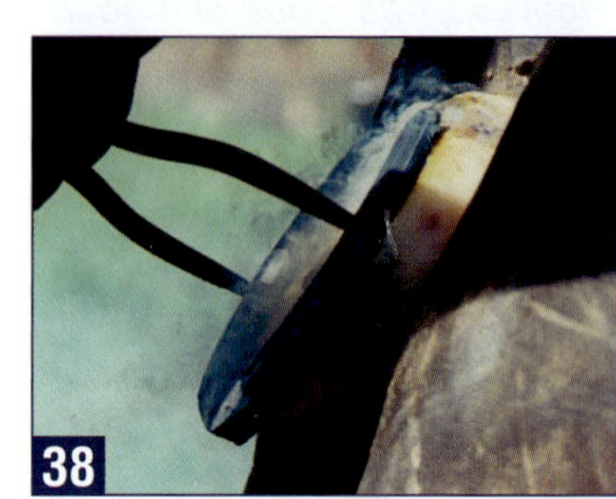

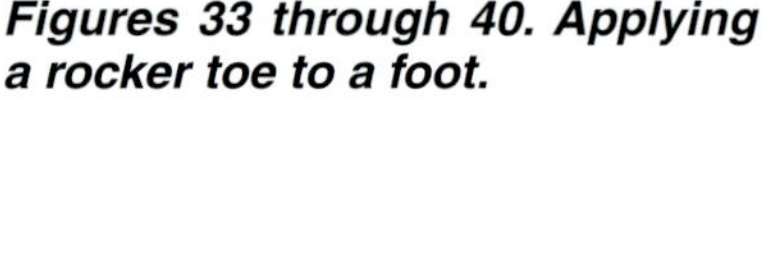

Figures 33 through 40. Applying a rocker toe to a foot.

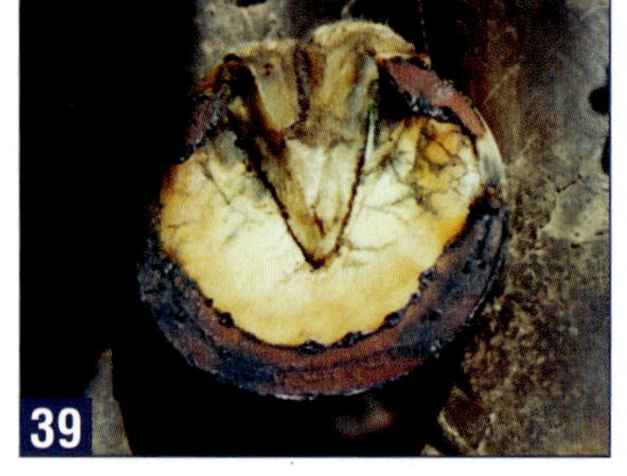

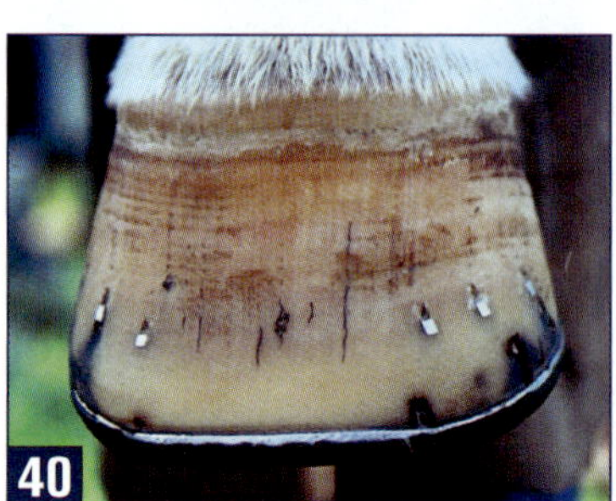

shoe more difficult to fit. When the rocker toe is complete, you want one, crisp line on the hoof surface of the shoe **(Figure 32)**.

To level a shoe with a rocker toe, hold the toe of the shoe over the near side of the anvil and level toward the heels with overlapping blows on the ground surface. Turn the shoe over and repeat the process on the hoof surface, hitting toward the inside perimeter of the web.

When fitting a rocker toe, you can start by drawing a line across the foot where you want the rocker toe to be **(Figures 33 and 34)**. Bevel the foot to that line to accommodate the level of the rocker toe. Burn the shoe **(Figure 35)** and evaluate where you need to remove horn by looking at the burn **(Figure 36)**. Lightly rasp the area that is burned **(Figure 37)**, avoiding the areas that did not burn. Burn again as in **Figure 38**, and you should end up with a nice full burn as shown in **Figure 39**. If everything is done correctly, you will end up with a tight and solid fit as seen in **Figure 40**. There are a lot of farriers that just accept gaps in a rocker toe as if they are unavoidable. Using the method described will help you stay out of that category. With a little experience, you will be able to forego using a marker on the foot and go straight to making the bevel at the toe.

ROLLED TOE

A rolled toe is similar to a rocker toe in application. A rolled toe is not as severe as a rocker toe, and the hoof surface remains level both on the shoe and the foot. Fitting a rolled toe is as easy as fitting any normal flat shoe, while it takes additional skill to fit a rocker toe.

Begin by heating the shoe and holding it so that one side of the toe is at the far edge of the anvil face **(Figure 41)**. By holding the shoe at the edge of the anvil, it is possible to hit the edge of the shoe with the center of the hammer. If this is done in the middle of the anvil, you will end up denting the anvil face with the edge of the hammer. Turn the hammer so that the head comes down at an angle, even though it is still a straight hammer swing **(Figure 42)**. Bevel an area on one side of the toe just

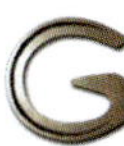

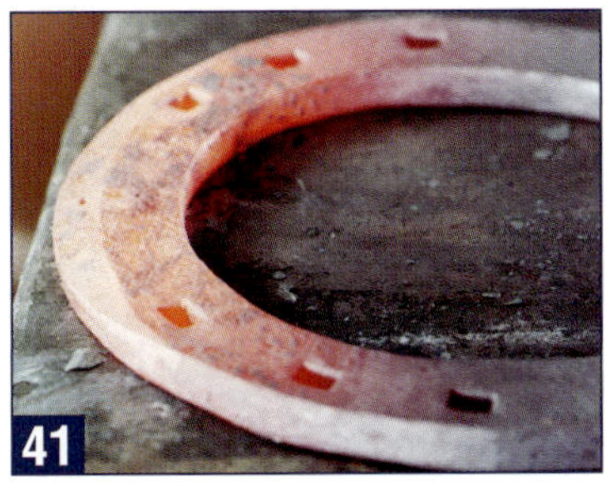

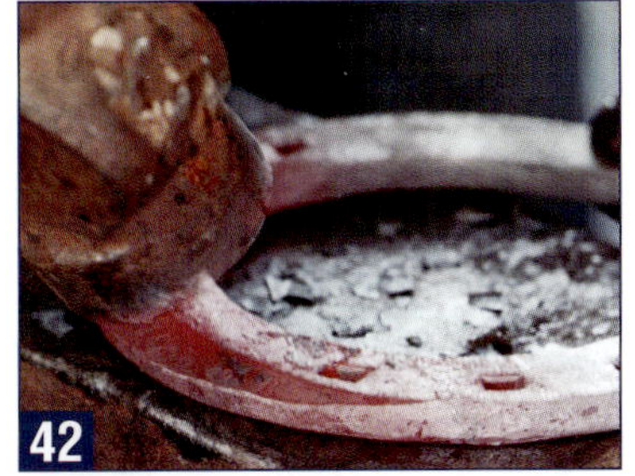

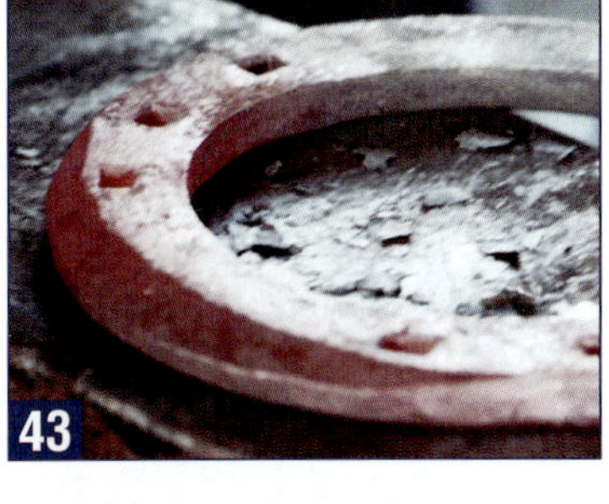

Figures 41 through 45. Making a rolled toe.

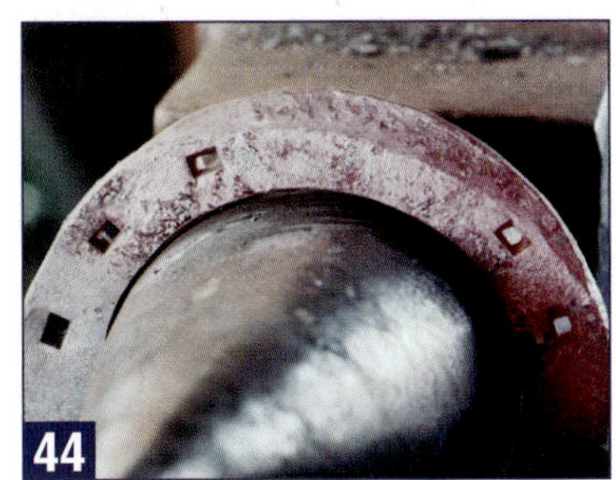

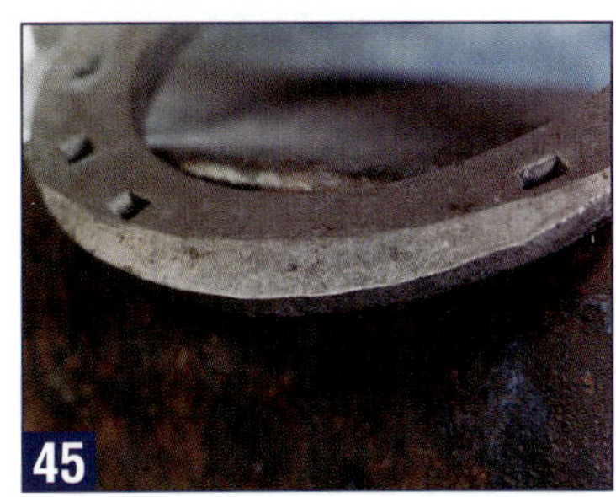

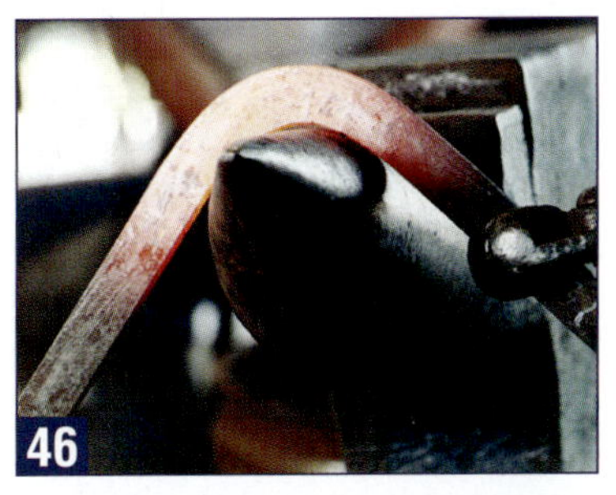

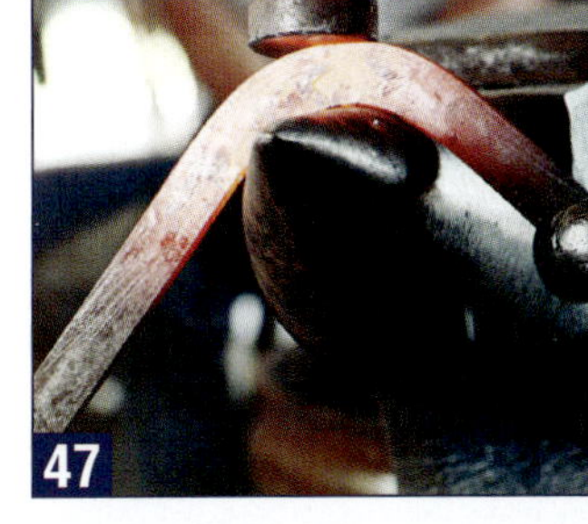

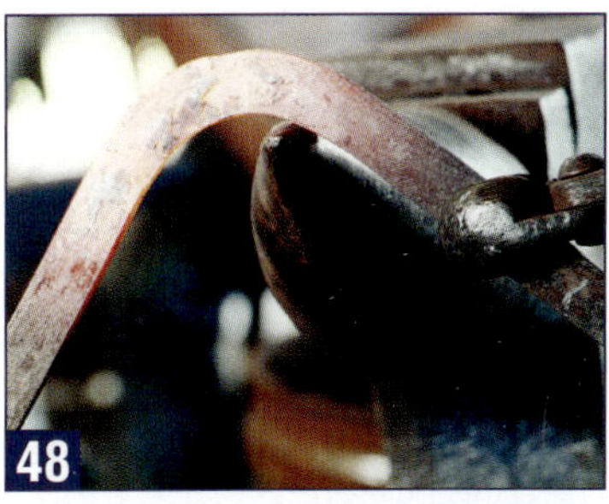

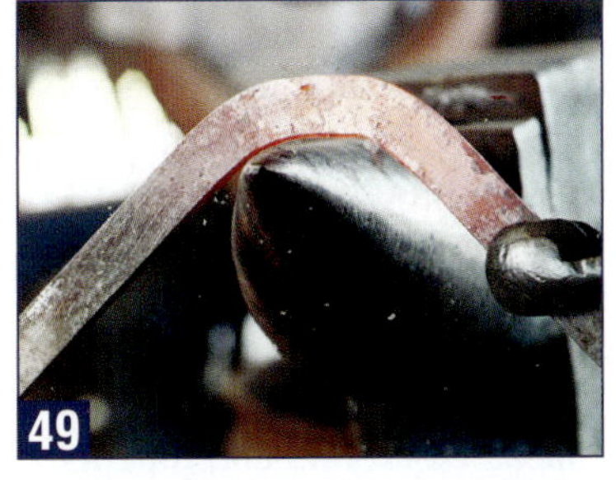

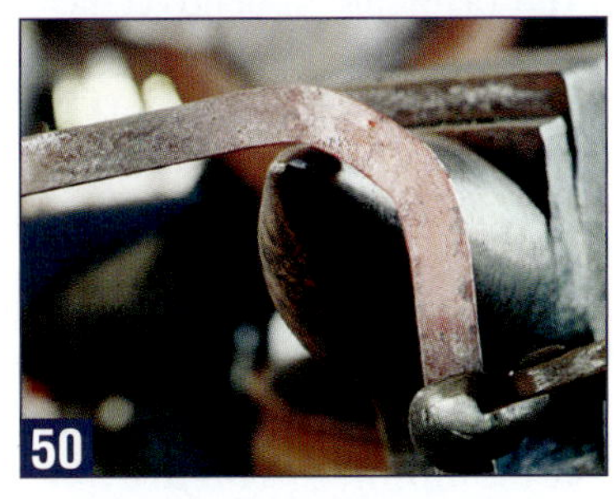

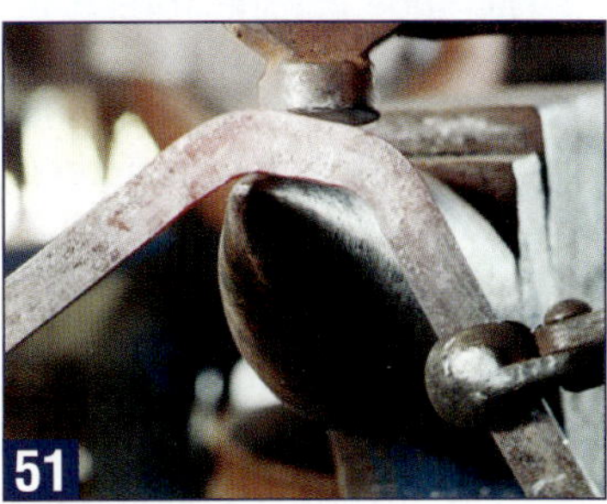

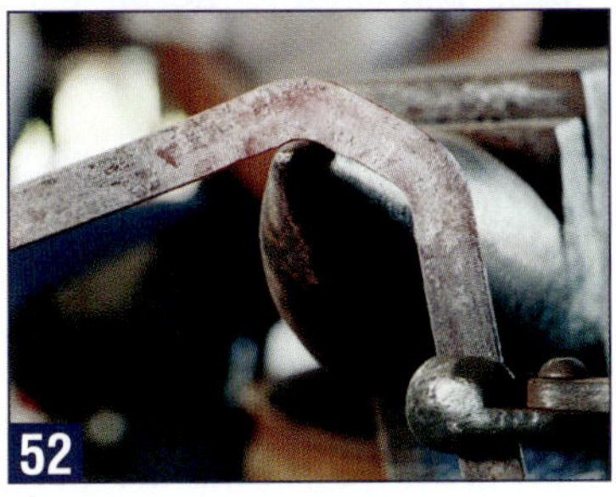

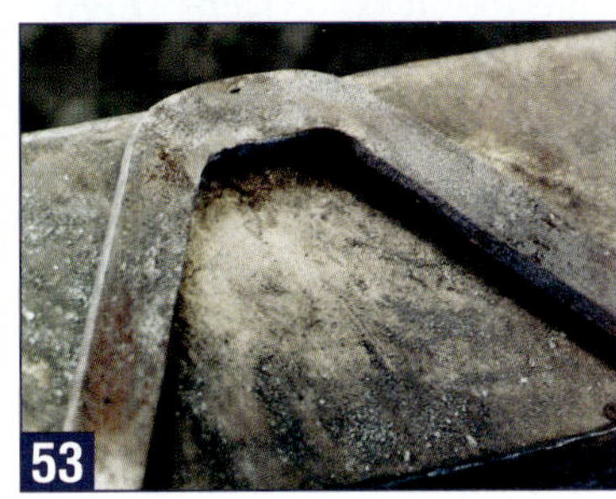

Figures 46 through 53. Forging a handmade square toe.

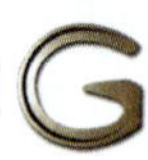

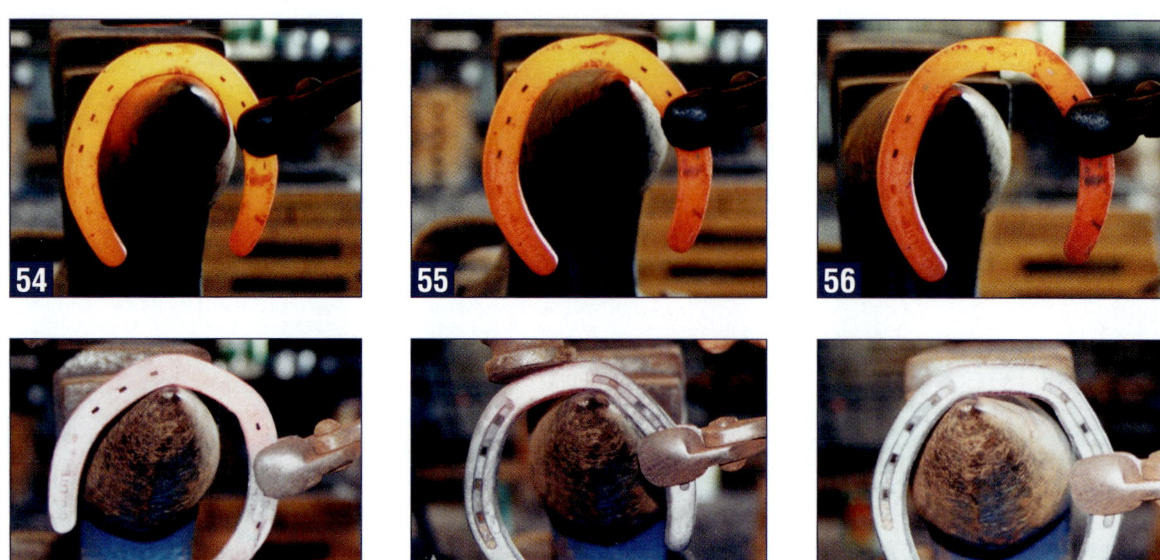

Figures 54 through 60. Forging a square toe on a keg shoe.

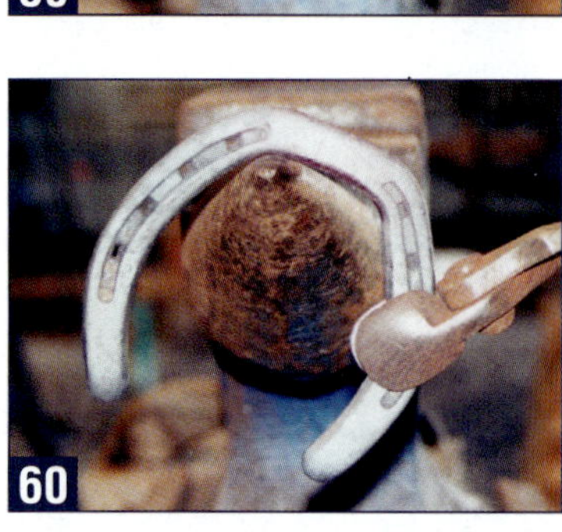

wider than the face of your hammer, then turn the shoe so you can repeat the process on the opposite side of the toe.

After a portion has been beveled on each side of the toe, simply connect the two bevels through the middle of the toe **(Figure 43)**. Try to control the hammer so that there is a neat clean line that defines the rolled toe.

The shoe can be forged back to the original width on the horn **(Figure 44)**. Once complete, the hoof surface will be flat, while the ground surface is forged to create a different breakover **(Figure 45)**. You can rasp the rolled toe to make it clean and crisp, but getting it that way with a hammer is generally not too hard to do either.

SQUARE TOE

There are three basic positions on the tip of the horn that are used to make a square toe. It is important that you work at the very tip of the horn so that the inside radius is small at each corner of the square toe.

Square toes are easiest applied to handmade shoes at the time when the toe bend is being made. It is a simple thing to square up and make crisp at this point in the process. Begin with a tight toe bend **(Figure 46)**, and move to the horn to begin forging the square portion of the toe. Center the toe bend on the horn and hit lightly **(Figure 47)**. Move to the tip of the horn and hit just past the point of contact **(Figure 48)**. Pull the shoe toward you so that the same amount is in front of the horn that was past it for the last hammer blow **(Figure 49)**. Hit the stock just in front of the point of contact. Lower your tong hand so that the branch extends straight out from the point of contact with the horn and hammer just past that point of contact **(Figure 50)**. Turn the stock around and repeat the steps **(Figure 51 - 52)**. You should end up with a well-defined square toe by using this process **(Figure 53)**.

If a square toe is going to be used on a keg shoe or a handmade that is already complete, the same positions on the anvil will make it easy. Heat the toe of the shoe and place it on the top of the horn in an area with a slightly larger radius than the one already in the toe **(Figure 54)**. Hammer directly into the top center of the horn until the inside of

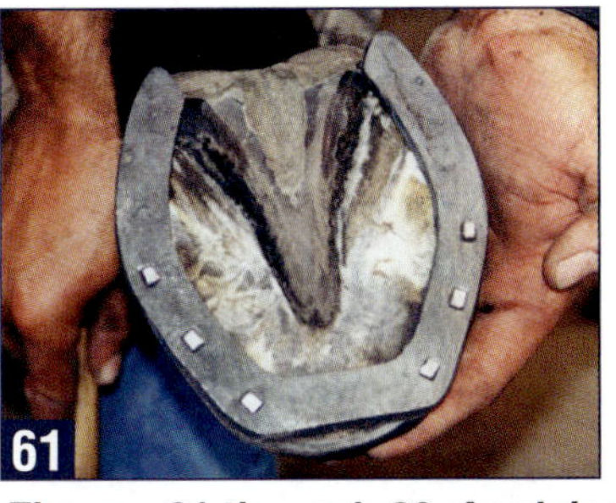

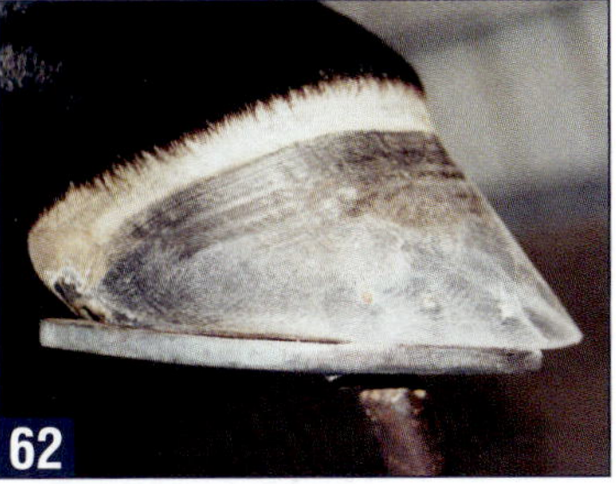

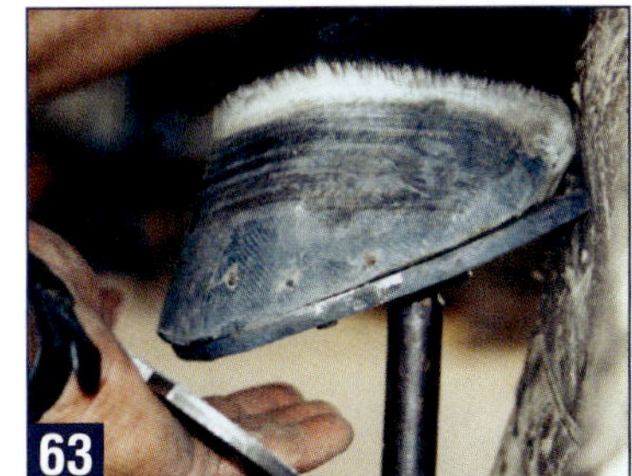

Figures 61 through 63. Applying a square toe to a foot.

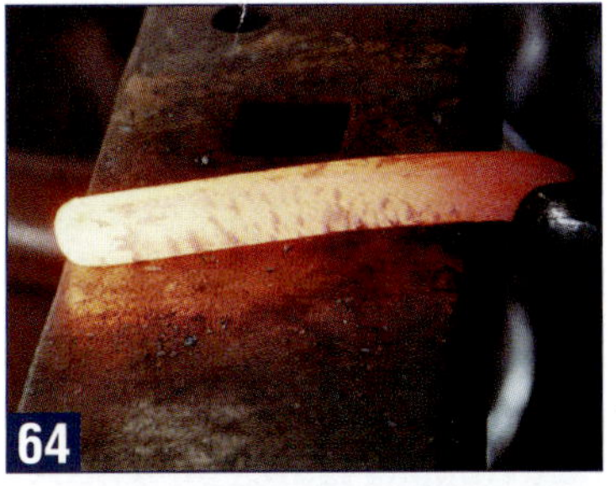

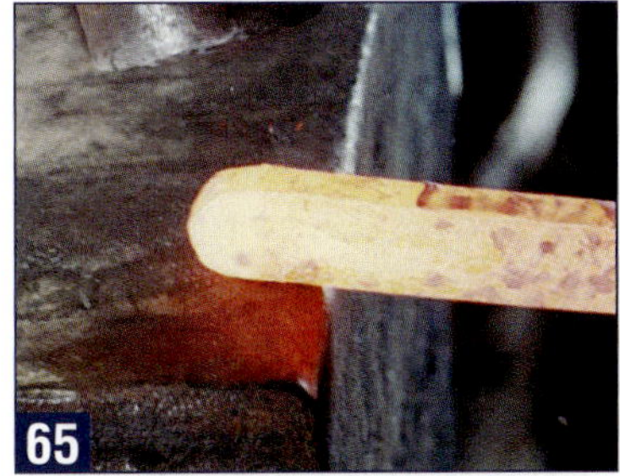

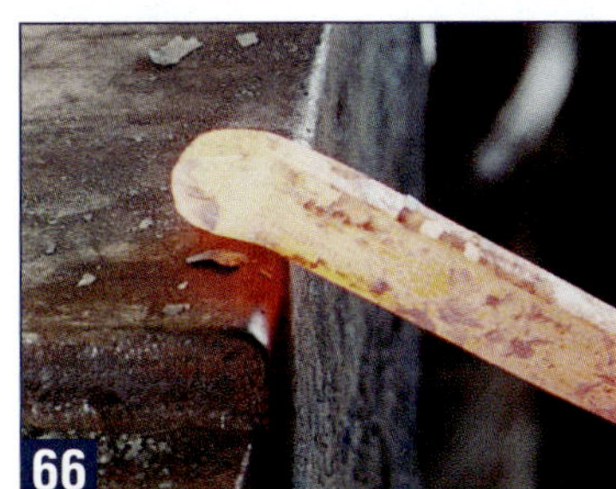

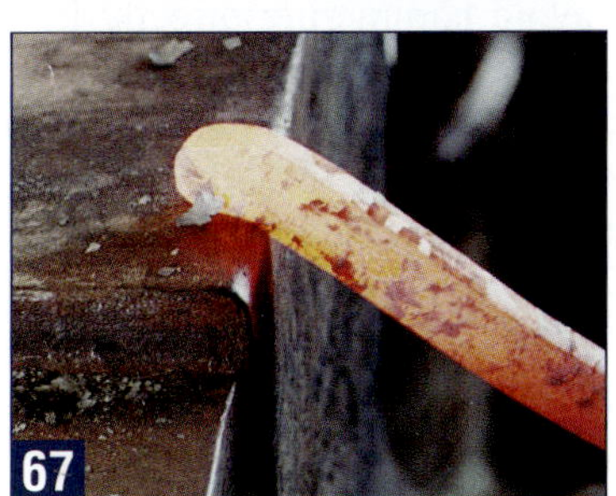

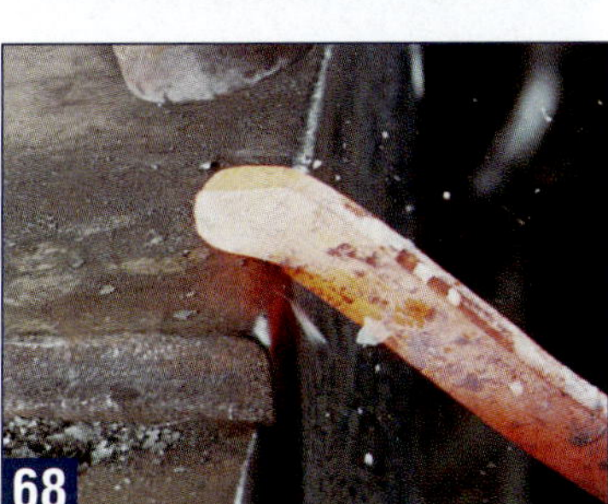

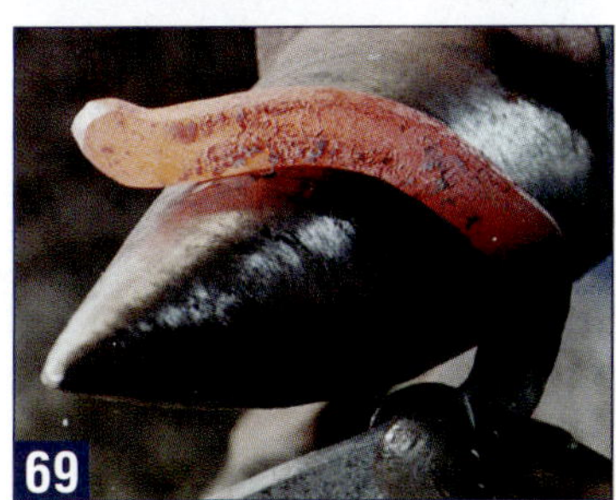

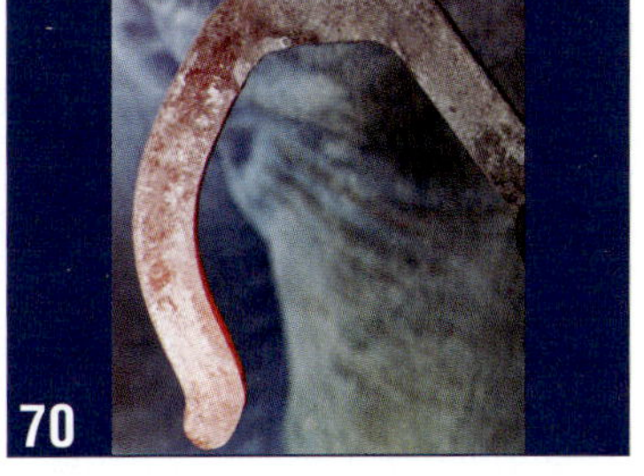

Figures 64 through 70. Forging a trailer on a handmade shoe.

the web makes contact with the horn. Move to the tip of the horn, and place the area of the toe that is to be bent on top of the horn. Hit beyond the point of contact on the horn to straighten the toe and start the initial bend **(Figure 55)**. Pull the shoe so that the area to be bent on the opposite side of the toe is on top of the horn **(Figure 56)**. Drive the hammer into the toe on the near side of the horn. Lower your tong hand, and hammer with an angled blow just beyond the bend **(Figure 57)**. Turn the shoe around and repeat the steps from the other side **(Figures 58-60)**. Take care to avoid hitting too hard, since nail holes are easily closed and the width of the stock can be compromised. While it isn't possible to make a truly crisp corner with this method, an adequate square toe can be accomplished.

A square toe should be fit where the corners of the toe fit the sides of the foot. You can see in **Figure 61** that the square toed shoe looks like a normal shoe on the foot with the toe moved back. Nail the shoe in this position, then take the foot to the stand.

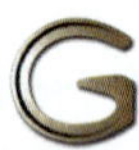

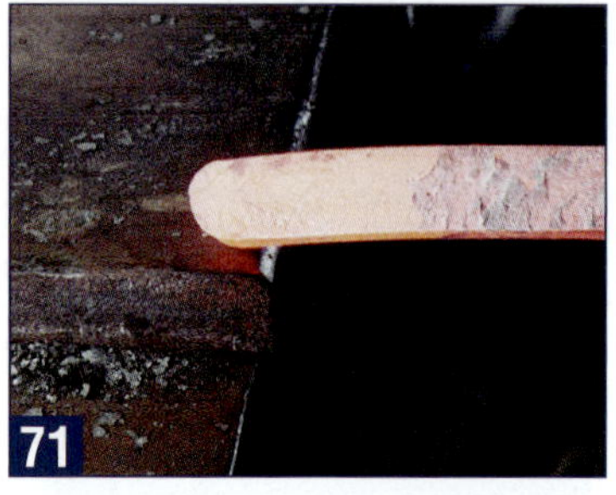

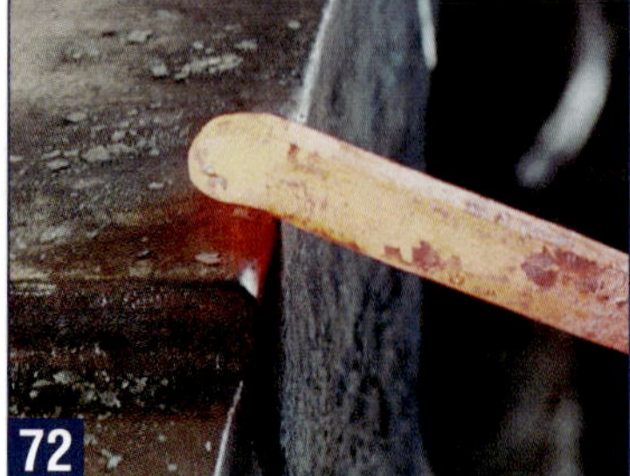

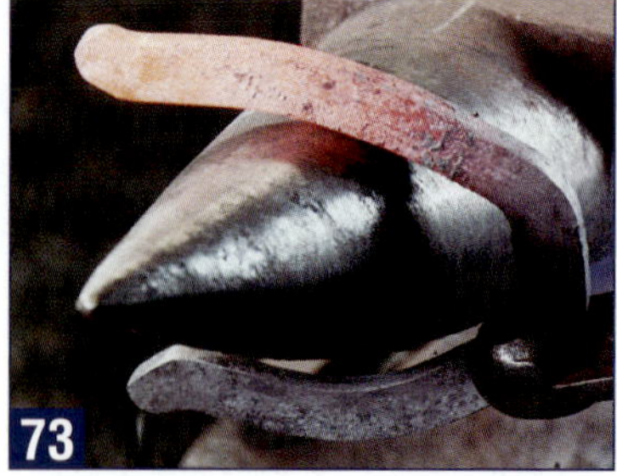

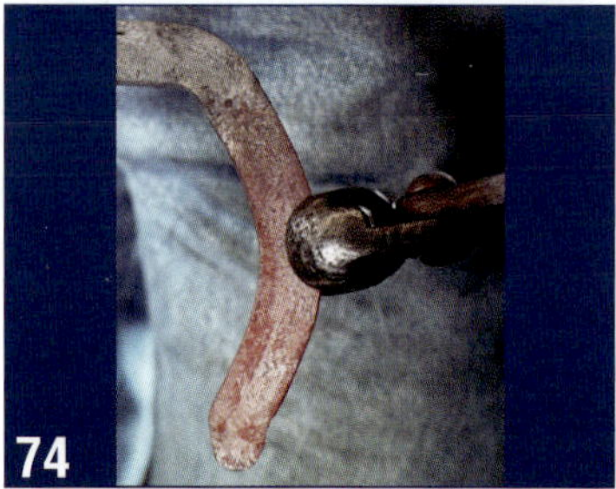

Figures 71 through 74. Forging an extended heel on a handmade shoe.

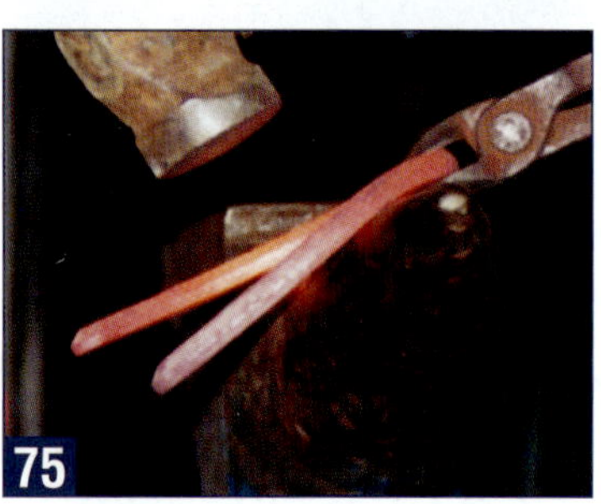

75. Bending the shoe to allow access to the heels

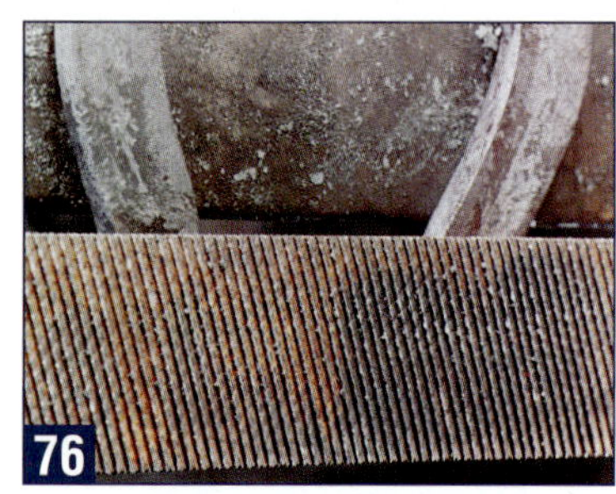

76. Hiding the extended heel and trailer so that you can see the shape of the shoe.

In **Figure 62**, the amount of foot past the shoe is evident. Rasp this portion at a bevel as in **Figure 63**. We call this the traveler's groove.

TRAILERS AND EXTENDED HEELS

These modifications are useful on many horses, and are often used in conjunction with a square toe. Like the square toe, they are easier to apply to a handmade while it is being made, but they can be forged on keg shoes and completed handmades when needed.

To make a trailer or extended heel on a handmade, begin by making a round heel while the shoe is being built **(Figure 64)**. The end of the stock can be upset in the straight to enhance the finished product if so desired. Once the round heel is forged, place the desired amount of stock past the near edge of the anvil face in an area where there is a good radius on the edge **(Figure 65)**. Hammer lightly as you allow the shoe to drop **(Figures 66-68)**. Try to avoid hammering directly into the corner of the anvil because it will cut deeply into the width of the stock. Continue to build the shoe normally, fine-tuning the angle of the trailer once the shoe is made **(Figures 69 - 70)**. There are three methods of defining a trailer that I know of. It can be at 45 degrees to the sagital plane of the foot; it can point to the toe nail on the opposite branch; or it can be parallel to the area of the opposite branch behind the quarter.

Extended heels are made the same way that trailers are **(Figures 71-74)**. The big exception is that the extended heel is not forged nearly as far as a trailer. To define an extended heel, it should be straight with the line of foot flight.

To apply extended heels or a trailer on a shoe that is already built, heat the shoe and hold by the toe. Place the shoe on the horn and bend the branch downward on the tong hand side of the shoe **(Figure 75)**. Flip the shoe over, and bend the opposite branch. Still holding the toe, build the extension just as you would with a handmade.

Trailers are found only on the lateral side, and they require more stock. For a handmade, mark the stock off-center in the straight to allow for the trailer. However far off-center a piece is marked,

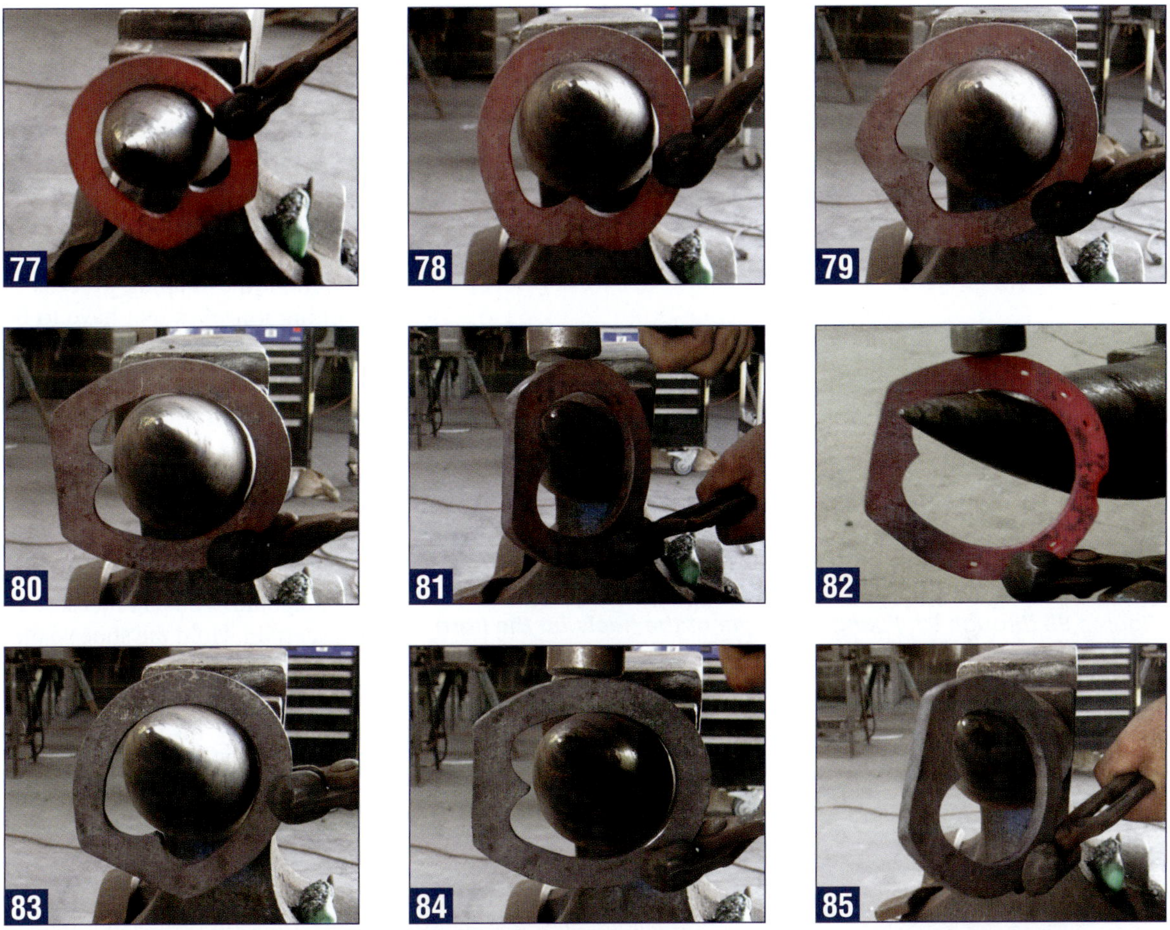

Figures 77 through 85. Steps in shaping a bar shoe.

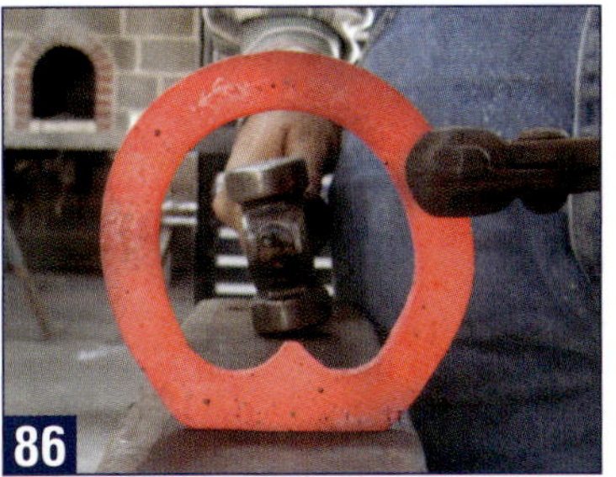

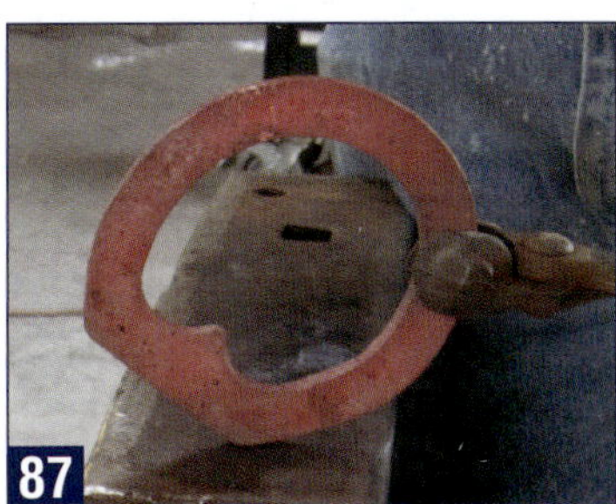

86 – 87. Hammering across the long diagonal.

the difference between the two branches will be doubled. With a keg shoe, there are two options. Either offset the toe to allow for the additional length needed, or build the trailer on the lateral side and cut the excess heel off the medial side. Once you have made these modifications, evaluate the shape of your shoe without including the modifications. You can see in **Figure 76** that I have placed a rasp over the extended heels so that I can see the shoe without having the modifications fool my eye.

SHAPING BAR SHOES

With time and practice, you will find that welding the bar shoe is the easiest part of the job. Making the

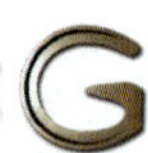

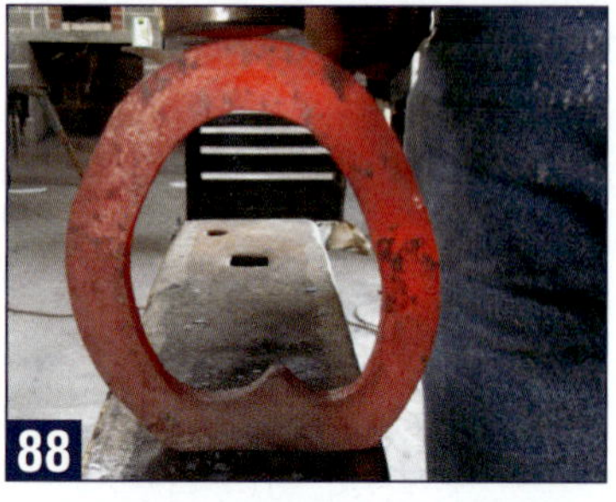

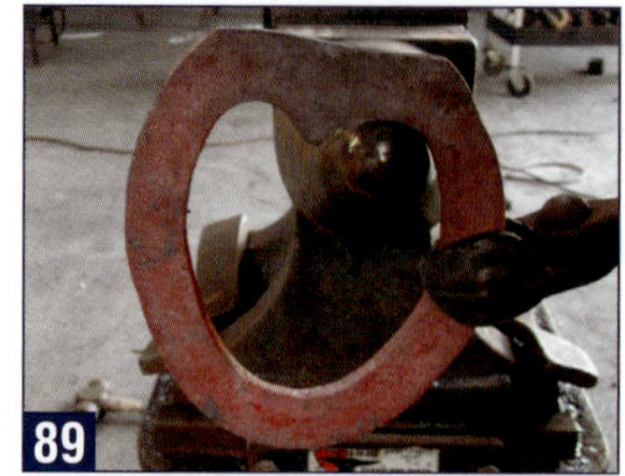

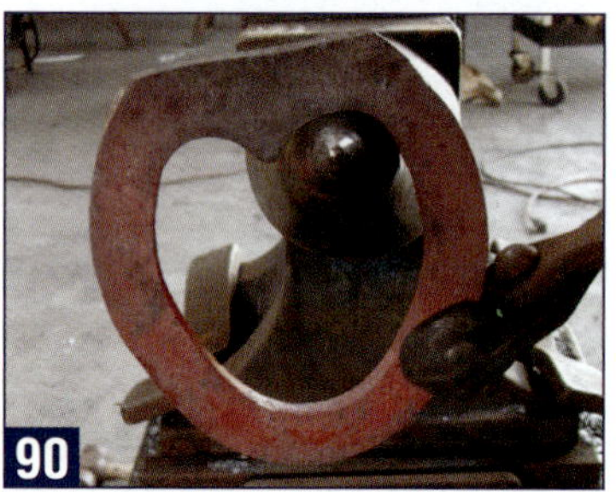

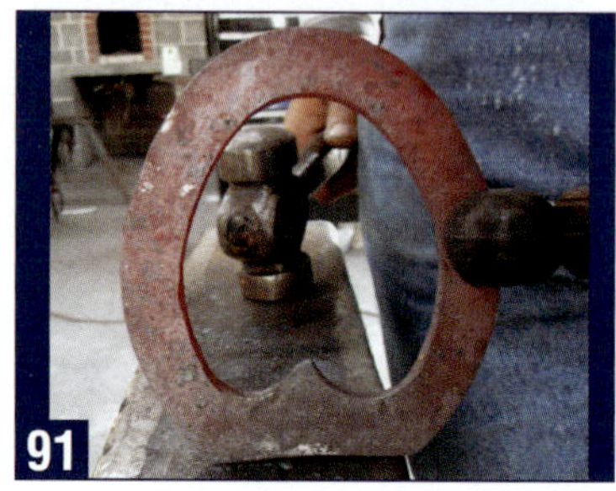

Figures 88 through 91. Fixing the angle of the heels on the horn.

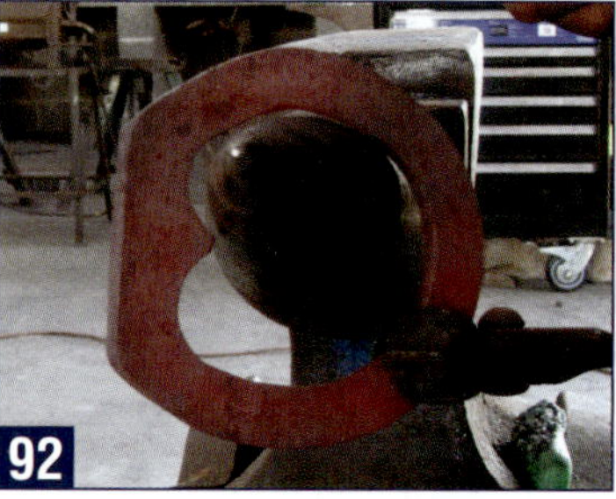

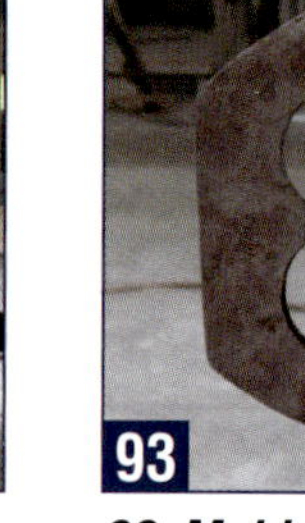

92. Finding a larger radius.

93. Making a tighter radius.

shoe the right size and shape is actually harder than the welding. Bear in mind that the bar connects both sides of the shoe. This means that anything you do to one side will affect the opposite side. With open-heeled shoes, it is possible to work one side of the shoe to where you want it and not worry about it changing while the other side is shaped. This just isn't so with a bar shoe.

Make sure that there is an even heat on the entire shoe, and work the shoe from widest point to widest point over the top of the horn **(Figure 77-80)**. Once you reach the widest part of the shoe, the bar should be perpendicular to the ground. From the widest part of the shoe to the bar, find a radius on the end of the horn that has the desired shape. **Figures 81 and 82** are of the ending position at the end of the horn from different angles. To shape this portion, you have to let your hammer travel over the shoe instead of moving your shoe under the hammer. Turn the shoe around, and repeat the entire process on the opposite side **(Figures 83-85)**. Hammer lightly throughout the shaping process to avoid big mistakes that have to be fixed.

A common problem with bar shoes is having a long diagonal **(Figure 86)**. If the bar is laid parallel to the near edge of the anvil, it will look like it is leaning to one side or the other. Whichever side it is leaning to will be the long diagonal. You can measure to make certain. Hold the shoe so that you can hammer across the long diagonal on the face of the anvil, and hit lightly on the other side **(Figure 87)**. This will shorten the longest diagonal while it lengthens the shortest diagonal. Often times it only takes a few well-placed blows to bring a shoe into symmetry.

Another method for dealing with a long radius is to determine where the tighter angle coming off of the bar in the heel is. You can see that the shoe in **Figure 88** has a tighter angle at the right heel than at the left. Place the bar on the tip of the horn so that you are holding the side of the shoe with the more open angle **(Figure 89)** and hammer just past the point of contact with the horn **(Figure 90)**. With just a few hammer blows, you can see the difference in the bar in **Figure 91**. This method is a more correct way than hammering across the long diagonal, but both methods have their merits.

The next thing to work on is radiuses in the shoe. You can forge these by finding a larger radius on the horn, and changing the radius of the shoe by forging it into the desired shape. In **Figure 92**, I am straightening a tight radius in the quarter, and in **Figure 93**, I am creating a tighter radius in the toe quarter.

If you need to crisp up the outside of the heels or decrease the width of your bar, there are a couple of

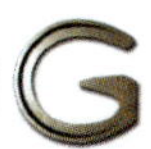

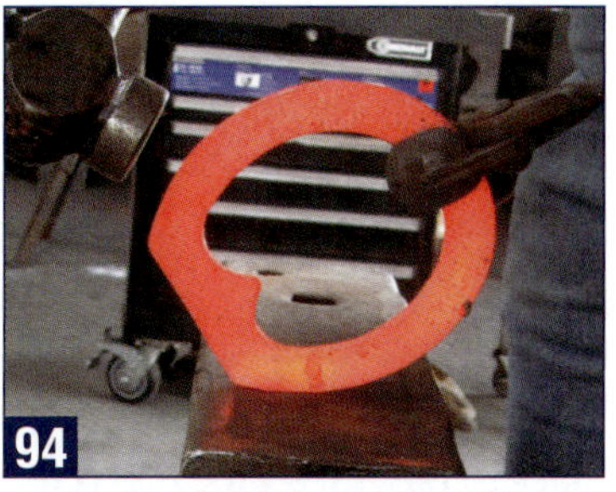

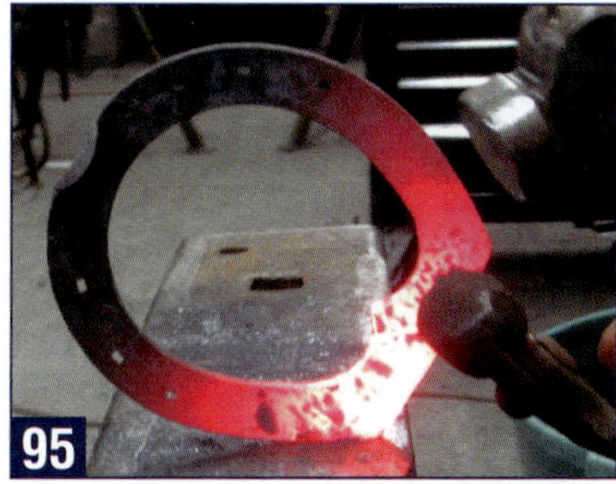

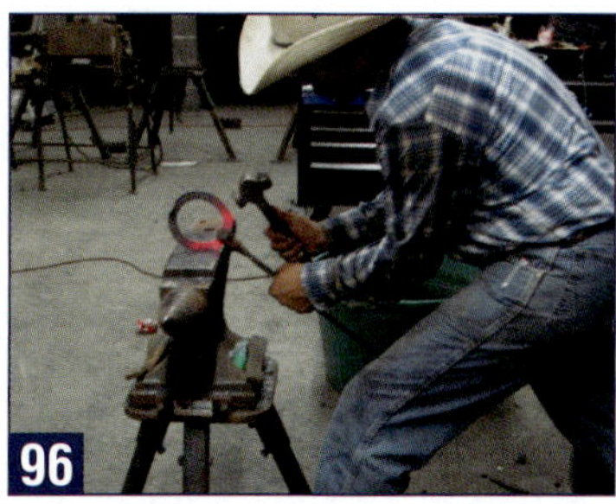

Figures 94 through 96. Crisping up the outside of the heels and shortening the bar.

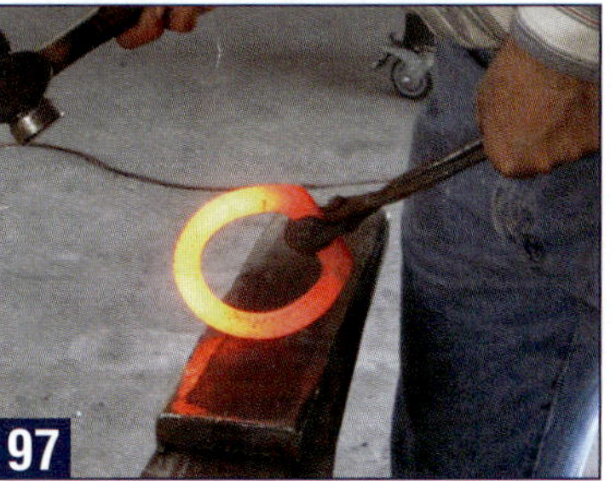

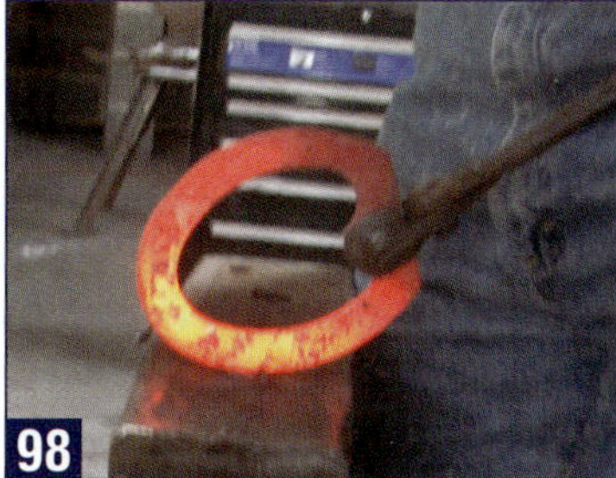

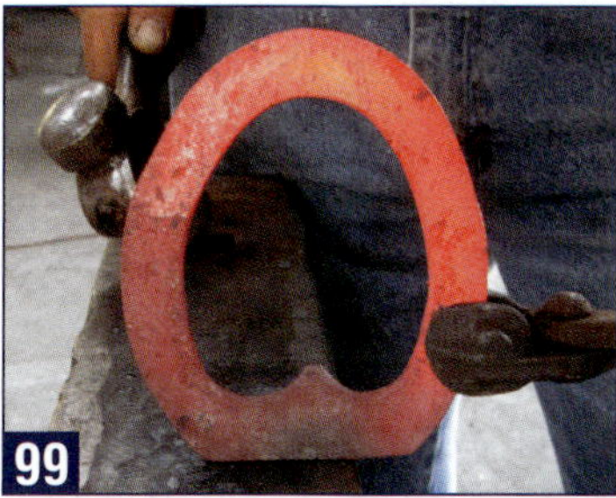

Figures 97 through 99. Steps in making a front bar shoe into a hind bar shoe.

good positions. First, you can hold the toe and place one heel on the anvil at an angle, then hammer into the opposite heel at an angle. You can see this in **Figure 94**. Another method is to hold the bar with the toe pointing away from you and hammer into one heel with an angled blow while the opposite heel is on the face of the anvil. **(Figure 95)** To do this move, you may have to lower your body to get the right angle as I am doing in **Figure 96**.

Finally, turning a front shoe into a hind shoe is easy with bar shoes. Simply heat the shoe and hold in the center of the bar. Place the shoe on the face of the anvil at an angle, and hammer at an angle from the opposite side **(Figures 97 and 98)**. Turn the shoe around and repeat from the other side. This is a fast and simple way to get a shoe close to a hind shape **(Figure 99)**, and you can move to the horn to finalize the shape.

We have covered a lot of ground in this chapter. Take each piece and work to master the techniques described. You will find that they are used constantly in the pursuit of becoming a great farrier, and everything that you can master and add to your skill set will bring you closer to that goal.

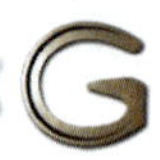

Chapter

28 CLIP FITTING

In some parts of the world, clips are as much a part of shoeing a horse as are nails. It makes sense to use clips if you have the skills to do it correctly. A well-clipped shoe that is nailed up and finished pretty on a good foot is the sort of thing that will set you apart from the competition.

The main function of a clip is to relieve the nails of shear forces. With the advent of pre-clipped shoes, many farriers are using clips without having the skills to use them correctly. Clips are not to be fitted cold or hammered in on iron shoes, yet this is a common practice now with such a large variety of products available. Clips should be angled to match the angle of the hoof wall, with a radius that matches the outside perimeter radius of the foot. They should be cut in and then burned into the outer hoof wall, and the final fit should be clean and completely smooth.

PROCEDURE FOR FITTING CLIPS

Begin by prepping the foot normally. Whether you pull your clip before or after shaping your shoe is a personal choice. Some farriers destroy the shoe shape when clipping, so they have to shape after clipping, whether they want to or not. See the section on pulling clips in Chapter 37, Forging Basics, for tips on how to avoid this problem.

With the clips pulled, place hot fitting tongs in the shoe. I personally like to use hot fitters that are attached to both sides of the shoe **(Figure 1)**, but you can get just as good a fit using a carrying pritchel or needle-nosed vice grips. Approach the horse with the shoe at a bright red heat. Clips are very thin, and if you try to fit with a shoe that is too cold, you will only end up cooling the clips off too soon to have them fit perfectly. The hoof wall is 25% water, and water is what we use to quench hot metal. Lift the foot you want to fit and put the shoe in position on the foot without actually touching the bottom of the foot with the hot shoe. Just touch the clip to the wall **(Figure 2)**. This is not to burn the clip into the foot, but rather to mark an area of the foot where the clip is going to be fitted. Your first touch is just to mark the foot.

Pull up on the toe of the foot so that you can get a good angle to cut out the area for the clip **(Figure 3)**. Place your off hand on the foot and use your thumb as a fulcrum for your knife. It is very similar to knifing the bottom of the foot. Trying to cut out clips without the aid of the off hand will generally lead to cutting out an area that is not the right exact size for the clip, and that leads to a bad clip fit. Cut to the depth that you think the clip needs to burn in to. If you want to move the shoe back with a toe clip, cut further to allow the shoe to move back. It is important to remember that this is not so much about burning the clip in, rather it is about cutting the clip in and sizing the area with a hot clip.

So far, the foot has not been exposed to too much heat. You have only touched it in one or two areas, depending on the number of clips. Now take the still hot shoe and burn it into position **(Figures 4 and 5)**. You may want to have a tool that you can push the shoe back into the foot with. The end of my hoof

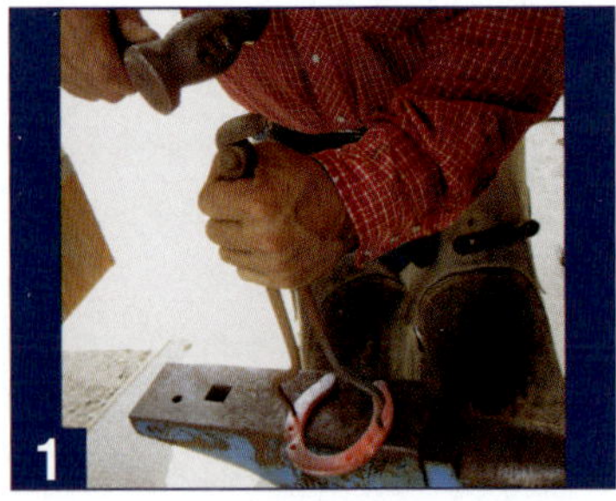

1 *Putting hot fitters into a shoe.*

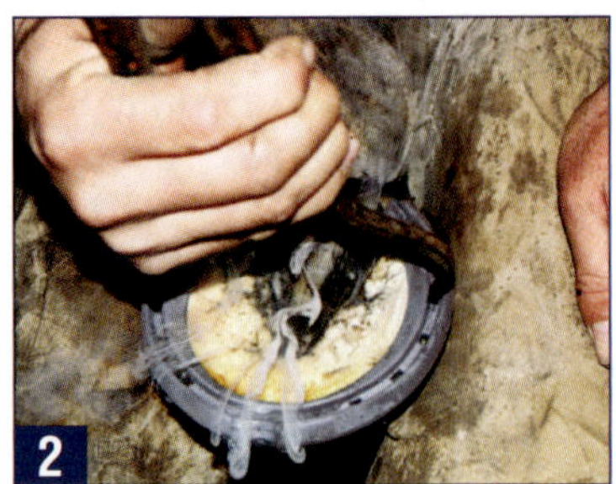

2 *Marking the toe clip.*

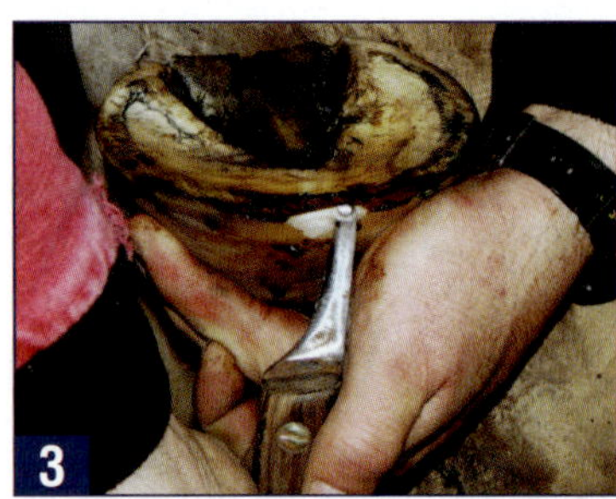

3 *Cutting the area that was marked.*

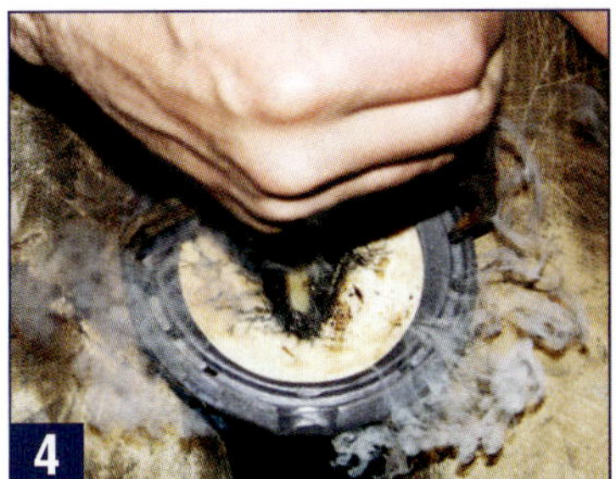
4 Burning the clip cut.

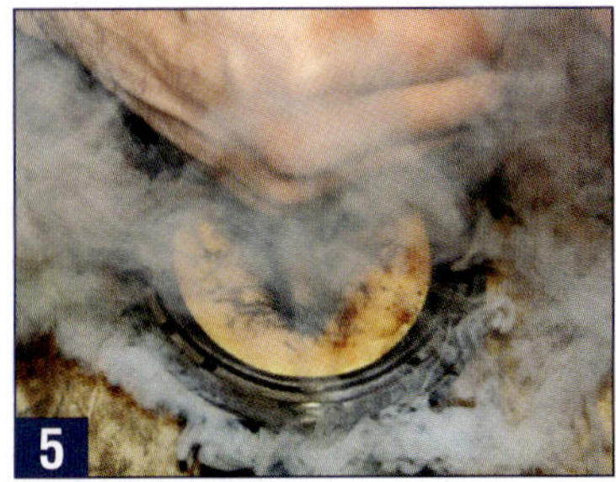
5 Finishing the burn on the clip cut.

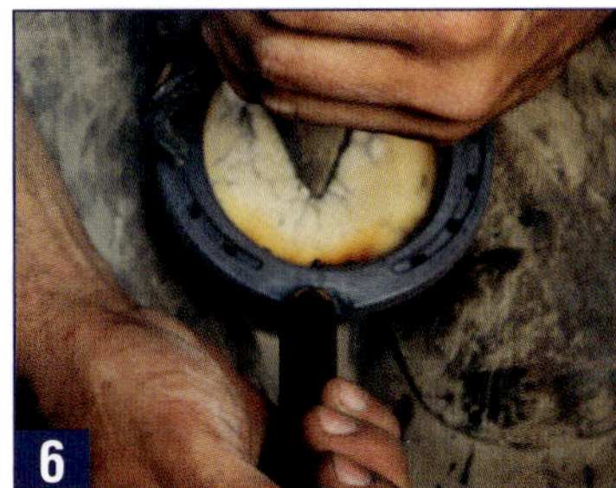
6 Pushing the shoe back into the clip cut with the end of my knife.

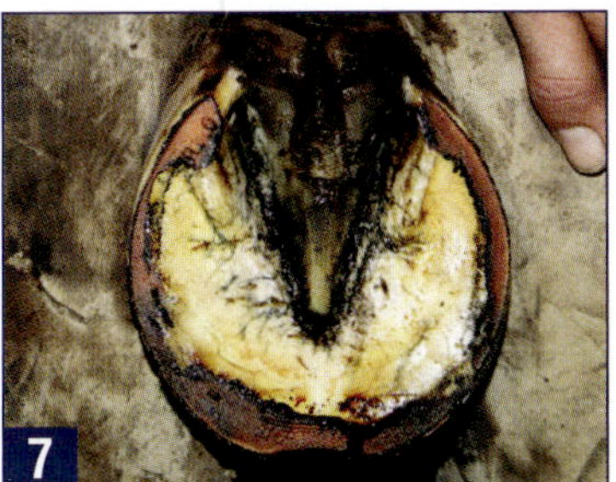
7 Burned foot with an even burn from heel to heel.

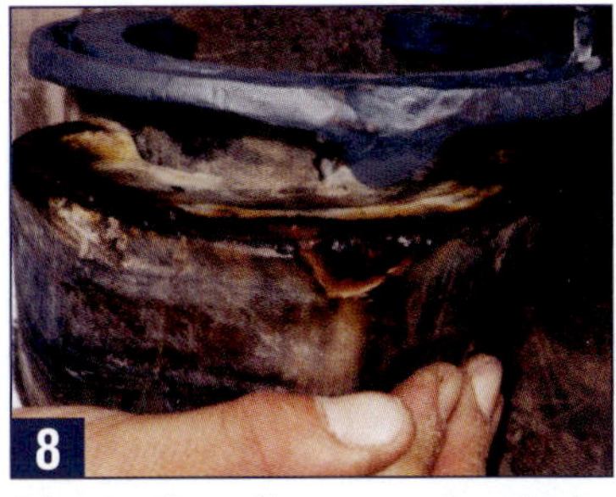
8 The entire clip area should be burned.

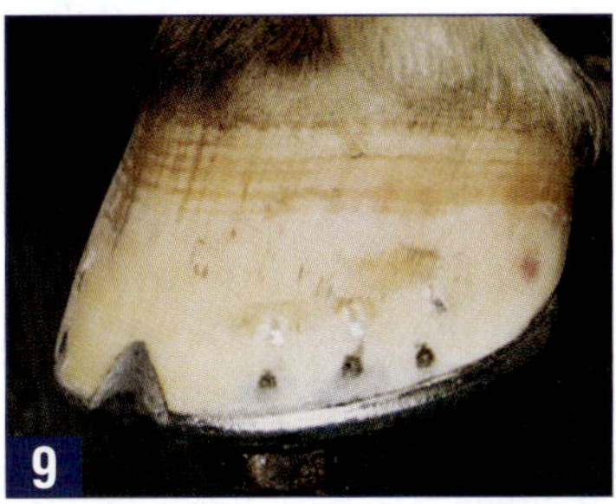
9 Finished foot with a good clip fit.

knives are brass or steel to allow for pushing on a hot shoe **(Figure 6)**, but you can use any piece of metal, such as the end of your rasp. This is a fast burn, and I count quickly to 4. I think if you were to time it, it would be at or just under 2 seconds. The final burn should be around the whole foot as in **Figure 7**, and the clip fit should be complete as in **Figure 8**.

The finished clip fit should be created with the hot clip. Cutting out the area again after the last burn will only serve to ruin the clip fit, so if you do have to cut some more, you will have to burn again. Ideally, clip fitting is a three-step process; there is a marking burn, a good clip cut, and a final burn. Sometimes the shoe needs to be moved back a little more, so you may have to repeat the cut and final burn, but that is an indication that something is not perfect in the job.

Problems include a foot that is not dressed properly, a clip that is laid down too far or not far enough, a clip that took too much material out of the shoe, or a shoe that has not been shaped correctly.

After the burn, you should make a habit of running your fingers across the clip fit, pushing towards the coronary band. I like to feel a ridge around the entire clip fit area, where there is a definite shoulder for the clip to fit in. This ridge, or shoulder, tells me a lot about the clip fit that I just burned. If it is deep, then the clip was laid down too far, or burned too hard. If there is no ridge, the clip was not laid down far enough or not burned back far enough. Paying attention to detail will help you learn to get a feel for what is exactly right with hot fitting a clip.

Doing everything right will create a clip fit that looks like the one in **Figure 9**. You should not be able to feel where the clip is on the foot. It should be like a nicely finished piece of furniture.

CLIPPING COLD

There are those rare occasions when you will have to cold fit a steel shoe with clips, but you always have to cold fit the clips on aluminum. Aluminum would melt before it got hot enough to hot fit the clips as just described. Following is a description of how I cold fit clips.

Begin with your normal hoof prep. Shape the shoe, but leave the clips standing up straight **(Figure 10)**. Take the shoe to the foot and place it in the position that you want to nail it **(Figure 11)**. This may

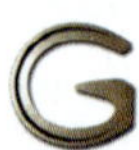

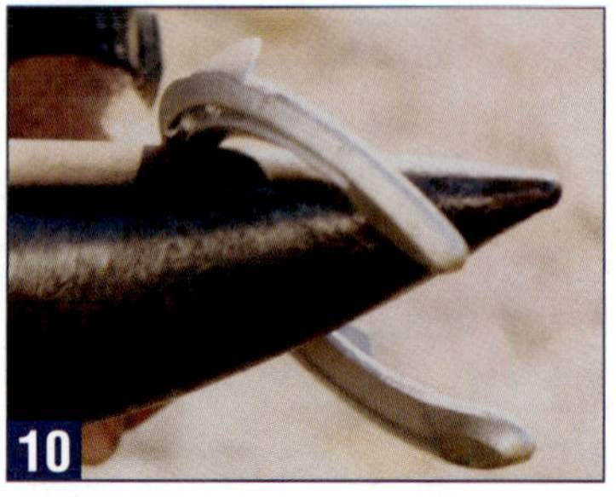

Cold shaping an aluminum shoe.

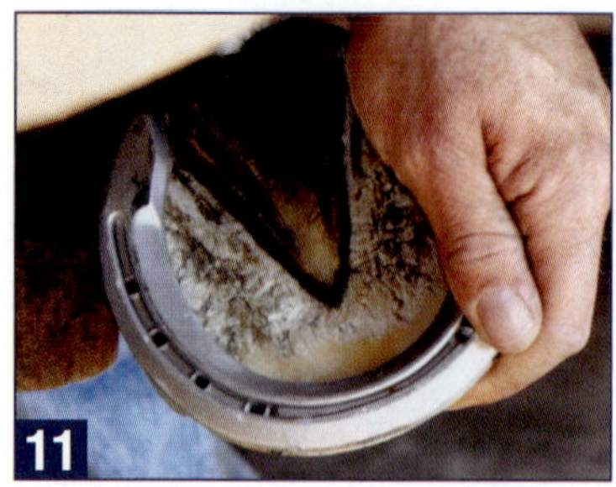

Placing the shoe on the foot.

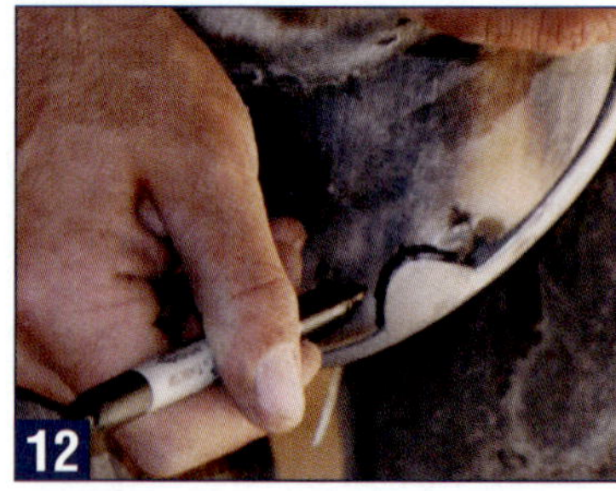

Marking the area for the clip fit.

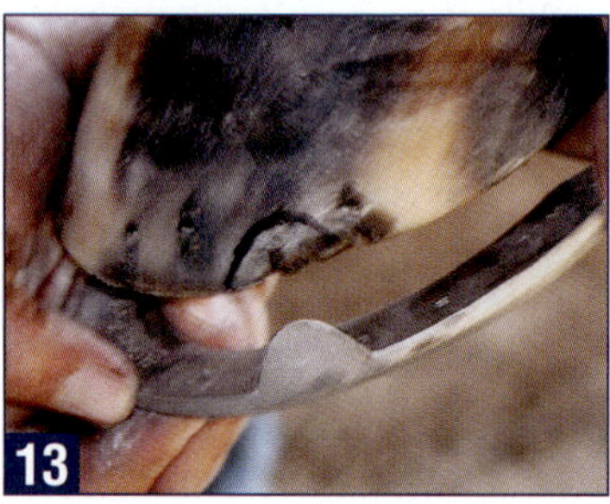

This is how the marked area will look.

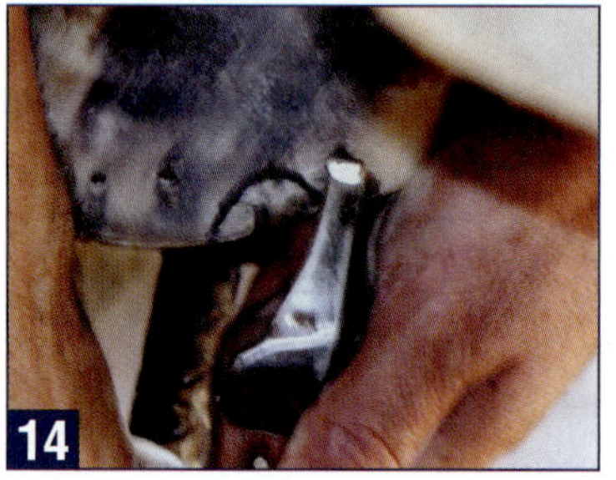

Cutting out the clip fit with a knife.

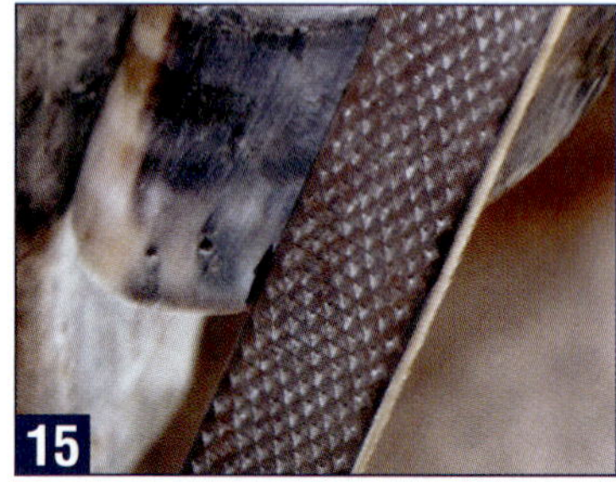

Cutting out the clip fit with a rasp.

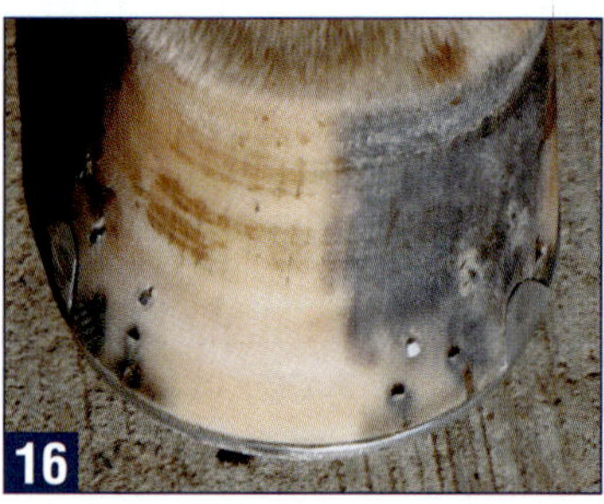

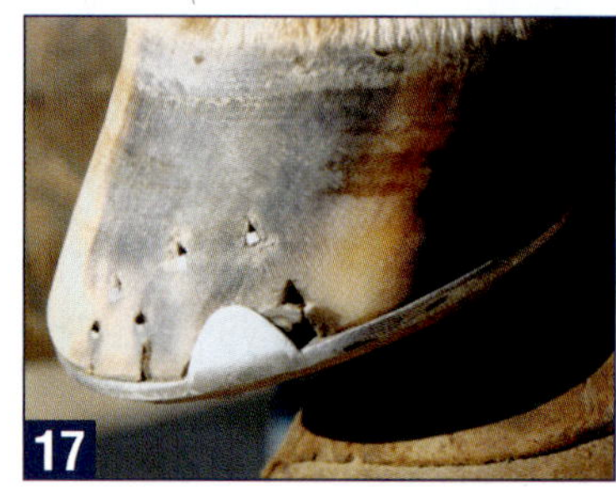

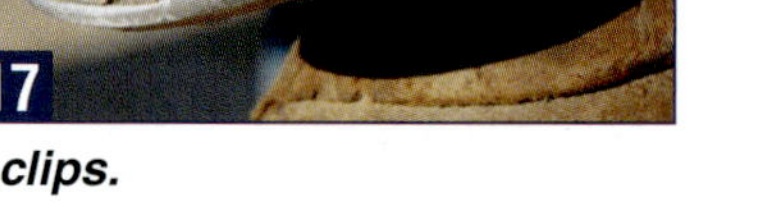

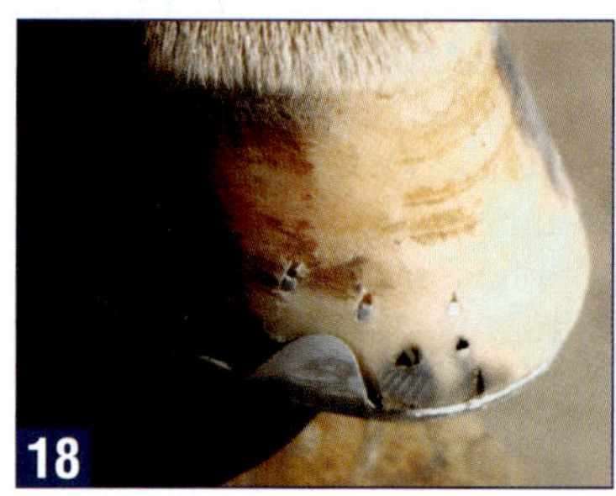

Finished foot with cold fit aluminum clips.

be difficult since you will be hampered by the clips, but you will have to get as close as you possibly can.

Take a marker and mark around the perimeter of the clips (**Figure 12 and 13**). Use either your hoof knife or a rasp to cut out the area of the clip (**Figures 14 and 15**). Go back to the anvil and lay the clips down to match the angle of the wall. Tap the shoe into position on the foot, and nail the shoe on. Generally speaking, the clips will require a bit of hammering to make them smooth, but this is not too big of a problem with aluminum.

The finished job will not be as nice as that of the hot fit clips, but it should look like those in **Figures 16-18**.

Another thing that you should know about aluminum pre-clipped shoes is that the clips are very easy to break off of the shoe. Place the clip on the face of the anvil, tilt the shoe slightly, and hit the base of the clip (**Figure 19**). It should break off at the base with a couple light hammer blows (**Figures 20 and 21**), and you can rasp up any sharp edges left behind.

When you are using pre-clipped shoes from manufacturers that make a large, thick clip,

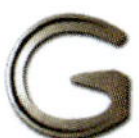

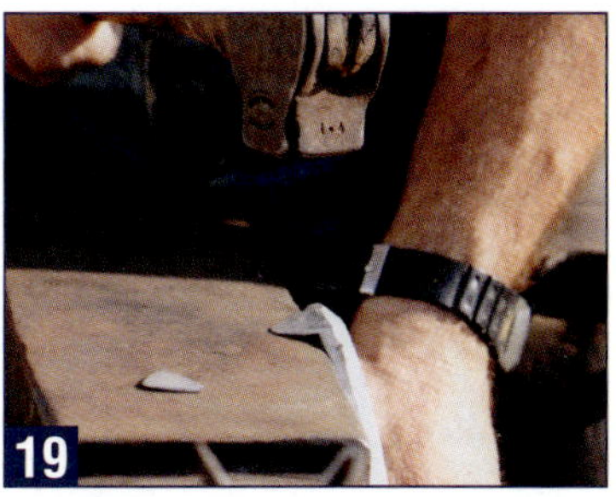

Breaking clips off of an aluminum shoe.

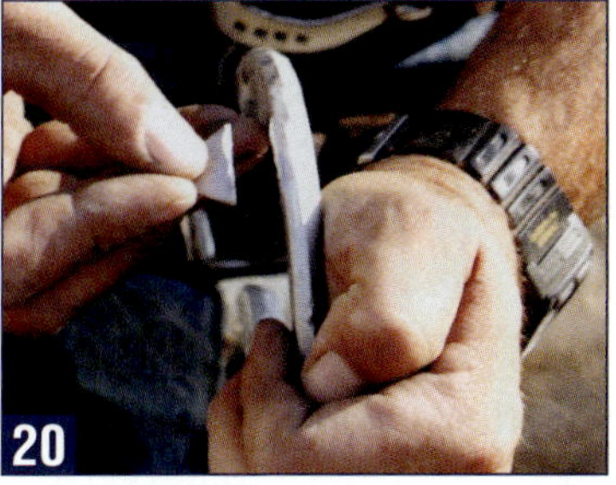

You can see how clean the break is.

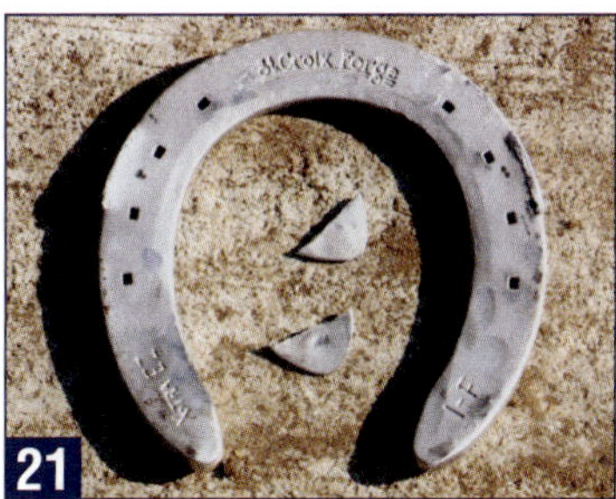

Shoe with the clips broken off.

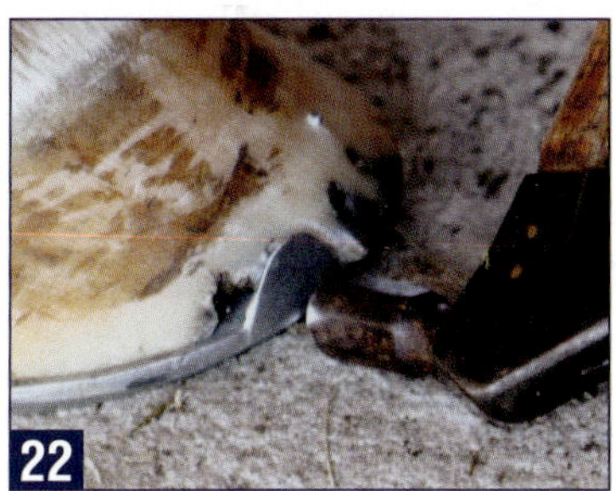

Hammering in a clip from the base of the clip.

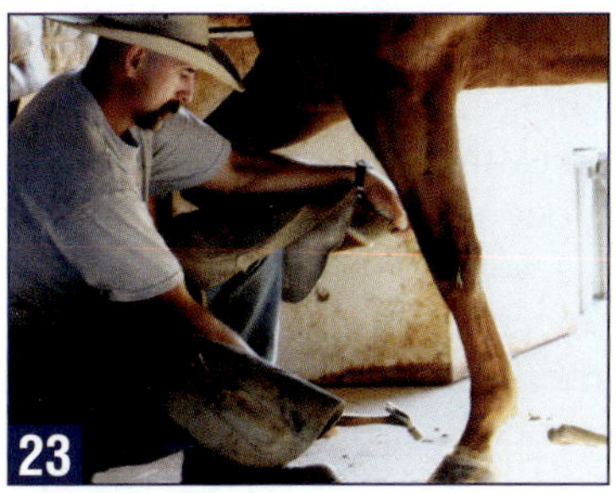

Loading the foot to have the clips hammered in.

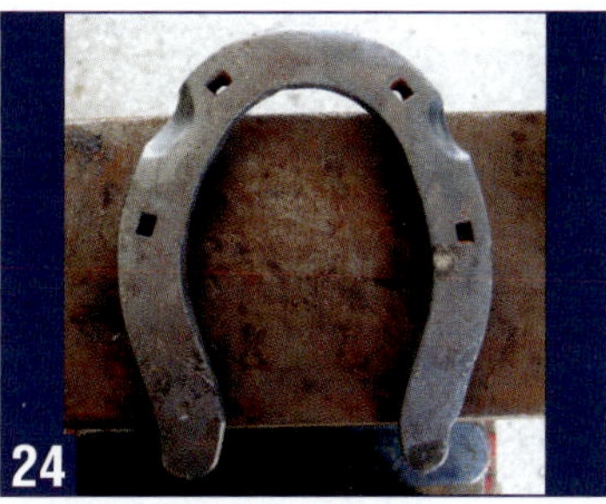

A common handmade shoe that we use on a lot of roping and cutting horses.

hammering on the clip will put stress on the foot. This happens because the large clips will pinch the area you hammered them into. If you are using quarter clips, they will place pressure across the whole foot. This can lead to some discomfort for that horse. You know what it feels like if your shoes are too tight and pressing across your foot. Now just imagine if they were made of steel and hammered into position. With aluminum shoes, the material is weak enough that you cannot get the same amount of pressure on the foot as you can with steel. It is not ideal to hammer on the clips, but it may have to be done on occasion.

If you do need to hammer on the clips, use your driving hammer, and start by hammering at the base of the clip **(Figure 22)**. Tap lightly, and work your way up to the tip. I like to have the foot that I am hammering on loaded, so I will hold the other foot in the air **(Figure 23)**. This causes the foot to be as expanded as I can make it and may help prevent the inherent problems of hammering clips into a wall in the first place.

Clips are an excellent way of improving shoe retention. Once you start using clips, you may find that a lot of feet do fine with only two nails per side, such as the handmade shoe in **Figure 24**. This can end up being a big savings by the end of your career. Clips also make a job stand out from the rest and help you to put your signature to every foot you shoe. Take the time needed to master pulling and fitting clips, and you will be doing one more thing that helps set you apart from the crowd.

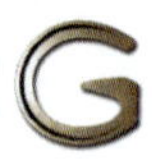

Chapter

29 HOT FITTING

There are a lot of myths surrounding hot fitting. When you read old textbooks on the subject, the authors seem to be pretty well split on the subject. Some of them have drawings to depict the damages that have been brought about by hot fitting, but those are only drawings, and you can draw anything you want to. You can also be wrong when you blame a problem on something.

Like many farriers, I began my journey through this trade doing some terrible shoeing out of ignorance. Although I was incompetent, I was thoroughly — and mistakenly — convinced of my skill. With some exposure to good farriers through clinics, contests, conventions and certifications, I was able to see what a good job was, I began to figure out how to accomplish that job. To achieve the level of shoeing that I wanted required that I learn to hot shoe. Once I saw the many benefits of hot shoeing over cold shoeing, there was no other choice for me. Complacency and laziness won't lead to great farriery, so I decided to learn just how to build and shape shoes to create the finished product that I wanted. The very best farriers in the world are mostly hot shoers. That fact alone should be an indication that there is a lot of merit to this method of shoeing.

The exact method for hot fitting that I use is as follows:

Heat the shoe to a bright red heat **(Figure 1)**. Secure hot fitters onto the shoe **(Figure 2)** using the type you like best. **Figure 3** shows a carrying pritchel and a pair of tongs that has been turned into hot fitters. I personally like hot fitters that attach to both branches of the shoe (the converted tongs). There are hot fitters that clamp on the shoe **(Figure 4)**, but they make it hard to see the shoe on the foot, and they also don't allow you to burn the shoe back, due to the prongs that hold the shoe. You can get good with a carrying pritchel, but it can distort nail holes and takes some practice to use it correctly. There are also other methods, including the use of vise-grips. The main priority is that you are able to get a good hot fit and not damage the hot shoe.

Pick up the foot you are going to hot fit and place the shoe in the exact place that you wish to nail it **(Figure 5 and 6)**. Press the shoe against the foot and count quickly to 4. This is just at, or slightly under, 2 seconds. There should be a lot of smoke **(Figures 7 and 8)**, but no flames. If you generate flames, the shoe is just a little too hot, or as in the case shown in **Figure 9**, there is chemical on the foot that flames up. The foot in **Figure 9** had just been treated with

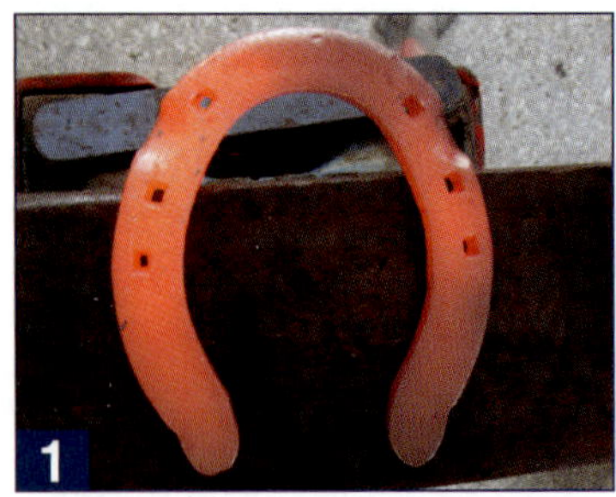

1 *Shoe ready to be hot fit.*

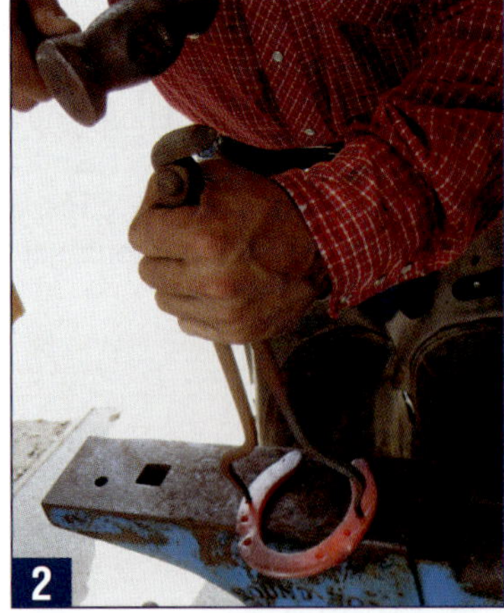

2 *Putting the hot fitters on the hot shoe.*

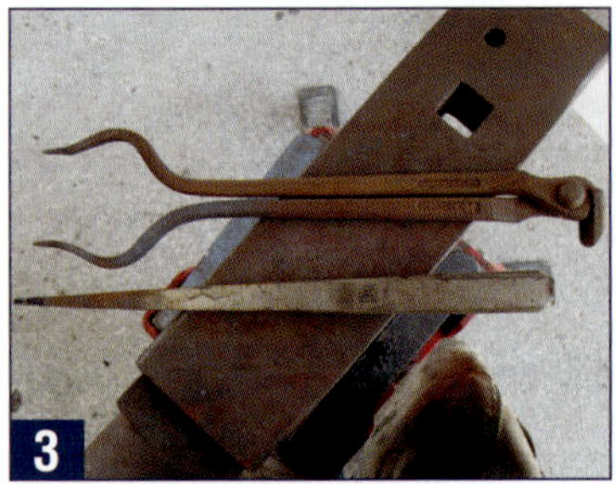

3 *Hot fitters made from tongs and a carrying pritchel.*

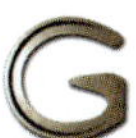

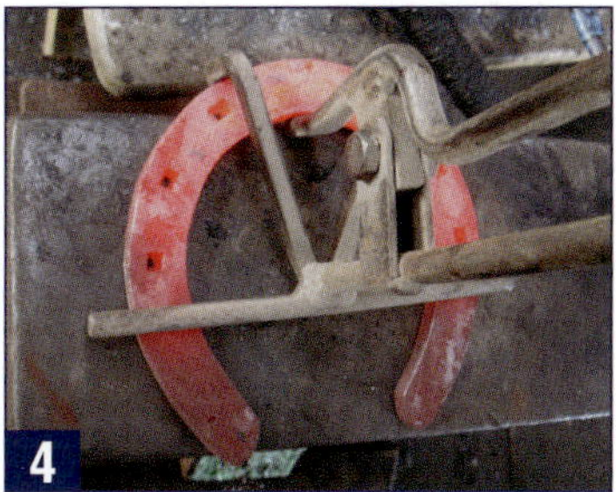

4

Clamp style hot fitters.

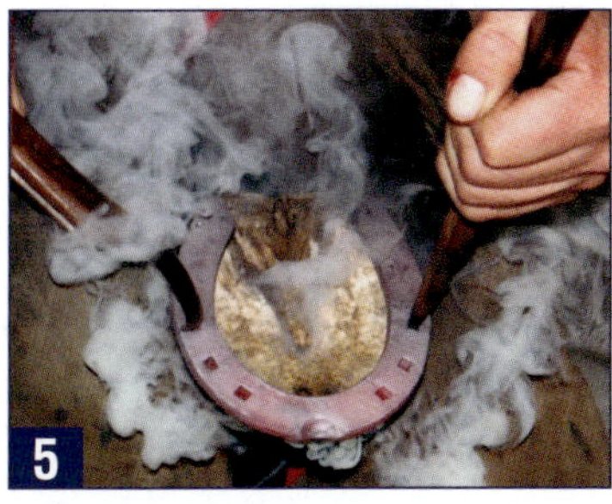

5

Carrying pritchel and hoof knife method of hot fitting.

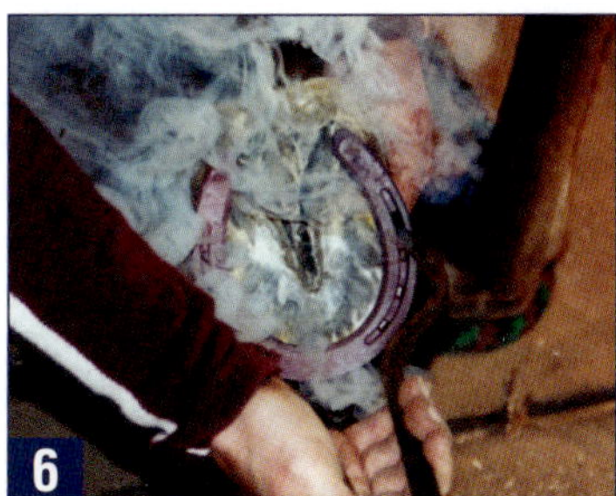

6

Kelly hot fitting in our normal method.

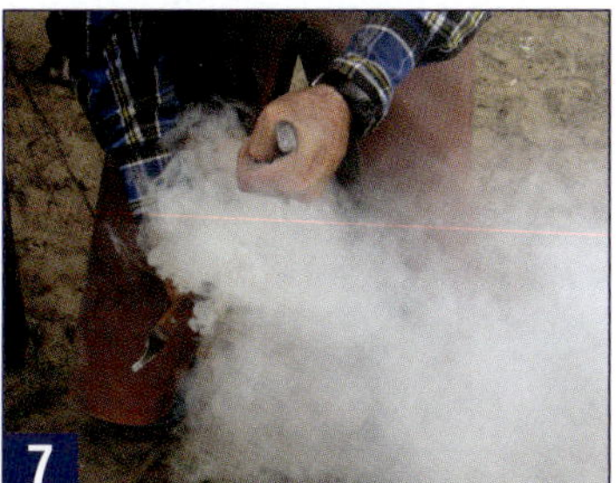

7

A lot of smoke

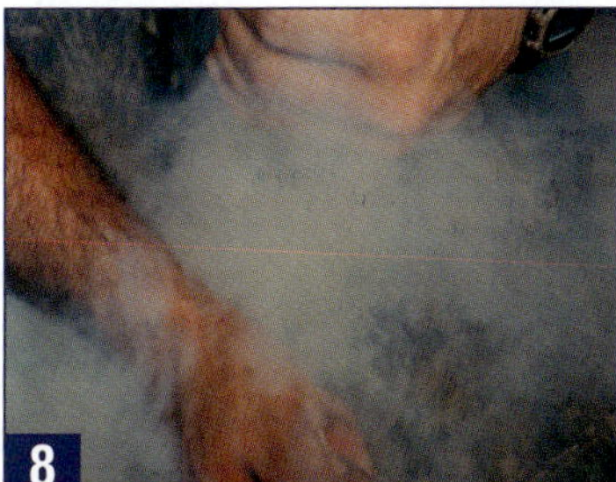

8

9

Hot fitting a foot with chemicals on it.

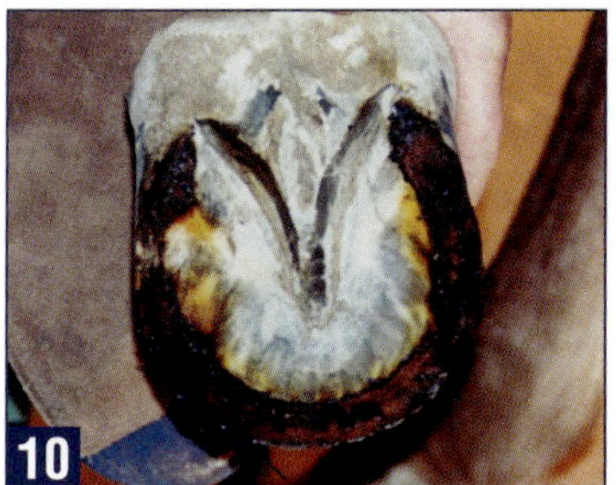

10

Foot after hot fitting.

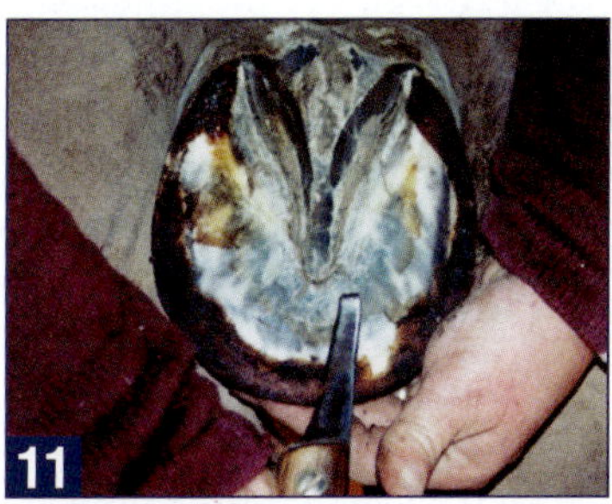

11

Removing the sole around the inside of the burn.

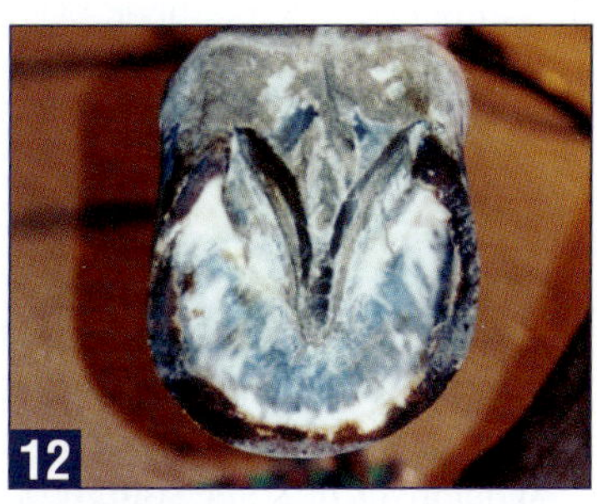

12

Foot ready to have the shoe nailed on.

chemicals, and we hot fit it to show what happens.

Once the fit is done, there will often be a slight area on the sole that needs removed with your knife to avoid sole pressure **(Figure 10-12)**. Right after hot fitting is the perfect time to do this, so set the shoe down in a safe place on the ground (where there is no dry hay, sawdust, or dead grass), and knife lightly across the sole and white line. Waiting to knife the burned sole away once it is cooled can be much harder to do since the foot will become tougher from the hot fit. This toughening, by the way, is one of the many reasons that I am such a fan of hot fitting.

When you are done relieving sole pressure, the hot fit is done. If there are any changes that are needed to the shape of the shoe, do them immediately when you go back to the anvil. Quench the shoe, and you are ready to nail.

Many farriers also use the softening of the hoof tissues from heat to help them knife out tough sole. Jeff Houston uses the following method quite often for trimming and finds it to be one of the handiest things he has learned. Once a foot is cleaned, take a small propane torch and heat the sole for a few

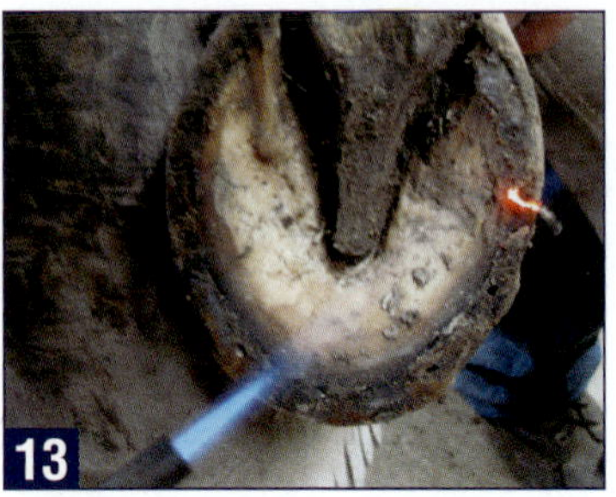
Using a torch to soften the sole.

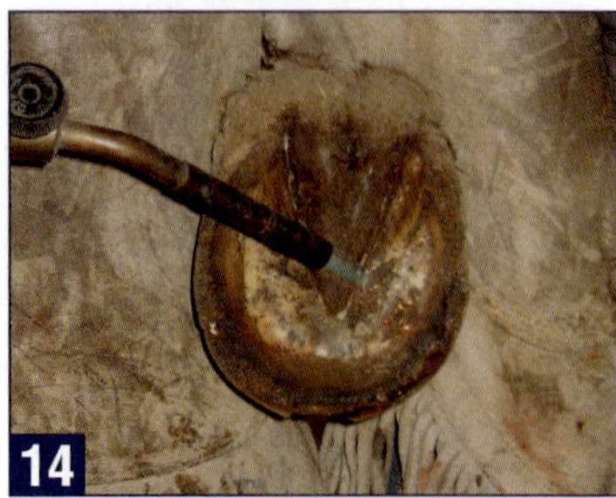
Heating a foot with a torch.

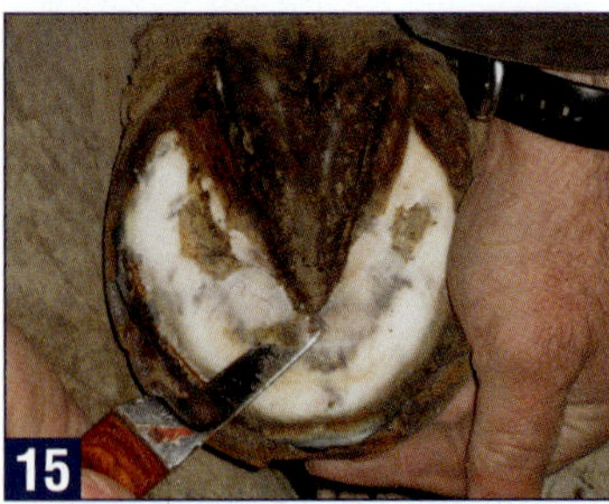
Knifing the hot and soft sole.

seconds **(Figure 13 and 14)**. Immediately knife **(Figure 15)** and you will be surprised how soft the sole has become. If you wait for the sole to cool, it will become harder than it was before it was heated in the first place.

It is difficult to find hard and fast proof concerning hot fitting. I was able to find one study. It was cited in a book by M.T. Richardson, and it is as follows.

Study reported in *The Practical Horse Shoer*, by M.T. Richardson. Pg. 101-102 A compilation of a bunch of articles from the magazine. Here is the study reported in summary.

In a 3 year study conducted at the Cavalry School of Saumur from September 22, 1841 to October 5th, 1844, "all of the near-sided horses of the school were shod cold, and the off-sided ones shod hot. In that space of time, out of 22,579 horses that were fitted in the cold state, 386 shoes were lost, detached or broken, and only 123 out of the same number were lost that were fitted while hot. That is, in the first case one shoe in 58 was detached, while in the second case one shoe out of 103 was lost."

That gives us some solid proof of the benefits of hot shoeing if the study is correct, and I personally believe that hot shoers lose a lot less shoes than cold shoers.

Since there is little else that can be found about hot shoeing, I decided to do this chapter in the form of a pros vs. cons list. As you look through these lists, think about the position of the horse. Many of the reasons farriers don't hot shoe have to do with themselves and not the horse. The horse does not care if it costs you more, required a lot of work for you to learn, or takes you more time. The horse only cares about how good a job is done.

By the same token, the horse is completely unimpressed that you are able to do the job with less equipment or skill. Again, the main objective for the horse is to have a competent job. So, as you read the rest of this section, try to look at this from the view of a hot shoer, a cold shoer and a horse.

Pros for hot shoeing:

- Anecdotally better for the foot
- Makes it easier to fit the shoe to the exact shape of the foot
- Makes fitting clips easier and precise
- Seals the tubules
- Kills bacteria
- Toughens the hoof tissue that has been seared
- Perfect union between the shoe and the foot
- Physically easier on the farrier's body
- Sets you apart from competition
- Can charge more

Cons for hot shoeing:

- Anecdotally bad for the foot
- Cost
- Time
- Skill
- Equipment
- Danger (being burned, breathing hoof smoke)
- May have to defend position on hot fitting

Pros for cold shoeing:

- Anecdotally better for the foot
- Fast
- Less equipment

Cons for cold shoeing:

- Anecdotally bad for the foot
- Harder to make the ideal shape in the shoe
- Modifications like clips and square toes are less likely to be used
- Difficult to fit clips
- Harder on your body

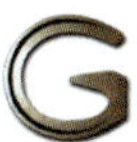

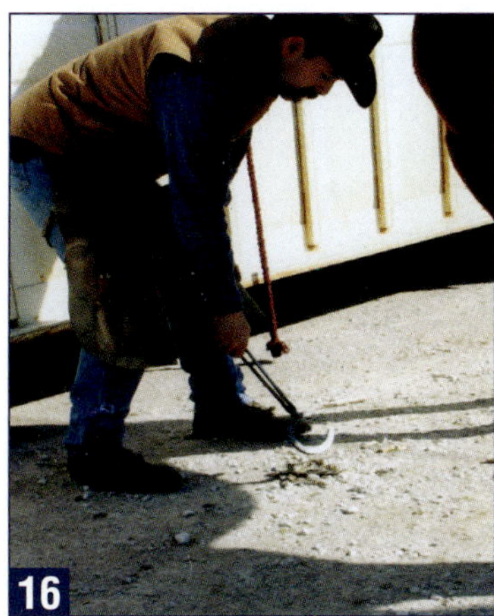

16

Placing a hot shoe on a pile of hoof trimmings.

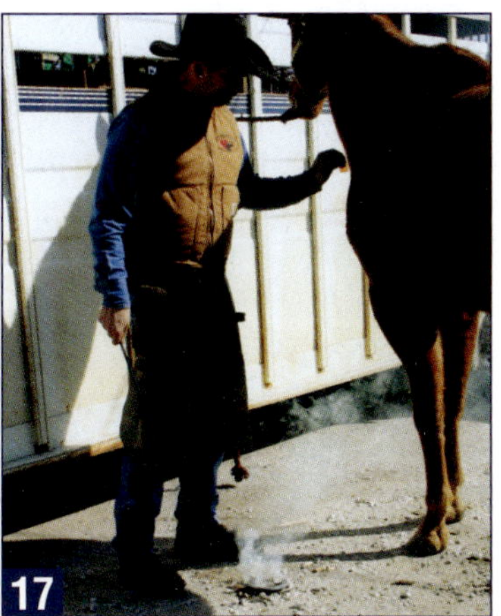

17

Calming a horse in a non-threatening situation while the smoke blows past him.

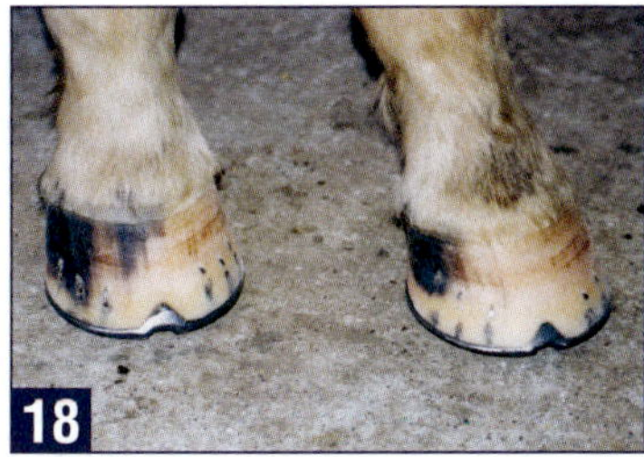

18

Clipped, clinched and finished feet.

- Bad for hearing

I don't think that these lists are complete, but they are well on the way to making the point. As you learn and grow as a farrier, try to make these lists longer in every category. I would appreciate seeing more in every category.

I often hear from cold shoers that horses don't like to be hot fit. That may be true of some horses, but some horses don't like to be shod at all, yet we shoe them anyway. It is just that with hot fitting, there is a sound and smoke that may make a horse nervous if not done properly. To prepare a horse for hot fitting, I like to place a hot shoe in a pile of hoof trimmings and calm the horse while there is smoke and the sound of burning going on **(Figure 16 and 17)**. You will find that most horses have no problem with hot fitting once you have done this.

Another item that I would like you to consider is that there is an accepted way of becoming great at anything that you wish to excel at. That method is to see what the recognized best in the world are doing, and then try to do the same. I think it is a bad idea to seek help and education from someone who is not at the top of his or her game, yet it is not uncommon for young farriers to be so eager to learn that they are led astray by older farriers who are not so smart or well respected, but more than willing to pass on their ignorance. If you apply this reasoning to hot shoeing, you will see that the recognized best in the world are mostly hot shoeing. It would be impossible to pass the AWCF, FWCF, ASF, or CJF exams without the skills needed to hot shoe, and I would venture that people with those credentials are among the best in the world. Results like those shown in **Figure 18** are not common with cold shoeing.

Hot shoeing is an old, established, traditional, and accepted method of shoeing horses. The majority of the best farriers in the world use hot shoeing as a regular tool to do the best shoeing that can be done. It is a simple way to do a better job and set yourself apart from the competition. The challenge is for you to learn these skills to help you achieve your goals of greatness in this amazing trade.

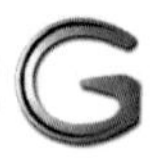

Chapter 30 NAILING

Once the shoe is fit, it is time to nail it on. A properly fit shoe will have all of the nail holes lined up over the white line of the foot. If it is too far inside the white line, the foot is quicked by the nail entering sensitive structures. If it is outside the white line, the nail is driven only into hoof wall, often breaking and cracking it in the process.

The act of nailing a shoe onto the foot of a living animal can be dangerous to both man and beast, and it should be done with great care. Nailing done correctly causes no problems, but done incorrectly, it can be the end of a horse. With that in mind, be certain that you understand the anatomy of the foot before you undertake driving a nail into it.

I like the nails to come out of the wall about one third of the way up the foot. This will cause the nail line to be parallel to the coronet. That is common for shoeing in the United Kingdom. In the United States, many like to have the nails parallel to the shoe. That is fine as well, and the difference comes down to style and what you think looks best. In reality, it is probably better to have a staggered nail line. “Staggered for strength” or “musical” nail lines are not parallel to anything. They are not pretty, but they do hold the horseshoe on the foot, and if a shoe is pulled, there is less of a chance of taking large pieces of hoof wall with it. I am not condoning or recommending musical nail lines, but they are not detrimental.

With the nail tip in the white line, you can hold the shaft of the nail with your thumb and index finger and use the rest of your fingers to feel the hoof wall to determine the angle that the nail should be placed. Generally speaking, the nail should be driven at the angle of the wall. The design of the nail should be facing the inside (the frog should always be able to see the pattern on the head), and the nail should be perpendicular to the shoe from a lateral view. As you drive the nail, it will sound dull at first, like it is being driven into soft wood. After a couple blows, the tip will enter the hoof wall, and it will feel like slightly harder wood. By the time the tip is exiting the foot, it will feel and sound like you are driving the nail through a piece of seasoned pine.

The angle of the nail should match the angle of the wall at that area. This will cause the nail to exit about one third of the way up the foot and hopefully in line with the other nails. The nail should be high enough that it can’t be bent over and have the tip touch the shoe, but not so high that the clinch will be in the taper of the tip. Most of the time when people have trouble with their nail lines, it comes down to the shape of the shoe. A well-made and properly shaped shoe makes nailing a breeze.

The type of nail that you use combined with the type of feet that you shoe will make a difference. Some nails are stiff (Capewell) and do well in harder, drier feet. Driving these nails in a softer, wetter foot will not have the same feel or same results. Being stiff, it will go higher in a softer foot. Some brands are softer (Delta) and work well on the softer, wetter feet. Again, these nails will act differently on a hard foot. Mustad seems to be in the middle as far as nail hardness is concerned.

Nails have heads and shanks that are mostly rectangular. There are categories of nails called city heads, race nails, and regular heads. They have a more rectangular shape when compared to an E-head nail (E stands for European). E-head nails look better in handmades than other types, at least in my opinion. You can see the most common nails in **Figures 1-4**. Beyond that, there are combination nails **(Figure 5)**, which are a race nail head with a city head nail shank, and slims. Slims are a lighter version of the size nail they resemble **(Figure 6)**. There are also nails that protrude past the shoe for traction and wearablity, such as the mud nails **(Figure 7)**, frost nails **(Figure 8),** and Duratrack nails **(Figure 9)**, which have borium brazed to the head. Since I have spent the majority of my career shoeing the American Quarter Horse, the most common nails I have used are the Capewell 4 1/2 Race nail, Mustad 5 City Head Slim, Mustad MX 50, and MX 55.

The main criteria for nail selection is that it lasts

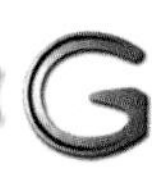

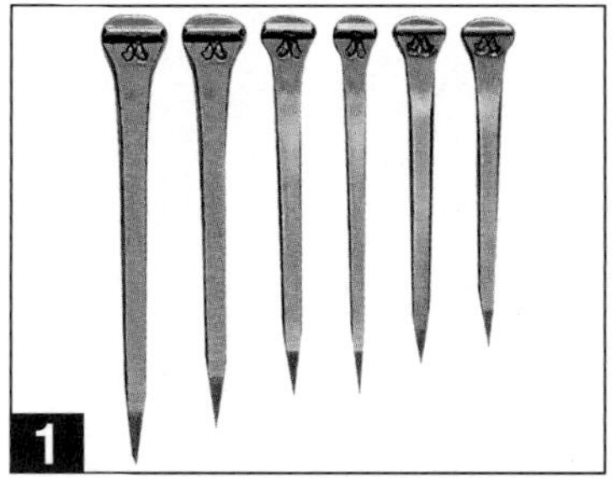

City Head nails.

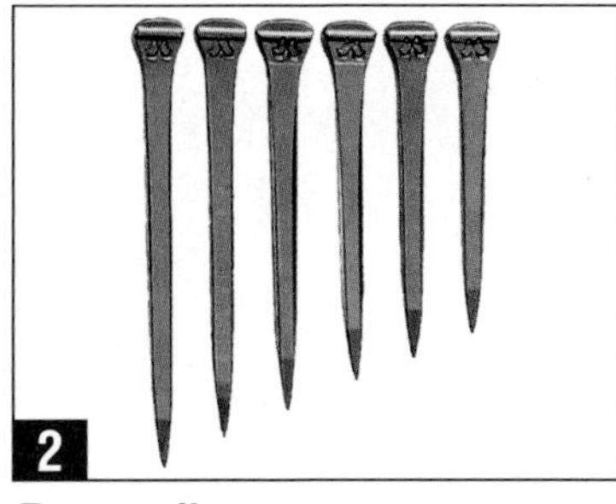

Race nails.

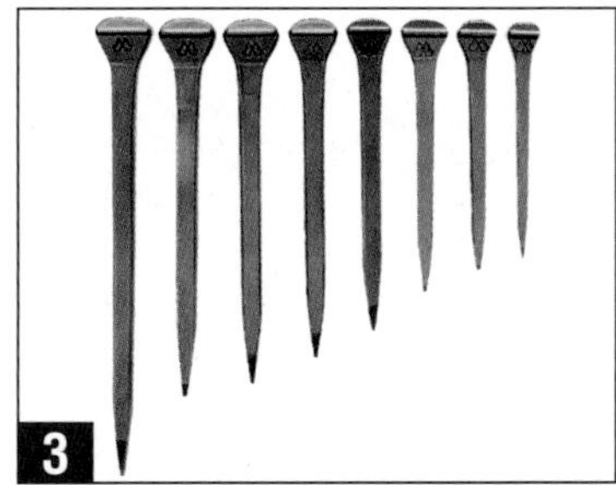

Regular Head nails.

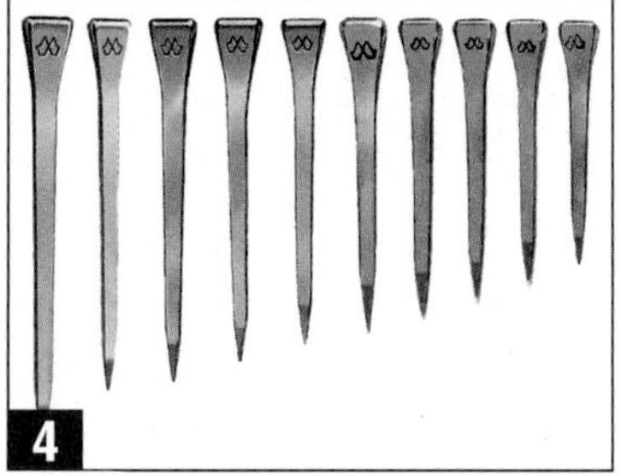

E-head nails.

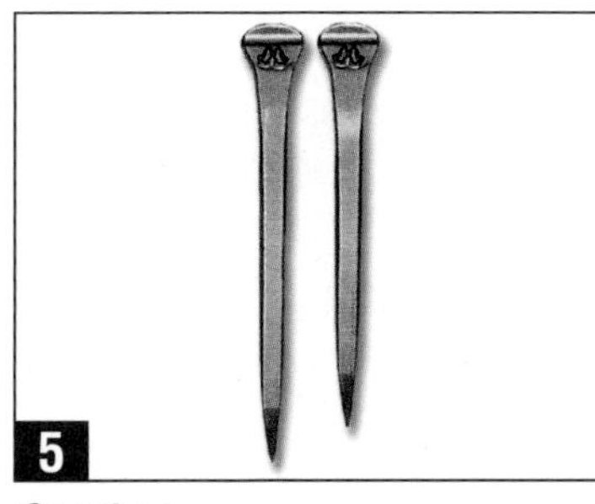

Combos.

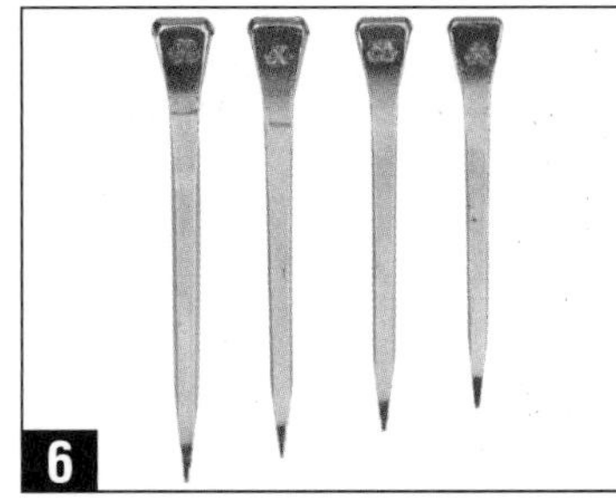

E-slims.

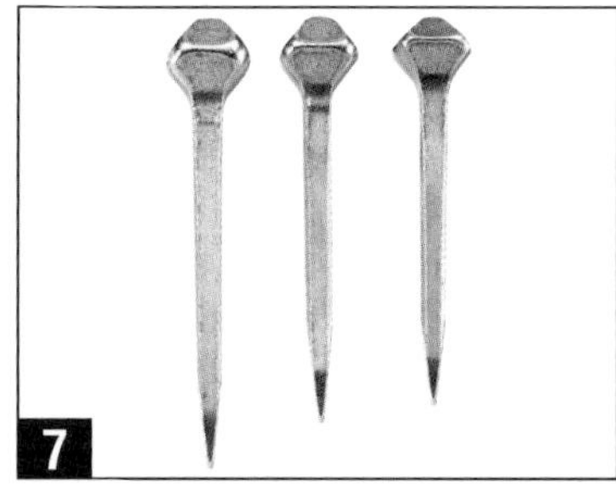

Mud nails.

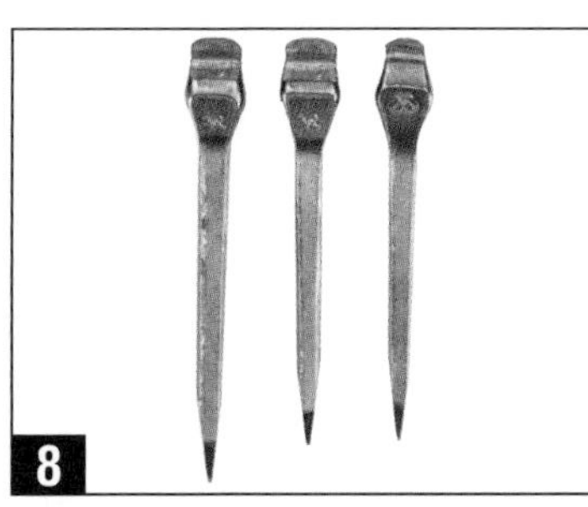

Frost nails.

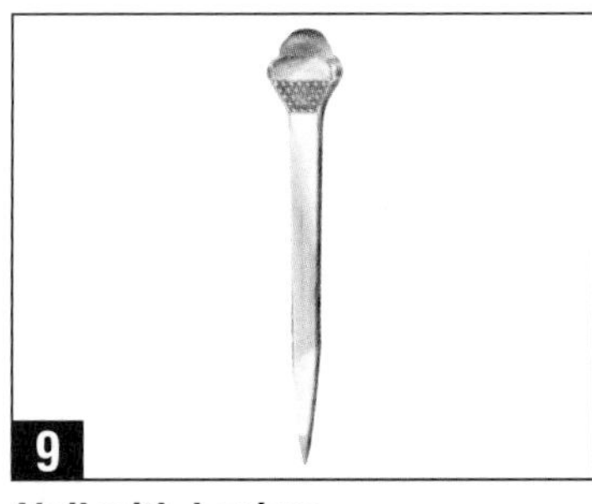

Nail with borium.

for the amount of time that you want the shoes to stay on. I have used nails that rusted too quickly for the feet in Missouri, and that causes a lot of weakness. I also want a nail that fits the hole well and does not shear easily.

When you look at what is holding a shoe on a foot, there is the area of the shank where it meets the head, multiplied by the number of nails that you put into the shoe. This means we are asking a lot of strength out of a small amount of material. It is not a wonder that horses lose shoes, rather a wonder that they don't lose more. Clips take the shearing force off nails, and if you are having shoes lost with the shank of the nails still in the foot, you should start clipping the shoes that you use.

SETTING WITHOUT CLIPS:

If you have clipped the shoe and fit it well, setting it is easy. Setting without clips can be more difficult, so here are a few suggestions to help you put the shoe where it goes on the foot.

Begin by placing the shoe on the foot exactly where you want it to be. Take a nail in your tong hand, and place it into a hole on your hammer-hand

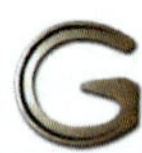

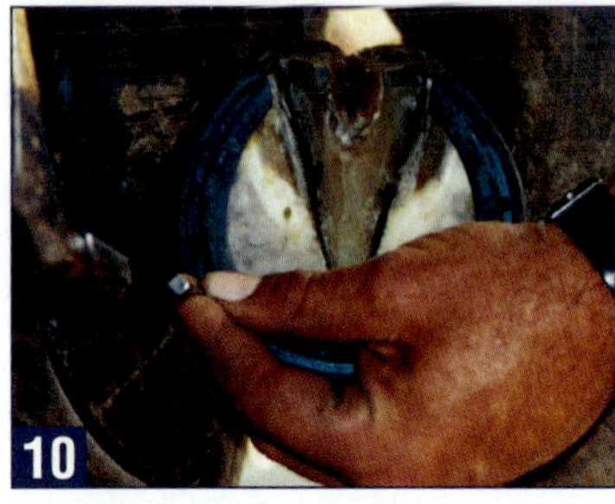

Positioning the shoe and holding it with my tong hand while putting a nail in the hammer-hand side.

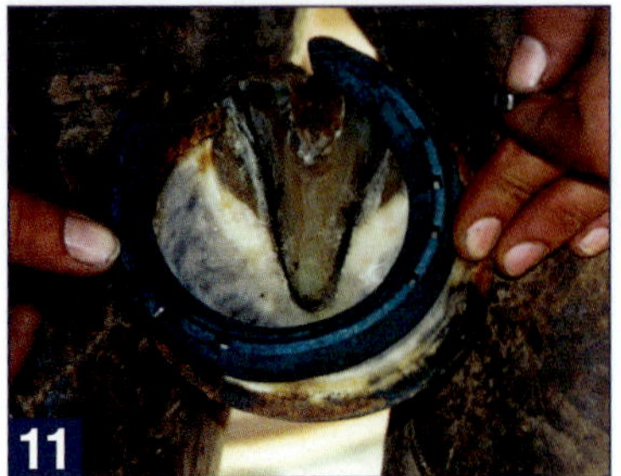

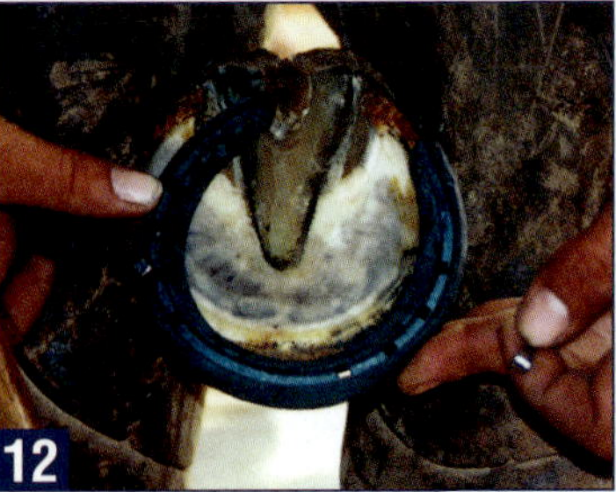

The shoe can be moved around at this point.

Find the perfect spot.

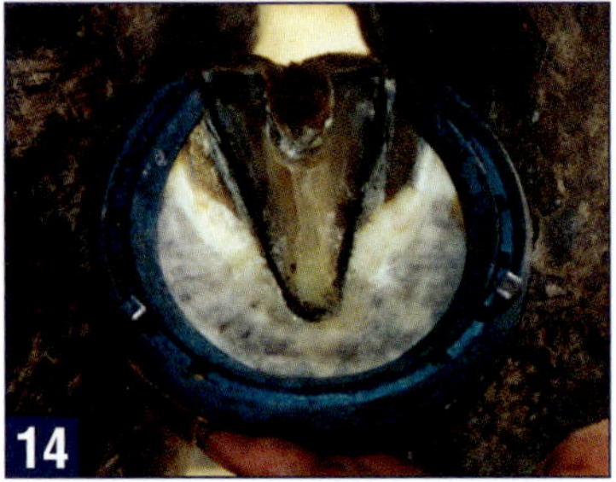

Driving the second nail in the tong-hand side of the shoe.

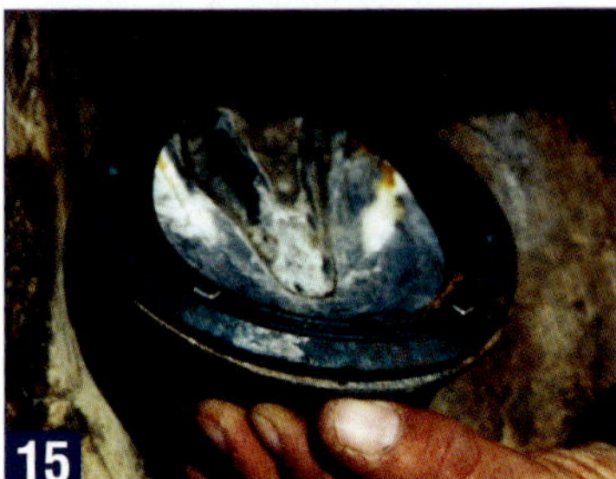

Shoe moved back from being set with toe nails.

side of the shoe. Place it toward the front outside corner of the nail hole. You can now hold the shoe in place against the foot with your tong hand while you drive the nail **(Figure 10)**.

The placement of the nail in the hole is important. It is similar to putting a hinge on a cabinet door with screws. When you place the screw toward one side of the hole in the hinge, the hinge will move that way. This will cause the gap between the door and the frame to become bigger or smaller, depending on where you put the screw. The same holds true for the nail in the nail hole of a shoe. The tip of the nail is quite small compared to the hole, so there are a lot of options for where the nail can be placed. Where you put the tip determines where the shoe is going to move when the nail is driven.

Drive the first nail about half way into the foot. The shoe is still loose and can be twisted around **(Figures 11 - 12)**. Position the shoe exactly where you want it **(Figure 13)** and put a nail in a hole on your tong-hand side. Again, place the tip of the nail toward the front outside corner of that hole as well. Drive the nail about half way **(Figure 14)**. You can now decide if you want the shoe to move to the left or to the right. If you want it to go right, drive the nail on the left side first, and vice versa.

Due to the shape of nail heads, they will push a shoe away from the side they are driven into. This allows the farrier to move the shoe a little when the nail is driven. The movement caused by horse nails can be used against you if you don't want the shoe to move. Because the shoe is shifted by the nail head, it is very hard to set unclipped shoes with the toe nails. In **Figure 15**, you can see that the shoe has been moved back from the perimeter of the toe by driving toe nails into the toe nail holes.

Once the nails are both driven, you can twist them off and evaluate the placement of the shoe on the foot **(Figure 16)**. If it needs to be moved slightly, you can do so by driving the right nails, and being careful about the placement of the tip of the nail in the hole.

SETTING CLIPPED SHOES

A properly shaped and fit clipped shoe is really easy to set. The clip puts the shoe in an exact position and makes the job of setting the shoe almost automatic. The important thing is to be certain that the shoe is fit well and the clip is burned or cut into the foot correctly.

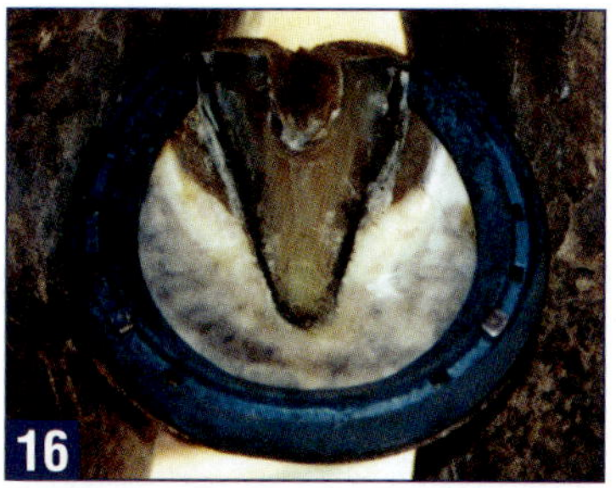
Properly set shoe, ready to be nailed down.

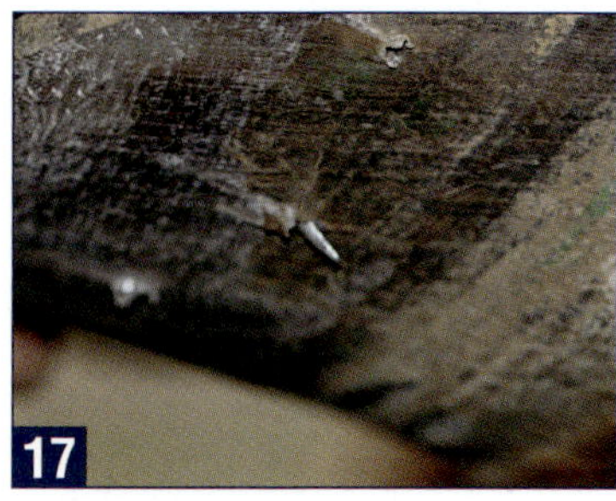
Tip of high nail.

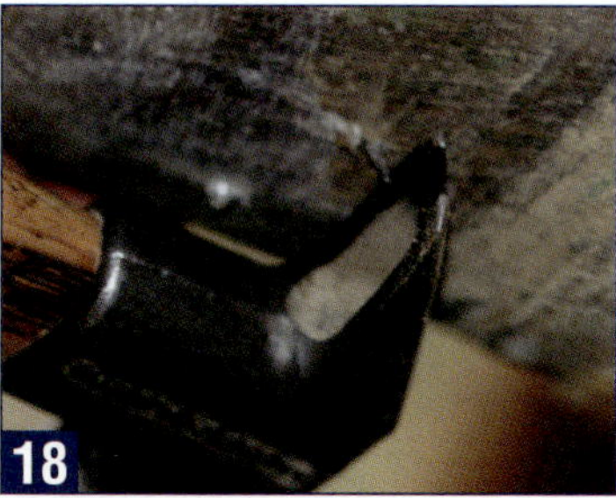
Bending the tip.

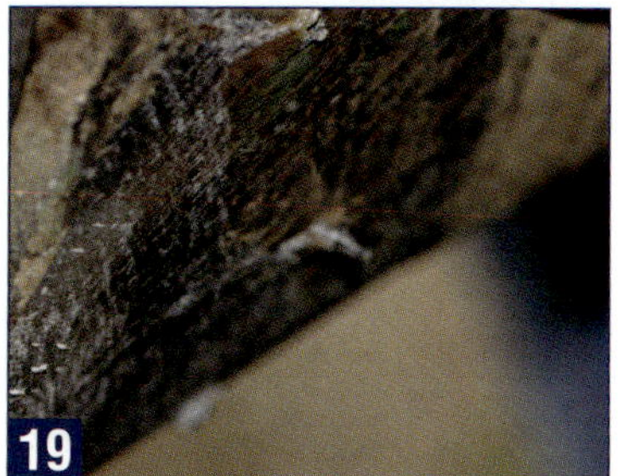
The tip is bent away from the wall.

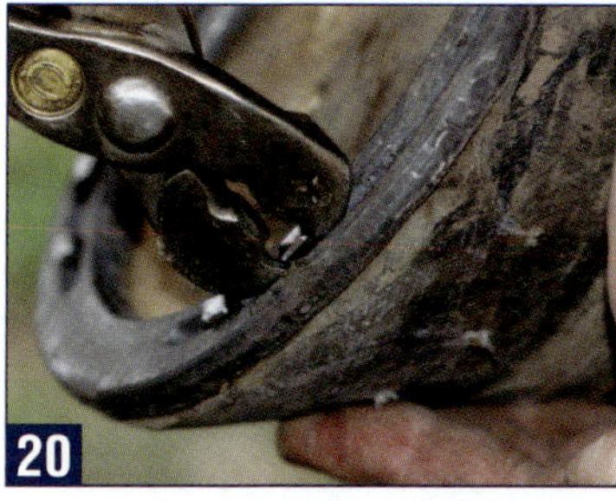
Pull the head free of the shoe.

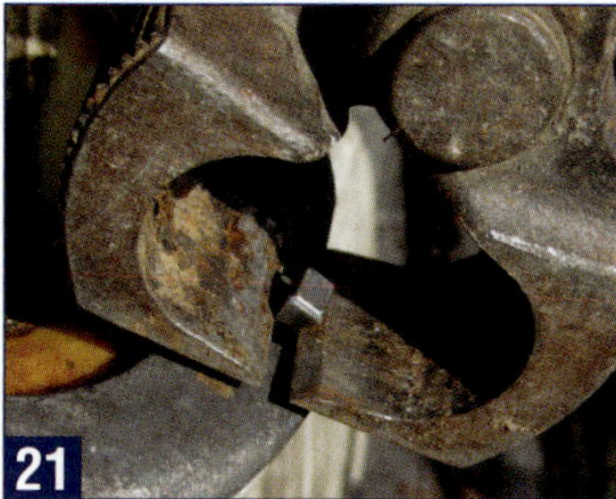
Grab the nail head in the middle of the jaws with your pulloffs.

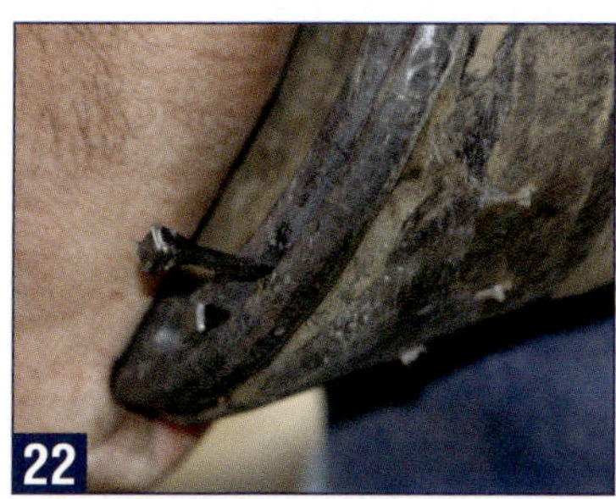
Pull the nail so that the bent tip is in the foot where you want it to exit the wall.

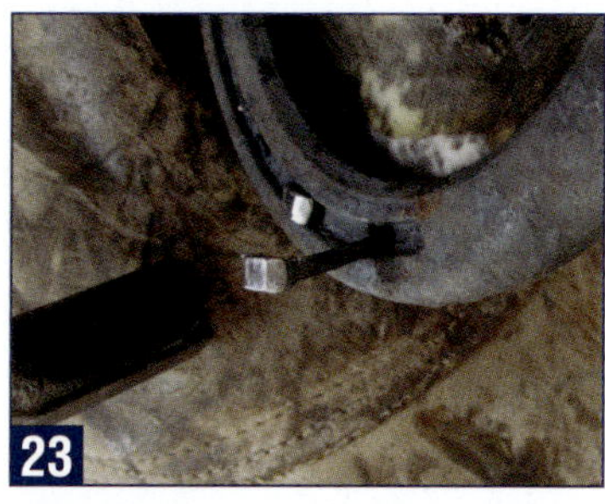
Hit sharply with the driving hammer.

I like to set clipped shoes with the toe nails. This drives the shoe back into the clip fit. With a toe clip, I will drive the toe nail on my hammer-hand side into the foot about half way. I then push the shoe toward my hammer-hand side and drive the toe nail in the tong hand side. The shoe can pivot around the clip, so I will evaluate where the heels of the shoe are ending up, and that allows me to determine which nail to drive all the way home first. If I want the shoe to move left, I drive the right nail, and vice versa.

When using quarter clips, I will drive a toe nail all the way home, and then follow up with the opposite toe nail. Quarter clips make shoe setting as easy as nailing on shoes that are already set.

SAVING NAILS

If you drive a nail that comes out too high, you can often save that nail with the following trick. In **Figure 17**, the nail has come out too high. Bend the tip of the nail away from the wall with your hammer **(Figures 18 and 19)**. Pull the head of the nail out of the shoe by grabbing it with your crease nail pullers,and moving the reins of the pullers towards the inside of the shoe **(Figure 20)**. With the head of the nail just clear of the shoe, grab it with your pulloffs **(Figure 21)**. Grab it in such a manner that the nail is in the middle of the jaws. Going too close to one end can make it hard to control how much of the shank is going to be pulled out of the shoe.

Pull the nail out of the shoe until the tip is where you want it to exit **(Figure 22)**. Strike the nail sharply with your driving hammer **(Figure 23)** ,

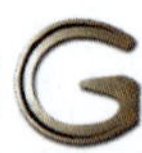

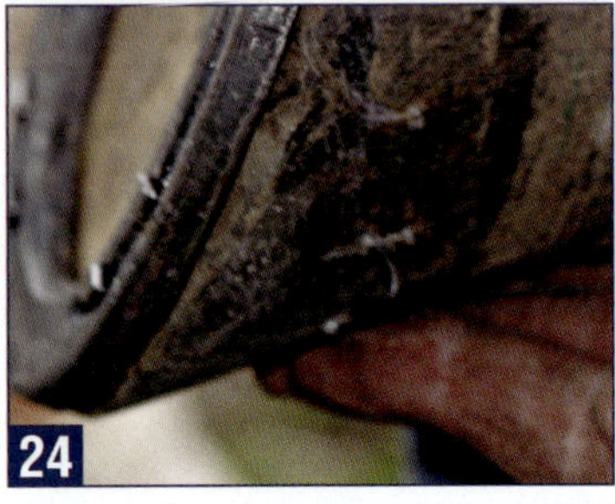

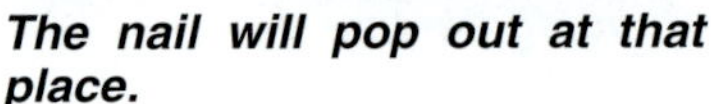
The nail will pop out at that place.

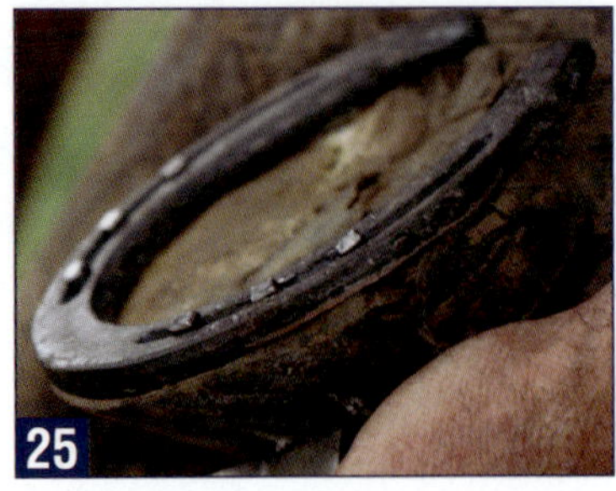

Set the nail and continue to finish the foot.

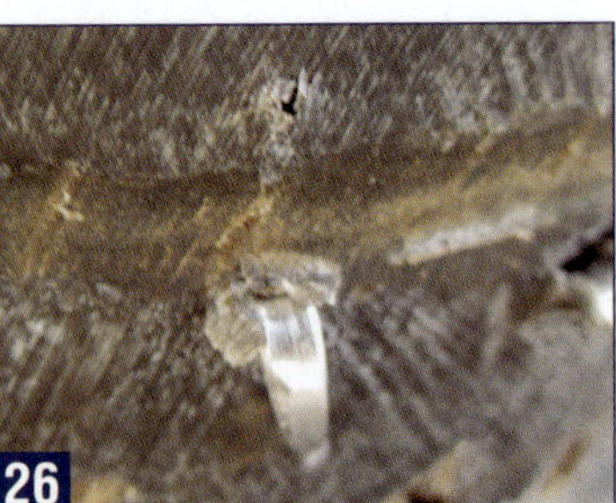

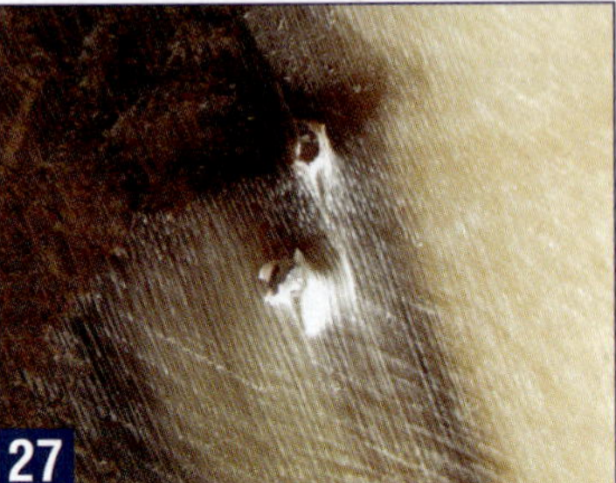

and the tip of the nail will exit the wall at that point **(Figure 24)**. Twist or wring it off and set it as you would normally **(Figure 25)**. Look carefully at **Figures 26 and 27**, and you can see where the nail originally came out of the wall above where the tip of the nail is now. The distance between those two points is determined by how far the nail is pulled out before it is driven back in. I have used this trick with great success for many years. I hope that you will get to do so as well.

Nailing is an essential part of shoeing horses. With time and practice, you may find that it is the part of the job that you enjoy the most.

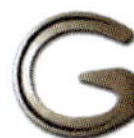

Chapter
31 CLINCHING 101

Clinching is an important aspect of shoeing a horse. If done improperly, keeping a shoe on the foot can become difficult. However, it is also a part of the job that is unlikely to cause damage to the hoof or horse, so it is often the realm of the apprentice or helper. There are a few principles involved in clinching that if understood, can make the job better and stronger.

I must begin by explaining that I finish very few feet in a year compared to many farriers. It has just fallen outside of my job description in the past several years, and I usually only finish a horse when competing or doing a demonstration. There have been many clinics where I really wish my wife, Kelly, were there to put the shine to the clinching.

When I first learned to shoe, it was common practice to take the edge of the rasp and carve a deep groove under the nail to bury the clinch in. The result of this practice is not attractive. **Figure 1** shows a clinch that was intentionally done with the line to show what it looks like. In **Figures 2 and 3** you can see what that sort of clinching will look like with a few weeks on it. For a contest or certification, doing this to a foot would result in a very low score. Today, most farriers have learned to get the proper amount of foot removed from under their clinches without making a groove that extends beyond the clinch.

A proper clinch will have as much nail thickness as possible in it. In order to get good thickness, the clinch should be imbedded in the wall. Modern clinchers make imbedding the clinch a little easier, and using a gouge makes it easier yet. To test the thickness of your clinches, try pulling some newly clinched nails **(Figure 4)** to look at the amount of material that makes the clinch. **Figure 5** is a clinch that was imbedded in a hole made by a gouge, and **Figure 6** is a clinch where only a rasp was used to

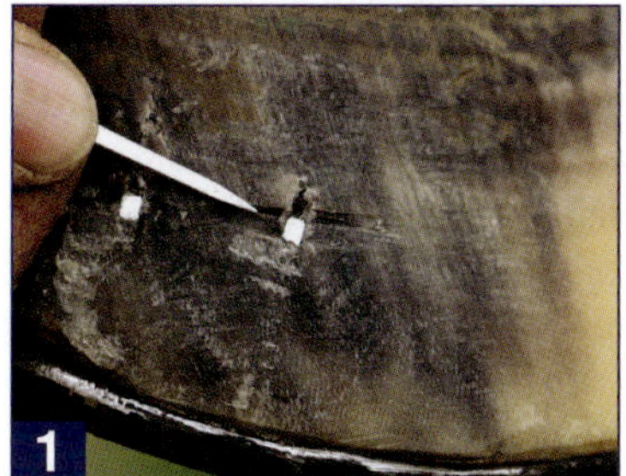
Bad clinching technique.

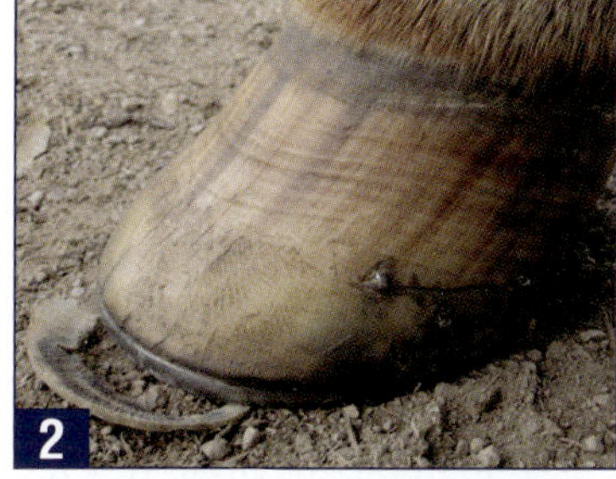
The results of bad technique.

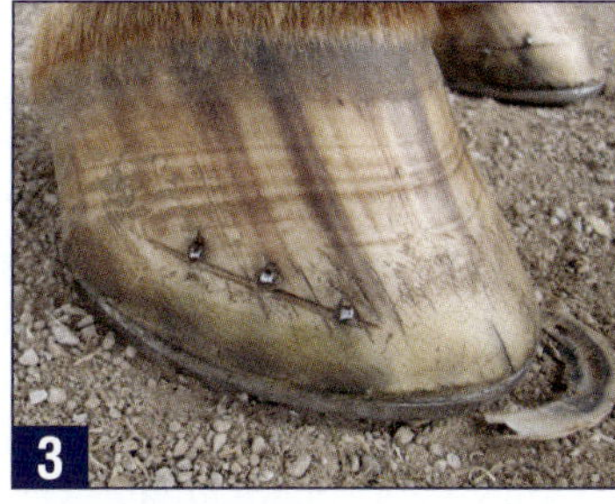
Bad technique.

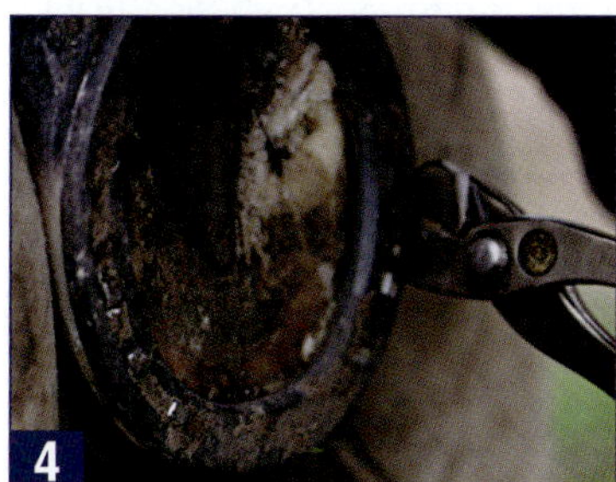
Pulling a nail to look at the clinch.

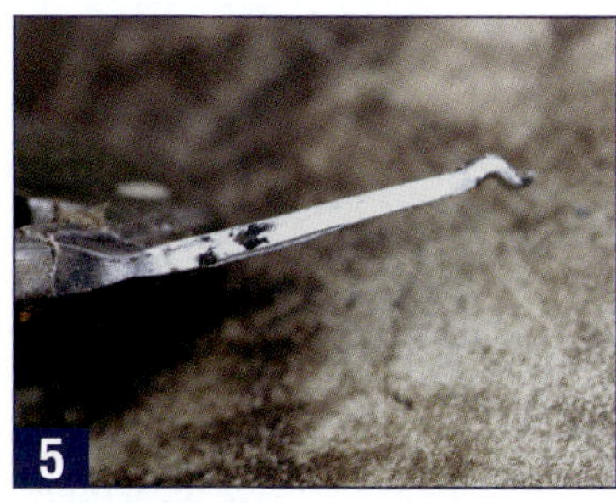
A strong clinch with a lot of material in it.

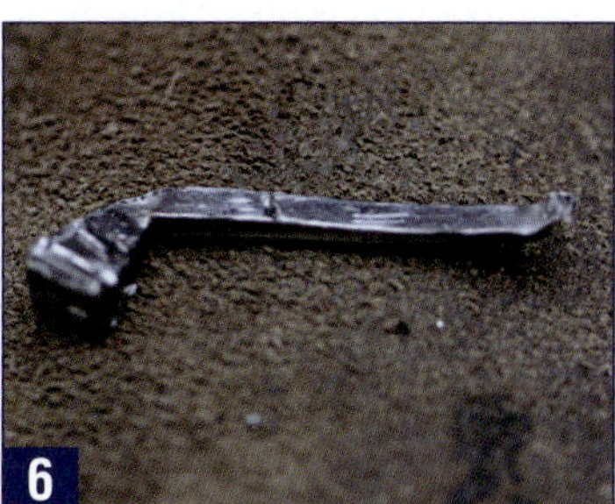
A weak clinch.

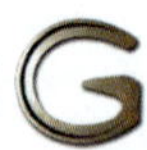

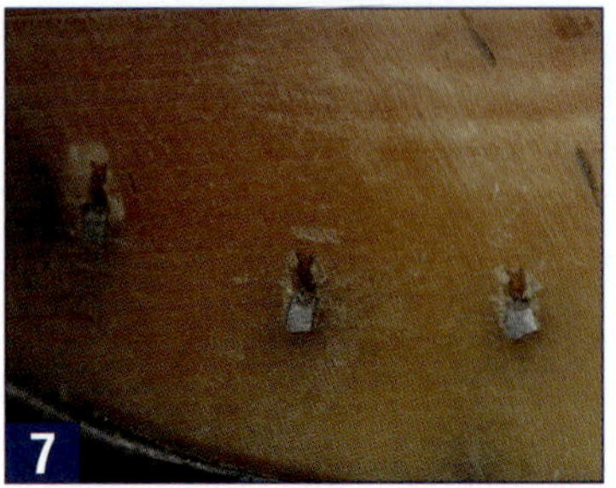
Different clinches.

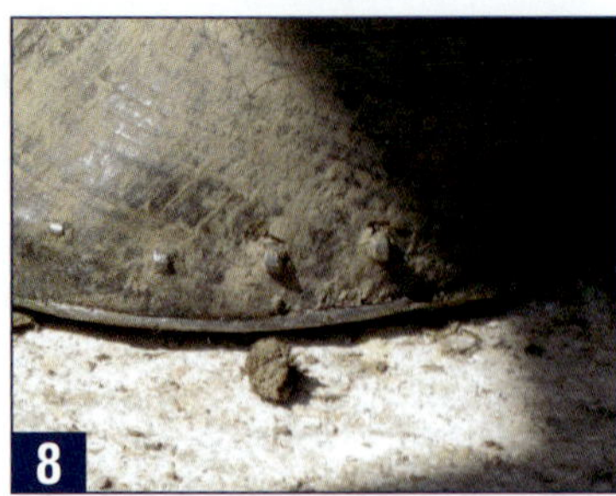
Bad clinching.

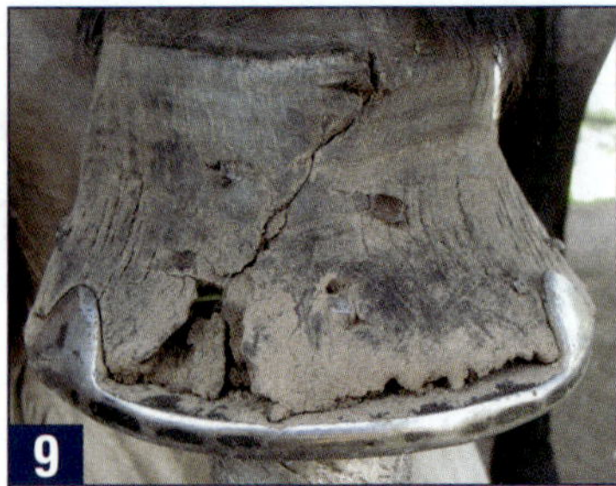
Popped clinches on a weak foot.

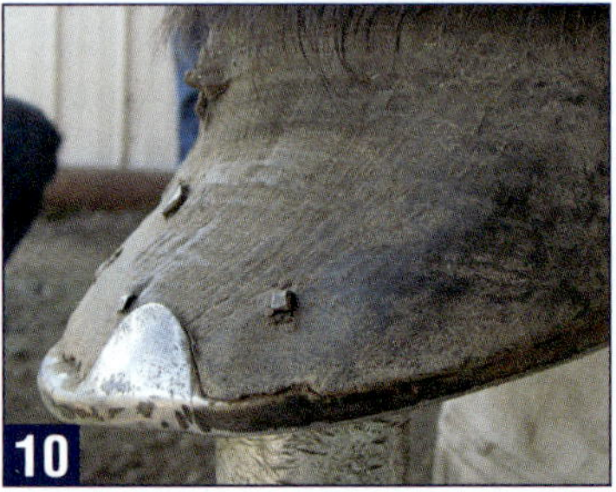
Same weak foot with popped clinches.

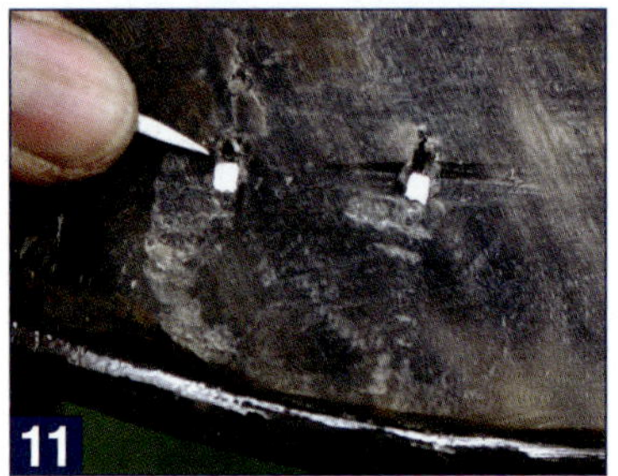
Gap above clinch when hammer clinching.

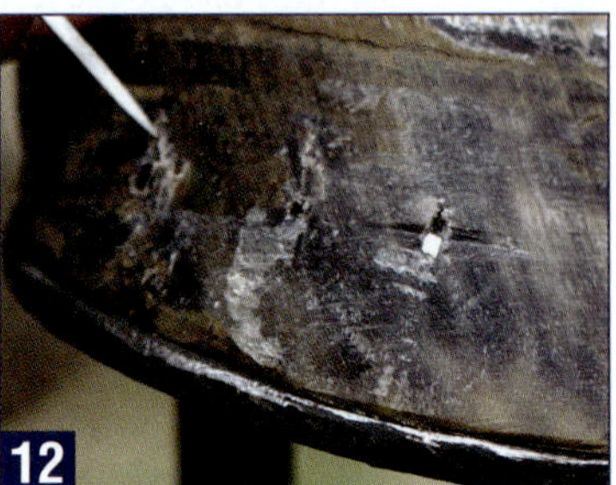
Gap above clinch when using clinchers.

remove the tissue under the nail. Notice the additional amount of steel in the first clinch as opposed to the second. There is no doubt about the abilities of the first to hold a shoe when compared to the second one.

Another thing to look for in a good clinch is a square shape. The clinch should be as long as the shank of the nail is wide. I try to achieve a square clinch. **Figure 7** shows good clinches on the second and third nail, while the toe nail is slightly short. By making a square clinch, you will have enough material to hold the shoe on the foot and also have a good-looking job. One of the most common things we see with bad clinches is that they have been left too long. Excess length will actually make a clinch weaker because you are not able to achieve as sharp an angle with the long clinch, and a short, sharp angle is stronger than a long, shallow angle. One reason for the long clinch is improper use of clinchers, and the other reason is not removing enough of the hoof wall under the nail before clinching.

Figure 8 is a foot that is seen elsewhere in this book under bad shoeing. This foot is two weeks into the shoeing, and you can see the toe nail clinch was rasped off, and the others are popped out and long. Really weak, long or wet feet will have the clinches pop out for a couple of reasons. First, the foot compacts every time the horse steps, and the nails stay the same length. With feet that are weak, this compaction makes the hole shorter than the nail. Second, as a long foot grows over the shoe, the clinches can be popped out as the shoe is sunk into the sole area of the foot. In **Figures 9 and 10**, you can see that this is a very weak foot. These clinches are at five weeks to the day, and they have popped out from the wall being so compromised.

The last thing that I like to see in a good clinch is a minimum of hoof wall being destroyed above the clinch. By driving a nail at an angle through the hoof wall then bending that nail back on itself, there is going to be an area where hoof is missing above the clinch. I have yet to see a clinch that is so precise that there is not at least a small gap. Generally, this gap will be about the size of the clinch when the farrier is using the technique of hammer clinching **(Figure 11)** and slightly longer when using clinching tongs **(Figure 12)**. However, we try to keep that gap as small as possible by using the clinchers with care.

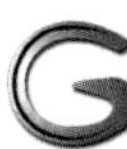

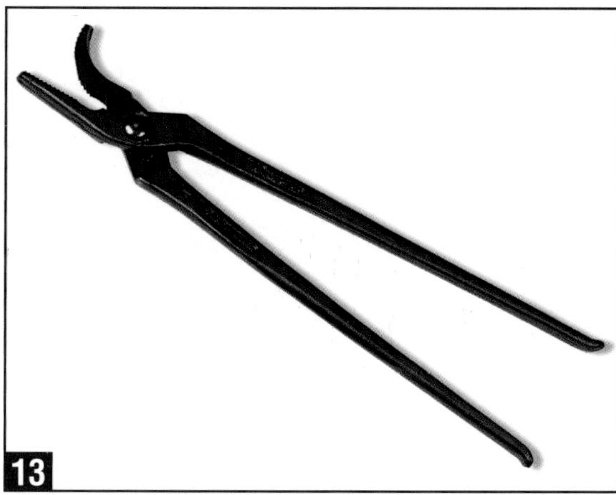

13

Alligator clinchers.

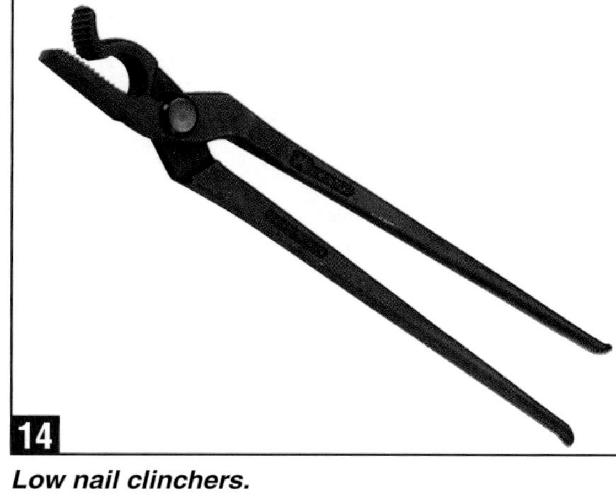

14

Low nail clinchers.

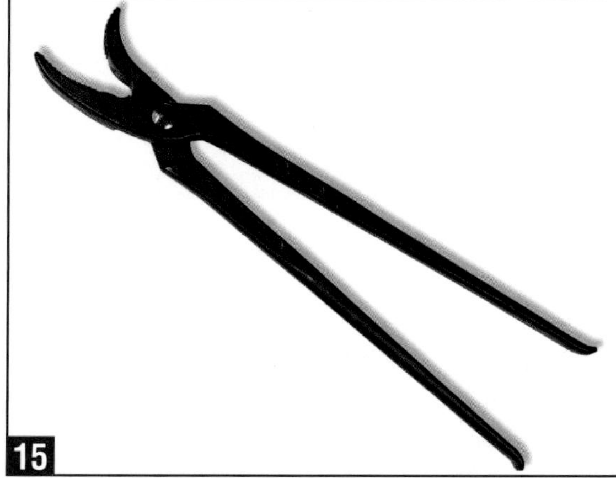

15

Delta-Mustad Hoofcare Center curved-jaw clinchers.

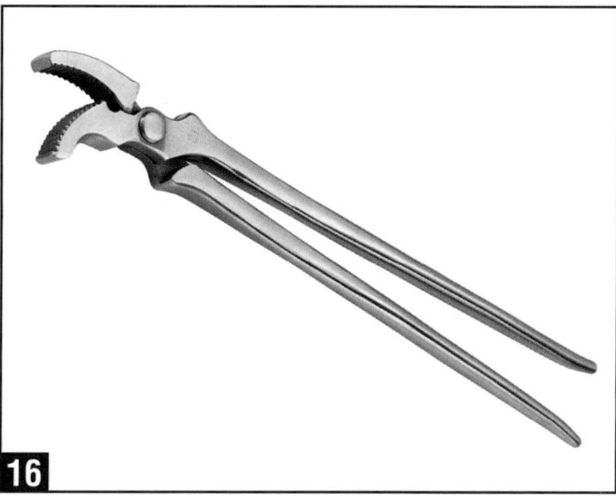

16

G.E. Forge and Tool curved-jaw clinchers.

METHODS

There are two basic methods that I know of to clinch a horse. Perhaps the most common in the United States is to use a pair of clinchers or clinching tongs. **Figures 13-16** show a variety of designs. The most common when I started shoeing was **Figure 13**, called an alligator clincher, although I never saw anyone use them on an alligator. **Figure 14** is for low nails, which you should never need, and **Figures 15 and 16** are of the curved jaw variety. There are other styles as well, such as the gooseneck and adjustable clinchers, but I find the curved jaws to be the best.

Currently, both Jim Keith Tools and G.E. Forge and Tool make a curved jaw clincher, with St. Croix and Delta Mustad Hoofcare Center offering a modified style of curved jaw that works quite well. The curved jaw is my favorite clincher design, but it took a few horses to get accustomed to the feel. With a curved jaw, you get more leverage than with normal clinchers. Without much effort, you can pull a lot of nail through a lot of foot. For this reason, many farriers do not like the way that curved jaw clinchers feel the first time they use them. However, most come to appreciate them once they have used them long enough to get a feel for them.

The clinchers pictured in **Figure 17** are one pair of a couple of curved-jaw prototype clinchers that were sent to me by Dan Bradley from G.E. before they hit the market. I think it was probably 1997 or 1998. At any rate, it is the same pair that Kelly still uses the most today. Talk about a bad deal for G.E. When you make tools, it is good for them to wear out at some point so that your customer will buy more.

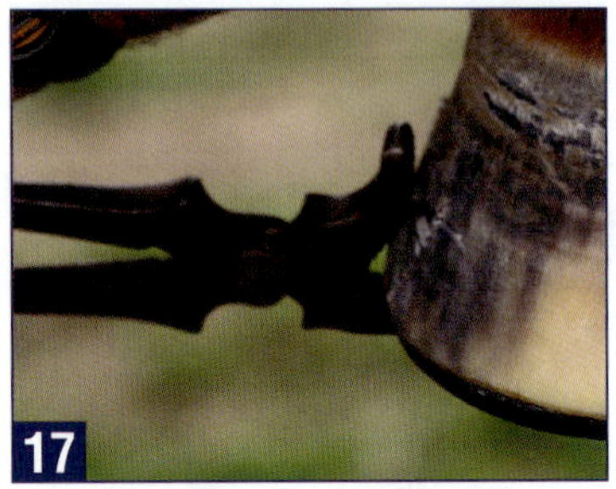

17

The G.E. prototype curved jaws that we have used for over 14 years.

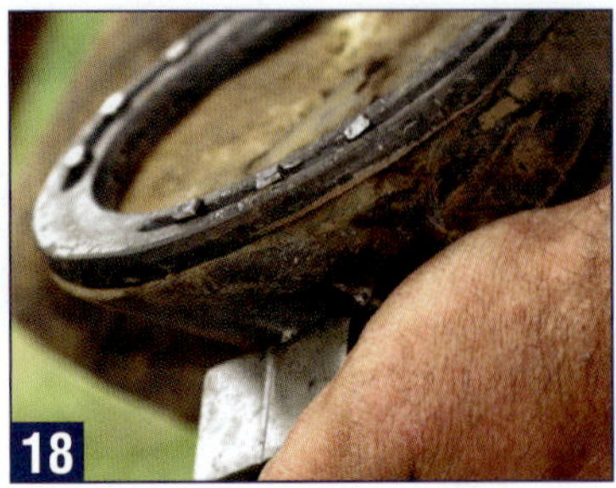

18

Setting or blocking nails with a pair of pulloffs.

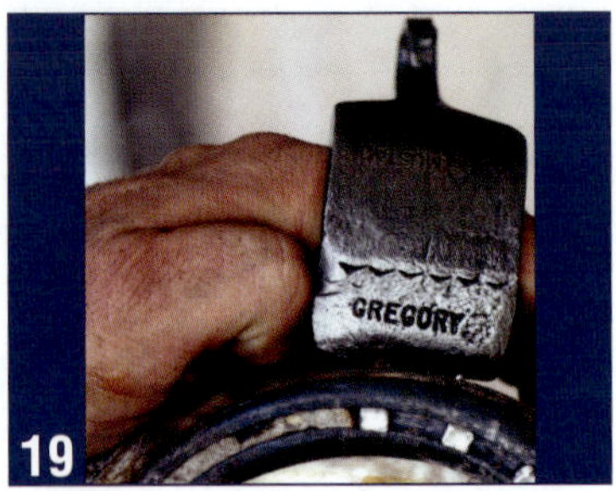

19

Blocking with a clinch block.

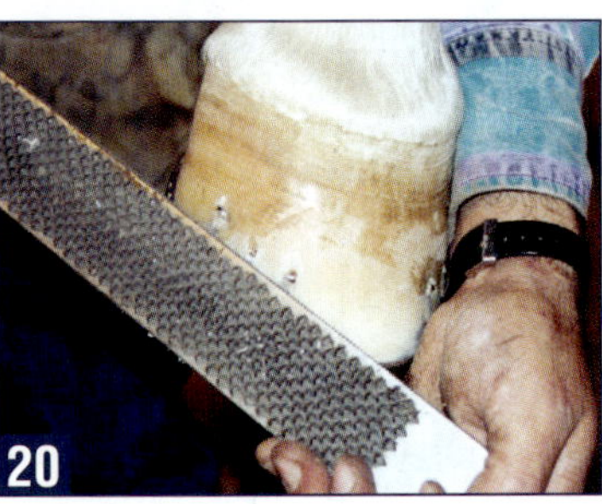

20

Rasping the burr off under a nail.

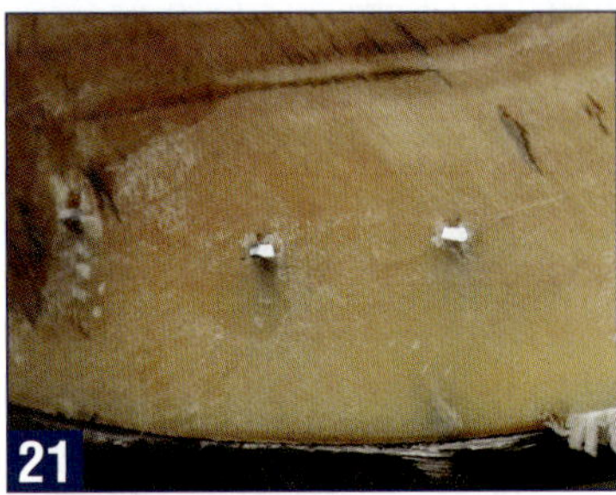

21

You can see that the burr is removed, but there is not a groove cut into the foot.

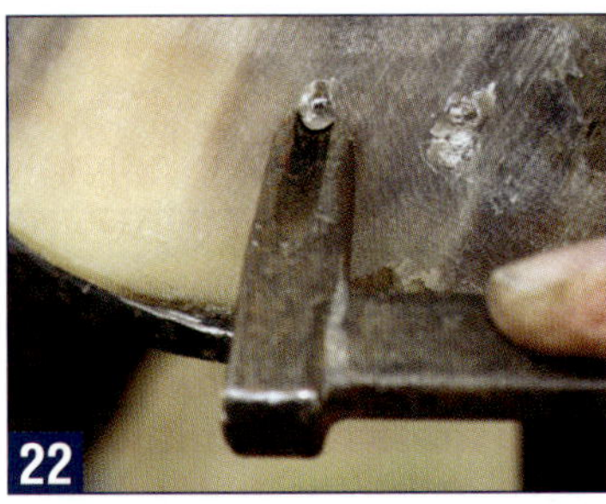

22

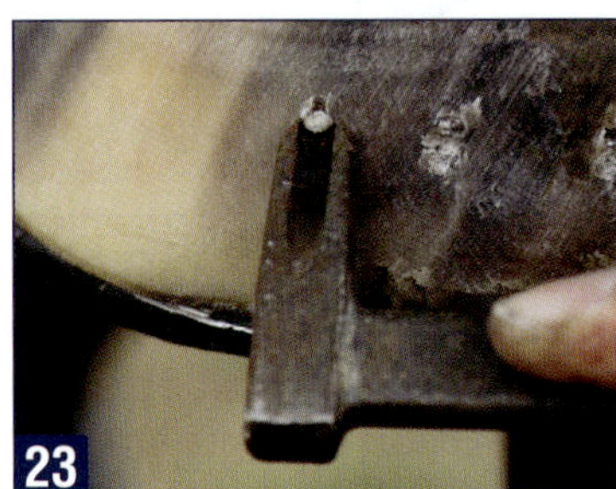

23

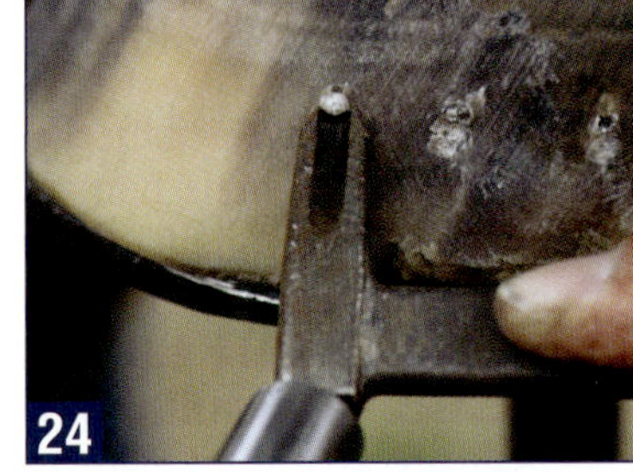

24

Using a gouge.

To properly clinch with a pair of curved-jaw clinchers, begin by setting, called blocking, the nail with your hammer and clinch block before bringing the foot forward. In **Figure 18**, I am using a pair of pulloffs, and in **Figure 19**, I am using a clinch block made from an old rasp as described in the forging exercise area of this book. Try to keep the edge of the block parallel to the shoe, and do not overdo this step. Blocking the nails too hard will make the gap above the clinch much longer. Set the nail hard enough that the portion sticking out of the hoof wall is at 90 degrees or less. Take the foot to the hoof stand and remove the small burr under the nail with the edge of the rasp **(Figure 20)**. Lay the smooth side of the rasp against the foot, and gently take the portion of hoof wall under the nail with the top edge (another thing to avoid overdoing). Look carefully at **Figure 21**, and you will see that there is not a deep line cut under the nail; just enough material was removed to make the wall flat where it was displaced by the nail being driven through it.

My preferred method of removing the material below the nail is with a gouge. Gouging will allow you to bury the clinch further into the hoof wall,

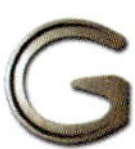

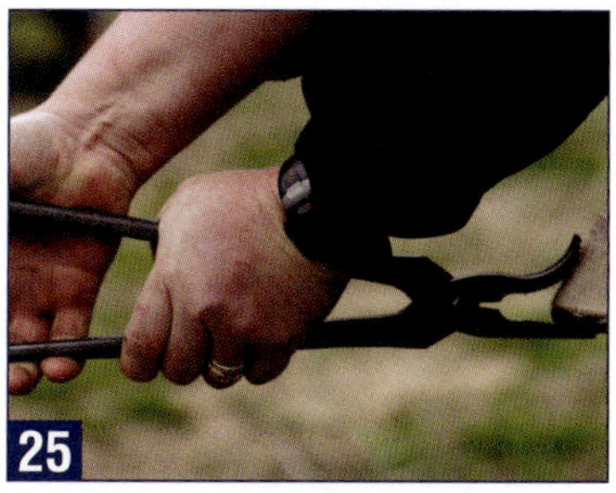

Clinching with clinchers. Comfortable hand position.

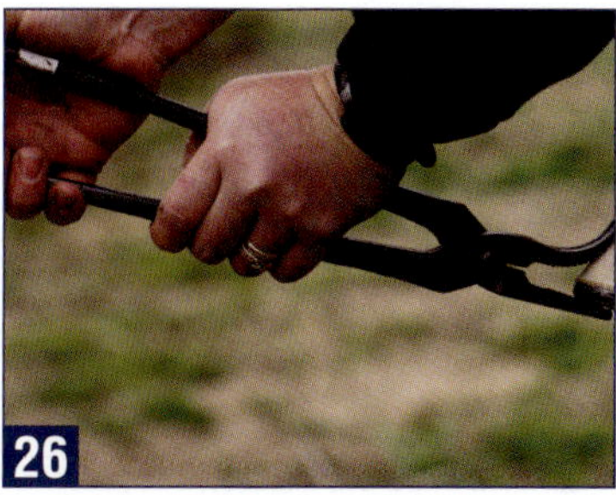

Squeeze lift and push.

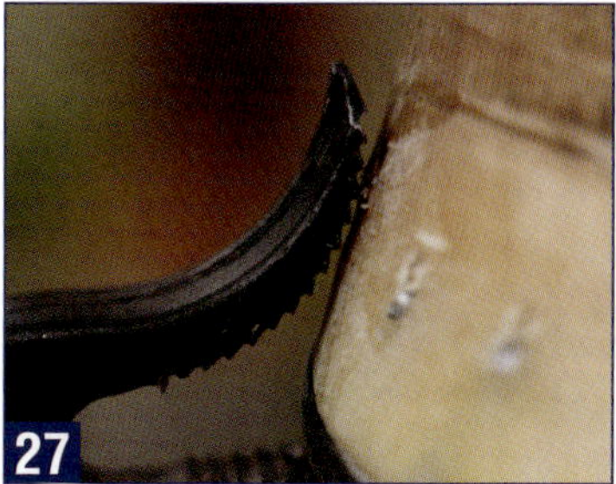

Detail of the nail being bent.

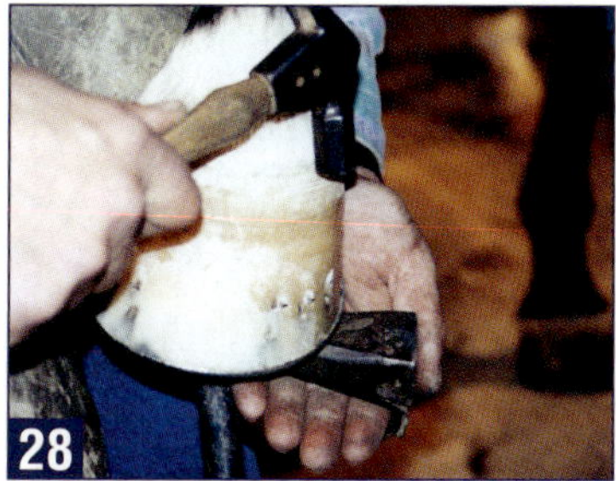

Hammer clinching.

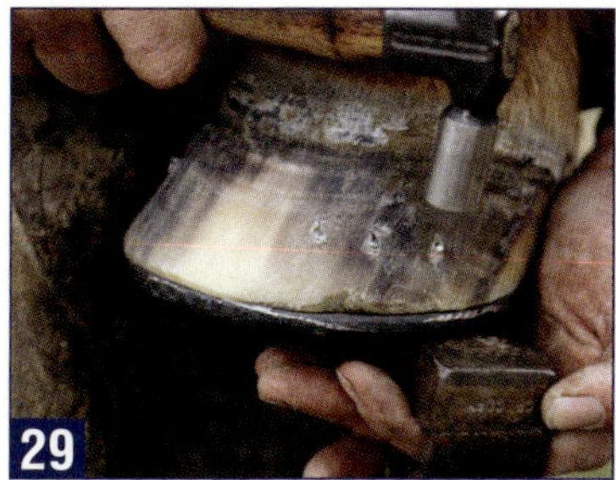

Hammer clinching.

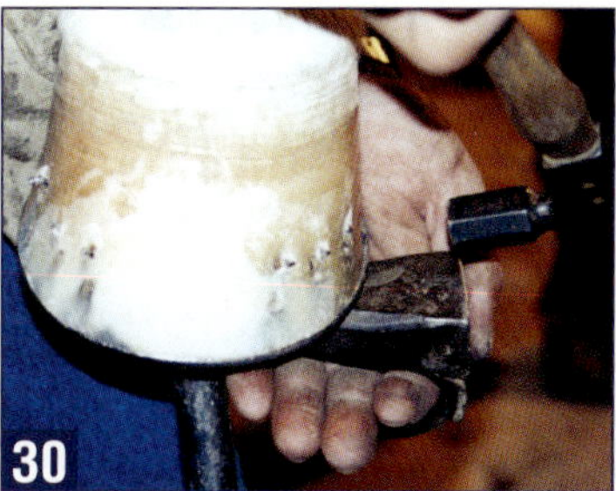

Hammering the clinch against the foot.

which results in a thicker clinch. To gouge, place the gouge under the nail and hammer it into the foot. As you hammer, twist the gouge downward while you continue to hammer from the same direction. Once the gouge has been twisted far enough, the last hammer blow will send the side of the gouge against the foot and the piece of material will be cleanly removed **(Figures 22-24)**.

Bend the clinch against and into the hoof wall with the clinchers. How you then squeeze and lift is important, and it takes a lot of "feel" to get good at. Here is a description that you can follow to develop that feel. Begin by placing the clinchers on the nail so that the jaws are open far enough that they will not close all the way when the clinch is finished, yet not so far apart that it is hard to get your hand around the reins. The bottom rein of the clinchers should be parallel to the bottom of the horse's foot **(Figure 25)**. Squeeze without lifting or pushing down on the reins as you feel the nail bend well past 90 degrees. Once the nail has bent to the proper angle, maintain the position of your hand nearest the foot as you lift with the hand furthest away from the foot. In **Figure 26**, Kelly is actually pushing down with her left hand while lifting with her right hand. This lifting motion will imbed the clinch into the hoof wall so that it won't be rasped off when the foot is finished. Pulling up too early will push on an incomplete clinch, so this is where the need for "feel" comes in. With practice, you will start to sense when and how hard to squeeze, when and how hard to lift, and develop that touch for a good clinch. **Figure 27** shows the clinch is bent enough, and this is the time to lift on the reins.

Everything is the same when clinching with alligator or gooseneck clinchers. The main difference is the amount of leverage generated by the design. Because less leverage is available with the alligator or gooseneck design, many farriers like them better. Less leverage means less chance of pulling the nail down the hoof and leaving a large gap above the clinch, but it also means more effort expended to get the same job done. Like most people, farriers tend to resist change. When the curved jaw came out, that was a big change.

One of the most common faults with clinching is leaving a big hole above the clinch. If you are having problems with that gap above the clinch, make certain that you are not pushing down on the clinchers when you first start to squeeze the clinch.

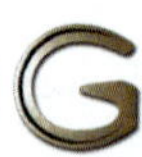

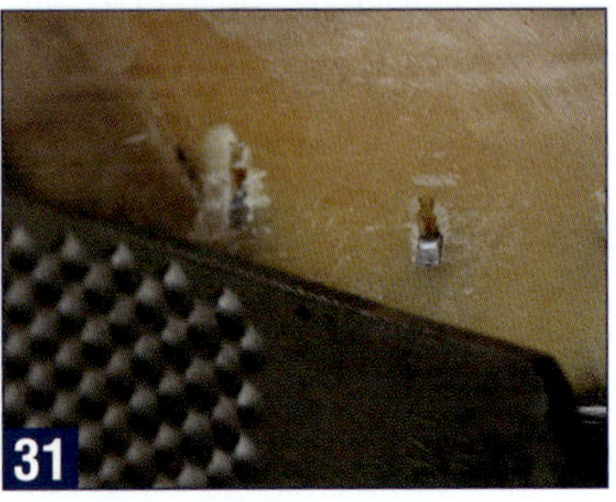
Rasping the clinches.

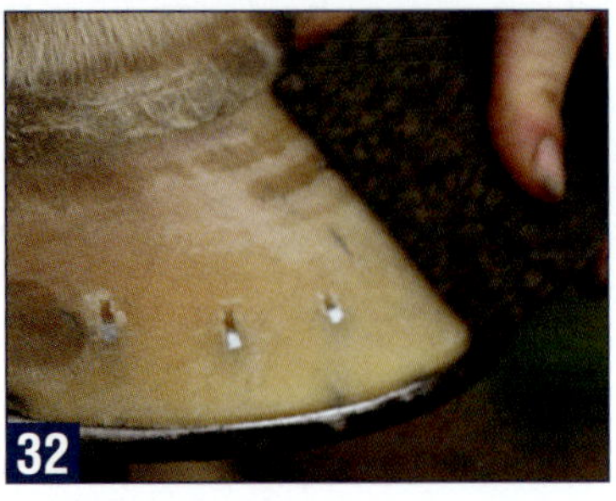
Sanding the foot.

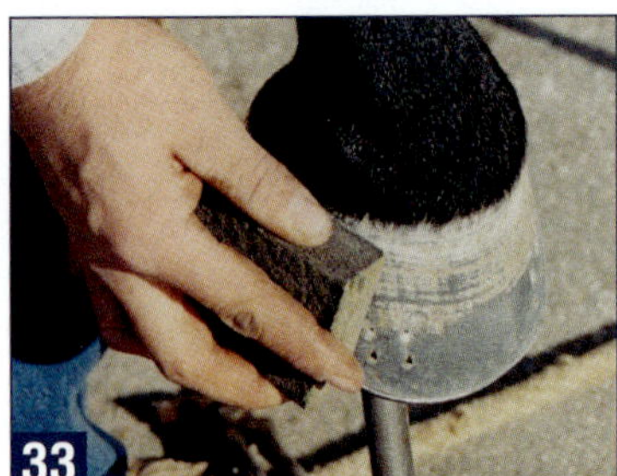

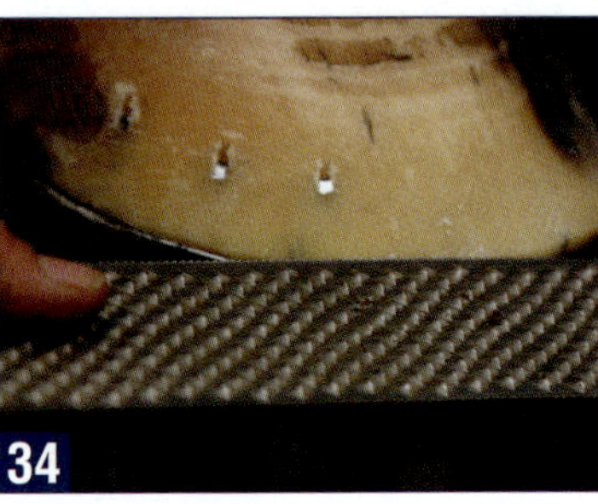
Filing the edge.

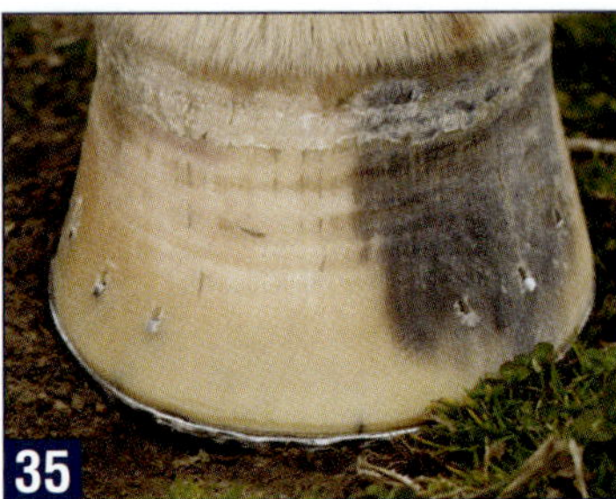
The results of good edge filing.

The act of pushing down will make the top jaw pull the nail out and down through the foot. This will result in a long clinch that is not easily imbedded in the hoof wall and large holes above the clinch. Even with the best clinching technique, the hole above the clinch is rarely smaller than the clinch itself.

Another good method of clinching is called hammer clinching. The resulting clinch from hammer clinching is often a better-looking clinch than most people can do with clinchers. For that reason, we use hammer clinches at most contests and certifications, and Cody hammer clinches all of his horses. A quick note about quality: If you strive for a high standard at all times, doing that high standard at a contest or exam is much easier than if you do average work every day and expect a high standard for only special occasions. Anything you want to get good at you should do often and make a part of your normal routine.

Begin by gouging the hoof wall below the nail as you did for using clinching tongs. Place your clinch block on the nail head, and then bend the clinch over by hammering from above. The first few blows will be with the edge of your hammer, and once the clinch is close to a 45-degree angle, you will drive it into the foot with the face of your driving hammer **(Figures 28-30)**. After you hammer the clinch into the wall, rasp lightly to clean up any burrs **(Figure 31)**, and sand with a sanding block to get a nice finish **(Figure 32-33)**. If done correctly, this method leaves the smallest gap above the clinch. The down side is that some horses do not appreciate the hammering on the outside of the foot, and you can potentially loosen the nail by driving the nail out of the shoe if the clinch block does not make contact with the nail head on the bottom of the shoe.

The final piece to finishing a shod foot nicely is to run the rasp around the perimeter of the shoe where it meets the foot. Hold the rasp with the smooth side down at the bottom of the foot. Using the edge of bottom edge of the rasp, run around the edge of the shoe **(Figure 34)**. This will make the edge of the shoe shine, and it will look like the foot grew a shoe. I call this portion of the job "edge filing." **Figure 35** depicts this pretty well. With practice, your feet should look like those in **Figures 36-39**.

Whatever style you choose to use, examine and judge the resulting clinches carefully. If you find a defect, go back through the process carefully to determine what is causing the problem. Break

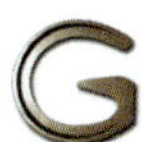

clinching down into the various tasks involved, and you can fix the individual task that is preventing a great clinch.

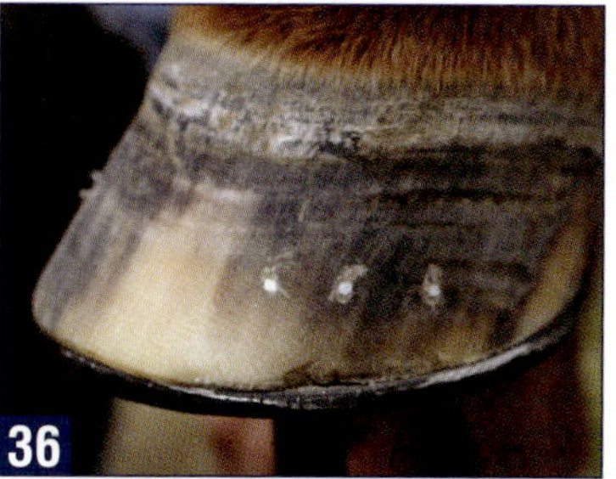

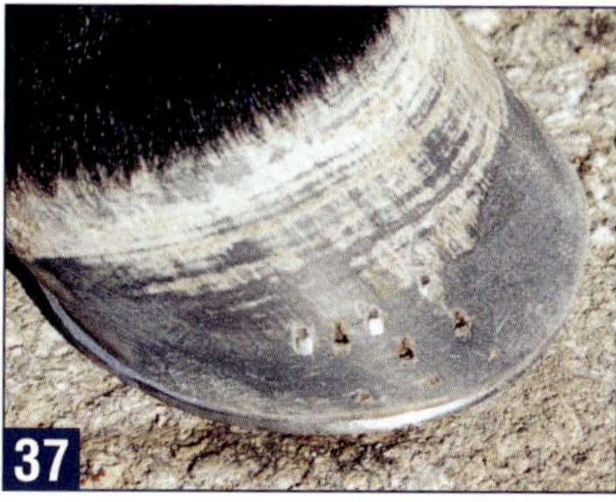

Nicely finished feet with hammer clinches.

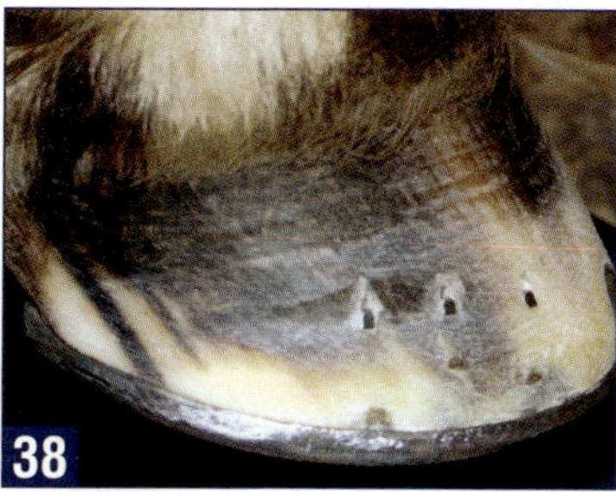

Finished foot clinched with clinchers.

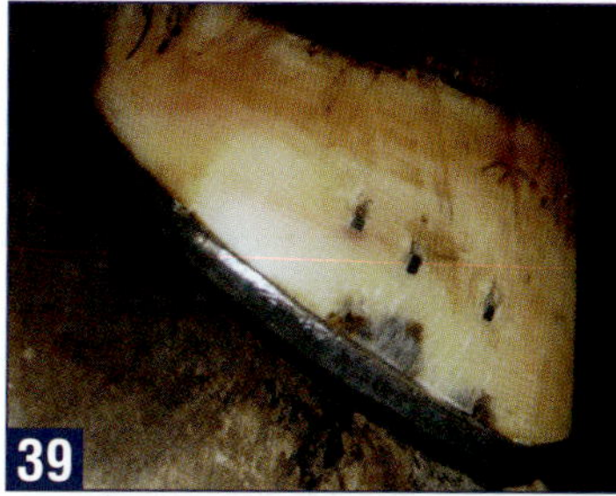

Finished foot with hammer clinches.

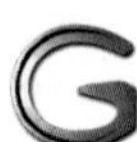

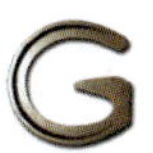

Section

8

Other Shoeing

Chapter 32: Modern Farriery 280

Chapter 33: Bad Shoeing 294

Chapter 34: Common Sense In The Shoeing vs. Barefoot Debate 302

Chapter 35: Myths of Farriery 306

" 27 "Look," says the Teacher,
"this is what I have discovered:
"Adding one thing to another to discover
the scheme of things. "

—Ecclesiastes 7:27
—New International Version

Chapter

32 MODERN FARRIERY

Just a quick note to start this chapter. There has been an amazing amount of technology that has been used to further the art of farriery over the last 20 years. A lot of this has been great for the horse, but overall, it has not been good for the skills of the farrier. At one time, if you did not have the skill to pull clips on your own, you did not get to shoe with clips. The same is true of so many things that can now be bought. The modern farrier can replace skill with product, and this leads to some farriers never developing those skills.

At times, this can be very bad for the horse. When pre-clipped shoes first appeared, I saw a lot of horses that had had shoes nailed on without proper trimming. I saw large clips being hammered over without being burned or cut in, and feet were drifting away from the center of the bony column. These shoes can be a problem because they place products in the hands of individuals who are not competent enough to use them — like a 3-year-old with a gun.

Conversely, there are things that we can do now that were all but impossible in the past. Primarily, extensions on foals are more common and easier than in the past, and this has been great for the horse and the farrier.

At any rate, there are a lot of modern materials available to use to shoe horses. I know that some think we won't be using nails at some point in the future, but I have to disagree. The nail will remain the cheapest and greenest way to shoe horses for a long time. There are a lot of resources involved in shoeing with glues, acrylics, and urethanes. These resources cost a lot of money, and there are thousands of horses that will do fine for their entire lives, shod skillfully with a simple steel shoe nailed on with a simple steel nail.

POUR-IN PADS

The main product that I have found to be a great thing in my practice has been the polyurethane pour-ins. The one I most commonly use is the Vettec Equi-Pak **(Figure 1)** and Equi-Pak CS **(Figure 2)**. The difference between the two is that the CS has copper sulfate in it to help with the prevention of certain bacteria and fungi. This product sticks to properly prepared hoof tissue really well, and it has done a lot of good for a lot of horses. It is a simple product to use, and there are measureable results in many cases.

Here is how we use Equi-Pak.

Begin by cleaning the foot as well as you can. Use a small wire brush to remove any dirt or manure, and knife away any tissue that should be knifed away anyway. Apply whatever shoe you are going to shoe with. Use a heat gun to dry and heat the hoof **(Figure 3)**, and then make a dam with Hawthorne's Sole Pack **(Figure 4)** or something similar, such as Play-Doh **(Figure 5)**, around whatever areas you don't want the Equi-Pak **(Figure 6)** to reach. Since I use this in almost every heart bar and W-shoe, I don't want the potential of pressure in the toe area where the coffin bone can be close to the surface on a foundered horse. I place the dam across the back of the bar where the Equi-Pak could leak out of the commissures. You can see this if you look closely at the back of the shoe in **Figure 6**. I also use it across the front of the frog plate.

While holding the foot in a position with the shoe close to parallel to the ground, I have someone squeeze the material into the cavity made by the shoe **(Figures 7 and 8)**. In most cases, it is important that the foot is not filled past the point where the Equi-Pak would protrude past the ground surface of the shoe. If it does, you may end up putting more pressure on the sole than you want to. Using the normal Equi-Pak will result in feet that look like those **Figures 9 and 10**. Equi-Pak CS will be blue as in **Figures 11 and 12**.

You can also use the styrofoam adhesive pieces that Vettec makes. These work really well, but if they are not necessary, there is no reason to spend the extra money on them. When working on feet that cannot be lifted high enough to get the shoe to parallel, the styrofoam is real handy.

To use the styrofoam, prepare the foot as

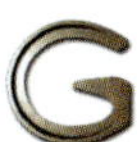

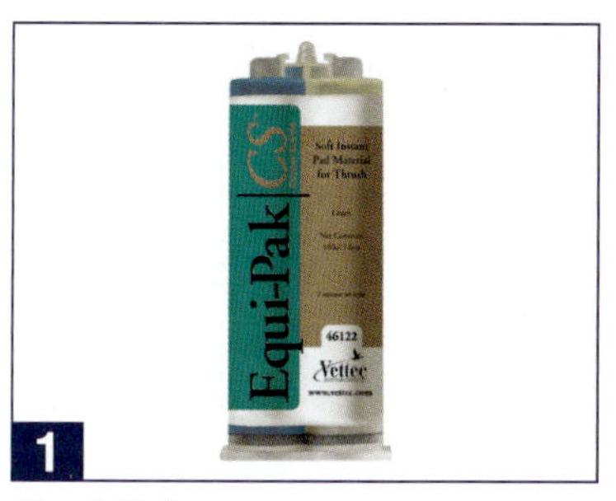

1 *Equi-Pak.*

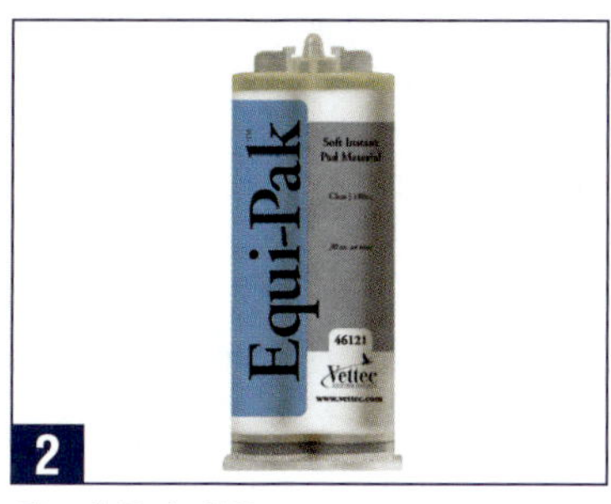

2 *Equi-Pak CS.*

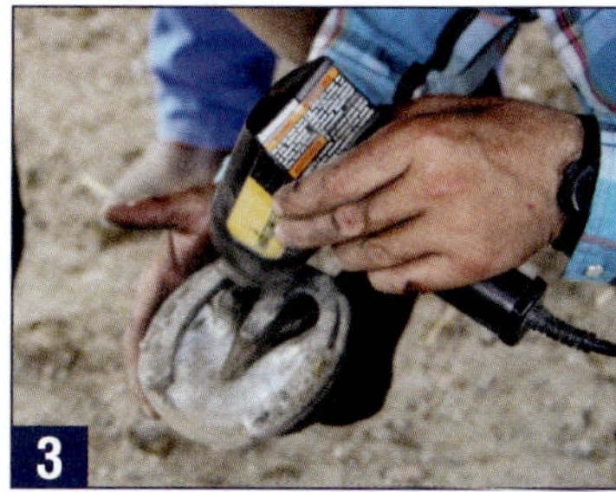

3 *Drying a foot with a heat gun.*

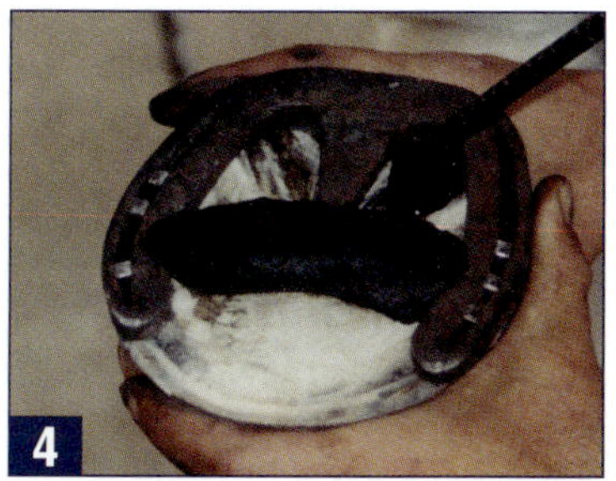

4 *W-shoe with Hawthorne Sole Pack to block the Equi-pak.*

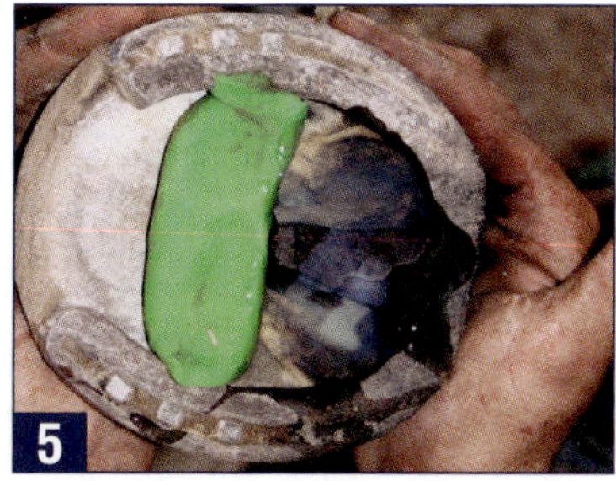

5 *W-shoe with dam made from Play-Doh.*

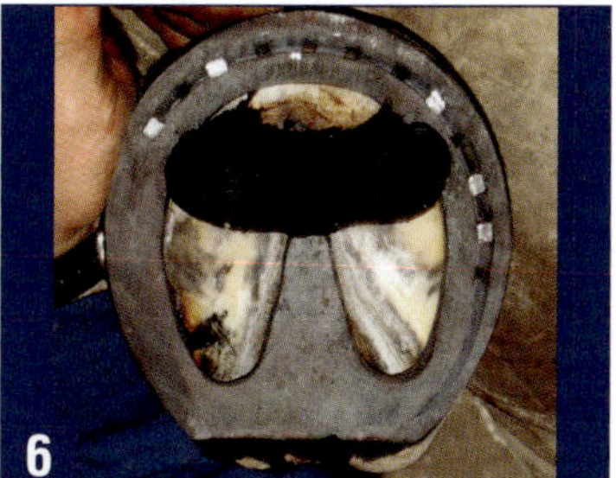

6 *Heart bar with Sole Pack blocking the toe area and the back of the heels under the bar.*

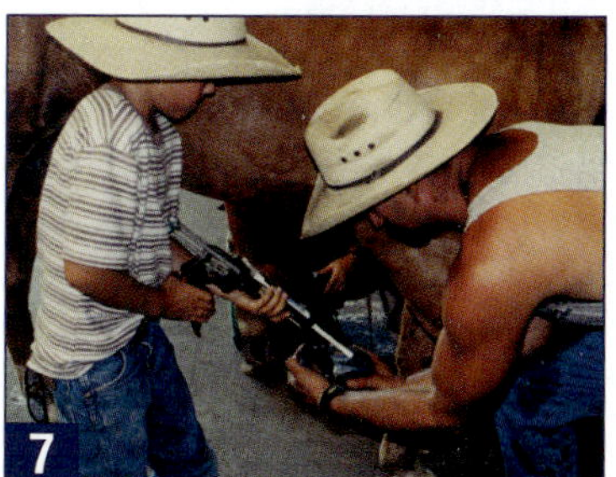

7 *Cody squeezing in the Equi-Pak for me.*

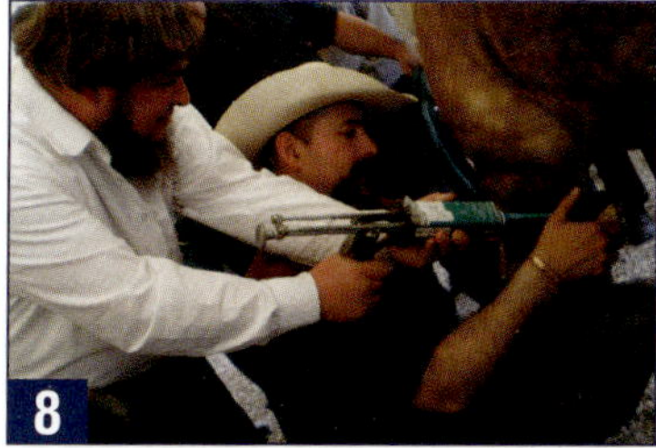

8 *Marvin Schwartz from Indiana putting the Equi-Pak in a foot for me when I did a clinic at his supply business, D. L. Schwartz Company, LLC.*

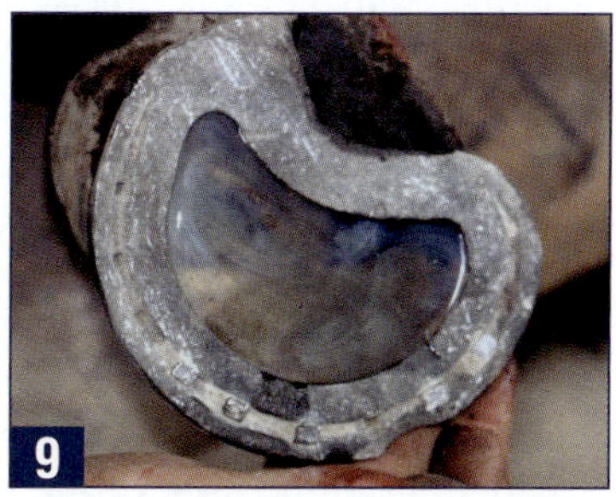

9 *Clear Equi-Pak in a Z-bar shoe.*

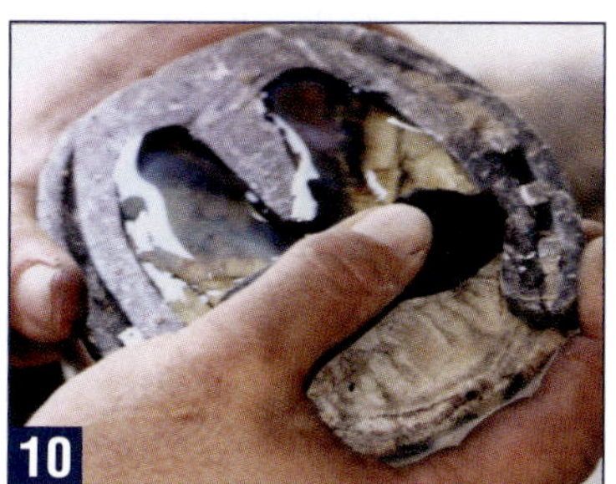

10 *Clear Equi-Pak in a w-shoe.*

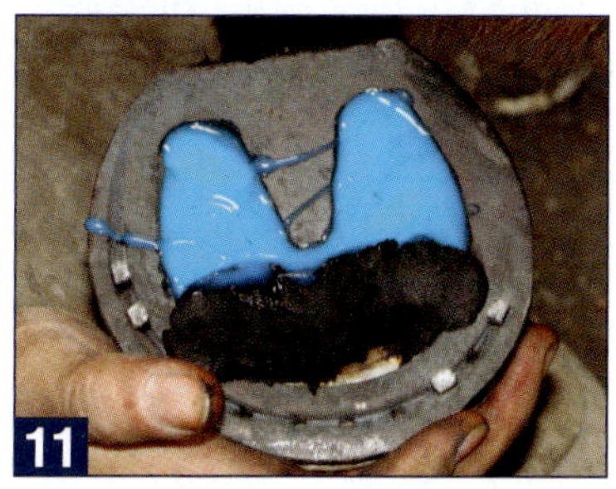

11 *Equi-Pak CS in a heart bar.*

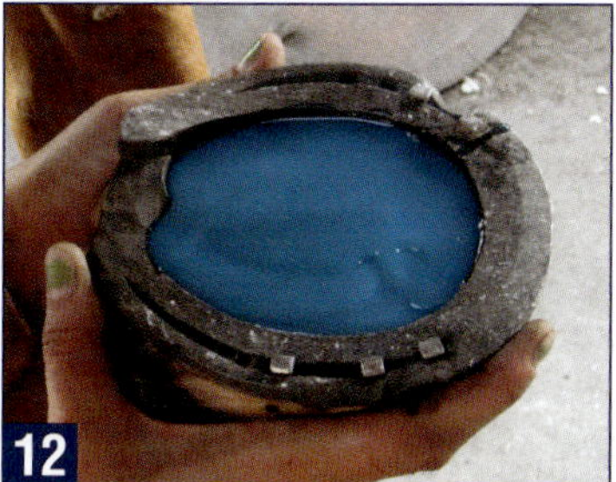

12 *Equi-Pak CS in a medial lift bar shoe.*

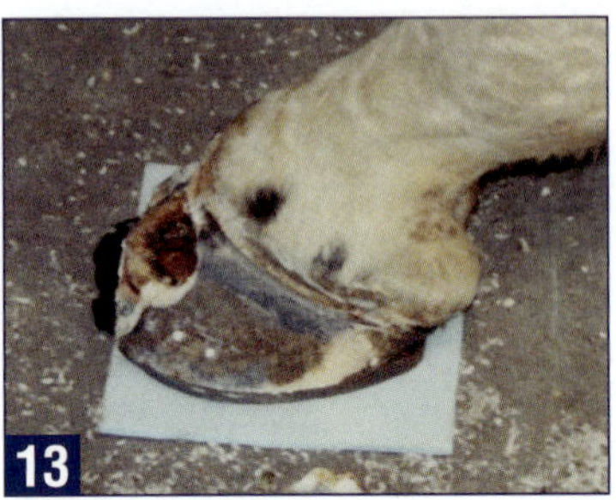

Styrofoam pad being compressed by the shoe.

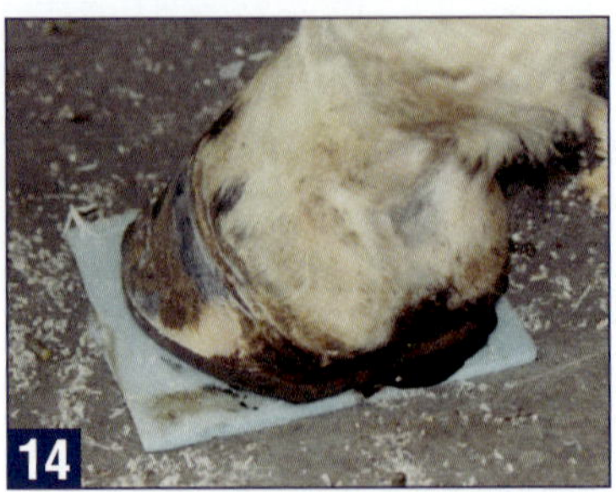

Small amount of leakage out the back of the shoe and Styrofoam pad.

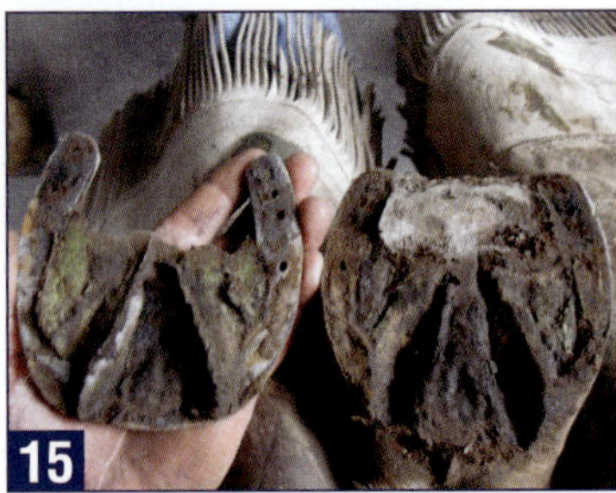

W-shoe with Equi-Pak attached to it next to the foot it came out of.

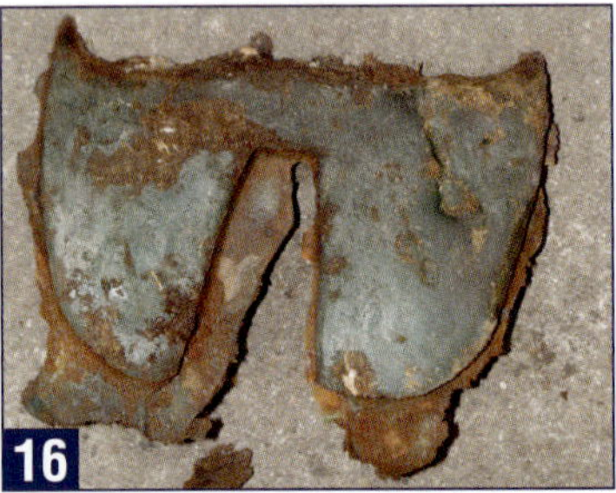

Piece of Equi-pak out of a foot after six weeks of wear.

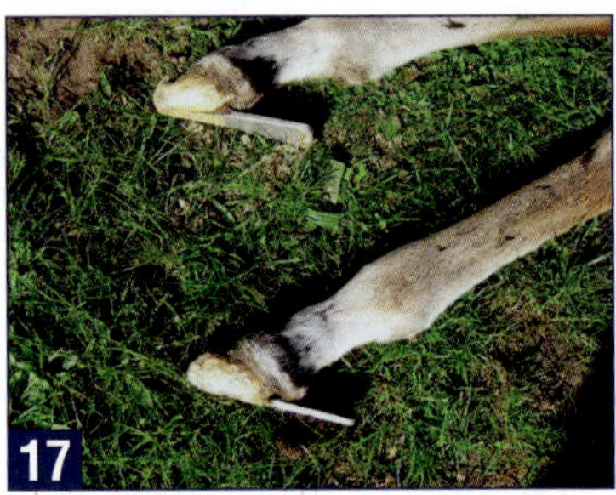

Heel extensions made from aluminum glued to a foal with flaccid tendons.

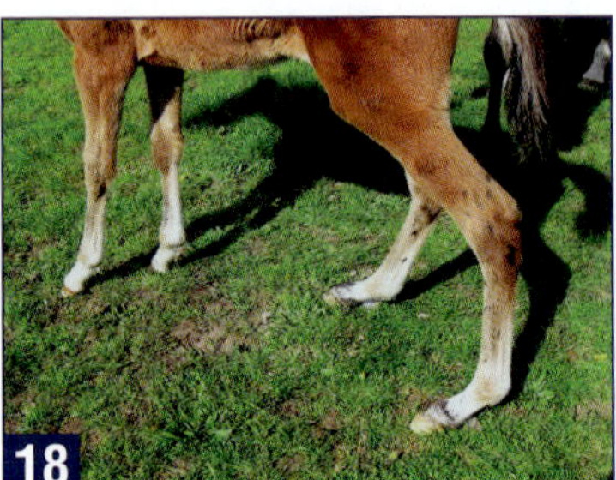

Same foal standing up.

described, and then place the styrofoam pad against the shoe. Allow the horse to stand on the pad so that it seals tightly around the shoe and makes a slight impression into the cavity formed by the shoe. This impression is what keeps the Equi-Pak from protruding past the rim of the shoe.

Lift the foot and pour the Equi-Pak into the back of the shoe. If you fill the cavity up all the way, you will have a fair amount of waste. Fill to about 3/4-inch from the back of the shoe, hold it up for about 30 seconds, and then place the foot on the ground **(Figure 13)**. When it loads, there will be just a little bit of Equi-Pak squeezed out the back. You can see a little bit of Adhere that has come out the back of the shoe in **Figure 14**. This is ideal.

If the foot has been properly prepared and the Equi-Pak applied correctly, when you come back to shoe the horse in six or seven weeks, you will find that the sole is nice and clean, and the Equi-Pak comes out as one piece **(Figures 15 and 16)**. When using a pad and packing alone, the area under the pad is often nasty and the sole is wet and dirty. Since the Equi-Pak actually adheres to the sole, it allows the sole to stay cleaner.

EXTENSIONS

Knowing the properties of potential hoof builders will help you make a choice of product that fits your needs. There are basically two ways of making a hoof builder stick to the foot. With acrylics, you will have a mechanical bond. This means that the product will fill whatever nooks and crannies it can find, and when it cures, the filling of those areas creates the bond. With polyurethanes, you have a chemical bond as well as a mechanical bond. This means that the urethane molecule will stick to the first molecule of something else that it contacts. However, you have the additional advantage of the mechanical bond. Each one has advantages in certain situations.

With a purely mechanical bond, you should clean with a solvent to dislodge any oild or dirt. With a chemical bond, those cleaners will leave a thin layer of film that will be what the product attaches to. For polyurethanes, the surface should be cleaned with a brush, and being dry is the most important factor. That is why a heat gun is used with polyurethane application.

I was having trouble using Super Fast at one point, so I called the Vettec rep and told him that

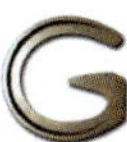

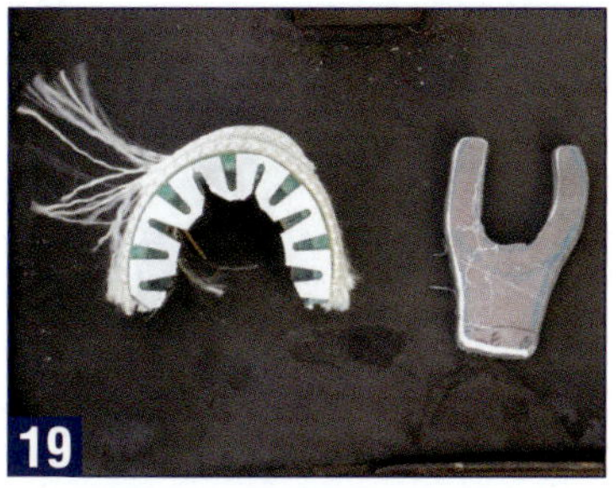

19 *Sound Horse system for a toe extension using a Series III universal cuff.*

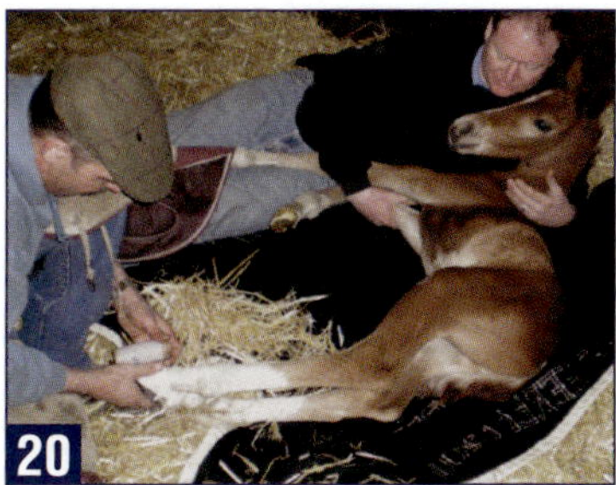

20 *Applying the toe extension to a foal.*

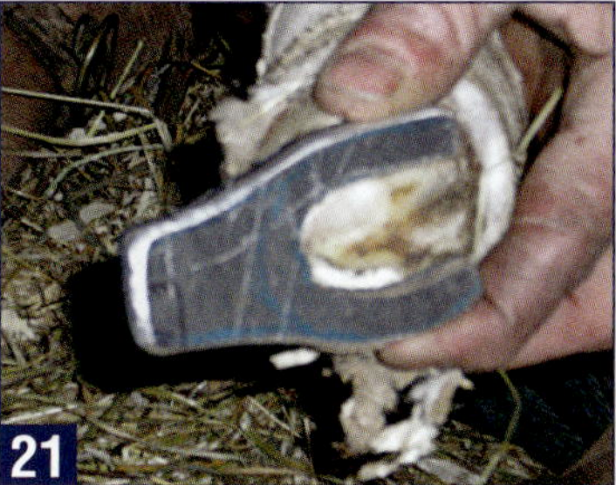

21 *The foot with the toe extension on it.*

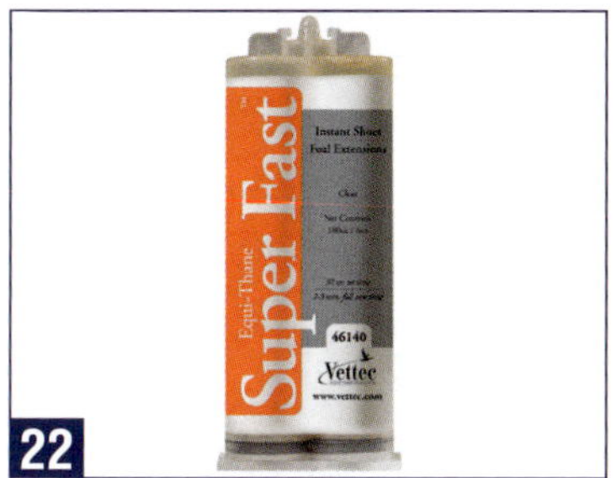

22 *Vettec Super Fast.*

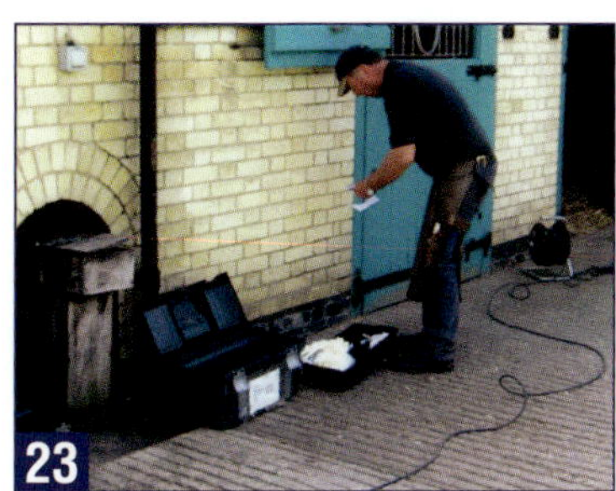

23 *Simon Curtis, FWCF, assembling equipment to apply extensions.*

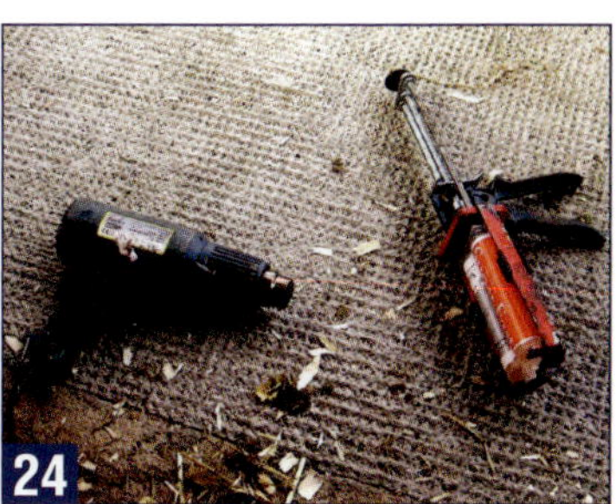

24 *Heat gun and loaded Super Fast in the applicator.*

the product just didn't work for me. First, he asked if I had read the directions. I said, "Of course … not." He asked how I was preparing the foot, and that part was fine. He asked how I was applying the polyurethane Super Fast, and here was the problem. Since I was trying to be cheap and not use any extra material, I had been applying the material, then feathering out the material with the plastic bag it came in. As I feathered it out, it became too thin to cure. The material has to be at least 1/8-inch thick to generate enough heat to cure properly. Who would ever have thought that little piece of information would be in the instructions? The thicker it gets, the hotter it gets. You need to be aware of that when using it over a crack or other potentially thin area. If the crack is deep, you can put a piece of wool felt in it to allow drainage, wick in medication, as well as provide a heat shield.

Extensions are often made from just the product, although it is not uncommon to glue on a piece of aluminum or other material to create a longer and stronger extension. In **Figures 17 and 18**, you can see the extensions that Simon Curtis glued on an expensive racehorse foal. In **Figures 19-21,** you can see the Sound Horse Technologies glue-on system being applied as a toe extension.

Since I don't do too much with hoof builders and extensions in my practice, it was great to spend some time with Simon Curtis, FWCF, who does a lot with them. Simon works on some of the best racehorses in Newmarket, England, and a large part of his business is taking care of foals and applying extensions. The primary product that he used while I was with him was Vettec Super Fast **(Figure 22)**.

Here is basically how this is done. Begin by trimming the foot so that there is new and clean tissue. Assemble all of the materials you will need. You should have the Super Fast in the applicator, heat gun, foam pad, tongue depressor, latex gloves, and an old rasp ready to go **(Figures 23 and 24)**. Prep the foot by trimming the side that you want to have the extension on. It is important to dress the outside wall of the foot as well **(Figures 25-27)**. Heat the foot **(Figure 28)** and apply some Super Fast to the bottom of the foot on the side you want the extension **(Figures 29 and 30)**. Put the foam pad over the Super Fast on the bottom of the foot **(Figure 31)**. The foam board should extend slightly further out than you want the extension to be. Pull the foot forward to put Super Fast up the side of the wall and

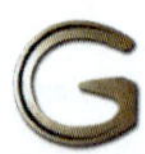

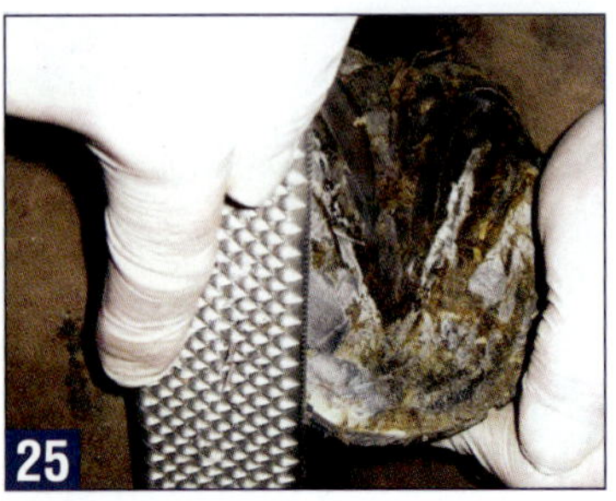

Trimming the foot.

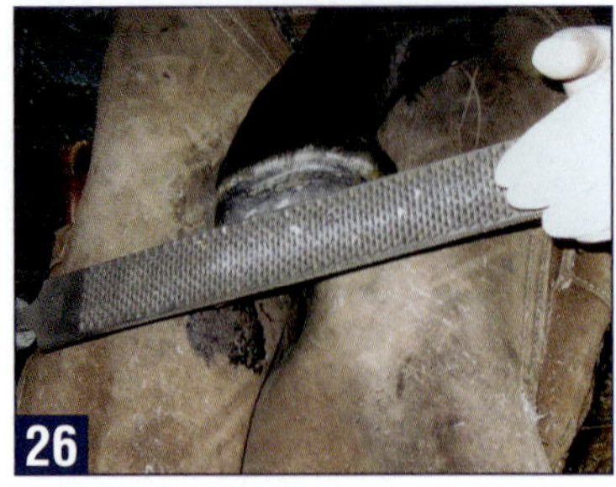

Dressing the foot.

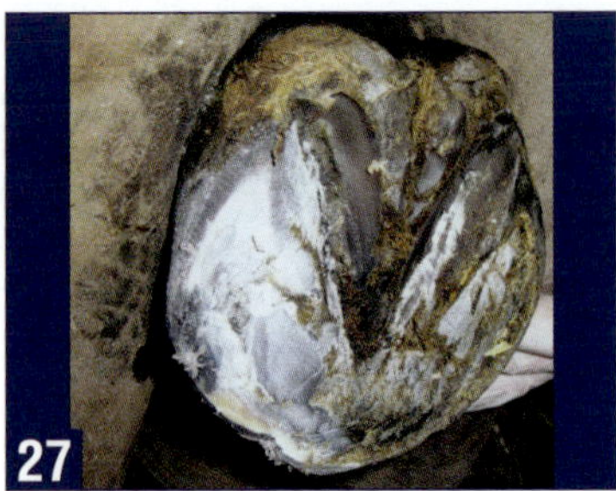

Foot ready for an extension.

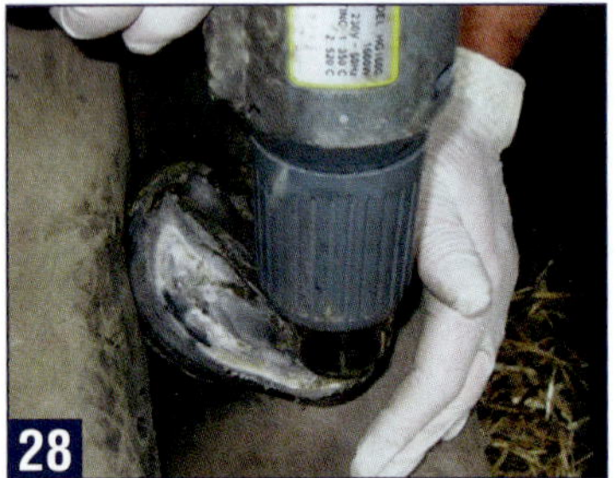

Heating up the foot.

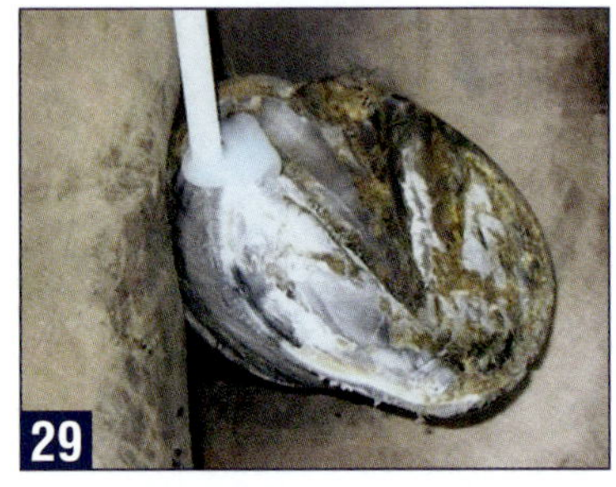

Applying Super Fast to the bottom of the foot.

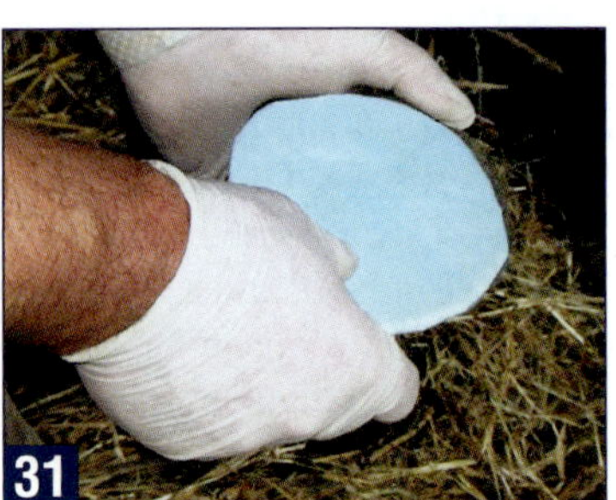

Placing the pre-cut foam pad on the foot.

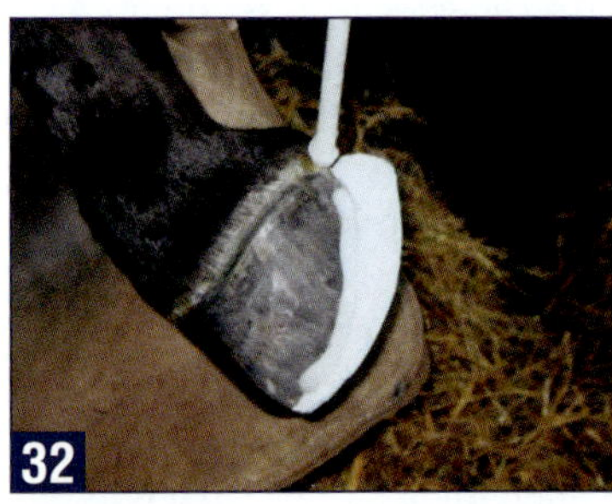

Pulling the foot forward to place Super Fast on the outside wall.

on top of the foam board **(Figures 32-35)**. Simon does this with only one mixing tip, but he has a lot of experience that allows him to be super fast with the Super Fast. There is no problem with having to use two, other than the expense of the extra tip and material.

As the Super Fast is curing, take a tongue depressor and smooth the outside of the extension **(Figures 36 and 37)**. You have to be fairly quick about this since the Super Fast can become too hard to spread in 60 seconds (thus the name, Super Fast). Do not feather it too thin at the end of the extension since it will not generate enough heat to cure properly. When you are done with this step, the extension should look like the one in **Figure 38**.

Allow the Super Fast to cure before setting the foot down. This should be at least 2 minutes. If you set it down too soon, you may break the bond as well as change the shape and position, so time it with your watch to maintain your patience. Once you set the foot down, it is ideal if you can give the Super Fast a few more minutes to cure before moving the horse on hard ground. Once it does, you can remove the foam pad and rasp to shape. It should look like the extension in **Figure 39**. You might also want to add a couple of grooves across the hardened ground surface to allow for a little traction.

On a trip to South Africa, I was lucky enough to spend a few days shoeing with Robbie Miller, CF. Like Simon Curtis, Robbie does a lot of racehorses and their babies. He uses Equilox and fiberglass fibers. His method is very close to Simon's, but the

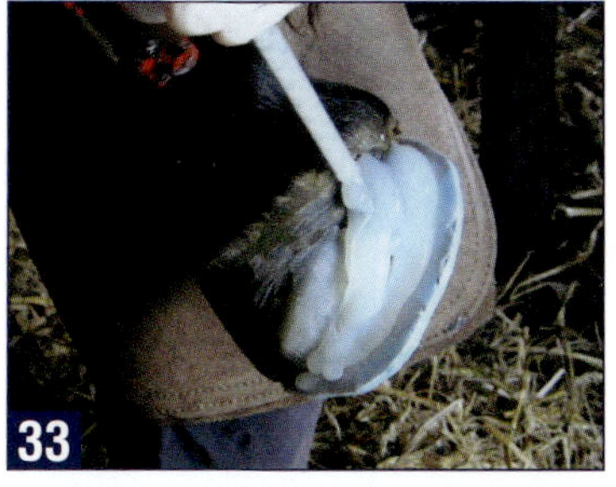

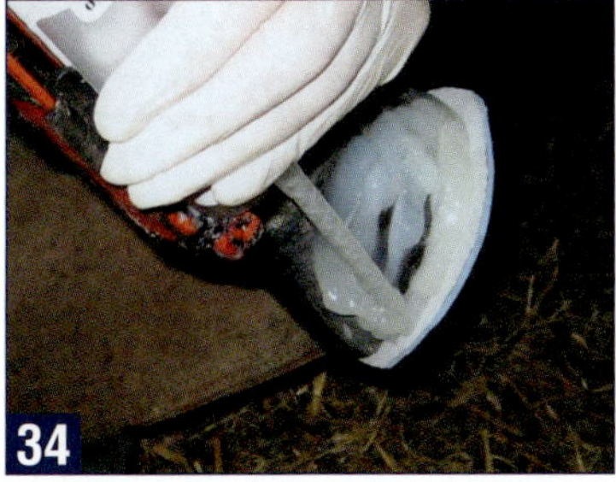

Building up the extension on the outside wall.

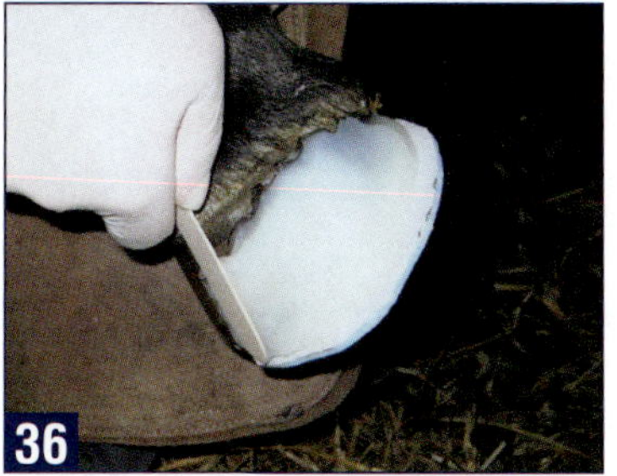

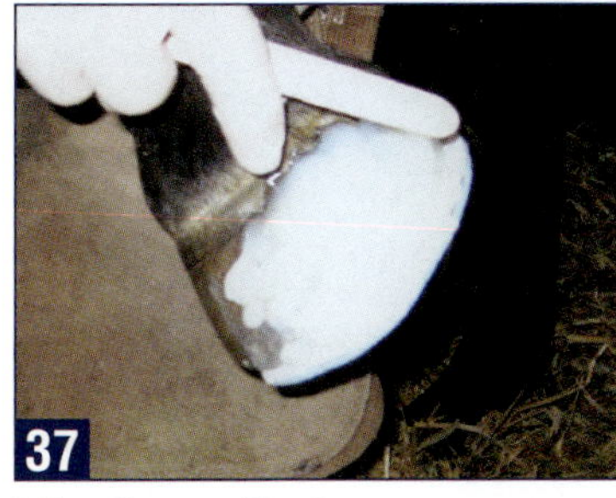

Using a tongue depressor to sculpt the Super Fast.

Allowing the extension to cure.

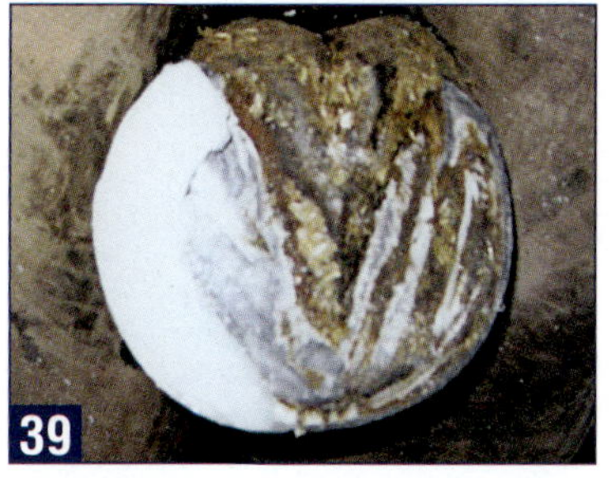

Finished extension from a solar view.

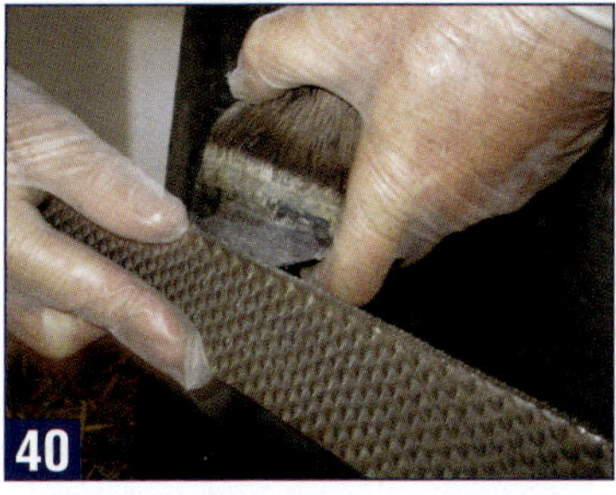

Robbie trimming a foot on a foal.

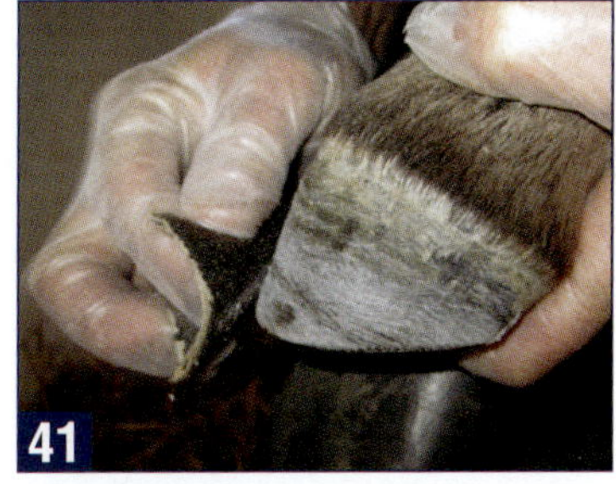

Sanding the foot with coarse sandpaper.

differences are worth mentioning.

Begin by prepping the foot so that there is good clean tissue to work with. Beyond just trimming, Robbie uses a coarse sandpaper to really clean the foot and give it an extra amount of tooth for the Equilox to stick to **(Figures 40 and 41)**. With the foot prepped, he puts a diaper on it to keep it clean and free of any contaminants **(Figure 42)**.

Figure 43 is the tray of all the

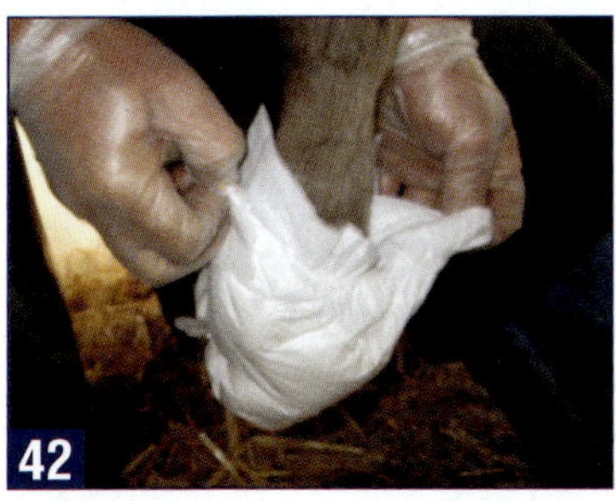

Placing a diaper on the foot to keep it clean.

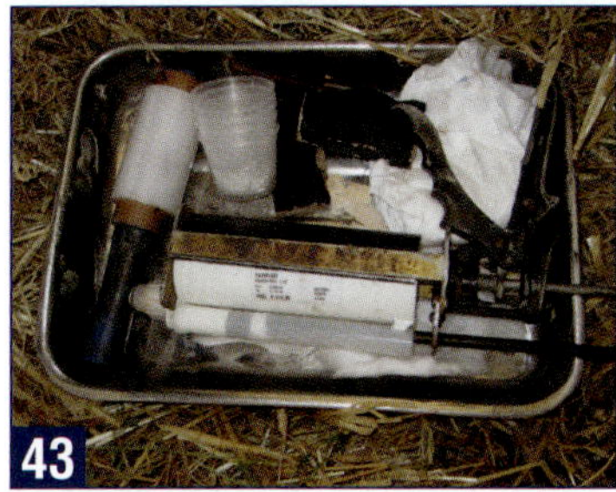

A tray full of the items that Robbie uses to make his foal extensions.

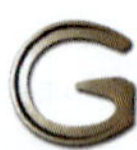

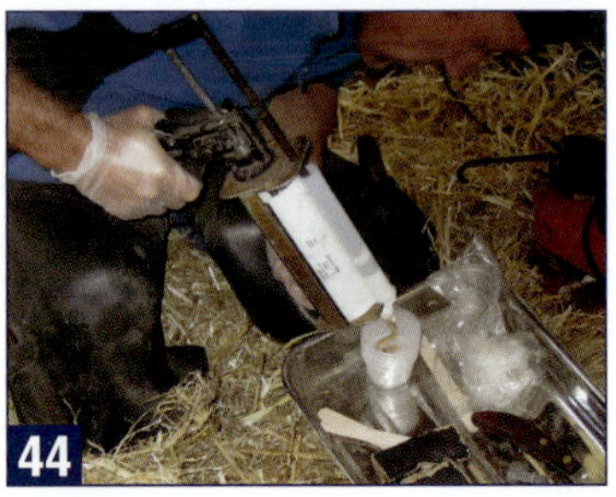

Filling a mixing cup with Equilox.

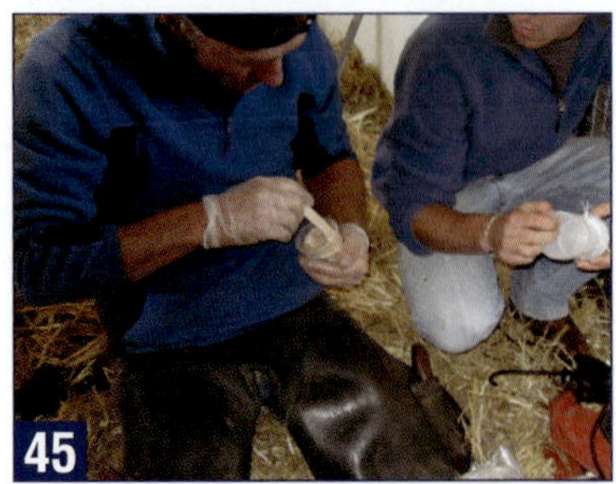

Robbie is mixing the Equilox while Calven adds fiberglass fibers.

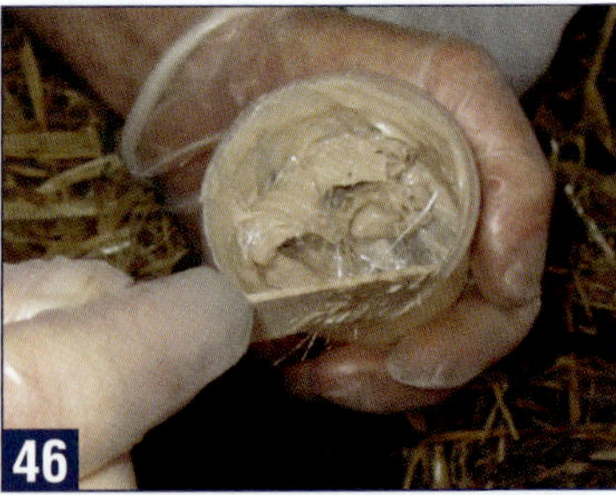

Mixing the material and waiting for it to get to the correct consistency.

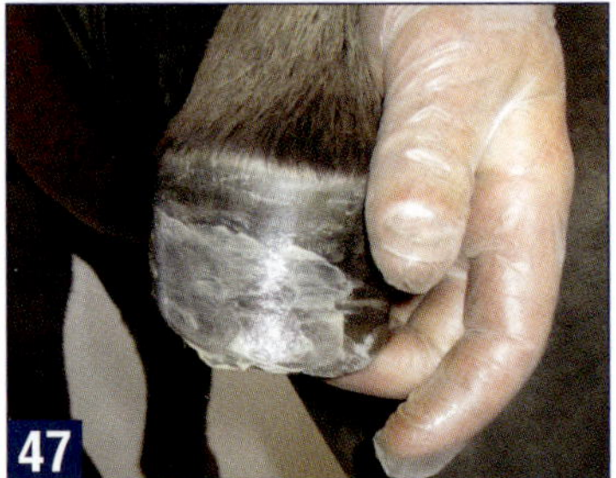

Thin layer of Equilox on the foot, called "buttering".

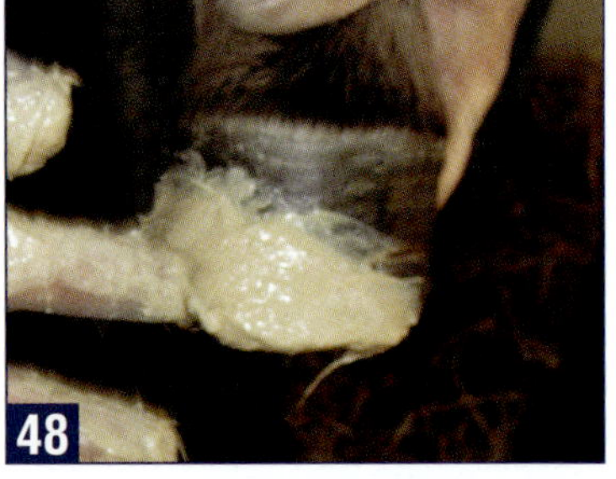

Applying the Equilox to the foot.

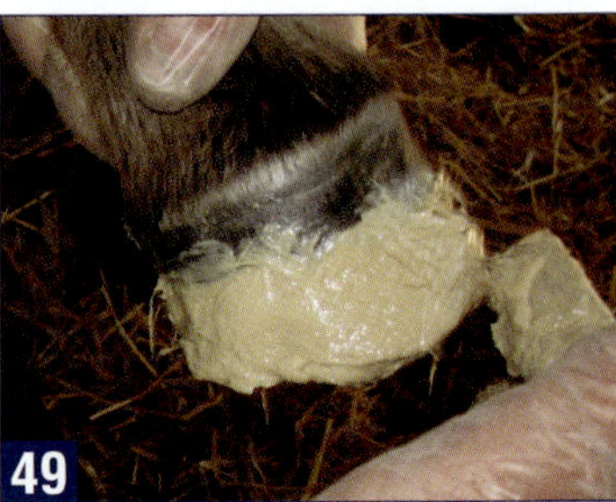

Shaping the Equilox extension.

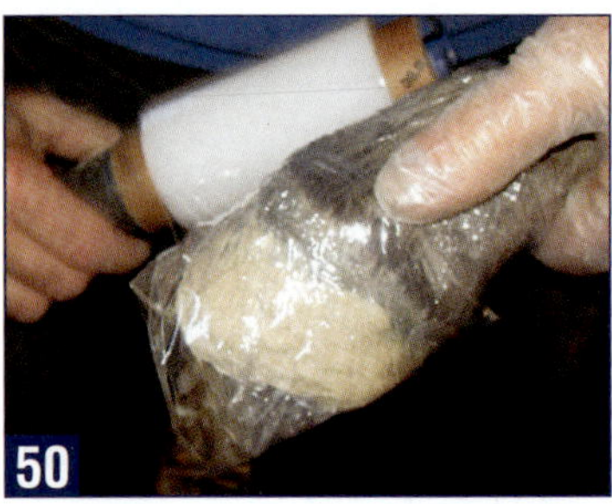

Wrapping the foot and extension in plastic wrap.

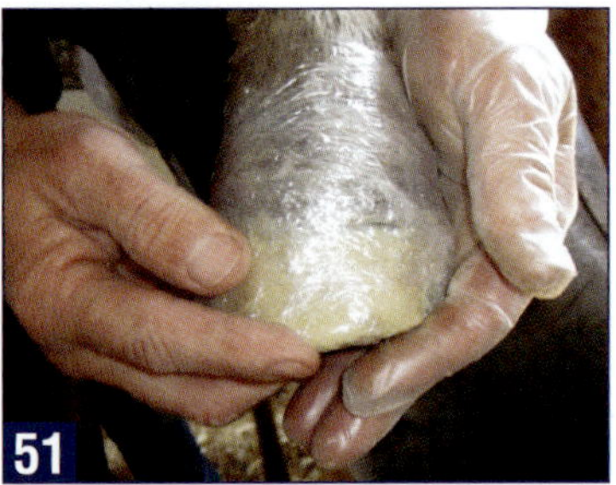

Shaping the extension through the plastic wrap and feeling to see when it gets hot.

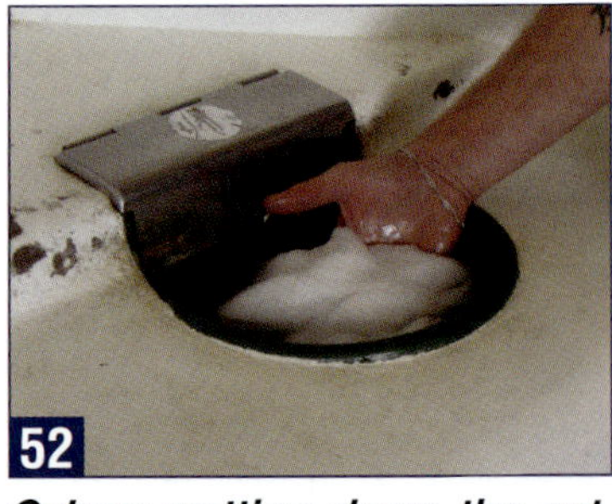

Calven wetting down the cotton batting.

items that he needs for the extension. He fills a mixing cup with the amount of Equilox that he will need **(Figure 44)** and then mixes it with a tongue depressor while his son, Calven, adds fiberglass fibers **(Figures 45 and 46)**. When the Equilox feels right to him (about a minute if you want to time it), he puts a thin layer of material on the foot **(Figure 47)** called 'buttering." Next, he applies the majority of the mixed Equilox to the foot in the area that he wants to have the extension **(Figures 48 and 49)**. Once it is close to the desired shape, he will wrap the foot and extension in plastic wrap **(Figure 50)**, and do some final shaping of the extension through the plastic **(Figure 51)**.

Robbie is careful to keep his hand on the acrylic as it cures so that he can tell what temperature it is at. When it begins to get hot, Calven wets down some cotton batting **(Figure 52)**, and Robbie places that on the extension so that the foot does not get too hot **(Figure 53)**.

Several minutes later, the extension is cured and unwrapped **(Figure 54)**. Robbie trims and shapes the extension as if it were a foot **(Figures 55 and 56)**, and the horse now has the support in the area

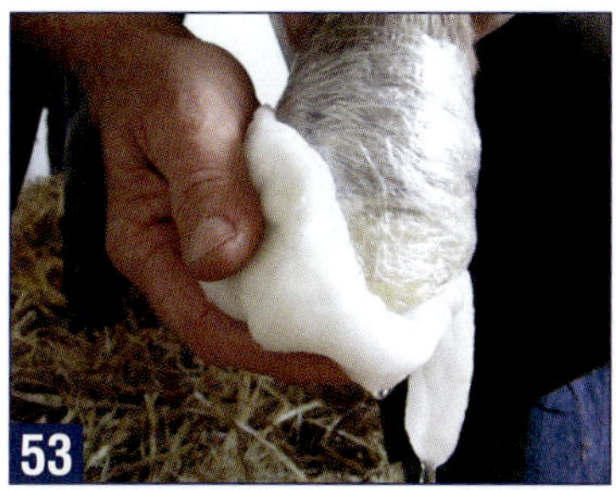
Applying the wet cotton to the extension to cool it down.

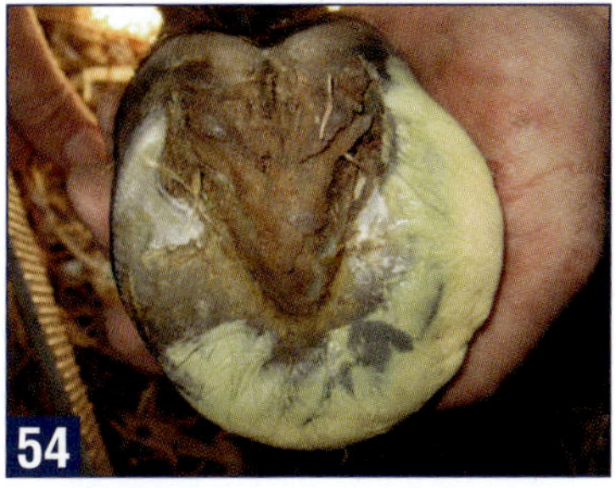
The extension, cured and unwrapped, ready to trim.

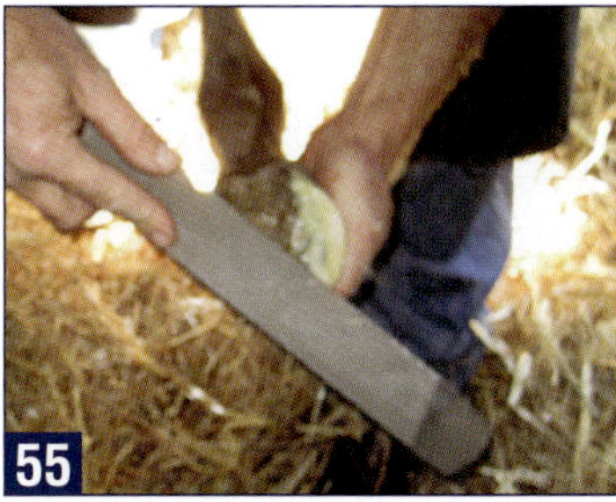
Shaping the extension with a rasp.

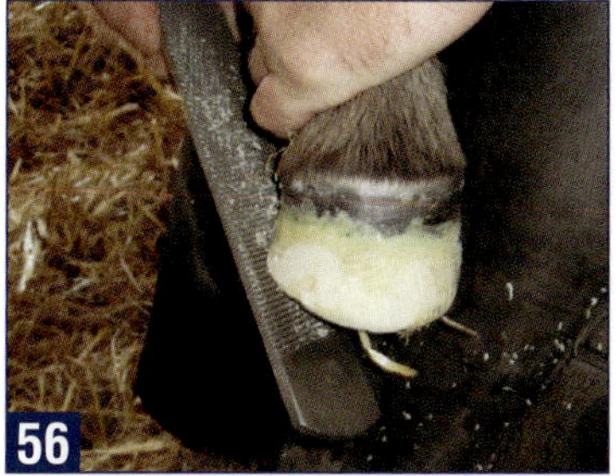
Shaping the extension with a rasp.

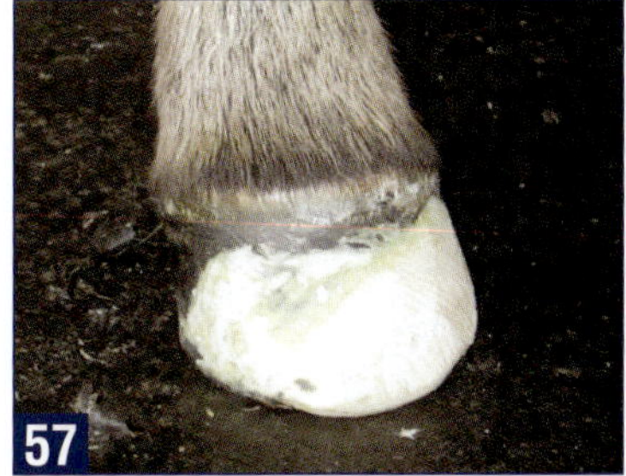
Finished extension.

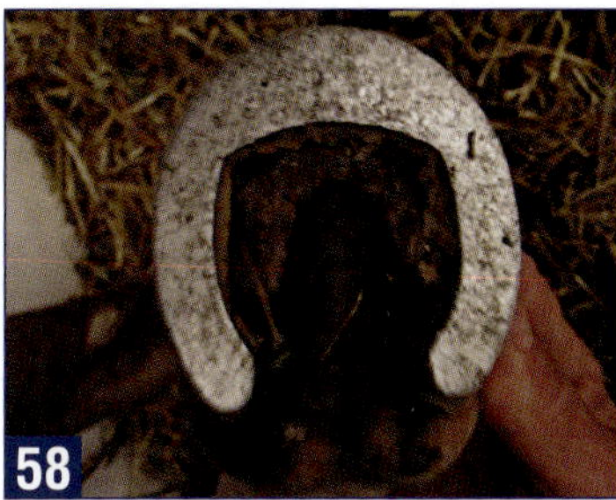
Aluminum shoe glued on a foot.

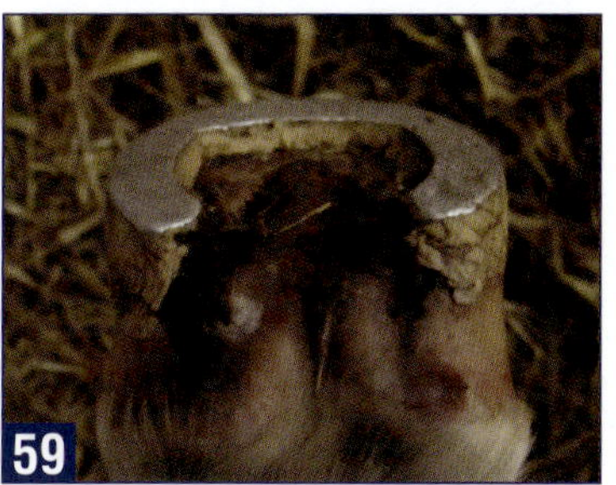
Aluminum shoe glued on a foot.

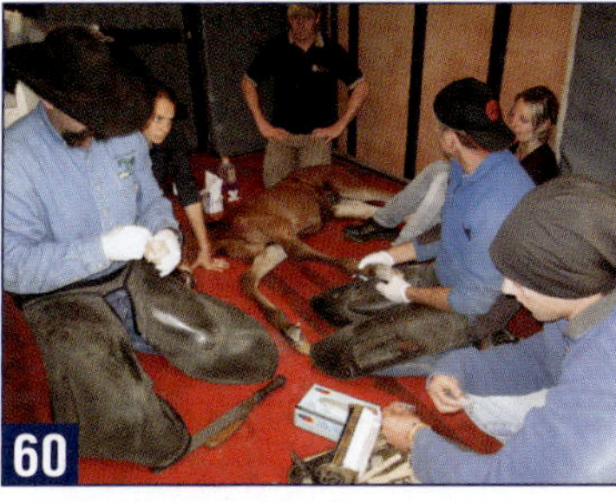
Robbie and I at Drakenstien Vet Clinic, working on a foal.

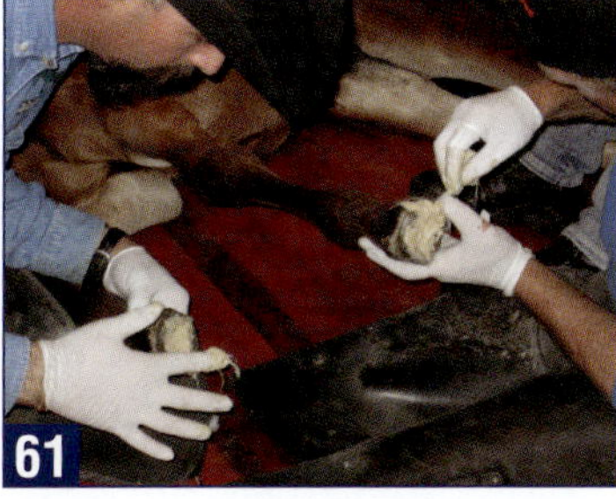
Applying extensions to the foal.

where it was needed **(Figure 57)**.

In **Figures 58 and 59,** you can see a small aluminum shoe that Robbie had glued to a foot to get the bearing surface he wanted on a foot that was too small to nail to. We did a lot of extensions that day, and we finished up with a foal at a vet clinic where Robbie and I both put on some extensions **(Figures 60-62)**.

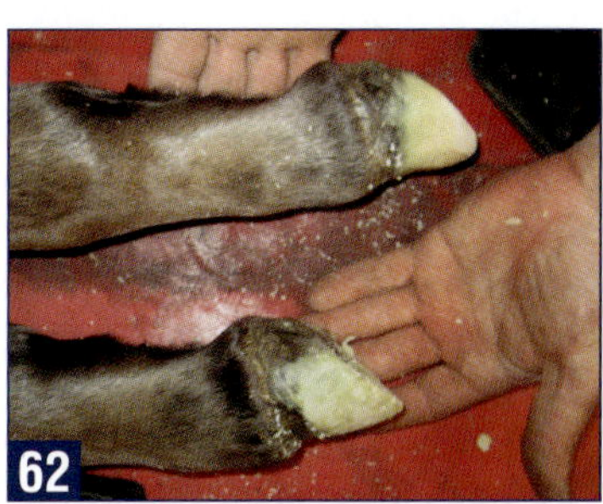
The extensions on the foal.

GLUE-ON SHOES

When it comes to gluing shoes on feet, the best results I have had were with Sigafoos shoes. These

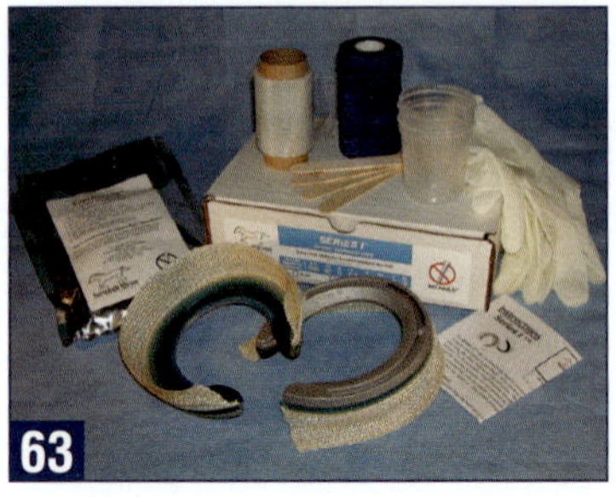

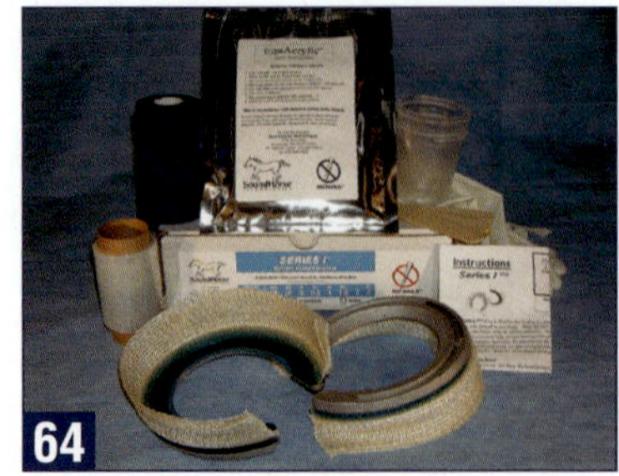

63 64

Sound Horse Sigafoos Shoe Sytem

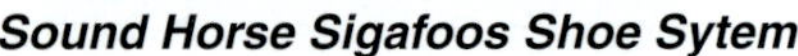

65

Front Sound Horse Sigafoos Shoes.

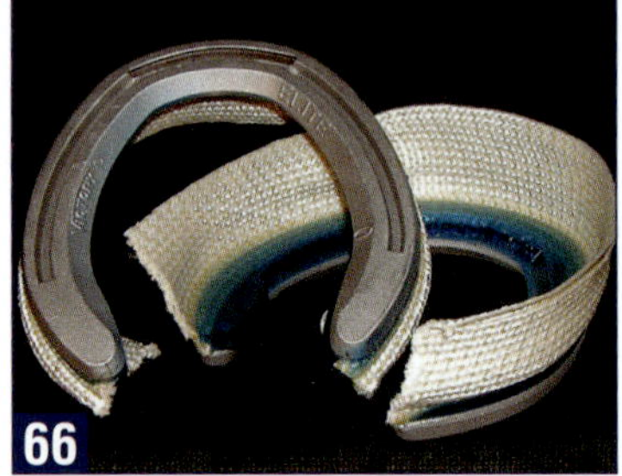

66

Hind Sound Horse Sigafoos Shoes.

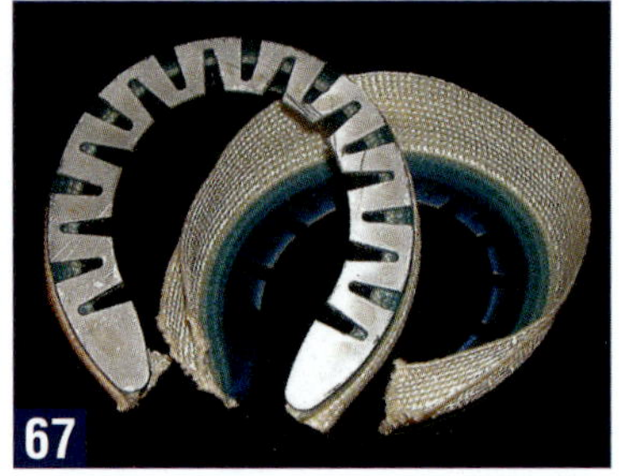

67

Another Sound Horse design product – Series III universal cuff.

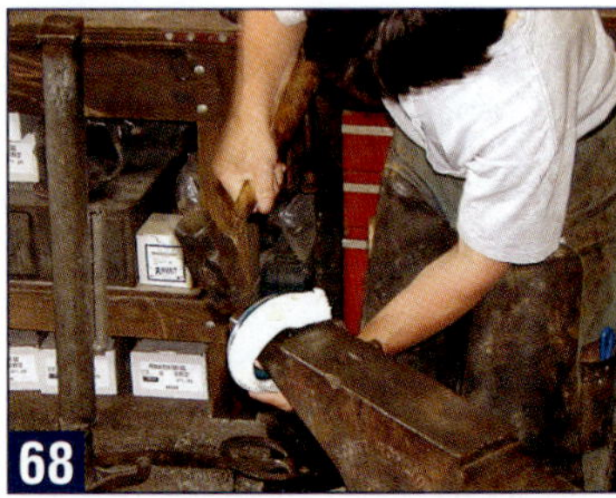

68

Cold shaping a Sound Horse Sigafoos shoe (forged aluminum).

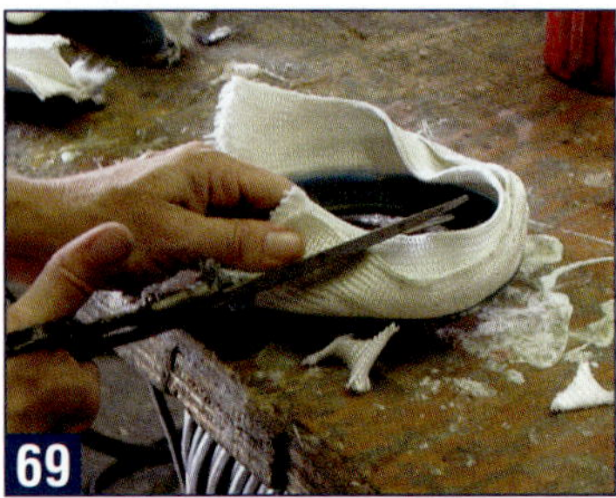

69

Trimming the fabric (Polyester – Vectran braided material).

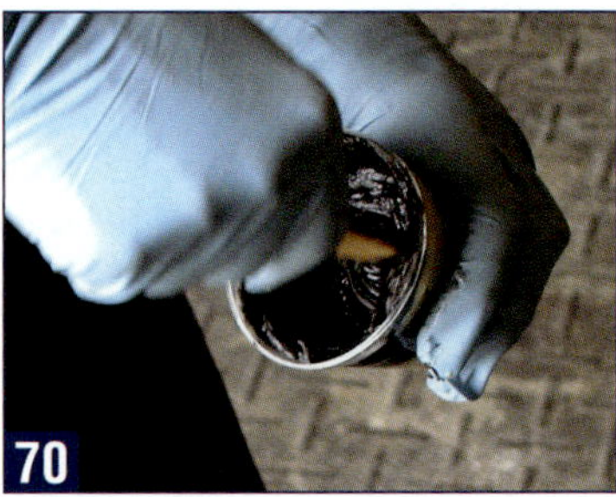

70

Mixing the Equilox (acrylic adhesive).

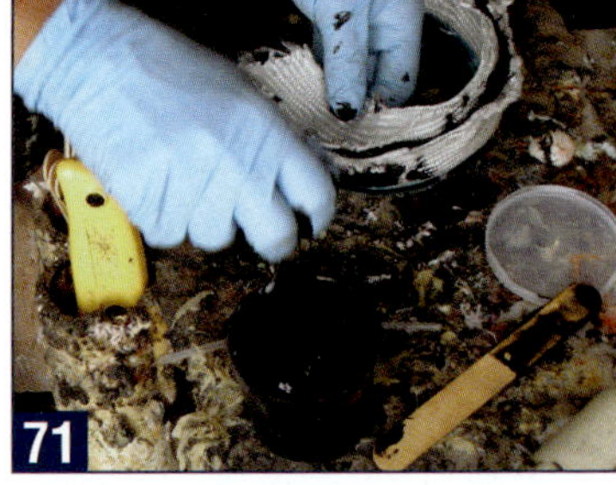

71

Working the Equilox into the Sound Horse fabric cuff.

are the invention of Rob Sigafoos, CJF, and they are a pretty brilliant method. **Figures 63 and 64** are of the Sound Horse Sigafoos Shoe Systems that come in kit form with a pair of shoes. Sigafoos shoes are an aluminum shoe with an attached fabric cuff made of a polyester braid called Vectran. These polymer fibers are much stronger than fiberglass and provide excellent resistance to abrasion **(Figures 65-67)**. The braided fabric is what is actually glued to the side of the hoof wall. These shoes are glued on with commercial acrylics, so you will be using a product with a mechanical bond instead of a chemical one.

The ones that you will come across for farriery are Equilox, Equibond, EquAcrylic, or Victory Hoof Life. It is important to note that the bond between the foot and the fabric has been proven stronger than 8 nails in some laboratory testing, and these shoes do stay on for a long time.

Begin by prepping the feet and cleaning them well. Shape the Sigafoos shoe to fit the foot a little full **(Figure 68)**. Trim the fabric with some good scissors so that it does not interfere with the coronary band at the heel **(Figure 69)**.

Mix the Equilox provided for at least a minute

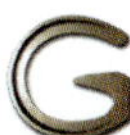

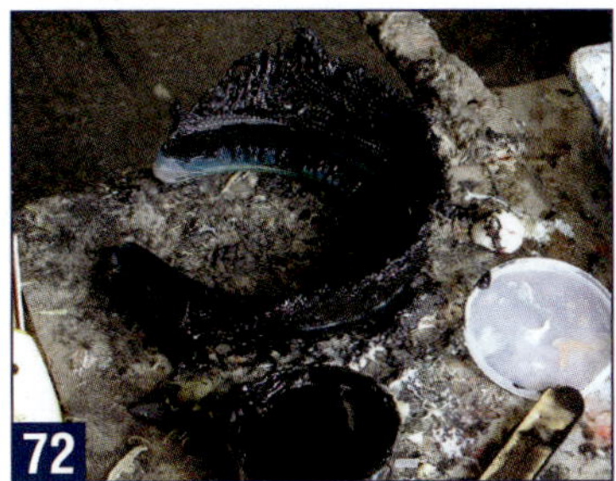

Sound Horse shoe ready to be applied.

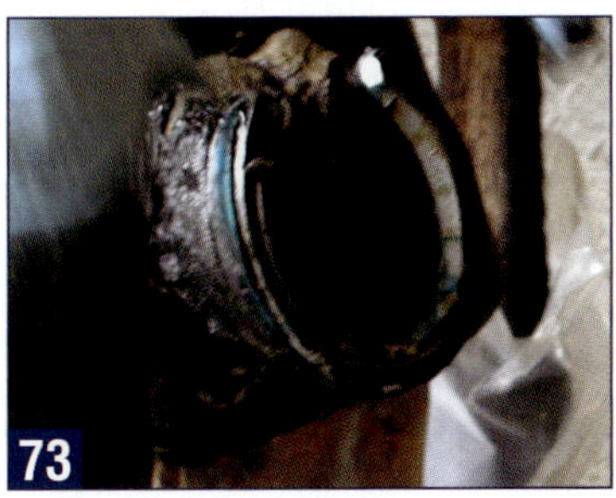

Placing the Sound Horse shoe on the foot.

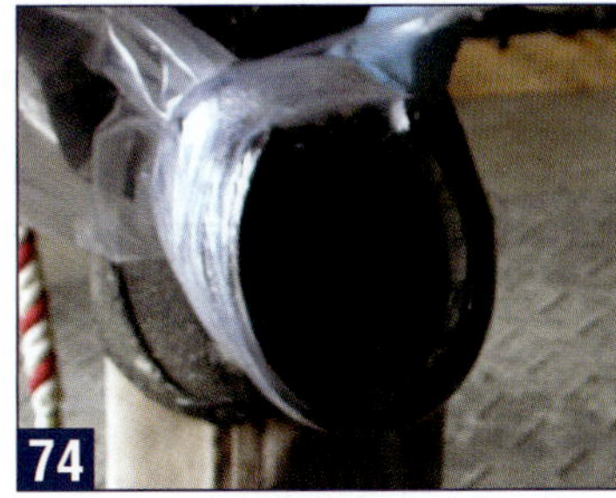

Wrapping the shoe and foot in stretch wrap.

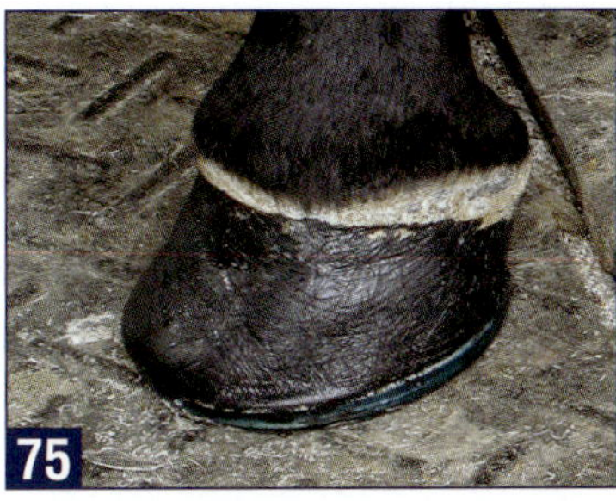

Finished foot from the lateral view (Sound Horse shoe).

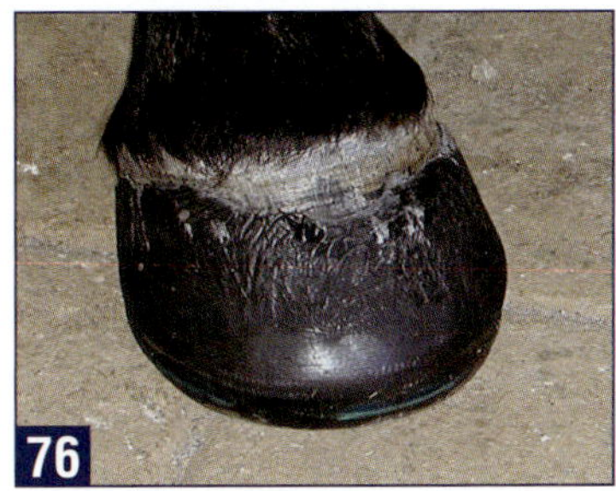

Finished foot from the dorsal view (Sound Horse shoe).

(Figure 70) and work it into the fabric on the shoe **(Figures 71 and 72)**. You should apply a layer of the Equilox to the foot, then slip the shoe on. Note that there is not fabric on the bottom on the hoof **(Figure 73)**. Wrap the whole thing in the plastic wrap provided with the kit, and set the foot carefully on the ground **(Figure 74)**. Once it cures, you will have a shoe glued on the foot for a long time **(Figures 75 and 76)**. The second one of these that I put on actually stayed on the foot for more than four months. Not really what you want to have happen, but it is a good example of the strength of the product.

When I was first introduced to the Sigafoos shoe, Bill Kirkpatrick gave me a pair at a clinic to take home and try. The glue would not cure for me, so I called and explained that there was a problem with the product. He asked if I had read the directions, to which I replied, "Of course … not." The glue has to be mixed for a full minute if you don't use Equilox in a tube with a mixing tip. He told me that an average minute to a farrier is actually only 17 to 29 seconds. When he graciously sent me another pair, sure enough, at 17 seconds of mixing, I thought a minute had passed. I should have had Kelly time the first attempt.

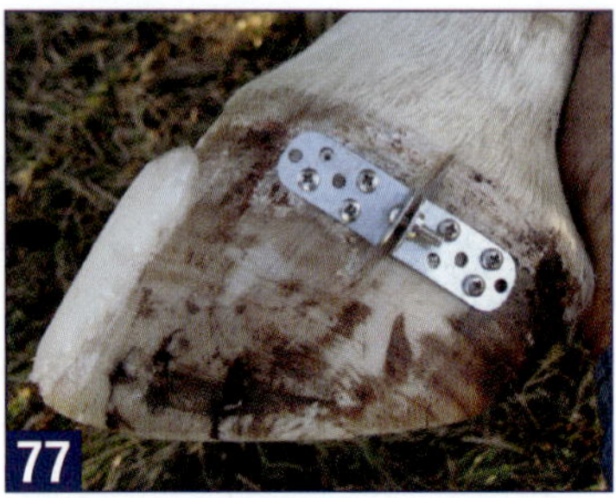

Quarter-crack repair system.

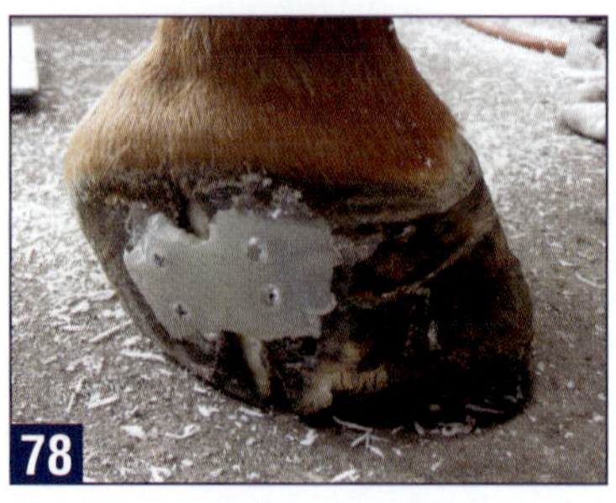

Quarter-crack repaired with screws and Super Fast.

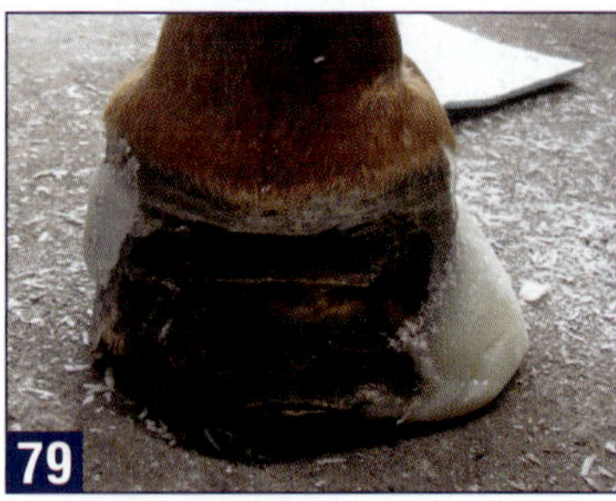

Lateral extension.

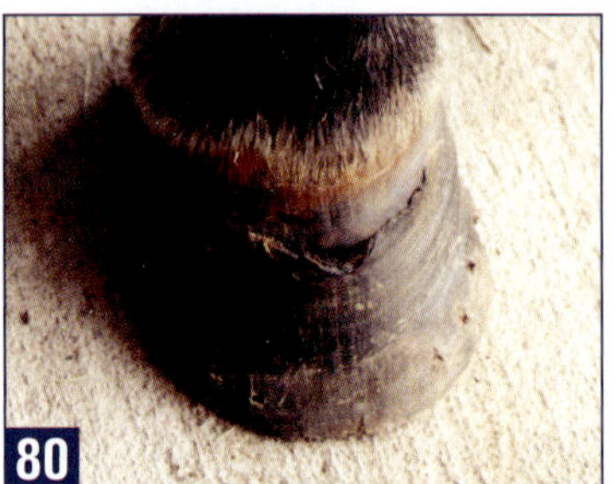

Dorsal Cleft.

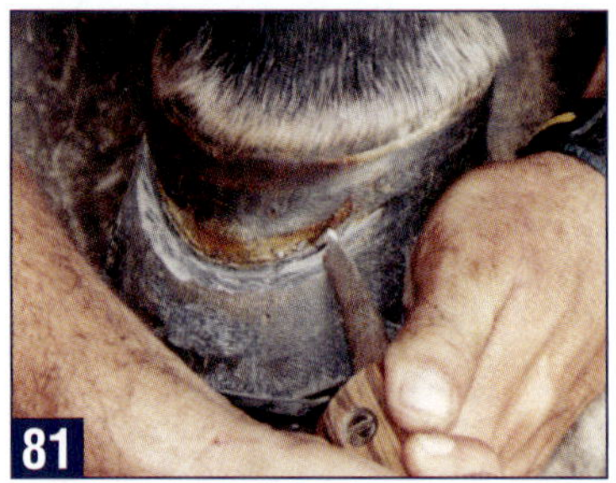

Cleaning up the cleft to apply Super Fast to it.

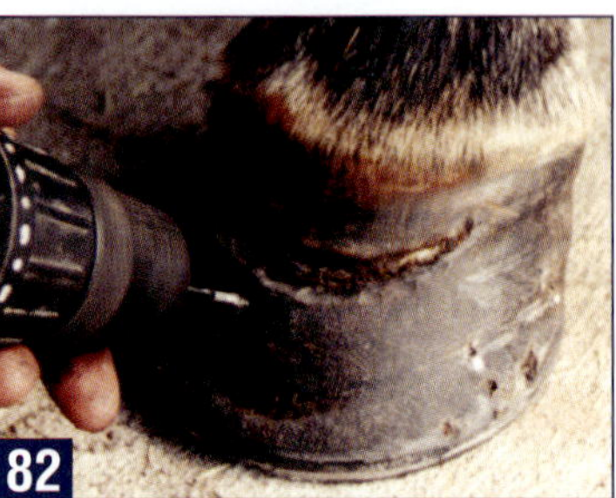

Drilling holes for screws.

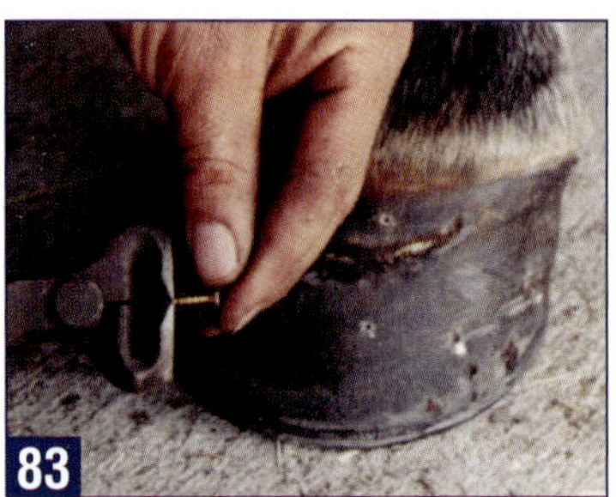

Preparing the screws to be placed in the foot.

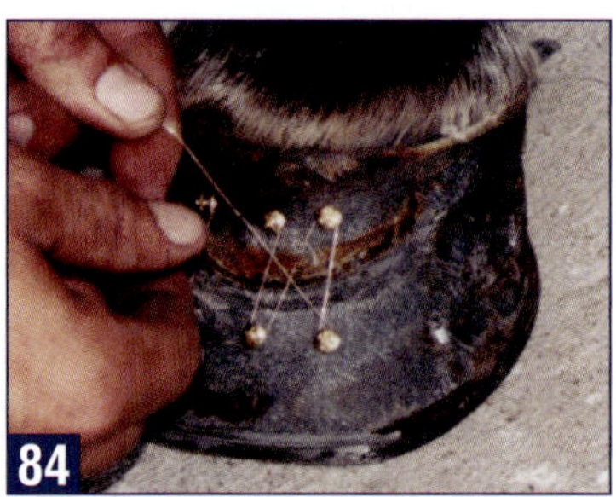

Putting wire on the screws in the foot.

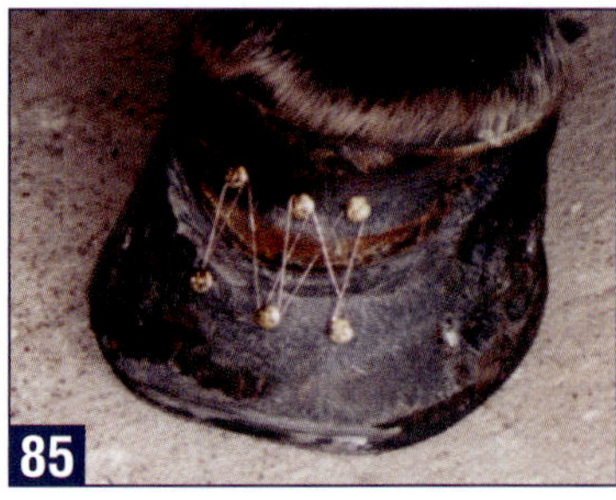

Foot ready to have the Super Fast applied.

CRACK REPAIR AND WALL STABILIZATION

The products mentioned can also be used to patch cracks in feet as well as strengthen the integrity of the hoof wall. When taking the AWCF Exam, there is a modern material component of the practical module during which a candidate is asked to apply some modern techniques to a foot. The task can be anything from a resection to a crack repair to finding a portion of the coffin bone from the sole in an abscess search. **Figures 77-79** are of some cadaver feet used as practice for the AWCF modern materials exam. You can see a couple of methods for fixing a quarter crac, as well as an extension made from Super Fast. It is important that a competent farrier be able to perform these tasks.

The horse in **Figures 80 and 81** had a bad cleft as the result of a large abscess breaking out of the coronary band a couple of months prior. There was enough movement in the wall that the horse was lame, so we decided to stabilize the crack. I began by drilling holes in the wall on either side of the crack **(Figure 82)**. There is tape on the drill bit to mark the depth that I want the drill bit to penetrate.

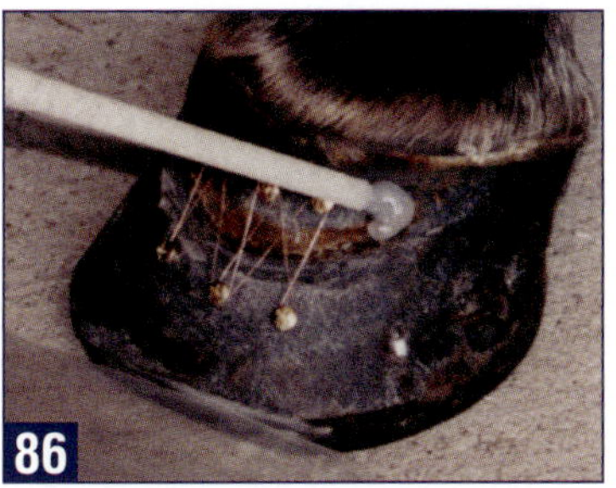
Putting the Super Fast on.

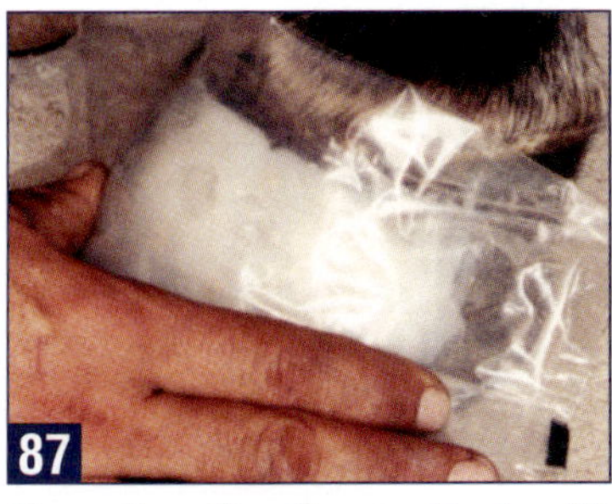
Covering the Super Fast with the bag it came in.

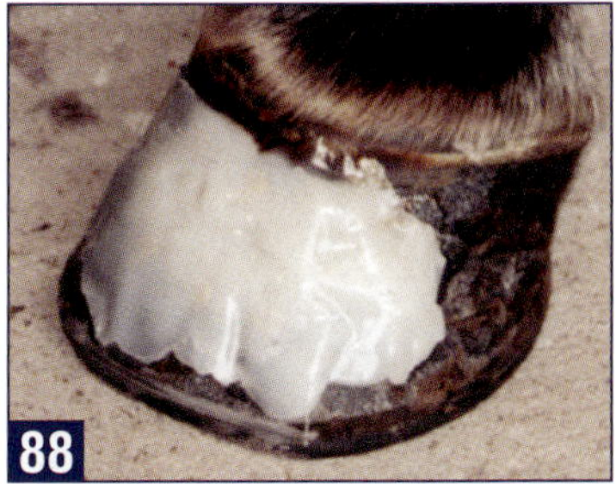
Once it is cured, remove the bag.

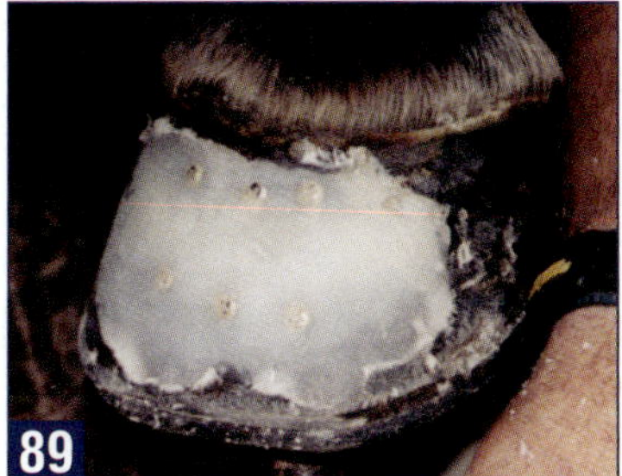
Dress the patch down to the screw heads.

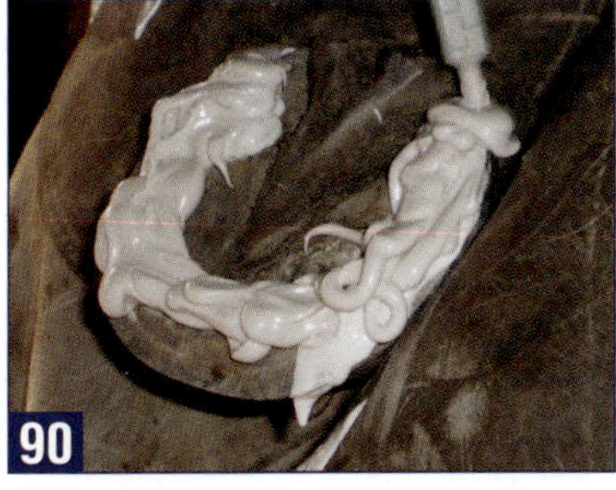
Applying an acrylic to the foot to glue on an egg bar.

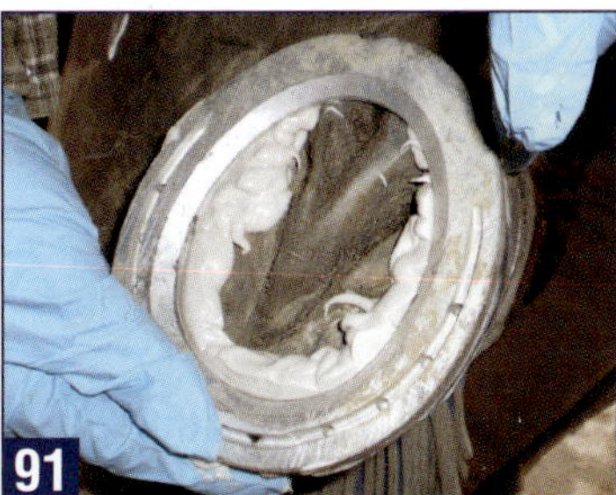
Placing the egg bar on the foot.

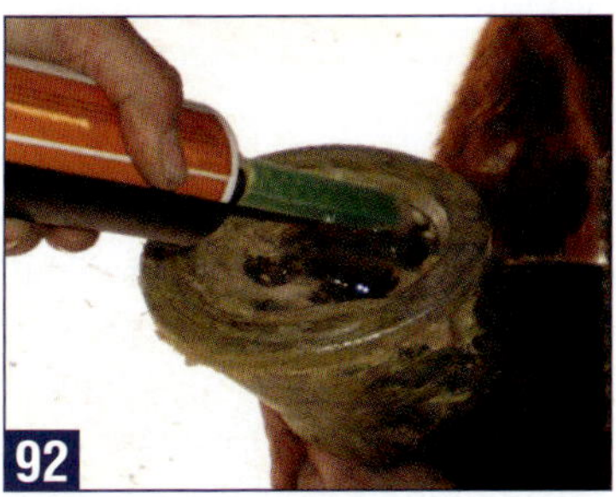
Filling the bottom of the shoe with a pour-in.

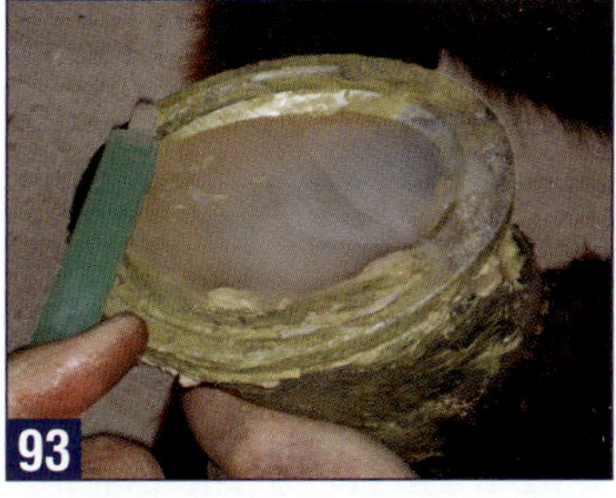
Egg bar glued to the foot with a pour-in pad.

I cut the tips off of some brass screws **(Figure 83)** and put them in the holes that I drilled. The next step is to wrap some wire around the screws to make a mesh that will help the Super Fast stay in place **(Figures 84 and 85)**. Liberally apply a thick coat of Super Fast **(Figure 86)** and use the inside of the bag that it came in to shape the Super Fast as it cures **(Figure 87)**. Be careful to avoid feathering it out on the ends. Once it is cured, remove the bag and let it stand for about 10 minutes **(Figure 88)**. The longer you can wait to finish, the better your finish will be. Eventually, you can rasp it until you just touch the heads of the screws **(Figure 89)**.

It is possible to glue ordinary shoes directly to the foot. In **Figure 90**, I am using an acrylic to bond a shoe to the foot. Begin by cleaning and drying the foot as you would for any of these applications. Apply a liberal amount of glue material **(Figure 91)** and press the shoe into the material. Allow the glue to cure, and use the heat gun if doing this in cool weather. As an added bonus to the horse, as well as an insurance policy to keep the shoe on, I am also applying a pour-in pad to the foot **(Figures 92 and 93)**. This particular horse was done as a product test for Mustad, so we were lax on all of the proper conditions so that the product could be tested against the worst scenarios. This shoe actually stayed on until I pulled it off about five weeks later. Needless to say, the acrylic used here was excellent.

I have used Super Fast to glue shoes on when there was no chance of a nail. In **Figure 94,** the

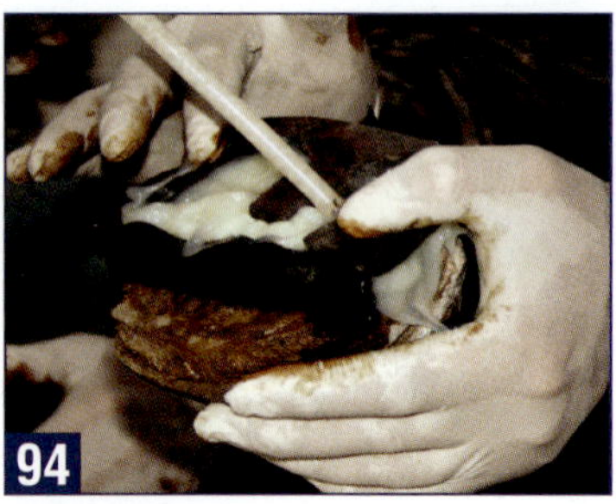
Gluing a w-shoe to a foot with Super Fast.

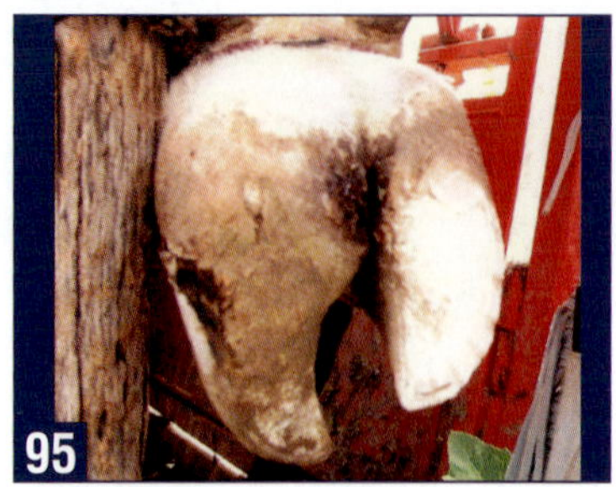
Trimmed claw next to the infected claw.

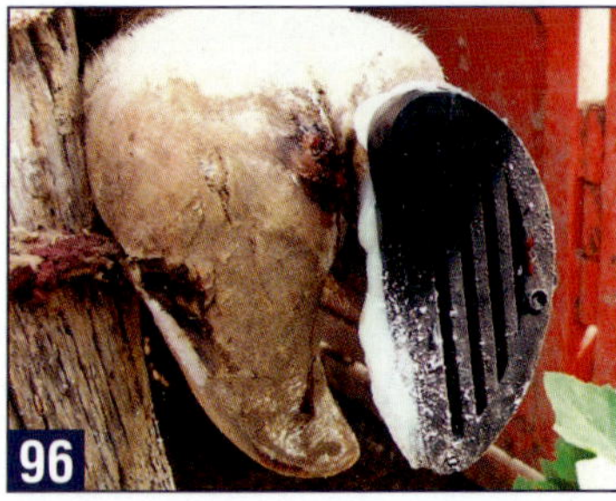
Shoe glued on to the good claw to allow the infected claw to heal.

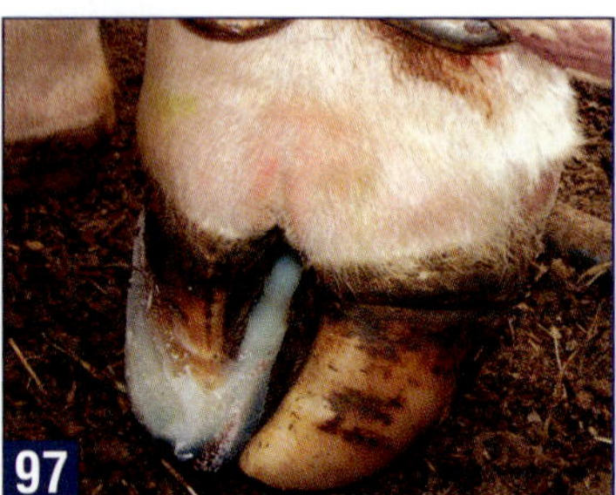
Dorsal view of finished job.

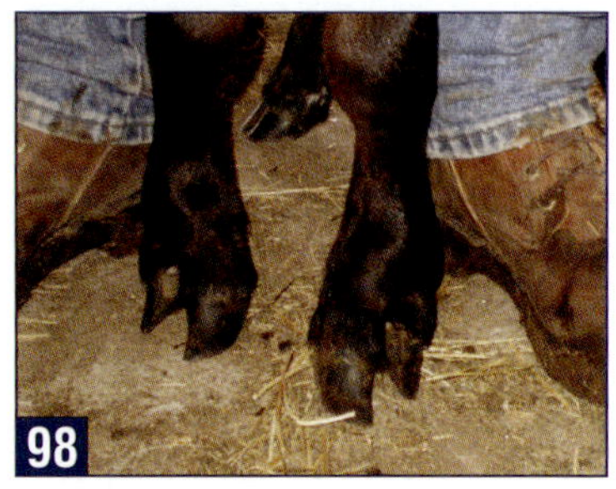
Calf with some bad conformational defects.

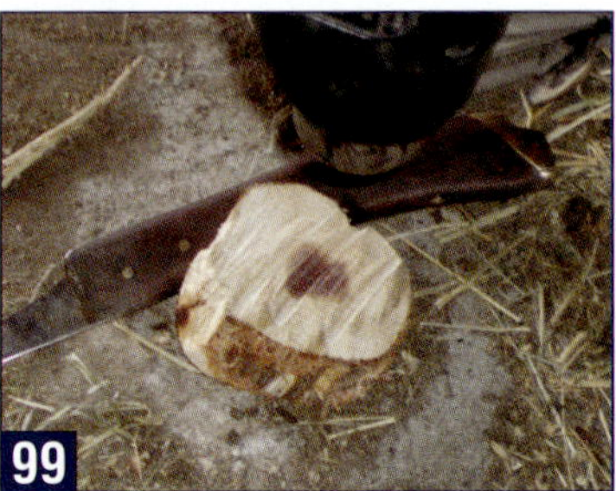
Heating the shoe made out of a cedar limb.

foot was broken away to the point that gluing on a shoe was the only chance of getting protection on the foot. Since I wanted to use a W-shoe as well, I simply made the shoe and glued it in place. It lasted for about six weeks, and we glued it on again. The main thing was that the horse was sound.

When you look at **Figure 94**, you will see that there is a lot of Super Fast all over the sole of the foot. That is not a recommended use of the product, since it can get so hard that it is like having a rock attached to the sole. Since this foot was so hard, so broken, and the horse lame, I was able to make an experienced judgment call that allowed me to use Super Fast here. You will gain that experience with time.

We have used Super Fast to glue shoes to cows on several occasions. In **Figure 95**, there is a bull that has an abscess in one claw. In order for it to heal, we glued a shoe to the opposite claw. The claw was cleaned well and heated with a heat gun. I applied the Super Fast and pressed a rubber shoe that was specifically made for that purpose onto the foot. You can see the results in **Figures 96 and 97**. The bull was able to walk better, allowing the infected claw to heal. After about a month, the shoe fell off and the bull was fine.

You can also use this product to glue corrective apparatuses on feet. In **Figure 98**, there is a very crooked-legged calf. I cut a piece of cedar at an angle, heated it up **(Figure 99)** and glued it to both claws **(Figures 100-102)**. To speed the cure time, we heated the glued-on shoe with a heat gun **(Figure 103)**. You can see the finished product in **Figure 104**. This allowed the animal to bear weight in such a way that the leg could grow straighter.

There are a lot of ways to use the different hoof builders, pour-ins and glues. You can use them to stabilize cracks, to attach shoes and other apparatuses, make the builder into a shoe of sorts on its own, and cushion the foot. I have found that all of these items have their place in shoeing horses, but please, don't let product replace skill. Learn to build any shoe for any foot, and you will be a long way ahead of the game. Put the use of modern materials on the list of things that you can do instead of the only thing that you can do.

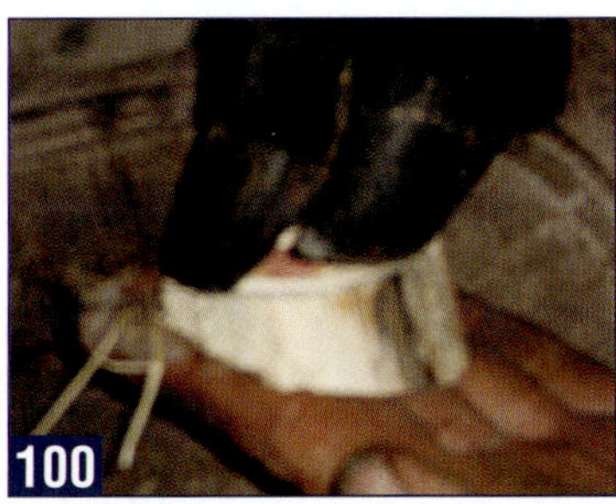

Placement of the wooden shoe on the foot.

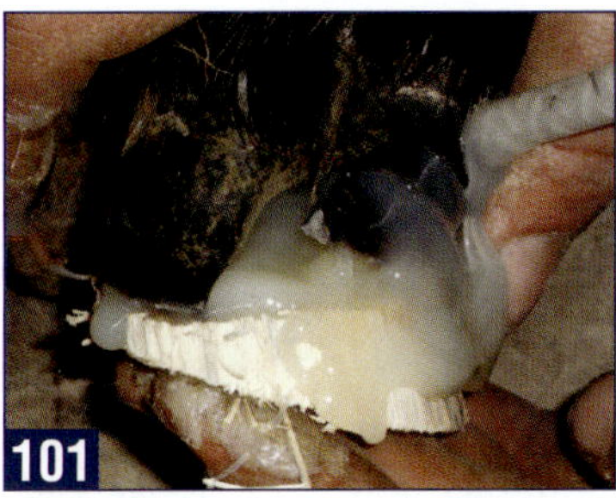

Gluing the shoe in position.

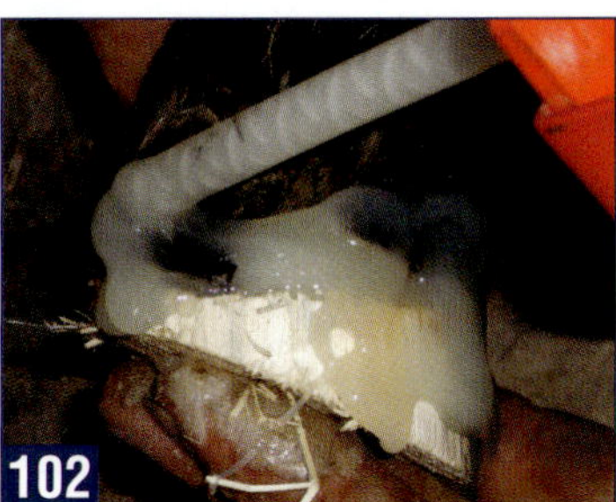

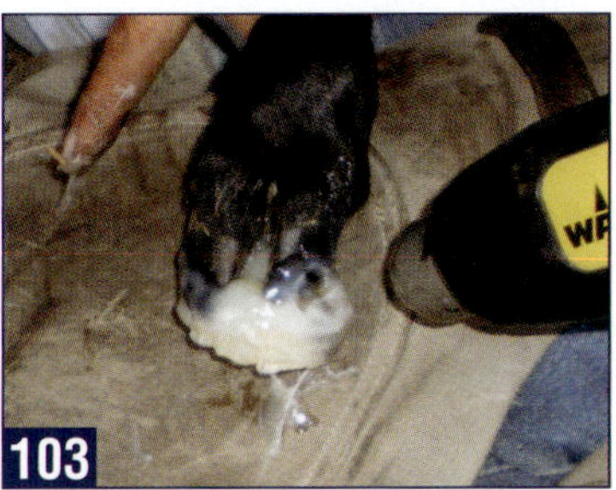

Heating the glue and shoe to cure.

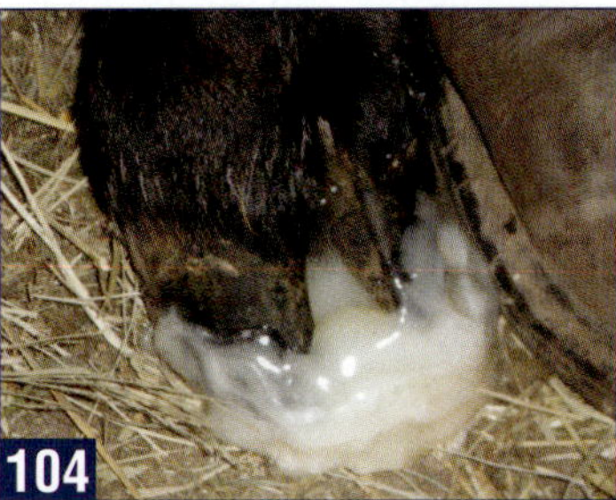

Finished job.

Chapter

33 BAD SHOEING

I have looked through many textbooks on the art of farriery, and it is rare to see anything written on bad shoeing. This makes sense, as you don't want to teach bad shoeing. However, through many years of teaching, I have found that you can teach a tremendous amount by looking at what is done wrong. For instance, if I happen to have a bad day at a clinic and miss my clip fit or have a sprung heel, the farriers that attended that clinic will remember those things that I did wrong better than what I did right — especially when I point out my mistake to them. They still learned. In fact, they probably learn even more, due to simple human nature. They learn what not to do.

This chapter is about that: What not to do. These are examples of some of the terrible things that are done to horses' feet out of ignorance. At least I hope it is out of ignorance. Ignorance can be fixed. An uncaring attitude of disregard and negligence, well, that can be harder to fix.

I've been running shoeing schools since 1992. That has given me the opportunity to see a lot of really bad shoeing. Some of the horses that we get to see at the school have been shod by folks who should not be shoeing horses. This has provided many learning opportunities, and I'm going to share some of those here.

Are you familiar with the term slipshod? If you look it up in the dictionary, you will find descriptions like negligent, shoddy, careless, and sloppy. Where do you think a term like that came from? It came from the word "shoe" and the word "slip;" directly from the world of farriery. Slipshod describes untidy work. It's not a word that you would ever want aimed at you or your shoeing.

The horse's foot is a remarkable structure, as we have already established. It can take a tremendous amount of abuse and still continue to function. I have seen shoeing that leaves me amazed to see the horse still walking. These are the sorts of things that make you get your camera out, while trying your best to keep the horse owner from knowing why you are taking pictures. Yet, often these horses are stoic. They refuse to limp.

Kelly and I have developed a theory over the years. I have heard it said that "God takes care of children and idiots," and the fact that some of the shoeing we see does not end up crippling a horse; well, it has to be the hand of God. If you do something to a horse that you know is bad and should make a horse sore, then you are going to have a lame horse. Sounds simple, right?

Here's the peculiar part. If someone who didn't know any better did that exact same thing to a horse, they often get away with it. Not always, but it is astounding how often we see things that just cannot be done to a horse without laming it, yet here that horse stands. Hand of God.

So far in this book, we have concentrated on what I consider to be good shoeing and sound shoeing principles. So we have in our mind what a good job consists of, and what it looks like. In summary, a good job will be:

- Sound horse
- Straight tubular horn
- Symmetrical
- Level
- Heels covered
- Good wall contact with the shoe
- No sole pressure
- Shoe shaped so nail holes are over the white line
- Straight, high clinches
- Balanced to achieve a straight hoof pastern axis (HPA)
- Clean and smooth finish
- Short, smooth, square clinches

These are most of the basic elements of a good shoeing job.

It is true that if you get 11 shoers and one horse together in a shop, there will be 12 opinions on what should be done. This is not a good thing for the farrier industry. With so many theories, ideas, methods, and opinions, a lot of bad is done to horses because of the blind leading the blind. For your part, take every decision on shoeing back to anatomy, and

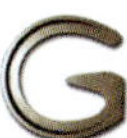

you will have your answer for what to do to a foot more often than not.

So here are several elements of a bad job:

- Lame horse from the shoeing
- Dubbed hoof wall
- Incorrect mediolateral balance
- Sole pressure
- Heels not covered
- Sprung heels
- Shape that does not have the same radiuses in it that the coffin bone does
- Shoe shaped so that nail holes are inside the white line
- Shoe shaped so that nail holes are outside the white line
- Large, long, rough clinches

As you go through this chapter, you are going to see that many of the bad jobs are also overdue to be shod again. I am fully aware that what was a good job on day one can look like a bad job 12 weeks later. The growth of the horse's foot does not allow it to wear the same shoe for that long without problems. As I was going through piles of photos, it became apparent that I didn't have many examples of freshly shod bad jobs. I am actually thankful for that, but I also have to be honest and say the reason is that I didn't take any pictures of my shoeing for the first 5 years of my career. We have all been there, and because I didn't know any better, the horses survived. Had I known better yet still did slipshod work, I probably would not still be a farrier.

I don't hold the results of these jobs against any of the horseshoers who did them, as long as they had the intention of doing right. You will see that many did, but were just a little further back on the road to becoming a good shoer. (At least I hope they are on that road, and not stuck in the ditch.)

Let's begin this by looking at the first picture of a well-shaped shoe on a long foot **(Figure 1)**. This foot needs to be reshod, and you can see that the majority of the problem with this job rests with the owner's neglect. The quarters of the foot are over the sides of the shoe, but the heels are still covered. Had this been a bad job on day one, it would look a lot worse now (as you will see with some of the following jobs).

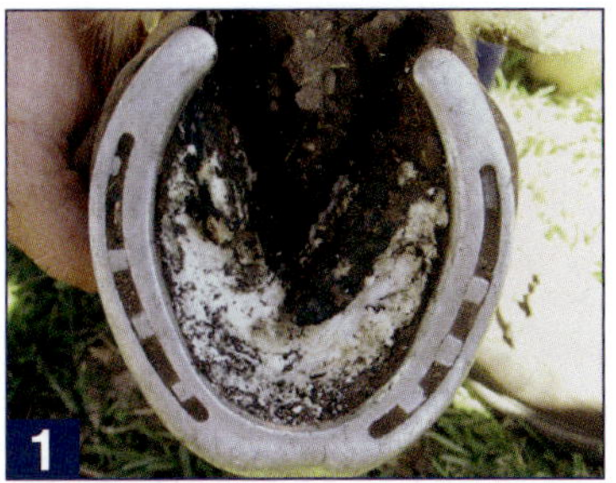

Well-shaped shoe on an overgrown foot.

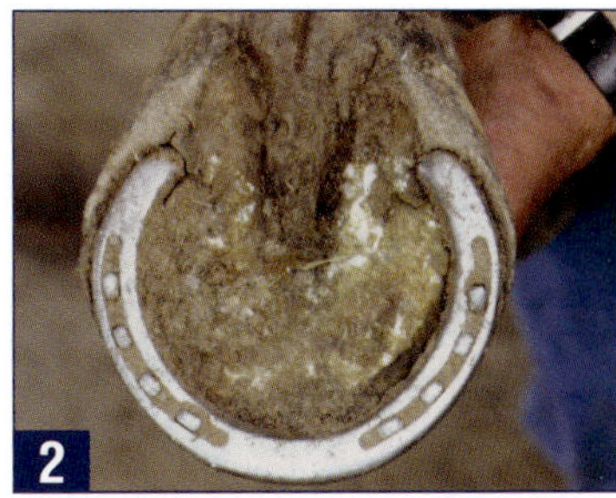

Shoe not properly shaped for the foot.

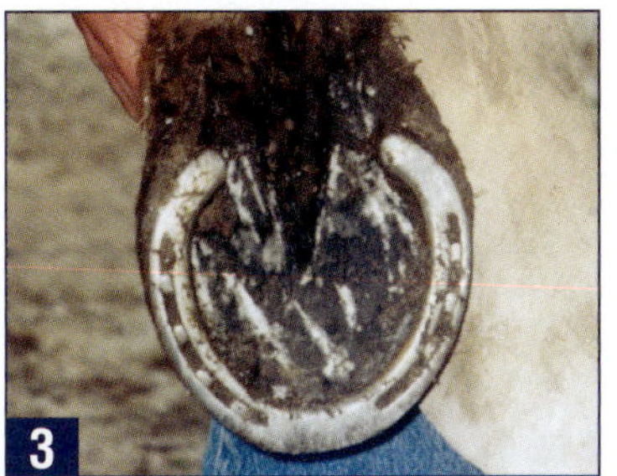

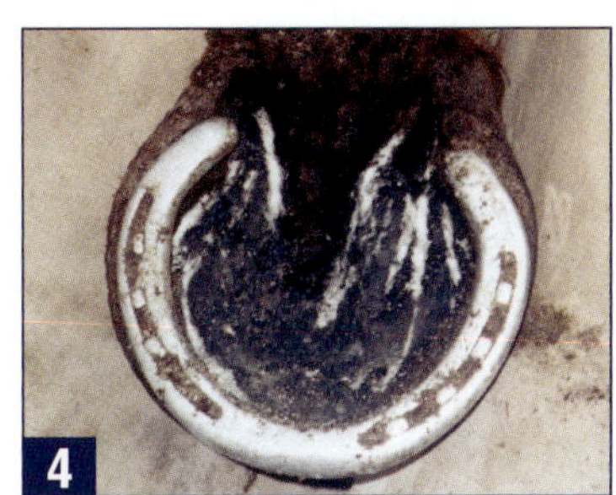

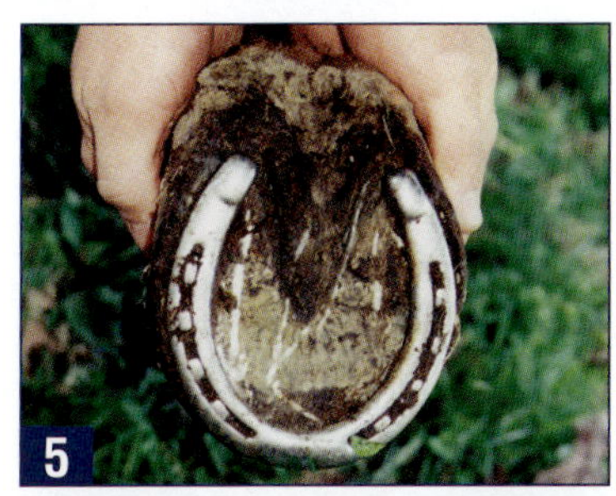

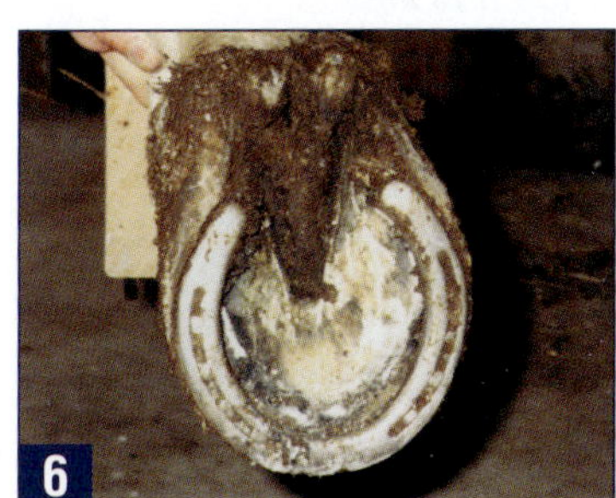

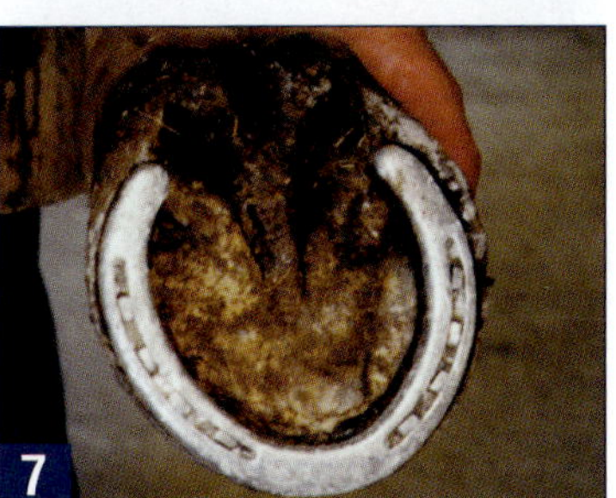

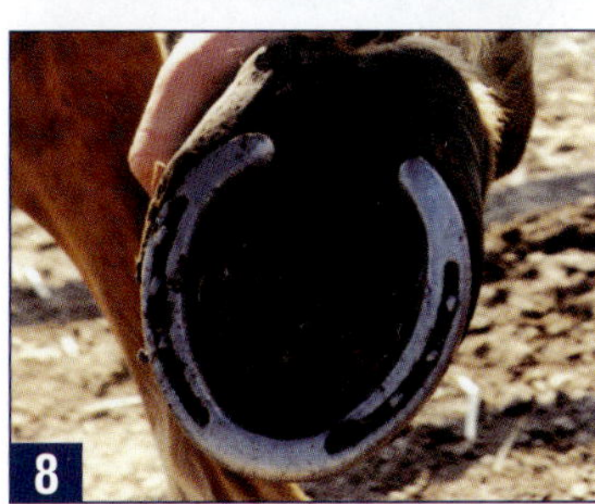

Figures 3-8 are shoes left on too long, and of questionable shape.

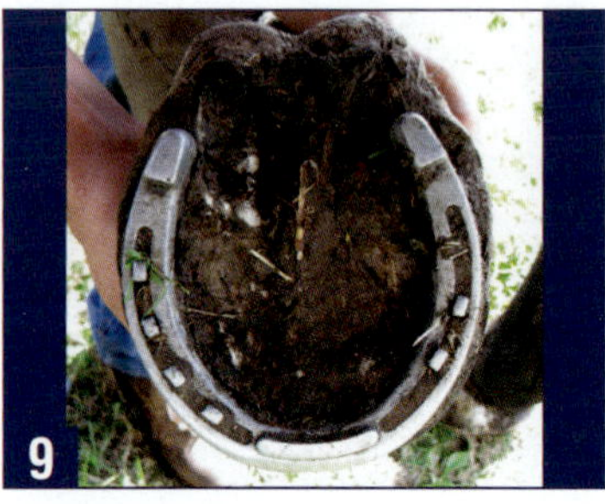

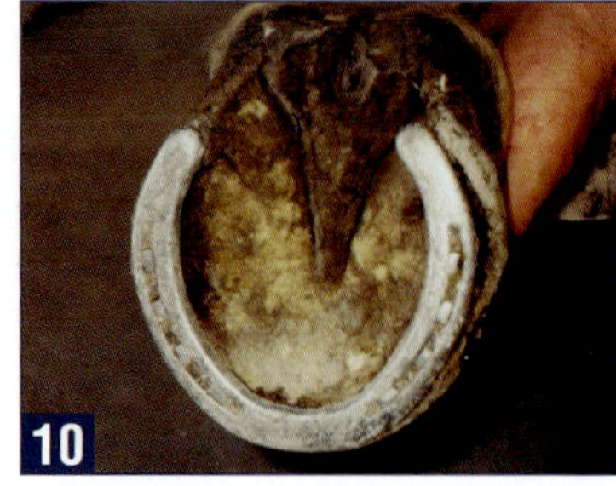

Twisted shoe.

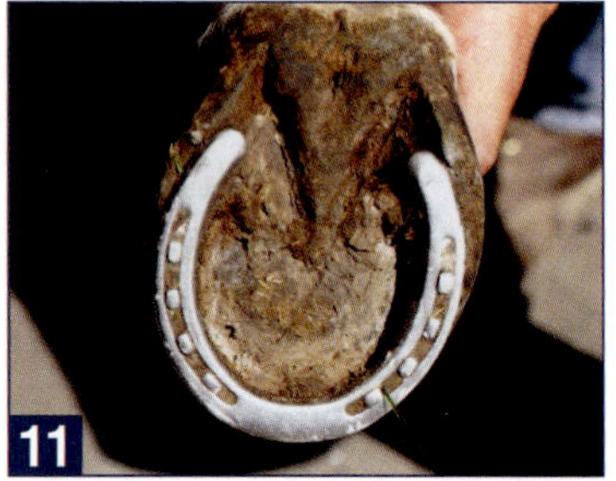

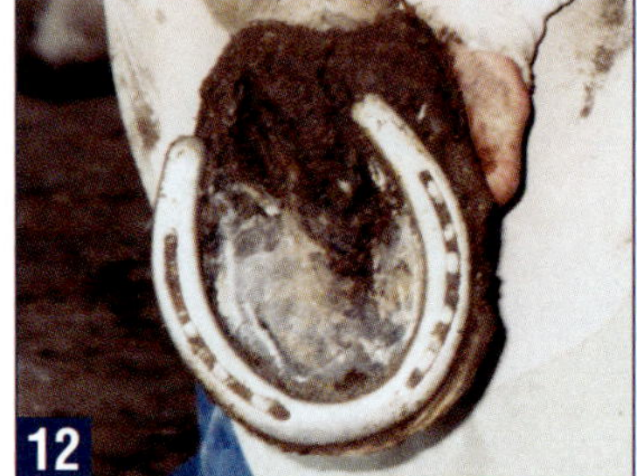

Shoe has slid

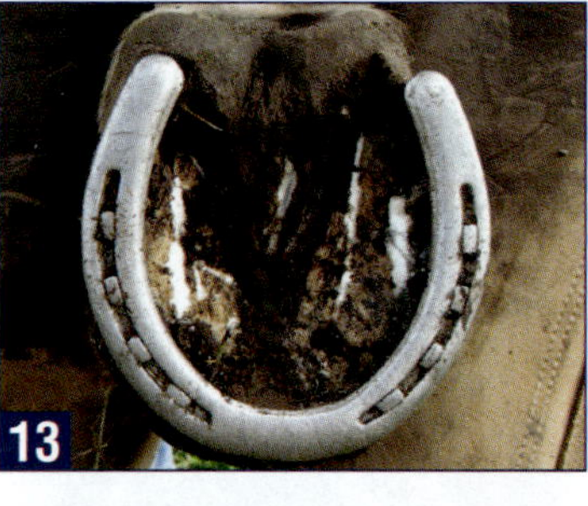

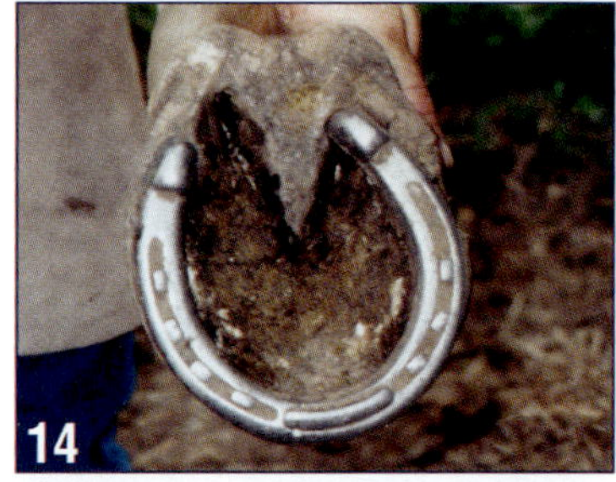

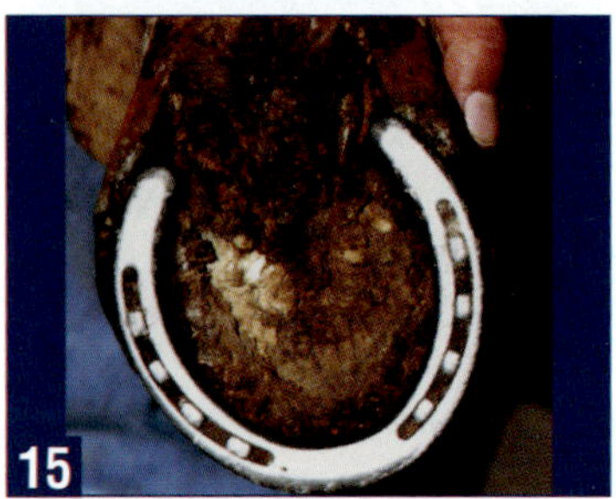

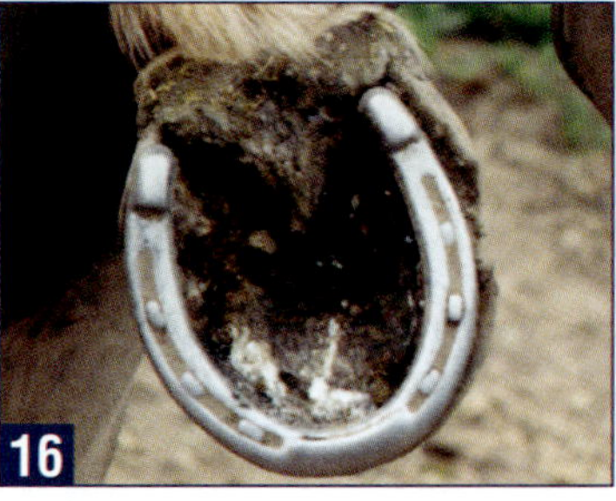

Shoes that were not set square on the foot.

Next, we have the shoeing that looks bad because of the shoe shapes and how long they have been on the feet. You will notice that the jobs in **Figures 2-8** are on very long feet. The shoes have been pulled forward because of hoof growth so that the heels are into the seat of corn, and many of these are front feet with hind-looking shoes on them. In fact, I think **Figure 8** may be the only hind foot in the bunch. Regardless, these jobs were probably on the bottom edge of average when they were new, but the horses were not injured. At least no short-term problems have been reported.

The average keg shoes of the late 1980s had a generic shape that was not a hind or a front but did favor a hind foot. The toe was fairly pointed, and the branches were straighter than most front feet. With the popularity of cold shoeing, many horses have been shod in front by the shoer simply opening up a generic keg shoe and leaving out the toenails to prevent a potential nail quicking.

Our next category is shoes that have shifted. Giving full benefit of the doubt, the shoes in **Figures 9 and 10** look like they may have been well shaped, but they have moved across the bottom of the foot. When I see this, I suspect that there is a mediolateral imbalance. If a foot is loading so that there is more weight on one side of the foot than another, it is common for shoes to shift around.

During fly season, horses will stomp their feet to shake flies off of their legs. This can put a lot of shearing force on nails, so we use a lot of toe clips in fly season.

There are times where shoes are moved a long way across a foot. When that happens, it is impossible to determine if there was anything done incorrectly when the job was new. **Figure 11** is one example, and the shoe in **Figure 12** is on the verge of being lost. Just a quick note here; if you have shoes that are moving, start clipping that horse. There is too much shear force on the shoe against the foot, and clips are designed precisely for taking that shear force.

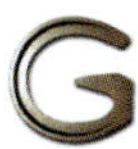

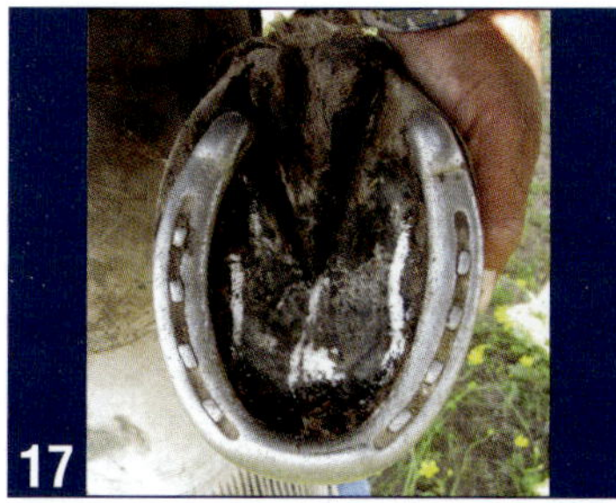

Badly shod near front.

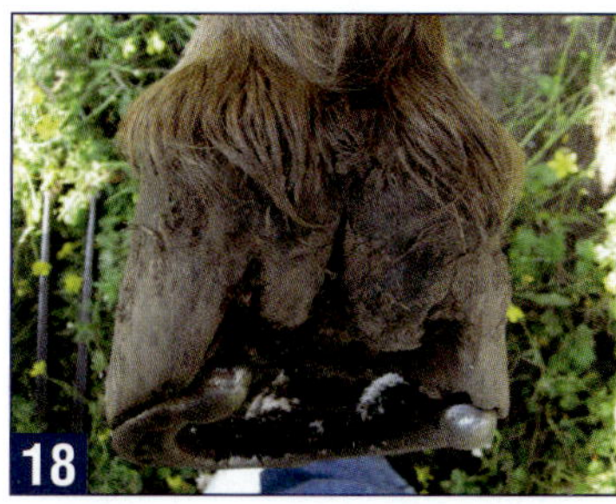

Near front. You can see the imbalance.

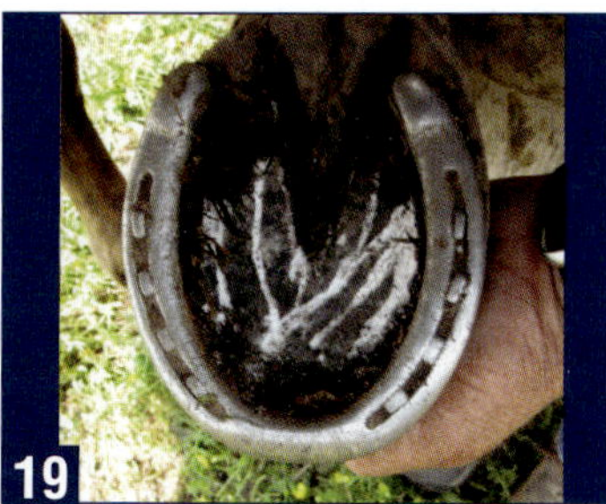

Opposite foot to Figure 17.

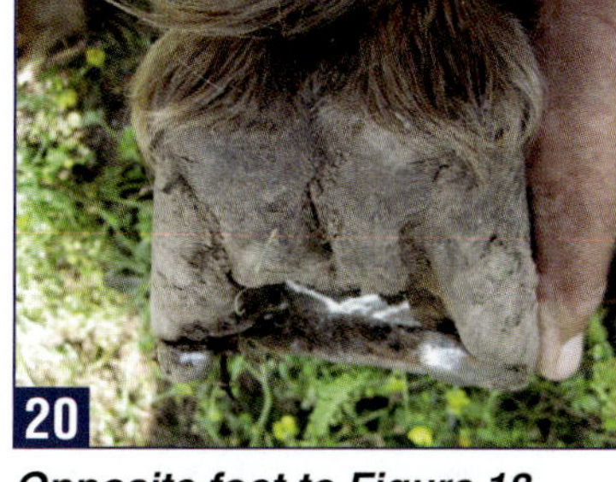

Opposite foot to Figure 18

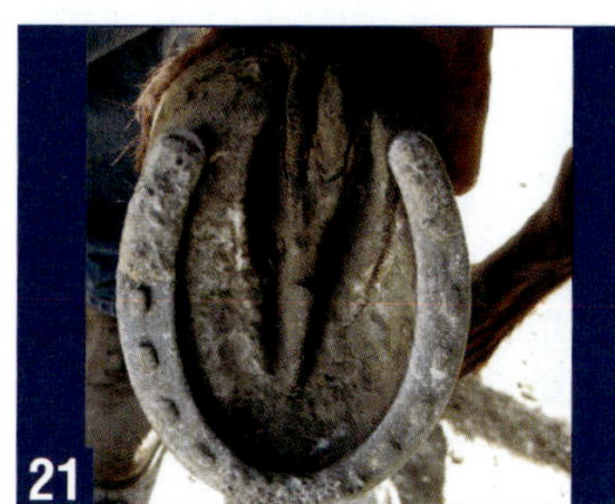

Short shod with Borium.

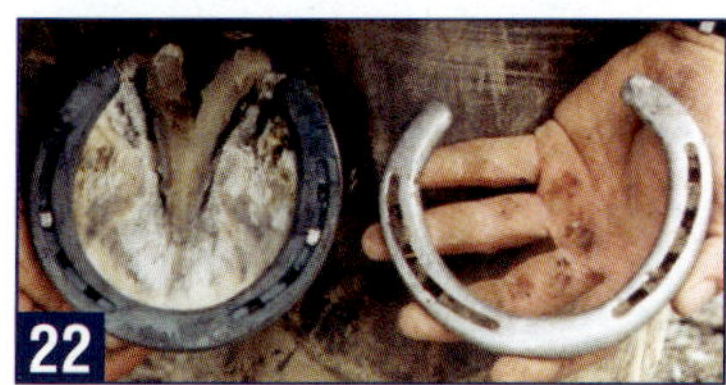

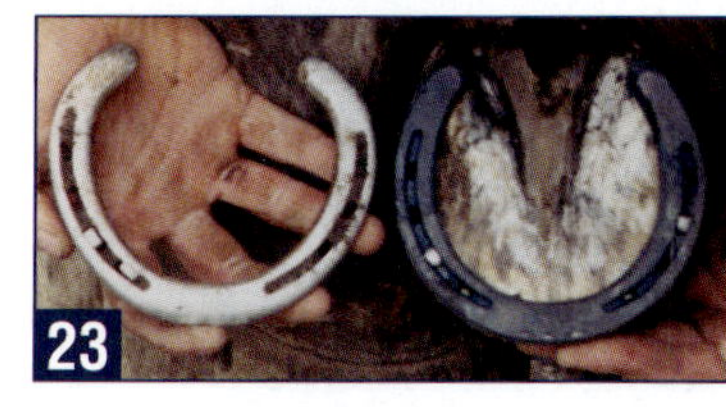

Before-and-after shoeing.

Our next category is just plain and simple, bad shoeing. The shoes in **Figures 13-16** were set twisted. When the job was fresh, the shoe was not centered on the frog. This was a problem on day one, and it is exacerbated because it was let go for a couple months. You can see that these shoes were nailed on without regard to good shoeing principles. There is a difference between shoeing a horse and just putting metal on feet. These are examples of metal on feet.

The front feet in **Figures 17-20** take a special spot. These are toed-and-heeled shoes that were nailed on with an intentional twist in the level. You can see from **Figures 18 and 20** that the shoes are more or less twisted from the medial heel through the lateral heel. These shoes were taken off a horse in 2010, and the shoer who did the work charged $45. The customer was happy with the shoeing because the shoes had stayed on. He even tipped the shoer to the tune of $50 per horse. That is practically criminal.

The next picture is some fresher shoeing in which the heels are not covered. Unfortunately, the photo does not really do it justice, so you need to study the picture closely to see what I am talking about. **Figure 21** was a horse that had only been shod for about 5 days. The lateral heel (the left heel as you look at the picture) is over an inch shy of the buttress. This foot has contracted heels, and you can see that neither one of them is covered. Needless to say, this horse was lame. The addition of borium to a bad shoeing only compounds the problem.

Coming up is the collection of work from farriers who are trying very hard to do the right thing; they are just in a situation where their ability is not up to the job at hand. That is okay. That can be fixed, and as you look at these pictures, it does not appear that any of these horses were shod by people afraid to work. I will say it again; we were all there at one point. Avoid getting in over your head, and get help on feet that you don't understand. There are a lot of talented people in this trade who are willing to help you.

Figures 22 and 23 show something you see a lot when a farrier starts losing shoes. The heels of the shoes have been bent around hard to keep any shoe from being stepped on. Often a farrier is judged solely on how well the shoes stay on. This causes people to do what these guys have done.

For the horses in **Figures 24-28**, I feel that the farrier just lacked vision. I have found throughout

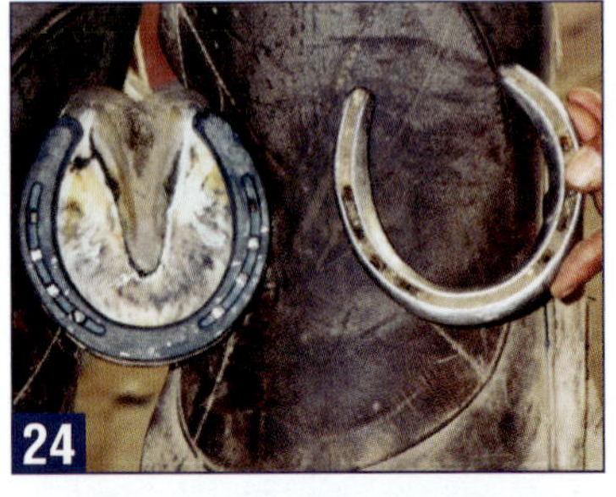

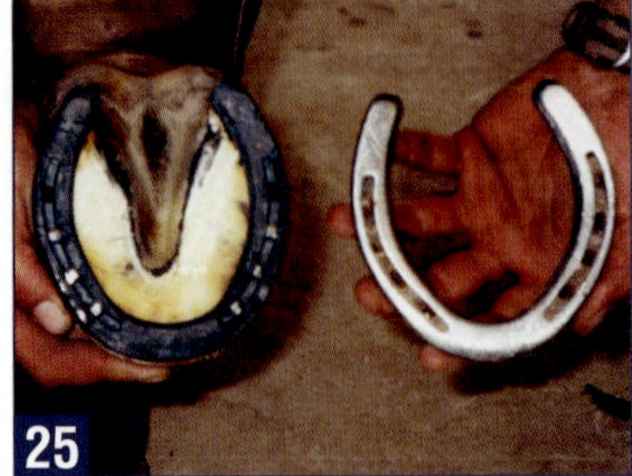

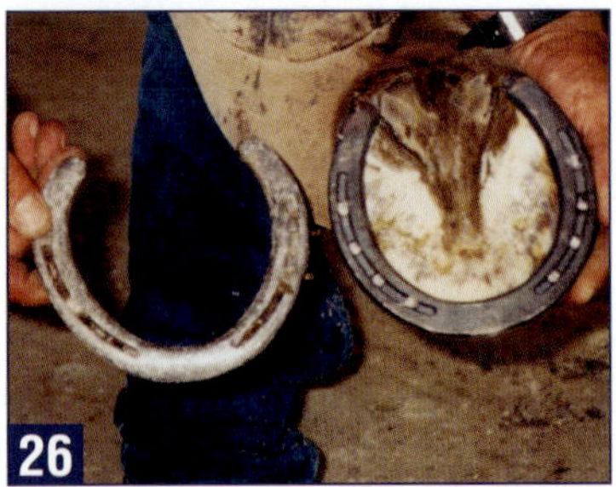

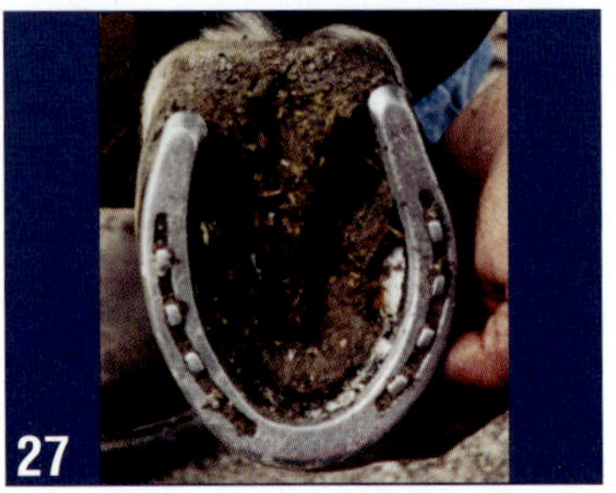

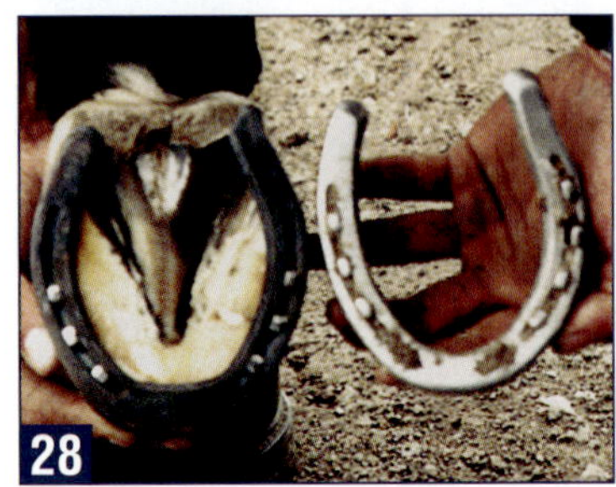

Before-and-after shoeing.

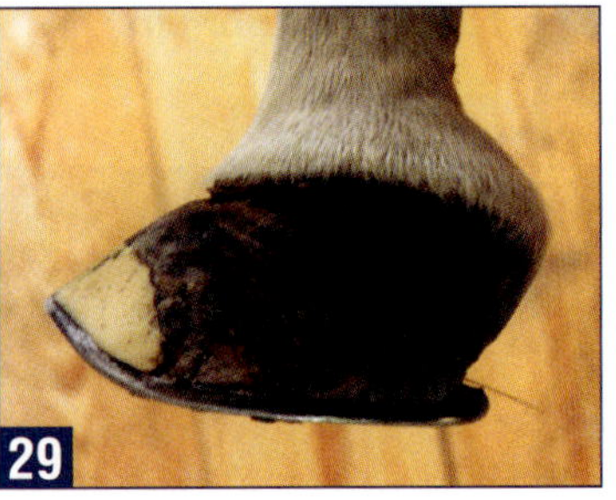

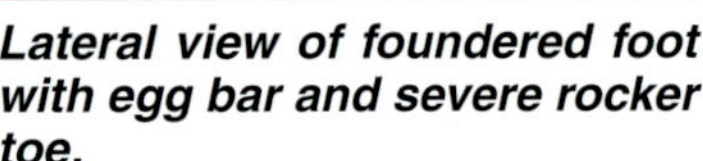

Lateral view of foundered foot with egg bar and severe rocker toe.

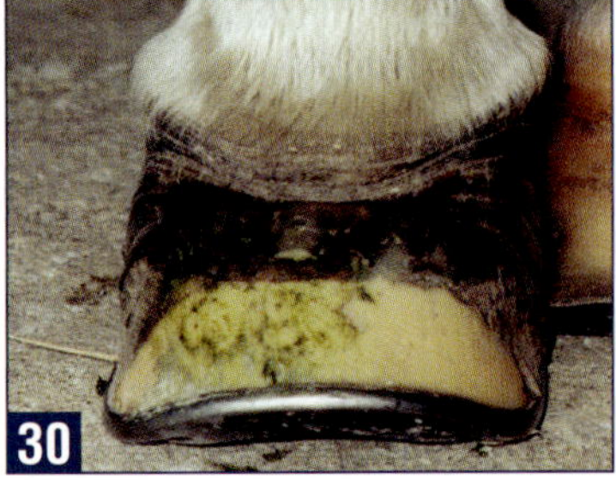

Dorsal view of the same foot.

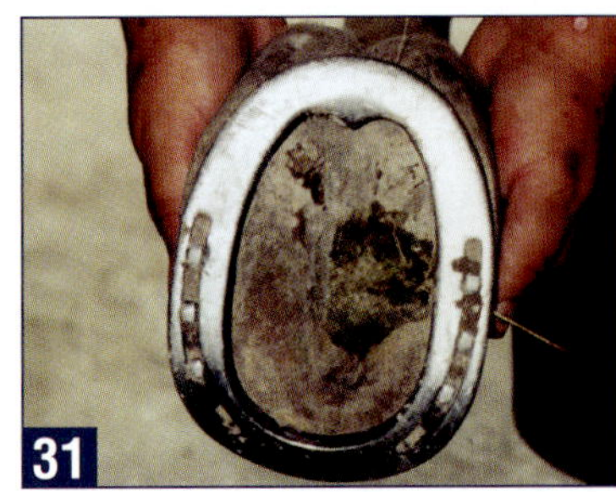

Solar view of the same foot.

my career, you should keep things simple. One of the simplest things is symmetry. It is quite controversial in this industry, and there are a number of what I consider good farriers and good friends who don't like the feet to be symmetrical. In my humble opinion, that is something you can decide for yourself once you have enough knowledge and ability to see the difference between symmetrical feet and the subtle differences these farriers see. But if you are teaching the art of farriery, teach symmetry to beginners. They can see it and understand it, while the idea of a slightly longer radius in the medial quarter vs. a shorter radius in the lateral quarter can be hard to define and see.

Case in point, **Figures 24-28**. Even those among my peers who see the most dramatic asymmetry would have difficulty arguing that the shapes of these shoes were what the feet in question needed.

Okay, now we get into the group of shoeing photos from those who have gotten in over their heads from a lack of knowledge and understanding. **Figures 29-31** are of a foundered horse that was done with an egg bar shoe with a rocker toe. To compound the problems for this horse, the front of the foot was then built up with acrylic so that there was pressure against a hoof wall that was not attached to the coffin bone. This farrier did a ton of work, and obviously has some mechanical ability. However, mechanical skills used without understanding can be a lethal combination, like a 3-year-old with a loaded gun. This is bad shoeing done with good intentions.

The next group is of a horse that came from several hours away as a referral from a veterinarian.

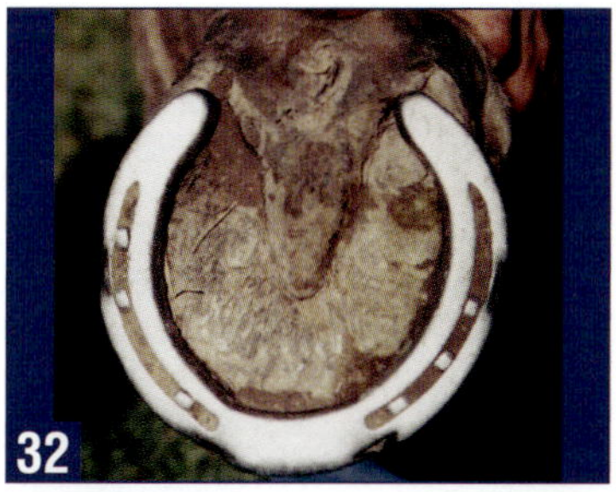

32 33 34 35 36 37 38 39

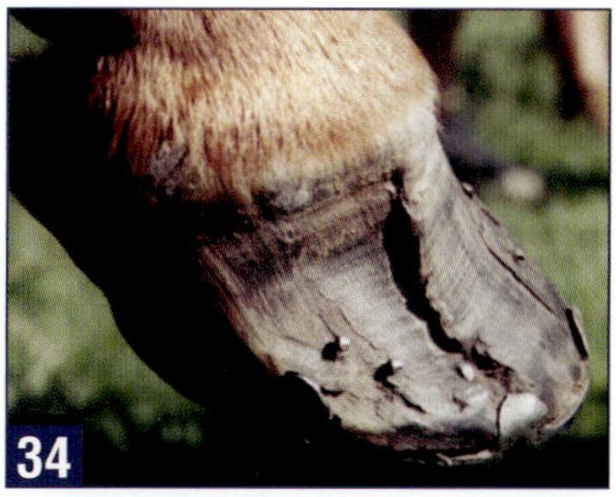

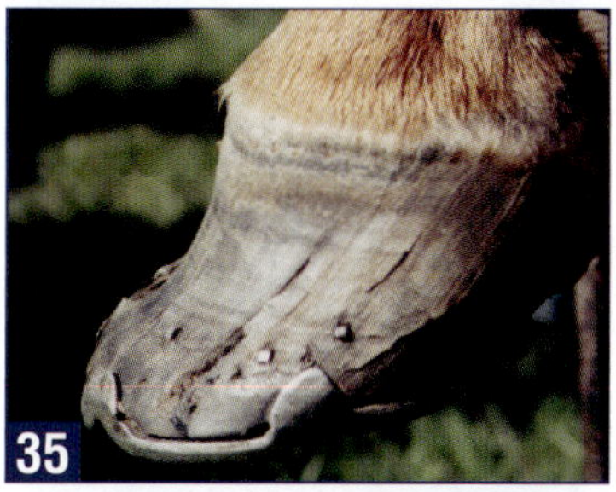

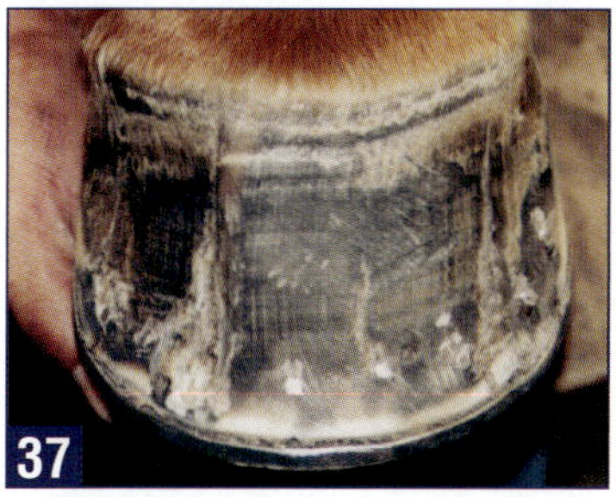

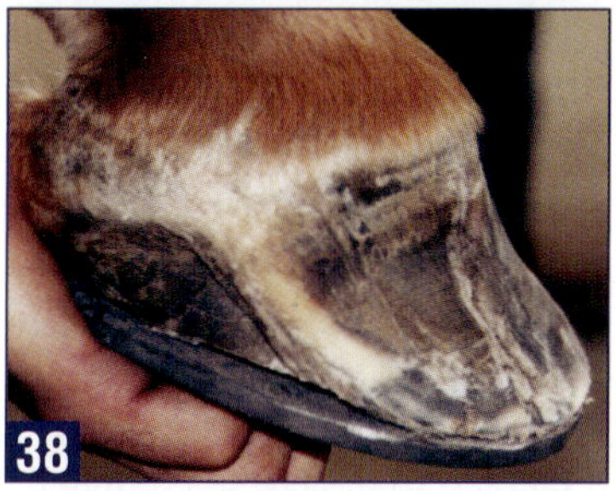

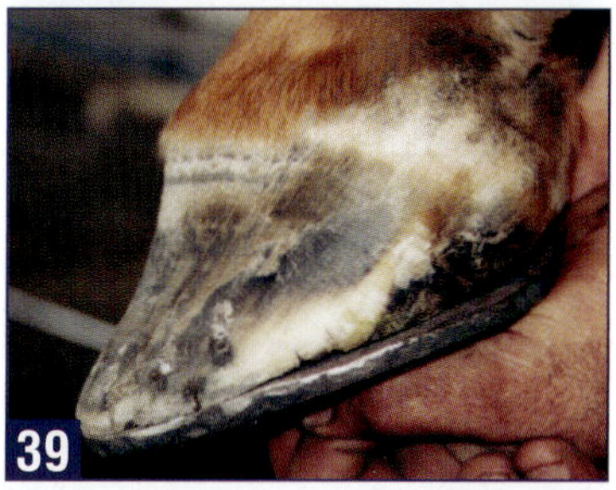

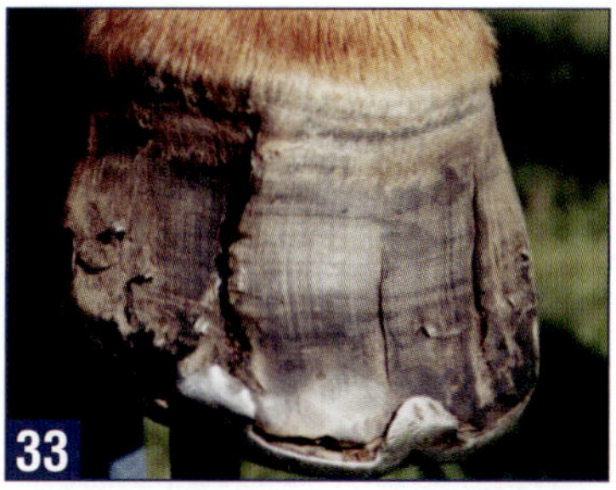

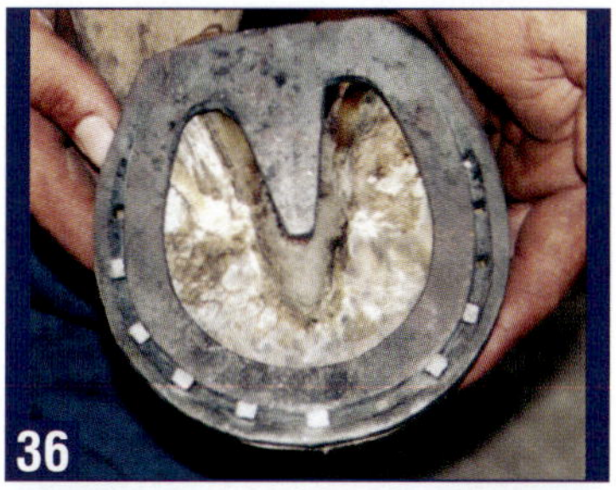

Before-and-after series of a horse with a bad foot and a lost farrier.

I told the owner to bring her farrier, and when she got to the shop, she said that he couldn't make it because he had a hair appointment that day. Unfortunate, because you can see that this guy was trying his hardest, he just did not understand some basic principles of good shoeing.

Figures 32-35 are what the foot looked like when the horse showed up. On the bottom of the foot **(Figure 32)** you can see where the guy pulled 4 clips. That takes some doing. However, when you look at the dorsal, lateral, and medial views, you can see that those clips were not effective. They are thin and only hammered over onto bent tubules.

Figures 36-39 show the same foot about an hour later. Compare **Figure 32 and 36**, and you will see a much different perimeter shape. Symmetry was applied to the foot, and the resulting shoe is now more appropriate for the foot. There are some non-traditional nails in the toe, and we used a heart bar to take some of the weight off of the weakened hoof wall.

Comparing **Figures 33-35** to **Figures 37-39** shows a dramatic change to the shape and strength of that foot. Even though a lot of tissue has been removed from that hoof wall, it is actually stronger from being straight. Think about a thick-but-bent pillar in a house that will have less strength than a thin pillar that is straight. Straight tubular horn is a basic principle of good shoeing. In fact, I think Edward Martin, FWCF, once said, "The answer is always straight tubular horn."

This leads nicely into talking about what bad shoeing looks like from the top. **Figure 40** is a lateral view of the horse in **Figure 21**. If you look at the dorsal wall, you will see that it has a very distinct dub to it. The farrier took his shoe with borium on it, nailed it somewhere on the bottom of the foot, then rasped off whatever foot stuck out past the shoe

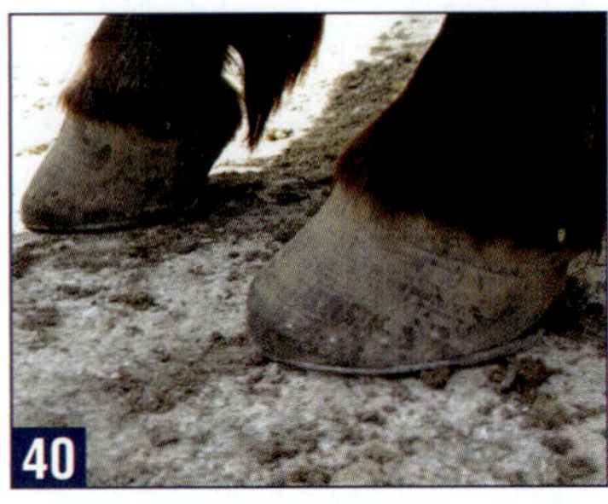

Lateral view of the foot in Figure 21. Horse is lame.

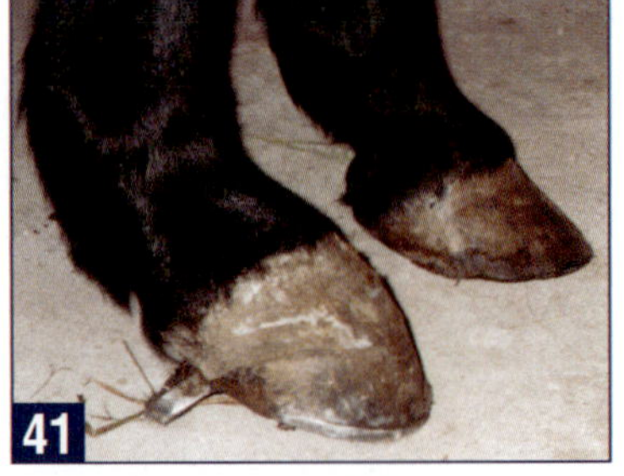

Bull nosed foot from past due reset on patten bar.

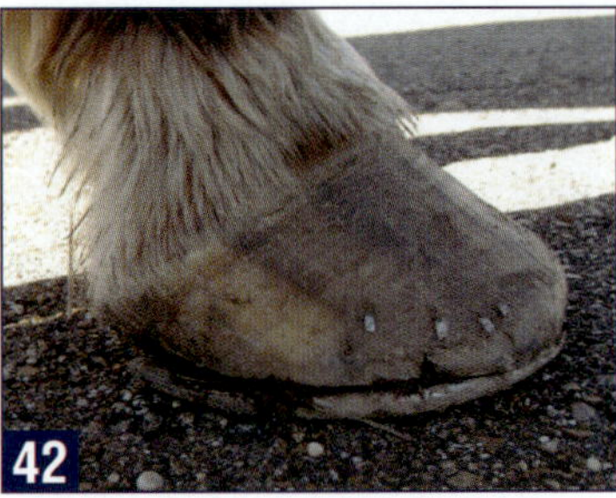

Lateral view of dubbed foot.

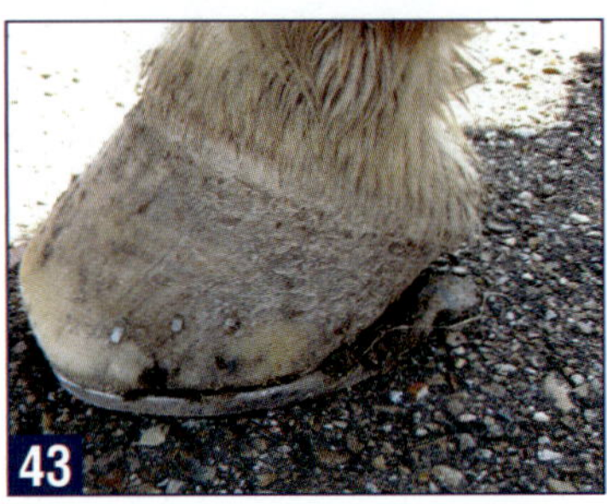

Lateral view of dubbed foot.

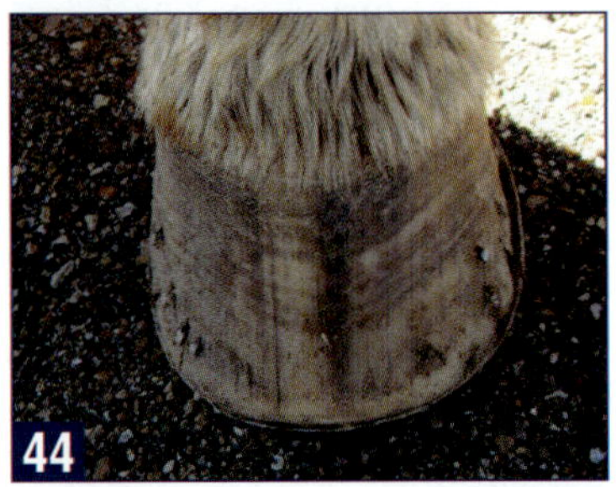

Dorsal oblique view of bad shoeing. Notice the unintentional extension.

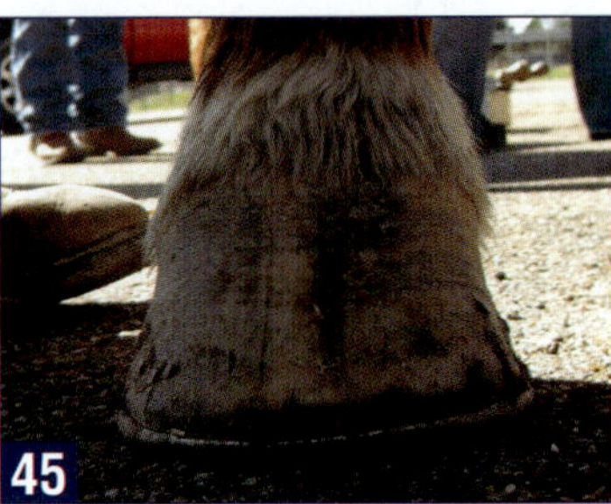

Dorsal view of bad shoeing.

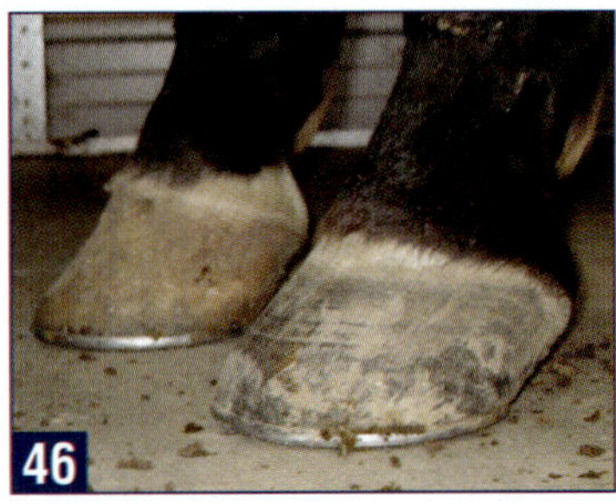

Lateral view of mismatched and dubbed feet.

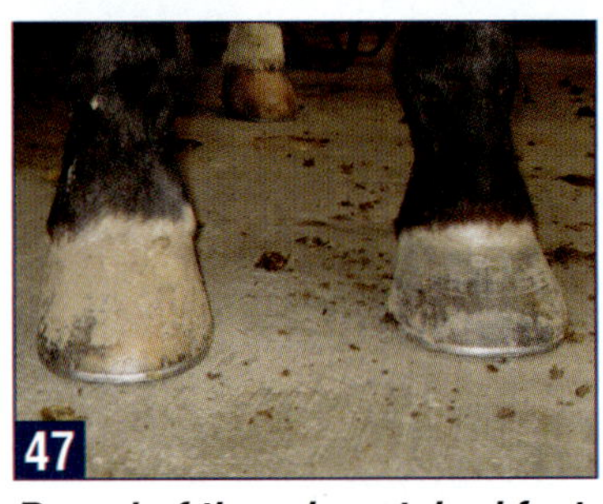

Dorsal of the mismatched feet.

when he was done clinching.

When a foot is dubbed, a corner is put into the tubules. A bull-nosed foot results from pressure against the tubules in an unnatural manner. **Figure 41** is an extreme example of a bull-nosed foot, where a patten bar was left on too long. Leaving a dub in the foot can also lead to this. The higher the dub gets on the dorsal wall, the greater the risk of it causing this bad bulge. You can see another low dub in a two-week old job that I saw at a rodeo in **Figures 42-45**. These are all the same horse, and you can get a feel for the mediolateral balance the horse was dealing with by looking at **Figure 45**. **Figures 46 and 47** are 4 weeks into the shoeing. With this horse, we also have the drastic angle and length differences to compound the problems, and the conformation of the horse did not call for the differences. What we are looking for in a good lateral view is demonstrated in **Figure 48**. You can see that natural angle has been achieved, and the dorsal wall is straight and strong.

From a dorsal view, you want to see feet that are the same length, and you want to see good balance. In **Figure 47**, you can see that these feet were trimmed to very different lengths. That is a common discrepancy when you have a wide foot vs. a narrow foot. This one is compounded even more by the fact that there is one black, one white, and a little bit of white in the coronet as well. When you come across feet that are this different, use your tape measure or dividers to compare them to each other.

From the front, you want to see work similar to what is pictured in **Figures 49 and 50**. The wall is nice and straight. The clinches are well made and

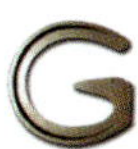

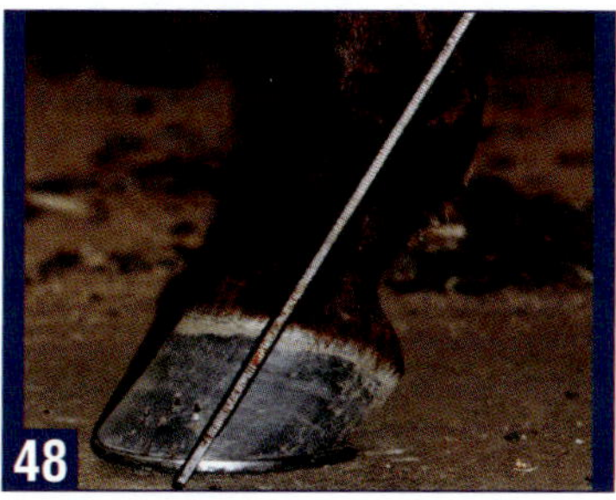

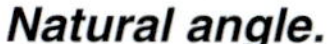

Natural angle.

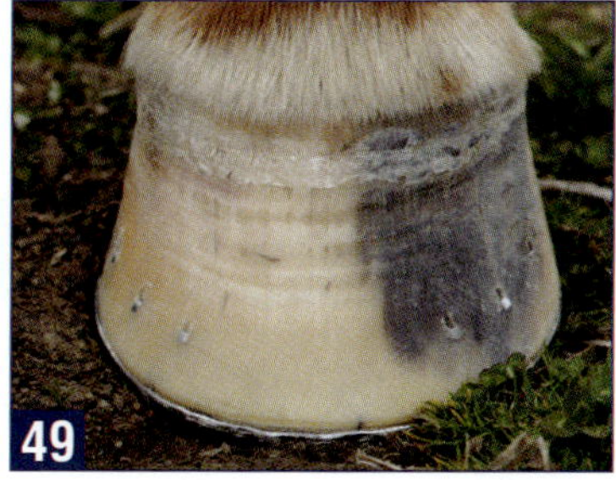

Figures 49 - 50: Dorsal views of good shoeing.

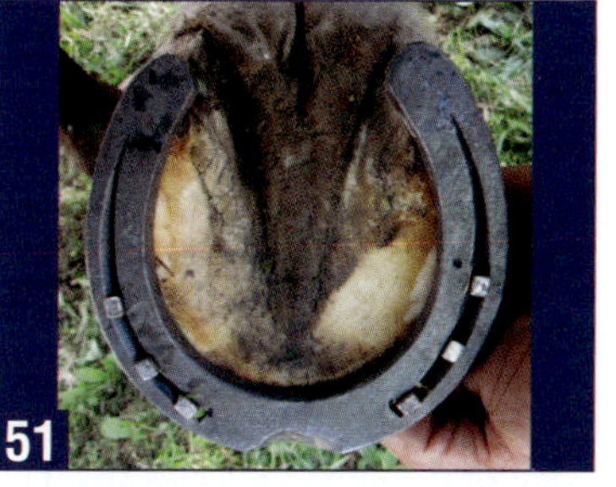

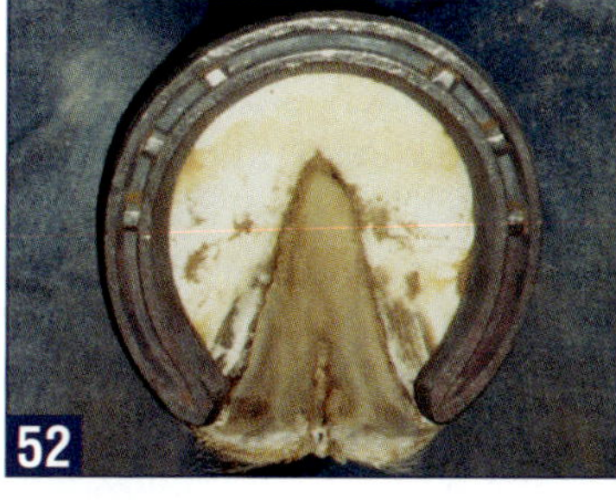

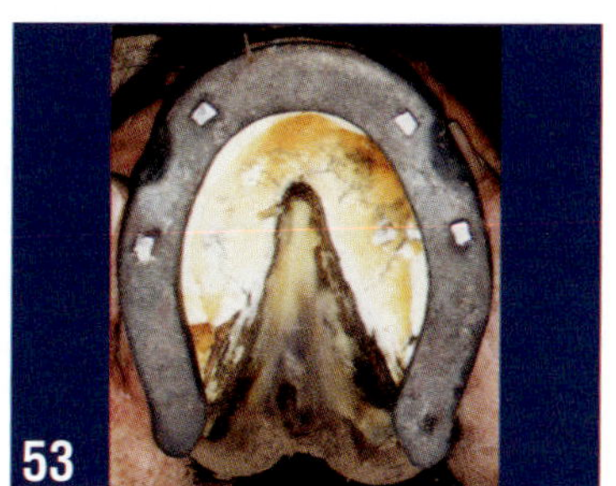

Figures 51 - 53: Solar view of good shoeing.

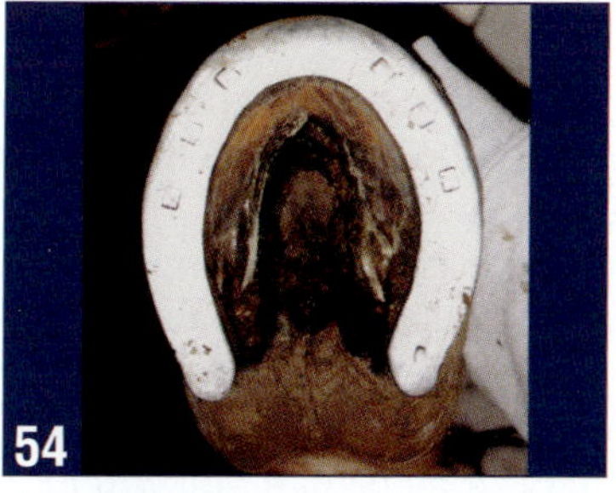

Good shoeing that is ready to be reset

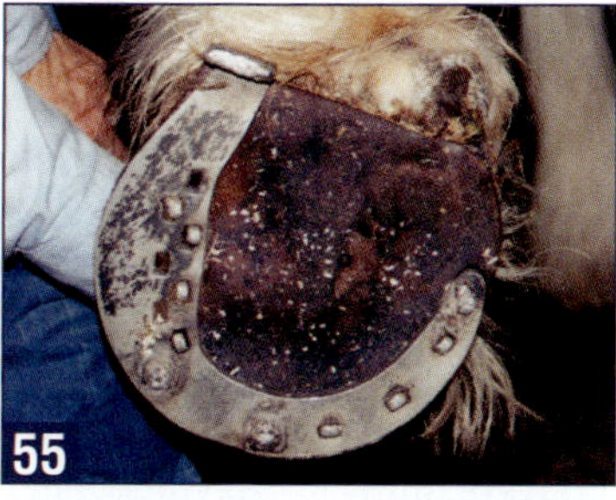

Shows shoeing for a draft at the expense of the horse.

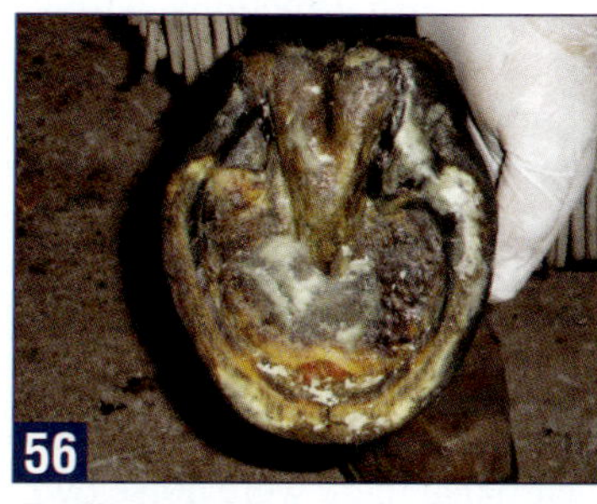

Badly infected foot from sole pressure.

strong, and the foot is under the leg. On the bottom of the foot you want to see well-made shoes shaped to complement the foot **(Figures 50-53)**. Even with the need of a reset, the foot should be covered, as is the one in **Figure 54**.

As we have been looking at these feet, you may have wondered to yourself what the big fuss is all about. At the beginning of this chapter we even talked about how often these horses stay sound anyway. Poor shoeing has resulted in what you see in **Figures 55 and 56**. Look closely at the draft foot in **Figure 55**, and you can see the damage to the bulb on the top right side of the photo. **Figure 56** is the result of sole pressure. On this particular foot, the vet estimated that over half of the attachment between the hoof and the coriums was compromised. Suffice it to say when you looked at the other shoes that were on this horse, the wonder was that the other feet were not in the same condition as this one.

Proper shoeing is not rocket-surgery. Good, solid, traditional and sound basics will serve you well. Your mission is to understand those basics, and then become good at applying them.

Chapter

34 COMMON SENSE IN THE SHOEING VS. BAREFOOT DEBATE

If you are new to this trade, you may see this as a new debate. In fact, it is not new at all. From the beginning, the benefits of applying shoes with nails to a living animal have been hotly contested by those who do not believe it is a good idea.

Unfortunately, the outsider would think that the participants in the debate were religious zealots or political rivals. At the heart of the matter is this animal we are all concerned about — the horse. Since the horse cannot verbalize a position in the debate in simple English, we have to read its response by its actions. A lame horse is telling you that there is something wrong in the locomotion system. If you caused that lameness intentionally based on a theory of trimming that does not make sense to the practical-minded person, then shame on you.

To me, there seems very little room for a debate. It is a simple matter that if the foot wears down faster than it can grow new horn, it needs protection. I have to admit that I was amazed the first time I heard that there were horse owners who were uninformed and gullible enough that they agreed their horse should suffer for a period of up to a year to get a foot that was tough enough to go without shoes. During this time, the horse needs to be trimmed at very short intervals as well as walked over gravel and hard surfaces to toughen up. That seems so much more callous than I thought anyone would want to be to a horse.

Regardless, I think that most of us would agree that the horse should not be made to suffer intentionally. (At least I hope we can all agree on that.) Does the application of shoes increase the potential for harm? Of course it does. You are about to drive nails into a foot. But, this only gives rise to the obvious need to be skilled at doing it. Bad shoeing is bad shoeing, and bad trimming can be just as bad — even more so when bad trimming is done intentionally through ignorance.

The horse is a noble and admired beast that has no say in how its own feet are treated. Based on geography, genetics, environment, ownership, farrier availability, farrier knowledge (or lack thereof), and other factors, the horse has to deal with how a human decided the feet should be. The horse is tied by a rope, then whatever style of hoof care is decided upon is applied. In a perfect world, there would have been some talking horses to lead us down the right path. This is not a perfect world. So, we have to decide what is best for the horse based purely on our experience and diligent study. For me, a sound horse is good; a lame horse is bad. It seems quite straightforward.

In all industries, there is a vocal minority that are incapable of good, sound, proper, and ethical craftsmanship. To the detriment of all, some of these are charismatic and talk a "good game" as they lead the innocent down the wrong path. If you will look at the farrier industry with an unbiased eye, you will see that the recognized experts (AFA Certified Journeyman Farriers, Associates and Fellows of the Worshipful Company of Farriers, and world-class-level competitors), all seem to have a similar stance. A well-made shoe applied by a skilled craftsman will have a huge beneficial impact on a horse. It can be the difference between a horse feeling good and being sound or being lame.

Taking a look at the crowd that is promoting named and fashionable trimming styles based on conjecture and fancy, and you will find that the ranks are filled with those who do not possess the skills needed to do a proper shoeing job. As such, they have found a niche in the industry, and they prey upon the horse owner who has a big heart but also a big lack of anatomical understanding to go with it.

There is a book that has come from the FWCF thesis written by Dr. Mike Miller, MD, CJF, FWCF. It is titled, *The Mirage of the Natural Foot. Science and Snake Oil in the Barefoot Trimming Debate.* This book **(Figure 1)** is based on the only controlled study of its kind where a number of horses at the same farm were trimmed with conventional methods, some with four-point trims and some with half four-point, half conventional. His study clearly indicates the harm that can come from a four-point trim. Regardless of your opinion in the matter, you owe it to yourself to read this book.

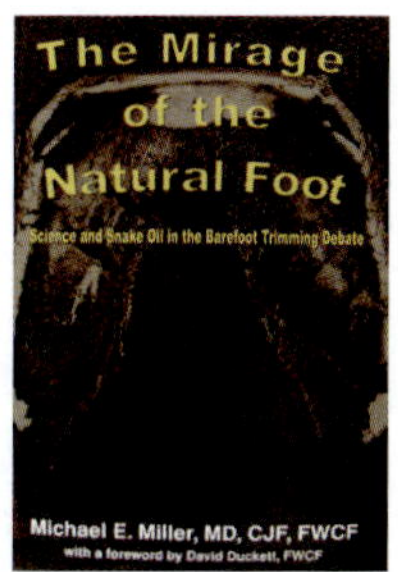

1 *Mike Miller's book cover.*

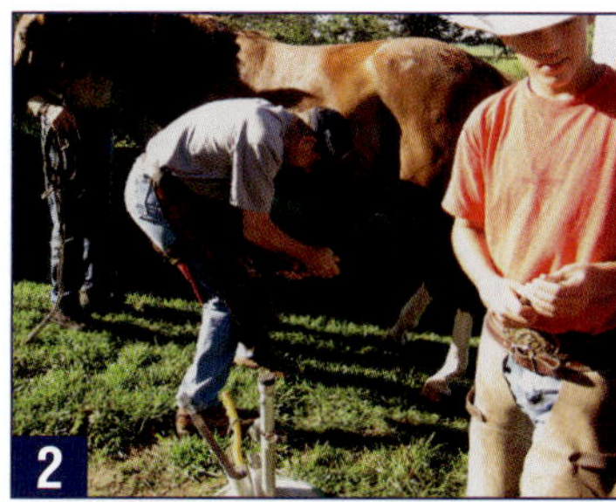

2 *Cody with Dr. Miller in the background at the start of the study.*

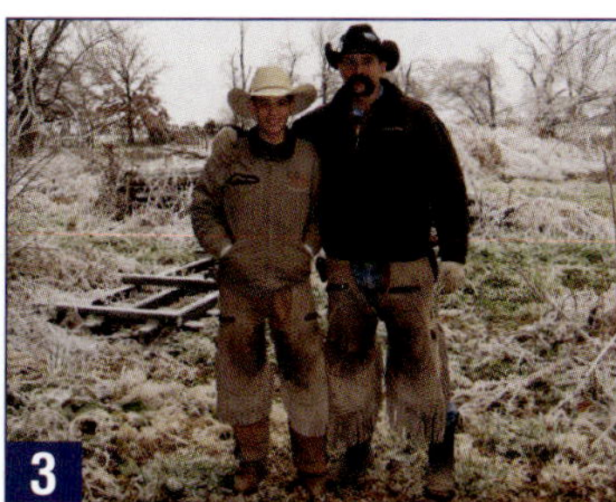

3 *Last trim of the study was done during a massive Missouri ice storm.*

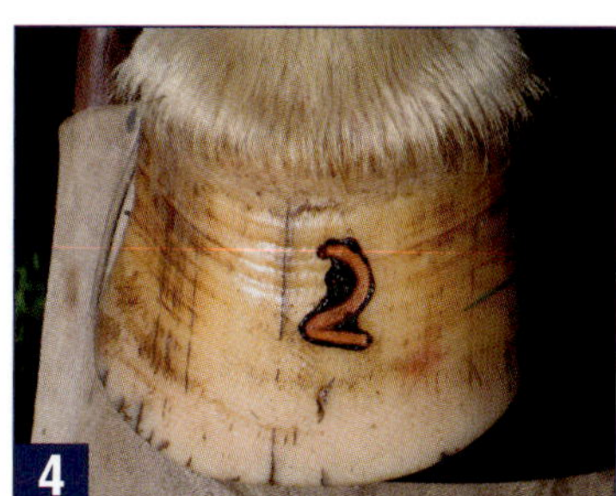

4 *Branded foot.*

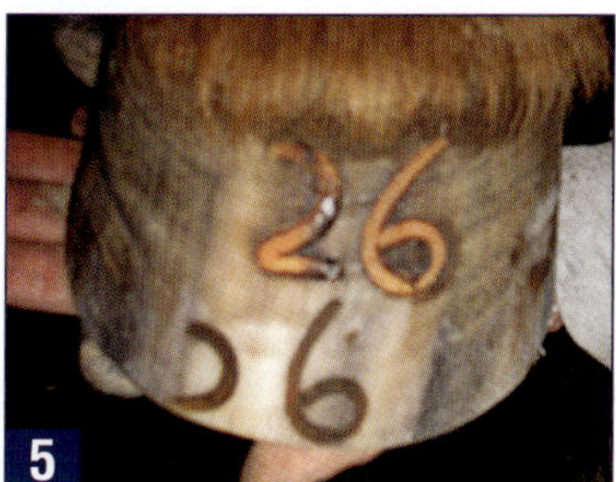

5 *Branded foot.*

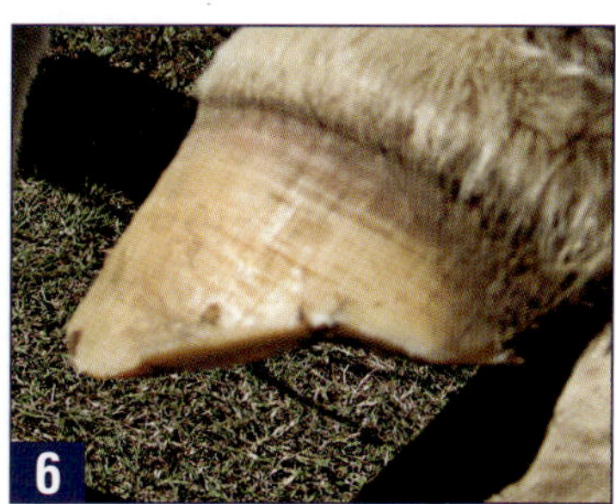

6 *Lateral view of first 4-point trim.*

Here is a basic overview of Mike's study. Kelly, Cody, and I were lucky enough to be a part of the trimming. As you can see from **Figure 2**, the weather was nice our first time to trim the 21 horses, and in **Figure 3**, you can see that our last outing was in quite the storm. All of the trimming was done by an AFA Certified Farrier; three AFA Certified Journeyman Farriers (one of whom was also an Associate of the Worshipful Company of Farriers), and another of the Journeyman being a Fellow of the Worshipful Company of Farriers. We all sat down to watch the video by Ric Redden concerning the four-point trim so that we could match the technique before commencing with the experiment. It was actually hard to make ourselves trim feet in the manner depicted on the video.

The horses were randomly selected from a list of twenty-one names. These were then put into three groups of seven. One group was trimmed with conventional methods, one with four-point technique, and the other group had one side trimmed conventionally, the opposite side with four-point. The changes wrought on these feet were amazing.

You can see in **Figures 4 and 5** how the feet were branded. **Figure 6** shows the lateral view of a four-point trimmed foot and **Figure 7** is what the bottom of a four-point foot looked like after its first trim. At this stage, the feet were all fairly similar, having been trimmed by the students in Heartland Horseshoeing School about six weeks prior to the start. **Figure 8** is the solar view of the off hind of a horse named Shipley. After three trim cycles (18 weeks), **Figure 8** is what that foot had become. You can see how much difference there is in the

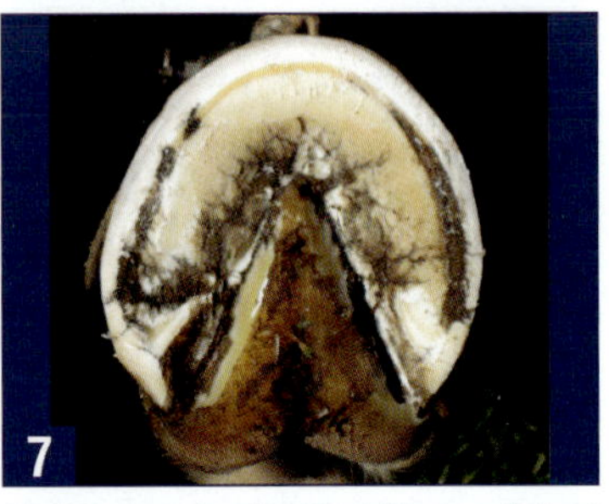

Bottom of a foot at time of first four-point trim.

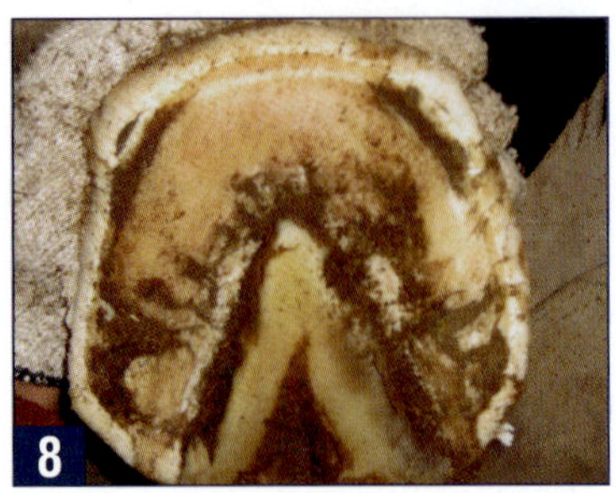

Bottom of the foot in Figure 7 after 18 weeks

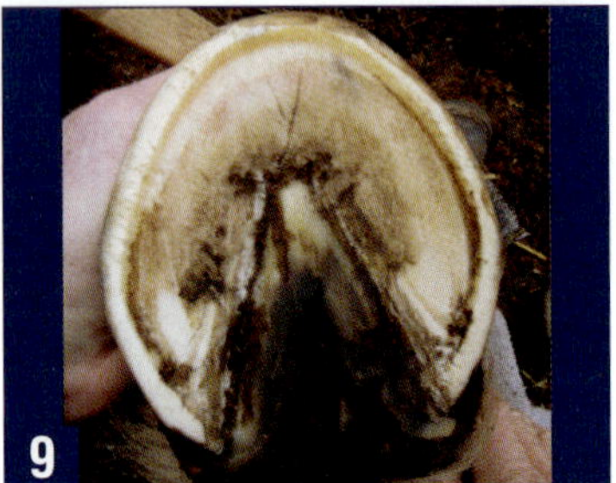

Conventionally trimmed foot.

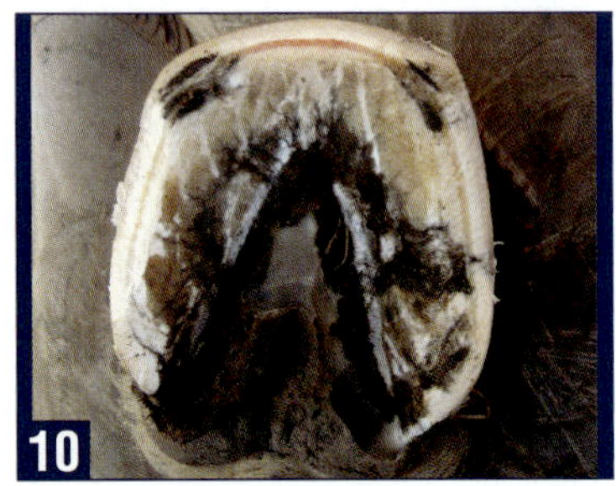

Same horse as Figure 9, only the opposite side with a four-point trim.

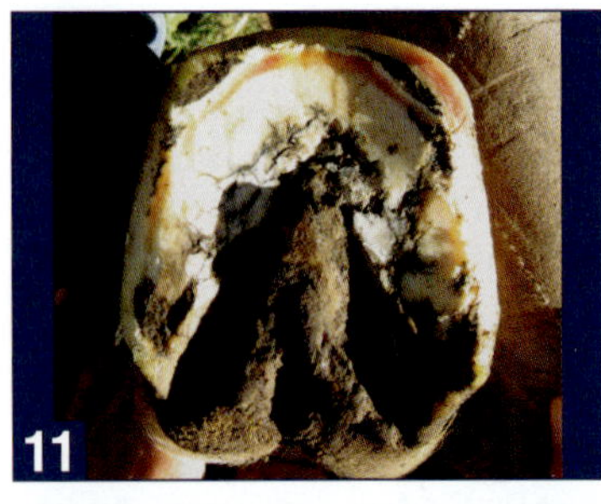

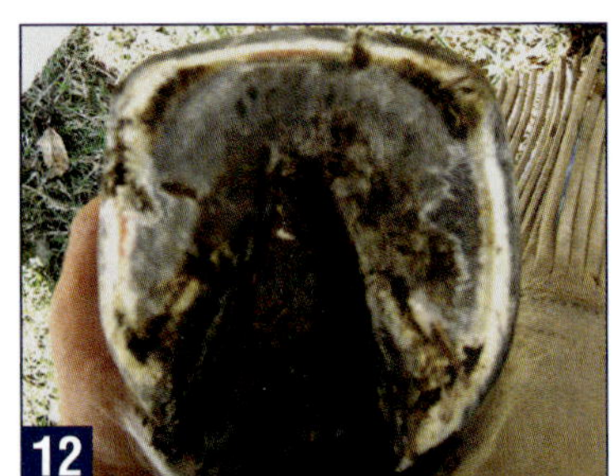

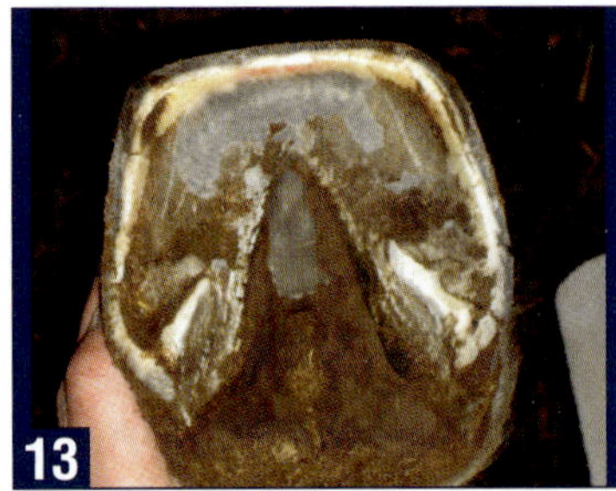

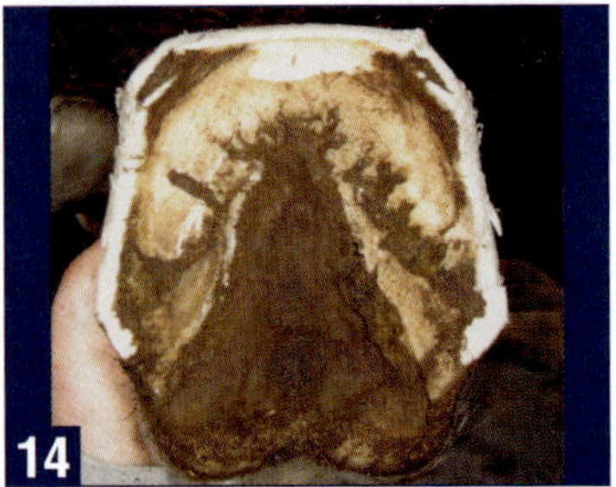

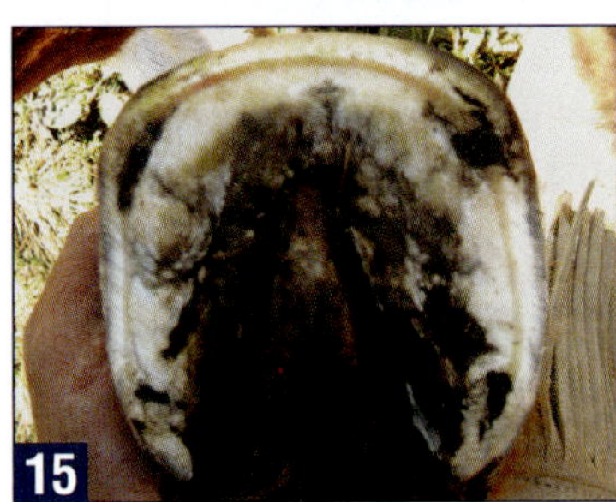

Figures 11 - 15. Damage done by four-point trims.

shape of the foot. The quarters have moved toward the heel, the foot is elongated, there are corners at both sides of the toe, and the toe-quarter area has a shorter radius in it with the white line stressed. **Figures 9 - 10** are of a combination horse that had 4-point on one side and conventional trim on the other. As you probably know from your studies of anatomy, this theory does not make any sense anatomically.

Foot after foot showed signs of major changes for the worse (**Figures 11-15**). You can see that bruising in the white line was common, and there was hardly a foot that the toe-quarter area did not get pulled and stretched out of shape. Another interesting thing that occurred

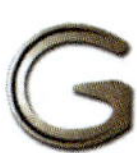

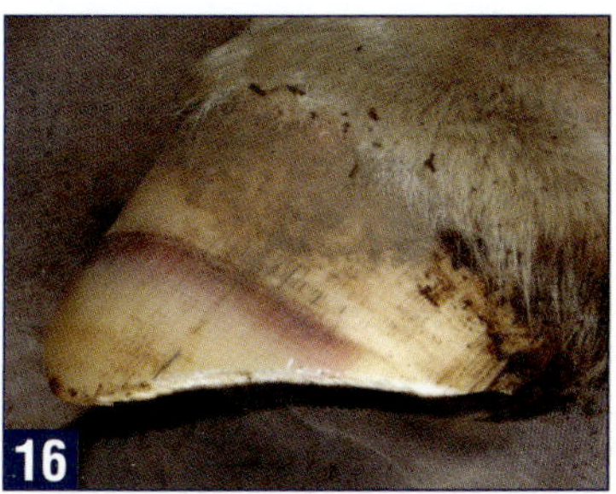

Lateral view of four-point trimmed foot with bruise that has a curve in it from the trim.

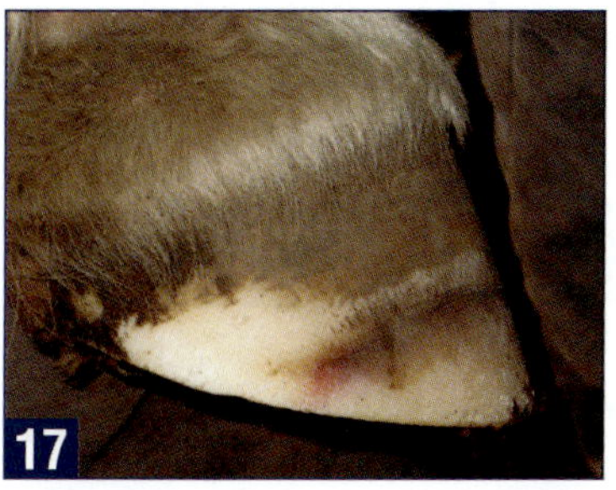

Opposite foot of the same horse. Notice the bruise is straight.

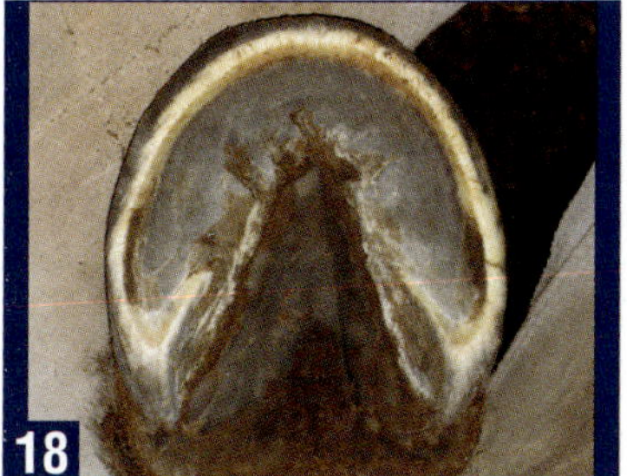

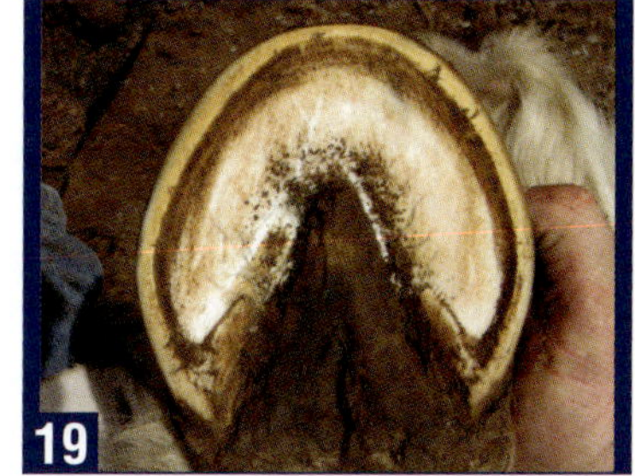

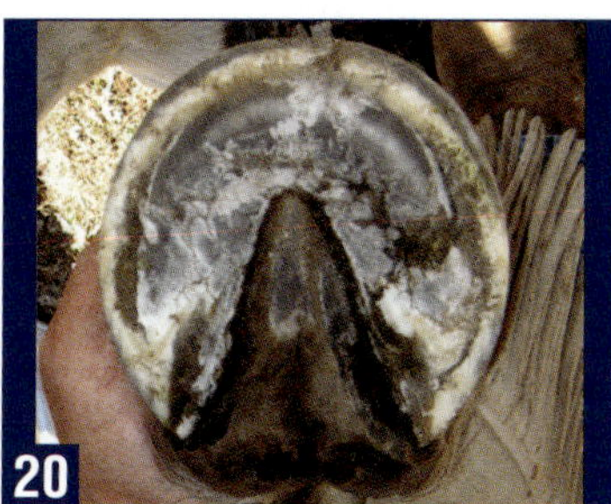

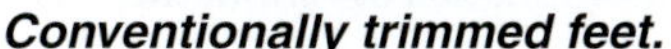

Conventionally trimmed feet.

was the shape of the wall and coronary band from a lateral view. This was most evident on one horse that had blood in the hoof wall on all four feet before the study began. Since one side was conventional on this horse and the opposite four-point, the differences were easily seen. You can see how the hoof wall has a much larger bow in it when you compare **Figures 16** to **Figure 17**.

My original notion was to continue the study once Dr. Miller was done, but I couldn't bring myself to do that to the feet any longer. You can see from the feet in **Figures 18-20** that this was a pretty good-footed group of horses, and destroying the feet for the sake of more proof did not seem like a good idea. Remember that you should always base your decisions about shoeing on good anatomy. When it doesn't make sense anatomically, it really doesn't make sense.

I have recently had the fortune to get some neat business insight from a farrier in British Columbia, Canada. This farrier had an interesting perspective on the recent "barefoot trimmer movement," and he made a great point about how many of the great farriers out there have really missed a big opportunity. All of the good farriers that are currently shoeing are also barefoot trimmers. There are horses in almost every practice that do not require shoes. Yet, we have allowed a group of people to out-market us by naming a service that we already provided anyway. The "Barefoot Trimmers" have found a niche in the farrier industry and have taken full advantage of it. Once they named it and made it seem like something different, the horse owning public was misled to think it is only one way or the other. We are all barefoot trimmers, it just so happens that some have skills beyond that level that allow the application of a shoe. As a result, we should also be advertising our barefoot trimming services. If it makes the customer feel better, you can charge more for the named trim, just make it a good, solid, tried and true, conventional trim.

My advice to any youngster who is trying to find their way in this trade is to find an excellent craftsman at making and applying horseshoes, one who is recognized by the farrier industry and his or her peers as being at the top of the trade. Emulate that craftsman so that you too can someday be among the ranks of those who know how a foot is made, how it works, and how they fit into that system to help the horse not hurt it.

Chapter 35 MYTHS OF FARRIERY

Thinking around things that you need to think around.

In the equine industries, there are often statements made that sound clever when first heard, but in reality make little, if any, sense. For some reason, when a nonsensical comment is made concerning a horse, it takes on a different air about it. Unfortunately for many beginners to the trade, these statements become fact without thought. It is my hope that this section can make you think about some of these pearls of wisdom in a new way.

I once read an article about a man who was well known for thinking about things in non-traditional ways. For instance, he talked about what we do when we want to put a hole in a piece of wood. We go to the store and buy a drill and drill-bit, but that is not what we really wanted. We wanted a hole. He also mentioned that we buy cars to get us from point A to point B, but the car spends only a fraction of its energy transporting us, and the bulk of its energy transporting the car. If we truly wanted only to get a person from point A to point B, cars would have a much different design.

Because of human nature, many of us like to have a powerful drill and accessories that give us the hole we want and the potential for future holes. We also like the status that driving a nice car allows, even though it may take more energy than required to do the main job we wanted done, getting us to where the car is going. Thinking about things from different angles can be really useful to the farrier who is trying to figure out how best to serve the equine and its owners.

Following is one of the most common foolish "pearls" of wisdom that often bounces around farrier gatherings: "To fix a horse that overreaches, speed up the front, and slow down the hinds." Not only did I hear this a lot when I was starting out, I have also read it in some of the more common and popular textbooks on horseshoeing. At first, this seems to make a lot of sense. And in fact, if it was possible to speed up the fronts and slow down the hinds, you would really prevent a lot of over-reaching. Although I have heard this from many farriers, I have yet to meet any who could tell me how to accomplish it. Pixar demonstrates the principle in the movie *Toy Story*. Remember the Slinky-dog grabbing onto the back of the moving van? As the van accelerated, the front went faster than the hinds, and the result was a longer Slinky-dog. Since horses lack the slinky in the middle, we have to deal with a backbone that makes the hinds go the same speed as the fronts. It is a guarantee that if the fronts of a horse are travelling at 10 miles per hour, the hinds will not be going at 9.9 mph, or 10.1 mph, they will be going at 10 miles per hour.

It is not a wonder that horses overreach, only that they don't overreach more. In **Figures 1 and 2**, you can get an idea of how a horse must be able to time the movement at speed of feet that it cannot see. In **Figure 3**, you can see a shoe that was lost from overreaching. That can create a dangerous moment for horse and rider.

Another gem that I used to recommend and think was pretty clever: "Horses will wear their feet to where they want them to be at." That sounds like it should make shoeing and hoof-prep a simple matter of following what the horse was doing to its feet naturally. I even used to advocate putting aluminum shoes on a horse to see where the feet wanted to wear. It was not until the Four-Point Trim theory really got some attention that I began to give this argument a lot of thought.

If you are involved in correcting any sort of angular limb deformity, you are aware that the lowest portion of the hoof will bear the most weight. For instance, a toed-out horse will wear the medial side of the hoof as the lateral side flares and gets longer. Why does the medial side wear more? Because, it is taking the most abuse from the conformational defect. As time passes without proper farrier intervention, the problem will get

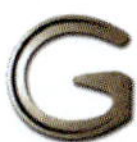

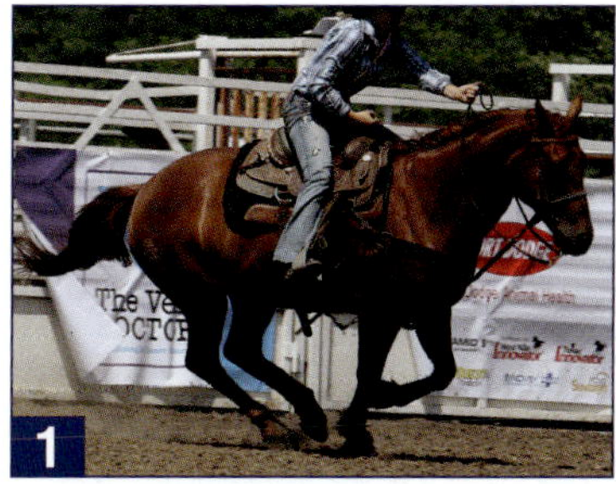

A Quarter Horse that is used for goat tying.

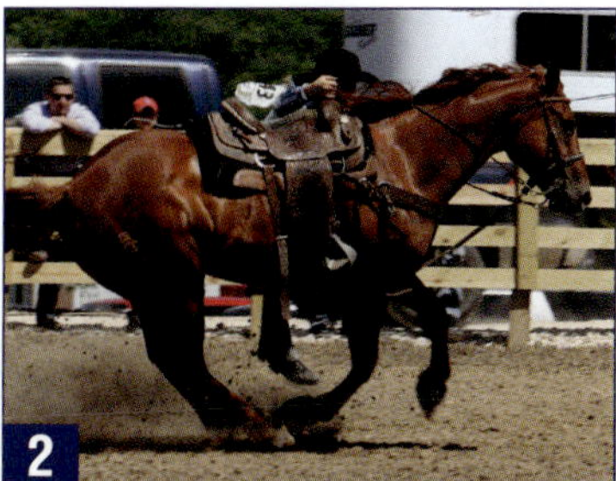

The same horse having to deal with the rider getting off at speed.

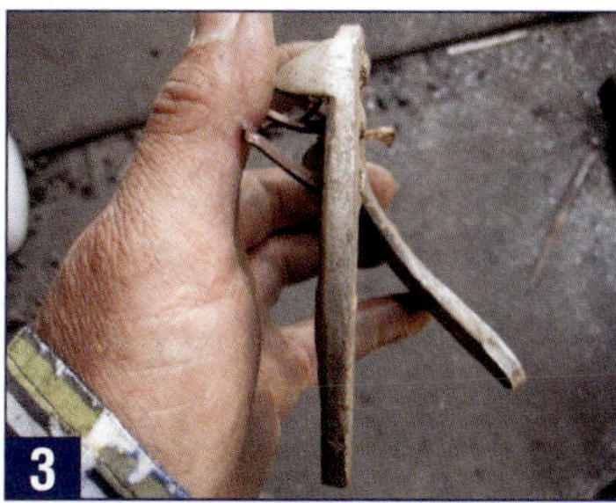

A shoe that was stepped off when the hind foot hit the front.

progressively worse. This would not be happening if the statement made was true, and the horse was wearing the feet to the level where it wanted them.

Now consider hearing this statement from a shoe salesman: "As a man walks in his boots over abrasive terrain for many miles, he will wear his boot to the level he wants his foot to be at. The posterior-lateral heel should be removed on all new boots, since studies have indicated that this is the area where most wear occurs in walking humans."

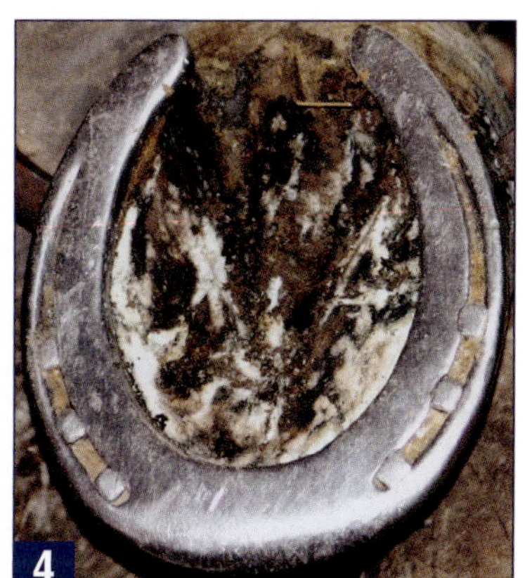

Toe-weight with wear on the lateral toe.

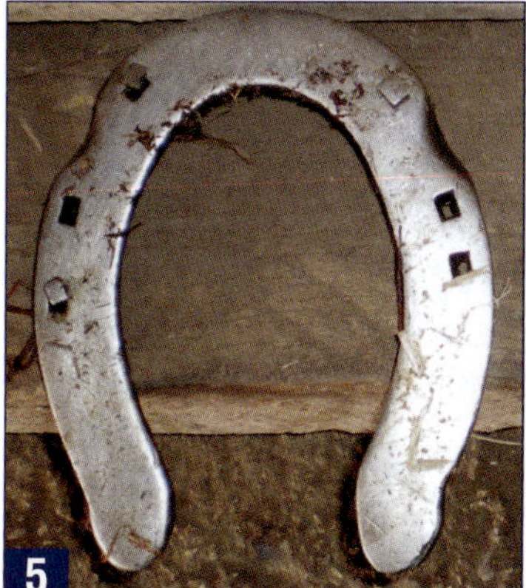

Evenly worn hind shoe.

Sounds pretty asinine when you think of it from that perspective. I don't think that the boot salesman would make a lot of sales if he rasped off the lateral heel of new boots because of the results of the study, and a lot of us would have backs that hurt even worse if we were to buy boots from that salesman.

In fact, the amount of the wear on my boots is in direct relation to how my back and hips are feeling. More wear means more aches, which means I need new boots.

The area that is wearing away is a high-wear area. As such, how does taking it away before the horse has a chance to wear it make any sense? Doing so makes as much sense as rasping the tread off of your brand new tires to make your truck go down the road better, based on the wear from the tires that were just removed.

Figure 4 shows a toe-weight with fairly common wear of the lateral toe. In **Figure 5** you can see the ideal even wear of a hind shoe.

When I was a kid at New Mexico Military Institute, I was on the rodeo team and had a horse with a crack in its foot. It was not much of a crack, but it was enough to bother me. I was about 16, so I was at that brilliant stage that only accompanies youth, and I had the horseshoer that shod the horses at the school rasp a line across that crack. He did me one better though, and rasped an X across it. He explained that an X dispersed the forces to 4 points. This was 1984, and that horse had that crack as long as I had him (sure wish I had a picture of that foot).

Anyway, I had been taught to deal with those pesky cracks with a little hash mark. When you think about it from an anatomical point of view, it is amazing that it was ever done the first time, much less on the thousands of horses it has been done to since. I have seen this on horses from Brazil to Africa to Australia, and I have yet to see one where the crack comes to a dead stop at the hash mark.

You would have to go through the entire thick-

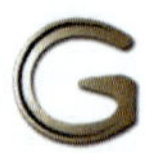

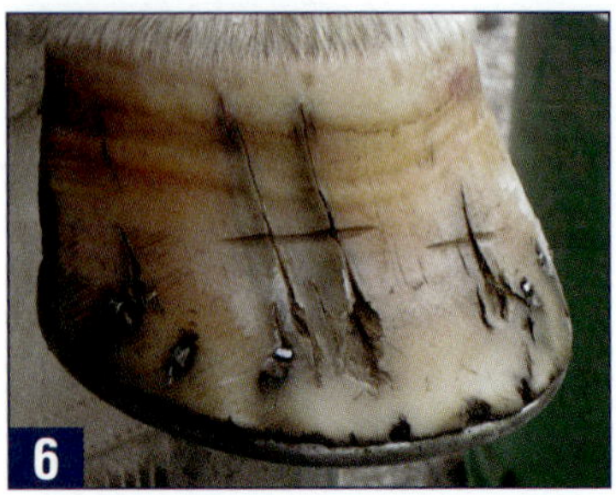

Cracks running through lines filed by a horseshoer or owner.

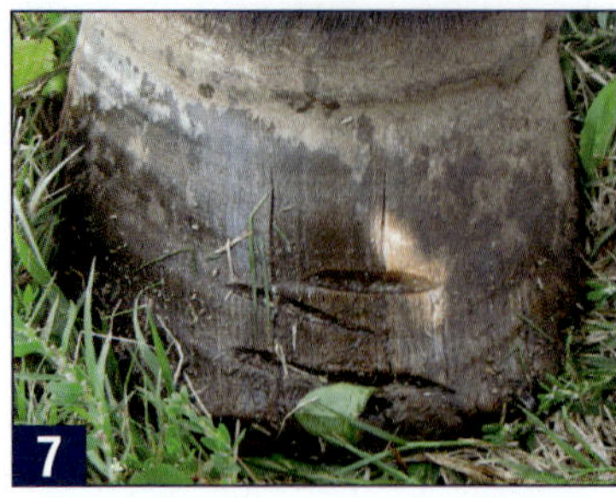

More cracks mean more lines to file.

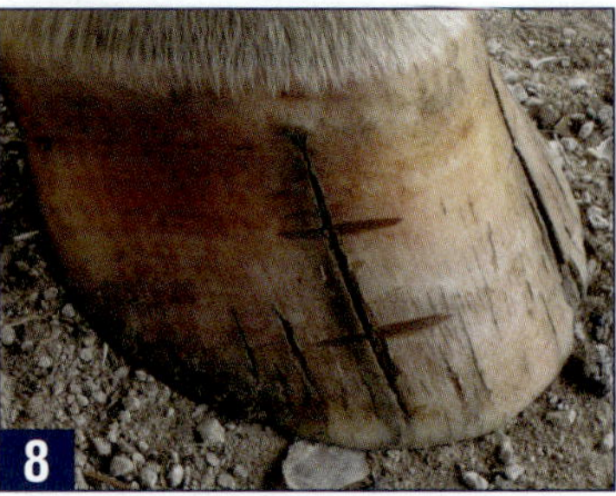

More hash marks with more cracks running through them.

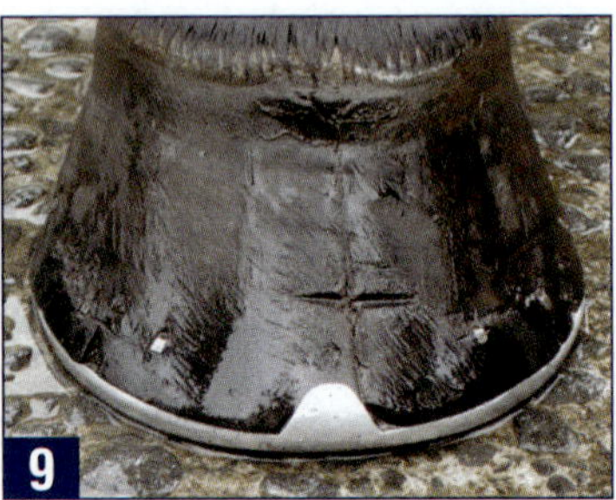

Racehorse in New Zealand with a line filed across the crack.

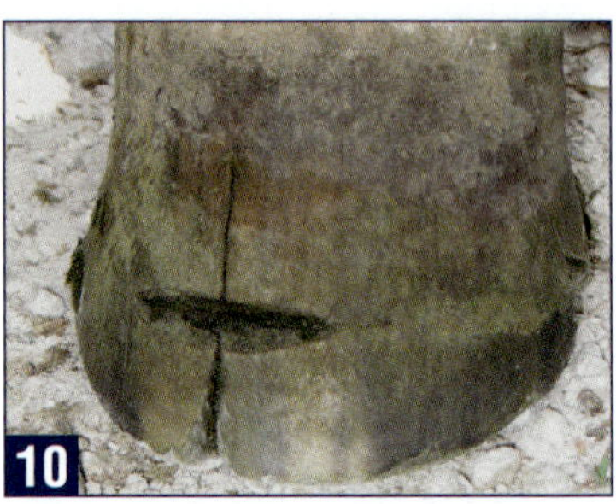

This one was filed deep — without success.

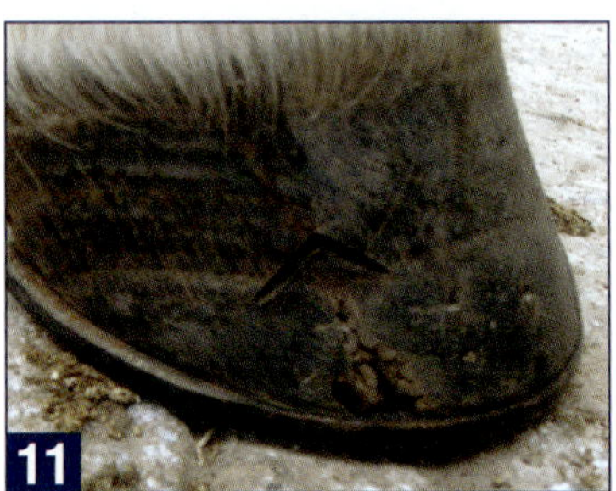

This is a horse in Brazil that the farrier burned an angled shape across the crack.

ness of the hoof wall to make that happen, and there is a bigger chance of harm from that fix than from most cracks anyway. Most of the time, the person filing the crack likes to file it at the very top of the crack. As such, you can often see that the lines were of no use since the crack continues through the line.

If you get clients who insists you file across hoof cracks, try telling them the tubular structure of the foot can be compared to the grains in a piece of wood. If you were to have a piece of 1-by-6-inch lumber that had a crack with the grain, do you think that carving a little line across it would help? Of course not! Yet many people think the same approach will help a horse. I am including several pictures **(Figures 6-11)** here so that you can show this to customers in the hope that they will quit asking farriers to do this. Perhaps we can kill this myth.

One that I have not heard in a long time — thankfully — is about full-fit shoes. It is true that the foot will expand when it bears weight, and a shoe should be wide enough on a foot to accommodate that hoof expansion, but there have been those who take it to the extreme. I have seen horses that were fit so full outside the foot that the buttress wasn't covered.

Putting a platform beyond the hoof capsule to the extent that the hoof capsule is not even completely on the platform does not make sense in a normal situation. There are lameness problems and situations where extreme fit is okay, but they don't exist on every horse.

When I asked a farrier at a clinic one time why he fit his horse so full, he responded by telling me that the full fit would put less weight on the foot. How can that be possible? If that worked, you could wear a pair of snowshoes when you got on the scales and lose all kinds of weight. Again, it is something that is said, sounds reasonable enough, but really does not make any sense.

Next we have the case of a horse that has graveled. The term "gravel" is actually used in veterinarian and farrier textbooks to describe what happens when an abscess breaks out the coronary band. The myth that a piece of rock has worked its way into the hoof capsule, and then migrated proximad to break out the coronary band has not been proven. What's more, the concept of that happening does not make much sense. What does happen is

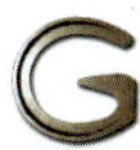

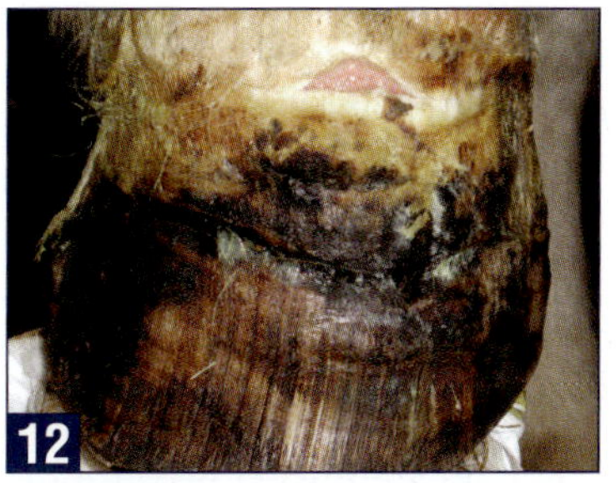

Foot with chronic infection breaking out the toe.

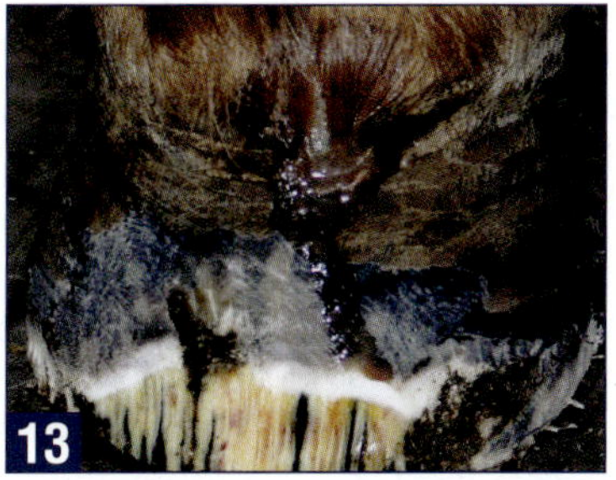

Pus discharge at the dorsal coronary band.

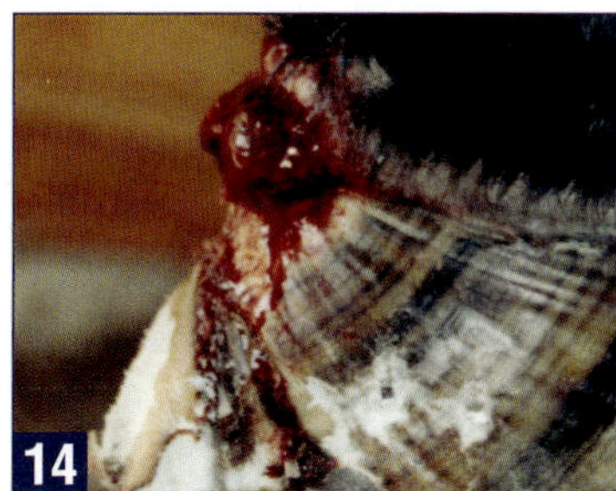

Infection that has broken out at the toe followed by blood.

that the bacteria in the abscess reproduces, releases gas in the process, and creates tracks that tear apart the path of least resistance.

When that path leads out through the coronary band, there is discharge present like that shown in **Figures 12-14**.

I can see where the idea of a piece of gravel came from. Horses are standing on dirt, sand and little rocks all the time, and the pus that drains will be sticky enough that a small rock could easily get into the wound and look like it was the cause. Even though it didn't cause the problem, it made itself look very suspicious by being there.

I don't know how many times I have heard someone watching a lame horse refer to the "short stride." Let us assume that we are evaluating a horse that is sore in the off front foot.

As the horse trots by, the off front is not hurting as much when it is in the air. However, it begins to hurt more as it hits the ground and hurts the most when it is completely loaded. To compensate for the pain, the horse will bob its head upwards as the off front becomes more loaded and the off front limb becomes perpendicular to the ground. The near front will come down closer to the off front foot, making it appear as if the horse has taken a shorter stride with the near front.

Here is what is really happening. There is a stance phase and swing phase to a stride. When the horse has contact with the ground, that foot is in the stance phase. As soon as the foot is no longer in contact with the ground, the foot is in the swing phase. There is also a dorsal and a palmar portion to the swing phase of each stride. As the near foot begins the stance phase, the off foot will leave the ground and begin the palmar portion of the swing phase. Once the off foot comes even with the near leg, the palmar portion of the swing phase ends, and the dorsal portion begins.

A horse that is lame on the off front will have a longer dorsal phase with the off front and a shorter palmar phase. In contrast, the near front will have a longer palmar phase and a shorter dorsal phase. However, each foot will end up traveling the same distance in its respective step, as long as the horse is moving in a straight line. It is guaranteed that if the off fore is travelling 6 feet per stride, the near fore is doing the same.

Try to imagine what would happen if it were physically possible for the horse to have different stride lengths. If there was a length difference of only 2 inches, within 12 steps, one foot would be 2 feet behind the other. The next time someone points out a horse that has a "short stride," ask them to give you lengths in feet or meters. They will say something like, "One leg is going 6 feet, and the opposite is going 5 feet."

Impossible. If the horse is walking in an arc, the inside stride will be shorter. In a straight line, the length has to be the same from side to side.

Added to the length-of-stride myth is the idea of breakover changing the speed and length of a stride. The myth is that if you stand a horse up steep, or use a rocker or square toe, the foot will break over faster and make a horse quicker, even though the length of the step will become shorter. This approach is popular among Western riders.

Conversely, the wisdom goes, if you lengthen the toe and lower the heels, the horse will get a longer stride due to the leverage that the longer toe provides. Racehorse trainers are fond of this theory. Both of these can sound plausible to the uneducated farrier or horseman, so they have gained widespread acceptance in a short time.

What often happens is that an incredibly athletic

horse wins some event, despite being shod poorly, and people credit the shoeing style for the win. Pretty soon, that shoeing style is a fad with a certain group. However, if you look closely at the theory, it doesn't hold up.

To disprove this theory quickly, nail a reverse wedge pad on one foot, and a normal wedge pad on the opposite. You now have one foot set up for a long, fast step, and the other set up to have a shorter, quicker step. If the theory was 100% correct, the horse would now have to move at different speeds with different stride lengths. I know this is impossible, but an ignorant farrier or horseman would believe it.

There are cutting horses that do quite well with a naturally low angle on pasterns and feet, and racehorses that win despite being a little bit too upright. The fact of the matter is that a horse is going to move at its very best when it is shod at its natural angle. If you create a situation where a horse is too steep or too shallow, you stress one part of the suspensory apparatus while relaxing another. The ramifications of doing so can be a disaster for that horse. See the section on Biomechanics in this book to explain in detail how angle affects tendons.

Throughout history, trades have evolved through the forward thinking of their craftsmen. By challenging what is the norm, you may find another way of thinking about some facet of farriery that makes more sense. By the same token, you can be led down a road of foolishness and ignorance. If a fool is also charismatic and a good speaker, he may develop a following of people who are misled because the fool is so convincing. It confounds those that have a greater understanding of the anatomy and the trade as a whole.

My suggestion to all the young farriers whom I encounter is to base their decisions about shoeing theory on anatomy. If it does not make sense anatomically, it probably does not make sense. Apply anatomical knowledge to the items just mentioned, and you may find what you thought was a good idea was in fact a theory based on guesswork and tradition. It is your responsibility to the horse to make certain that you are doing what is in that horse's best interest. Become educated and thoughtful to avoid the traps that lay in wait for the average horseshoer.

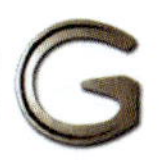

Section

9

In the Fire

Chapter 36: Intro to Forging 312

Chapter 37: Forging Basics 322

Chapter 38: Exercises in the Forge 336

Chapter 39: Tong Making 354

Chapter 40: The Basic Hind 359

Chapter 41: The Basic Front 371

Chapter 42: Using Concave to Make Shoes 381

" 25 Thy shoes shall be iron and brass;
and as thy days, so shall thy strength be. "

—Deuteronomy 33:25
—New King James Version

" 10 Beat your plowshares into swords and your pruning hooks into spears: let the weak say, I am strong. "

—Joel 3:10
—New King James Version

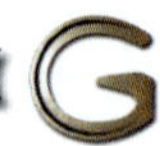

Chapter

36 INTRO TO FORGING

Forging is basically changing the shape of a piece of metal by heating it and applying force. As it pertains to the farrier, we are using a forge to heat the steel, an anvil and a hammer to apply the force needed to alter the shape, and sometimes a tool like a punch or creaser to make specific changes.

Most horseshoes are made from bar stock. When discussing dimensions of bar stock, it is referred to by the thickness and width. The width is always the largest measurement. A piece of ½-inch by 1-inch would have a thickness of ½ inch and a width of 1 inch. In the United States, we tend to say the thickness first, followed by the width. In the United Kingdom, the thickness is often stated first, so they would describe the same piece of stock just mentioned as 1-by-1/2 inch.

There are basically four things that a blacksmith can do with hot steel: cut, draw, upset, and weld. Let's look at each one.

Cut: This application is done with either a hardy that fits in the accommodating hole in the anvil for that purpose, or with a handled tool of transmission.

Hardies and cutting tools come in a variety of shapes and sizes for many different applications. **Figures 1-3** show cutting hot steel, and **Figure 4** shows cutting the frog plate in an aluminum heart bar. Once the cut is made most of the way through the piece, it can be moved to the hardy hole **(Figure 5)** or the edge of the anvil **(Figure 6)** to finish the cut without damaging the sharp end of the cutting tool. It is handy to have a copper plate to put on the anvil for cutting.

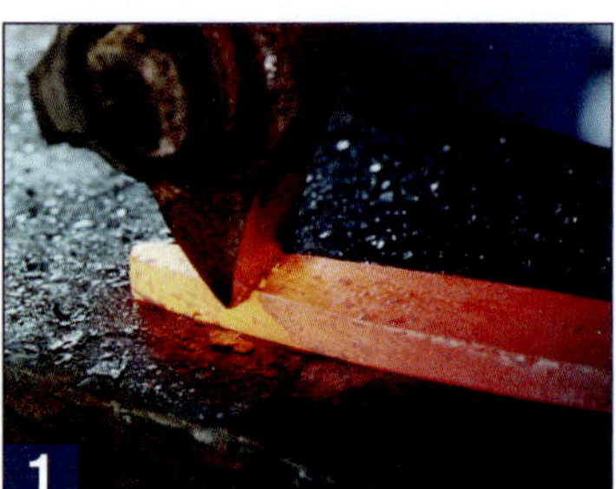

1 *Cutting hot steel.*

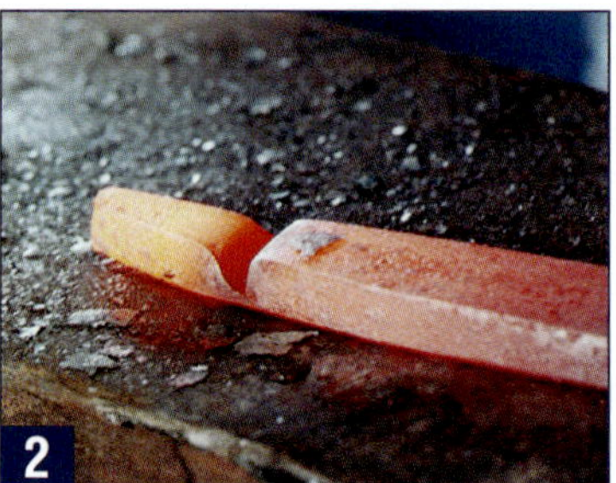

2 *The cut is most of the way through.*

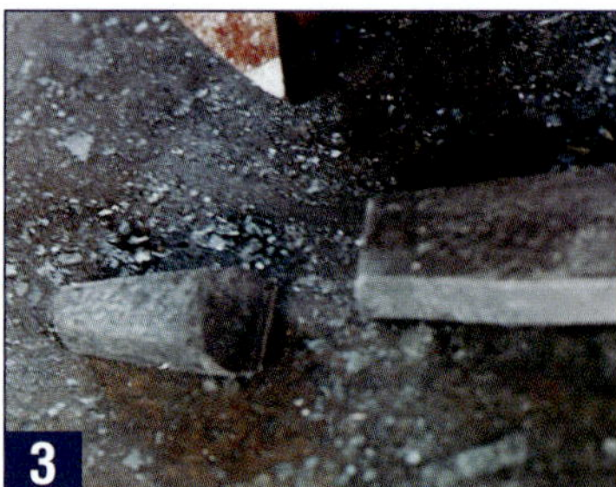

3 *The piece is cut off.*

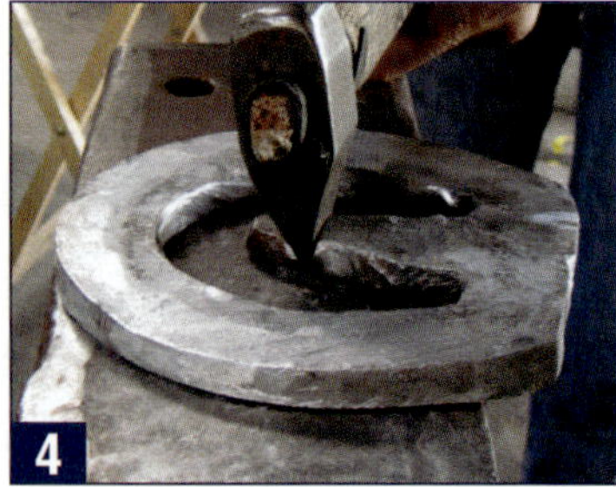

4

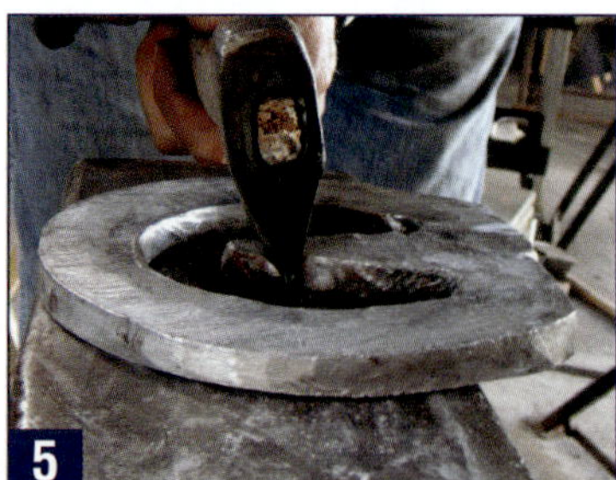

5

Cutting the frog plate on an aluminum shoe.

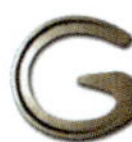

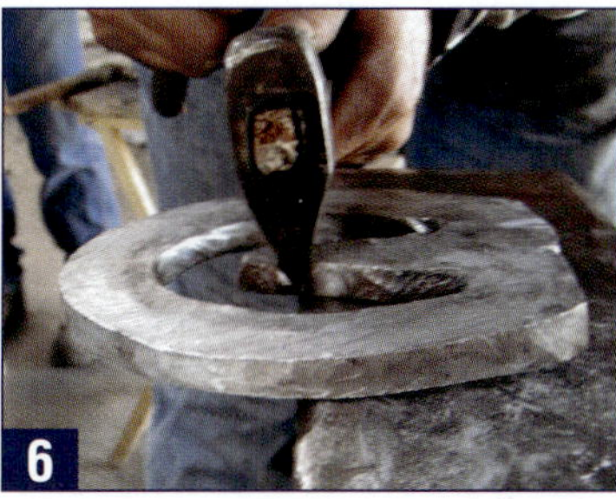
Moving to the edge of the anvil to cut through the piece without hurting the anvil or the cutting tool.

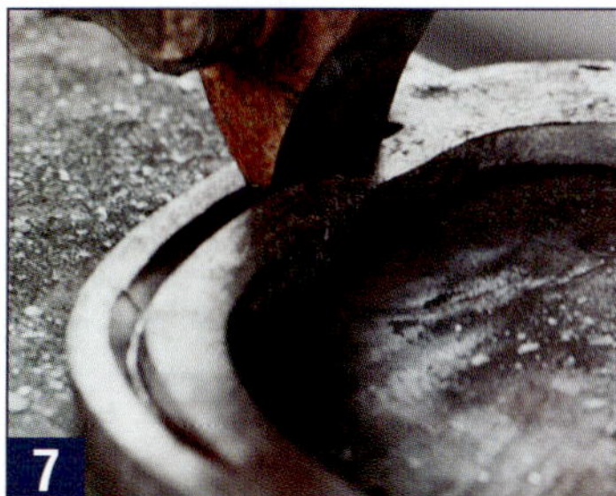
Fullering.

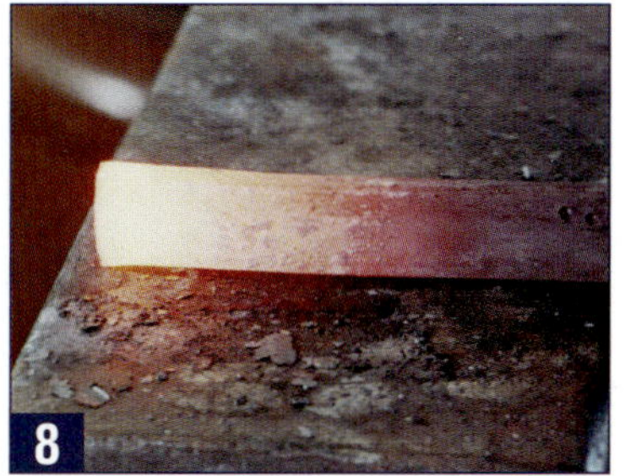

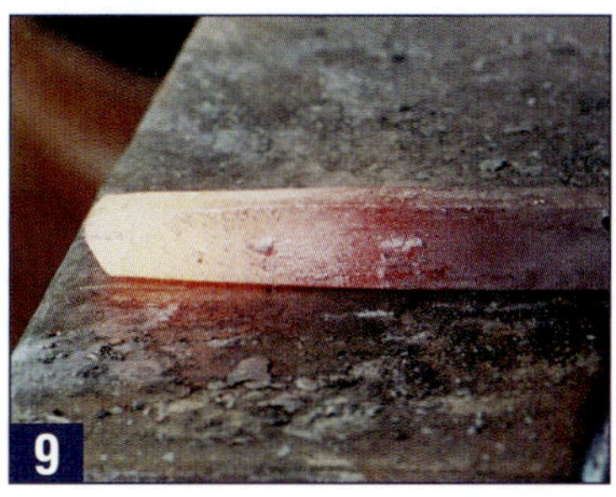

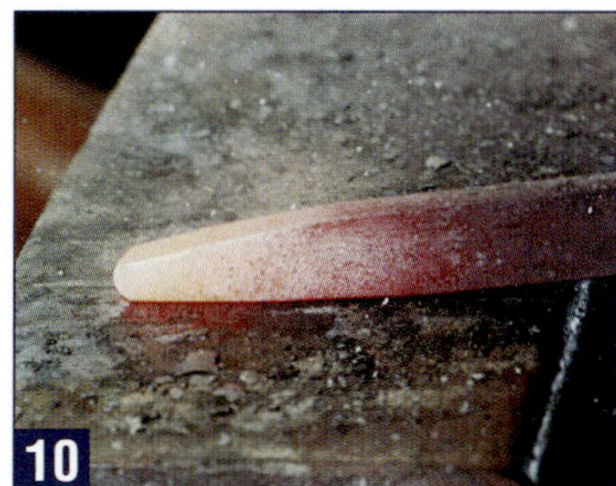
Drawing out a piece of hot steel.

A creaser, or fuller, is a shoemaking tool of transmission that is designed to cut hot steel. However, it is a controlled cut that is intended to leave a mark in the metal of a predetermined shape and depth **(Figure 7)**.

Draw: Stock is drawn when a given piece is made longer while the cross-section of the piece is diminished. For instance, a 10-inch piece of 1/4 by 1 inches will become 11 inches of 1/4- by 3/4 inch if it is drawn to that dimension. **Figures 8-10** show a piece of bar stock that is being drawn out on the anvil by repeated hammer blows. **Figure 11** shows the steps used to forge a hoof pick. A horseshoe is cut, drawn to the correct dimension, then bent into shape. In **Figure 12**, the edge of the hammer is being used to draw a clip.

Upset: This is the opposite of draw. When a piece of stock is upset, the length is diminished

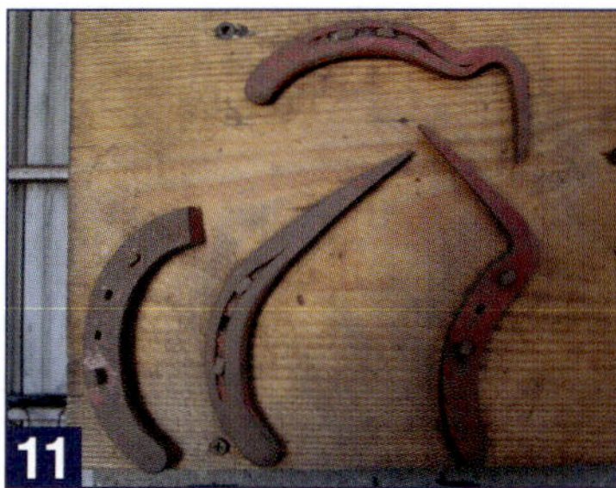
Steps in making a hoof pick.

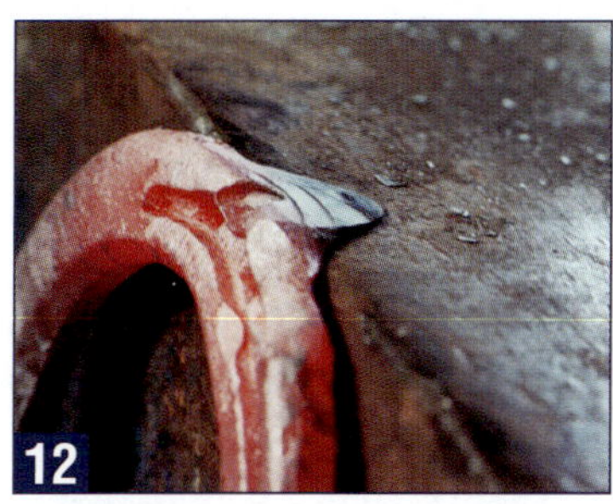
Drawing a clip with the edge of the hammer.

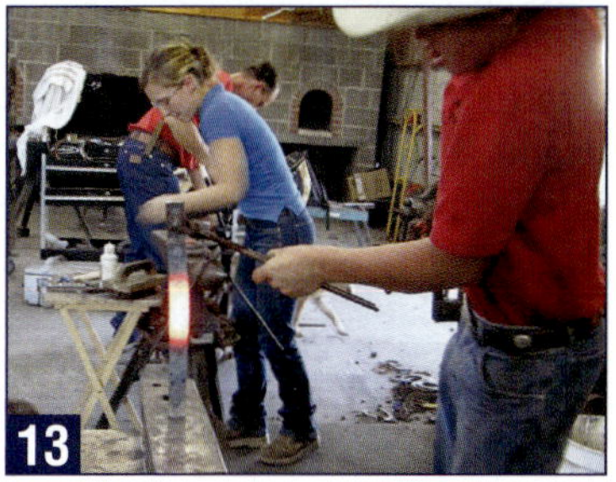

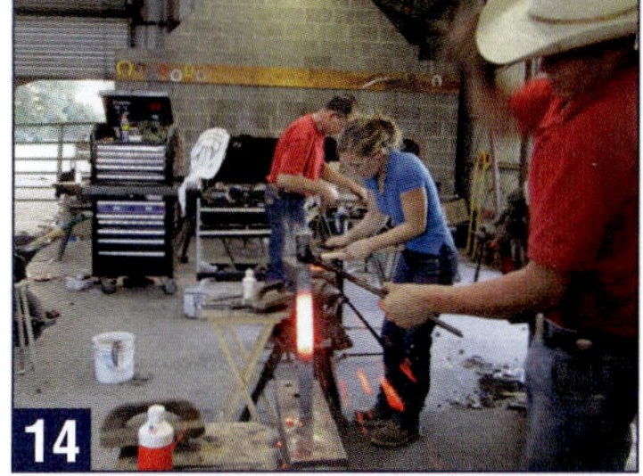
Figures 13 - 14: Cody bumping the toe of a shoe.

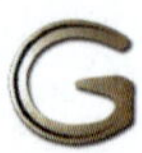

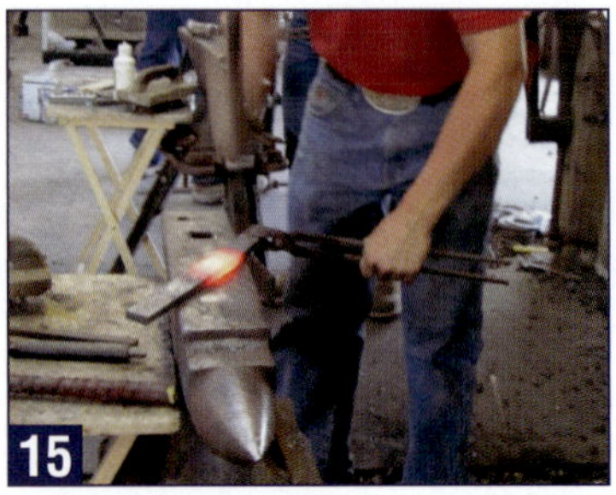

15

Leveling the piece during the bumping process.

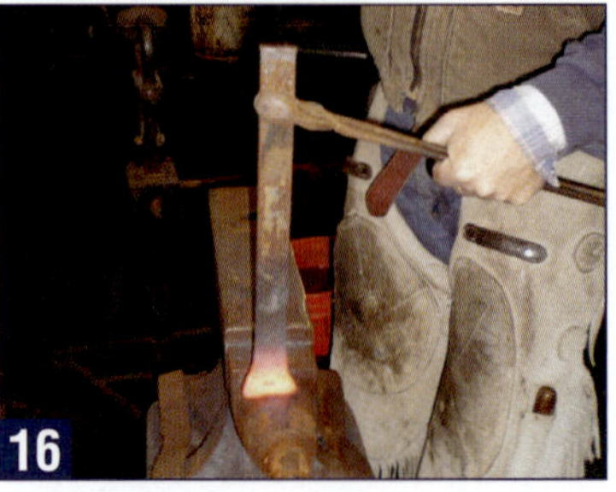

16

Bumping on the horn to make the bottom of the piece spread faster.

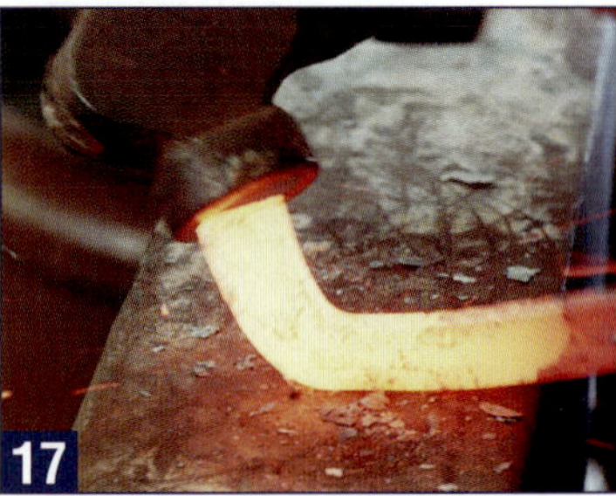

17

Upsetting the steel to make a "hockey stick".

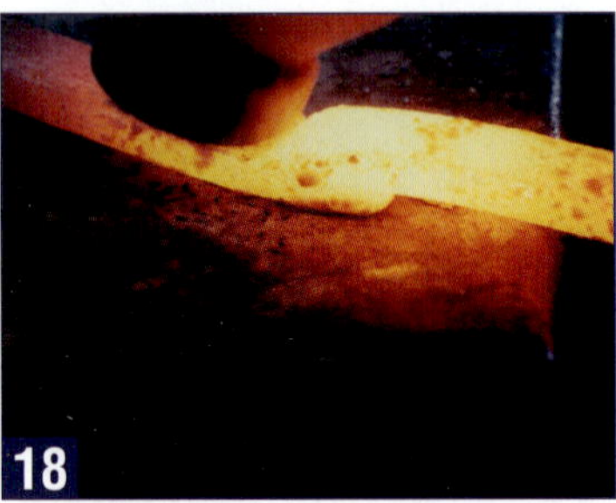

18

Welding with the corner of the hammer.

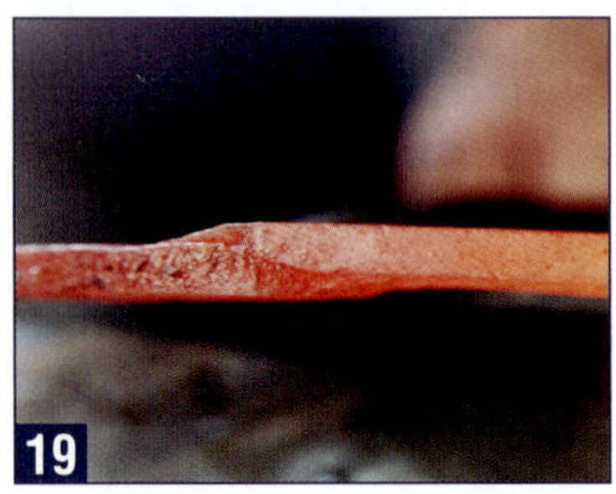

19

The pieces after the first jump weld.

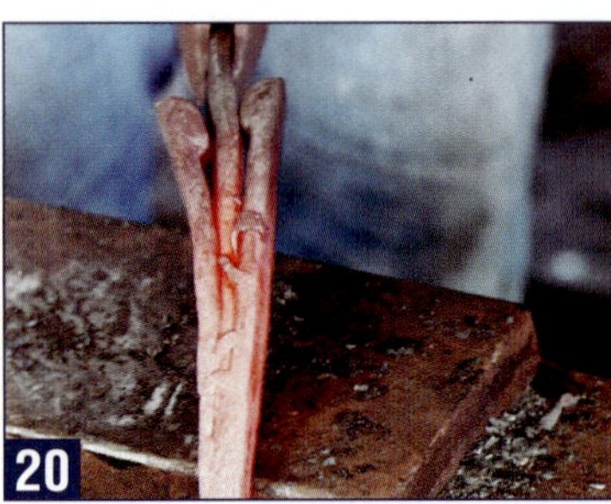

20

Early in the process of making a horseshoe sandwich.

while the cross-section is increased. For instance, a 6-inch piece of 5/16-by-3/4 inch can be upset into a 3-inch piece of 5/8-inch square. In **Figures 13 and 14**, Cody is bumping the center of a piece of bar stock to make a stronger toe in a shoe. When the steel bends, it has to be straightened **(Figure 15)** so that the force of the blow is driven into the steel and not dissipated by the bend.

Figure 16 is a picture of a piece of steel that is being upset on one end on the top of the horn. By quenching the area of the steel that is the correct dimension, upsetting can be directed to only a portion of the stock. Using the horn makes the piece spread more in 2 directions. Upsetting is the basis of making a hockey stick on a bar shoe **(Figure 17)**.

Weld: Welding occurs when two pieces of metal are joined together by heat and proper hammering. Many believe that welding is the most difficult task that a blacksmith has to do, but that is a fallacy. **Figures 18 and 19** show a forge weld between 2 separate pieces of steel, and **Figure 20** is the beginnings of a horseshoe sandwich.

Bend and Twist: Bending or twisting is considered by some as an additional application that a blacksmith can do to hot steel, but when bending, the inside of the stock is being upset and the outside is being drawn. **Figure 21** shows a toe bend being made in a piece of stock, and **Figure 22** is the beginnings of a heel caulk being bent over the edge of the anvil. When twisting stock of any shape other than round, the outside is being drawn. If twisting round stock, there should be no visible change in the metal.

There are several types of forges used by blacksmiths. In the United States, the common ones found in farrier shops and shoeing rigs are either propane or coal/coke. It is not overly important which type of forge you prefer as long as it is able to consistently heat steel to the desired temperature. My personal favorite is a side-blast coke forge. Due to the availability of firepots versus a side-blast tuyere, I use a bottom-blast coke forge for 75% of the work that I do. For the majority of the work done in the field, I use a propane forge. You can find out more about forges in Chapter 5, Your Shoeing Shop.

BUILDING SKILLS

Every horseshoe can be broken down into a series of tasks. If you approach your forging with that in mind, it will be easier to practice individual

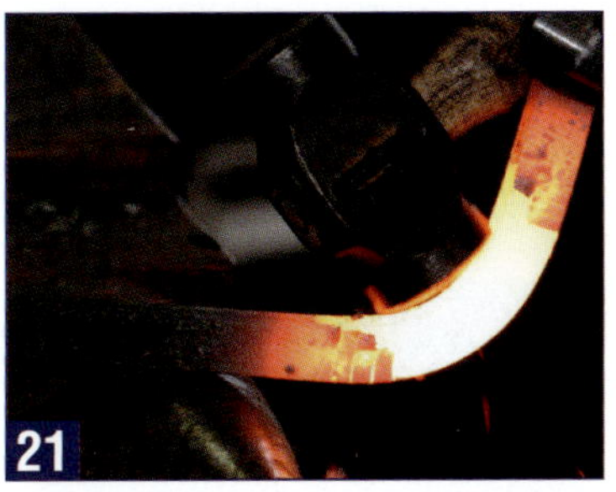

Making a toe bend with an angled blow and the round side of the hammer.

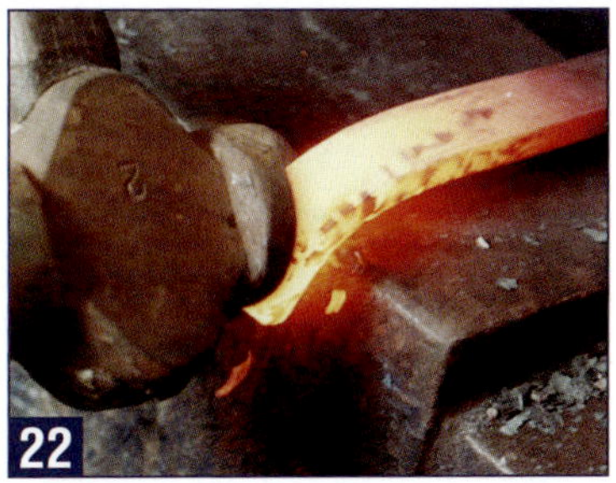

Bending the stock to make a heel caulk.

tasks on a repetitive basis in order to complete an entire project as a better piece. For instance, if you are having trouble with building heels, practice just building heels until they have become quick and easy. This practice will pay off when you are making the heels on a shoe.

Mastering each individual task in the shoe making process is the method I use to teach my students to build the final product.

The same holds true for most of the skills needed by a farrier. There are some farrier businesses that are run with several farriers working together. For efficiency, there will be one person assigned to a particular task in the shoeing process, and many horses can be shod with superior quality and speed.

It works like this; one farrier will pull shoes and do knife work, the next will trim while another is building the shoes. There will be one to nail and one to finish. The work of 10 individual farriers can be done in the same amount of time by 5.

This is the principle of the assembly line applied to shoeing, however, the quality is top notch. Each person on the team becomes extremely competent at one individual task. Every so often they will shift and each move to another position. In this way, they are able to eventually become very good at the whole job.

Approach any new skill you are trying to master from this perspective. Break it down into simple tasks, master each of those tasks, and finally put the individual tasks together to master the whole job.

KNOWING YOUR ANVIL HORN

All of the skills presented in this text are being done on a round-horn anvil. Having a round horn is perhaps the most important aspect of a good anvil. The shoes you will be building are actually forged into the shape of the horn, and the shape can be predicted and controlled when the horn is round. With flat-horned anvils, the metal has to be forged in the air to a perceived correct shape, instead of using the horn for an exact die of the desired shape. Forging on a flat horned anvil is often referred to as working on the "mystery tour."

Using your horn correctly can be difficult, especially for those who have been forging for some time without having been taught to efficiently use the horn. I fell into this category and had been competing for several years when Bob Marshall began to show me the correct way. I was ready to kill something out of frustration after that first clinic. You have to go backward a long way to finally begin going forward.

Having a complete understanding of the principles involved is the best place to start. If you can wrap your mind around the concept, you will be better able to apply it once you hit the shop. Study this section carefully and stay true to form. You will learn what you practice, so practicing with attention to detail and discipline will advance your skills faster than just spending time spinning your wheels.

With a round-horn anvil, the shape of the horn goes from a tight, consistent radius at the tip, to a larger, consistent radius at the step where the horn meets the anvil body. There are literally thousands of radiuses from the tip to base. Add to that the radiuses that exist if the horn is approached from an angle. By turning slightly, a larger radius can be achieved, all the way to a straight line across the top dead center of the horn. Every hoof, from the pony to the draft, has radiuses that can be found on a proper round-horn anvil.

Divide the horn into three separate regions by drawing a line along the top and a line from the

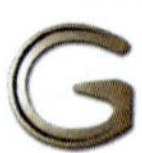

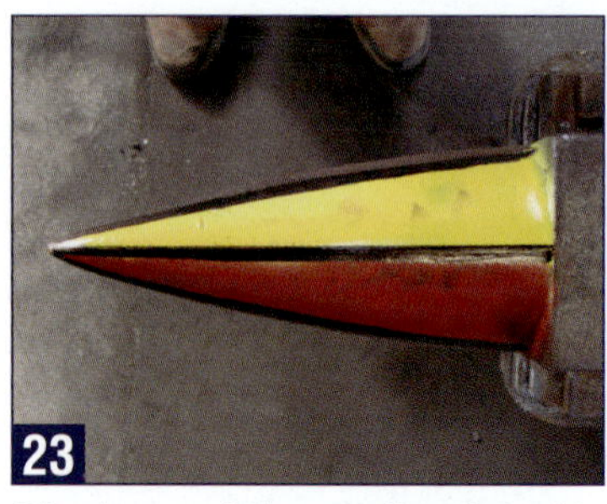

The horn of the anvil painted to define the forging zones.

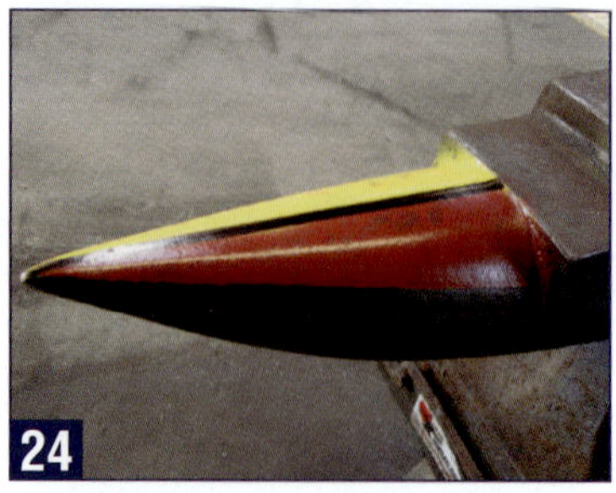

Near side of the horn, red, which would be the straightening side.

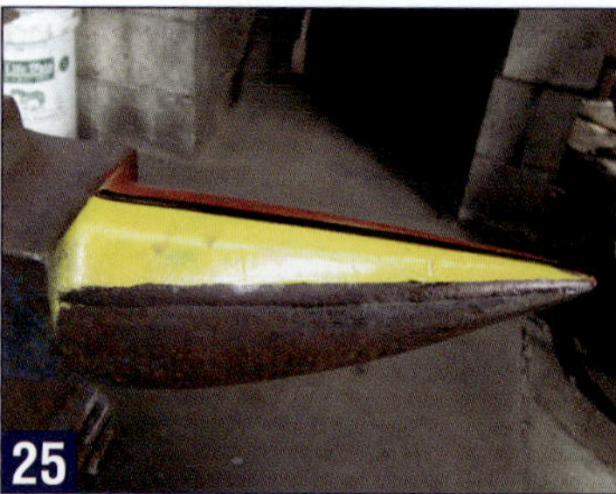

Off side of the horn, yellow, which would be the bending side for a right-handed person.

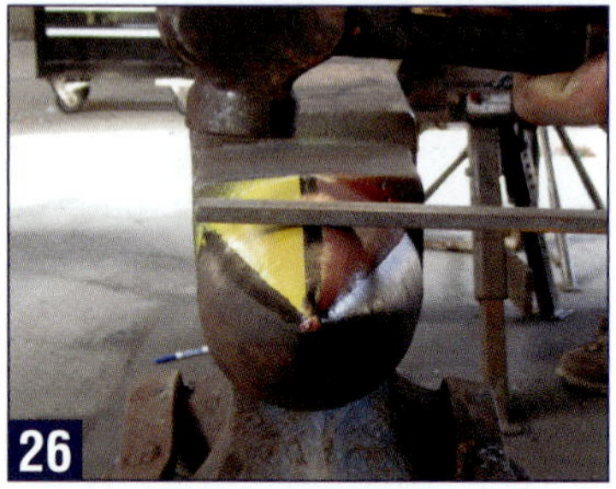

Cold stock in position to be bent with the hammer coming down in the bending zone.

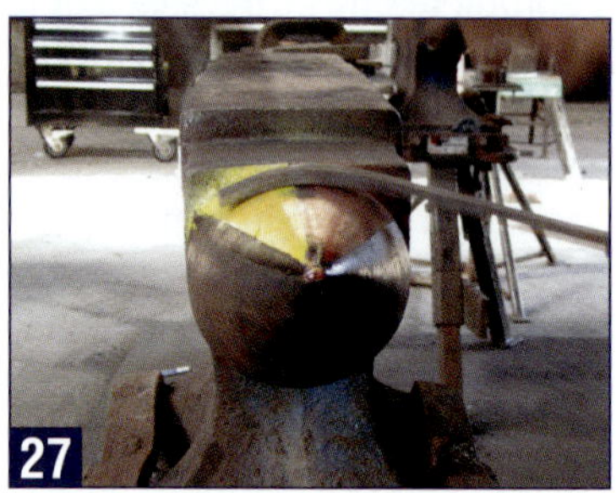

28

The stock is bent by driving it into the die of the round horn and dropping the tong hand.

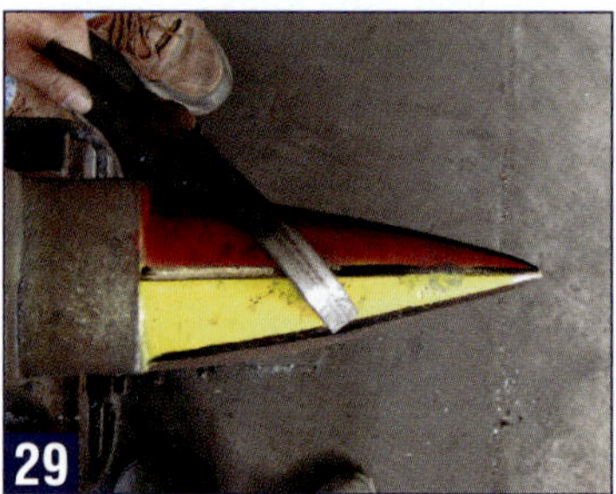

Placing the stock on the horn to straighten it, bird's eye view.

base of the horn to the tip on each side. There will be two triangles defined on top of the horn **(Figure 23)**. The one on the near side is the straightening zone, the far side is the bending zone, and the top dead center (anvil ridge) is the maintenance zone. Being right handed, I stand at the anvil with the horn facing toward the left. **Figure 24** shows the horn pointing left. The red side of the horn is the side I use for straightening. **Figure 25** is the opposite side of the horn, and the yellow portion would be my bending zone.

Ninety-nine percent of your forging should be done within these zones. There are exceptions, however they are few. Frank Turley once told me that there is an appropriate time to drill a hole in a piece of metal without first using a center punch, he just didn't know when that appropriate time was. I feel the same way about the forging zones.

If a piece of metal is pressed (with a hammer blow) into the shape that the horn provides, the shape can be predicted and controlled. By knowing the radius that the horn represents, a consistent shape can be made time after time. If the metal is being forged in the air, or over a flat spot, the blacksmith has to stop where it "feels" right, and consistency is lost.

The horn on the anvil does not change. The radiuses are always there, waiting for the forger to put the metal in the correct position. When bending a piece of steel around the horn to a particular shape, we only want a very small gap to occur in the bending zone beyond the ridge of the horn. Move the steel just a little at a time. By getting into a rhythm where your tong hand and hammer hand are in sync, moving slowly with precision, a shoe can be made quickly and consistently. It just takes practice.

To test the power of using the forging zones, try

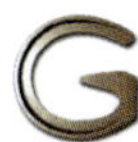

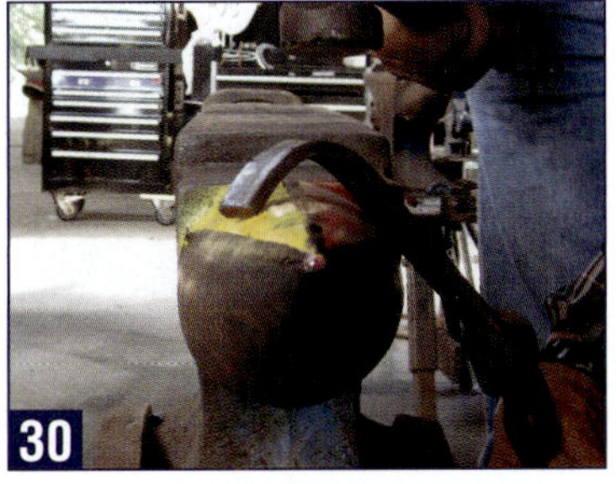

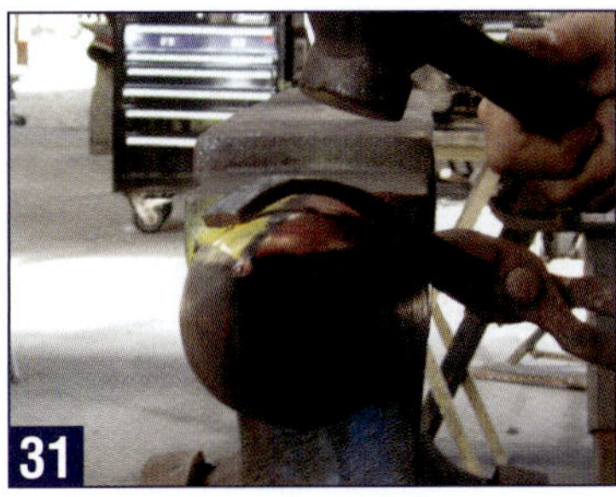

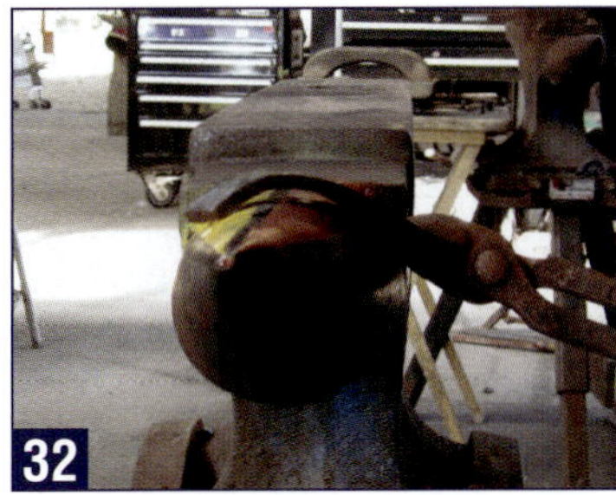

Straightening the stock by hammering into the near side of the horn.

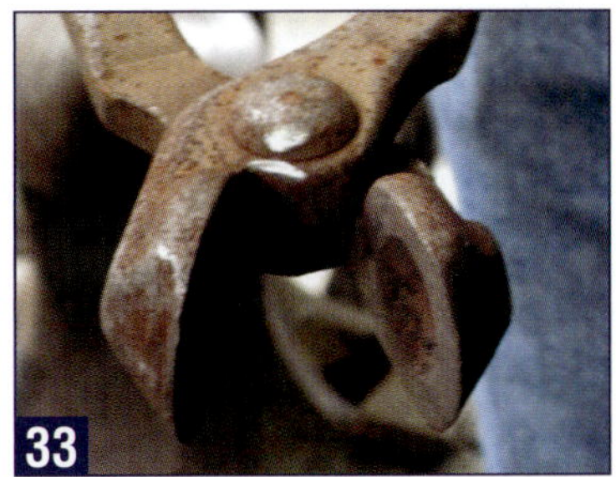

Inside of the tongs, notice the shiny spot on the corner of the boss.

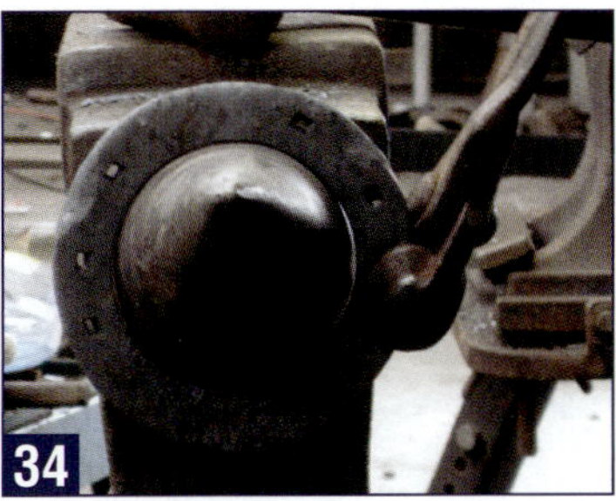

Tong position with three points of contact with the tongs.

taking a length of 5/16-by-3/4-inch bar stock and lay it on the horn so that only a short piece of the bar stock extends past the top centerline of the horn **(Figure 26)**. Hammer lightly so that the heel of the hammer is in line with the anvil ridge and the force of the blow is directed into the bending zone. It will take only a few hammer blows, and not much power, to make the cold stock bend to the radius of the horn **(Figure 27 and 28)**. If this works so easily on cold stock, imagine how well it will work on hot steel when it is done with skill and precision.

To straighten the piece I just bent, I turn so that I find a longer radius on the horn. **Figure 29** shows the angle that I am at from above. In **Figures 30-32**, the piece is being straightened by my hammer coming down on the straight side of the horn, with the piece being held so that there is a gap on that side for it to be pushed into.

The method being described can be compared to martial arts, while forging on the mystery tour can be considered street fighting. For a street fighter, power and strength are more important than skill, while a skilled martial-arts expert can be smaller and much weaker than the opponent that is defeated. Forging is not about strength or power. It is about technique, skill, practice, and ability to apply some practical physics.

TONG POSITION

A lot is happening when a shoe is being made. Competent craftsmen can make it look simple and easy. The work flows off the anvil with the speed and grace that is the definition of poetry in motion. Because so much is going on, spectators often focus on just what is happening to the metal being forged. It is bright, giving off light and changing color as it changes shape. No wonder that it is such a draw for the eye. But there are a lot of things that the observer should be focusing on.

As you gain experience, you will start to notice what is happening in the periphery: Where the smith stands behind the anvil; where the tongs are being held; where the piece is being held by the tongs; what heat each task is being done at; why certain things are done in a special order; etc. Try to see the whole picture the next time you have the opportunity to watch a skilled forger.

The position of the tongs is as important as how the hammer is wielded. There are three areas of contact that can be used with most common farrier

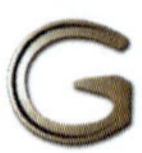

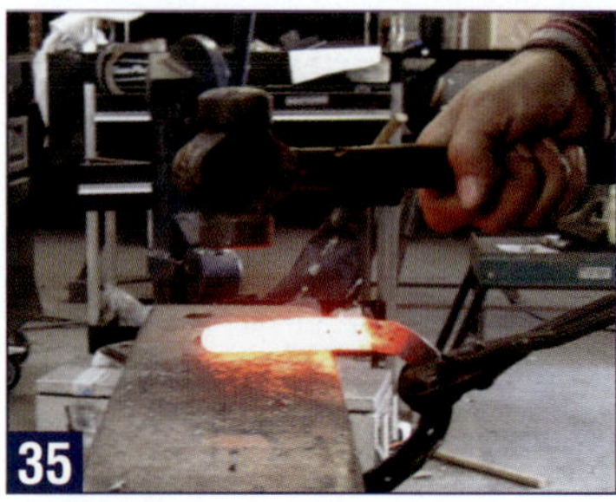

Flat hammer blow.

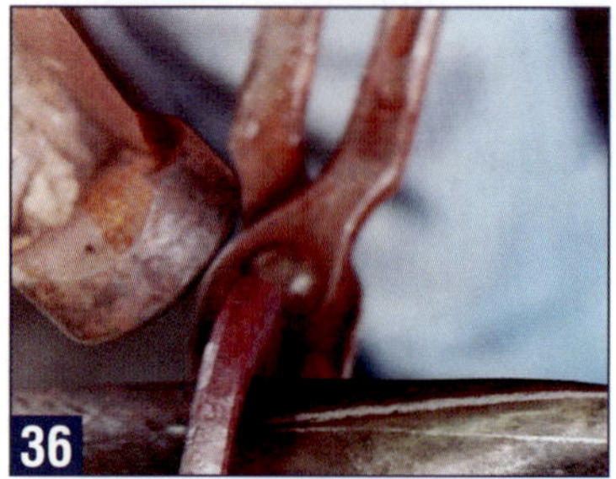

Angled hammer blow made by turning the hammer in your hand, hemming a shoe.

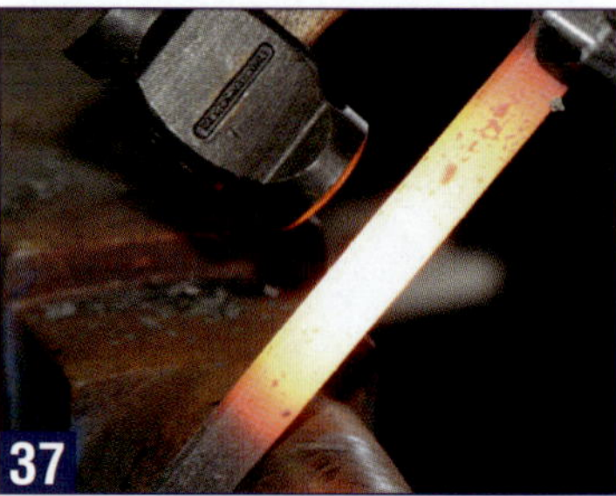

Angled hammer blow to make a toe bend.

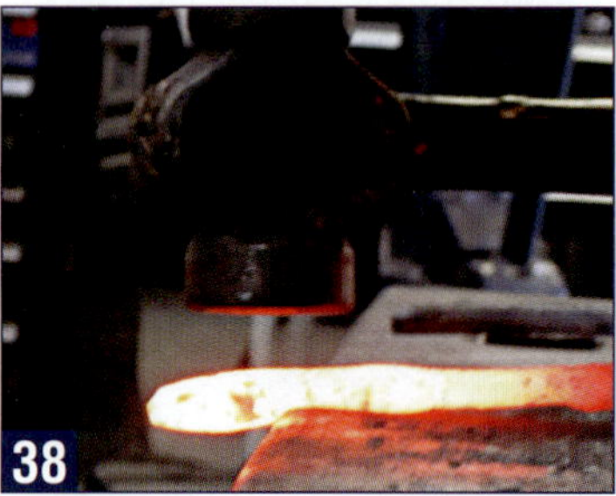

Half face or shouldering hammer blow.

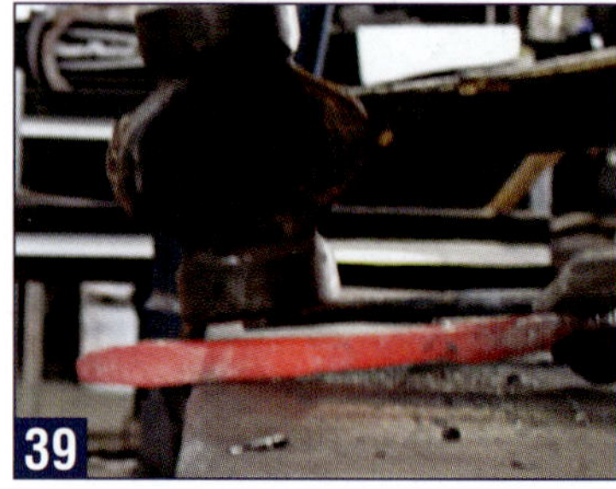

Edge-to-edge hammer blow.

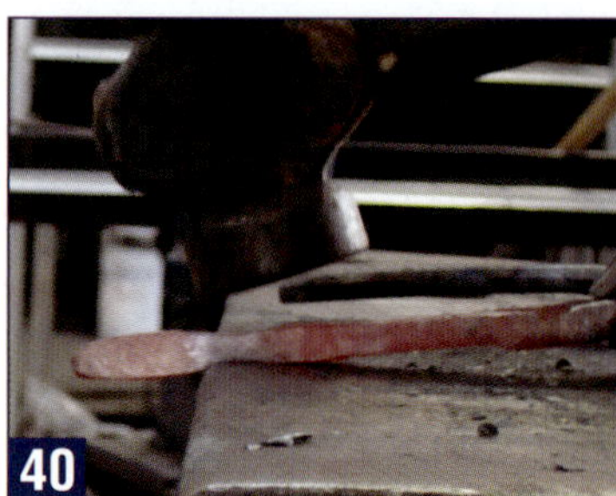

tongs. These areas are both jaws and the inside of the boss. **Figure 33** shows the inside of the boss is shiny from being in contact with the shoes being worked, and **Figure 34** shows the proper position of the tongs on a ring. Knowing how and when to apply the leverage available from the tongs is important. Most of us hold our tongs in our "off" hand. That means those who are right-handed swing the hammer with the right hand as the left hand manipulates the steel and tongs. It takes a long time to get the right and left hands to work well together. Pay close attention to the pictures in this book that include the tongs. Try to stay strict to form and make your tong hand work for you, not against you.

Roy Bloom, CJF, said it best when he said "this is labor," holding up his hammer hand, "and this is management," holding up his tong hand. "Labor and management don't get along unless you make them."

HAMMERING

The amount of power that comes from a well-delivered hammer blow is quite amazing. When you think about it, there are an almost infinite number of variables when it comes to hammering. The weight of the hammer, angle of the blow, height of the anvil, strength of the smith, hammer control, design of the hammer, length of the handle. The list goes on. Every forger needs to find a hammer design and weight that is appropriate. Bear in mind, that what works for some, may not work for others. In my early career, I tried to copy the styles of some folks with such different and opposing styles that I ended up actually setting myself back. You need to find someone who you respect enough to spend time with and who has a body type and forging style that you can mimic.

A basic farriers rounding hammer will weigh from 1 lb, 12 oz, to 2 lb, 8 oz. One face will be flat, and the opposite face will have a convex surface. The majority of hammering is done with the flat side. I tend to use the round side for hitting on the inside of a bend (such as a toe bend) and for striking the top of punches or upsetting stock.

While hammering, accelerate the upward swing from the level of the anvil to about half way through the swing. Once the hammer reaches the apex of the swing, accelerate for about the first half of the down swing. Allow yourself to relax as much as possible so that you will be able to forge for extended periods of time. Don't grip the hammer and tongs with a

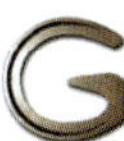

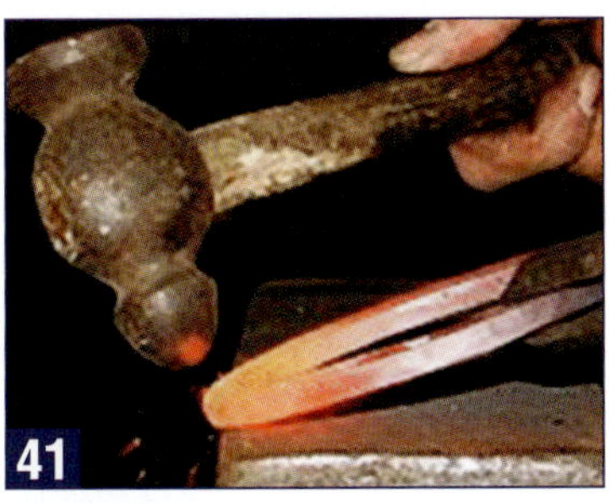

Shearing hammer blow to make a clip.

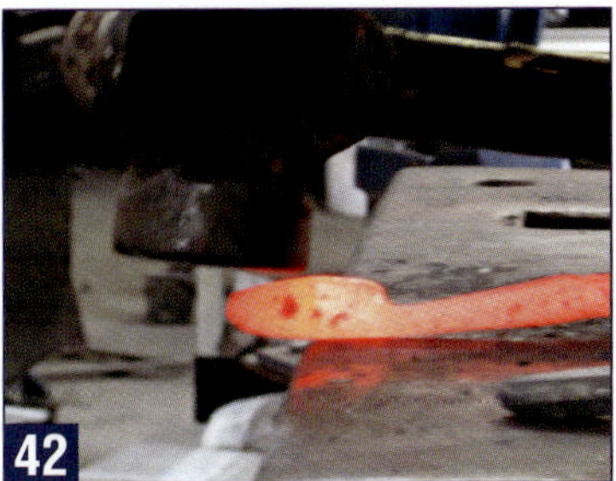

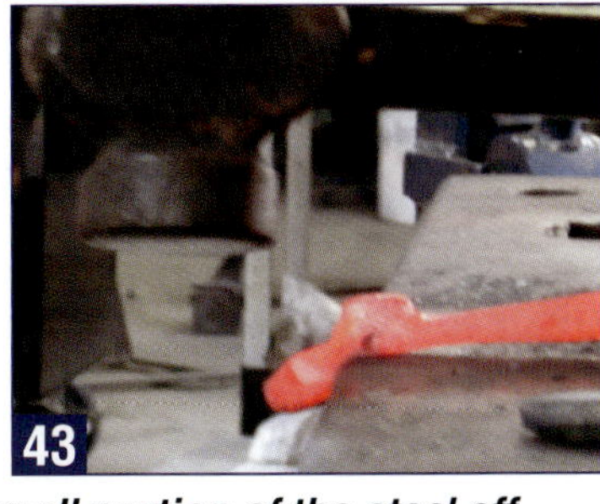

Shearing hammer blow cutting a small portion of the steel off.

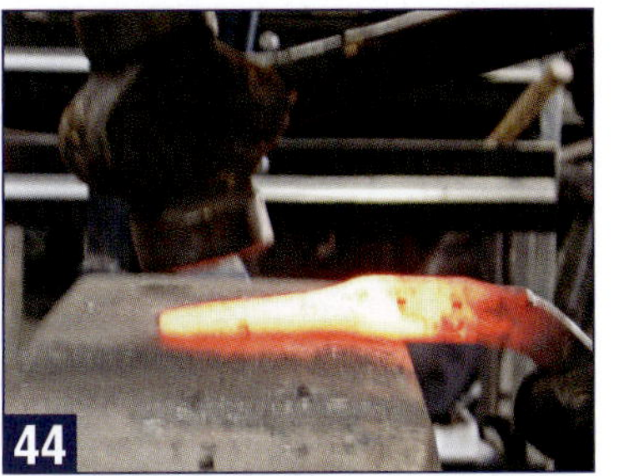

Drawing the steel out to make a jar caulk.

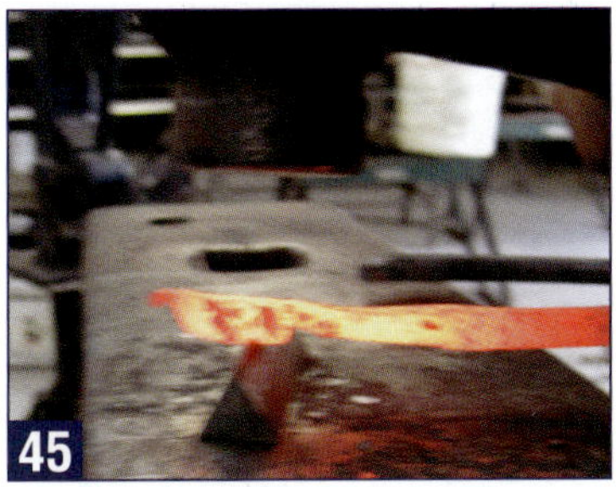

Cutting through the steel with an anvil devil to make the caulk.

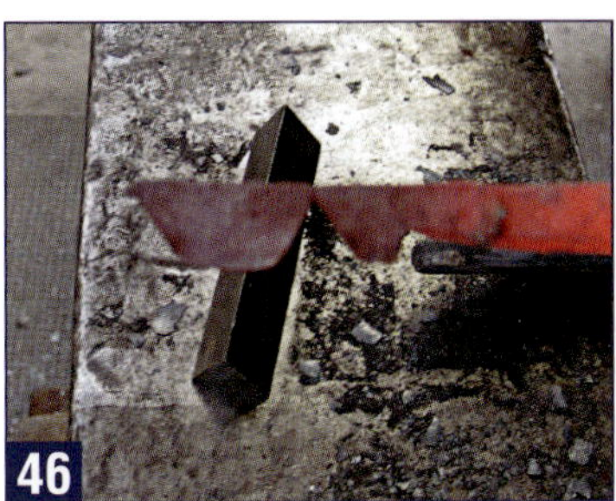

Caulk is formed and cut.

tight grip. Use the loosest grip that will still allow you to control the hammer and tongs.

When the hammer strikes the hot metal, allow all of the power of the swing to be used. If you watch people forging, you will see that some hit the steel and get the hammer back in the air immediately. Much of the blow is wasted. Others have an almost indiscernible pause once the hammer hits the steel. Those who have that slight pause will get more done with less work because they are allowing the entire energy of the blow to be used. You can do a simple test of this by driving some nails into a board or hoof. Don't fight the hammer, let it work with and for you. Again, (I know you're sick of this word) practice.

There are a few different types of hammer blows that you should be acquainted with. The ones used most for forging horseshoes are:

- **Flat:** The hammer is coming down so that the hammer face is parallel to the anvil face **(Figure 35)**.
- **Angled:** The hammer is being swung at an angle to the face of the anvil, or the hammer handle is held in the hand with a slight turn to allow the hammer face to hit the stock at an angle. **Figure 36** shows a shoe being hemmed on the horn, with the hammer being brought down straight, but the head turned to create the angle. **Figure 37** shows hammering at an angle on the inside of a toe bend.
- **Half-faced:** Sometimes called a "shouldering blow", the hammer comes down so that only half the face is over the top of the anvil. The other half is beyond the edge of the anvil **(Figure 38)**.
- **Edge-to-edge:** An edge-to-edge blow is one where the edge of the anvil is lined up exactly with the edge of the hammer **(Figures 39 and 40)**. This type of blow is generally used for making nails, rivets, or other shouldered types of projects. It takes considerable hammer control to master this type of hammer blow.
- **Shearing Blow:** This is accomplished by hammering with the head of the hammer coming down just beyond the edge of the anvil. It is a common type of hammer swing for clipping **(Figure 41)** or to cut off a small piece of steel at the edge of the anvil **(Figures 42 and 43)**. As with the edge-to-edge blow, this takes a lot of hammer control.

It may be useful to evaluate the height of your

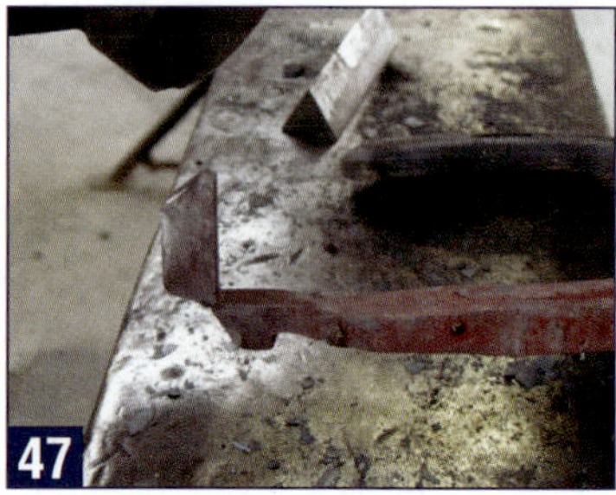
Bend it back on itself.

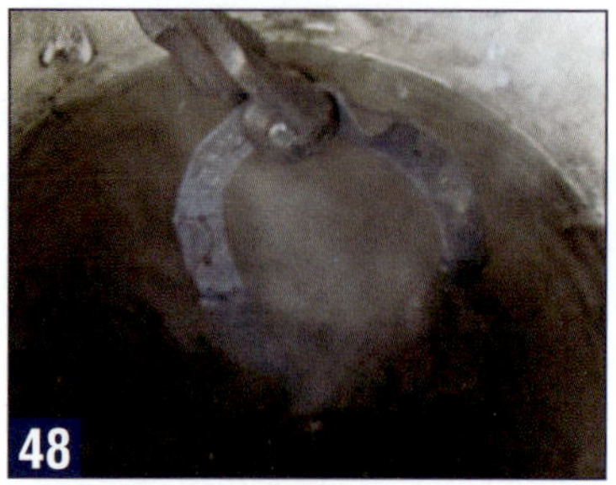
Quench the caulk.

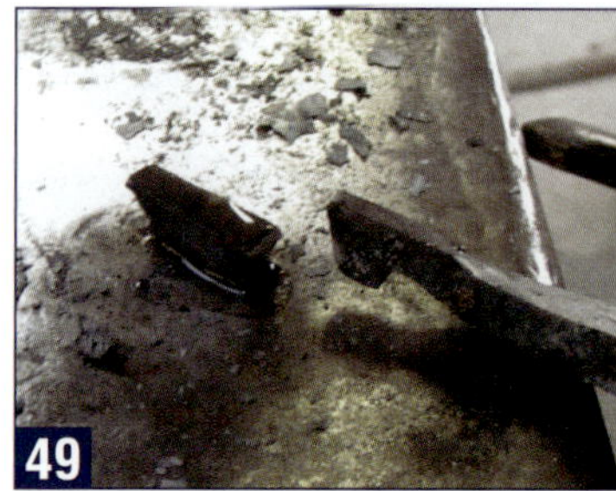
Break it off.

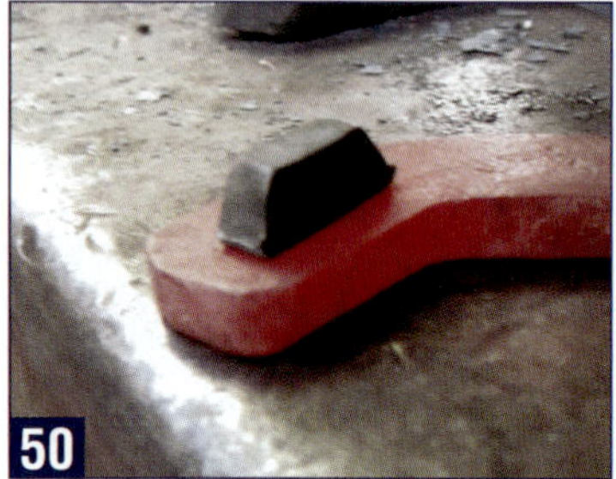
Place the caulk on the brushed and heated shoe.

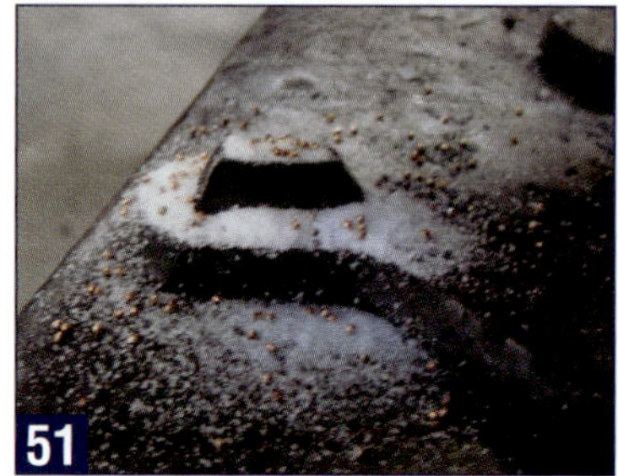
Apply flux and copper.

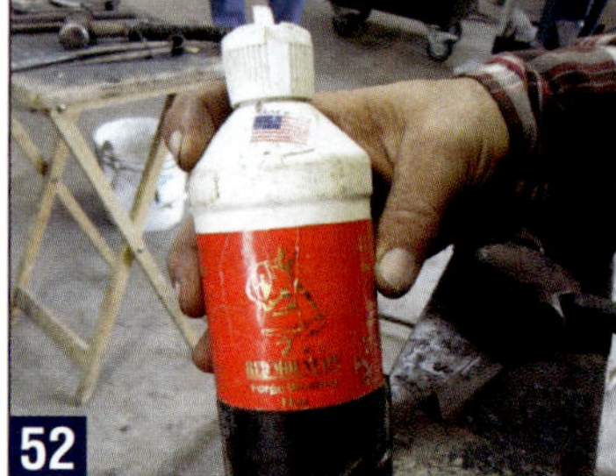
Red Mountain Brazing Flux.

anvil if you are having any problems hitting your work with flat, level hammer blows. My anvil is higher than most in consideration of my back. I want the face of the anvil to be at a level that is comfortable for my tong hand. My hammer will stop where it does, but the tong hand has to steady the piece on top of the anvil. To begin, place your anvil so that the face is even with the bottom of your knuckles when you stand beside the anvil with your feet together making a fist. Adjust the height from there if you find that something else is more comfortable for you. Some say that the higher anvil will cost some power, but forging is not a game of power. It is all technique and skill.

BRAZING

Brazing in the forge is actually a pretty easy thing to do. It is basically joining two pieces of metal with another metal. In this demonstration, I am brazing a jar caulk to a shoe with copper.

Make the jar caulk by forging the shape **(Figure 44)** and cutting it for the caulk. Cut most of the way through **(Figures 45 and 46)**, and then bend it back **(Figure 47)**. Cool it, **(Figure 48)**, and it can be broken off easily **(Figure 49)**. Heat, brush, and level the shoe that is going to get the caulk, and then place the caulk on the shoe where you want it to be brazed **(Figure 50)**. Flux the shoe and apply copper **(Figure 51)**. You can use copper wire and Borax, but I really like the Red Mountain Brazing Flux **(Figure 52)**. It has little pieces of copper in it that melt faster then most wire. Place the shoe on top of a hot fire **(Figure 53)**, and then only look at it in short intervals unless you have dark glasses. If you look at it directly for any length of time, you can flash burn your eyes, the same way you could by welding without a facemask.

Once the copper melts and puddles, you can see it run under and around the caulk. Pull it out of the fire slowly and steadily. At this point, the copper is molten, so the caulk is sitting there from gravity, not from the strength of the copper **(Figure 54)**. Carefully place the shoe on the anvil and press on top of the caulk with your hammer **(Figure 55)**. Cody likes to give it a light tap, but if you hit it very hard, the copper will be squeezed out of the joint. I prefer to press until the copper is no longer molten.

Quench the caulk and shoe **(Figure 56)**, and then brush vigorously. The joints between the caulk

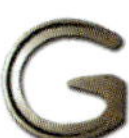

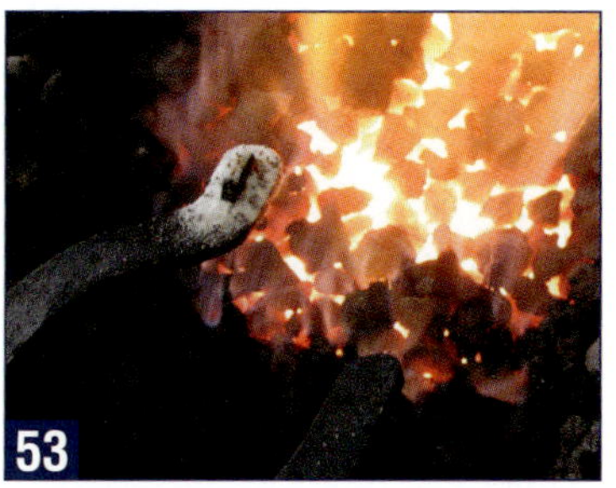

Place the shoe on top of a hot fire.

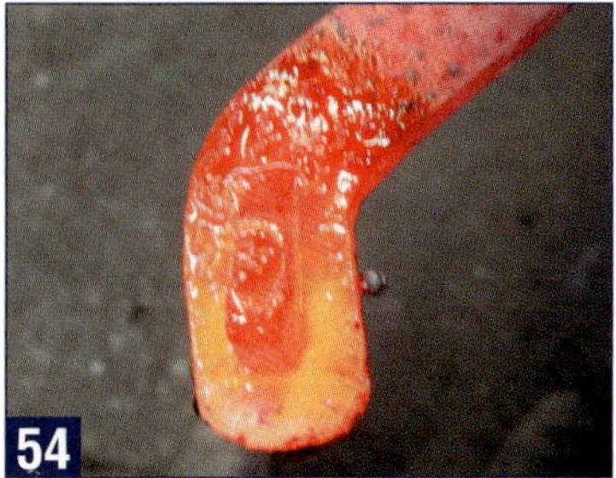

Molten copper.

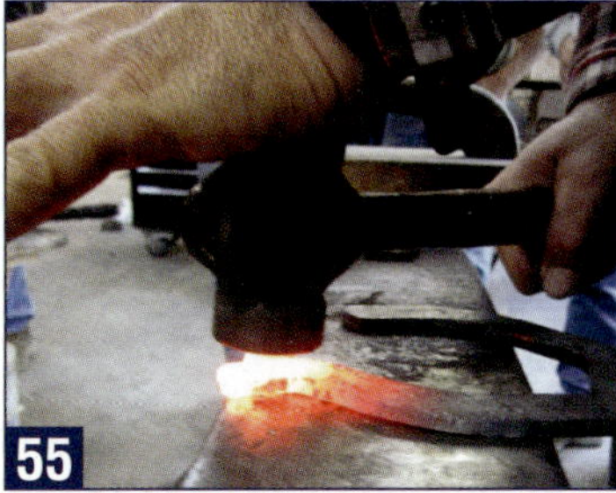

Press on the caulk as the copper cools enough to no longer be liquid.

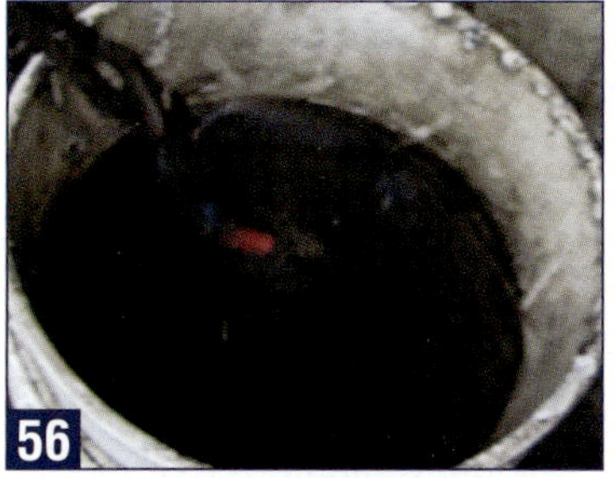

Quench the caulk once the copper is no longer molten.

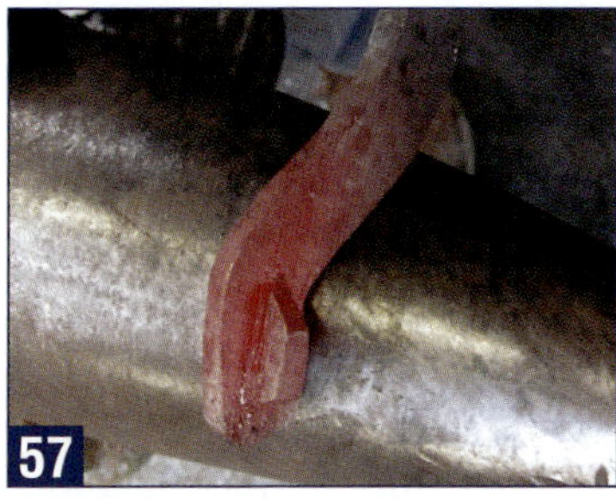

Brush the piece and look at the joint.

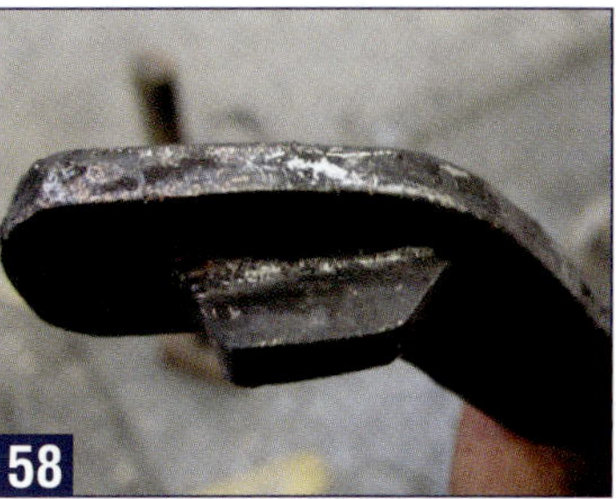

The joint is strong and complete.

and shoe should look like the ones in **Figures 57 and 58**. If you break the caulk off of the shoe, the amount of copper that ran between them is evident **(Figure 59)**. This happens from a process known as capillary action, or capillarity. This is a phenomenon of liquids where they rise in a narrow space and may move against gravity. There is a lot to the capillary action, but all you need to know here is that it describes why hot copper flows between the caulk and shoe.

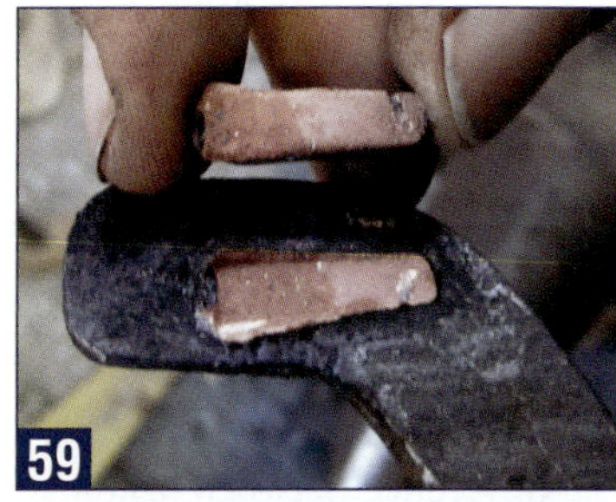

Breaking off the caulk reveals the amount of copper between the shoe and caulk.

PRACTICE MENTALITY

For years I practiced for contests with the idea that I needed to be fast enough to get done. To date, I have always finished the class. However, there are countless times that I finished the class only to turn in ugly and useless shoes. Because I was so intent on just getting done, I sacrificed a lot of quality. When the time came that my skills were sufficient to make nicer shoes in the time allotted, I struggled with making a good, quality, usable shoe.

A friend of mine named Steve Hayes approached his forging from a different perspective. Being a perfectionist to the extreme, Steve practiced quality above all else. Many the times we would forge together, and I would time him with a sundial. After years of building beautiful shoes, Steve came to a point where he could make the shoes in time. Since quality was his priority from the beginning, he was next to unbeatable in a contest situation.

Having a chance to do it over, I would forget about the clock and concentrate on building as good a shoe as I could during practice. Speed will come eventually, you just can't rush it. Approach every shoe as if it will be the best shoe ever made. The mentality you develop early in your forging career will haunt or help you throughout the rest of your career.

And finally, choose your mentors carefully.

Chapter 37 FORGING BASICS

This section is dedicated to some of the basic projects and processes that come into play when using a forge to perfect the art of farriery. We will begin with a discussion of some of the tasks that combine to make a horseshoe. From there, we will move to some exercises that you can do to make you a better blacksmith. Take this chapter with you to the shop and refer to it as you build your forging skills. Try to get each segment of the project correct so that the next segment will follow correctly. One of the key principles of blacksmithing is that one step leads to another. Doing each task properly is essential to moving on to the next task.

Learning to forge can be painful. You may become frustrated and disgusted, but you can work through that. When you finally build these skills, you will find that you are a farrier who is in demand. You will be doing what the best in the world do when they shoe a horse. There is no better company.

THE FOUNDATION

There are some facets of shoe building that should be mastered as individual tasks. Portions of the shoe, such as punching nail holes or building heels, are common on most shoes. Learning how to punch holes and build heels consistently can be the difference between usable and unusable shoes.

Jim Keith taught me a superb way of teaching a student to forge, and I use his method constantly. With beginners, I like to assign a project, then have the student cut several pieces of stock for that one project. Each task involved in that project is done individually on each piece of stock, one piece after another. They then do the next task in the process on each piece until they have completed the project in multiples. This method of teaching allows the student to do repetitive practice and master their projects by mastering the individual tasks. I have found this method to be far superior to having students just build one shoe after the other from start to finish. One person using this method for six shoes would be a better forger after those six shoes were completed than a person who was building six shoes, one after the other.

Here is how I have my students build their first shoes. Cut six 12-inch pieces of stock and mark each piece for the desired shoe. Heat the first piece and make a toe bend. Heat the second piece, and make a toe bend to match the first. Repeat the toe bends on each piece of stock until all six are laying one on top of the other as matched pieces.

Take the first piece and make a heel on the end of it, as well as the slight bend to counteract inertia. Do the same to all the other pieces until they are once again all matched and at the same point in the shoe making process. Take the first piece and turn the branch. Repeat for the remaining five pieces. Continue with the other branch, making the heel, and bending the branch, doing the same to all the pieces. When the students are done with this step-by-step process, they will have six completed shoes. The students will have learned twice as much as if they had made one shoe at a time from toe bend to finish with all six pieces. Try this with any shoe or forging that you are struggling with to determine if it will work for you, and I bet that it will.

BASIC TASKS

Punching Nail Holes

The thickness of the stock should be appropriate for the size of the nail that will be driven into the foot. It would not be appropriate to be nailing a shoe made of 1/2- by-1-inch bar stock on a foot with MX50 nails. On the other hand, an E10 Slim will not fit 5/16-by-3/4-inch bar. If the nail is appropriate for the stock, the same punch should work for every thickness. If you are driving an E5 in 5/16-inch stock, the same punch can be used to punch a nail hole for an E9 in 1/2-inch stock. The important aspect is the angles on the sides of the punch, and the dimensions at the very end of the punch. The end of the punch should exactly match the end of the pritchel (**Figure 1**).

The fore punch aspect of making nail holes is best done in stock that is red (**Figure 2**). Much hotter

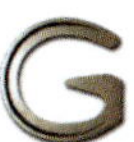

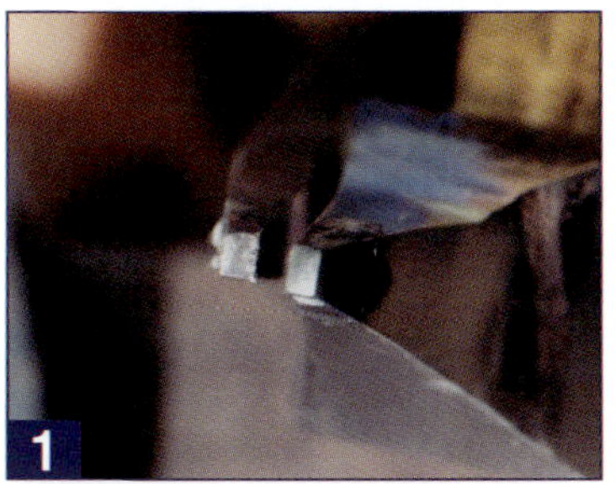

Detail of the end of a fore punch and matching pritchel.

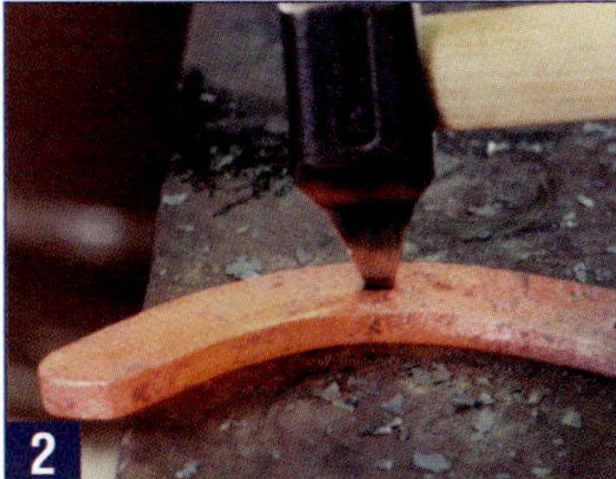

Correct color for using the fore punch.

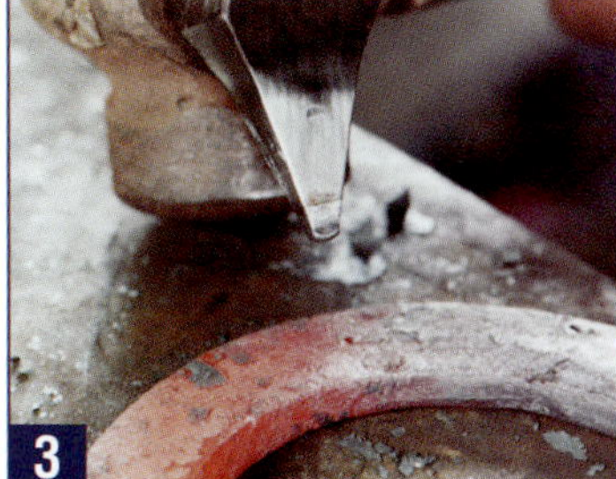

Moving to another hole using the hammer as a guide.

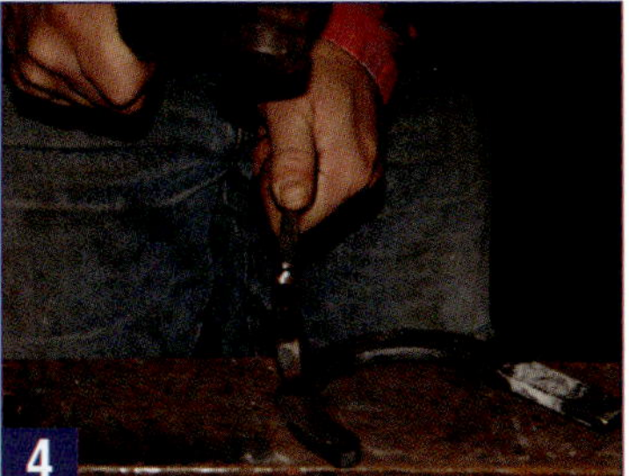

Holding the punch upright.

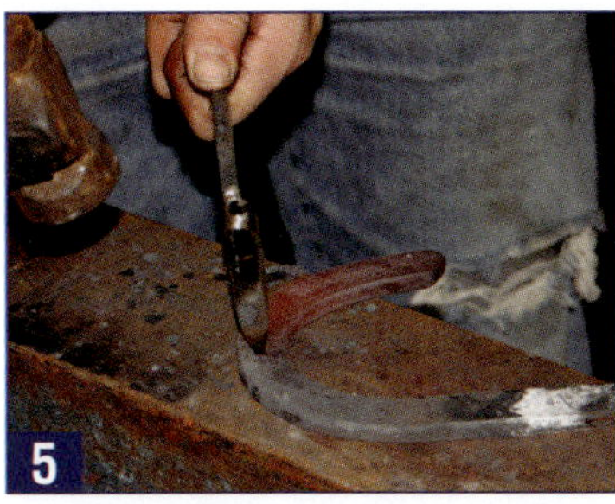

Holding the punch at an angle.

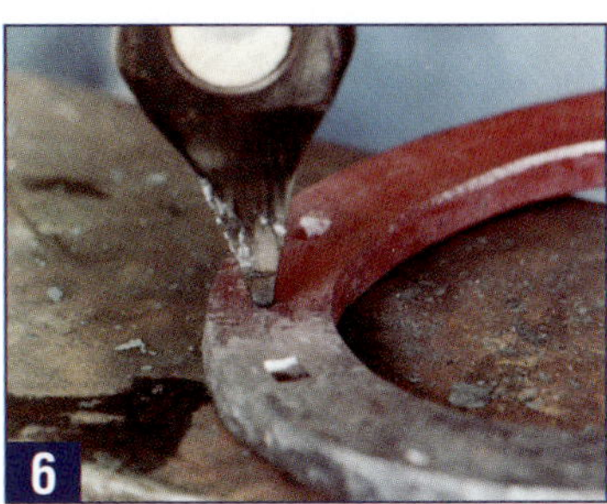

Punching

will displace too much steel, while much cooler can be hard on the punch. Place the punch in position, using your hammerhead to help guide the punch to the exact placement **(Figure 3)**. Hold the punch so that it is perpendicular to the stock **(Figure 4)** In a few instances it may be desirable to angle the fore punch to achieve pitch on the nail, **(Figure 5)** however, the pitch is mainly achieved with the angle of the pritchel.

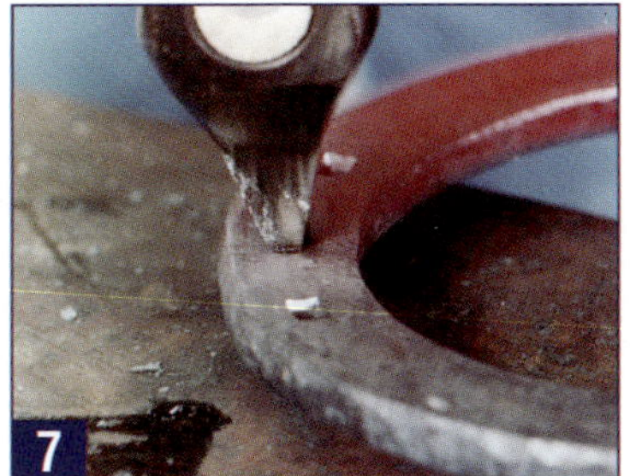

Punching

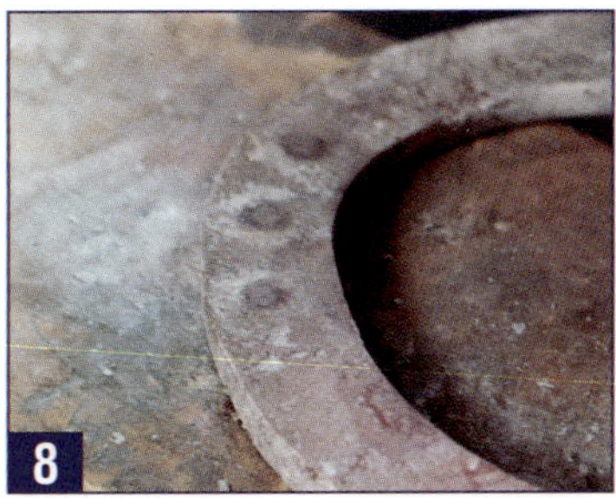

Shiny spot on the hoof surface of the shoe where the punch was used.

Strike the top of the punch with two or three solid hammer blows, or until the desired depth is achieved **(Figures 6-7)**. It will take some time to develop a feel for the correct depth. Remove the punch from the hot steel as quickly as possible to avoid overheating. Punch the appropriate number of nail holes in the ground surface of the shoe.

After using the fore punch, hammer with flat blows on the hoof surface of the shoe. There will be a shiny gray area where the punch was driven into the stock on the ground surface **(Figure 8)**. By hammering on the hoof surface at this time, two things are accomplished. First, the small piece of metal that is about to be sheared out by the pritchel is cooled, making it easier to pritchel. Secondly, the edges around the bottom of the nail hole are crisped up and stressed, making it easier to punch out the little piece with a pritchel. You can try pritchelling without first hammering the hoof surface flat, then compare it to the holes that you punch after hammering. I think that you will see a big difference.

Now, move to the horn to forge the stock back to the original width where it was displaced by the fore punch **(Figures 9-10)**. The bumps that you are forging out of the width of the shoe are called "frog eyes." A good method to forge out frog eyes is to hammer lightly over the outside edge of the shoe

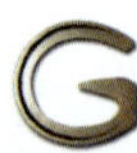

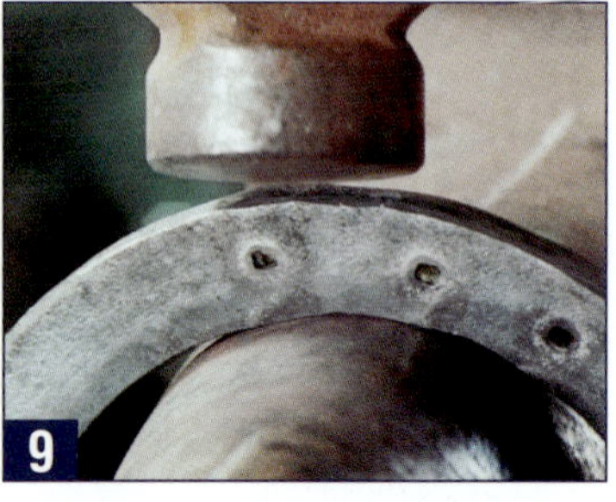

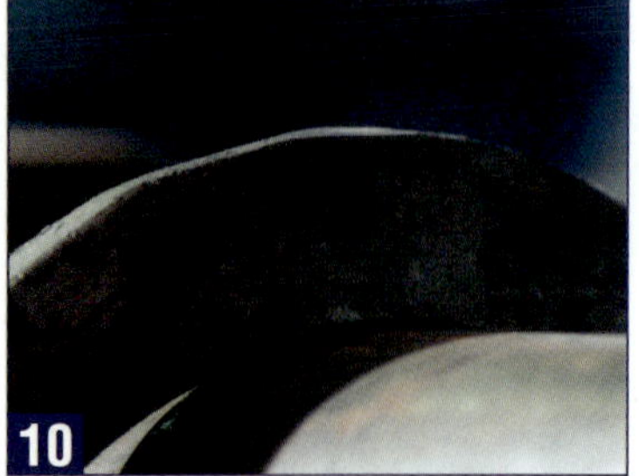

Forging out the frog eyes.

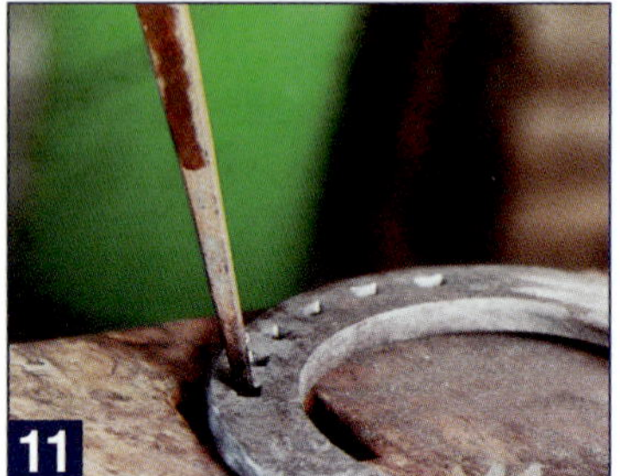

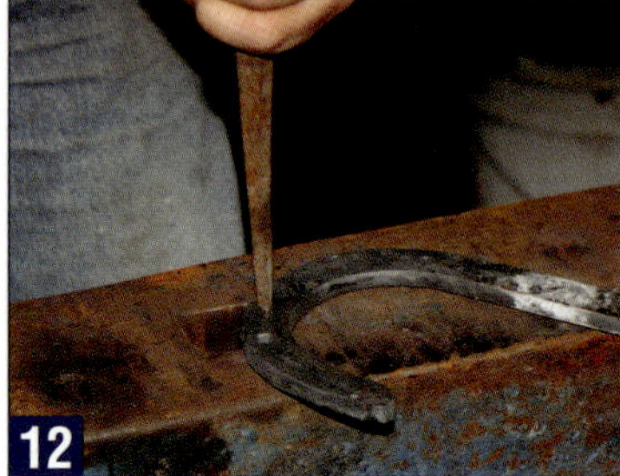

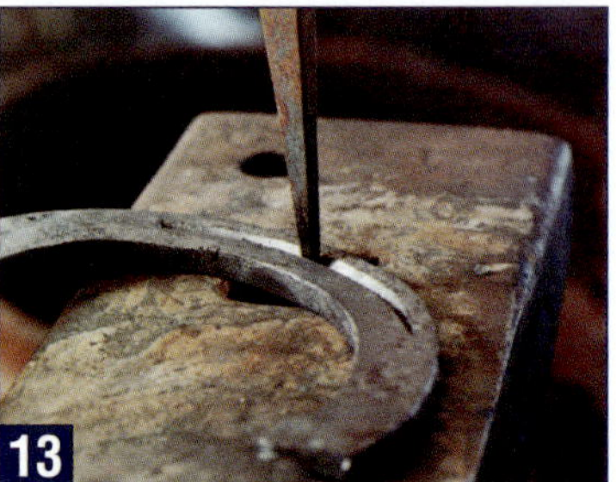

Pritchel angle.

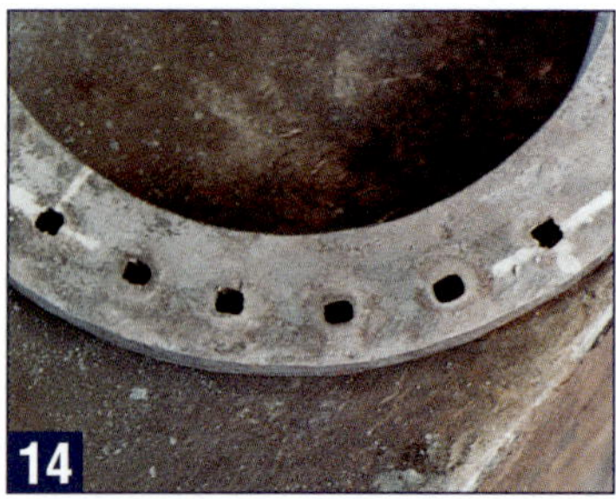

Punched holes. Coarse to fine, left to right.

on the horn, making three passes. First, concentrate on one edge, then the opposite edge, and finally, hammer through the middle. The shoe should be fairly cool for this process so that you don't end up closing the nail hole that you just punched.

The stock is cooling during this time and should now be at a dark red to black heat. If everything has been done correctly, the shoe is now ready for pritchelling. It is not desirable to have the stock too hot when using the pritchel, because hot steel will not sheer out of the bottom of the hole like it does when it is cool. When hot, it is more likely to draw. This leaves pieces of flashing around the hole that will interfere with proper nail fit.

Place the pritchel in the nail hole and move the shoe over the hardy or pritchel hole on the face of the anvil. When pritchelling the toe nail, try to drive the pritchel at an angle to match the angle of the hoof wall at the toe **(Figure 11)**. There is less of an angle at the second nail **(Figure 12)**, and pretty much straight up and down at the heel **(Figures 13)**. The pritchel should be hit with one or two sharp, solid hammer blows. The position of the nail hole on the hoof surface of the shoe is known as nail exit depth. Holes that are closest to the inside of the web are known as coarse, and holes toward the outside edge of the web are called fine. If you carefully study **Figures 14**, you will see that the holes on the left side of the shoe are coarse, and they are progesively finer as you look to the right.

The pitch of these nails was determined by the angle of the pritchel, not the placement of the punch in the ground surface.

Get the pritchel out of the shoe quickly, dipping it into a bar of soap to cool and lubricate the working end. There are a variety of products that can be used for lubricating the pritchel. Beeswax, tallow, saddle soap, hoof packing, and other similar substances will work just as well as soap. I don't use beeswax since it makes the face of the anvil slick. My prefer-

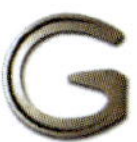

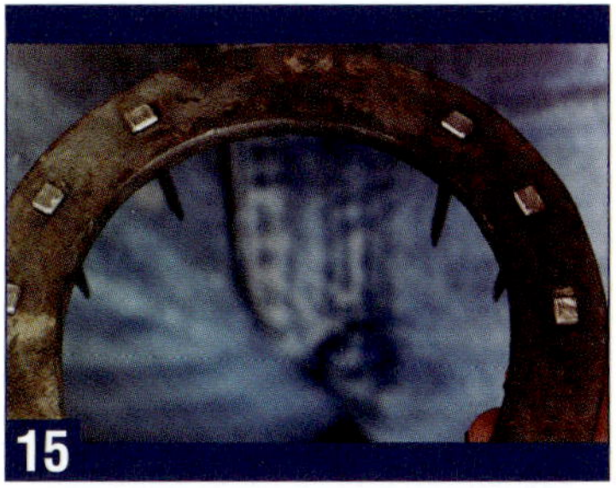

Nails in a plain stamped shoe.

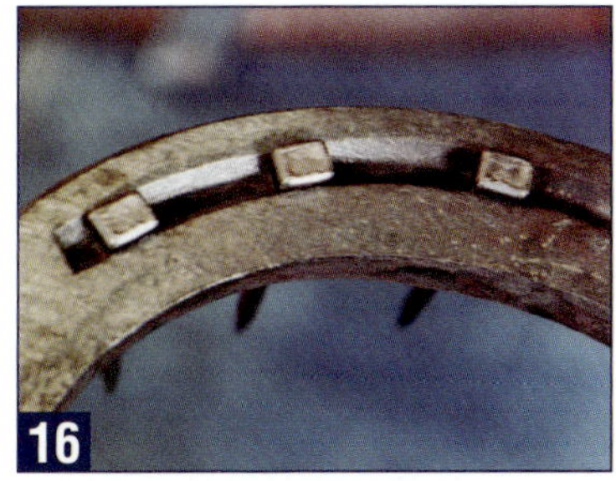

Nails in a fullered shoe.

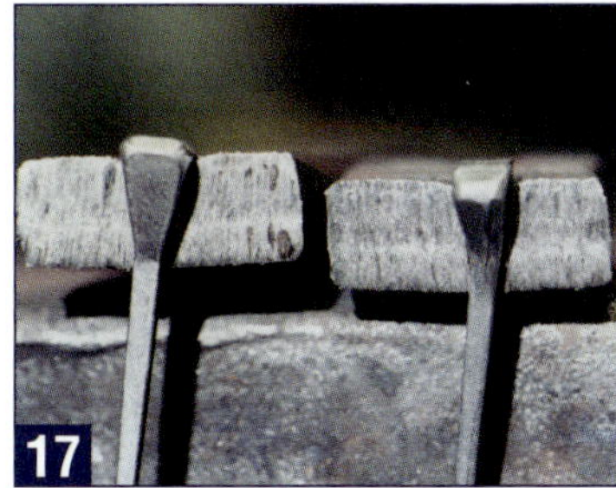

Cross section of nail holes.

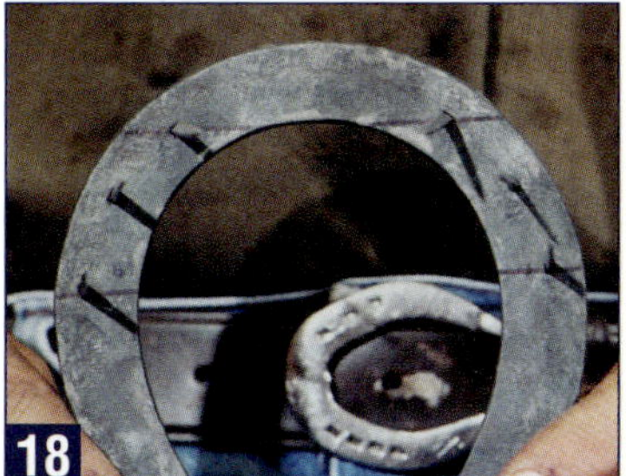

Pitch in a shoe.

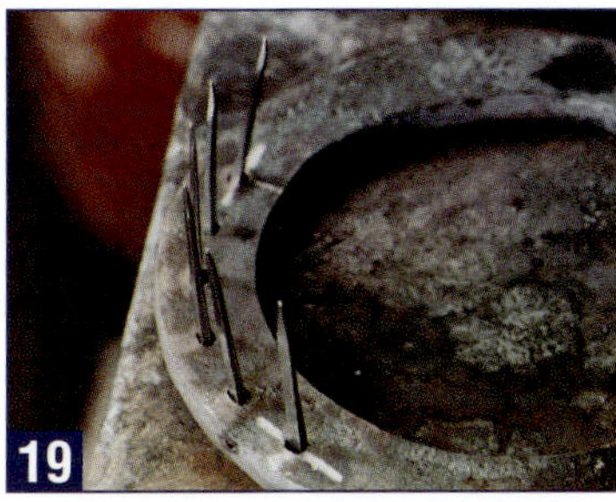

Demonstrating pitch in a ring.

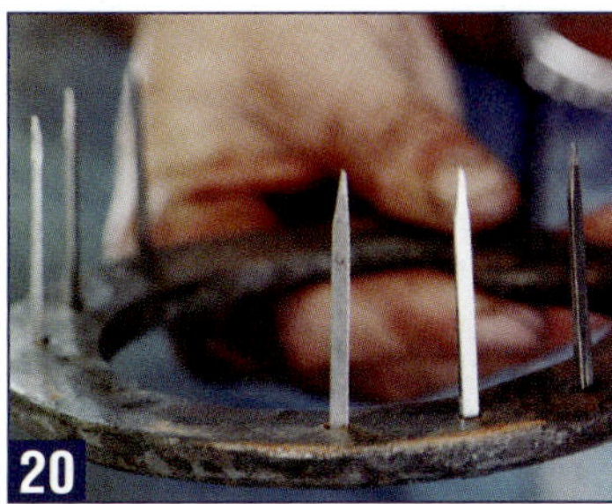

Nails stay in the holes when the shoe is turned upside down.

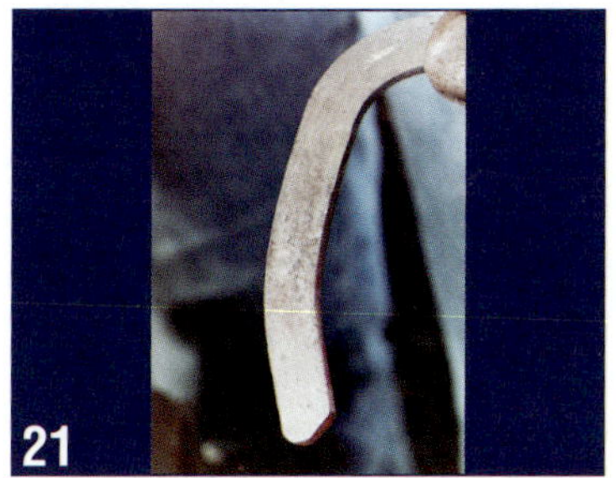

Heel check.

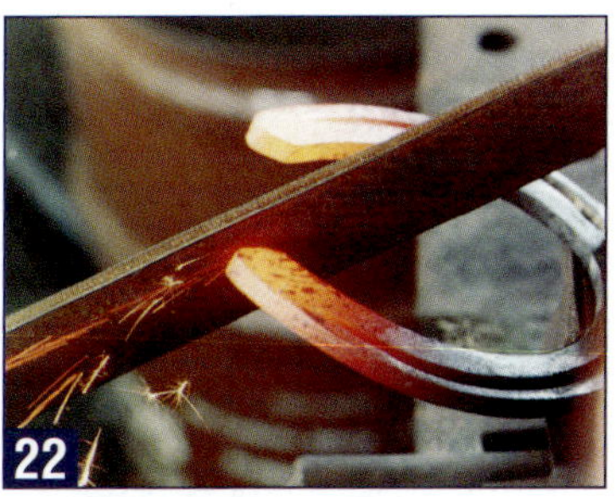

Rasping the check.

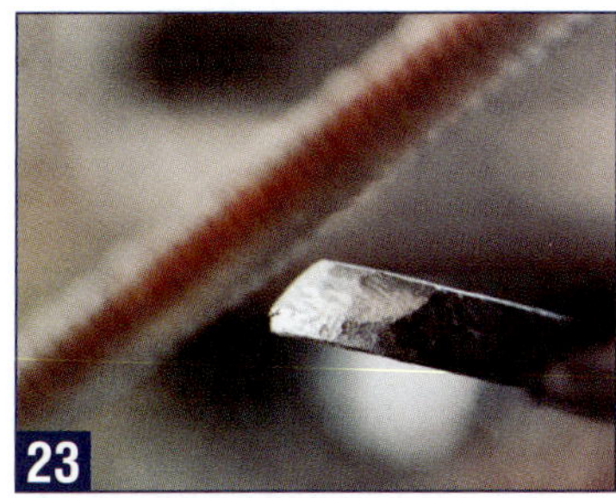

Rasping the heel cut.

ence is saddle soap.

Nail fit and pitch are essential items when judging handmade shoes. **Figures 15 and 16** show proper nail fit in a plain stamped and fullered shoe, and **Figure 17** is a couple of nail holes that have been sawed through so that you can see the pitch of the nails as well as how tight the head fits the hole. The nail on the left is an MX50, which is an E-head design, while the nail on the right is a City Head Nail. Pitch can be seen in **Figures 18 and 19**. Ideally, the nails will fit securely enough that you can turn the shoe upside down without the nails falling out of the shoe as in **Figures 20**.

Heels

Heels can be broken down into two parts. When viewed on the width of the stock, the angle of the heel is called "heel check." You can see how this would cover the heel of a hoof where the angle of the bar comes off the angle of the hoof wall **(Figure 21)**. The heel check can be forged or rasped on a shoe **(Figure 22)**. When viewed on the thickness of the stock, the angle at the end of the shoe is called "heel cut" **(Figure 23)** and this is usually rasped on a handmade. Several years ago, the heel cut was actually cut by a V-hardy. This was a traditional way of making a heel in the United States in the 1980s and before, especially when hot shoes were common.

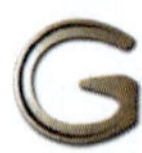

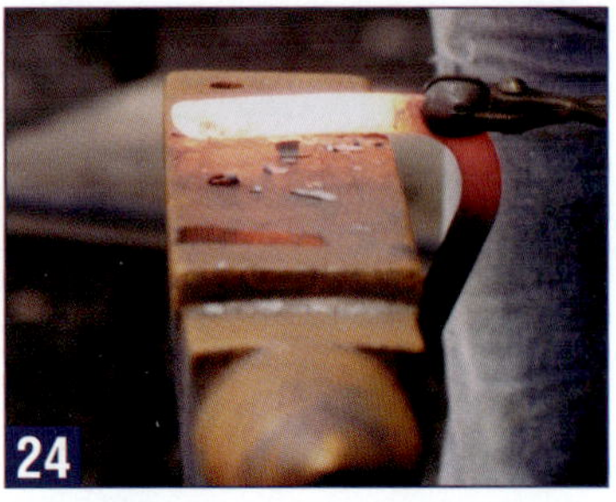

Position for beginning a heel.

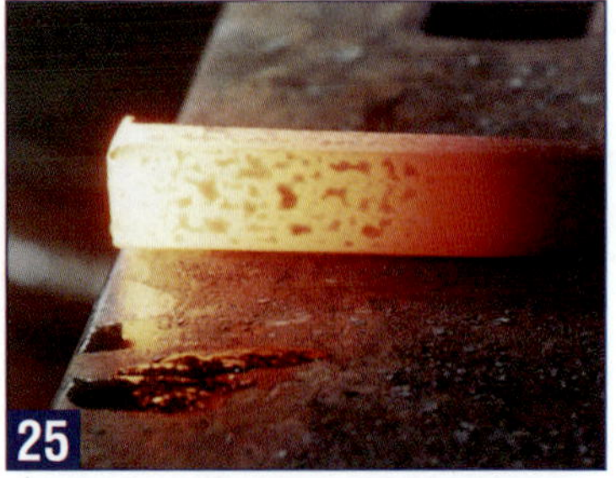

Stock at the edge of the anvil.

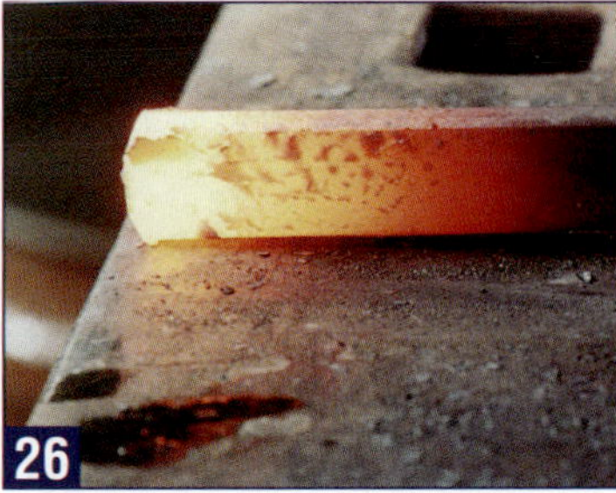

Pulling the corners back.

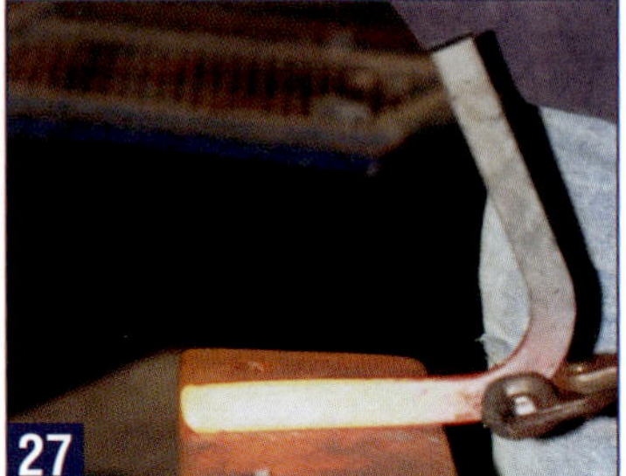

Working the inside of the heel.

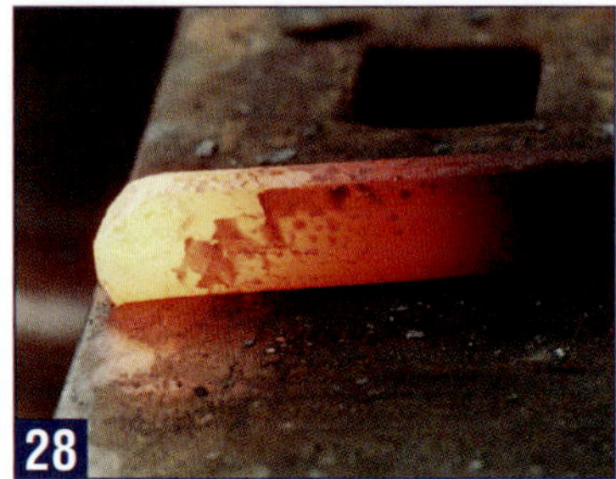

Forming the check.

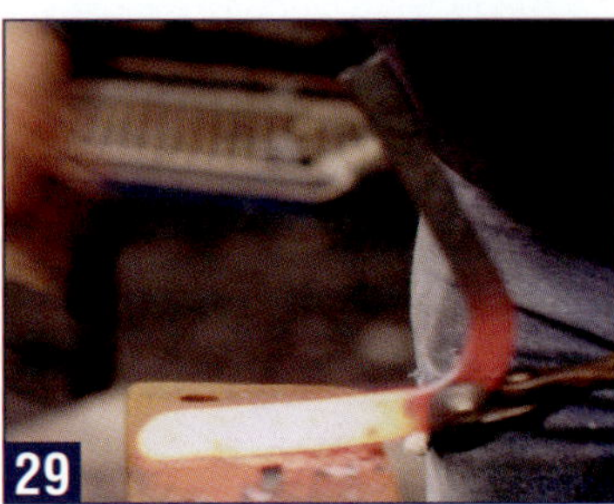

Finishing the heel.

Hot shoes were keg shoes with really long heels so that the farrier could mark the length, and then cut off the excess. They were also handy for making heel caulks or bar shoes, and they made stocking a shoeing rig easier, since you really only needed one size.

A note on forging: When you forge the end of a wide piece of steel, there is a tendency for the outside of the steel to move under the hammer the most; the edge in contact with the face of the anvil to move a little less; and the middle to remain static. As you continue to hit the steel, the outside draws and lengthens, creating a cavity where the inside is not moving. This can be seen when making punches and heels. In order to keep this cavity from occurring, you need to reduce the width on the end of the stock. You can do this by pulling the corners back, which effectively makes the end of the stock narrower.

Making a heel is simply changing the angle on the end of the bar stock. Try not to make this harder than it is. The angle we are after is one that matches the buttress and bar at the heel region of the hoof. How you hold the shoe to make a heel is also a crucial part of making a good heel. You need to hold it in a manner that will allow it to stay solid and stable while you hit it yet do the least amount of damage to your shoe. With a toe bend made, place your tongs in the area where a toe nail would be punched. The stock should look like it is a straight piece of metal sticking out of the tongs **(Figure 24)**. One problem that a lot of people have with making heels is that they hold the wrong part of the toe with their tongs. This makes the toe warp badly when the heel is hit. There will be some damage done to the outside of the shoe by the boss of your tongs, but these little dents can be easily forged or rasped out of the shoe.

Begin by heating the end of the stock, and placing it at the edge of the anvil **(Figure 25)**. Placement is important so that you can have clearance for the hammer head when you hit with the angled blows. The corner that you are working on is the outside of the shoe. Hammer at an angle toward the end of the stock, pulling the outside corner back **(Figure 26)**. Turn the stock over and repeat the same hammer blows from the same angle on the other corner **(Figures 27-28)**. It should only take about 3 hammer blows on each side to achieve the desired shape. These hammer blows change the width of the stock at the very end, taking it from 3/4 inch to somewhere around 3/8 inch. If this is not done, there

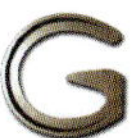

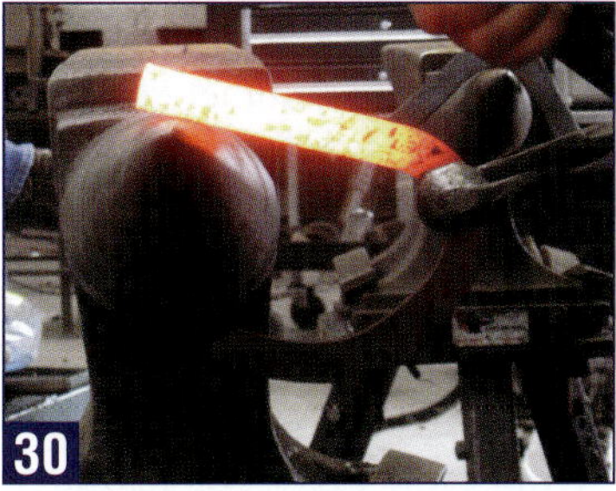
Bob Marshall style, first bend.

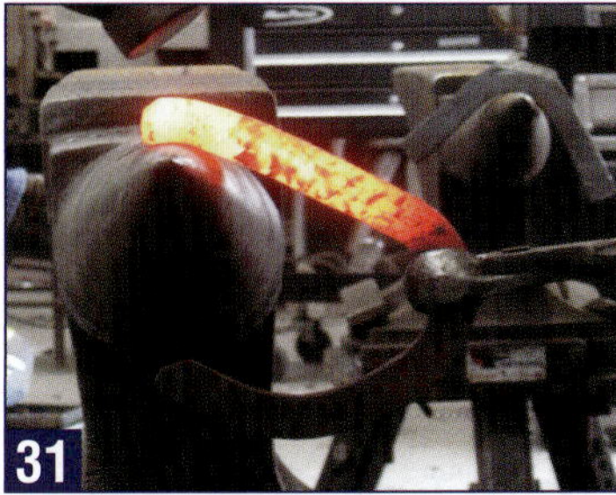
Finishing the first bend.

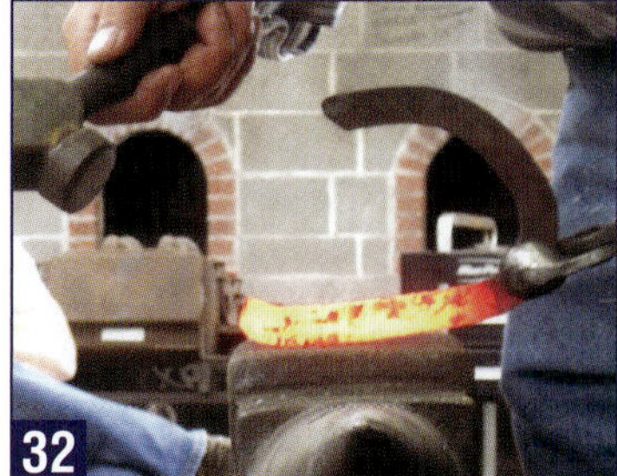
Moving to the inside of the check.

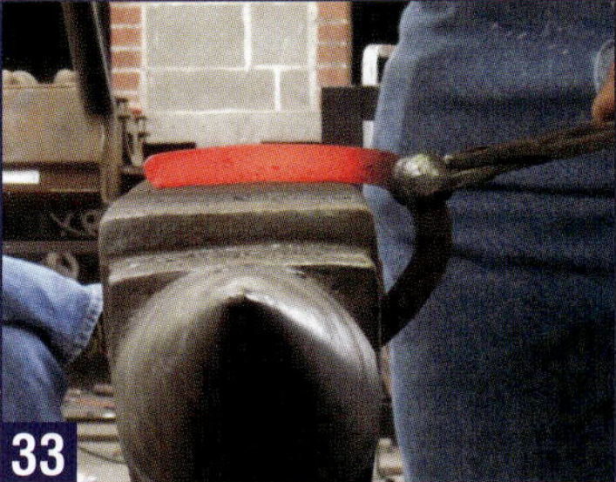
Cleaning up the outside of the heel.

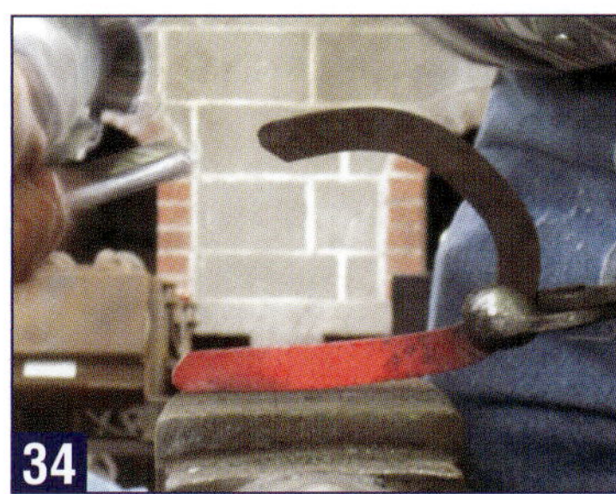
Finshing the inside.

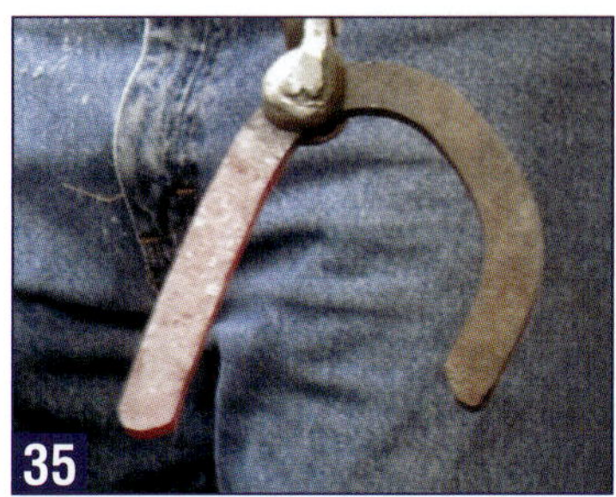
Finished heel.

is a good chance that the end of the heel will have "fish lips." *(See Note On Forging)*

Leave the stock in the same position and hammer with angled blows that will forge the appropriate angle to make the desired heel-check **(Figure 29)**. The hammer should be driving toward the middle of your thigh on your tong hand side. If your heel-checks are too long, try moving your body so that you can see the far side of your anvil. Being in this position allows you to bring the hammer in at the proper angle. I sometimes draw an X on this portion of the anvil for students and don't let them make the heel unless they can see it.

The thickness of the stock will be greatly increased from the forging of the heel. Lay the stock flat on the face of the anvil and forge back to the original thickness. Bring the stock back to the edge of the anvil and repeat the previous steps to make the perfect heel-check.

Bob Marshall developed another method that provides some outstanding results. Begin by bending a short portion of the stock over the top of the horn, bending toward the inside of the shoe **(Figures 30-31)**. Turn the shoe over, and hammer at an angle into the inside of the heel to make the check **(Figure 32)**. Take the stock back to the original thickness, and repeat the last steps of the first heel described here **(Figures 33-34)**. **Figure 35** shows the finished product.

It does not matter which method you use, the importance is in the finished product. My suggestion is to pick one to master, make it your style, and stay with it for quite a while. Once you can make a consistent heel in fewer than 20 hammer blows, learn the other style.

Clips

Clips are an integral part of shoe building and a necessary skill for anyone who wishes to be a good farrier. There are a wide variety of methods for pulling good clips. The method used for pulling the clip is irrelevant, as long as the outcome is a quality clip. A quality clip, as defined for contest and certification judging, has no loss in the width dimension of the parent stock the clip has been pulled from **(Figure 36)**, the clip is clean and crisp on the inside edge **(Figure 37)**. and the shoe is level behind the clip. The clip should also be symmetrical and have an attractive shape **(Figures 38-39)**.

To begin a clip, draw the source material from the outside edge of the shoe. This can be done several ways, using everything from bob punches to

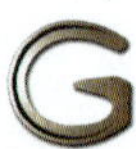

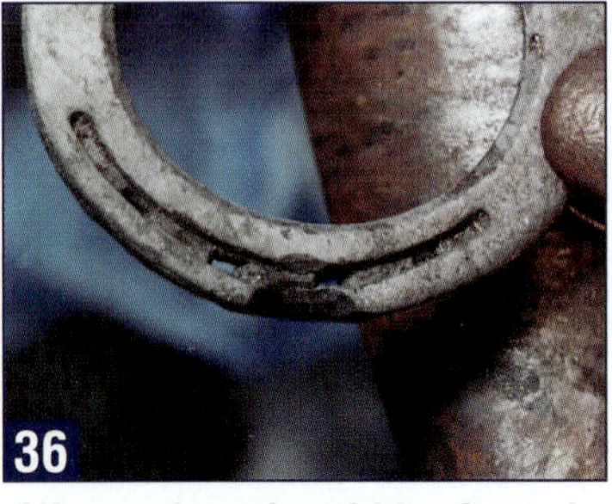

Clip, no loss in width of stock.

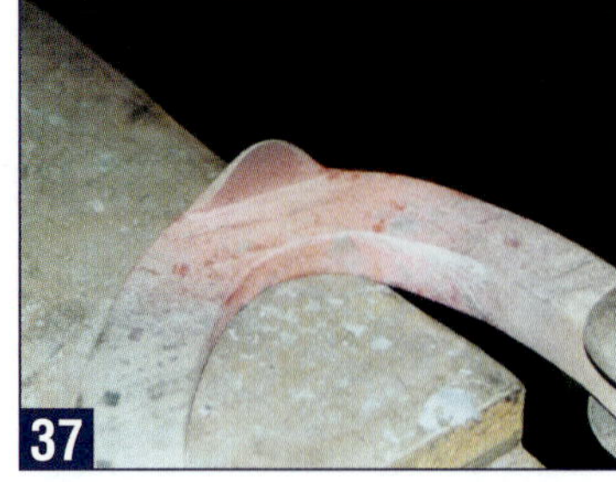

Clean in back of the clip.

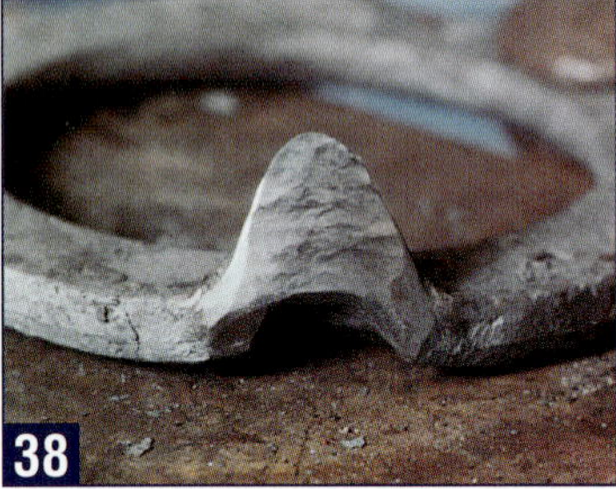

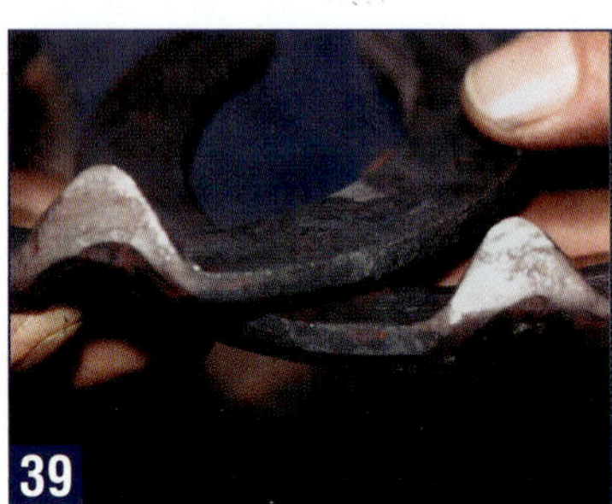

Good, solid clips.

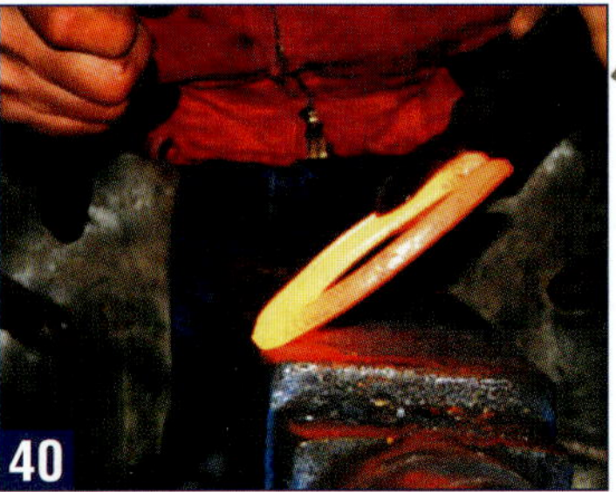

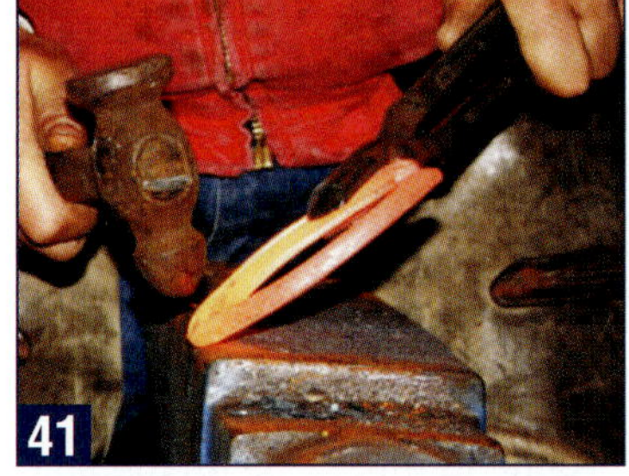

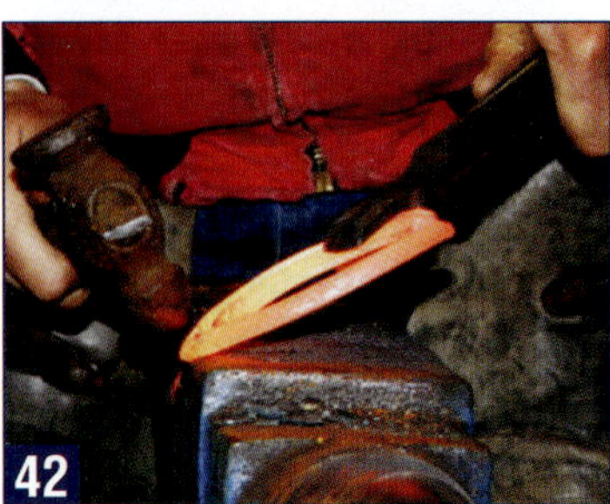

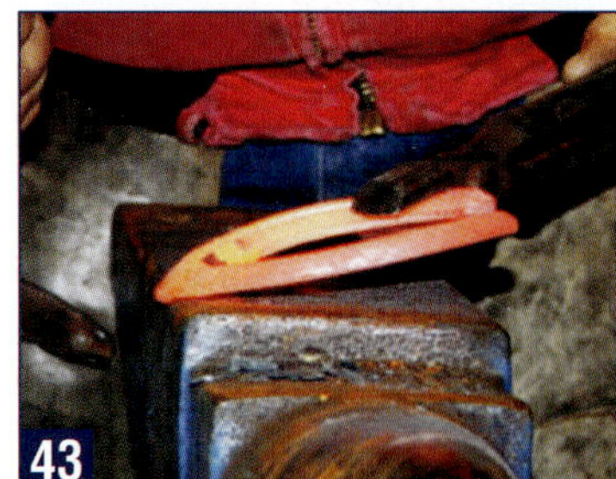

Pulling the source material.

specialty hammers. In my everyday shoeing I use a clipping hammer, which is just a fancy sort of ball peen. This is my everyday hammer that I use for shaping and clipping keg shoes when I am not using hand-mades. For the clip pictured, I am using a clip hammer designed and built by Dave Showen.

Draw the source material by holding the shoe over the edge of the anvil at roughly a 45-degree angle to the face of the anvil **(Figure 40)**. I like to have the shoe over the radius edge of the anvil instead of a sharp corner. The shoe should be approximately 3/16-inch past the edge of the anvil for the average saddle-horse shoe. Angle your hammer blows at 90 degrees to the shoe, or 45 degrees to the face of the anvil. The trick is not to hit where you are looking, but to look where you want to hit. Look directly in the middle of the area you wish to pull the clip from. As you hammer, drop the shoe to a lesser angle as you continue to swing your hammer at 45 degrees to the face of the anvil **(Figures 41-43)**. The size and position of the source material is important. Make certain that the inside edge of the source material is parallel to the web of the shoe and is large enough to get a proper clip. It should look like **Figures 44-46**. I cannot emphasize enough how important it is that you make a good source. Like many things in blacksmithing, you have to get the current step correct for the next step to work.

Turn the shoe over and level around and behind the source material **(Figure 47)**. Another method is placing the source material over the edge of the anvil, or in the hardy hole, and hammering on the ground surface of the shoe **(Figure 48)**. My friend Jeff actually likes to give the source a little tap here to help level the shoe around the clip. He says that it is the best hammer blow in clip building.

Hold the shoe so that the source material is on the face of the anvil at a crisp corner. Maintain down-

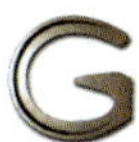

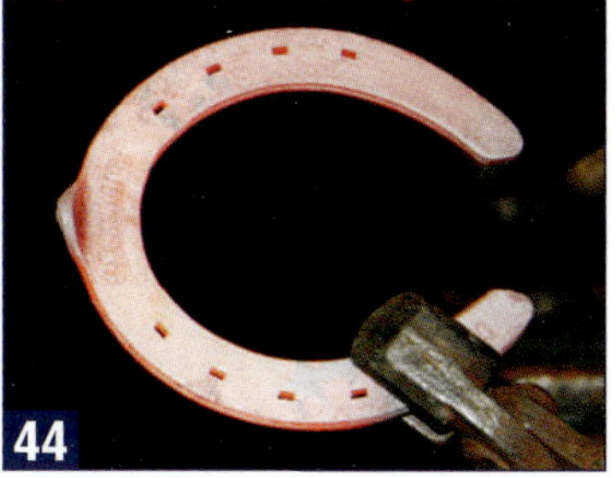

44

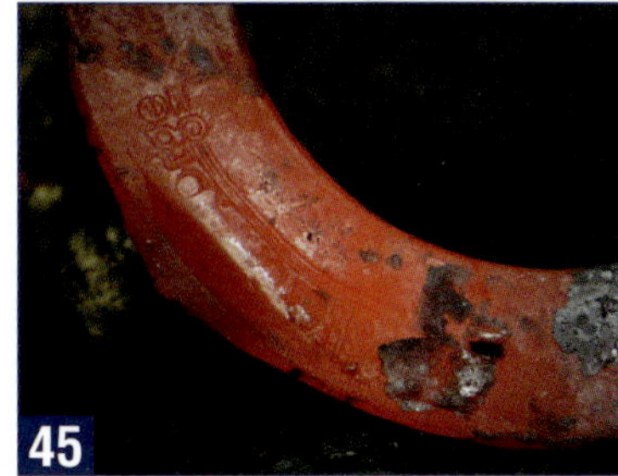

45

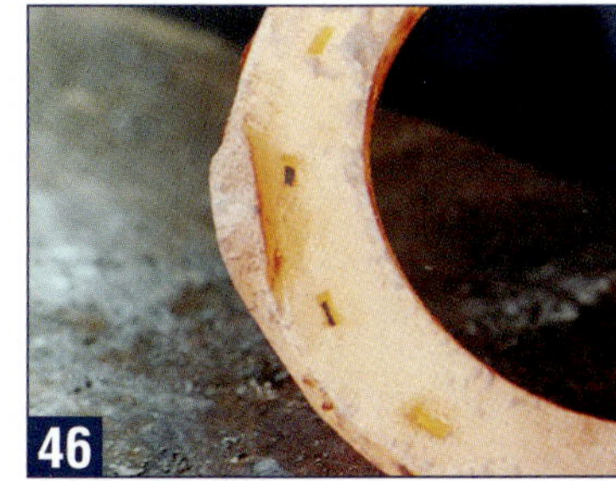

46

How the source should look.

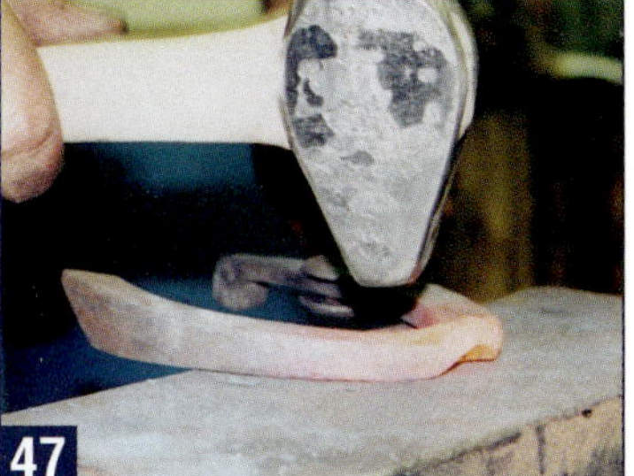

47

Level around the source.

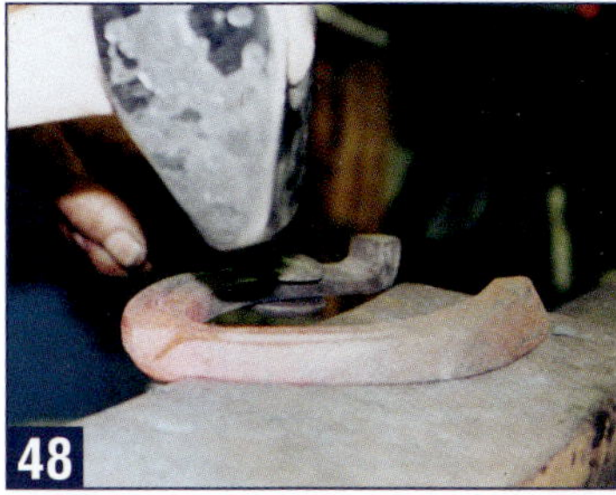

48

Using the edge of the anvil to clean up around the source.

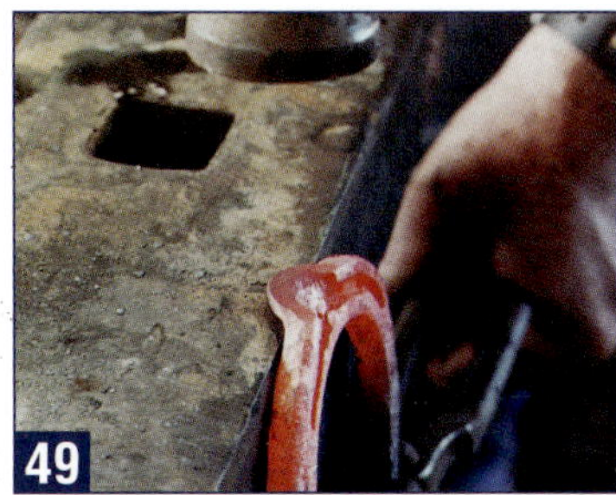

49

Starting the base of the clip.

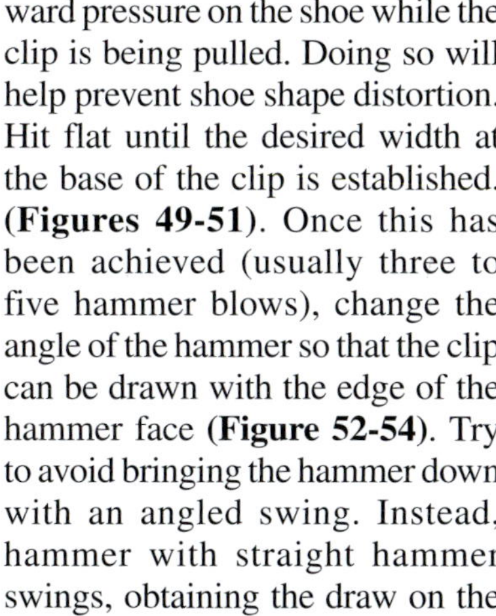

ward pressure on the shoe while the clip is being pulled. Doing so will help prevent shoe shape distortion. Hit flat until the desired width at the base of the clip is established. **(Figures 49-51)**. Once this has been achieved (usually three to five hammer blows), change the angle of the hammer so that the clip can be drawn with the edge of the hammer face **(Figure 52-54)**. Try to avoid bringing the hammer down with an angled swing. Instead, hammer with straight hammer swings, obtaining the draw on the

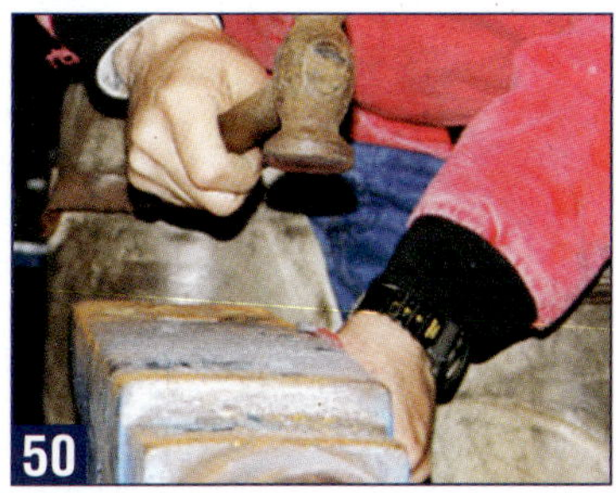

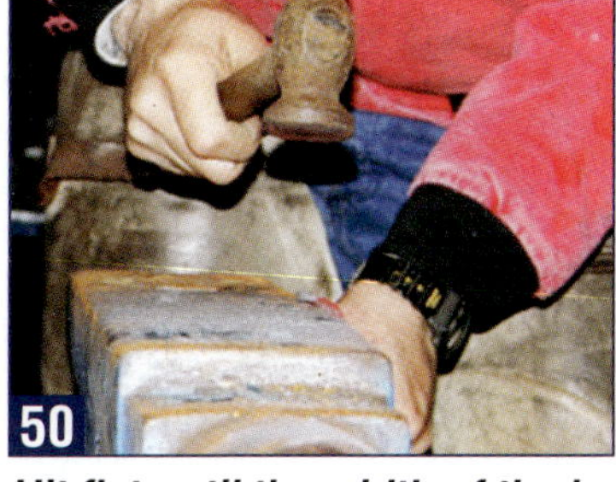

50

51

Hit flat until the width of the base is established.

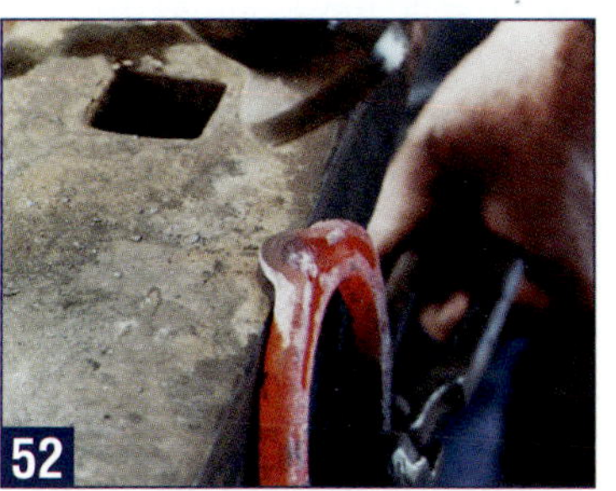

52

53

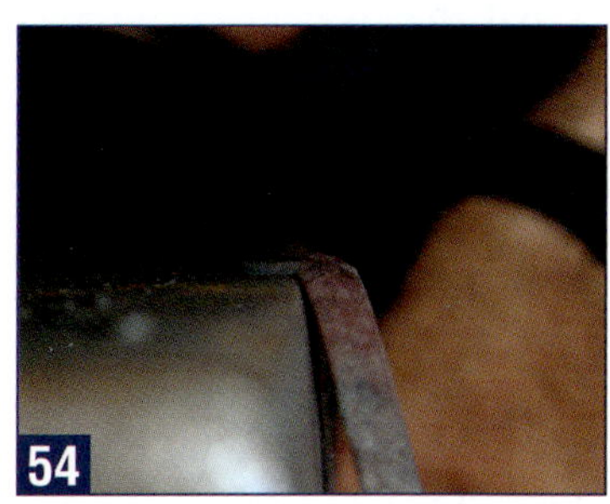

54

Draw the clip with the edge of the hammer.

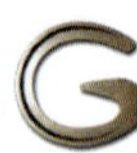

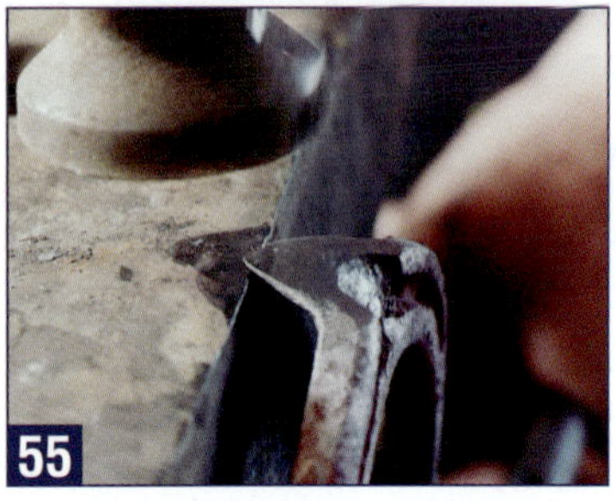

Finishing the clip.

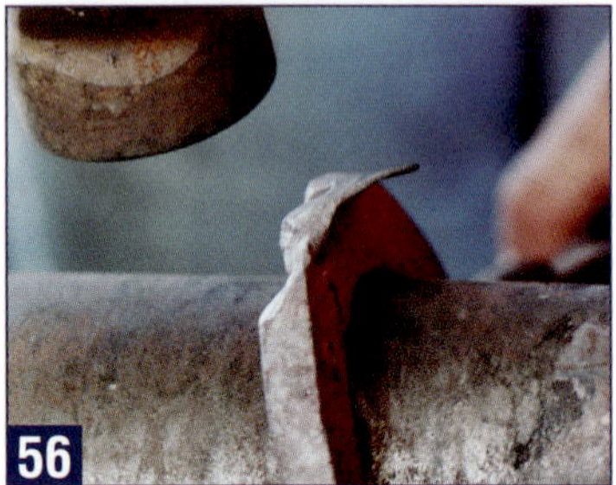

Laying the clip down.

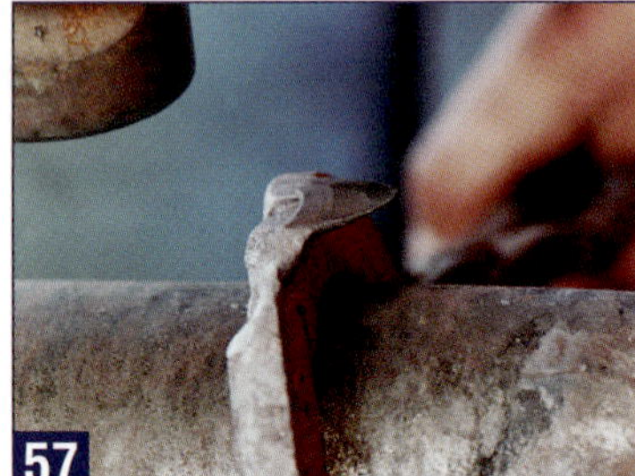

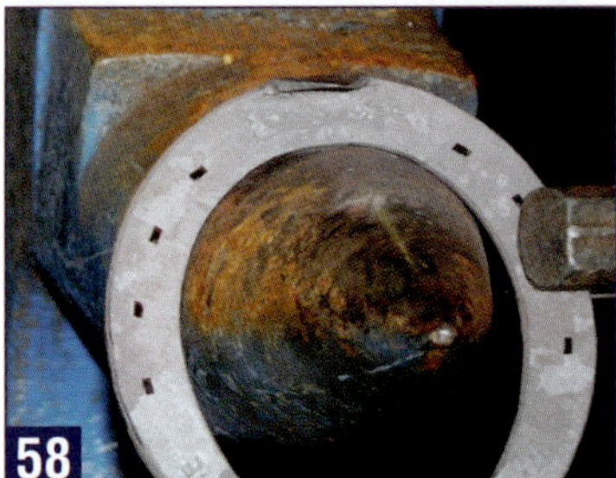

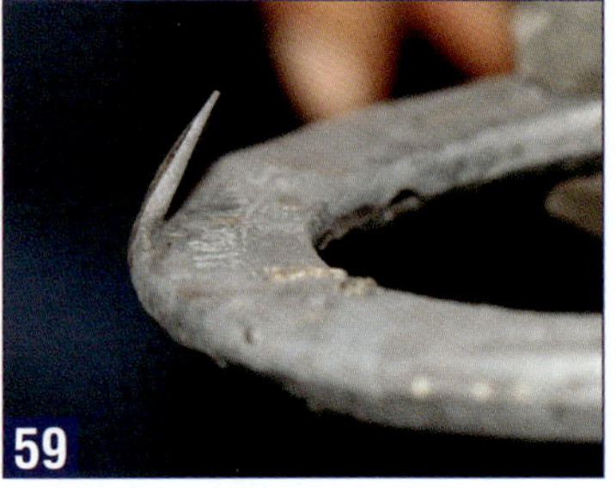

Side view of the clip.

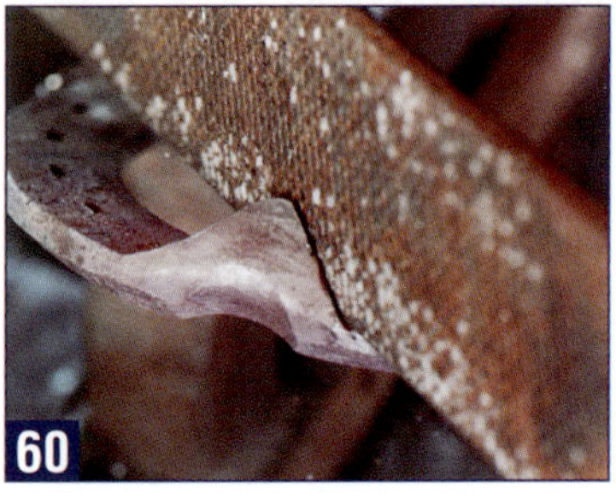

Cleaning the clip up with a rasp.

clip by hitting with the edge of the hammer face. Hammering with straight hammer swings will greatly increase accuracy and hammer control, even though you are not hitting with the face of the hammer in a flat manner.

As you draw the clip, a line will occur on the material. Chase this line with the edge of the hammer, following it until the clip is drawn to an appropriate height. Finish the clip with light, overlapping, flat hammer blows to forge out any of the lines remaining on the outside surface of the clip as you slowly allow the clip to slide off the anvil **(Figure 55)**.

I like to draw the clip from the side in my everyday work. I stand behind the heel and place the clip source on the near side of the anvil, drawing the clip from left to right. By pulling a clip in this manner, it is easy to see exactly how the clip is being drawn.

Once you have a clip, no matter how it was pulled, you need to lay it down so that it is at the angle of the hoof wall. It should also have a radius in it to match that portion of the hoof wall. To do this, place the shoe on the matching radius of the horn, and tilt it slightly so that you are able to see the hoof surface of the shoe. Tap the side and base of the clip with your hammer **(Figure 56)** and move across the base of the clip until is matches the angle and radius you are trying to achieve **(Figures 57-58)**.

There are two reasons for the radius. The first is so you can finish the clip perfectly smooth against the foot. If it were laid down flat, you would have a radius in the foot and a flat spot at the clip. The next reason you want a radius in the clip is so that it will appear a little thicker when it is being judged. Looking across a clip with a radius gives a false impression of mass **(Figure 59)**.

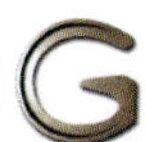

For the times that you need to rasp your clips, rasp from behind the clip at an angle **(Figure 60)**, being careful to prevent gouging the hoof surface of the shoe.

Finally, if you are pulling a clip on a rim shoe, you need to hold it at a higher angle so that you can get your hammer to the inside of the outer rim. **Figures 61-64** show how to start a clip on a rim shoe, and **Figure 65** is how the clip should look from the ground surface.

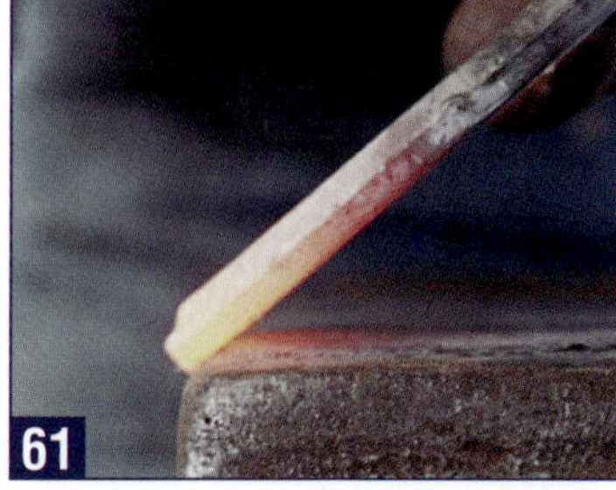

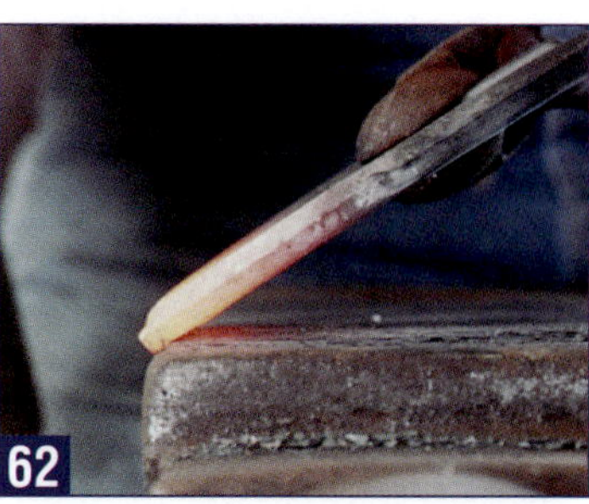

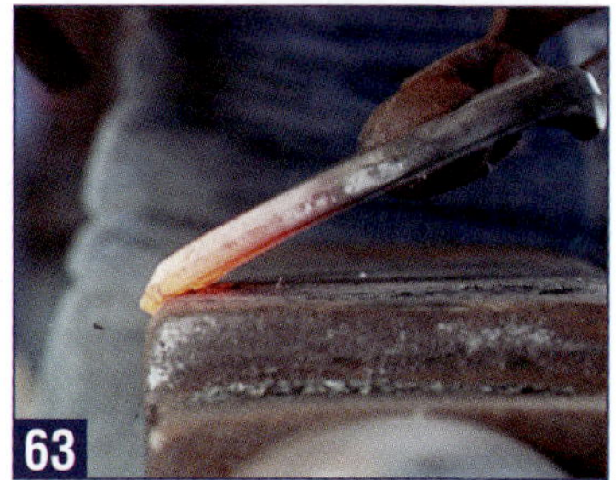

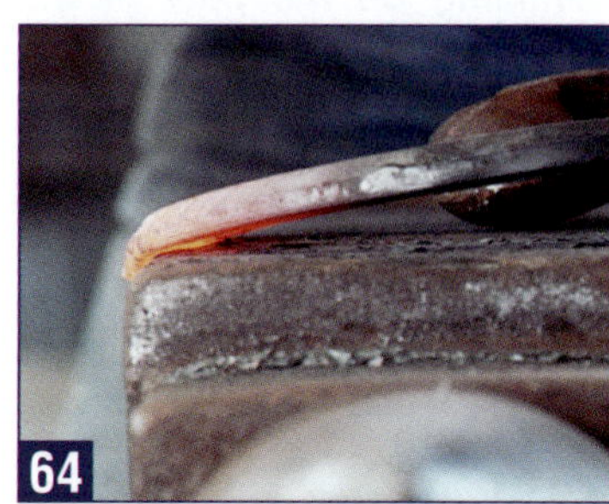

Series for a rim shoe clip.

Creasing/Fullering

Fullering (or creasing) are the terms used to define the cut put into a shoe for the placement of the nails. These two terms are used interchangeably, and you may find that the preferred term is based more on geography than anything else. In the United Kingdom, you are more likely to hear fullering, and in the United States, you are more likely to hear creasing. For this reason, I try to mix it up as much as possible so that my students will have the benefit of using the terminology. The same goes for the use of anatomical terminology.

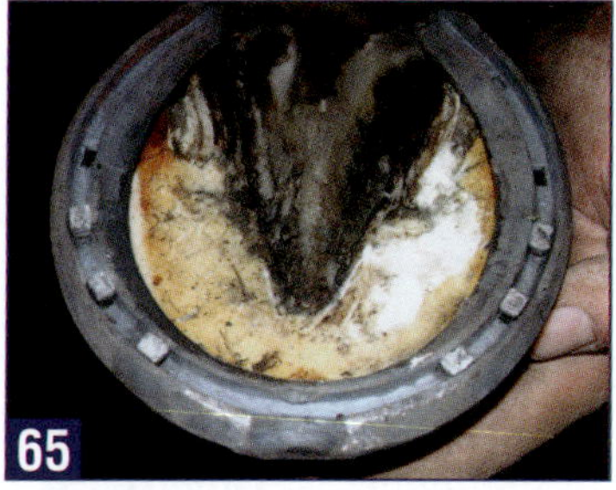

Toe clip on a rim shoe.

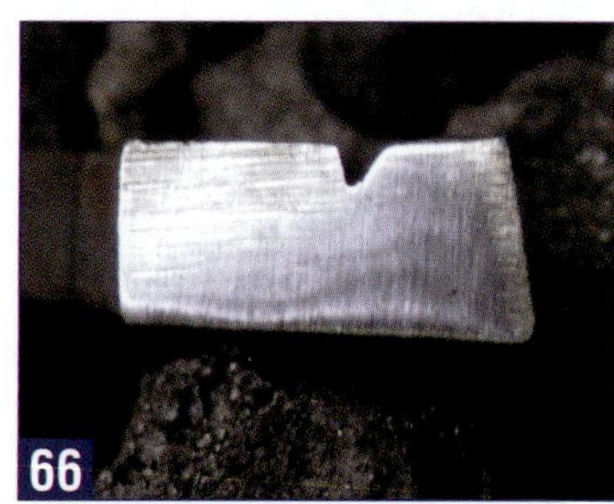

Cross section of hemmed steel with the fullering marked.

One of the advantages of creasing a shoe is that the nails are easy to remove one at a time. This is something that is difficult with a plain-stamped shoe. Due to the fact that metal is not removed from the crease, only displaced, shoes that are fullered will be somewhat longer than shoes that are only punched. The displaced material translates into a longer branch.

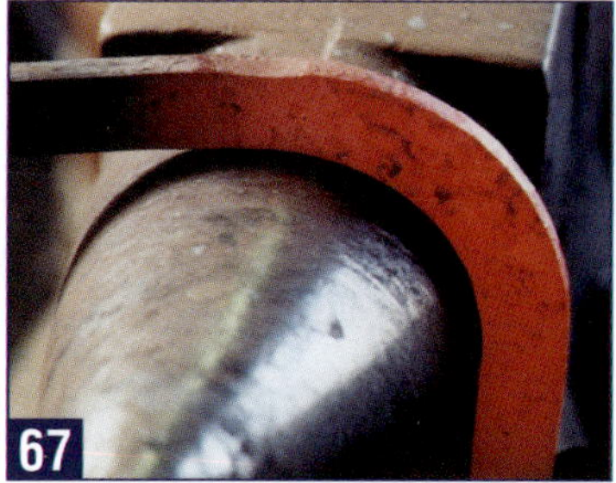

Starting the hemming.

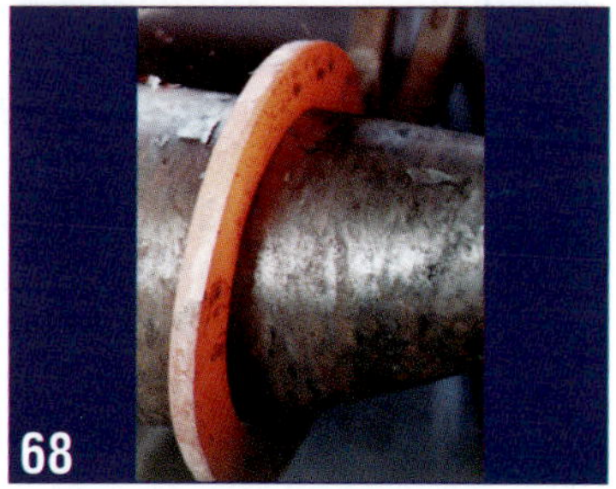

Hemming on the horn.

To prepare the shoe for creasing, we want to decrease the width on the ground surface of the shoe, as well as increase the thickness on the outside edge, and thin the metal on the inside thickness. This is called hemming, and **Figure 66** shows a cross section of a piece of steel that has been hemmed and had the fullering marked. As you look at it, the outside edge is on the right. You can see how it is thicker, and the top, which would be the ground surface, is not as wide as the other side.

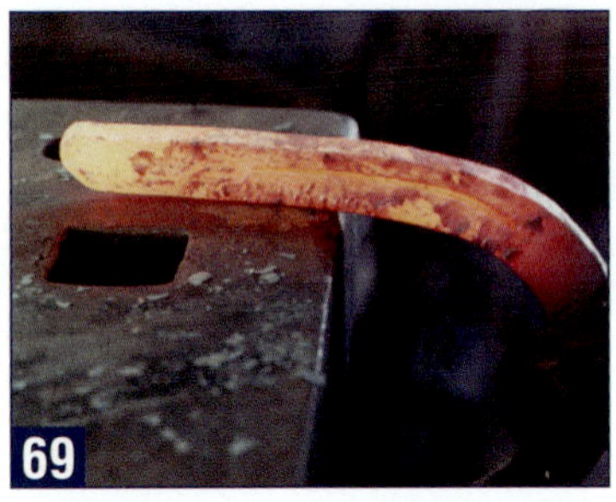

Hemming on the heel of the anvil.

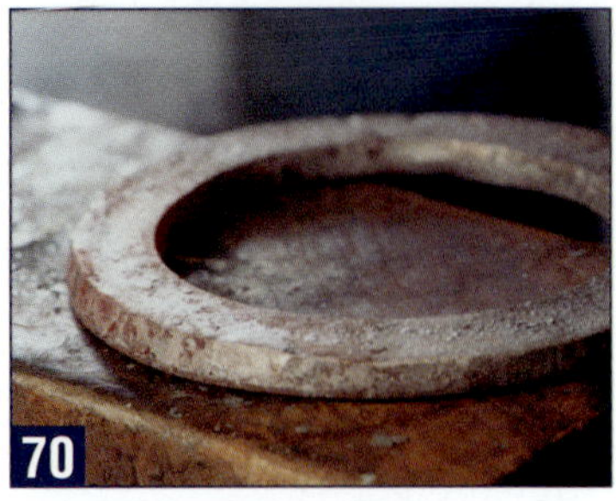

Side view of what the hemming should look like here.

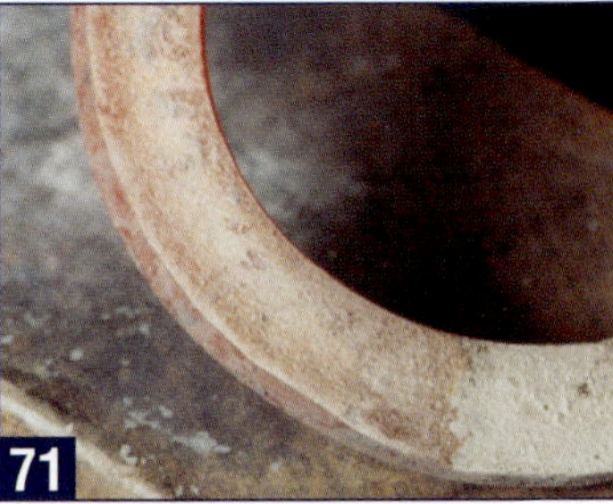

Ground surface of proper hemming.

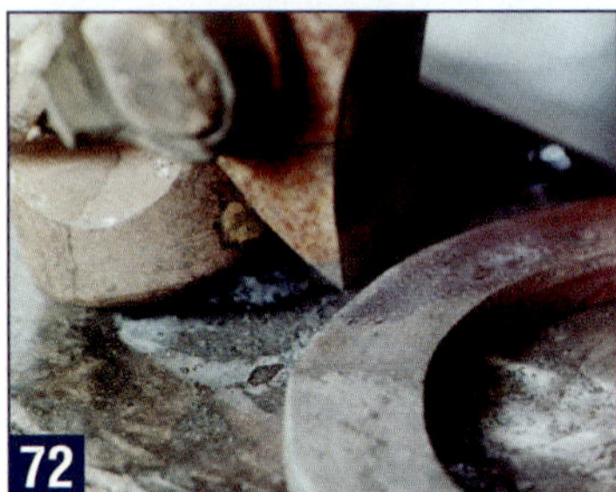

Guiding the fuller into the shoe.

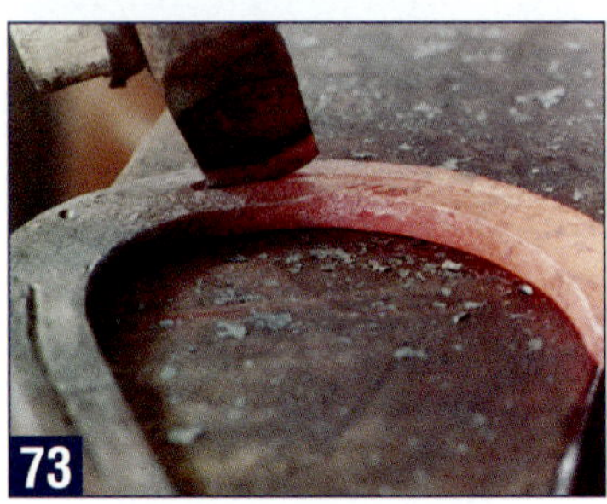

Start by angling the fuller.

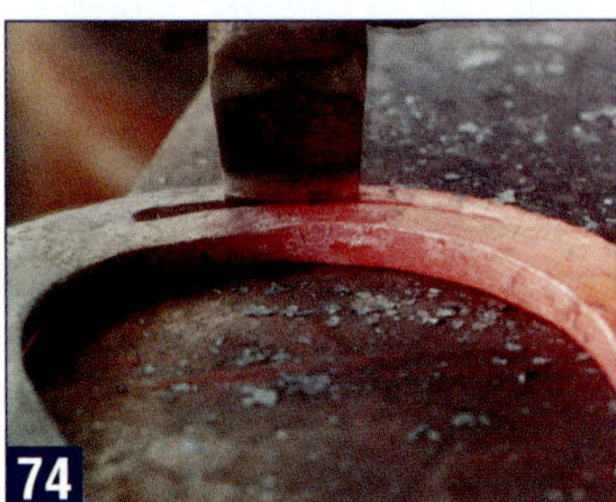

Move around the shoe.

When creasing a shoe, begin by marking the place where the crease will begin. This is usually done in the straight with a center punch before the shoe is turned. Place the shoe on the horn and twist the hammer handle in your hand to make the face hit at an angle. Carefully use the edge of the hammer to begin the hem where the crease will start in the toe **(Figure 67)**. It will take a lot of practice and hammer control to master this. Roll the shoe around the horn as you continue to hit with the angled hammer blows as you can see on the ring in **Figure 68**. I generally begin the hem on the horn and move to the heel of the anvil to hem the remainder of the branch when possible **(Figure 69)**. With some shoes, such as bar shoes that are already welded, all the hemming is done on the horn.

The hem should cause the outside of the stock to become thicker **(Figure 70)** as the ground surface loses width **(Figure 71)**. The hoof surface should remain unchanged, although we want the hem to extend the complete thickness of the stock. Some people will only hem half the thickness of the stock, which is not enough to accomplish what you are trying to achieve. If the hem is not done to at least the depth of the crease, there will be a lot of distortion in the section of the stock. If you study these figures closely, you will see that the hem is pretty close to the full thickness of the stock.

Place the fuller at the mark, using your hammerhead as a guide **(Figure 72)**. Be steady as you place the fuller where you want it, and angle it so that it will form a crisp cut at the beginning of the crease **(Figure 73)**. Hit the fuller two or three times as you drop the handle to a position parallel to the shoe. After the fuller is hit, raise the handle and walk the fuller about half the width of the blade before you hit it again. Continue with this motion of walking the fuller and hitting it when it comes to parallel until the crease is the desired length **(Figures 74-75)**. Most shoes will have the fullering taper out at the heel of the shoe and have a sharp, crisp corner at the toe **(Figure 76)**. With some diligent practice, you will find that in no time you will develop a rhythm that makes creasing easier.

After the crease is marked, if the shoe needs leveled, hit the hoof surface, being careful to hit only the inside of the web to avoid destroying the hemming. Run the fuller through until the crease is 3/4ths the thickness of the stock in depth. Use a drift punch to bottom out the nail holes in the bottom of the crease **(Figure 77)**. Move the shoe to the horn and forge out any frogeyes or other discrepancies in

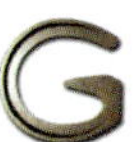

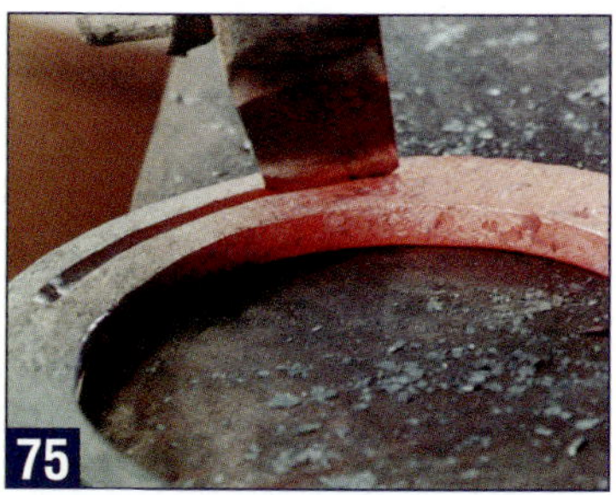
Use rocking motion to move the fuller.

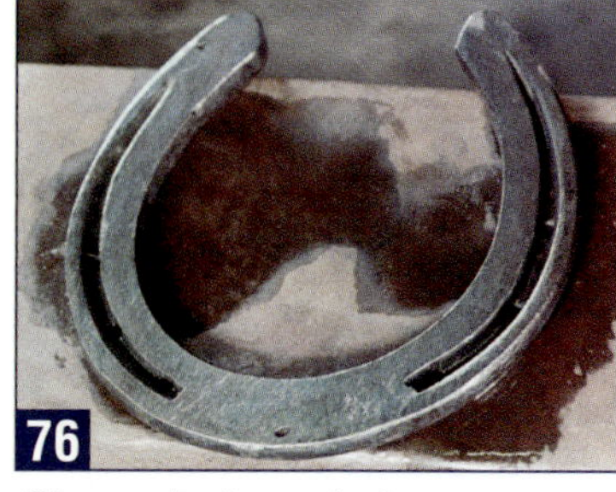
Clean starts and stops.

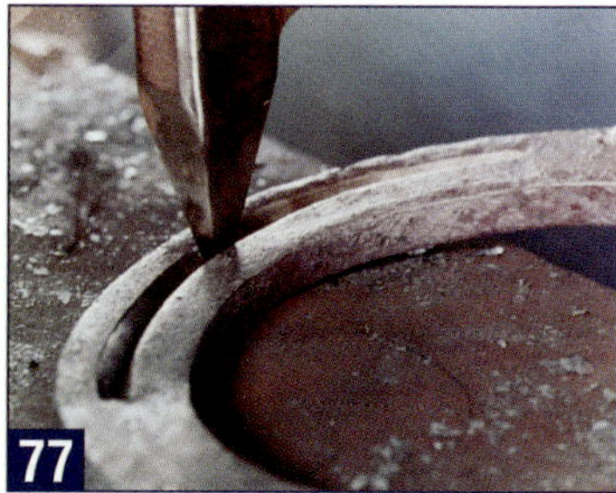
Using the drift.

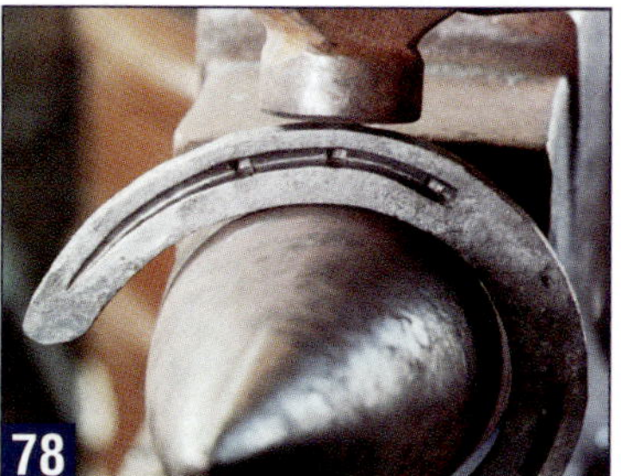
Clean up frog eyes.

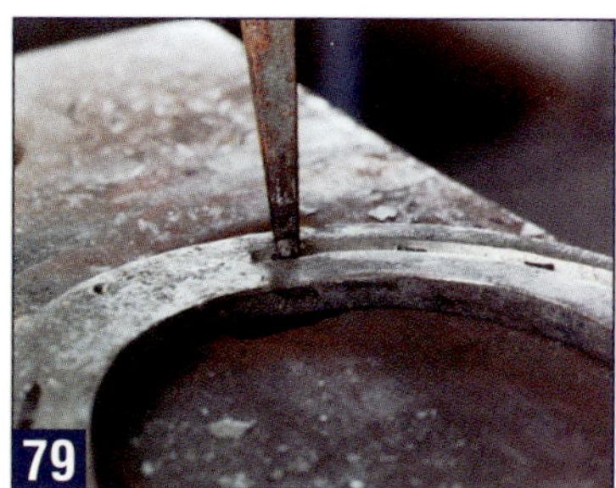
Pritchel.

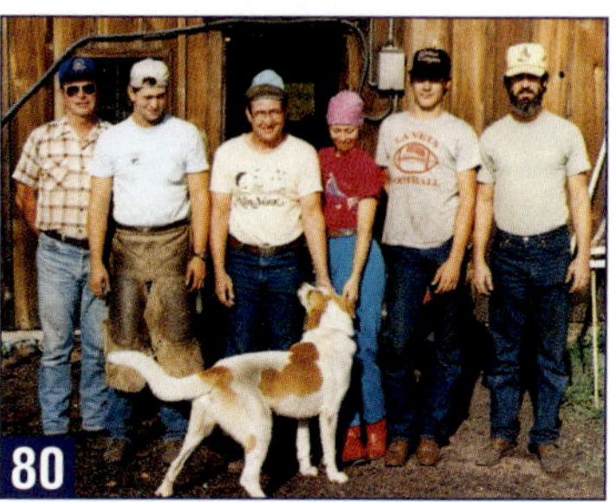
Frank Turley's Blacksmith School, Fall class of 1990.

the width of the stock **(Figure 78)**. Place the shoe on the face of the anvil with the hoof surface up, and hammer with overlapping hammer blows from toe to heel, and pritchel as you did with the plain stamped nail holes **(Figure 79)**.

By this description, fullering sounds deceptively easy. Like most of the tasks you will find when learning to forge, they are all easy once you master them through hours of practice.

Welding

Welding is the joining of two or more pieces of steel to make one piece. Forge welding is the process of using a forge and pressure to join the metal. The forge provides the heat, and the hammer-anvil combination provides the pressure. Everything just has to be set up right for success.

Many farriers think that welding is the most difficult skill to achieve in the fire. It is with this in mind that I have my students weld on the first day of class. At that point, they don't know that it should be difficult. I would like to suggest that if a student that is new to the skills of blacksmithing can weld on the first day in the fire, welding can not be that difficult. Frank Turley taught me to do this with beginners when I took his course in 1990. You can see Frank in the middle of his group of blacksmith students in August of 1990. I am second from the left, then Frank, and the only other one I remember is Stuart Greenburg on the far right **(Figure 80)**. I thought welding was hard before he showed me how simple it really is. Think of welding as like cooking. If the oven is right, the ingredients are properly mixed, and the chef knows what to do, the end product is good.

It is easier to weld two pieces that are holding themselves together than it is to weld two completely separate pieces. For this reason, I recommend beginning with a project that allows you to bring both ends to be welded out of the forge with one pair of tongs. Chain links and bar shoes are a couple of examples.

Welding occurs when the surface of the metal becomes hot enough for the molecular structure of the metal to join another piece of steel at the same temperature. Flux is applied to prevent the surface of the metal from getting scale on it. Scale is the result of oxygen coming in contact with the hot surface of the metal. Propane forges cause a lot of scale because the oxygen is not being consumed by the fire the way it is in a coal or coke fire. I have never been able to weld in propane without flux,

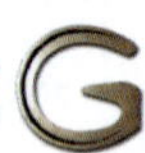

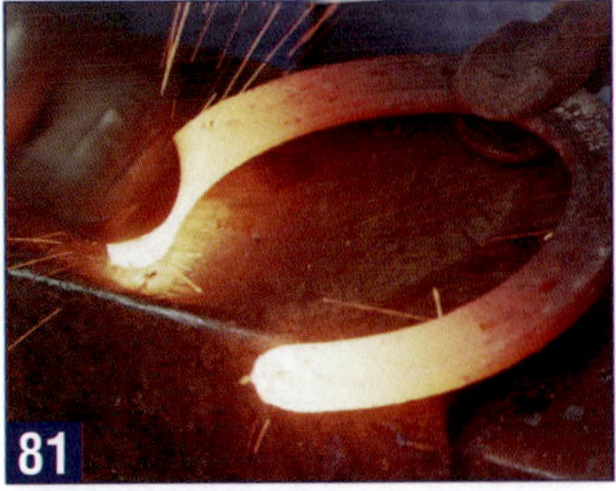

Scarfing the heels.

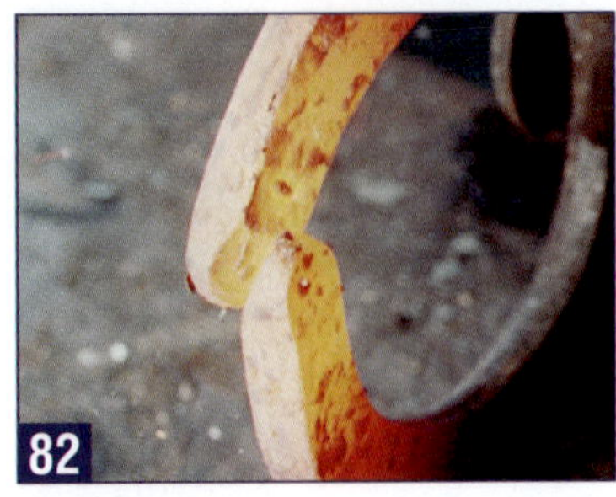

Overlap.

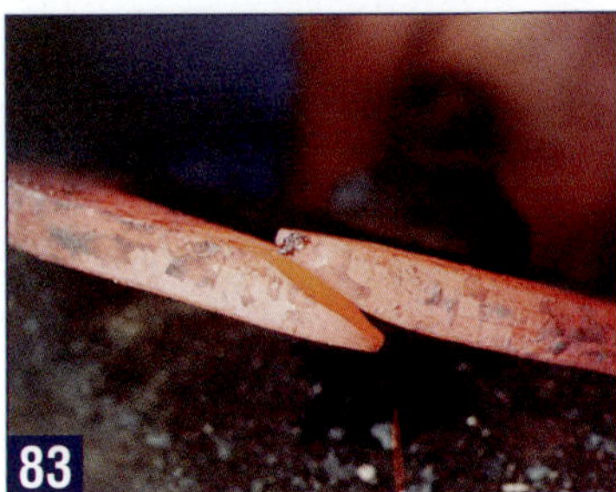

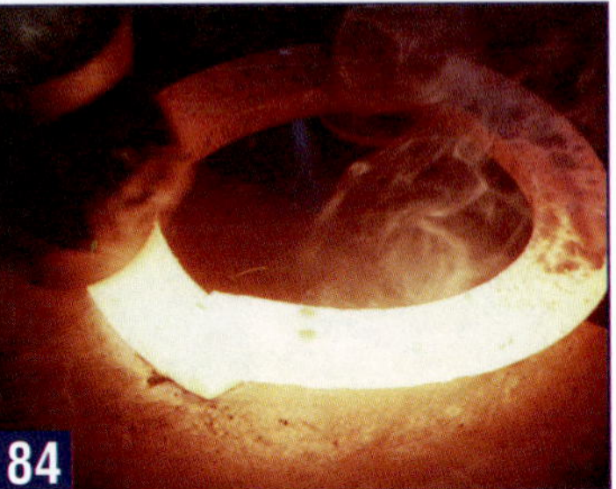

Weld with the toe of the hammer.

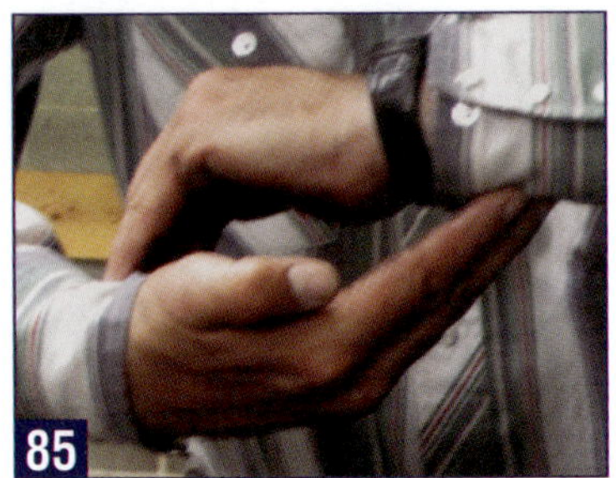

Hands depicting the areas that are welded in the first welding heat.

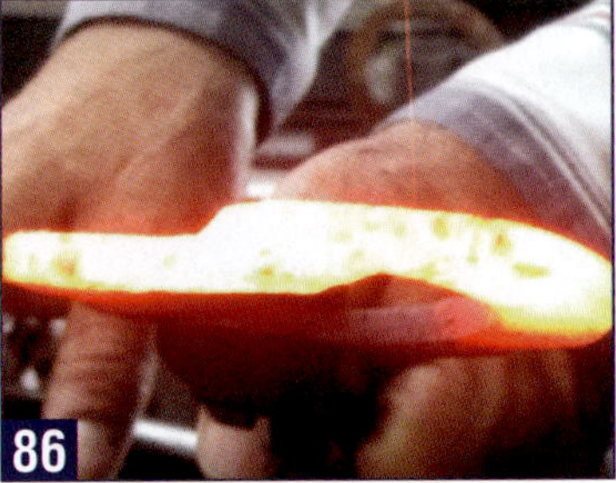

It should look like this after the first welding heat.

but it can be done with ease in a coal or coke forge. The reasons for this are twofold. First, there is more oxygen consumption by the coke forge, and second, the coke forge is much hotter than a gas forge.

To weld, the metal must be prepared correctly. It must be clean of scale, and forging a scarf on the edge to be welded is helpful for beginners. With most propane forges, the pressure must be turned up to achieve enough heat, usually 12 to 15 pounds on the pressure gauge. For this demonstration we are going to weld a simple ring out of an old horseshoe.

Begin by heating the shoe and brushing it with a butcher-block brush right out of the fire. Sharpen the heels on the width of the stock at the end of the anvil face **(Figure 81)**. The sharpened area is called a scarf, and there are many different ways to scarf for different applications. Repeat the same steps to the opposite branch of the shoe. Close the shoe so that the heel on your tong side when holding the toe of the shoe is on top of the heel on your hammer side **(Figures 82-83)**. Add flux, then place the shoe back in the fire. Wait until the shoe is hot enough to weld. In propane, the shoe will disappear in the fire. This means that it will take just a second for your eyes to focus on the shoe in the fire if you have been looking away. When a shoe disappears in the fire, it is as hot as that particular fire is going to get it. In coal or coke, it will be a yellow heat. Disappearing in a coke fire is really disappearing because it is burned away.

Remove the shoe and hammer with one quick, light, flat hammer blow directly over the weld. Change the angle of the hammer so that the toe of the hammer is coming down directly over the seam of the weld **(Figure 84)**. Hammer quickly until the seam disappears, turn the shoe over fast and repeat the process on the opposite side. In **Figure 85**, I am holding my hands together to depict the portion of the weld that has been accomplished in the first heat. You can see the piece after the first welding heat in **Figure 86**.

Brush the weld, flux, and return to the fire. Once the shoe is at a welding heat, come out of the fire and hammer directly on top of the weld with quick, light, flat hammer blows **(Figure 87)**. Move to the horn and forge the outside perimeter of the weld **(Figure 88)**. If done correctly, you will end up with a seamless weld **(Figure 89)** You can use this piece to make a ring as the one in **Figure 90**. Look at the detail of my tong boss in **(Figure 91)**. If you are using your tongs correctly to achieve 3 points of contact, the boss will be shiny.

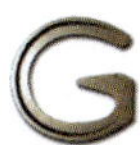

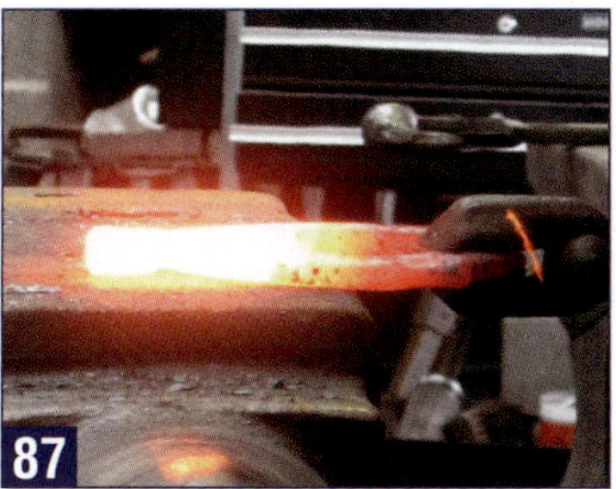

Fast, soft, and flat blows on the second heat.

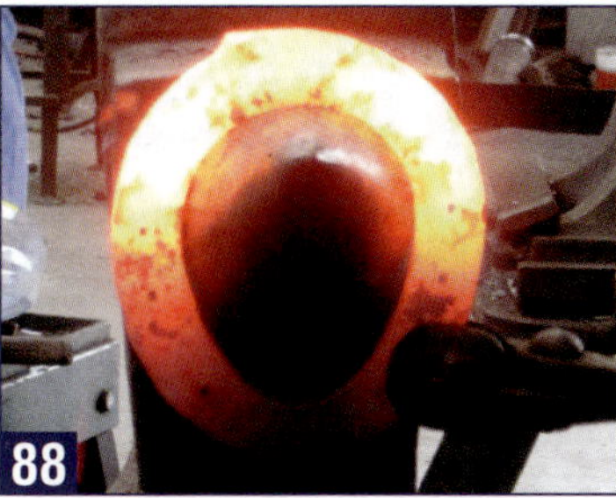

Forge the weld on the horn.

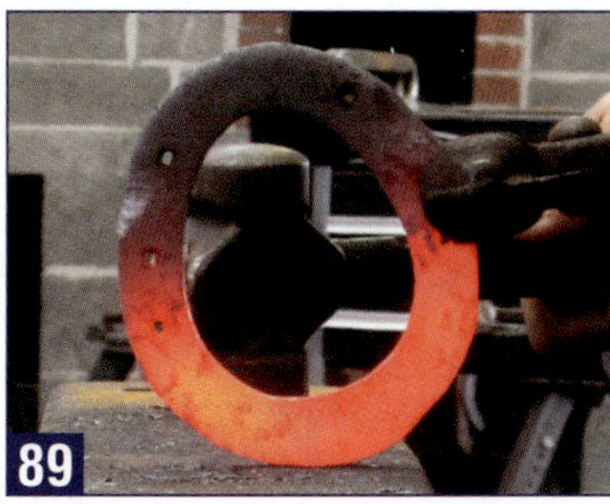

Finished with the second welding heat.

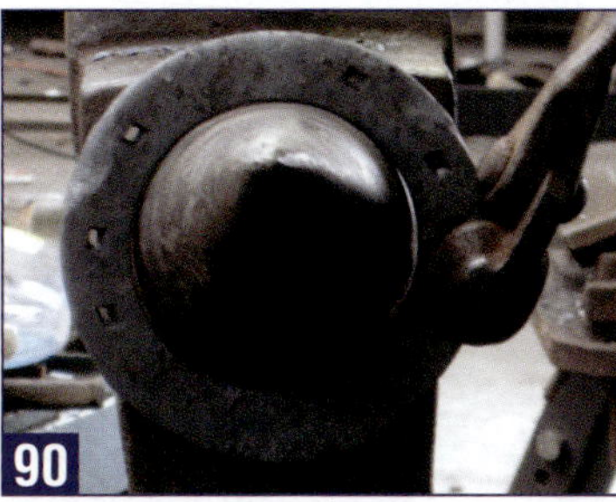

Shape the piece into a perfect ring.

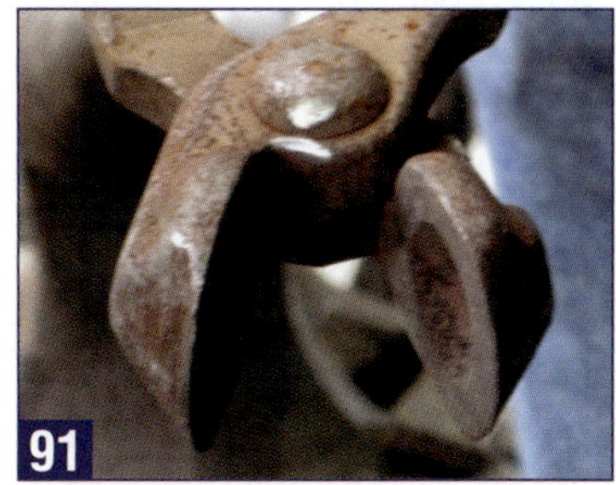

The shiny area of my tong boss from using three points of contact with the shoe.

Troubleshooting The Welding Process

When welding is unsuccessful, it can be traced to a few mistakes made by the blacksmith. The most common is trying to weld too cold. Be patient with the forge. It will only heat at a certain speed. If this is the problem in a propane forge, try working two projects at the same time. While one is being worked on the anvil, the other is being heated, and you aren't standing there waiting impatiently for the appropriate heat.

Sometimes the steel is being left in the fire too long. In propane, the flux will no longer be molten after a certain point, leaving a thick scale. Commercial flux will stay molten longer in the forge than borax, and gives you a longer window of opportunity. In coke, the piece of steel can be burnt away if left too long. Another common problem is hitting the steel too hard while trying to weld it. If the steel is hit too hard, it will draw faster than it can bond. Welding is best done with quick, light hammer blows. Try using a lighter hammer if this is a problem for you.

With beginners, the anvil, hammer, and thought process are not always ready when the steel is ready. Once the steel is at the right welding heat, bring it out of the fire and hit the weld as quick as possible. The environment outside of the forge draws heat from the steel at an extremely fast pace, and the welding heat is quickly lost if the blacksmith is not ready when the steel is. You can't take the piece from the fire and spend several seconds looking for your hammer when you need to be swinging.

Another important aspect of forge welding is confidence. Like many things in life, if you believe that you can, you can. If you believe that you can't, well you are probably right about that as well.

This chapter covered a lot of tasks and processes that come together to make basic horseshoes. Once you learn what is in this chapter, you will find that the skills will transfer to the majority of the horseshoes that can be made. There is another chapter that covers some exercises you can do to increase your skill level. You will get further faster by breaking down the whole into tasks, then mastering each task in turn. Give it a try, and good luck on your American Farriers Association Certified Farrier and Certified Journeyman Farrier tests as well as your FITS Exams, and the Diploma, Associateship, and Fellowship of the Worshipful Company of Farrier exams.

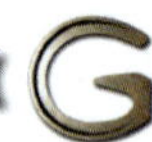

Chapter 38 EXERCISES IN THE FORGE

Exercises Designed to Improve Your Skills

RING EXERCISE

Making a welded ring from bar stock or old shoes is perhaps one of the best all-around exercises that you can do. Even if you are an advanced forger, there is a tremendous amount that you can learn from building rings. Many of the elements of shoe building are utilized when you build a ring, and you can use that ring to practice fullering, nail holes, clips, shaping, forging, and welding.

To build one out of bar stock, simply heat most of a 13 to 15 inch length of steel. Practice a toe bend, **(Figure 1)** and then bend the hot branch around the horn, staying on top of the horn. **(Figure 2)** It should come around like the stock in **Figure 3**. Once you have it bent around, heat the opposite branch and bring the two together. **(Figures 4-5)** Arrange the ends of the stock so that when you hold the "toe" area, the branch on your tong hand side is on top of the branch in your hammer hand side **(Figure 6)**. This will allow you to get rid of the seams with the toe of your hammer on the first welding heat.

Flux the weld site, heat, hit quick and lightly, and use the toe of your hammer to blend away the seams. Once the seam disappears on one side, quickly flip the piece and blend away the seam on the other side **(Figure 7)**. After the first welding heat, it should look like **Figure 8**. On the next heat, hit fast and light in the middle of the weld on the anvil face **(Figure 9)**. Move to the horn and forge the stock to the original dimension **(Figures 10-11)**. You are now ready to make it into a perfect circle, which is the next great bit of practice you get when

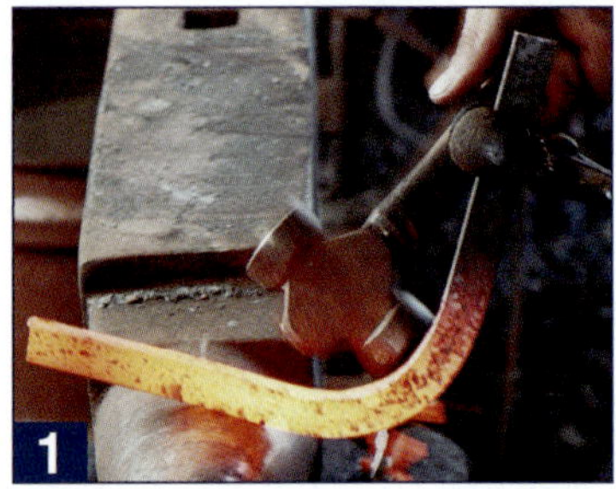

1 *Make a bend in the stock as if it were a toe bend.*

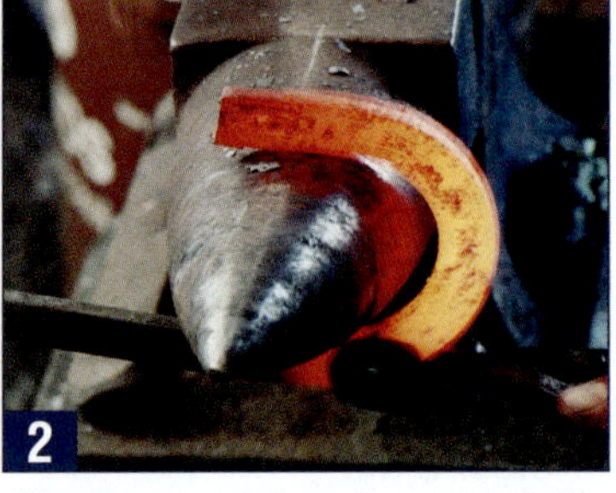

2 *Continue to bend around the horn.*

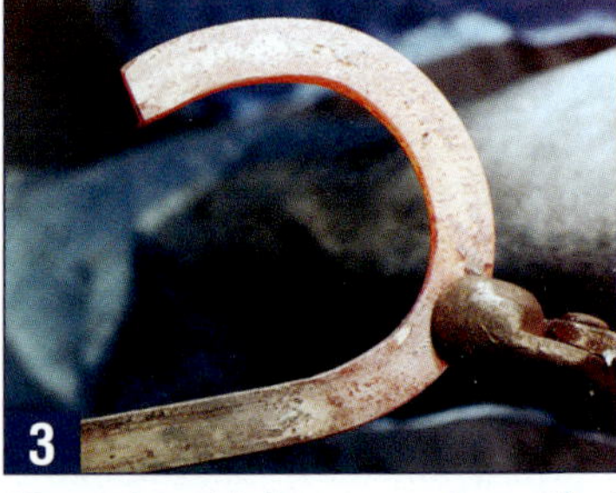

3 *You should have a piece that looks like this at the end of heat one.*

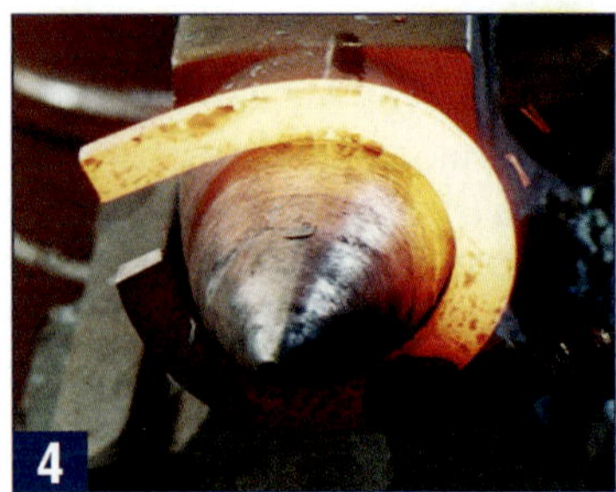

4 *Do the same thing to the other side.*

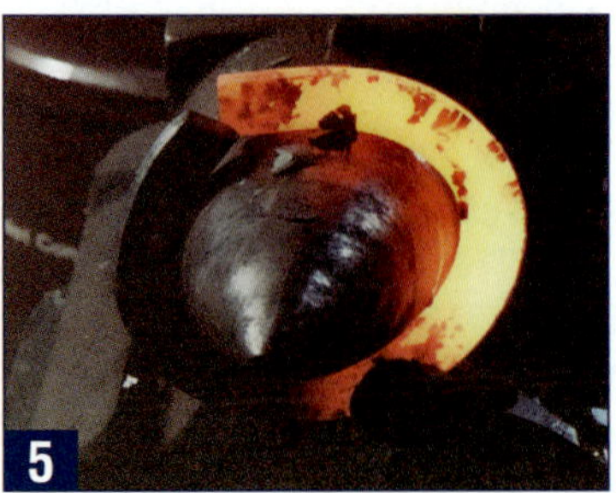

5 *Stay on top of the horn.*

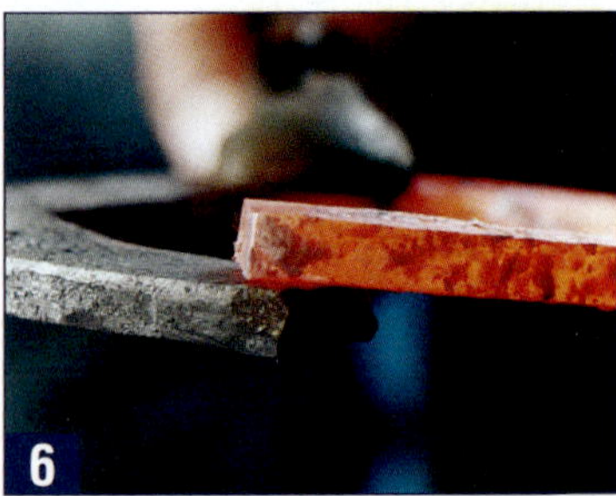

6 *Overlap the pieces with your tong hand side on top of your hammer hand side.*

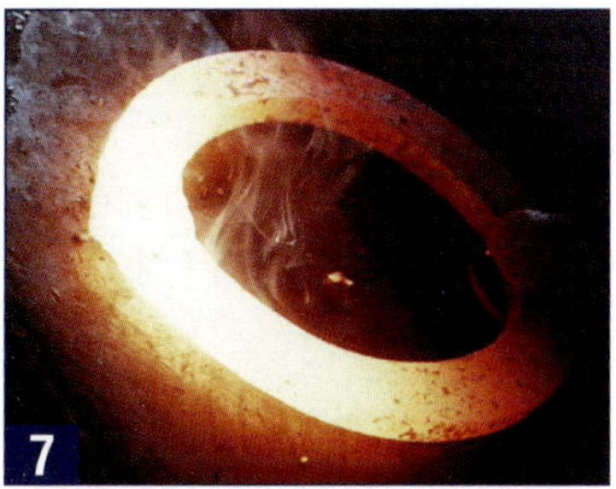

First welding heat.

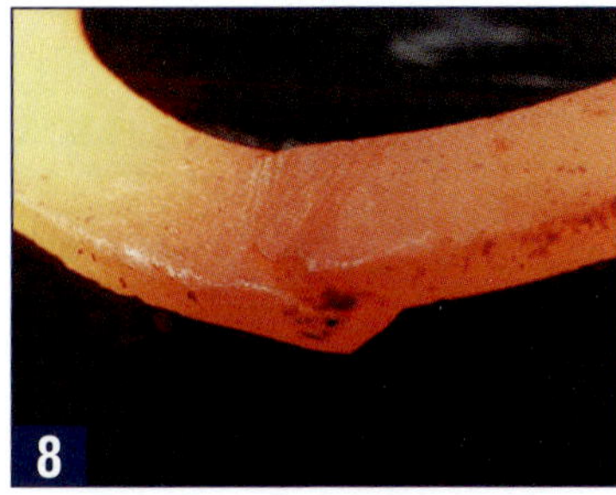

The seams should be gone.

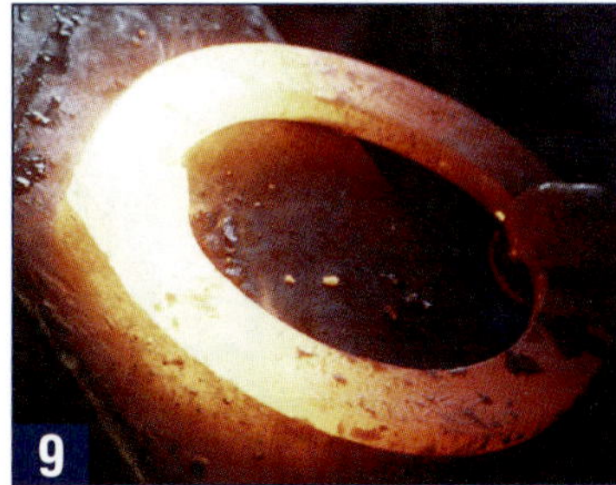

Second welding heat.

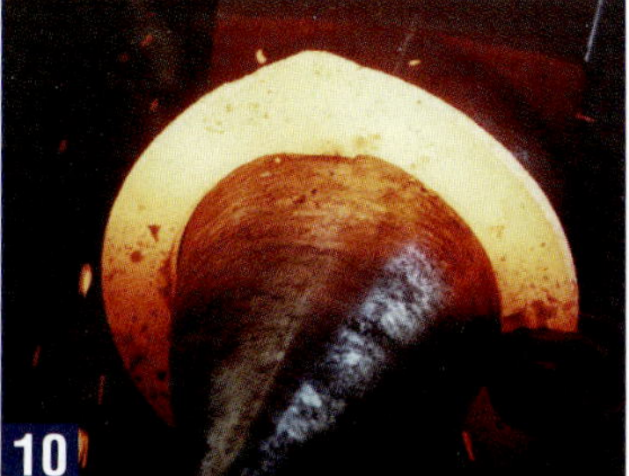

Forge the weld on the horn.

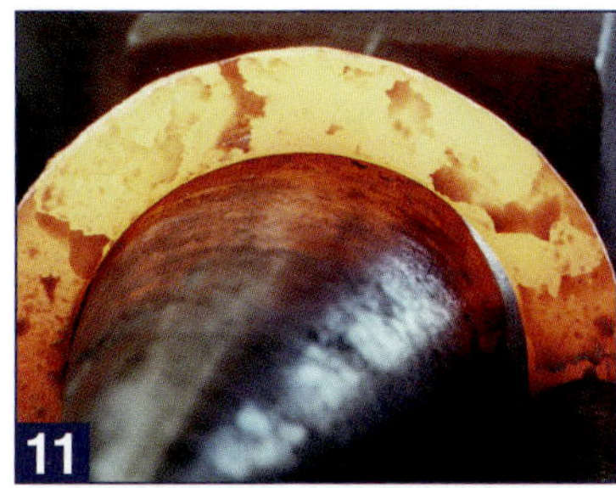

Forge the stock back to original width.

building rings.

To do this, hit just beyond the top of the horn as you roll the shoe around. As you study **Figures 12-16**, you can see that the ring is getting rounder. Take a good look at the tong position, and be strict with your tong position as well as where your hammer is hitting. Don't hit too hard. The reason we get this stuff hot is so that we don't have to hit it too hard. Just roll it around and around until it is perfectly round. Now you have something to play and practice with.

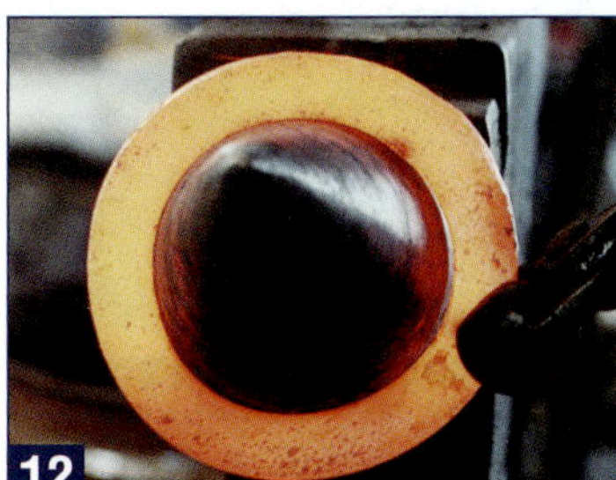

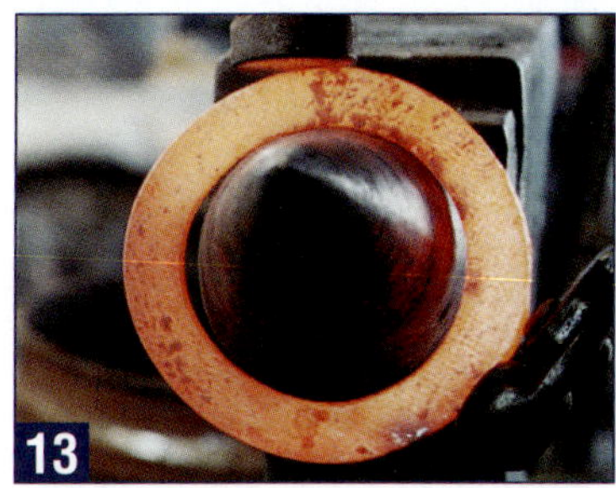

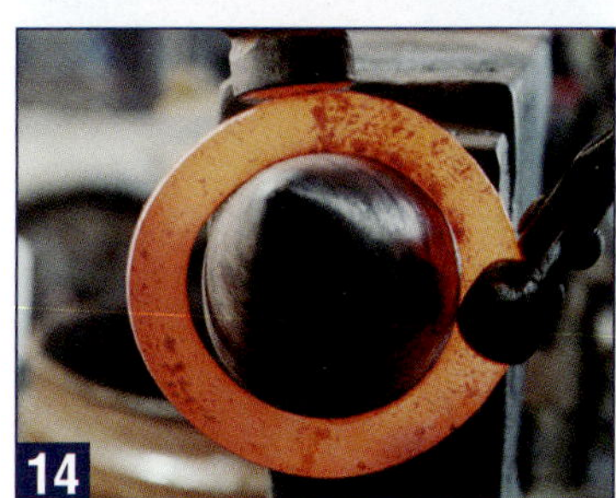

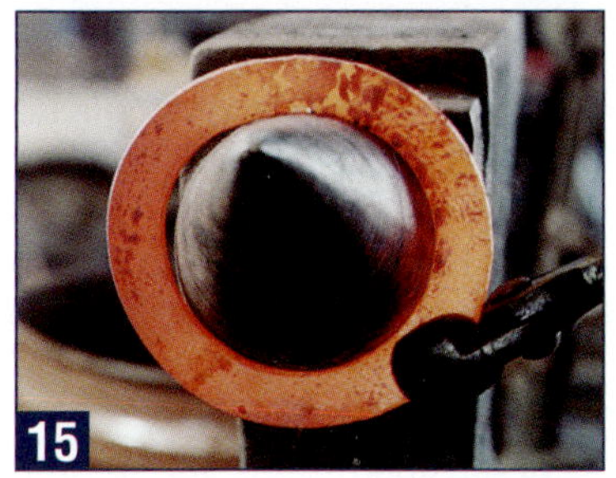

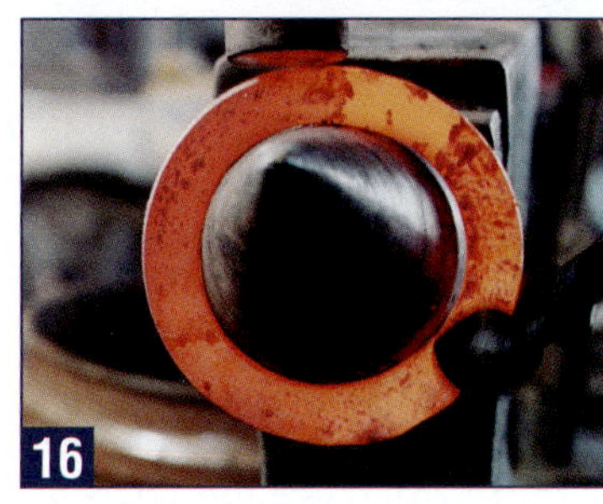

Move around the horn, shaping the ring into a perfect circle.

TOE BENDS

Begin by cutting as many pieces of stock as you feel that you can handle. The more the merrier **(Figure -17)**. Mark each piece with training wheels (see Chapter 40), or toenails for the desired shoe **(Figure 18)**. Make the first toe-bend so that it is as near to perfect as you are able. Repeat on each piece after that, laying them on top of each other to determine any discrepancies **(Figure19)**. You can continue from there to make the rest of the shoe, one task at a time **(Figure 20)**. **Figure 21** shows the three stages of a 3 heat, plain-stamped front shoe.

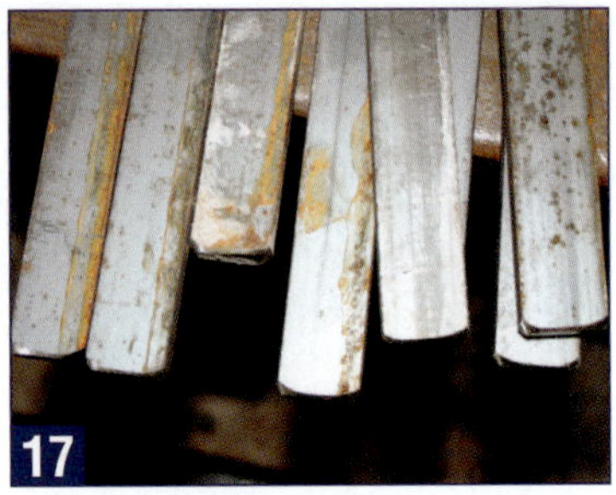
17 Stock ready to play.

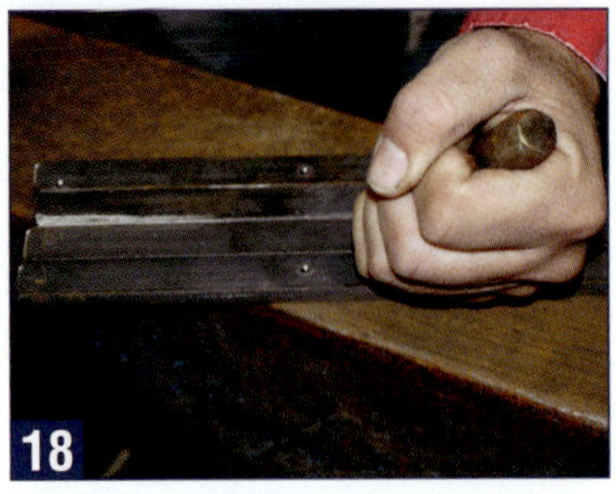
18 Mark the stock to make the toe bends.

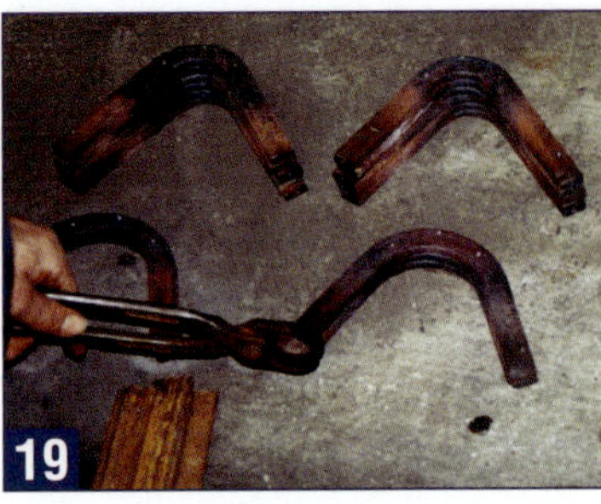
19 Make and stack the toe bends.

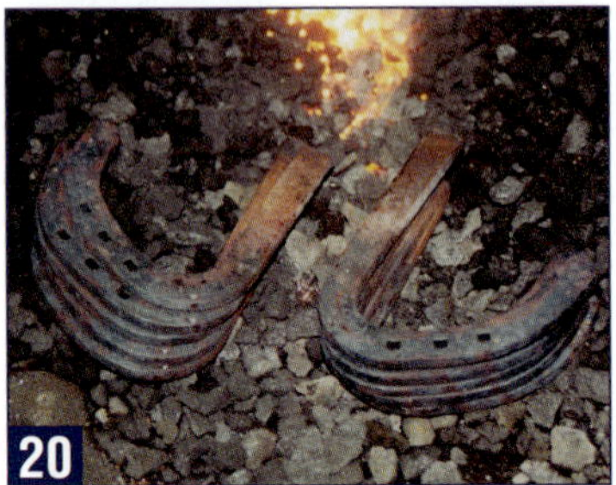
20 Shoes ready for their third and final heat.

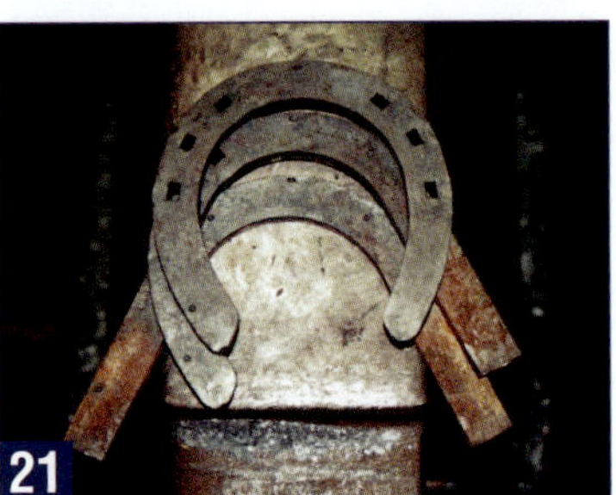
21 The three stages of a three-heat plain stamped front shoe.

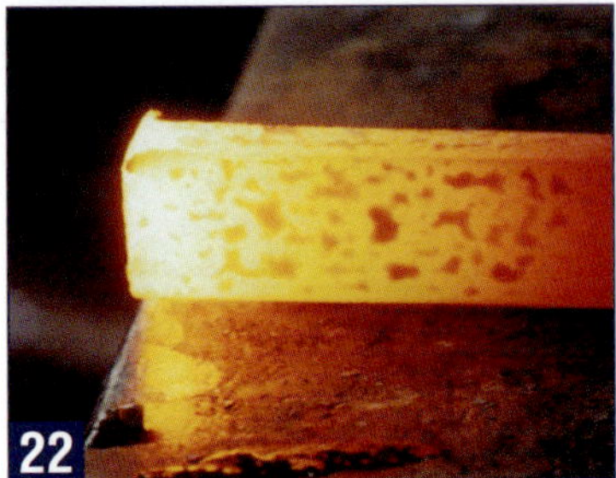
22 Pull the outside corner back towards you.

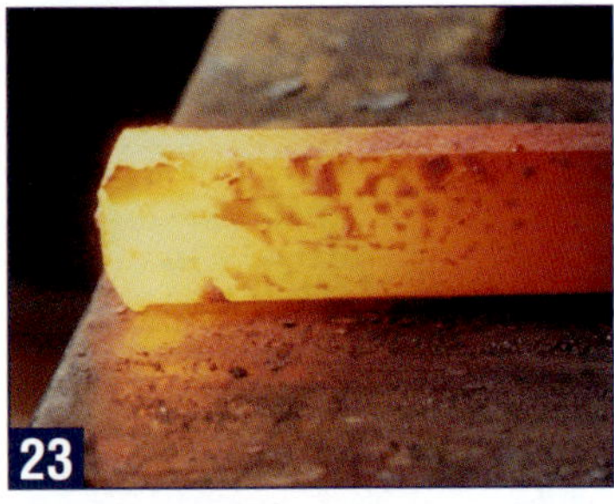
23 Do the exact same move to the inside corner.

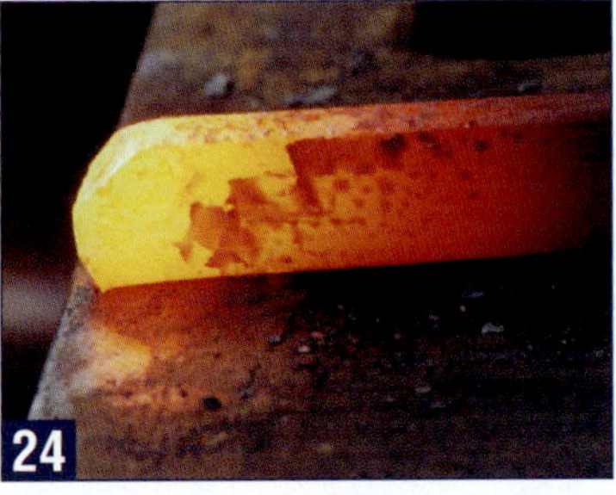
24 Hammer at an angle to establish your heel check. Finish the heel.

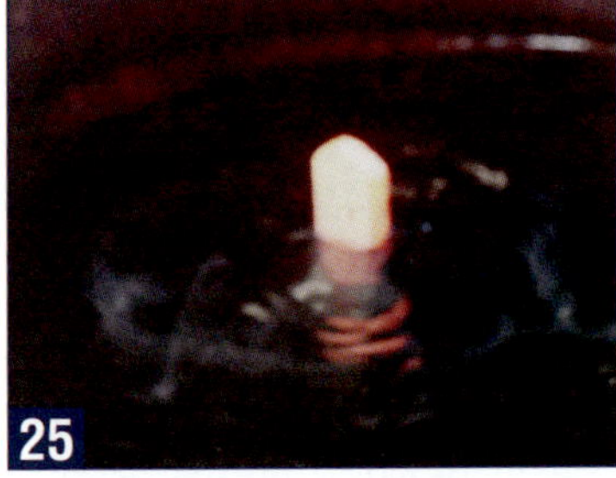
25 Quench to the tip of the heel to upset it back to square.

HEELS

Cut a ten-inch piece of stock that is the desired cross-section for the typical shoes that you will use. For most saddle horses, this will be 5/16 by 3/4 inch. Make a heel on one end of the stock **(Figures 22-24)**. Reheat the stock and quench till there is only about an inch on the end with the heel hot **(Figure 25)**. Upset this area on the face of the anvil until it is back to the original dimensions. **(Figures 26-28)** The side of the stock that you strike with the hammer will upset slightly, preventing proper tong fit. Simply smash it back to flat on the face of the anvil **(Figure 29)**.

Every time you build a heel, mark the stock with a center punch **(Figure 30)** so that you can keep track of the number of heels you are building. Try to reach a goal. Build another heel **(Figures 31-33)** and upset back to square. Try to work this so that you are able to build the heel and upset the stock in one heat.

NAIL HOLES

Begin by making a ring. Once the ring is made, punch a bunch of nail holes in a row about 1/4" apart on one side of the ring **(Figures 34-35)**. By this time, the steel should be at an appropriate pritcheling temperature. Pritchel out the holes and check with a nail. **(Figures 36-37)** Reheat and punch more holes. After a while, try placing the holes an

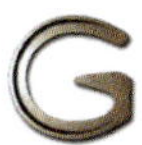

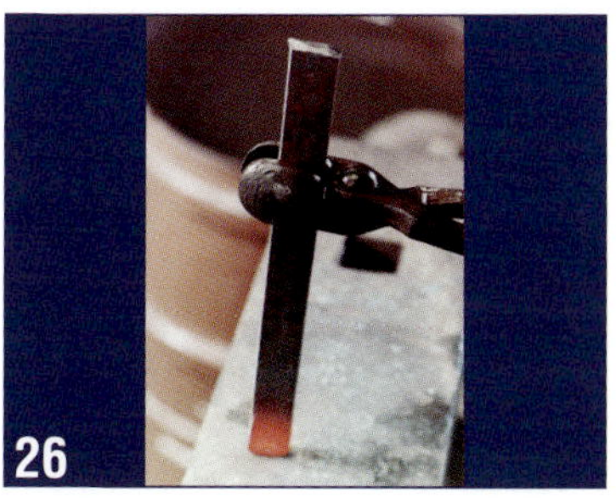

Upset the heel.

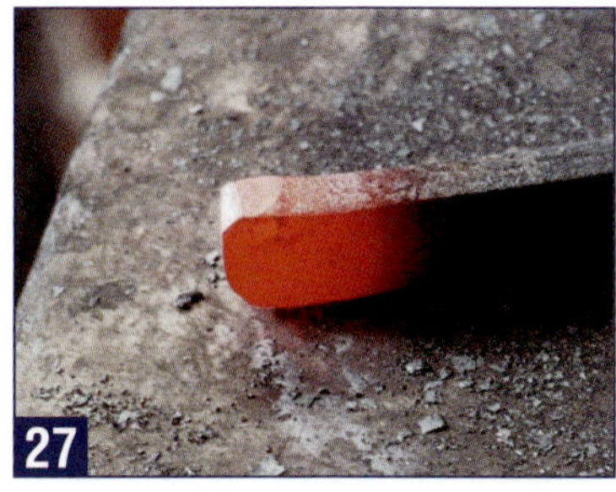

Forge the stock back to square.

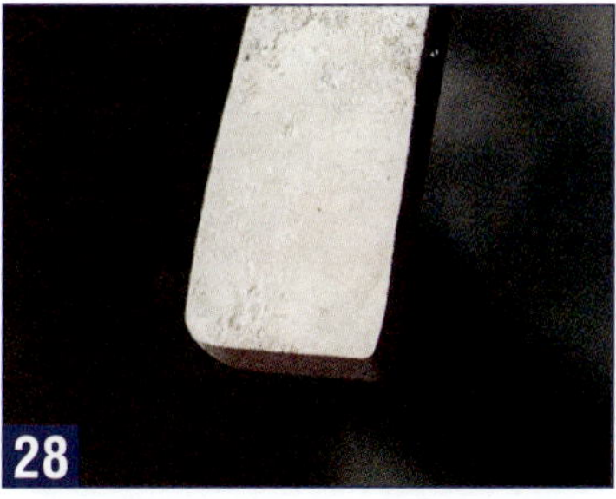

The end is now ready to heat and make another heel

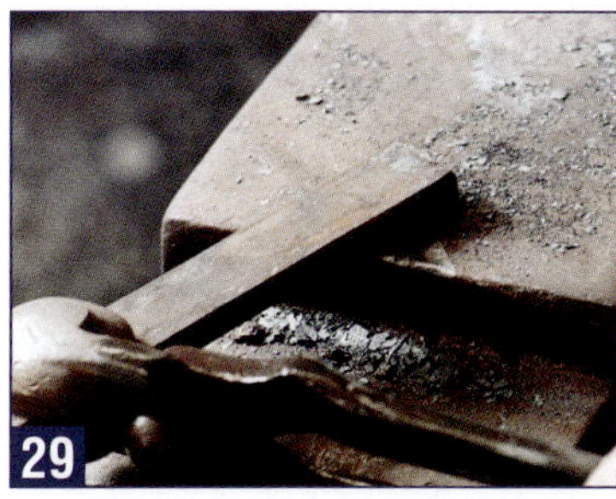

Smash the cold end that you hit with your hammer.

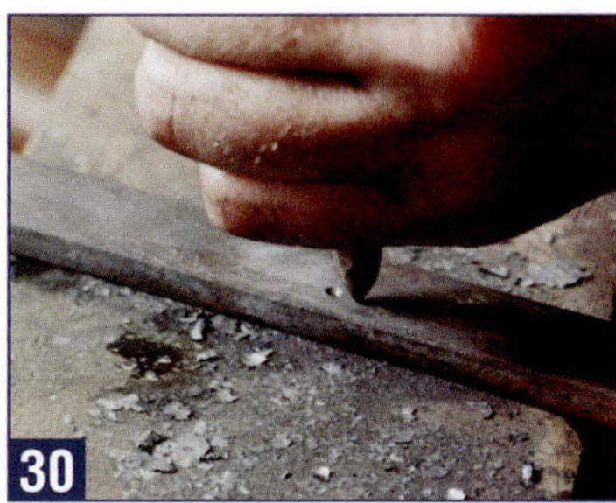

Mark the stock so that you can keep track of the number of heels you have made.

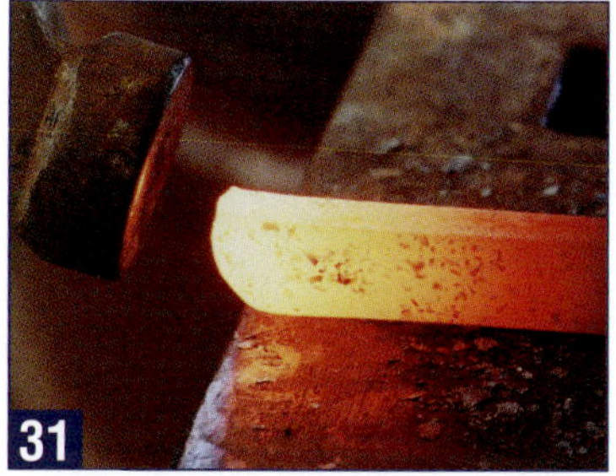

Make another heel.

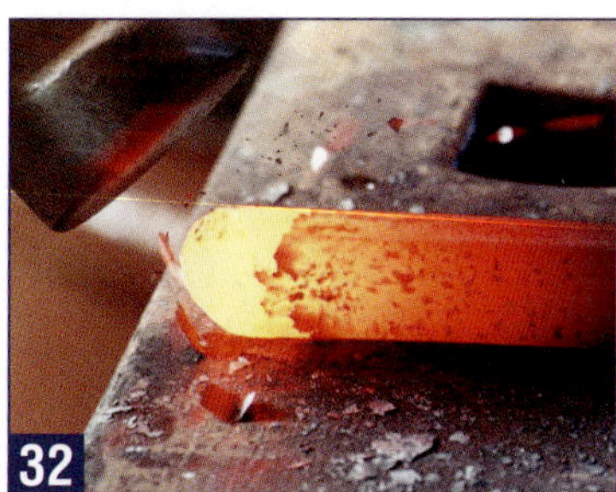

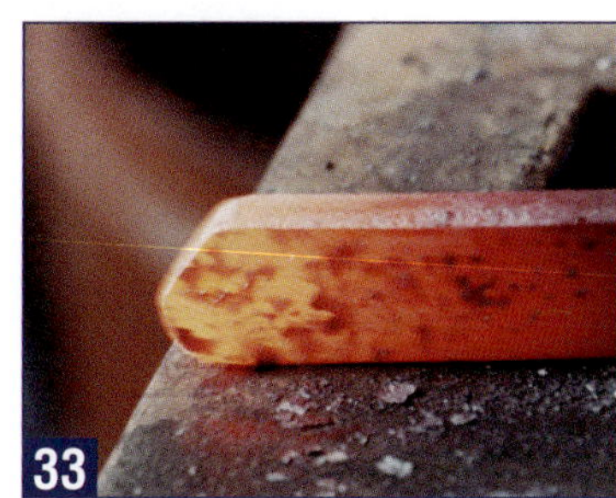

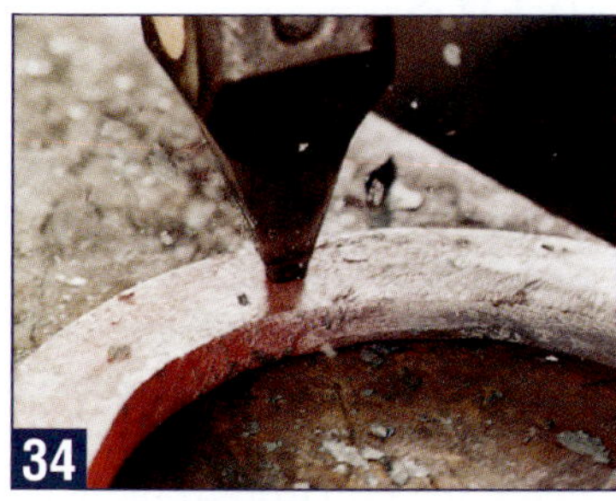

Place your fore punch on the ring.

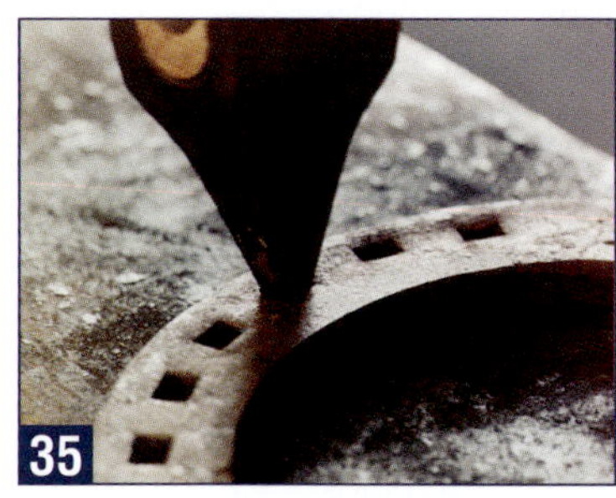

Make several holes in the ring.

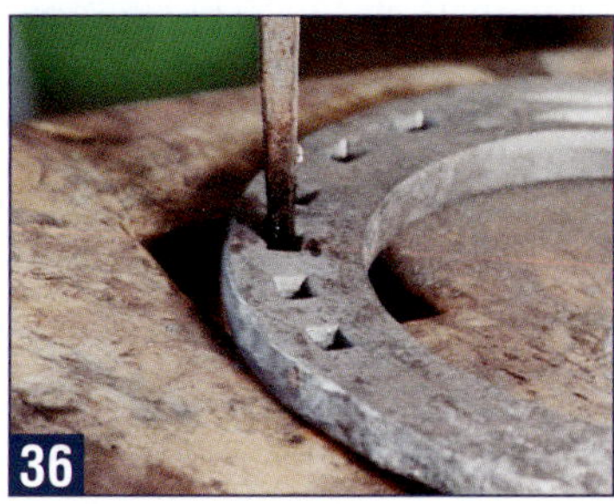

Pritchel the holes.

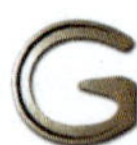

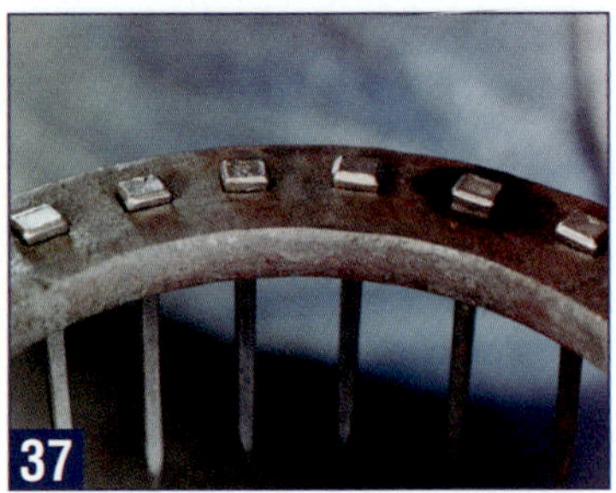

Check the nails.

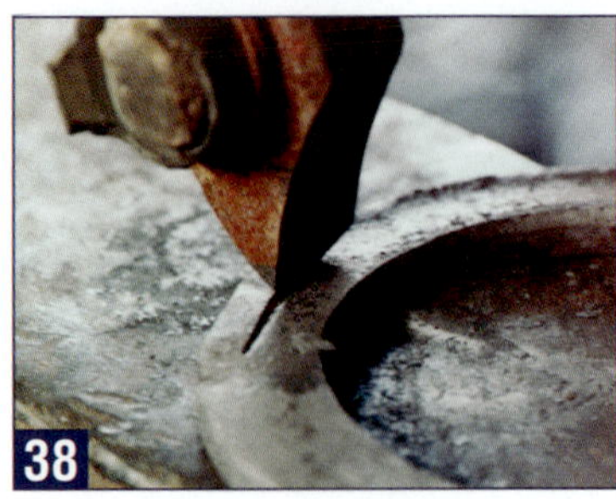

Run the first fullering.

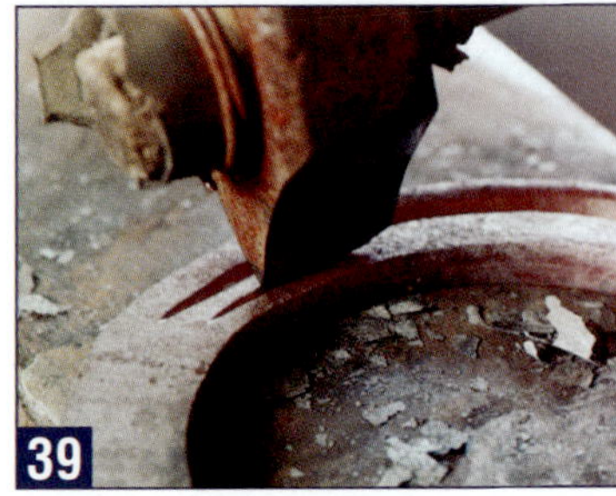

Run another fullering inside the first.

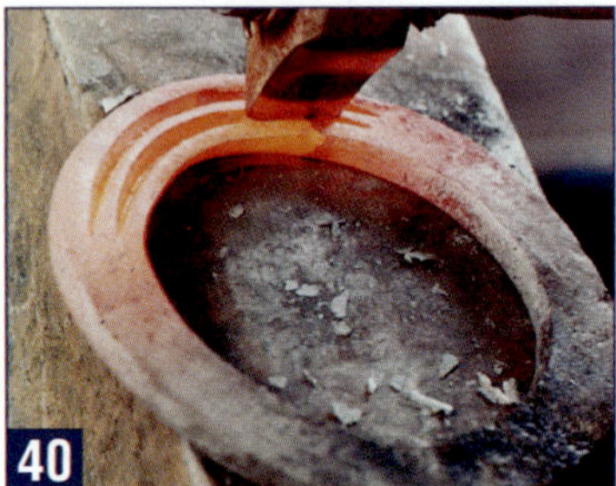

Run another fullering inside the first.

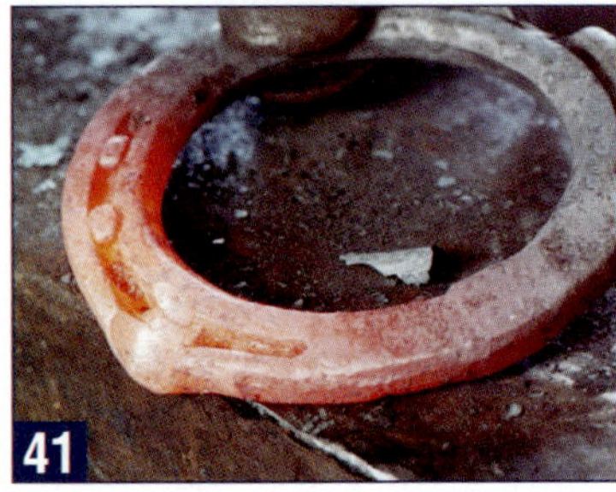

Start of the clip source with a cross peen.

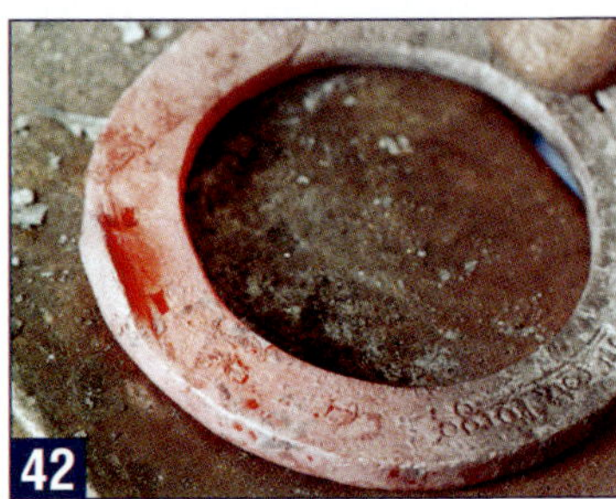

How the source looks with a cross peen.

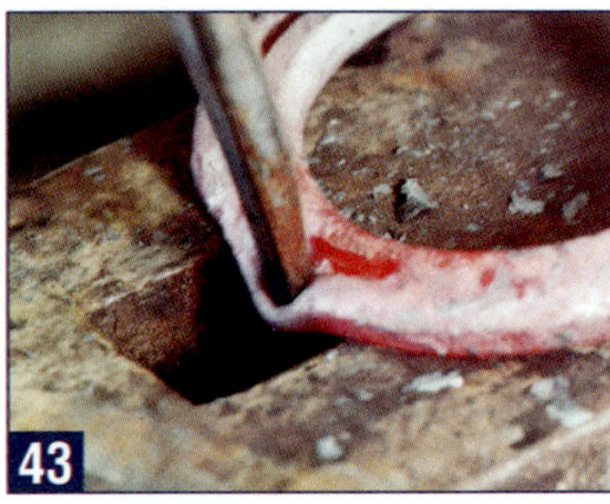

Starting a clip with a bob punch.

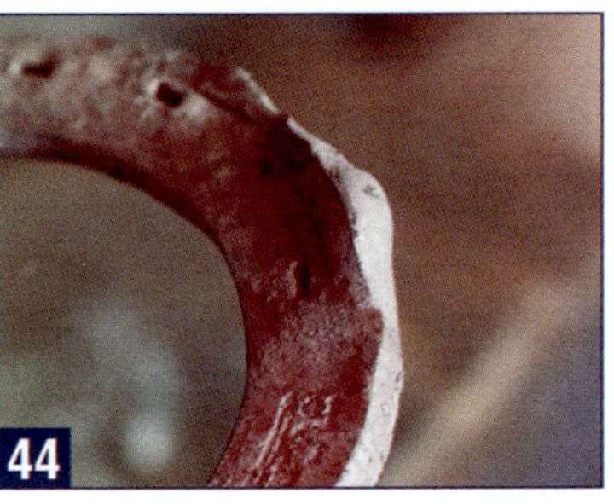

How the source looks with a bob punch.

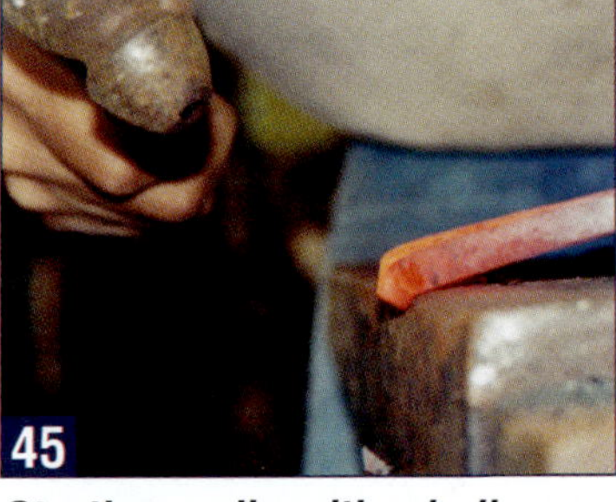

Starting a clip with a ball peen.

inch apart and then practice splitting the distance between the holes with another hole. You can also experiment with changing the location on the stock where you wish to punch the holes. The closer to the inside edge is called coarse, and the closer to the outside edge is called fine.

This exercise is an excellent way to become proficient with a creaser as well. Instead of punching the nail holes, use the ring to practice fullering. Fuller one crease **(Figure 38)** and try to place another crease inside of the first **(Figures 39-40)**.

CLIPS

Make another ring and practice just the clip source with whatever method you deem appropriate. The source in **Figures 41-42** is pulled with a cross peen, and the source in **Figures 43-44** is pulled with a bob punch. My favorite method of using the ball peen clipping hammer **(Figure 45)** producing the source in **Figure 46**. Once you have this task down, draw the clips from the source. In **Figure 47**, I am drawing the clip toward me with the peen on the cross peen. In **Figure 48**, the clip is being drawn toward me with the heel edge of

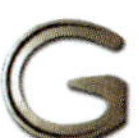

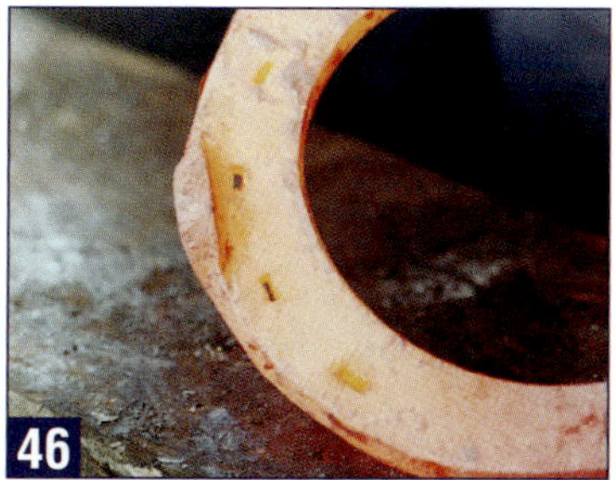

Source with a ball peen.

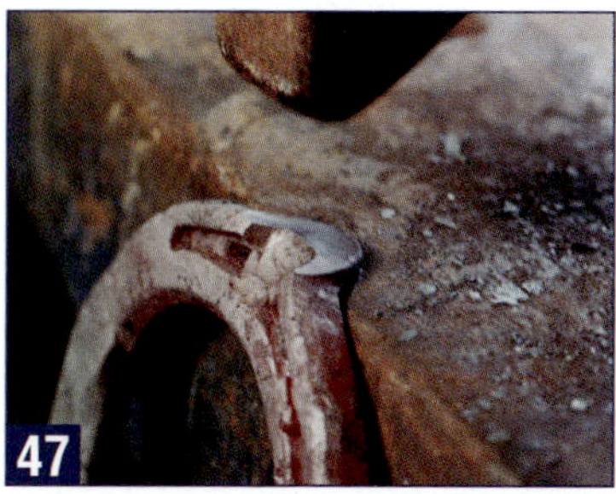

Pulling the clip toward me with the cross peen.

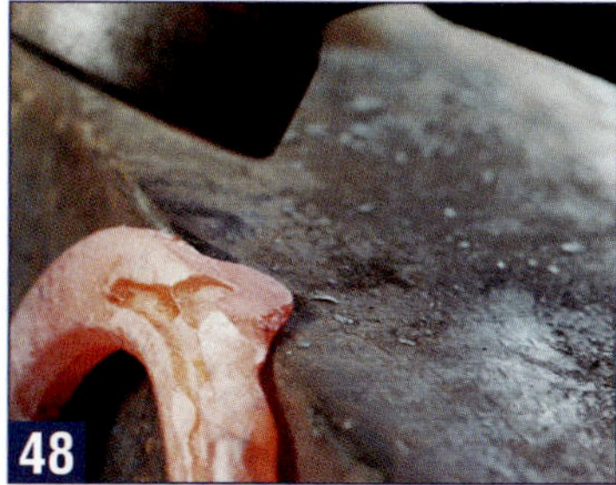

Pulling the clip toward me with the heel of the hammer.

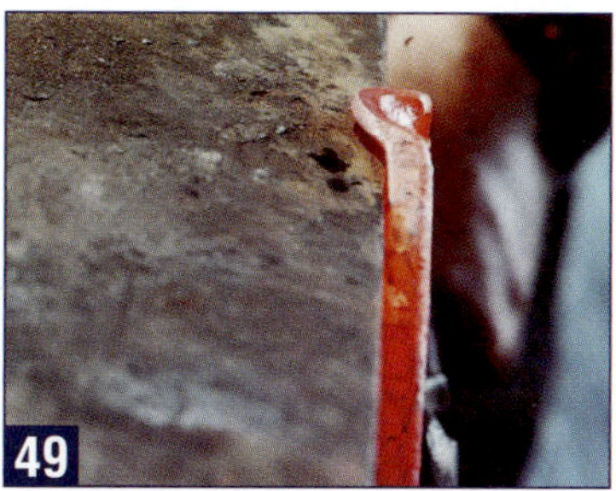

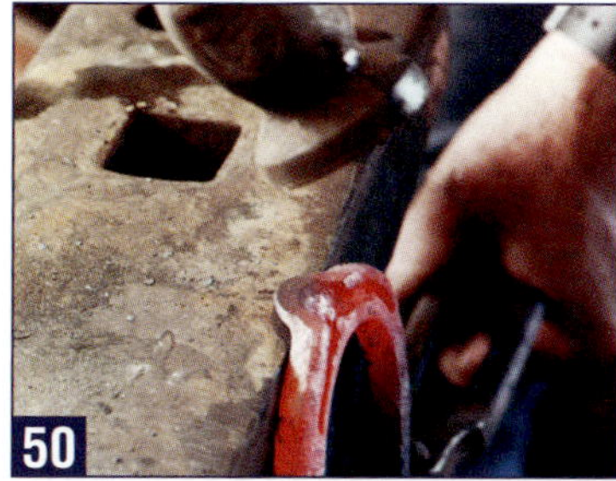

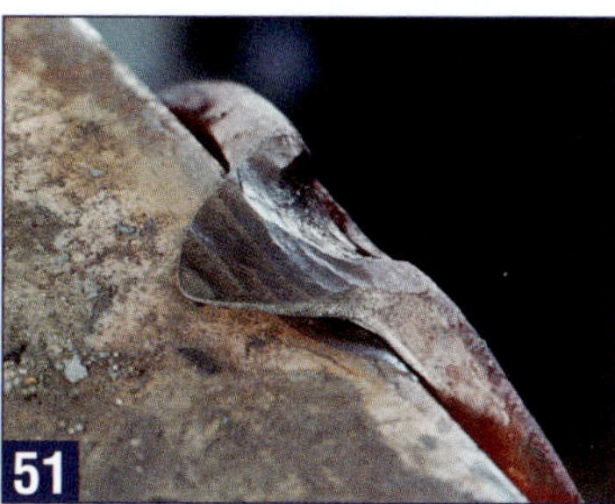

Pulling the clip from the side of the anvil with the side of the clipping hammer.

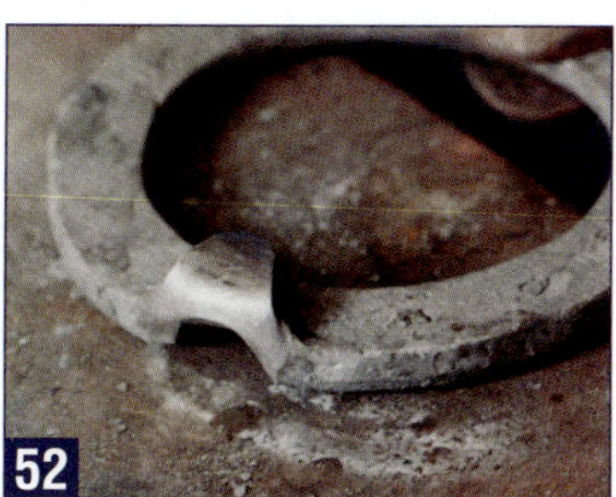

Smash the practice clips to pull more.

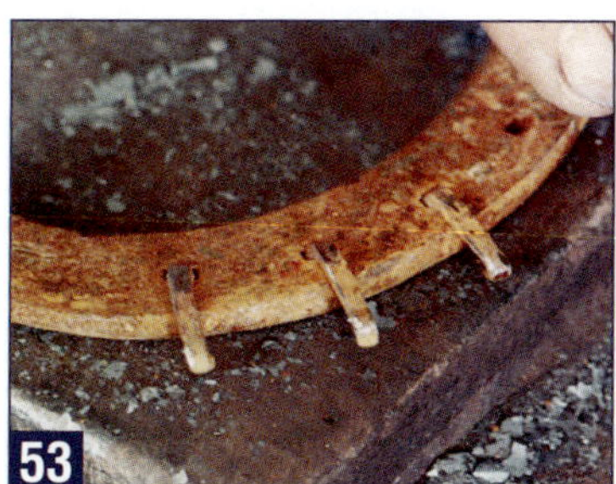

Bend the nails over.

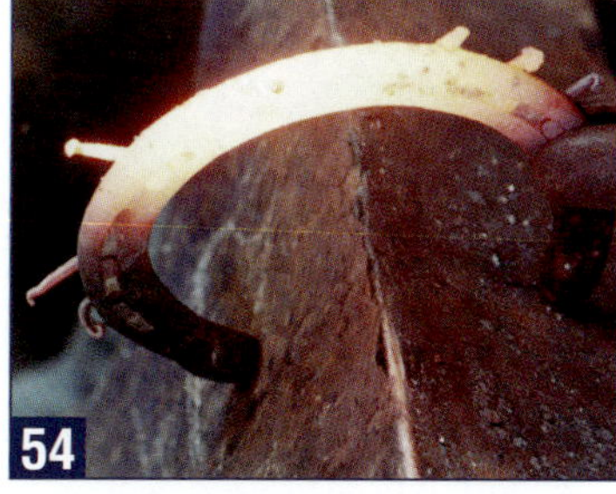

Open the toe of the hot shoe.

a rounding hammer. In **Figures 49-51**, the clip is being drawn from the side with the edge of the ball peen clipping hammer. You can then smash the clips down and pull another clip for continued practice **(Figure 52).** After several hours, put both tasks (the source and drawing) together to form a clip. Practice until you can shape a shoe and place two clips on it in one heat.

WELDING

Making a horseshoe sandwich is a great project for a beginner to learn. There are a lot of forging skills used to make a horseshoe sandwich. Begin by taking two old horseshoes and heating the toe of one shoe and one branch of the other. If there are old nails in the shoe, leave them there and bend them over flat before you begin. **(Figure 53)** They will end up welding into the nail holes, which make it easier to have a clean, crisp final piece.

The shoe that is hot at the toe should be opened at the toe, **(Figure 54)** and bent over on itself towards the ground surface. **(Figures 55-56)** If you bend towards the hoof surface, there will be a crease in the shoe that has to be welded up, instead of just a

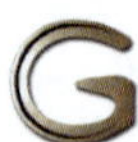

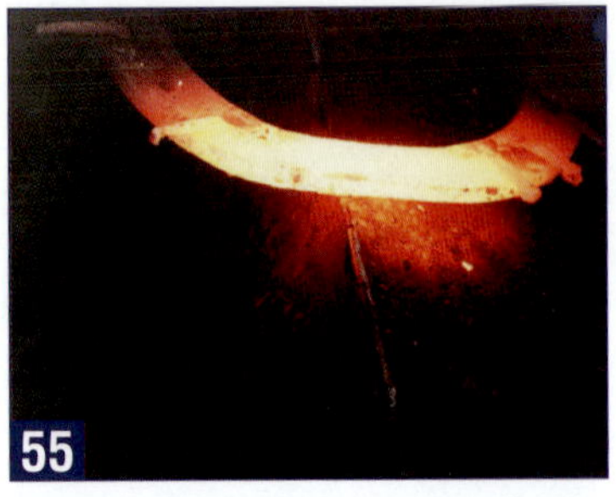

Bend the shoe toward the ground surface.

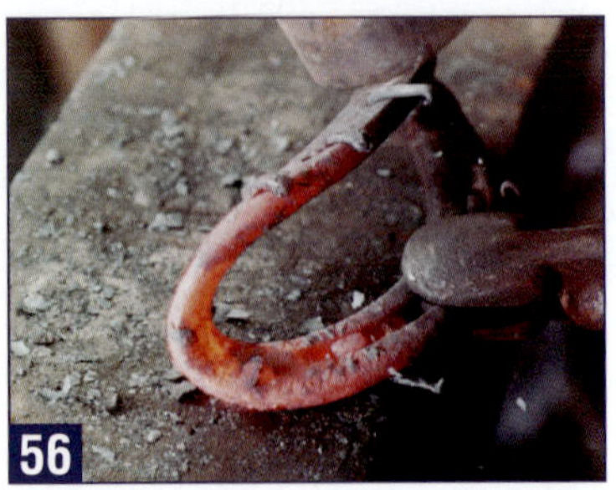

Bend it so that there is still room for the thickness of another shoe.

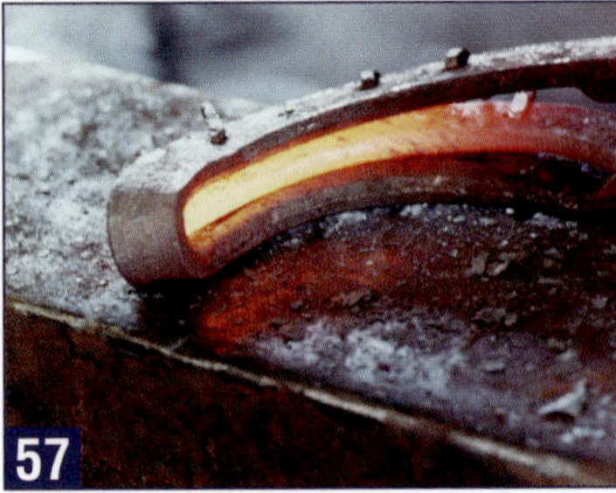

Insert the other shoe into the center of the first shoe that was bent.

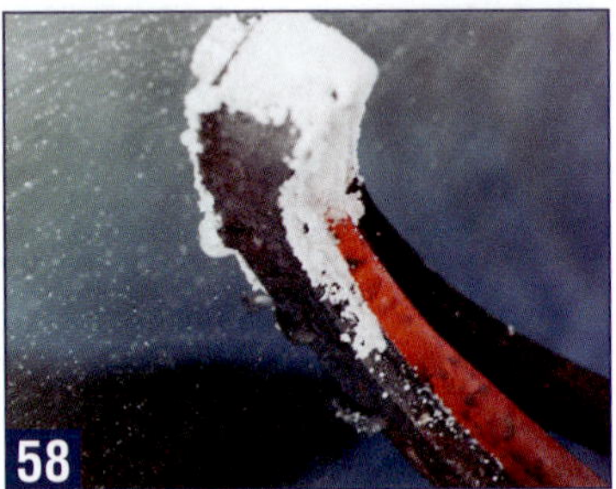

Flux and put into the fire.

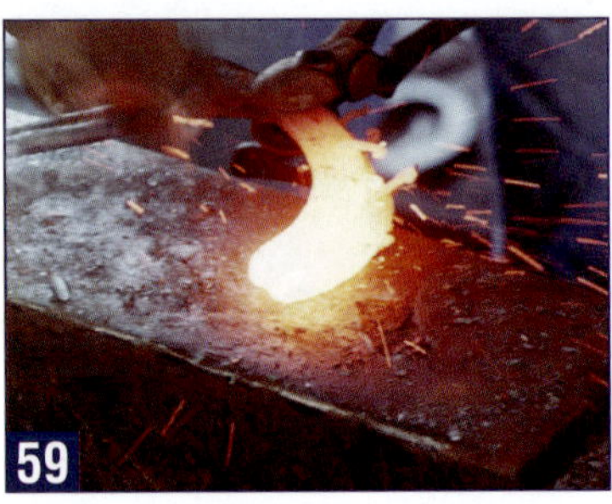

Fast, soft hammer blows to start the weld.

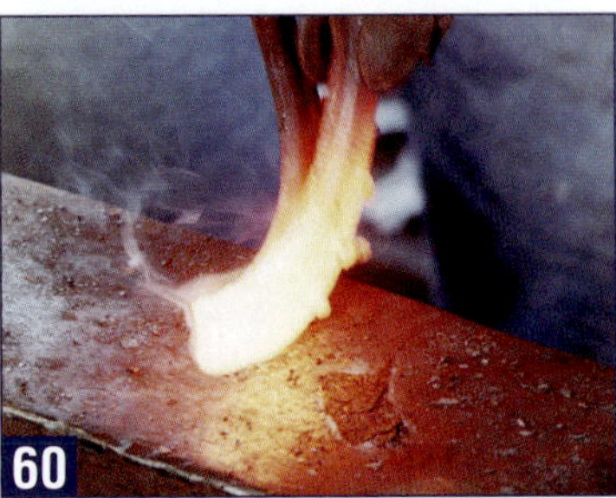

Get the second welding heat and continue to weld.

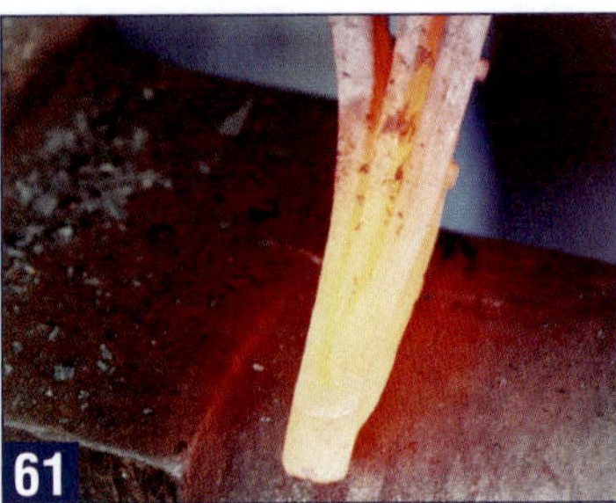

Straighten as soon as you can.

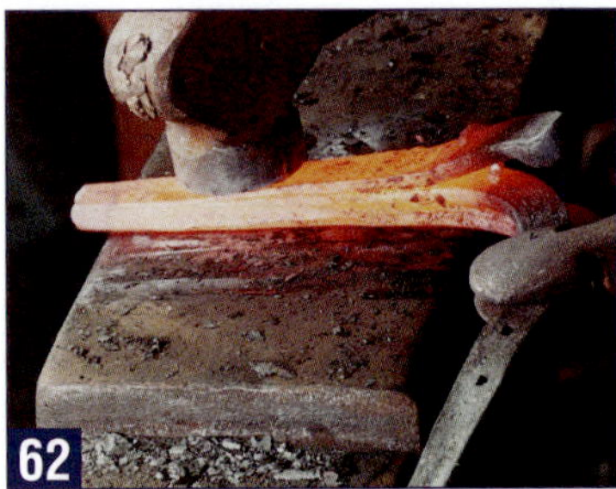

Hammer from all sides.

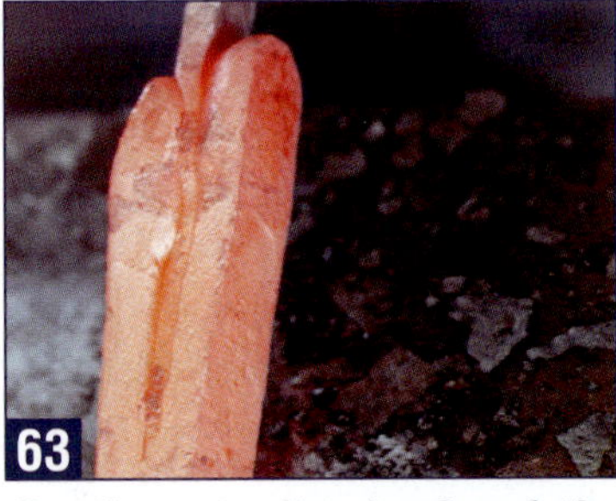

Continue to the heels of the bent shoe.

small nail hole when bent the other way. Straighten out the hot branch on the other shoe and place the curved side of the shoe back in the fire.

Take both pieces from the fire and insert the curved portion of the one shoe into the shoe that is bent **(Figure 57)**. Close up the bent shoe on top of the curved shoe with a couple of medium hammer blows. Flux the end of the piece and place it back into the fire **(Figure 58)**. Once a welding heat is achieved, come out of the fire and quickly hammer with quick, light, flat blows on the width of the piece **(Figure 59)**. This is the most critical welding heat. Stop hammering once the piece has welded enough to hold itself together, brush, flux, and return to the fire.

Continue welding and forging the piece, working only a small area every heat. **(Figures 60-63)** Once you reach the heels of the bent shoe, bend the straight piece of the shoe in the middle back over, bending towards the ground surface. **(Figures 64-65)** Continue welding and forging until there is a completely welded piece of bar stock. **(Figures 66-67)** Forge to the desired dimensions by upsetting the end to a perfect section, **(Figures 68-69)** and

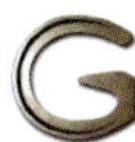

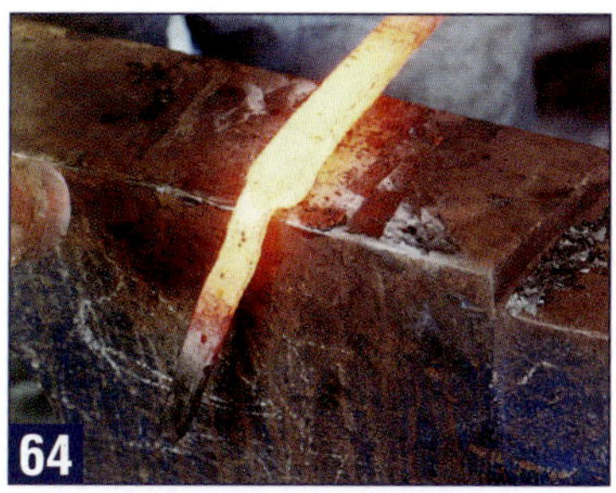

Bend the unwelded piece back over the welded pieces.

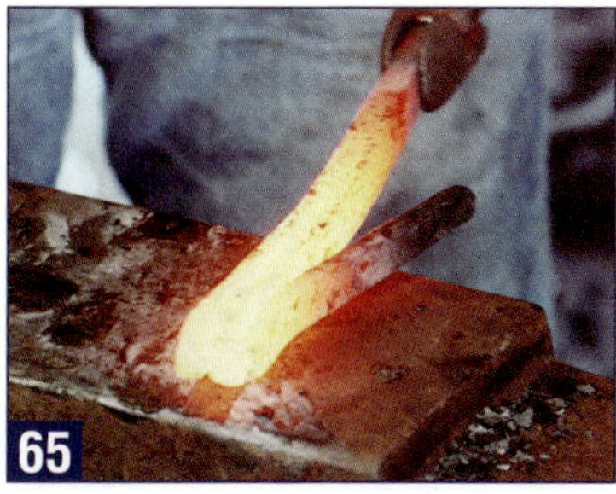

Bend toward the ground surface of the shoe.

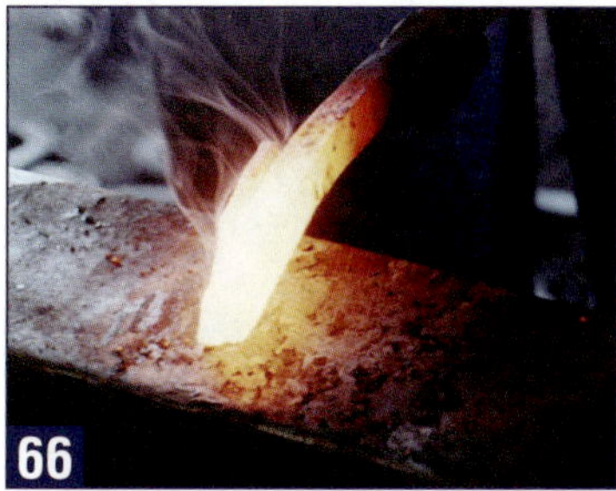

Weld.

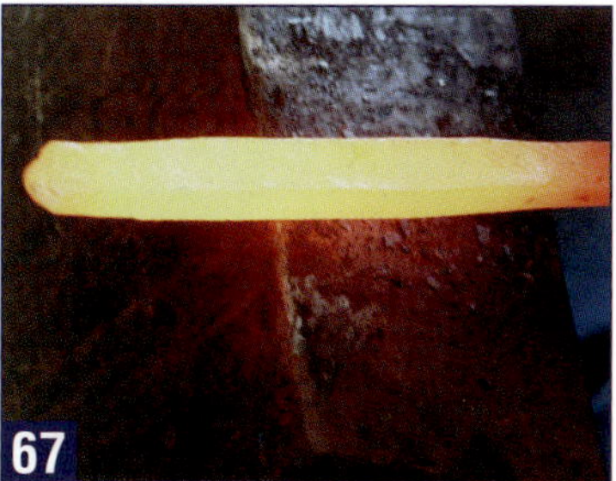

Continue welding throughout the piece.

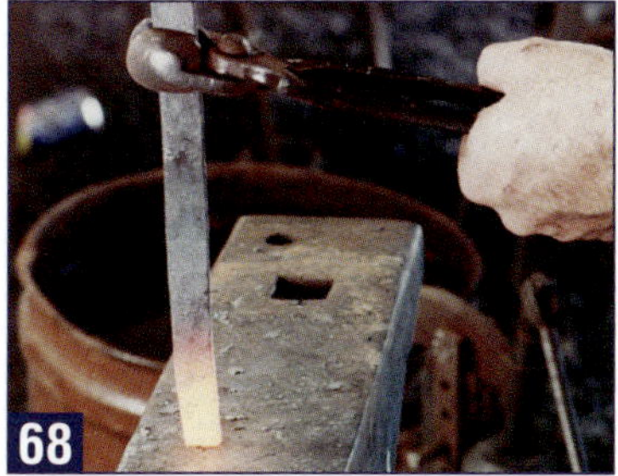

Upset the end to make it square.

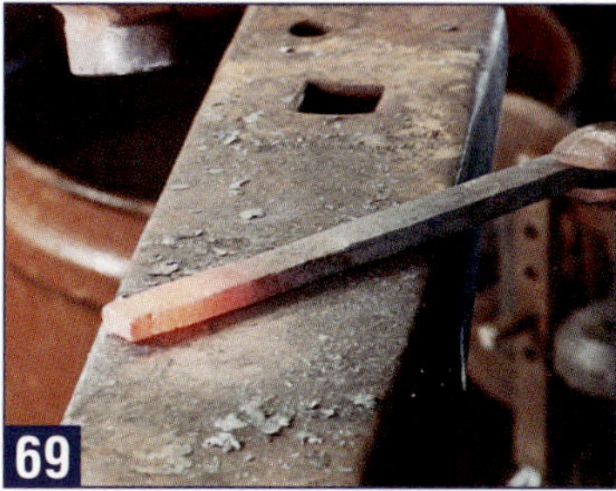

Forge it rectangular.

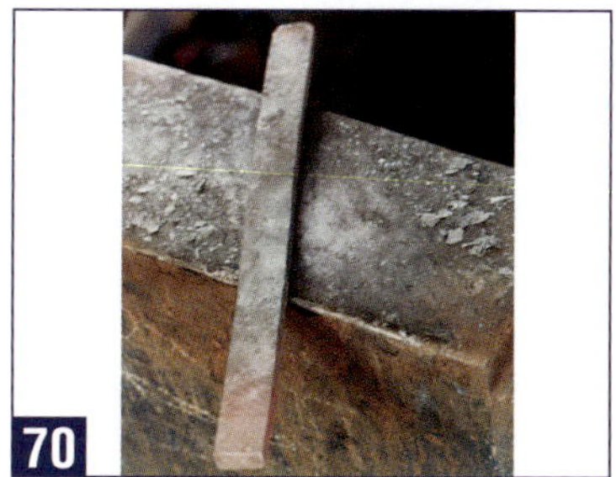

Finished piece of bar stock.

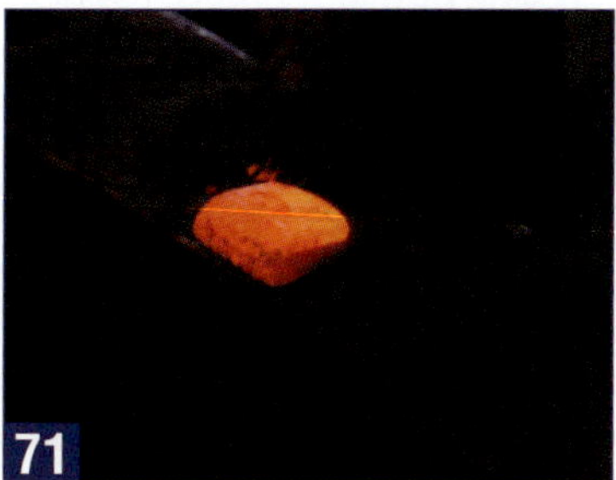

Make the first bend in the end of the rasp.

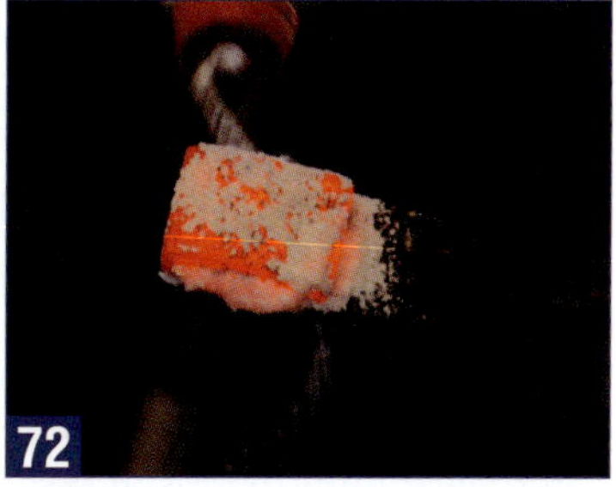

Flux.

working towards center until you have what you are looking for **(Figure 70)**.

Be forewarned, this is a lot of work and it will test your skill. Once you are finished, you will be proud of it. However, when you show it to your spouse, it just looks like a piece of metal. There is no indication of the work that went into it, and your spouse may disappoint you with a noticeable lack of enthusiasm. Don't let it bother you. This is just the natural response from someone who is looking at bar stock.

CLINCH BLOCK

Now that you have made a horseshoe sandwich, you can make a clinch block out of an old rasp. Starting a clinch block is easier than starting the horseshoe sandwich, but there are some potential pitfalls.

There is something special about making and using your own tools. The following project is a clinch block made from a rasp. Making this clinch block will help develop your welding skills as well as result in a very usable item. It is the sort of tool that you will never wear out, so if you do a good job, you will have a tool to last for several careers.

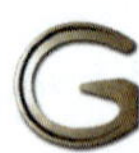

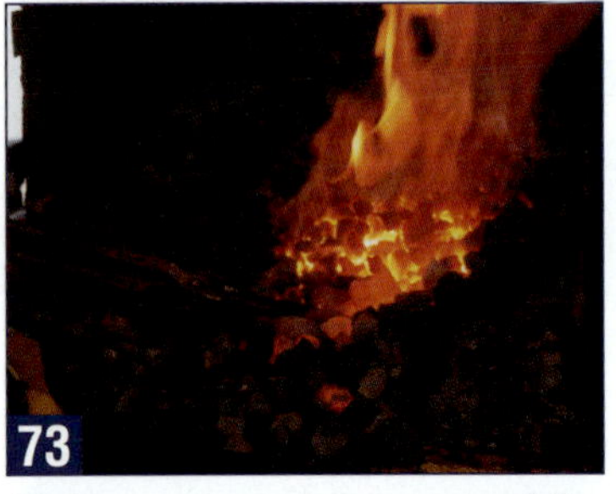
73
Make sure you have a good fire going.

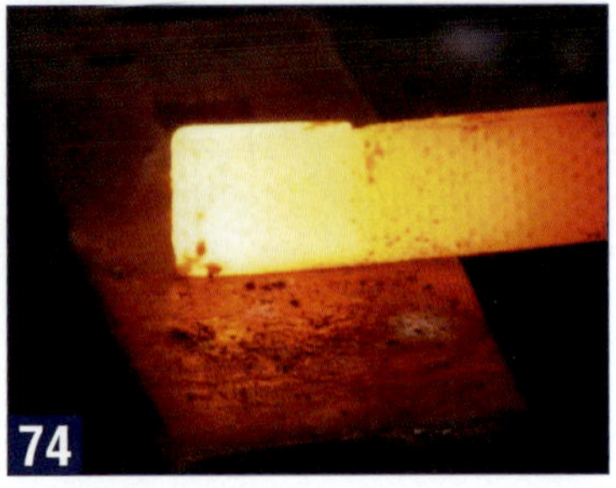
74
Weld the piece.

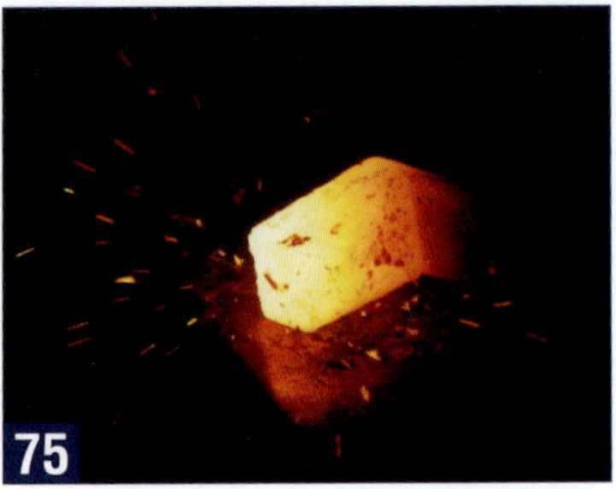
75
Continue to weld and shape.

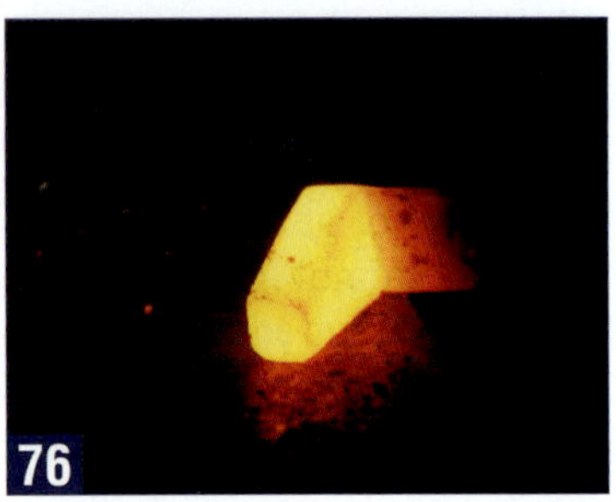
76

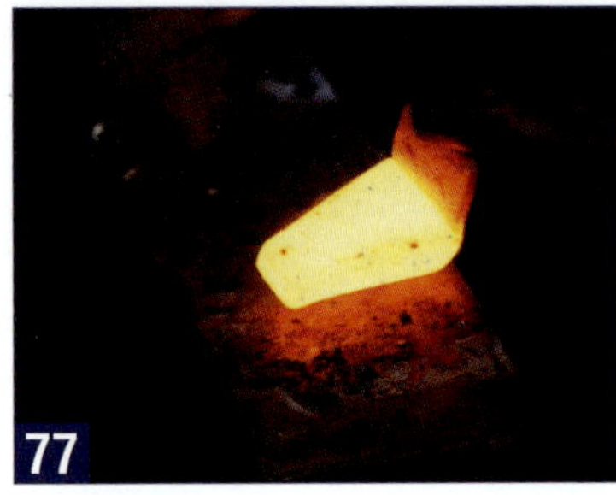
77

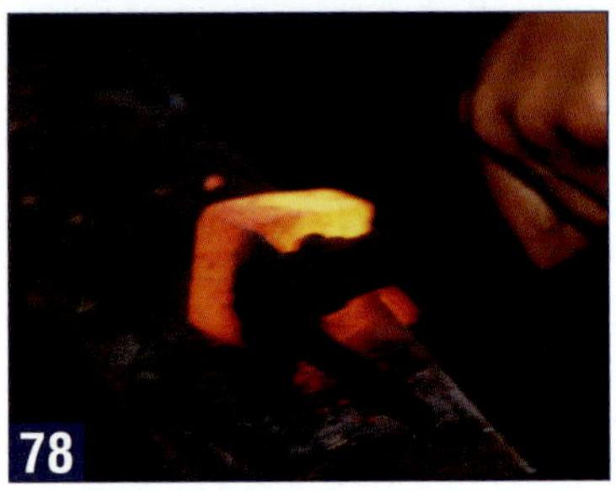
78

Taper the block for a good fit in your hand.

To begin with, heat the end of the rasp and bend about 2 inches over the corner of the far side of the anvil **(Figure 71)**. I personally like to make the bend with the rough side of the rasp out so that the finished product will have a texture. Bend the piece flat against the rasp, and apply flux **(Figure 72)**.

Heat to a welding heat. In coke, this will be a bright yellow, just before or at a light spark. Spend the time needed to make a good fire like the one in **Figure 73**. If you are doing this in a propane forge, heat until the metal disappears in the forge but before the flux is no longer molten. Bring the piece out of the fire and hit with quick, soft hammer blows, just like when you started the horseshoe sandwich **(Figure 74)**. Bend the piece back onto itself, and continue to weld until there is only a small amount of rasp and tang left.

As the welded portion continues to get bigger **(Figure 75)**. The difference in mass between the welded and unwelded portion can now cause some problems. Since there is so much large mass (the welded portion), and we are covering it with the thinner piece (the unwelded portion), achieving a good heat can be difficult. To deal with this in a coke fire, prepare the piece for welding the same way you have been. Place the piece in the fire with the largest portion down and get a slow heat. Once the large mass is hot enough to weld, turn the piece over to get the thin piece hot enough to weld. Getting your heat slowly is important. If you rush this part of the job, you can burn the thin piece before the large piece is hot enough to weld. If you are working in propane, put the piece in the fire and turn it every once in a while to get an even heat.

When welding, you can always tell where the bond is good by the way the metal cools. It will darken faster in an area of less mass that is not completely welded to the larger mass. The last weld can be tough because there is such a difference in the large and small pieces left to be welded. Place the piece in the fire in such a manner that the block is getting hot without burning off the tang. Forge the block with a slight taper to fit your hand more comfortably **(Figures 76-78)**. Forge the top corner (or working corner) as square as possible, and you may find that it is easier to hit if you put the edge on the anvil, and hit the bottom of the block **(Figure 79)**. You can place the tang in a vice and rasp the working corner square and sharp if you are not able to forge it.

The last step is forging the shape of the handle. I like to have a slight scroll on the end of the tang, but that is a personal preference. You can design

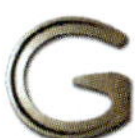

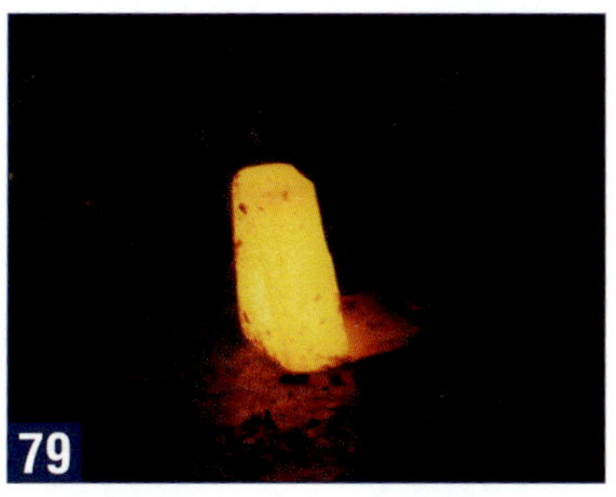
79 Clean up and sharpen the working end of the block.

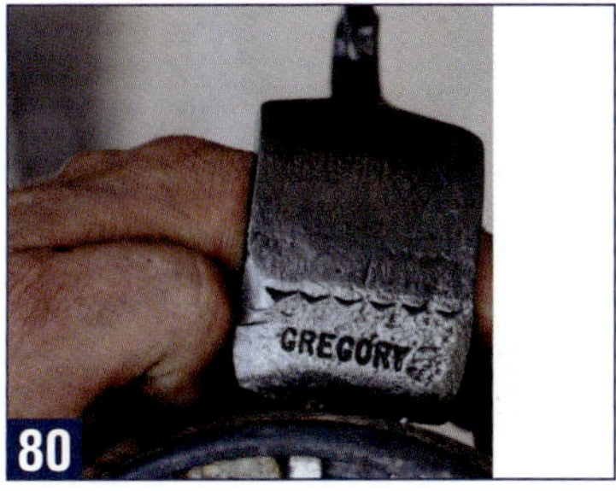

80 Finished product ready to serve.

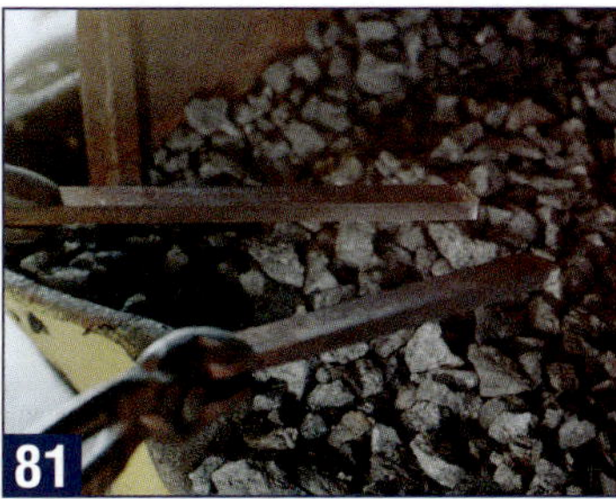
81 2 pieces of stock that I am using for a practice run.

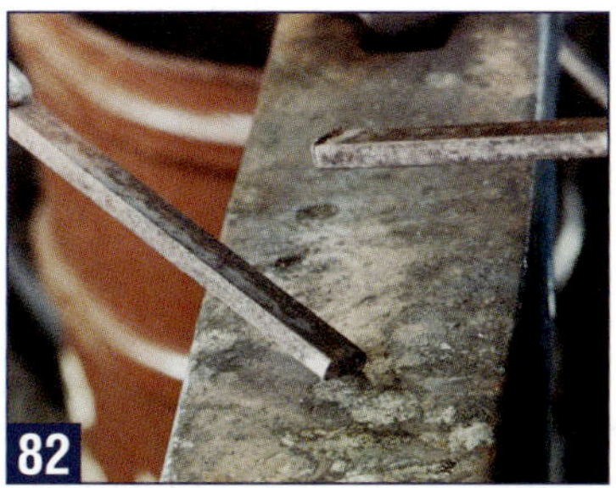
82 Go to the anvil.

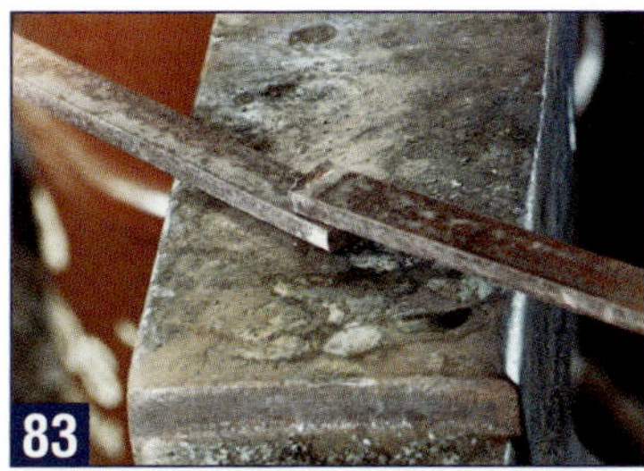
83 Drop my tongs from my hammer hand as I place the piece on the anvil and pick up my hammer. Place the other piece on top of

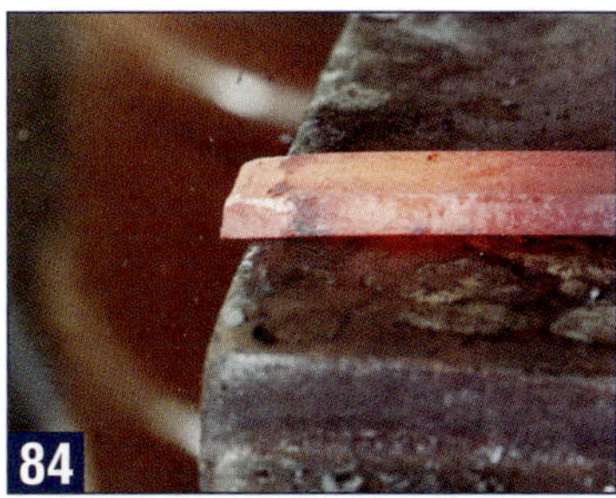
84 Placed over the edge to make the grab.

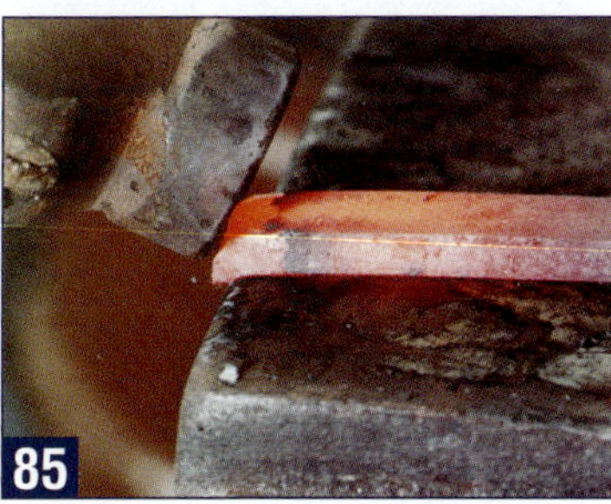
85 Forging the scarf and grab.

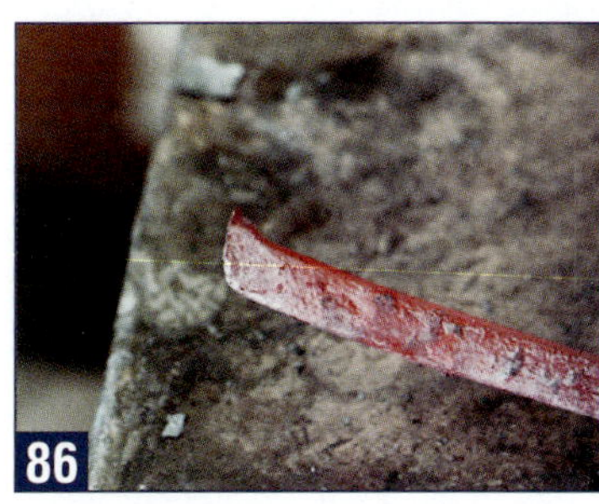
86 This piece is ready for jump welding.

this any way you want. To make the scroll, heat the tang and bend it around the end of the horn, then bend the piece over so that there is a large enough gap to fit your hand comfortably. Allow the piece to air cool. DO NOT QUENCH! Most rasps will become brittle if quenched while hot, and you will break the handle off if it is hardened from quenching.

When it is done, hold it in your hand to get a feel for the tool **(Figure 80)**. Take it to the next horse you shoe and put it to work. This is a solid clinch block with a design that sets nails well. It is also perfect for hammer clinching. Kelly is still using one I made for her in 1995, and I hope you can use the one that you make until your last horse.

DROP-TONG OR JUMP WELDING

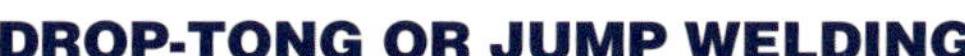

Jump welding implies welding two dissimilar pieces of steel together with a forge, anvil and hammer. This is more difficult to do since the pieces are not being held together for you. Choreograph the moves needed with cold steel as practice before actually trying to weld. In **Figures 81 through 83**, I am going through the motions to practice exactly how I will jump weld once the steel is hot. The window for welding is so small that you need to have this all figured out before it is hot.

Heat the pieces to be welded. Brush the piece and then scarf the end over the edge of the anvil, making a little grab. **(Figures 84-86)**. Do the same to both pieces, then flux them before returning to the fire. The little grabs that are part of the scarf are going to be facing each other when you do your first weld **(Figure 87)**. Bring both pieces up to the same temperature. Hold the piece that will be placed on

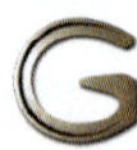

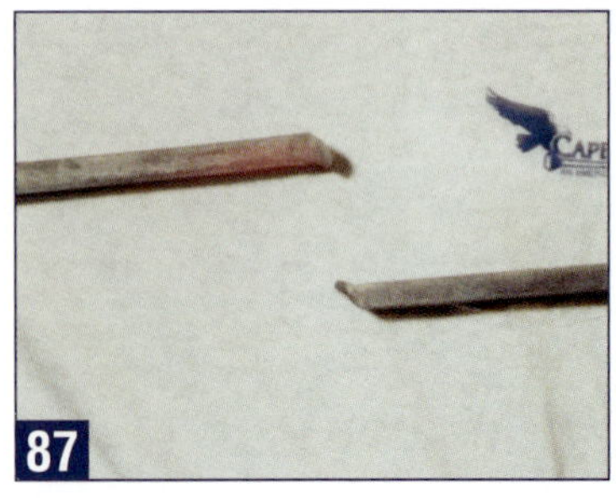

The pieces will go together with the grabs toward each other.

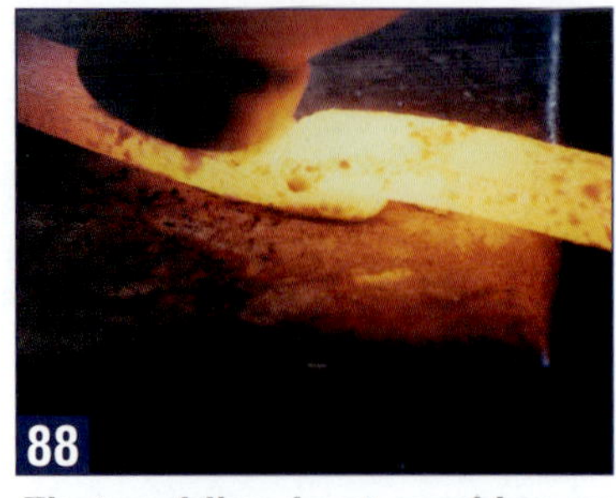

First welding heat, working on the seams.

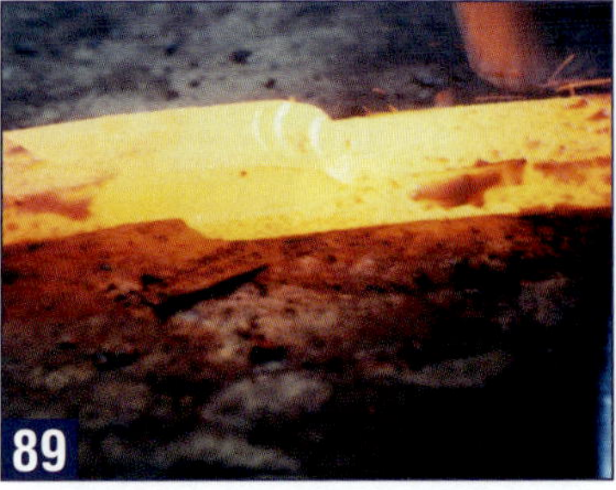

Hammer until the welding heat is gone.

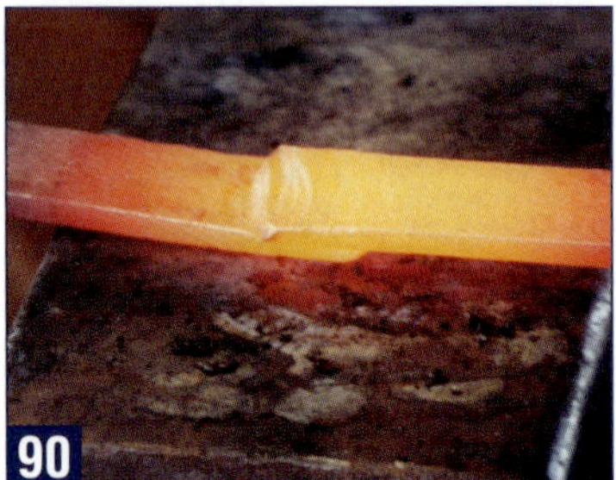

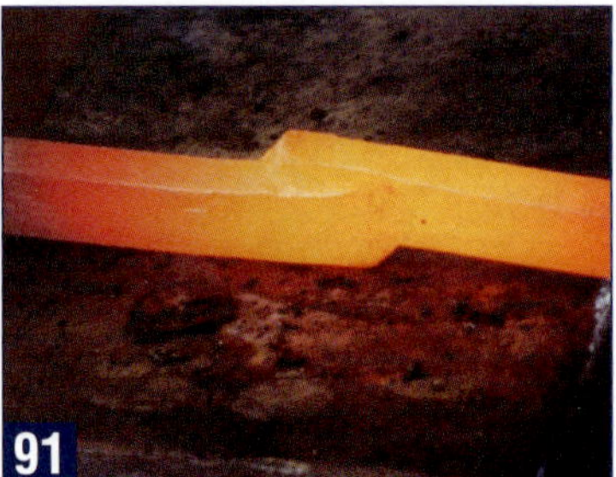

Should look like this after the first heat.

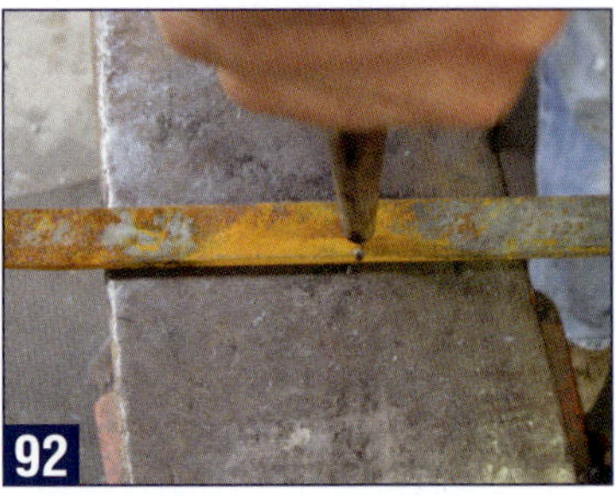

Mark center on the stock.

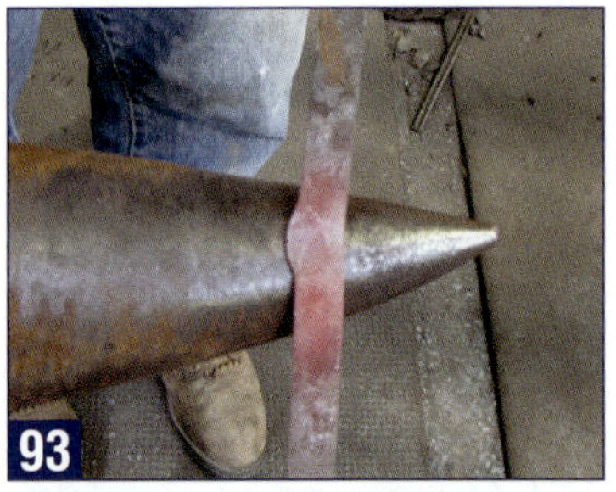

Scarf by hammering on the horn.

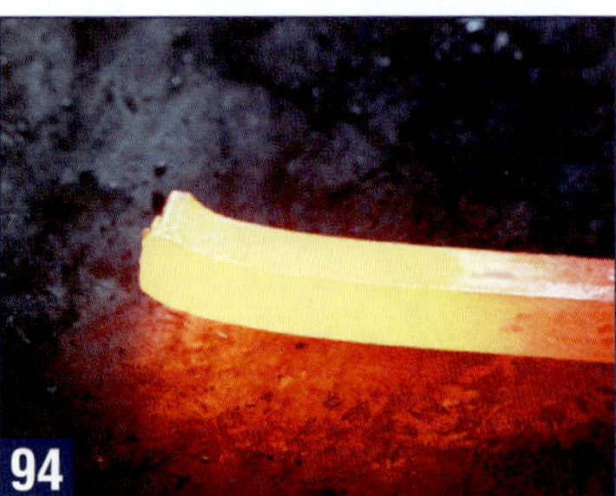

Make a scarf and grab on the piece that is going to come in at 90 degrees.

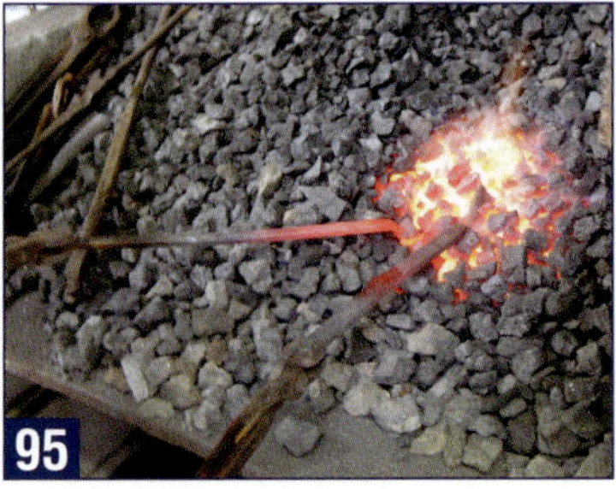

Get a good heat.

the face of the anvil with the tongs in your hammer hand. Bring both pieces from the fire and place the piece in your hammer hand on the anvil. As you drop the tongs and grab the hammer, place the piece in your tong hand on top of the first piece and hit with a quick, light blow. Don't over forge at this point, just try to get rid of the seams. If it all went well, you should have just seen what you are seeing in **Figures 88-91**. Brush, flux, and return to the fire as quickly as possible for the second welding heat. From this point on, it is just like welding the ring or horseshoe sandwich. You want to achieve a welding heat, hit light and fast to weld, and then hit harder and flat to shape.

MAKING A T-SQUARE

This next series is making a weld at an angle. For this project, we are going to make a T-square to use when learning to level front feet. Begin with a couple of short pieces of scrap. Mark center **(Figure 92)** and then make a small scarf on that piece over the horn **(Figure 93)**. Forge a grab on the end of the other piece, just like you did when jump welding straight **(Figure 94)**. Bring both pieces to a good welding heat **(Figure 95),** and come out of the fire to make your first jump weld. **(Figures 96-97)**

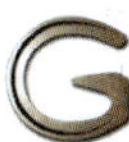

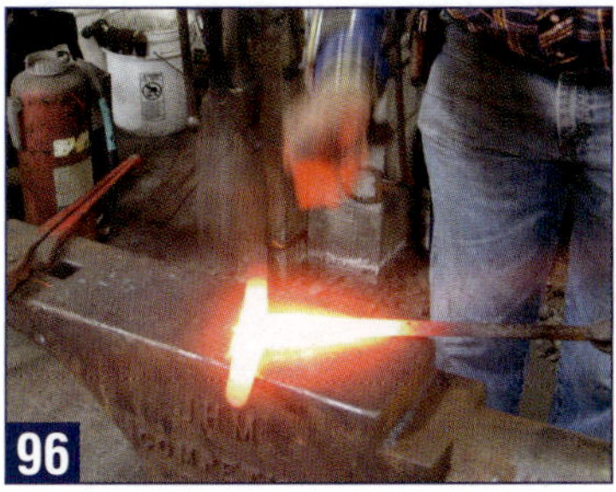
First welding heat.

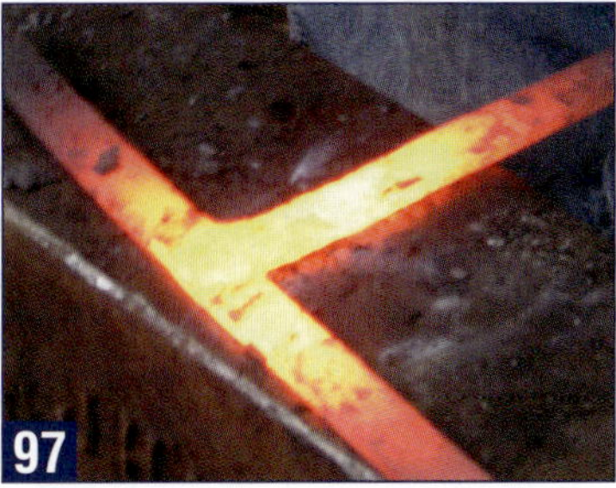
Work until the stock is no longer hot enough to weld.

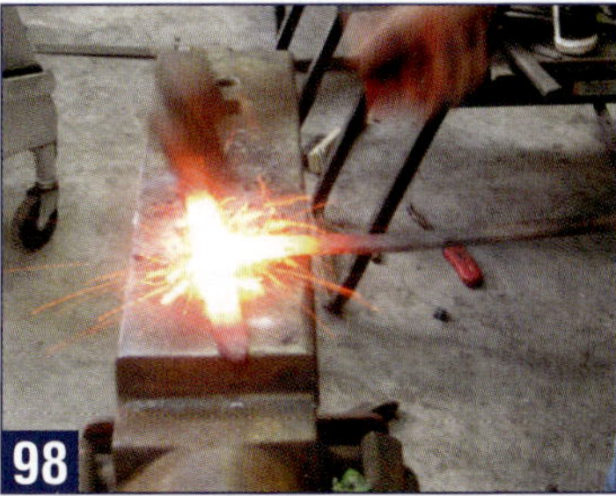
Second welding heat.

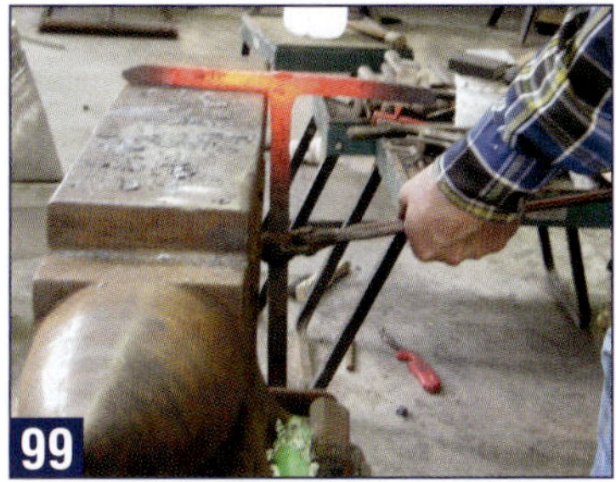
Clean up the weld on the corner of the anvil.

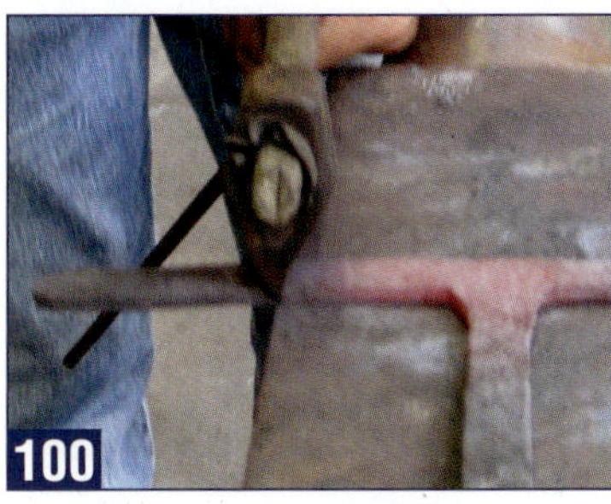
Cut off excess material.

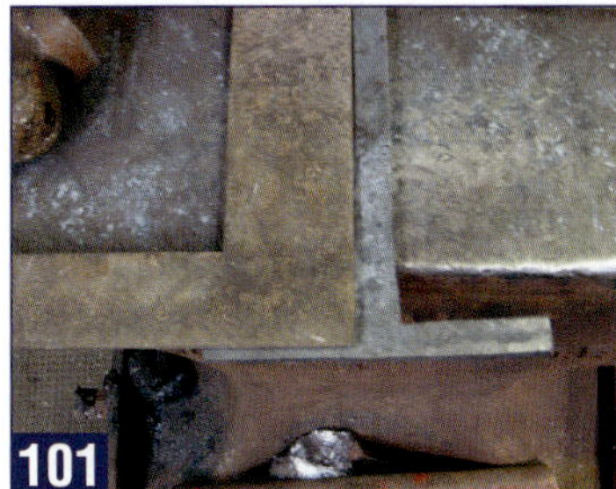
Check with a square.

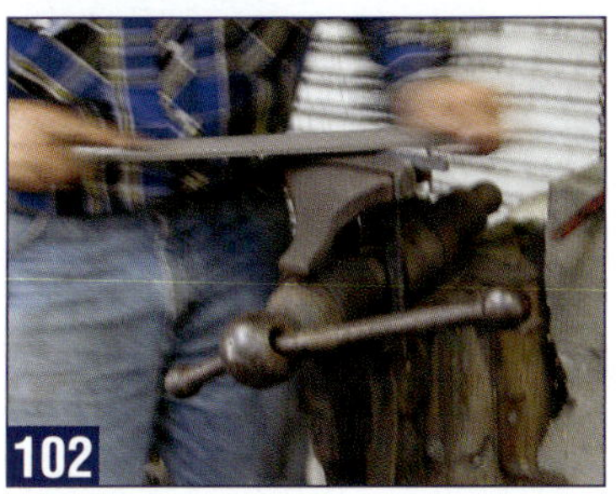
Clean it up with a rasp in a vice.

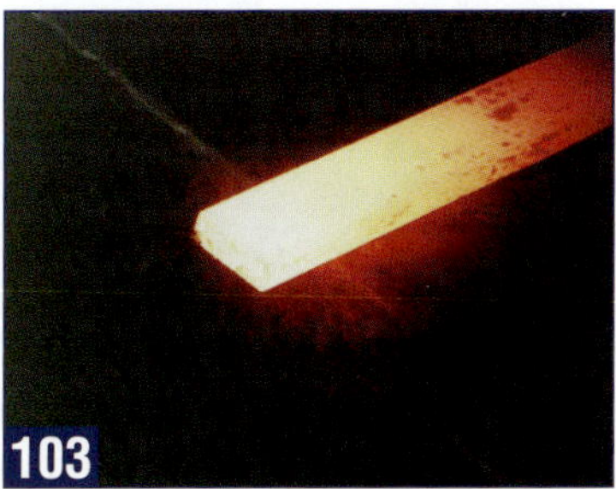
Place stock past soft corner to be bent.

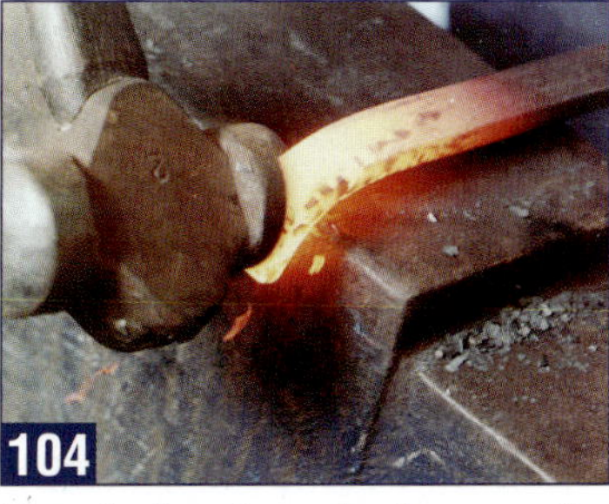
Bend about an inch over the edge.

Take a second welding heat and weld as in **Figure 98**. Square the piece up **(Figure 99)** and cut off any excess **(Figure 100).** Check it with a square, **(Figure 101)**, and finish the project by rasping the end smooth **(Figure 102).** This is an excellent way to practice a jump weld as well as end up with something that is useable.

HEEL CAULKS

If you decide to compete in farrier contests, you will find that there are a lot of competition shoes that have heel caulks on them. There are a variety of sizes and shapes, but the most common are like the one found on the lateral heel of a roadster. Besides being good for traction, wear, and increasing the hoof angle on hard ground, they are an excellent forge practice.

Begin by bending around an inch of stock over a corner of the anvil that has a radius **(Figure 103-104).** Turn the stock so that the bent piece is straight away from you and you are hitting with your hammer handle at 0 degrees to the bent piece **(Figure 105).** Repeat that exact blow about three times, then turn the piece a half turn so that the caulk is facing you and your hammer handle is still at 0 degrees to the caulk **(Figure 106).** Again, hit about

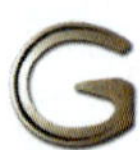

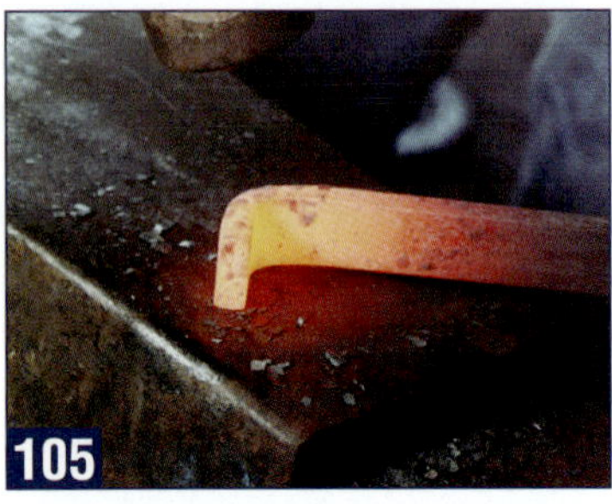

105

Point away from you.

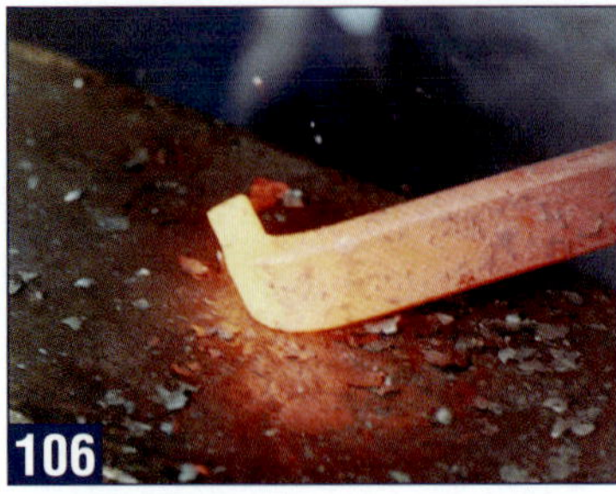

106

Point toward you.

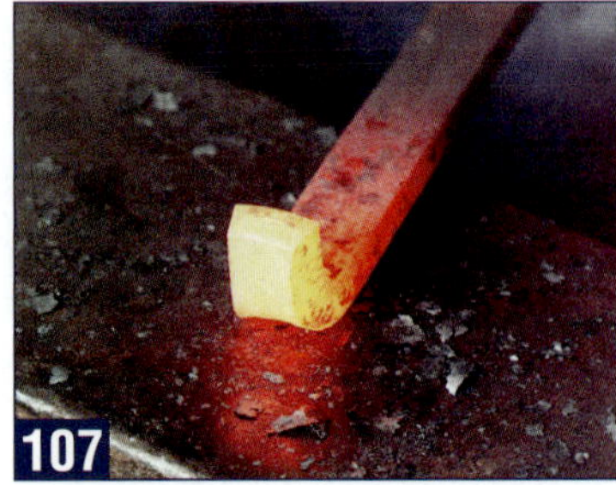

107

Point the caulk up.

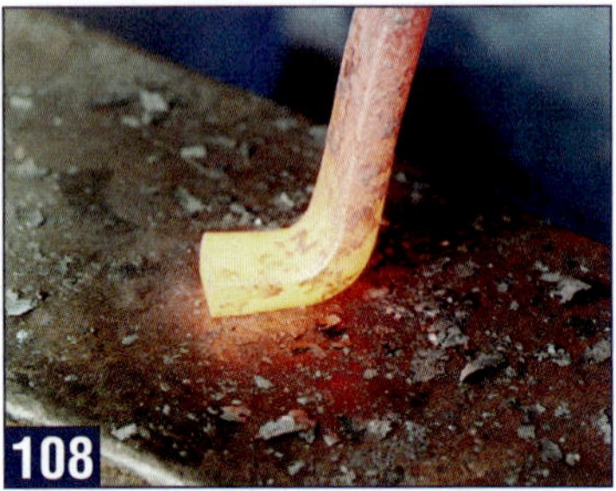

108

Stand the stock up so that you can hit the inside of the caulk.

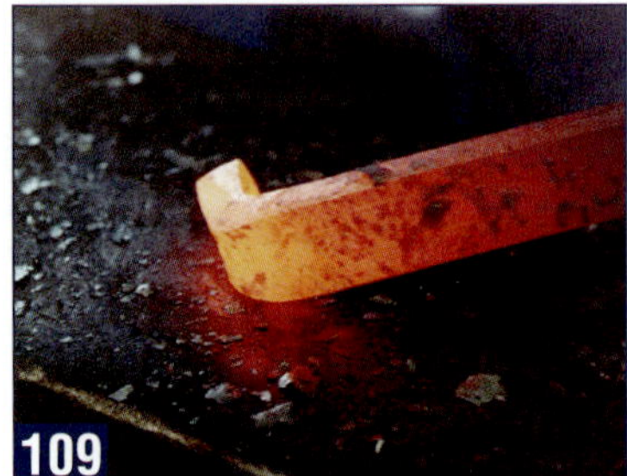

109

Repeat the process.

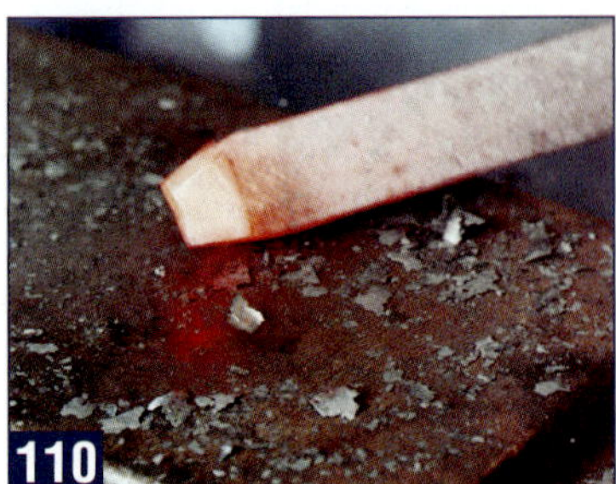

110

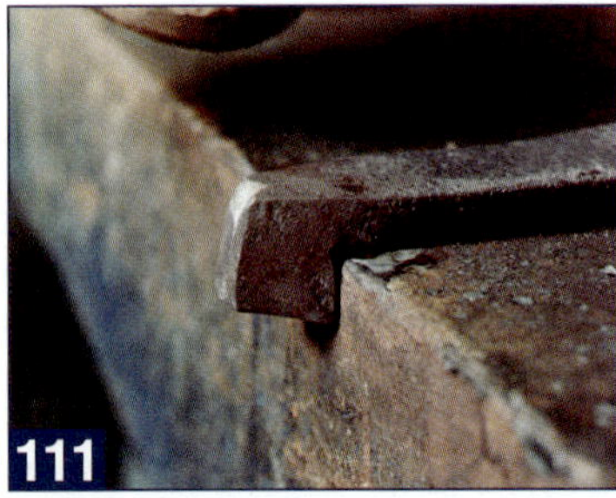

111

Finish the caulkin over a clean edge.

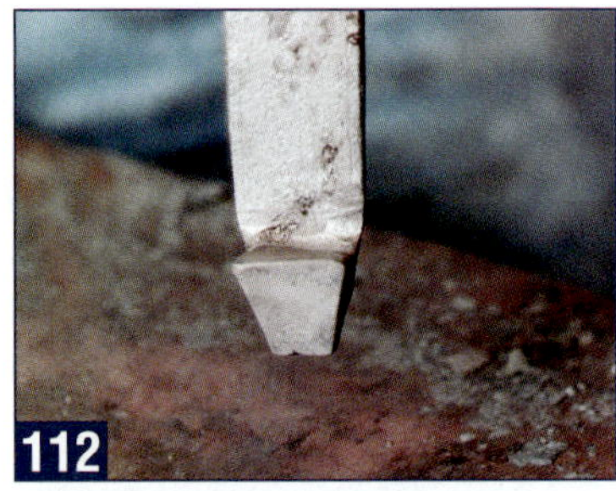

112

It should look like this from the ground surface.

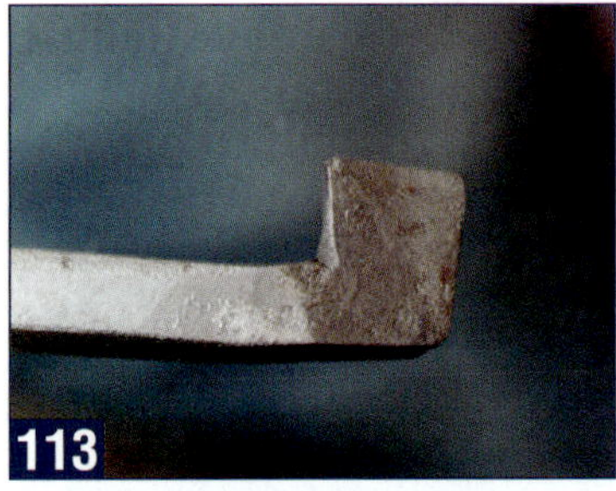

113

From a lateral view, you should have crisp straight sides.

three times. Turn the caulkin up on the anvil and hit once on the ground surface of the caulk. **(Figure 107)** Lift on the stock so that the back edge of the caulk is on the face of the anvil, and hit the inside of the caulk to keep it from folding over on itself. **(Figure 108)** These are the four main positions to forge a caulk. Try to develop a rhythm and hit each side the same number of times. That should be about three times on each side for every once on top.

While you are forging the caulk, lift on the stock so that the back edge of the caulk becomes tapered **(Figures 109-110).** Continue to shape the caulk using the hammer blows described above. To finish, place the caulk over a clean edge of the anvil and forge lightly into the corner **(Figure 111).** Keep the last move to a minimum, and you should end up with a caulkin like that pictured in **Figures 112 - 113**.

If you are building a caulk on stock that has a 1 to 2 ratio, you can shoulder the stock to make a nice corner. Begin with the shoulder on the hoof surface of the shoe over a soft corner of the anvil **(Figure 114-115).** Bend the caulk away from that shoulder as seen in **Figures 116-118**. Forge the caulk as described for the previous caulk and shown in **Figures 119-125**. You will find stock with this ratio is much easier to make a caulk on than other bar stock with a larger difference in the ratio of

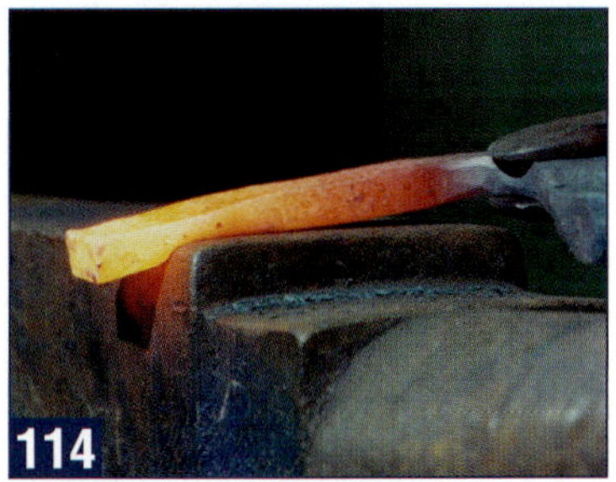

Shoulder the stock.

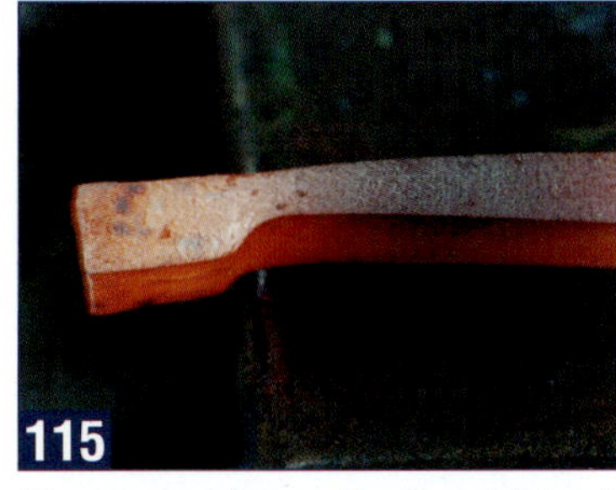

For a roadster, it should look like this.

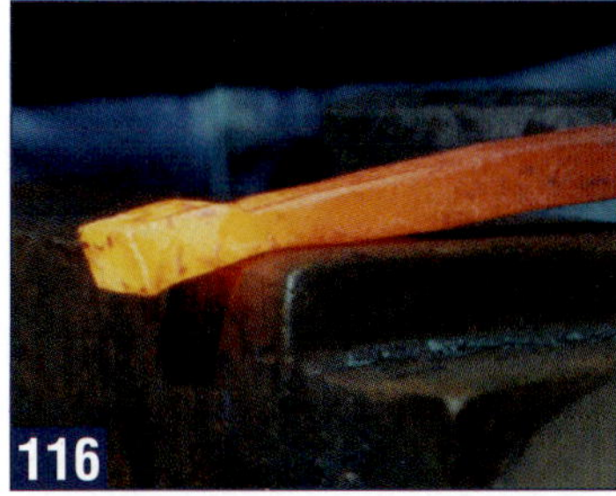

Bend away from the shoulder.

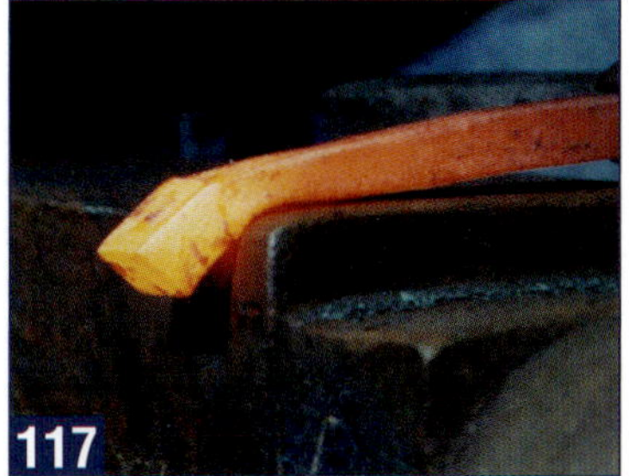

Bend away from the shoulder.

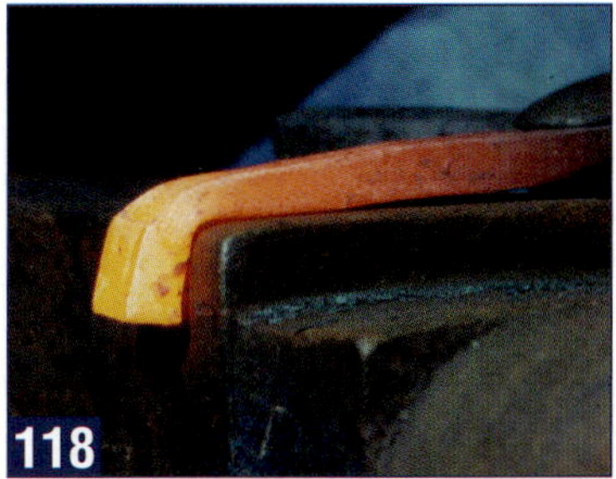

119
Point toward you.

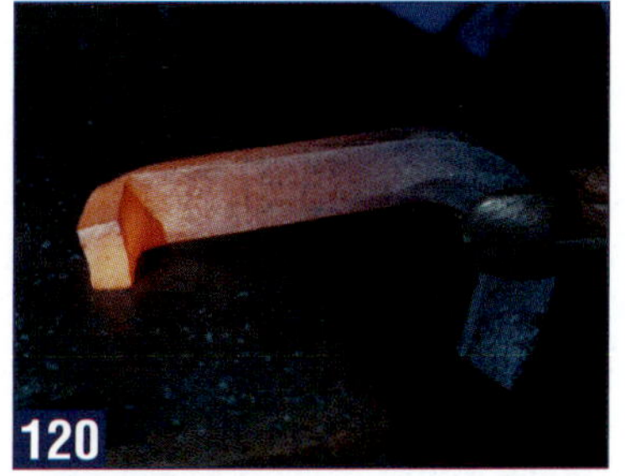

Point away.

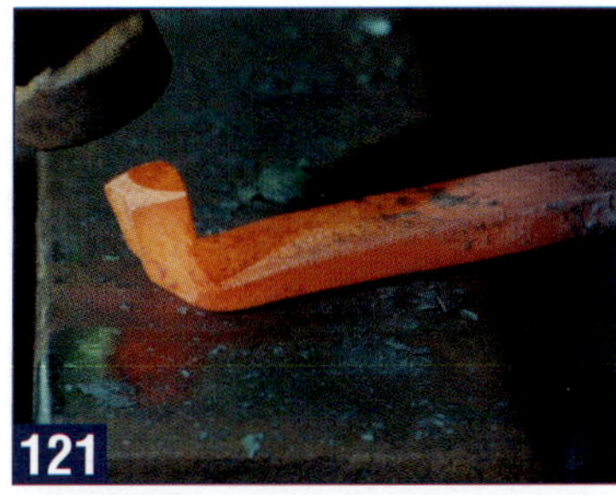

Point up.

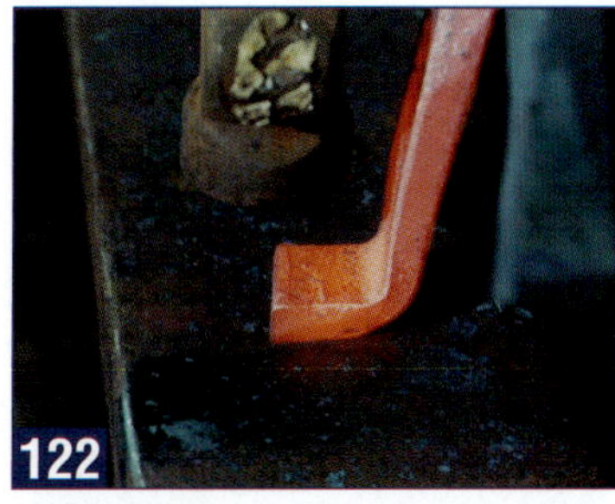

Hit inside.

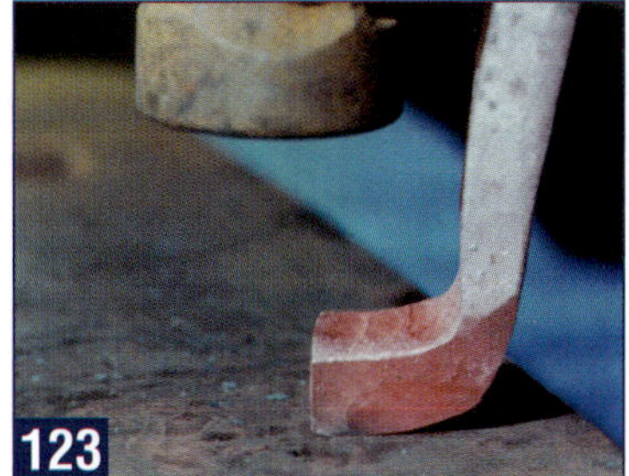

Hit inside.

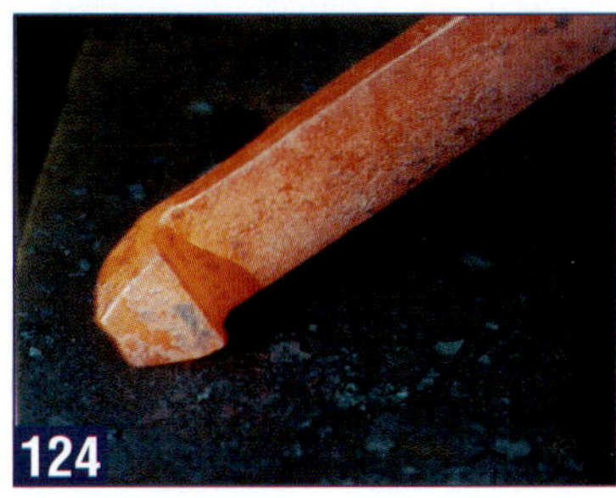

Finish from the side.

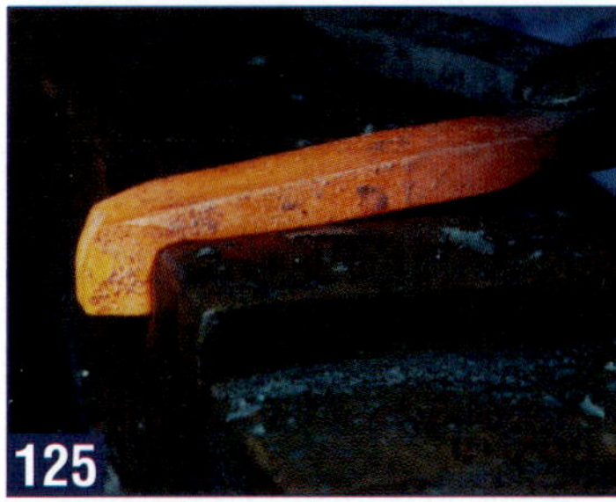

Clean up over the edge of the anvil.

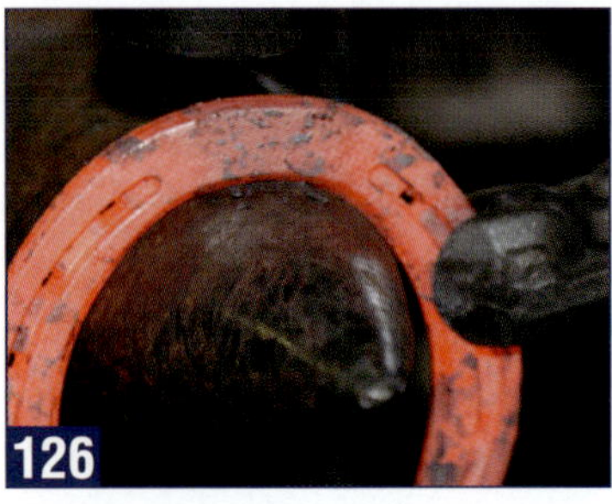

Notice that the tongs are not past the inside of the shoe.

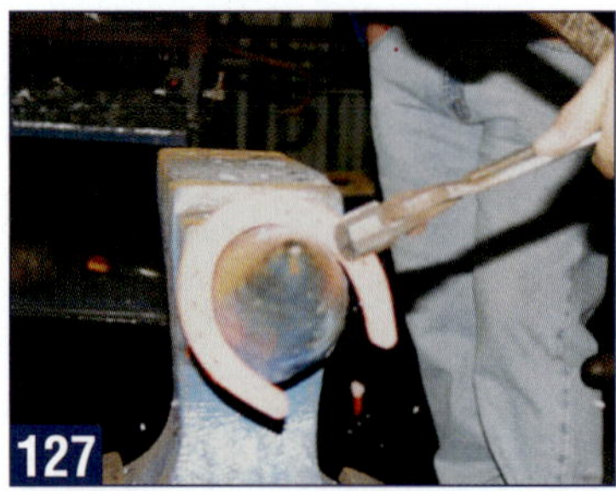

Start on the side of the horn that is closest to you.

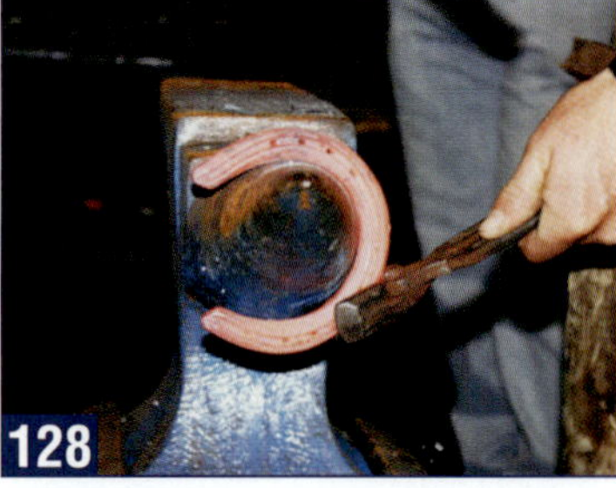

Pull the shoe around the horn. three points of contact between the tongs and the shoe.

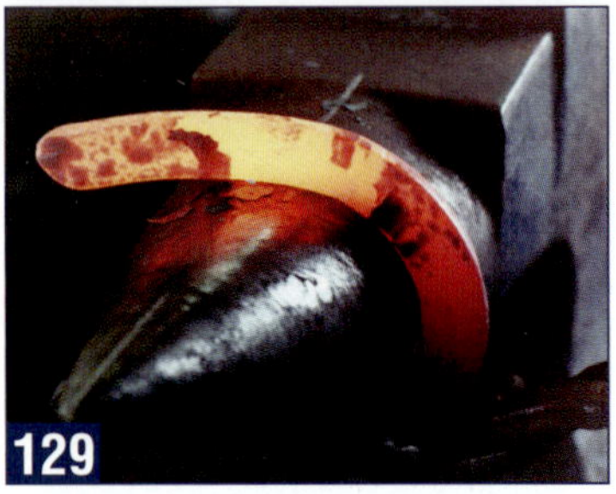

Achieve good tong position.

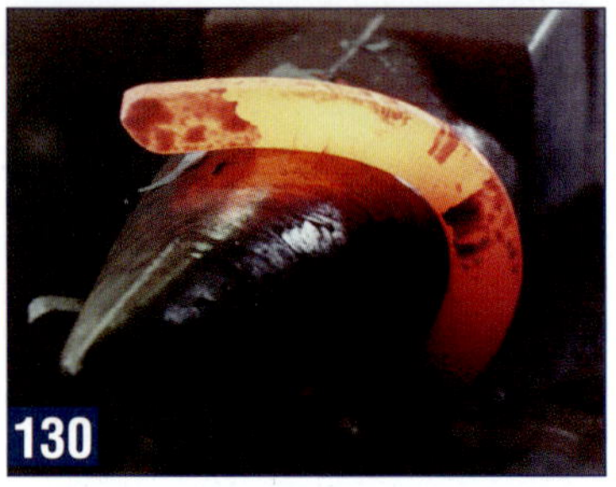

Continue through the heels.

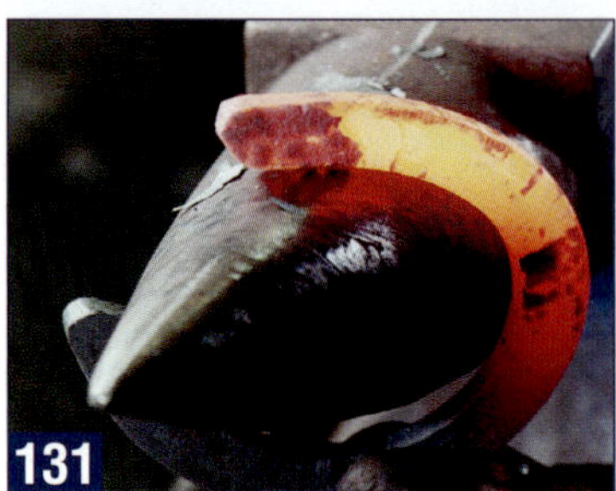

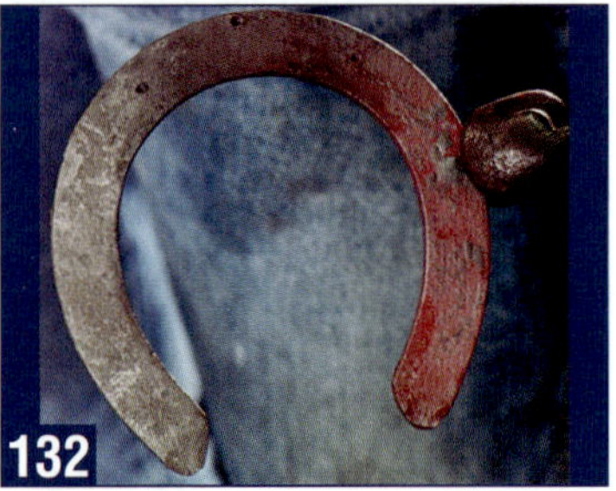

The finished shape should look like this.

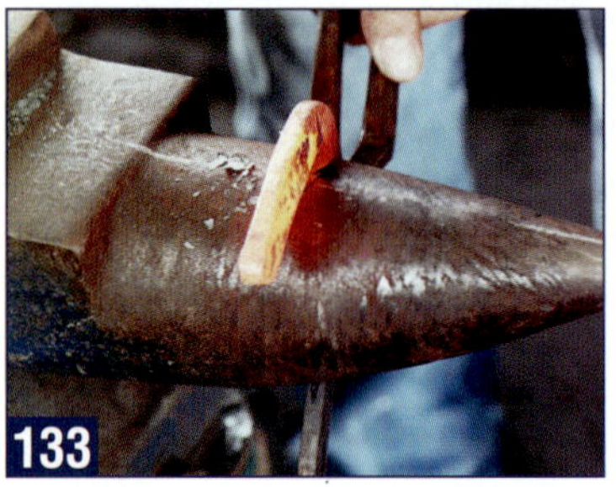

View from the other side of the anvil.

width to thickness.

SHAPING

In the journey to become a farrier, there is perhaps nothing harder to learn than the art of shaping. Trimming a good foot is part of the equation, as is making a good shoe. However, to make a good shoe that matches and enhances the foot just trimmed, that is a critical element of good shoeing.

There are some rules to shaping that it would serve you well to know. First, try to avoid letting the jaws of the tongs interfere with the inner perimeter of the shoe **(Figure 126).** Next, try to do as much shaping on the horn as possible, always pushing the shoe into the shape of the round horn. Third, tong position is critical. It may even be more critical than the hammer, although there is a debate there.

Look at **Figure 127**. Here the shoe is being held from the side and pulled around the horn as the hammer shapes the toe of the shoe to match the horn. In **Figure 128**, the tongs have pivoted on the shoe but are still in the same location on the shoe. The big difference now is that there are three points of contact with the shoe. One point is on each jaw, and the third point is at the base of the boss. This is a powerful way to hold any hot metal. **Figures 129-131** show how to finish that branch through the heel. Turn the shoe around, and do the same moves from the other side to make a symmetrical front shoe. **(Figure 132)**

Seen from the other side of the anvil, study **Figures 133-135** to see that the shoe is not only being rolled around the horn, it is also being twisted

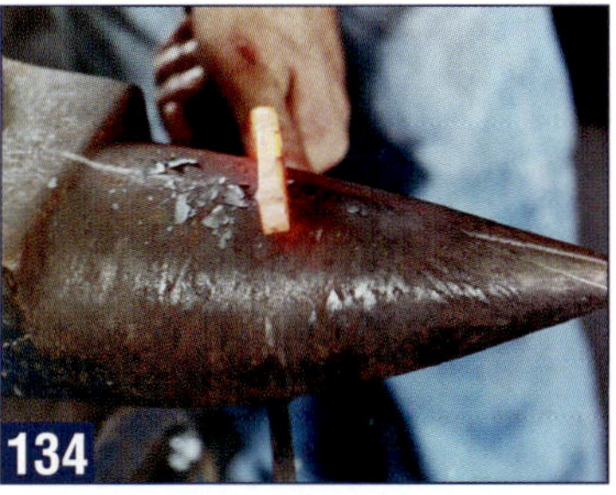

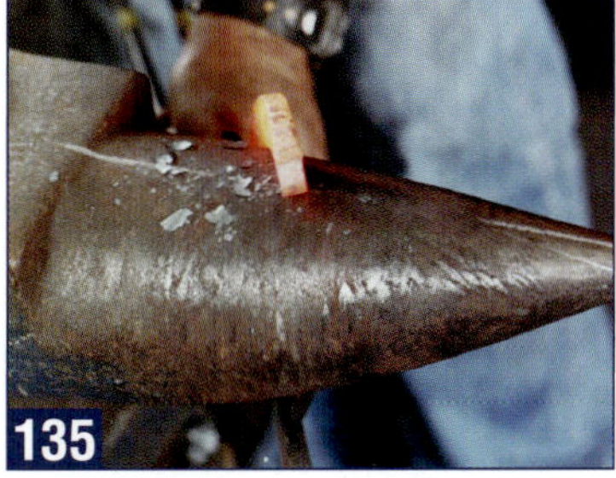

See how the shoe is being rotated and twisted.

Set the toe of the hind.

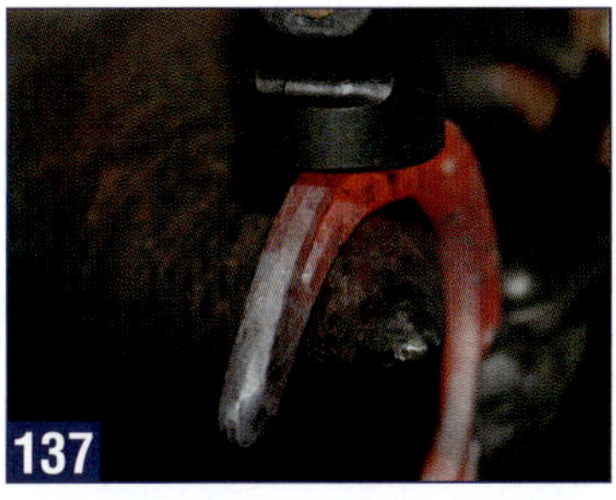

Turn the shoe to find a long radius as you hit the near side of the horn.

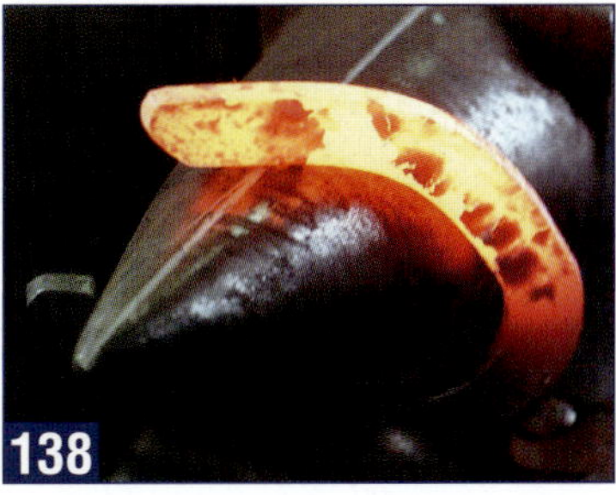

Twist to find the radius of the quarter.

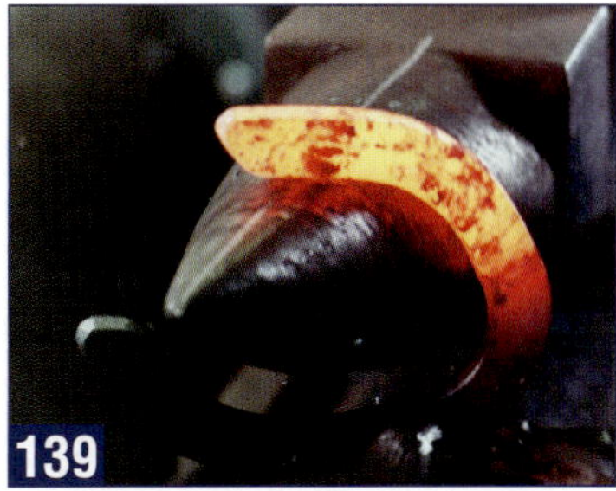

Roll the shoe off the anvil as you form the quarter.

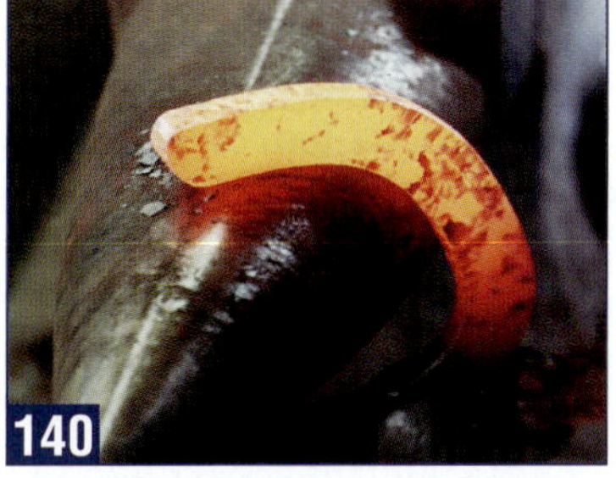

Continue through the heel of the shoe.

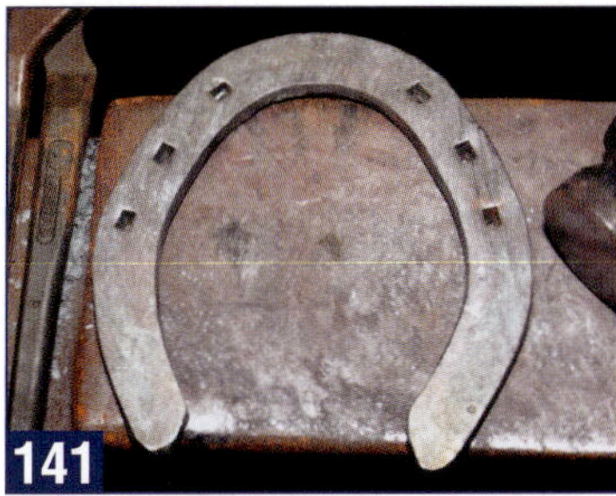

This is a good shape.

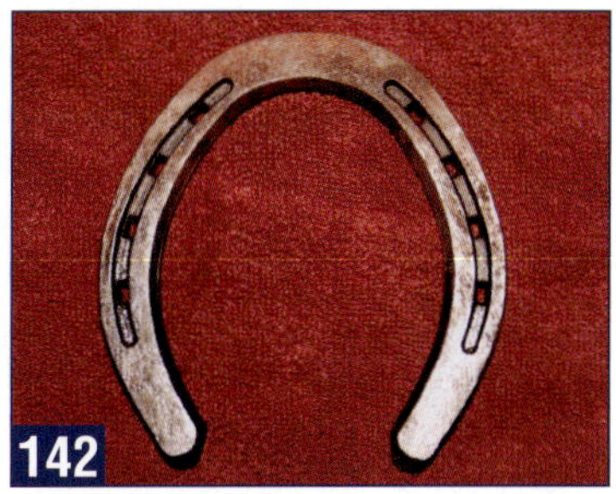

This is also a good hind shape.

so that the radius of the shoe is changed. As the tongs are moved toward my right, the radius of the shoe becomes longer, making a blunter curve.

To shape a hind, set the toe as in **Figure 136**. From this point, turn the shoe to find a long radius on the horn from the toe quarter to the quarter. **(Figure 137).** Hit on the near side of the horn to straighten the shoe, then turn back to gain a shorter radius as you rotate the shoe off of the horn as in **Figures 138-140**. The desired end result will look like the shoes in **Figures 141 or 142**. Try to achieve symmetry and a good shape every time, even when you are just having fun in the shop.

Assemble a pile of used shoes with the nails removed. Shape them from fronts into hinds and back again. Continue this process until the shoes are completely dead. At this point, grab the next two shoes and keep shaping. I encourage students to spend six hours straight at this process to teach them how to shape. Those who refuse to make the effort are generally the ones who do not go home with a diploma.

THE FIGURE-EIGHT

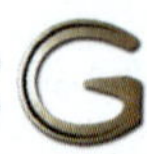

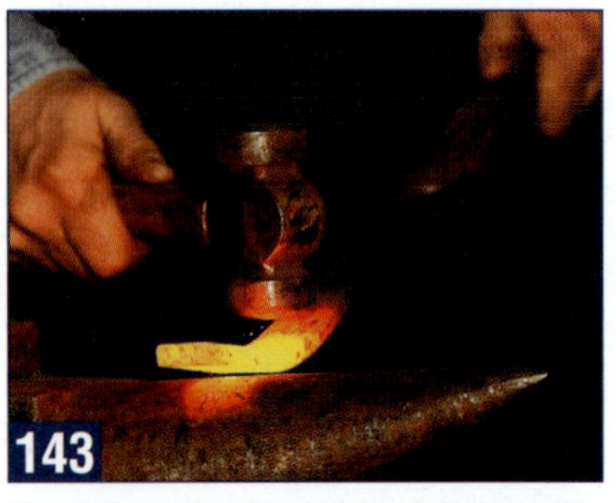

Starting the bend by hitting the stock that is bridged between my tongs and the horn.

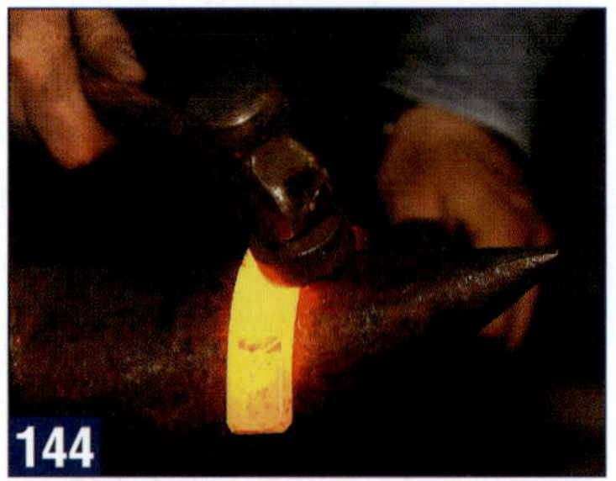

145

Moving to the horn to bend the first part of the figure-eight around.

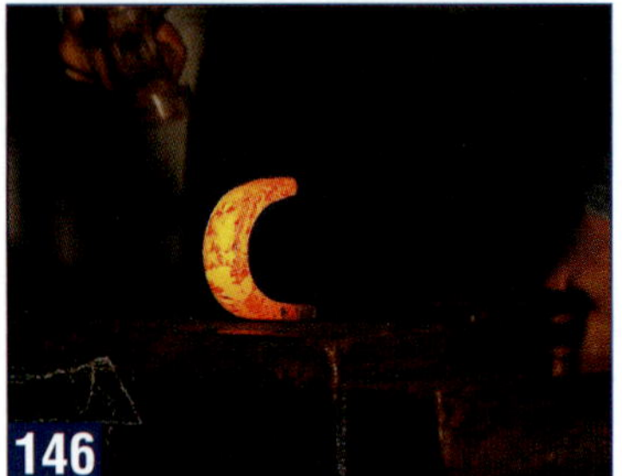

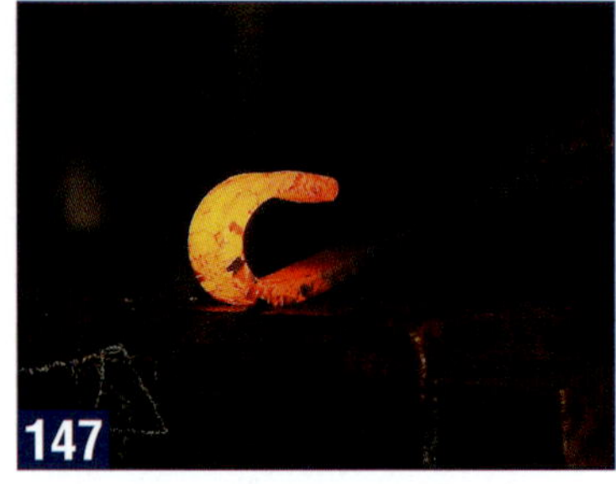

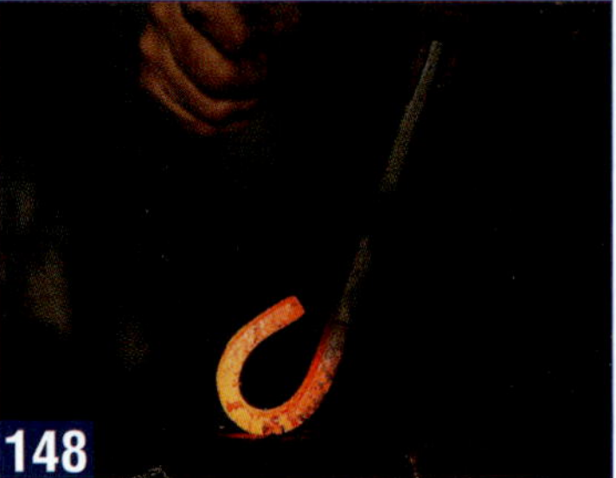

Bending the piece back into itself on the face of the anvil.

One of the final items I suggest that you make is a figure-eight out of 1/2-by-1-inch bar stock. This little item will allow you to punch holes in items that may not easily fit on the anvil in a way that makes punching a hole easy. For instance, pritcheling a nail hole in a shoe that already has clips drawn on it, or punching the rivet hole in the boss of a pair of tongs. **Figures 143 - 155** were taken by Mark Rikard, CF, of Alabama at a clinic I did for Mike Miller, MD, CJF, FWCF.

The figure-eight is easy to make, and when needed, you will be happy that you made it. Begin with a 12-inch piece of 1/2-by-1-inch bar stock. Mark both sides of the steel in the center with an anvil devil. Balancing the steel on the anvil devil is an easy way to find center.

Heat a little more than half the piece, and bend a loop in the stock, bringing the end of the bar stock to the mark you made in the center. This is done partly on the horn **(Figures 143-145)**, and partly by hammering the steel lightly into itself **(Figures 146-149)**. With one side complete, heat the straight branch and bend it the opposite direction to match the first side that you made **(Figures 150-153)**. **Figure 154** shows the complete figure-eight item.

There are a lot of ways to place an item on the figure-eight to allow you to punch a hole through your project. In **Figure 155**, I am pritcheling out the holes in a shoe that has quarter clips already pulled. This is perhaps the most common use for a farrier who has made one of these figure-eights.

This chapter has covered a large number of fun and useful things that will increase your skills and forging ability if you will do them. Practice with a purpose and take the time to do it correctly. If you learn to forge correctly in the beginning, speed will follow. I hope you enjoy the art of forging as much as I have throughout my career. It will make you a better farrier.

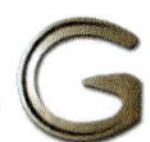

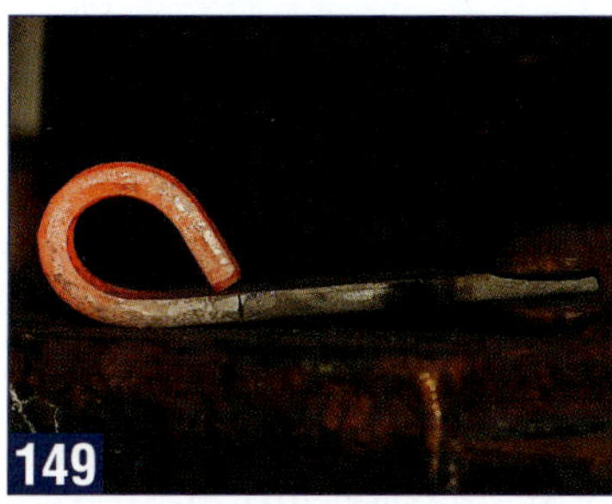

149

Stop when you get it to the center mark made by the anvil devil.

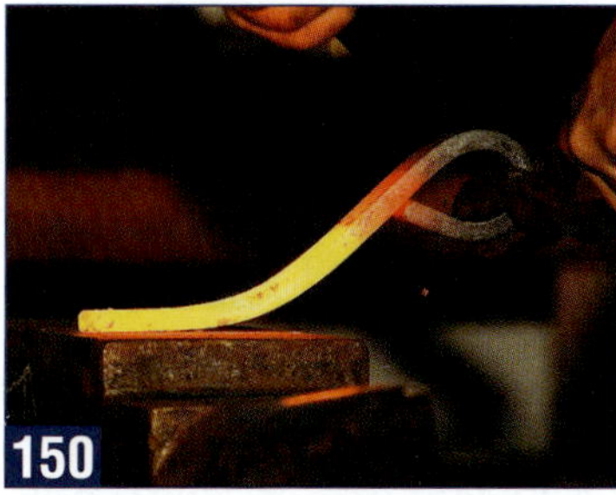

150

Starting the bend on the opposite side.

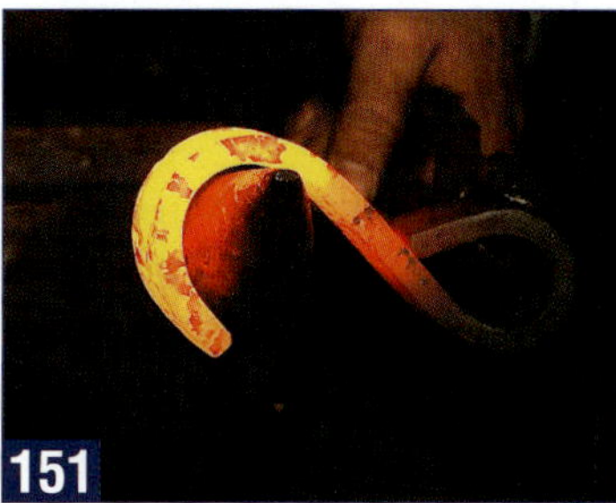

151

Shaping around the horn.

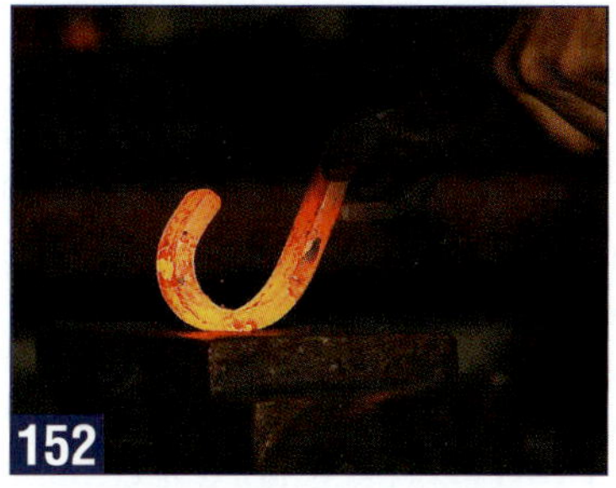

152

Bending it back into itself.

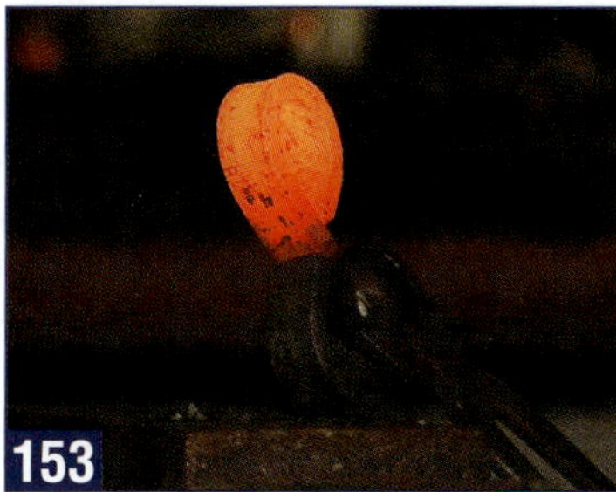

153

154

The finished figure-eight.

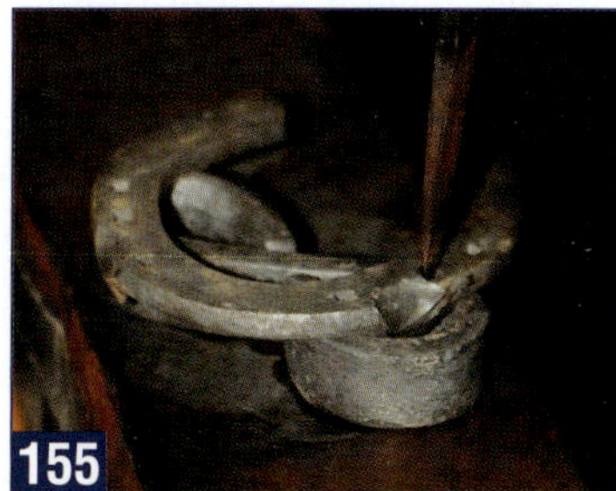

155

Pritcheling out a hole in a shoe with quarter clips already pulled on it.

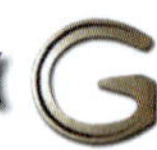

Chapter 39 TONG MAKING

Making your own tongs is something that every farrier should at least learn how to do. It is a great forging exercise, and there is just something about using a pair of tongs that you made for yourself.

In this section, I am going to do a brief description of making bolt tongs. However, you can make any sort of tong you wish. The jaws will just need to be made appropriately for whatever style of tong you wish to make. I strongly advise that you get an old pair of tongs and grind the rivet off so that you have a rein and jaw to look at. That makes it easier to see where you want to go with the pair you are making.

To make this pair of tongs, start with some 3/4-inch round bar stock, about 8 or 9 inches long **(Figure 1)**. Heat one end, and place it over the near edge of the anvil. Forge this area down with half-faced hammer blows until you have forged the jaw to your desired dimension **(Figure 2)**. The one pictured is about 3/8-by-1 inch **(Figure 3)**. Turn the steel a quarter turn counter-clockwise, and place the stock so that the portion you already forged is beyond the off side of the anvil **(Figure 4)**. You will now create the area of the boss. The boss is the part of a pair of tongs that the rivet goes through. Forge this area with half faced blows **(Figure 5)** and you will end up with a piece that looks like **Figures 6-7**.

Take another heat and move to the horn. Define the boss by making a notch with a cross peen or similar tool **(Figure 8)** and you will end up with what you see in **Figure 9**. Forge on the horn just behind the notch that you just made to form a sharp beginning to the rein **(Figures 10-11)**. This is not a necessary thing and can kind of be considered sex appeal. It does enhance the look of a pair of tongs and shows an extra level of skill of the maker.

For making bolt tongs, you will now bend over

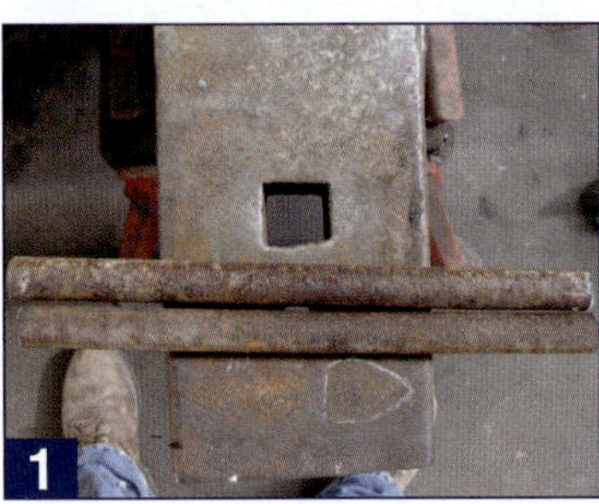

1 *Bar stock to make tongs. Here I am using old sucker-rod from an oil well.*

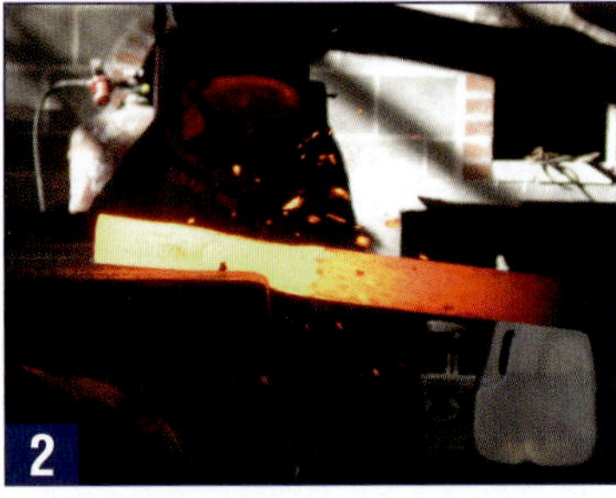

2 *Half-face hammer blows to make a shoulder.*

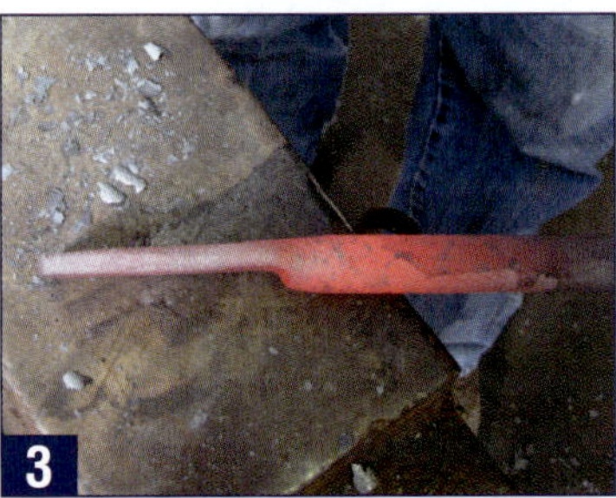

3 *Shouldered area for the jaws.*

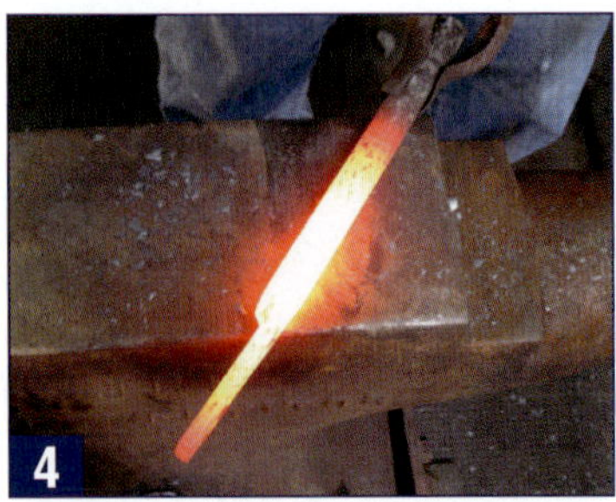

4 *Stock turned 45 degrees to the edge of the anvil.*

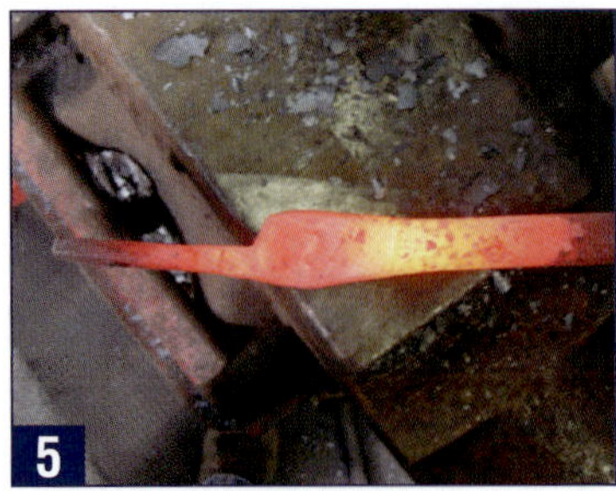

5 *Forge the boss.*

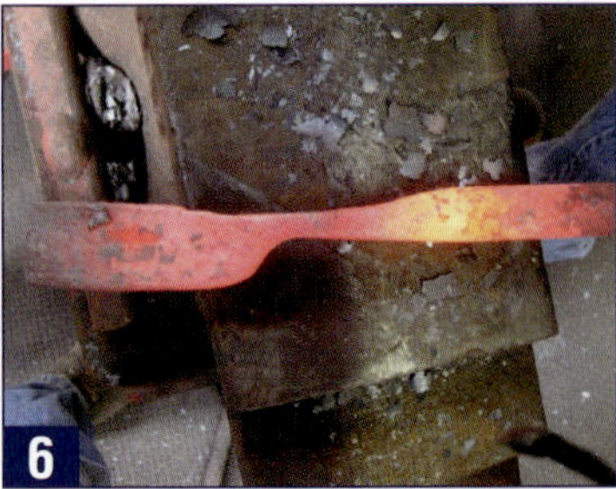

6 *Your piece should look like this.*

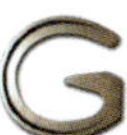

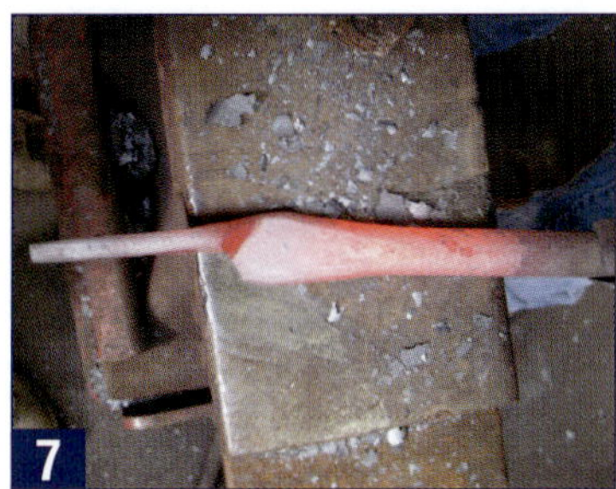

Side view of piece.

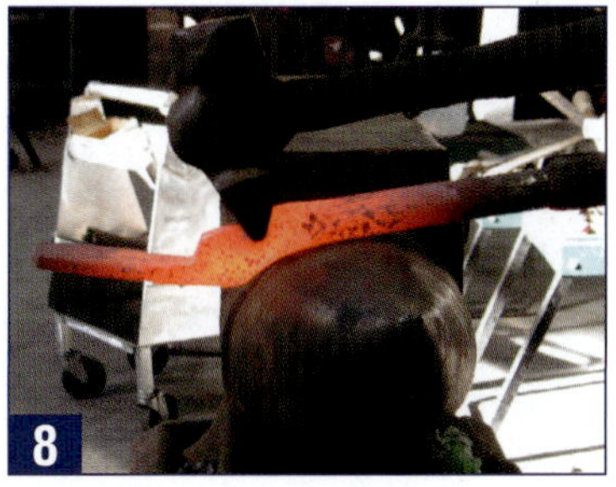

Move to the horn and use a cross peen to start the reins.

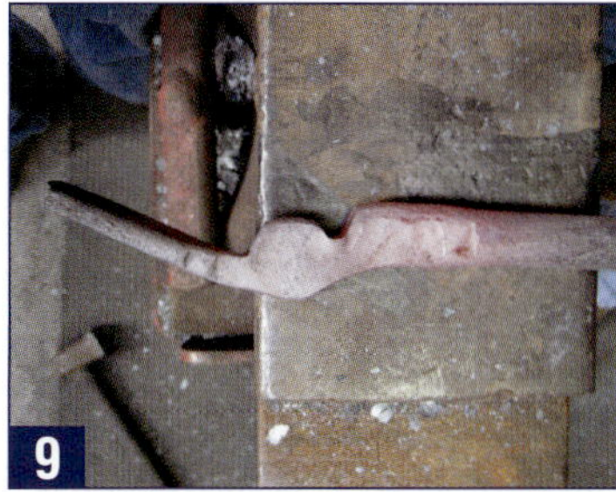

It should look similar to this.

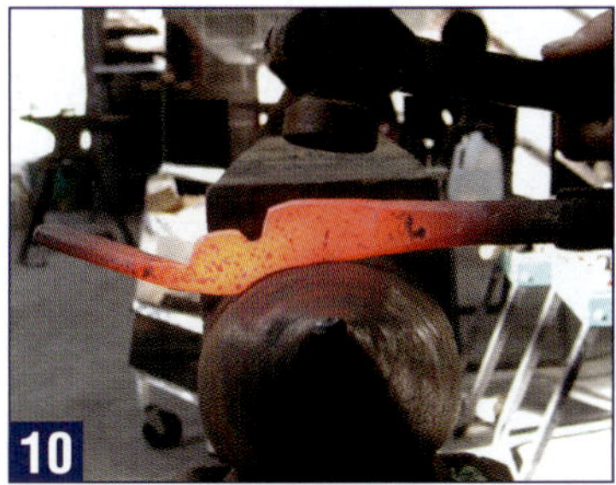

Forge on the horn.

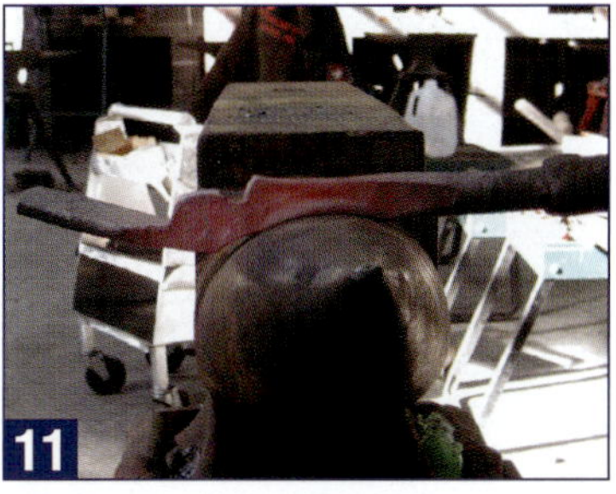

Continue to make the sex appeal at the beginning of the rein.

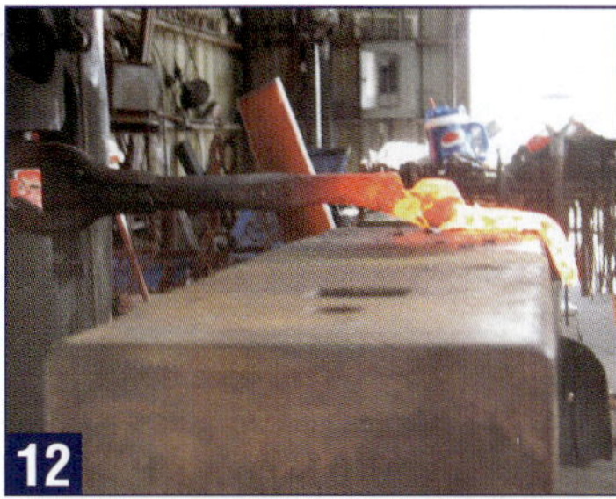

Bend the end of the jaw away from the boss.

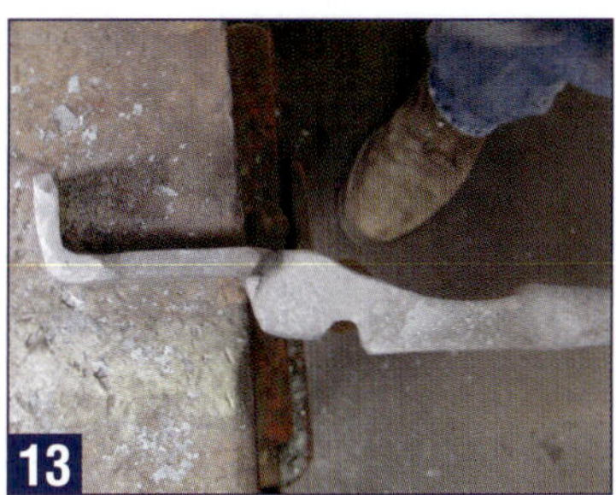

Here is the first jaw.

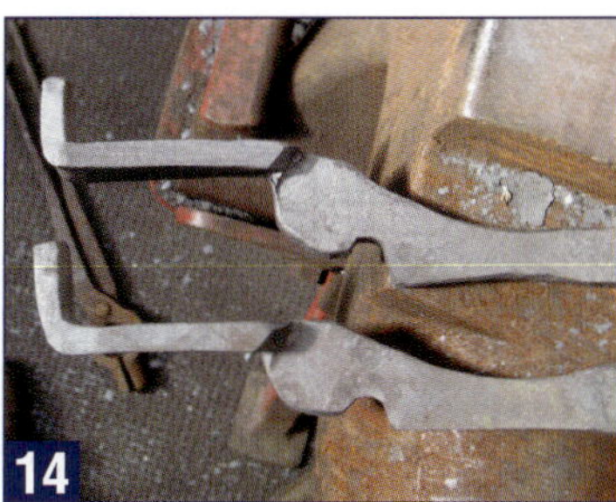

Make another just like it.

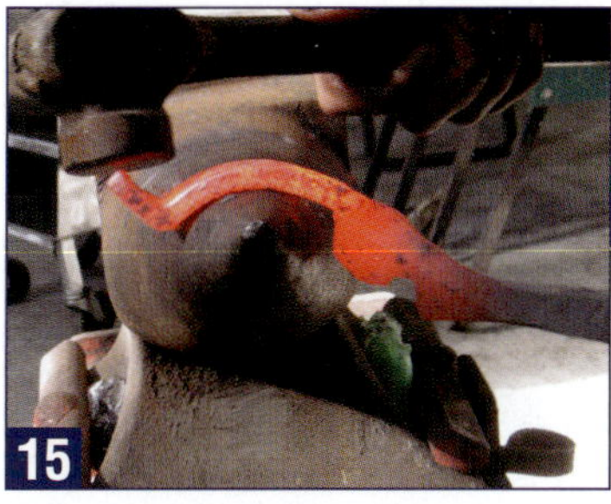

Bend the base of the jaw around the horn.

an inch or so on the end of the jaw **(Figures 12-13)**. Make another that looks exactly the same out of the other piece of stock **(Figure 14)**. Same shoulders, same bends, same size, all forged exactly the same way. These two pieces are not mirror images; they are supposed to be identical.

Bend a radius into the jaw around the horn **(Figure 15)**, and then use the cross peen in the step of the anvil to begin forming where the jaw will be round to hold round stock **(Figure 16)**. Take another heat and punch a hole in the middle of the boss with a stud punch. To do this, drive the punch

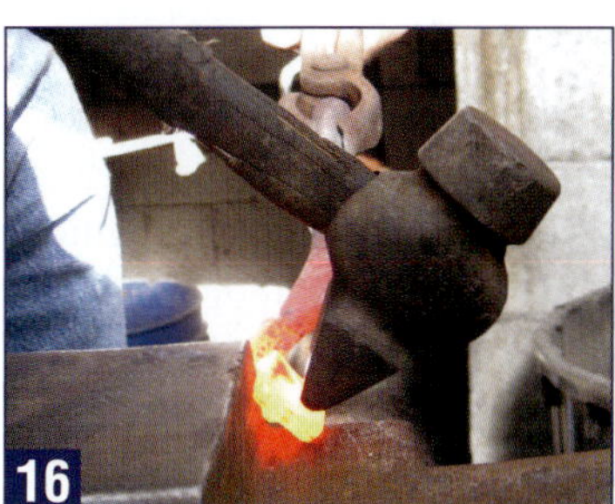

Start the rounded area here to shape for bolt tongs.

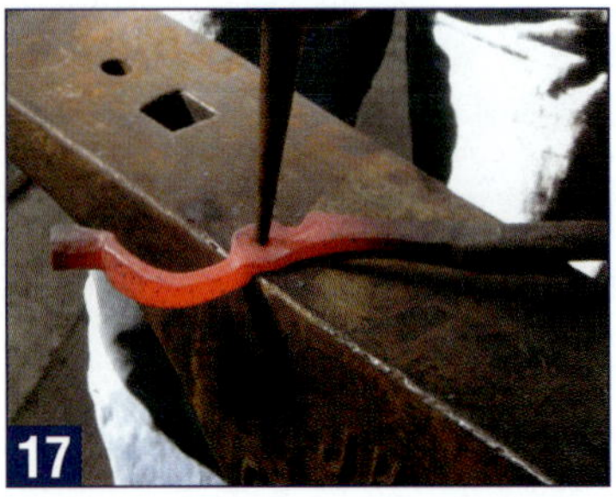

Punch the rivet hole from one side.

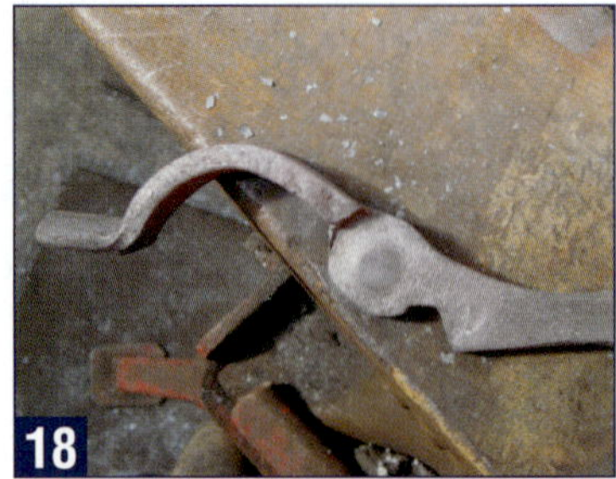

You should be able to see a shiny area where the stud punch was driven.

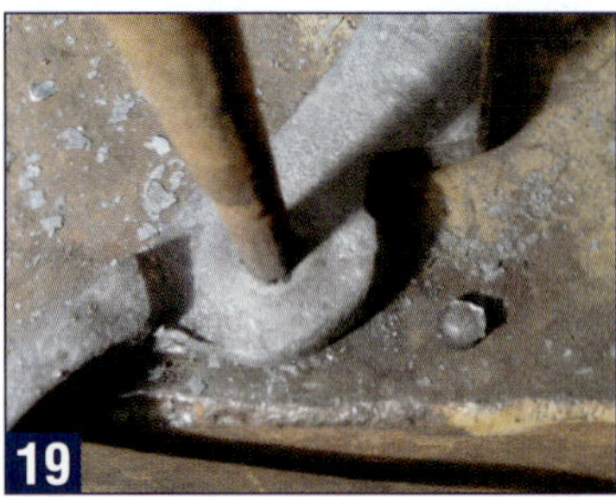

Punch out the plug from the other side with the stud punch.

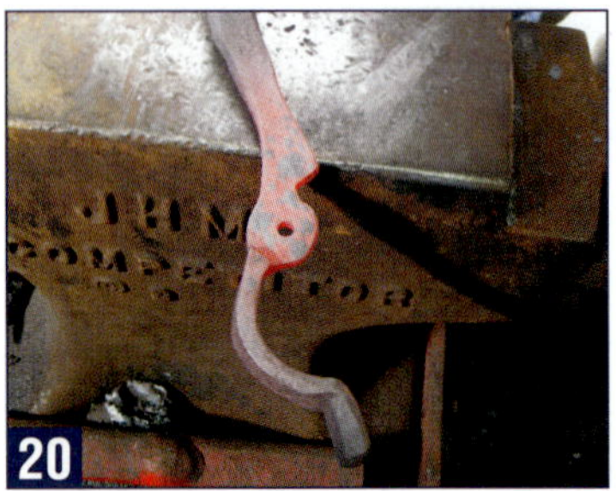

Place the jaw past the edge of the anvil at an angle.

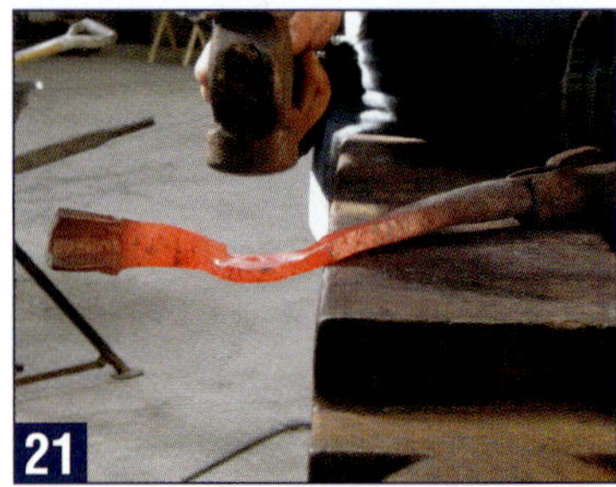

Forge the offset to line the jaws up.

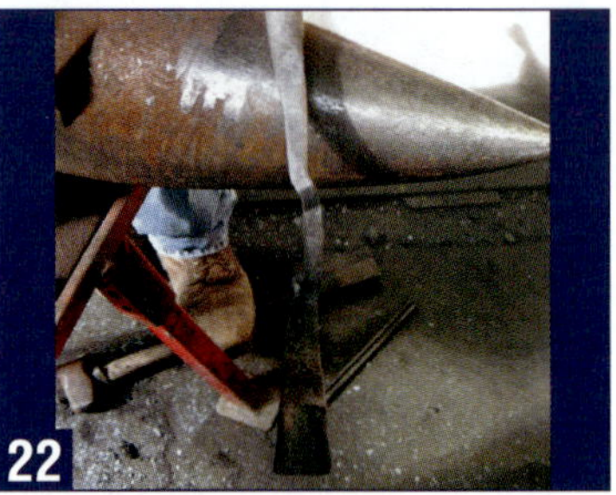

Your tongs should be at this point now.

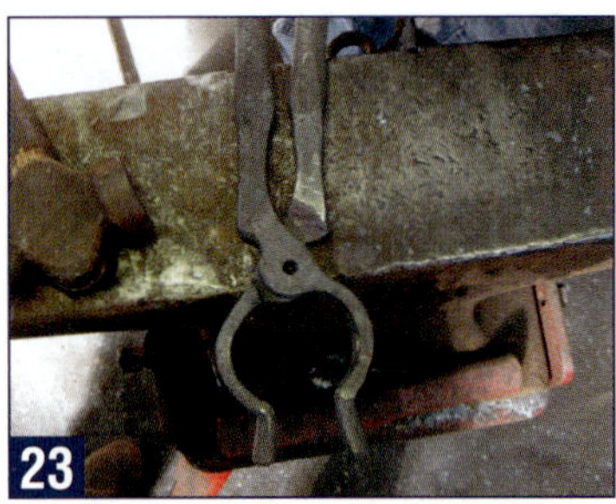

Place the two pieces together to see how they line up.

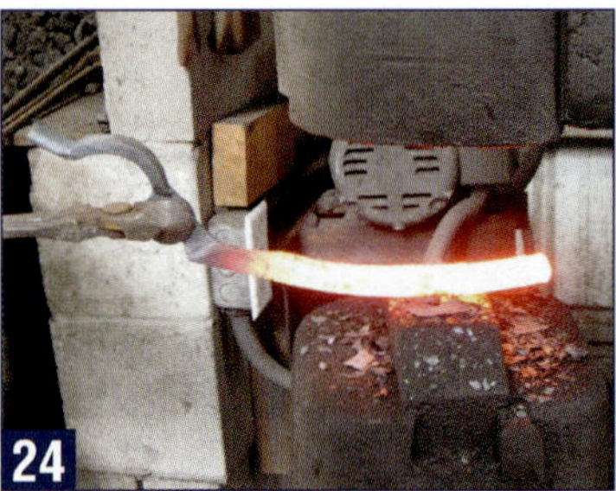

Draw out the reins.

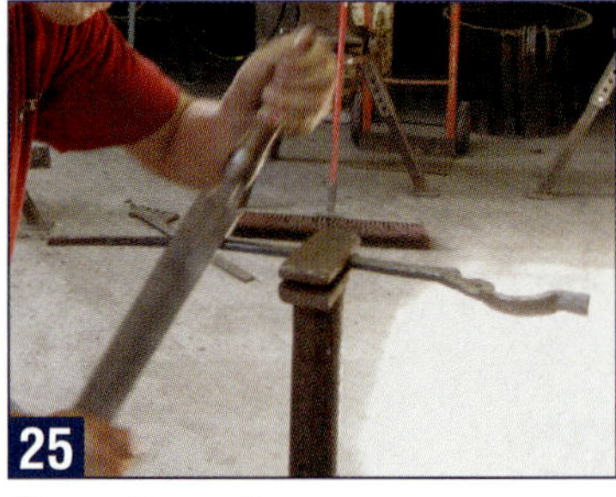

Rasp the reins.

into the red-hot boss about 80% of the way **(Figure 17)**. You want the opposite side to have the same shiny spot that we have when punching nail holes in a shoe after just using the fore punch **(Figure 18)**. Put the stud punch in the middle of the shiny spot and drive out the little slug that is blocking the hole **(Figure 19)**.

The next step is to make the offset that will put the reins on top of each other when the tongs are put together. By doing this, you make it so that these tongs are ambidextrous. In some brands of tongs, the reins lay beside each other because the offset is not made. These types of tongs are easier to use in one hand or the other, making them more right- or left-handed. The offset in the rein eliminates this problem. Hold the tongs at about 45 degrees to the off side edge of the anvil, **(Figure 20)**, hit beyond the point of contact **(Figure 21)**, and try to make it look like **Figure 22**. Repeat with the other piece, making sure that you offset the same way on each. The two pieces should now fit together as shown in **Figure 23**.

The next step is to draw out the reins. In **Figure 24**, I am doing it with a trip hammer. My cameraman

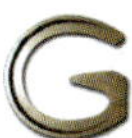

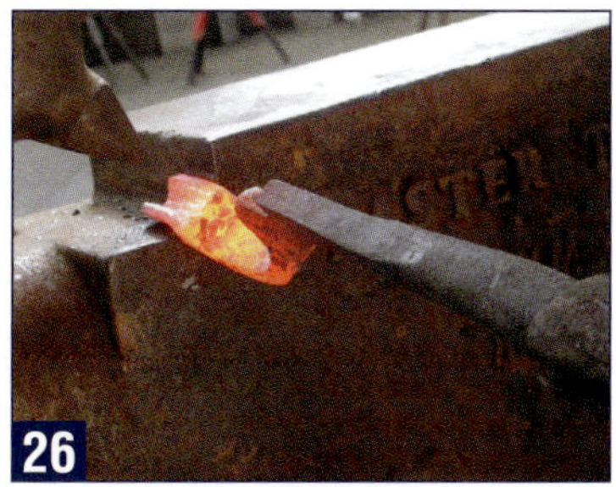

26

Refine the jaw shape.

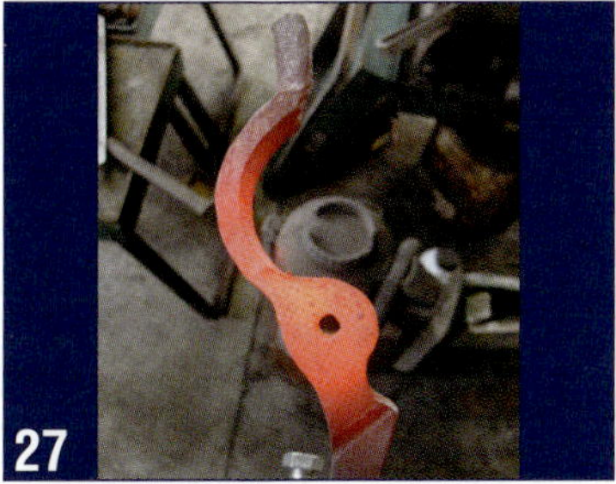

27

You should spend enough time to get everything right at this stage.

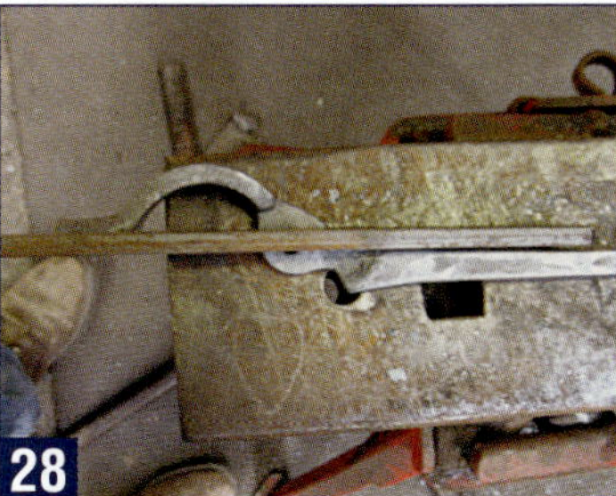

28

Check the alignment with stock going through the rivet hole, parallel to the jaws and the reins.

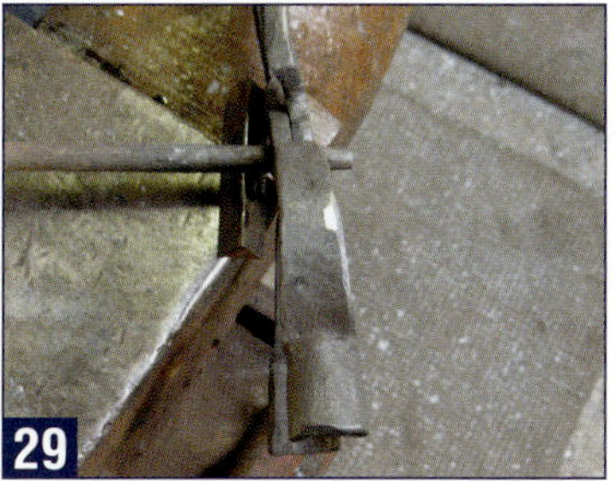

29

Place rivet stock through hole to check size.

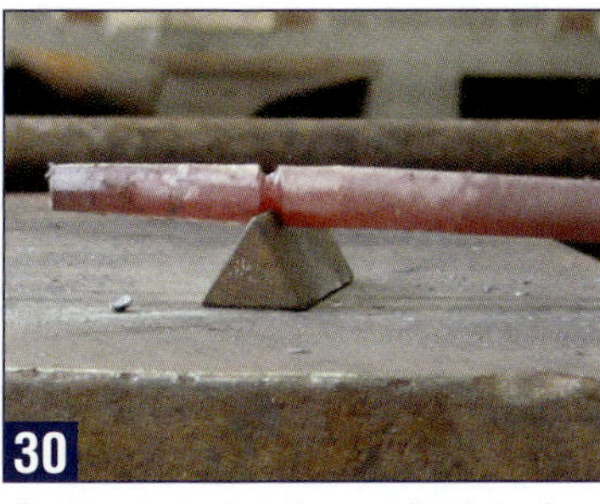

30

Cut part way through the rivet stock.

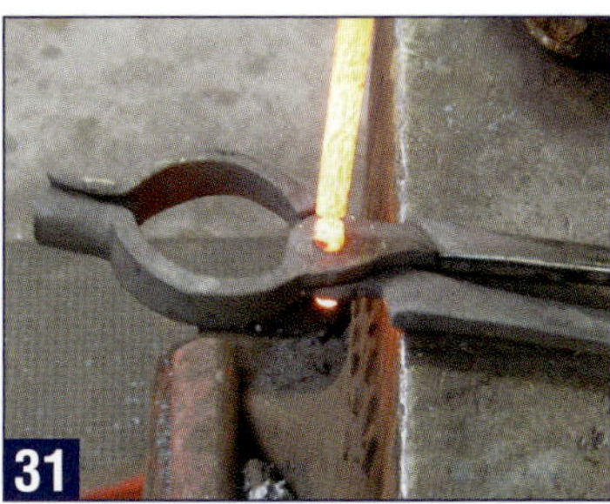

31

Heat the rivet, place it in the hole, and break it off.

Cody is usually my striker, but he has not mastered striking and taking pictures at the same time. After drawing the reins out, it is time to grind them. I like using a 14-inch straight grinder powered by a 17-year-old boy **(Figure 25)**. Spend the time to clean and crisp up all the surfaces at this point since it will be hard to do once the tongs are put together **(Figures 26-27)**.

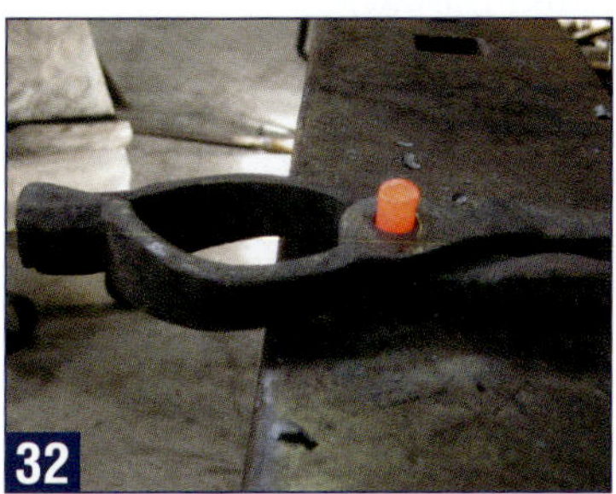

32

Forge the rivet.

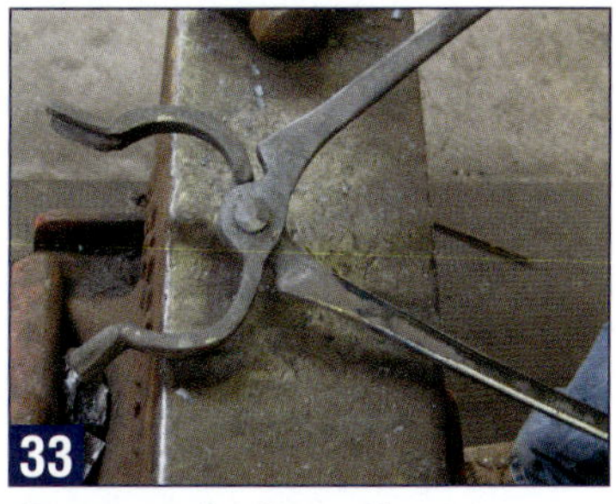

33

Open and close the tongs at this point.

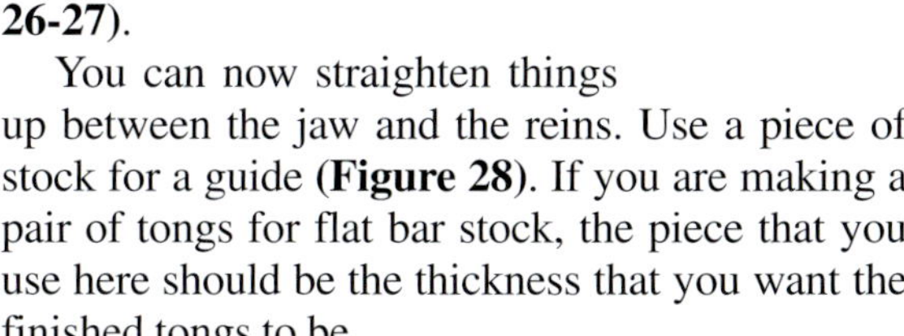

You can now straighten things up between the jaw and the reins. Use a piece of stock for a guide **(Figure 28)**. If you are making a pair of tongs for flat bar stock, the piece that you use here should be the thickness that you want the finished tongs to be.

The next step is to rivet the two pieces together. You can buy commercial rivets, you can make good rivets, or you can use the method that I show here.

I show this method because it can easily be done with any large enough stock, and it is quite easy. It was shown to me by the late, great Eddie Watson, CJF. Forge a round taper in the stock so that it fits sufficiently through the holes in the bosses **(Figure 29)**. Cut the piece with an anvil devil **(Figure 30)**, rolling as you cut so that it is cut through to the middle. Don't break off the rivet, just cut most of the way through.

Heat the end of the stock and place the rivet into the 2 holes **(Figure 31)**. Break off the piece of bar and forge the rivet head while it is still hot **(Figure 32)**. Work the tongs while the jaws and reins are still cool, and the rivet is still warm **(Figure 33)**. Heat both jaws to size the tongs with the stock that they are designed to hold **(Figure 34)**. Send them back

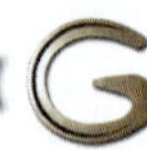

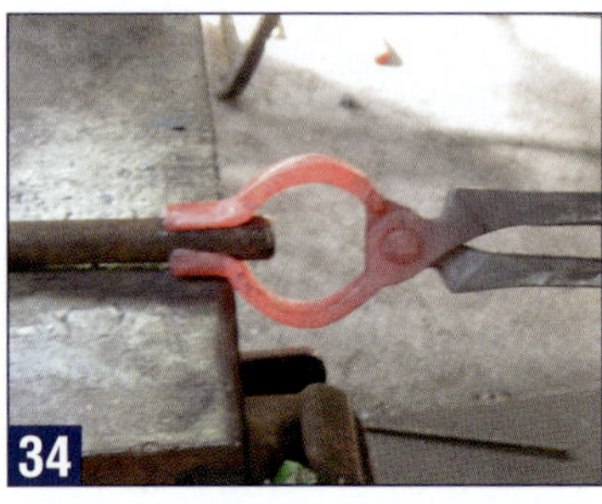

Heat everything and shape the jaws.

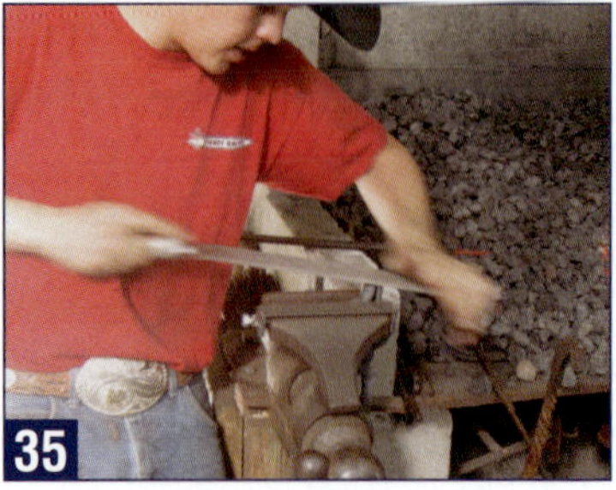

Back to the grinder.

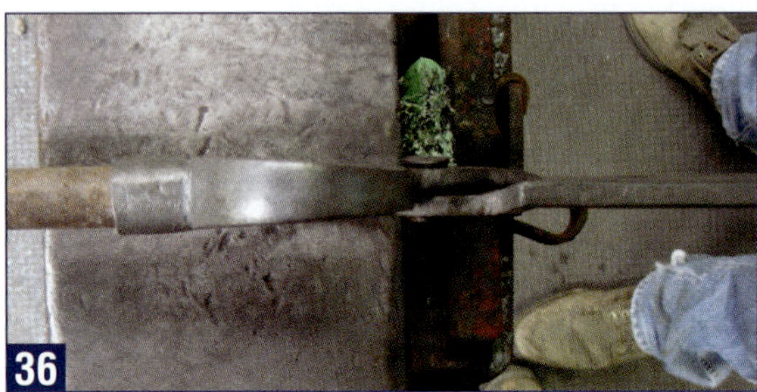

Finished tongs.

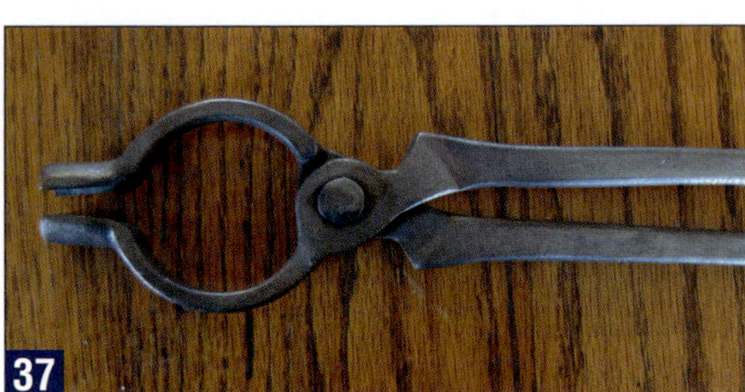

to the grinding department **(Figure 35)** and you will have a pair of tongs **(Figures 36 -37)** that should give good service for years to come.

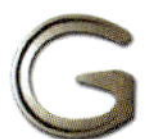

Chapter
40 THE BASIC HIND

In Five Heats to a Blank

This is perhaps one of the best shoes to introduce you to the world of shoemaking. Like most shoes, having the right toe-bend is paramount. The formula is straightforward and simple, and following strict form is important.

TOOLS NEEDED

- Hammer
- Appropriate tongs
- Center punch
- Silver pencil
- Anvil devil

SETUP

Make this shoe out of 11 1/2 inches of stock that is 3/4-inch wide. The choice of thickness is at your discretion, but the shoe in the pictures is 5/16-inch thick. Find center and mark with a silver pencil or soapstone. Draw a line across the width of the stock 1 1/4 inches from center (**Figure 1**). This mark is the area where the training wheels will be, and it corresponds to the location of the toe nail holes, which can be marked at this time with a center punch (**Figure 2**).

Lay the stock over an anvil devil and mark both edges of the stock. These marks are what we are referring to when we talk about training wheels (**Figure 3**). It is important that there are training wheels on both the inside and outside edge, since they will both be needed as reference points.

PROCESS

HEAT 1

Heat the center of the stock and hold with the width of the stock past the jaws and the tongs at a 90-degree angle to the stock (**Figure 4**). Position the

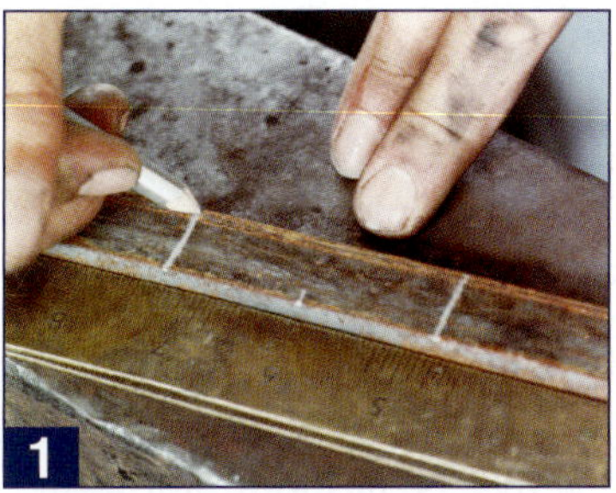

Marking the steel to begin the blank.

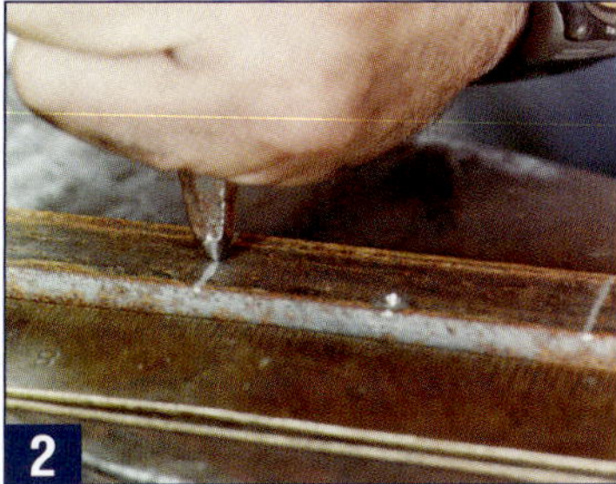

Using a center punch.

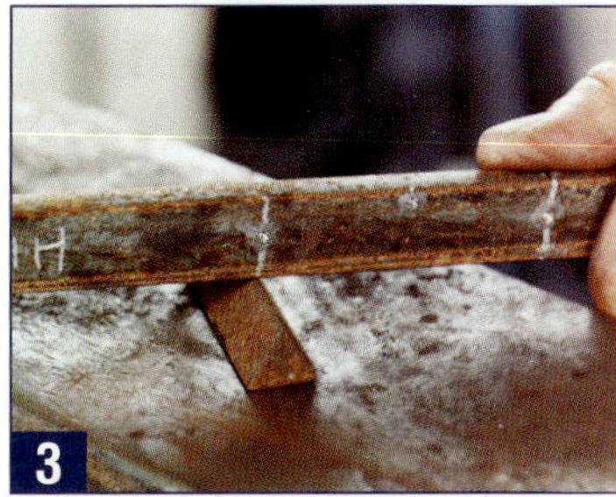

Marking the training wheels with the anvil devil.

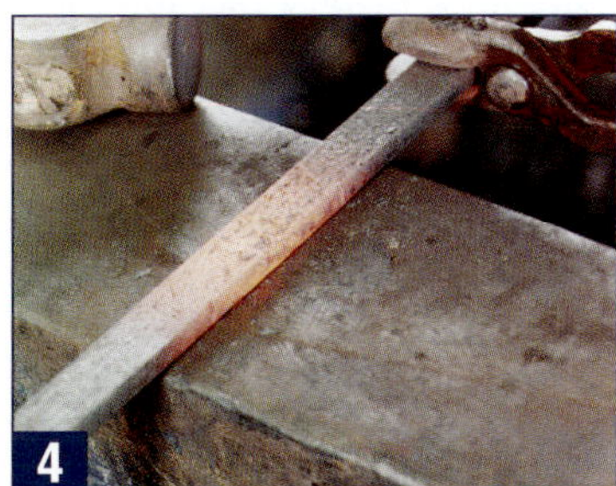

Heat in the center of the stock.

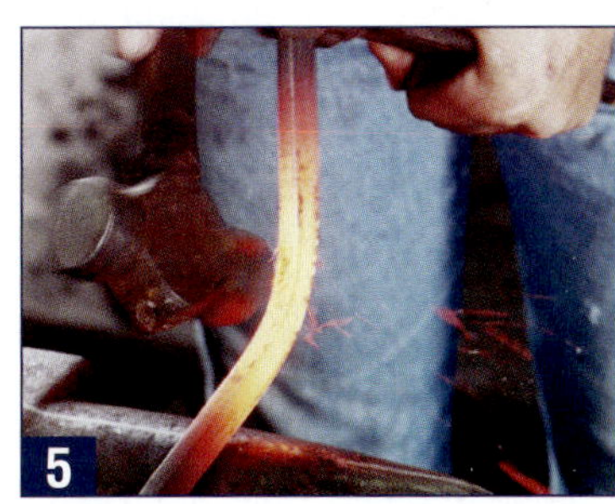

Begin the toe bend.

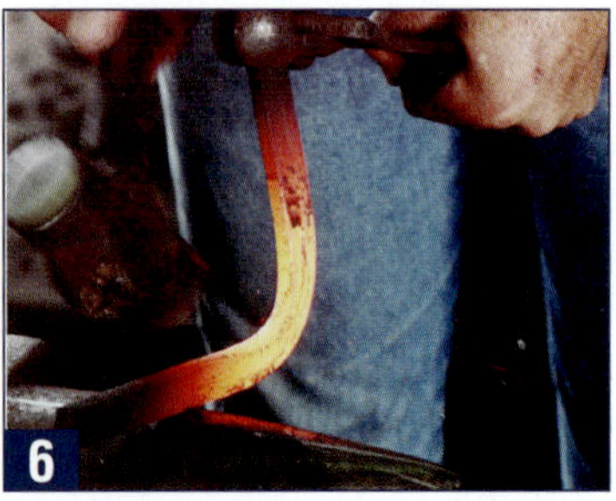

Continue past 90 degrees.

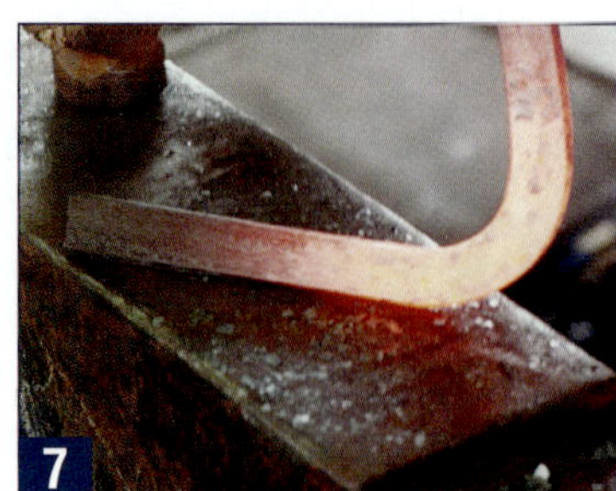

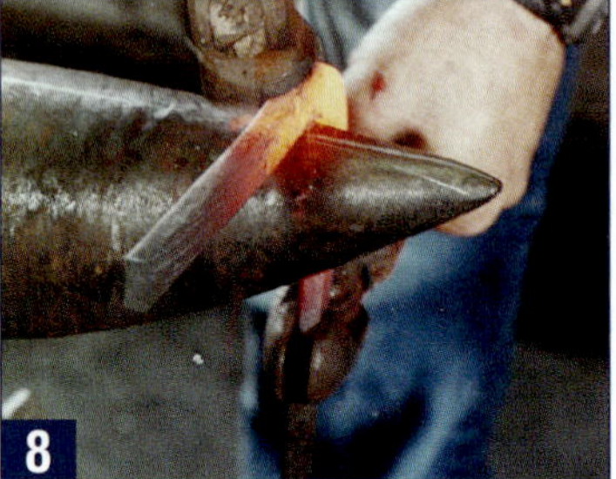

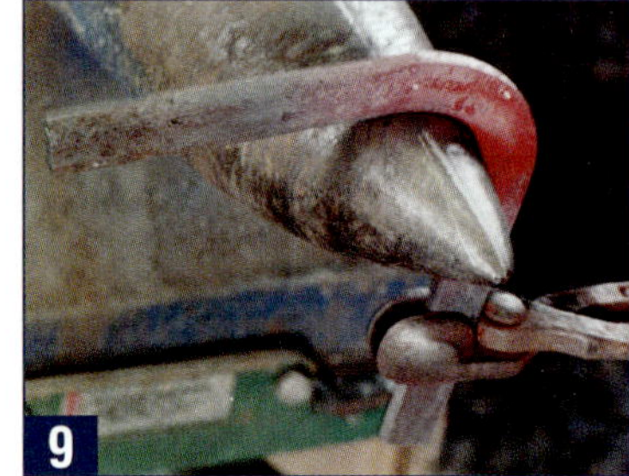

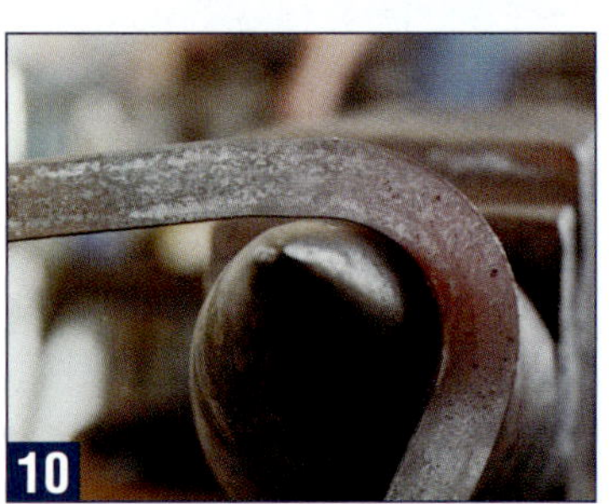

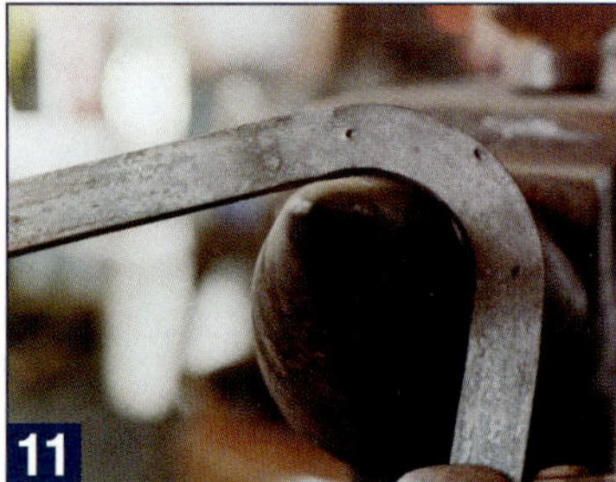

Set the toe.

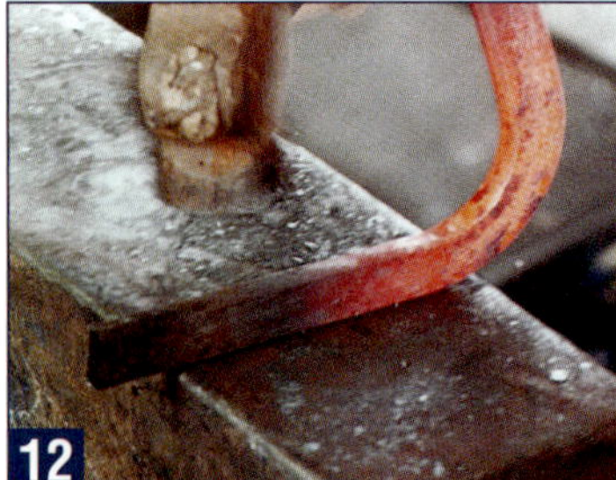

Straighten the branch by hitting the inside of the shoe.

stock on the horn and hammer in the center of the piece between the training wheels **(Figure 5)**. This will create a rough toe bend.

Once you have bent the stock to an angle tighter than 90 degrees **(Figures 6-7)**, turn the stock over and place the toe bend on the horn **(Figure 8)**. Move toward the tip of the horn far enough that you have a radius on the inside of the stock that is appropriate for the size of the desired hind shoe. The smaller the toe, the further toward the tip of the horn the toe should be made. Push downward with the tongs so that the training wheel is now over the dead center top of the horn **(Figure 9)**. Hit the stock so that your hammer would land with three-quarters of the hammer face beyond the centerline or ridge of the horn. Hammer until the toe is in contact with the horn **(Figure 10)** and turn the shoe around and do the same to the opposite side of the toe **(Figure 11)**. This is called setting the toe and gives the shoes you build a consistent radius appropriate for the foot. Stop once you have achieved this position so that the width of the stock is not compromised.

After setting the toe, inertia will often cause the branch of the shoe to bend away from the toe. When this happens, turn the piece in such a way that you are able to hit the inside of the branch with your hammer **(Figure 12)**. This will straighten the stock back out.

When bending the shoe on the horn, you can tell if the stock is bending or being forged by what you feel in your tong hand as well as what you hear. If you have direct contact with the horn, the stock will be thinned by hammering it against the horn, and there will be a solid sound when it is hammered. There will be little, if any, shock transferred to your tongs. You do not want to hammer too hard once you have contact since the stock width dimension will be lost. If your tongs are jumping in your hand with every blow and it doesn't sound solid, the stock is being bent, not smashed and forged.

Once this is done, place the shoe on the face of the anvil and hammer the inside of the web to relieve

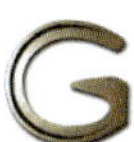

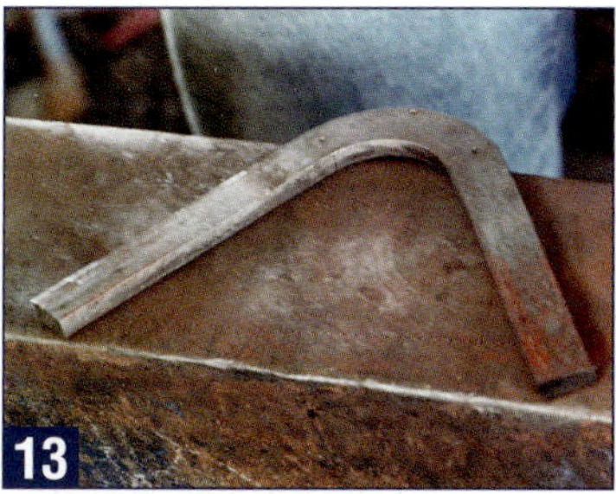
Finished toe bend.

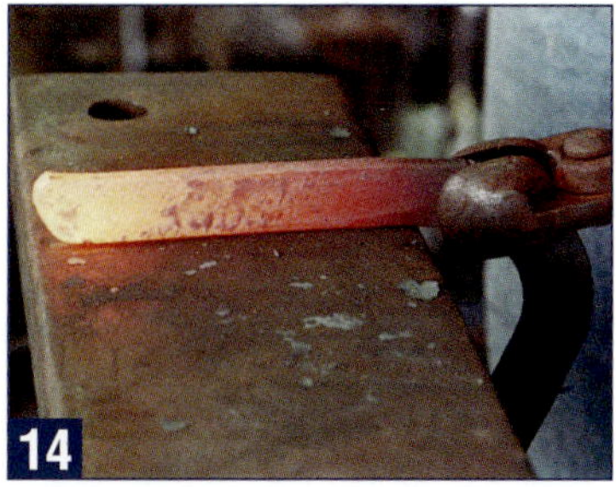
Start heel.

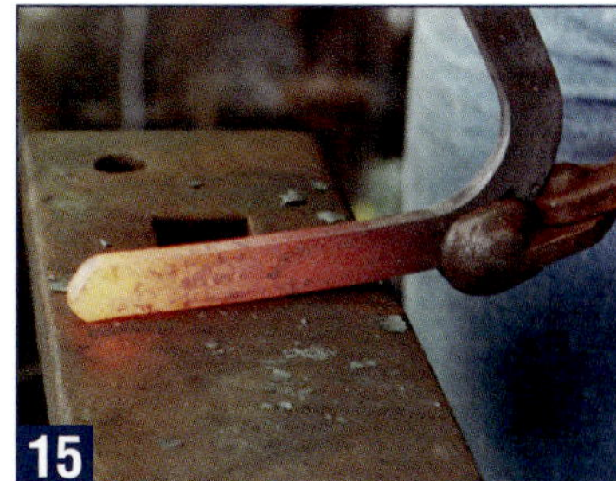
Finish heel.

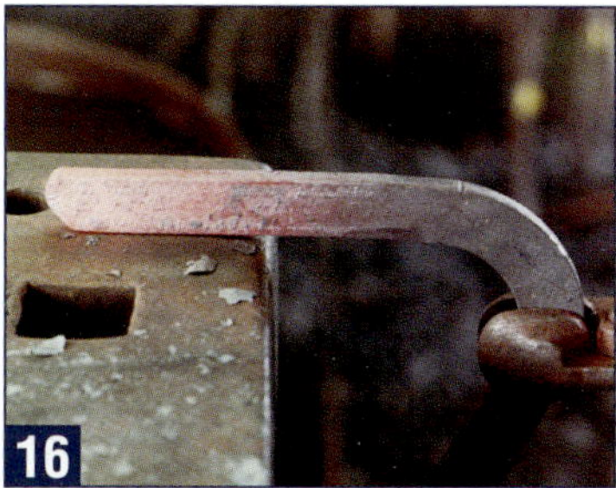
Move to heel of anvil to counteract inertia.

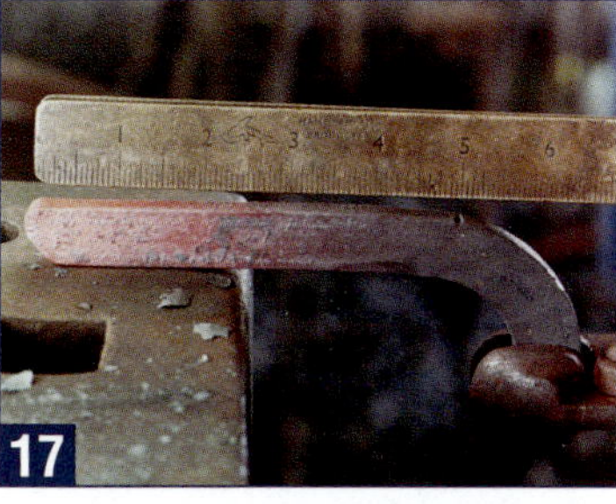

Locate the area between the heel and the training wheel.

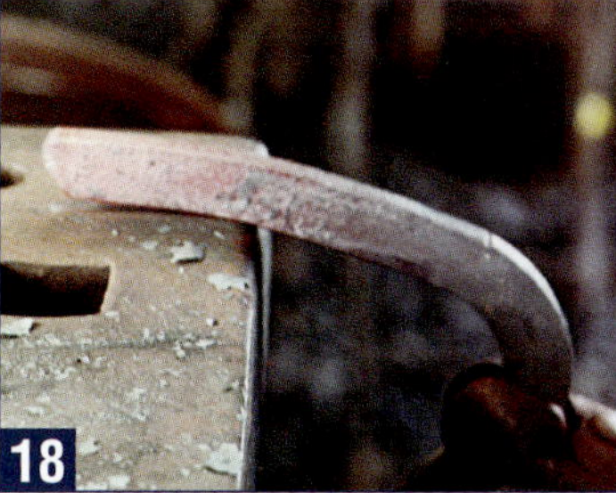
Counteracting inertia.

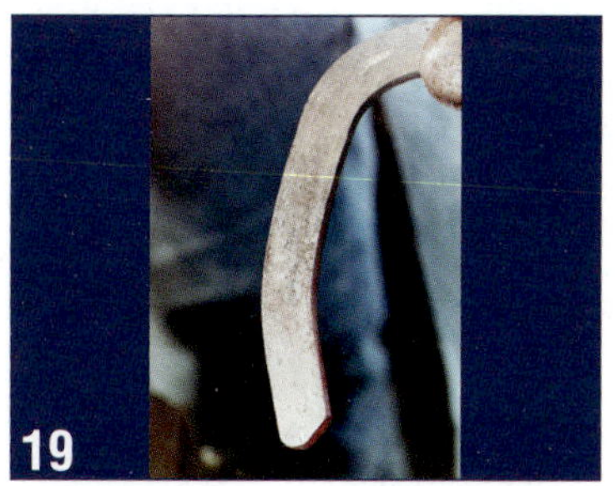
The end result of Heat 2.

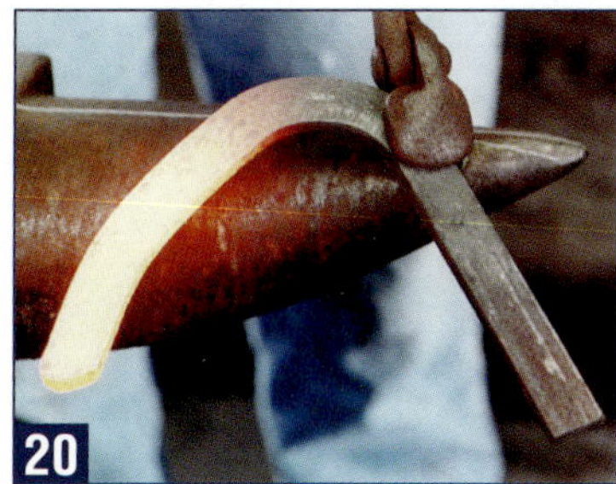
Heat through the toe.

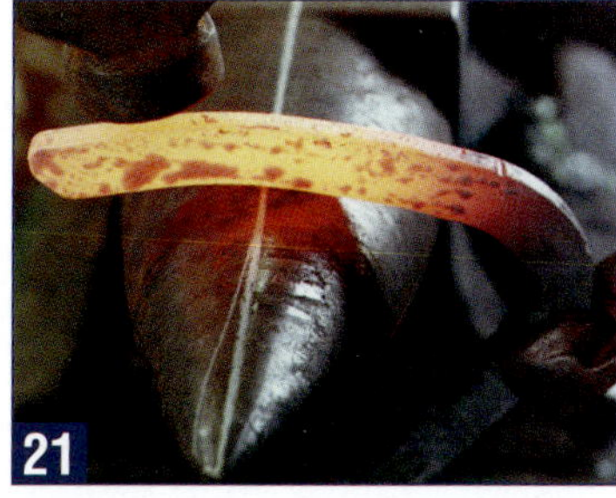
Move to horn so that the middle of the branch from heel to training wheel is on the horn.

sole pressure and remove the added thickness that results from bending a piece of hot steel. Roll the toe of the shoe around the horn while hammering with light, over-lapping hammer blows, working in the area of the horn that the toe was created on.

Once this heat is complete, you should have a proper hind toe bend **(Figure 13)**.

HEAT 2

Heat one branch to a good forging heat, bring it out of the fire and build the heel **(Figures 14 and 15)**. (Refer to the Basic Tasks Section for tips on making the heel) Place the end of the shoe over the heel of the anvil so that the middle of the branch between the heel and the training wheel is lined up with the near edge of the anvil face **(Figure 16-17)**. Hammer with light blows as you let the weight of the shoe fall off the anvil **(Figure 18)**. This makes a slight bend in the branch at the area of the quarter **(Figure 19)**, which aids in counter-acting the effects of inertia when the branch is bent around the horn.

HEAT 3

Heat the branch with the heel on it all the way

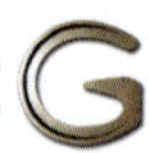

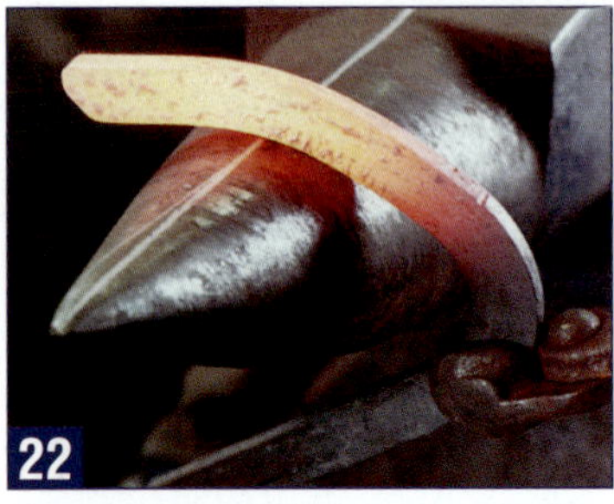

Bend the stock into the radius of the quarter.

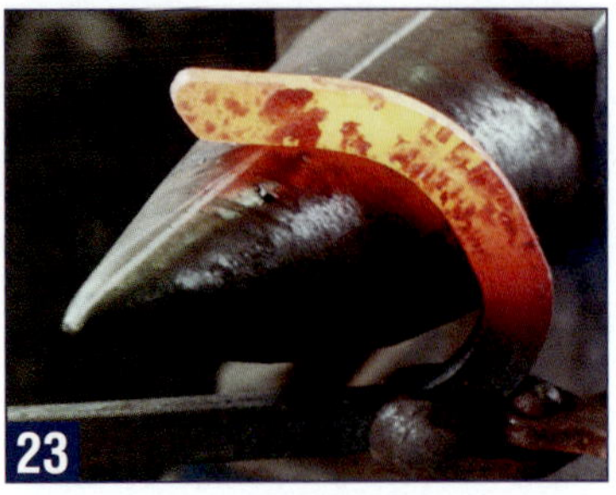

Drop your tong hand to create the bend.

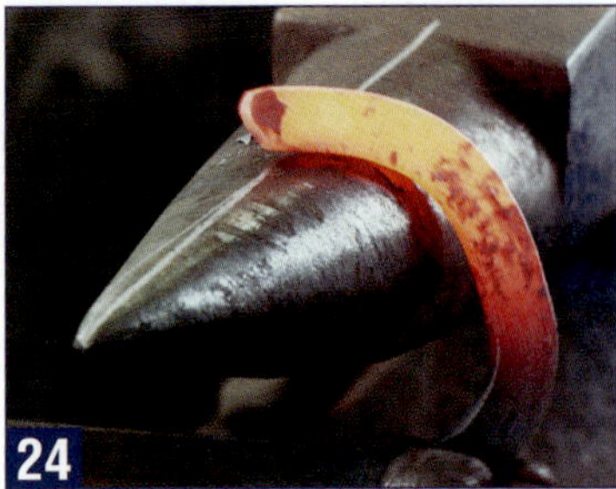

Continue through the end of the heel.

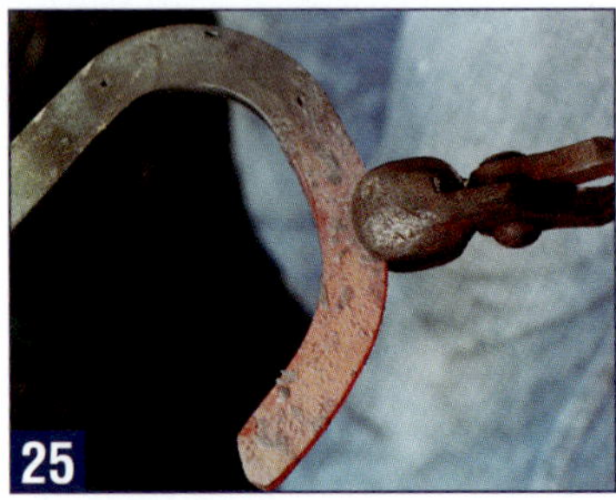

You should have half a shoe at the end of Heat 3.

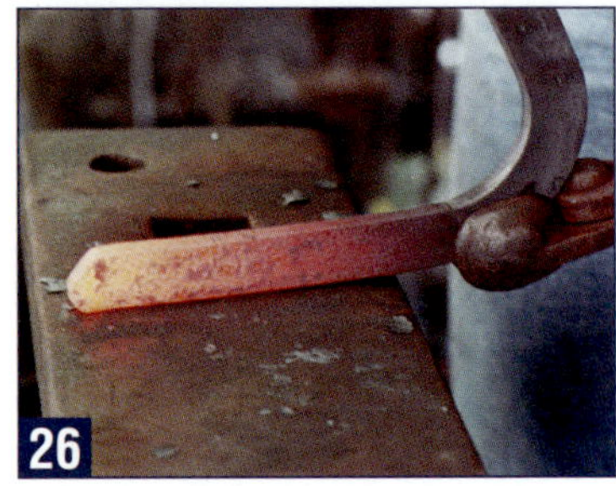

Heel.

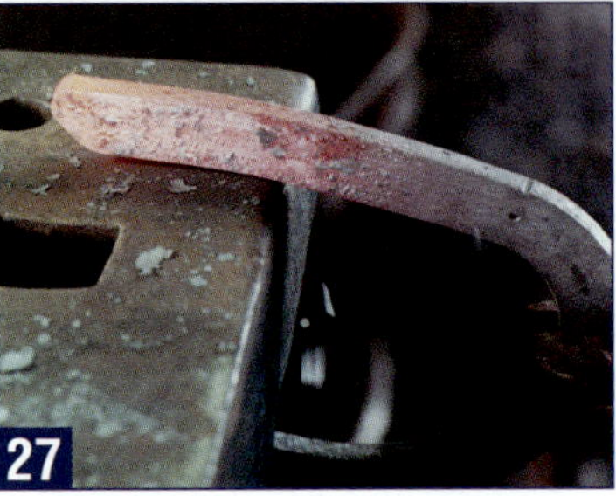

Move to counteract inertia.

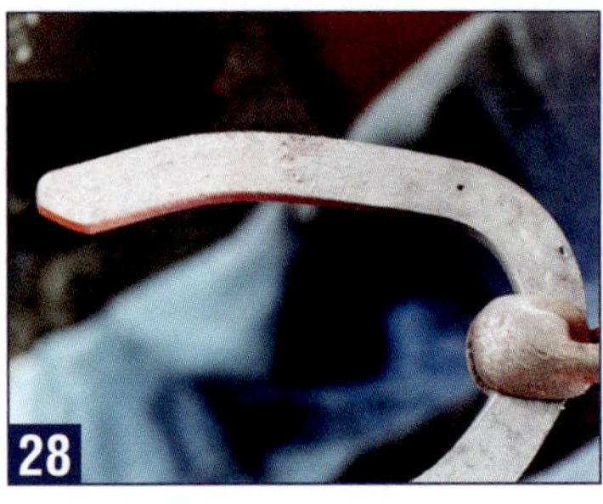

End of Heat 4.

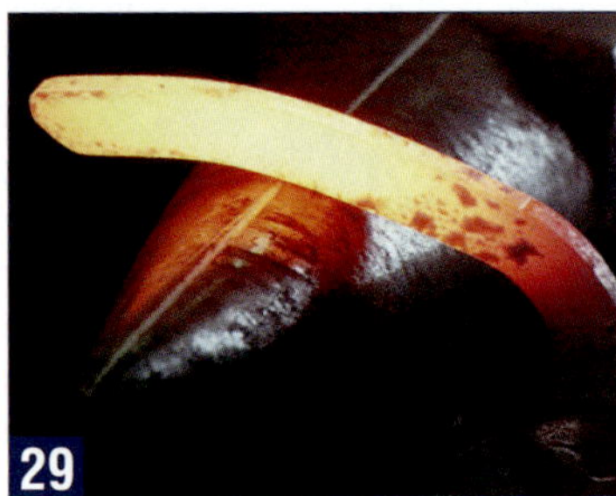

Bend on the horn.

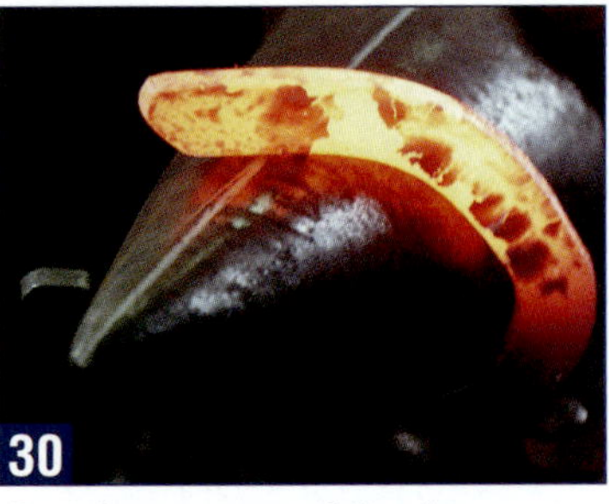

Continue around the horn.

to the toe **(Figure 20)** and place it over the horn in an area with a large enough radius to fit the quarter **(Figure 21)**. Estimate the middle point between the heel and the training wheel. This point should be dead center top of the anvil. Push down with your tong hand to create a gap beyond the ridge, and lightly hammer so that the hammer is forcing the steel to take the shape of the horn in that area **(Figure 22)**. The shoe is being forged in the bending area of the forging zone on the far side of the horn. Having the tongs positioned so that you have the three points of contact is helpful at this junction. If there is not a gap beyond the center of the horn, the steel will be smashed and lose dimension. If you don't have a gap, readjust tong position and maintain strict form.

As the steel bends, slightly move the reins of the tongs toward the near side of the anvil to find a longer radius by twisting the shoe. Lower the reins at the same time to keep the gap open on the bending zone of the horn **(Figures 23-24)**. Forcing the shoe into this gap and around this particular radius is what determines the final shape of the quarter. Continue through till the end of the heel comes

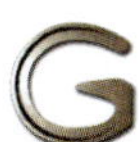

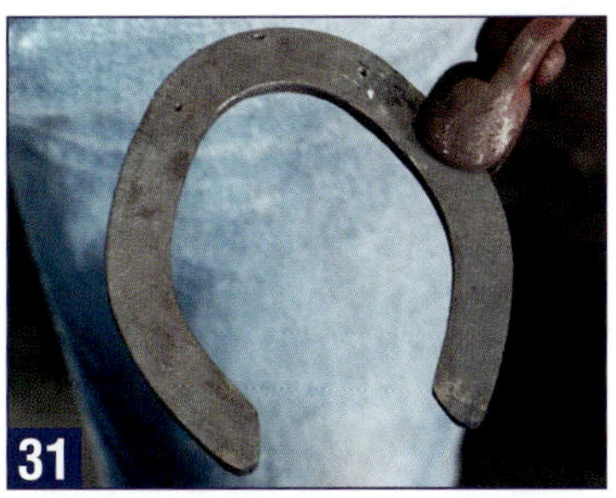

Finished blank.

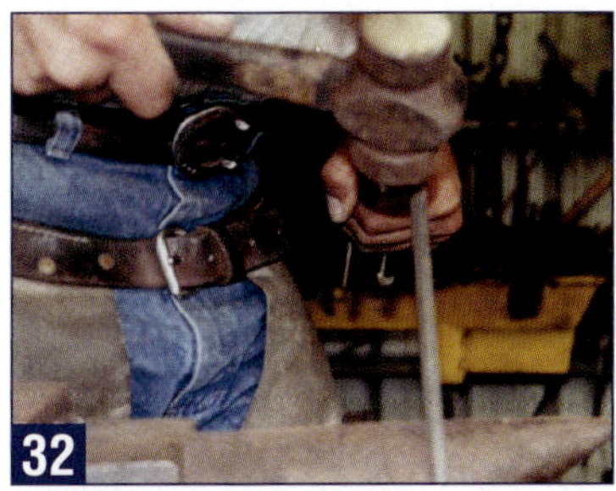

Making a toe bend with the hammer, stock, and tongs out of alignment at 0 degrees.

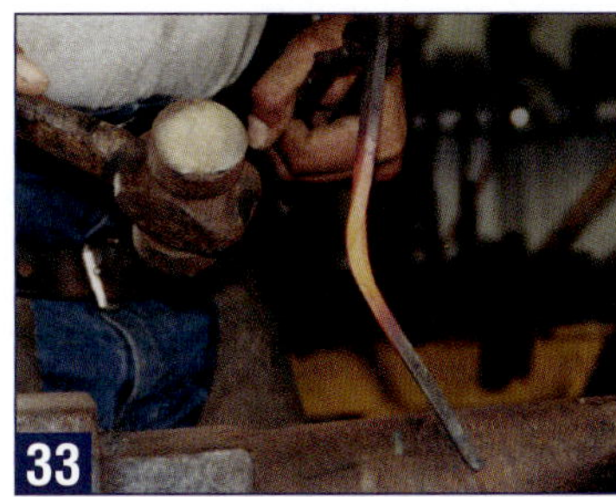

Warping from bad technique.

past the centerline of the horn as in **Figure 24**. This will keep the heel of the shoe from being "Muley", which is a shoe with heels that do not come around from the quarter.

At this point you will have half of a hind shoe complete **(Figure 25)**.

HEATS 4 AND 5

These heats are repeats of Heats 2 and 3 **(Figures 26-30)**. Now you have a blank hind shoe **(Figure 31)**.

With practice, you will find that the shoes are coming out symmetrical with little effort. If you are able to do the same moves around the horn on each side of the shoe at the same heat, you will end up with a shoe that has all the bends and curves in the right places. Lots of practice is the key to success when it comes to any forge project.

BASIC HIND IN THREE HEATS WITH NAIL HOLES

Once you have practiced the previous exercise to a level that it comes out correctly consistently every time, you will be ready to leave the training wheels behind and begin to make shoes for everyday use.

Shoes that are made in three heats are really more efficient for me than shoes made in one or two heats. The reason for this is that the shoe is going back into the forge while it is still a little bit hotter, plus the various tasks needed to produce the shoe are happening at the right heat. For instance, the nails are being punched at a red heat, while the pritcheling is being done at a black heat. With a two-heat shoe, the first heat requires you to make the heel, bend the toe, bend the branch and then punch the nails. The second branch and nails are done at a slightly hotter temperature, since the toe is already done, and that difference can be enough to cause inconsistent shoes.

SETUP

Begin by cutting the desired length of stock. The shoe pictured is made from 11 1/2 inches of 5/16-by-3/4-inch bar stock. Mark center of the stock, mark toe nails at 1 1/4 inches from center, and the lateral branch. Later, you may want to mark off center in order to allow enough difference for thinning (sweetening) the medial branch. For now, we will make a generic shoe that is neither a near or off hind, other than the fact that the lateral heel has a mark in it.

PROCESS

HEAT 1

Heat the stock in the toe and hold at a 90-degree angle with the width of the stock past the tongs and the other end of the stock roughly 3/4-inch past the horn. Metal moves the most where it is the hottest, so be certain that there is a uniform heat through the toe. Hammer directly into the middle of the stock, trying to keep the hammer, tongs, and stock all lined up as close to straight as possible. In **Figures 32-33**, I am making a toe bend in a slider plate with my hammer coming in at an angle. If you hammer across the stock with the hammer and tongs out of alignment, you run a greater risk of warping the steel. The greater the width of the stock, the greater the problem from warping as shown in **Figure 33**. In **Figures 34-35**, I am making the toe bend with everything at 0 degrees. This allows for a straighter toe bend without the warping problems.

Once you have a rough toe bend, lay the steel on the anvil with the ground surface down. Look at the inside of the web as you relieve sole pressure

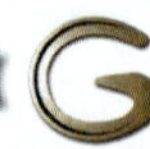

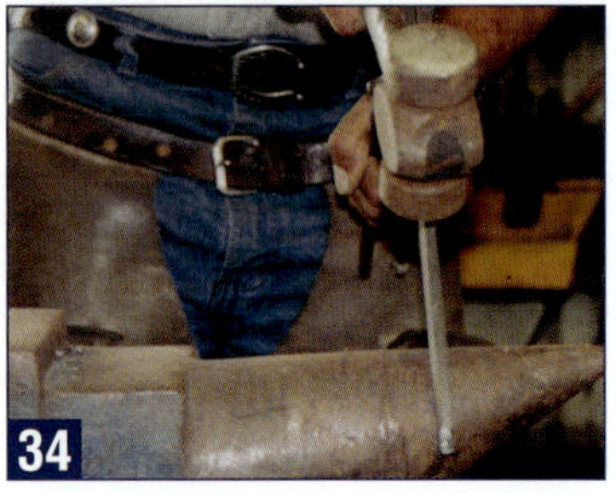

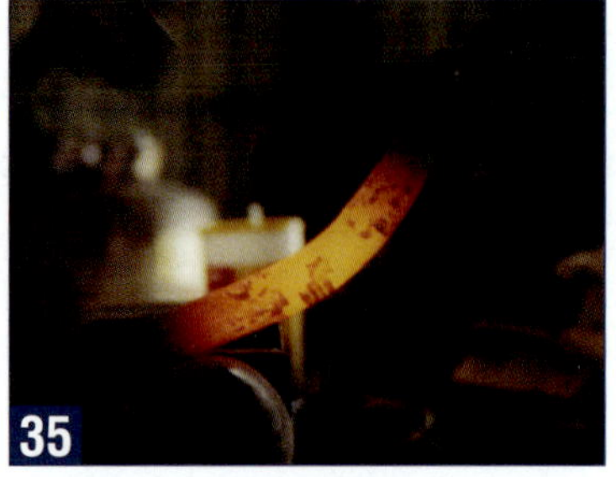

Good positioning and technique for making a toe bend.

Relieve sole pressure.

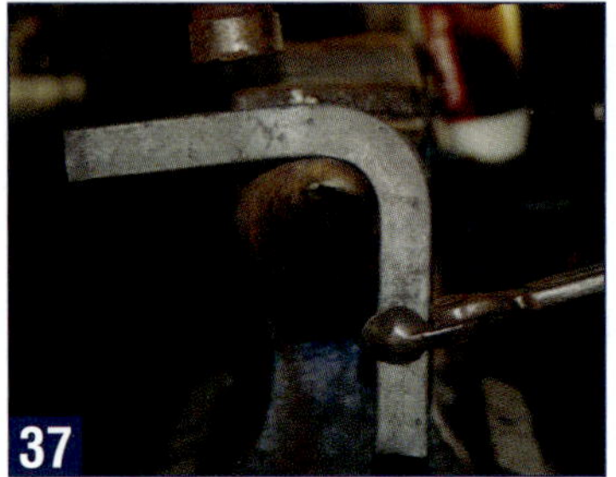

Set the toe.

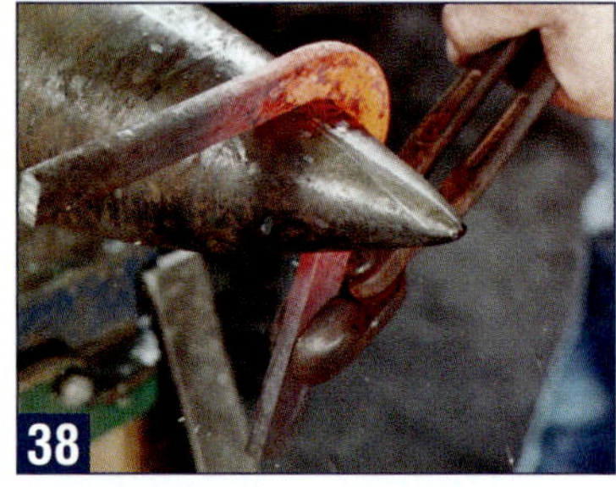

Set the toe.

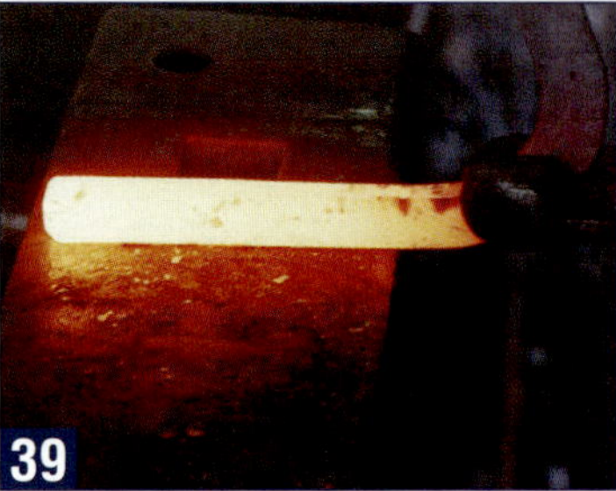

Make a heel.

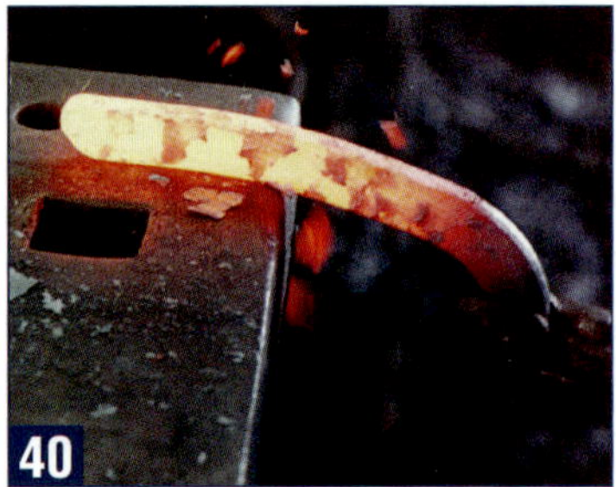

Counteract inertia.

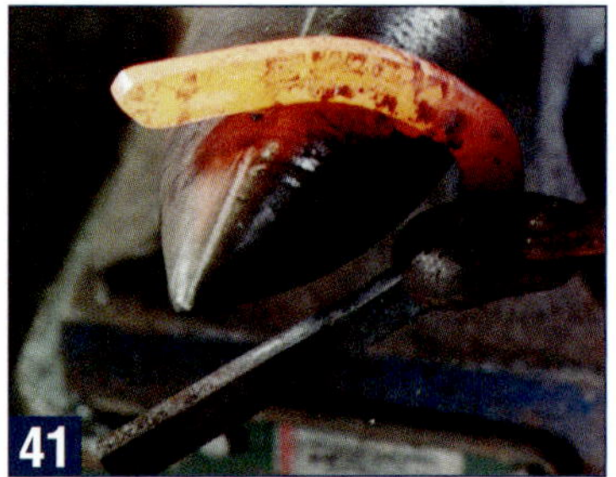

Bend the branch on the horn.

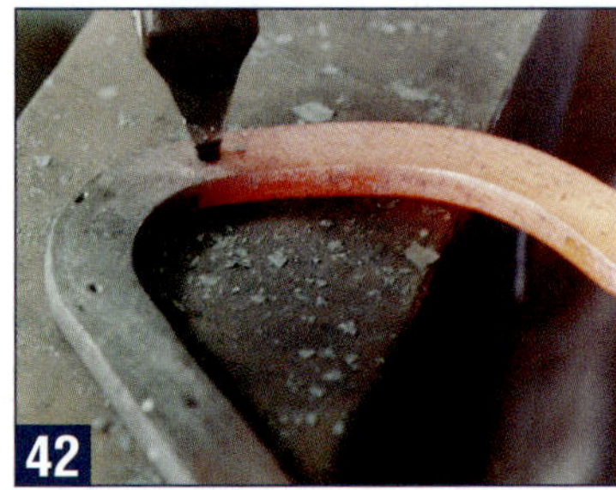

Punch toe nail.

and thin out the thickness on the inside of the toe bend **(Figure 36)**. I like to use the flat side of my rounding hammer for this. Move to the horn and forge the exact size and shape of the toe that you are trying to achieve, using the moves that we used when we had training wheels **(Figures 37-38)**. Since the toe nails are marked in the same area that the training wheels were located, it is possible to use these marks for training wheels when setting the toe. This first heat should be a fast heat, so the shoe will come to the next forging heat quicker in the fire.

HEAT 2

Heat the lateral branch to a good forging heat. Once it is out of the forge, build a heel **(Figure 39)**, counteract inertia **(Figure 40)**, and move to the horn to build the rest of the branch **(Figure 41)**. The shoe is at the right heat to fore punch. Punch the toe nail where it is marked **(Figure 42)**. Move toward the heel (about 1 3/4 inches from the toe nails for this size of shoe) and punch the heel nails **(Figure 43)**. A divider can be useful for determining this position. Punch the second nail directly between the toe and heel nails **(Figure 44)**. If the shoe is to have quarter

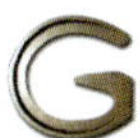

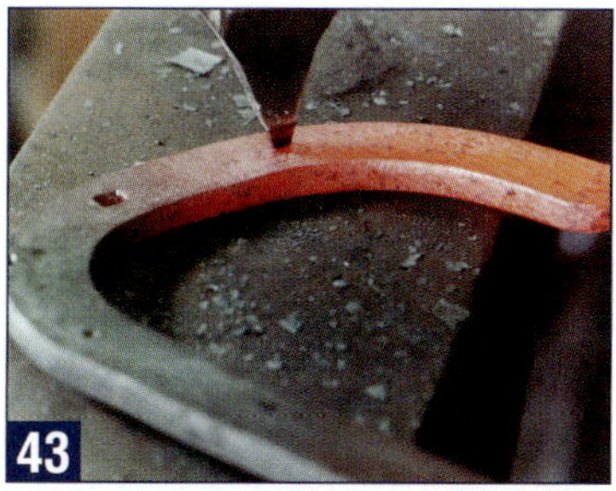
Punch heel nail.

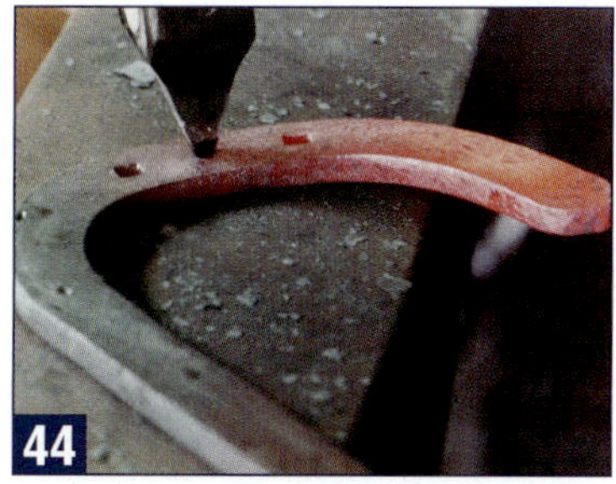
Make second nail between toe and heel nails.

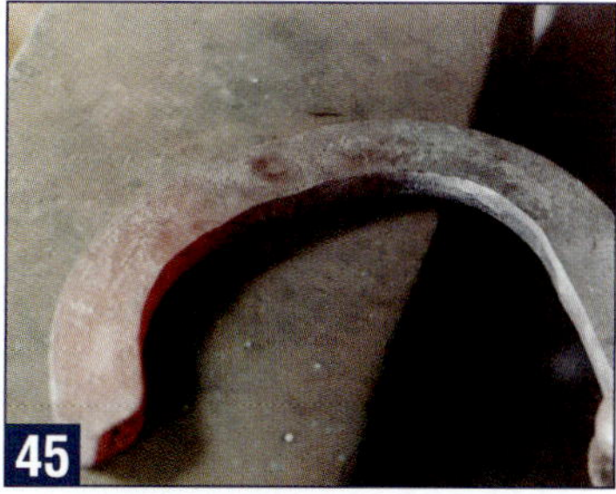
Hammer across the hoof surface of the shoe.

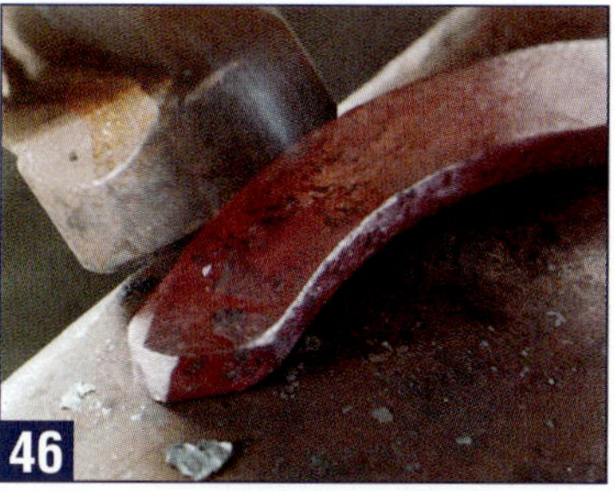
Box from the heel nail through the heel of the shoe.

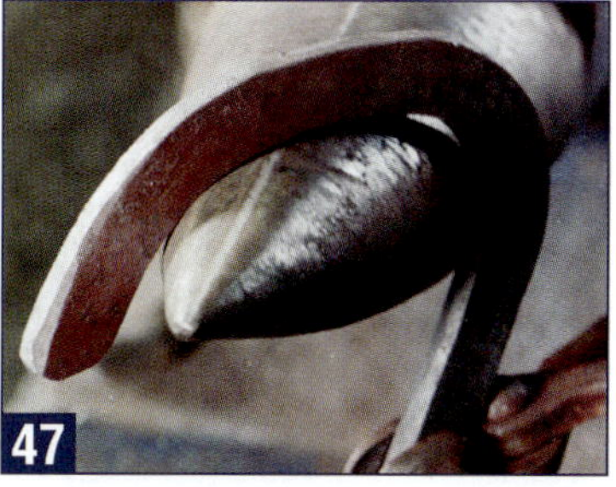
Perfect the shape and forge out the frog eyes.

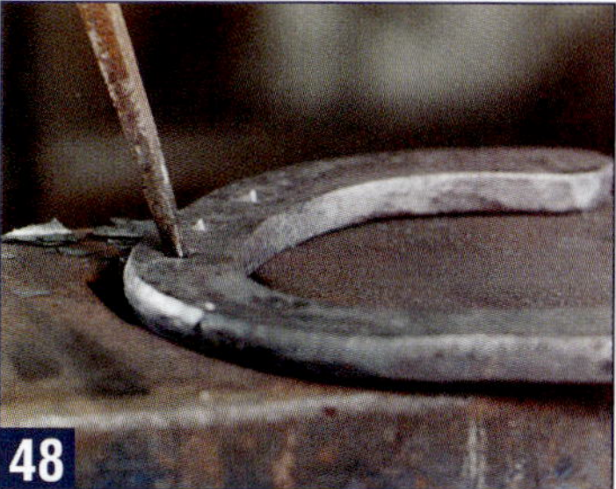
Pritchel.

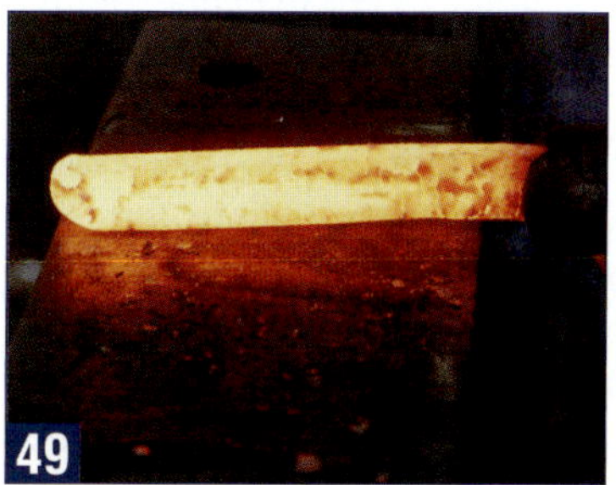
Make medial heel.

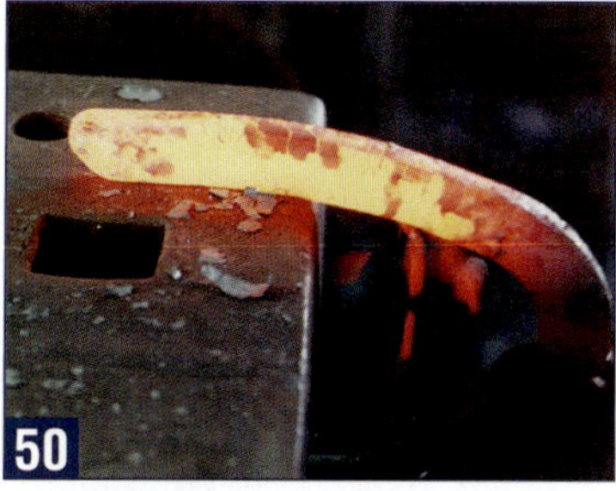
Counteract inertia.

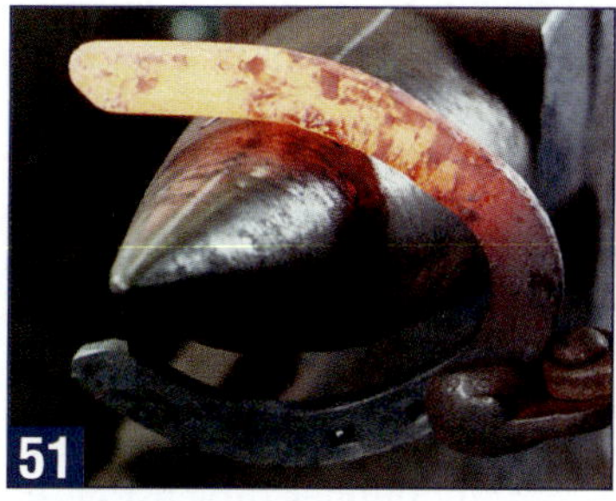
Bend around the horn.

clips, leave a larger gap between the first and second nail holes. See the Basic Tasks Section for more information about punching nail holes.

Turn the shoe over and hammer using overlapping blows from the toe to the heel **(Figure 45)**.

This is an excellent time to do any required boxing **(Figure 46)**. Boxing is defined as putting a slight bevel on the edge of the hoof surface of the shoe. Boxing is often done from the last nail hole through the heel. Safing is beveling the ground surface of the shoe. Any frog eyes can now be forged out of the shoe and the shape can also be fixed at this point **(Figure 47)**.

By now, the shoe is at a black heat. Place the ground surface up and pritchel out the nail holes **(Figure 48)**. Remember to angle the pritchel to take care of the nail exit depth. Lay the pritchel at roughly 65 degrees for the toe nail, 80 degrees for the second nail, and 90 degrees for the heel nail.

Once the holes are pritchelled, hammer the hoof surface from toe to heel again to level and crisp the branch. Check the fit of the nail holes and pritchel again if there is any problem with your nail fit. You will not continue to do this once you become

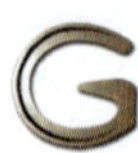

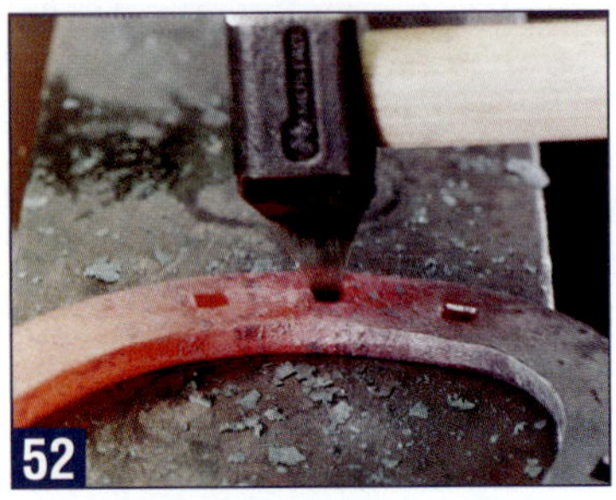

52 *Punch medial nails.*

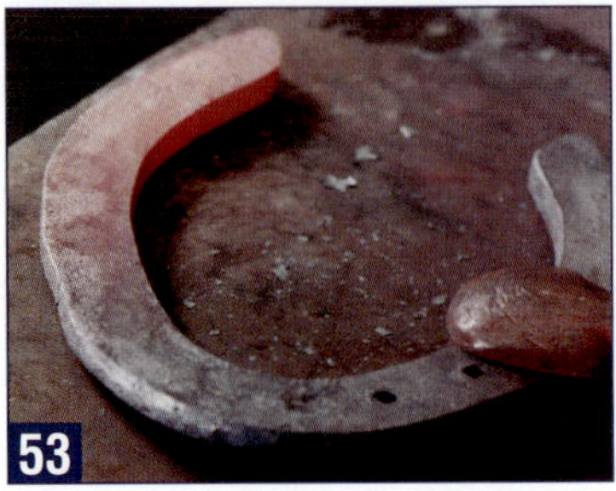

53 *Hammer on hoof surface.*

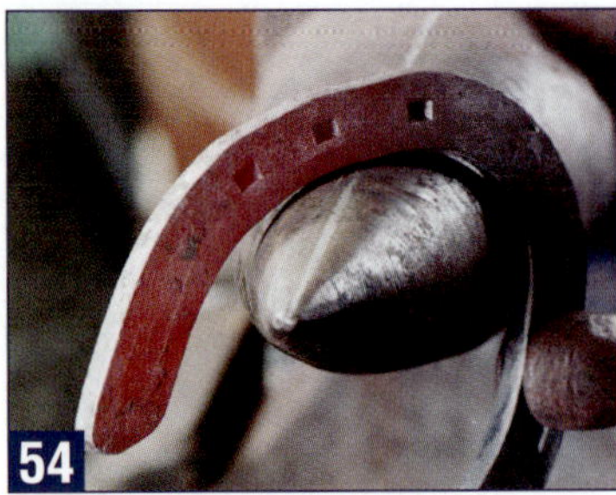

54 *Shape and forge out frogeyes.*

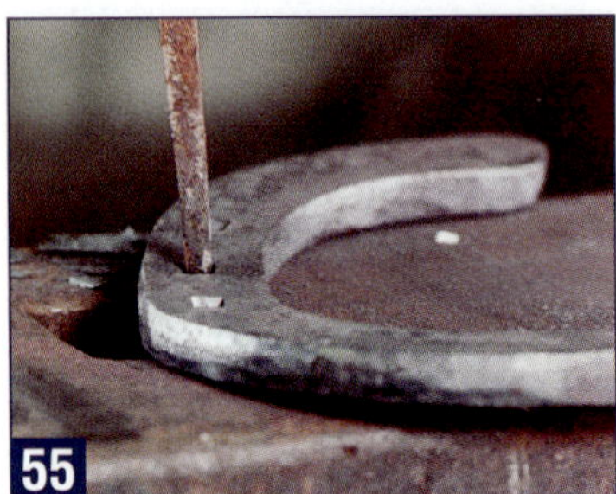

55 *Pritchel.*

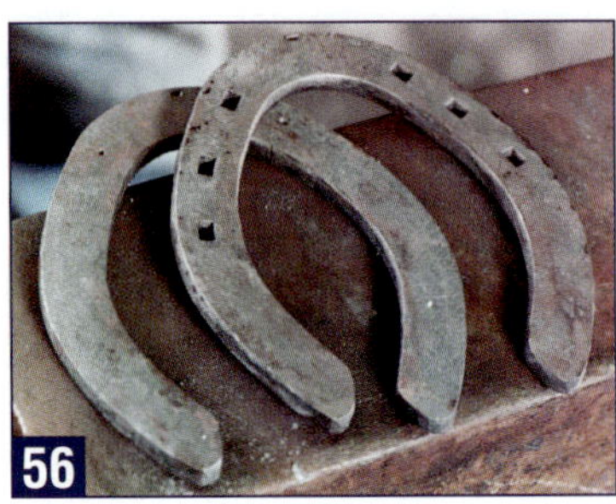

56 *Finished plain stamped shoe with the blank.*

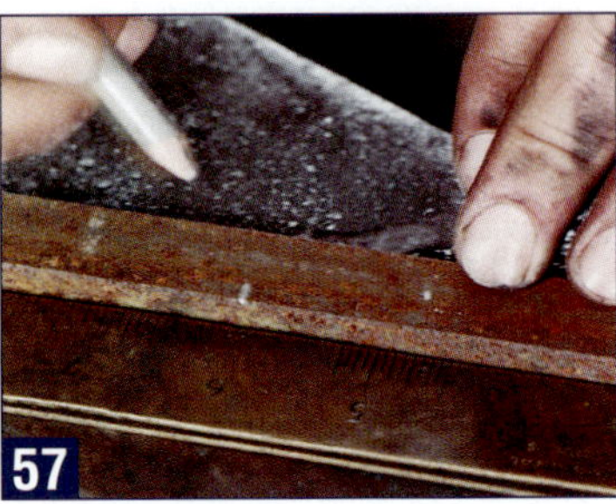

57 *Mark 1/8 inch off center to make a left or right shoe.*

proficient at punching nails. Eventually you will only check the nail fit after the entire shoe is built.

HEAT 3

This heat is a repeat of the second heat. The only difference will be if the shoe has been marked off center to allow sweetening of the medial branch. If this is the case, build the heel to a rough shape and then forge the last 1 1/2 inches of the branch to a slightly thinner dimension. Finish the heel, then build the second branch just as you did the first branch in Heat 2 **(Figures 49-55)**.

If all went well, you now have a nicely made hind shoe that is a match to the blanks you have been practicing **(Figure 56)**.

This is a very efficient and easy method for building shoes. When the shape is not exactly what you want, take a light fourth heat and shape the shoe to the foot you are working on. You may be able to clip and fix the shape in the same heat if you are proficient at clipping.

BASIC HIND FULLERED IN THREE HEATS

After practicing building the hind shoe as well as the fullering process, you can put the shoe and the crease together.

SETUP

By this point you should be making lefts and rights, so we will mark the shoe slightly differently than we did for the plain stamped shoe **(Figure 57)**. Begin by determining which foot you are making the shoe for. If it is a left, move the center punch mark toward the left side of the branch 1/8 inch. This causes the shoe to be 1/4 inch out since the lateral branch is 1/4 inch longer than the medial branch. Mark the right side (lateral branch) of the stock and mark the nail hole location at 1 1/4 inches from the center mark.

HEAT 1

Heat the stock and make a hind toe bend **(Figure 58-59)**. Relieving sole pressure is extremely important for fullered shoes and I often thin the inside of the web a little extra to widen the stock. Since the fuller will be driven into the shoe and displace some of the width, having a toe that is wider than the original width is helpful. This is the same move as seen in **Figure 36**. We sometimes upset the stock in

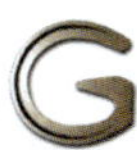

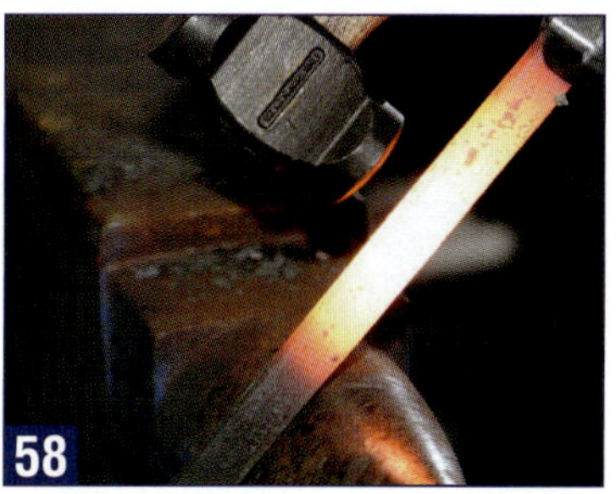

58 *Make toe bend.*

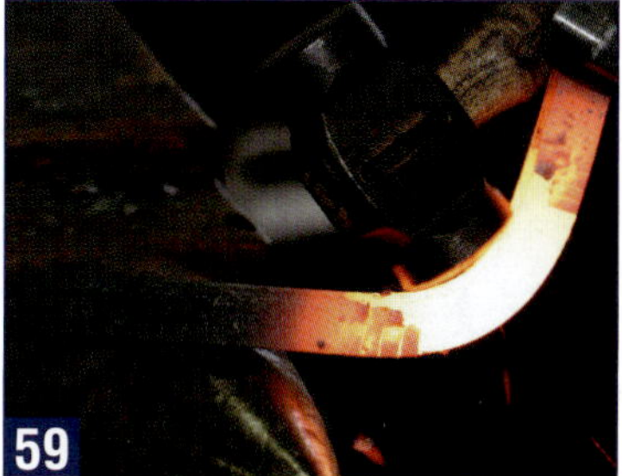

59

60 *Begin hemming at the beginning of the crease.*

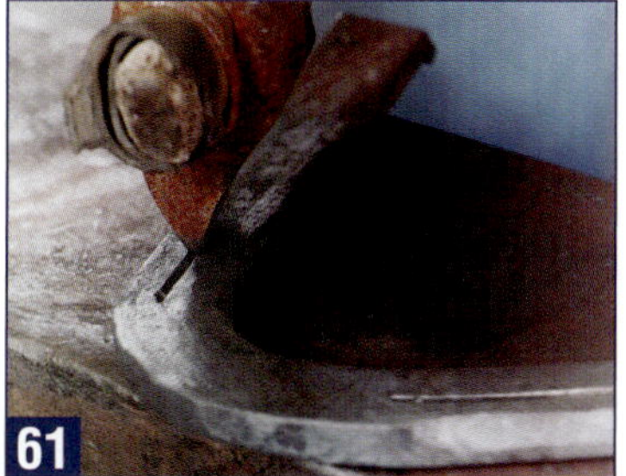

61 *Mark fullering.*

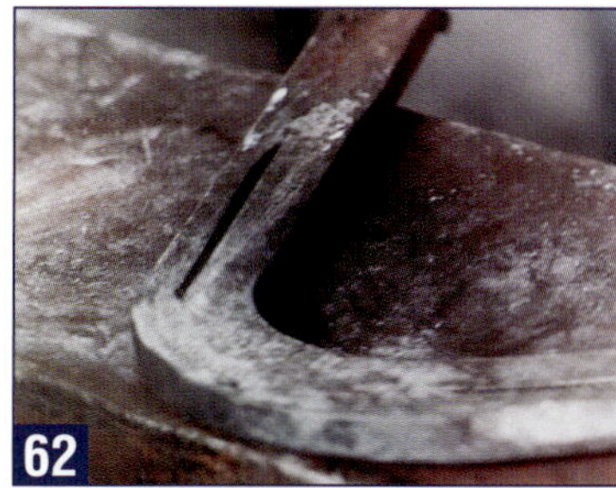

62 *Fullering marked.*

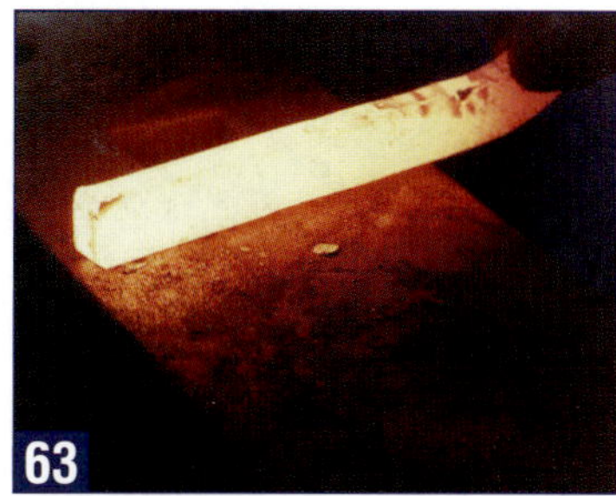

63 *Make lateral heel.*

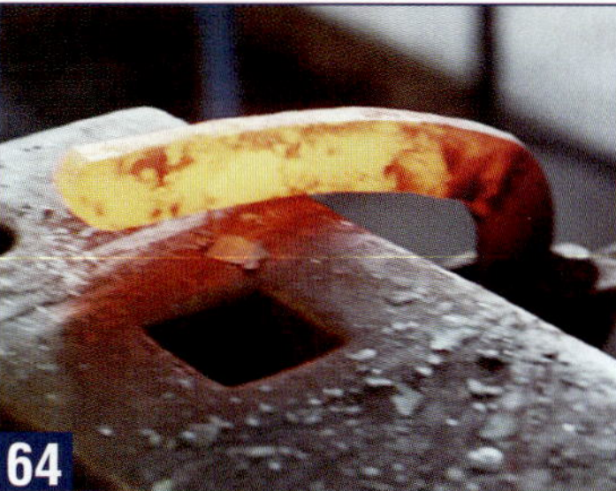

64 *Counteract inertia.*

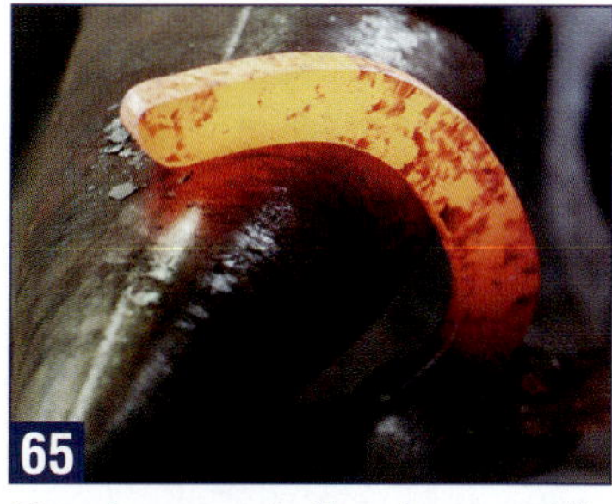

65 *Bend around the horn while finishing the hemming.*

the toe to enhance the wider stock in the toe.

Begin hemming the stock on the horn at the area marked for the toe nail **(Figure 60)**. Once you have hemmed about half inch of the branch, move to the opposite branch to hem it as well. You should be able to set your toe at this point and mark your fullering **(Figures 61-62)**.

HEAT 2

Build the lateral heel **(Figure 63)**, counteract inertia **(Figure 64)** and turn the shoe on the horn **(Figure 65)**. You can finish the hemming when you turn the branch. Crease the lateral branch **(Figures 66-68)**. At the toe side of the crease, you will want to create a crisp, sharp edge. To accomplish this, position the creaser at an angle so that the toe side corner of the creaser blade lines up vertically with the diagonal top corner of the creaser where you are going to hit it **(Figure 68)**. Hit the creaser in this position, and lower about half way to level for the second hit. Lower so that the handle is level for the final hammer blow **(Figure 69)**.

Place the drift or fore punch in the crease to make the nail holes **(Figure 70)**. Forge out frog eyes, box,

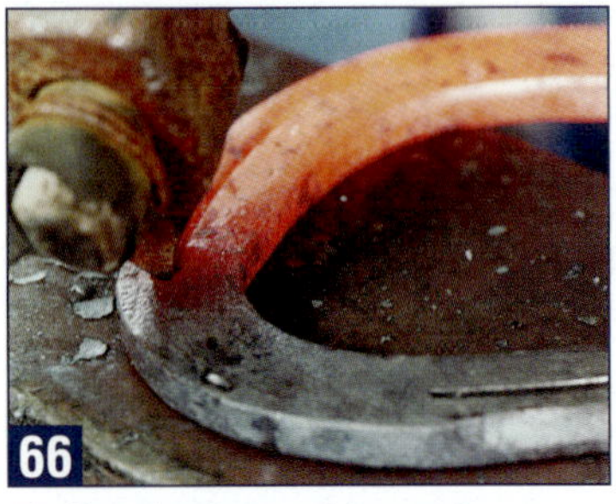

Fuller the lateral branch.

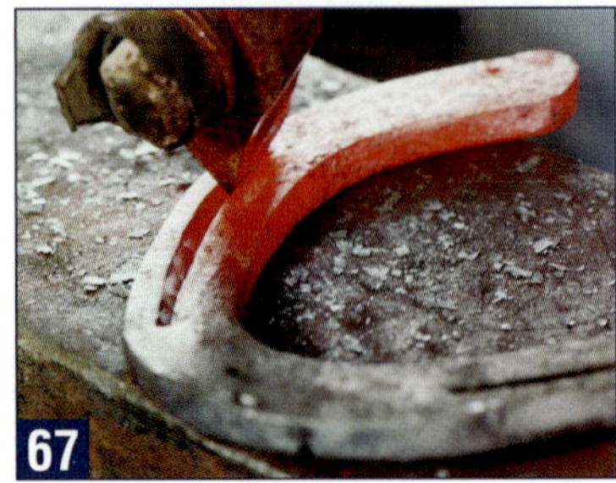

68

Make a crisp start at the toe.

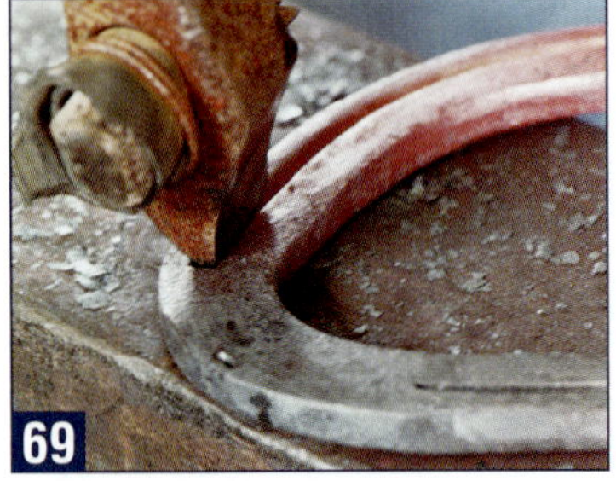

Drop fuller handle to continue fullering through the branch.

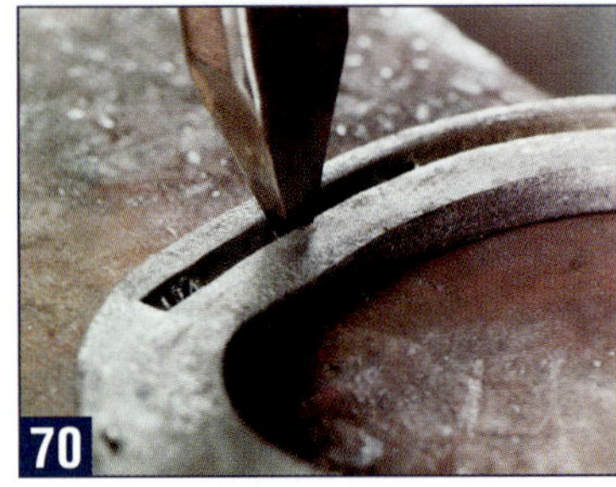

Drift nail holes.

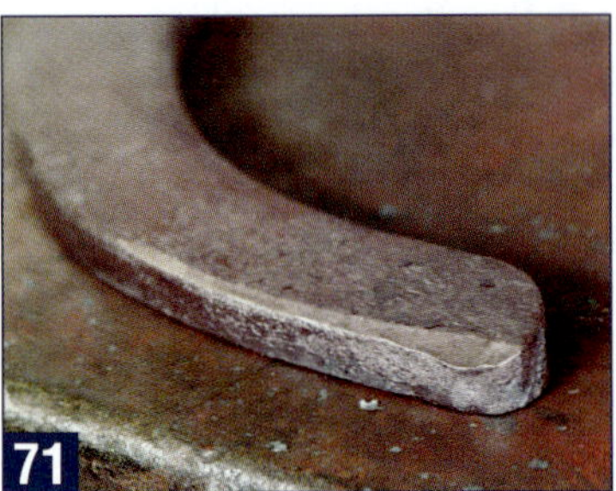

Box heel.

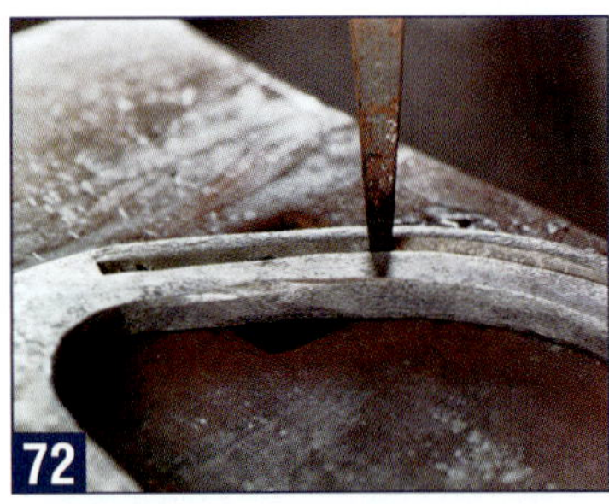

Pritchel.

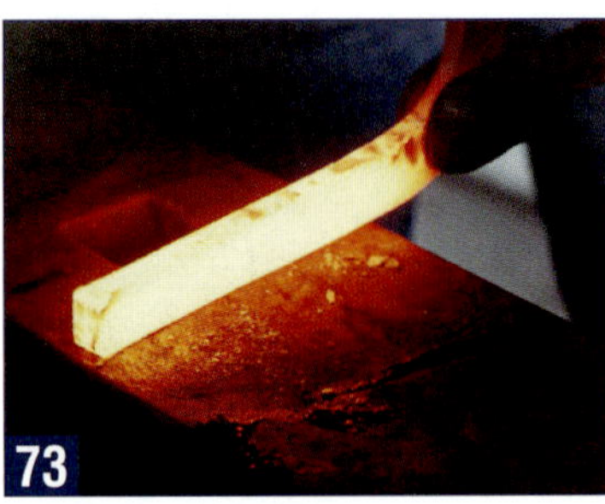

Make medial heel.

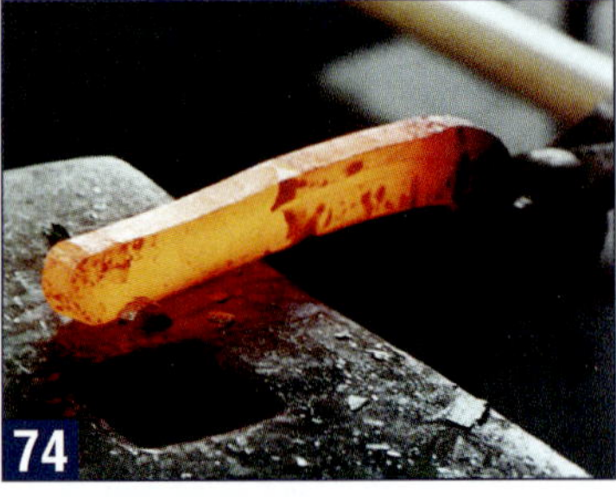

Sweeten by thinning the width of the branch.

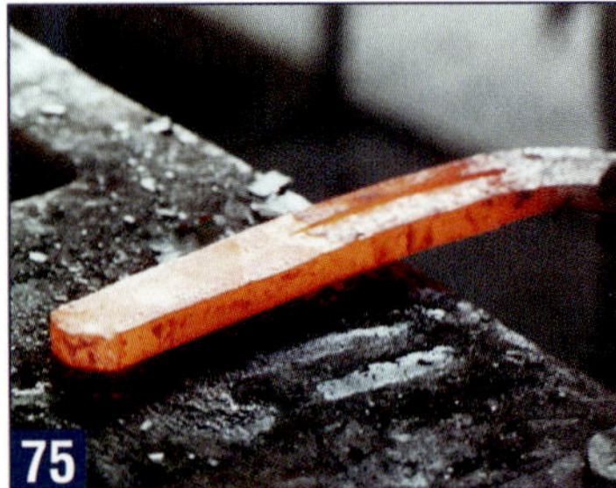

Forge back to original thickness.

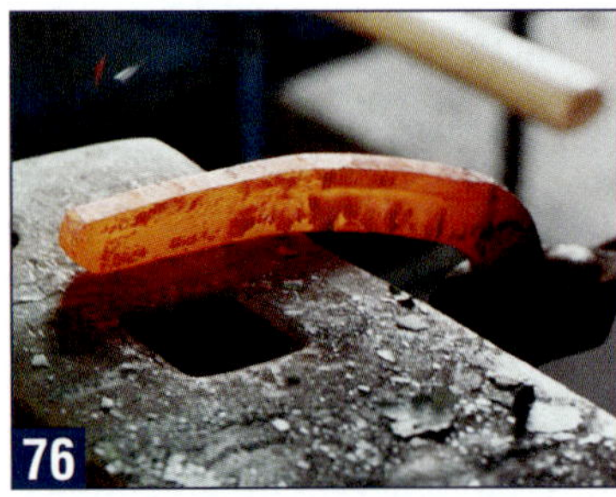

Counteract inertia.

(Figure 71) and pritchel the branch **(Figure 72)**.

HEAT 3

Heat the medial branch, build the heel to the first phase **(Figure 73)**. At this point, you will taper the end of the branch (called sweetening) **(Figure 74)**. This will cause the thickness of the stock to increase, so you will have to draw

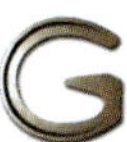

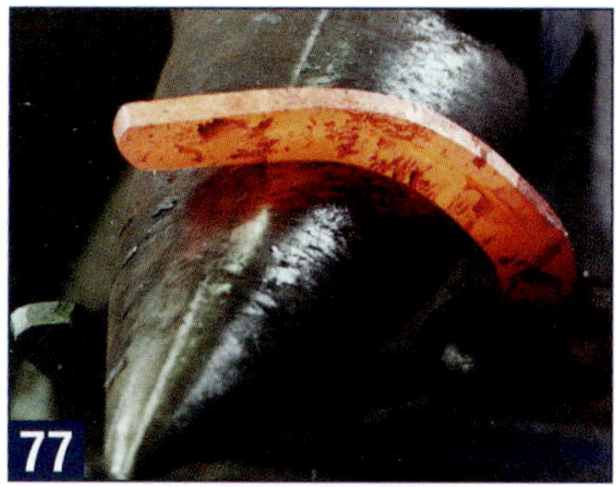
77
Bend quarter on horn.

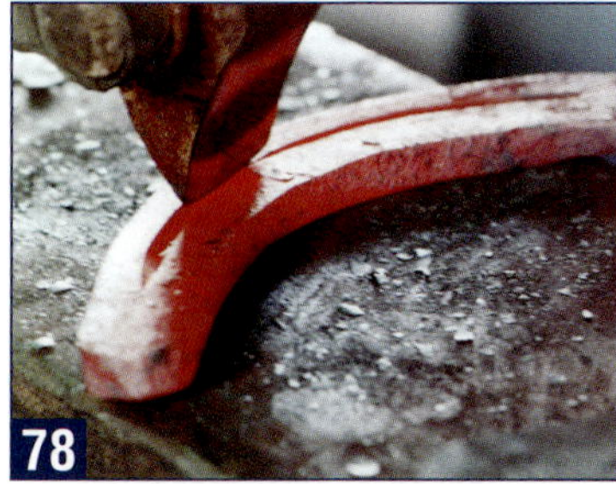
78
Fuller medial branch.

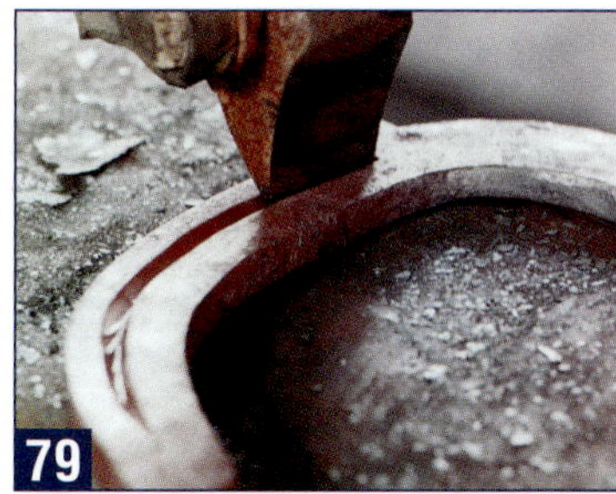
79
Come to the end of the fullering.

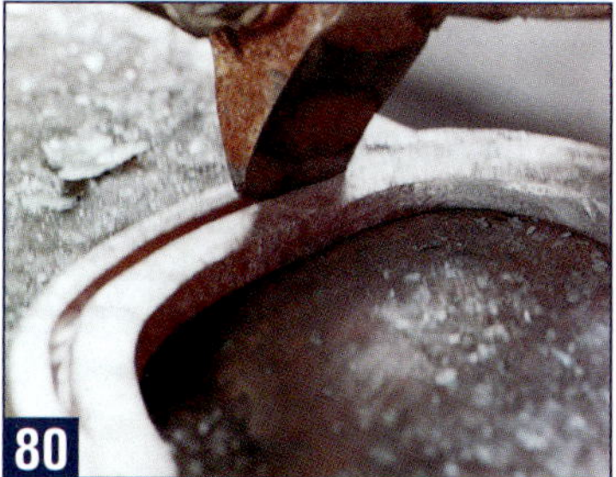
80
Drop the handle of the fuller to create crisp corner.

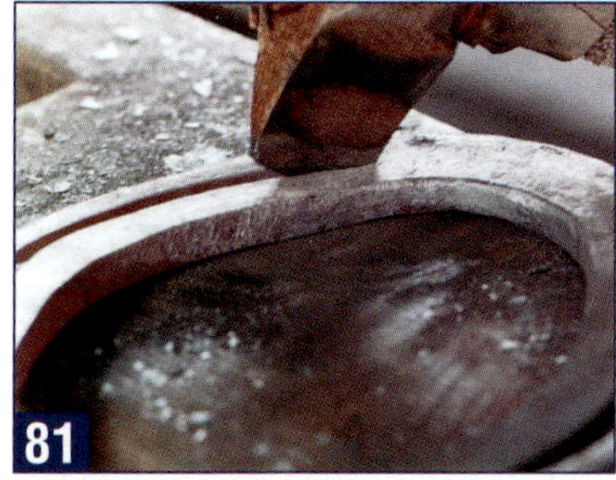
81
Drop a little further to finish the crisp corner.

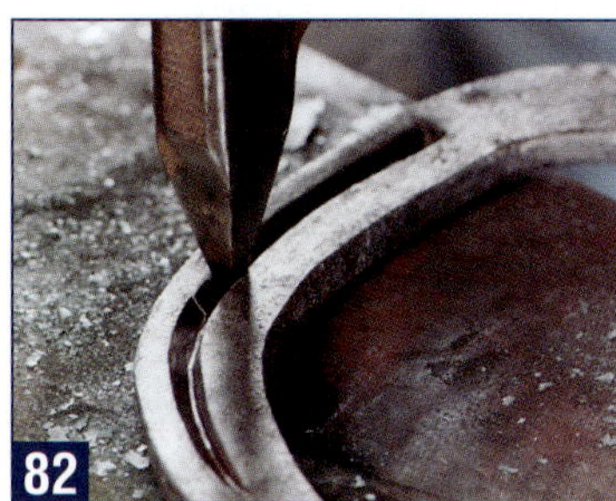
82
Drift.

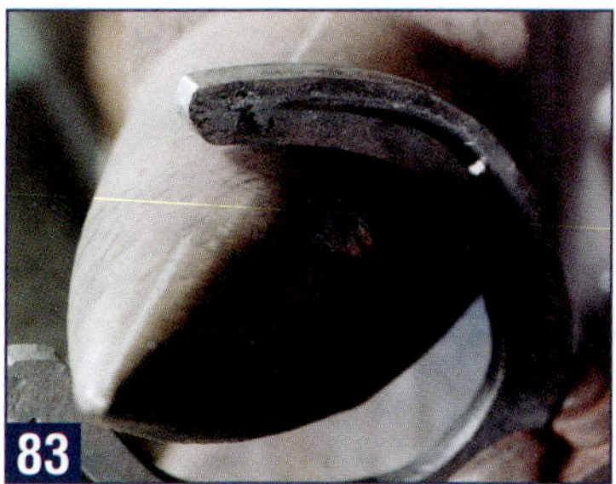
83
Clean up shape and frog eyes on the horn.

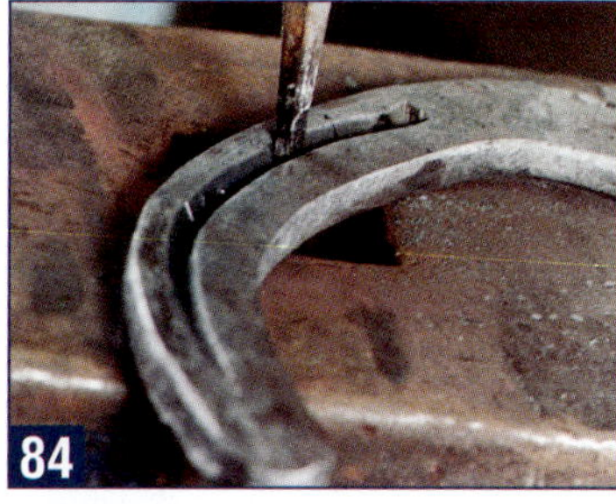
84
Pritchel.

the end of the branch back to original thickness **(Figure 75)**. When the sweetening is done, you can finish the heel and counteract inertia **(Figure 76)** before you turn the branch on the horn **(Figure 77)**. To fuller this branch, you will have to turn the shoe so that the heels are facing the opposite direction than on the lateral branch. In this example, the lateral branch fullering began at the toe, meaning that the fullering will begin at the heel for the medial branch **(Figure 78)**. It would be exactly the opposite if you were building the shoe for the other foot. The crease will end at the toe, where we want to have a defined, crisp stop. To make the crisp corner, fuller to the desired area at the toe **(Figure 79)**. Drop the handle of the fuller so that the corner you are striking is lined up directly over the leading corner of the fuller **(Figures 80-81)**. It is the same move as the opposite side, with the primary difference being that the leading edge of the fuller is toward you instead of away. This means lowering the handle instead of lifting it in order to make the corner. Finish the branch the same as you did for the lateral side **(Figures 82-84)**.

Now you have a blank, a plain stamped hind, and

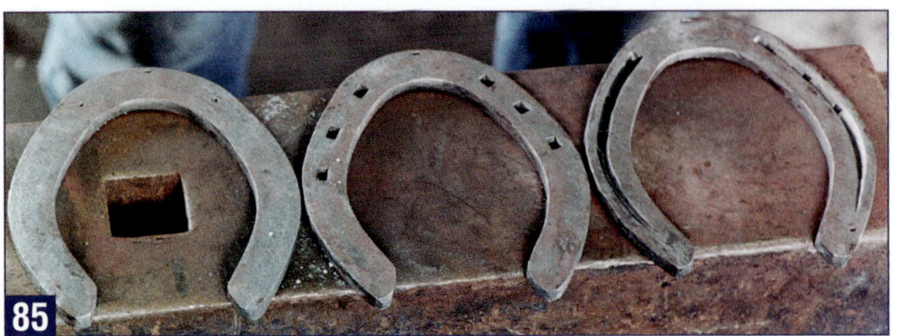

Finished shoes. From blank, to plain stamped, to fullered hinds.

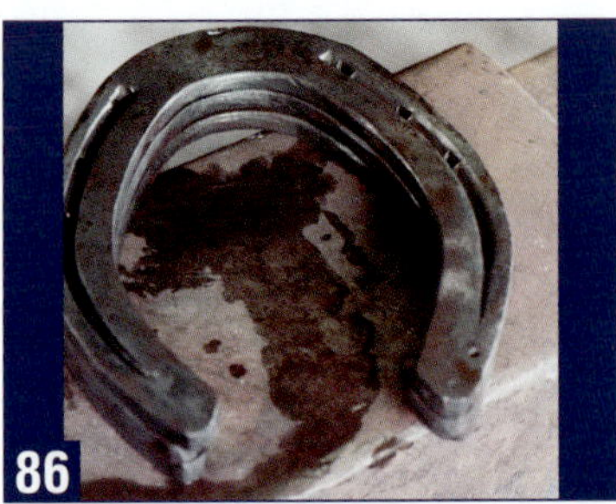

Shoes in a pile. The fullered shoe is the largest of the three.

a fullered hind **(Figures 85-86)**. You will find that the fullered hind is the largest of the three if you have made them from all the same length of stock. Fullering generally causes about 1/4 inch of growth per branch. If you are measuring a foot, you can fit the same foot with 1/2 inch less steel if you are fullering. Due to the additional amount of forging required in punching nail holes, the plain stamped shoe will also be larger than the blank.

Both punching and fullering are efficient and easy methods for building shoes. When the shape is not exactly what you want, take a light fourth heat and shape the shoe to the foot you are working on. You will be able to clip, fix the shape, and fit the shoe in the same heat with practice.

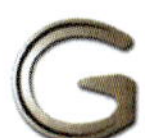

Chapter

41 THE BASIC FRONT

Five Heats to a Blank

If you are doing these in order, you should have already learned how to make the hind shoe. There are enough similarities between the two that we can pick up the speed in the description of the front in the interest of not wasting time. The tools you need will be the same, and we will make the front shoes using the same processes for the most part, with the major difference being the different shape that each possesses. We will also cover the process for rasping up and finishing a shoe at the end of this chapter. This method of shoe making is an adaptation of what Bob Marshall taught me.

Begin with cutting a piece of stock. We are using a piece of stock that is 12 inches of 5/16-by-3/4 inch. Divide the stock into fourths (3 inches, 3 inches, 3 inches, 3 inches) and mark center **(Figure 1)**. From the outside 3 inch line, measure toward the center width of the stock. In this case, that would be 3/4 inches since we are using 5/16 by 3/4 inch stock. **(Figure 2)**. This is the area for marking your training wheels for a front shoe. The measurements should have you ending up with training wheels that are 2 1/4 inches from center, or 3 3/4inches from the end.

HEAT 1

Heat the stock and get a toe bend. You can see from **Figures 3-5** that I am working in the area between the training wheels. Bend until the stock is bent just past 90 degrees **(Figure 6)**. Move to the horn and work around a larger radius than you used for the hind shoe to make a broader, larger radius in the toe of the shoe. I begin in the middle of the toe **(Figure 7)** and roll the shoe around the horn while

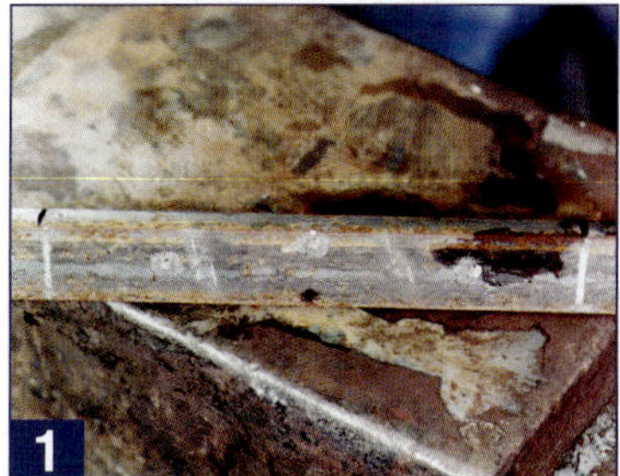

1

Marking the steel for training wheels.

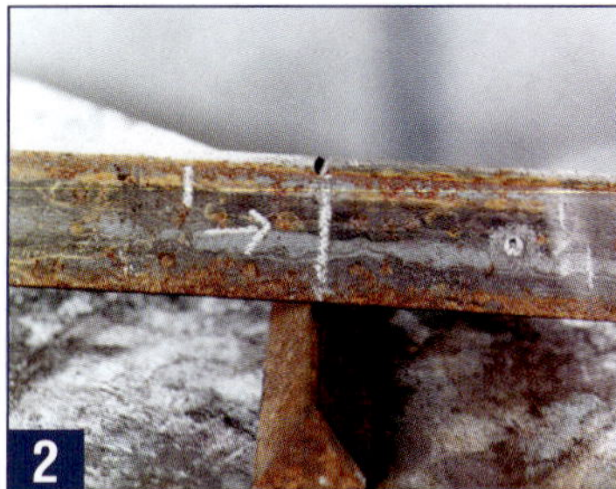

2

Marking training wheels.

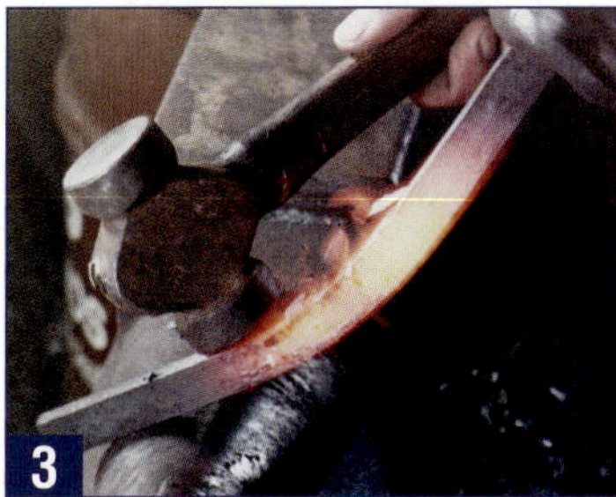

3

Starting the toe bend.

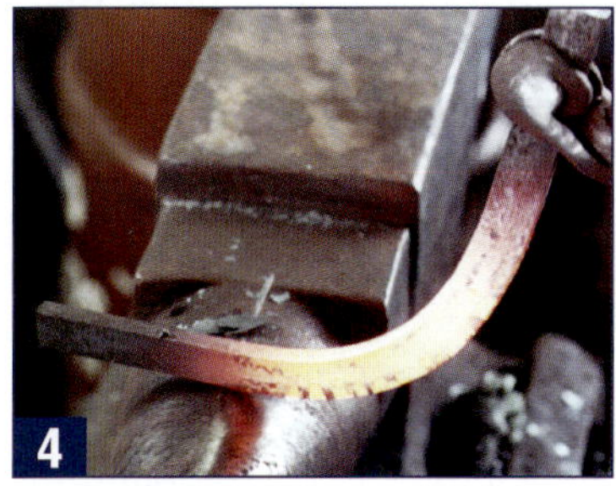

4

Keep bending.

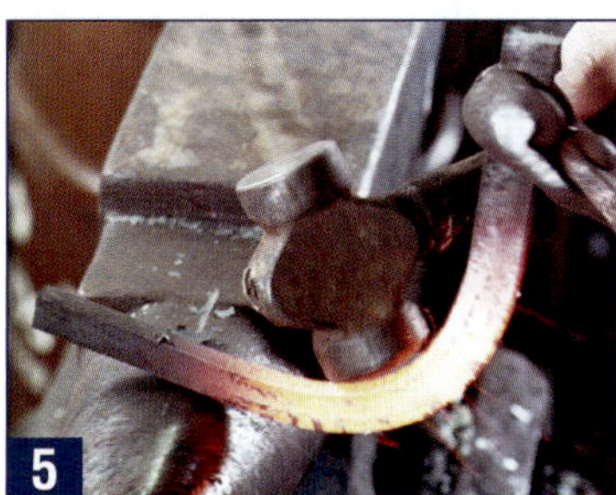

5

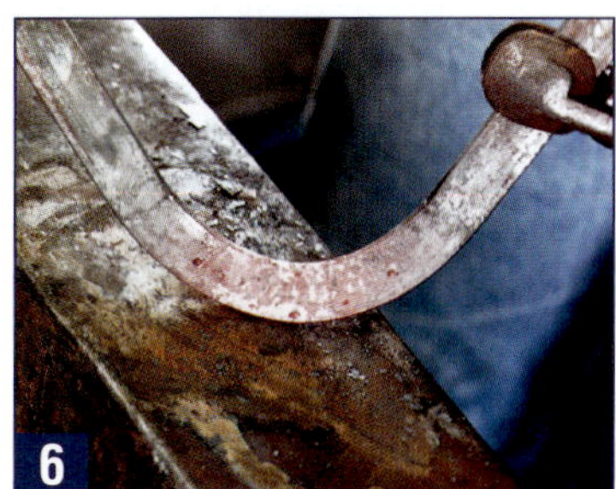

6

The toe is bent past 90 degrees, so it is ready to be seated out and set.

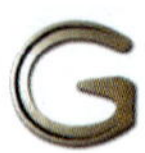

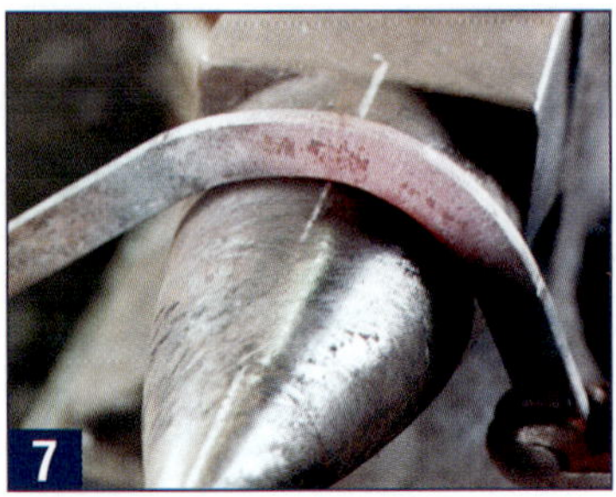

Move around the horn.

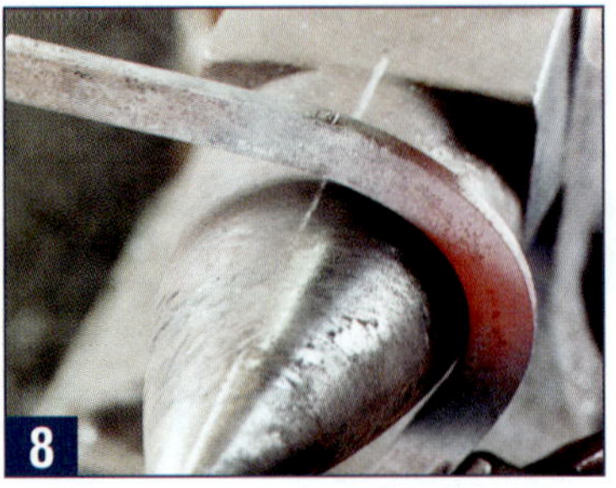

Stop when the training wheel gets to top dead center.

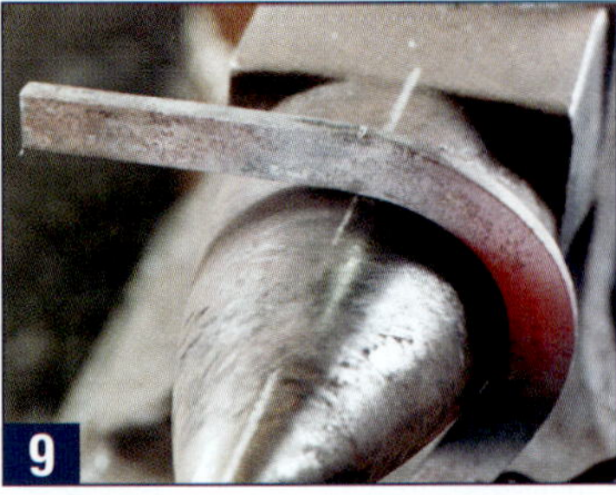

Hammer just beyond the point of contact to make the toe-quarter.

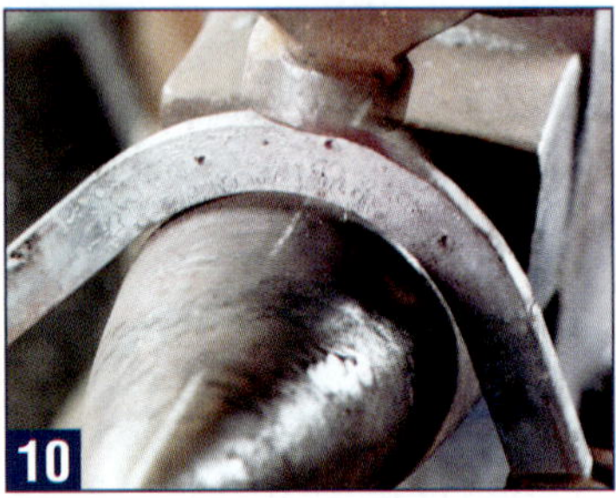

Turn the shoe around to do the same to the opposite side.

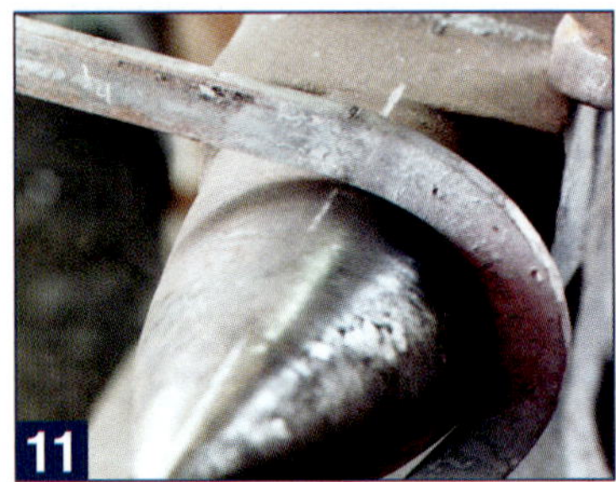

Move around the horn.

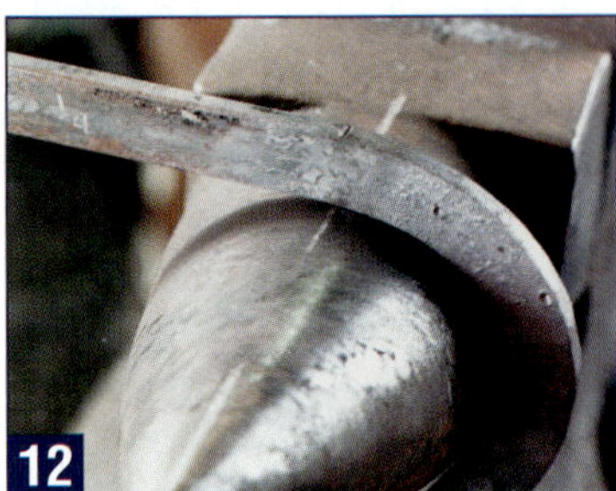

Set the toe.

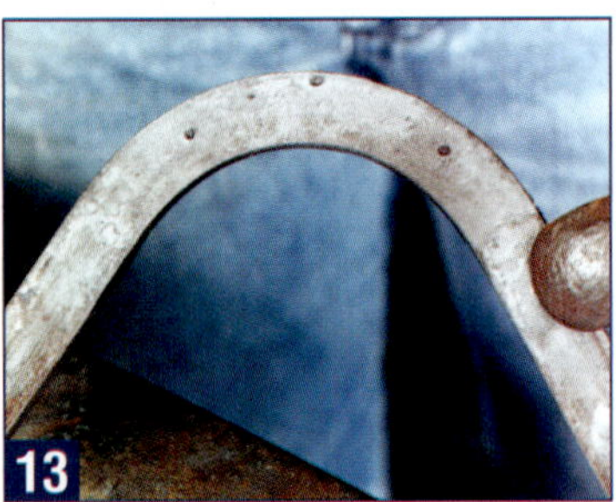

Finished toe bend, first heat done.

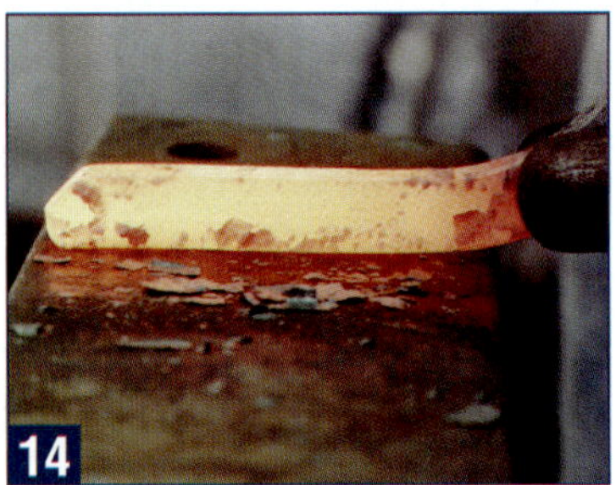

Make the heel.

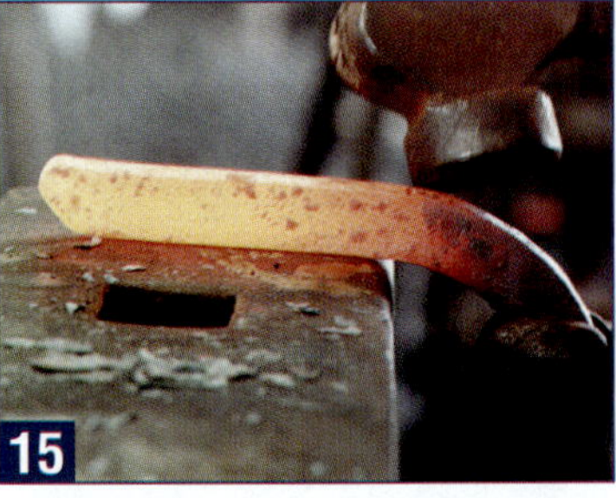

Place in position for counter inertia bend.

I hammer just past the center of the horn (**Figure 8**). Once the training wheel gets to the top center of the horn, I stop rolling with my tong hand and set the toe (**Figure 9**). Turn the shoe around and repeat through the other side (**Figure 10-12**), and you should have a toe bend like the one in **Figure 13**.

HEAT 2

Make a heel like you learned with the hind shoe (**Figure 14**). The counter move to inertia is a little different on the front shoe. Begin by placing the training wheel at the near edge of the heel of the anvil (**Figure 15**). Pull the shoe back and down slowly as you hammer towards the heel of the shoe. You can see this in a series in **Figures 16-24**. There is not a big gap between the shoe and the anvil face, just enough to cause the bends you see at the end of Heat 2 in **Figure 25**.

HEAT 3

This next part is where you can really get good at making front shoes. You have to have a round-horned anvil, but by rolling the shoe around the horn while also changing the radius from moving

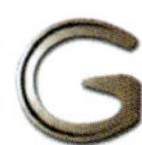

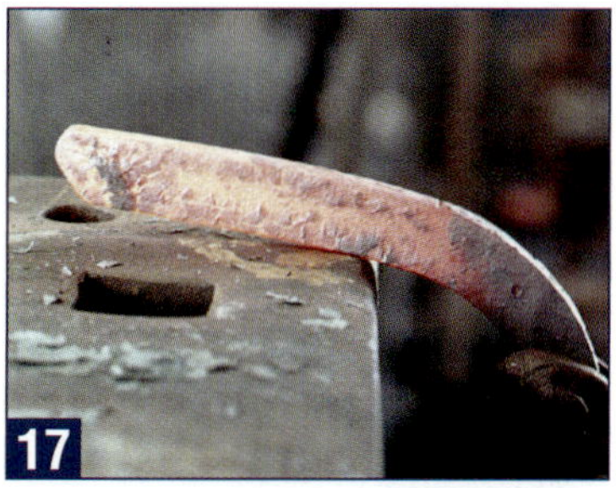

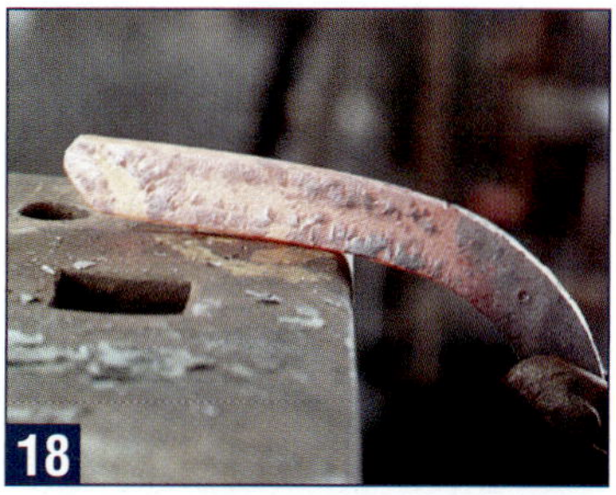

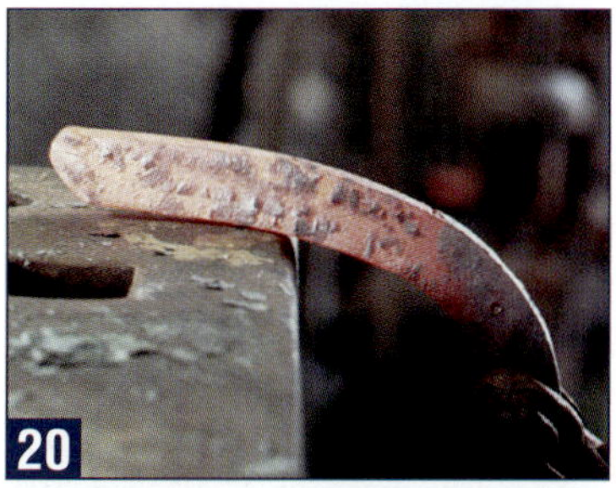

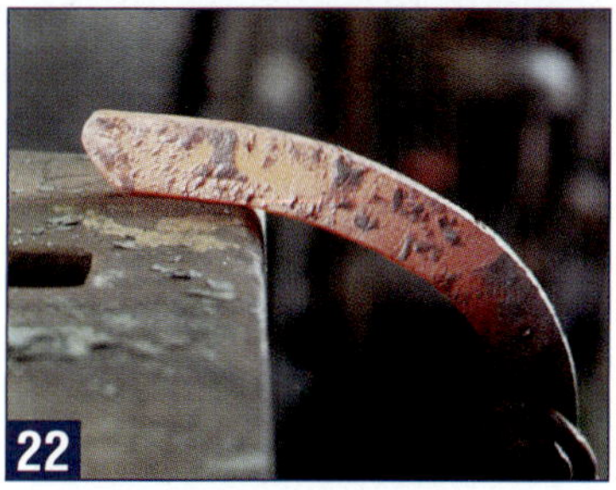

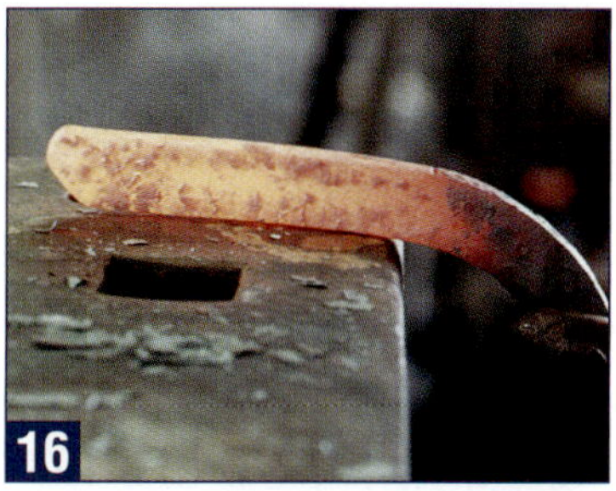

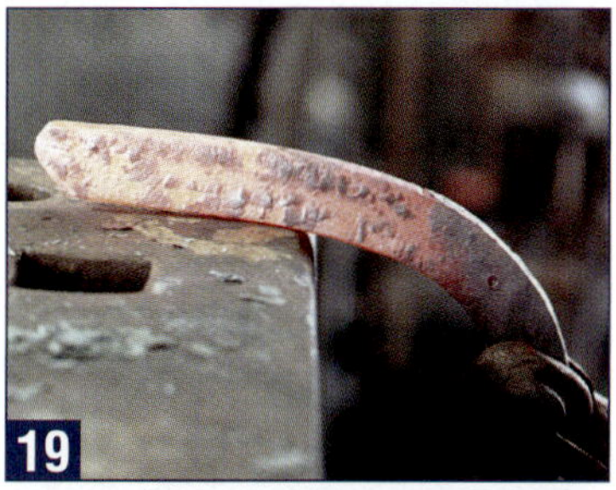

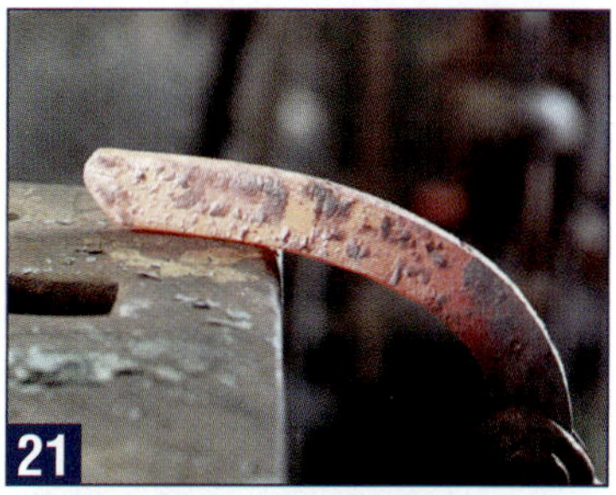

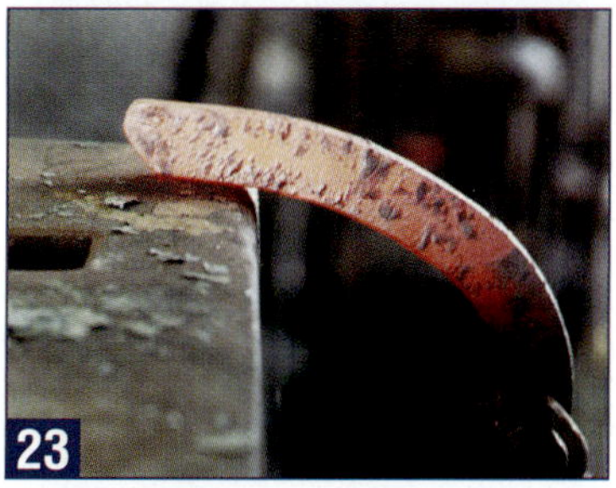

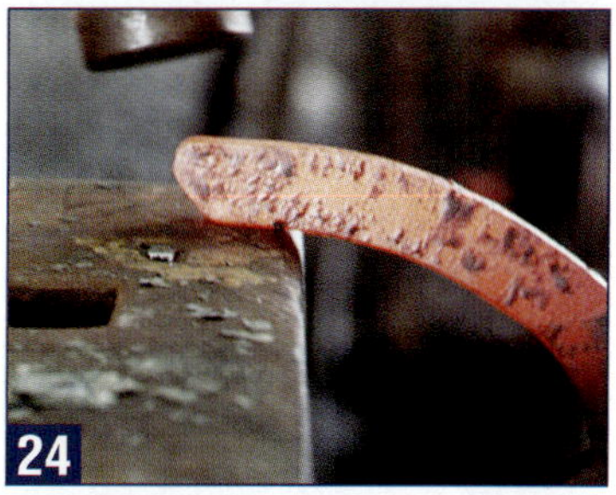

Hammer lightly while the shoe is pulled toward you and lowered at the same time.

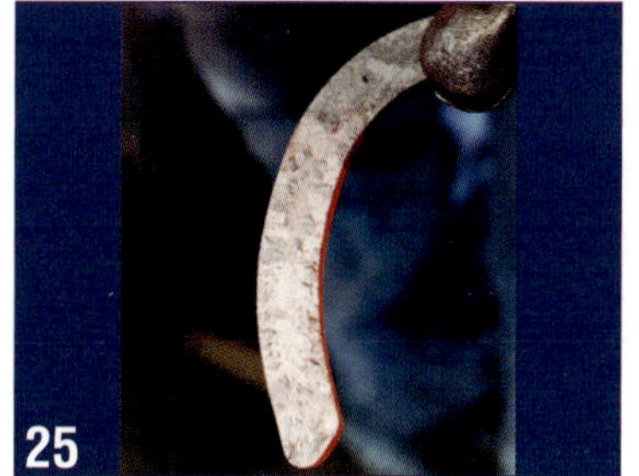

Second heat finished.

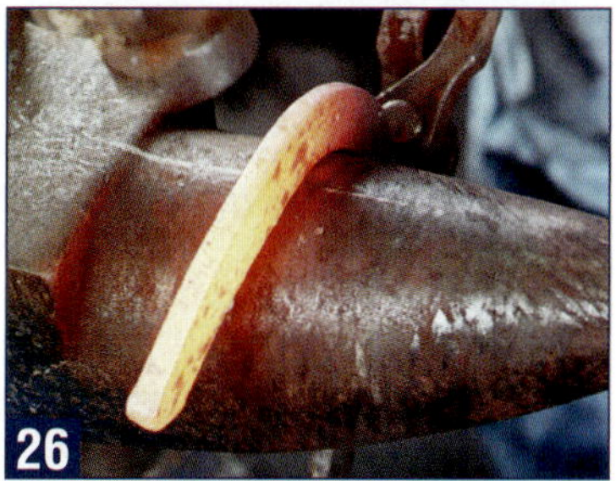

Heat through the toe and move to the horn where the radius of the toe fits the radius of the horn.

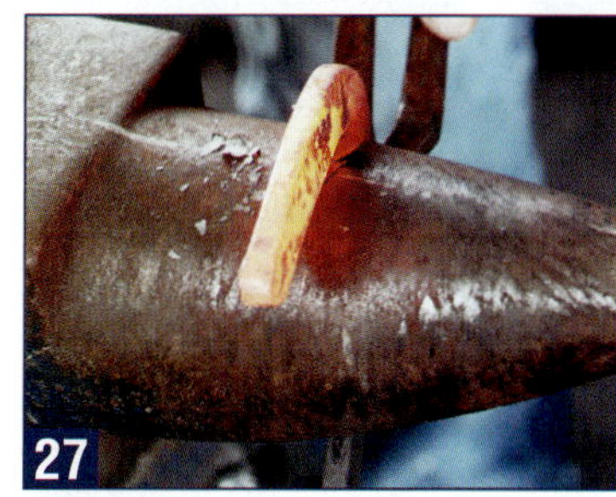

Drop the shoe as you bend it around the horn.

your tong hand towards your hammer hand, you can make a perfect shape in one trip. Begin by heating to the toe. Place the shoe on the horn with the training wheel on the hot side up **(Figure 26)**. Now hit just beyond the top center of the horn while you roll the shoe around. **(Figure 27)** When you get to the widest part of the shoe (about where the heel nail will be and about 3/4 inches past the training wheel), move your tong hand toward your hammer hand while still dropping your tong hand. This should be a smooth and fluid movement while still hitting past the top center of the horn **(Figures**

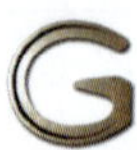

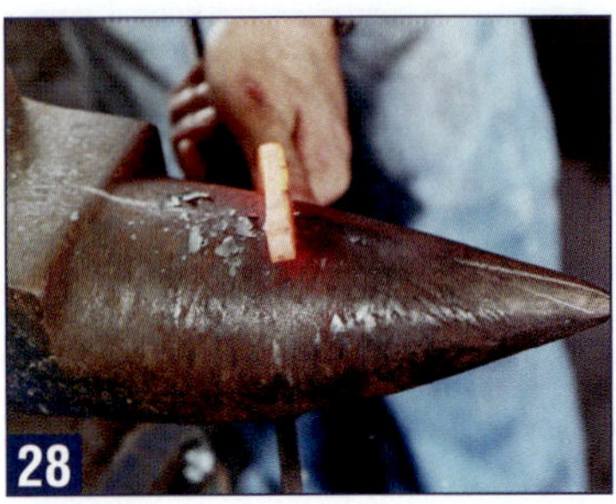
Change radiuses to make the branch.

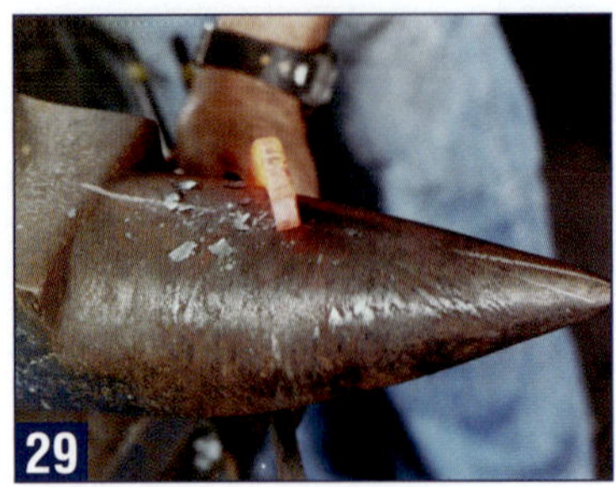
Go all the way through the heel.

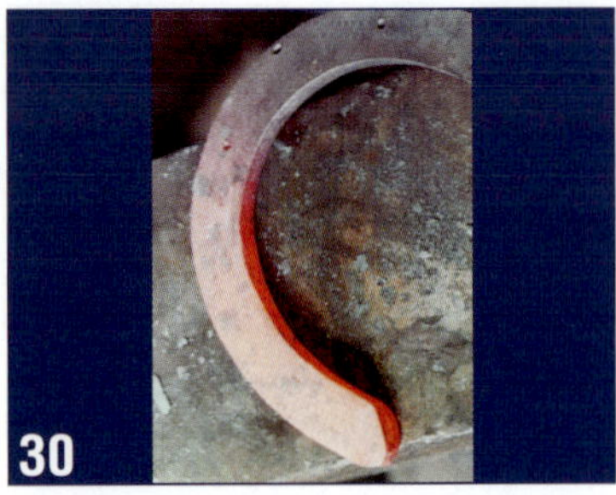
Finished with first branch and third heat.

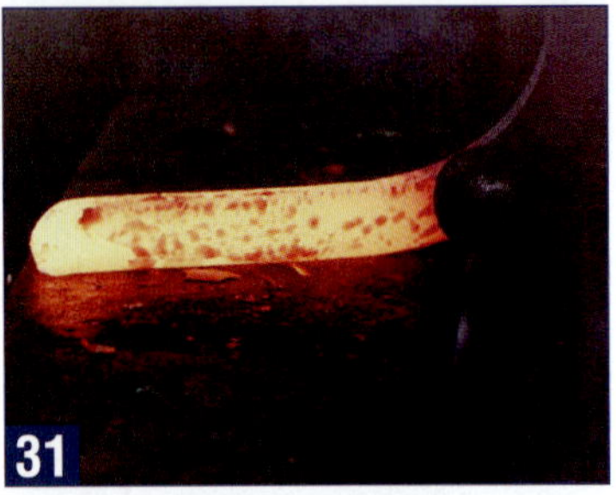
Make the inside heel.

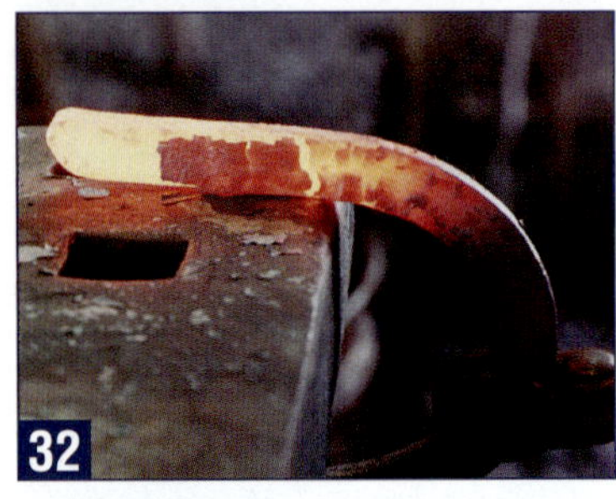
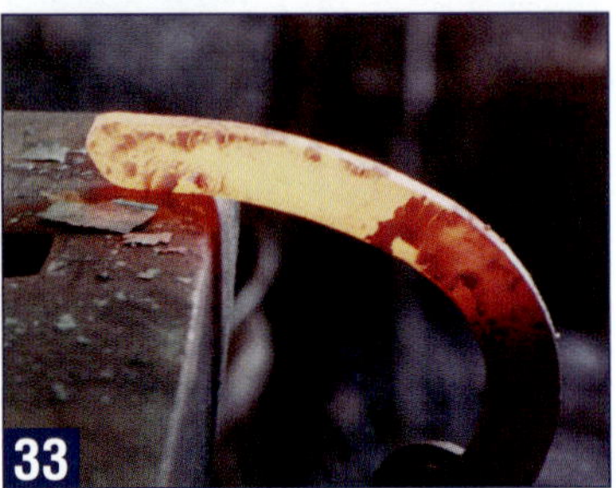
Counteract inertia bend.

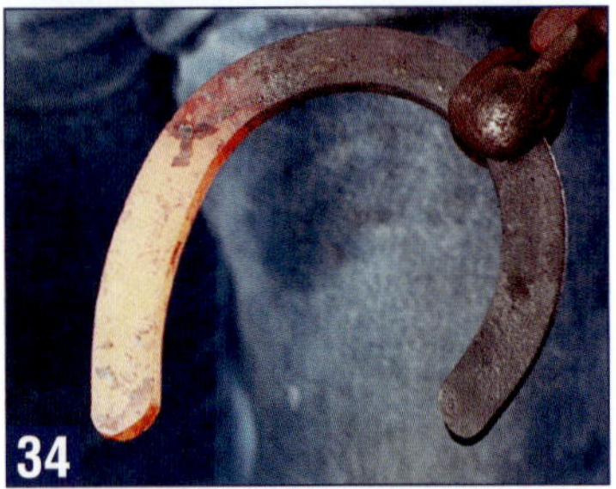
Fourth heat finished.

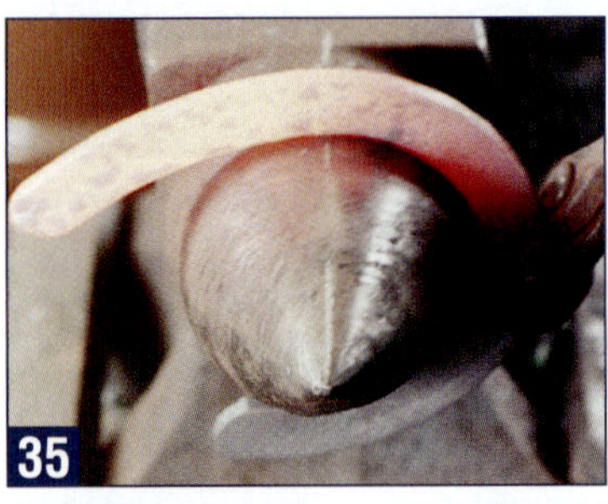
Heat through the toe and start the bend.

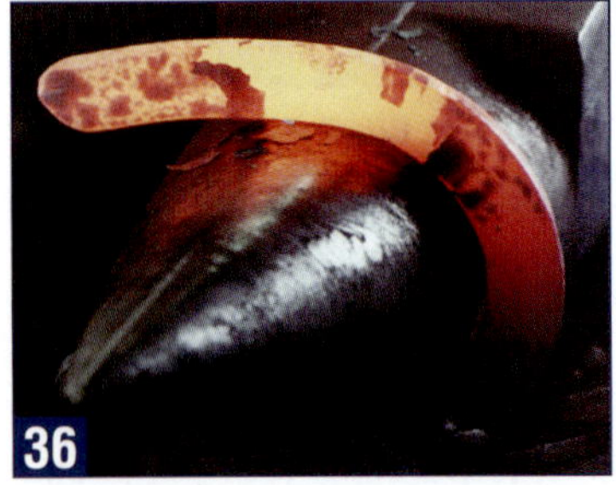
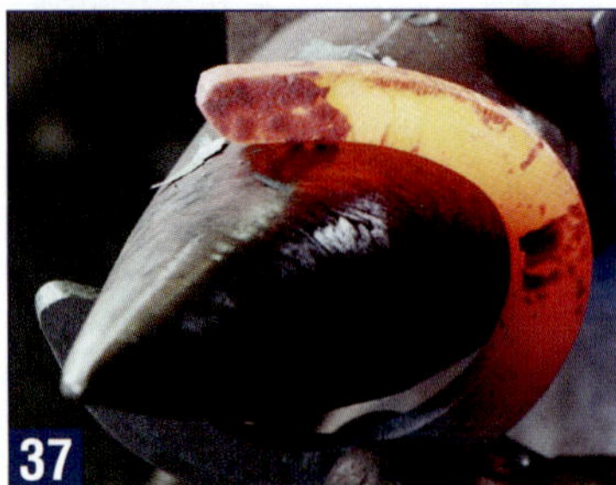
Shape the second branch.

28-29). With practice, you should end up with half a shoe like the one in **Figure 30**.

HEAT 4

This is basically a repeat of Heat 2, just as we did in the hind shoe. **Figures 31-34** depict Heat 4.

HEAT 5

Heat 5 is a repeat of Heat 3

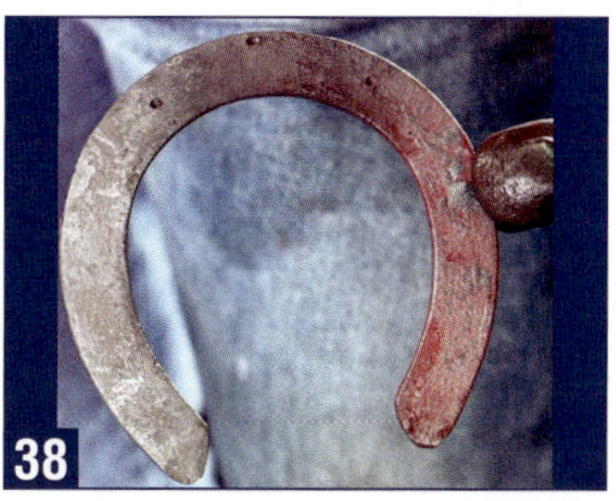
Finished blank, fifth heat done.

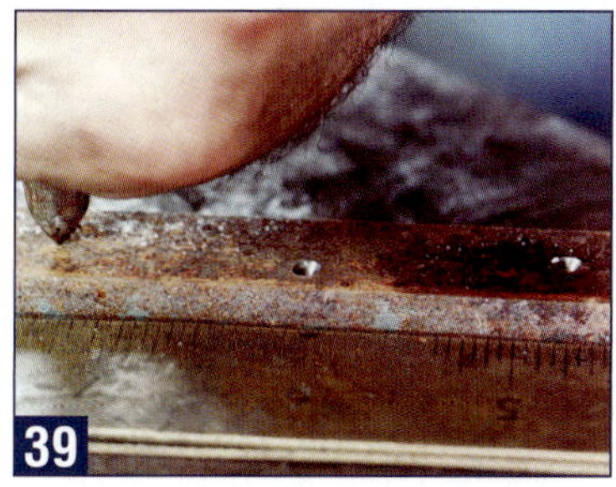
Mark 1 5/16 inch from center on most saddle-horse-sized shoes.

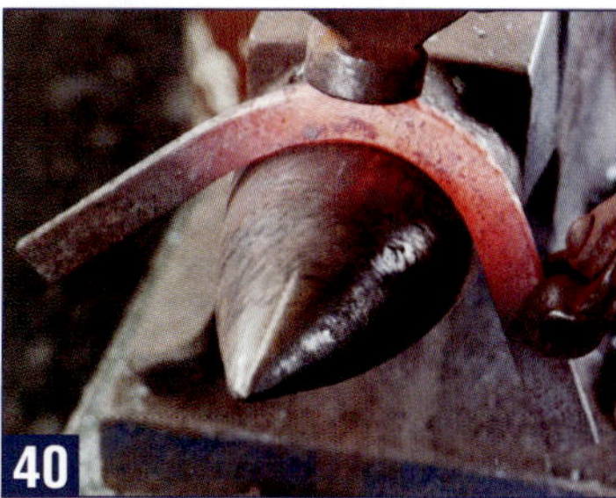
Make the toe bend.

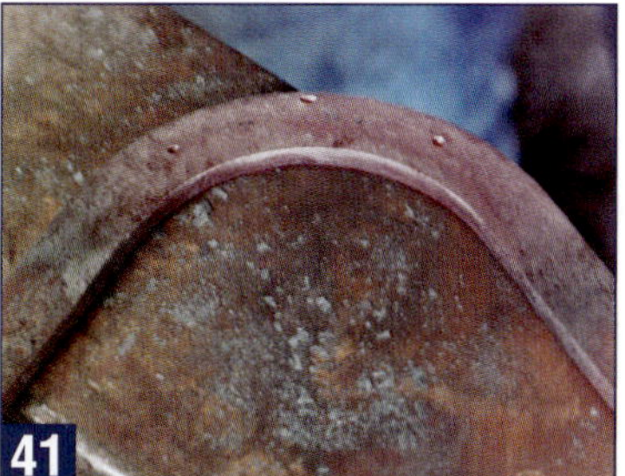
Finished toe bend.

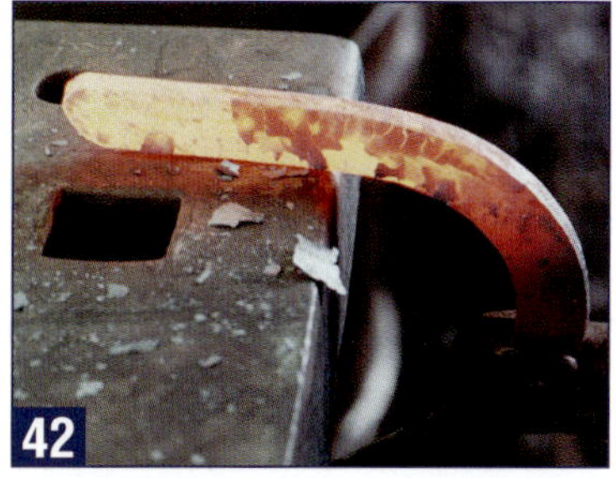
Second heat. Counteract inertia bend.

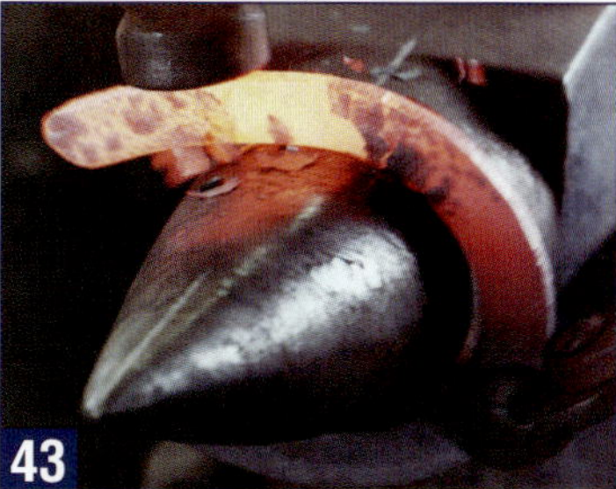
Shape branch.

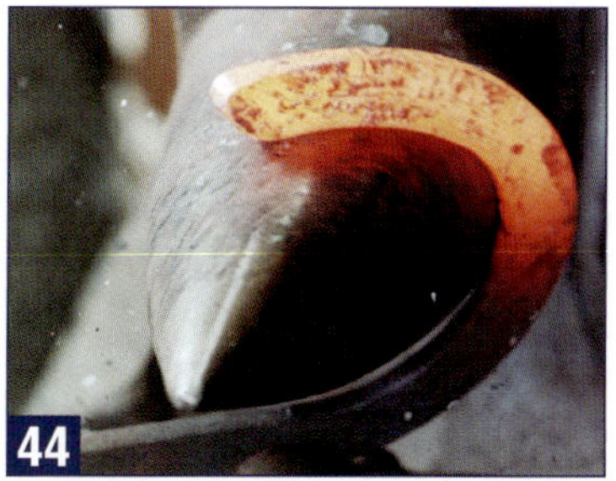
Shape branch.

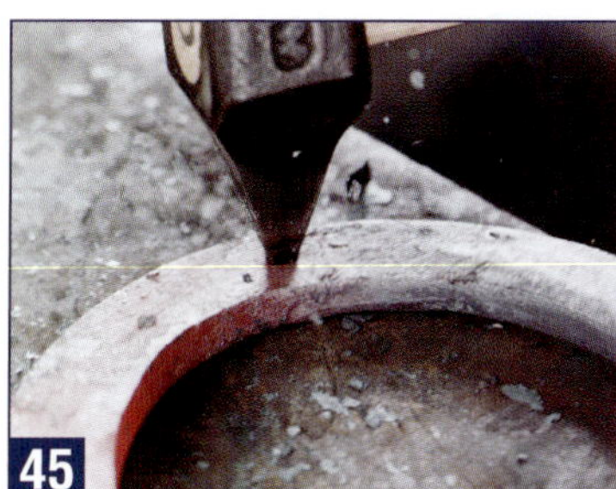
Make toe nail.

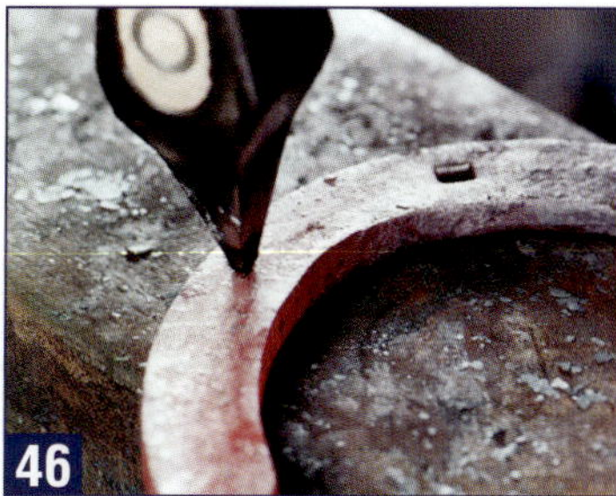
Make heel nail.

(Figures 35-37), and you should end up with a shoe like the blank in **Figure 38**.

PLAIN STAMPED FRONT SHOE IN THREE HEATS

If you are building this shoe without the training wheels, concentrate on working the center third of the stock when making the toe bend. The way that I like to lay out a front shoe is to mark center, then I place the marks for the toe nails at around 1 5/16 inches from the center for most saddle-horse feet **(Figure 39)**. I will go wider if the foot is wide or narrower if the foot is narrow. In either case, simply punching the nail hole to the inside or outside of the center punch mark for the nail hole should be sufficient to move the location of the hole to accommodate the width of the toe.

HEAT 1

Take a heat in the center of the stock and make a toe bend as you did for Heat 1 of the blank. Seat it out, and set the toe **(Figures 40 and 41)**.

HEAT 2

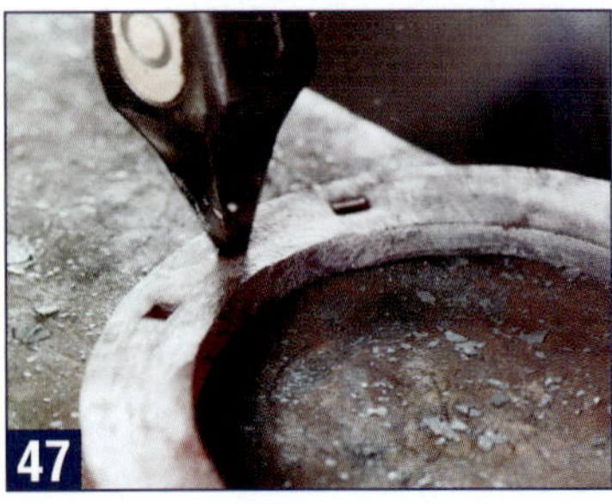
Place second nail between the two.

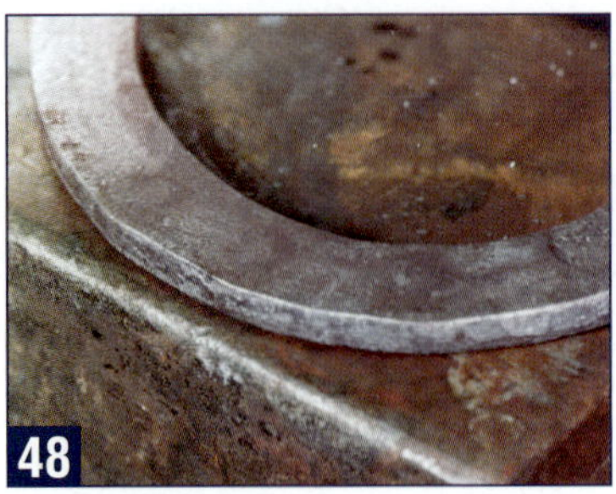
Hammer along the hoof surface of the shoe.

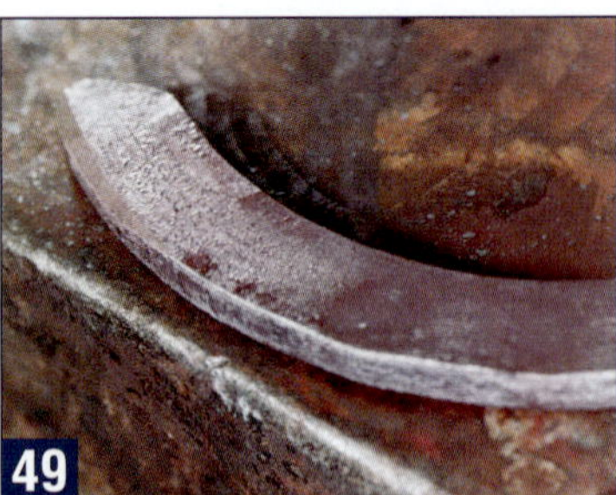
Box from the heel nail back.

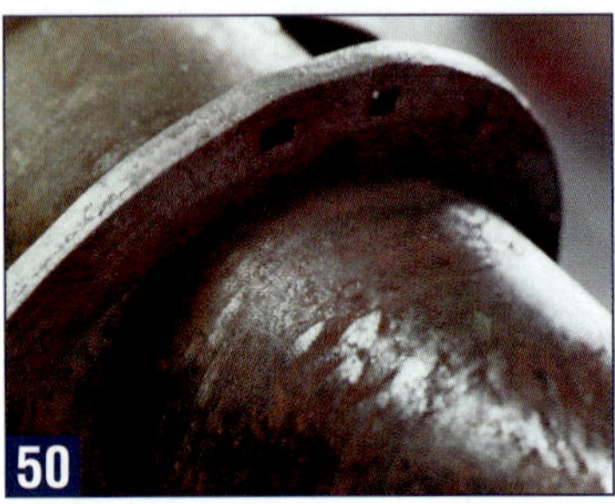
Forge out frog eyes and shape the branch.

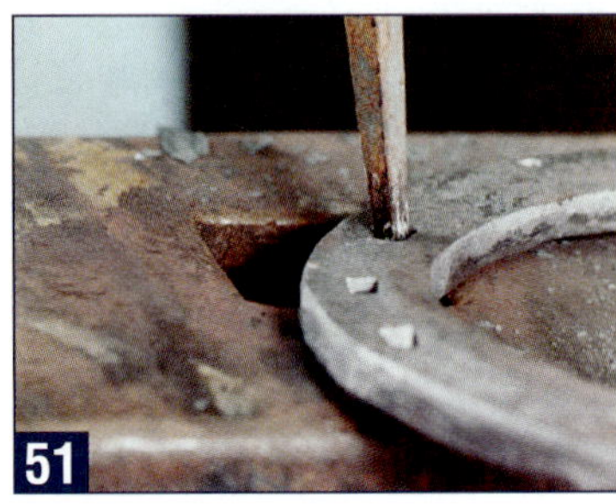
Pritchel. Second heat done.

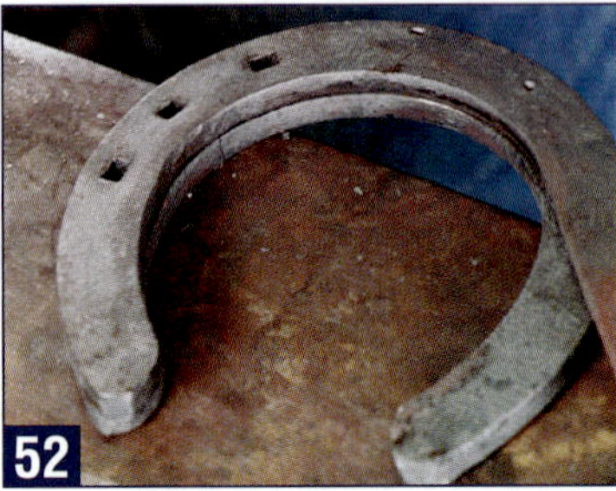
Compare half the shoe with a finished front horseshoe.

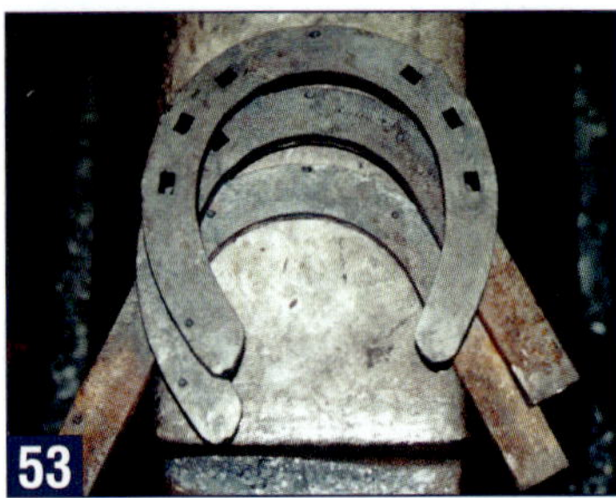
The three steps of the front shoe.

Heat one branch through the middle of the toe and make a heel as you have already learned to do. Create the counteract inertia bend on the heel, then move to the horn. Start at the toe, then drop your tong hand to form the branch. I only allow myself one trip to the horn at this point. Taking a lot of pains to shape the perfect shoe at this point is a waste of time **(Figures 42-44)**.

Move to the face of the anvil and drive your fore punch for the toe nail **(Figure 45)**. Make the heel nail **(Figure 46)**, and then split the difference for the second nail **(Figure 47)**. Hammer across the hoof surface of the shoe **(Figure 48)**, box from the heel nail back **(Figure 49)**, and take care of frog eyes on the horn while you perfect the shape of the branch **(Figure 50)**. Pritchel the nail holes (a lot of angle at the toe, less at the second nail, and straight up at the heel nail as with the hind shoes) **(Figure 51)**. Make the branch flat, but don't get too fussy about perfect level at this juncture.

This is a good time to compare what you have made to a finished shoe. You can use your blank for this process. In **Figure 52**, you can see that the half of the shoe just made matches the blank that

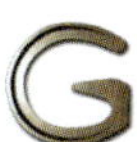

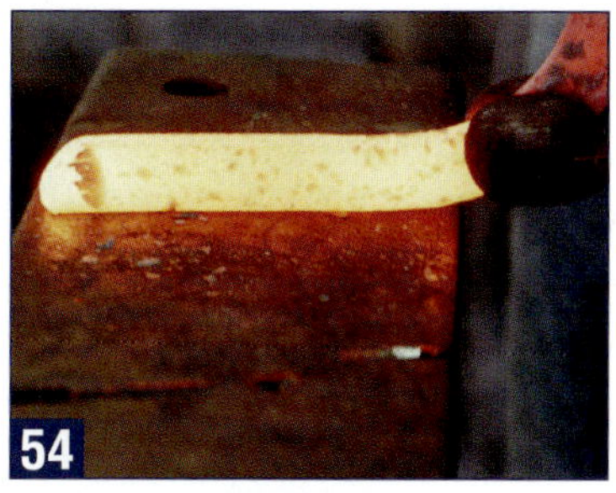

Make the inside heel.

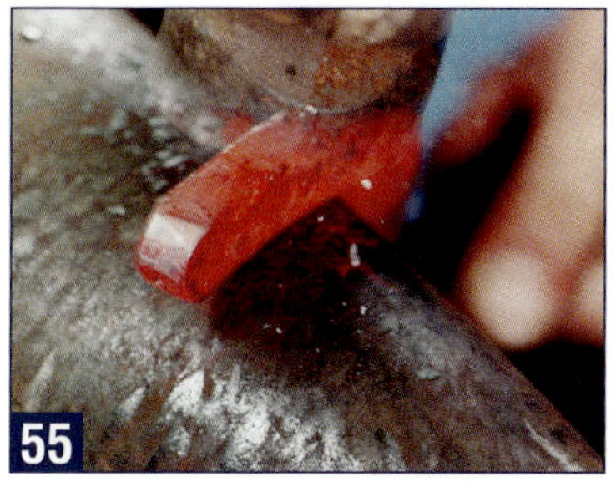

Bend the branch.

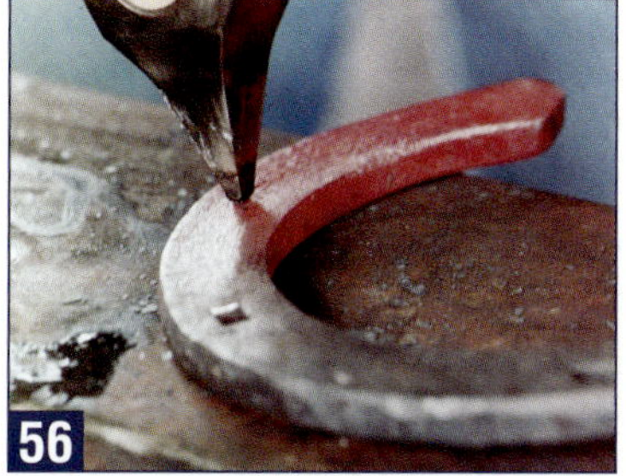

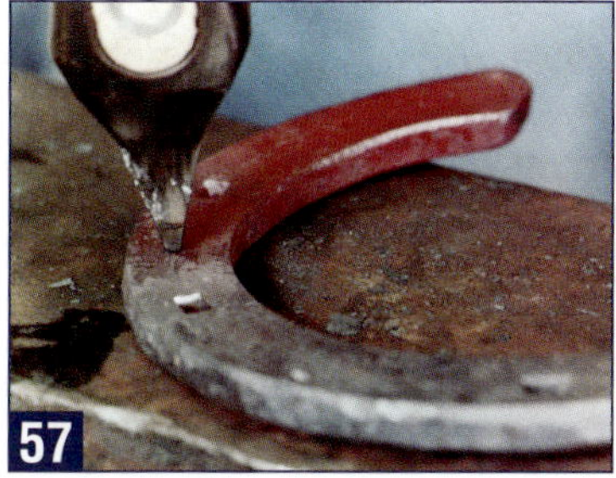

Make the nail holes with the fore punch.

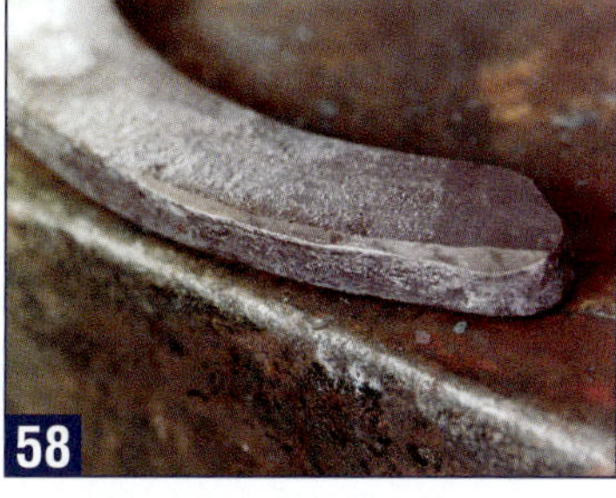

Box from the heel nail back.

we made before. It is a good idea to know what a shoe should look like in each phase, as you can see from **Figure 53**.

HEAT 3

This will be an exact duplicate of the second heat. The only difference might be if you are making a left or right, and you would sweeten the inside branch. If so, you will be adding about 10 hammer blows to the process, and you should have offset the center punch to allow for the length gained from sweetening.

Figures 54 through 59 depict the process of Heat 3.

At the end of Heat 3, you should have a good shoe that is ready to clip and hot fit **(Figure 60)**. If all went well, it will be a replica of the blank, with nail holes.

The fullered front in three heats is going to be just the same as the shoe just described, with the addi-

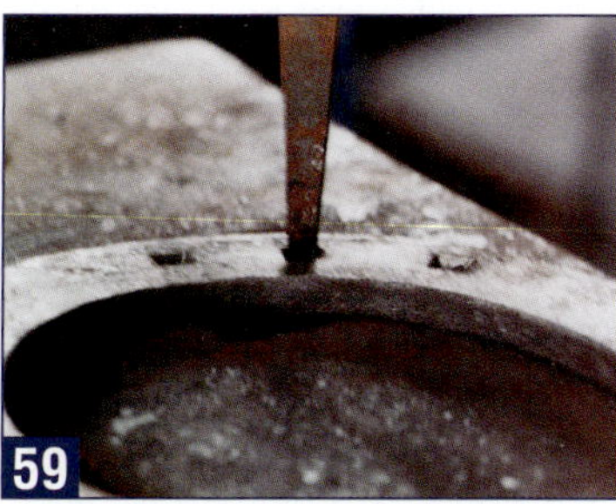

Pritchel. Third heat done.

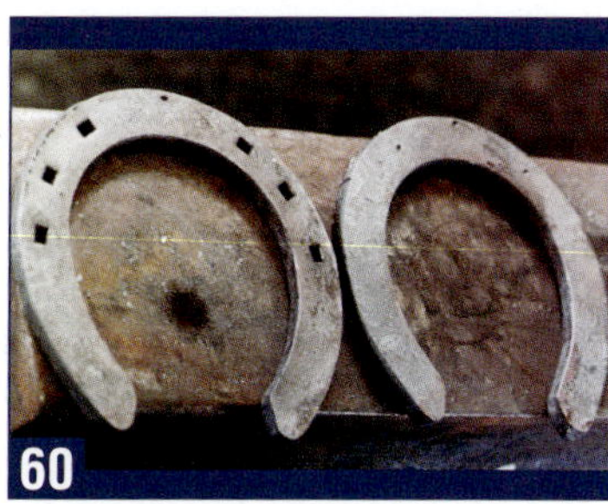

Finished shoe next to the blank.

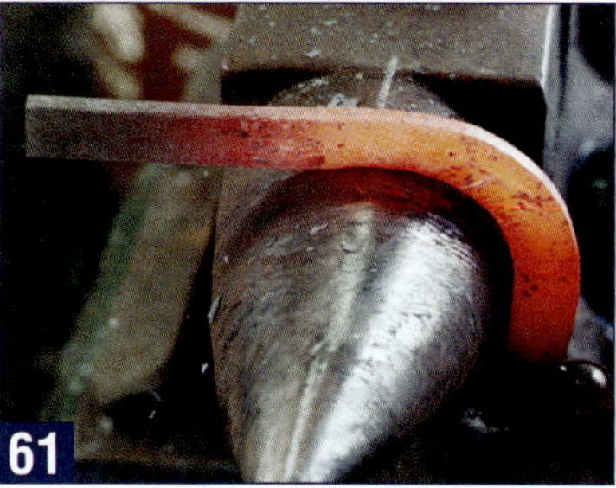

Start hemming on the horn after making the toe bend.

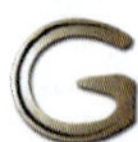

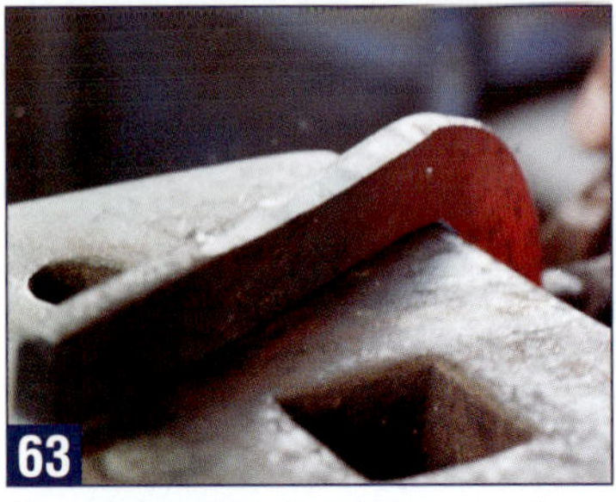

Move to the heel to continue the hemming.

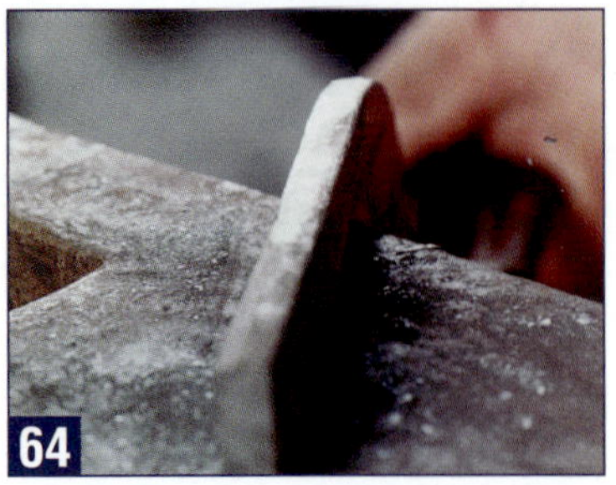

You can see the angle on the edge of the stock if you look closely at Figure 64.

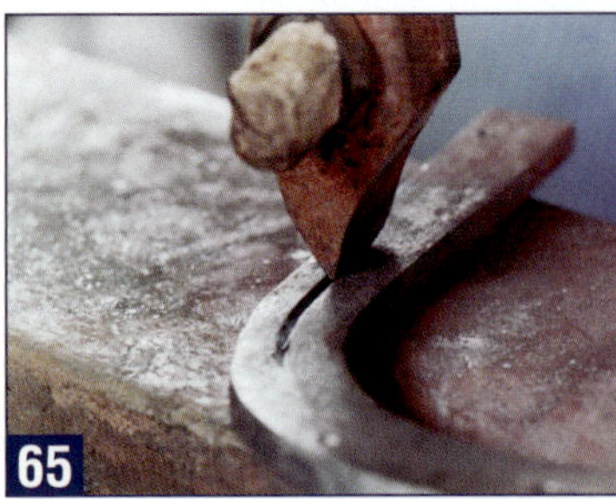

Mark the fullering. First heat done.

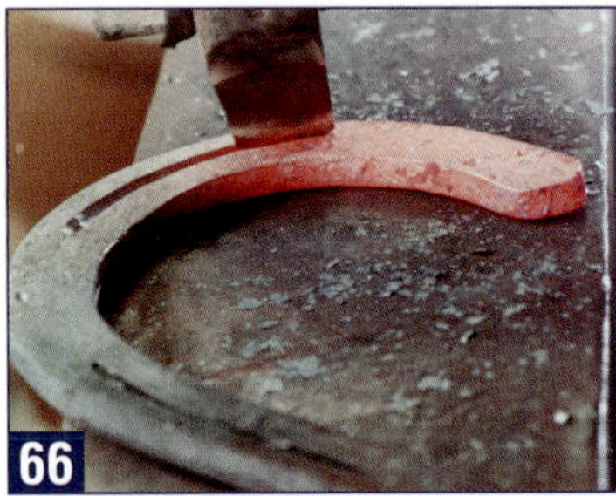

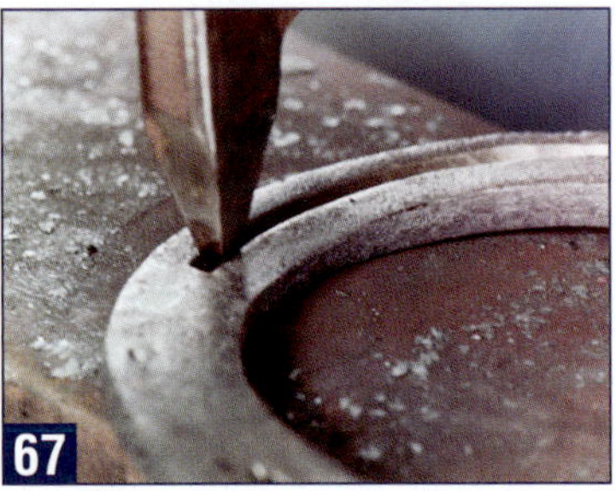

Heat through the toe and make the first branch.

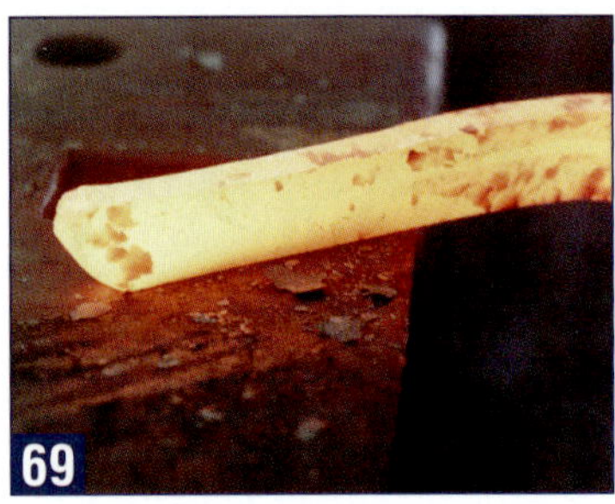

Sweeten the branch by thinning it slightly.

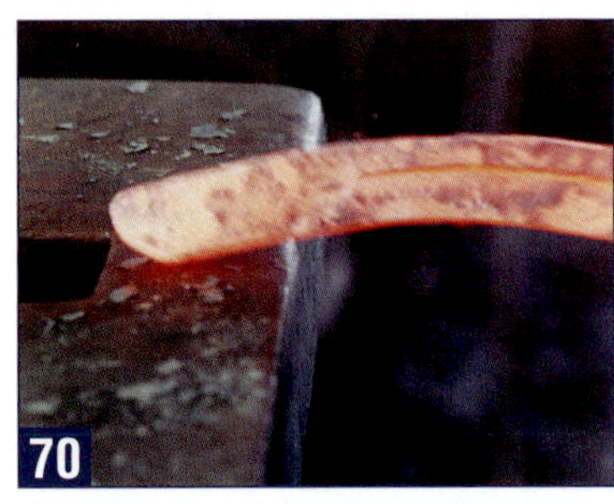

Counteract inertia at the same time.

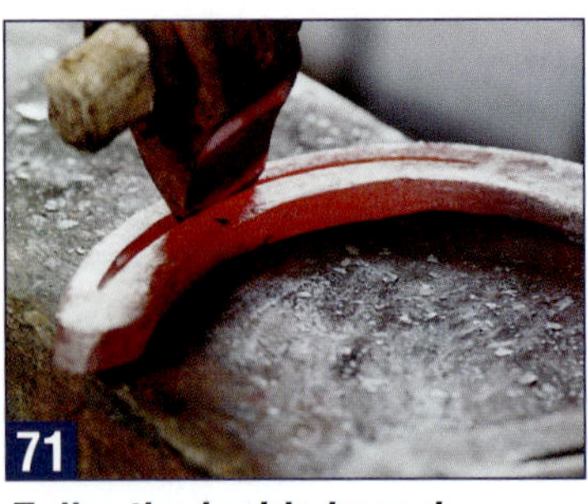

Fuller the inside branch.

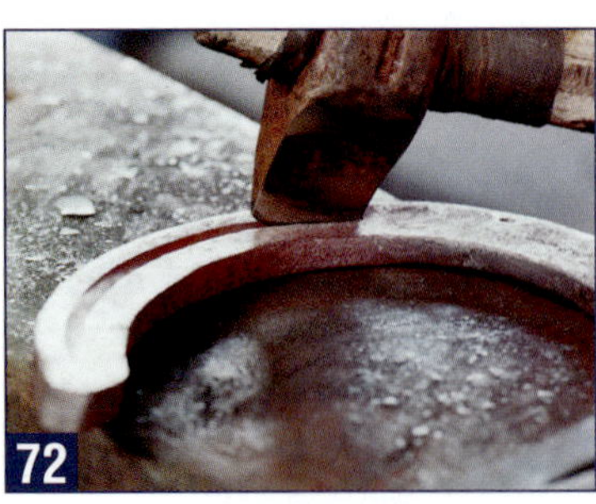

Second heat done.

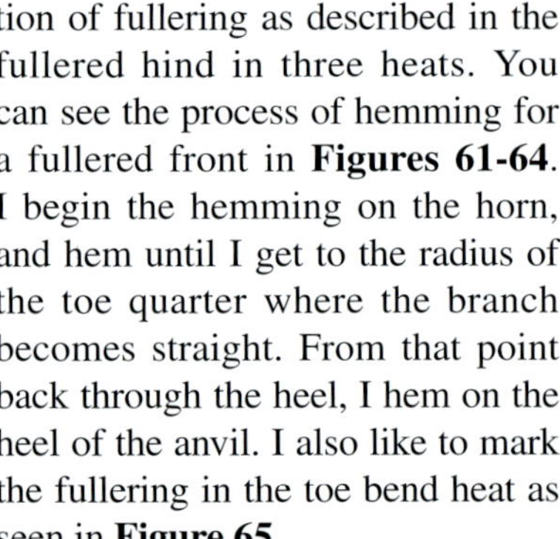

tion of fullering as described in the fullered hind in three heats. You can see the process of hemming for a fullered front in **Figures 61-64**. I begin the hemming on the horn, and hem until I get to the radius of the toe quarter where the branch becomes straight. From that point back through the heel, I hem on the heel of the anvil. I also like to mark the fullering in the toe bend heat as seen in **Figure 65**.

Figures 66-68 show making the outside branch during Heat 2. The exact steps are not shown in pictures, since they have been already explained and detailed elsewhere.

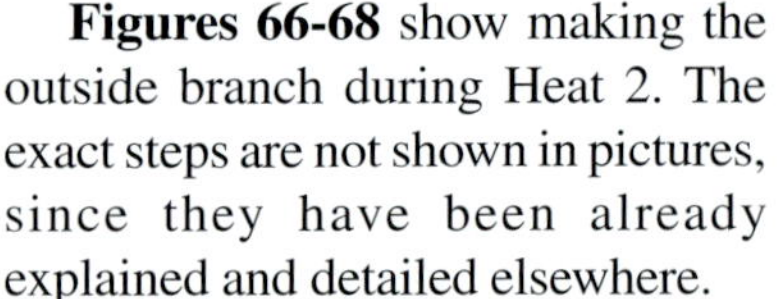

In **Figure 69** I am sweetening the inside heel, and in **Figure 70**, I am also making the counter inertia bend while sweetening the heel. **Figures 71-76** finish the inside branch to finish the shoe in three heats. In **Figure 77**, you can see the three shoes just made on top of each other. The fullered

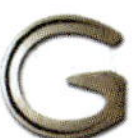

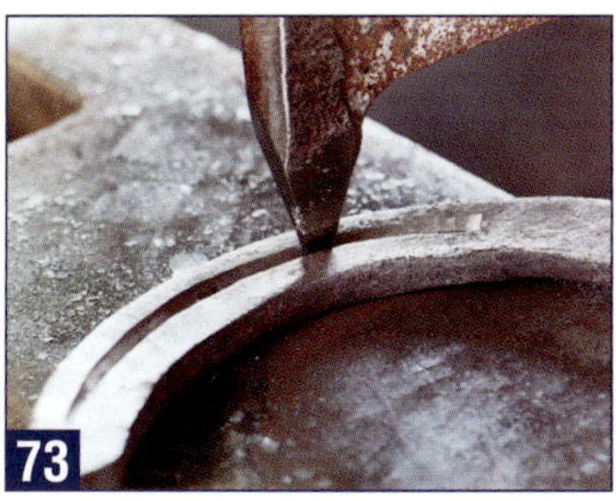
Punch.

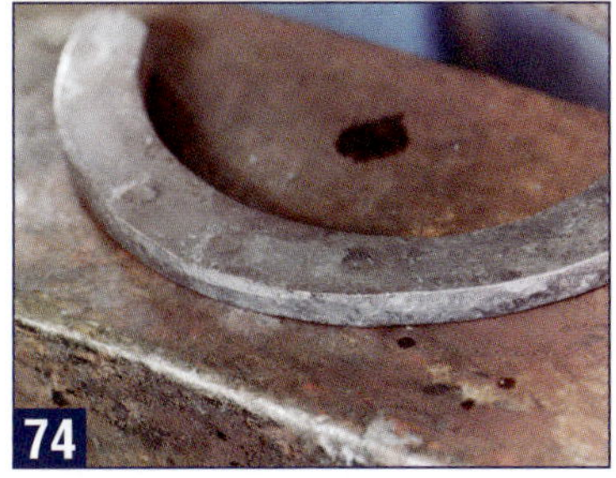
Hammer along the hoof surface;

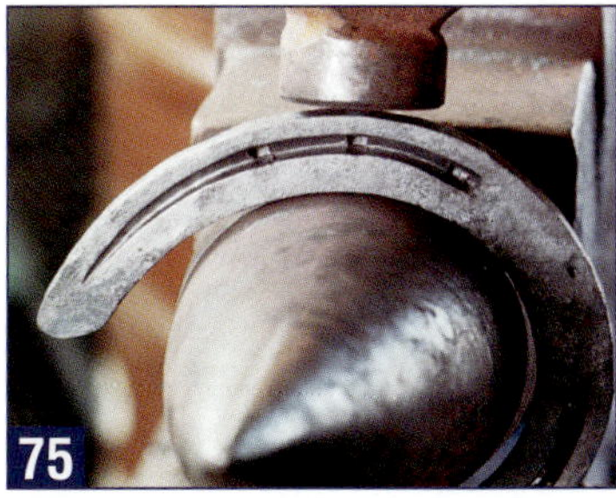
Shape and forge frog eyes on the horn.

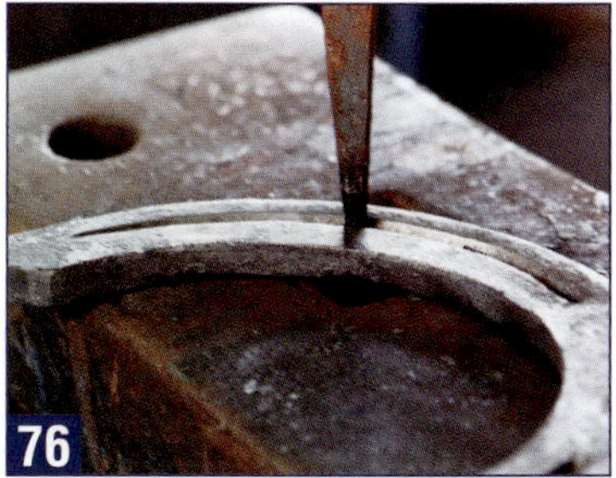
Pritchel, and the shoe should be finished.

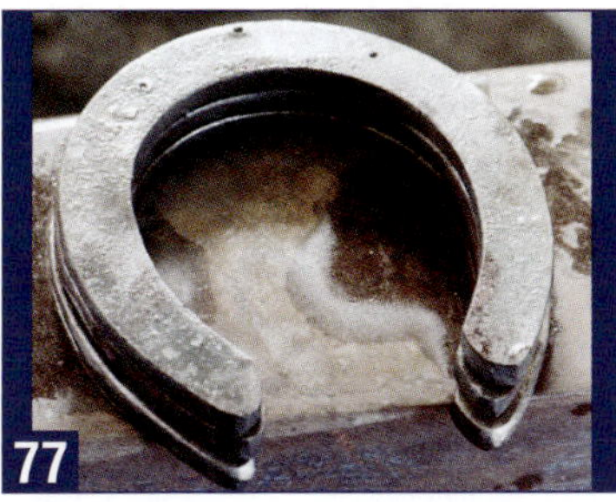
Three shoes stacked to compare.

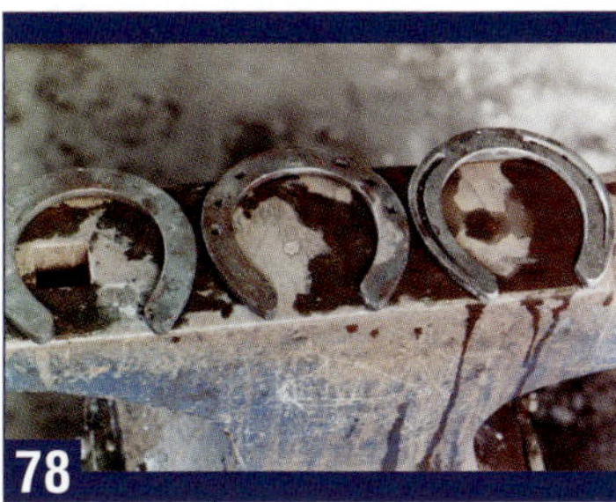
Siide by side blank, plain stamped, and fullered front shoes.

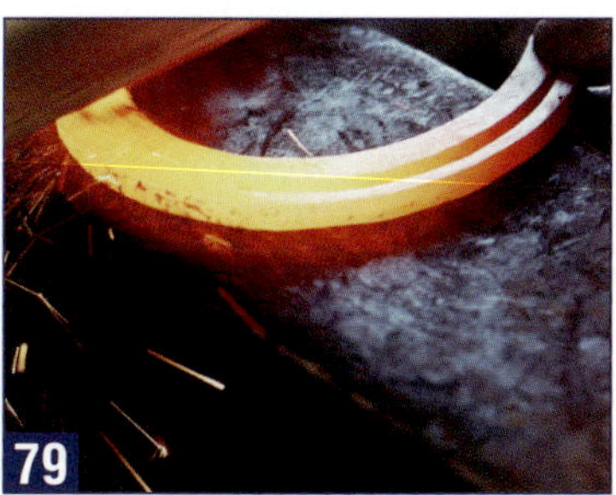
Brushing a hot shoe.

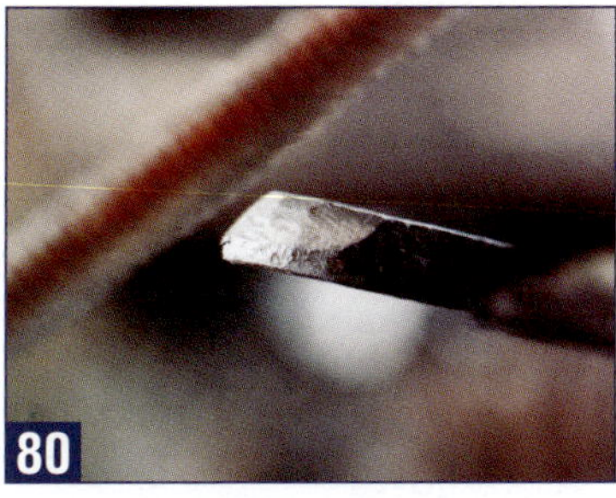
Rasping the heel cut.

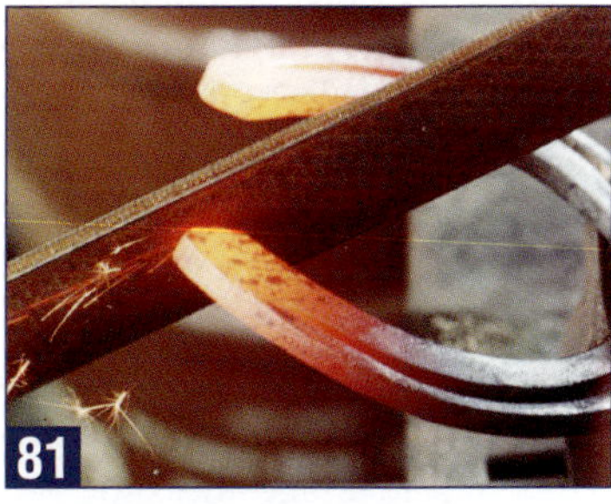
Rasping the heel check.

shoe is on the bottom, and you can see that it is the largest of the three. **Figure 78** shows the three shoes next to each other.

To get a good finish on the shoe, it is a good idea to brush the shoe every heat throughout the building of the shoe **(Figure 79)**. This prevents hammering the scale into the surface of the steel, and there is also a safety aspect to keeping the scale from breaking off and landing on you.

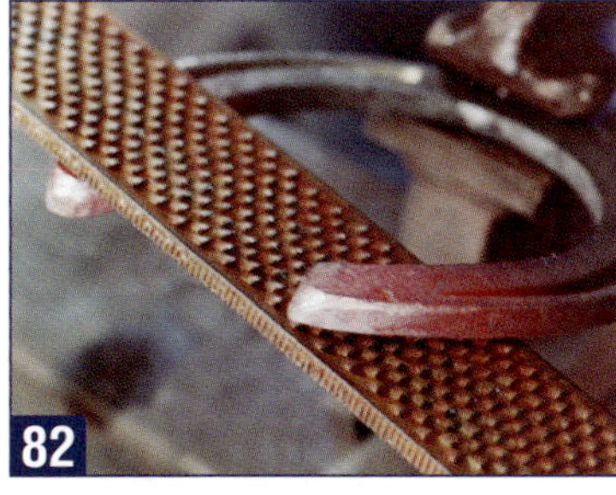
Moving the heels.

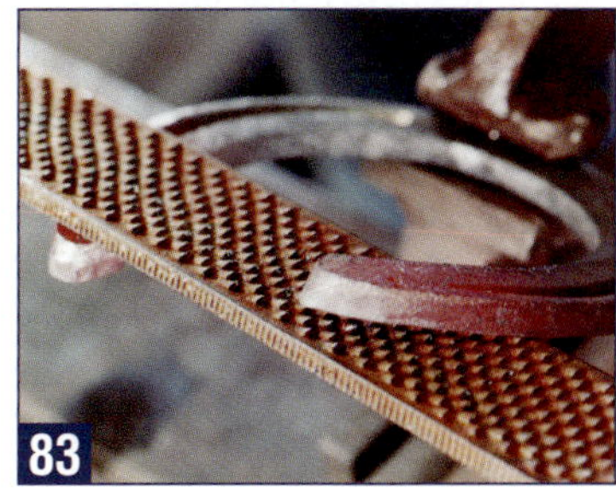

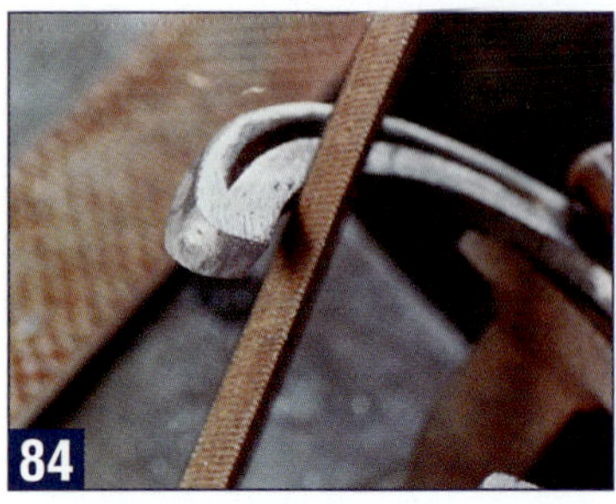

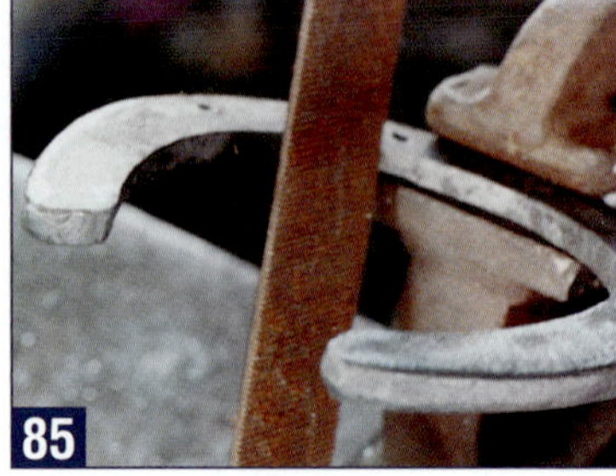

Half-round file on the inside of the shoe.

Rasp the edges.

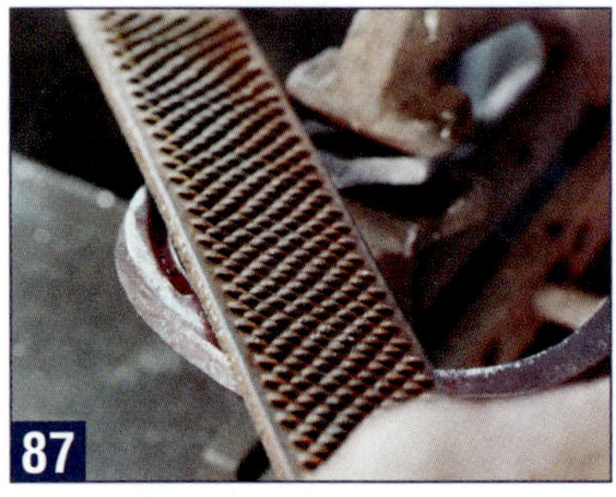

Rasp the surfaces.

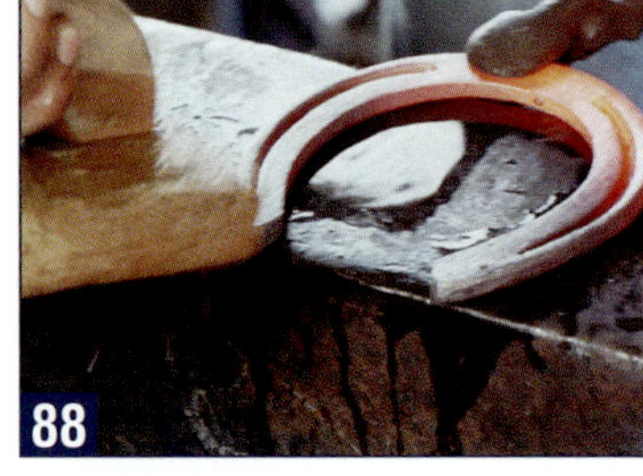

Wet brush.

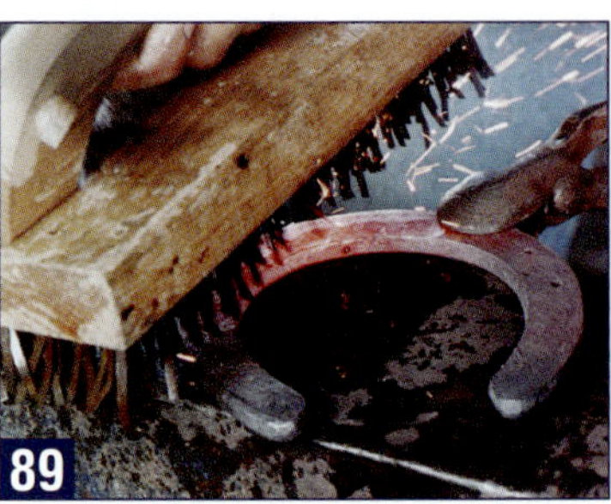

Once the shoe is built, place it in a vise and file the heels. In **Figure 80**, I am rasping the heel cut. That is the angle on the thickness of the stock. The check can also be rasped into the shoe at this time **(Figure 81)**. The check is the angle on the width of the stock,and should not take much to rasp correctly if you forged your heel the right way. You can bend the shoe out of level with your rasp if you need to in order to obtain better access to the heels. Put the rasp between the heels and leverage the shoe out of level **(Figures 82-83)**.

Next, file the inside of the shoe with the half-round file **(Figures 84-85)**, and then move the shoe in the vise to rasp the other surfaces **(Figures 86-87)**. With the rasping complete, level the shoe and get another light heat. Bring the shoe out of the fire, and brush it vigorously with a wet brush **(Figures 88-89)**. The water helps to break the small scale off the surface of the shoe, and the brush finishes the job. Continue to brush until you have achieved the finish you are after. This is a good way to finish a contest specimen shoe. If the shoe is going into a display, you may want to wipe it down with a rag that has Vasoline or oil on it.

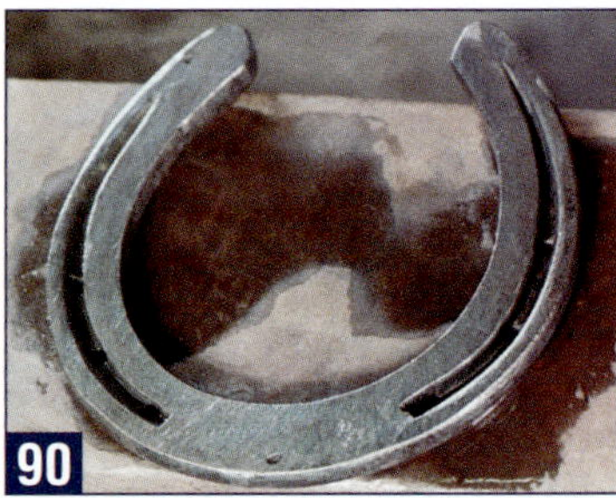

Finished shoe.

With all of that done, you should have a shoe that resembles the shoe in **Figure 90**. Practice regularly, diligently, and correctly to become competent at shoe building. If you start building these shoes and nailing them on feet, you will find that your ability to make shoes will increase almost daily. It is a fun and rewarding process, and I wish you all the best with it.

Photos in this chapter were taken by Jonathan Brisbin.

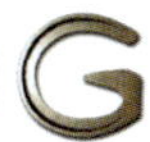

Chapter

42 USING CONCAVE TO MAKE SHOES

Concave is a type of bar stock that is very popular in the United Kingdom. It is a section of steel that is similar to what we refer to as a rim shoe in the United States. This is a great section of steel to make shoes out of, and these shoes provide more traction.

You can make your own concave section through a process known as tooled and fullering. When doing this, you begin with a piece of square bar and run it through a swage block to make a triangular cross section. The next step is to run a fuller through the section to make a groove. This is a lot of work, but the resulting shoes are great.

Generally, concave bar stock is made by passing hot steel through rollers that make the section. This can be an expensive process, and the only people that really buy concave stock are farriers. As such, concave will cost you a bit more, but I think you will find that the amount of skill you build by using it, and the way your horses will move, make it worth the price.

When making a normal concave shoe, it is important to bear in mind that concave stock does not move or stretch like regular bar stock. You will have to determine what your particular measurements are, but if you make a few shoes and measure them, you will find out how it moves for you. In general, I would suggest that you use half an inch more concave stock to cover the same amount of foot that you would with a plain stamped shoe made from flat bar stock. Also, concave does not have the structural strength that normal stock does, as can easily be seen just looking at the portion of material missing from the stock. You can see this well in **Figure 1**. A little bit of hammer will go a long way when you are making concave shoes. They are easily wrecked if you are too aggressive.

For this chapter, I decided to make a quarter-clipped hind shoe for a left foot. Cody is demonstrating his method with a toe-clipped front shoe.

To begin, mark the stock in the center, or off center if you are making a left or right **(Figure 1)**. Here is the first trick I know of for using concave. When you make the toe bend, hold the stock at just enough of an angle that the stock will appear as solid bar when you hammer through it **(Figure 2)**. This means that the inside hoof surface corner is now lined up with the outside ground surface corner. Doing this allows you to make the bend with less warping, which is a big problem when making concave shoes.

When leveling the toe bend, try to avoid hitting on the ground surface of the stock. Hammer on the hoof surface with light blows and set your toe as you would normally for the shoe you are making **(Figure 3)**. In **Figure 4**, you can see the toe bend at the end of the first heat.

On the second heat, begin your heel on the outside of the stock and collapse the groove in the middle of the concave, taking it to just past center. Turn the stock over and work the inside corner, eventually collapsing the groove from the inside **(Figure 5)**. Keep your hammer blows light and easy as you forge a good heel on the end of the

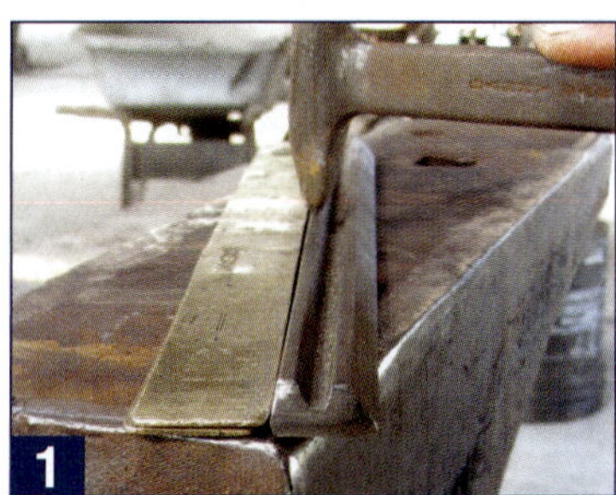

1

Marking the concave stock to make the shoe.

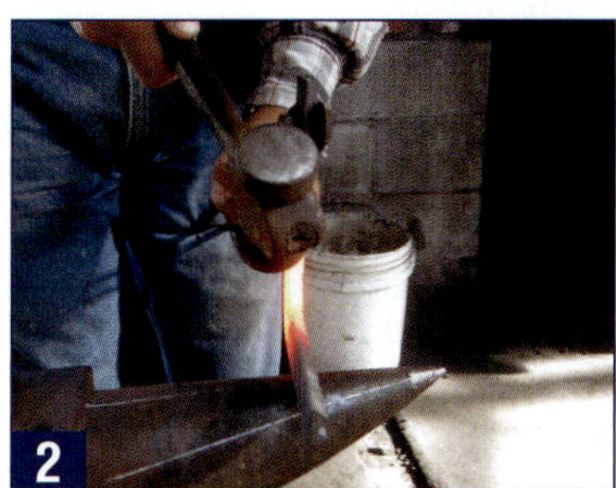

2

Making the toe bend. Stock is turned in the tongs.

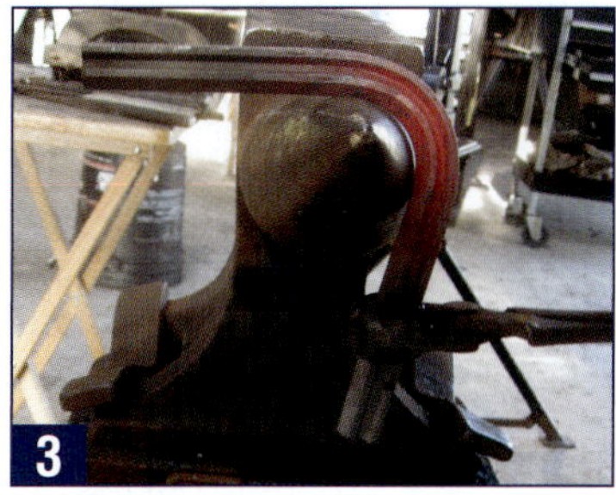

3

Setting the toe.

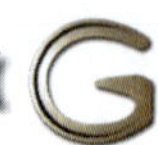

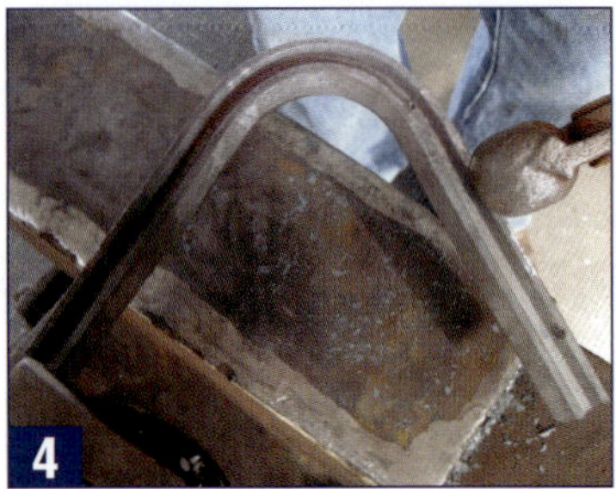
Finished toe bend for a hind shoe.

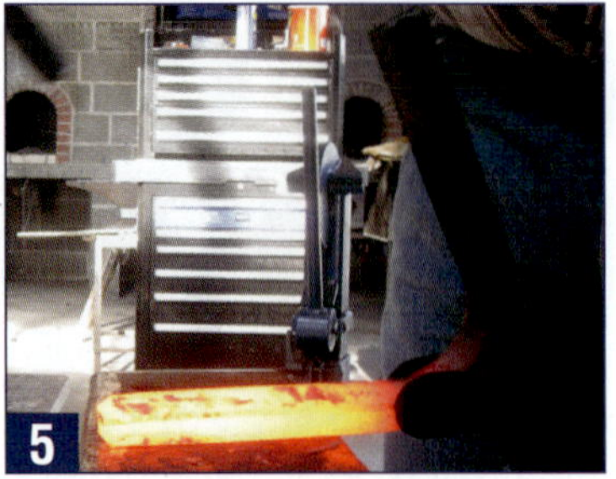
Making the outside heel.

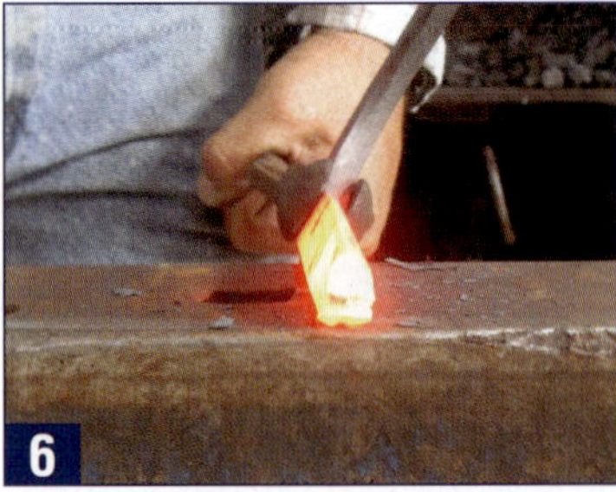
Stock being held twisted so that the flat side is visible to me.

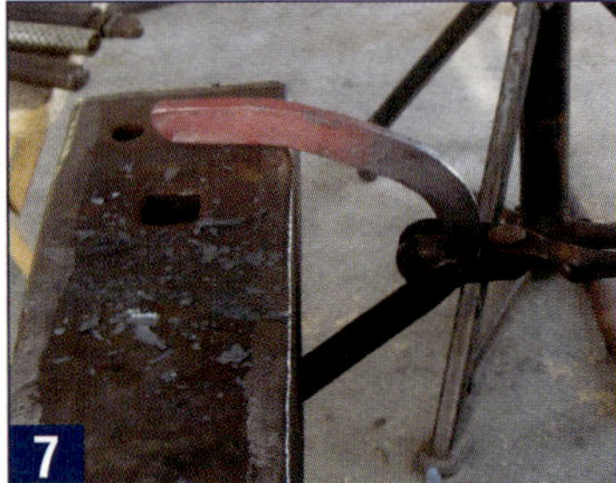
Move to counteract inertia.

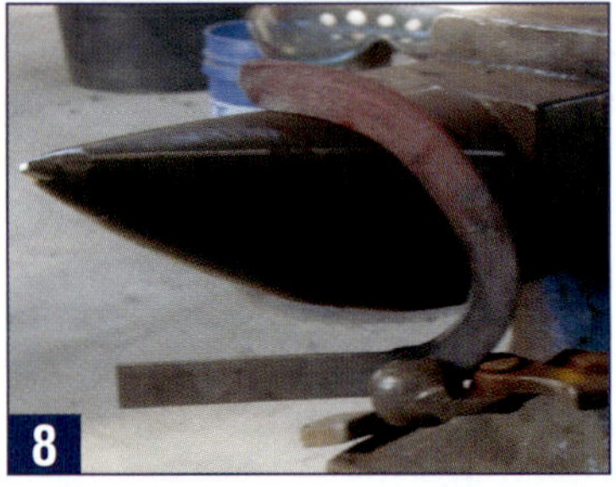
Bending the shoe around the horn.

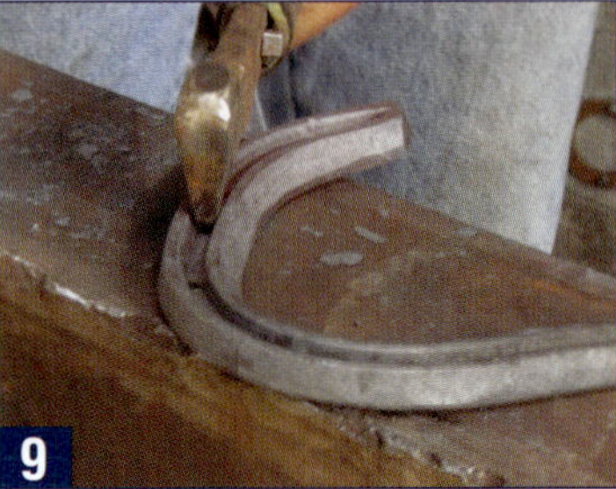
Punching nail holes.

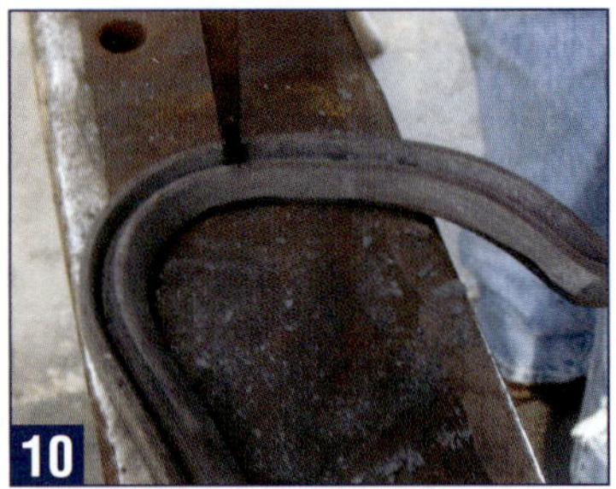
Pritchelling.

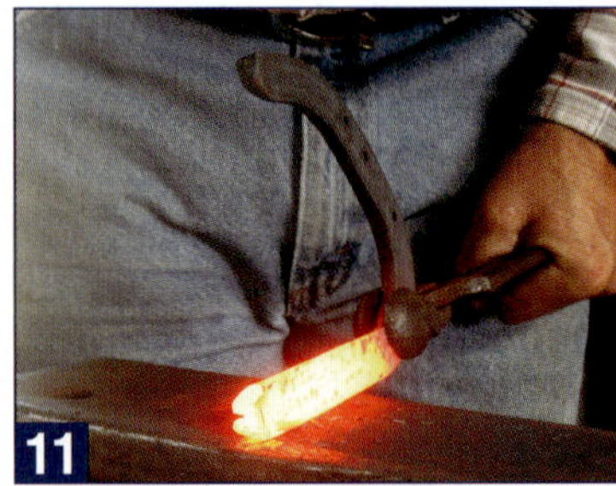
Making the inside heel.

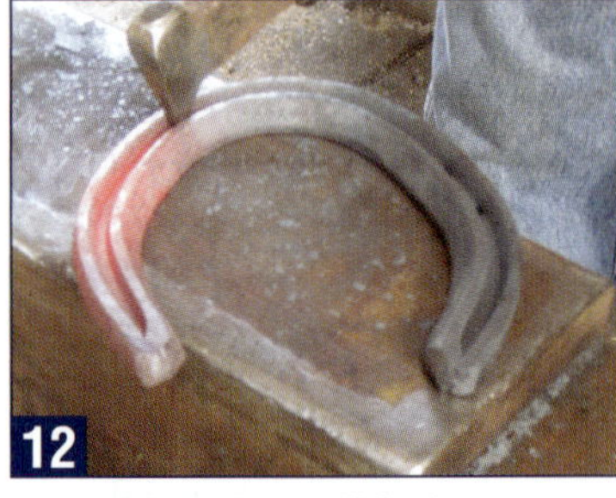
Punching the nail holes.

stock. You will see in **Figure 6** that I am keeping the stock twisted slightly, so that it appears as a piece of solid bar. That helps to forge through the strength of the stock, as we did with the toe bend, as well as to maintain the foot-bearing surface at the heel. Put a slight bend in the branch to counteract inertia **(Figure 7)**.

Bend the branch around the horn and punch your nail holes **(Figures 8-10)**. You may have to make a punch that has a longer neck on it to get to the bottom of the crease. Your normal fore punch may be too thick to bottom out the hole without affecting the sides of the crease. Forge the hoof surface, work out frog eyes, box, pritchel, and finish the branch.

As you are used to doing, repeat the steps on the second branch to make the shoe **(Figures 11-13)**. Just a quick note on sweetening the inside heel; with light blows, try to collapse the crease slightly toward the ground surface to make the inside ground surface of the shoe narrower than the hoof surface. Creating a big divot in the shoe is a fault that a lot of farriers have on the hoof surface of the heel. This can be avoided by keeping the stock twisted as discussed earlier. Since concave does not move as much as normal stock, you don't need to offset the toe as much to make the heels come out evenly.

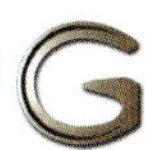

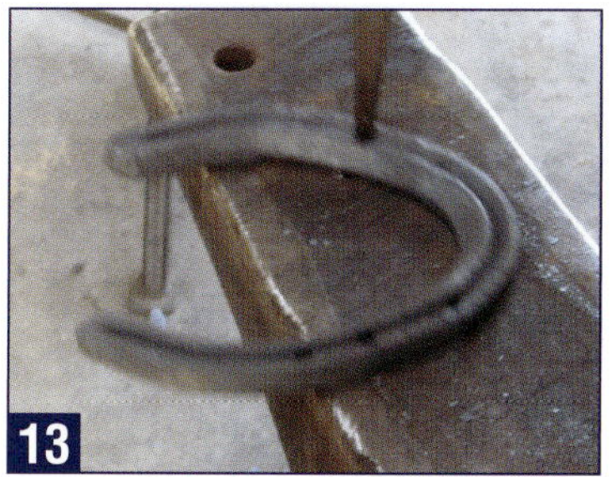
Pritchelling.

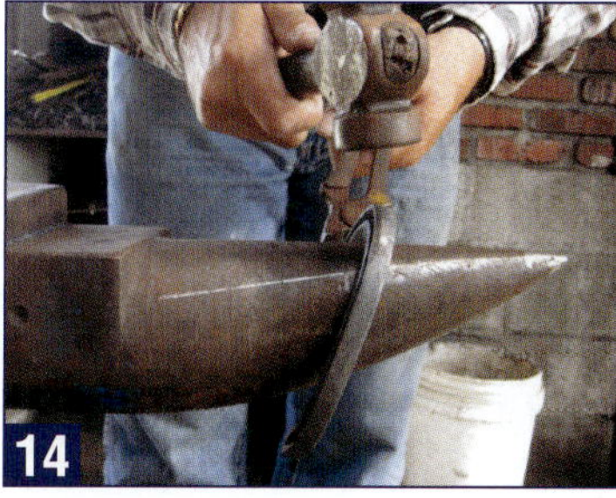
Safing the toe.

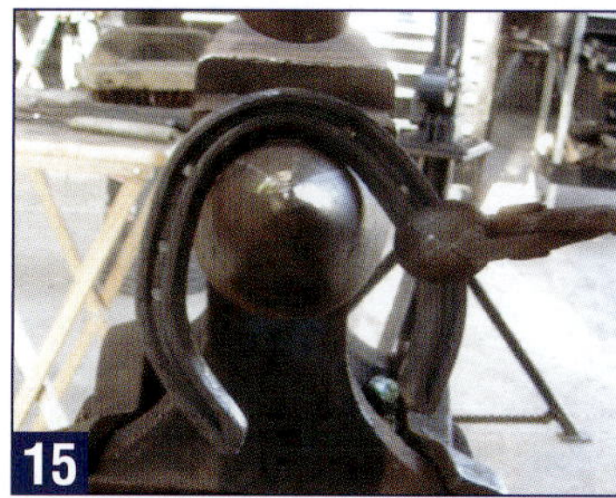
Another view of safing the toe.

In **Figures 14-15**, I am safing the toe. To do this, forge exactly as you would for hemming a shoe that you are about to crease. The amount that you safe is up to you. I generally like to collapse the groove in the shoe about half way. **Figure 16** is the unclipped three-heat shoe off the hammer.

This shoe is quarter clipped, and I am going to draw the clips with a ball peen clipping hammer. I have seen a lot of people invade the inside ridge of the groove when pulling their clips on concave, so be careful to avoid that. The method for clipping is the same as discussed in the forging exercises, but you can see the sequence in **Figures 17-19**. **Figure 20** is a detail of the clip, showing the inside edge of the groove.

With the clips pulled, all that is left is rasping it to finish. You can use a half-round file to clean up the inside edge of the shoe **(Figure 21)**. **Figures 22-23** are detail shots of the hoof surface at the heels. It is imperative that you keep that flat and clean. **Figure 24** is the finished shoe.

Cody uses almost all handmades on the horses he shoes, and almost all of the front shoes are concave. He makes the concave shoes in two heats with a toe clip, and the process he uses deserves demonstrating here.

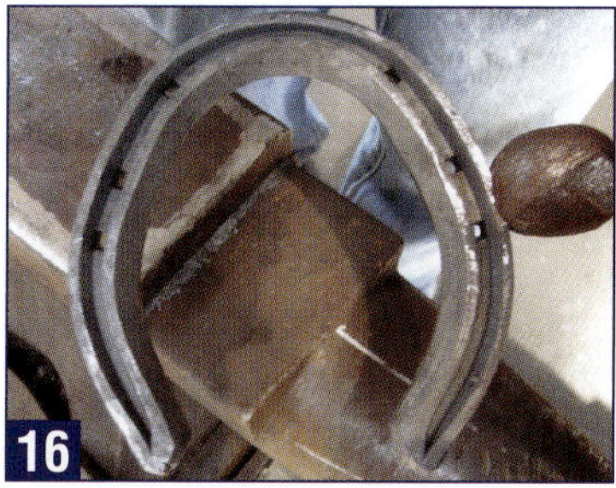
Hammer-finished shoe.

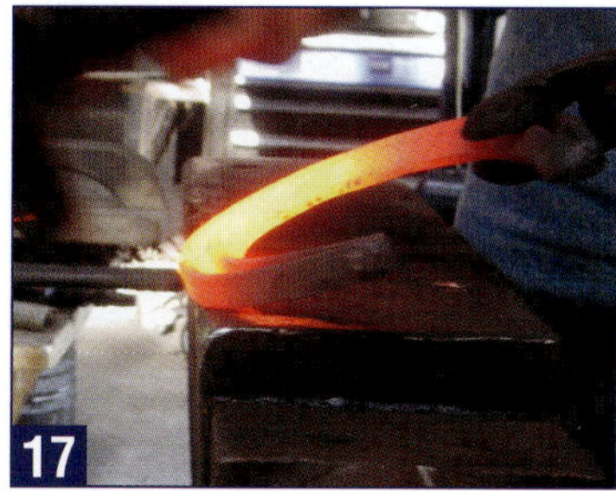
Pulling source for clips.

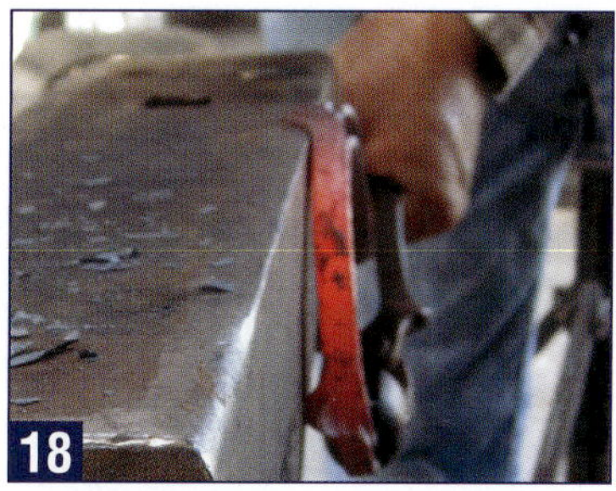

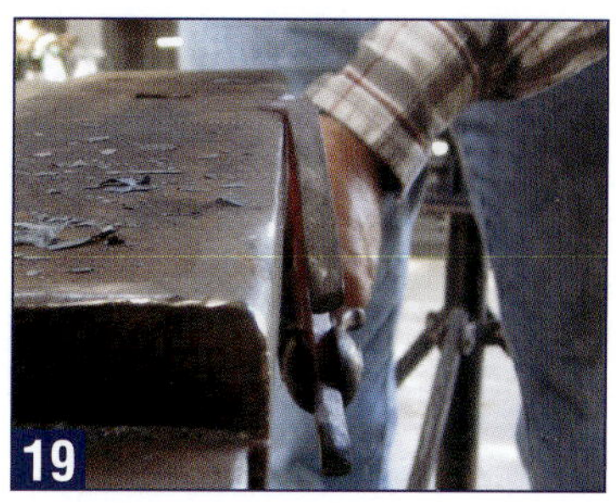
Pulling clips.

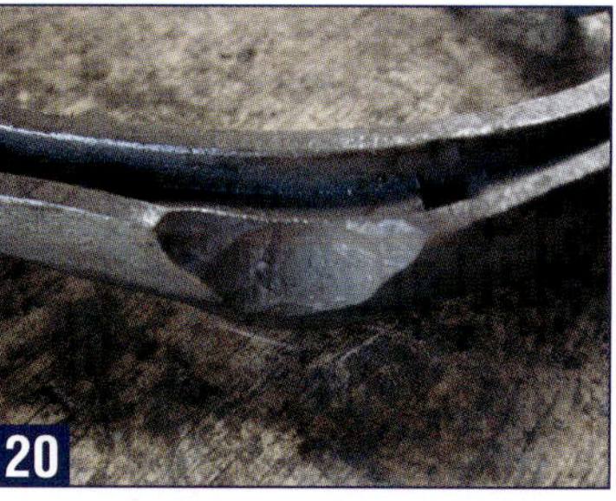
Detail of the area from where the clip was pulled.

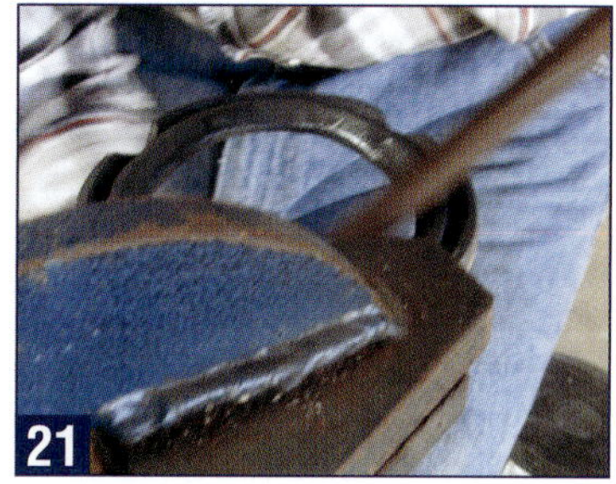
Rasping the shoe.

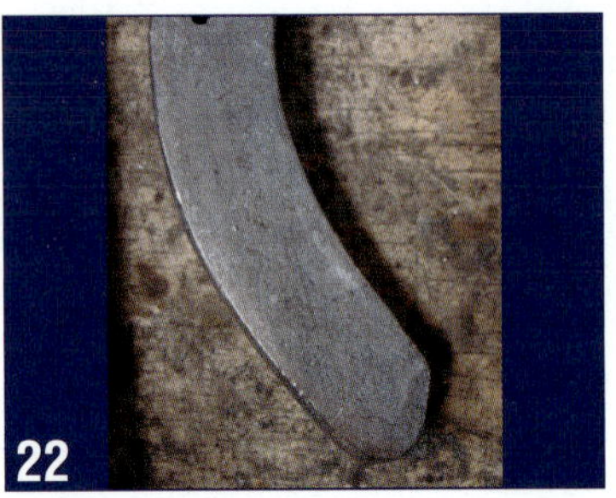
22 Detail of lateral heel.

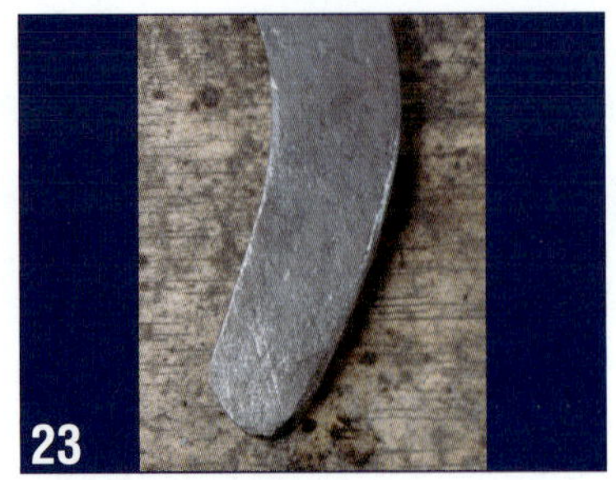
23 Detail of medial heel.

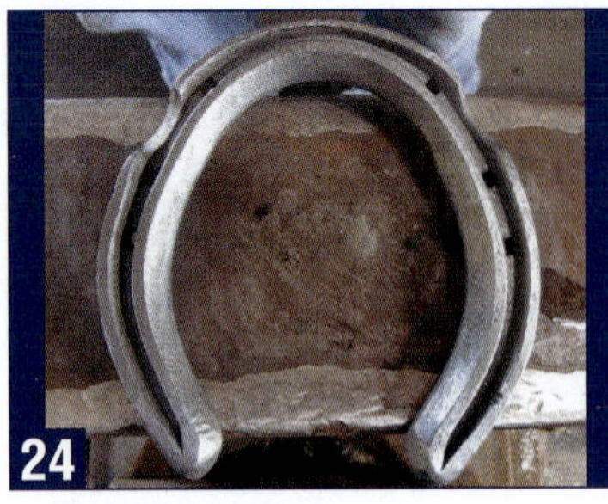
24 Finished shoe.

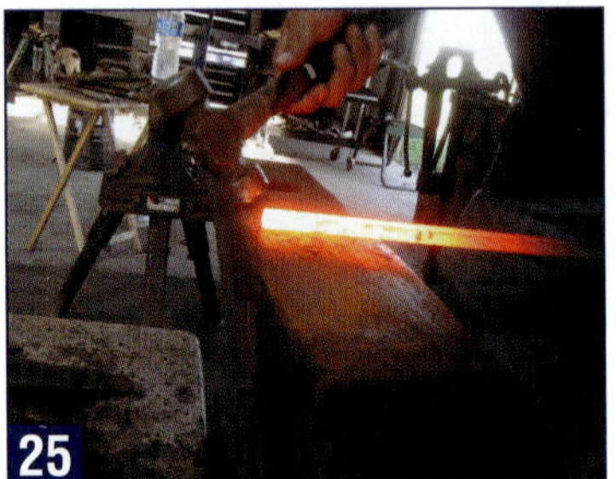
25 Cody making the first heel.

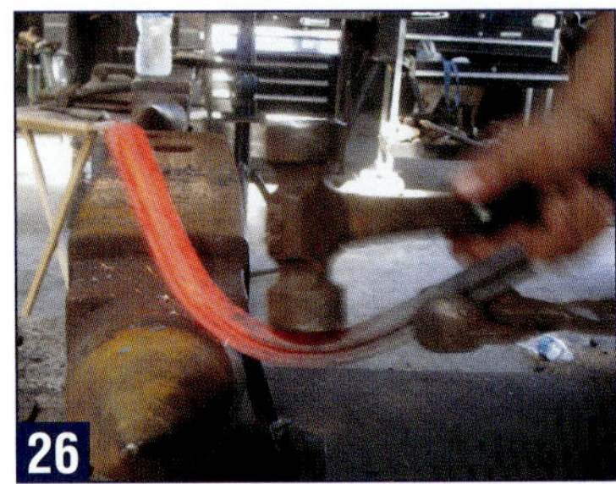
26 Toe bend.

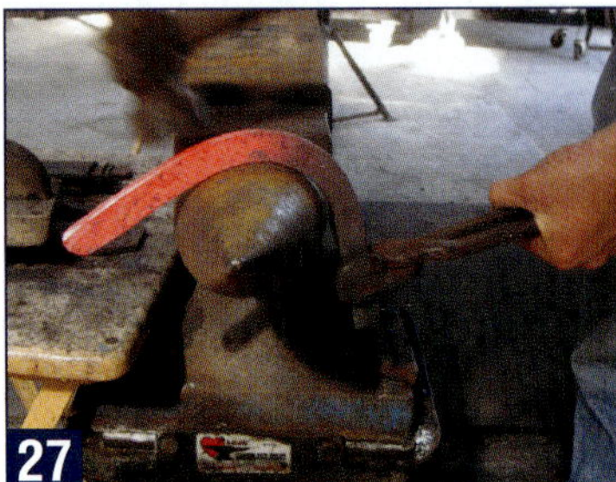
27 Setting the toe.

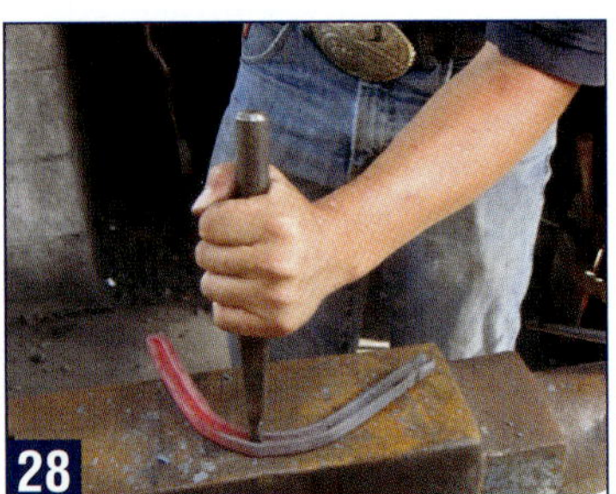
28 Placing the bob punch.

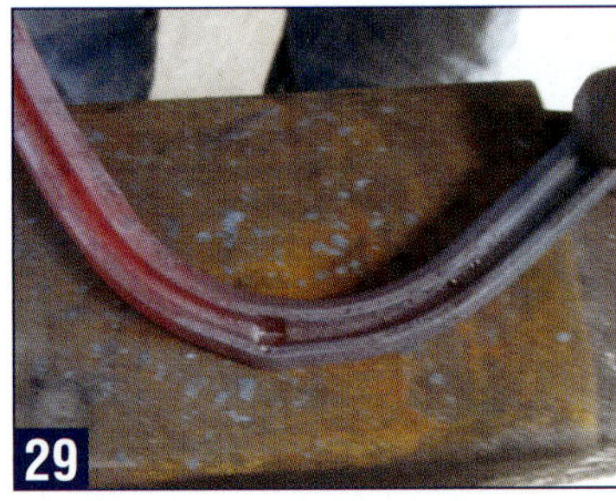
29 Source from the bob punch.

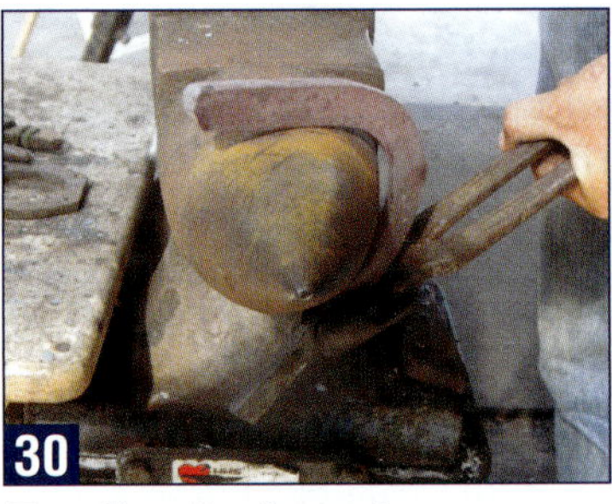
30 Bending the branch.

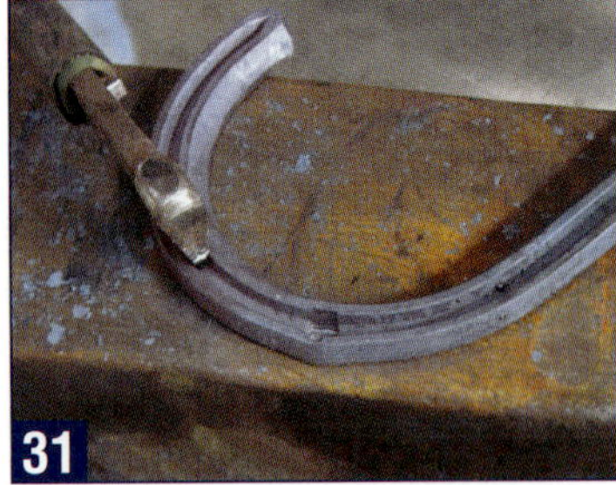
31 Punching the nail holes.

On the first heat, he heats up at least three quarters of the stock. He comes out of the fire, makes his outside heel **(Figure 25)**, cracks the toe and sets it **(Figures 26-27)**, puts the bob punch in the center of the toe for his toe clip **(Figure 28)**, and turns that branch **(Figures 29-30)**. He still has enough heat for the nail holes and pritcheling to finish the first heat **(Figures 31-32)**. The half-made shoe looks like **Figure 33** at this point.

Cody is making a pair of shoes in this series, and you can see from **Figures 34-37** that he has consistency in his shoe building. That is an important part

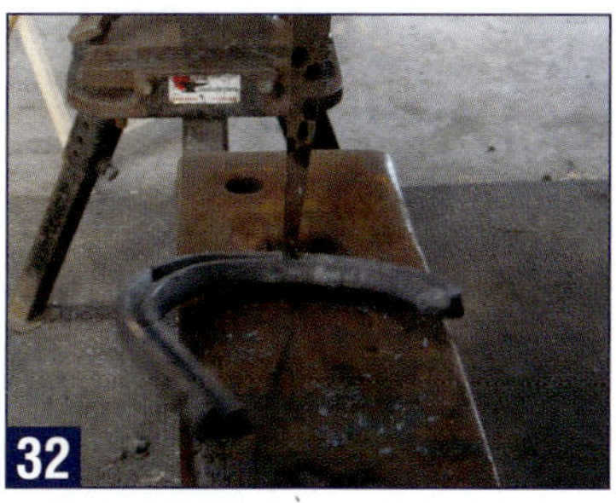

Pritchelling.

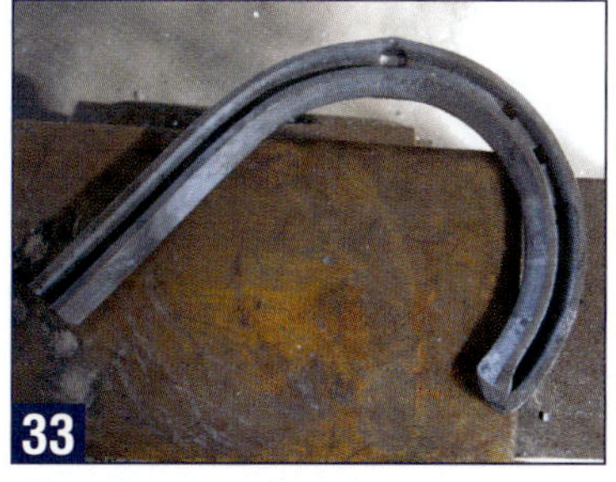

First heat complete.

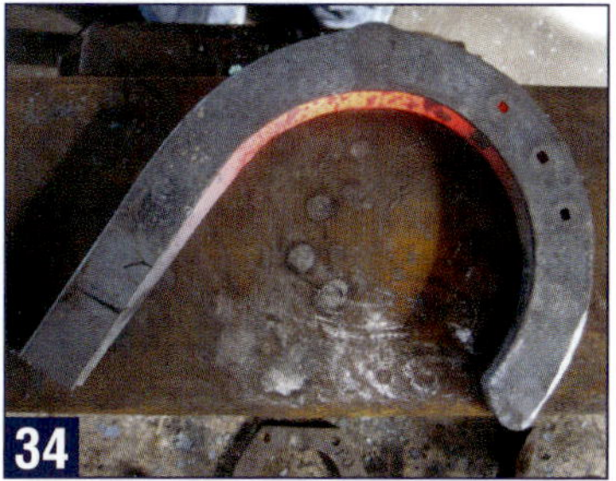

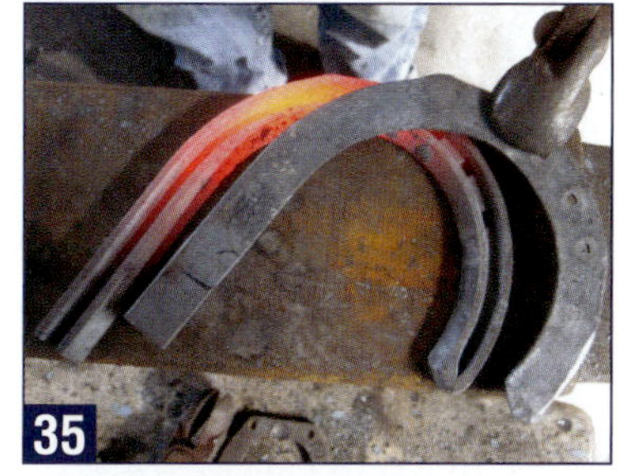

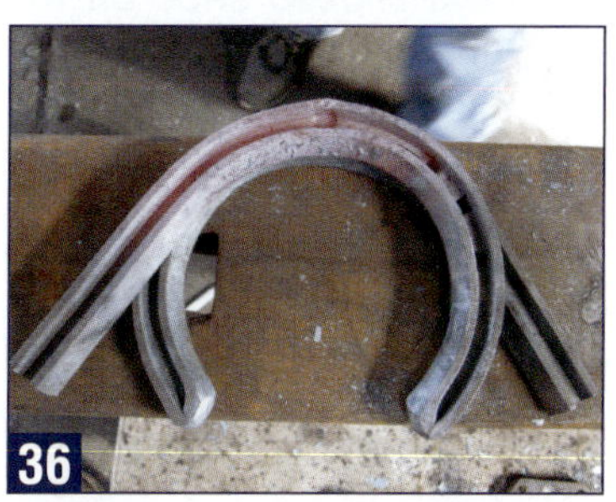

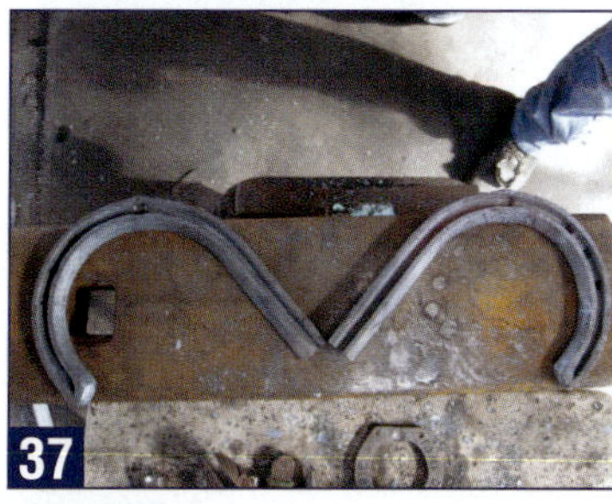

Comparison to the second shoe of the pair.

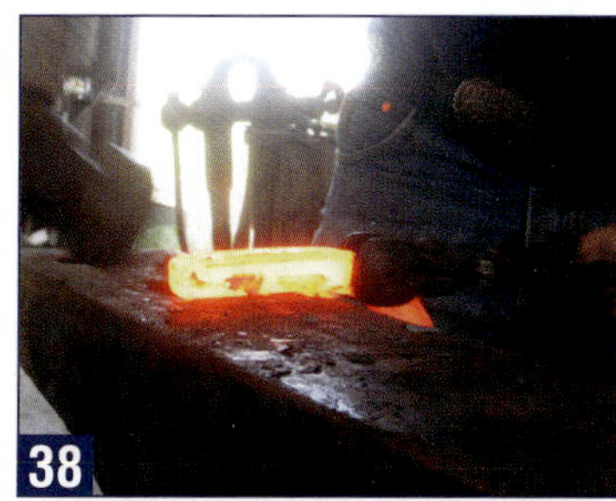

Making the inside heel, beginning of second heat.

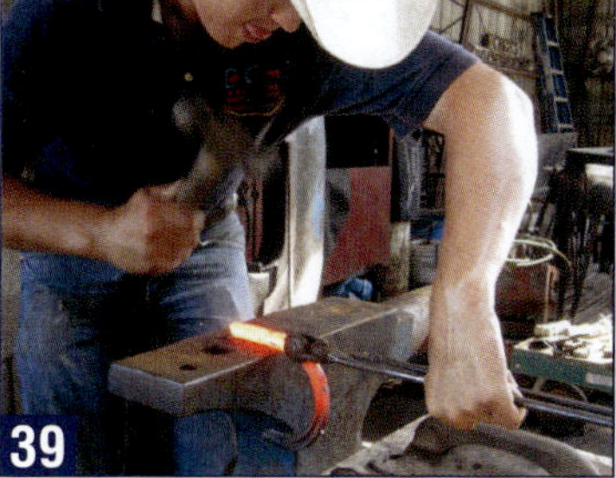

Cody's move for the inside heel of his left shoes.

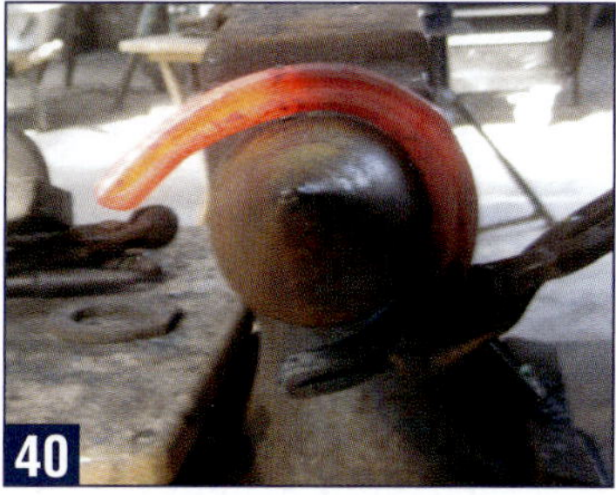

Bending the branch around the horn.

of any forging; knowing what it should look like at each stage and being able to reproduce it every time.

On the second heat, he makes the inside heel **(Figure 38)** and uses an unusual way to achieve the safing and sweetening on the inside heel of his left shoes **(Figure 39)**. Next, he wraps the branch **(Figure 40)** and pulls his clip before punching the nails **(Figures 41-42)**. Now that he has a toe clip on

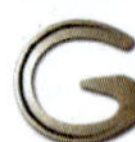

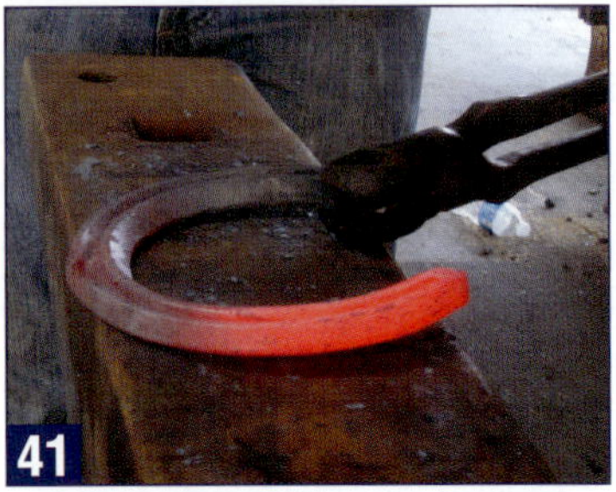
Pulling the toe clip.

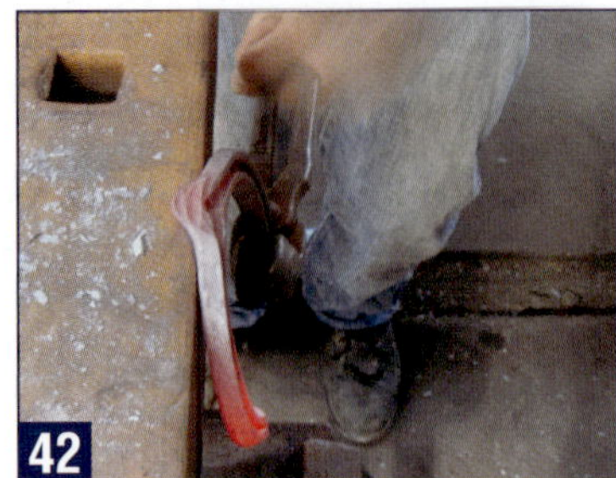

Punching nail holes.

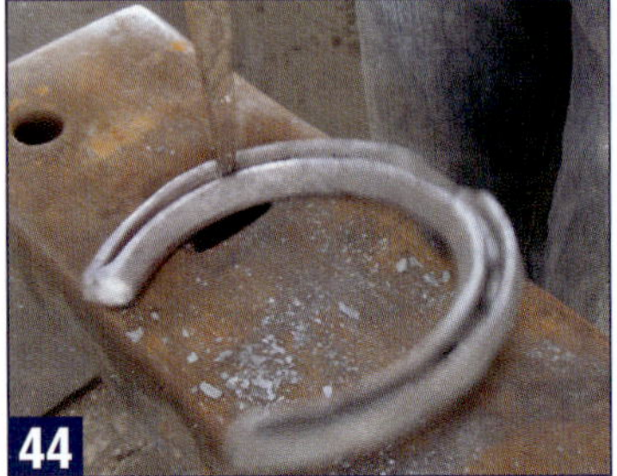
Pritchelling in the hardy hole.

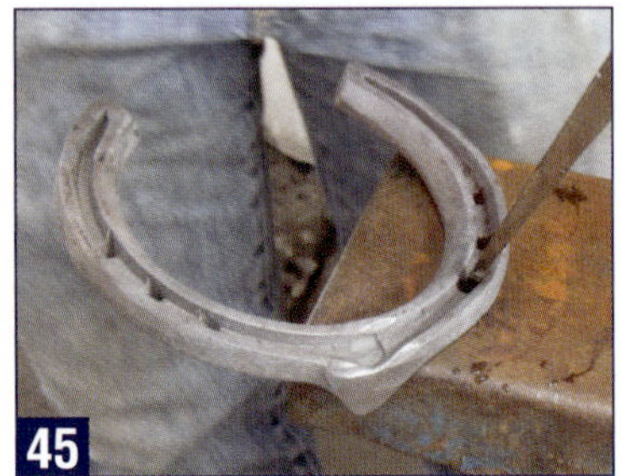
Pritchelling in the pritchel hole.

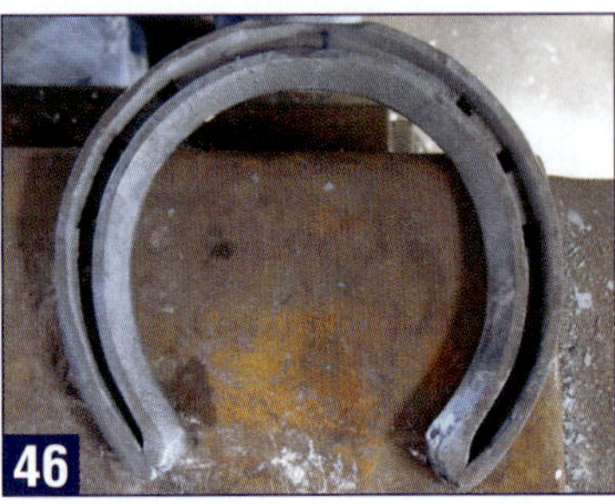
Two-heat clipped shoe off the hammer.

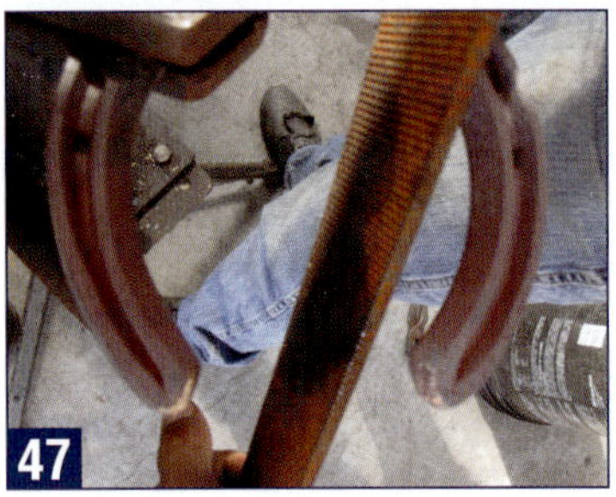
Rasping the shoe.

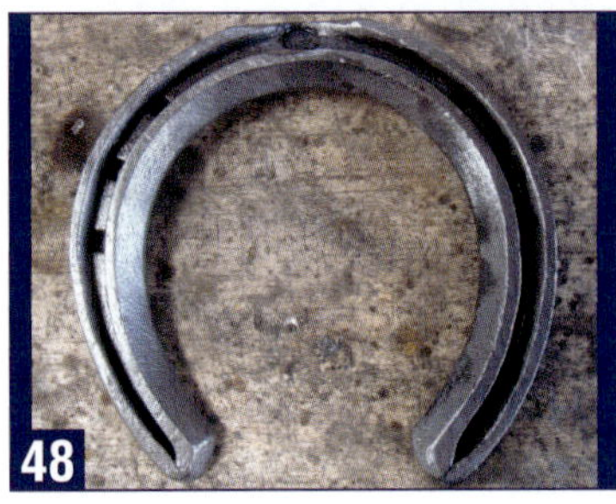
Finished shoe.

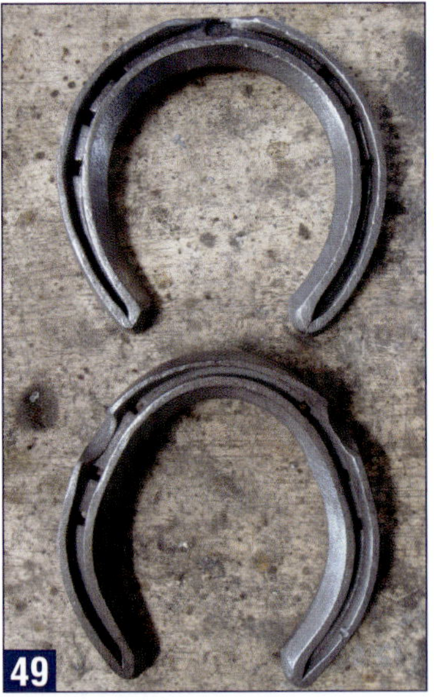
Our finished shoes.

the shoe, he has to be careful when he punches the nail holes since there is a clip in the way **(Figure 43)**. Some of the holes can be pritcheled in the hardy hole **(Figure 44)**, but he has to use the pritchel hole for the toe nail **(Figure 45)**. **Figure 46** is the two-heat shoe off the hammer.

Next he will rasp up the shoe as I did on the previous shoe **(Figure 47)**. A little brushing and you have a shoe like the one in **Figure 48**. **Figure 49** is the shoes we made together.

This is a very efficient and effective way to make a concave shoe. Once you get handy with it, you will be making a pair in 15 minutes or less. Since Cody makes the majority of his shoes at the horse, having an efficient method is crucial. Whatever your method or style, I think you will find that concave bar stock is a fun and easy material to make shoes out of.

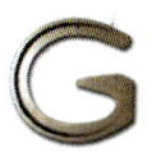

Section

10

Lameness and Pathology

Chapter 43: Lameness 389

Chapter 44: Causes of Lameness.......................... 401

Chapter 45: Pathologies of the Horse's Foot

-1 Abscess 403

-2 Canker.. 413

-3 Club Foot.. 415

-4 Coffin Bone Fractures 418

-5 Corns 422

-6 Cracks 425

-7 Dropped Sole 435

-8 Founder and Laminitis 438

-9 Hoof Avulsion 450

-10 Keratoma 452

-11 Navicular 455

-12 Pedal Osteitis 461

-13 Quarter Cracks 463

-14 Quittor 468

-15 Sheared Heels 470

-16 Sidebone 473

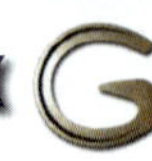

-17 Soft Heel Cracks 477
-18 Sole Bruises 479
-19 Thrush 482
-20 White Line Disease 484

Chapter 46: Pathologies of the Horse's Limb

-1 Bowed Tendons 491
-2 Broken Bones 493
-3 Bucked Shins 495
-4 Capped Hocks and Elbows 496
-5 Carpitis 498
-6 Curb 501
-7 Osselets 503
-8 Radial Nerve Paralysis 505
-9 Ringbone 506
-10 Severed Tendons 511
-11 Spavin 515
-12 Splints 519
-13 Sprained Suspensory Ligament 521
-14 Stifled and Stifle Lameness 524
-15 Stringhalt 526
-16 Thoroughpin 527
-17 Windpuffs 528

" 30 And great multitudes came unto him, having with them those that were lame, blind, dumb, maimed, and many others, and cast them down at Jesus' feet; and he healed them "

—Matthew 15:30
—King James Version

Chapter

43 LAMENESS

To start this chapter, let's define a few of the terms that get thrown around in this industry. Vocabulary is a great place to begin any discussion in farriery, so here it is:

TERMINOLOGY

- **Lameness:** Abnormal gait due to pain.
- **Pathological Shoeing:** Farriery strategies aimed at helping horses with diseased or damaged limbs.
- **Therapeutic Shoeing:** Farriery strategies aimed at preventing a potential injury, or managing chronic lameness issues.
- **Surgical Shoeing:** Farriery related to repairing hooves following surgery.
- **Corrective Shoeing:** Farriery applied to improve the condition of a foot toward an ideal. By this definition, every time a farrier removes a piece of hoof for any reason, it is corrective in nature. If you are not taking the foot toward an ideal, why should the piece of hoof be removed?

As a farrier, you will often be a part of helping a horse recover from lameness. What exactly causes a horse to limp? Lameness itself is basically a change of gait due to pain. A horse will limp for the same reason that you or I would. We are trying to protect an anatomical structure in our bodies that has suffered injury. It is an effort to keep that part from becoming hurt worse that causes the limping. Since horses are not able to speak with words, a good horseman learns to listen to what a horse has to say with body language and behavior. If you are lucky enough to shoe for experienced horse owners, they can be invaluable in helping to determine what is wrong with a given horse. For your part, you have to not only be able to read a horse, you have to distinguish between the owners that know something and those who don't.

Carefully study the common lameness problems that horses face, and you can be a huge asset to the veterinarian-farrier team. A competent vet working with a competent farrier on a horse that is owned by a conscientious owner is the best situation for a hurting animal. Take the responsibility seriously, and build your skills so that you are a valuable part of that team.

There are a series of criteria that must be met before you begin shoeing any lame horse. The first question to answer: Is what you are trying to do anatomically possible? For example, if you have a horse with a fractured coffin bone, it would not be anatomically possible to implant a healthy coffin bone from a donor horse at this time. This may seem like a silly example, but if you stay in this industry long enough, you will find people who apply some silly shoeing strategies based on an ignorance of anatomy.

The next question: Is the procedure financially viable for that particular horse? Some horses have a value that is well beyond what they cost. For these lucky "family member" horses, some owners will spare no expense. Other horses may have a distinct dollar value to their owner, and the shoeing proposed may be worth more than the horse.

I always try to let customers know ahead of time what they are about to spend. If you tell them the cost after the shoeing and they get mad, both parties can be upset. The customer may think you are charging too much, and you will be offended because they are basically telling you that you are not worth what you are charging. Lose–lose situations are never good. By telling them ahead of time, they can make an informed decision about proceeding or look elsewhere.

The last criterion is perhaps the hardest one to determine. It is your ability and skill to do the job. Your personal skill level can be hard to determine for a multitude of reasons, but one reason is that your skills should always be improving. A job that you could not do a month ago may not be any problem now — if you have been practicing your forge work, reading this textbook, or spending some time with a mentor. Avoid making yourself look bad by getting in over your head. Doing so will only make your customers lose faith in you, and the outcome for the horse is not likely to be good.

You will find that the best farriers in the world are very secure in their abilities, and most will willingly help any other farrier that asks. Another fact about these competent farriers is that they are probably not looking for business. Competent farriers usually have more work than they can get done anyway. The fact that they are so busy means you generally won't have to worry about these great farriers taking business from you if you call on them for help with a problem horse.

It seems to me the farriers that won't ever help or show anything to another farrier are usually the ones that can't help or show you much anyway. Keep pushing so that the limits of your skill are always changing for the better.

LAMENESS DIAGNOSTICS

One of the first steps in diagnosing lameness is to gather some historical data. There is a series of questions that I recommend when dealing with a lame horse. Answers to these questions may prove invaluable to arriving at an accurate diagnosis. This is the list I use, but it may not be comprehensive to your situation. If you can think of any additional questions that will help, be sure to add them.

- What is the horse's age?
- What breed is the horse?
- What are its living conditions? (Stall, paddock, large pasture, with other horses, etc.)
- Are any stable mates exhibiting similar symptoms?
- What is the horse used for?
- When did lameness first occur?
- Was there any incident that led to the lameness?
- Was lameness gradual or sudden?
- Has this horse ever had similar lameness issues before?
- Has the feed, stabling, use, or training of this horse recently changed?
- Is the lameness constant or does it fluctuate at certain times of the day or with use?
- Has anything been tried already for this lameness?

Answers to these questions and any other question that occurs to you may lead you in the right direction to help this horse. Be aware of who is present when asking these questions. If you are going with a customer that is looking at buying a horse, the seller may not reveal everything they know. If you ask your questions in front of a trader trying to make a sale, you are likely to be told that the horse was been owned by a little old lady, was always kept inside, and was only ridden to church on Sunday.

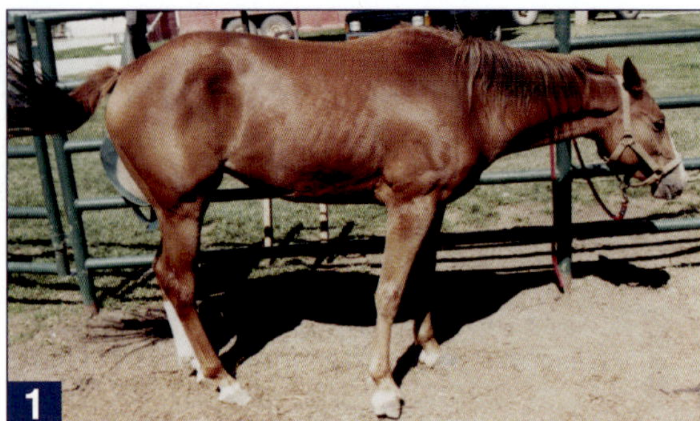

A horse in obvious discomfort.

The next step in the process of diagnosing lameness is to observe the horse at rest. I have to admit that I do not always put the time in for this step that I should. If there are other horses to be shod, I will have the customer tie the lame horse somewhere where I can see it, and look over at the lame horse while I get the other horses shod. If I am there just for the one lame horse, I will have the horse brought out before I begin taking the history, so that I can watch the horse while talking with the customer.

When you are looking at the horse at rest, you are looking for several things. Body language will show you when a horse is in misery. Ears back, wringing tail, squinting, head posture, and other signs can be seen with some practice. Try to determine if a horse is avoiding the use of one limb or another. Look for any asymmetry that you can see in the feet, legs, or musculature. Walk around the horse so you can see it from several angles and try not to jump to conclusions. Sometimes an old blemish will draw your attention, and you may overlook the real lameness issue.

Figures 1-3 are of horses that are in obvious distress. The horse in **Figure 1** has a badly crippled leg that was injured when she was a foal, and the good foot has developed an abscess. You can see by how her back is hunched, her tail is wringing, and the look in her eyes that she cannot get any relief. The horse in **Figure 2** is in a similar state. You can see by how she is leaning to the rear that she is trying to get as much weight off of the front feet as

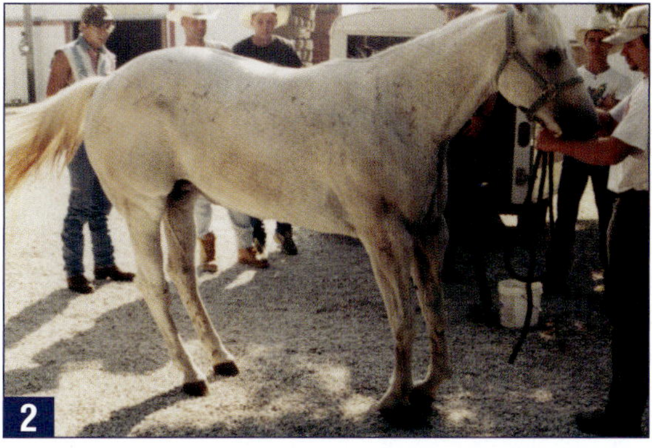

2 *A horse with lameness in both front legs. The tendon contracture is so severe that both legs*

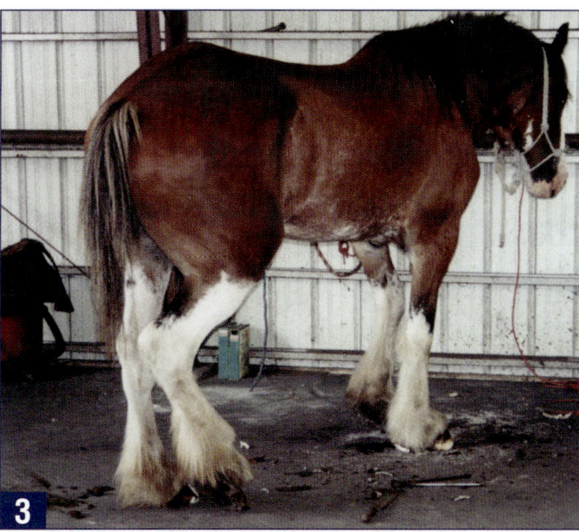

3 *A horse trying to relieve diagonal feet.*

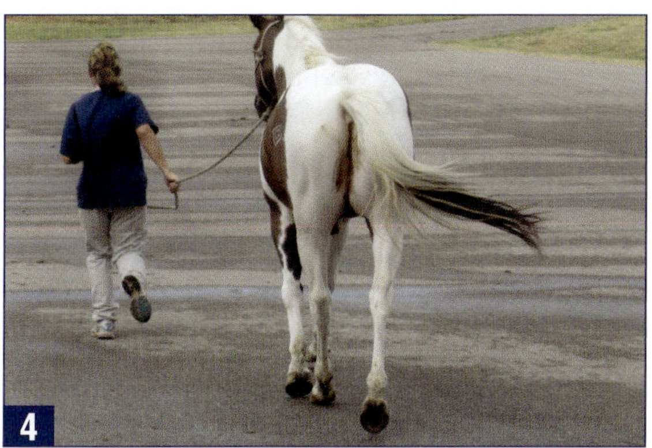

4 *Trotting the horse away.*

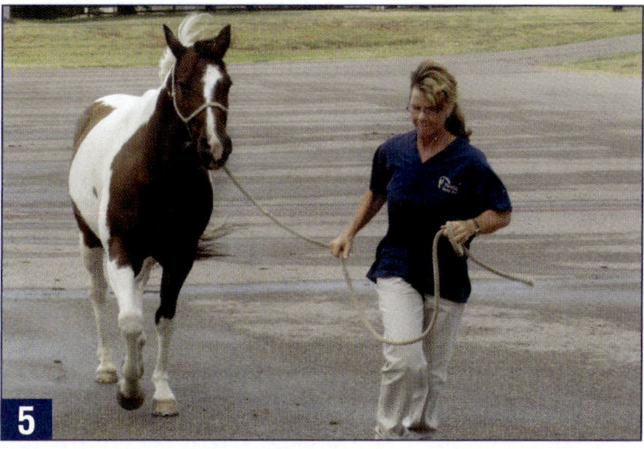

5 *Trotting a horse toward you.*

possible. The Clydesdale in **Figure 3** is attempting to relieve two diagonal feet, although this can only be accomplished for brief periods.

I try not to say too much to an owner at this point, even if I think I know what the problem is. Doing so can be embarrassing when you pick up the foot and find a nail sticking out of the commissure. Be patient and continue with the exam in an orderly fashion.

The next step in the process of diagnosing a lameness is to examine the feet. Start by cleaning the feet. If the horse is barefoot, do some very light knife work to see the sole and frog and look for any obvious hoof conformation abnormalities. The longer you are a blacksmith, the harder it will be to feel temperature differences, but you can feel heat with the inside of your forearm.

The medial and lateral palmar arteries pass over the sesamoids, and you can find a pulse at this point. If a foot has any sort of inflammation or infection, it will have a bounding pulse. While this does not tell you exactly what is going on in a digit, it is a valuable indicator that there is indeed a potential problem below the fetlock of that limb.

After the hooves have been examined, have the owner move the horse. I like to watch a horse at a walk and then at a trot on firm, even footing (**Figures 4-5**). If you will have the horse led in a triangular pattern, you will be able to watch the horse move away from you, from the side, and then back toward you. Horses that are only lame when ridden should be ridden in the tack that is generally used and by the rider that usually rides them. Improperly fitted tack and poor horsemanship can be the cause of many lameness problems that do not present themselves at other times.

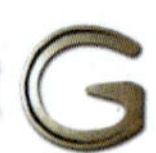

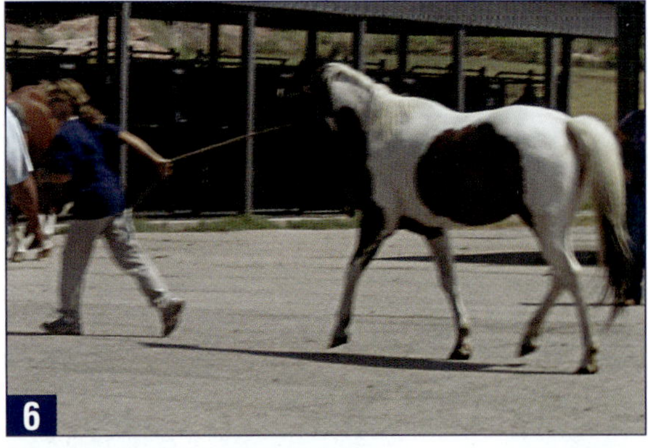

Moving the horse in a circle.

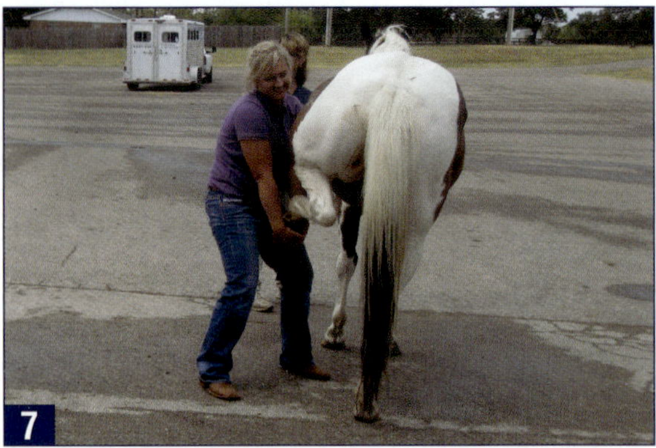

Flexion tests.

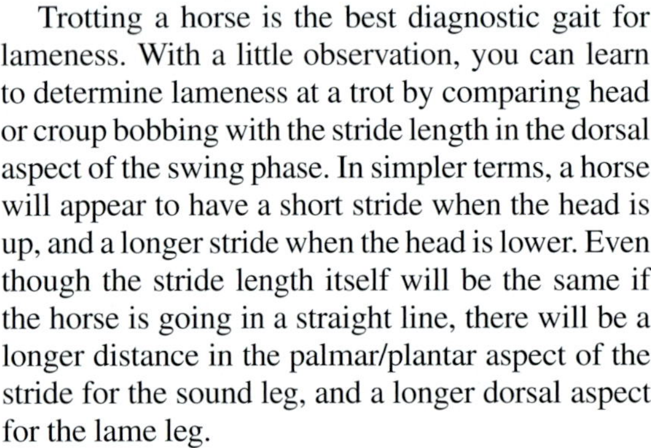

Trotting a horse is the best diagnostic gait for lameness. With a little observation, you can learn to determine lameness at a trot by comparing head or croup bobbing with the stride length in the dorsal aspect of the swing phase. In simpler terms, a horse will appear to have a short stride when the head is up, and a longer stride when the head is lower. Even though the stride length itself will be the same if the horse is going in a straight line, there will be a longer distance in the palmar/plantar aspect of the stride for the sound leg, and a longer dorsal aspect for the lame leg.

Take the example of how you limp right after a horse has smashed your foot. If the hoof lands on your right foot, your foot will hurt the most when it is on the ground, and the least when it is in the air. As you walk, you will stride forward with a long stride on that hurt right foot, but the pain will intensify as it hits the ground. When your body weight gets over the top of the hurt foot, you will bob your head upward in an attempt to lessen the weight, and put your left foot down in a hurry. Your left foot will have traveled as far as your right foot in the air (if you are going in a straight line), but it will look like a shorter stride from a lateral view because you put it down closer to the toe of your right foot in an effort to get some relief. Horses do the same when they have pain in a foot.

Longeing a horse, or working the horse in a round pen, may also show lameness that is not present elsewhere. Working a horse in a circle can also make a subtle lameness more evident. In **Figure 6**, you can see a horse being examined at Oakridge Equine in Edmond, Oklahoma. He has been walked and trotted in the straight and is now being made to go in a circle in opposite directions.

The next step is to do flexion tests on individual joints **(Figure 7)**. Be careful to avoid a false positive, which can occur if a flexion test if done too forcefully. If you over bend any joint with excessive force, you can cause pain that was not present before you bent the joint. Place the joint in question in a flexed position for around 45 seconds. Determine if the horse tenses during this period, or if there are any spasms in the upper limb. Drop the foot, and immediately trot the horse off. The flexion test will often aggravate lameness, and the horse will take several lame steps. Most of the time, the lameness will lessen within 8 to 10 steps and the horse will return to its pre-flexion test condition. On the hind limb, the reciprocal apparatus can make it hard to flex only one joint. The position of your hands is important if you want to flex the fetlock joint more than the hock.

Finally, I like to lead the horse myself and make the horse pivot on the hind legs while the front end is brought around. Think about turning a horse at the end of a narrow alley. If the horse will not cross the near front foot over the off front foot when turned to the right (and vice versa going left), then I will be suspicious of the planted foot. For instance, a horse moving to the right in this manner will lift the near front foot and place it beyond the off front. If the horse is unwilling to do this, the lameness will often present in the off front foot.

After seeing the horse in motion, it is time to re-examine the feet. Use hoof testers to find the area of the foot that is in the most pain. I will generally begin this part of the exam by using the hoof testers on the sound foot. By testing the sound foot first, you can get a determination of how the horse is going to react to hoof testers. There is a lot of

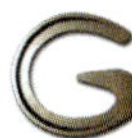

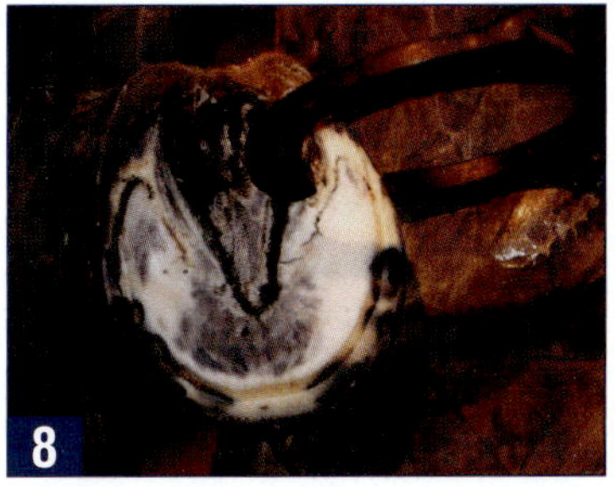

Hoof testers starting on one heel.

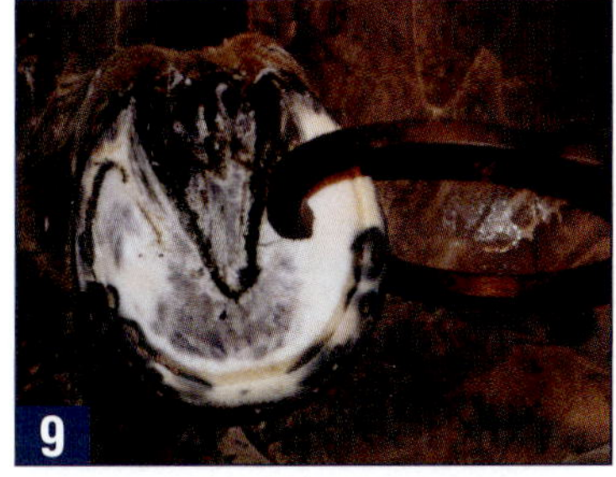

Moving around the quarter.

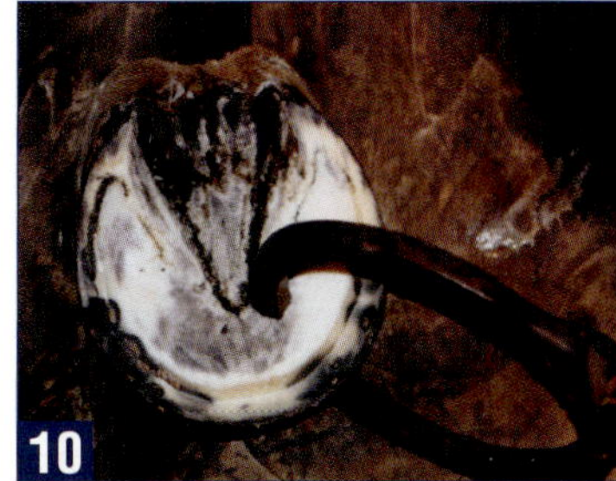

Toe quarter.

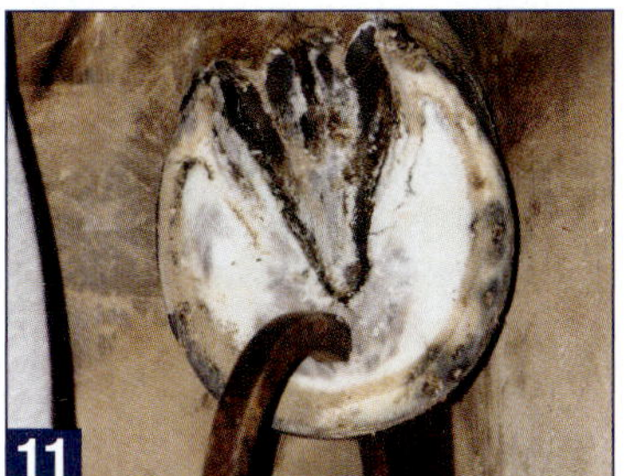

Toe.

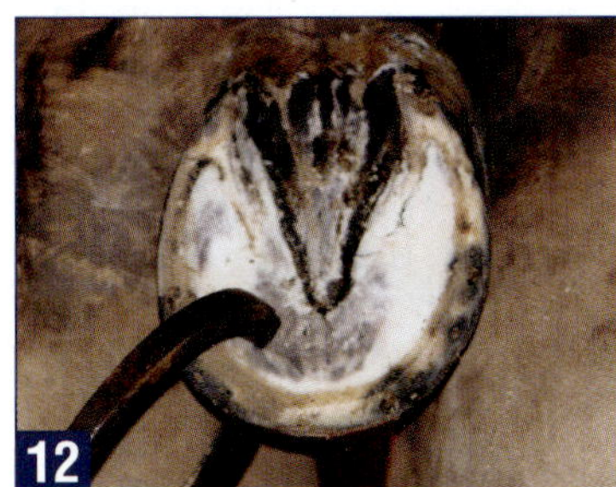

Toe quarter.

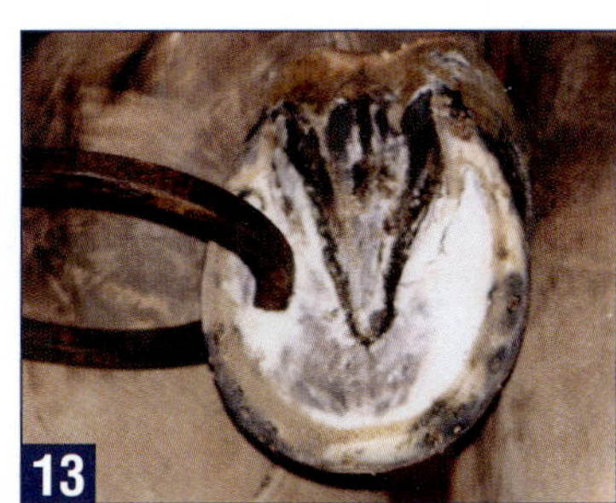

Quarter.

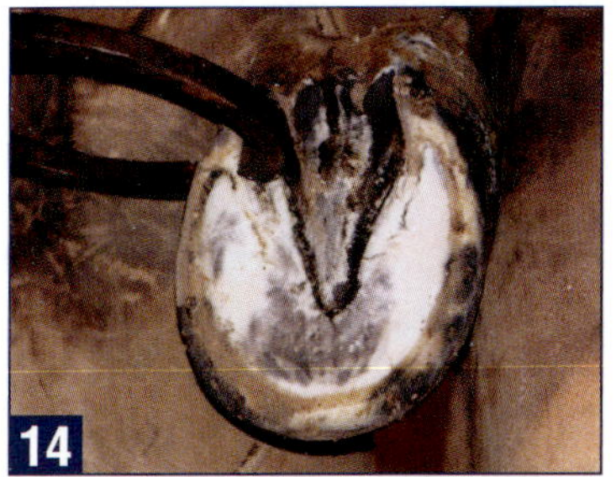

Heel.

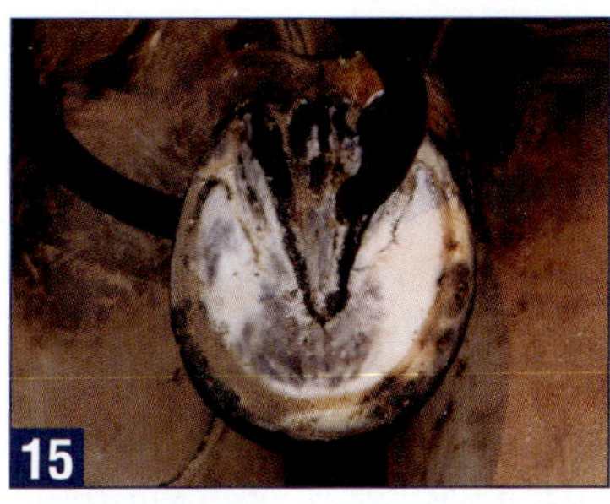

From one side of the frog to the opposite wall.

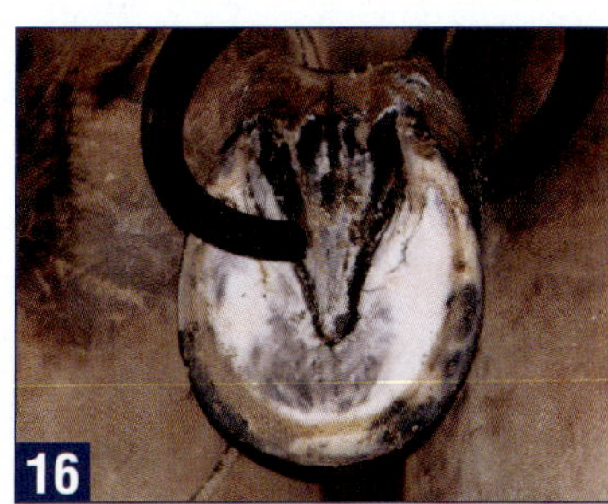

Repeat the last step on the other side.

leverage that can be applied with hoof testers, so even a sound horse can be made to flinch if the testers are used incorrectly. I like to use both hands, and move around the foot in a methodical manner. Start at one heel with one jaw of the testers on the bar and the other jaw on the outside of the hoof wall, about an inch from the bottom of the foot. Squeeze and release, being aware of any sign the horse may give you that it is in pain. Move forward the thickness of the jaw and repeat. Do this around the entire foot. Then place the jaw on the medial side of the frog at the widest part of the foot, and other jaw on the lateral side of the hoof wall at the widest point, about a half-inch below the coronary band. Squeeze there, and then move to the lateral side of the frog and medial side of the hoof wall. These last two positions are the ones most commonly used to determine navicular pain, but it is important to have the jaw on the wall close to the coronary band if you are going to affect the navicular region at all. **Figures 8-17** show the general method for using hoof testers around a foot. They can be used with shoes on **(Figures 18-19)**, but shoes add stability and strength to a foot, so they may make it harder to get a good reading with the hoof testers.

After I have a base line for how the horse will react to hoof testers on a sound foot, I will move to the lame foot and repeat the process. If all goes

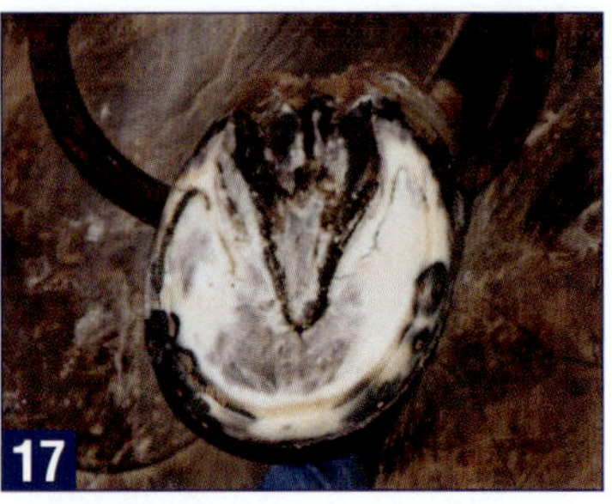

Across the heels.

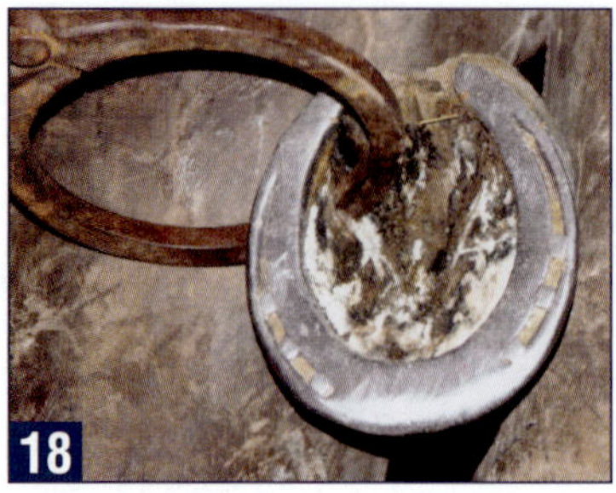

Hoof testers on a shod foot.

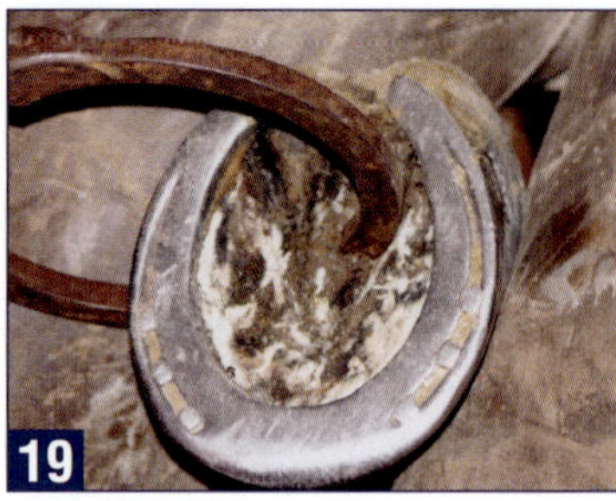

Hoof testers in use.

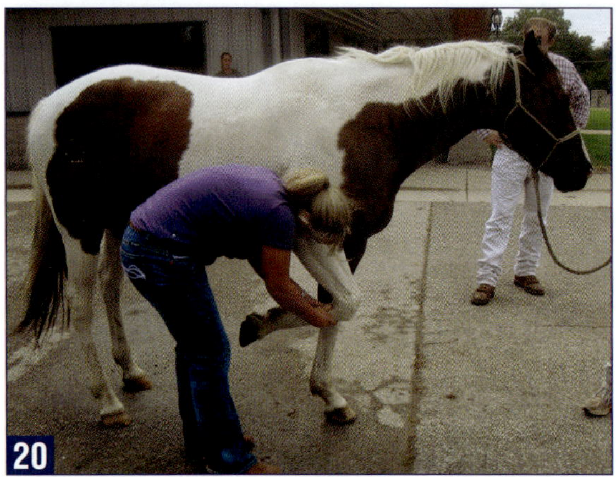

Examining the leg.

well, you will find what you are looking for when the horse exhibits more pain in one area of the hoof than another.

Be aware that some horses are hard to shoe and jump around all the time. This can make it hard to interpret a flinch from the pressure of hoof testers. By the same token, some horses are so well trained that they do not react as much as you would expect for the injury they are dealing with. This is where your ability to read an individual horse will come in handy.

Once the feet have been carefully examined and the hoof testers have been used, it is time to examine the rest of the limb. Run your hands up and down all the limbs and palpate any area that may seem swollen. Feel for any asymmetry and inflammation. Pick up the feet and move the limb through a range of motion. Be careful to avoid being too rough at this stage, since most horses will have pain if their joints are aggressively bent **(Figure 20)**.

Once you are done with the exam, be certain of your diagnosis before expressing an opinion. I am very careful to remind the customer that I am not a vet and what I am telling them is only my opinion. Since we live in a rural area, there are many times when decisions must be made on a horse without the advice of a vet. This is not legal in some parts of the world, but it is fairly common in the United States. If at all possible, you should try to find a competent vet that you respect.

One item I tried to always bear in mind is that it is better to paint a less favorable picture than a favorable one. I have seen horses that appeared to have a very slight problem. Experience would have led most to claim that the horse would be fine in no time, only to have the horse get worse and have to be put down. When something like this happens, the farrier loses. The owner's hopes are up, only to be smashed; and the farrier was obviously no good, or the horse would have been saved.

If, on the other hand, the farrier would have said that the horse was certain to have complications, then the farrier turns out to be very intuitive when complications arise. If the horse recovers, then the farrier is an outstanding practitioner, because the horse was saved against all odds. This is something to think about.

As a farrier, you have to be very careful with diagnosing any lameness. You can identify a lameness and act as an extremely important advisor and member of a vet-farrier-owner team that is working to get the horse sound, but there is a line you have to be careful not to cross. As you gain experience, you will also gain respect from the vet and equine community. Sometimes, you may be in situations where you are asked to do things that are in the veterinarian's realm. The rule of thumb to remember when dealing with somebody else's animal is that voluntarily entering the sensitive structures without a license to practice veterinarian medicine is against the law in the United States.

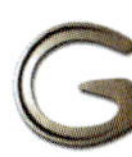

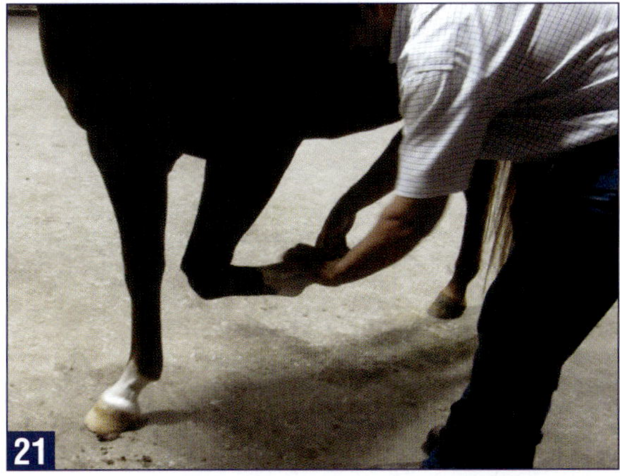

Dr. Lamb administering the palmar digital nerve block.

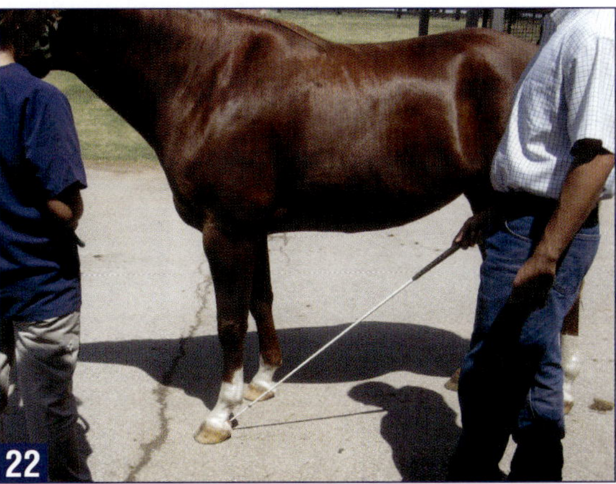

Testing for sensitivity after the nerve block.

This includes giving shots, and technically, cutting abscesses out of feet.

I have always followed my instinct when it came to working on the border of the vet-farrier realms. If a customer makes me feel even slightly uncomfortable, I will not go beyond the strict definition of my farrier duties. On the other hand, some customers would rather have a farrier go after an abscess than a veterinarian, and with those whom I am comfortable with, that is what I do. I'm not recommending that you do this, I'm just telling you how I handle it. And by the way, anytime I dealt with a customer who told me about suing anyone for any reason, I would get that customer off the books immediately.

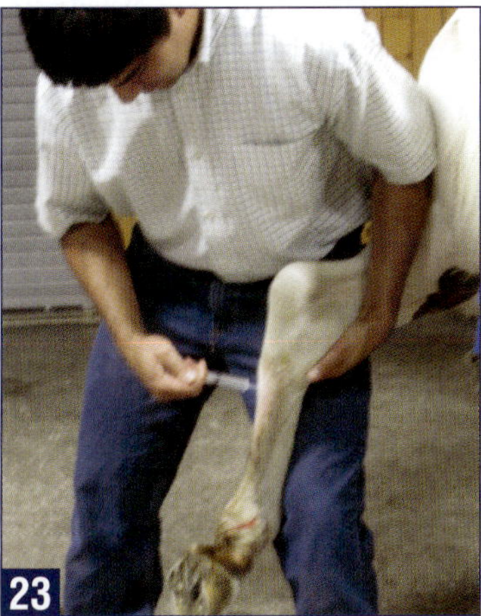

Dr. Lamb placing a nerve block higher up the leg.

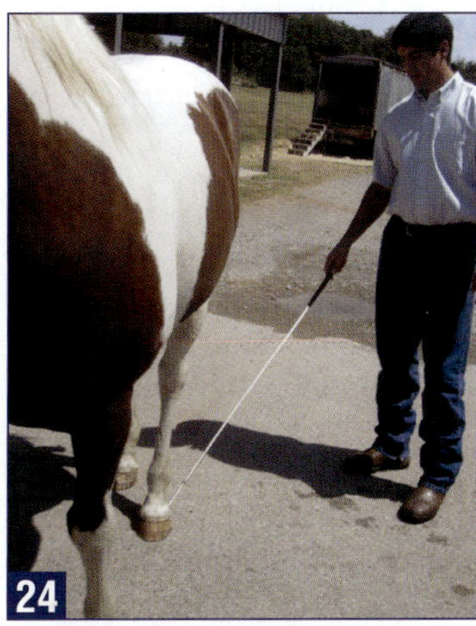

Testing for sensitivity.

There are a lot of things that a vet can legally do that the layman — including farriers — cannot. Here is a partial list with a brief description so that you can be familiar with some of the techniques that are common in identifying the location of lameness.

Regional Anesthesia: A technique of deadening a portion of the limb to determine if the horse will be sound when there is no sensation in an area. This is one of the best tools that a vet has to really pinpoint an area of pain, but it can be time consuming to do correctly. Most of the time, the vet will begin with a distal palmar digital nerve block (plantar on the hind limb), and wait a few minutes before moving the horse to see if lameness subsides. If the horse becomes sound, the pain is in the palmar aspect of the foot (caudal heel pain). If not, the vet will continue with the next block. In **Figure 21**, you can see Dr. Lamb of Oakridge Equine putting the palmar digital nerve block in.

Once the nerve block has had time to work, the vet will check the block by poking the foot to see if the horse reacts to the sensation. This allows the vet to be certain of where exactly the nerve block is working and where it is not **(Figure 22)**.

The next blocks will generally be above the bifurcation of the digital nerves to deaden everything from the fetlock down. If the horse becomes sound, then it is likely the lameness is from pain in the pastern region. If the horse is still lame, the vet

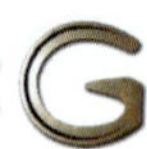

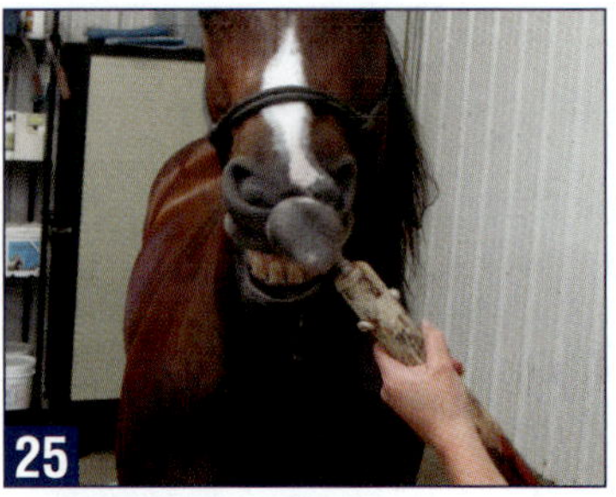
Applying a twitch.

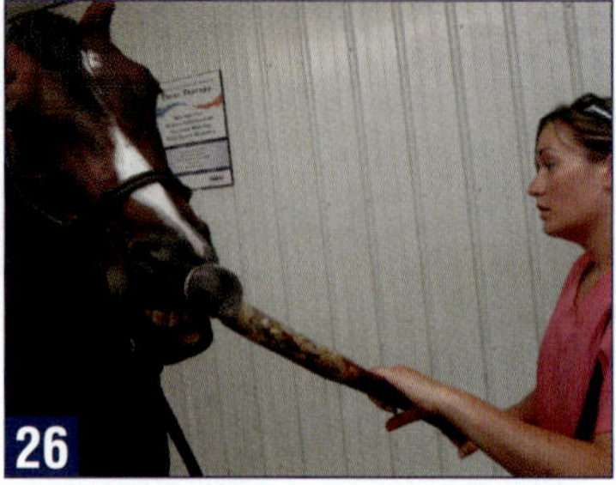
Applying a twitch.

Most blocks can last one to two hours; do not let an injured animal injure itself further by using a damaged limb that should be rested. Since the horse will feel no pain for a time, it may do a lot of damage to itself if not confined.

A quick note here: It is customary to twitch a horse to administer a nerve block (**Figures 25-26**). When the leg is first penetrated with a needle, a lot of horses will react by stomping or kicking, which may cause injury to the vet doing the work. When you see the twitch being applied, don't be concerned. It is the safest way to accomplish the task.

will continue proximal to just below the knee or hock. This process can take a long time and requires a vet with a good technique to make certain that the horse is injected in the exactly right spot (**Figures 23-24**).

Ultrasound: A technique that uses ultra-high-

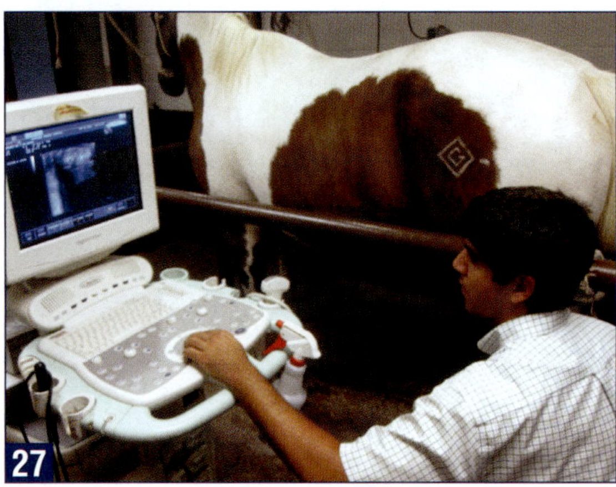
Dr. Lamb using the ultrasound machine at Oakridge Equine.

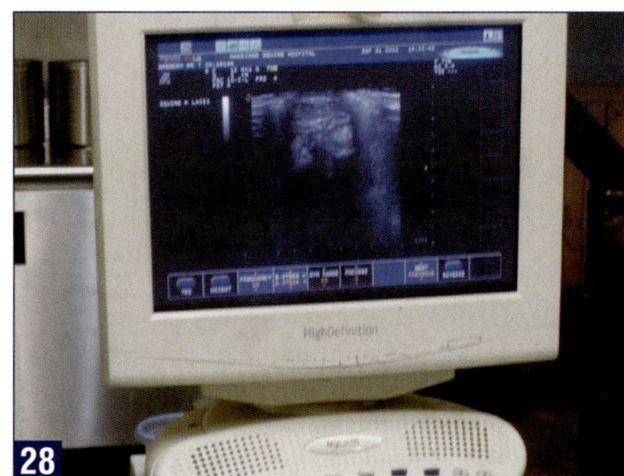
Ultrasound display.

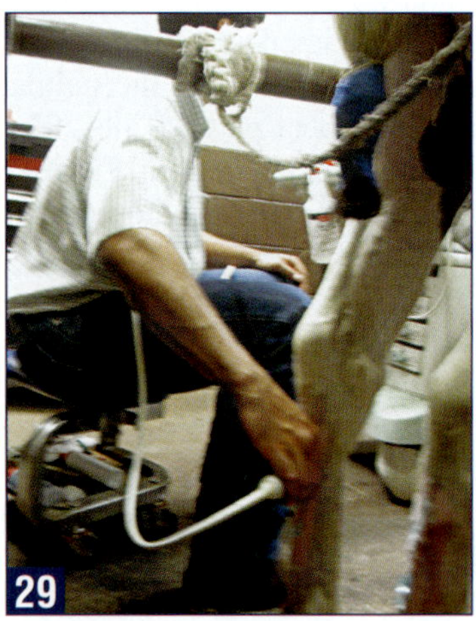
Looking for lesions and damage with the ultrasound.

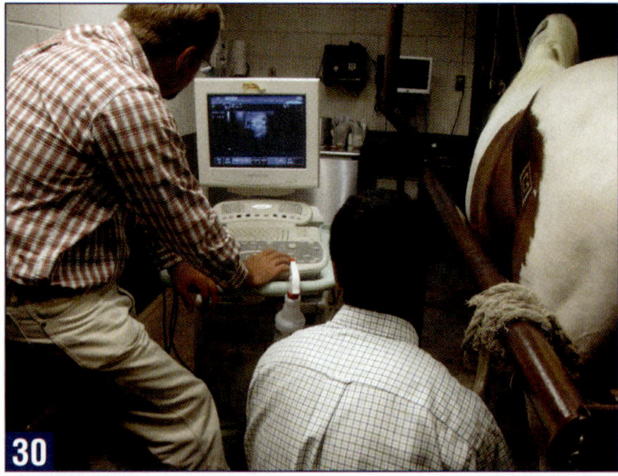
Dr. Zubrod looking at the ultrasound with Dr. Lamb.

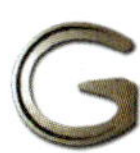

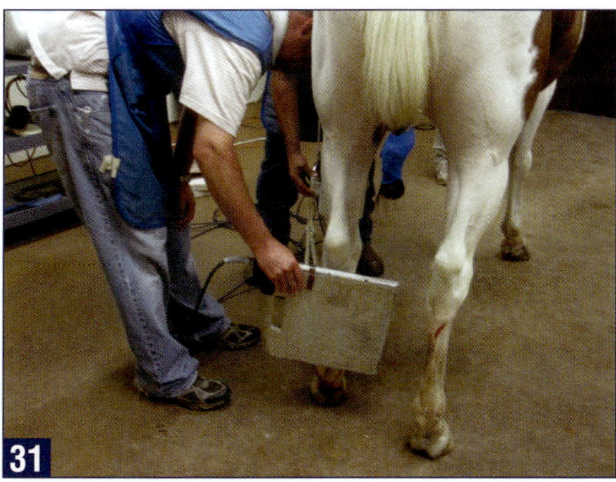

31

Radiographs being taken.

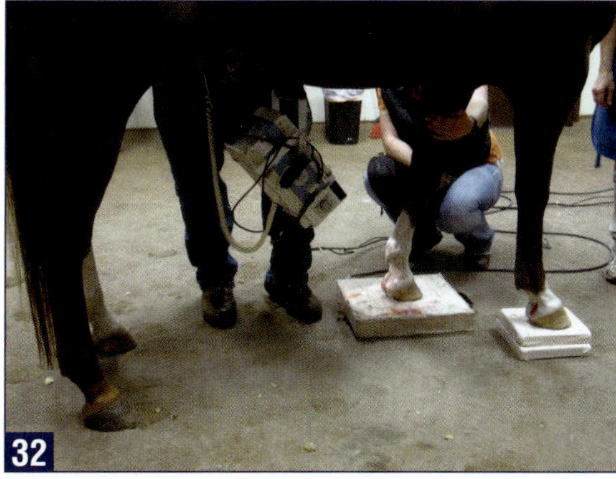

32

Good technique is essential in taking radiographs.

frequency sound waves to examine soft tissue **(Figures 27-30)**. A probe with a vibrating crystal in it emits the waves through the soft tissue, and some of the waves are reflected or echoed back. The main goal of ultrasound is to determine the density of different soft tissues to find any abnormality that may indicate the reason for a lameness issue. Artifacts are common, so any suspected areas of interest should be looked at from several different views to be certain that the lesion is indeed real.

Interpreting the results from an ultrasound takes experience and a high level of anatomical knowledge. In my experience, the method can be very useful in determining how well a problem is healing as well as being a good additional diagnostic resource when used with other techniques.

Radiography: Commonly called an X-ray, a radiograph is an image that is produced by passing gamma rays through an object. The resulting picture **(Figures 31-33)** is an indication of the density of the object being X-rayed. The denser an object — for instance, bone — the whiter the image. This makes X-rays less useful for soft tissue lesions, but very useful for seeing bone changes or abnormalities.

The image is basically an indication of how many gamma rays were able to make it to the film. Bone will block a lot of the rays, so the film behind bones stays white. Air will block none of them, so the film where the rays pass through air is black, or exposed. The middle of the cannon bone is hollow (medullary cavity), so it shows up with less white than the cortex around it. When bones are broken, have osteophytes, or any other potential density changes, those changes can often be seen with a radiograph.

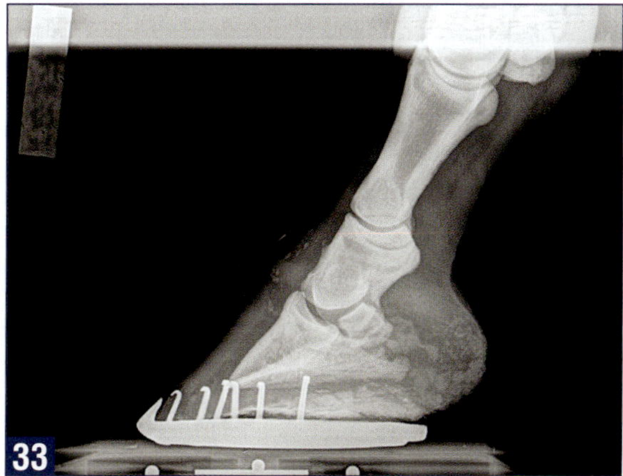

33

Radiograph.

Good technique is a must with radiographs. The feet must be cleaned and the horse must hold still, as must the technician taking the image and the one holding the film. Everyone in the area should be protected from radiation with the proper lead vests and gloves.

Radiographs are common enough that most farriers will look at quite a few during their careers. If you know anatomy, you can be a big asset in determining what is being looked at and how best to treat it.

Nuclear Scintigraphy: This is commonly called a bone scan and is a process that involves injecting radioactive particles intravenously, then measuring their uptake in the tissue. The uptake is determined by using a gamma camera.

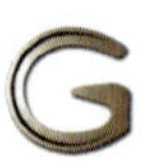

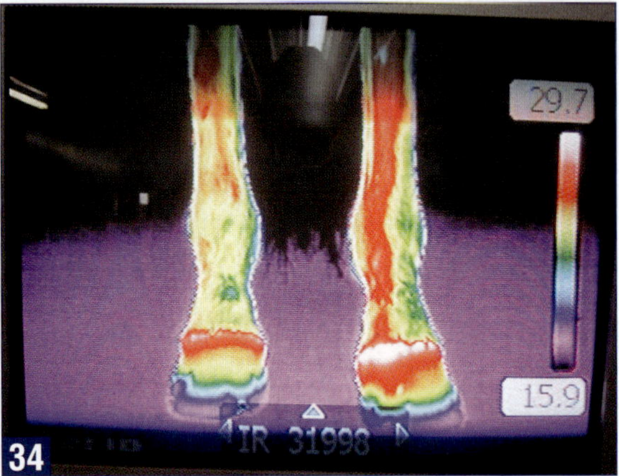

34 *Picture of a thermography camera image.*

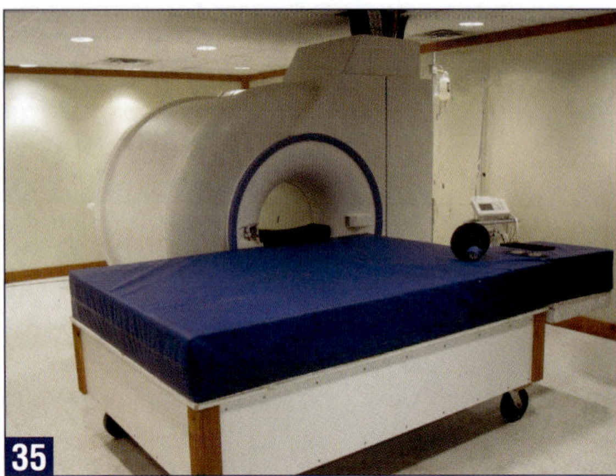

35 *The equine MRI at Oakridge Equine.*

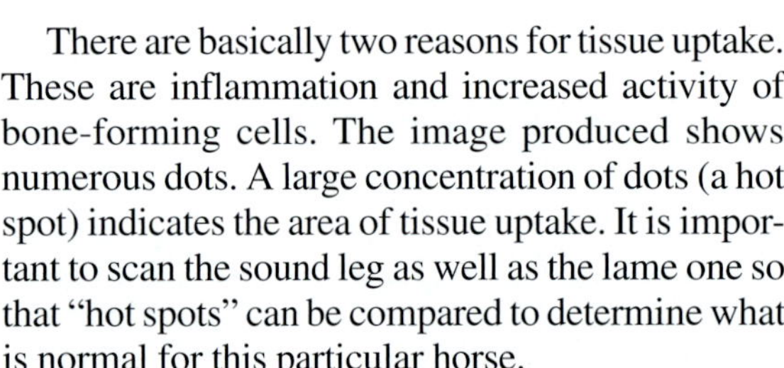

There are basically two reasons for tissue uptake. These are inflammation and increased activity of bone-forming cells. The image produced shows numerous dots. A large concentration of dots (a hot spot) indicates the area of tissue uptake. It is important to scan the sound leg as well as the lame one so that "hot spots" can be compared to determine what is normal for this particular horse.

This technique can often find problems before a radiograph and is a good method for finding multiple lesions and identifying pain. However, it does not give detailed information about the lesion, only that there is an abundance of blood flow or cell activity present in an area.

It is costly and time consuming, and there are a lot of regulations regarding the handling of the equipment as well as the handling of the horse once the procedure has been done. This is going to be found mainly at universities.

Arthrocentisis: This is the collection of synovial fluid, often called a joint tap. Synovial fluid can be collected for analysis to determine if there is any joint damage, infection, or inflammation. Collection should be done in the most sterile way possible to prevent introducing infection in to the joint.

The color of the fluid, its texture, and whether it forms a clot are all things a trained person can determine without a lab report. The lab will be looking for bacteria, white blood cells, and protein as well as the viscosity of the synovial fluid.

Thermography (Figure 34): This is the detection of small changes in heat caused by an increased blood flow to an area. If a horse has an inflammation, thermography can often find it quickly, allowing for earlier treatment. As with many of the tools veterinarians use, the skill of the interpreter is important.

Magnetic Resonance Imaging (MRI): MRI **(Figures 35-37)** is becoming a common diagnostic tool in human medicine, but for horses, it requires general anesthesia as well as quite a bit of equipment. MRIs will give you more information about a potential soft tissue problem than you can get from other diagnostic equipment. However, it is expensive and only available in a few of the larger and more modern clinics.

These are several of the more common diagnostic tools available to the modern veterinarian. Learn enough about each so that you can understand how each works to help you and the vet help the horse.

Lameness Grades: Most vets that I have worked with use a numbered grading system to describe the amount of pain that a horse is exhibiting. One system is called the Obel Lameness Grades, based on the work of Dr. Niles Obel in the late 1940s, and the modern system is the American Association of Equine Practitioners (AAEP) Lameness Scale. Here are those two systems:

OBEL LAMENESS GRADES

- **Grade 1:** At rest the horse will alternately and incessantly lift the feet. Lameness is not evident at a walk but a short stilted gait is noted at a trot.
- **Grade 2:** Horses move willingly at a walk, but the gait is stilted. A foot can be lifted off the

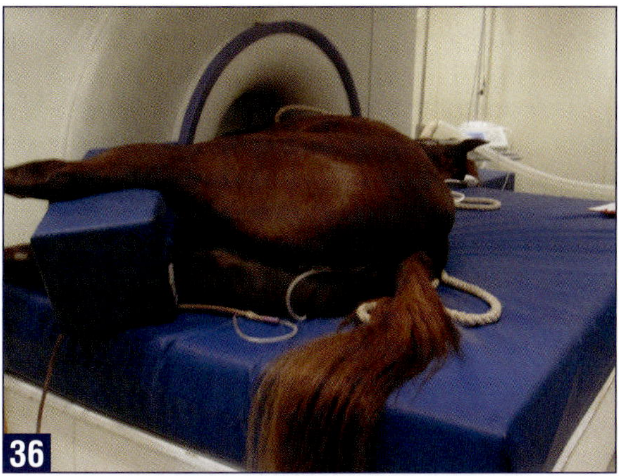

A horse with its leg in the MRI machine.

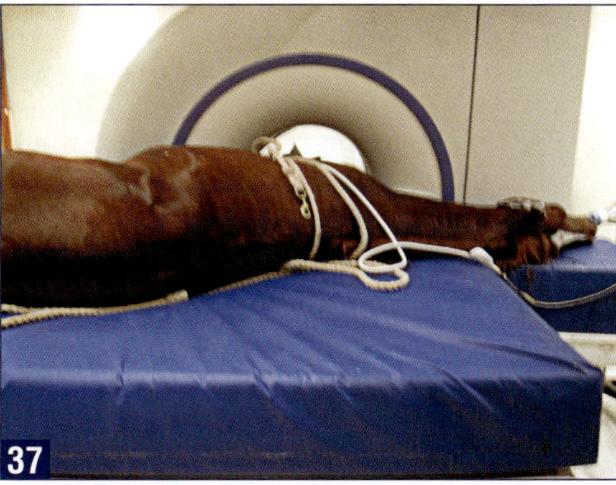

MRIs are particularly helpful in diagnosing soft-tissue injuries.

ground without difficulty.

- **Grade 3:** The horse moves reluctantly and vigorously resists attempts to have a foot lifted.
- **Grade 4:** The horse refuses to move and will not do so unless forced.

AAEP LAMENESS SCALE

- **0:** Lameness not perceptible under any circumstances.
- **1:** Lameness is difficult to observe and is not consistently apparent, regardless of circumstances (eg, weight carrying, circling, inclines, hard surfaces, etc.)
- **2:** Lameness is difficult to observe at a walk or when trotting in a strait line but consistently apparent under certain circumstances (eg, weight carrying, circling, inclines, hard surfaces, etc.)
- **3:** Lameness is consistently observable at a trot under all circumstances.
- **4:** Lameness is obvious at a walk.
- **5:** Lameness produces minimal weight bearing in motion and/or at rest or a complete inability to move.

Once a diagnosis has been reached, it is time to advise the client on how to deal with the problem. I like to use the acronym DRASTA to categorize each part of a problem so that I remember every aspect that I am supposed to tell the customer about.

The acronym DRASTA stands for:

- Definition
- Reason
- Anatomy
- Symptoms
- Treatment: Farrier, veterinarian, owner
- Anticipated outcome

This is a simple adaptation of the British system that used the acronym DACCT. That is a great system, but I changed it to suit my purpose of teaching. I always felt that an added category for anticipated outcome was a good addition, and I like to divide the treatment options between the farrier, vet and owner. There are many instances in the text where I do not completely cover the veterinarian options, since this book is mainly aimed at farriery. Besides, one of the remnants of my time with the military makes me like an acronym that makes a word that can be pronounced.

Once you have a diagnosis, the next step is to determine in which direction you want to go to achieve good results for the horse. Keep your goal realistic, especially when dealing with a customer. Be certain that you discuss what the intended long-term use of this horse is so that all parties involved have realistic expectations.

The four main categories that pathological shoeing principles fall into are:

- **Support:** This is achieved by placing the platform (shoe) for the bony column in such a way that the forces on injured structures are minimized. A good example would be using an egg bar shoe on a horse with a bowed tendon.
- **Foot Load Transfer:** When a foot has an injury in a specific area, shoeing can be aimed at relieving stress on one portion of the foot and making another part of the foot take up the slack. The heart bar is one of the best examples

of a shoe that will transfer load from one area of the foot to another, taking stress from the wall and placing it on the frog.

- **Protect:** Protecting a damaged foot would entail putting a shoe or foot covering on the foot to prevent damage from the environment. Examples would be pads, hospital plates, or even wide-webbed shoes.
- **Angle/Balance Change:** Changing the angle of the foot will alter the hoof-pastern angle. With many suspensory related lameness issues, changing the angle of the hoof will change the stress on individual tendons or ligaments. For example, if you have a horse with pain in the deep flexor tendon, increasing the angle of the hoof can alleviate some of the stress on the deep flexor tendon. Making a change to the mediolateral balance will have an impact on how and where the foot loads, and may affect how it lands as well as how the bones are stressed and the joints are loaded.

MOVING THE STONE

There is an old saying that Jeff Houston, a good friend of mine, shared with me. "You can get used to anything except for a stone in your shoe." If you've ever had to deal with a stone in your shoe and were unable to do anything about it, you'll probably agree it's a pretty apt saying.

I often compare shoeing lame horses with moving the stone in my shoe. If there is a rock in the heel of my shoe, and I have to live with it for a time, I become quite lame after a while from the pressure from that stone. At some point, I'll shake my boot and get the rock to move to the toe of my boot. I still have a rock in my shoe, but I feel so much better because it is in an area that is not already sore. The relief is so great that I actually look sound for a time, until my foot gets sore from having a rock in the toe of my boot. Shoeing lame horses can be like this.

Sometimes you will shoe a crippled horse, and they will immediately go sound: Limp in-leap out. Of course you feel like a hero, and the customer is pleased. If this happens while you are doing a clinic, you look really good in front of the crowd. However, the horse may slowly become lame again, because there is still a problem. At first, the stress on the foot has been changed so that the foot is relieved and the lameness — temporarily — vanishes. In other words, the shoeing has only moved the rock from the heel of the shoe to the toe.

This is an important concept to understand when shoeing lame horses. It tells you why very different theories of shoeing can work from shoeing period to shoeing period on the same horse. I find that sometimes by simply changing the style of shoe on a horse every few shoeing cycles — say shoeing with an egg-bar shoe, then moving on to an onion-heel shoe — I can keep a horse more comfortable.

This anecdote also explains why some really crazy theories of shoeing can realize short-term success. I have been to clinics where the clinician will shoe the horse with some sort of contraption that should not work. Yet, the horse looks better right away. I have made it a point to follow up on a few of those clinics, and it turns out that a lot of the horses will become lame again. A change at that point may make the horse feel better again for a while. A good rule of thumb is to not use anything on a foot that you don't fully understand or that looks crazy. There are a lot of products on the market that allow some guys to use stuff that they don't have the skill to use. As I explained this to Dr. Marcotte, "If you hand a gun to a 5-year-old, you can't be surprised when someone gets shot".

A friend of mine, Phil Fisher, CJF, told me about a horse with navicular syndromw that he had in his practice when he was a young farrier. He would stand that horse up when he shod it, it would do well for a while, and then when it got sore, the customer would take it to another farrier. This other farrier would chop off the heel, and the horse would be sound again for a while. Once it got sore again, the customer would bring it back to Phil and he would stand it up again. He said this happened many times over the career of this horse, and the back and forth kept the horse going for many years.

Keep this in mind when shoeing lame horses, and understand what is happening when they go good or bad. Try to apply good basics in all your shoeing and stay within the principles of anatomy, physiology and biomechanics that you understand. If you are nailing on a shoe that you cannot explain, you are exposing yourself to all sorts of problems. Study anatomy diligently so that you can make a decision about shoeing that makes good, anatomical sense. You will find that superior anatomical knowledge leads you further in the direction of basic shoeing than it does in the direction of space-age apparatuses.

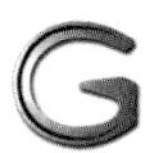

Chapter

44 CAUSES OF LAMENESS

A horse can become lame and sore for a multitude of reasons. A large part of good diagnosis is to determine cause.

The most frequent causes are going to fall under these categories:

- Genetics
- Environment, including feed, injury, and neglect
- Shoeing/trimming
- Occupation

GENETICS

It is unfortunate, but too often, horses are bred for the wrong reasons. Breeding for color or head size or other traits that are only aesthetic but ridiculous, has led too often to horses that have conformations that predispose them to lameness. A pretty paint horse with calf knees and tiny feet is only a pasture ornament. Another thing that happens is that the horses that are too lame to be used are the ones that get bred. I have seen many cases where a mare had some genetic problem that prevented her from being usable, which put her in the category of brood stock. This is irresponsible, yet it happens a lot.

ENVIRONMENT

Horses do not come with owner' manuals, although they should. It is not a wonder when a horse that is not fed or watered has problems. There are some things that are unavoidable, and it has always surprised me how there are horses in the best settings that have the worst injuries, while others are turned out in a minefield stay safe.

I have a wonderful customer of over 20 years by the name of Tanya Haubein. She is a horseman's horseman and has a degree in equine husbandry. Tanya had a really nice mare in a pipe corral that had held many horses before and since. This mare was feeling frisky, and she kicked and bucked, fell against the pipe, and broke her back. It is one of the safest horse environments you can have, yet the horse still got hurt.

By the same token, we see horses that live in a junkyard of old farm equipment, surrounded by low-lying barbed wire fences, and they are not injured nearly as often as you would expect.

Some customers do not understand the maintenance that comes with horse owning. As a farrier, it is important that you help these folks in a respectful and kind manner. They already feel like outsiders, and if you are being helpful now, it will pay dividends later. Horses that have regular foot care are more likely to stay comfortable and sound, and you may have to let the customer know that regular foot care means at least every 8 weeks.

SHOEING AND TRIMMING

Here is a big one. Way too often, poor and ignorant horseshoers are the cause of lameness. As a horseshoer, you will get blamed for some problems that you are innocent of. But there is a good reason this happens. It happens because so many bad shoers have given the trade a bad name, and the first thing a person with a lame horse is going to think is that the last person to work on the feet is at fault. Just remember what it was like to be a consumer instead of a farrier.

In the short term, if lameness happens more than about 10 days from shoeing, the farrier is probably not at fault. In fact, 10 days is a stretch. More likely, acute lameness from shoeing is going to present within the first 48 hours, if not immediately. Issues such as close nails, sole pressure, quicks, imbalance, short-shoeing, and drastic change can fall within the farrier's realm of responsibility, and some of these can cause long-term problems. However, many things that you will be blamed for are not your fault (and occasionally some of the good you get credit for is due to reasons beyond your control as well).

I have a good friend named Dr. John Marcotte, a veterinarian, who provided several of the radiographs for this book. He contends that mediolateral balance is a huge contributor to lameness, yet is often overlooked. Since the advent of digital X-rays and some of the software that goes with it, it is possible to see the bones and joints in a whole new way. There are quite a few feet in which a radiograph shows that the coffin bone is not level, although the foot appears level externally. This is abnormal anatomy since the coffin bone should be balanced within the foot in the normal horse, but it brings up some interesting concerns.

OCCUPATION

Once you begin to shoe horses in an area, it is quite likely that you will start to have more customers in one equine discipline than another. Pretty soon, you may find that you shoe 90% jumpers, while only 10% of your clientele is made up of mixed disciplines. Once you reach that stage, you will start to see lameness that is associated with that type of horse use. In my case, I see a lot of hock problems, navicular problems, and some suspensory apparatus problems. This is due to the fact that I am shoeing more cutting and rodeo horses than anything else.

With the school, we get to see a lot of problems like founder, thrush, and abscesses. Again, it goes hand-in-hand with the type of horse and clientele that you service. With some experience, you will begin to notice trends, and you will become good at shoeing horses that fall into those categories.

A quick thought on this subject: Every time you read an article in a trade journal about shoeing, take into account the experience of the author in respect to the type of horses they shoe. An article about racehorses in England is not going to have a lot in common with an article about roping horses in the United States. Since that farrier sees problems that are related to that type of horse, you have to be aware that a lot of the observations come from the job that horse does.

While this is only one piece of the puzzle when it comes to understanding what makes any individual horse limp, it is an important piece. Take the time to carefully consider some of these points when you are dealing with a lame horse. There are things that can be fixed, and things that can't. Knowing the difference will help you help the horse.

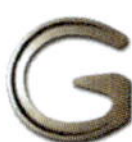

Chapter

45-1 ABSCESS

DEFINITION

An abscess is a cavity filled with pus and necrotic (dead) tissue. The farrier's concern is an abscess or infection inside the hoof capsule.

REASON

An abscess occurs because bacteria have penetrated the horny (epidermal) regions of the hoof, invading the sensitive (dermal) portion of the foot. Bacteria thrive in areas with damaged tissue and poor blood supply. Bacteria can enter through various routes. Often, the horse has had a wound such as a nail quick, sole quick, or rock puncture. A large entry point may also become a good drainage point. Drainage prevents the severe pain that is associated with abscesses.

A bruise or area of sole pressure can turn into an abscess, and cracks in the hoof wall can also become an entry point for the bacteria that causes them. With bruising, there will be stagnant blood in an area, and with that blood, there will also be blood serum, a favorite food supply for bacteria. All it takes is the smallest fissure — to allow the bacteria access to the bruised area — for a bruise to become an abscess.

In **Figure 1**, you can see a foot in which a rock had been trapped under the shoe. That can lead to some bad bruising, which can easily become an abscess. **Figure 2** is a foundered horse with some sole bruising. This is common with founder, and the cavity made between the wall and coffin bone, as well as the sole bruising, often lead to abscesses. The foot in **Figure 3** has some unusual cavities in the toe area, but they did not end up becoming infected. The lack of black material or discharge and no lameness indicates that there is not an abscess.

Large entry points allow easy drainage, so the feet in **Figures 4-5**

1

Rock lodged in foot under the shoe.

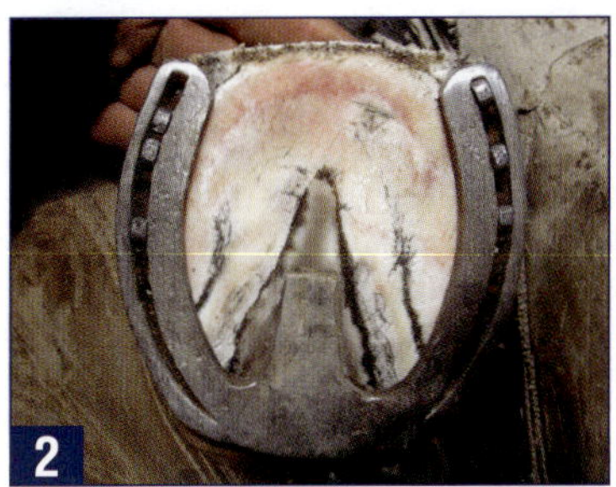

Bruising is evident at the toe of a foundered horse.

3

Unusual cavities in the toe of a foot that are not infected.

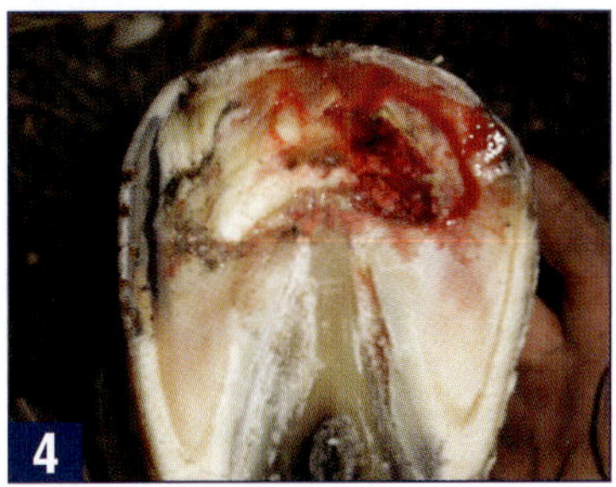

Large area of bleeding in the sole of a foundered horse.

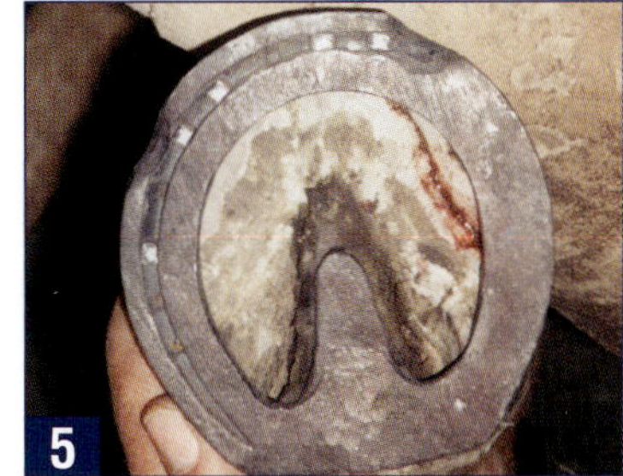

A horse suffering with a major cut to the sole.

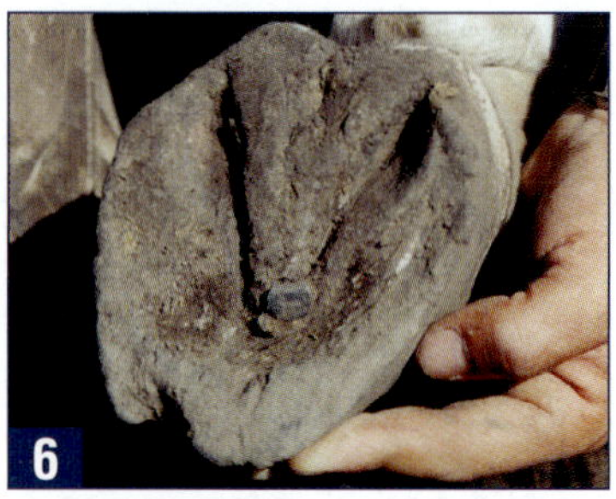

Nail in the point of the frog.

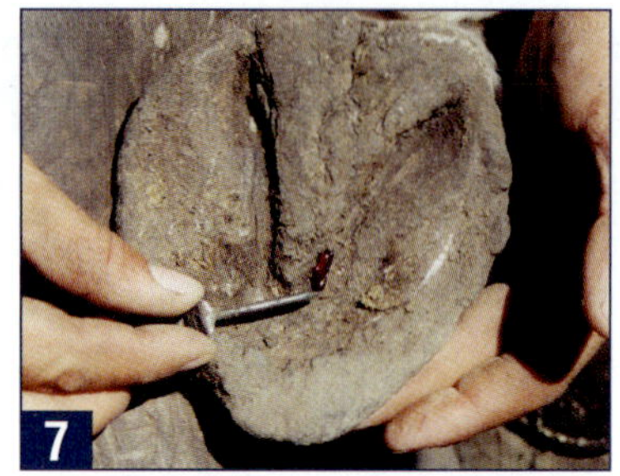

The nail after removal.

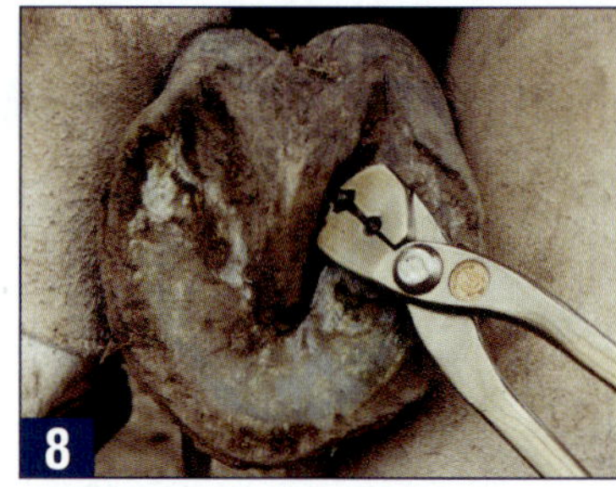

Nail in the commissure.

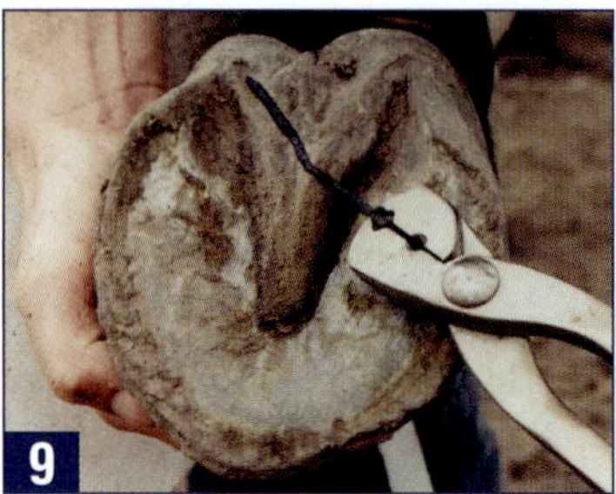

After removal.

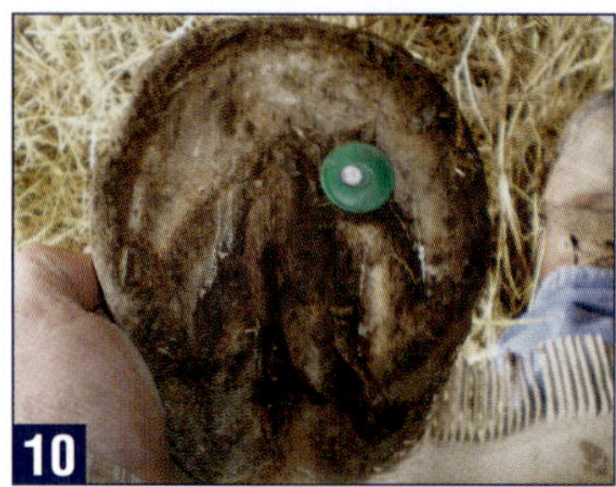

Nail in the sole.

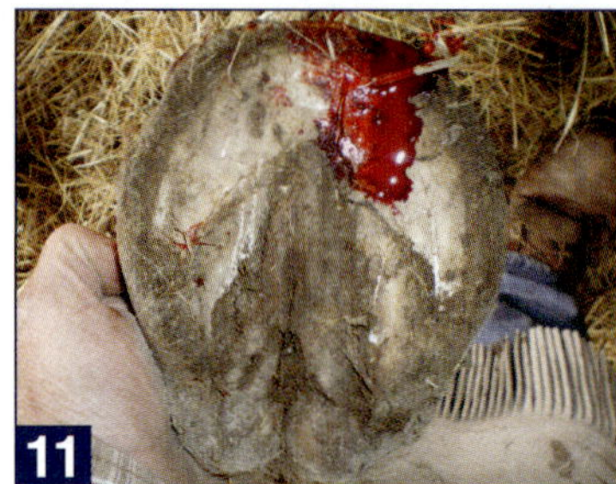

Lots of bleeding after removal.

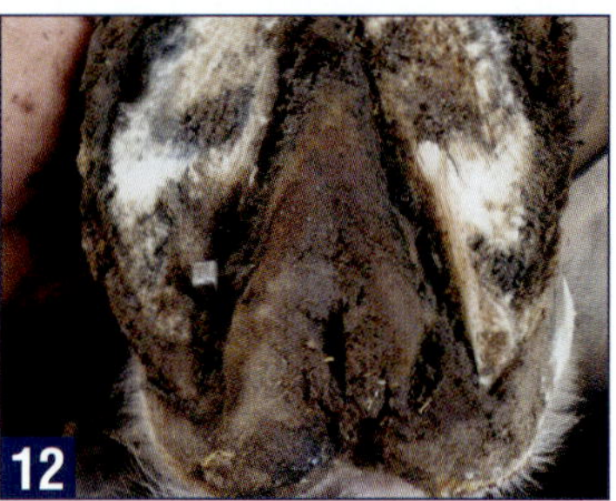

Horse nail in the commissure.

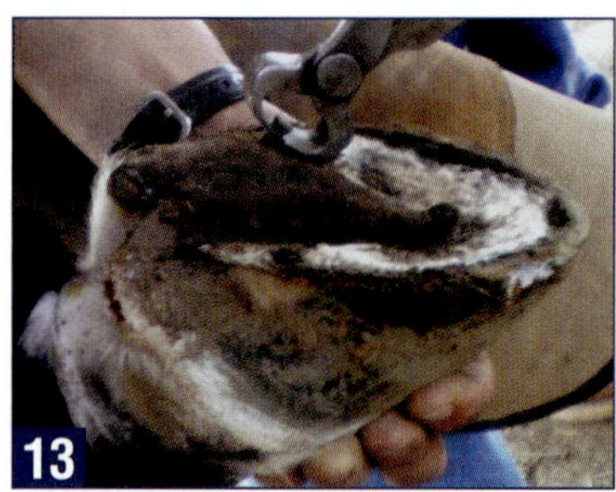

Removing the nail.

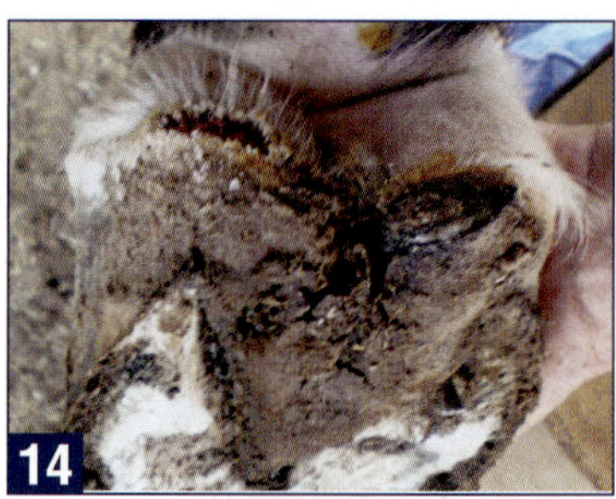

Area at the bulb where the abscess caused by the nail broke out.

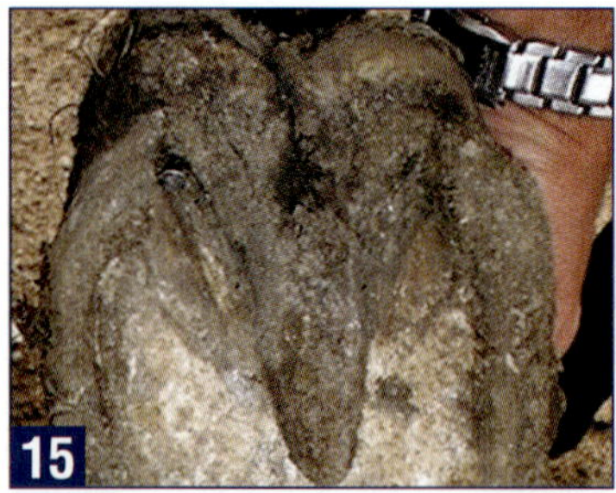

Another nail in the commissure.

are not likely to have major problems with lameness from infection, since the size of the injuries will make it unlikely that pressure will build up in the feet. The feet pictured in **Figure 6-11** are from horses with nails that have been lodged deep within the foot. I strongly urge you to have a veterinarian take an X-ray before removing nails like these. Knowing exactly to where they have penetrated is very important to the proper treatment. If a nail has reached the joint capsule or navicular bursa, the horse has a greater chance of this injury becoming life threatening.

The horse in **Figures 12-14** has a horseshoe nail

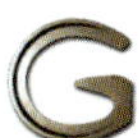

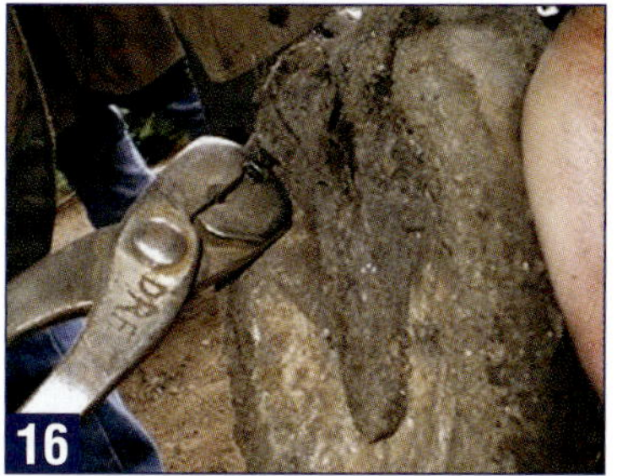

16 *Removal.*

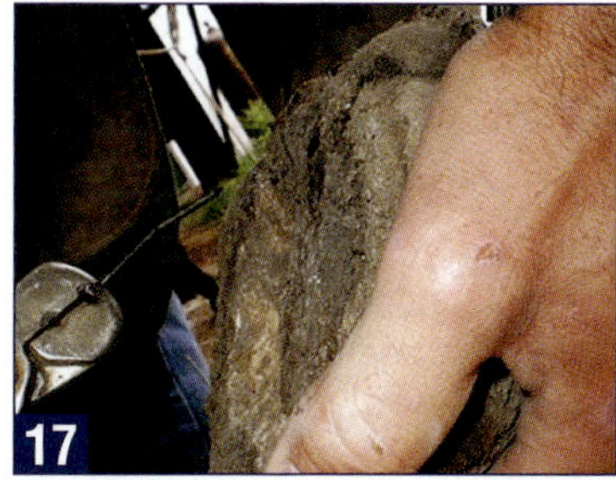

17 *The length and track of the nail.*

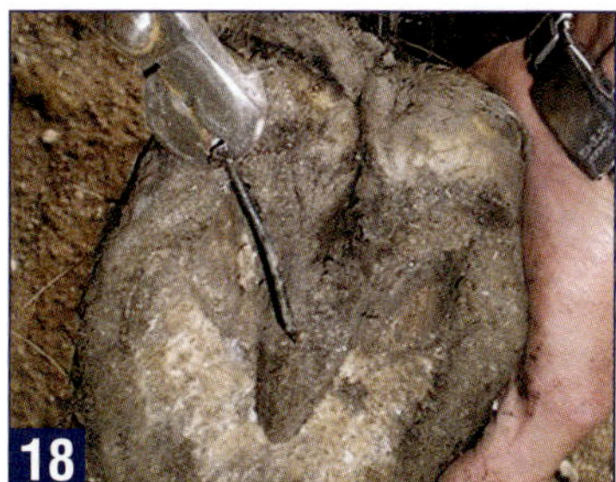

18 *The nail.*

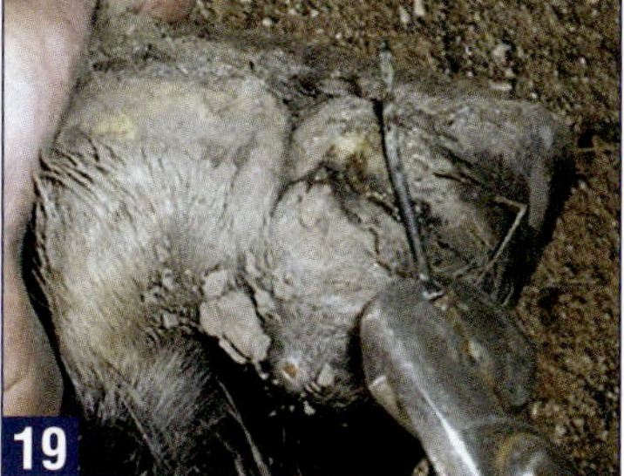

19 *Where the abscess broke.*

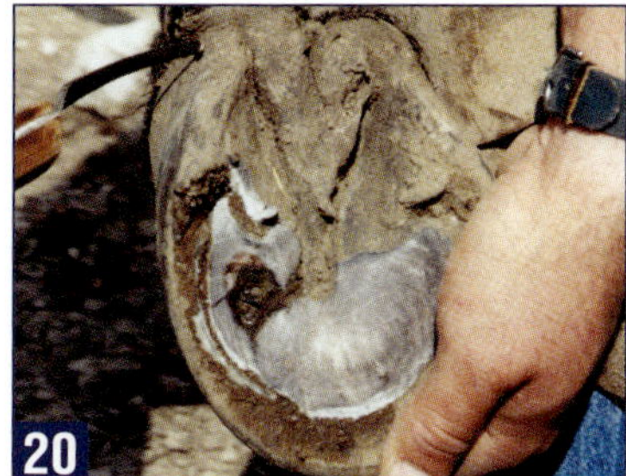

20 *Abscess in quarter.*

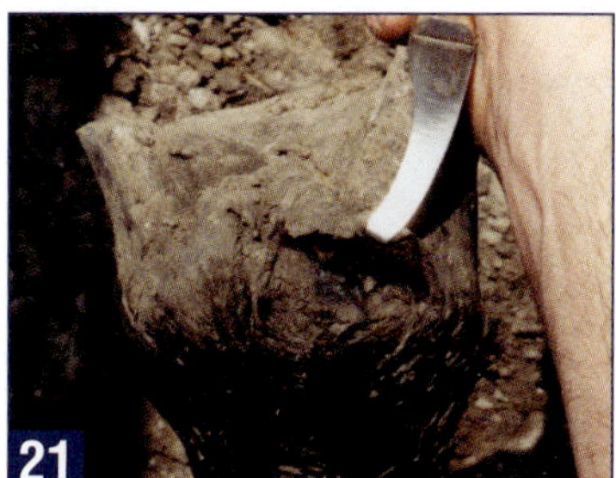

21 *Gravitated to the bulbs.*

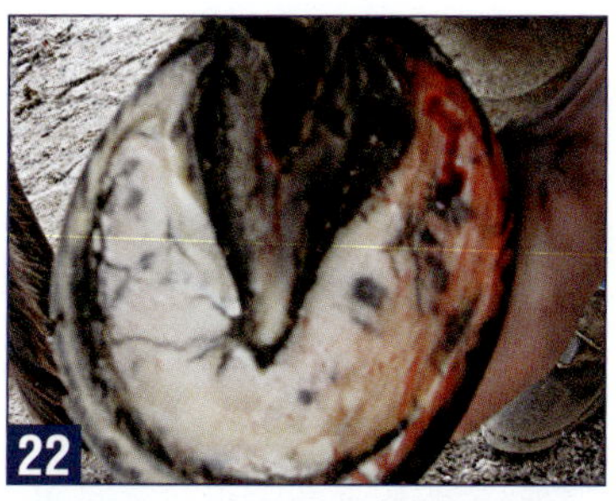

22 *Unusual anatomy, bleeding in the seat of corn on a long foot.*

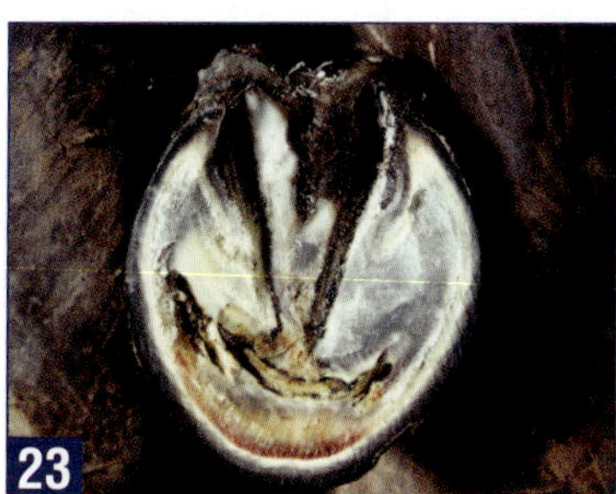

23 *Results of an abscess.*

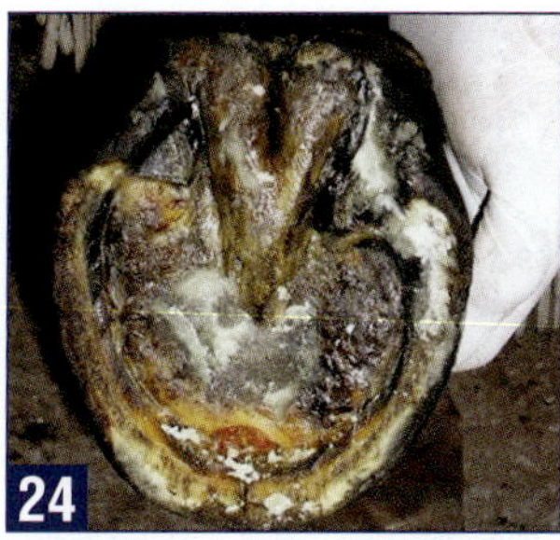

24 *Large infection in the foot.*

lodged in a commissure. In **Figure 14**, you can see that an abscess has already formed and burst from the back of the foot at the bulbs. **Figures 15-19** are a similar case. It is not uncommon for a horse owner to miss the fact that there is a nail in the foot, even though the horse is lame. This gives the wound time enough to become infected and burst an abscess. **Figures 20-21** are of a horse that developed an abscess in the quarter, which then spread under the foot to the bulbs as well.

Figure 22 shows a foot that is bleeding in the seat of corn area, even though the foot is not short enough to bleed. In rare instances, I have found abnormal anatomy. With a situation like this, you may find blood supply where you don't expect it. When this happens, you still have a good chance of an abscess.

Abscesses can do a little damage or a lot, depending on the amount of time it takes for them to find a drainage point. In **Figure 23**, you can see a foot that has suffered a fairly large abscess by the look of the size of the resulting cavity. In **Figures 24-25**, the entire sole has been compromised. These horses really suffered while the abscess was tearing the foot apart. Once they have resolved themselves, the sole will peel away to reveal newer sole as in

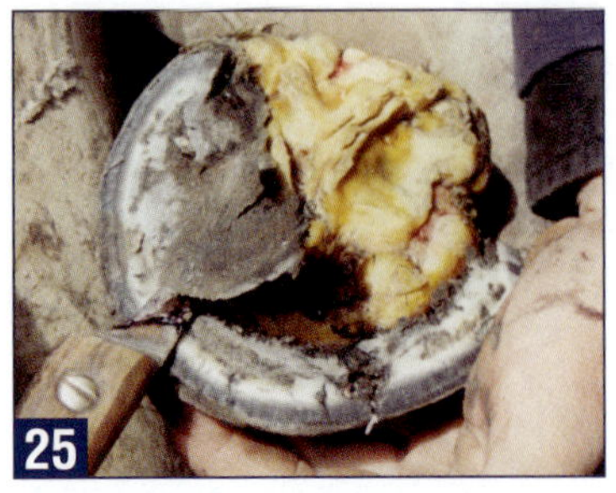

25

Results of a huge abscess that suppurated across the entire sole.

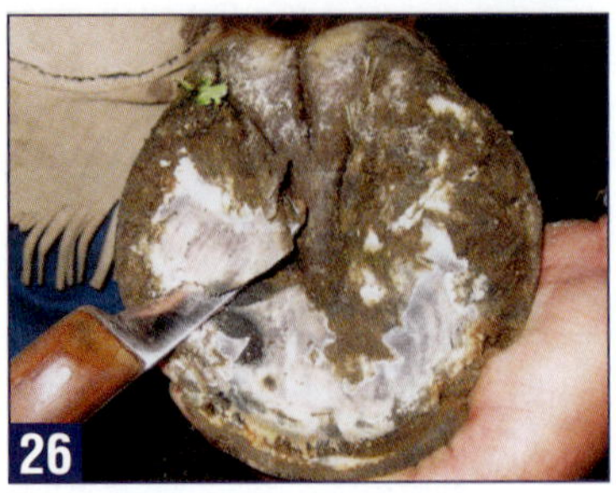

26

Evidence of old abscess.

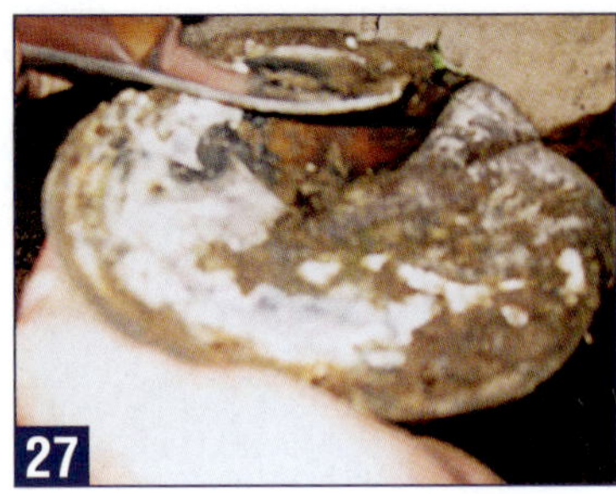

27

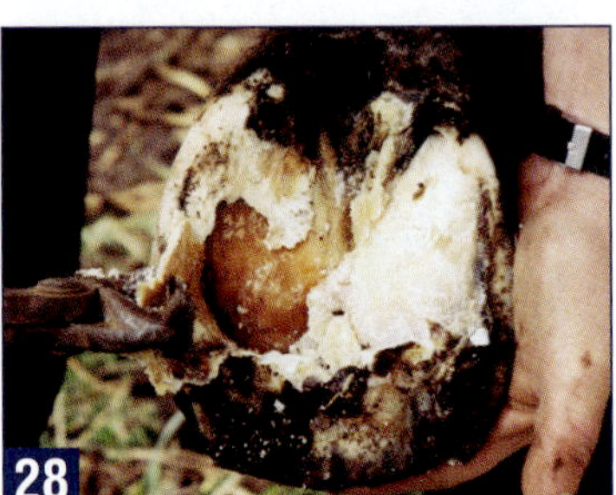

28

Evidence of old abscess.

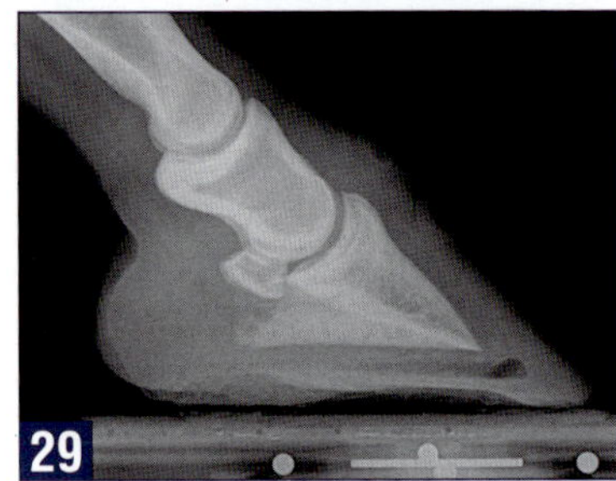

29

Lateral radiograph of an abscess at the tip of the coffin bone.

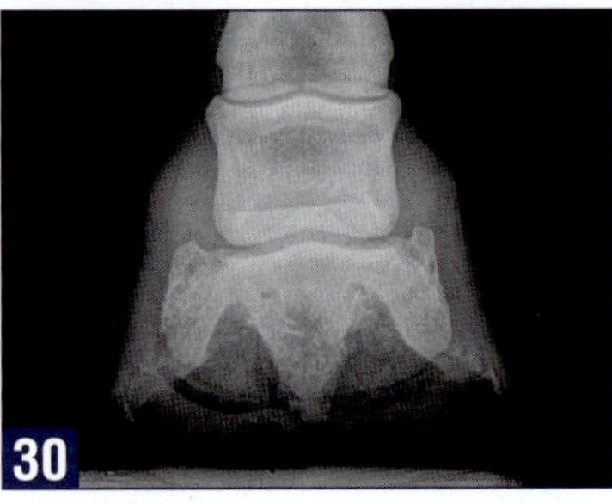

30

Dorsal/palmar view of the same abscess.

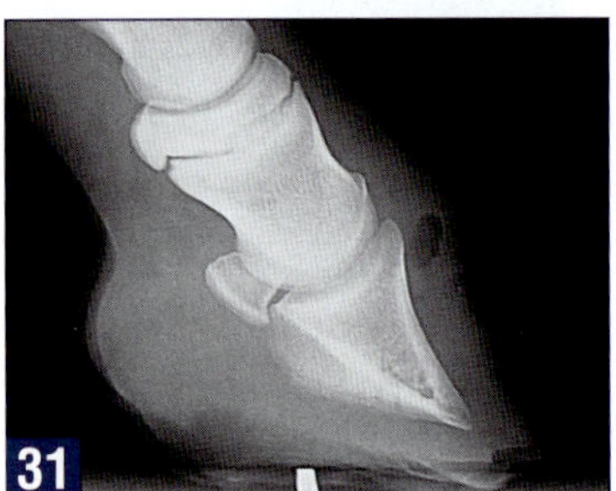

31

Abscess at the coronet.

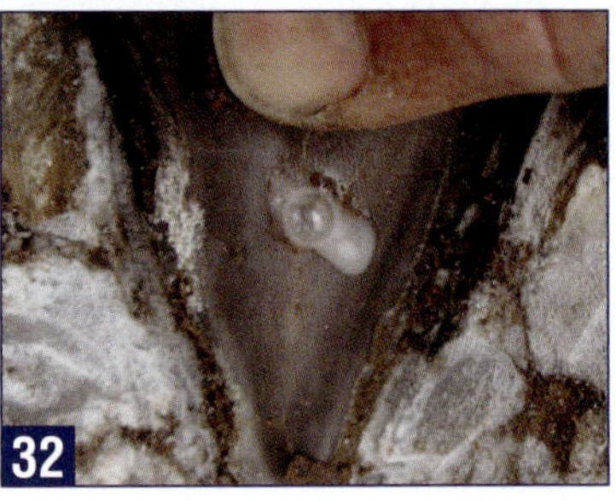

32

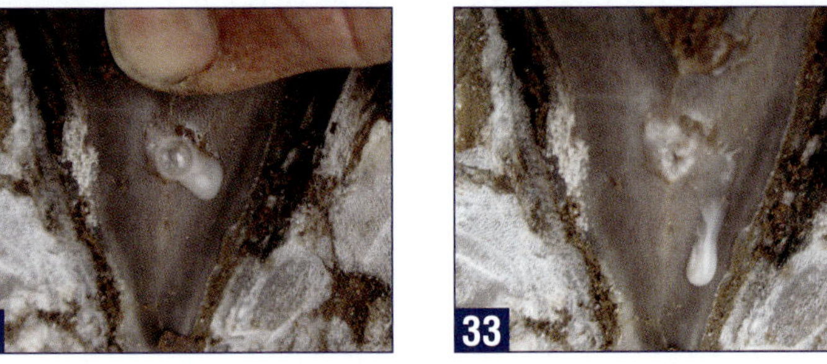

33

Drainage from a fat pocket deposited by the merocrine gland.

34

Drainage from a fat pocket deposited by the merocrine gland.

Figures 26-28.

Abscesses are visible as a black spot of radiolucent space on radiographs in **Figures 29-30** (taken by Dr. John Marcotte) of an abscess around the distal tip of the coffin bone. **Figure 31** (taken by Dr. Scott Morrison) is of an abscess at the coronet.

There is an anatomical structure in the digital cushion known as the merocrine gland. This gland secretes fat into the frog, and this fat can become a pocket of whitish, greasy fluid in the frog. When trimming the frog, the pocket can be hit, and the fluid can drain. When that happens, novice farriers

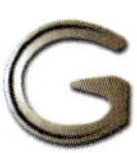

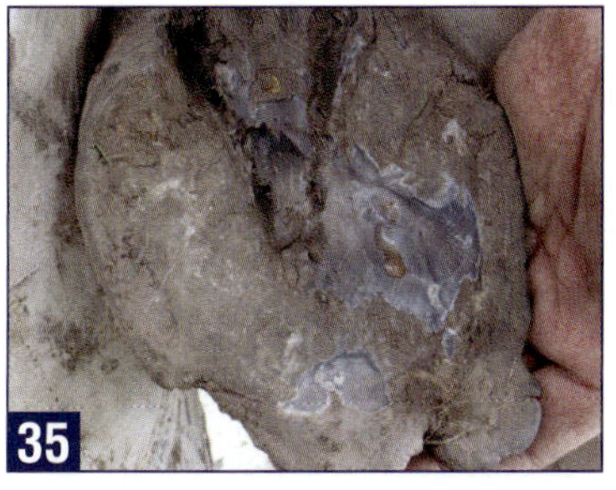

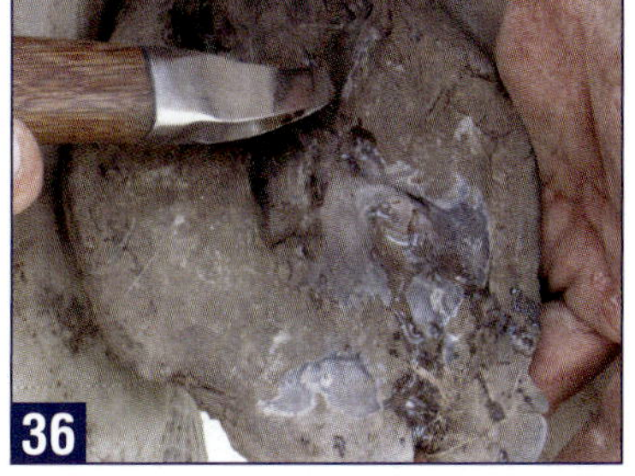

Abscess draining from the sole.

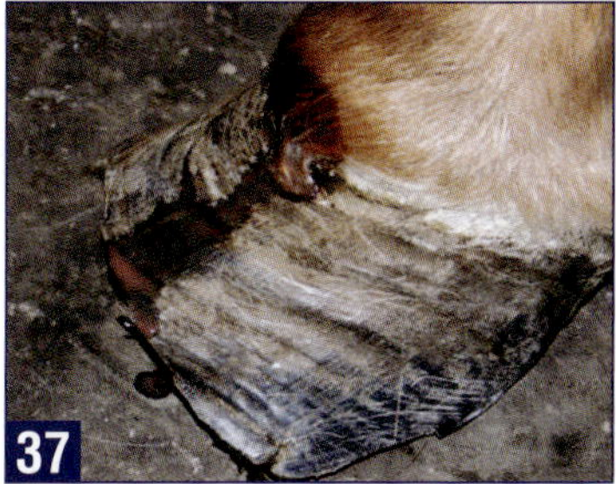

Abscess that has broken out at top of the hoof wall in the toe.

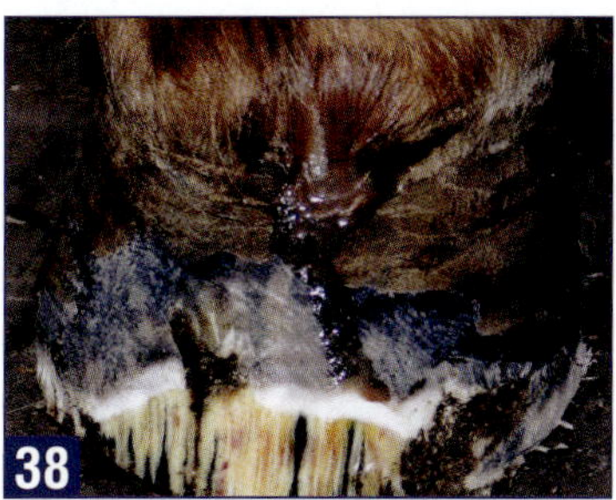

Abscess that has broken out at top of the hoof wall in the toe.

are often fooled into thinking they have hit an abscess **(Figures 32-34)**. They haven't. The pus draining from an abscess is often darker, sometimes black, and may have a pinkish hue to it from blood. In **Figures 35-36**, I have cut through the sole to locate an abscess, and the drainage is almost brown. The pus draining from the coronet in **Figures 37-38** is also of a darker tint.

ANATOMY

The infection in the hoof can involve any portion of the foot, but the areas most commonly involved are the horny and sensitive sole, horny laminae, sensitive laminae, and coronary band. Depending on the area of the insult, the horny and sensitive frog can be involved as well. That type of abscess often breaks out from the back of the heels at the bulbs, as in **Figures 14-19**. It is not uncommon for the fetlock and pastern areas to swell with untreated abscesses.

SYMPTOMS

Abscesses are extremely painful for a horse, with Grade 4 lameness common. The horse holds the foot in the air, and will be extremely reluctant to bear weight on it. You can often find one spot that is more sore than another with a pair of hoof testers, but the foot is so painful that you can get a reaction in most areas of the foot.

I believe the pain can be compared to what we suffer when we crush the end of our finger and the fingernail turns black from bleeding. The pressure of the blood under the fingernail can be quite painful.

The classic signs of inflammation include heat, pain, redness (in bare skin), swelling, and loss of function from pain. Inflammation may be a result of physical injury, bacterial or viral infection, or reaction to poisons or toxins. Infection may cause more heat and pain than physical injury. With an abscess, you should be able to feel increased heat in the foot as well as a bounding pulse in the digital arteries from increased blood flow.

The area to check for a bounding pulse is at the back of the fetlock over the sesamoid bones, just below the bifurcation of the artery.

Bacteria invading sensitive structures may reproduce rapidly. This process causes a gas, usually only seen in anaerobic infection. Anaerobic infection is the worst kind of infection, and the buildup of gas places pressure on the sensitive structures. As it continues to grow, the horny and sensitive structures are separated and torn apart.

The bacteria provoke a response from the immune system of the horse with white blood cells arriving through the circulation. The white cells ingest the bacteria and may die in the process. The resulting mixture of live and dead white cells, dead tissue, bacteria, and serum is commonly known as pus. The collection of pus expands and causes pressure that is painful for the horse. The abscess then expands along the line of least resistance. Production of gas in the abscess cavity increases the pressure and is typical of anaerobic bacteria that do not need oxygen to live and thrive in dead tissue.

The abscess may spread across the sole until it

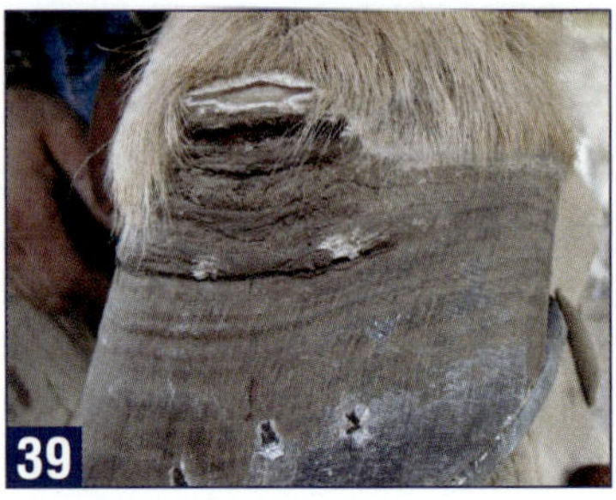

Cleft.

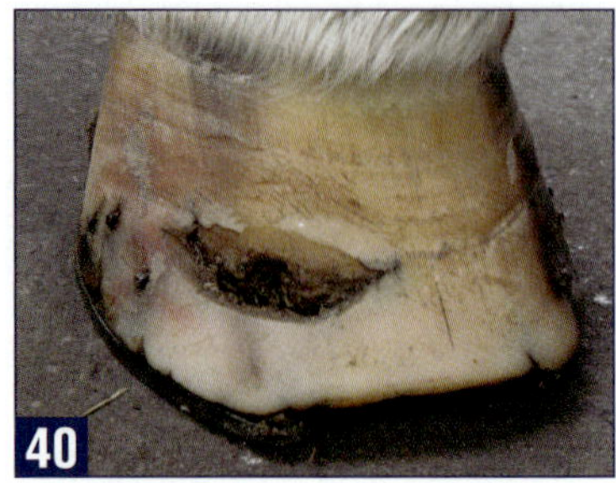

Cleft that has grown down.

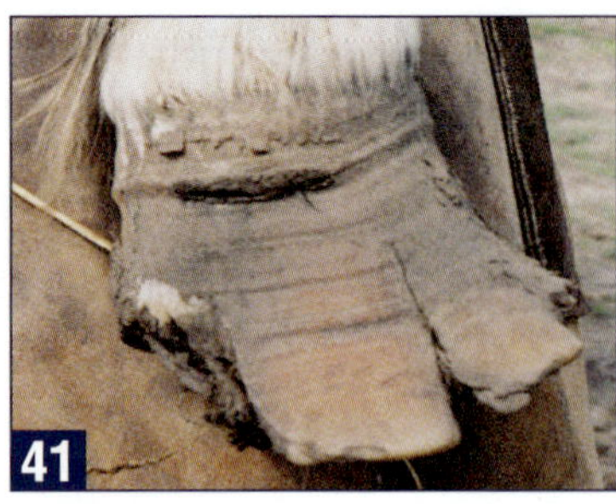

Cleft.

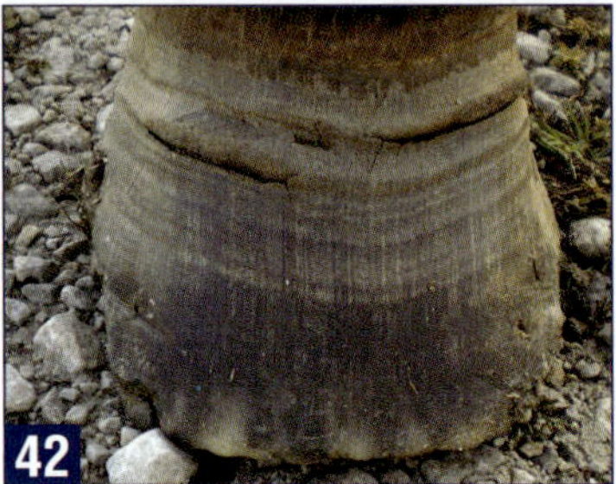

2 Clefts.

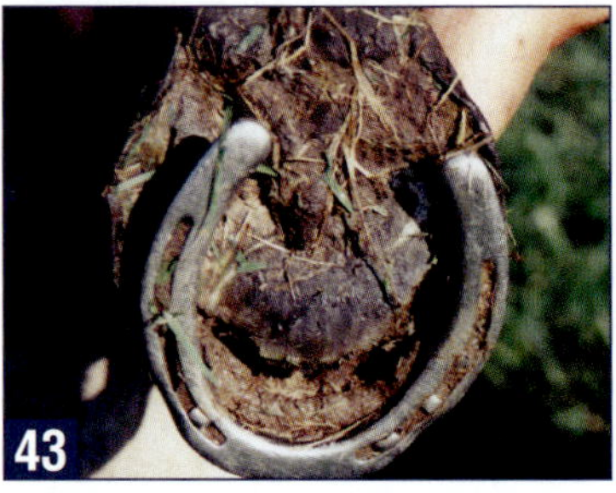

Shoe barely hanging on to just a small part of the foot still connected.

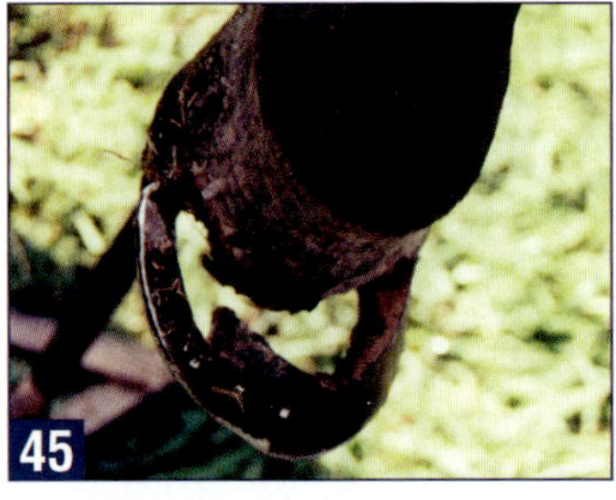

Shoe barely hanging on to just a small part of the foot still connected.

reaches the hoof wall at the wall-sole junction. Here, the white line is stronger than the bond between the horny and sensitive laminae, and the abscess can move proximad toward the coronary band. Once it reaches the coronary band, it will break out of the hoof and drain. If this happens, the horse will generally feel some relief.

Traditional teaching was that a piece of rock penetrated the foot, then moved up the hoof wall and broke out at the coronary band. Thus, an abscess is still often referred to as "gravel" and you will still hear some folks refer to a horse as "gravelling." Rocks do not travel through, up, or around a horse's foot; this is myth. Although most horse professionals know this, the name "gravel" remains.

As the pus is draining, hoof wall production in the abscess area of the coronary band is interrupted. The rest of the hoof wall is still growing, so once the drainage area resumes hoof wall production, there will be a gap in the hoof. It will appear as a horizontal crack that is the length of the area where the drainage happened. This crack is known as a cleft. It will grow down from the coronary band and finally make its way to the ground. If you have a really long cleft from a bad abscess, you may have to deal with a large area of foot that tends to break off when it gets closer to the ground.

Clefts come in various sizes **(Figures 39-42)**. In **Figures 43-45**, the cleft was large enough that a large section of the foot broke away with the shoe still on it. Luckily, the cleft had grown down far enough that the breakage did not extend into sensitive structures. To strengthen a large cleft and prevent the breakage that you see in **Figure 43-45**, the area can be strengthened with some of the

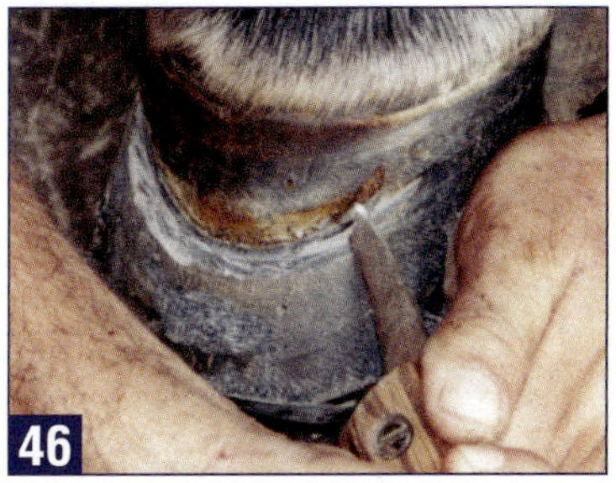

Cleft that was causing lameness. Cleaning it out to prepare it for a patch.

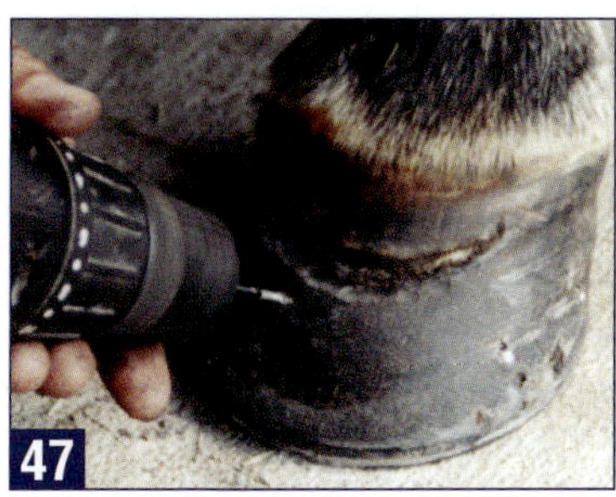

Drilling pilot holes.

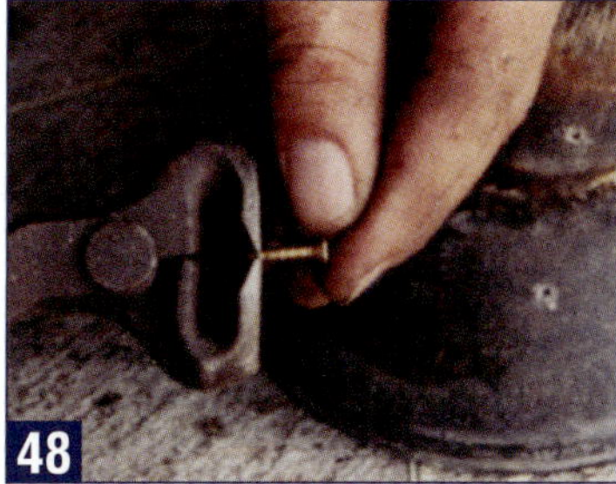

Cutting the screws so that they don't invade sensitive structures.

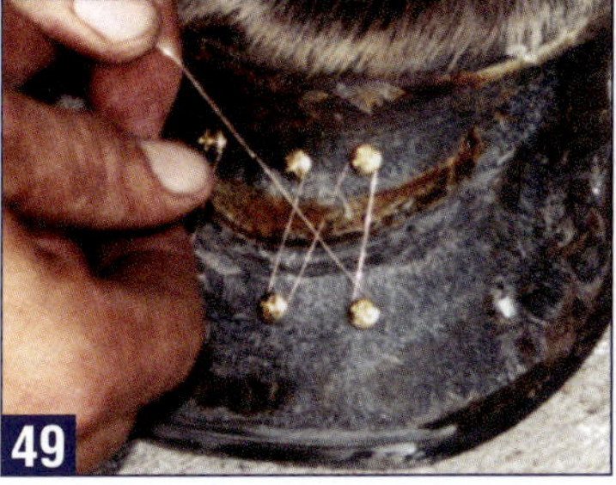

Lacing the wire around the screws.

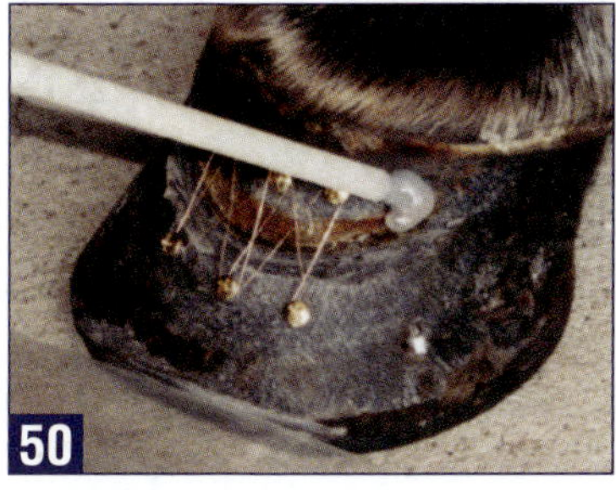

Covering the crack with Super Fast.

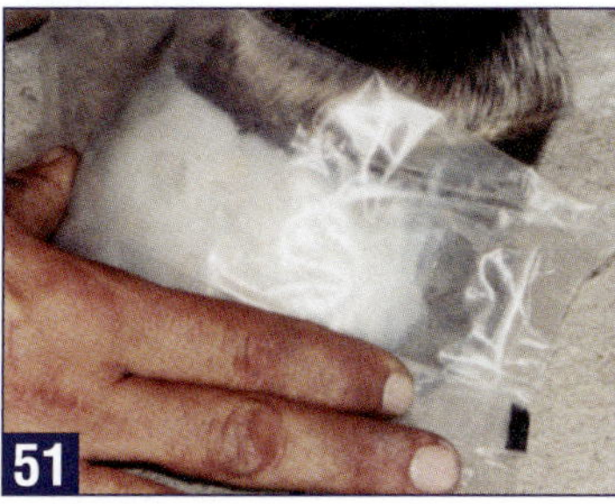

Putting plastic on the Super Fast.

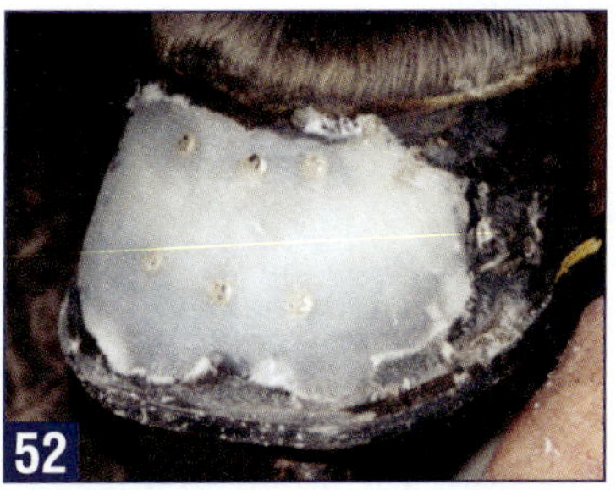

The patch has been rasped to the screw heads.

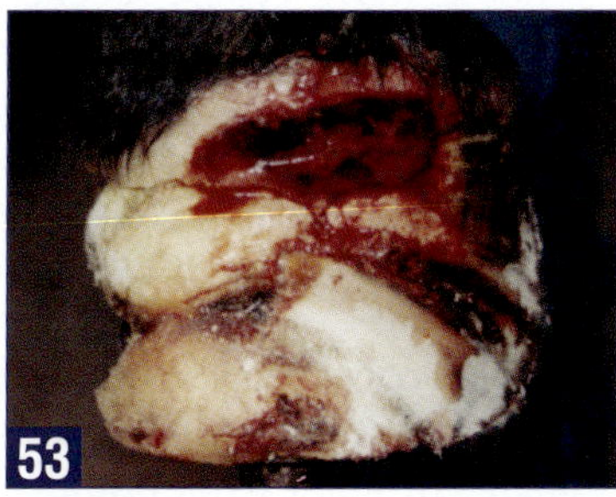

Bad abscess at the toe.

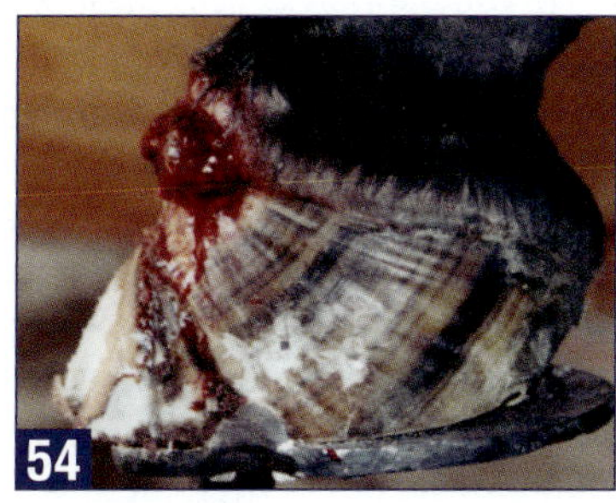

Lateral view.

commercially available acrylics and polyurethanes. To do this, begin by making certain that sensitive structures are not exposed **(Figure 46)** and clean out the area to be strengthened. Drill a series of pilot holes on either sides of the crack **(Figure 47)**. Notice the tape on the drill bit to determine depth. Use zinc-coated or brass screws, and cut them if they are too long **(Figure 48)**. Once the screws are in, wrap wire around them to act as net for better adhesion of the material that is about to be applied to the foot **(Figure 49)**. In **Figure 50**, I am applying Vettec Super Fast to the cleft. Cover it with plastic **(Figure 51)**, and once it cures, you can rasp down to the screw heads **(Figure 52)**.

This particular horse was lame until I did this. Strengthening the wall made the horse sound again, and the cleft grew out successfully.

The next three pictures are from a horse that had badly foundered on one foot. It developed an abscess at the toe, which broke out the coronet. **Figure 53** is a dorsal view of this foot with a bloody mess where the abscess broke. **Figure 54** is a lateral view of that foot, and **Figure 55** was taken several weeks later when the abscess was calming down.

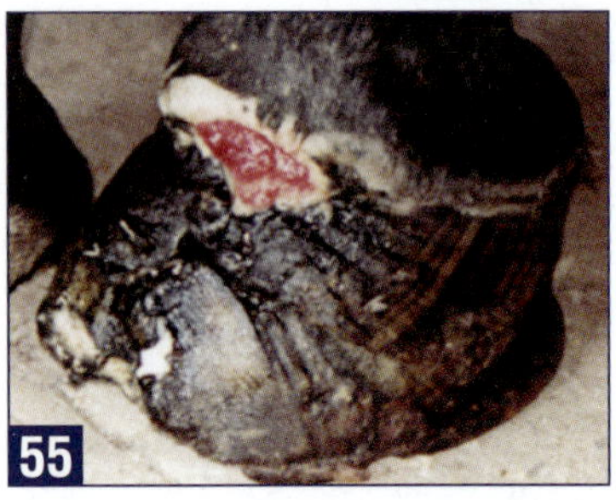

Several weeks after the initial insult.

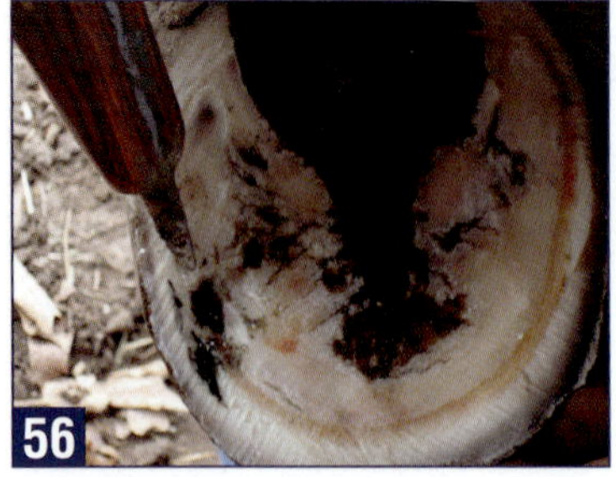

Abscess on the side of the foot.

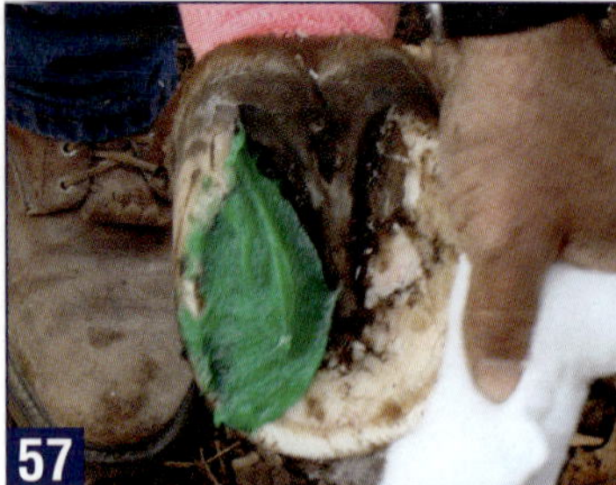

Applying the Epson salt poultice and cotton batting.

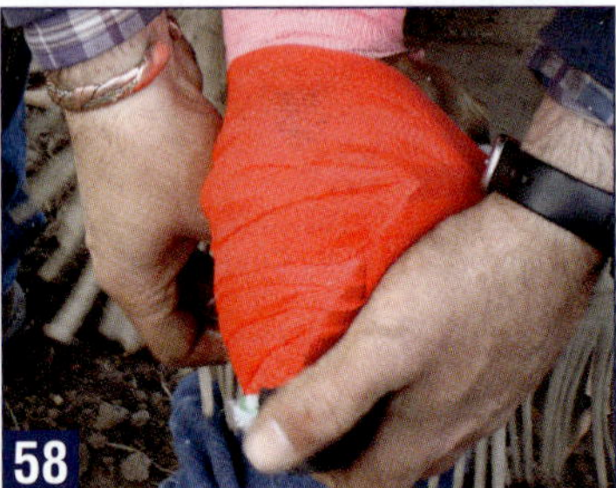

The foot is wrapped in an Elasticon bandage.

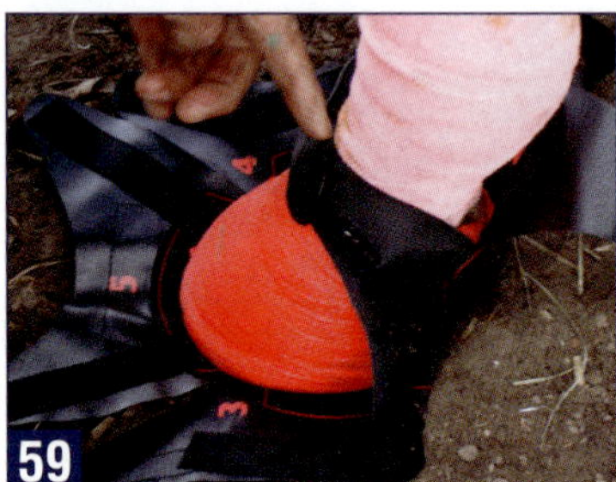

Applying the boot.

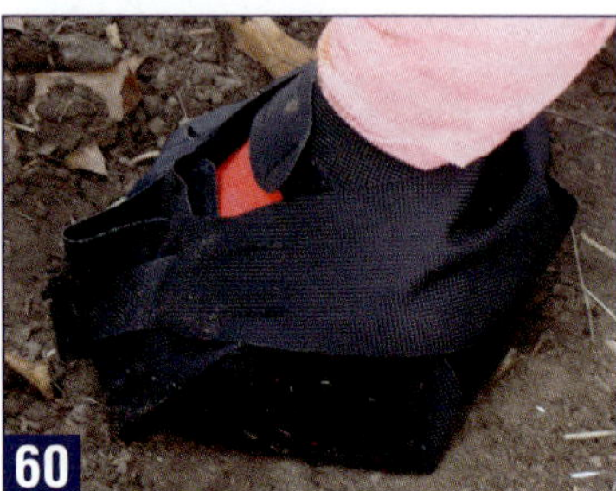

Lateral view with the boot on.

TREATMENT

If you happen to be the cause of the introduction of bacteria, for instance from driving a bad nail when you shod the horse, it should be an easy matter to treat the infection with an Epsom salts poultice. The poultice will stimulate drainage. The common scenario for a shoer-caused abscess is: Shortly after shoeing, the horse seems fine. In 3 to 7 days, the horse becomes Grade 4 lame. If caused by a bad nail and the nail is still in the foot, the farrier will pull the bad nail. Often there will be drainage from the nail hole.

If not a bad nail and you don't know exactly where the abscess is, start by placing thumb pressure around the sole as you would with hoof testers. If the horse does not react, use real hoof testers. Use the hoof testers carefully, with lighter pressure than might be routine for a non-abscess exam.

Look closely at the coronary band. It will often bulge and the hair will stand on end in the area that the abscess is likely to drain from. If at all possible, I like to cut out an area of the hoof wall itself to allow the drainage. Just go up about an inch from the bottom of the foot and cut a little window into the wall with an abscess probe or your loop knife. Since this hole is on the side of the foot instead of the bottom, it is less likely to pack with debris and cause secondary problems.

Sometimes an abscess will drain; the horse is recovering but then suffers a reccurrence. If the abscess has walled off an area with bacteria behind it, a secondary abscess may have developed. It will be just like the first, and you will deal with it just as you did the original abscess.

To establish drainage on the bottom of the foot without cutting the sole, I generally use an Epsom salts poultice with a boot for about a week. In **Figure 56**, an area inside the white line indicates where the abscess is. I clean out the area as much as possible. After cleaning, I apply the poultice **(Figure 57)**, cover with cotton batting, and wrap with an Elasticon bandage **(Figure 58)**. Cover the bandaged foot with the boot of your choice **(Figure 59-61)**. In this series of photos, I am using a really neat product that is made by Kaeco. It is an abscess kit that should be in the every tack room and horse trailer.

In many areas, it was, and still is, common practice to soak a foot in warm water and Epsom salts twice a day for 15 minutes at a time when dealing with an abscess. That is fine, but with the poultice, I have continuous exposure to the Epson salts to draw

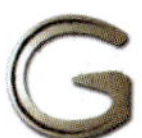

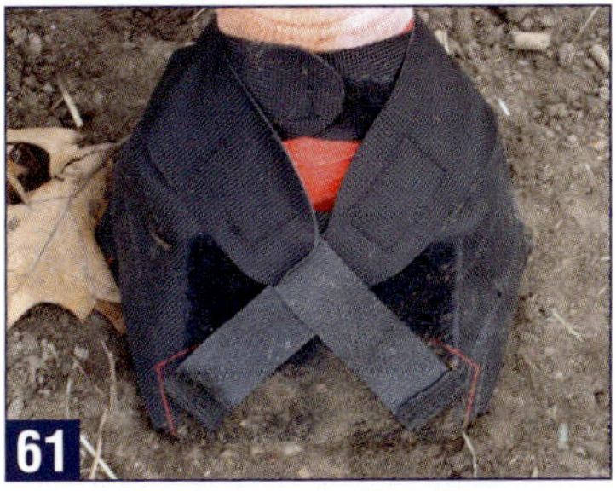

61

Dorsal view with the boot on.

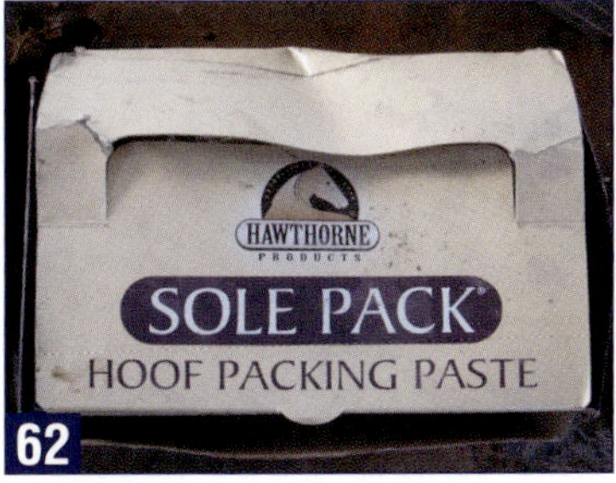

62

Hawthorne Products Sole Pack.

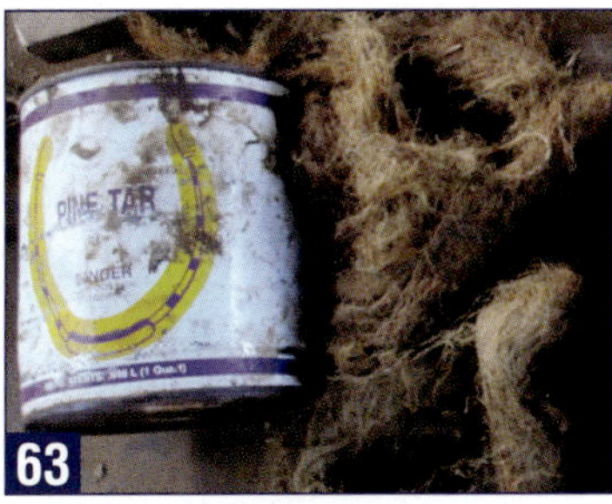

63

Pine tar and oakum.

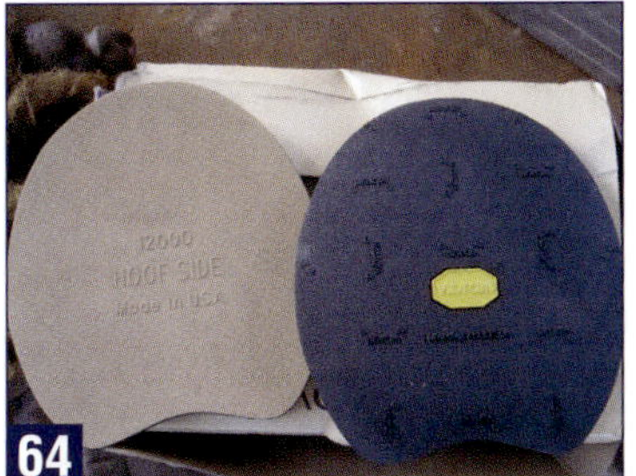

64

Vibram hoof pads.

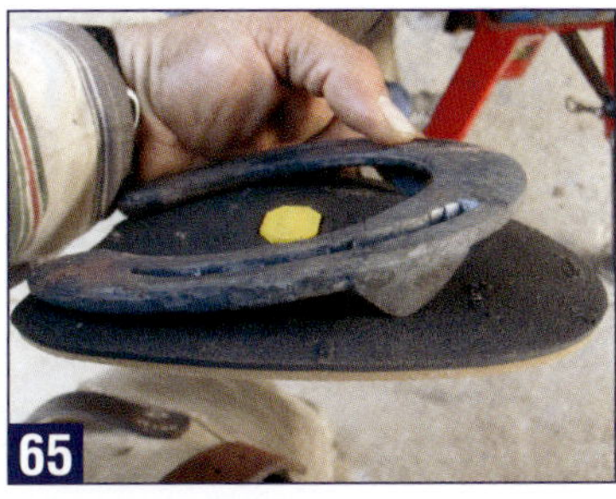

65

Shoe on pad to locate area to cut for the clips.

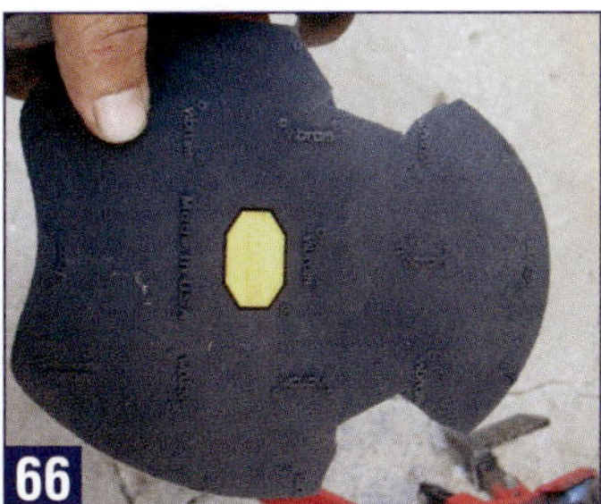

66

Pad ready for clipped shoe.

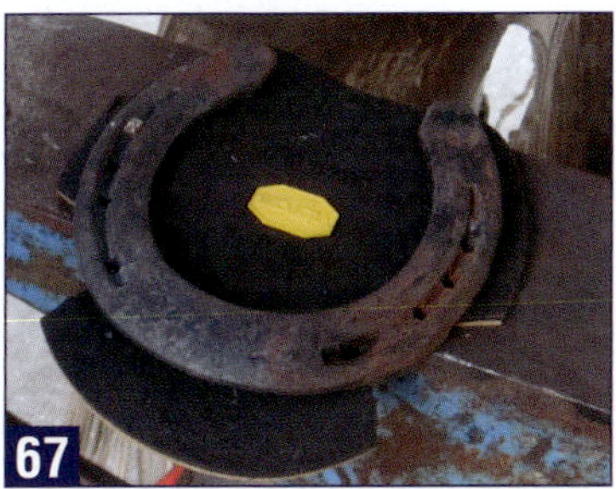

67

Putting nails in the shoe to hold the pad in place.

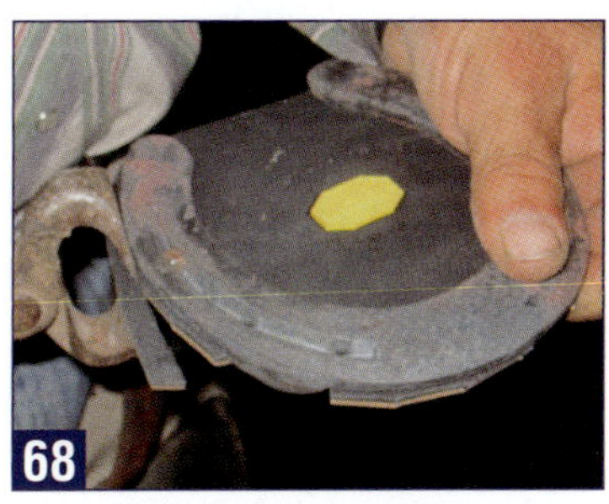

68

Cutting around the pad.

the abscess out. I have found the poultice to be superior to soaking. 3M Animal Care's Animalintex also works well as a poultice material, according to Dr. Mike Miller.

When I create drainage on the bottom of the foot but the horse has to go into work without the benefit of constant care, I will put a shoe on with a pad. Under the pad I like to use Hawthorne Products Sole Pack **(Figure 62)**. It is medicated,

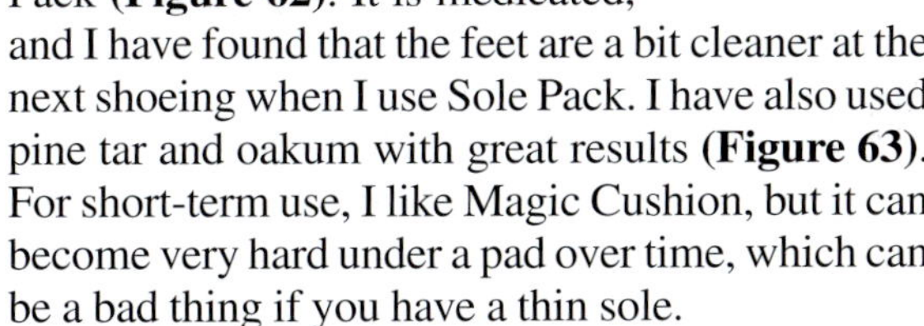

and I have found that the feet are a bit cleaner at the next shoeing when I use Sole Pack. I have also used pine tar and oakum with great results **(Figure 63)**. For short-term use, I like Magic Cushion, but it can become very hard under a pad over time, which can be a bad thing if you have a thin sole.

I follow these steps to use a regular pad. Since I only put on a few pads a year, I don't have a pad cutter, band-saw, drill press, rivets, or a lot of the other things that you will want to have if you are doing a lot of pads. This method works in a business like mine that doesn't require a lot of pads.

In this series I am using Vibram Pads **(Figure 64)**, which are incredibly strong.

After hot fitting the foot, place the shoe on the pad so that you can see where the clips are going to be located **(Figure 65)**. Cut the pad to accommodate the clips **(Figure 66)**. Place the shoe on the pad and drive the heel nails into the pad **(Figure 67)**. Cut out around the pad with nippers **(Figure 68)**, and the pad and shoe are ready to be nailed on **(Figures 69-70)**.

Prevention is worth a lot, so if I happen to know that I have quicked a horse, I will apply Hot Nail to the area immediately. Hot Nail is another great product from Hawrhone Products. I also use it anytime that there is a fresh injury on the bottom of the foot as in **Figure 71-74**. Here, there was a thorn

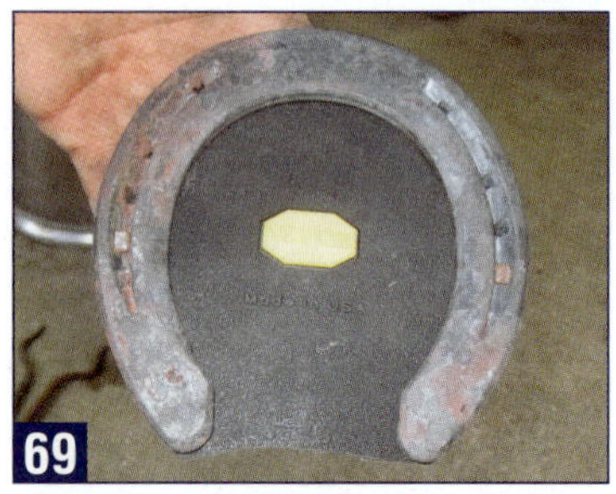

Shoe and pad ready to be nailed.

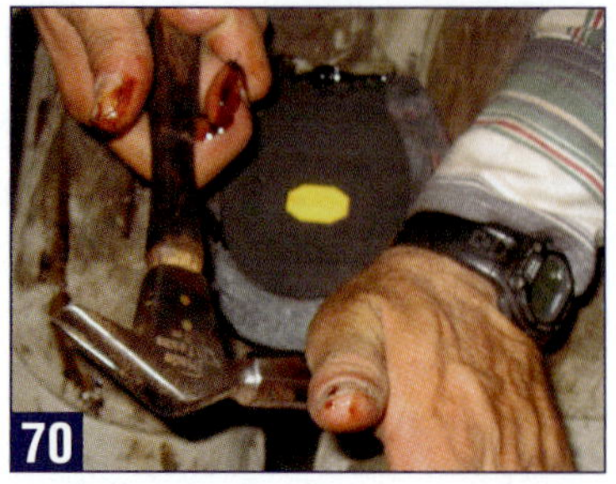

Nailing on the shoe with the pad.

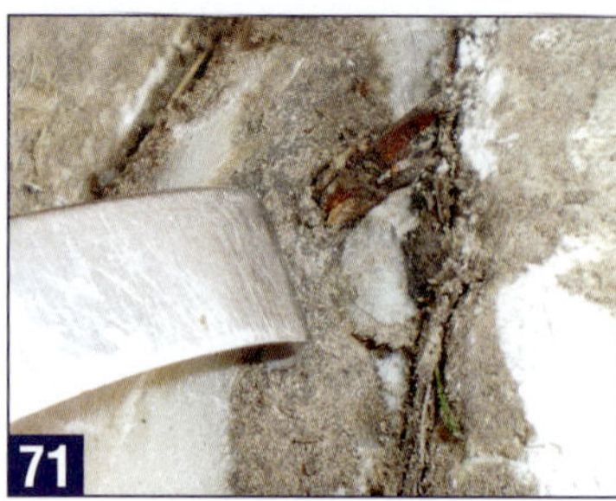

Thorn in the frog.

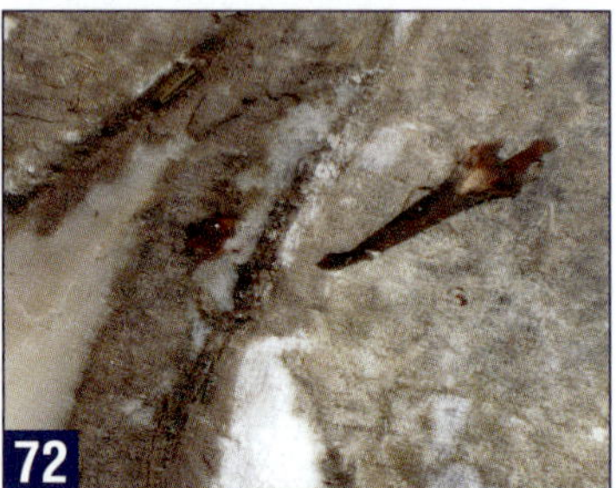

After the thorn has been removed.

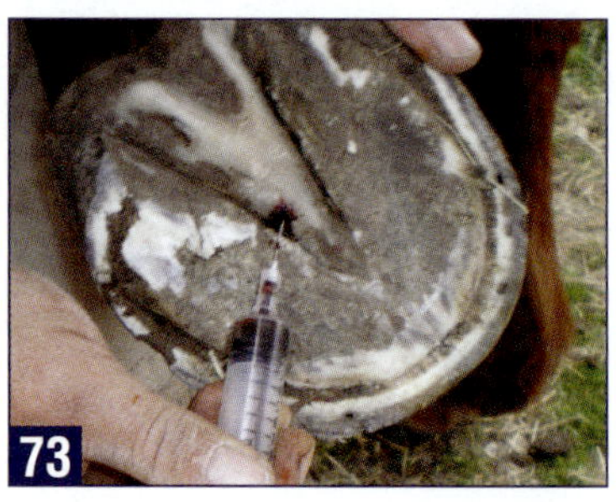

Putting Hot Nail into the thorn hole.

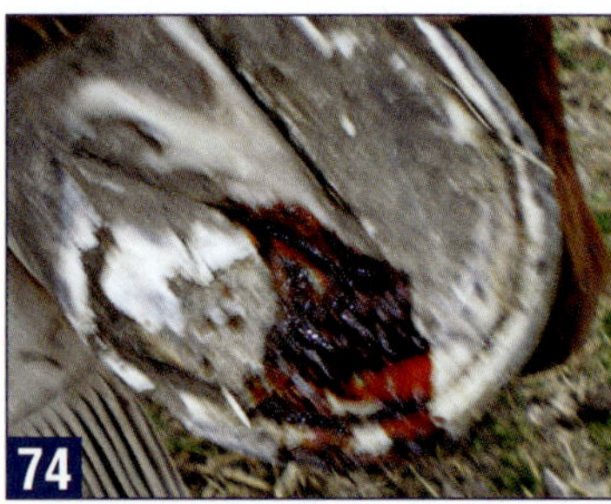

Treated area.

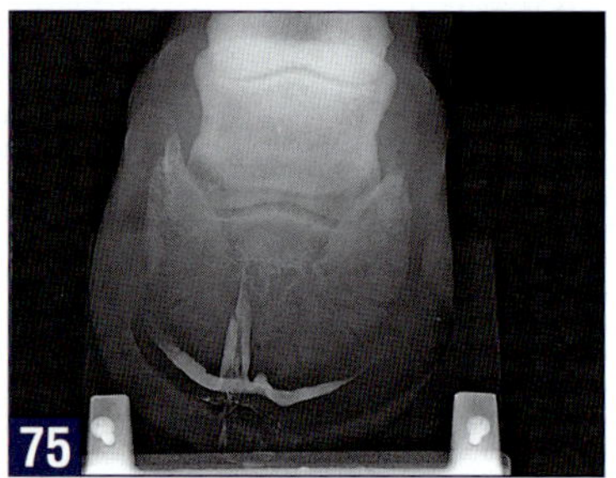

in the frog. Once it was extracted, I put some Hot Nail in the wound with a syringe. Pure iodine is too caustic, so it should not be used on fresh injuries.

Finally, the farrier should advise the customer of the danger of tetanus from any sort of injury, especially in the case where the farrier has accidentally quicked the horse. Tetanus is easily guarded against but potentially fatal if not vaccinated.

Since horses are so lame when they have an abscess, vets are often the first ones called by the owner. The vet will often explore the foot with a hoof knife to cause drainage. This can be good or bad, depending on the experience of the vet. Once this is done, they will often bandage the foot with Epsom salts poultice or Icthamol and send it home to be treated for a few days until it can be shod again.

The use of antibiotics or anti-inflammatories is done on a case-by-case basis. Failing adequate drainage, antibiotics alone cannot succeed; the selection of medications should be left to the vet.

Abscesses cause such severe pain that a horse will seem to make a miraculous recovery within a few days after establishing drainage. Depending on the extent of tissue that has been damaged, the owner can start using the horse again once it is no longer lame. I prefer that the owner change the bandage system and reapply the poultice every day for at least three days — more if the horse is still not sound. It is also helpful if the horse can be kept in dry stabling. Wet footing enhances bacterial growth. If owners are able to obtain a Kaeco Abscess Kits, they can often do the horse a lot of good before the farrier even arrives.

ANTICIPATED OUTCOME

Even though an abscess causes major lameness, recovery is often quick. I expect a horse to suffer until the abscess is draining. From that point, lameness should decrease for the next two to five days until the horse is as sound as it was before the abscess.

IN SHORT:

D – Infection in the foot.

T – Cause to drain, draw with Epson salt poultice, protect with pad or boot.

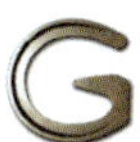

Chapter

45-2 CANKER

DEFINITION

Canker is an abnormal and accelerated growth of tissue from the sensitive frog. It can also involve the sole, hoof wall, bulbs, and coronary band in severe cases. Most of these begin in the frog and move to the rest of the foot.

REASONS

There is very little agreement on the cause of canker. It was long thought to be a result of exposure to ammonia compounds, especially from urine. Canker is found most often in hind feet but may occur in any foot. Wet and filthy stabling has also been implicated as the cause, but it can be found in horses that live in above average conditions. At present, the true cause of canker is unknown. Draft horses seem to be more susceptible than smaller breeds.

ANATOMY

The sensitive frog is certainly involved. The canker will grow from the sensitive frog and be covered with the horny frog in the early stages. In severe cases, the growth will include the sole, bulbs, wall, and coronary band.

SYMPTOMS

With mild canker in the early stages, an area of the frog may seem to have a different consistency than a normal frog. This unusual appearance may have an ammonia odor, and it will bleed easily. The canker may have a whitish covering, and it may also have a structure to it that resembles a cabbage.

Large cankers bleed very easily, and the affected horse may be quite sore when the canker is abraded or stressed.

Figure 1 shows a small canker that looks like the leaves of a cabbage. In **Figure 2**, the canker is being cut away from the frog. **Figure 3** shows the

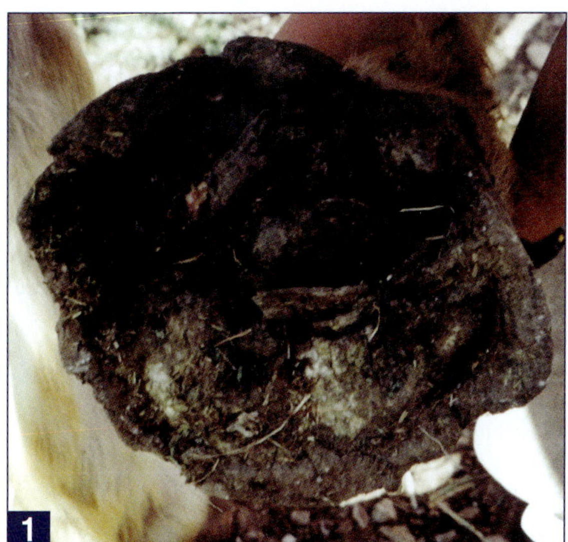

1

Canker in the frog.

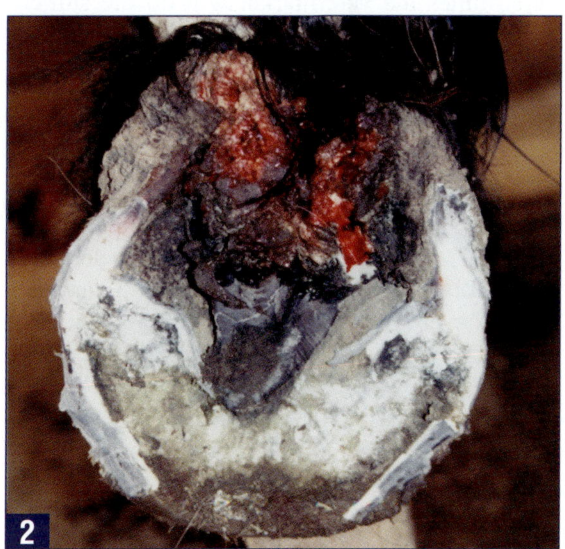

2

Canker that is being cut off of the frog.

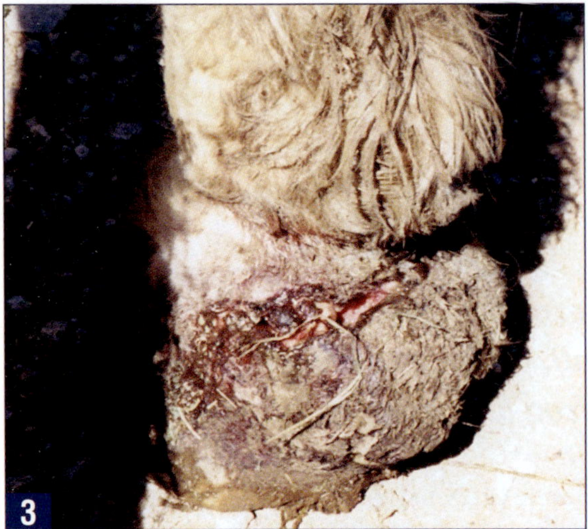

Medial view of a massive canker that has gone beyond the bottom of the foot.

medial view of a canker that, became so severe that it invaded the bulbs entirely, as well as the sides of the foot above the coronet. Finally, **Figure 4** shows a canker that has grown to immense proportions, taking over the back of the foot entirely. All of these are in the feet of draft horses.

TREATMENT

Treatment of canker involves the removal of all of the growth. This is a surgical procedure, as the lesion will bleed profusely as well as hurt the horse. Often times the veterinarian will do the surgery using a tourniquet at the fetlock, after administering local anesthesia. It will generally be necessary to cauterize the area. The surgical removal should be precise so that only abnormal tissue is removed, and healthy tissue left.

After debridement, a topical solution of 10% benzoyl peroxide in acetone should be applied as a local antiseptic treatment, and then a powder made from ground up metronidazole tablets is applied. This is covered with bandages.

You will probably be making a bar shoe with a hospital plate for this kind of problem. This will allow the owner to take the plate off every day, clean the area, and then apply the benzoyl peroxide/ acetone mixture followed by the ground up pills and gauze.

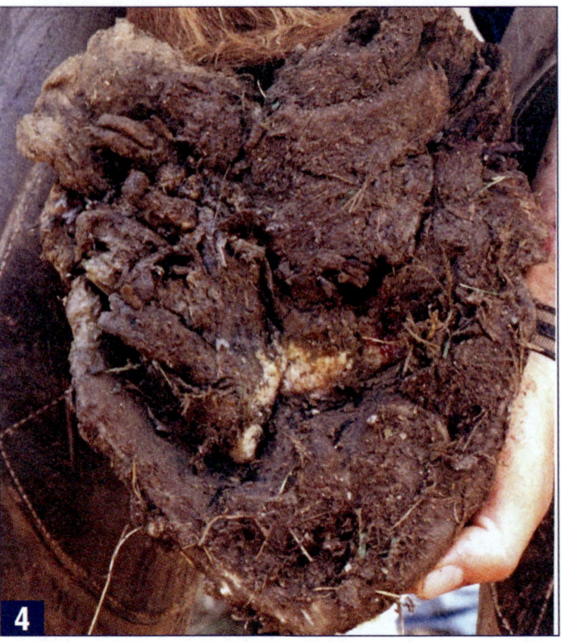

Large canker that involves the entire frog, bars, heels, bulbs, and hoof wall from the widest point back.

The hospital plate can be made in a variety of ways, but a one-bolt plate makes it easier for the owner to treat the horse daily.

ANTICIPATED OUTCOME

Despite the general belief that canker is incurable, the method mentioned has been very successful.

IN SHORT

D: Fast-growing abnormal tissue in the foot, mainly the frog.

T: 10% benzoyl peroxide mixed with acetone, applied to the foot after removal of growth and then sprinkled with metronidazole pills ground up. Bandaged and covered with a hospital plate.

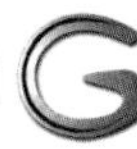

Chapter

45-3 CLUB FOOT

DEFINITION

A club foot is one that is abnormally steeper than it should be based on the rest of the horse's conformation. This problem is graded by degree by many, going from Grade 1, least severe, to Grade 4, knuckled over.

REASON

There is a lot of conjecture about the cause of a club foot. In many instances, it is an inherited trait. There is good evidence to suggest that the breeding practices of selecting horses with a shorter head and neck have caused foals to feed with one foot forward and one foot back in order to get their mouth to the ground. Over time, one foot becomes steeper and one becomes shallower, resulting in what is commonly known as high-low syndrome. These horses can be considered to have a club foot on the steep side in most cases. Young horses that are fed an inappropriate diet of too much grain and supplements are also prone to a club foot as the cannon bone grows faster than the deep flexor tendon.

Young horses that wear their toe down excessively can develop a club foot as the deep flexor tendon shortens to its resting length. There are also horses that have been injured in the flexor muscle mass. This can cause the contracture of the muscle and tendon from a pain response, resulting in a club foot. Founder can also result in a shortening of the tendon from the new position of P3 inside the hoof capsule.

Regardless of the cause, the end result is a foot that is overly steep, and something that the farrier, veterinarian, and owner need to deal with.

ANATOMY

The deep flexor muscle and tendon, coffin bone, cannon bone, and possibly the superficial flexor tendon and suspensory ligament.

SYMPTOMS

There is one front foot that is at a steeper angle than the opposite foot. A Grade 1 will be about 5 degrees steeper, but the foot will otherwise be normal. A Grade 2 will be between 5 and 10 degrees steeper, and if there are growth rings, they will be wider at the heel and narrower at the toe, indicating that the heel grows faster than the toe. Grade 3 is going to have a dish in the toe, and the coronary band will be close to parallel to the ground. If the heels are trimmed to where they should be on this type of foot, they will not touch the ground when the horse is standing square. Grade 4 is going to present with the coronary band higher at the heels, dish in the toe, and the fetlock knuckling over. Of course, there are varying degrees within each Grade.

Figure 1 shows a horse that I would consider a severe Grade 3. The coronary band is not quite parallel to the ground, but the toe is dished and the fetlock is on the verge of knuckling over. **Figure 2** is about the same. **Figure 3** is a horse that is a Grade 4 on both feet, with the near being a more severe degree of Grade 4 than the right. **Figure 4** shows a better view of this poor horse's conformation.

TREATMENT

The treatment in the early stages is to determine the cause and aggressively treat it at that time. If it is feed-related in a young horse, change the feeding immediately. When I did a lot of halter horses, the youngsters were allowed unlimited feed. We battled a lot of club feet, and the owners were hesitant to change anything about their management. I got out of doing that type of horse. It was too hard to battle for the horse when the owners were unwilling to do what was right. They had what they considered an acceptable amount of loss that they saw as just part of raising halter horses. It was a very asinine way of doing things.

For horses that are developing a club foot as

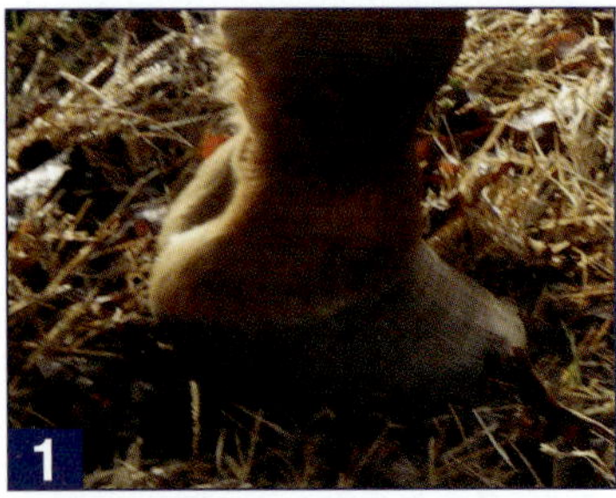
Severe Grade 3 club foot.

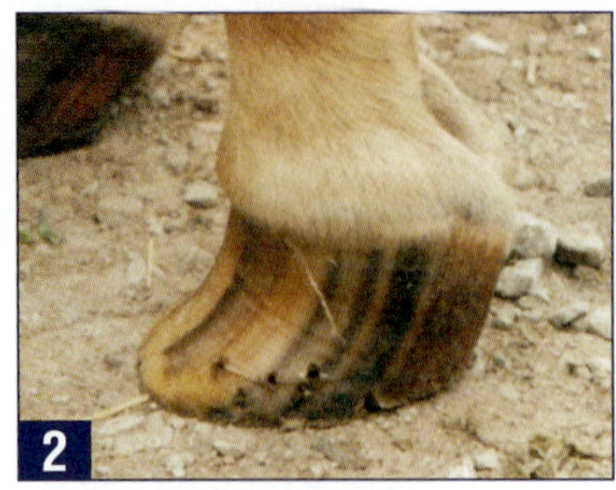
Grade 3 club foot.

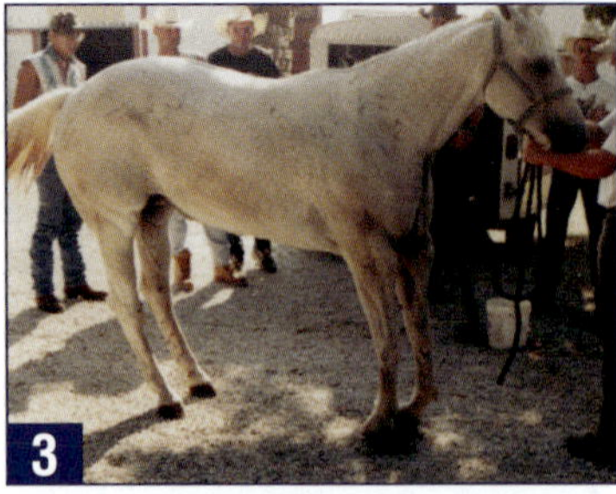
Horse with Grade 4 club feet on both legs, with one more severe than the other.

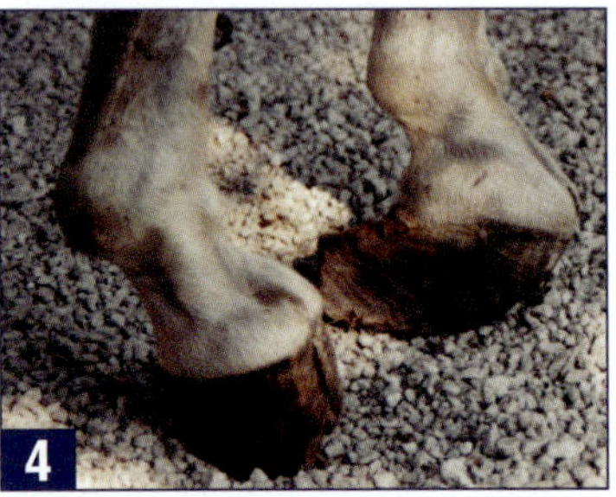
Closer views of the crippled horse from Figure 3.

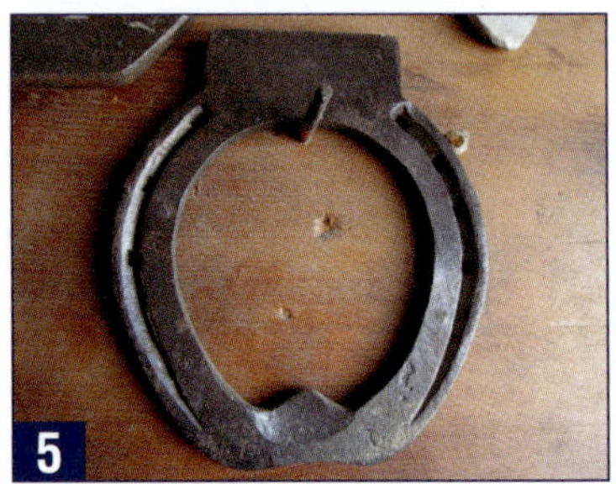
Toe-extension bar shoe.

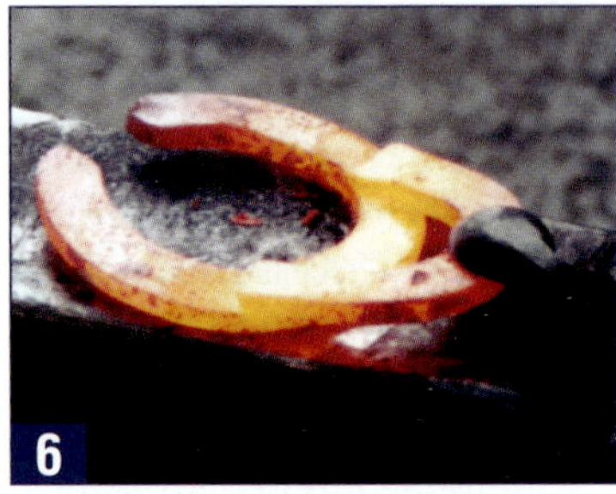
Making a toe extension by welding on the extension.

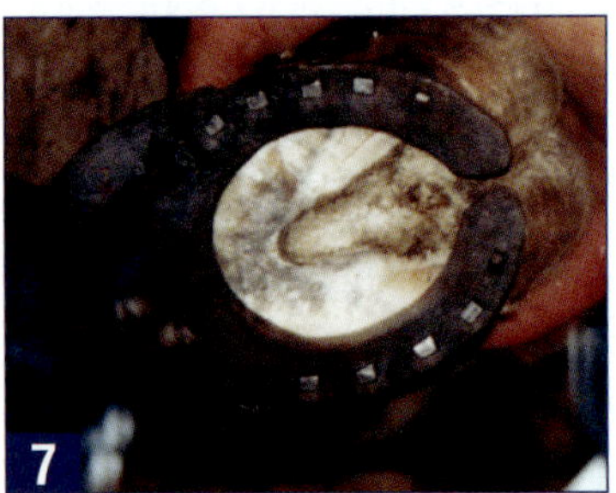
Putting the extended-toe shoe on.

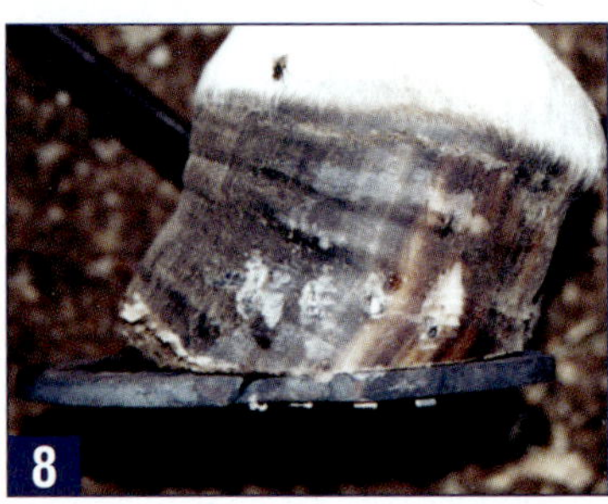
Lateral view of the shoe on the foot.

result of grazing on the ground, providing feed in a bunk that is a foot off the ground may prevent the high-low syndrome. With flexor muscle injury, get a vet involved immediately so that the recovery process does not result in a club foot.

With Grade 1 and Grade 2, approach the horse as a foot-shoer instead of a horseshoer. The reason for this is that you can't match both feet up in most cases without causing problems. Accept the fact that one is steeper and trim it so that the bones of the digit are aligned correctly for that leg. Explain to the customer that there will be a difference between the two feet, but that is the best strategy for keeping the horse sound. Trying to trim the club foot to an angle as shallow as the other foot is likely to result in lameness and potentially mechanical founder.

For Grade 3 and Grade 4, trimming and shoeing alone is not likely to fix the problem. For these horses, a vet must be involved to do surgery if there is any hope of a sound horse. The most common surgery is a tenotomy of the deep flexor tendon. This allows the coffin bone to change position without the extreme amount of pull coming from the deep flexor tendon. This should be followed by the application of a toe-extension shoe possibly with a reverse wedge if the foot cannot be trimmed shallow enough **(Figure 5)**.

The horse in **Figures 3-4** was shod on the worst foot with a toe extension shoe that was made by jump welding a piece to the toe **(Figures 6-8)**. This is one way to make any kind of extension, and it is a fast and easy way to make them in the field.

Figure 9 is a badly foundered horse that has

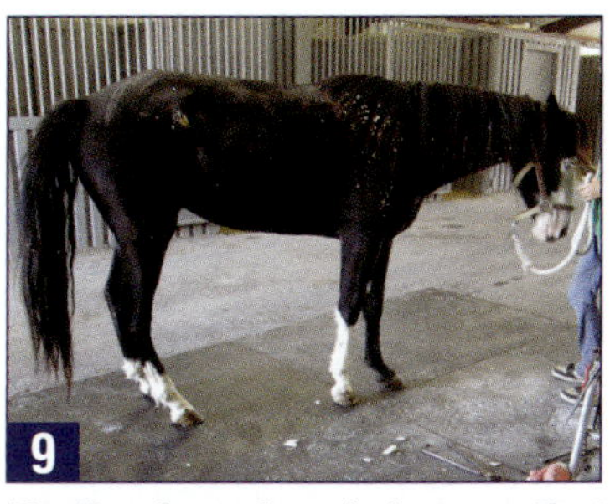

Badly foundered horse that had been knuckling over prior to deep flexor tenotomy.

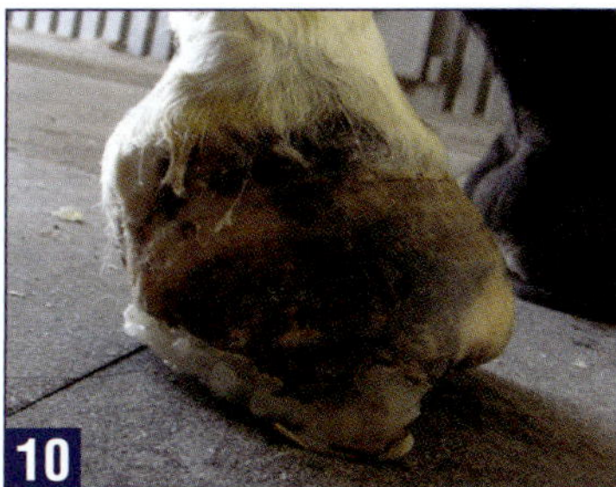

Lateral view of one of the feet with a Super Fast W-shoe on.

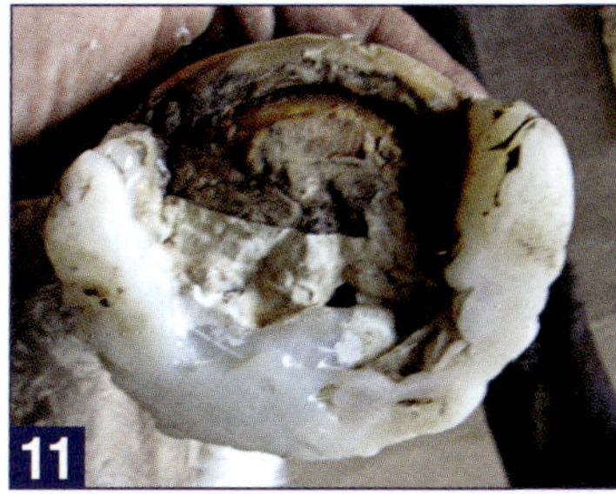

The more foundered foot with the Super Fast W-shoe.

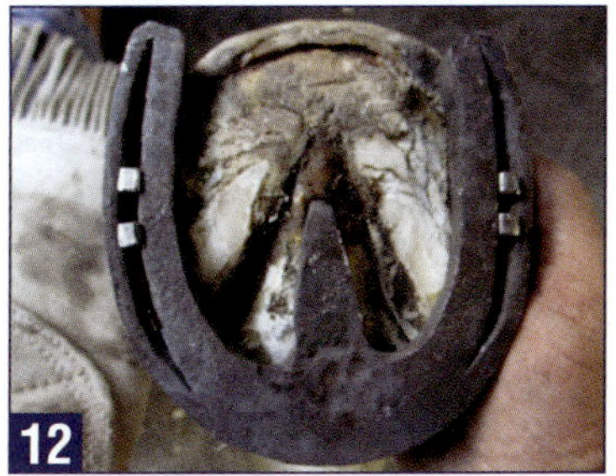

Reverse wedge steel W-shoe on the bottom of the foot.

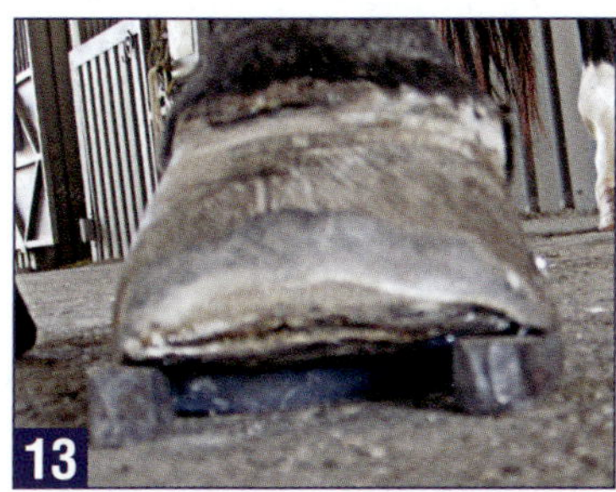

Dorsal view showing the gap at the front of the toe from the reverse wedge W-shoe.

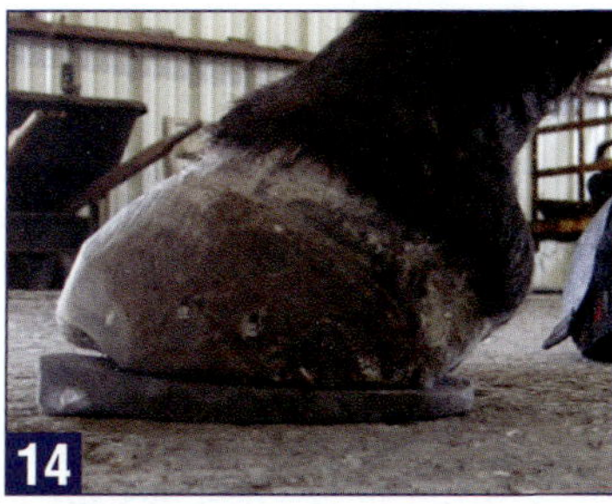

Lateral view of the foot with the W-shoe.

had the deep flexor tenotomy. Then Dr. Marcotte made a W-shoe out of Super Fast **(Figures 10-11)**. This worked well for a temporary measure until we could put on a reverse wedge W-shoe with a slight toe extension compared to the coffin bone. **Figure 12** is the shoe on the foot and **Figure 13** is a dorsal view on the ground. **Figure 14** is a lateral view of the foot on the ground, and **Figure 15** shows a radiograph of the alignment of the bones in the digit and the reverse wedge. Before the surgery, this horse was unable to stand on one leg while the other was worked on.

The owner has to be willing to follow the advice of the vet and farrier if the horse is to end up comfortable enough to use or live a content life.

ANTICIPATED OUTCOME

Depending on the severity of the club foot, many horses will end up being usable. They may have a greater tendency toward stumbling. Horses that are a Grade 3 or 4 are not likely to become rideable, but they may be managed to the point where they can live without discomfort.

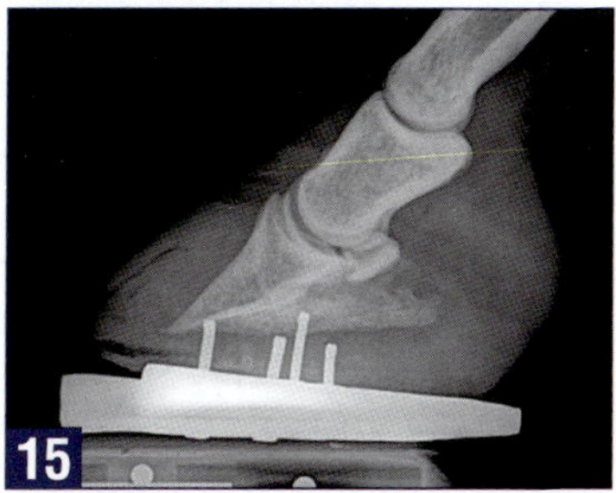

Radiograph showing the angle of the digit with the reverse wedge W-shoe.

IN SHORT

D: One front foot is steeper than the other, from slight degree to the point of knuckling over.

T: Trim and shoe for proper hoof pastern axis (HPA) in mild cases, tenotomy and toe extensions, in more severe cases.

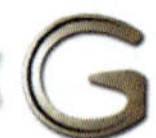

Chapter

45-4 Coffin Bone Fractures

DEFINITION

The distal phalanx has been chipped or suffered a break.

REASON

P3 fractures are generally caused by trauma from repeated concussion or may occur in coffin bones that have been weakened by pedal osteitis, bone cysts, or other causes. If a horse is bearing a lot of weight on a foot and twists hard, that action can also lead to a fracture.

ANATOMY

All coffin bone fractures are going to involve the coffin bone. There are articular and non-articular fractures, depending entirely on if the break involves the coffin joint. Fractures are labeled based on their location and the plane that they lie in, such as sagittal fractures, distal margin or rim fractures, wing fractures, and fractures of the extensor process. **Figure 1** depicts these fracture sites.

SYMPTOMS

Depending on where the fracture occurs, the horse may be mildly to severely lame. Fractures that involve the joint (articular) will cause a horse to be a Grade 4 lame. An example of a sagital articular fracture is shown in **Figure 2**. **Figures 3-4** are P3 fractures of lesser severity, and **Figures 5-6** show wing fractures. **Figure 5** shows a non-articular wing fracture of a foal, and **Figure 6** shows an articular wing fracture. Sometimes fractures may present as milder lameness. If you are using hoof testers with certain fractures, you may think that the foot is simply bruised. A radiograph is necessary to determine where and how bad a break in the coffin bone is.

TREATMENT

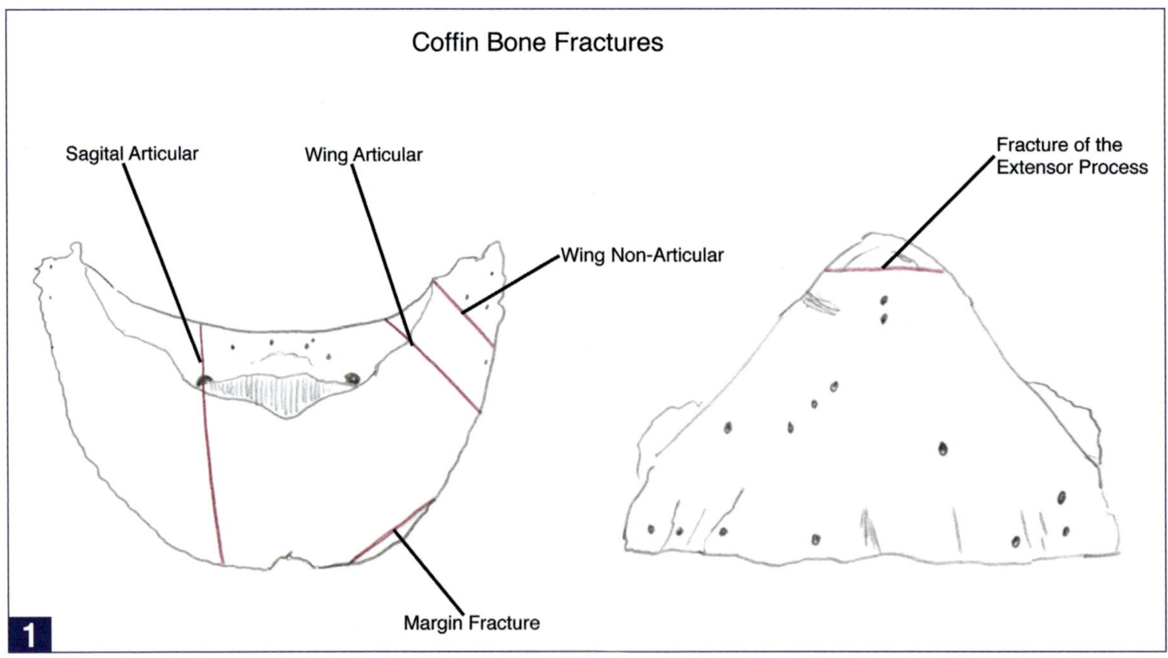

Drawings of the coffin bone to represent the different types of fractures.

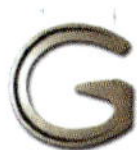

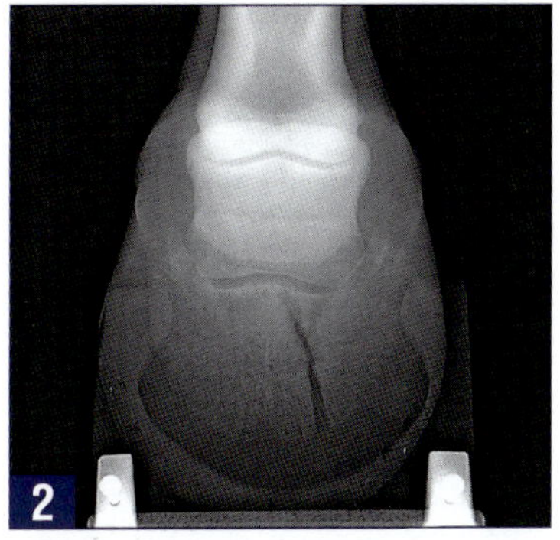

Radiograph of an articular sagital fracture, courtesy of Dr. Scott Morrison.

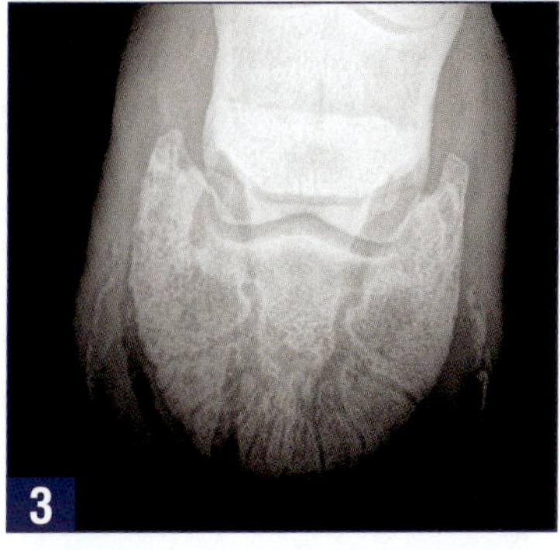

Fractured P3 with an abscess present, courtesy of Dr. John Marcotte.

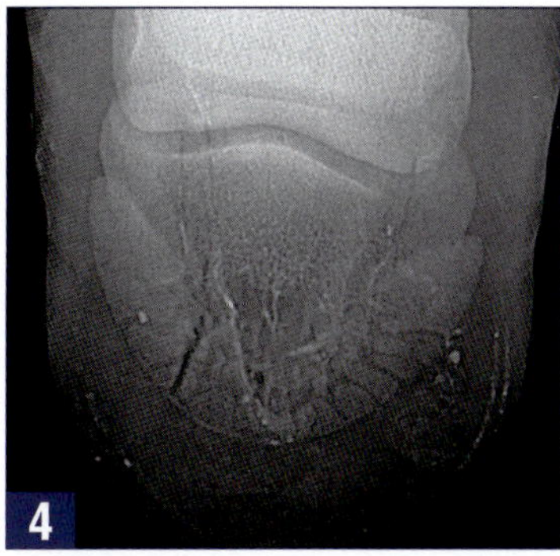

Fracture of P3 from Dr. Morrison.

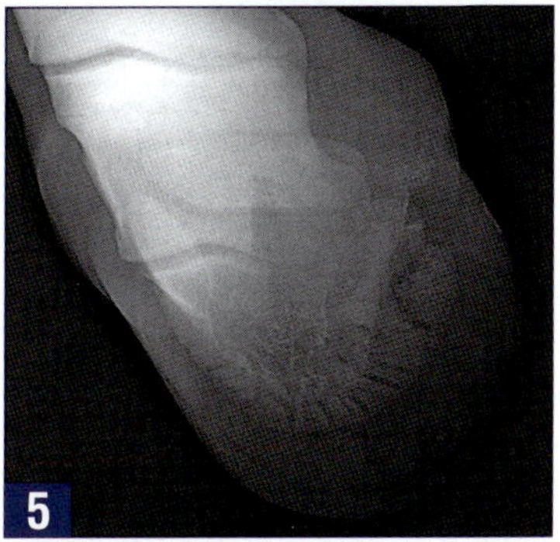

Non-articular wing fracture from Dr. Morrison.

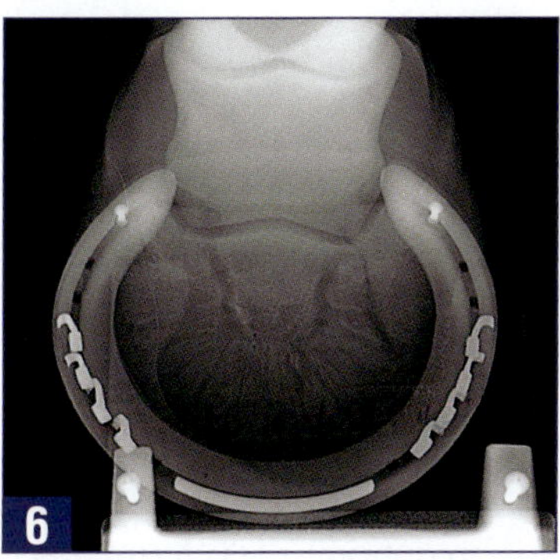

Articular wing fracture from Dr. Marcotte.

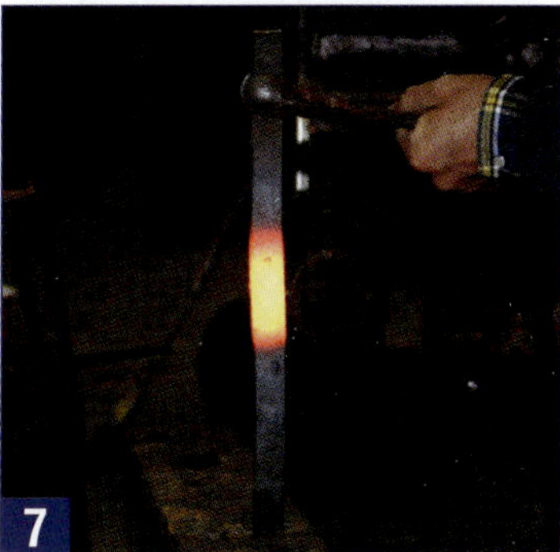

Bumping the toe for a wider web on a bar shoe for a P3 fracture.

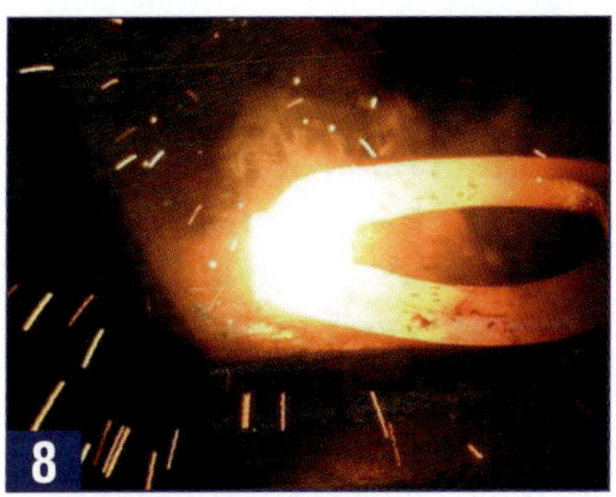

Welding the bar shoe.

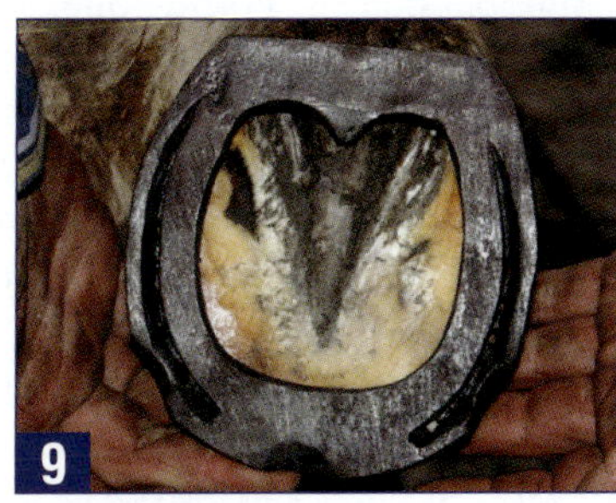

Bar shoe in position.

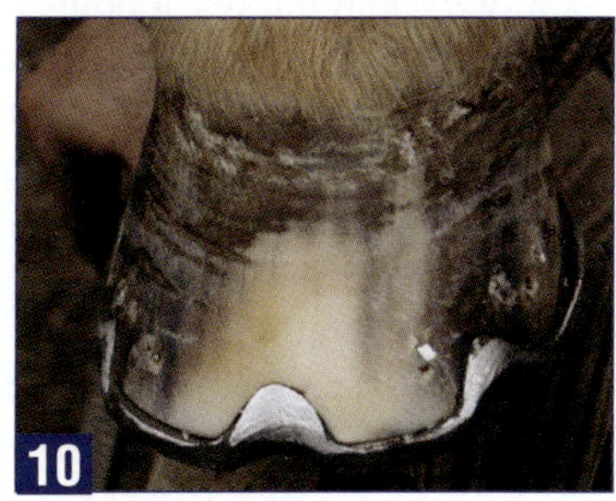

Clips fit properly.

The first thing that a farrier wants to consider with a coffin bone fracture is protection and stabilization of the hoof capsule. With this in mind, a wide-webbed bar shoe with several clips or a continuous clip is called for. I prefer just using well-placed clips if the fracture is not extreme. You should also use a pour-in pad if there is no sensitive structure involvement, but make certain that it does not protrude past the ground surface of the shoe.

Make the bar shoe using either a wide stock, or by bumping the stock for additional width **(Figure 7)**. The wider the stock, the better protection you can provide for the fractured coffin bone. In **Figure 8**, I am welding the bar shoe that you see in **Figures 9-12**. The clips are burned in and flush with the wall **(Figure 10),** and I block the back of the bar with Hawthorne's Sole Pack **(Figure 11)** before applying the pour-in pad **(Figure 12)**. **Figure 13** shows a

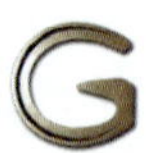

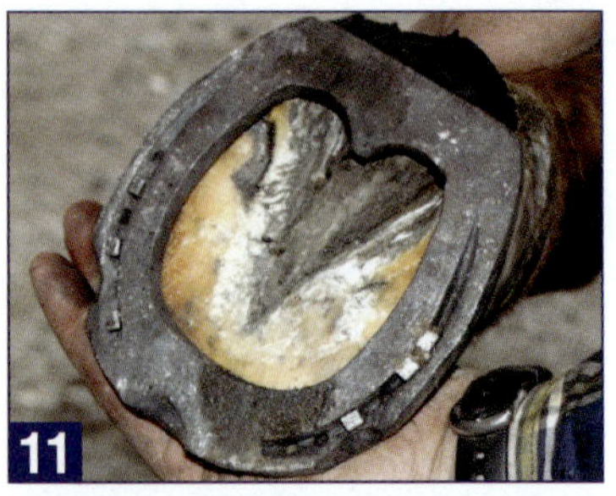

Damming the back of the shoe with Sole Pack

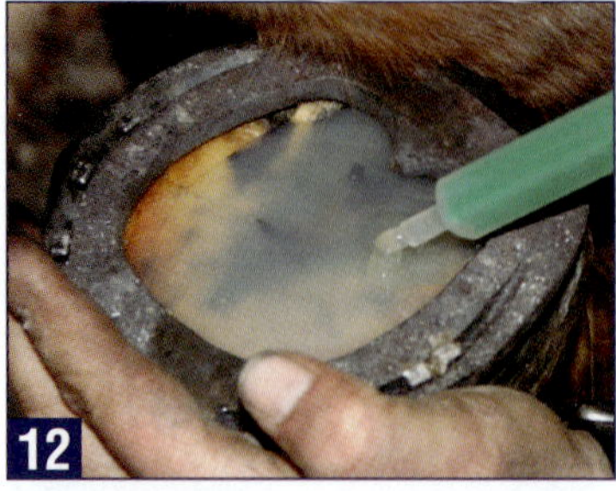

Pour-in pad.

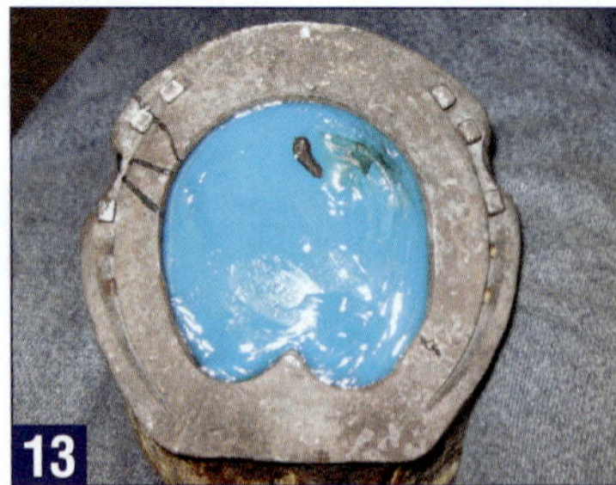

Equi-Pak CS pour-in.

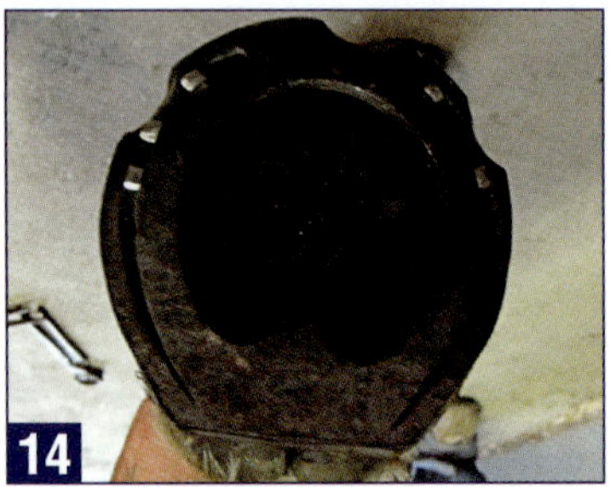

Bar shoe with pad.

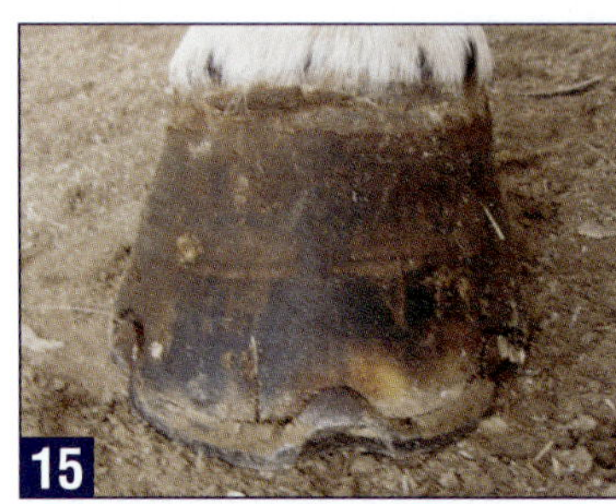

Shoe on the foot at 6 weeks.

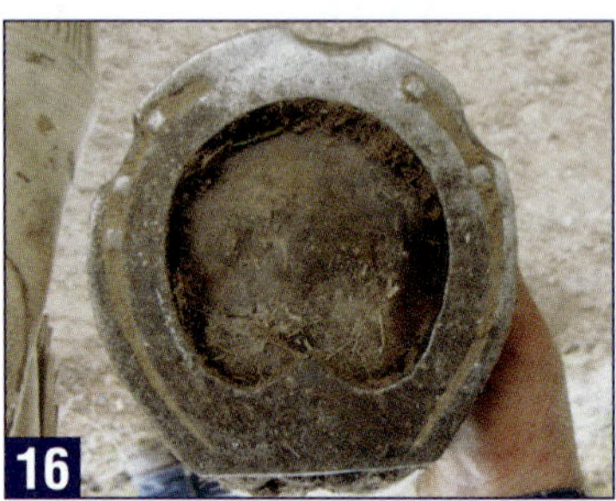

Shoe on the foot at 6 weeks.

different horse where a pour-in pad was an option, and here I used Equi-Pak CS.

The next series is a horse that not only had a fractured coffin bone but also had an abscess. As such, we could not use a pour-in material, but had to use a regular pad. When I first saw this horse, he was Grade 4 lame. A radiograph for this horse can be seen in **Figure 3**. The shoe was made and the pad applied **(Figure 14)**. When the horse came back for a reset at 6 weeks **(Figures 15-16)**, he had grown some pretty good length and lameness had decreased to about Grade 2. After trimming the foot **(Figures 17-19)**, I decided to go with the same shoe and pad for another 6 weeks **(Figure 20)**. At 12 weeks from the first shoeing **(Figure 21)**, the horny sole that had separated from the abscess pulled off **(Figures 22-23)**. The horse was sound at this point, so I shod him with normal open-heeled shoes. This was a very successful abscess and fractured coffin bone treatment.

Horses with coffin bone fractures need stall rest, so the owner will be involved with keeping this horse from being overly active as well as monitoring for any possible infections or complications. Veterinarians play a big role in diagnosis, since they take the radiographs and have the expertise to read them. For horses that have an articular fracture, vets may have to do surgery to place screws in the coffin bone.

For fractures of the extensor process, the pieces of P3 can be surgically removed or, if large enough, be reattached to the coffin bone with screws. This type of fracture can happen from too much pull on the main extensor tendon and can be unilateral or bilateral. The primary indication that this type of fracture has occurred will be a foot that develops more of a hind shape as well as a bulge just proximal to the dorsal coronary band. This is know as buttress foot. Shoe normally and allow the horse to rest for 6 months.

ANTICIPATED OUTCOME

This horse is looking at about 8 to 10 months of recovery, but if it goes well, there is a better than average chance of making a full recovery.

IN SHORT

D: Broken coffin bone.

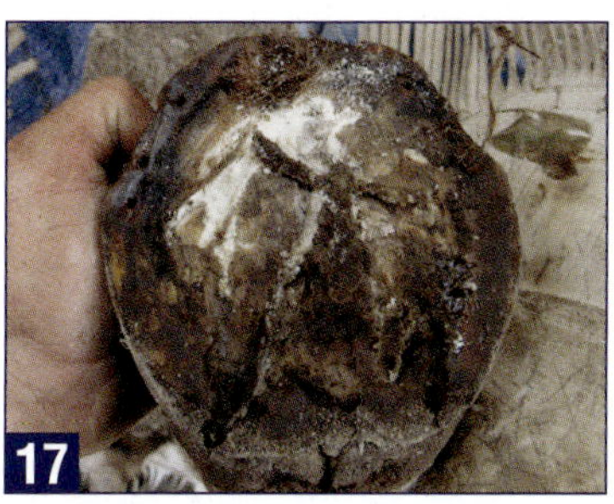

The bottom of the foot at 6 weeks.

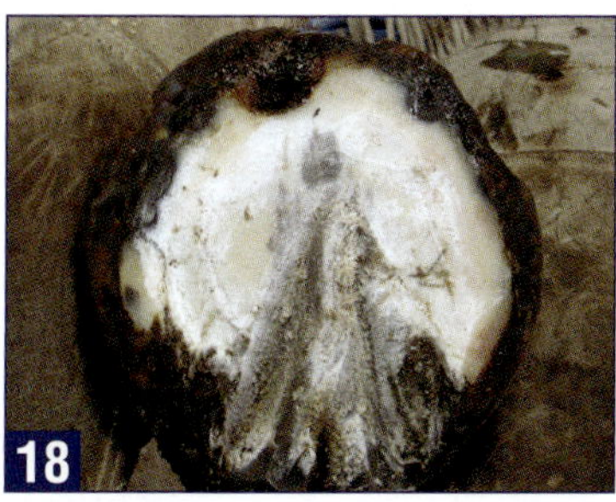

Initial knife work on the foot at 6 weeks.

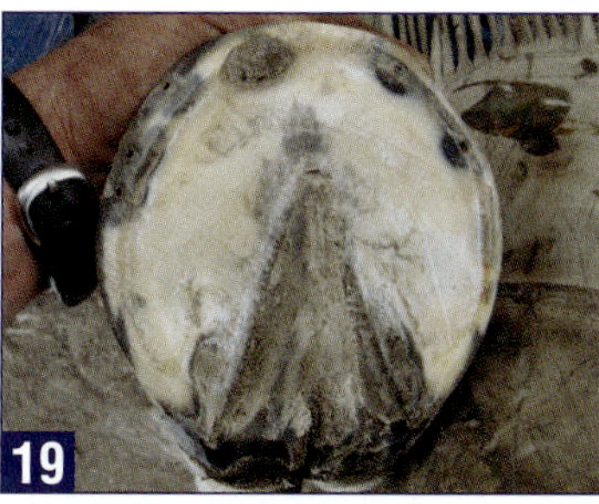

Trimmed at 6 weeks.

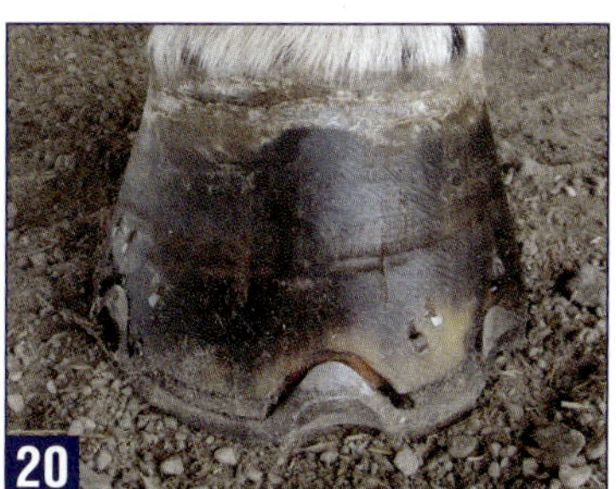

Shoe reset.

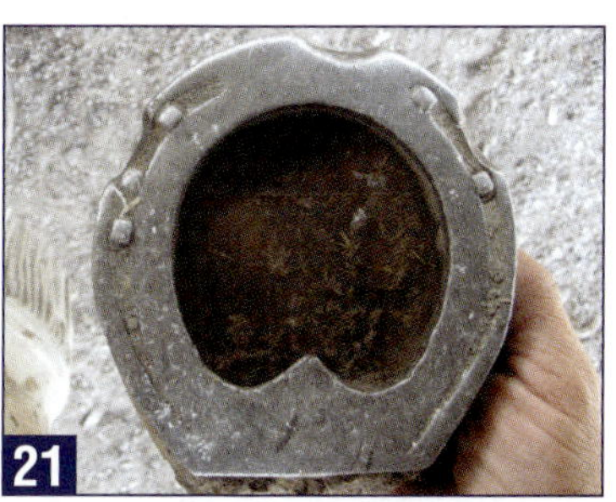

Shoe on the foot after first reset, 12 weeks from first application.

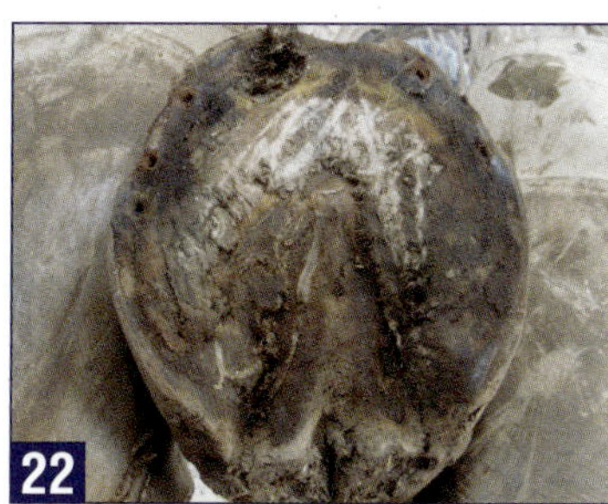

Bottom of the foot at 12 weeks.

T: Stall rest, wide-webbed bar shoe with side clips and a rocker toe with a pour-in pad, or use a regular pad if infection is present.

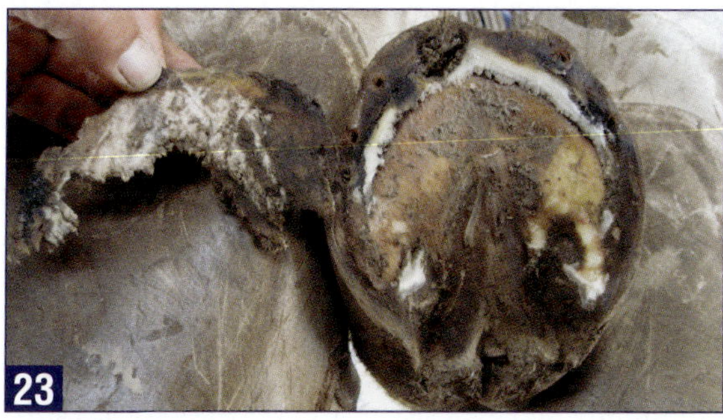

Large portion of horny sole pulled off of the foot at 12 weeks.

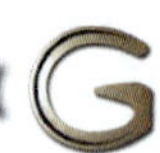

Chapter

45-5 CORNS

DEFINITION

Corns is the common name given to damage in the area of the foot known as the seat of corn. The seat of corn is the sole that is between the angle of the bar and the hoof wall in the heel.

REASON

Corns are thought to be caused by pressure in the seat of corn area. This pressure can come from debris getting between the shoe and the foot in this area, or more commonly from leaving shoes on too long. Since a lot of feet grow faster at the toe, the shoe can be pulled forward on the foot with time. As the shoe is pulled forward, the heel region often expands beyond the shoe, and the new position of the shoe places the heels directly into the seat of corn area. Tight shoeing or shoeing with heel caulks can also cause corns. **Figure 1** is typical of the type of shoeing you would expect to see on a foot with corns.

ANATOMY

The anatomy involved with corns is the seat of corn, almost always on the front feet.

SYMPTOMS

There are three types of corns that you will commonly see. These are the dry/red corn, moist corn and infected corn. Each involves injury to the seat of corn, but they all tell a slightly different story. Since this is a problem in the heel region, there is the potential for this to be misdiagnosed as navicular or other heel lameness problems.

The red or dry corn is a bruise. It will appear as a red bruise in the seat of corn, and horses can have a varying degree of lameness. Hoof testers will tell you how bad the bruise is affecting the horse. **Figure 2** shows the common look of a dry corn.

If it is a moist corn, serum will be present. This will appear as a thick liquid that seeps from the seat of corn. On occasion, you will see a hole in the area that will look like a puncture wound. **Figure 3** shows what was once a moist corn but did not turn into an infected corn.

With an infected, or suppurating corn, the horse will be sore, and you will in effect be dealing with an abscess. **Figure 4** is of an infected corn, and this horse does have a deep abscess and lameness that are a direct result of this corn. In **Figures 5-6**, you can see the results of an infected corn that has

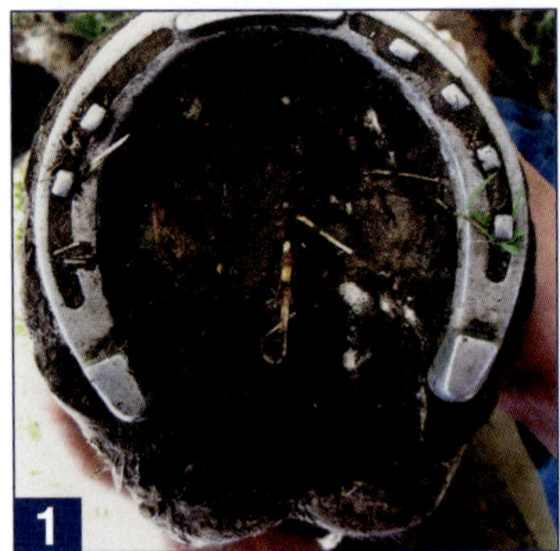

Type of shoeing that can cause corns. Heel caulks fit tight and left on for too long.

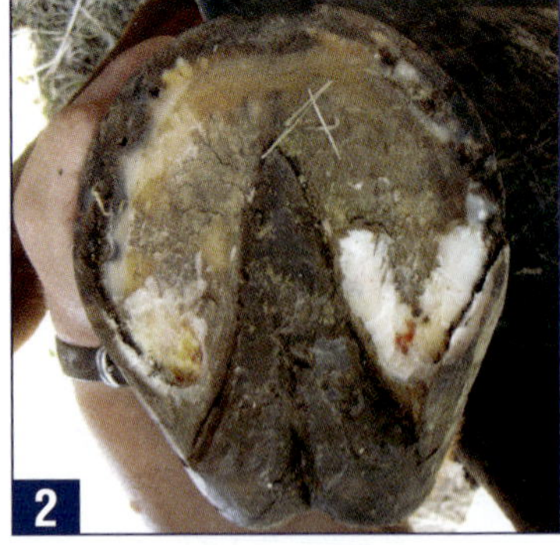

Dry corn.

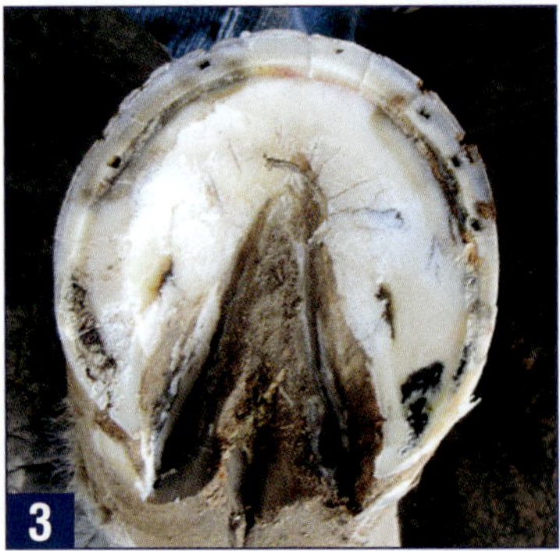

Remnants of a moist corn.

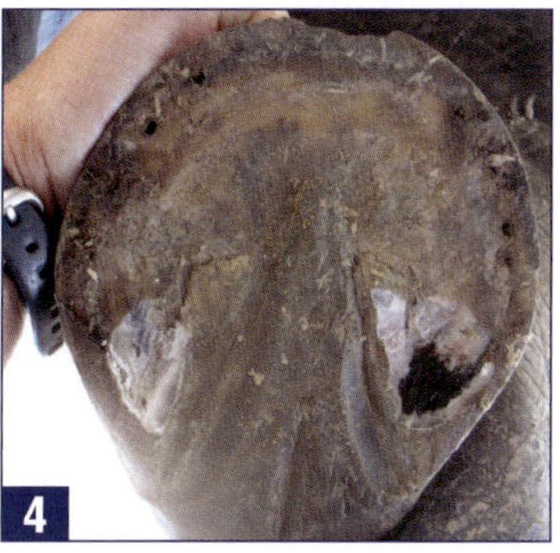
4
Infected corn.

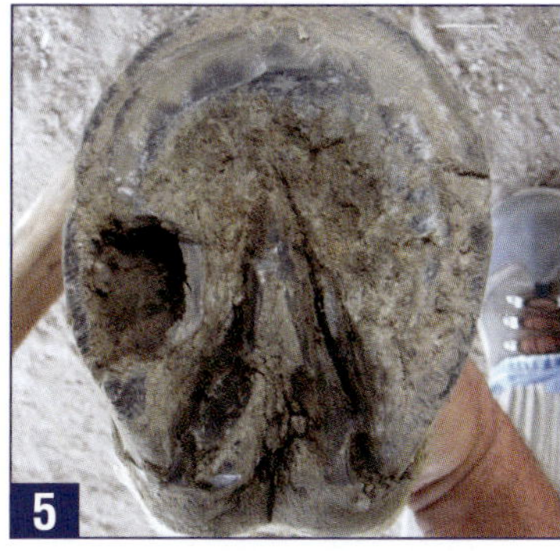
5
Results of an infected corn.

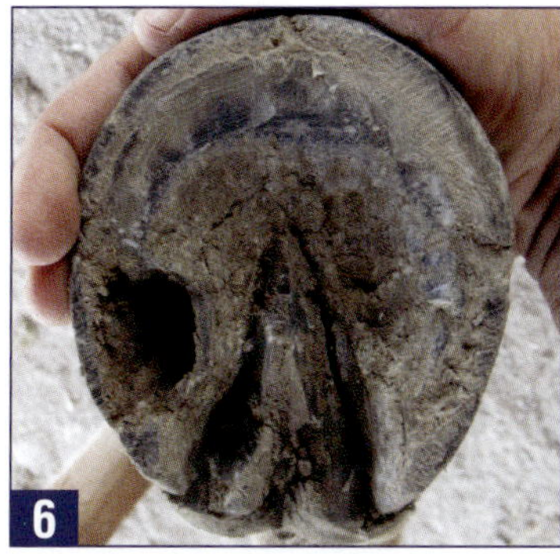
6
Foot held at an angle to show how deep the infected corn went.

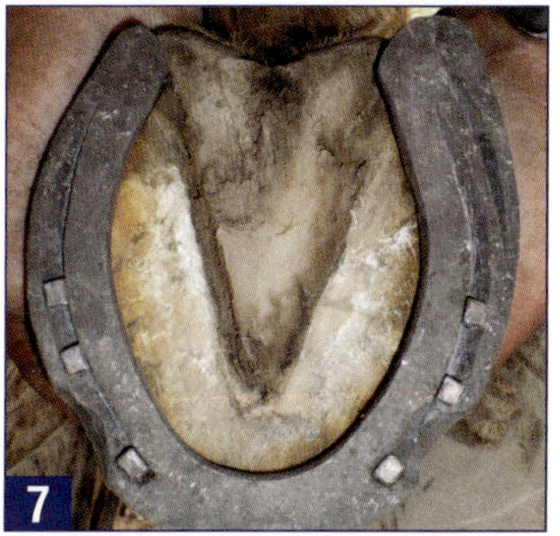
7
Bumped up heel that can give coverage to a corn if needed.

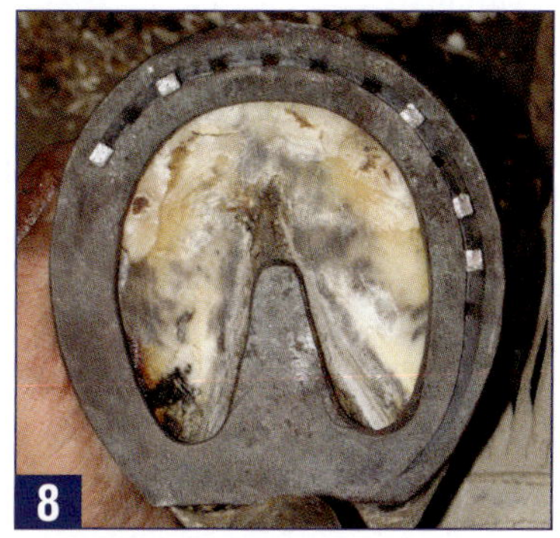
8
Heart bar on a foot.

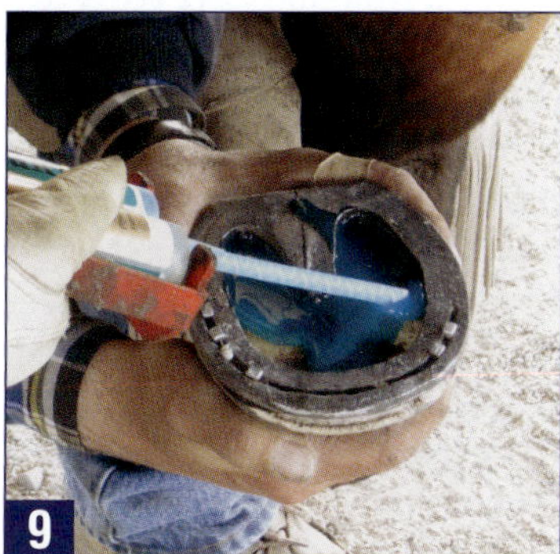
9
Putting Equi-Pak in the foot with the heart bar.

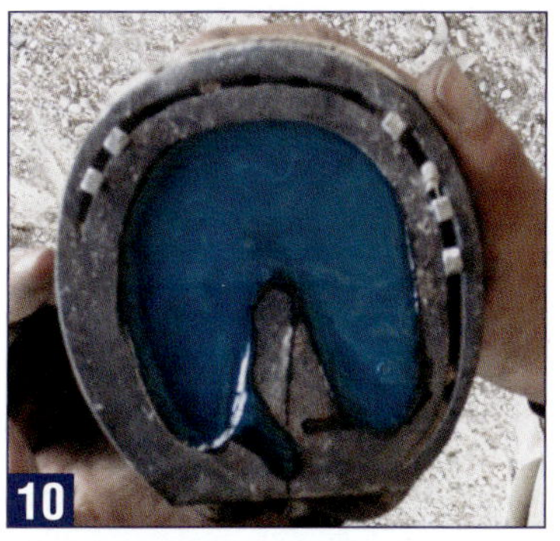
10
Shoe on foot with Equi-Pak.

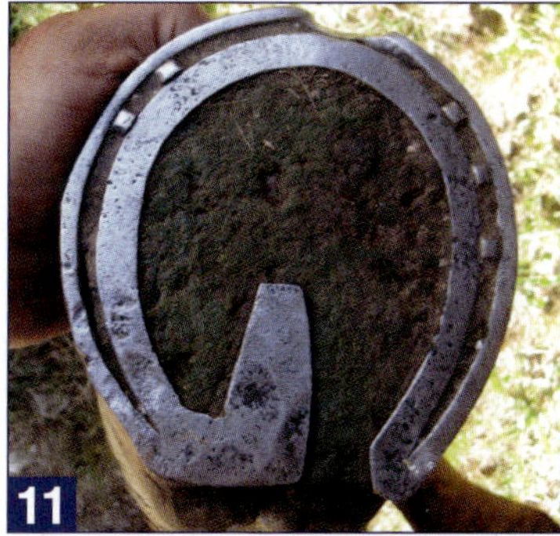
11
G-bar.

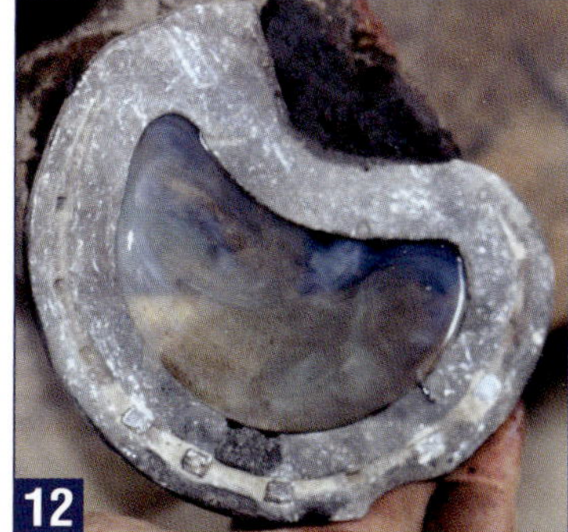
12
Z-bar.

drained. This foot just needs time to grow back out to become normal again.

TREATMENT

For a moist or red corn, shoe with a wide-webbed shoe, possibly adding width in the heel of the corn **(Figure 7)**. Make certain to have good expansion of the shoe in the heels and avoid sole pressure in the seat of corn. With lame horses, you may find that a heart bar and Equi-Pak are a necessity to make the horse comfortable **(Figures 8-10)**. Other good options are a G-bar **(Figure 11)**, a Z-bar **(Figure**

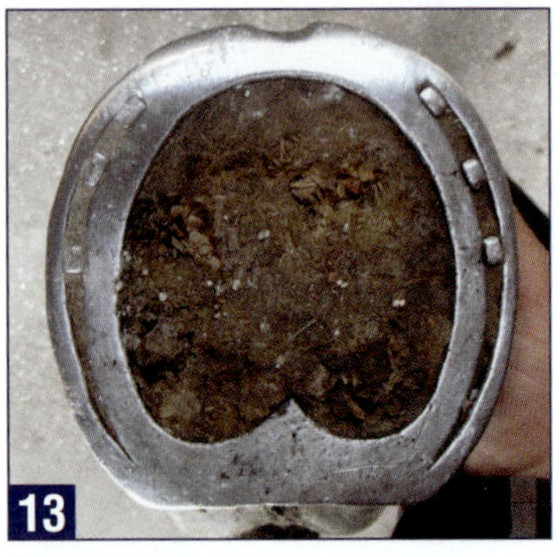

13 *Straight bar.*

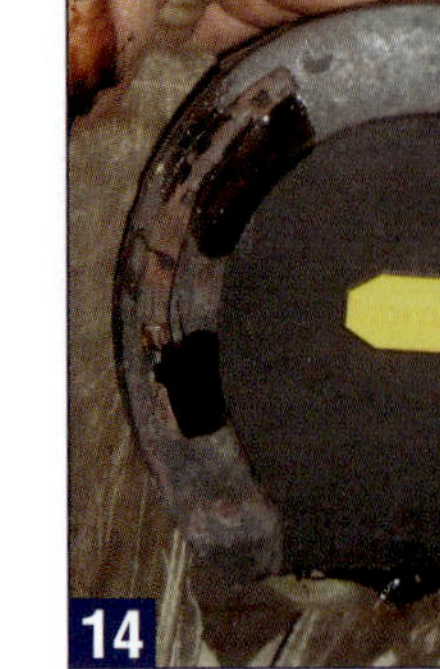

14 *Shoe and pad on foot.*

12) or a straight bar **(Figure 13)**. You can also use a pad if that seems called for in any particular foot **(Figure 14)**.

If you are dealing with a suppurating corn, treat it as an abscess. Apply an Epsom salts poultice and bandage for several days until the infection has resolved itself. Once it has cleared up, shoe as if it were a dry or moist corn. Be certain that the infection is cleared up before you cover it.

A vet and horse owner may have the same involvement as if they were dealing with an abscess.

ANTICIPATED OUTCOME

Most of the corns I have dealt with were easily taken care of, but there are some horses that suffer from chronic corns due to their conformation or other factors. With this type of horse, be certain to always fit with adequate length and expansion.

IN SHORT

D: Bruise or damage in the seat of corn.

T: Full fit wide-webbed shoe, G-bar, Z-bar, heart bar, or straight bar, and possibly Equi-Pak

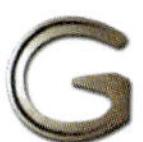

Chapter

45-6 CRACKS

DEFINITION

A crack can really be any long opening in the hoof wall, but for this particular DRASTA, we are concerned with cracks that are parallel to the tubules in the hoof wall. We will also deal with quarter cracks specifically in a different area. So the definition we are going with here is: A split or fissure in the hoof wall that is more or less vertical.

REASON

A crack can happen for a lot of reasons; drastic moisture changes, uneven weight bearing, coronary band injury, weak hooves, improper nutrition, white line disease, keratoma, flared and dished horn, or just overall poor horn. Regardless of the cause, the treatments are going to be pretty much the same.

The most common reasons I see cracks happen are neglect and flare. In **Figures 1-5**, there is a foot that has flared, resulting in a crack. In **Figure 2**, I am trimming a lot of the flare with my nippers, and in **Figure 5**, the white coloration at the bottom of the foot indicates that I have dressed to the non-pigmented inside of the stratum medium.

Figures 6-7 are of a foot with flare on one side that has pulled the foot apart and made a crack. In

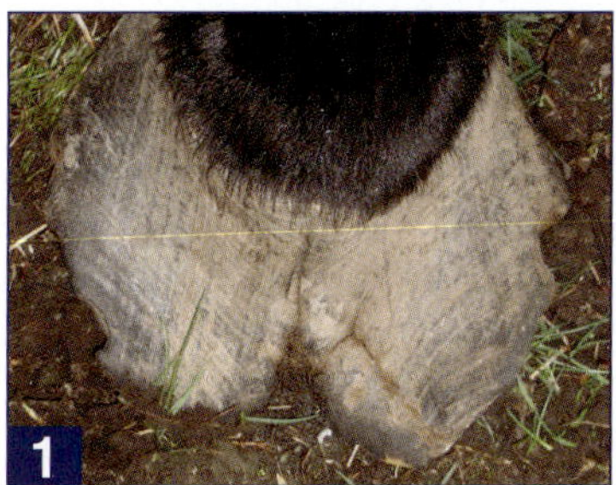

Flare causing a crack in the foot.

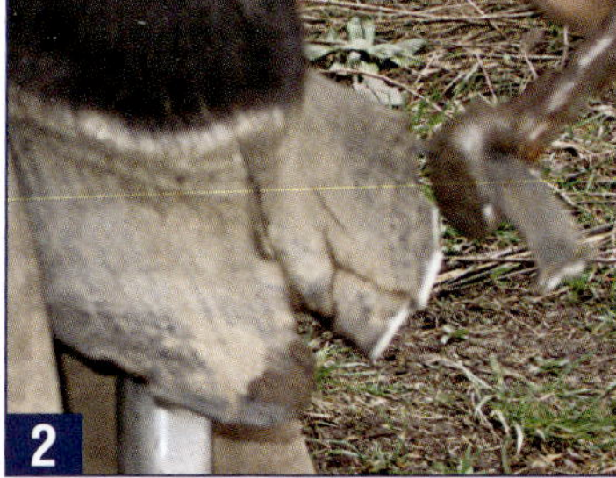

Trimming around the flare.

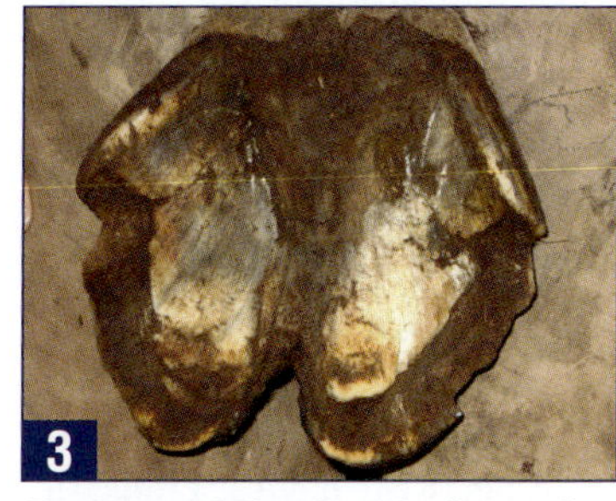

Bottom of the foot before trimming.

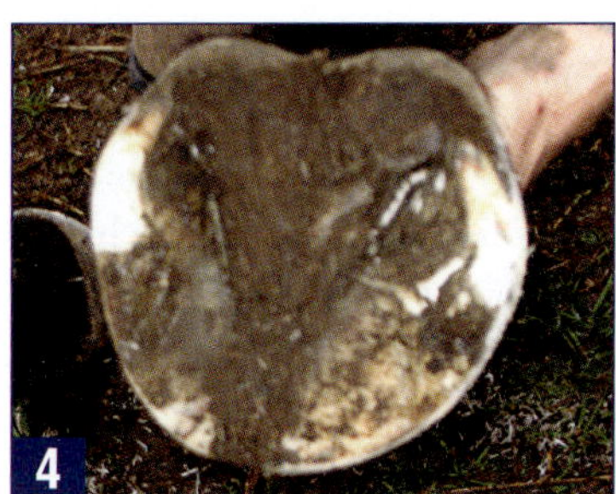

After trimming.

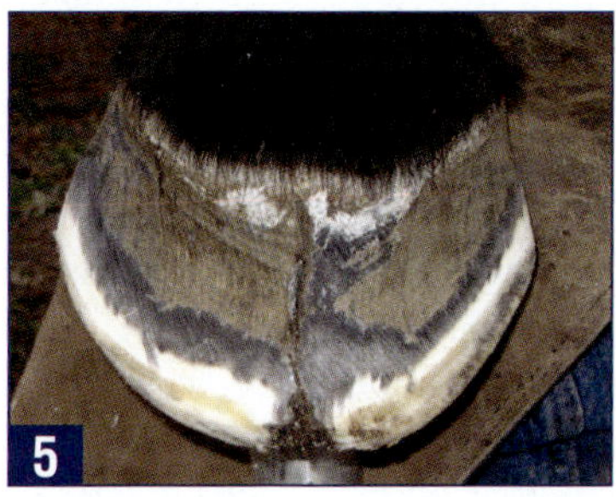

Dressed after trimming, notice the non-pigmented stratum medium.

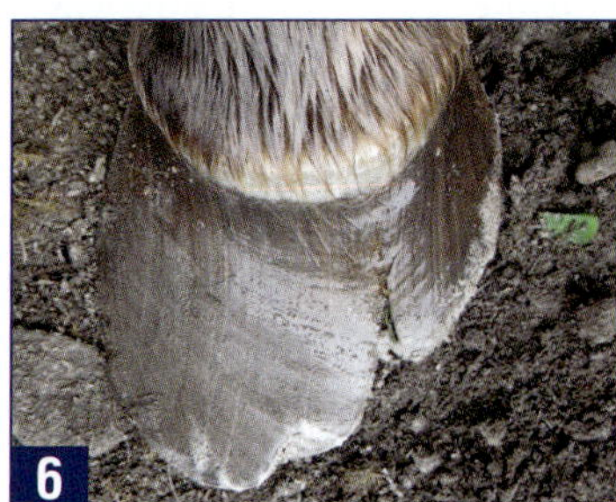

Flare causing crack.

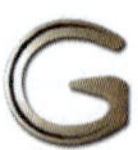

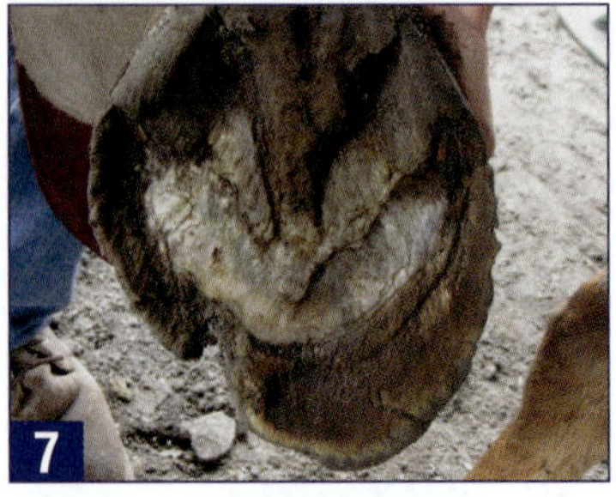

7 *Bottom of foot before trimming.*

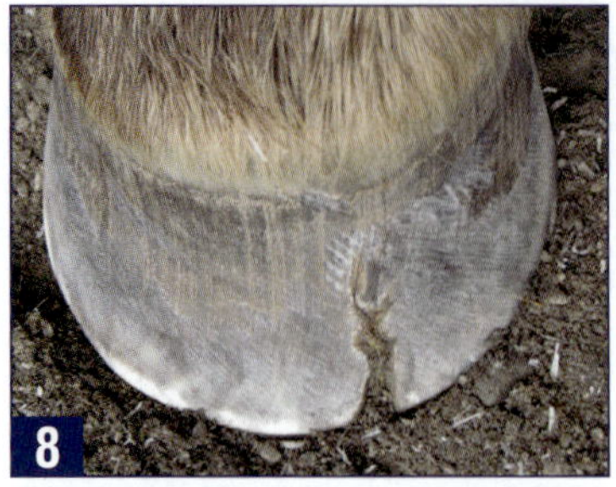

8 *After trimming, the forces that caused the crack are gone.*

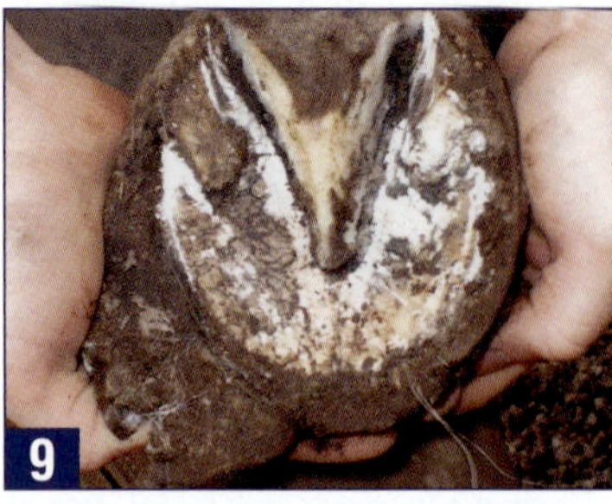

9 *Another flare that caused a crack.*

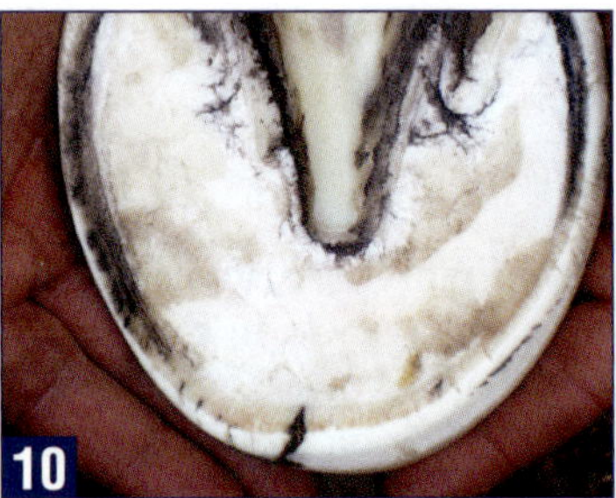

10 *Once the foot is trimmed, the crack can easily be seen.*

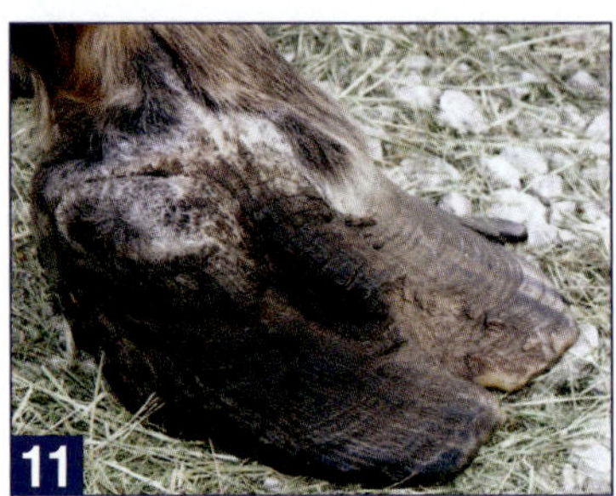

11 *Injury to the coronet that caused a crack.*

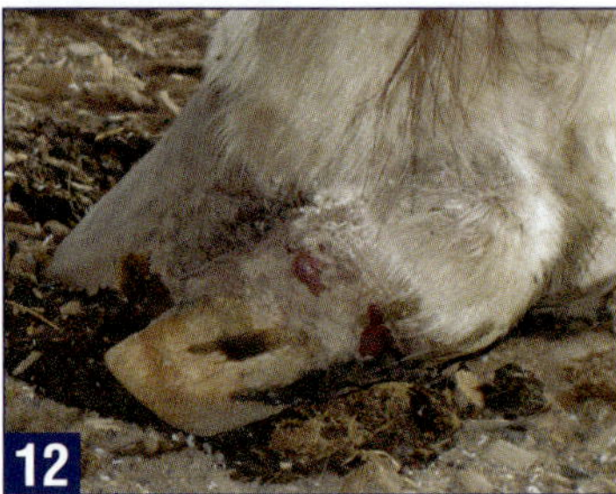

12 *Injury related crack.*

Figure 8, you can see the trimmed foot, and just trimming this foot will allow it to grow normally. **Figures 9-10** show a similar foot, and the depth of the crack is easily seen on the bottom of the trimmed foot in **Figure 10**.

Cracks often accompany an injury. This is readily apparent in **Figures 11-12**.

ANATOMY

When you have a crack in the hoof wall, the obvious anatomical structure is going to be the hoof wall. However, there can be more involved, depending on the severity and location of the crack. A deep crack can involve any portion of the foot under the hoof wall such as the coffin bone, lateral cartilages, and laminae. If an infection results from the crack, the entire foot may become involved.

SYMPTOMS

You will often have customers point out superficial shallow cracks that are only in the outside of the stratum medium, and these are of little consequence. The ones that are serious are the ones that allow bacteria into the sensitive structures, or worse, allow different parts of the foot to move independently of each other.

With shallow cracks, there is no problem or lameness. The foot just has a look that a customer would prefer not to see. These will often dress out of the foot with very little effort. Farriers who do not understand anatomy, or sometimes customers themselves, will often rasp a little hash mark across the crack. This only serves as an advertisement of ignorance. I could not help putting some of these photos in here to show how little success this method offers, so here is a medley of cracks with hash marks through them **(Figures 13-19)**. This even persists internationally. **Figure 16** is of a racehorse in New Zealand.

From an anatomy perspective, it should be easy to see why this crosshatch line does not work. The only way that the hash mark could work is if it were deep enough to involve the entire hoof wall, in which case it would be worse than most cracks anyway.

With cracks that allow movement of different regions of the hoof wall, you will have lameness. If there is an infection to go with it, you will have severe lameness. In **Figure 20**, there was a crack in the quarter, and it led to the entire piece being torn away from the rest of the hoof. Carefully examining

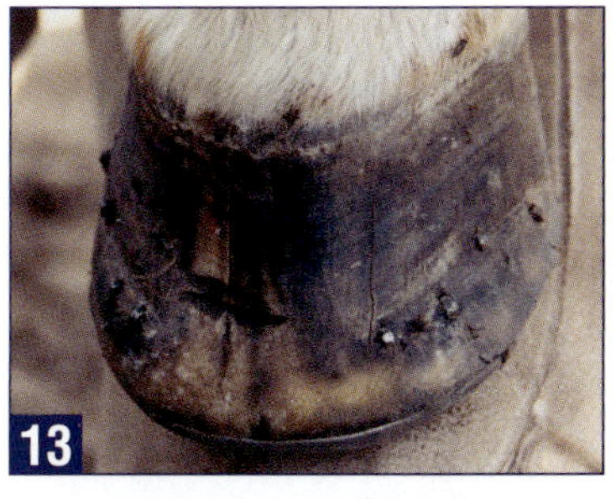

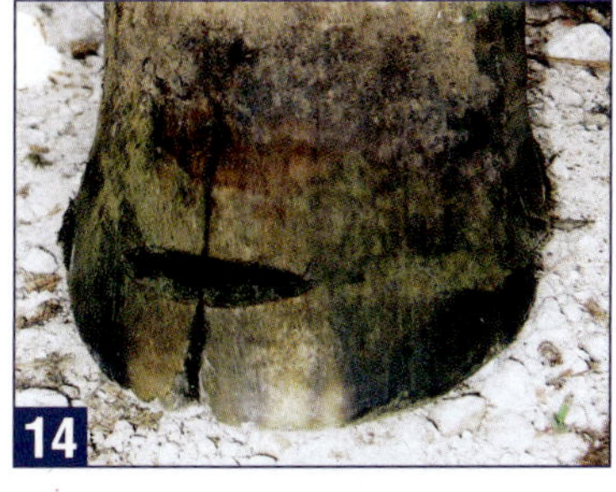

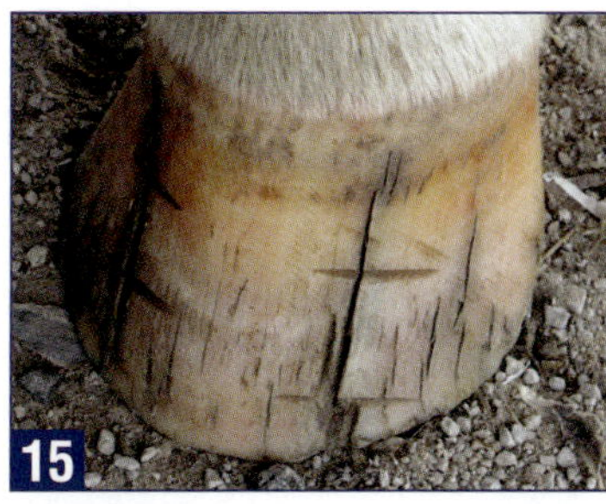

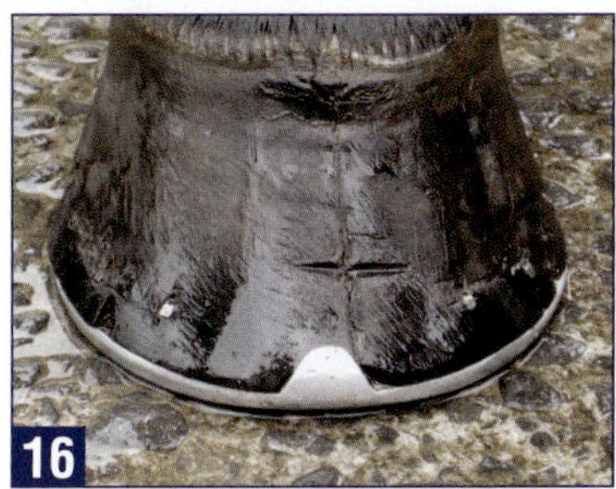

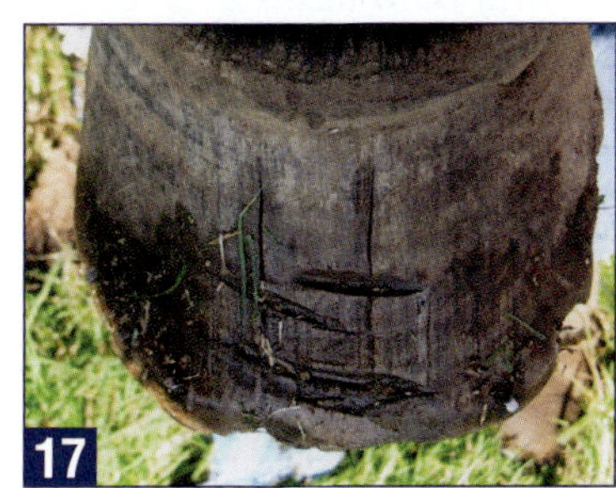

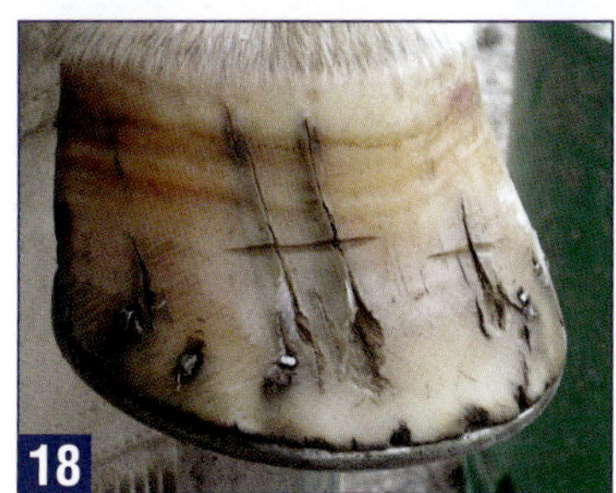

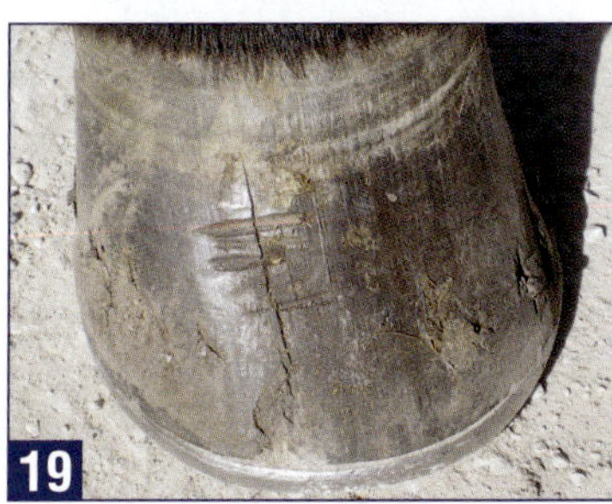

Hash marks in feet and the cracks that run through them.

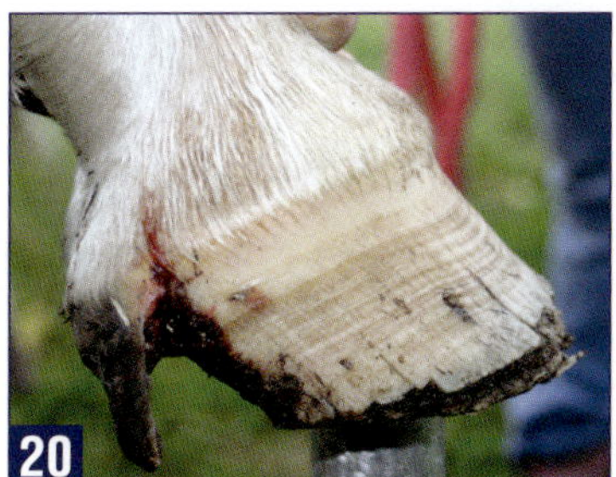

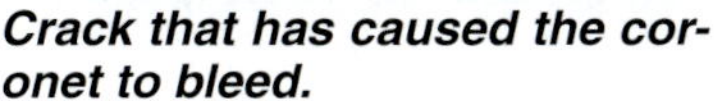

Crack that has caused the coronet to bleed.

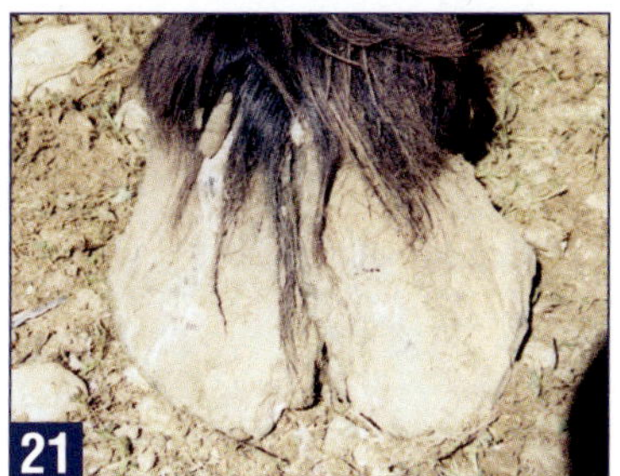

Severe crack through the entire thickness of the wall.

the photo will show the blood at the top of the crack, and every time this piece of wall moves, the horse is in pain. In **Figures 21-22**, there is a crack that is so deep and chronic that the horse is Grade 4 lame. The foot has been trimmed in **Figure 23**, and the wall has been so deformed by this crack that the non-pigmented stratum medium is revealed down both sides of the crack from the top of the hoof wall on down. This indicates that the coronary band has been disfigured.

TREATMENT

As a farrier, begin treating a crack by trying to figure out what has caused it. If there is something

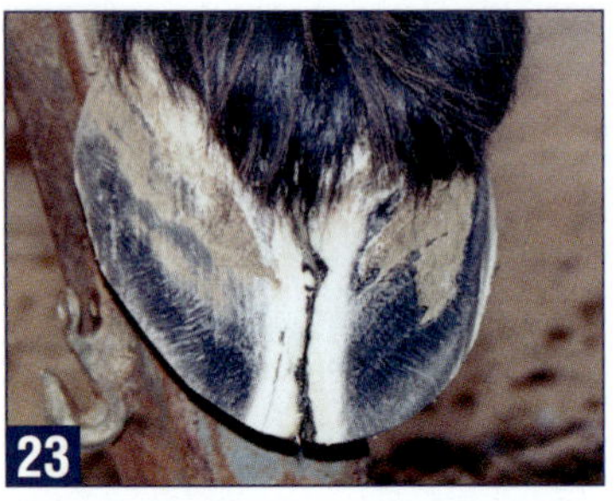

23 *Once the foot is dressed, the non-pigmented stratum medium is revealed down both sides of the crack.*

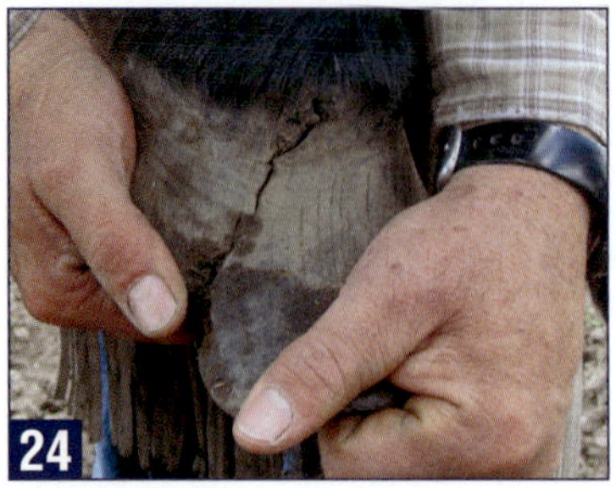

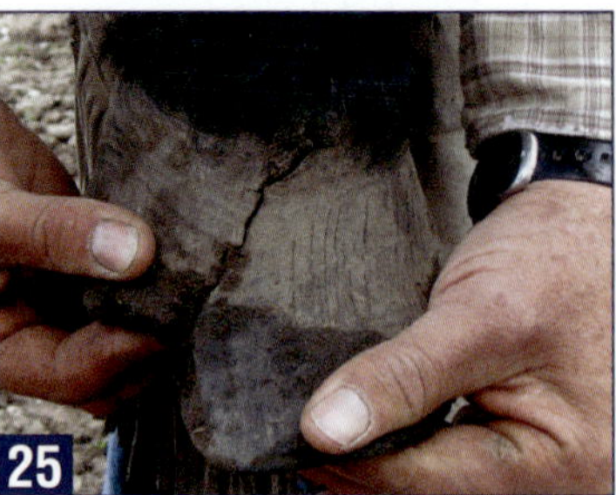

24 **25** *Moving both sides of a foot, separated by a crack on a neglected foot.*

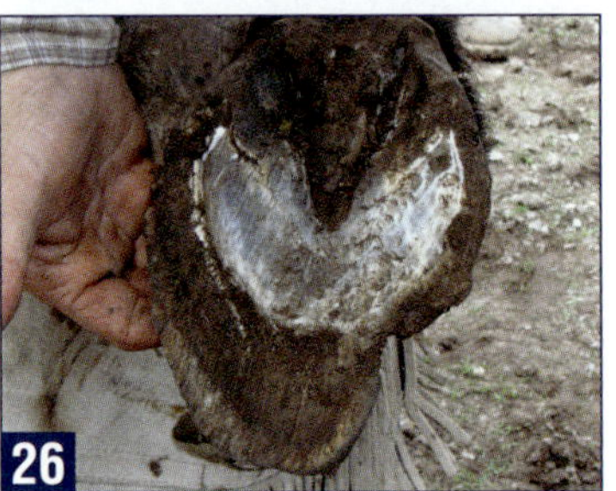

26 *Bottom of the neglected foot.*

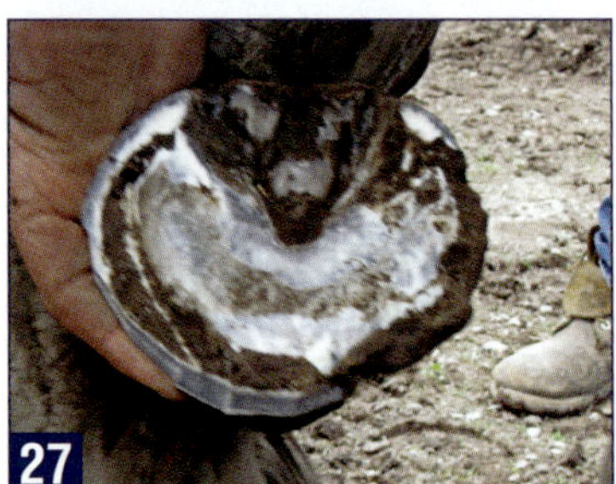

27 *The foot after trimming.*

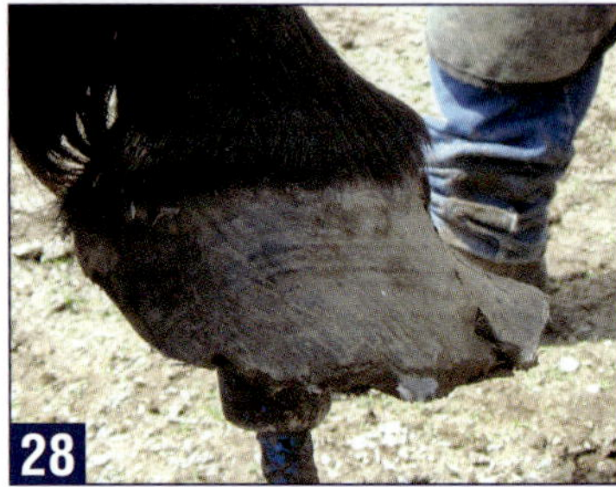

28 *Lateral view of the foot from the outside after the bottom has been trimmed.*

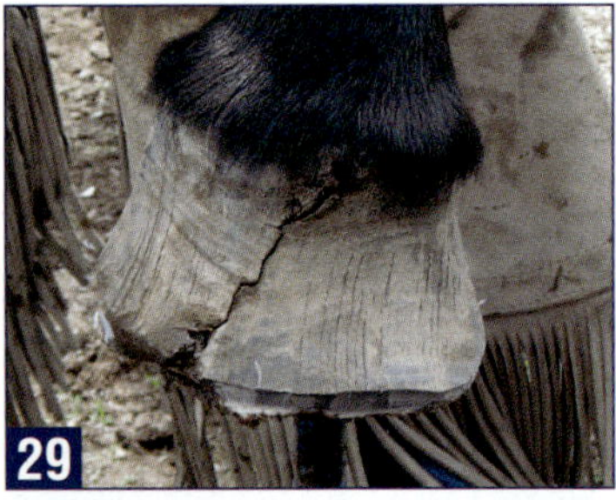

29 *Dorsal view of the foot before dressing.*

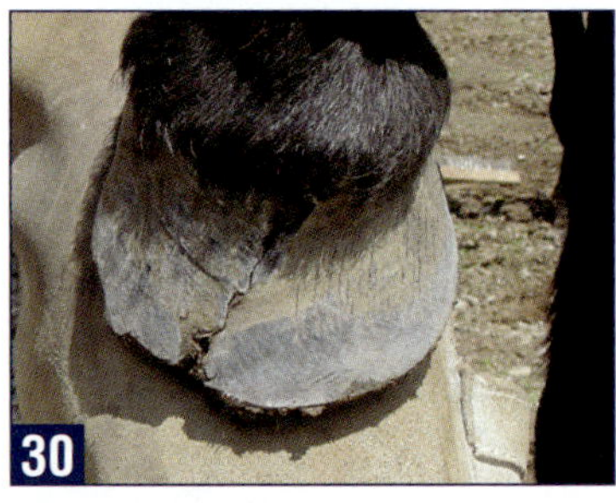

30 *The foot dressed.*

that you can do to treat the cause, the crack will grow out and be gone. For instance, if a crack has happened from bad nutrition, starting the horse on a good supplement or diet may take care of the weak hooves. It is also imperative that the foot is dressed to create as straight a hoof wall as possible. There are some instances where it is not possible to dress enough horn away, but the closer you can get, the better.

Often the crack will still need to be stabilized for enough time to grow new strong hoof wall. There are quite a few options for reinforcing a weak hoof wall at a crack; a farrier just needs to decide which one fits which circumstance. Here are my favorites:

Lace nail. I use lace nails when there is good thickness of hoof wall, a deep toe crack, for instance. This will allow the foot to be strong enough to grow out without further cracking. Once the lace nail gets to the ground, simply trim it out. Here is a series of a successful nail lace job on a horse that was Grade 4 lame when presented and was Grade 1 lame immediately after the first treatment.

In **Figures 24-25**, the two sides of the foot are

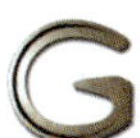

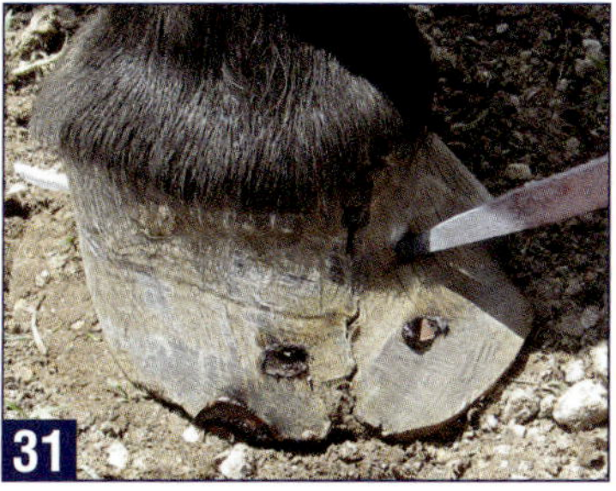

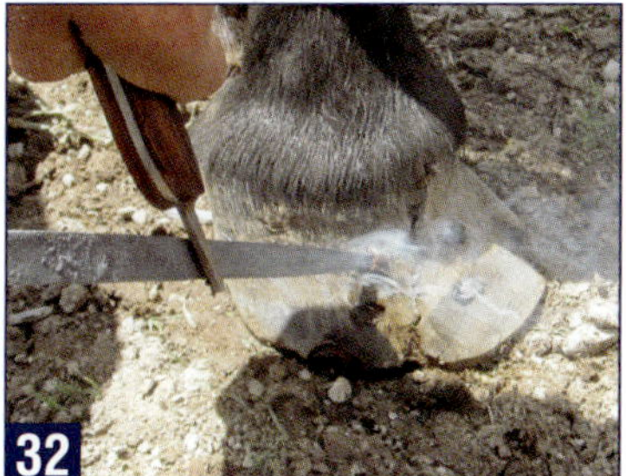

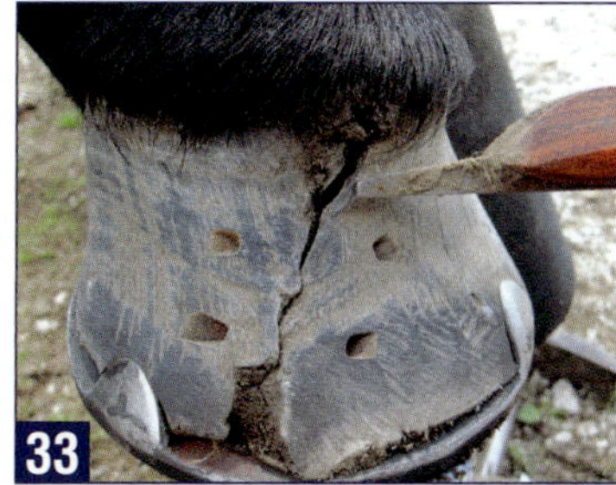

Burning holes for the lace nail.

The foot has been shod with clips and the holes for the lace nail are burned into it.

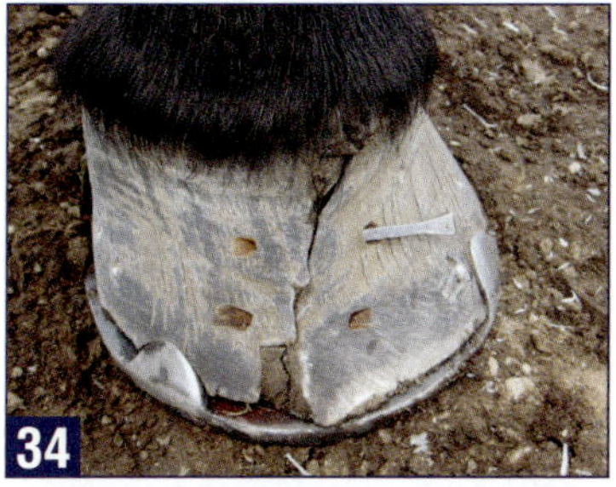

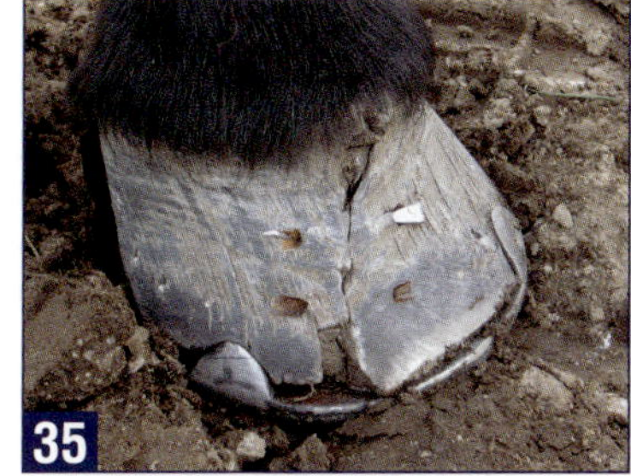

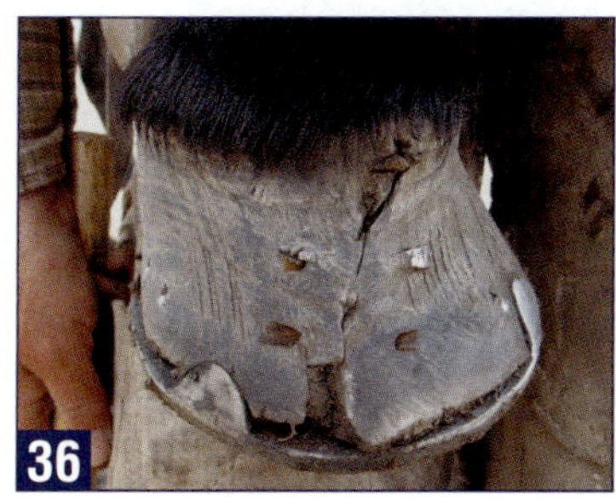

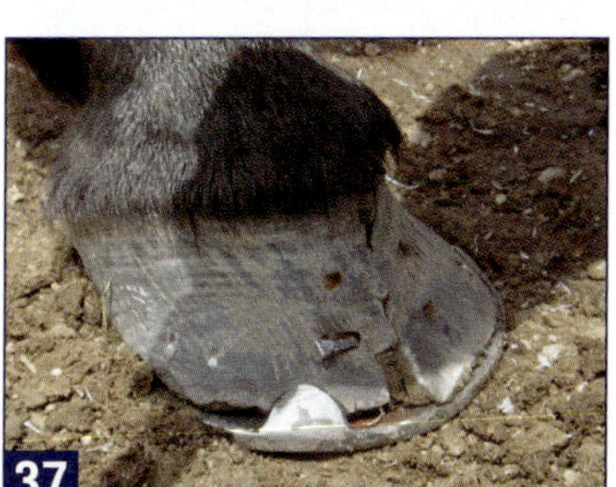

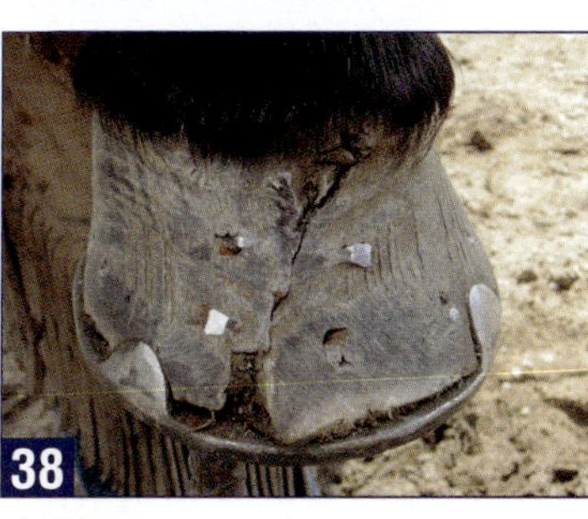

Driving nails across the foot and finishing.

being moved independently of each other. Being able to move the sides by hand indicates that the crack has really weakened this foot. **Figure 26** is a picture of the bottom of the foot, and the amount of foot that has grown into a flare shows the neglect that caused this crack. Begin by trimming the foot as close to a normal shape as possible (finding the wooden Indian) **(Figures 27-30)**. Fit a shoe with clips on either side of the crack, and burn them in correctly to stabilize the hoof wall as much as possible.

I burn holes on either side of the crack with a hot pritchel **(Figures 31-32)**. These holes are going to be where the nail is driven through and allow for the head to set in the foot on one side and the clinch on the other. **Figure 33** shows the foot with the holes burned into it and the shoe nailed on.

The next step is to drive the nails across the crack. In **Figures 34-36**, I am driving and clinching the top nail, and **Figures 37-38** show the bottom nail. This foot is now treated for the crack the first time the horse was presented.

Six weeks later, the horse is returned for another shoeing. The foot was in much better shape, as

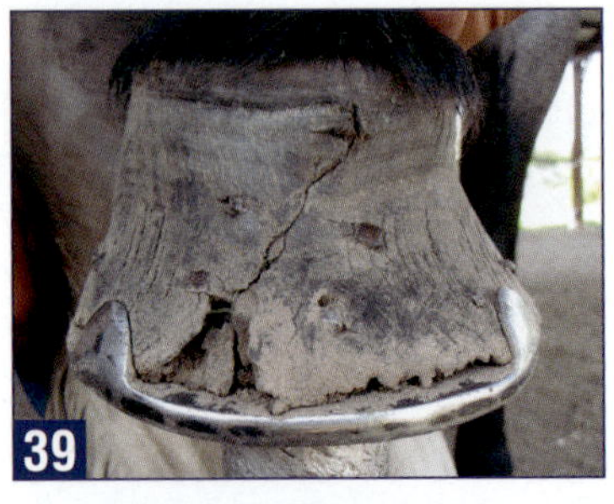

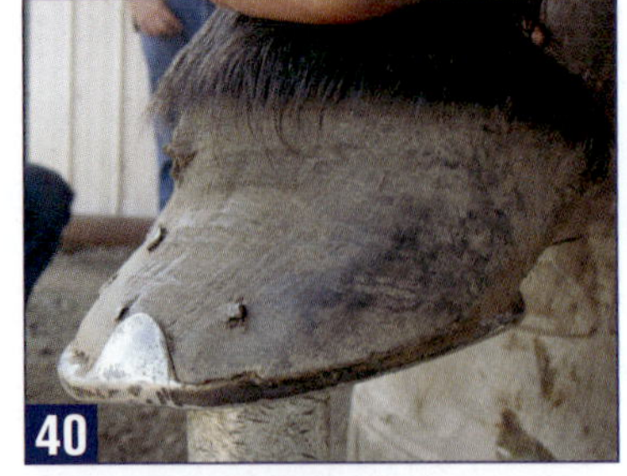

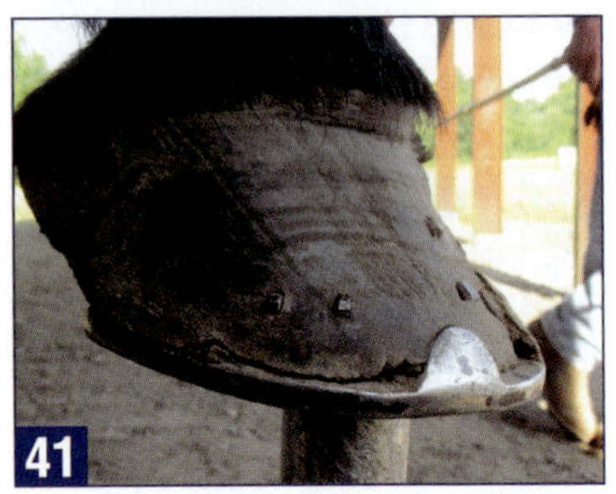

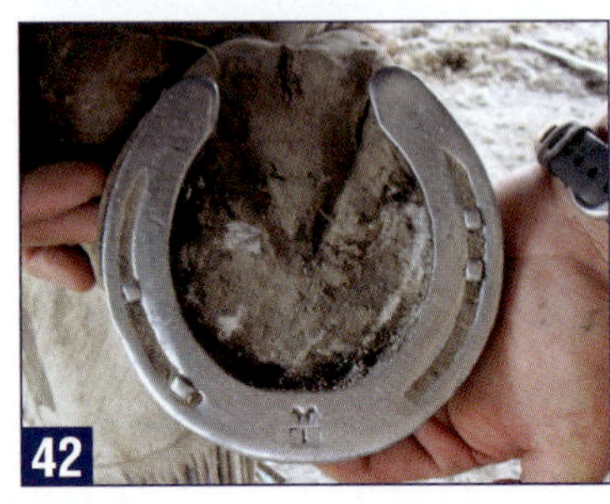

6 weeks later, this is how the foot looked.

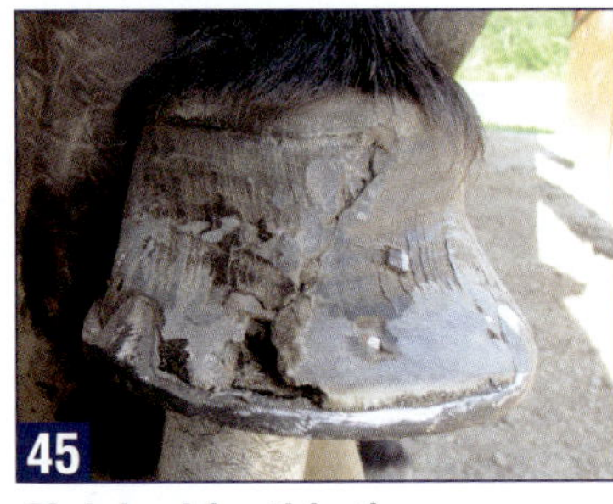

Notice the amount of good wall that is being created at the top of the crack.

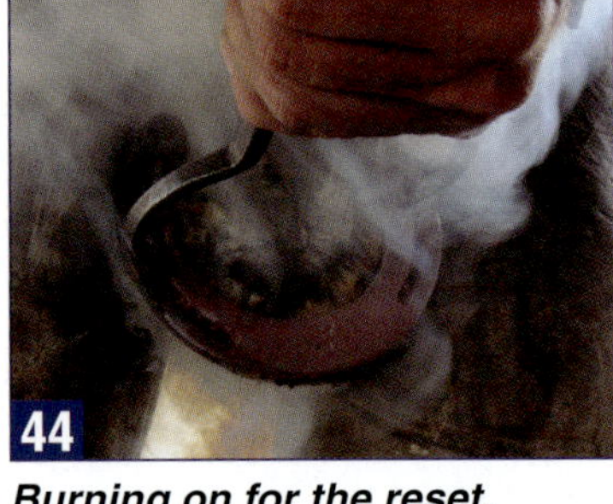

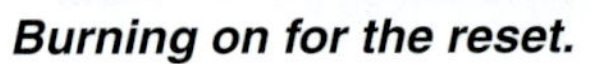

Burning on for the reset.

Finished for this time.

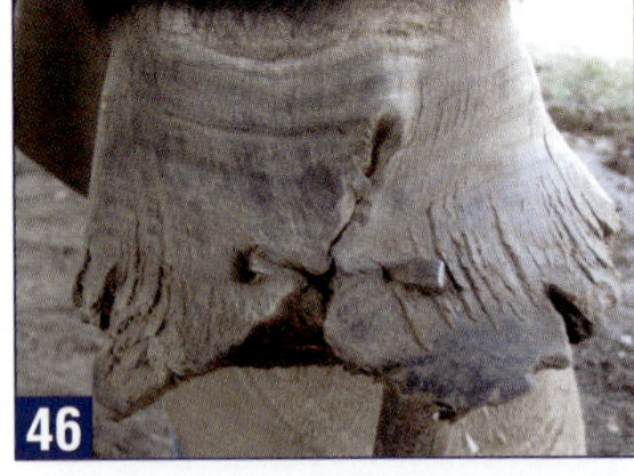

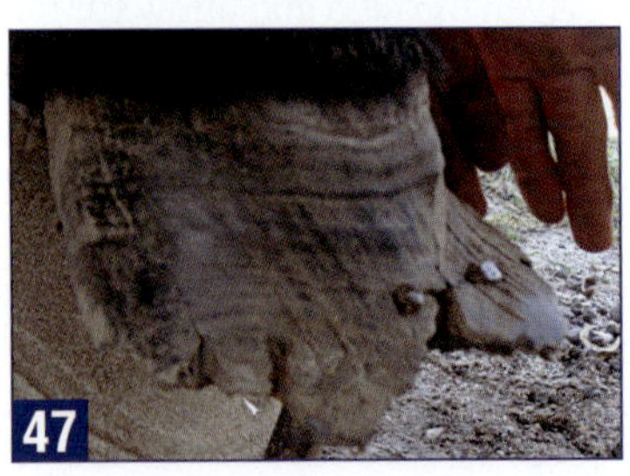

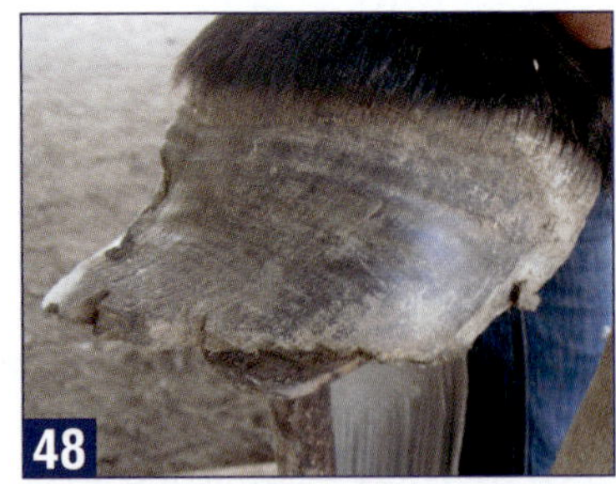

What the foot looked like 10 weeks after the second treatment and losing the shoe.

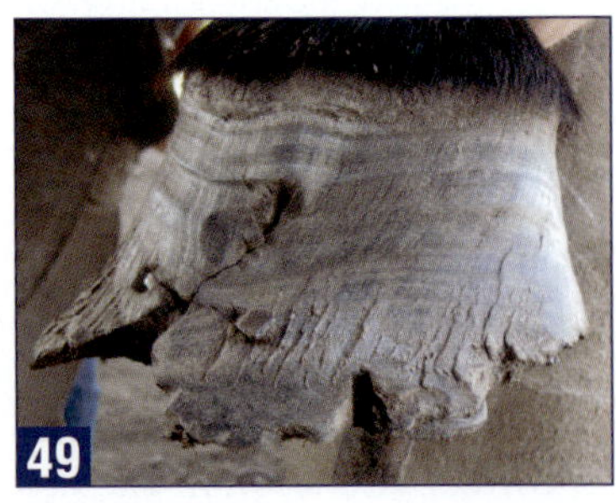

The amount of good foot at the top of the crack is amazing.

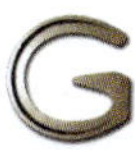

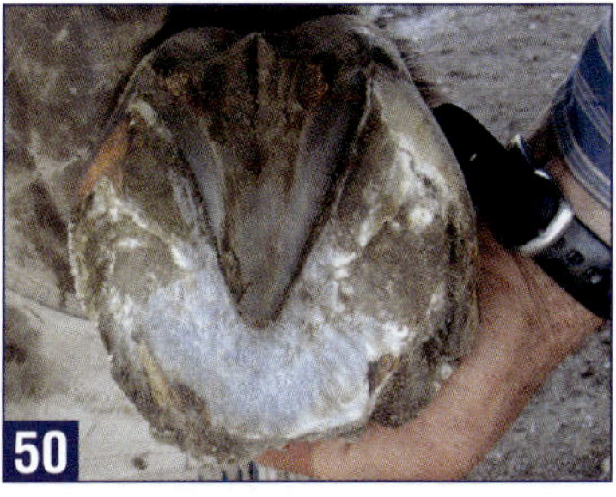

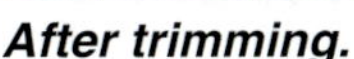

After trimming.

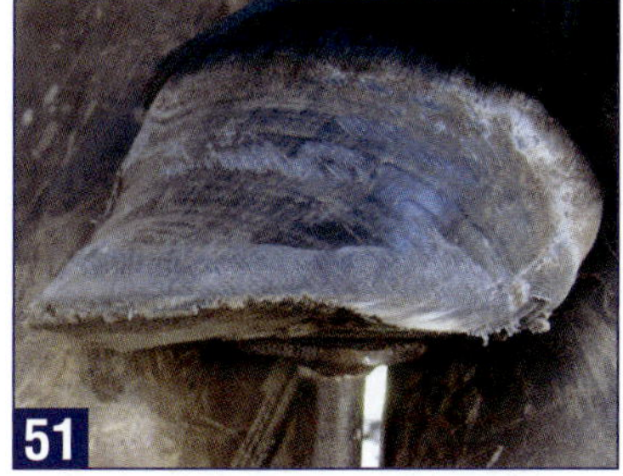

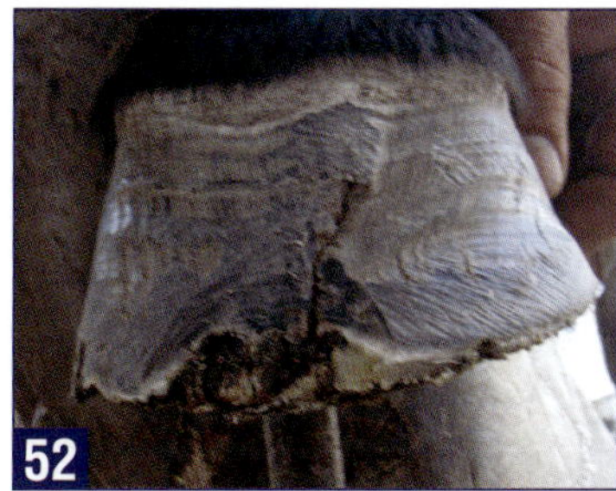

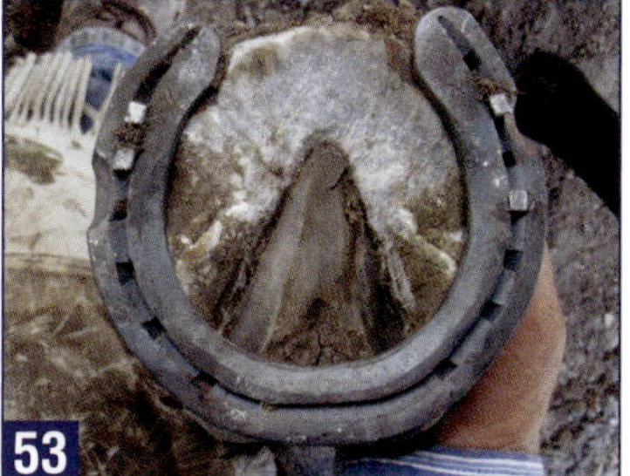

Reverse shoe nailed on.

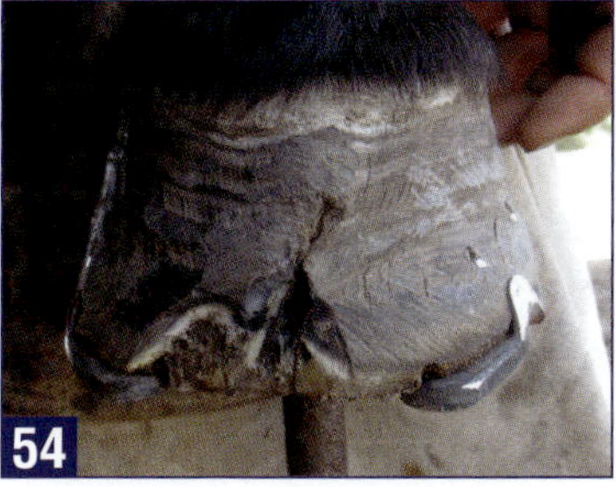

Dorsal view after being shod.

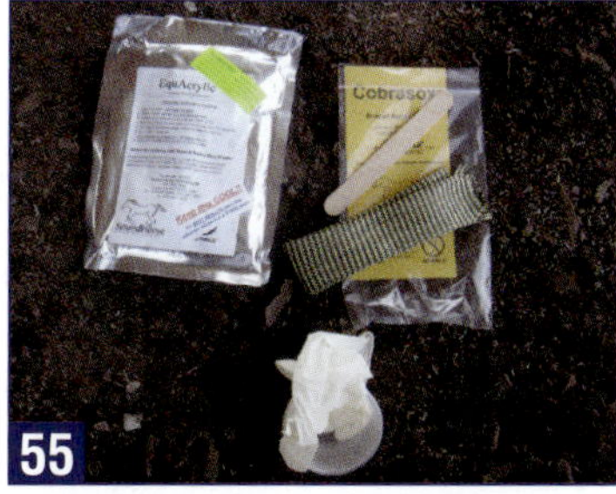

Cobrasox from Sound Horse.

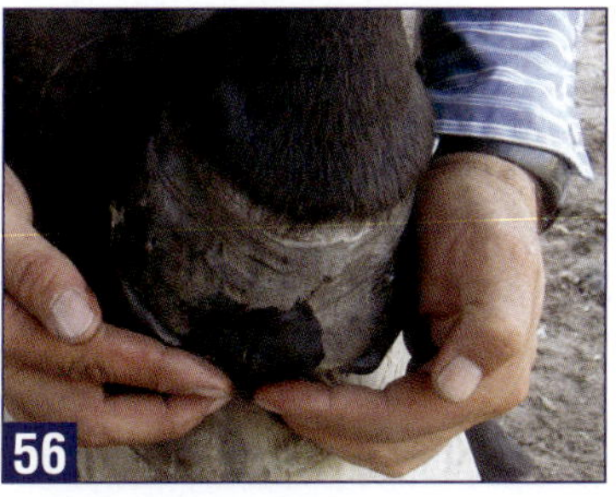

Putting Sole Pack in the bottom of the crack.

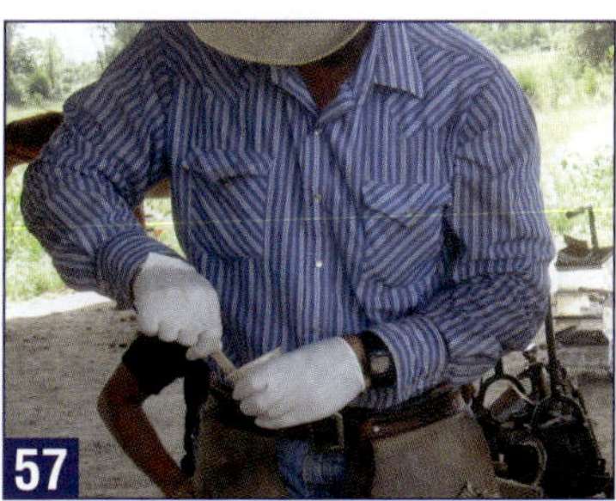

Mixing the acrylic.

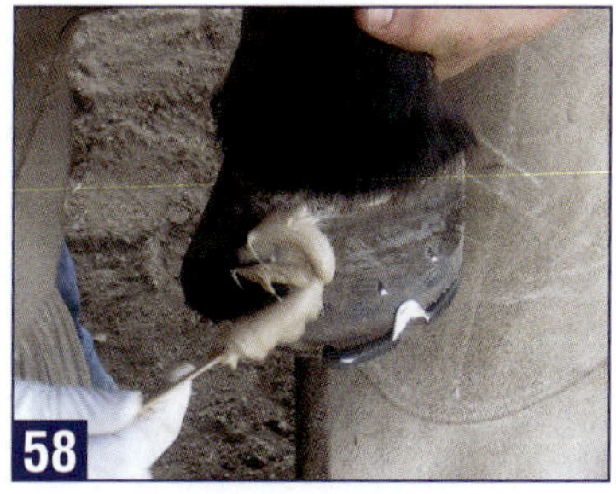

Putting acrylic on the foot.

Figures 39-42 show. In **Figure 43**, the top of the hoof wall is starting to grow solid, and the top of the crack is not moving. All that is required on the second visit is to reset the horse **(Figures 44-45)**.

The third time the horse is presented has taken the customer about 10 weeks. **Figures 46-49** show the condition of the foot, and the horse is just about Grade 3 lame at this time. However, notice the amount of good foot that is above the crack. I trimmed and dressed the foot **(Figures 50-52)** and decided to go with a reverse shoe at this time, since the toe of the foot was so damaged at the ground surface **(Figures 53-54)**. The lace nails have been completely trimmed out at this stage.

I decide to use a product called Cobrasox from Sound Horse Technologies **(Figure 55)**. This is a weave of polyester and carbon fiber that creates a strong patch. The foot is prepped by dressing it with the rough side of the rasp. The area that I don't want any acrylic in is blocked with some Sole Pack, as I am doing in **Figure 56**. I then cut a length of the Cobrasox and mix the acrylic as per the instructions **(Figure 57)**, smear some of the acrylic on the foot **(Figure 58)**, and work some of

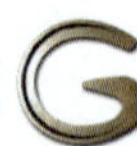

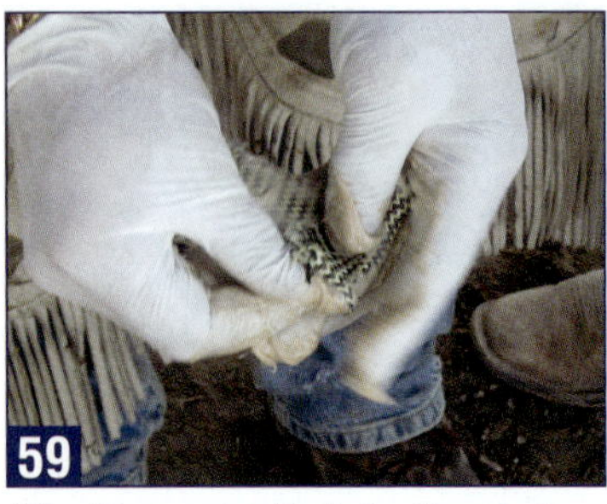
Working acrylic into the Cobrasox.

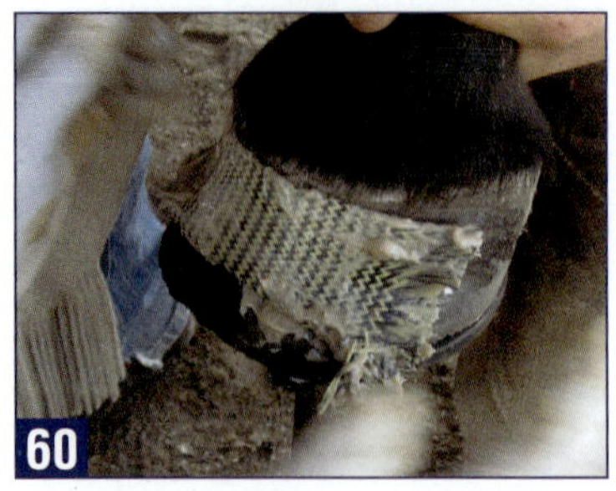
Putting the Cobrasox on the foot.

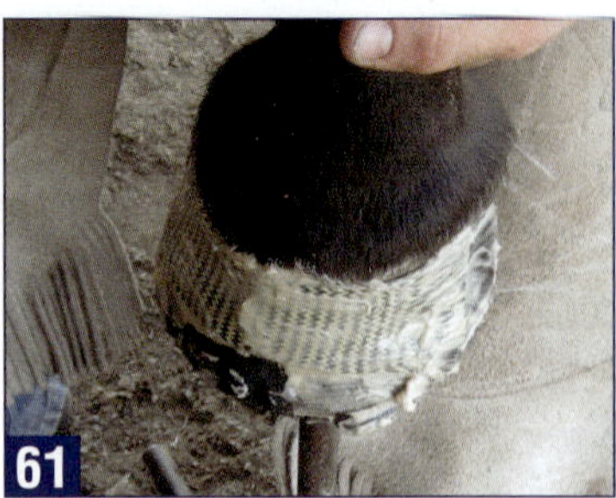

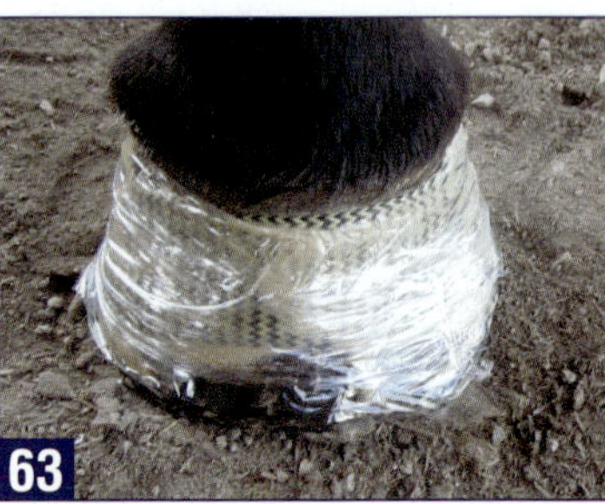
Wrapping the foot in plastic wrap.

Give it several minutes to cure.

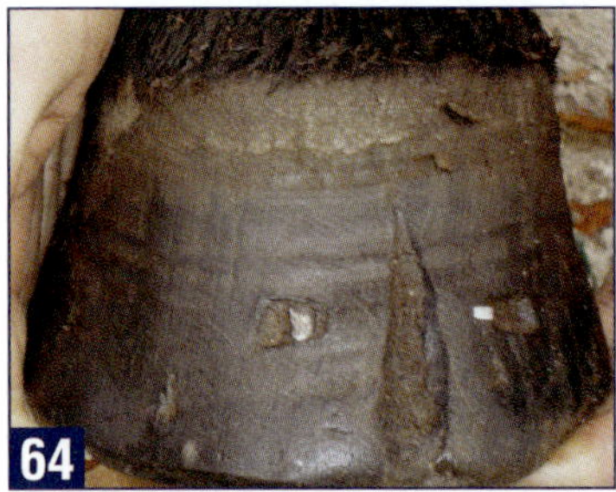

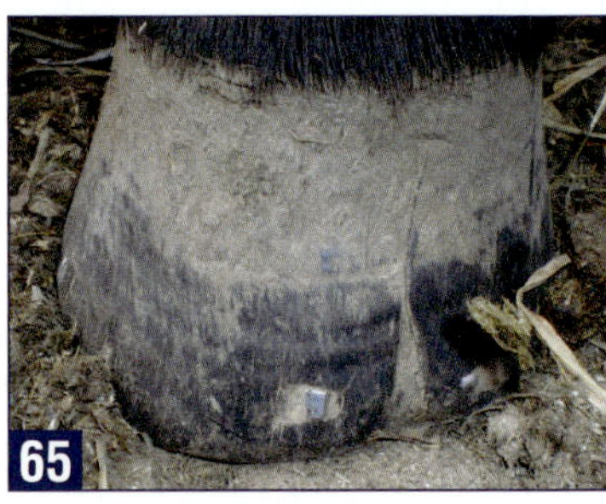

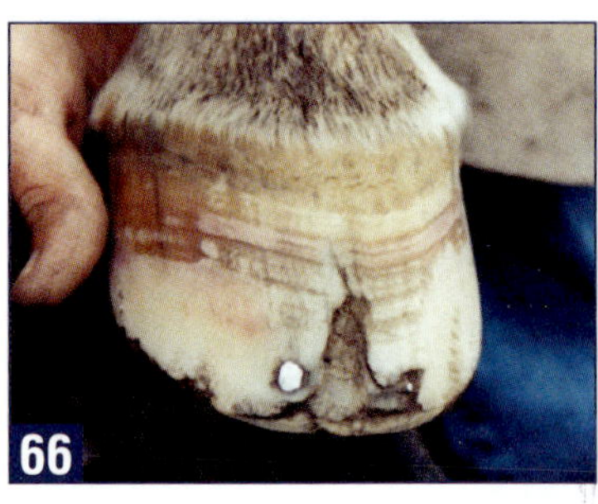
Nail laces showing how the crack has been stabilized.

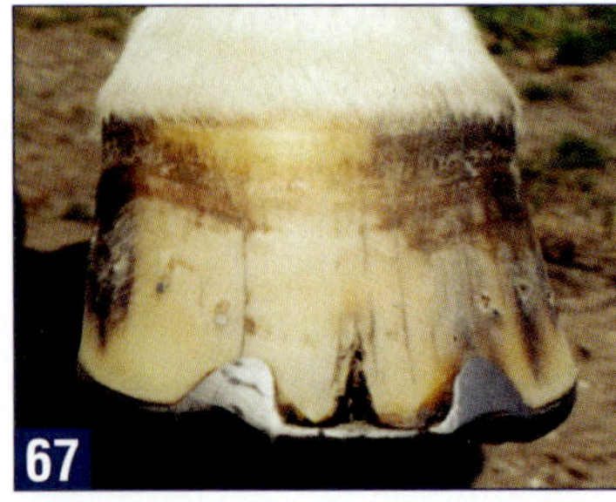
Foot with clips on either side of the crack.

it deep into the Cobrasox **(Figure 59)**. I place the Cobrasox over the crack **(Figures 60-61)**, and then wrap the whole thing in plastic wrap to allow it to cure **(Figures 62-63)**.

The Cobrasox replaced the lace nails at this point in the treatment of the horse, and the horse was sound again when it left the school.

Lace nails have proven themselves to me time after time. **Figures 64-66** show cracks that have been laced, and the crack has disappeared at the top. This is an indication of how much those lace nails stabilized the crack.

Using screws, wire, and Super-Fast is also a handy way to stabilize a crack. For a lot of cracks that do not involve sensitive structures, you can put a series of screws down both sides of the crack, then run a thin wire between and around the screws. Determine how long the screws have to be by measuring the thickness of the hoof wall at the ground surface, then put tape on the drill bit to avoid drilling too deep. The wire around the screws will give the acrylic or urethane something else to bond to. Once you have made this matrix with the screws and wire, place your hoof builder over the area. Let it cure, then rasp till you just touch the screw heads. For times when sensitive structures are involved, you can put a drain in the crack. Without a drain, you will end up with a painful infection. A complete series of this process can be seen in Chapter 32, Modern Materials and Methods.

With most cracks, I will also place clips on the shoe that help to fortify the strength of the hoof wall **(Figure 67)**. I find that using a bar shoe can also be helpful, and as with most hoof problems, a good, solid trim that observes traditional principles of balance can really help. There are other methods, but the ones stated will generally take care of most cracks. One of the big things is time, and if you can make the wall grow faster, you will heal the crack that much sooner, so a good feed supplement is a good idea.

From a veterinarian's perspective, the main thing that can be done is surgery on the coronary band or the keratoma if that is the cause of the crack. Otherwise, working hand in hand with a competent farrier is recommended.

The owner simply needs to watch the crack and advise the farrier if there are any problems. They also need to stay on a good schedule to prevent length of foot becoming leverage.

ANTICIPATED OUTCOME

If you stabilize a crack, the horse should become comfortable pretty quickly. Be sure that you let the owner know that there is a certain amount of time that has to pass, and that is just part of dealing with a crack. However, if dealt with correctly, most cracks will improve.

IN SHORT

D: Vertical break in the hoof wall.

T: Stabilize the hoof and allow time to grow.

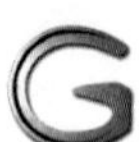

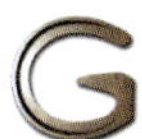

Chapter

45-7 DROPPED SOLE

DEFINITION

This refers to a sole that is prolapsed below the border of the hoof wall. The sole appears convex instead of concave. Figure 1 is a picture of what you will often see with a dropped sole.

REASON

A dropped sole is not an uncommon conformation on wide, flat feet that have a lot of angle to the side wall at the quarter. These types of feet tend to flare excessively, which leads to the sole becoming prolapsed. Dropped sole can also develop when the hoof wall becomes overly worn or broken off, similar to breaking a fingernail into the quick.

Dropped sole may develop from extremely thick shoes and hard work. I once worked on a carriage horse from Denver that had worn shoes with a thick rubber insert that was required by the city. This insert caused the shoe to actually be about 2 inches in total thickness. When the shoe was pulled, the sole and frog was so prolapsed that the bare foot had a 1-inch gap between the heels and the ground.

Dropped soles are extremely common on foundered horses and sinkers. A sinker is similar to founder. The difference is that all the laminae have let go, not just at the toe region. When a horse sinks, the hoof capsule is actually now in a more proximal position than before. With founder, the detached laminae at the toe allow the foot to pull away from the coffin bone. This creates a situation where the horse may be walking completely on the sole, which is now considered dropped or prolapsed. In **Figure 2**, the separation of the laminae has resulted in this horse having a dropped sole. It may be hard to see in this photo, but the sole on this foot is actually about 3/8 inch lower than the hoof wall at the toe. Since the laminar attachment is so compromised on these types of feet, the remedies for a dropped sole are not recommended. This places the weight back on the wall, which cannot take the weight. So, if you are dealing with founder, refer to the section on founder in this book.

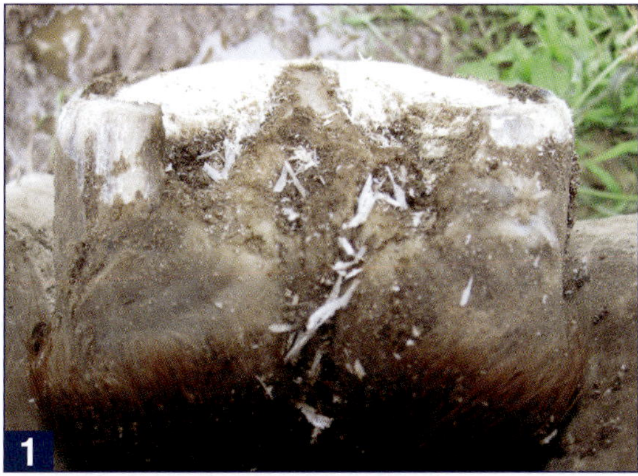

1

Palmar view of a dropped sole.

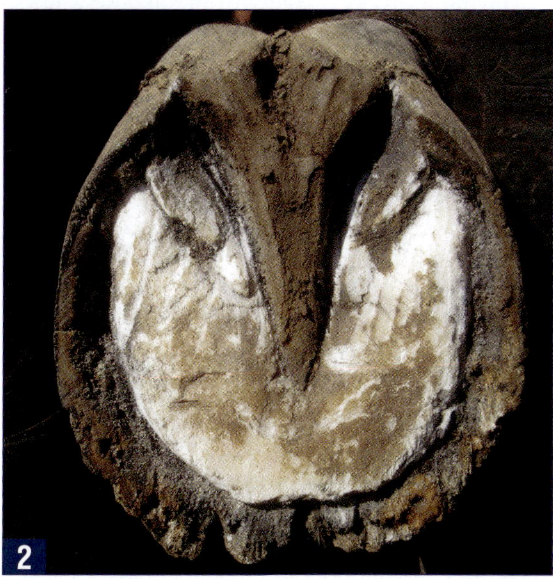

2

Solar view of a foundered foot with a dropped sole.

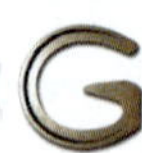

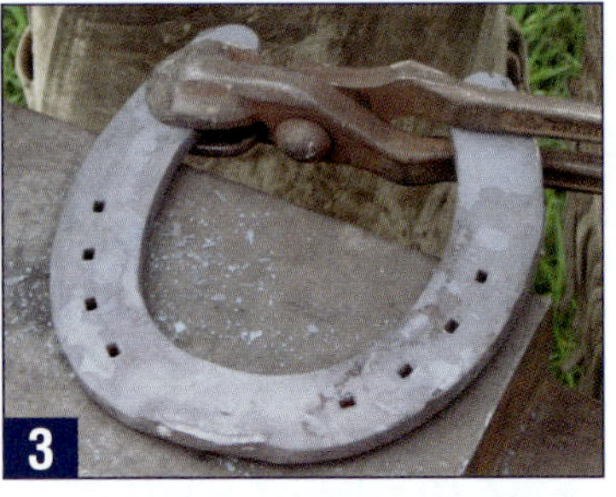

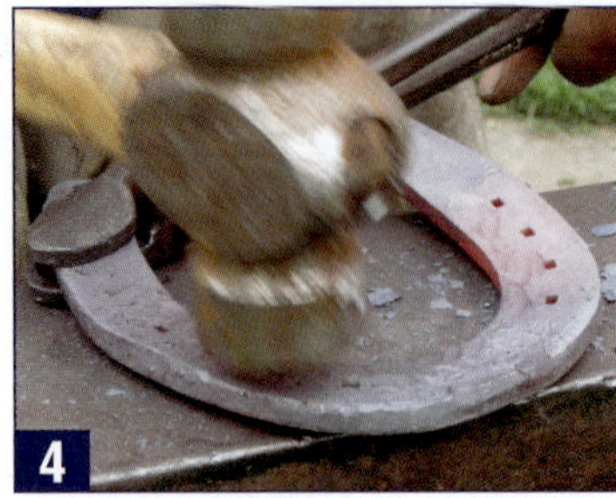

Forging the cup into the shoe on the hoof surface.

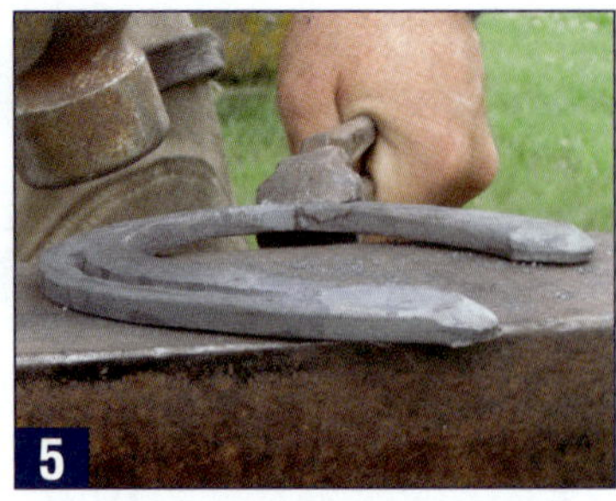

Leveling around the outside of the ground surface.

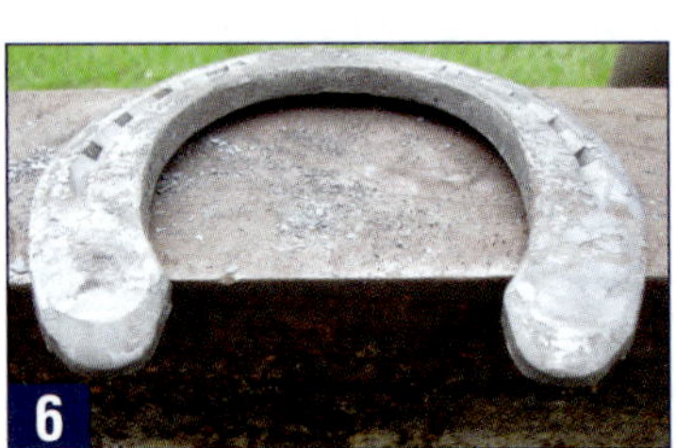

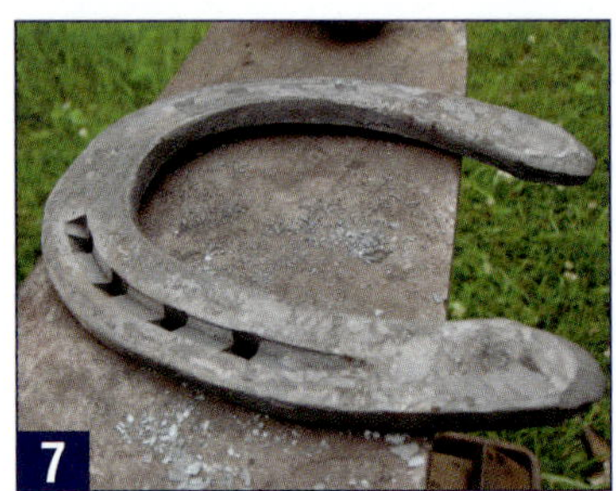

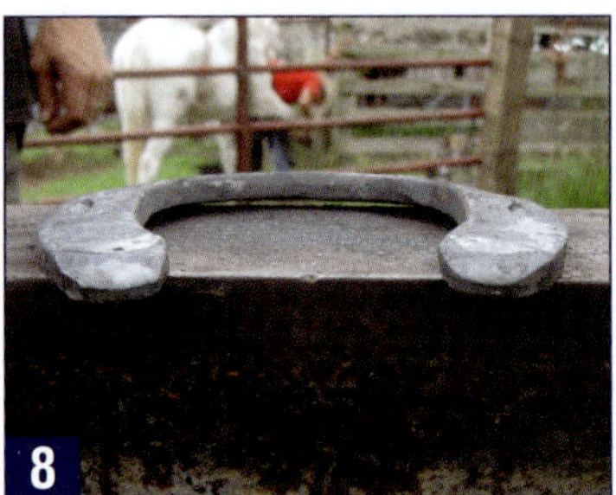

Views of the cupped shoe showing the detail of the twist in the web.

ANATOMY

Sole, hoof wall, and, in the case of a foundered horse or sinker, the laminae.

SYMPTOMS

Having a dropped sole will predispose a horse to bruising. This in turn will predispose to lameness from the bruised sole. If you are dealing with a sinker, the horse will be Grade 4 lame.

Visually, you will have a horse that bears weight on its sole if barefoot. The sole just protrudes too far distally.

A dropped sole by itself will not make the horse sore, but the fact that the sole is much more likely to be injured from concussion can make the horse footsore.

TREATMENT

The primary principle to think about when shoeing a horse with a dropped sole is protection. You can protect this sole in a number of ways. A wide-webbed, deep-seated shoe is one option. You may want to use aluminum to really get good shoe thickness without too much weight. Pads and rim pads are also a common option that provides protection to the foot, especially combined with shoe thickness to get the sole away from the ground.

Another shoe that we use is one that we call a cupped shoe. This is one where the web actually has a twist in it so that the outside hoof surface contacts the foot, but the inside ground surface contacts the ground. This allows the effects of a major deep-seated shoe made of steel without too much weight. In some instances, you might want a heart bar so that the frog can bear some of the weight that the sole has been taking.

To make the cupped shoe, hold the tongs so that one heel is in the jaws, and the other between the reins **(Figures 3-4)**. Lift on the shoe as you hit around the inside hoof surface of the shoe. Turn the shoe over and hammer around the outside edge of the shoe to level it **(Figure 5)**. When it is finished, the shoe should have a cross section like the shoe in **Figures 6-8**. The inside of the web on the ground surface will be on the ground, and the outside of the web on the hoof surface will be against the hoof wall. Just a quick note: When you do this to a shoe, you will change the pitch on the nails. This can make it easier to quick a horse, so be aware of the change.

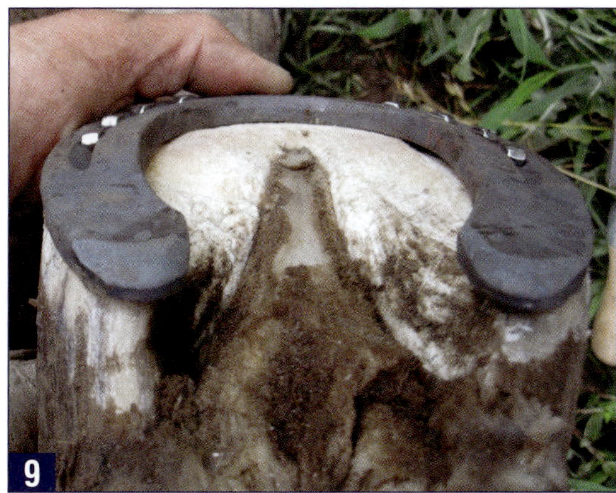

Cupped shoe on the dropped sole foot.

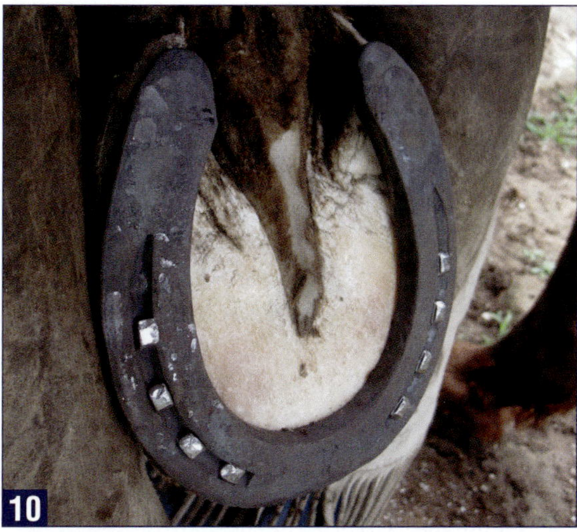

Cupped shoe on the dropped sole foot.

In **Figures 9-10**, the foot from **Figure 1** has had the cupped shoe applied. Even though it has had a major cupping, the inside of the shoe is still in contact with the sole. While this is not ideal, if the sole is tough enough to take it, it is not a problem.

For dropped soles that have become bruised enough that the horse is dealing with abscesses, a hospital plate would be quite useful. This will allow the owner to change out the Epsom Salt poultice as well as provide superior protection. You may want to use an Equi-Pak pour-in if the horse is a little sore but does not have an abscess.

For flat and flared feet, dress the flare as much as possible to achieve straight tubular horn. With regular hoof care, these feet generally come around. Putting these horses on a good supplement is also recommended.

The veterinarian will not have a big role in most dropped soles, but they will be immensely important if you are dealing with a sinker. A sinker requires continuous care and medication.

Horse owners should try to avoid rough and rocky terrain as well as monitor the horse to avoid lameness.

ANTICIPATED OUTCOME

For horses that suffer only from the environment, shoes of any sort will allow the hoof wall to grow down past the sole. In the case of founder, there are other problems that get in the way of recovery. For flared feet, a tight schedule and good shoeing can bring the foot into a much healthier position.

IN SHORT

D: Sole on a lower plane than the bottom of the hoof wall.

T: Protect with deep-seated shoe, cupped shoe, Equi-Pak, or pads or hospital plate.

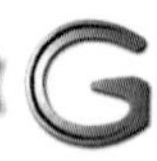

Chapter

45-8 FOUNDER AND LAMINITIS

DEFINITION

Founder is the separation of the coffin bone from the hoof wall.

It is important to understand the difference between the terms laminitis and founder, even though the two terms are used by most as if they meant the same thing.

Looking first at the term founder, in the dictionary, there are several words used to describe it. Break-down, sink, crumple, and fall all come up under the heading founder, and these are pretty good descriptions of what is happening to a foundered foot. When talking about the foot, founder is referring to the coffin bone actually being separated from the hoof wall, and the dorsal aspect of the bone is in a different plane than the dorsal plane of the hoof wall. This means that there has been tearing of the laminae in the dorsal foot, resulting in a lot of movement of the coffin bone in an area that does not allow for that kind of movement.

Laminitis basically means inflamed laminae. Anytime you see the suffix "itis," it means inflammation, such as in bursitis, tendonitis, dermatitis, etc. When a horse is suffering from laminitis, the dermal laminae are inflamed. This can lead to the separation that becomes founder. However, it is important to note that a horse can be afflicted with laminitis even if it does not founder. But, if a horse does indeed founder, you can bet that there is laminitis present. The separation of the laminae could not happen without becoming inflamed.

Unfortunately, founder is one of the problems that you will see and have to deal with the most in many farrier practices.

REASON

I have a good friend, Mike Miller, MD, CJF, FWCF. He was able to give me as good a description for the reason that horses founder as I have heard, so I include it here.

"Among the many risk factors and etiologies for laminitis are: genetic (breed) disposition; overfeeding on some carbohydrates (spring grass, grains); incomplete delivery of the placenta after foaling; excessive watering of hot stock. There are many other suggested causes, but they ultimately converge in a ***final common pathway*** of destruction of the lamellar bond. Purely mechanical causes such as road founder or well-leg breakdown opposite a lame foot are not really part of this pathway.

"Maintenance of the lamellar bond requires delivery of oxygen, glucose, and other nutrients to the basement membrane and dermal lamella. Lacking this support, there is a breakdown of the desmosomal bonds between the lamina, and release of such factors as membrane metalo-proteinases (MMPs) which appear to further degrade the lamella."

However, even with all of the science and information that we are able to gather, the actual cause of founder is still not completely known.

Basically, there is a failure of the bond between the laminae. The weight of the horse, the pull on the deep flexor tendon, and the upward pressure on the toe from the ground can cause the foot to be pulled apart at the dorsal aspect.

The final common pathway shown in this section is a concept in medicine that describes many different ways that you can end up with a problem. The end result is that problem. Mike made a flow chart to show a few of the reasons for founder and the final result. The chart is shown on the next page.

Simplified Flow Chart: Cascade Towards the Final Common Pathway of Laminitis

ANATOMY

During the initial stages of a horse becoming laminitic, the anatomy is going to be the digital

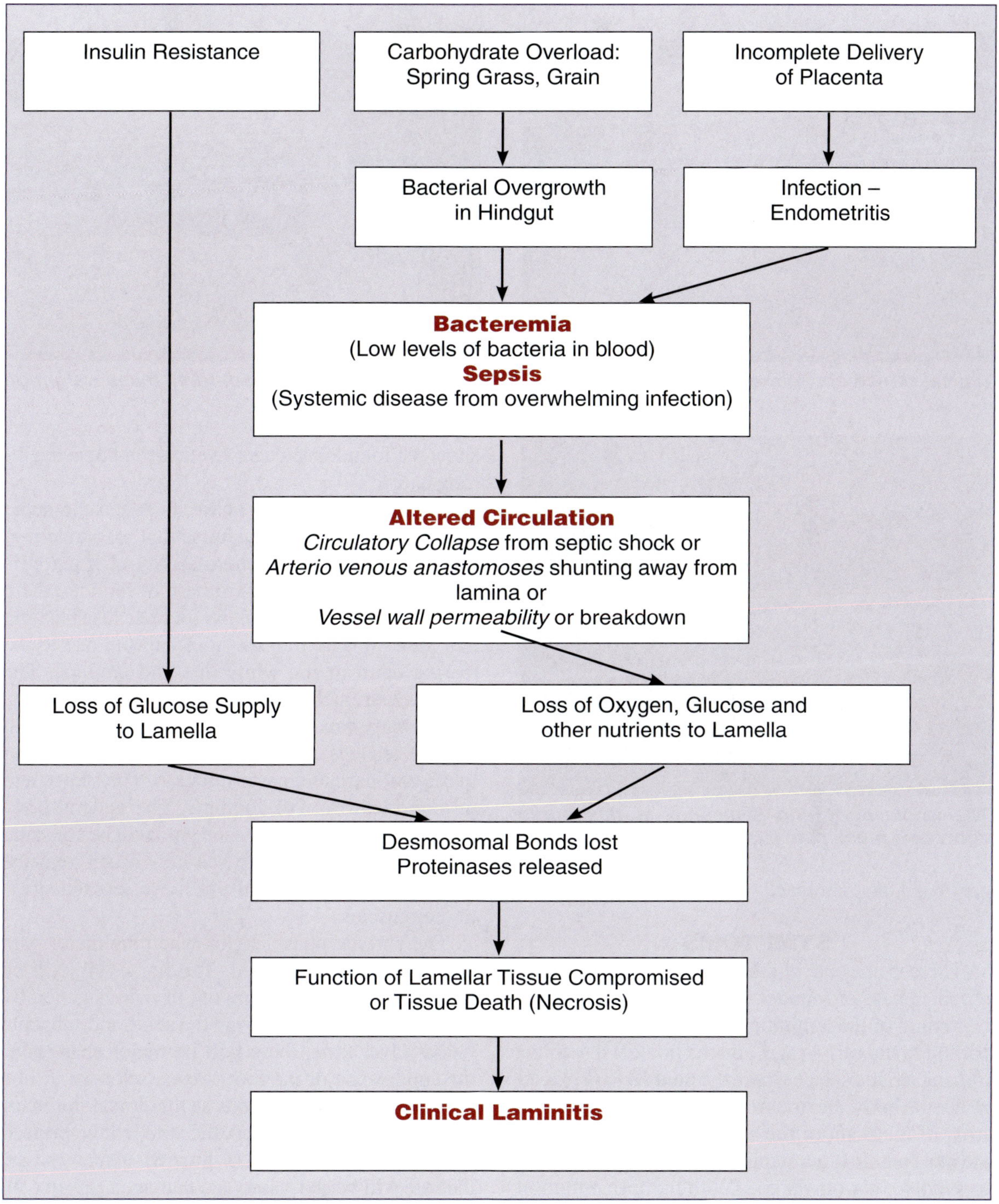

Insulin Resistance

Carbohydrate Overload: Spring Grass, Grain

Incomplete Delivery of Placenta

Bacterial Overgrowth in Hindgut

Infection – Endometritis

Bacteremia
(Low levels of bacteria in blood)
Sepsis
(Systemic disease from overwhelming infection)

Altered Circulation
Circulatory Collapse from septic shock or
Arterio venous anastomoses shunting away from lamina or
Vessel wall permeability or breakdown

Loss of Glucose Supply to Lamella

Loss of Oxygen, Glucose and other nutrients to Lamella

Desmosomal Bonds lost
Proteinases released

Function of Lamellar Tissue Compromised or Tissue Death (Necrosis)

Clinical Laminitis

arteries, veins, arterio venous anastamoses (AVAs), and basement membrane. Once the inflammation begins, we enter the actual laminitis stage.

When a horse has laminitis, the main anatomy involved is the dermal and epidermal laminae. All of the laminae around the foot may be involved, but due to the stress placed on a foot, the laminae at the toe is generally what becomes damaged the most.

If the laminitis leads to founder, then the anatomy becomes: Deep flexor tendon, sole, P3, dorsal coro-

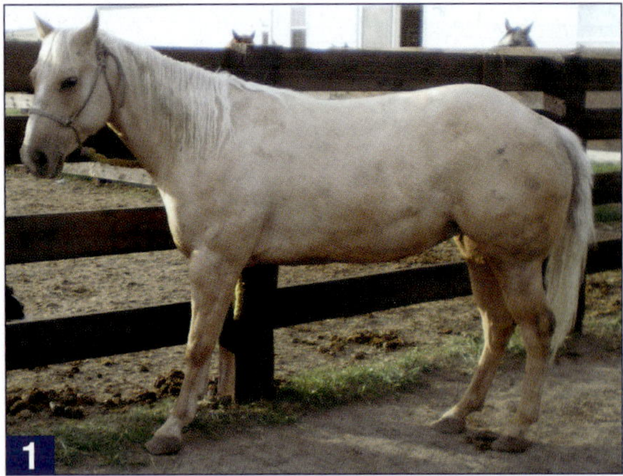

Typical stance of a foundered horse.

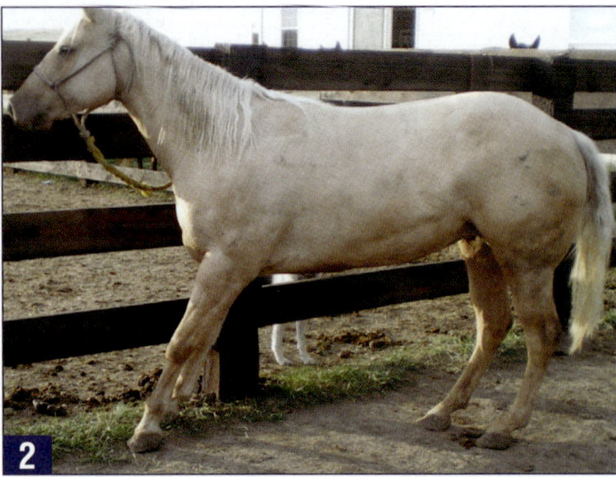

The way that a foundered horse takes weight off of the front feet to turn.

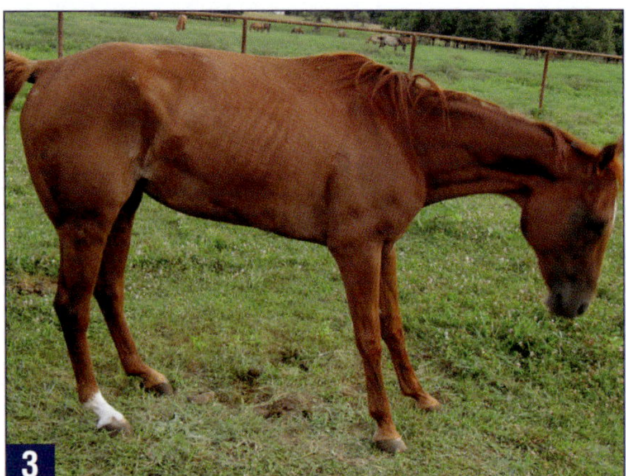

The whole body and demeanor of this horse show how much pain it is in.

nary band, and laminae.

SYMPTOMS

There is an acute phase, a subacute phase, and a chronic phase of founder. The acute phase is at the beginning of the laminitic episode. It is severe and painful in the early stage, and the horse will exhibit a characteristic stance where the hind feet are placed under the body, and the front feet are placed well in front of the point of the shoulder. Since the toe is the most painful area at this stage, the horse is trying to keep weight off the toe. With the inflammation in the foot, there will be pain, heat and swelling, primarily at the toe and dorsal coronary band. When the foot is this sore, the horse will actually try to rear slightly and twist when it wants to turn, utilizing its hindquarters to the utmost. Forward motion while turning will exacerbate the pain. **Figures 1 and 2** show the founder stance as well as the horse beginning a turn.

Next is the subacute phase, between the acute and chronic phases. For a horse that is foundering, this is the stage where the majority of rotation is going to occur. During this phase of founder, there will often be infections in the foot because bacteria has been allowed into the hoof capsule due to the tearing apart of the white line and laminae. The horse is extremely lame, the hair will stand out on the coronary band, you will feel a bounding pulse in the affected legs, and there will be heat and swelling in the coronary and pastern region. The stance and turning methods will continue. The general body condition will deteriorate, and pain will be constant. In **Figure 3**, it is easy to see how much pain the horse is in. Just look at the tail, eye set, and stress of the muscles.

The chronic phase begins when the major pain and rotation has subsided. The horse will still be lame and sore, but the amount of pain is generally less than experienced during the acute and subacute phase. Over time, there will be major changes in the appearance of the foot. Abscesses may still be forming and can break out at the dorsal coronary band **(Figures 4-6)**. Often, the sole will be bruised **(Figure 7)** and prolapsed **(Figure 8)**. In many cases, the sole will be abscessed and damaged (**Figure 9**), and the coffin bone can penetrate it **(Figure 10)**. Sole thickness (called sole depth) can be very thin when the coffin bone is pressing on it from above, and these feet are easily quicked **(Figure 11)**. There is also a dip in the coronary band, just above the hairline.

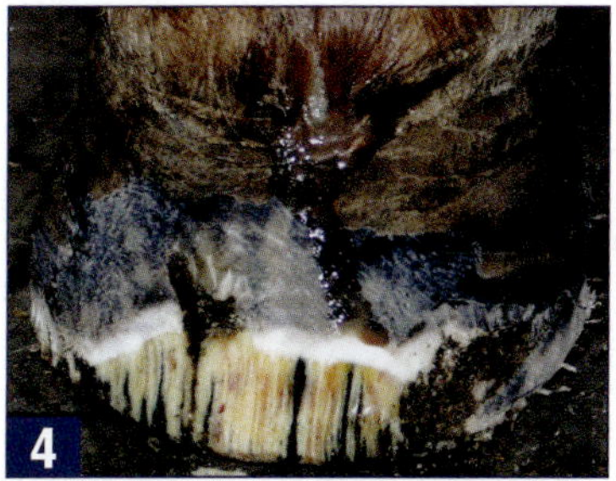

Abscess on a foundered foot breaking out the toe.

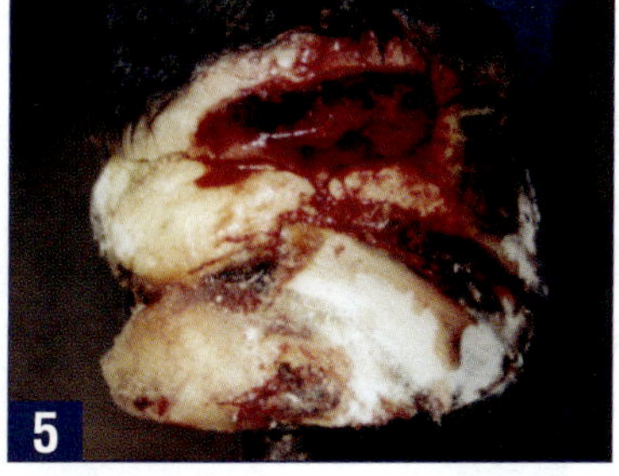

Abscess breaking out the toe.

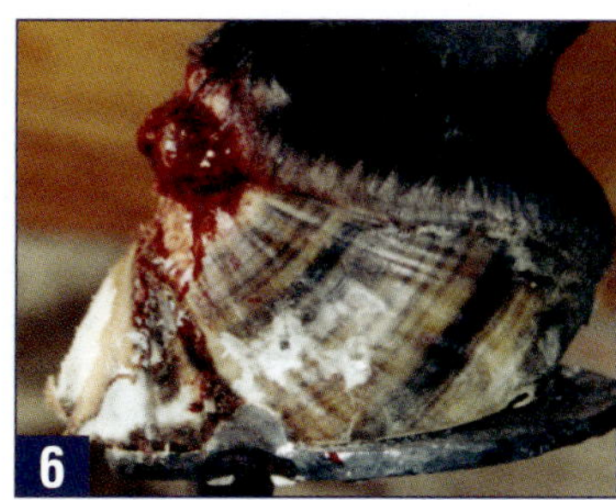

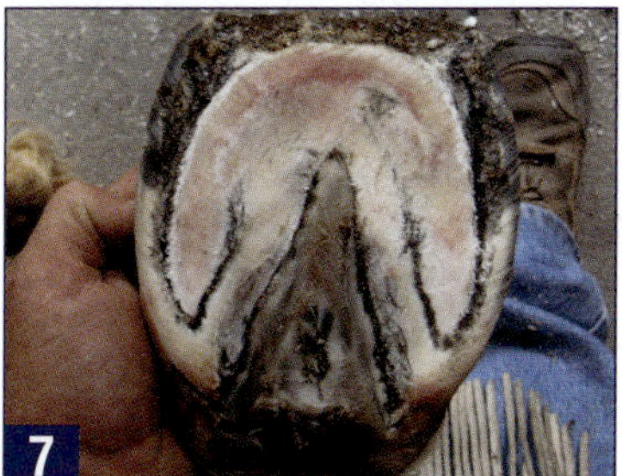

Bruised sole.

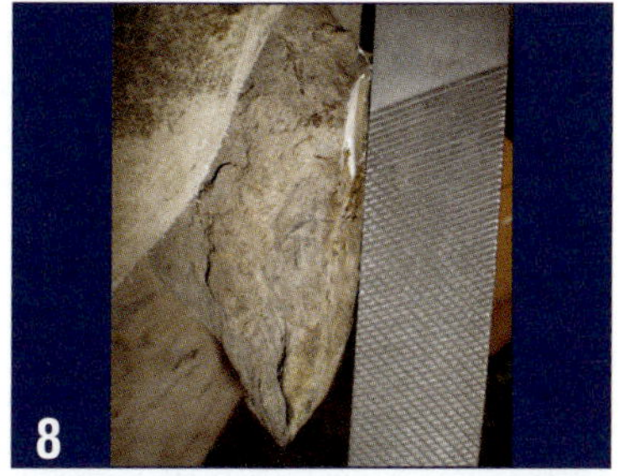

Lateral view of a foundered foot with the rasp laying across it to show the prolapse of the sole.

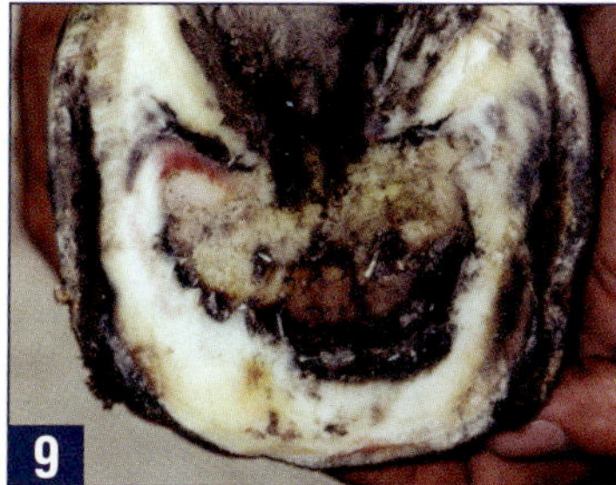

Thin and damaged sole.

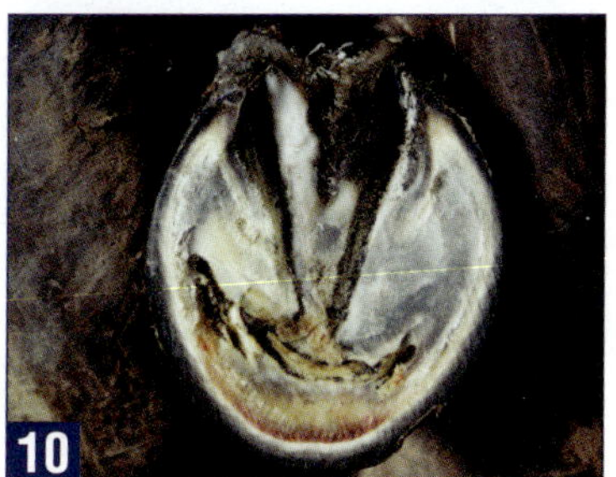

Thin and damaged sole.

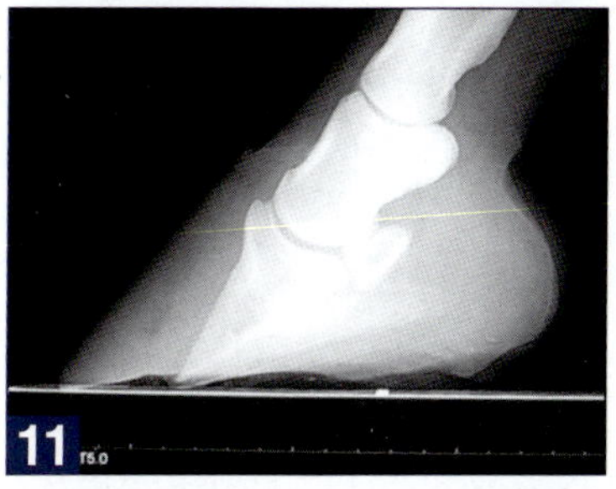

Sole that has been penetrated by the rotation of the coffin bone.

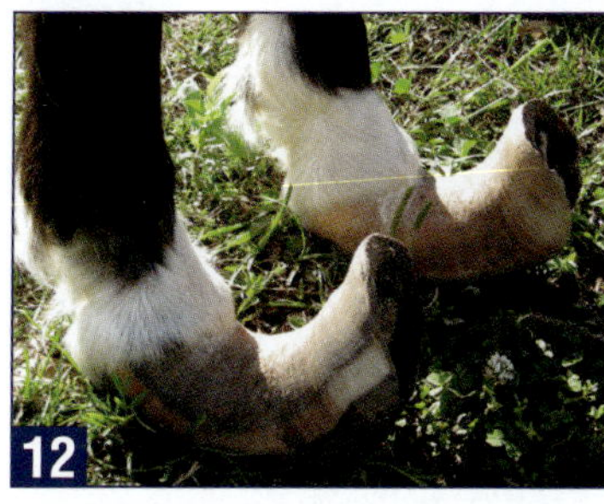

Toes curling up on a foundered pony.

There can be a curling in the hoof capsule caused by the heels growing faster than the toe **(Figure 12)**. If fever lines are present (and they usually are), they will be wide at the heels and converge at the toe **(Figure 13)**. The white line will be stretched and look like the underside of a mushroom cap **(Figure 14)**. Given enough time, the deep flexor tendon and subcarpal check ligament will become shorter,

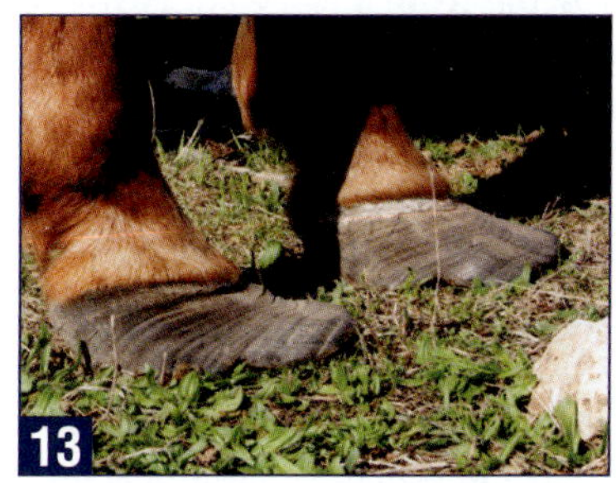

Fever lines in foundered feet. Wide at the heels, converging at the toe.

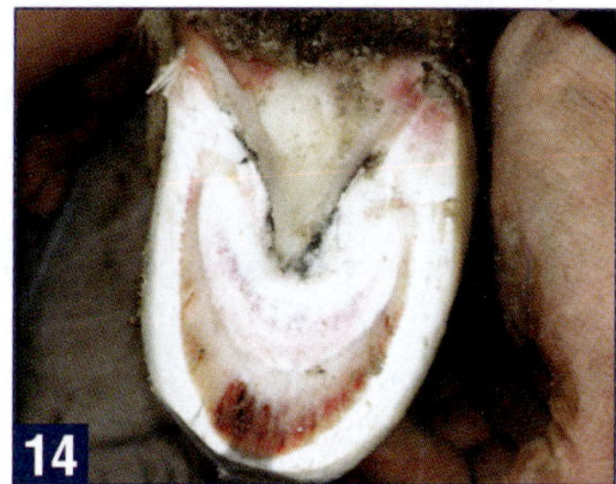

Stretched white line that resembles a mushroom.

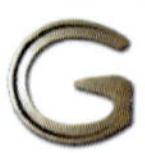

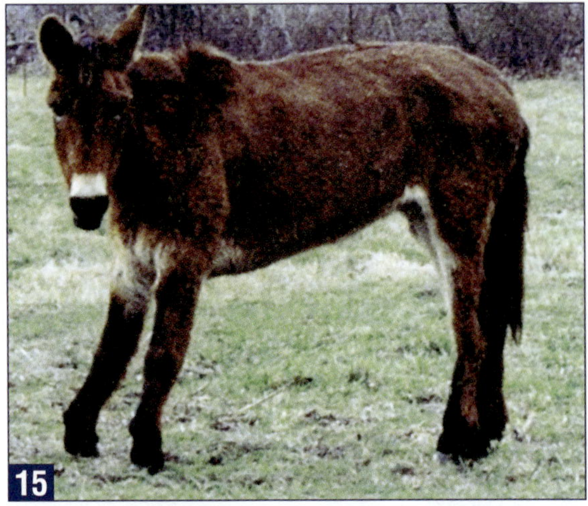

The fetlock is knuckling over from the pull of the deep flexor tendon.

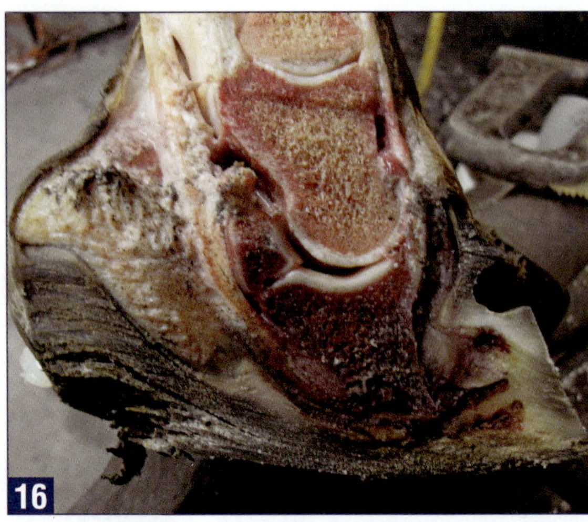

Sagittal section of a cadaver foot that was severely foundered.

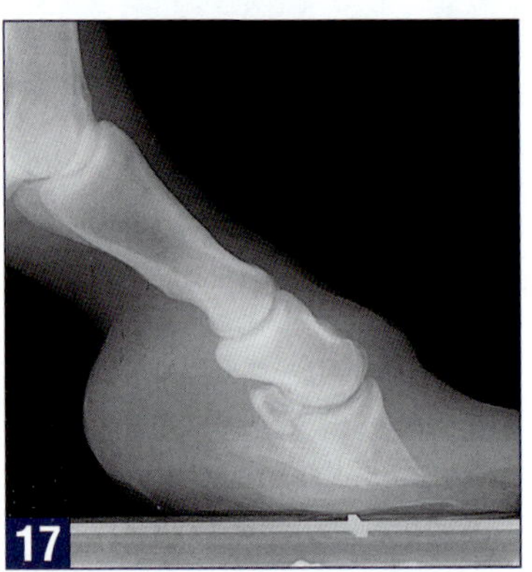

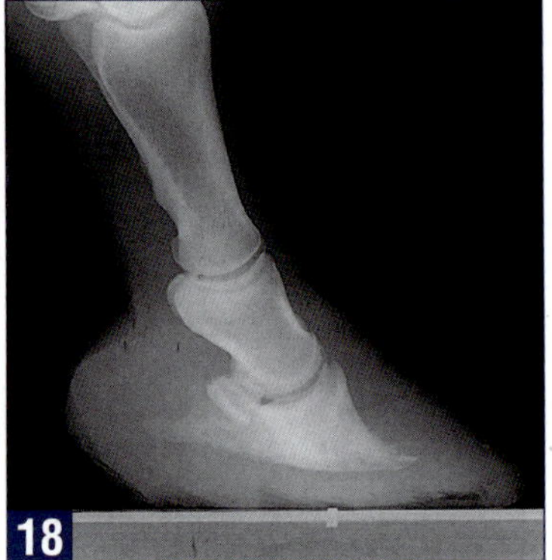

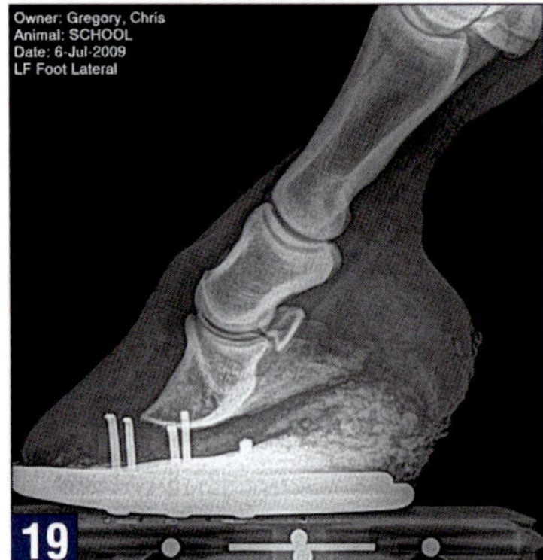

X-ray showing remodeling of P3.

causing the feet to knuckle over at the fetlock **(Figure 15)**.

Radiographic changes on a foundered foot are easy to see. **Figure 16** shows a sagittal section of a severely foundered foot. Notice the shape of the coffin bone, the way that the wall is growing from a deformed coronary band that is in the wrong place, and the amount of sole depth that was available on this foot. Now, when looking at an X-ray, you can remember what the sagittal section looks like.

All of these films are from either Dr. Morrison or Dr. Marcotte. **Figures 17-19** are the ones that are easiest to compare to the sagittal section because the coffin bone has changed so much. **Figure 20** is a bad case, as there is no sole depth at the point of the coffin bone. **Figure 21** shows some changes in the coffin bone with a lot of damage and change to the hoof wall. **Figure 22** is what we see most often when looking at a chronic foundered foot. Some vets will talk about the degree of rotation. This is determined by comparing the angle of the dorsal coffin bone to the angle of the dorsal hoof wall. However, this information can be misleading, and a comparison to the pastern bones should be considered as well.

TREATMENT

There is no such thing as a mild case of founder. Regardless of the degrees of rotation or the amount of pain, founder is a serious problem.

As soon as there is any suspicion of founder or laminitis, a veterinarian should be called out. The vet will often treat the cause; for instance, a horse that has gotten into grain will have oil and charcoal pumped

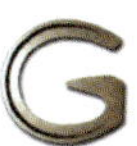

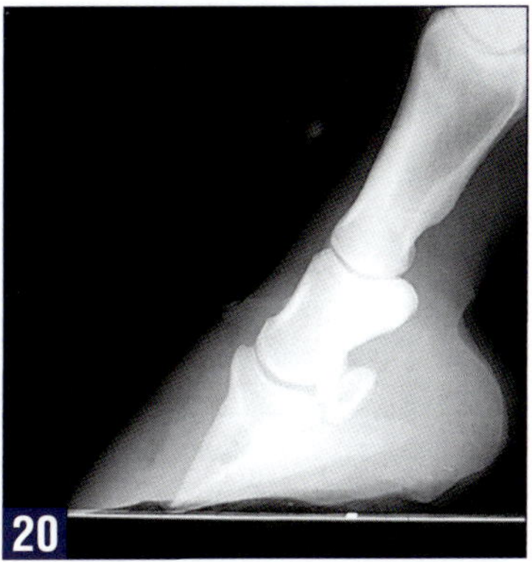

X-ray showing no sole depth as P3 pushes through the sole.

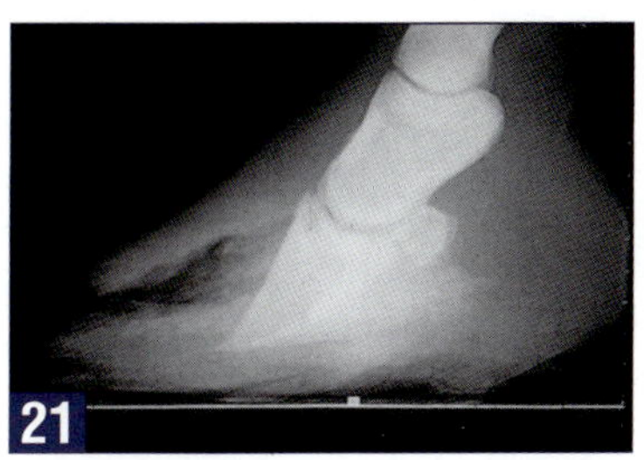

X-ray showing a lot of changes to the hoof wall.

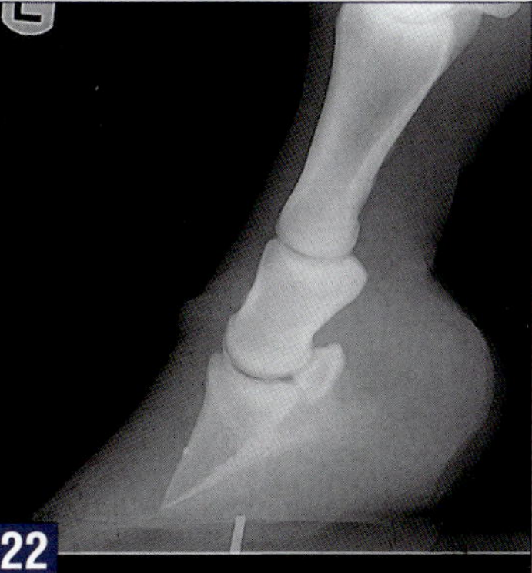

Common look to a foundered foot in X-ray.

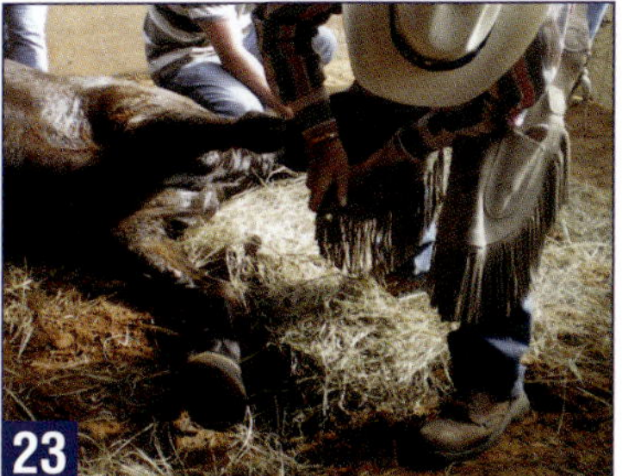

Working on a horse that is too sore to stand.

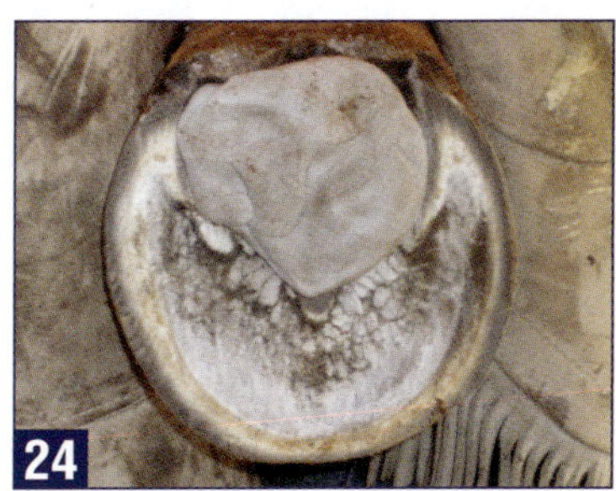

Impression material on the frog.

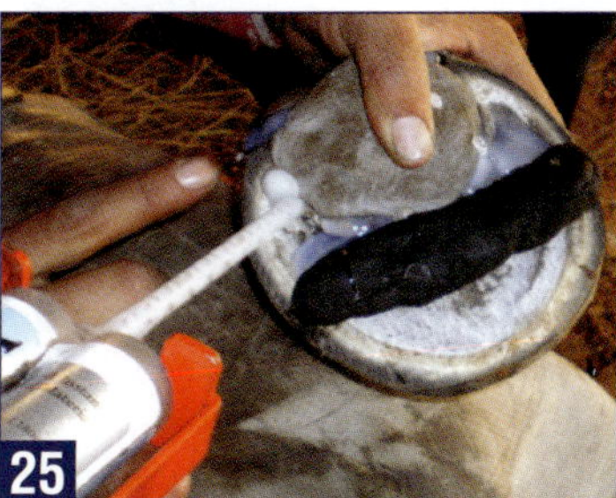

Equi-Pak around the impression material.

into its stomach through a tube inserted in the nose. There are a number of drugs that can be administered, but I will leave those to the vet.

From the farrier's viewpoint, if the horse has been recently trimmed or shod, the feet should be left as is, and you should use an impression material, Sole Guard, Equi-Pak, or similar substances attached to the rear half of the foot to exclude the toe from weight bearing. Sole Guard or Equi-Pak will adhere to the foot. Impression material will have to be taped on. With horses that need to be trimmed, try to trim normally, leaving as much sole as you can. At this point, the look of the bottom of the foot has not had time to change too much, and it is not uncommon for an inexperienced farrier to take too much sole. This only compounds the problem and makes abscesses even more likely.

The horse in **Figure 23** is so sore from an acute case of founder that it is reluctant to stand. Go ahead and work on horses like this while they are lying down, if possible. I put some impression material over the frog **(Figure 24)**, put Equi-Pak around it to recruit some of the bars and heel **(Figure 25)**, and covered the whole thing with duct tape. While that will not stay on the foot for turn out, a horse that is hurt this bad is not going to be moving too much.

The horse should be placed in extremely deep bedding. I recommend a stall with soft shavings that are 12 inches deep. The feet and legs from mid cannon bone down should be iced as much as possible for the first 72 hours. I had always heard from the old-timers that you should make the horse stand in a fast flowing river, and that would do the trick of icing the legs if it is cold enough. Horses do not have the same reaction to cold and ice on their feet that we do, and it will not cause discomfort to have their feet and lower legs iced.

Getting some weight off the feet for a few hours a day is also a good idea. You can use an animal harness and take a few hundred pounds off of the horse by hanging it from a rafter, the bucket of a tractor, or a tree. With the perfect facilities, you may want to back a flatbed trailer into a pond, tie the horse to the end of it with the water up to the middle

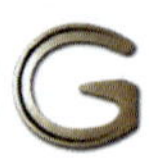

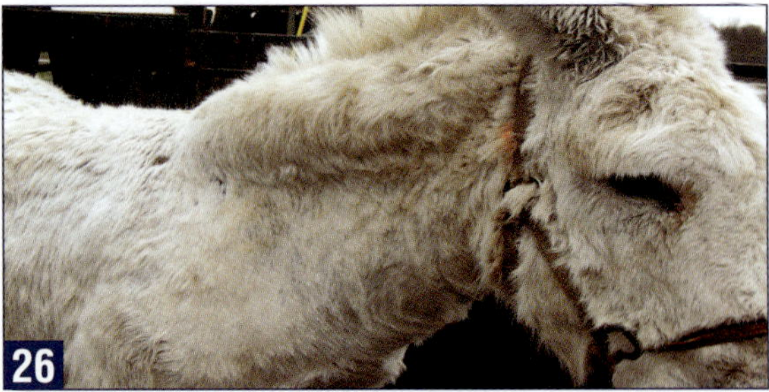

26 *Cresty neck on a foundered donkey.*

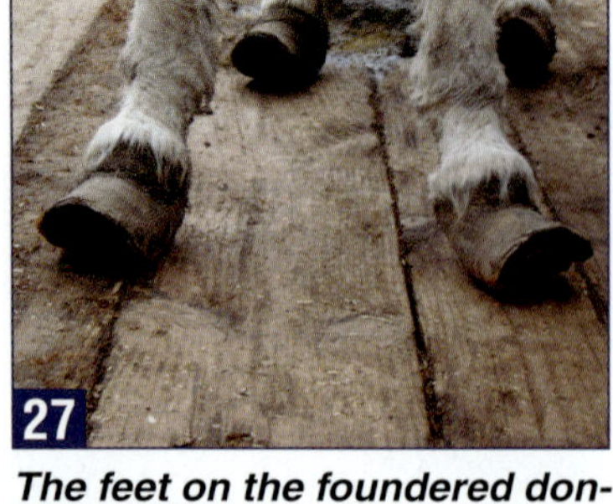

27 *The feet on the foundered donkey before trimming.*

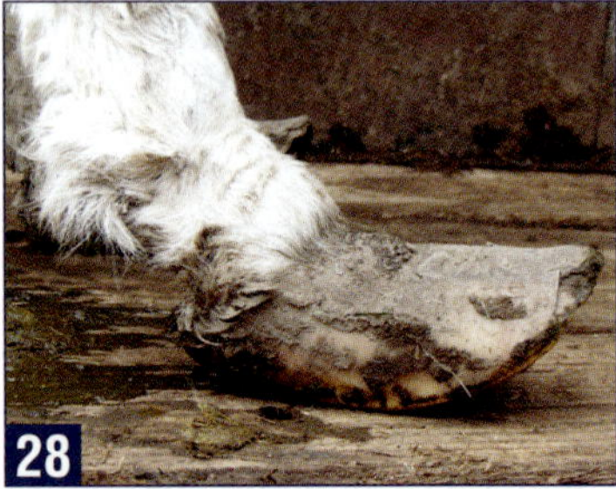

28 *The feet on the foundered donkey before trimming.*

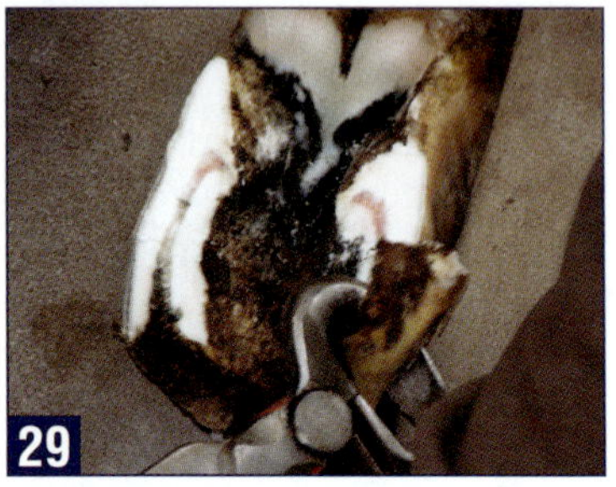

29 *Removing the heels.*

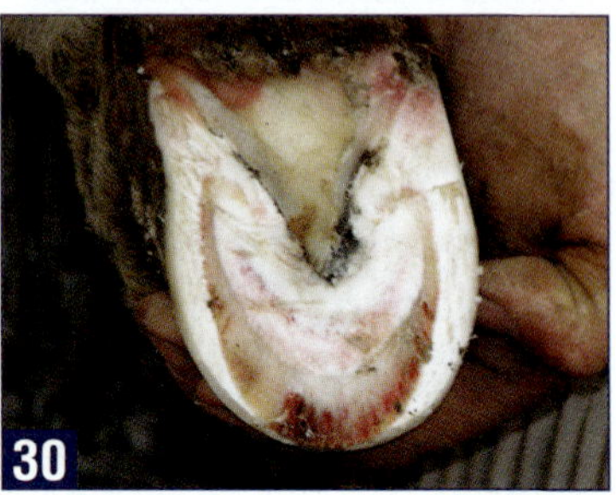

30 *Bottom of trimmed foot.*

of its trunk, and feed it on the end of the trailer. The water will provide buoyancy, and the silt will allow the feet to find their perfect comfort level without too much resistance. This is not something that you can keep a horse in or doing for 24 hours, but a few hours of relief every day will really help. Read the horse to see if its comfort level improves and tailor the treatment to that particular horse.

Although these recommendations require the horse to have wet feet for an extended period of time, the potential damage from that is minimal compared to the complications of full-blown founder. While I understand that doing all of the mentioned things for the acute and subacute phase can be difficult, you need to do as much as the horse, the owner, the facilities, and the season allow. I wouldn't put a horse in a pond in the middle of winter or hang it in a weak tree.

Chronic Phase

After the infections and severe pain have run their course, the horse has entered the chronic phase. It has probably been 10 days to 3 weeks from the onset of the founder, depending on how bad the horse has foundered.

The trim is the foundation for success at this junction. Knowing the sole depth and position of the coffin bone is helpful, so get X-rays if possible. You can put a thumbtack in a thick part of the frog and tape a nail or piece of wire to the dorsal wall to give you guides to measure to. Generally, the heels need to be lowered, the toe backed up, and the sole in front of the frog left alone. Of course, each case is an individual, and excessive growth in front of the frog may need to be removed in some cases.

Figure 26 shows the cresty neck of a foundered donkey. Fat pockets on the neck and rump are common on some of these foundered animals. The donkey's feet prior to the trim can be seen in **Figure 27-28**. In **Figure 29**, the heels are being trimmed, and **Figure 30** shows what the foot looks like on the bottom after being trimmed. **Figure 31** is a post-trim lateral view of the off front foot, and **Figure 32** shows the position of the legs and feet after trimming.

Figure 33 is of another neglected animal with severe changes in the hooves. The feet have been trimmed back as far as possible, and the horse is more comfortable, despite a little blood showing on the dorsal wall **(Figures 34-35)**. **Figure 36** is the pre-trim picture of another case of neglect and founder. Again, trim the heels back **(Figures 37-38)**. In **Figure 39**, it is evident that the toe is backed up

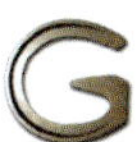

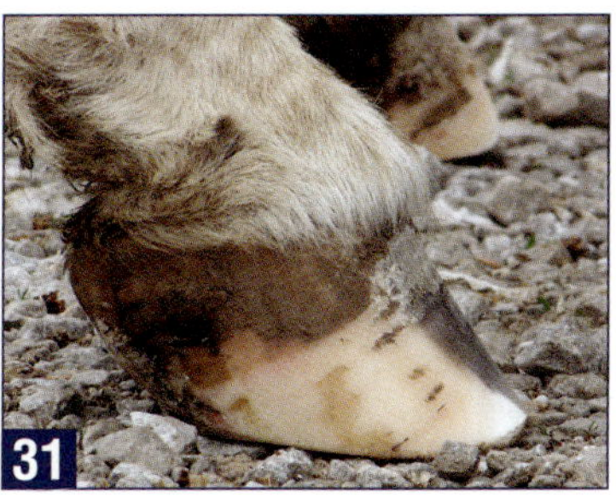

Lateral view of trimmed foot.

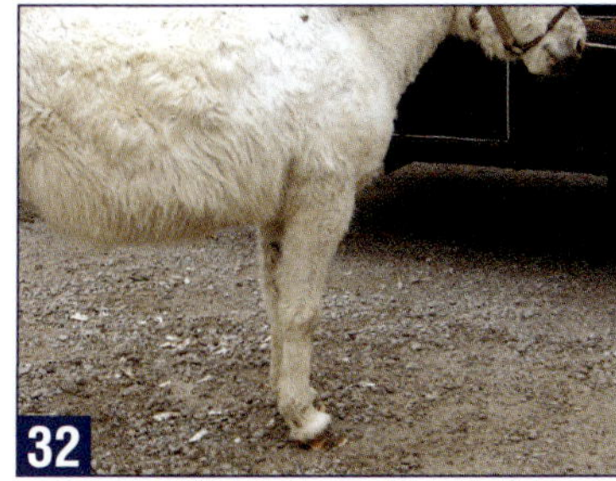

The front end of the donkey after trimming.

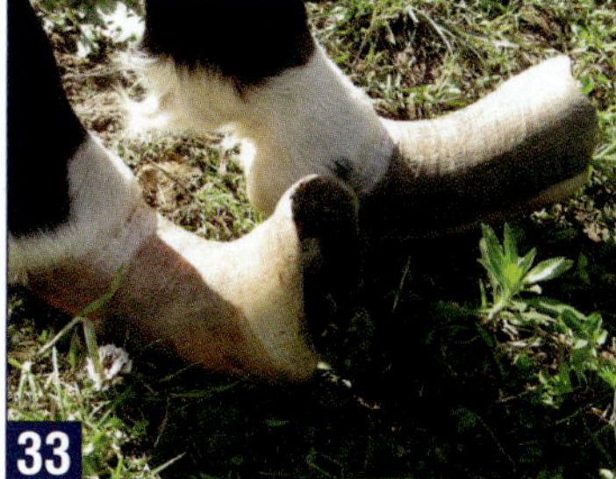

Curled and neglected foundered feet.

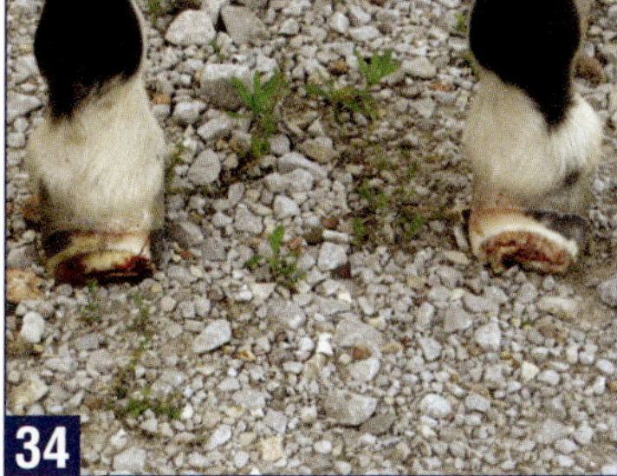

After trimming.

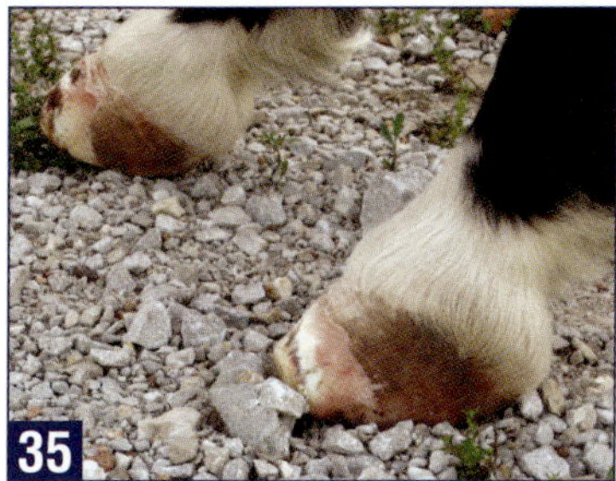

36

Neglected foundered feet.

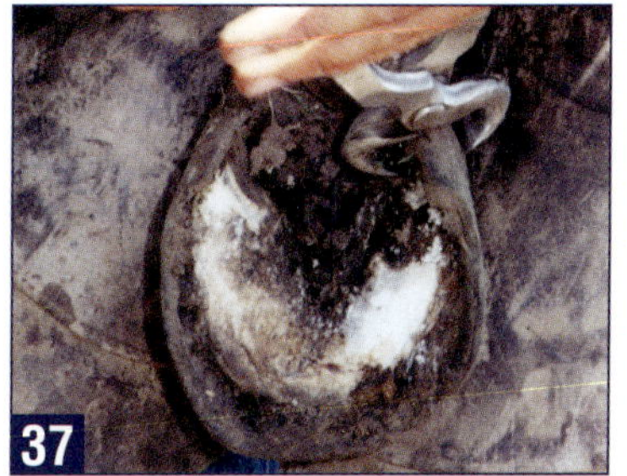

Trimming the bottom of the foot.

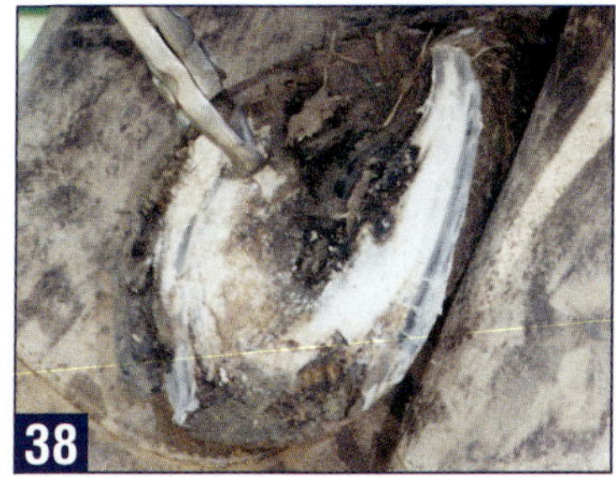

39

The bottom trimmed.

through the entire thickness of the hoof wall, right into the white line. **Figures 40-41** show the foot on the ground after trimming. Notice that the foot is not in contact with the ground in a normal position.

In cases like this, we often leave the animal barefoot. Since the owners have already shown that neglect is part of this animal's life, putting shoes on will only make the animal worse in the long run. Shoes can stay on feet like this for a very long time, and when there is excess growth, there can be excess force on an already damaged laminar junction.

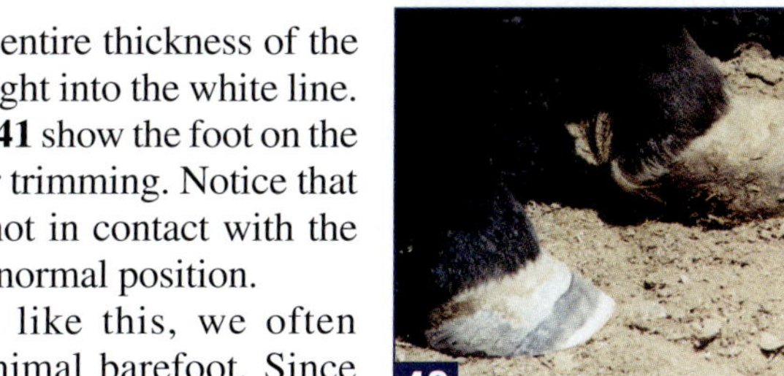

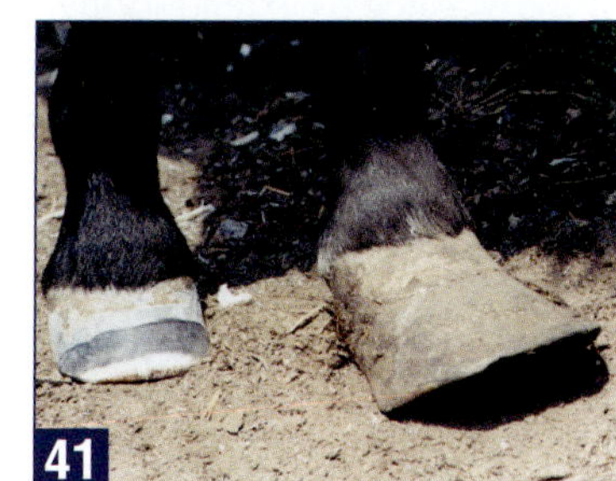

Lateral view of the trimmed foot next to the one that is not yet trimmed. Notice that the dressing went right through the wall into the stretched white line.

In the ones that are going to get shod, at this point you can apply a shoe. My favorite is a W-shoe. This shoe is also known as an open-toed heart bar,

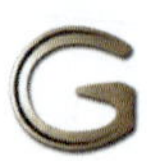

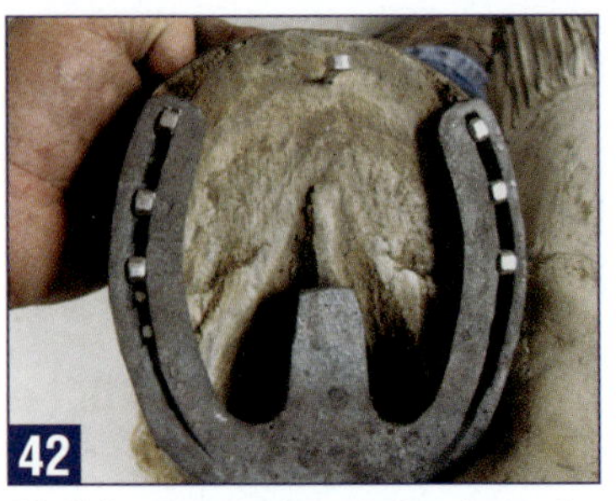
Nail in the sole of the foot, inside the white line.

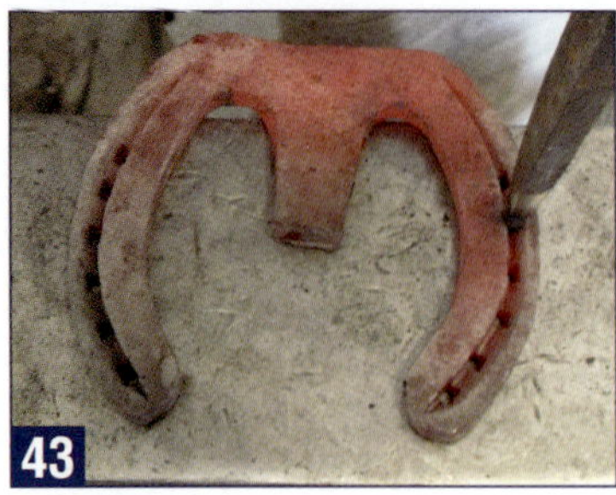
W-shoe being made.

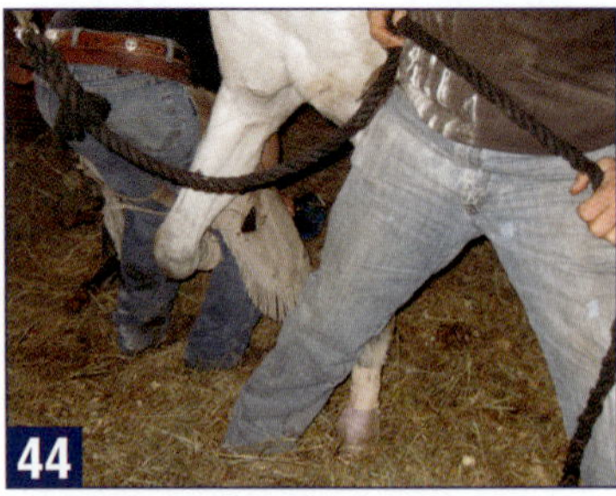
Bracing the opposite leg so that the other foot can be worked on.

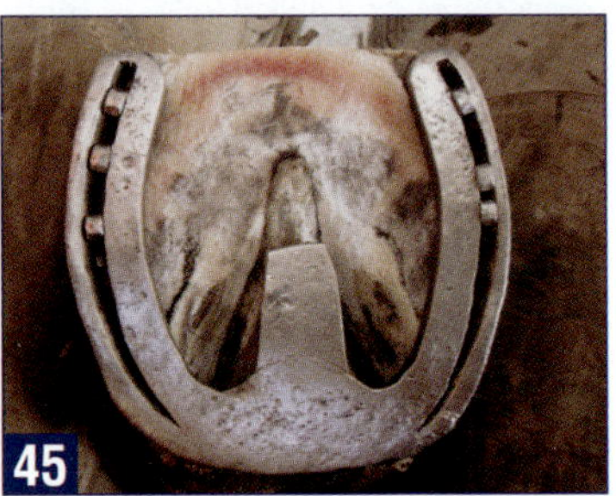
W-shoe on foot.

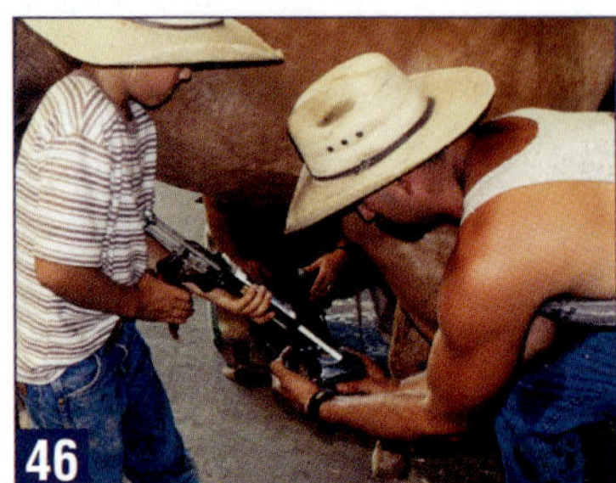
Cody putting Equi-Pak in a W-shoe for me.

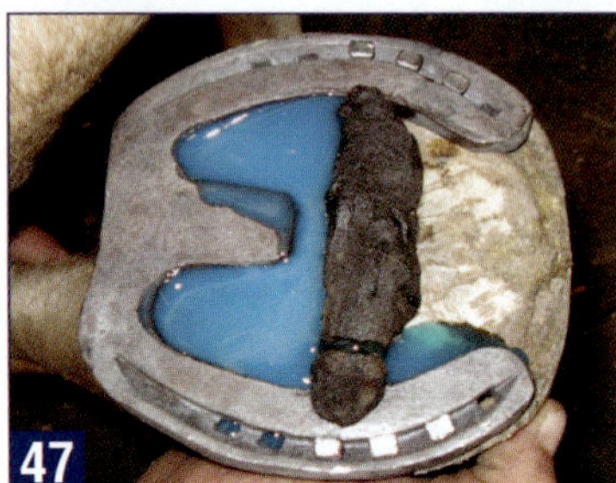
W-shoe with Equi-Pak.

and you can place weight on the frog but keep the injured toe area from having to bear weight. To apply this shoe, I will trim the heels as needed and build a shoe so that the frog plate is just touching the frog when the shoe is nailed on. Positive frog pressure has not been successful when I have used it. The tip of the frog plate should not be any further forward than 3/8 of an inch behind the apex of the frog unless X-rays tell you different. I like the ends of the W-shoe to extend to the last point of horny tissue in front of the tip of the coffin bone. Look at **Figure 42**. Notice that there is a nail driven into the sole inside the white line. This indicates that the white line is not a good representation of the position of the coffin bone, and there is horny tissue where it is not expected. Radiographs will show this. If needed, I will have a vet tranquilize the horse for me so I can get the shoe on the foot. It can be glued to the foot, but that is not something that I do a lot of. I have had so much success with this shoe, that it is usually my first choice when working on a foundered foot.

Look at the Chapter 50 in the **Shoe Arsenal** section of this book for specific instructions on making the W-shoe. Make it with a lot of nail holes so that when it is being nailed, a good spot can always be found **(Figure 43)**. For horses that are knuckling over, the holder may have to brace the opposite leg while the horse is being worked on **(Figure 44)**. Once the shoe of choice is nailed on, I will make a dam of Sole Pack in front of the tip of the frog plate and fill the back portion of the shoe with Equi-Pak (**Figures 46-47**). This helps keep the shoe on the foot, puts some pressure on the bars and sole that is not damaged, and keeps the area under the bar clean. In the days before Equi-Pak, it was hard for owners to keep the area around the frog and commissures clean, and most heart bars would result in a case of thrush.

If the frog is recessed, I can change the plane of the frog plate **(Figure 48)**. An easy way to do this is by placing the reins of a pair of tongs under the bar on either side of the frog plate and hammering the center of the bar **(Figure 49)**. A piece of pad can also be inserted or riveted between the frog plate and the frog **(Figures 50-51)**.

In some cases, I will use a full heart bar **(Figure 52)**, but I don't put too much pressure on the toe. One problem with a full heart bar is that a gap at the toe can trap debris that may cause problems, and if it

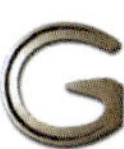

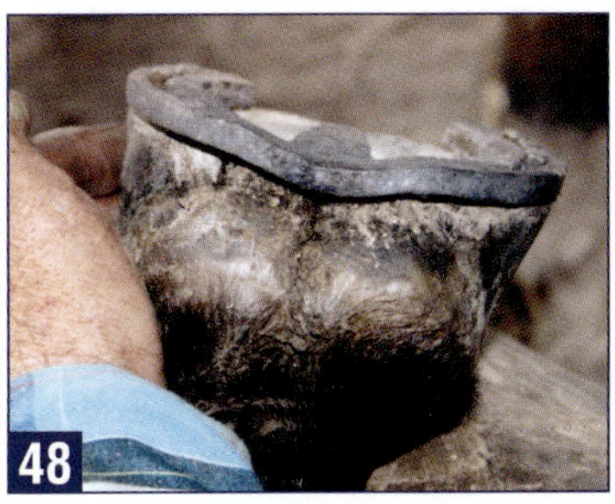

Frog plate in a different plane than the shoe for a recessed frog.

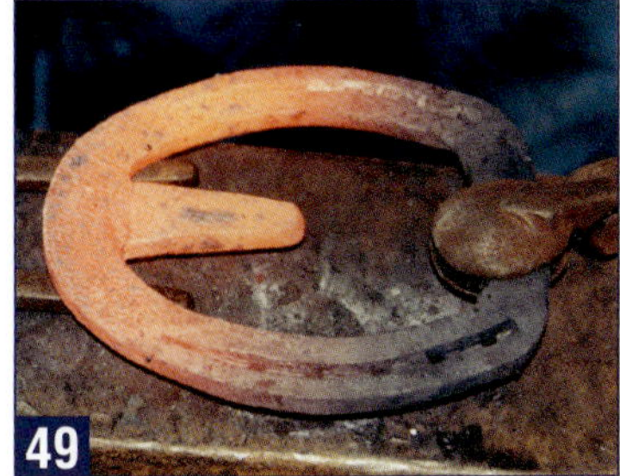

Method of changing the plane of the frog plate.

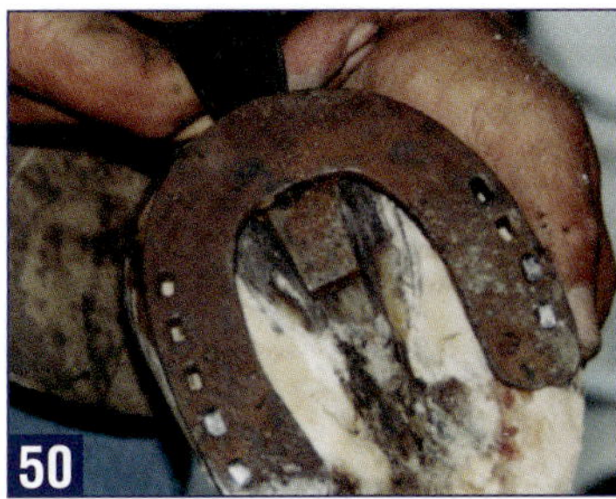

Inserting a piece of pad under the frog plate.

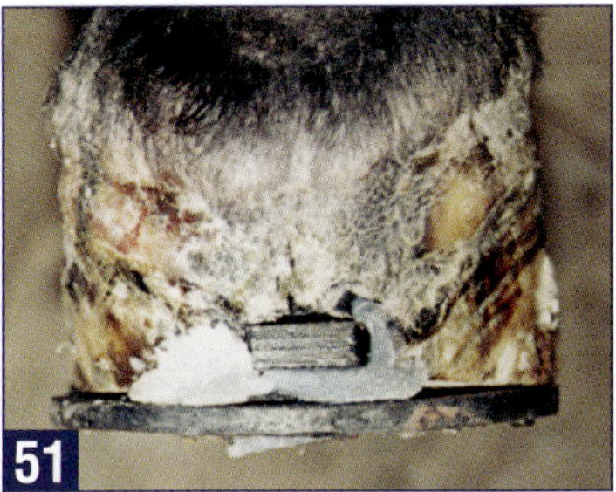

The pad after it is placed between the frog and shoe with Equi-Pak around it to secure it.

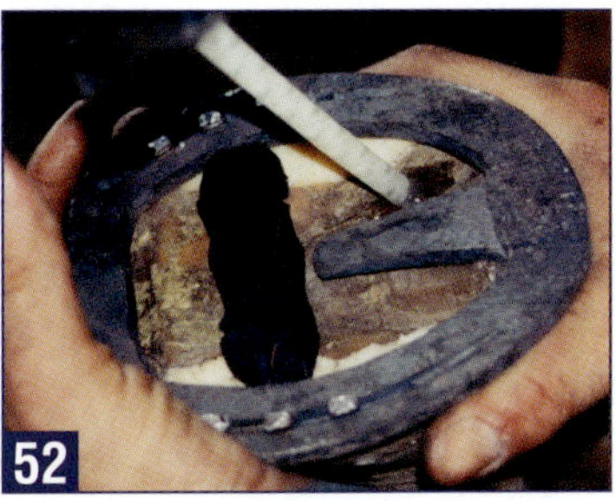

Full Heart bar with Equi-Pak being put in.

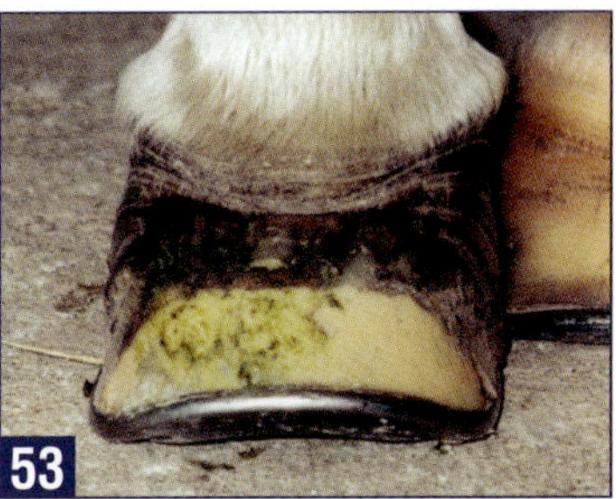

Acrylic building up the toe of a badly foundered foot. Done out of ignorance.

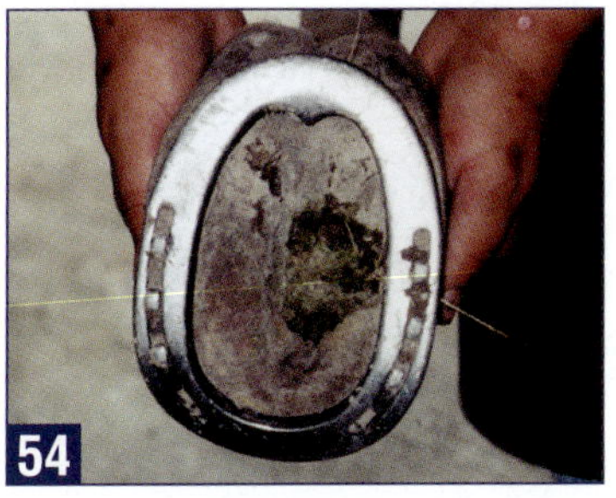

Keg shoe Egg bar on the foundered foot.

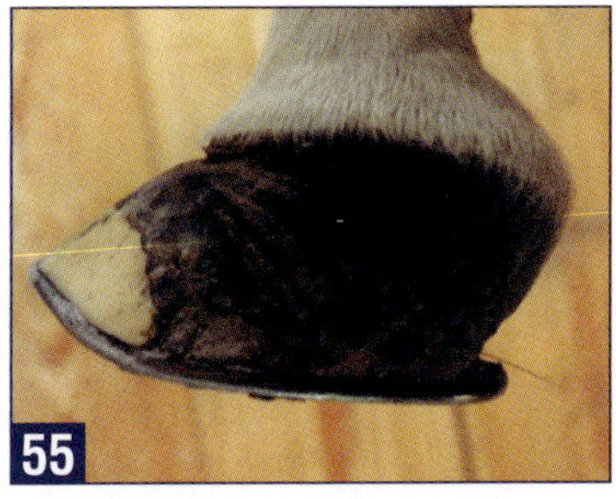

Rocker toe with the acrylic putting a lot of pressure on the toe where it is not needed.

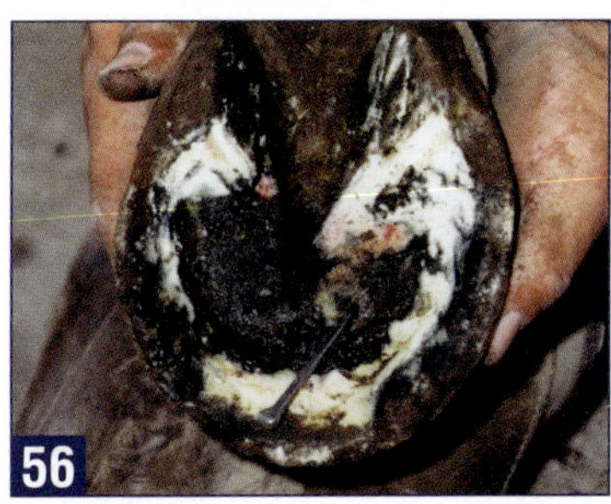

Abscess on foundered foot.

is tight against the toe, it may cause pressure on the toe that I don't want since the toe is so weakened. Speaking of pressure at the toe, **Figures 53-55** show the work of a horseshoer that did not understand what founder was. This guy did a lot of work, using an egg bar, Equilox, and putting an extreme rocker toe on the shoe, all in an effort to make the toe of the foot bear weight, which is exactly what it should not be doing in its damaged condition. Just look at how much pressure is on the dorsal coronary band in **Figure 55**. Needless to say, this horse was extremely lame.

A lot of foundered feet should be bandaged when sensitive structures are exposed, or when abscesses **(Figure 56)** are present. We like to use a diaper covered with elastic wrap, then covered with a boot **(Figures 57-59)**. Another option is to bandage without the boot. Begin with the diaper and elastic wrap **(Figure 60)**, then make a pad out of duct tape **(Figure 61)**. Place that over the bottom of the foot and tape it in place **(Figures 62-63)**. The boot is more durable, but either way will work to allow the foot to heal.

In some cases, I have done resections of the

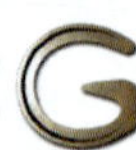

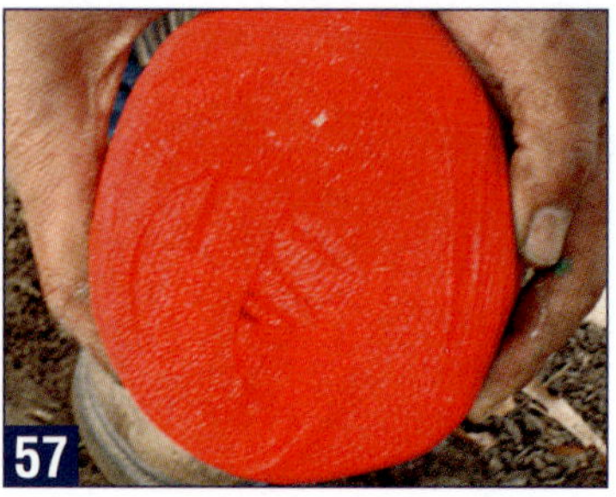

Foot wrapped in elastic wrap.

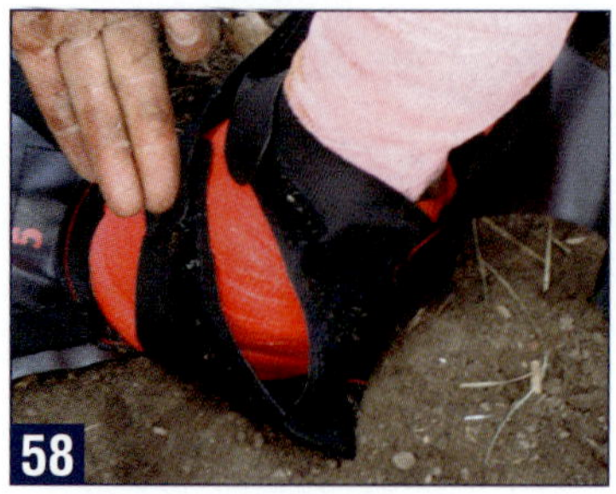

Putting on the boot.

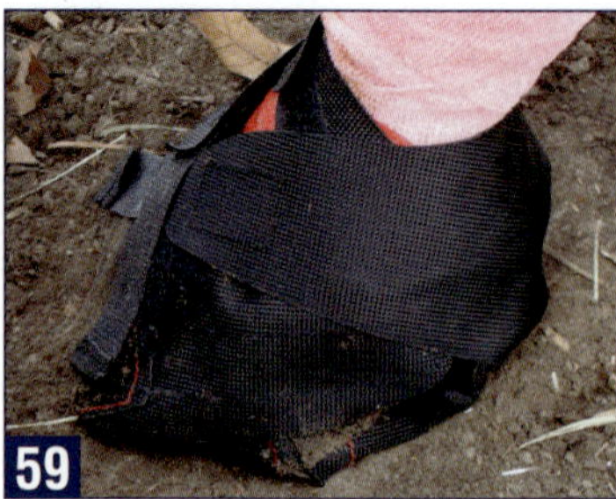

The boot placed on the foot. Part of the Kaeco Abscess Kit.

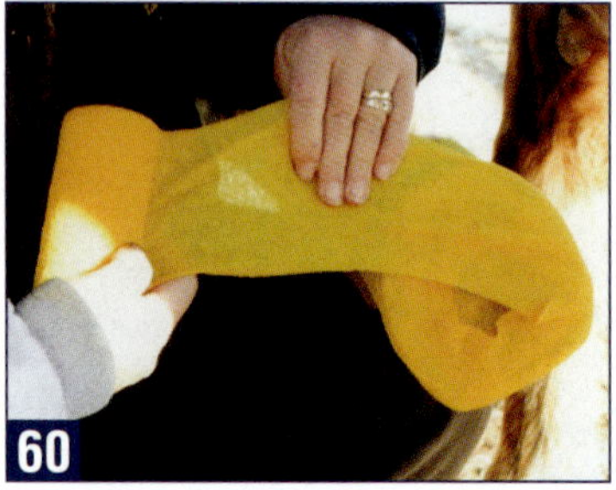

Wrapping the foot in elastic wrap.

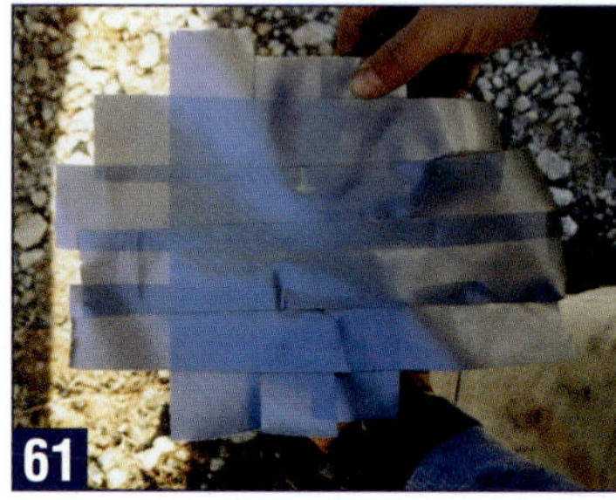

A pad made out of duct tape.

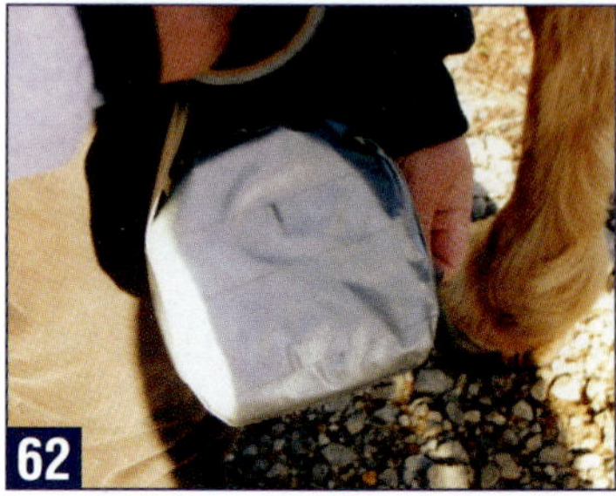

Taping the pad to the bottom of the foot.

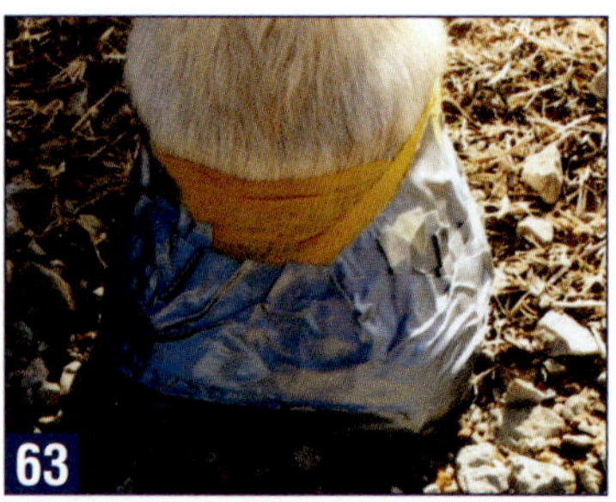

The foot that has been bandaged.

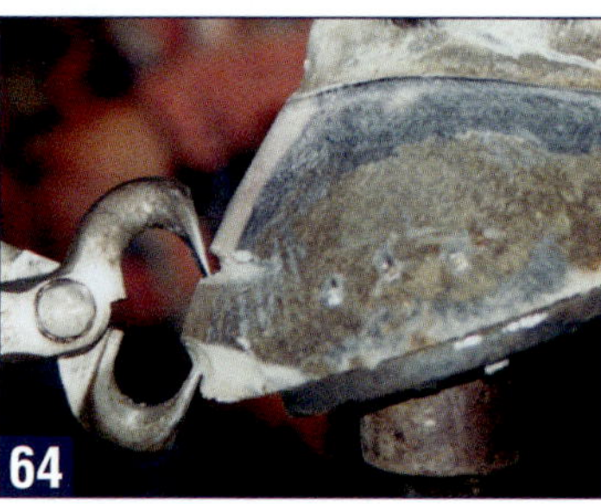

Doing a resection.

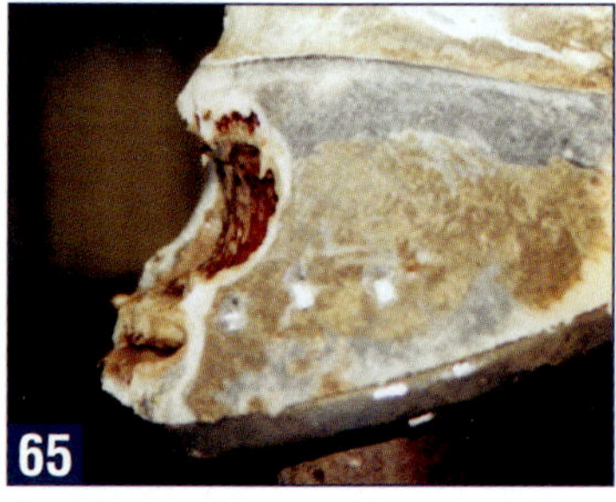

Doing a resection.

dorsal wall. I like to do this with my knife, nippers, and rasp rather than with a Dremel tool, but that is my own bias, and the horse won't care as long as it is done correctly **(Figures 64-67)**. When you do a resection, you should remove hoof wall just to the point of bleeding. Try to keep it from bleeding if you are working without a vet, but when a vet is there, they don't mind seeing and working in blood. Another option besides the resection is to groove the foot **(Figure 68)**. This is done very easily with the edge of the rasp, and you can cut through the outer hoof wall into the stratum internum to take pressure off of the coronary band at the toe.

In the farrier market, there are a lot of options and products designed for shoeing foundered horses. Be certain that you understand the mechanics and principles behind whatever item you decide to put on a foot. One that has really become popular lately is the clog. This is a block of wood that is screwed to the foot. In my opinion, this is the same as moving the rock as discussed in the introduction to lameness chapter. It can also be dangerous if not done correctly when the screws enter sensitive structures, but so can nails that are driven without

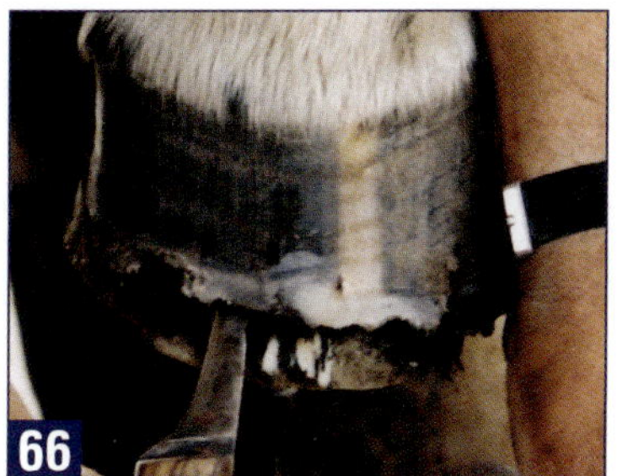

Doing a resection.

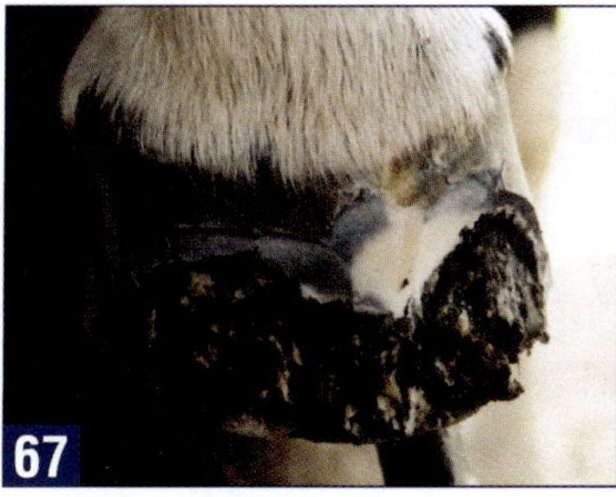

Doing a resection.

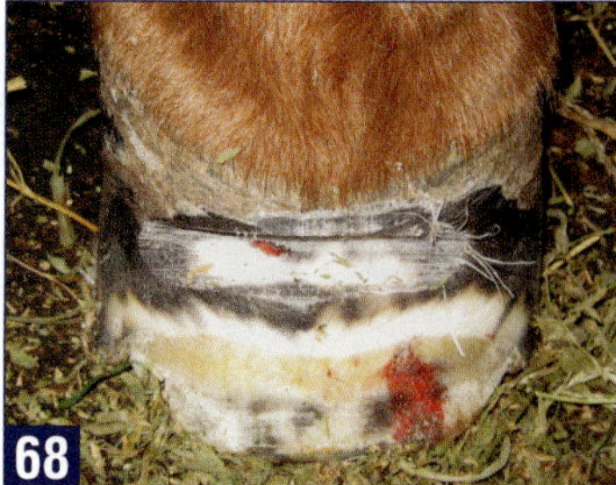

Groove in the wall below the coronary band at the toe.

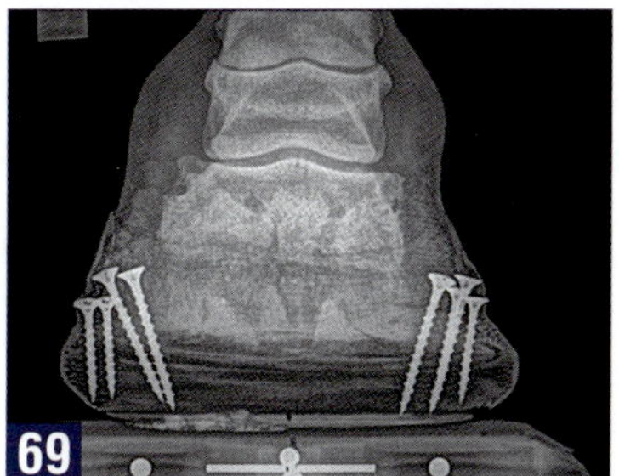

Dorsal/palmar X-ray of a clog screwed to a foot with incorrect mediolateral balance.

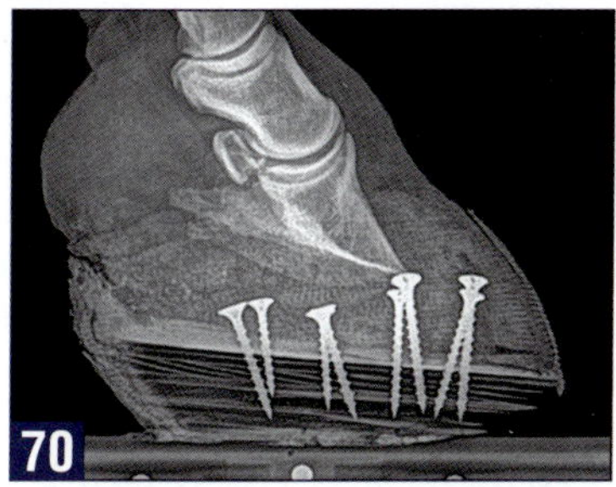

Lateral view of foundered foot with clog. Same foot as figure 69.

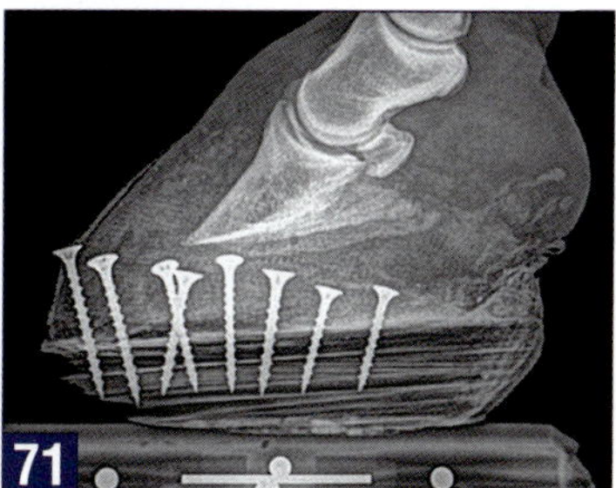

Lateral view of the other foundered foot on this horse.

skill and experience. One of my biggest concerns with the clog is mediolateral balance. **Figure 69** is a dorsal/palmar X-ray of a foot with a clog, and the incorrect balance of the coffin bone is immediately evident. **Figures 70-71** show the different feet on this same horse, and there is quite a difference in the hoof-pastern axis as well. If you use these, just be certain that you are careful in the application. I have had a lot of success with foundered feet and have yet to need the clog.

There are a lot of variables in the chronic phase. You may end up with a neglected foundered hoof with the toe completely off the ground and the heels growing straight forward. You may have twists in the hoof capsule. Some feet may have very little depth of sole, while some may have a lot. The horse may or may not be lame. Each horse will be different. When I deal with these feet, I try to imagine the coffin bone and determine where it would be if the hoof capsule were not so distorted. Once I have figured out where I want to go with that foot, I begin trimming. From here on, it is wooden Indian time. Drop the heels, back up the toe, and if you are shoeing, try to avoid putting pressure on the toe of the foot or the sole.

Keep these horses on a tight schedule to improve your chance of bringing them back to soundness. The longer they go between shoeing and trimming, the greater the change that you have to make each time. These drastic changes can cause the horse more pain.

ANTICIPATED OUTCOME

Anytime that you are dealing with founder, the outcome is guarded at best. Even the least amount of separation can become fatal to the horse, given the wrong set of circumstances. While it is possible for a horse to recover fully, I would be careful in predicting which horses fall into that category. Explain the seriousness of this problem to the owner, attack the problem aggressively, and add this horse to your prayer list.

IN SHORT

D: Inflammation of the laminae, may lead to separation of the coffin bone and hoof wall.

T: Impression material or polymer urethane in the rear half of the foot for the acute and subacute phase, followed by a W-shoe or similar shoeing strategy to place weight on the frog in the chronic phase.

Chapter

45-9 HOOF AVULSION

DEFINITION

The hoof capsule has come off of the coffin bone. Figures 1-4 show an avulsion a couple of months after the initial insult.

REASONS

This can happen from an infection in the foot bad enough to destroy a lot of the bond between the dermal coriums and the epidermal horn. It would be quite a bad infection.

Another potential reason is a horse that has been badly foundered or possibly endured an advanced case of white line disease. In cases like these, there could be enough of the bond missing to allow an avulsion.

Horses that have been nerved, especially a high nerving, are more susceptible to avulsion because if they get their feet caught in something, they may continue to pull without a pain sensation.

Finally, there is the potential for horses to get their foot caught tight enough in a rock crevice or possibly a cattle guard. If they are moving at speed when the foot gets caught, it is possible for the momentum of their body to go forward and leave the hoof capsule behind.

ANATOMY

The obvious anatomy will be the hoof capsule and the coriums.

SYMPTOMS

This is not a hard problem to diagnose. The hoof capsule will be missing from the bottom of the leg. There will be Grade 4 lameness present, and the horse will be in severe pain.

TREATMENT

One of the first things that a farrier should do here is explain that this is a bad problem that — even if successfully treated — will result in a horse that will likely not be sound. Establish the financial limitations of this animal. For some brood stock with great bloodlines, going through the rehab and expense of surviving an avulsion may be viable. For most others, it is not.

If the horse is younger than 2 years old, there is also the problem with the way that the rest of the body will have to develop while the new foot grows back on the injured leg. We have seen hips, hocks, knees, shoulders, and opposite feet get completely destroyed by being asked to do the job of two limbs.

In a perfect world, the horse will be lying down long enough for you to apply a heart bar to the opposite foot as a preventive measure against founder and other stress-related problems. You won't be able to pick up the good foot to work on it, and it is likely to have problems. The photos in this section show the good foot is quite long and needing a trim. Notice how the wall has changed in the top inch of the foot, indicating the time of the avulsion to the near front.

For horses that the owner wishes to save, the veterinarian will be the first person involved. Generally speaking, for the first three months or so, there are going to be bandages, medicine, soakings, antibiotics, and stall rest for this horse. The owner will have to doctor this horse as per the vet's instructions for at least six months, and there will be at least a year until the foot is grown back. Infection is a big risk in the early days of an avulsion.

As soon as there is good enough horn on the ground to apply a shoe to, you may want to get something on that foot. It will probably be a W-shoe since the heels will get to the ground before the toe. You should also have a pretty decent horny frog and sole by the time the heels grow out. If at all possible, you will want to glue the W-shoe to the foot with only one or two nails actually driven.

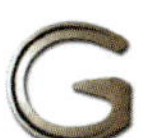

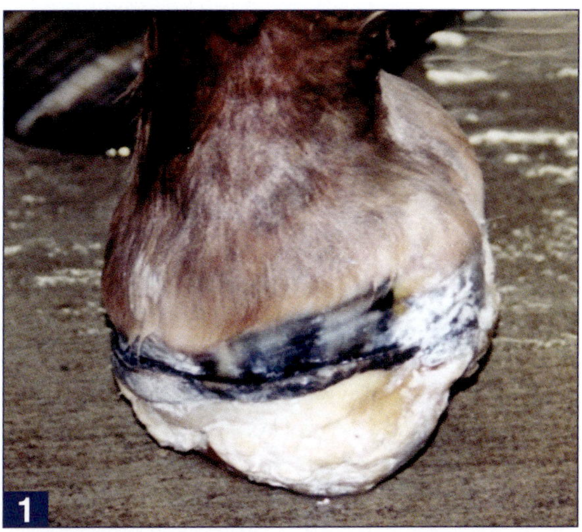

Lateral view of injured near front foot.

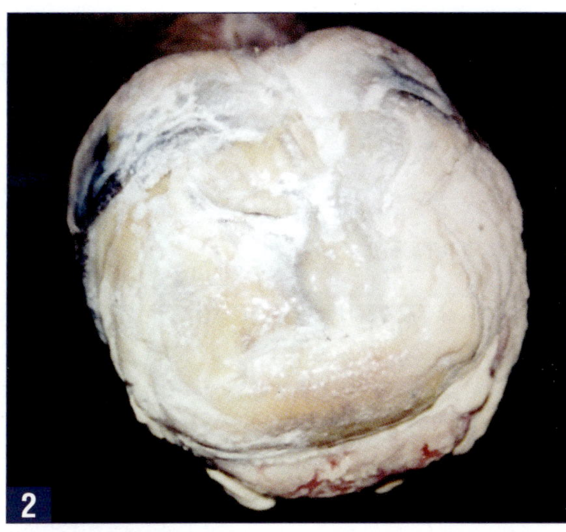

Solar view of injury.

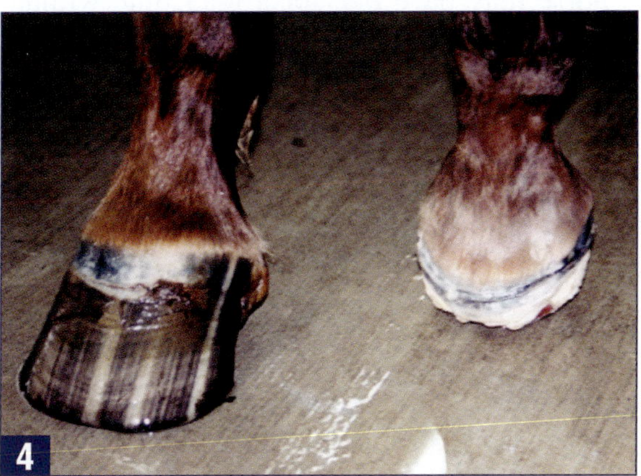

Dorsal view of both feet on injured horse.

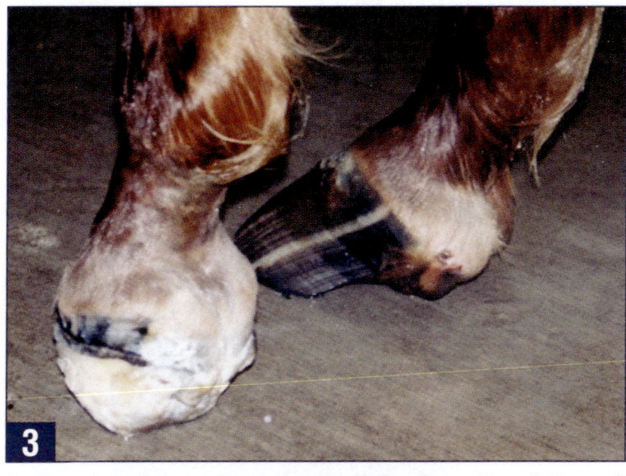

Lateral palmar view; notice the length of the off front foot.

Getting something on this foot should go a long way toward increasing the comfort level for this horse.

One other thing to mention is that this horse should certainly be on a good supplement for hoof growth. The faster the new foot grows, the better.

It will take from nine months to a year to get a new foot on this horse. Once you do, the new foot will probably be smaller than the opposite foot, and there is a good chance that the horse will still be sore, especially if it is ridden or used hard. Most horses that suffer an avulsion are destroyed instead of going through what it takes to get over it.

ANTICIPATED OUTCOME

I would not hold out too much hope for this horse. Even if it does survive, there is little chance of it being sound.

IN SHORT

D: The hoof capsule has come off the end of the leg.

T: Bandaging and doctoring continuously until some foot grows out. At that point, a W-shoe may be partially nailed and glued to the foot.

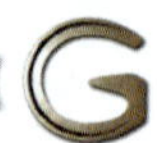

Chapter

45-10 KERATOMA

DEFINITION

This is a tumor of the horn that generally involves the stratum internum.

REASON

A keratoma can occur from continuous irritation to the hoof from injury or just be excess keratinization.

ANATOMY

Since the keratoma is on the inside of the hoof wall, it will involve the hoof wall and laminae, and in severe cases, the coffin bone can be remodeled. I have seen cases where the white line deviates toward the frog or the hoof wall has a ridge or bulge in it. In some severe cases, several keratomas have occurred in the same foot, causing it to become infected and separated from the coffin bone **(Figures 1-4)**.

SYMPTOMS

The keratoma can grow slowly enough that a horse may have one for a long time without suffering any lameness. It can also cause a horse to be extremely lame, depending on how aggressive it

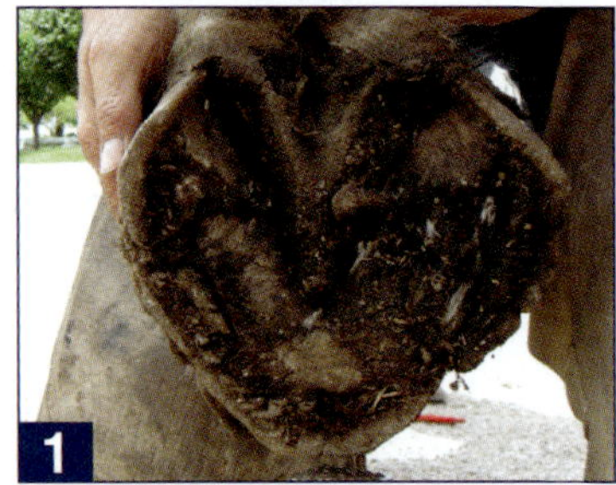

Untrimmed foot with keratomas in the lateral wall.

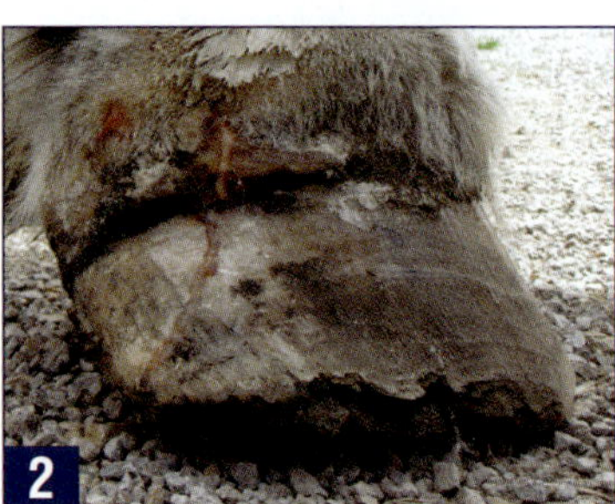

Damage and defects apparent from the keratomas.

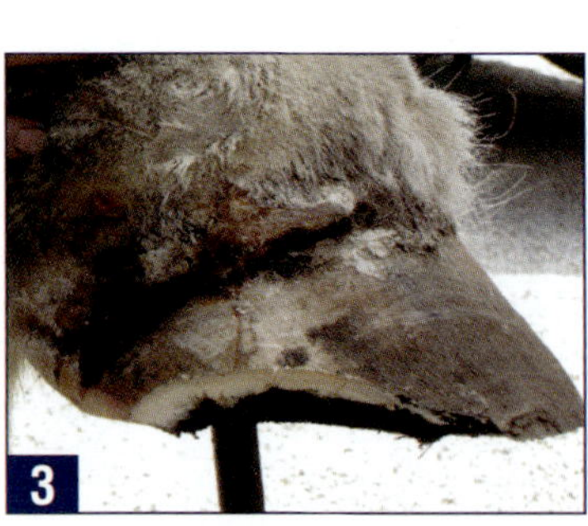

Damage and defects apparent from the keratomas.

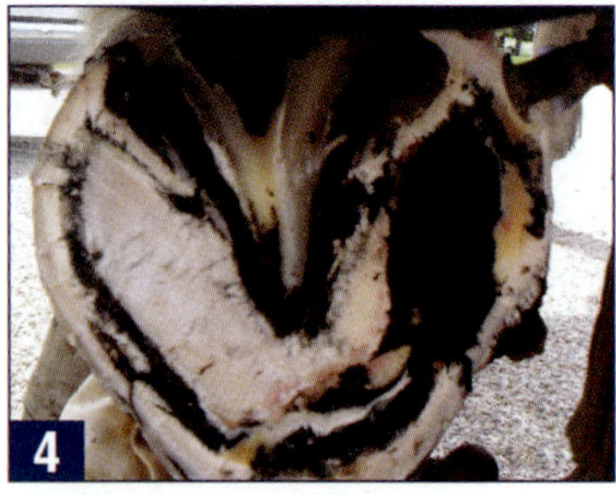

Bottom of the foot has been trimmed.

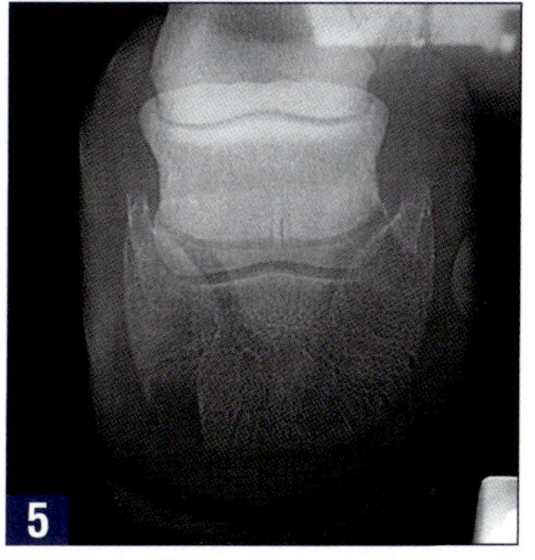

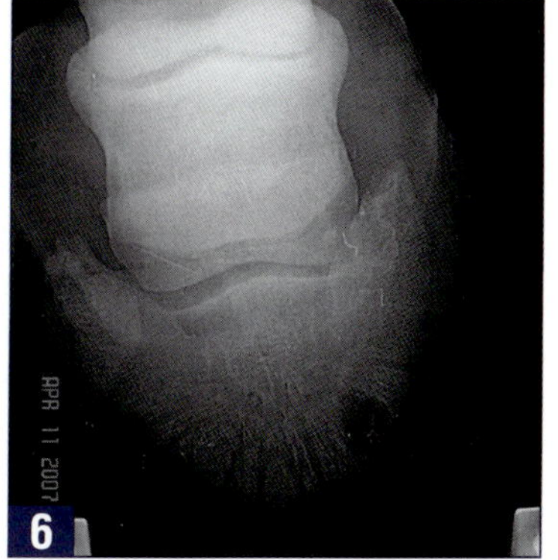

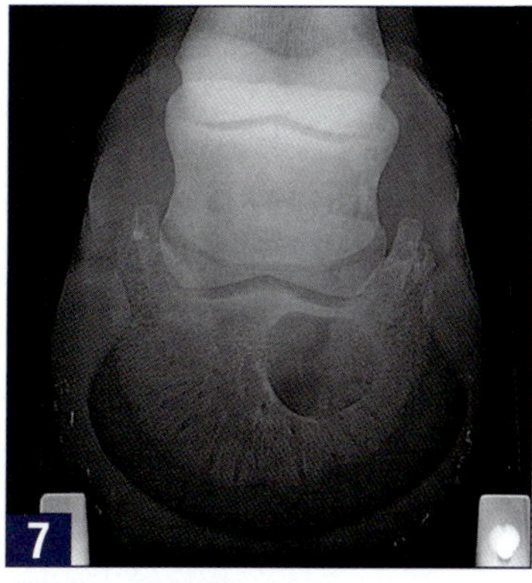

Radiographs showing the amount of damage a keratoma has done to different coffin bones.

is, how much damage it is causing, and its location. Keratomas can be hard to diagnose, but good radiographs at the right angle will often allow the veterinarian to give a good diagnosis. Dr. Scott Morrison has provided me with several keratoma radiographs (**Figures 5-8**). **Figures 7-8** are different views of the same foot.

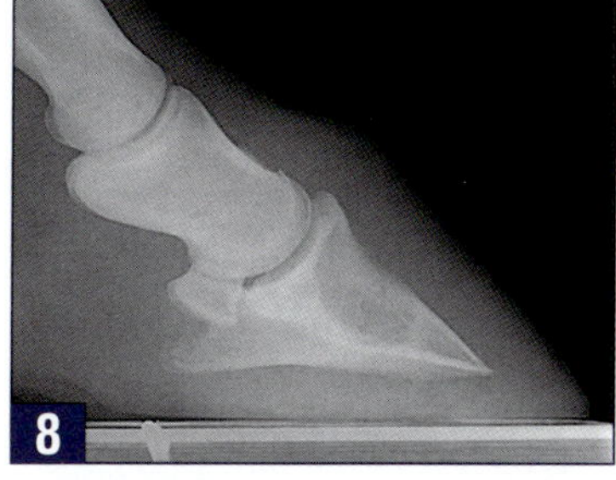

The lateral view shows that P3 is less dense from the keratoma.

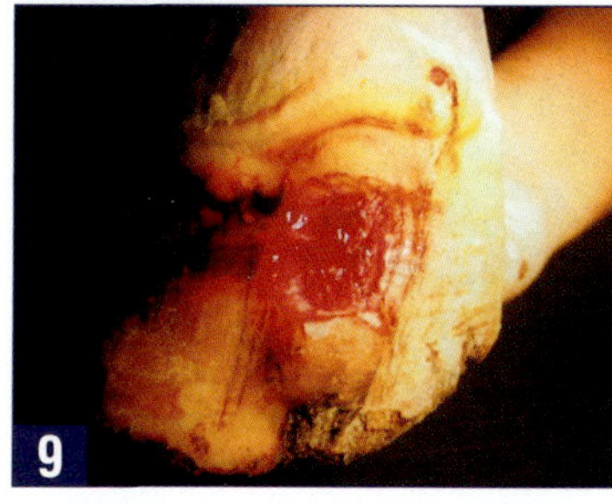

Hoof wall removed showing a keratoma underneath.

TREATMENT

Keratomas generally need to be surgically removed by a vet. The farrier's role is providing technical support and assistance, and you may have to invent a shoe that will support the foot once the vet has done surgery. Depending on location and size of the keratoma, it may have to be removed from the top of the wall, through a resection cut into the wall, or from the bottom. **Figures 9-12** show a keratoma being cut out of the side of a foot by Dr. Brent Hague at Oakridge Equine. In **Figure 12**, the size of the hole left behind is pretty large, and **Figure 13** shows the actual keratoma that has been removed.

The foot in **Figures 14-15** was

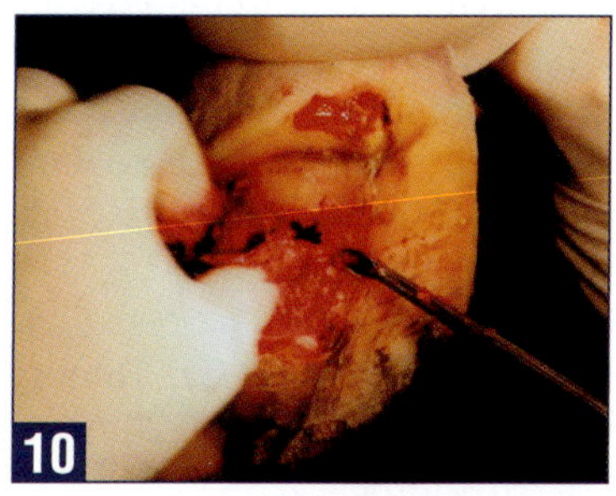

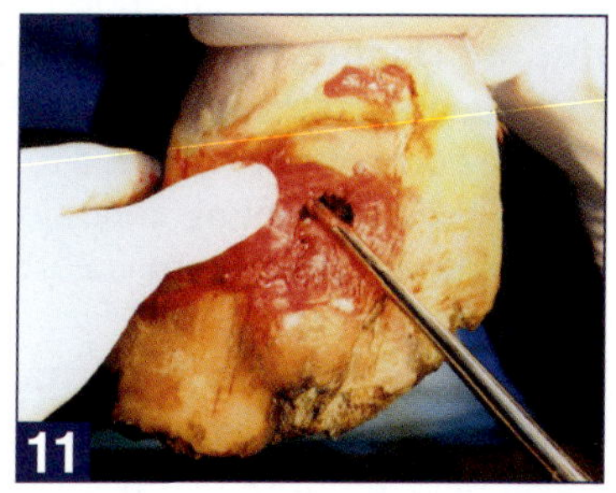

Removing the keratoma.

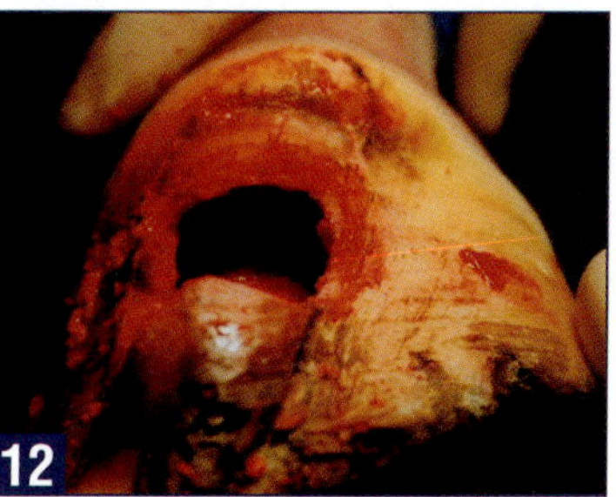

Hole left in the foot after the keratoma is removed.

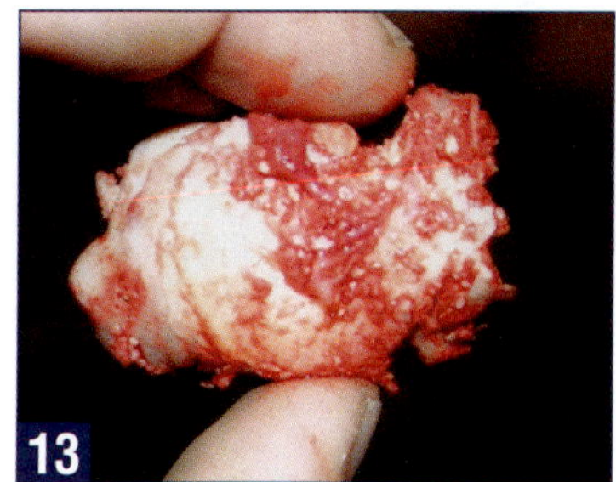

The keratoma that was in the foot.

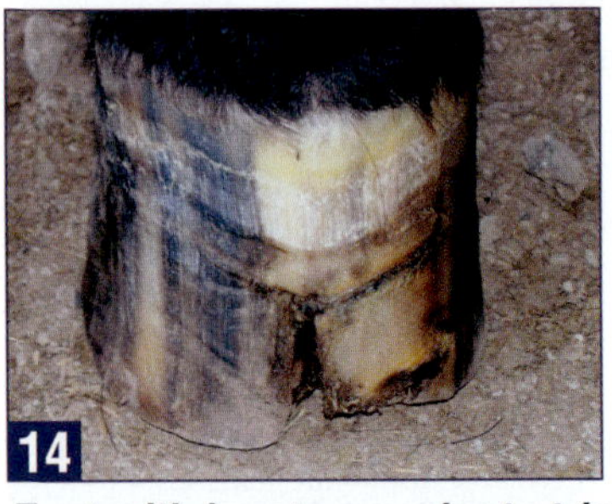
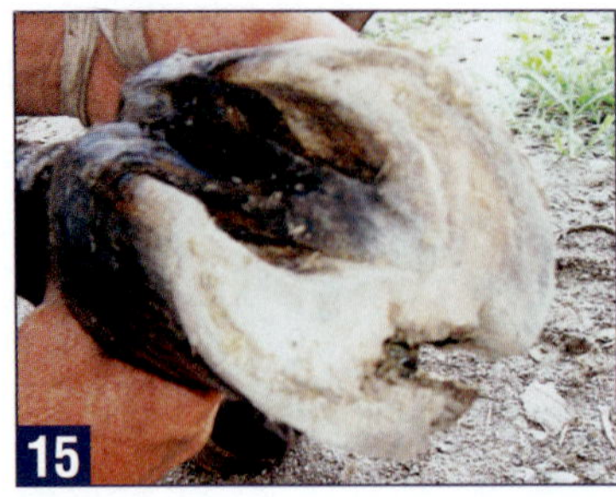

Foot with keratoma prior to trimming.

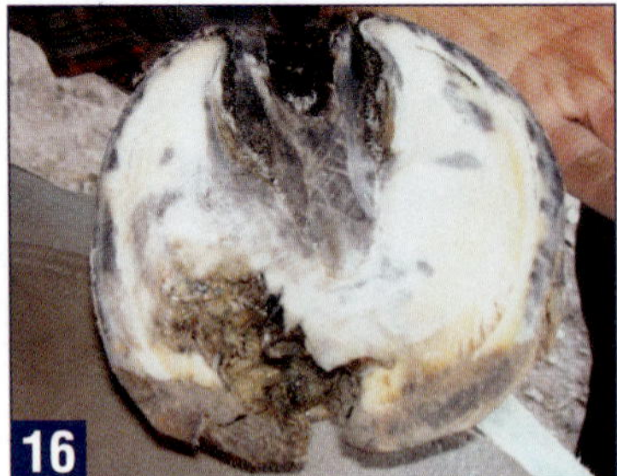

Bottom trimmed.

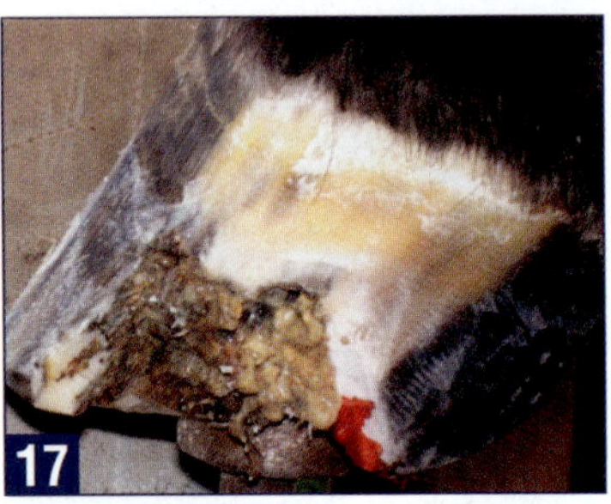

Start of resection.

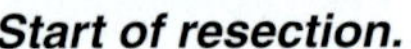

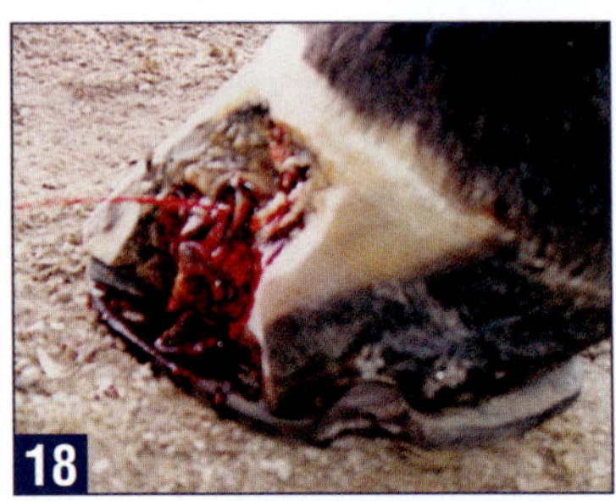

Blood squirting from the foot.

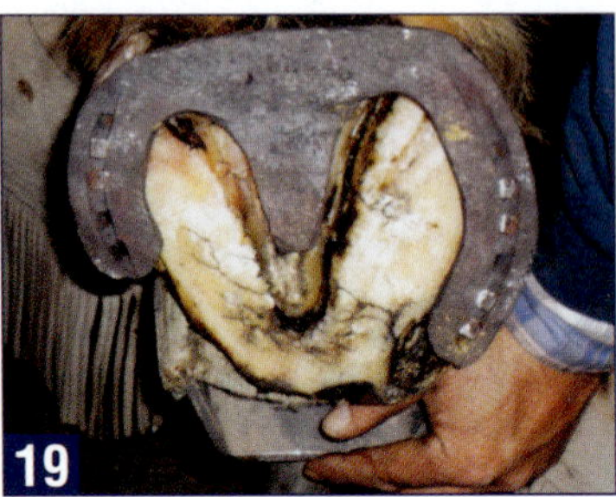

W-shoe on a draft horse with keratomas.

pretty well damaged, so I trimmed it **(Figure 16)** and shod it with a bar shoe. The hoof wall was resected **(Figure 17)** and a stream of blood can be seen shooting out of the foot in **Figure 18**.

The horse owner will need to be sure to keep the horse in clean stabling conditions to help prevent infection anytime there are sensitive structures exposed.

Typical shoes may be a straight bar, heart bar, W-shoe, or Z-bar. **Figure 19** is a W-shoe on a draft horse once the foot had been resected. With time and support, the foot can grow back normally, and the horse return to work, depending on the amount of damage that has been done.

ANTICIPATED OUTCOME

There are a lot of potential results from a keratoma, so each case must be evaluated individually.

IN SHORT:

D: Tumor in the hoof wall.

T: Surgical removal varied shoeing.

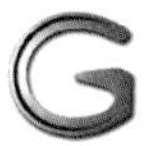

Chapter

45-11 NAVICULAR

DEFINITION

Navicular, navicular syndrome, or podotrochleosis is referring to lameness that is caused by pain in the navicular region.

This is a very broad definition, and because of this broad definition, a lot of horses that have heel pain (caudal hoof lameness) are diagnosed incorrectly as suffering from navicular syndrome. Since the horse will present with soreness in the heel region, shoeing to alleviate that will often help horses with navicular syndrome as well.

Navicular syndrome usually affects only the front feet. I have never personally seen it diagnosed in the hind feet, but that is not to say that it would be impossible. The anatomy of the horse places more weight on the front feet, and the way that fronts are used compared to hinds means that navicular is much more likely in front.

REASON

There has been quite a bit of research into the cause of navicular syndrome, but a definite cause has yet to be identified. The following is conjecture based on experience.

I have found that cases of navicular syndrome will fall under two basic categories, primarily caused by conformation and the use of the horse. These are:

Concussion Related: Often found on steep and upright horses, the conformation of the horse causes the navicular bone to be repeatedly hammered by the 2nd phalanx above. Repeated stress can cause material fatigue and eventual failure. These horses will often develop a narrower foot with deeper commissures and a weak frog.

Suspensory Related: Found in horses that are shallow, the deep flexor tendon is extremely tight as it passes over the podotrochlear (navicular) bursa. Because it is so tight, the pressure and wear over the navicular bone causes the navicular bursa to become inflamed (navicular bursitis), which leads to full blown navicular lameness.

Most likely, navicular syndrome is caused by a multitude factors including: use of the horse, conformation, terrain the horse lives and works on, balance problems, heredity, age. The navicular bone can also be broken.

The classic belief of the cause of navicular syndrome was that it was due to lack of circulation. It was thought to begin as a lack of blood supply to the navicular region (thrombosis). This leads to sub-cartilage bone change (osteochondrosis), which results in bone loss and demineralization of the navicular bone. However, most recent research discounts this as a cause of navicular lameness, and the radiographic changes that were once thought to be indications of navicular syndrome seem to be as common in sound horses as in lame ones, which means that the remodeling may be completely normal.

ANATOMY

Navicular bone, navicular ligaments, coffin joint, deep flexor tendon, podotrochlear (navicular) bursa,

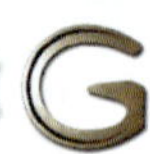

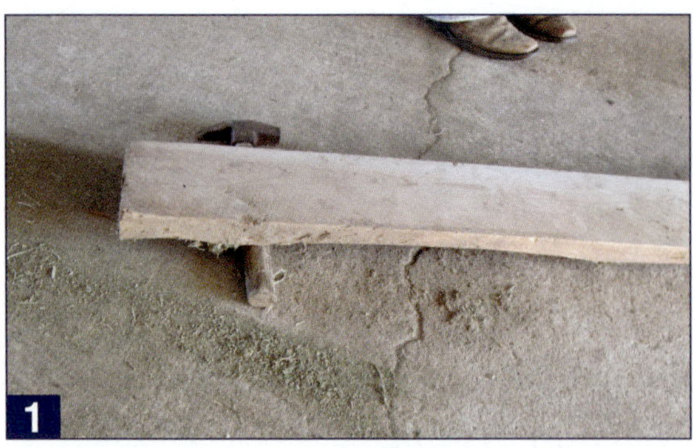

For the board test, I've placed the hammer handle under the end of the board so that I can get my fingers under it to lift.

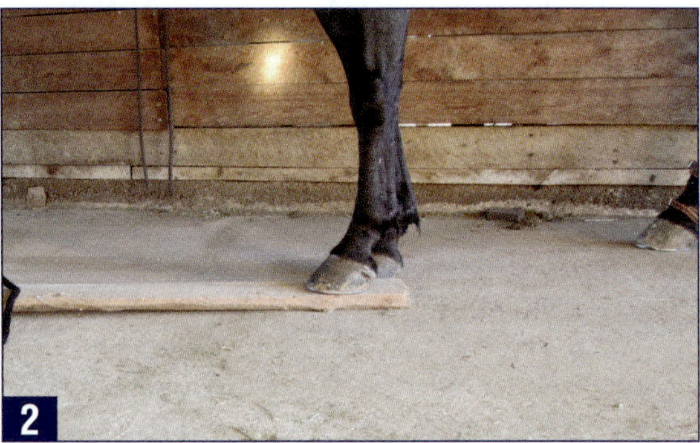

Placing the foot on the end of the board.

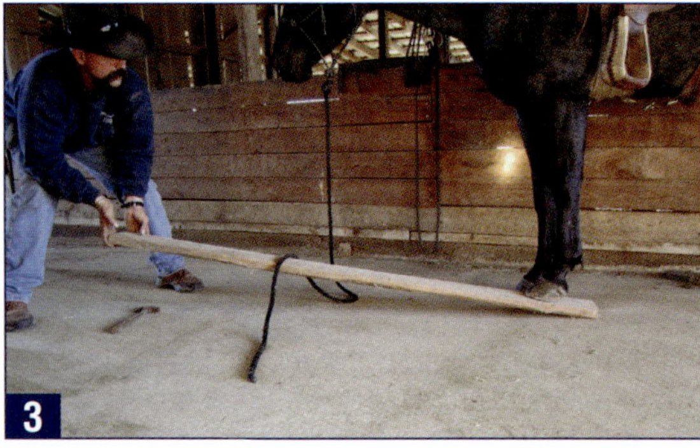

Lifting the board to put stress on the deep flexor tendon as it passes over the navicular bone.

may all be involved

SYMPTOMS

The symptoms of navicular are fairly universal, regardless of the cause. The primary difference will be in the conformation of the individual horse, not necessarily in the way the horse moves or responds to hoof testers and other navicular tests. With the upright and shallow horse, the conformation will be obvious.

The common symptoms with navicular syndrome are:

- A short choppy stride after being immobile for a while.
- Sensitivity to hoof testers when they are applied across the frog, to the opposite wall at the widest part of the foot, and when used across the foot from quarter to quarter.
- Radiographic evidence of bone change.
- Horse will often place one foot in front of the other when tied, and place more weight on the toe of that foot. This is called "pointing."
- Horse is lame on one leg, but becomes lame on the other leg when the worst foot is blocked. Navicular is rarely unilateral, so this is one of the best diagnostic tools available.
- The horse does not like to stand with a wedge placed under the toe and will walk off lame from doing so.
- If you place the handle of your knife under the frog, the horse does not want to stand on it.
- Flexion tests on the coffin joint illicit a lameness response.

The board test, in which the foot is placed on a board, then the board is lifted so that the toe is raised, will cause worsening of pain in the navicular region. Place one end of the board on something so that you can get your fingers under it to lift **(Figure 1)**. Lift slowly to put pressure on the deep flexor tendon. You can see this being performed on a horse in **Figures 2-3**.

Here are several radiographs showing the navicular bone and the changes that can take place. The first five are courtesy of Dr. John Marcotte. I will begin with what could be considered a normal picture **(Figure 4)**. This view is called a skyline view, and it allows us to see a good picture of the navicular bone. The cortex around the bone looks strong and symmetrical. The medullas in the bone are fairly symmetrical, and there aren't more than

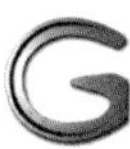

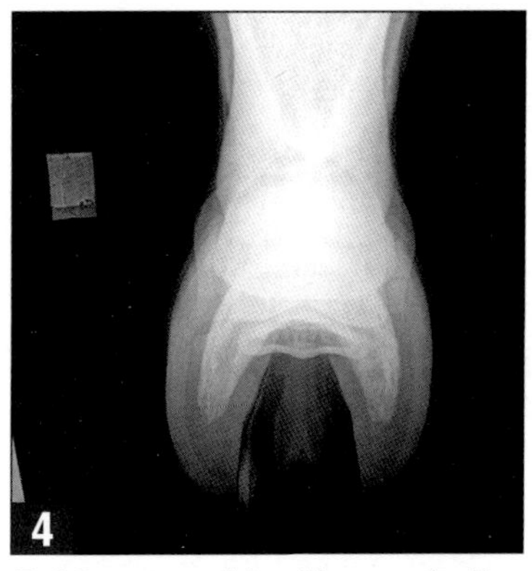

Fairly good-looking skyline view of the navicular bone.

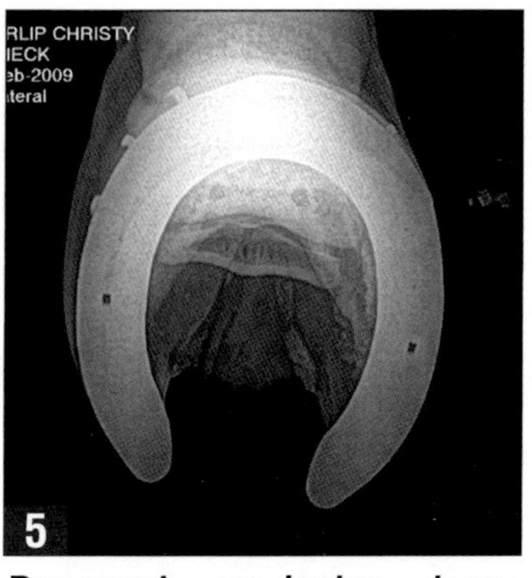

Damaged navicular bone, showing the uneven cortex.

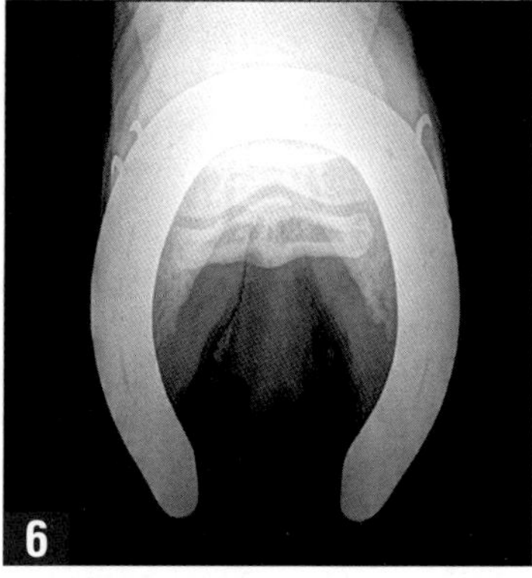

Navicular bone with slightly unusual ends.

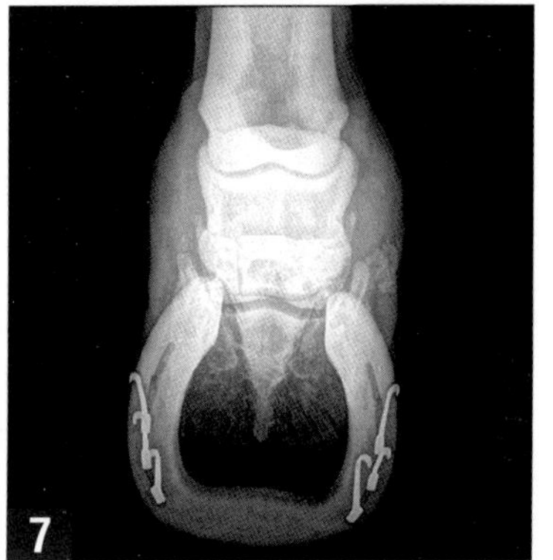

Broken navicular bone.

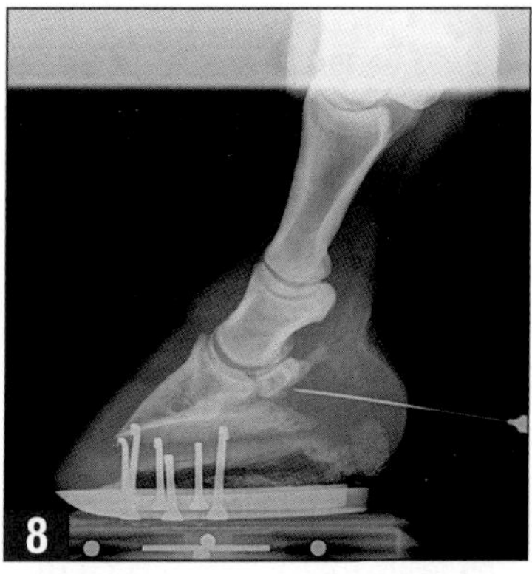

Injecting the navicular region.

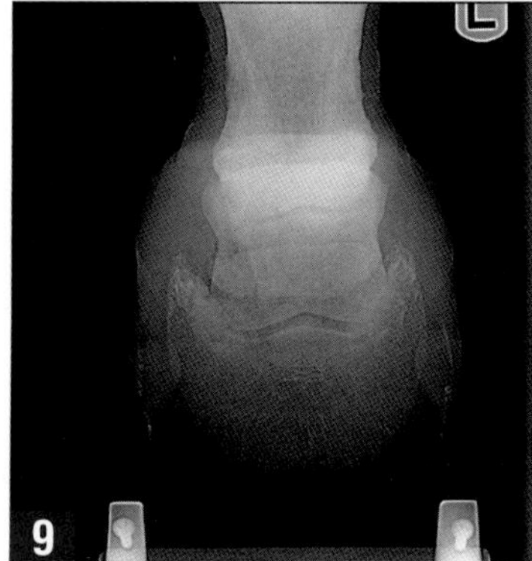

Broken navicular bone.

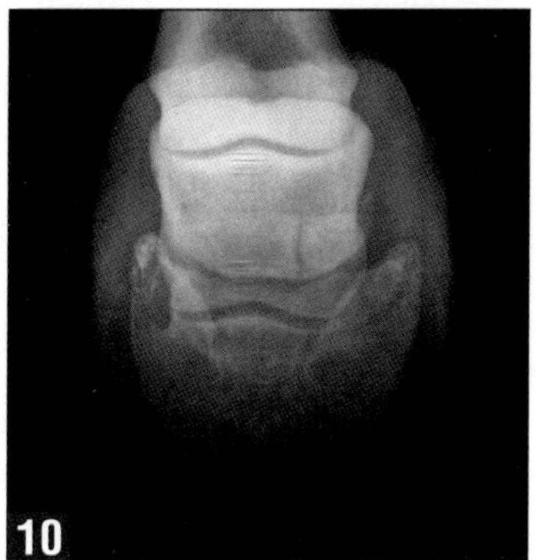

Broken navicular bone.

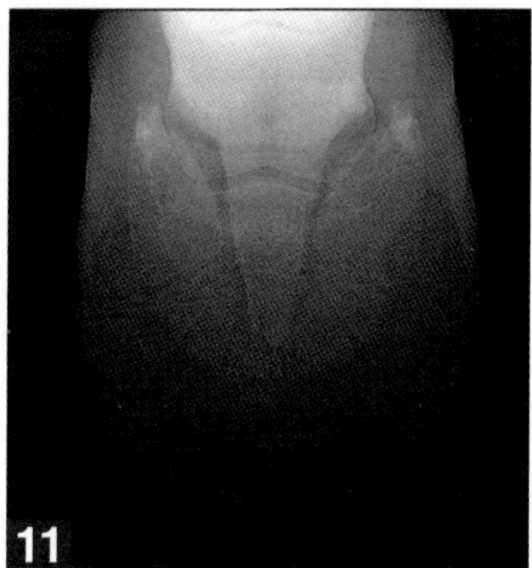

Bone cyst in the navicular bone.

seven, which is traditionally the number most clinicians use as a normal amount. If you compare that to **Figure 5**, the difference between the bones is evident. Look toward the top left side of the navicular bone, and you will notice that the cortex becomes misshapen. **Figure 6** shows a navicular bone that is a different shape on the ends, even though the cortex does not look too asymmetrical.

Figure 7 shows a navicular bone that has been broken. Look at the left side of the X-ray to see the break. In **Figure 8**, Dr. Marcotte has placed a needle in the navicular bursa as a last attempt to give the horse some relief. Notice the bone changes on the navicular bone that are evident in this lateral view where bone is extending proximal from the navicular bone.

Figures 9 -11 are from Dr. Scott Morrison. They are a dorsal oblique view. In **Figures 9 and 10**,

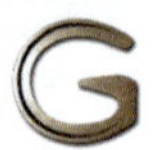

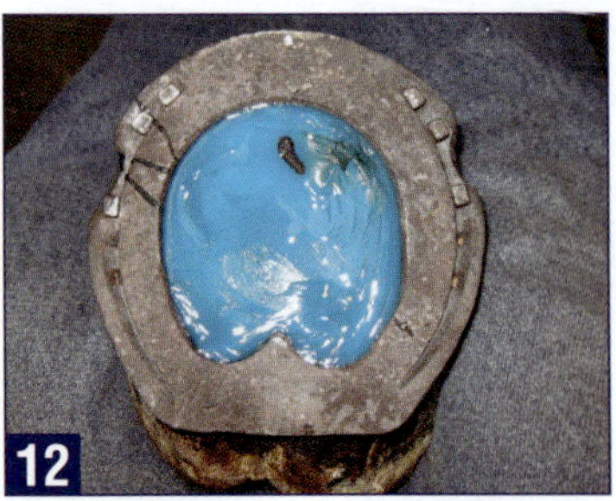

Clipped straight bar filled with Equi-Pak.

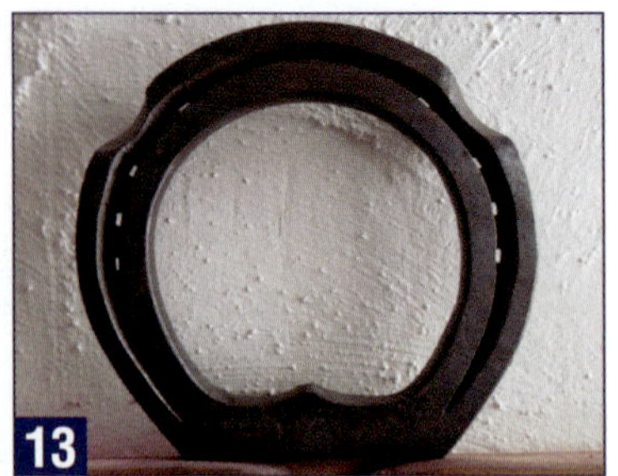

Fullered straight bar with quarter clips and a rocker toe.

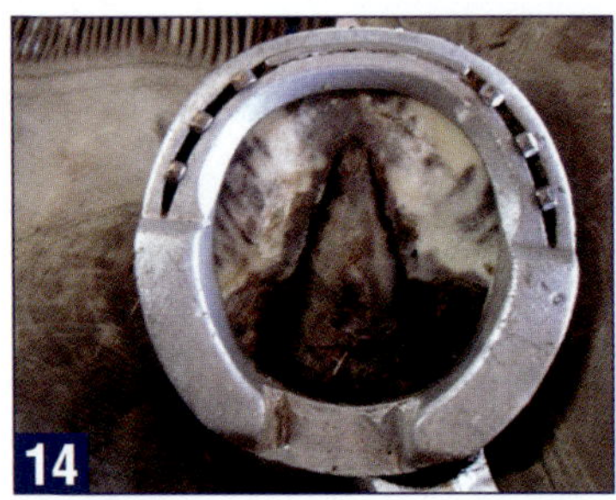

Aluminum navicular bar shoe on a foot.

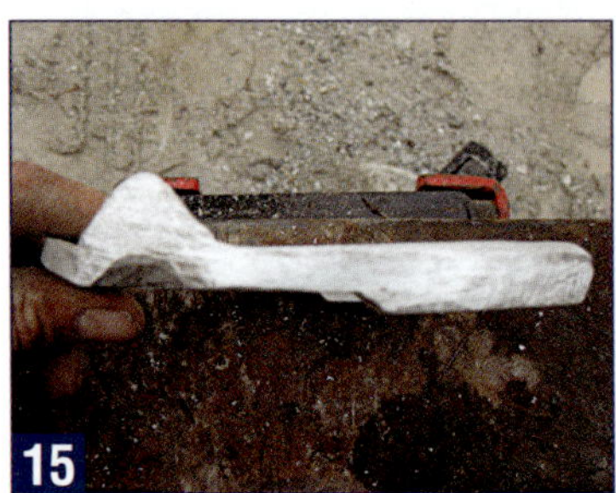

Lateral view of an aluminum navicular bar shoe.

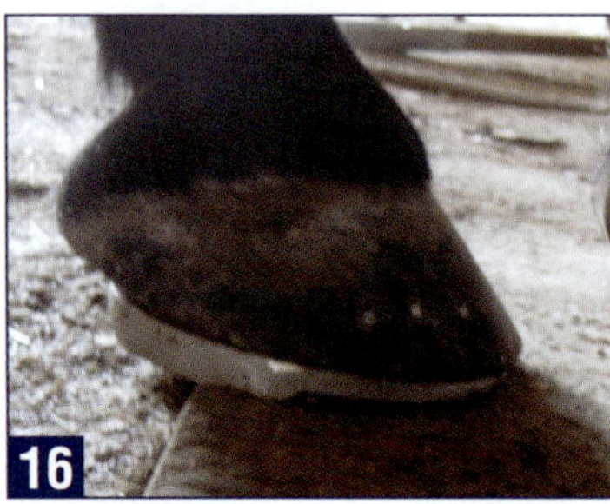

Medial view of the aluminum navicular bar shoe on a foot.

the navicular bone is broken. This is more evident in **Figure 10** than **Figure 9**. **Figure 11** shows a circular area in the middle of the navicular bone that would be consistent with a bone cyst.

The radiographs should give you a pretty good idea of the anatomy of the navicular bone and the navicular region as well as what is seen on some of these horses that are suffering from pain in this region.

TREATMENT

The first thing to consider for treatment is the conformation that you are presented with. Shoeing will be different for a horse that is suffering from concussion-related navicular than one that is dealing with suspensory-related problems. As such, the treatment for each type needs to be covered.

With any type of navicular problem, mediolateral balance is key. Uneven weight bearing will only cause more stress on an already sore bone and joint. Moving the point of breakover back is also universally accepted as a benefit to horses with navicular syndrome. This does reduce the amount of stress on the deep flexor tendon when the horse is moving.

Concussion related: With this type of conformation, you should concentrate on trimming to the natural angle that is appropriate for the horse. Making the foot steeper will only cause the navicular bone to be placed more directly under the bony column.

Once natural angle is achieved, I like to make a straight bar shoe with quarter clips and a rocker toe. The bar shoe will stabilize the foot and make it stronger. The quarter clips add to that, and the rocker toe allows the horse to move with less stress on the deep flexor tendon. If there is not a lot of frog sensitivity, I like to use a pour-in pad in the bottom of the shoe. This dissipates shock and changes the way that the sole, bars, and frog bear weight. Make certain when using pour-ins that you do not allow the material to project beyond the ground surface of the shoe. If it does, the sole can end up bearing more weight than intended. **Figure 12** shows a common sort of bar shoe that I would use for this problem, although a rocker toe is recommended. **Figure 13** is of a clipped straight bar with a rocker toe.

Suspensory Related: For a horse suffering from navicular lameness with a shallow angle, increasing the angle can often cause some relief. If there is enough foot to do it with the trim, I prefer trimming the foot more steeply. If the foot does not allow it, then I will use a wedge shoe, navicular aluminum

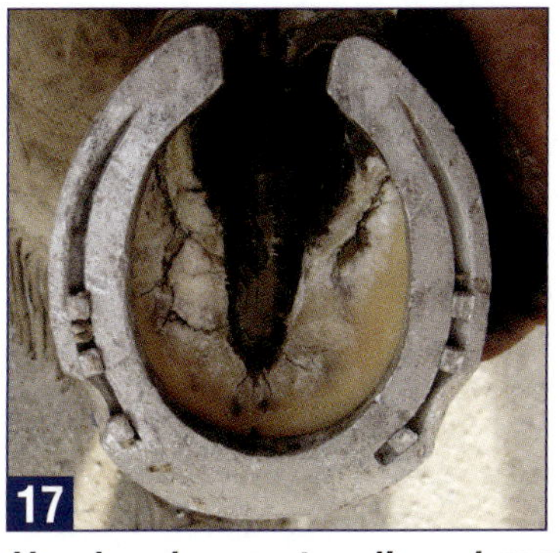

Handmade, quarter clipped, rocker toed, aluminum wedge shoes on the front feet of a naviculared horse.

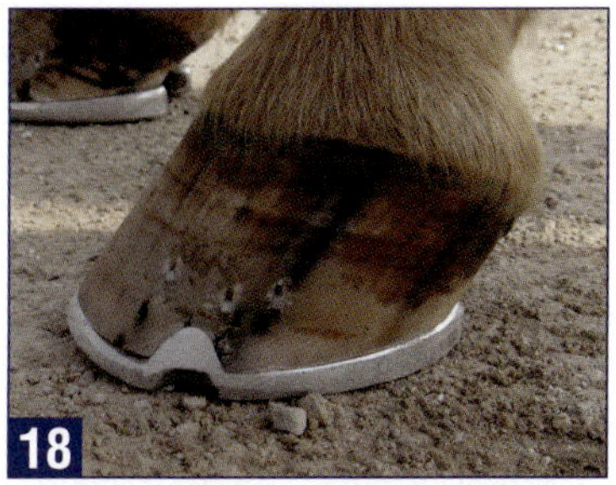

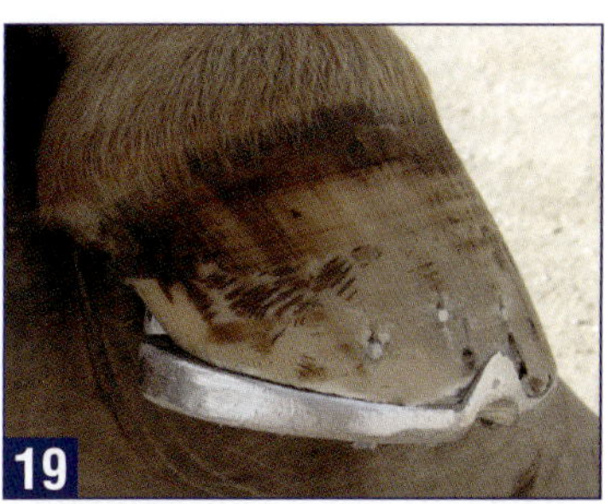

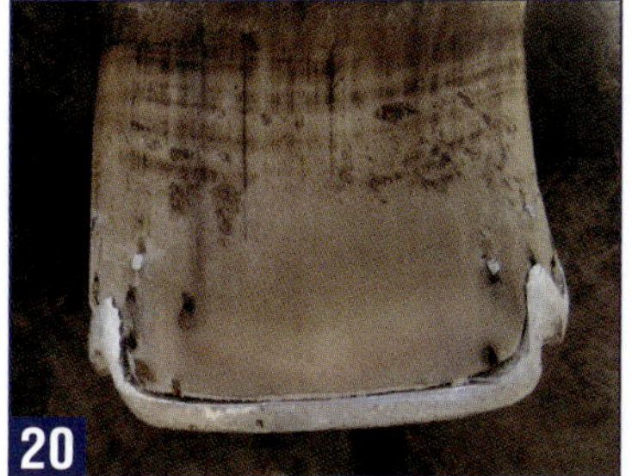

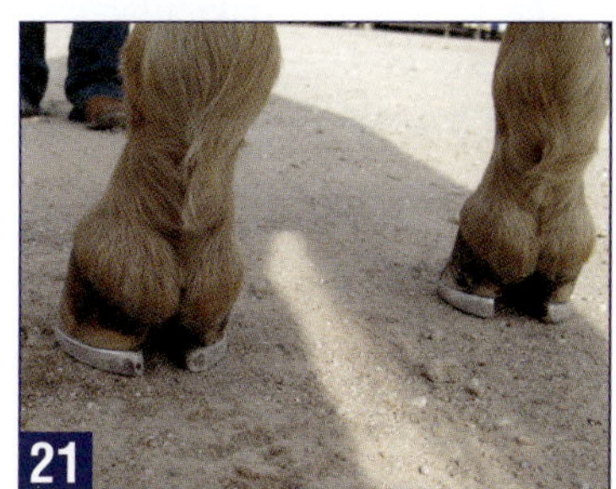

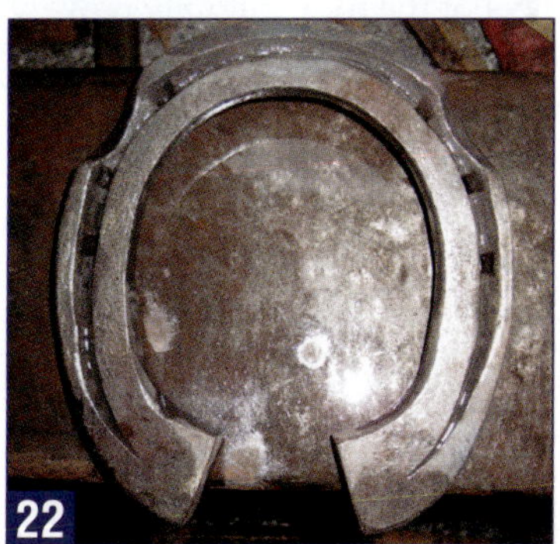

Fullered onion heel shoe.

bar shoe, or wedge pad.

Figures 14-16 are of the commercially available aluminum navicular bar shoes. These are easy to use and light, offering a lot of support without a lot of weight. That is the benefit of aluminum. **Figures 17-21** show some handmade, rocker toed, aluminum wedges that can be used if you do not want to use a bar shoe.

The amount of angle change does not have to be drastic. Just a couple of degrees will allow enough of a change to provide increased comfort. The principle being applied here is explained in depth in chapter 12 **Biomechanics**. Making the foot steeper takes stress off of the deep flexor as it passes over the navicular bone, right in the area where the podotrochlear bursa is located to provide lubrication.

With any type of navicular lame horse, I take the current conformation and stance into account. If the foot is overly shallow for the hoof pastern axis, I will increase the angle of the hoof. If the foot is at a correct hoof pastern axis, I may increase the angle slightly. For horses that are already a little steep, I will leave the angle where they stand.

After the straight bar is used for a couple of shoeing cycles, I often like to use an onion heel shoe. When using this shoe, I don't use the Equi-Pak. I think that the way this shoe works is that the heels will float in soft terrain, and the toe will penetrate. This means that the hoof bears weight in a steeper position when the horse is being used in soft terrain, thereby relieving stress on the deep flexor tendon as well as the navicular bursa. If you use a pour-in, the float vs. penetration aspect of this shoe will be negated. Using the onion heel shoe falls under the category of "moving the stone" as discussed in the first chapter on Lameness. **Figure 22** is a handmade onion heel shoe. The toe can be made thinner, or the heels wider, to make this shoe do more of what it is designed to do.

I have had vets want me to use a heart bar on horses with navicular in the past, but I find that this is not generally a good idea. When you think about how a horse responds to hoof testers when applied to the frog in the navicular test, you can see how frog pressure from a shoe could be the wrong tactic. On the occasions where I did use the heart bar out of situation political correctness, I made certain to avoid frog pressure. This means that the heart bar was simply a straight bar with a little more protection in the frog area.

Egg bars are also used frequently with navicular syndrome, and I find them to have very little advantage to offer over straight bars. An egg bar will place more stress on the heel of the foot, but may prevent the sinking of the heels into the ground as much as a straight bar. However, this is going to be a very small benefit when compared to the pressure it will add to the heels.

There are a lot of things that a vet can do, including prescribing drugs, injecting the navicular region, and performing a surgery. The most common surgery is a neurectomy, which is the removal of a portion of the digital nerve.

If a horse has a neurectomy, there is a chance that the it will become more dangerous to ride. Without feeling in the foot, a horse will not be as aware of exactly where their foot is on the ground, making it likely to stumble. Make sure that the customer is aware of this if you are part of advising them on what to do with the horse.

Check with a vet to see if they recommend anti-inflammatories for the horse, and do not over-use the horse.

ANTICIPATED OUTCOME

Navicular syndrome is one of those lameness problems that tend to degenerate with time. Even in best-case scenarios, I would be very guarded about holding out much hope for this horse. That is not to say that the horse cannot be used, it just means that it will always have lameness issues related to this problem, and it is expected to get worse.

IN SHORT

D: Lameness from pain in the navicular region.

T: Straight bar, quarter clips, rocker toe, Equi-Pak. Increase angle on horses that are not overly steep. Onion heel shoes may also be used.

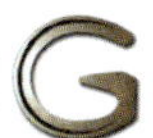

Chapter

45-12 PEDAL OSTEITIS

DEFINITION

If you break down the term pedal osteitis, the definition is clear. Pedal refers to the coffin bone; oste refers to bone; and itis means inflammation. Pedal osteitis is inflammation of the coffin bone.

REASON

This is thought to be primarily a problem that arises from lack of blood supply to the coffin bone. Concussion, sole pressure and chronic bruising are thought to be the primary causes of pedal osteitis.

ANATOMY

The main anatomy will be the coffin bone, but the blood supply to the distal border of the coffin bone should also be included.

SYMPTOMS

Often both front feet are affected, which can make diagnosis a problem. The horse may have a shuffling gate similar to that of a navicular horse. This happens because both feet are hurt, and the horse cannot limp on just one bad foot.

The foot or feet may show soreness over the entire sole. However, radiographs are a necessity to have a competent diagnosis. In an X-ray, you will see a jagged and uneven border of the coffin bone as well as shadows in the bone that show the demineralization. In the radiograph from Dr. Morrison, the ragged edge is evident, and there is also a margin (rim) fracture on the left side of the coffin bone **(Figure 1)**.

TREATEMENT

From a shoeing perspective, the main thing that we want to do is protect the bottom of the foot,and insure that there is no sole pressure. I shoe horses with pedal osteitis just like I do horses with a fractured coffin bone **(Figure 2)**. I like to use a wide-webbed, deep-seated bar shoe. Quarter clips will also stabilize the hoof capsule more, and a rocker toe will not hurt anything here. I will also use a Vettec Equi-Pak pour-in, being careful to avoid

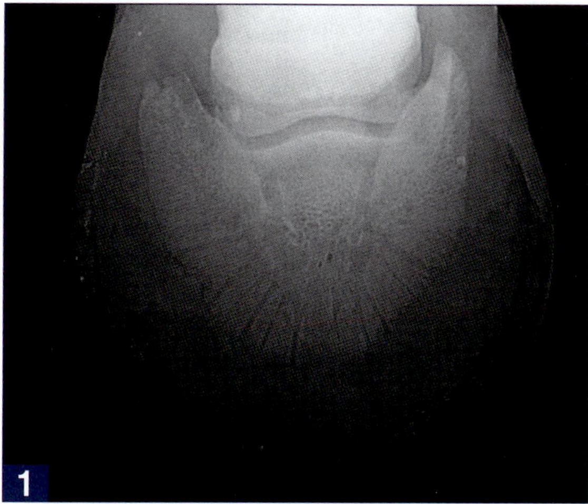

1

Radiograph of pedal osteitis.

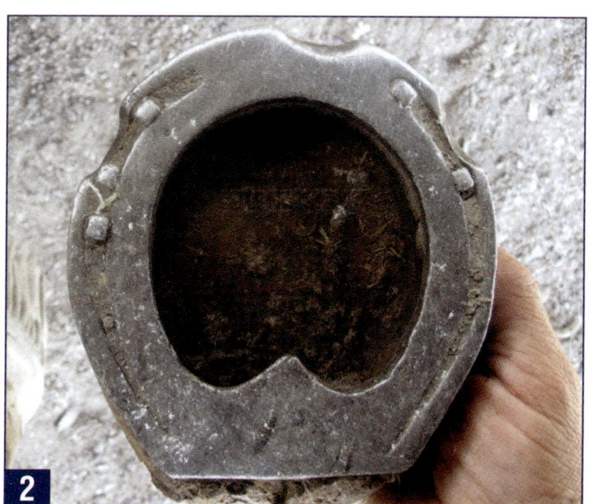

2

Shoe on a foot with a broken coffin bone, but the same sort of shoe used for pedal osteitis.

letting the Equi-Pak get past the ground surface of the shoe.

Many vets will prescribe anti-inflammatory medication for horses with pedal osteitis. The ability to take and interpret X-rays is critical in the correct diagnosis, so the vet is a very big part of dealing with this problem.

The main thing that an owner can do is provide rest for this horse. A stall with a medium run would be a good place for this horse to stay for the next six months.

I once had a customer with a horse that suffered from pedal osteitis. The horse was quite lame when it came into the shop, and I shod it with a bar shoe that had a diagonal bar across it and riveted a pad to the bar. This was in the days before we had stuff like Equi-Pak. The horse was immediately sound. I made an appointment for the horse five weeks later and told the owner that the horse needed rest.

This owner was a shoer's wife, and I ran into him about two months later. I asked about the horse, and he said it was doing great. In fact, it was so good after I shod it, that six weeks later he had pulled my bar shoes and shod it with rim shoes so that it could go to a rodeo or two. His wife had just won at a pro show the night before.

I was glad for them, but ambivalent as well. The next time I saw him, he told me that they had had to put the horse down. Had the horse been given enough time to recover at the onset, it might have gone on to have a lengthy career.

Sometimes it is a good thing for a horse to stay a little bit lame for long enough for it to heal.

ANTICIPATED OUTCOME

In my experience, these horses are not often fixed to the point that the coffin bone looks normal in a radiograph. They may be sound enough to be used, but it is important for the owner to stay ahead on hoof care and keep a close eye on the way the horse moves. I tend to keep these horses in straight bar shoes.

IN SHORT

D: Inflamed coffin bone.

T: Deep seated straight bar, quarter clips, rocker toe with Equi-Pak.

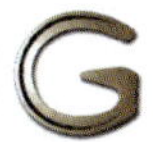

Chapter

45-13 QUARTER CRACKS

DEFINITION

Quarter cracks are cracks in the hoof wall that begin at the coronary band and split downward, parallel to the tubules in the quarter region of the hoof.

REASON

Quarter cracks can be caused by imbalance in the trim. Oftentimes you will find a certain type of foot (narrow, upright, and too small) will get a quarter crack on the low side. A foot will bear more weight on the side that is short or low, and this can cause the foot to develop a quarter crack.

Trimming a foot so that it is high in the quarter can also cause a quarter crack. When the foot bears weight, the high quarter area will end up under too much of a load, and when the toe and heels try to find the ground, it can pull the foot apart at the coronary band. **Figure 1** is a drawing that depicts how that can occur.

Another potential cause is a hoof with proximal coronary band displacement. When the coronary band comes high in the quarter area, there can be a lot of trauma in that area from the expansion of the collateral cartilages when the foot bears weight. As the fetlock descends, the pastern can be pushed against the collateral cartilages, and they will hit the inside of the coronary band with every step. This can lead to inflammation and eventually a crack.

Finally, you can have a coronary band that has

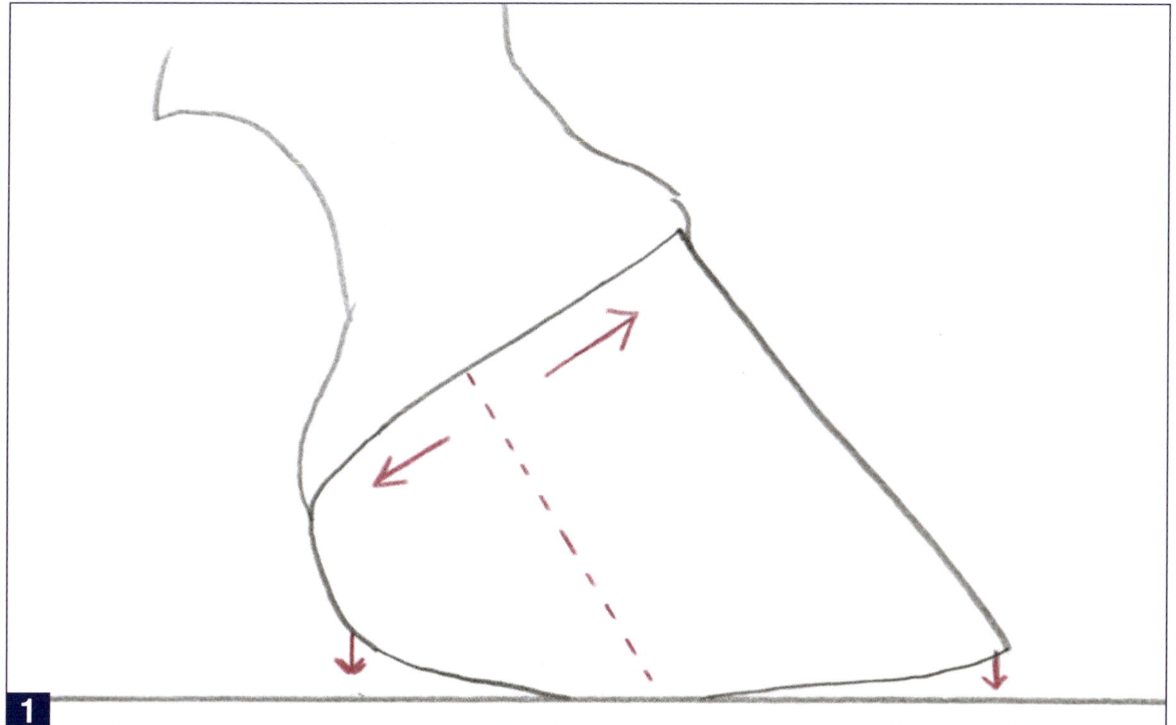

1

Drawing to show how a foot that is high in the quarters can get a quarter crack.

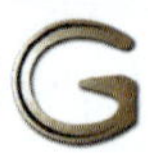

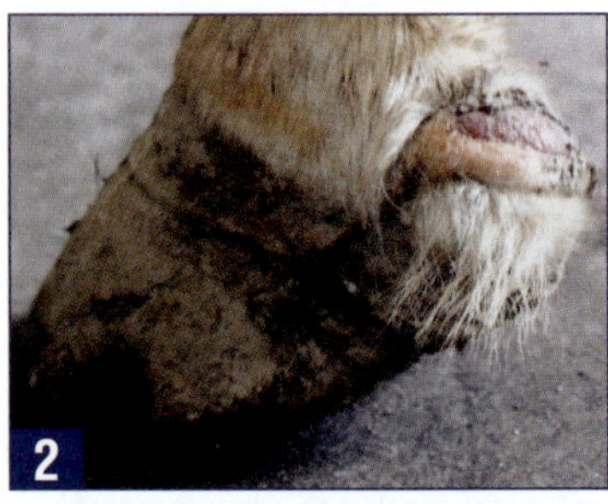
Injury across the bulbs that will result in a damaged coronary band and the potential for chronic quarter cracks.

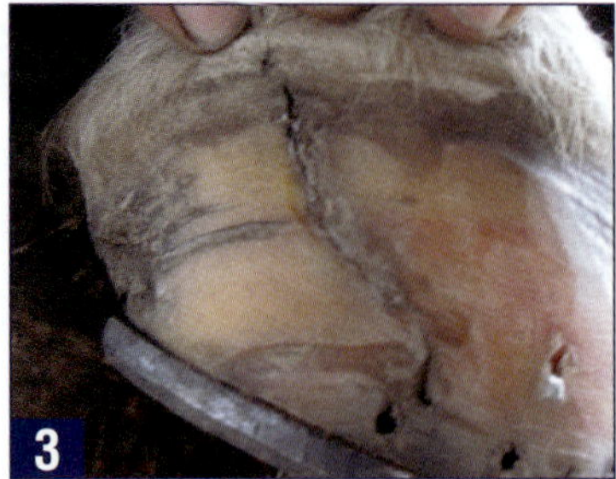
Quarter crack that is about 3 weeks old.

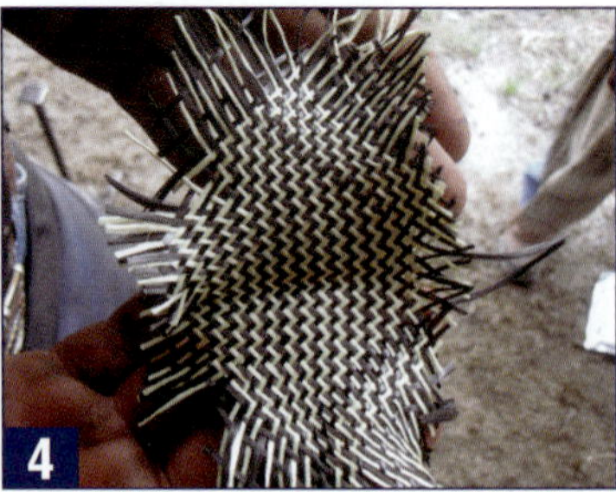
Cobrasox.

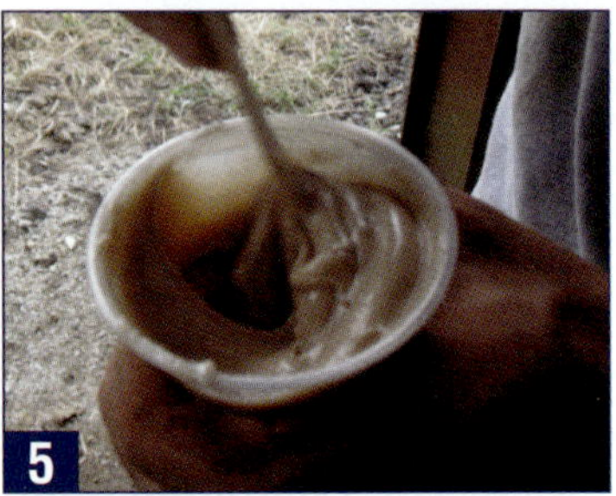
Mixing the acrylic. Make sure to time it for one minute.

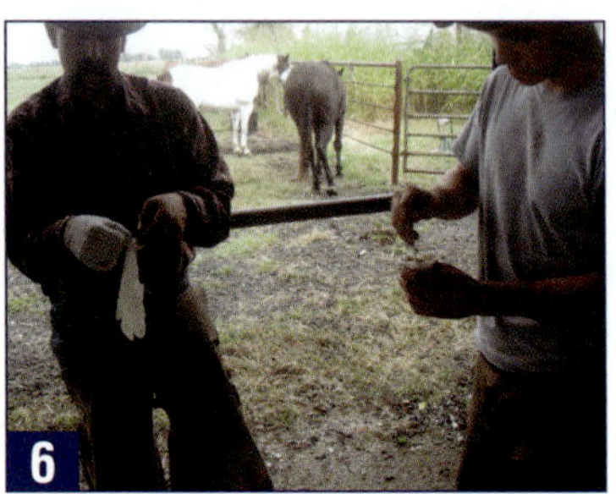
Putting on gloves while Riley mixes the acrylic.

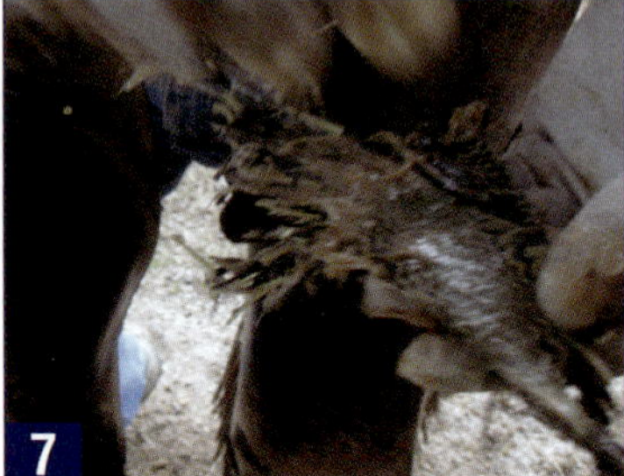
Impregnated Cobrasox.

been injured. Often you will see a scar across the bulbs and through the coronary band from an injury by wire, rope, or tin (**Figure 2**). Once the coronary band is cut, it can heal with a permanent change in the hoof wall below that area. Sometimes this scarred area will cause the foot to be weaker there, and when it is, a quarter crack is common.

ANATOMY

The primary anatomy will be the hoof wall and the coronary band in the quarter region. The laminae under that region of the foot are also involved.

SYMPTOMS

When a horse is suffering with a quarter crack, they are often lame from the movement of the foot where it should not be moving. I have heard it said that the horse gets pinched from quarter cracks, but I am not certain that this happens. You will see the split in the foot moving distad from the coronary band, and sometimes it will bleed. In the event that the crack becomes infected, the horse may become quite sore.

TREATMENT

There are a couple of strategies that you can employ when it comes to quarter cracks. The most common (and the one that I would most often recommend), is to stabilize the crack with polyurethane or acrylic. My preferred method is to use Super Fast by Vettec, or the patch kit from Sound Horse Technologies.

Begin by trimming the foot and dish the quarters. Apply your shoe and leave a gap in the quarters that is below the crack if you follow the tubules down. The foot in **Figure 3** had a gap in the quarters that was about 3/16inch when the shoe was applied. It took less than 30 minutes for the quarter to descend to the shoe, and I only regret that I didn't take a before and after photos of that movement.

For this particular patch, I want a foot that is not too sore, and does not have an infection or any seepage. Begin by cleaning out and debriding the cracked area of the foot. Rasp the area so that there is clean hoof wall to attach your patch to. I am putting on the Cobrasox for this patch **(Figure 4)**. Mix the acrylic and put on gloves **(Figures 5-6)**. Impregnate the polyester and carbon-mesh patch material with the acrylic **(Figure 7)** and put some of the acrylic over the area of the foot that you want to patch **(Figure 8)**.

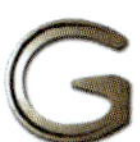

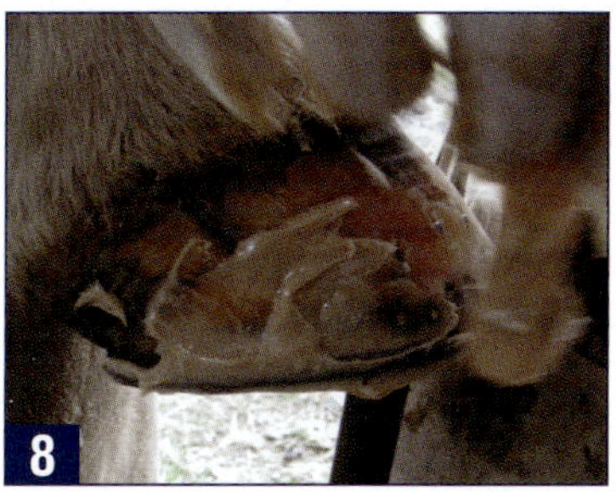

Putting acrylic on the foot.

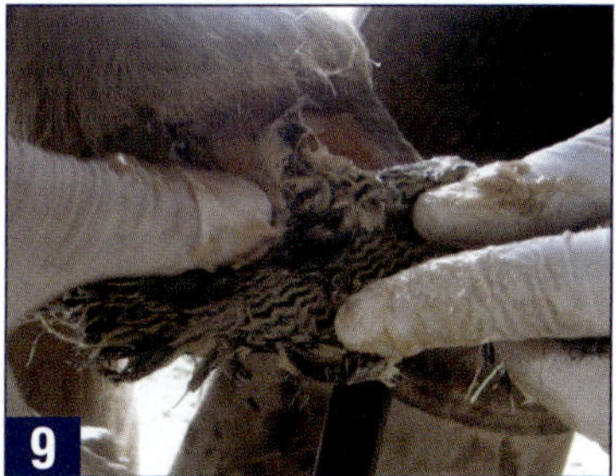

Placing the patch on the foot.

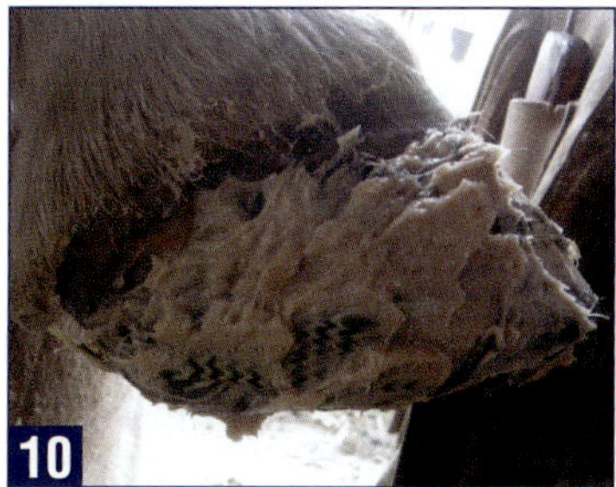

Covering the whole thing with acrylic.

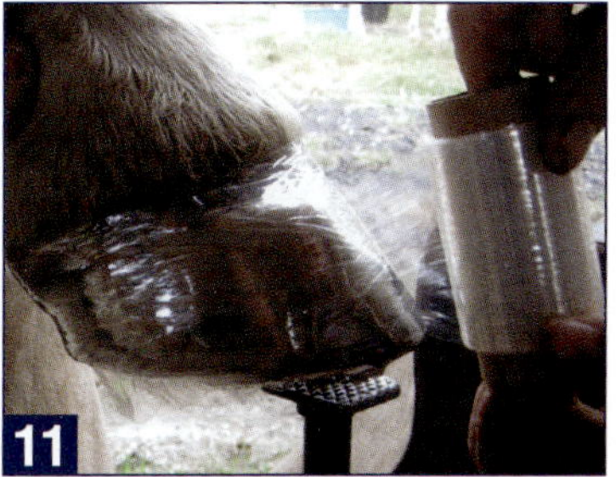

Wrapping the foot with plastic wrap.

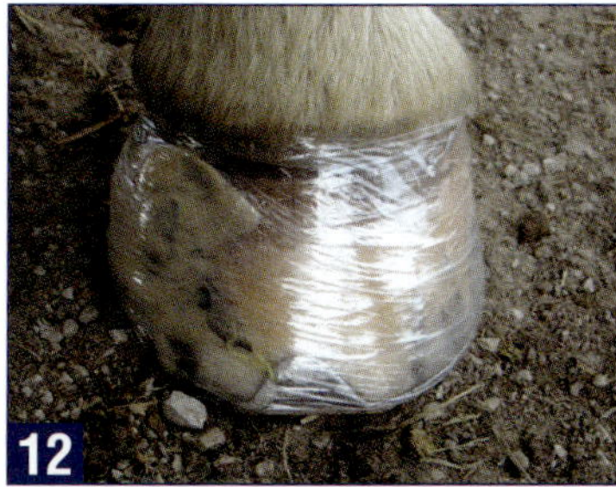

Allowing it to cure.

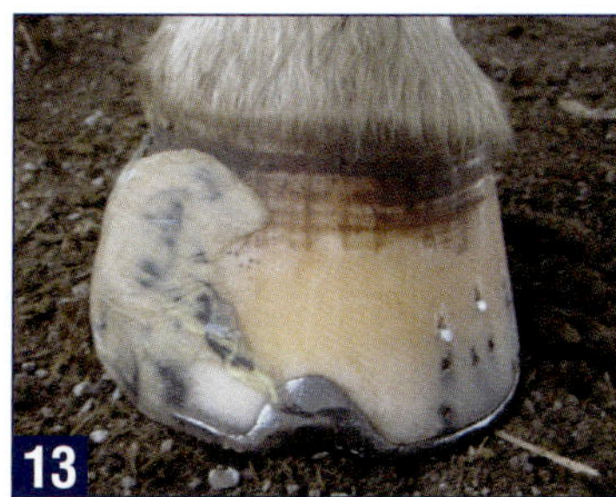

Finished patch.

Place the patch on the foot and cover it with more of the acrylic **(Figures 9-10)**. Wrap the whole foot in plastic wrap **(Figure 11)** and let it cure **(Figure 12)**. If you can work on other feet or another horse, let the patch cure for as long as you can, a minimum of 5 minutes. When it has stood for a while, take the plastic off, and you should have a much stronger area of the foot and a more comfortable horse **(Figures 13-14)**.

If there is any seepage or blood, you will also have to have a drain under the patch. Without a drain, this will turn into a very sore infection. Make the drain with felt wool, then cover the area with the patch material. The felt wool will not only keep the material from sealing in bacteria, it will also act as a heat shield while the material cures and provide a wick to get medication into the crack. The urethane has to be at least 1/4inch thick to generate enough heat to cure. In the cold season, I will also use the heat gun on the urethane.

Another strategy is to use small wire and the double-drilled washers. Make the washers by cutting small pieces of tin. For the wire, you can use stainless steel suture. There are now kits available from Sound Horse that include washers with the wires already placed. Drill very small holes that go toward the inside of the crack. Place the wires and washers on either side of the crack and twist the wires up in the middle of the crack. Once this wire lace is done, you can choose to cover it with Super Fast or the patch pictured. Depending on the nature of the crack and the use of the horse. The shoe and trim on the foot will stay the same as mentioned.

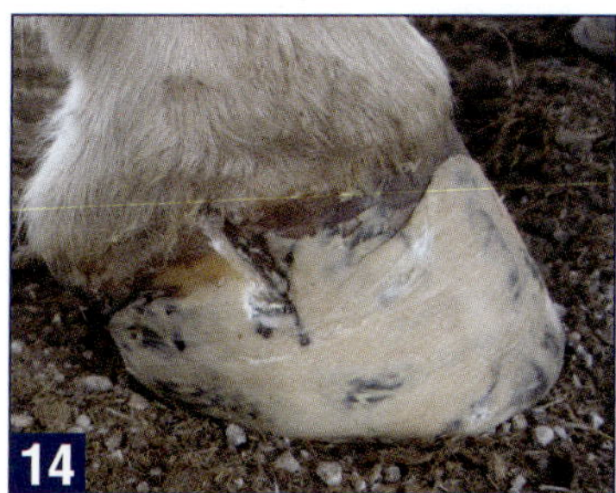

Finished patch.

This next horse has an older quarter crack that is due to a defect in the coronet, as well as neglect **(Figures 15-16)**. With a foot like this, constant and proper hoof care is a necessity. This particular horse

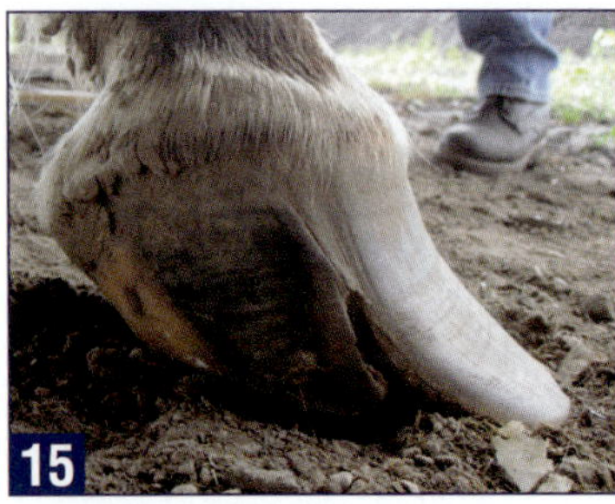
Foot with chronic quarter crack issues.

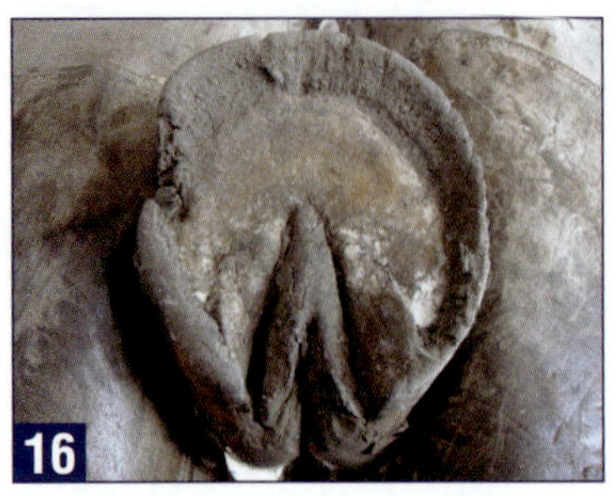
The foot before trimming, solar view.

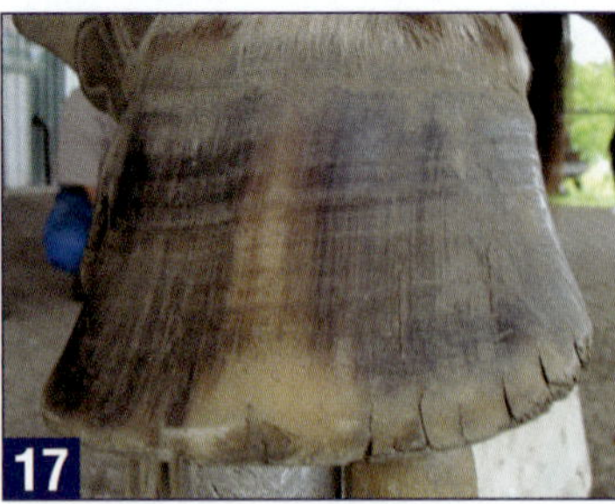
Dorsal view showing uneven growth.

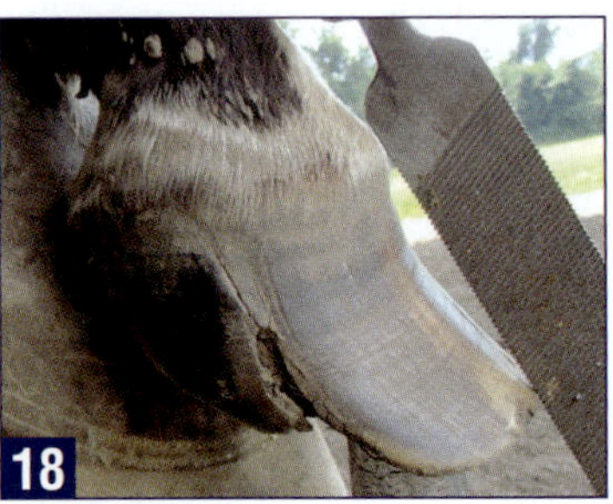
The dish present in the toe of the foot.

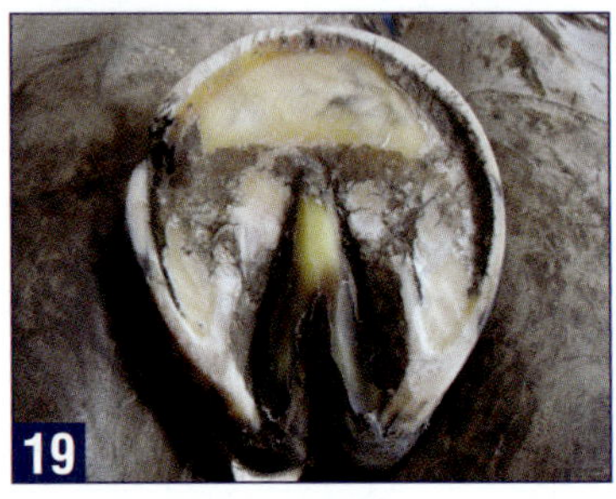
Solar view trimmed.

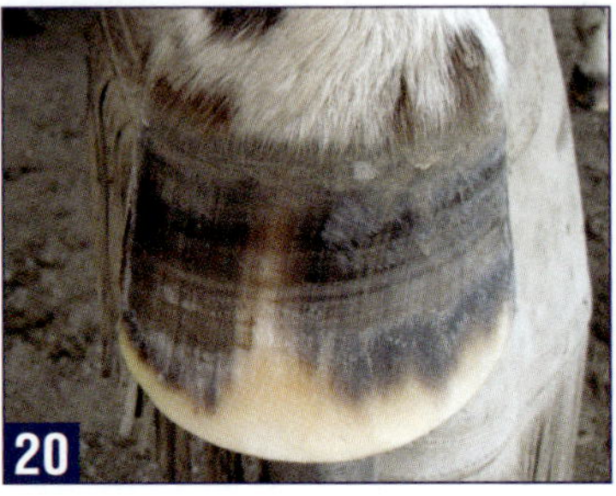
Dorsal view trimmed.

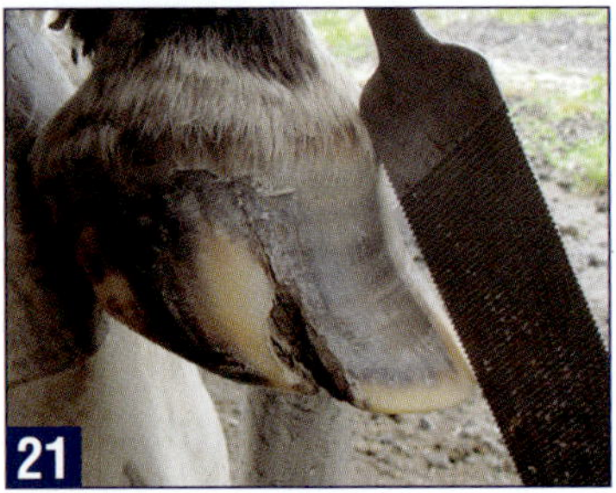
Lateral view trimmed.

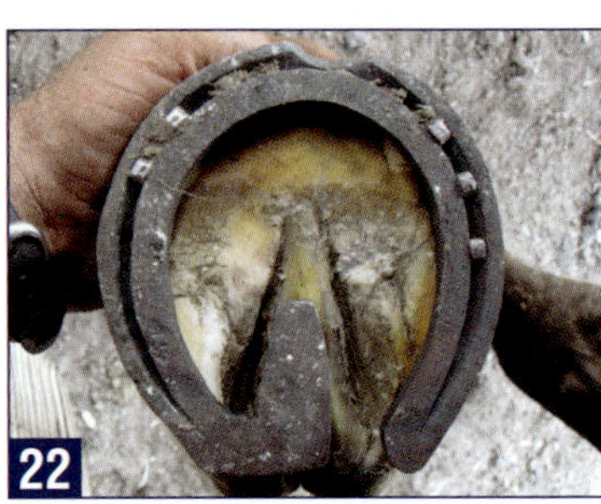
G-bar shoe.

was a Grade 3 lame, and probably had been for some time. If you look at the dorsal view **(Figure 17)** the growth rings in the foot indicate that there is an imbalance in the actual growth of the foot from medial to lateral. The rings are wider on the lateral side and converge toward the medial side. This is most likely a response to inflammation on the lateral side where the quarter crack is. More blood supply has resulted in more growth on one side.

Figure 18 shows that the toe has a large dish in it. This sort of foot conformation only serves to pull the foot apart at the quarters with every step, so it must be addressed in the trim. **Figures 19-21** show the foot after the trim. It was not possible to get the entire dish out of the toe on the first trim in **Figure 21**. Since this horse was a donated project, he did not get a patch, just a G-bar shoe, shown in **Figure 22**. After shoeing, this horse was Grade 1 lame (only evident at a trot) and much happier.

On the next shoeing, the horse was reset, but continued as a Grade 1 lame. Cody decided to put a handmade cupped breakover shoe that has a higher inside and the breakover sloped off from heel to heel. Several views of this shoe are seen in **Figures**

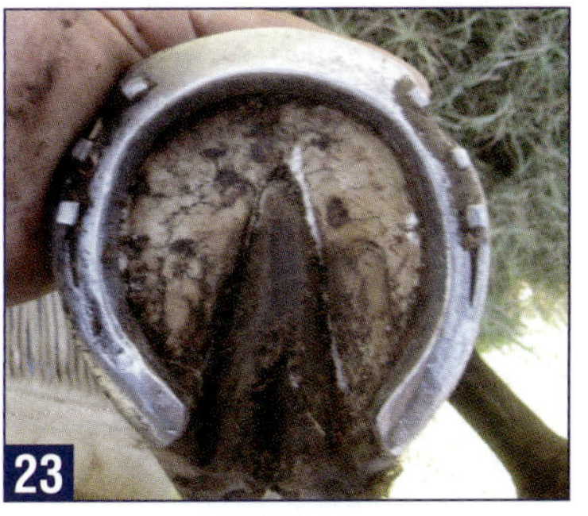

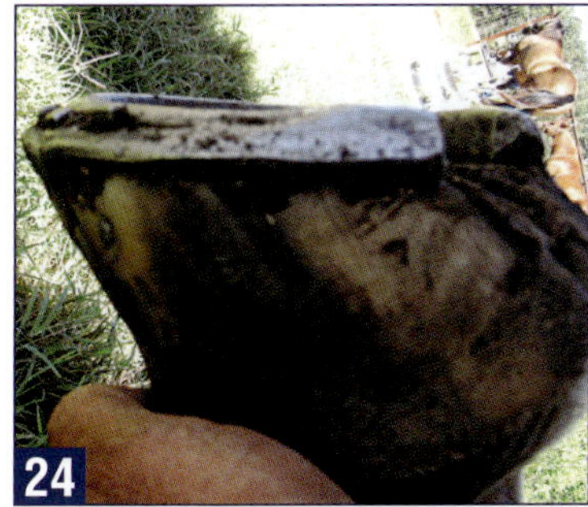

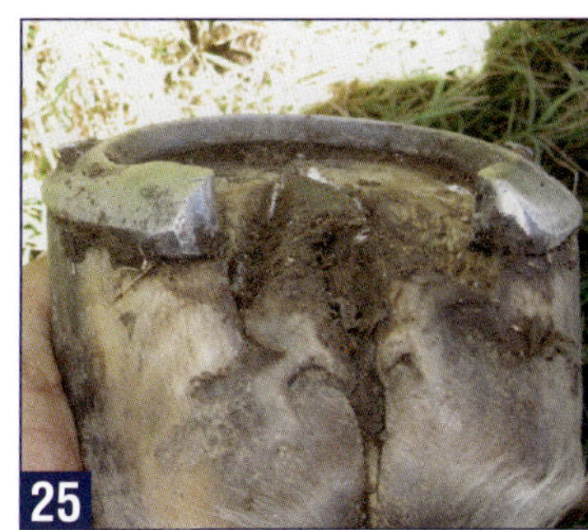

Handmade cupped breakover shoe.

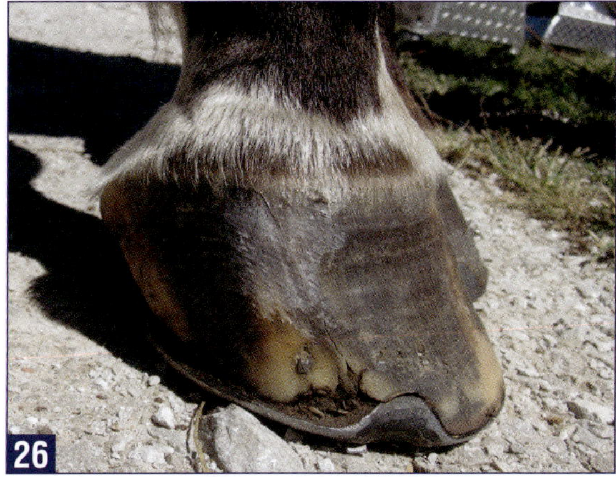

Lateral view of the foot 14 weeks after first presented.

23-26. This made the horse sound, and he has been ever since. In **Figure 26**, the transformation of the foot is readily apparent at 14 weeks from the first shoeing.

I have also had success with using a Z-bar shoe, but I have found the heart bar or G-bar to be better with quarter cracks.

From the veterinarian realm, you may find a horse that needs to have surgery on the coronary band. Most of the time, this will be with horses that are dealing with a quarter crack that has come on from the scarred hoof or possibly a keratoma. The vet can also be helpful with the administration of anti-inflammatory medicine or antibiotics if an infection is part of this problem.

The owner needs to keep the horse out of really wet conditions when there is any sort of patch as well as monitor to make certain that there are no setbacks. I would also recommend that this horse be fed a hoof supplement so that the crack can grow down as fast as possible.

ANTICIPATED OUTCOME

One problem with quarter cracks is that they can recur in certain horses. As such, I am always guarded when dealing with these horses. For preventive measures, I will dip the quarters on purpose most of the time when I trim that foot. Once the crack is stabilized, the horse is generally much more comfortable. I would expect the crack to grow out and the horse to return to use.

IN SHORT

D: Cracks in the quarter of the foot, originating at the coronet.

T: Stabilization with polyurethane or acrylic, trim and shoe to relieve stress in the quarter area.

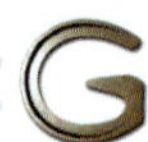

Chapter

45-14 Quittor

DEFINITION

Quittor refers to an infected or necrotic collateral cartilage.

REASON

Quitter can be caused by anything that allows the lateral cartilages to become infected. This can be an abscess that gravitates that far, or a direct injury such as a wire cut or puncture. This seems to be another one of those problems that is more common in draft horses.

ANATOMY

The primary anatomy will be the collateral cartilages.

SYMPTOMS

A horse with quittor will usually develop drainage in the quarter region, either at the coronary band or just above it. Most often, the horse will be lame until the drainage occurs, then the lameness will subside until the next episode. The primary diagnosis for quittor is the constant development of abscesses.

The foot in **Figure 1** has had chronic abscess problems for some time, and the drainage is above the coronary band, as is often the case with quittor. On the bottom of the foot, there is an obvious area of chronic abscess **(Figure 2)**, and in **Figure 3**, the foot is trimmed so that the quarter is floated (taking it out of weight bearing) while the horse awaits veterinarian care.

TREATMENT

Think of treatment for quittor as if it were a keratoma. This means that treatment for the most part is in the vet's realm. The vet will surgically remove the infected cartilage. Surgery is delicate since the joint capsule for the coffin joint is just axial to the collateral cartilages, and removal of all the infected material can be difficult. Injection of a contrast medium can assist the vet in determining the amount of infected cartilage, as well as the location of the drainage tract. **Figures 4-5** are courtesy of Dr. Morrison. They show the drainage tract in the lateral cartilages that have been injected with the

1

Lateral view of infected foot.

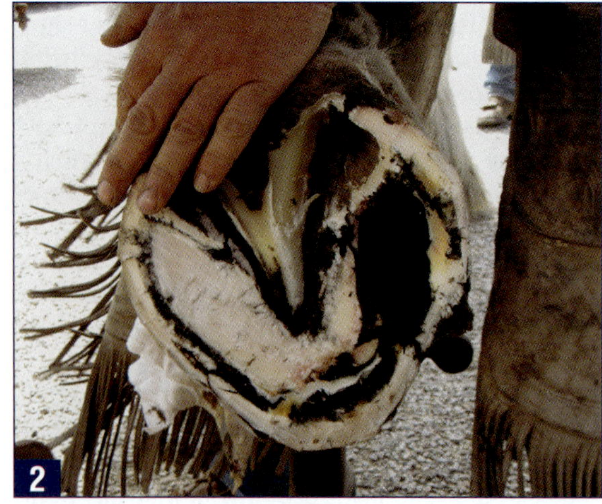

Solar view showing the area of damage in the quarter.

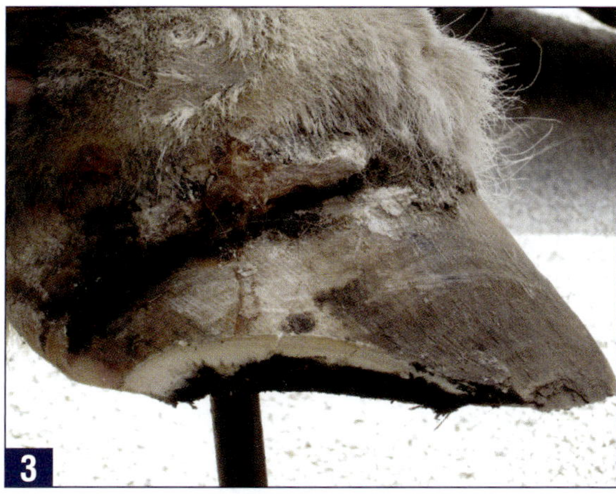

The foot is trimmed with the quarter floated so that the damaged area of the foot does not have to bear weight.

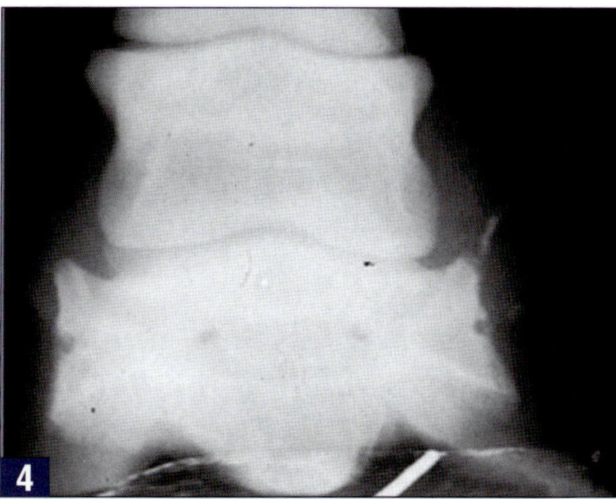

Radiograph showing the extent of a quittor.

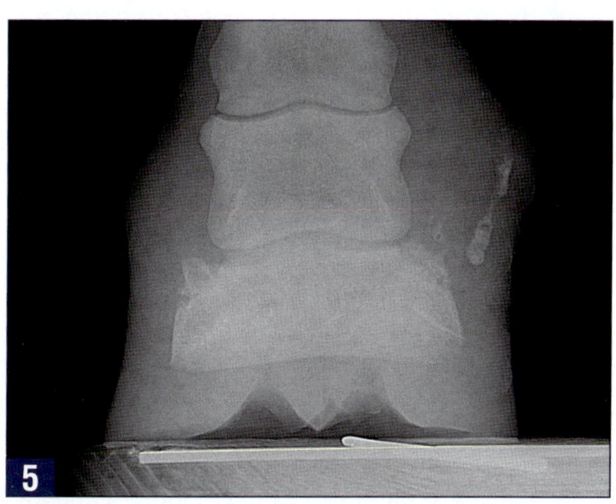

Radiograph showing the extent of a quittor.

radiopaque dye. Farrier involvement may include designing a shoe to support a foot that has been traumatized by surgery. In the event that the surgery can occur above the hoof wall, shoeing — if needed at all — may be normal. A G-bar **(Figure 6)** or heart bar **(Figure 7)**, can be very helpful when trying to shift weight off of a foot that has been compromised by surgery.

Since the lateral cartilages do not have a tremendous amount of vascular supply, they do not respond well to antibiotics. Low volume of blood to the tissue means that the antibiotics are not being delivered as easily as they would be to highly vascular areas. The horse owner will generally have to change dressings and bandages on the foot after surgery on a regular basis as well as monitor the recovery of the horse.

ANTICIPATED OUTCOME

Surprisingly, once the infected cartilage has been removed, most horses make a full recovery. However, it is very difficult to get all of the infected cartilage tissue, and if the coffin joint pouch is damaged during surgery, the prognosis becomes much worse.

IN SHORT

D: Necrotic collateral cartilage.

T: Surgical removal, shoe to stabilize foot post-op.

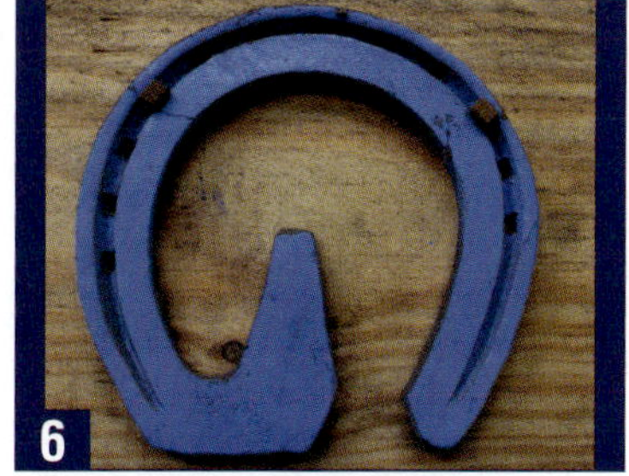

G-bar that can take weight from the wall after surgery, transferring it to the frog.

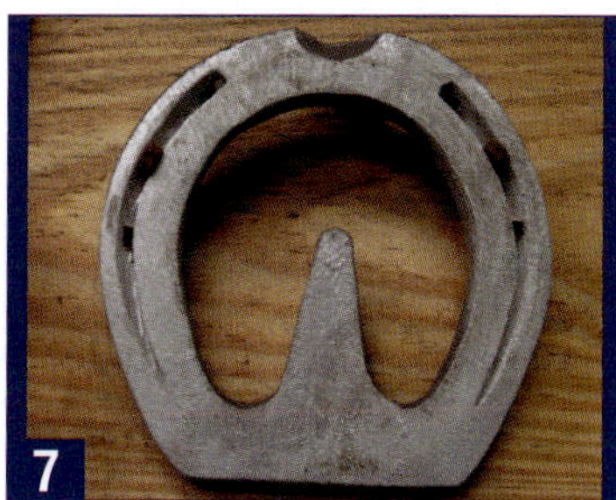

Heart bar can work like the G-bar if more support and foot stabilization is required.

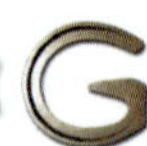

Chapter

45-15 SHEARED HEELS

DEFINITION

Sheared heels refers to a situation in which the bulbs of the foot are in different planes.

REASON

Sheared heels almost always occur from imbalance, however, the condition can be the result of an injury. When imbalance is the culprit, the bulb that is proximal has often been shoved into that position from being on the side of the foot that was shortest. When you have one side of the foot longer than the other, the short side will end up being closer to the axis of the limb when it is under load. For this reason, the short side takes more punishment.

Weak feet are prone to develop sheared heels. This can also happen when not supporting the frog and sole when using a graduated (wedged heel) shoe. According to Jim Ferrie, FWCF, the frog will prolapse through the shoe and the heels will become weakened and more damaged. This weakening will predispose the horse to developing a sheared heel. Pour-in pads or frog pads help prevent this by supporting the center of the foot.

ANATOMY

With sheared heels, the anatomy affected will be the bulbs, heels of the foot, and coronary band. Bear in mind that the heel area of the wall will have some attachment to the collateral cartilages, and not just to the coffin bone.

SYMPTOMS

There are a lot of horses with sheared heels that do not have any lameness or soreness related to the sheared heels. They may have some issues in the early stages of the sheared heel development that occurs simply from the inflammation of the workload on that side of the foot.

Sheared heels may lead to soft heel cracks between the bulbs. If that happens, lameness is a good possibility. Refer to the section on soft heel cracks if you end up dealing with one of those cases.

Figure 1 shows a sheared heel with the heel length from the bulb to the ground a similar length.

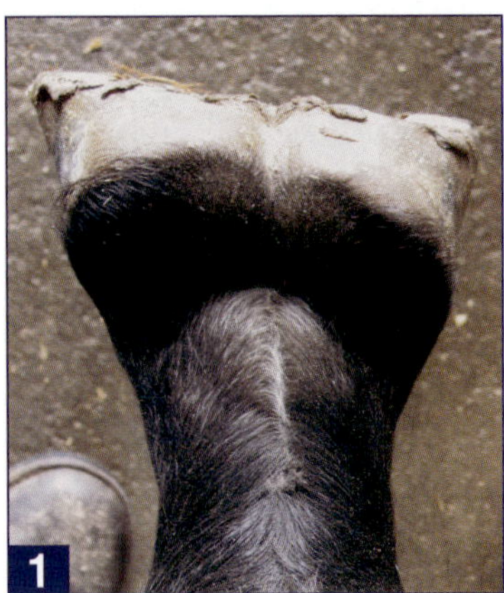

1 *Foot with sheared heels and bad balance.*

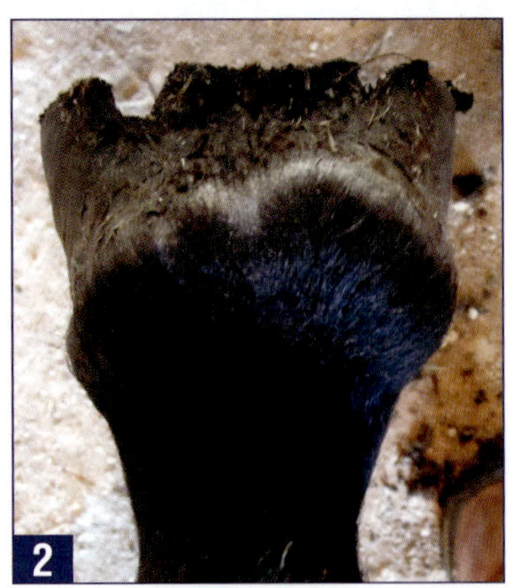

2 *Untrimmed foot with sheared heels.*

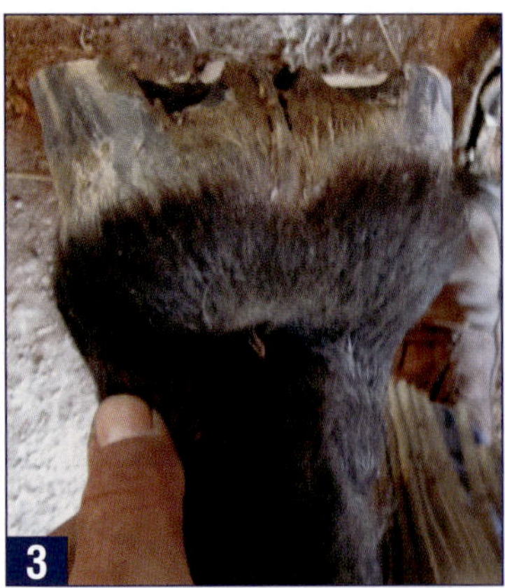

3 *Trimmed foot with sheared heels.*

That makes the mediolateral balance of the foot as incorrect as the bulbs. Inexperienced farriers may try to trim the foot at the level of the bulbs and cause the sheared heels to actually become worse. The foot will end up looking like **Figure 1** after trimming to the level of the bulbs. This is an incorrect method of balancing this particular foot.

Figure 2 shows an untrimmed foot with sheared heels, and **Figure 3** shows a foot after trimming. Notice the different length of wall from the bulbs to the ground in **Figure 3**, which results in good mediolateral balance that is not related to the bulbs, but rather to the long axis of the bony column.

TREATMENT

If there is not a lameness issue, I generally do not try to fix the horse with a sheared heel. It is important that you watch beginning farriers carefully when they trim feet with sheared heels. Since the bulb is higher on the one side, the length of wall at that heel will be longer. If the shoer is balancing the foot to the bulbs or coronary band, they will make that heel short again, which is what led to the problem in the beginning, and the side with the sheared heel will be loaded and damaged more.

If the sheared heel is indeed something that you want to fix, begin by trimming the foot normally, which would be level on the long axis. Make and fit a heart bar shoe, and then float the sheared heel before nailing the shoe on. (Floating refers to intentionally leaving a gap between the foot and the shoe.) I like to fill the back of my heart bar shoes with Equi-Pak, so I will place Sole Pack in any area that I am trying to float between the foot and the shoe. The Sole Pack will keep the Equi-Pak from getting in the floated area and supporting the section of the foot that I am trying to leave unsupported.

When you are determining exactly where to float the heel from, look at the side of the foot and follow the tubules down from the point of the coronary band that is most distal in the quarter area of the foot. Start the float at this point, and make it wider as you get to the heel. It would be rare to float more that 1/4 of an inch. **Figure 4** is a drawing

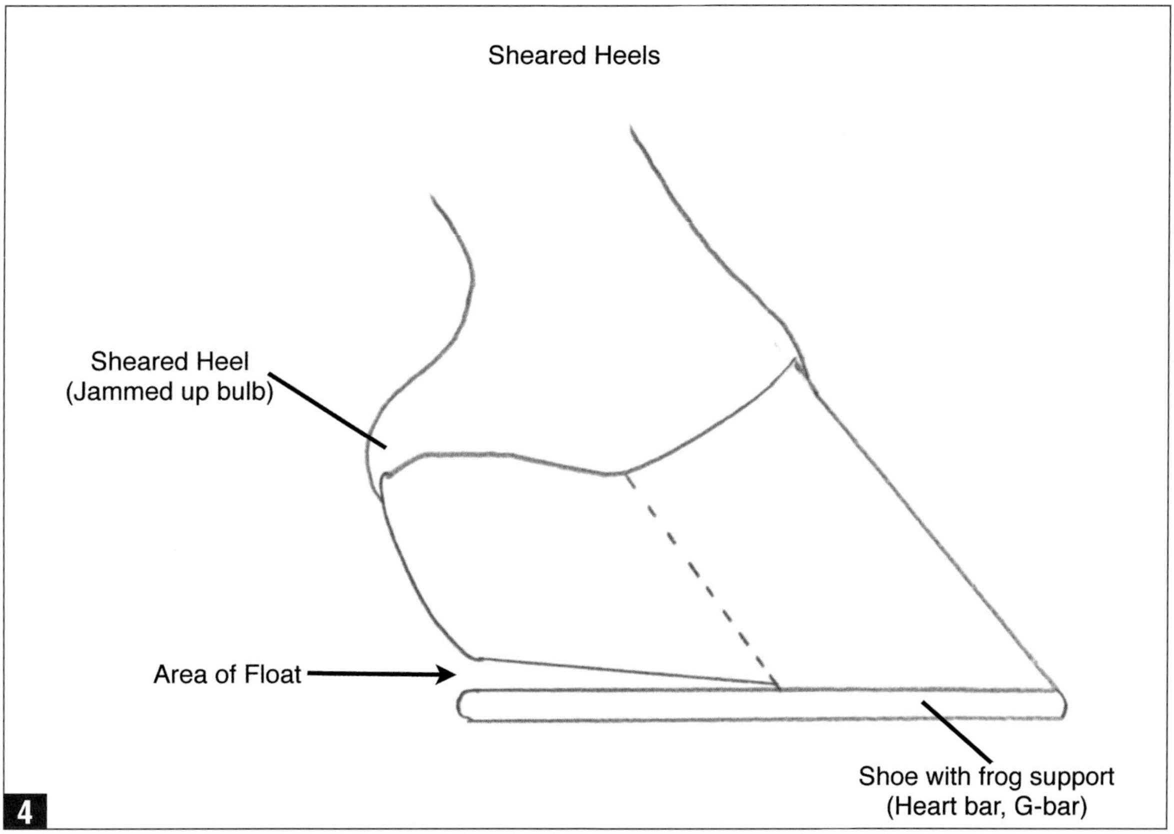

Drawing of a foot with sheared heel and where it would be floated.

depicting the sheared heel and the area that would be floated.

The reason I use a heart bar is that I want the frog to take some of the load. I have tried to do it with a straight bar in the past, and it has caused quite a bit of distortion at the toe on the side that was floated. Also be aware that there may be some soreness as the heel and bulb are moving into the new position. It is similar to having braces on your teeth, which is commonly done for aesthetic purposes, but causes pain while the teeth are moving from the inflammation of being forced around.

The shoe should be reset at as short an interval as possible so that the float can be re-established regularly. You can also have the owner use a hacksaw blade every week or so to make a slight float again without pulling the shoe.

Due to the fact that there is hoof wall attachment to the collateral cartilages in the heel region of the foot, the heels are more flexible than the wall at the toe would be. This allows the region to move more than other areas of the hoof wall without causing as much pain as would be caused if the movement were in another area. What this means to the farrier is that a sheared heel does not always cause pain, and fixing it can also be accomplished at times without pain. Not always, but often.

Treatment by a veterinarian does not really apply. The vet can advise the use of an anti-inflammatory if needed. The owner needs to watch the horse for soreness as well as possibly re-establishing the float on the heel.

ANTICIPATED OUTCOME

Sheared heels rarely cause much in the way of lameness, so I would not anticipate that a horse is lame when dealing with the problem. Bear in mind that my experience is primarily with Quarter Horses, and these horses have a smaller and more upright foot than many other breeds. I have heard from many of my colleagues that they have to deal with a lot of sheared heels. The horse may become sore when you are trying to fix it, but that should also pass. If you fix the blemish, it should stay fixed, and the horse should be sound.

IN SHORT

D: The bulbs are in different planes.

T: Shoe with a heart bar shoe and float the heel on the side that the bulb is higher or leave alone if aesthetics are not a problem for you or the owner.

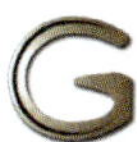

Chapter

45-16 SIDEBONE

DEFINITION

Sidebone is the term used to describe the ossification (turning into bone) of the collateral cartilages.

REASONS

There are several potential reasons for sidebone. First is the type of work that a horse does. Horses that are used on hard footing are prone to sidebone from the concussion of their occupation. A lot of carriage horses will develop sidebones from a life of pulling a cart over hard terrain.

Another common cause is conformation. Mediolateral imbalance will place more weight on one side of the foot than another, and this leads to what is known as unilateral sidebone. With unilateral sidebone, just one of the lateral cartilages is affected. Bilateral sidebones refers to both collateral cartilages becoming bone. **Figures 1-2** are of a coffin bone with unilateral sidebone.

Injury can also lead to the lateral cartilage turning into bone. A common injury is for a horse to have a wire or rope cut that involves the collateral cartilages. This can make it ossify when it is healing. **Figures 3-5** show some feet with injuries that could easily lead to sidebone.

Displaced coronary bands may play a part as well, just as they do in quarter cracks. If there is a proximal displacement at the quarter, the collateral cartilages are being smashed into the top of the hoof

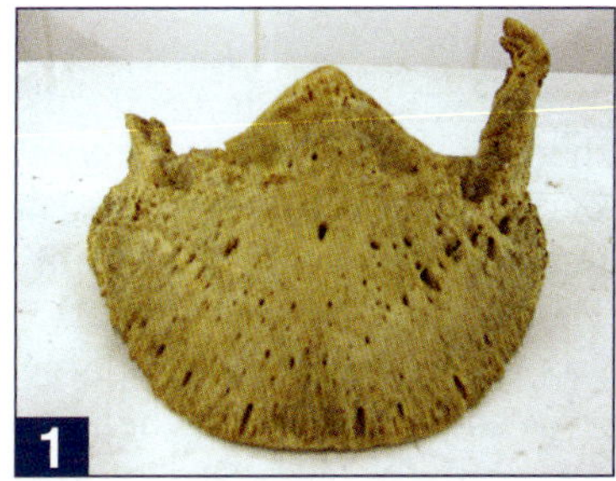

Dorsal view of a coffin bone with a unilateral sidebone.

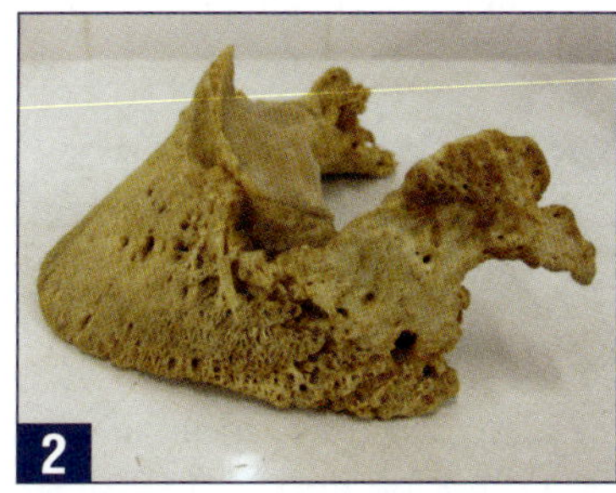

Lateral view of the same coffin bone.

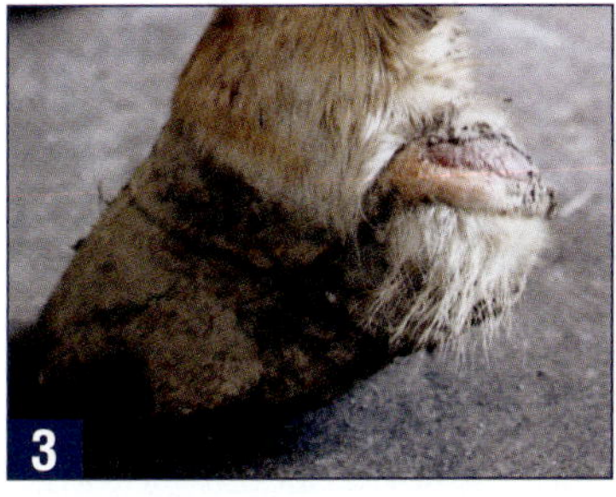

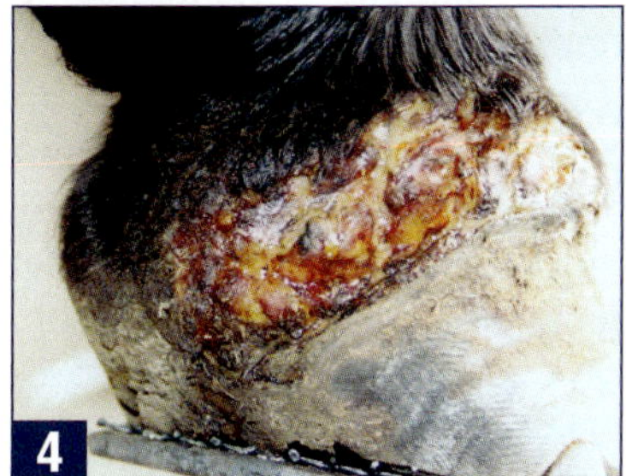

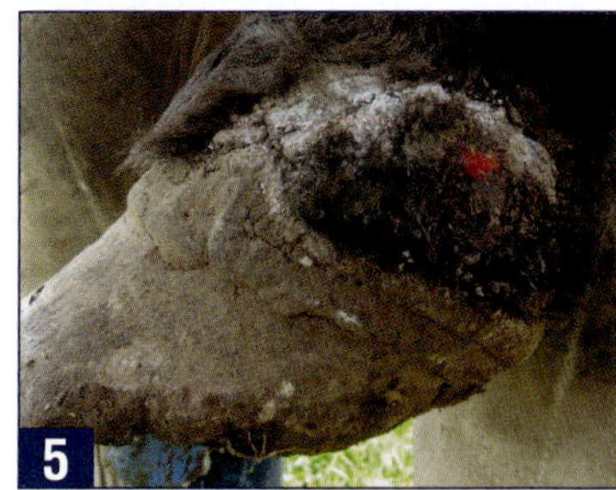

Injured foot that can lead to sidebone.

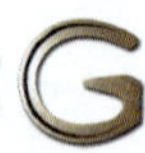

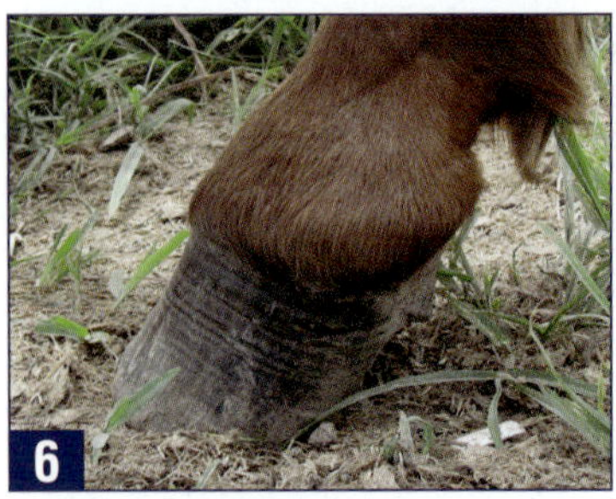

Lateral view of a foot with a large sidebone.

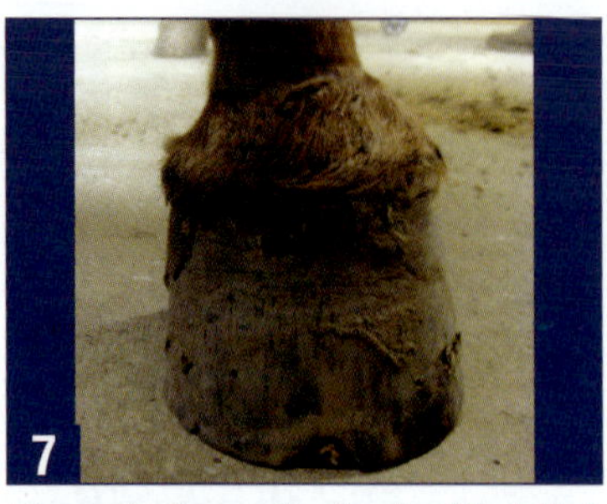

Dorsal view of a foot with bilateral sidebones.

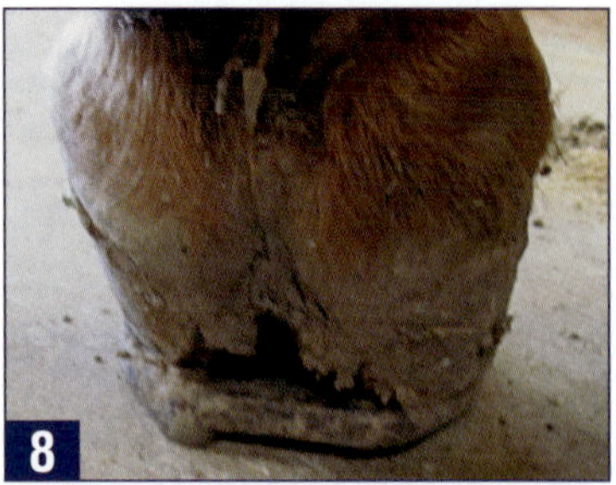

Palmar view of a foot with bilateral sidebones. Notice how small the foot is compared to the area at the coronet.

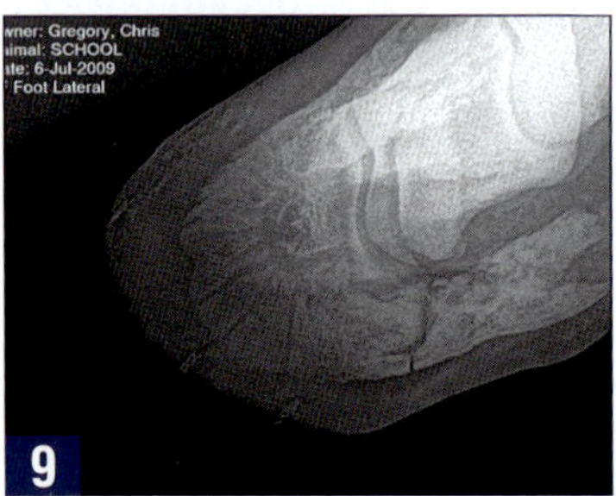

Radiograph of sidebones showing a clear break.

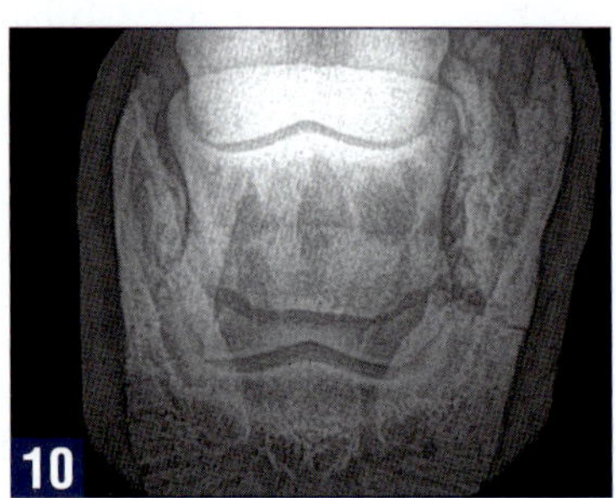

Radiograph of sidebones.

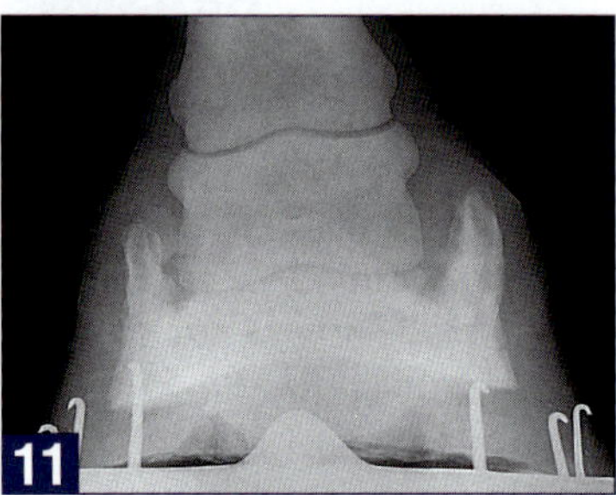

Dorsal/palmar radiograph of bilateral sidebones.

wall where there should not be hoof wall. This will cause trauma to the collateral cartilages, which may lead to sidebone.

ANATOMY

The anatomy for this will be the collateral cartilages.

SYMPTOMS

When sidebone is first forming, a horse may be quite lame. It would not be uncommon to see a Grade 2 lameness that lasts several months as the lateral cartilage goes through the transformation from cartilage to bone. In many cases, though not all, the horse will return to soundness once the change is completed. If you are certain of the diagnosis in the early phase of sidebone development, the horse should be shod with a rocker-toe shoe, or — in the cases of unilateral sidebone — a sidebone shoe.

After the collateral cartilages have completed the change to bone, it is rare for the horse to be sore from the sidebones themselves. However, sidebones can lead to other problems. The shape of the feet will often change from sidebones, since the coronary band may now be a new shape. It is difficult to change the shape of the foot back toward ideal when dealing with sidebones, so I will often just shape my shoes to the shape that the foot presents. **Figure 6** shows a large sidebone on the lateral side of the foot. **Figures 7-8** show a foot with bilateral sidebone. The coronary band is larger than the bottom of the foot from the development of the sidebone.

With a radiograph, the extent of the sidebone can easily be seen. It is also possible to feel the sidebones above the hoof wall at the back of the foot. With normal feet, you can palpate and feel the malleable collateral cartilages. Once they have ossified, this area is hard and immobile. **Figures 9-10** are from radiographs by Dr. Marcotte of the foot in **Figures 7-8**. Notice that they have been fractured. **Figure 11** shows another horse with bilateral sidebones, with the radiograph taken by Dr. Morrison.

TREATMENT

In an ideal situation, a horse should be turned out to rest if it displays lameness in the early phase

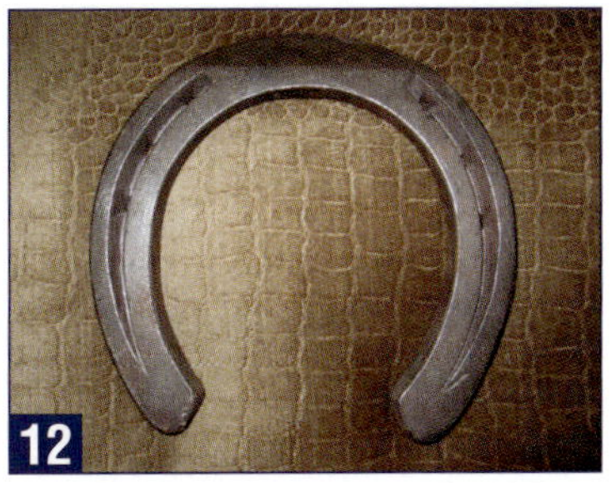

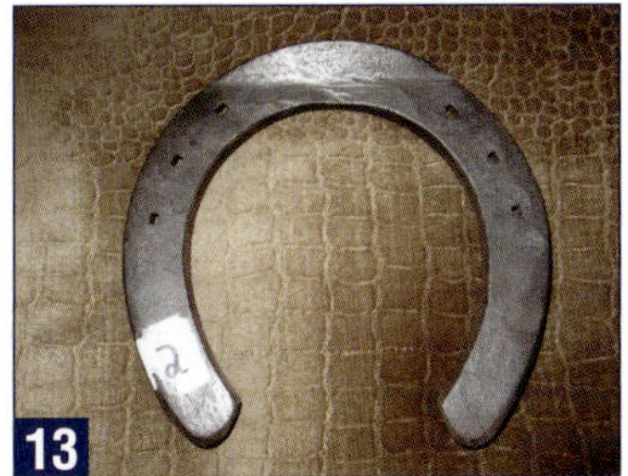

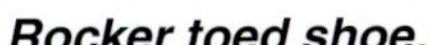

Rocker toed shoe.

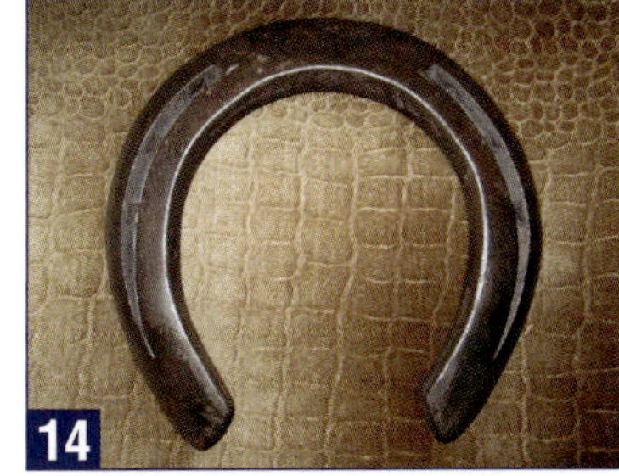

Cupped breakover shoe.

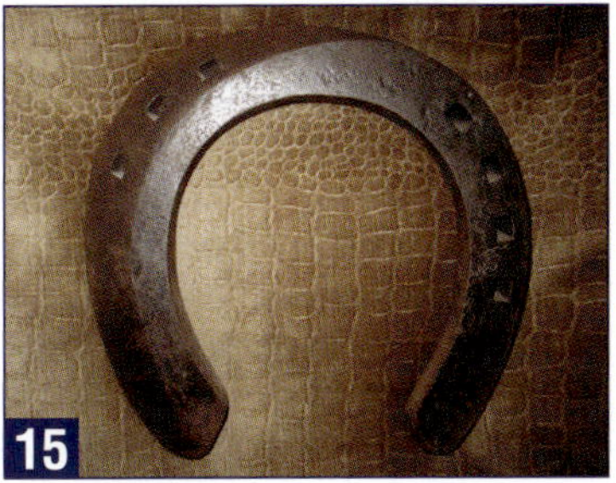

Sidebone shoe.

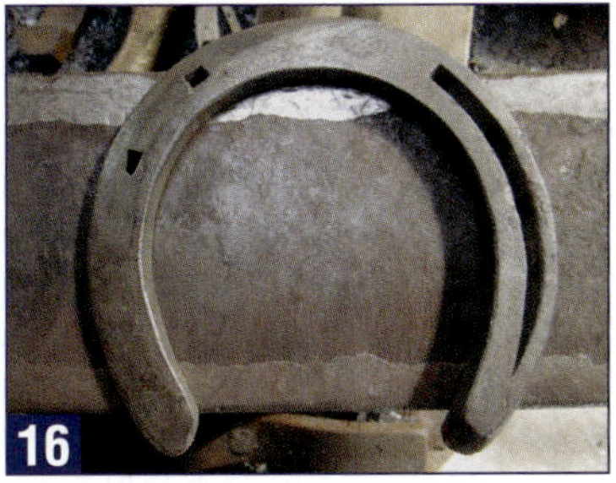

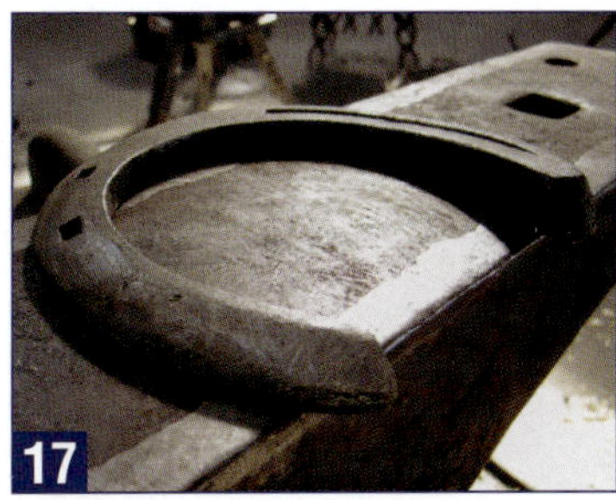

Detail of a sidebone shoe showing the wedged branch and the bevel.

of sidebone development. Once the sidebone is completely formed, the horse can be brought back in and shod normally without pain. This is not always an option since people want to use their horses. I recommend that you shoe with a severe rocker toe **(Figures 12-13)**, or a cupped breakover shoe **(Figure 14)** for bilateral sidebone. There is a classic sidebone shoe for unilateral sidebone and a rocker-bar shoe if these shoes don't work. A sidebone shoe is simply a shoe that has a long rolled toe from the good side of the foot through the end of the heel on the side that is developing the sidebone. **Figures 15-17** show sidebone shoes.

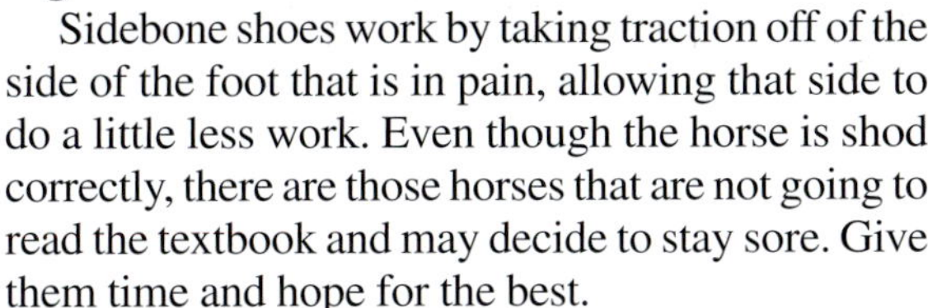

Sidebone shoes work by taking traction off of the side of the foot that is in pain, allowing that side to do a little less work. Even though the horse is shod correctly, there are those horses that are not going to read the textbook and may decide to stay sore. Give them time and hope for the best.

Another thing worth trying with a sore horse is to groove the foot where the sidebone is developing. I have had one FWCF Examiner recommend grooving horizontally, and another recommend grooving vertically. I think either way may provide some relief as you weaken the wall that the lateral cartilage is being jammed against. Grooving can be done in several different ways, but I find using the edge of my rasp to be the easiest for horizontal grooving **(Figure 18)**. I have seen grooving also done with a hot iron as well as with a Dremel tool.

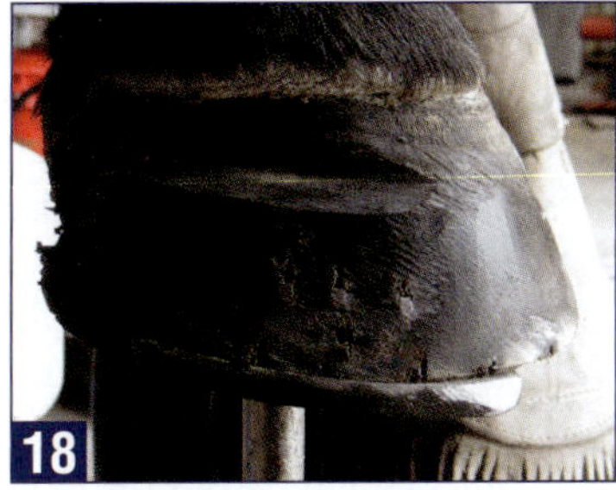

Foot that has been grooved with a rasp.

I have had to deal with broken sidebones on an overreaching barrel horse. The sidebone does not heal easily once it is broken, so that horse did have to deal with lameness issues. Mediolateral balance is critical when dealing with this problem. Due to the way the foot grows out of balance on this horse, there are times where the only option to achieve

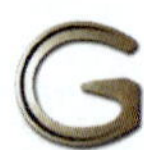

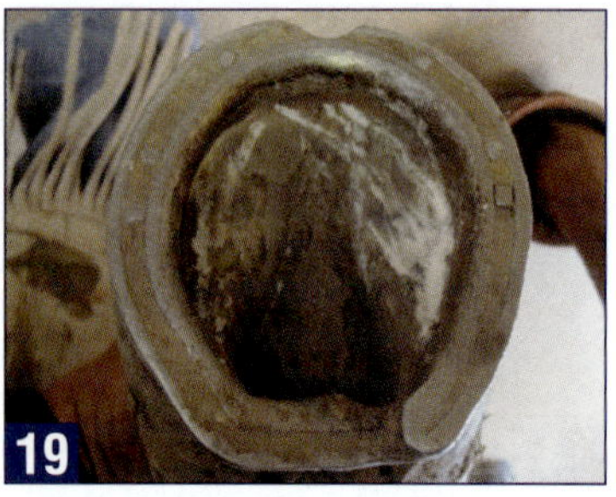

Medial lift bar shoe on the foot.

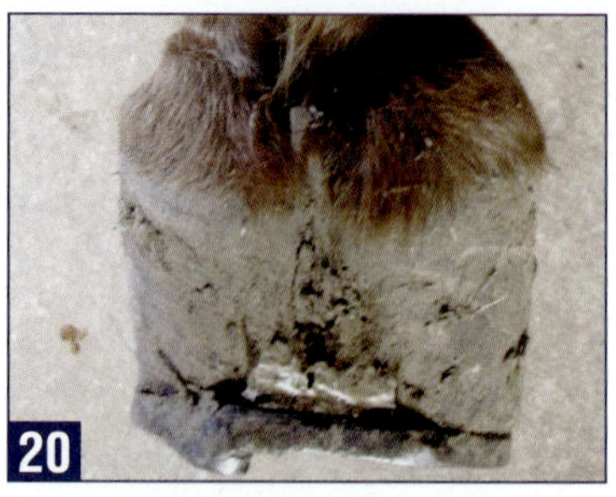

Medial lift bar shoe showing how it changed the mediolateral balance on this foot.

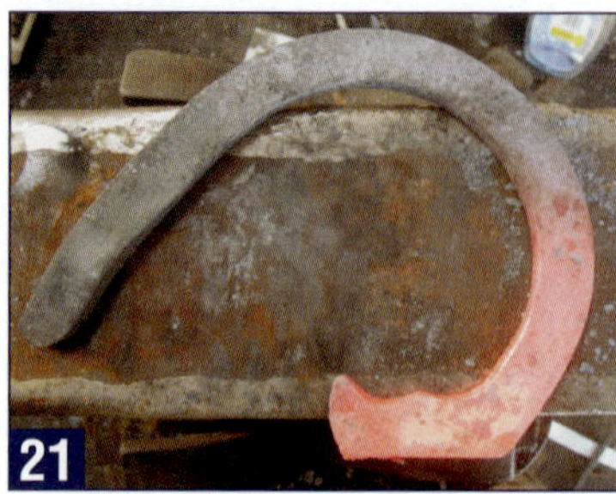

Setup for a whip across medial lift bar shoe.

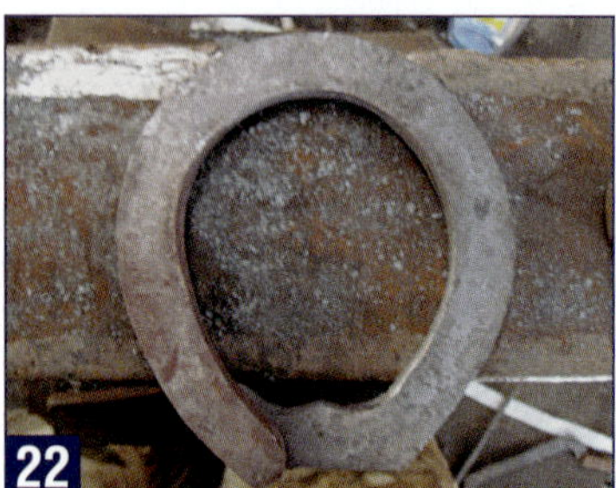

Bringing the heel into the bar.

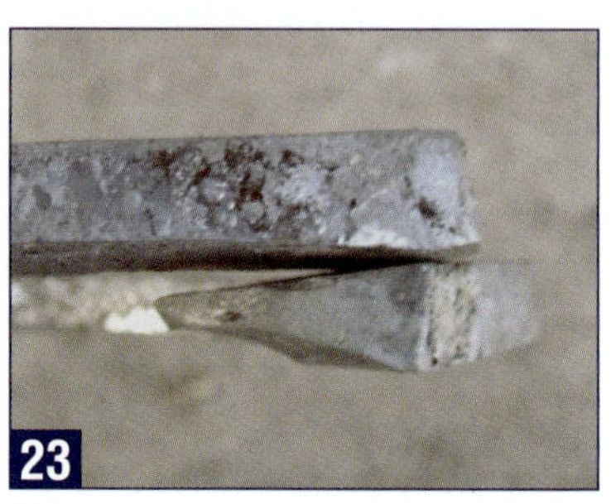

The overlap of the heel and bar.

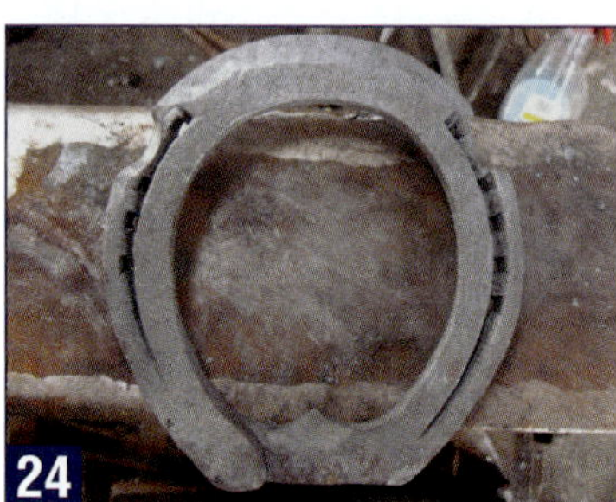

Finished shoe with rolled toe.

mediolateral balance has been through the application of a shoe. The shoe I like the best to wedge across the foot is called a medial lift bar shoe, and it is done with a whip-across bar. This shoe can be seen in **Figures 19-20**. This particular horse went from lame to sound when the bar shoe was applied, and the bar shoe was used until the foot had grown enough that I could restore balance with the trim.

Figures 21-24 should give most readers a pretty good understanding of how to construct this shoe.

The vet will be a big part of the diagnosis. Radiographs can tell so much about sidebone that can't be seen without them. The customer should avoid using the horse when it is lame. This can be harder to get a customer to do than you might imagine, so spend some time with them describing what to look for.

ANTICIPATED OUTCOME

Most horses should be sound eventually, even though the sidebone will be a permanent blemish.

IN SHORT:

D: Ossification of the collateral cartilages.

T: Rocker toe, sidebone shoe, rocker-bar shoe.

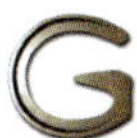

Chapter

45-17 Soft Heel Cracks

DEFINITION

This is referring to the area between the bulbs becoming inflamed and infected. I refer to this as a soft heel crack.

REASON

Some feet are predisposed to have problems in this area from conformation. Sheared heels, weak heels, or a deep central sulcus of the frog will predispose a horse to problems with soft heel cracks.

ANATOMY

The crease between the bulbs that separates the bulbs is the area that is involved.

SYMPTOMS

Feet with these soft heel cracks can be intermittently lame. There will be discharge from these cracks, and it easily becomes infected. This area will stay constantly moist, which causes it to become weaker and more susceptible to damage and infection. A tool can be inserted into the area, and it will go deep between the bulbs. If the horse has lameness, the insertion of the tool will cause the horse to flinch. In **Figure 1**, there is a foot that is still pretty strong with a soft heel crack. In **Figures 2-3**, there is a foot with a soft heel crack with a hoof pick being inserted into the crack itself.

TREATMENT

The first thing that a farrier must do is to stabilize the foot as much as possible. This will require a bar shoe, and I like to place clips well back on feet that have a lot of movement in them. Not behind the widest point, but perhaps at that point. The same sort of bar shoe that you might use for a horse with a fractured coffin bone is great for stabilizing a foot. The bar shoe will also have the advantage of protecting this area of the foot from getting stuff stuck in it like grass or other debris.

At one time we would treat this area by flossing it with gauze that had been soaked in full strength Lysol in the old glass bottle. Most horses would recover, but not all. In later years we have used the antibiotics used for mastitis in cows. This product can be placed between the bulbs to clear it up. **Figures 4-6** show a soft heel crack being treated with the mastitis antibiotics. It is running out of the central sulcus in **Figure 6**. Alternatively, metronidazole tablets can be crushed, mixed with water into a paste, and used the same way. Since I do so many more Quarter Horses than other breeds, this is not a problem that I see too often.

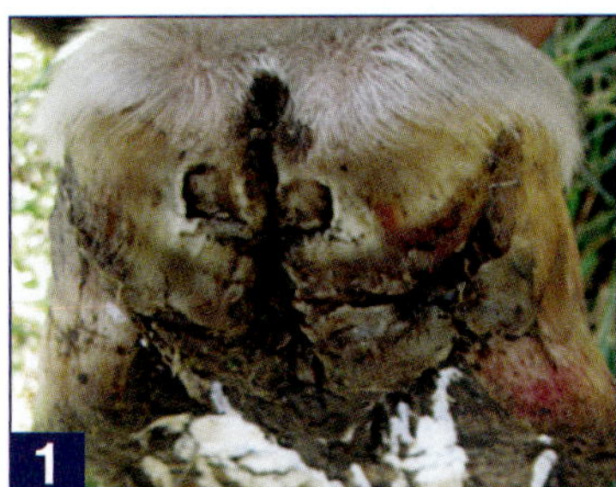

Foot with the beginnings of a soft heel crack.

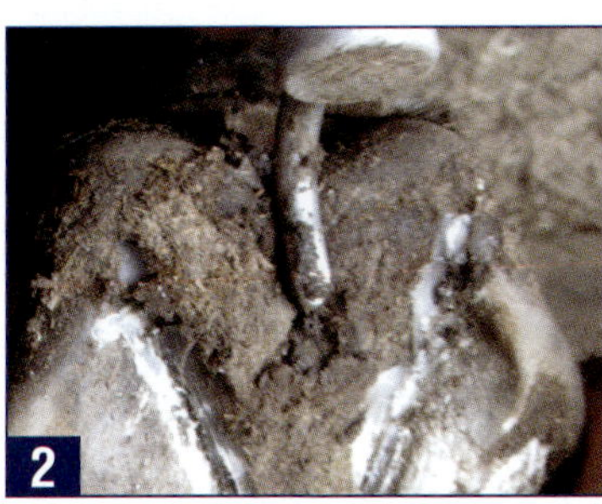

Soft heel crack with a hoof pick just outside of it.

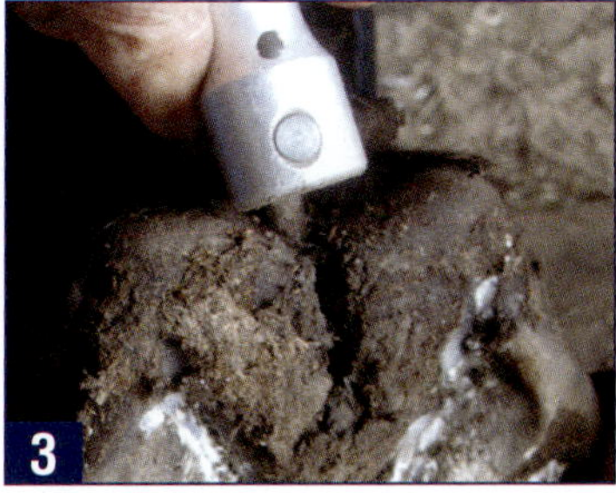

The hoof pick has been inserted so far that it can't be seen in the soft heel crack.

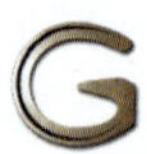

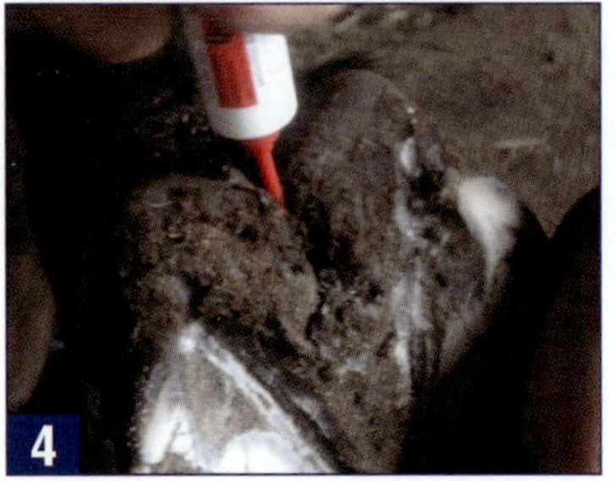

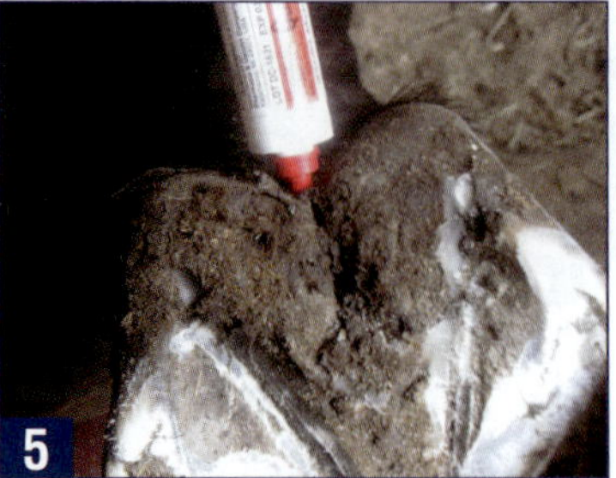

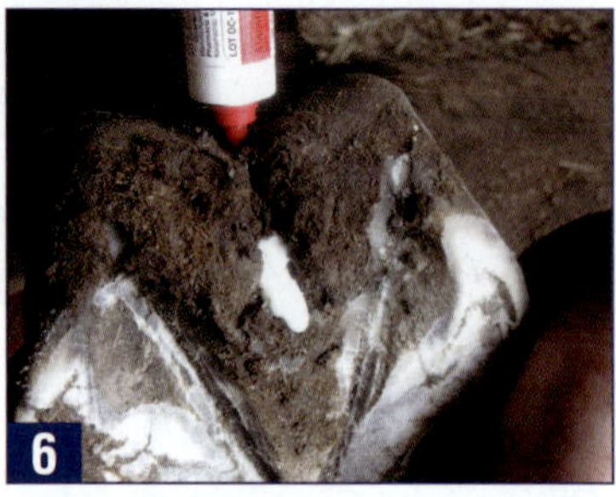

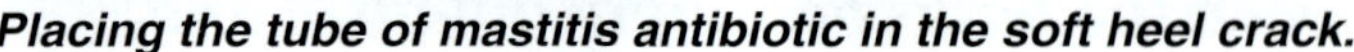

Placing the tube of mastitis antibiotic in the soft heel crack.

The medicine is running out of the central sulcus of the frog.

The veterinarian may have another topical solution for you, and the owner's primary job is to keep this area clean and apply whatever you decide to suggest. I would have them clean and doctor the area every other day for the first week, and then go to a twice a week schedule after that until the next shoeing.

ANTICIPATED OUTCOME

If you are able to keep this foot from moving, this problem tends to go away. However, it is the type of problem that recurs in some horses quite easily.

IN SHORT

D: Crack between the bulbs.

T: Stabilize foot with bar shoe and apply topical solution of mastitis ointment.

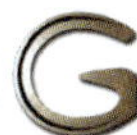

Chapter 45-18 SOLE BRUISES

DEFINITION

A sole bruise is a discoloration of the sole from damage to the sole. They are often dark red and sometimes have a bluish tint.

REASONS

Bruises in the sole are caused from trauma to the sole. Horses with flat soles are more prone to sole bruises, but any foot can become bruised under the right conditions. Riding a horse without shoes in rough terrain is a common cause of sole bruising. Other common causes are large gravel and frozen mud.

If a rock or other foreign body gets trapped in the sole **(Figure 1)**, the horse will be bearing weight on a small area of the foot, which can easily become bruised.

Poor shoeing technique that causes sole pressure is also responsible for a lot of sole bruises.

ANATOMY

The horny sole will show the results of the sole bruising, but the sensitive sole has been damaged for the bruise to be showing up in the horny sole.

SYMPTOMS

When you see the bruise in the horny sole during trimming, you are looking at the history of the sole. **Figure 2** is a common look to a sole bruise that is from two weeks to a month old. The bloody marking happens while the sensitive sole is producing the horny sole. You will find horses that have bad looking bruises in the horny sole, yet they are not lame **(Figure 3)**. Conversely, you may find horses that are sore from bruising in the sole, yet there is not yet the discoloration in the horny sole. This means that the sole bruise is quite new, and you will see the resulting bruise sometime in a future trim.

Neglected feet, like the one in **Figure 4**, will often have quite a bit of bruising. Since the foot is also white, a ring of blood can be seen in the hoof wall as well. The bottom of this foot is seen in **Figure 5**. Notice the amount of bruising all around this foot from the white line to the wall to the sole and frog. **Figure 6** shows another foot on this same donkey.

1

Foot with a rock stuck in the bottom of it.

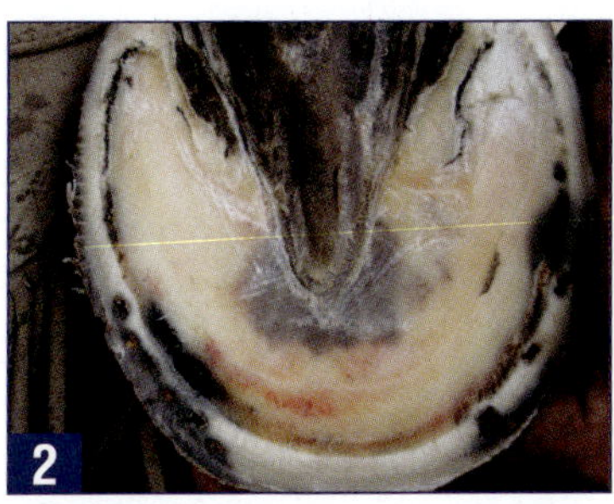

Normal look to sole bruising.

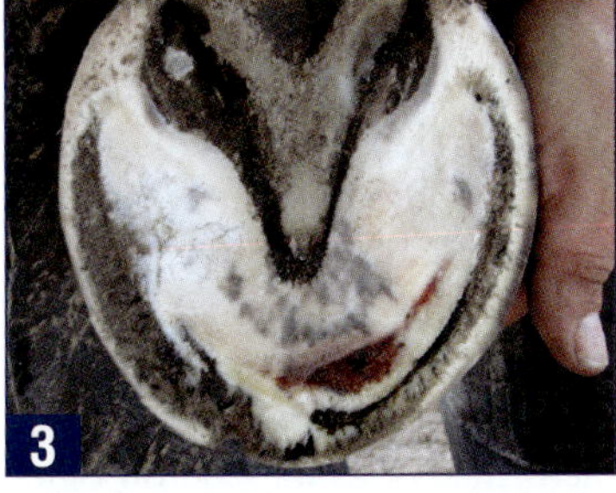

A recent and deep bruise with a lot of coagulated blood present.

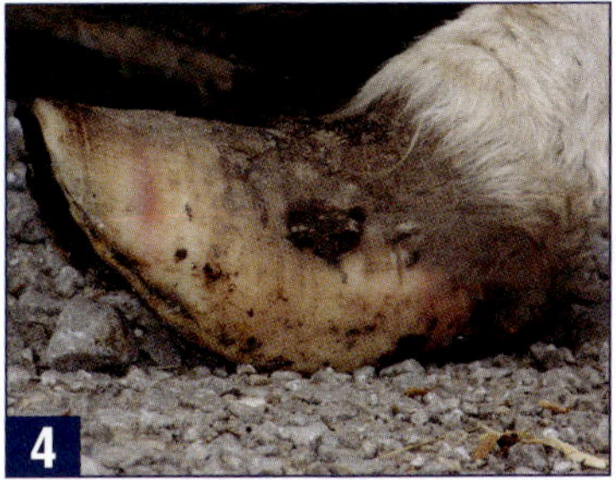

Lateral view of a neglected foot.

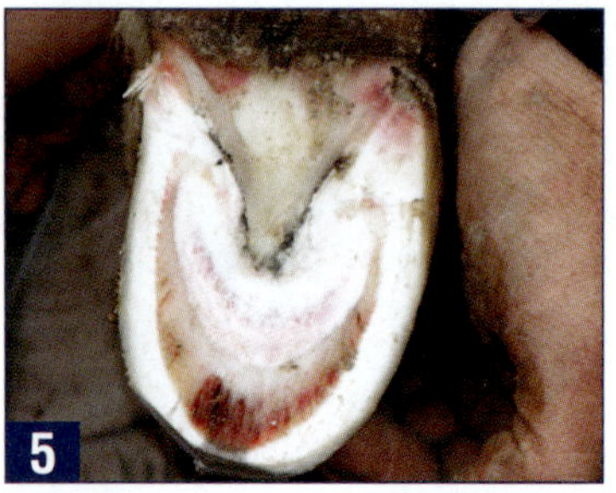

Bottom of the neglected foot from Figure 4.

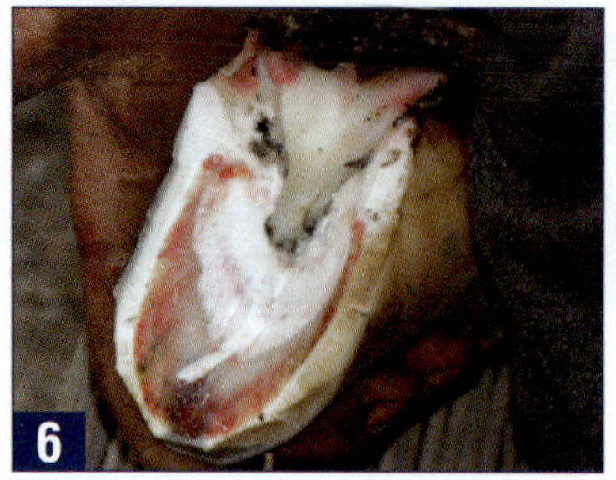

Another foot on the same animal. Notice the bruising all around the foot.

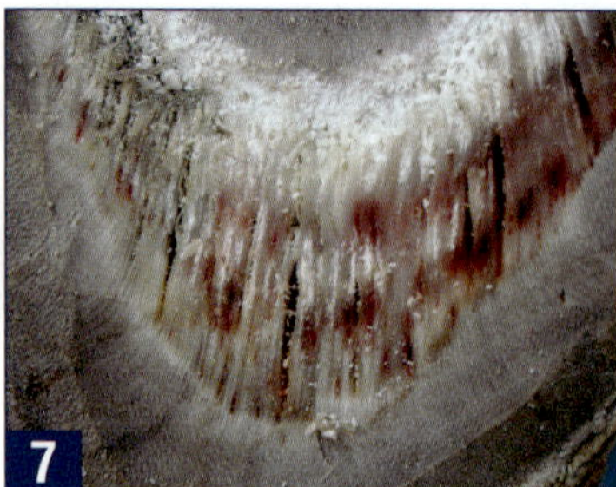

The stretched and bruised white line on a foundered hoof.

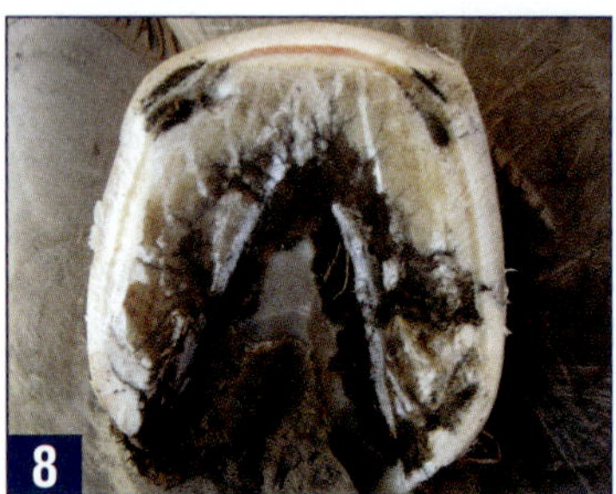

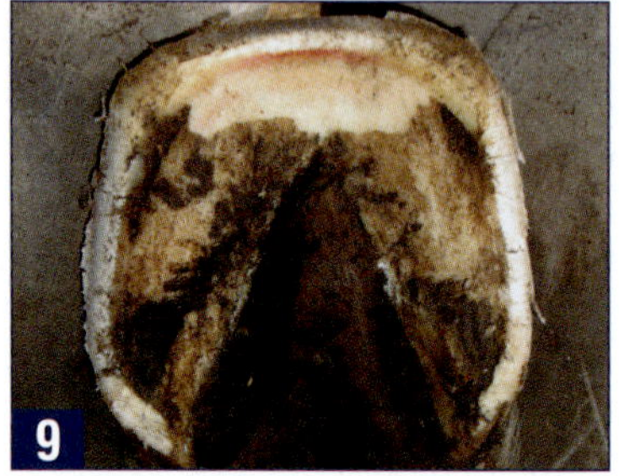

Bruising in the white line from stress caused by the four-point trim.

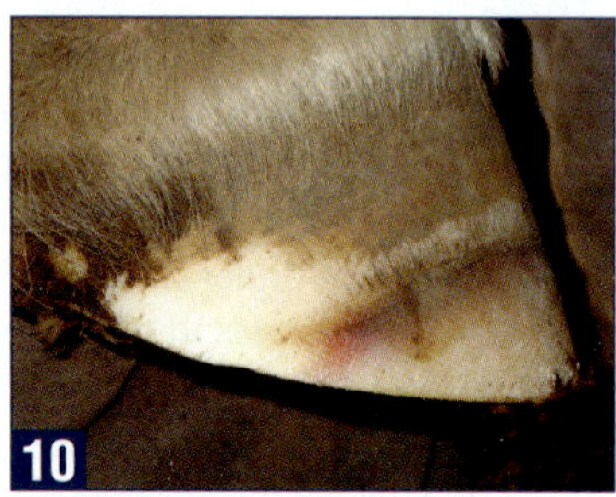

Bruise on the outside of the hoof that is parallel to the coronet on a traditionally trimmed foot.

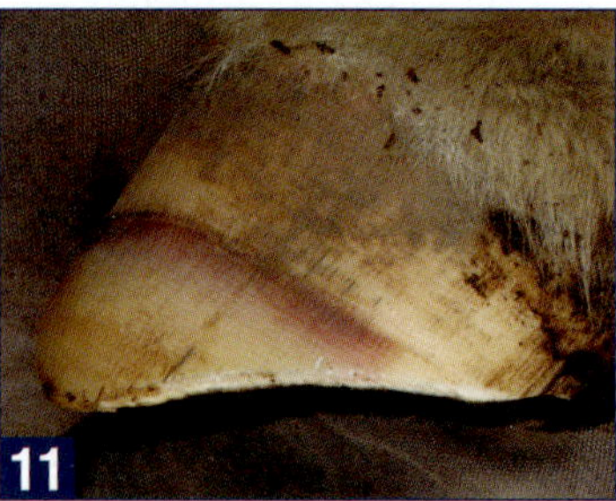

Bruise on the outside of another foot on the same horse that was trimmed using the four-point method.

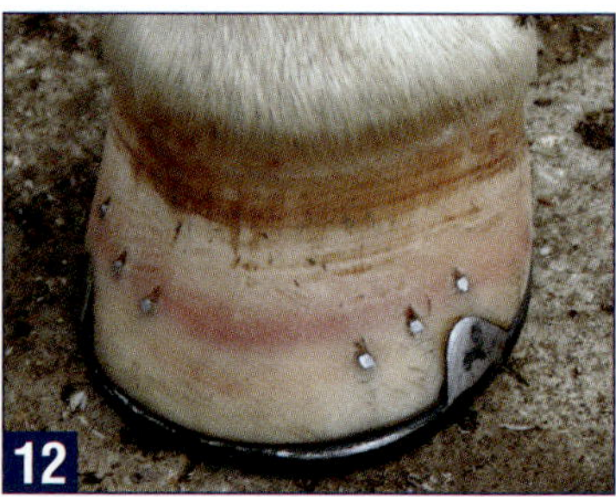

Bruise around the outside of a white foot.

Bruising in the white line is a sign of undue stress. It is common in the white line of foundered feet, as **Figure 7** shows. When we did the study with Dr. Miller on the four-point trim, we caused a lot of white line stress on these horses that they didn't have before **(Figures 8-9)**. Bruising in the hoof wall can give a history of how the foot grows. One of the horses from the study that was a four-point trim on one side and a conventional trim on the other shows how the line of bruise around the foot changed over the course of being trimmed with the four-point style. Notice in **Figure 10** that the bruise is straight, and in **Figure 11**, it has a wave in it from the 4-point trim. This type of bruising happens when the foot is being produced at the coronary band. Blood is deposited in the stratum medium for a lot of reasons, most of them systemic issues such as sickness or stress. **Figure 12** shows another bruise in the hoof wall. Notice that all of these are being shown on white feet. While the bruise does happen on black feet, it is not as apparent as it is on white feet.

Bruises in the sole mean that blood serum

is present. Since serum is such a good food for bacteria, it is not uncommon for a bruise to end up being an abscess.

TREATMENT

When you are dealing with sole bruises, treat the horse as you would for a dropped sole. You may need a deep-seated shoe, bar shoe, pad, pour-in, hospital plate, or some shoe of your own devising that will protect the sole. See the section on dropped sole for pictures of the cupped shoe. Allow the horse enough time to become sound again and be aware that abscesses are common on bruised feet.

The veterinarian should be wary of over trimming soles on horses that are only bruised. Removing the horny sole over a bruise that is not yet an abscess is not recommended, however it is done from time to time by over-zealous vets. Veterinarians don't mind seeing blood in a foot, but farriers are trained that this is a bad thing.

Owners should watch for potential abscess lameness and avoid using horses in rough terrain without proper protection.

ANTICIPATED OUTCOME

Most of the time a horse with a sole bruise will be comfortable as soon as the foot is protected. Since abscesses do happen with bruising, you may have to deal with an abscess, which may make the healing time a little longer.

IN SHORT

D: Damage and discoloration in the sole from direct trauma.

T: Protect with wide webbed shoe, pads, pour-in, or similar shoeing strategies.

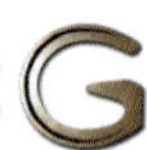

Chapter

45-19 THRUSH

DEFINITION

Thrush is an infestation of the foot by anaerobic bacteria.

REASON

Thrush will occur primarily in feet that are not well cared for in damp and unsanitary conditions. Feet with imbalances such as sheared heels are more prone, as are feet with deep sulci and smaller frogs. There is also some anecdotal evidence to suggest that some horses are just more susceptible to thrush than others.

ANATOMY

The frog can spread over the commissures if it does not shed or get trimmed away. When this happens, it creates an area that is perfect for thrush. That is why the frog is the primary structure that gets eaten by thrush, especially in the commissures under the side of the frog. In severe cases, thrush consumes enough of the horny frog that sensitive structures are exposed, and the horse is likely to have infections.

With soft heel cracks that extend between the bulbs as extensions of the central sulcus of the frog, the bulbs and digital cushion can be added to the anatomy that is affected by thrush.

SYMPTOMS

Thrush is easy to recognize. It is black, thick, slightly oily, and has a distinct unpleasant odor. The frog will become raggedy where the thrush has eaten away the horny tissue, and occasionally you will see black holes in the sole as well, where the thrush is damaging horny sole. I have seen cases of thrush in which the bottoms of the commissures actually bled when I cleaned them out. When it becomes that severe, it is likely that the horse will develop an infection. The foot in **Figures 1-2** is bleeding from the tip of the frog, which has deteriorated due to thrush.

Figures 3-4 show what thrush commonly looks like on a frog. Notice how in **Figure 4** the bulbs are unbalanced and there are cracks on the palmar aspect of the frog. **Figure 5** shows early development of thrush in an otherwise nice foot. This thrush was deep in the commissures and would not be a problem if the owner kept the foot clean. **Figure 6** is another foot with thrush in the fairly early stages, and **Figure 7** is a foot that is long and has a frog compromised by thrush.

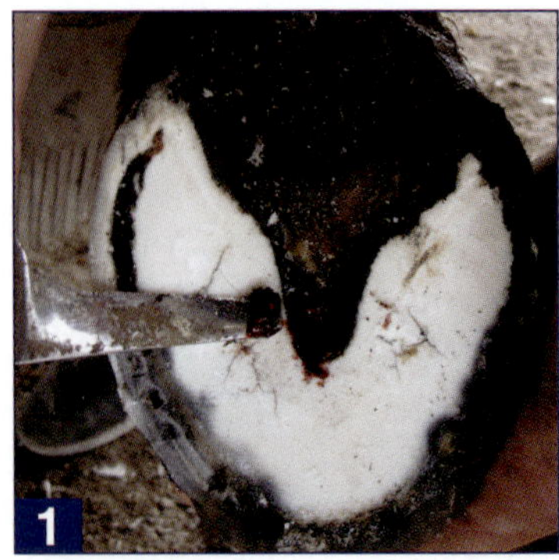

1

Foot with thrush that has been deteriorated through to sensitive structures.

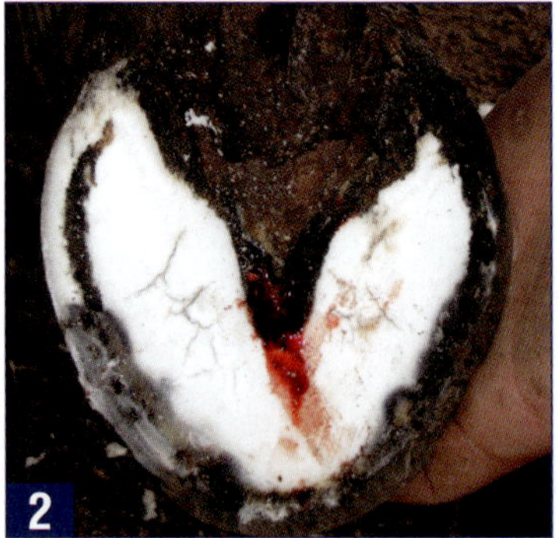

2

The blood that is coming from the damaged area is evident at the point of the frog.

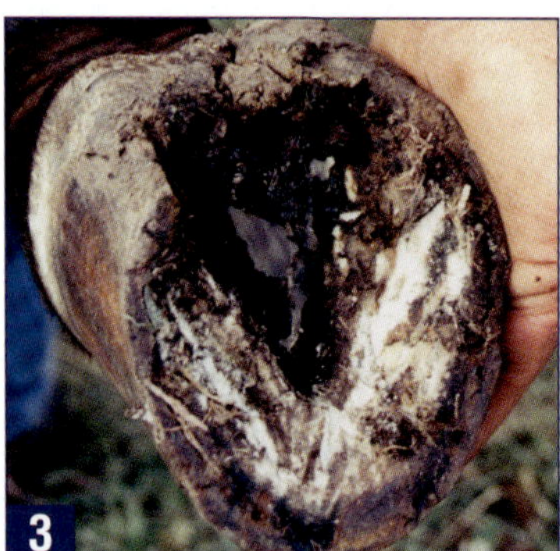

3

A foot with thrush.

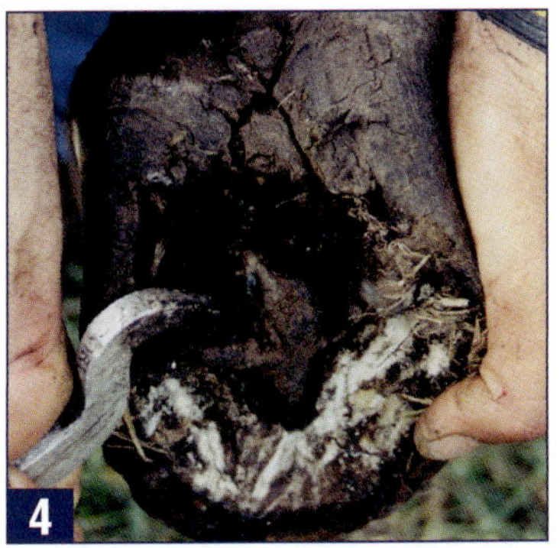

Same foot showing the depth of the damage under the frog.

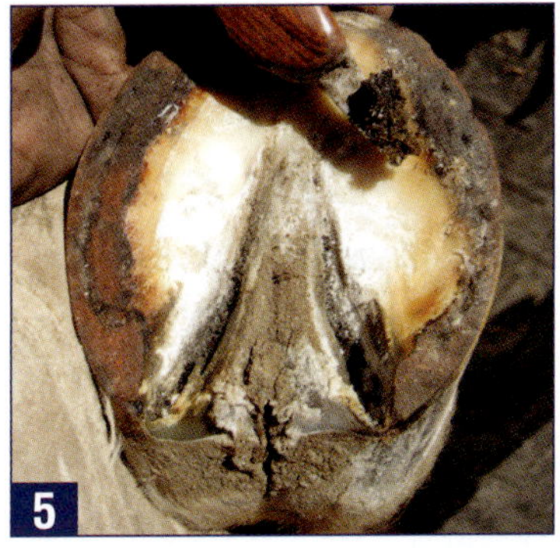

Deep thrush, but not yet severe.

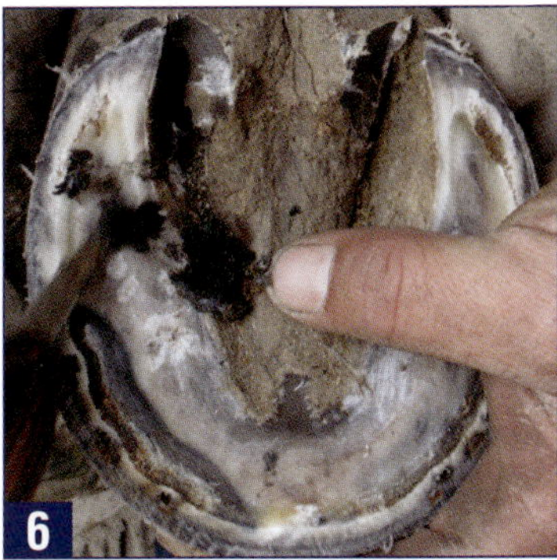

Digging out thrush from the commissure.

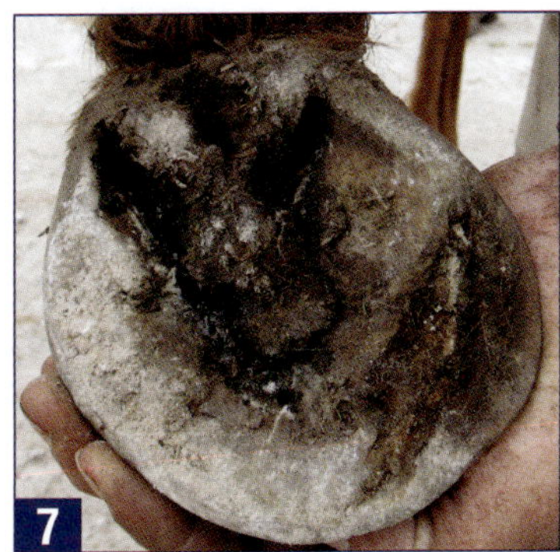

Typical look to a thrushy foot.

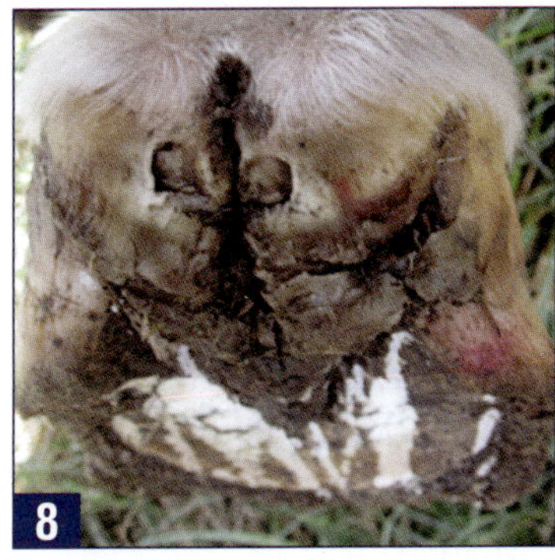

Soft heel crack extending between the bulbs.

Feet that develop soft heel cracks often look like **Figure 8**. However, this seems to be more common in feet with more badly sheared heels than the one in **Figure 8**.

TREATMENT

Mild thrush can generally be dealt with by simply knifing away the damaged frog and having the owner follow up by cleaning the foot regularly, as well as improving the stable conditions. With consistent hygiene and proper trimming, the thrush will die from the exposure to oxygen.

When thrush is severe, you will need to cut away the damaged horny frog, then apply a topical thrush remedy. There are several commercial thrush remedies available. I prefer Mustad Thrush Buster, but there are a lot to choose from.

In the event that sensitive structures are exposed from the damaged epidermal horn, you may need to treat this foot as if it had an abscess.

For soft heel cracks, the medicine used to treat mastitis in cows is excellent, and it even comes in an applicator that is ideal for use in between the bulbs. Crushed metronidazole tablets, diluted 1% povidine iodine, and 0.5% chlorhexidine are also popular antiseptic treatments.

The owner needs to clean the foot out daily and treat with the thrush remedy that you recommended. After about two weeks, the application of topical solution can be reduced to every third day, and finally to use as needed. Couple the foot treatment with keeping the environment clean and dry as well as regular farrier visits, and thrush should clear up pretty quickly.

ANTICIPATED OUTCOME

Thrush is rarely a big problem, and following the above steps should clear it up nicely in the majority of cases.

IN SHORT

D: Anaerobic bacteria damaging the frog.
T: Regular cleaning, topical thrush remedy.

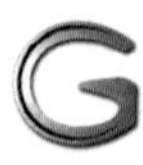

Chapter

45-20 WHITE LINE DISEASE

DEFINITION

The term white line disease is a bit of a misnomer. On the bottom of the foot, the white line is consumed, but once the disease progresses past the origin of the white line (terminal papillae at the distal end of the sensitive laminae), it becomes a disease that consumes the stratum internum. The definition is: The destruction of the white line and stratum internum by bacteria and fungus.

REASON

Typically, white line disease (WLD) will begin as a separation in the zone between the wall and sole that allows the bacteria and fungus to enter. Once the separation occurs, we don't know if a bacterium starts it and is then joined by an opportunistic fungus, or vice versa. Both bacteria and fungi are present.

Originally wet, humid, and unsanitary conditions were thought to be the culprit. However, the disease has been found in all sorts of climates and conditions. Some horses seem to have a predisposition to white line disease. The bacteria involved is anaerobic, so once it gets inside the hoof wall, the oxygen in the outside environment cannot get to it.

ANATOMY

The white line and the stratum internum of the hoof wall.

SYMPTOMS

On the bottom of the foot, the white line will be a cavity filled with a black, mud-like, and possibly cheesy substance. As you dig it out, you will find that this crevice can be quite deep. In advanced cases, you will hear a hollow sound if you tap on the wall with the handle of your hoof knife or driving hammer. **Figures 1-4** are of feet with white line disease before any treatment. In **Figure 1**, you can see that there is a large area at the toe that is separated from the sole. **Figure 2** shows a donkey hoof with separation from quarter to quarter. **Figure 3** is looking into the separation that a hoof had at the toe quarter, and **Figure 4** is a small area right in the center of the toe. There is also a nail sticking out of the damaged area to show the depth.

This problem does not make a horse sore until it gets bad enough that the remaining laminae are no longer enough to support the horse's weight. White line disease is quite similar to the fungus that some people develop under their toenails and fingernails. The nail is separated from the finger, but there is not any pain associated with this. There is only pain if the attachment is made so small that the fingernail is ripped away from the remaining attachment. For a horse, there is not any pain or lameness while the separation is happening, but if it is made weak enough that it rips the foot apart, there will be lameness. You can end up with a foundered foot or even a sinker or hoof avulsion.

TREATMENT

When you are dealing with a new case of white line disease, it might be treated as easily as doing a small resection. If you are removing less than 10% of the foot, you can shoe with clips and a normal shoe, and even leave barefoot in a lot of instances. It is very important that all the infected hoof tissue be removed. Leaving any of the cheesy, gray and granular hoof tissue will allow the white line disease to continue. **Figures 5-6** are of the small area seen in **Figure 4**. Once this was removed, the base of

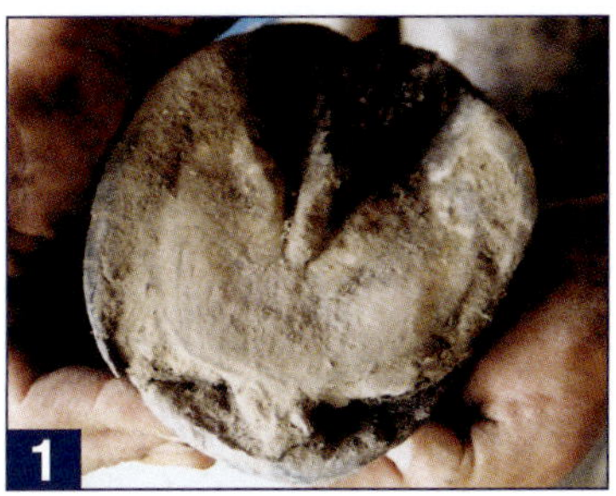

Separation around the toe.

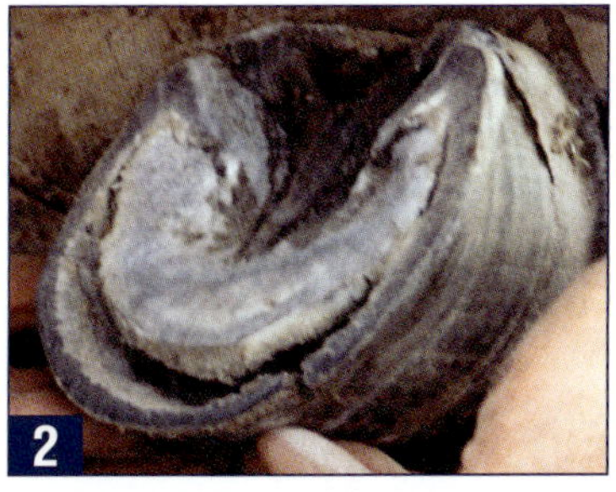

Donkey foot with separation from quarter to quarter.

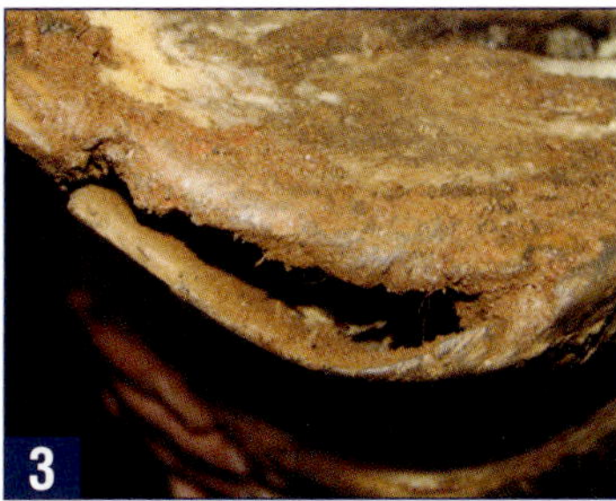

Separation at the toe quarter.

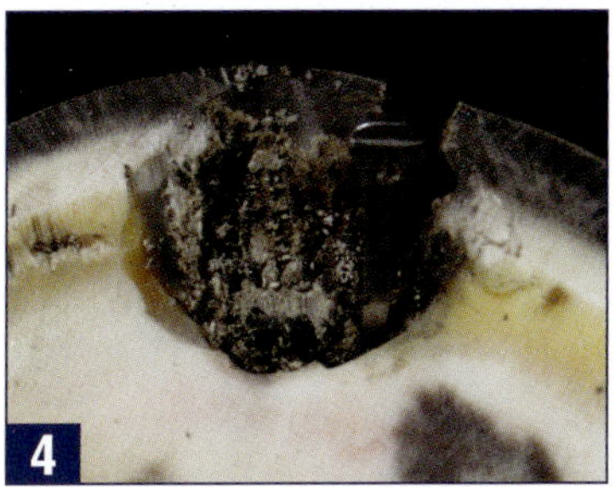

Small pocket of WLD at the toe.

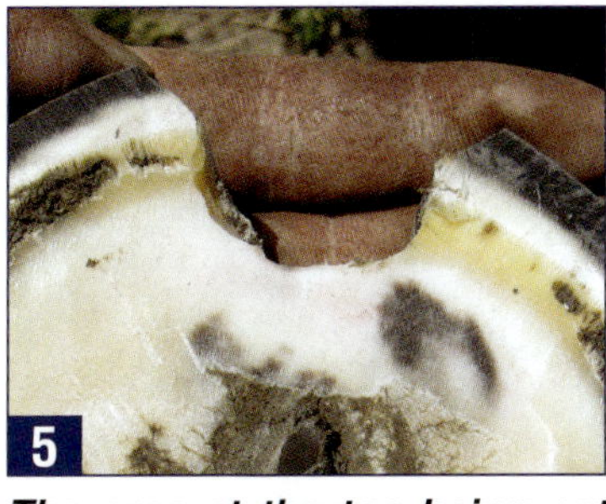

The area at the toe being cut out.

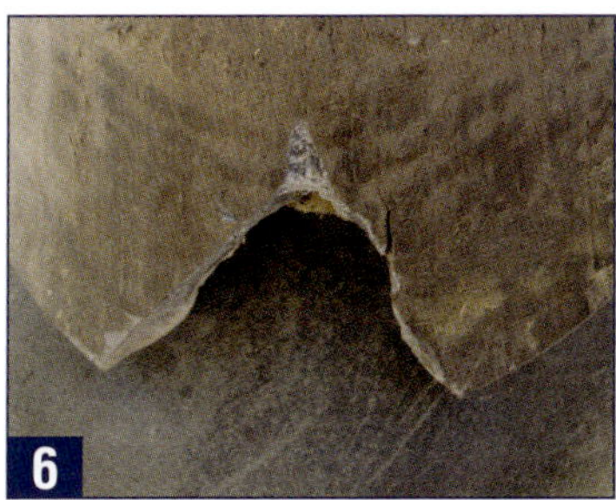

Dorsal view after the area was removed.

the problem was exposed, and the horse was shod with a normal shoe with quarter clips.

Once you start removing more than that, you will need to consider using bar shoes and Vettec Equi-Pak. The W-shoe and heart bar can be very useful on a foot that has a compromised laminae attachment between hoof wall and coffin bone. The main use of the heart bar is to place weight on the frog while relieving some of the weight on the hoof wall. What better shoe could there be for this problem?

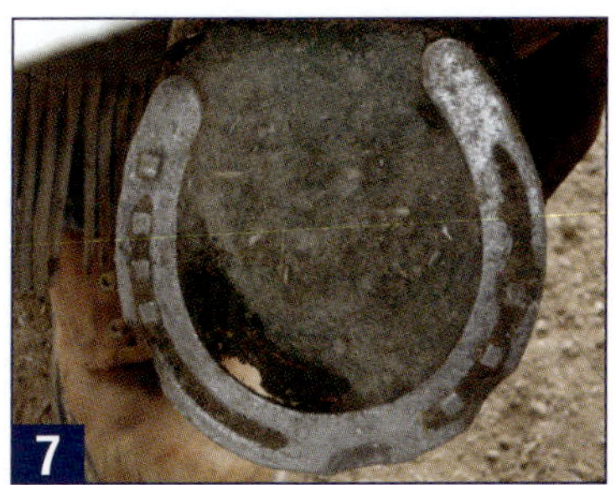

Shoe that Cody put on a horse that lost a shoe and had WLD.

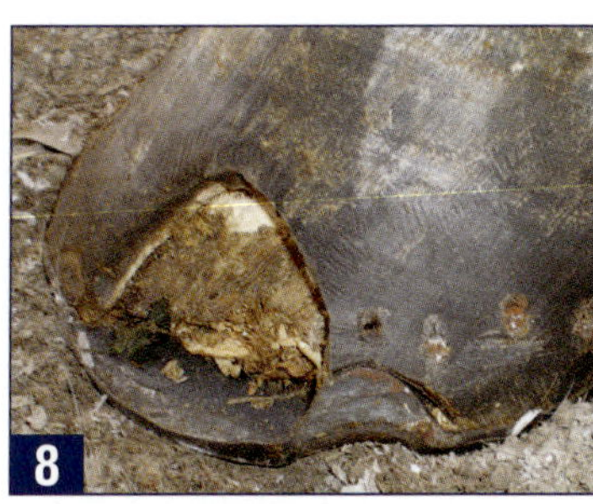

Lateral view of same foot.

Here is a series on a horse that made a complete recovery. First, a little background. We have a long-standing and fantastic customer that rides cutting horses. His top horse had always struggled with WLD, but we had kept it at bay with regular shoeing and small removal of infected material that didn't really involve much of the foot at all. The horse ended up having a major episode occur in a short span of time and lost a shoe. Cody had just turned 16, so I sent him to meet the horse and customer at a cutting to put the shoe back on. He ended up removing quite a bit of horn and creating a shoe that would do the trick. Needless to say, a 16-year-old boy doing that to your top horse would make you a little nervous, so the customer called and said I needed to see the horse right away. Cody also called to let me know that there was a lot going on with the foot. Cody did a great job of doing what the foot needed to get through the competition. Anyway, **Figures 7-8** show the shoe that Cody put on the foot, and the next photos are what I ended up doing to that foot.

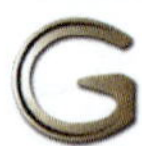

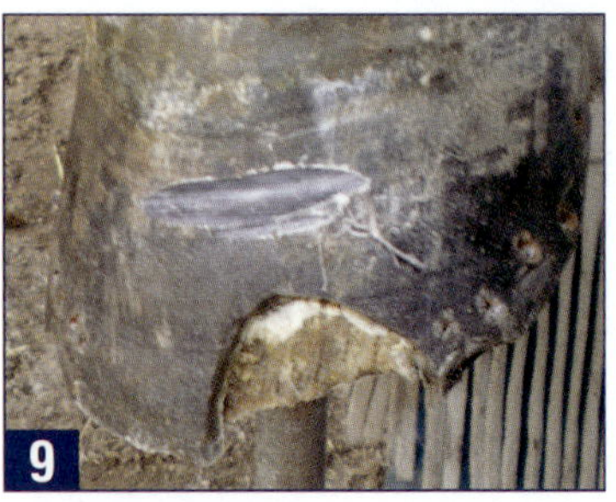

Foot scored with a rasp to start the resection.

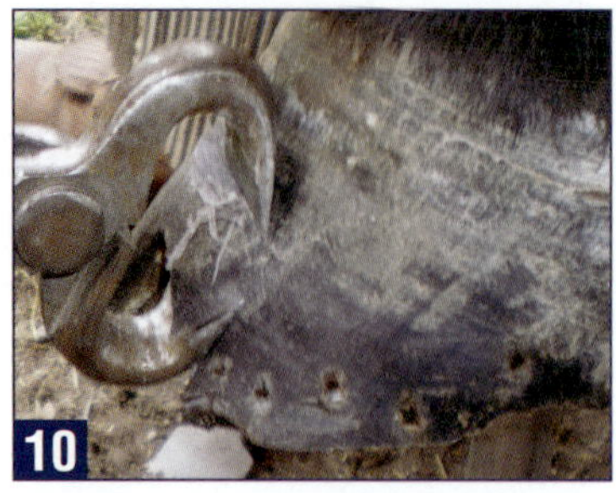

Cutting the outer hoof wall with nippers.

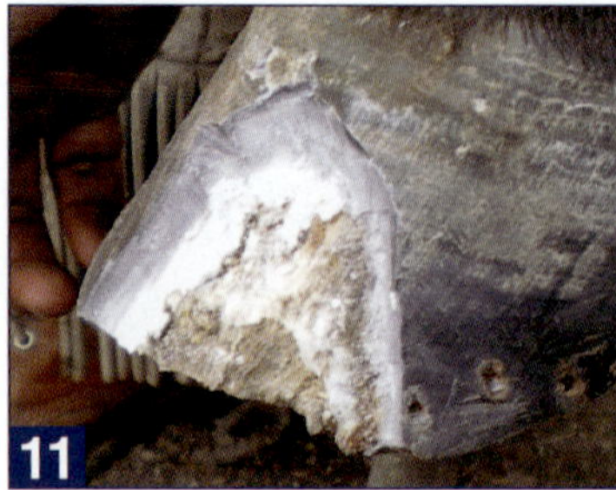

Resected as far as nippers will go.

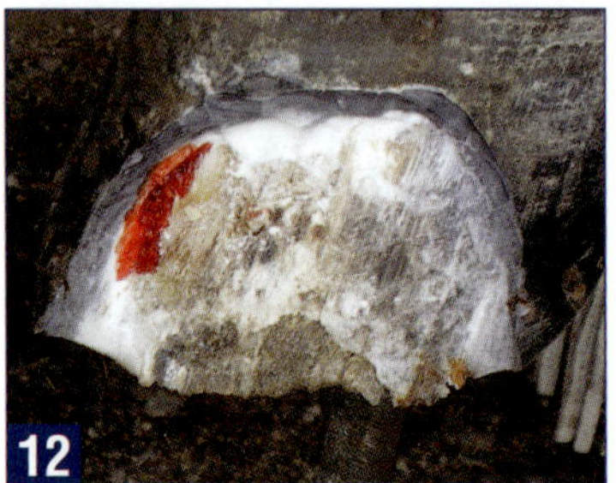

Finished resection with knife until blood was reached.

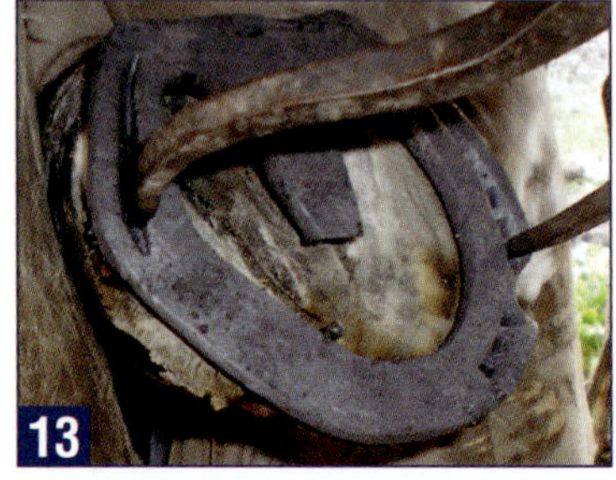

Heart bar being hot fit.

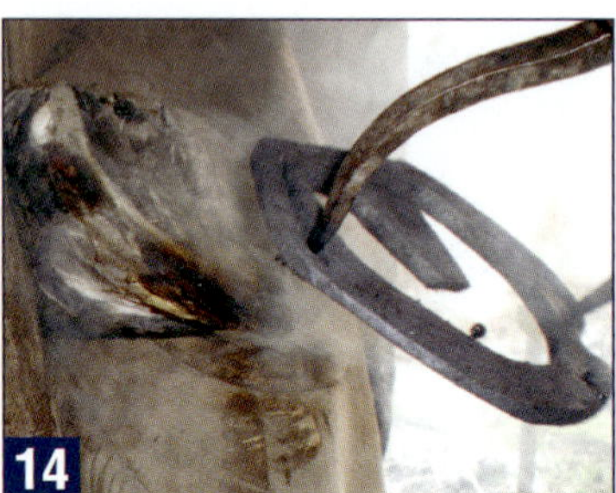

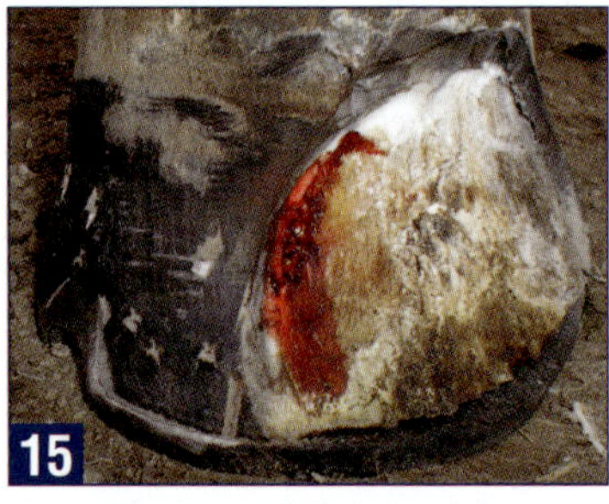

Dorsal view of finished foot.

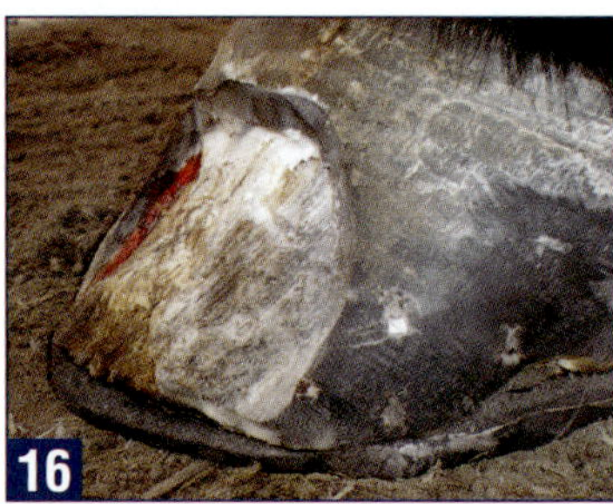

Lateral view of finished foot.

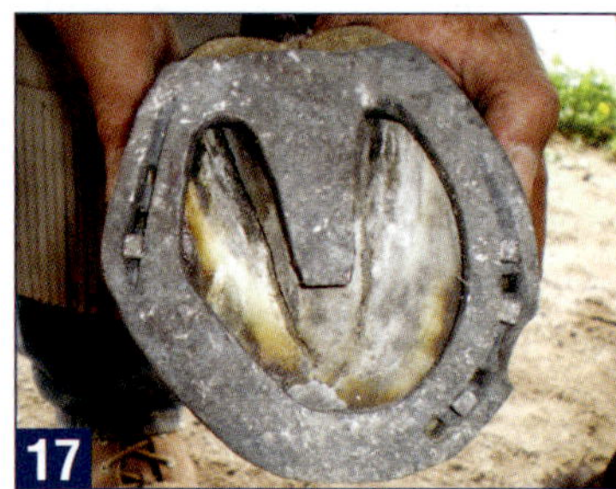

Heart bar on the foot.

In **Figure 9**, I have trimmed the bottom of the foot, and rasped a line in the wall to allow my nippers a place to grab to start the resection. In **Figure 10**, I am nipping the outer wall. Nippers get most of the wall removed **(Figure 11)**, and I use my knife on the rest until I hit blood **(Figure 12)**. Getting to blood in a WLD resection lets you know that you have reached the end of the infestation. However, it also increases the chance of getting an infection. A farrier should never voluntarily enter sensitive structures without a veterinarian's supervision.

I made a heart bar for the foot, and fit it up. In **Figures 13-14** the heart bar is being fitted. Notice that it is quite cool for a hot fit. The reason for this is that we are burning over the frog, and I do not like to put too hot a shoe on a structure with such high moisture content. It has the potential to transfer a lot of heat into the frog, like when a wet rag is used to pick up a hot plate. The heat can get through the wet rag easily. **Figures 15-16** show the outside of the foot with the shoe on, and **Figure 17** shows the bottom of the foot with the heart bar on it. This heart bar is made specifically for this foot, so it is shaped

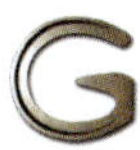

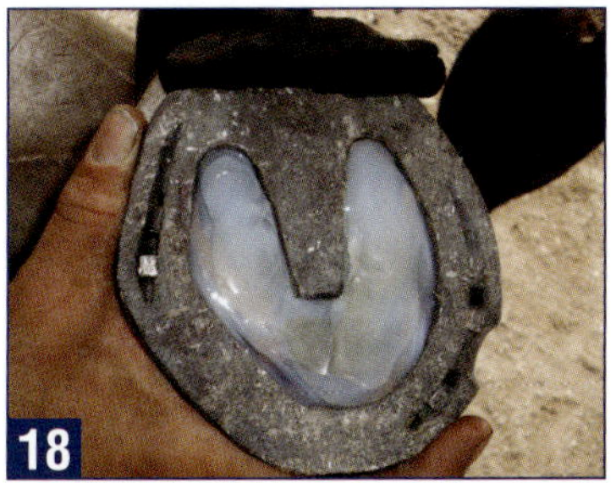

Filled with a pour in of Equi-Pak.

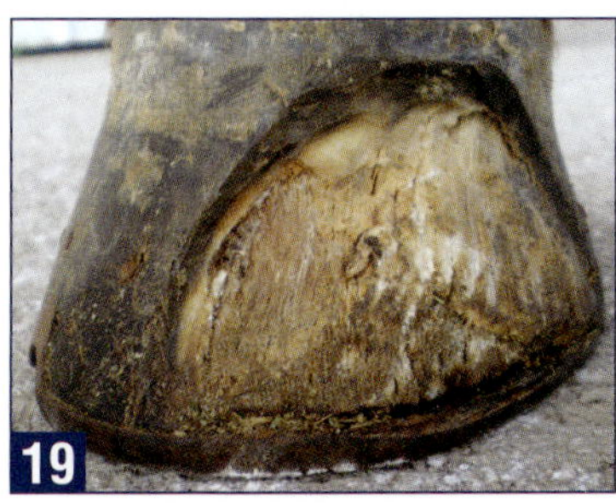

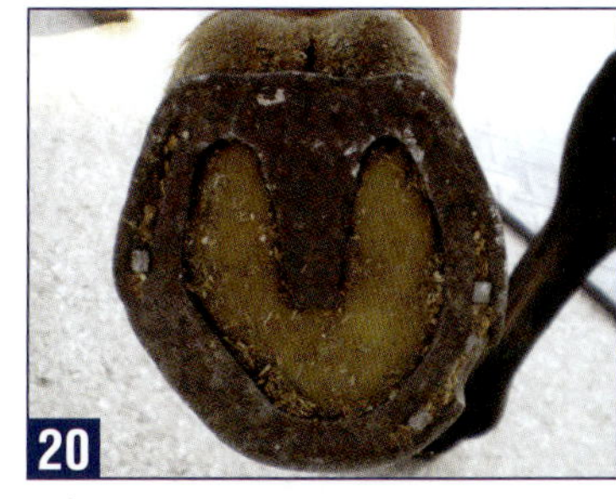

The foot at the next shoeing, well on its way to recovery.

exactly where I want it, and only has holes where I have foot that can take nails. The job is finished with Equi-Pak **(Figure 18)**, which I put in almost all heart bars to distribute weight as well as prevent the inherent problems of trapping debris that exist with a bar over the frog and commissures.

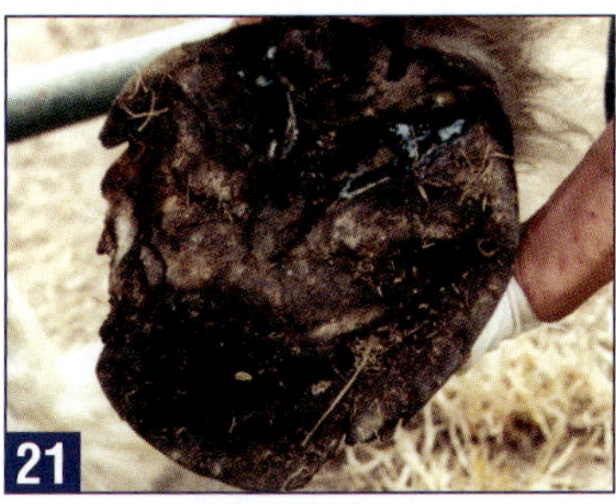

Sarah's foot when first presented.

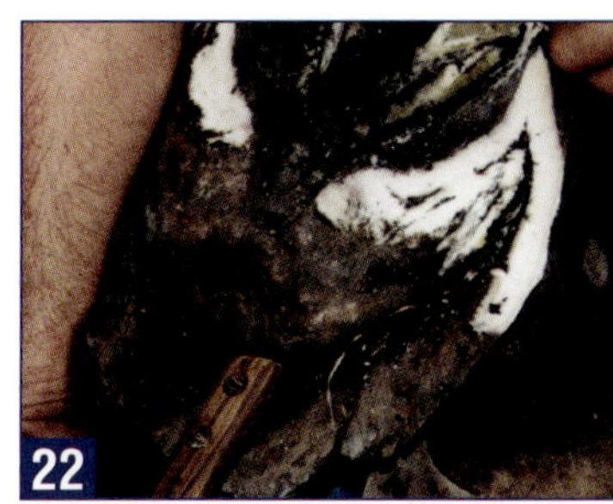

Hoof knife in the white line.

Resecting the hoof wall allows oxygen access to the bacteria, and this will kill it graveyard dead since it is anaerobic. To give me some insurance, I like to add the use of some commercial white line disease remedies to the equation. Grand Circuit makes a product known as White Lightning, which is a sodium chlorite. It is a bit labor intensive for the customer, but I have had good success on some bad cases with it. White Lightning requires the customer to mix the remedy with vinegar and place the foot and mixture in a bag that can be sealed at the top, and then left for 45 minutes per treatment. Grand Circuit makes a bag, but you can use a saline I.V. bag. When the White Lightning and vinegar is mixed, there is a chemical reaction that creates a vapor of chlorine dioxide. Chlorine dioxide is a gas that can't be stored, so it has to be created on site. The vapor is what you are trying to get into the white line disease, not the liquid. **Figures 19-20** are the foot on the next visit. This horse was shod with the heart bar for three shoeing cycles and fed Farriers Formula. He made a complete recovery.

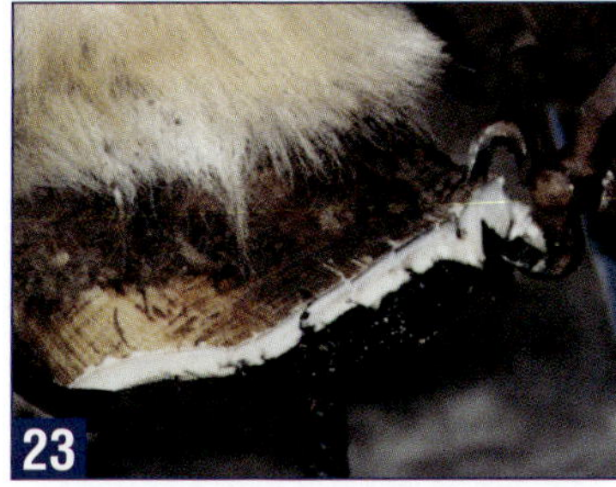

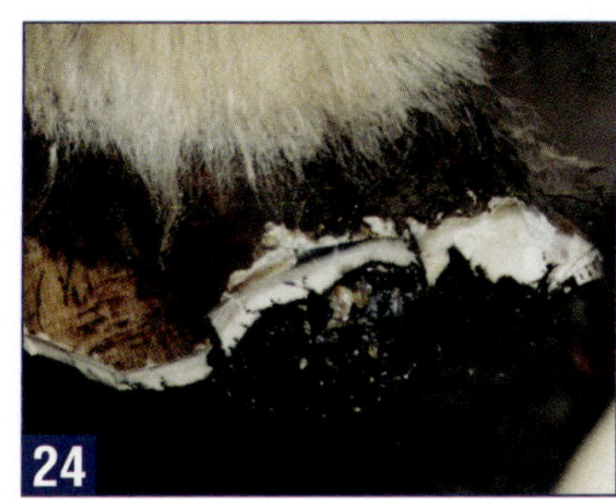

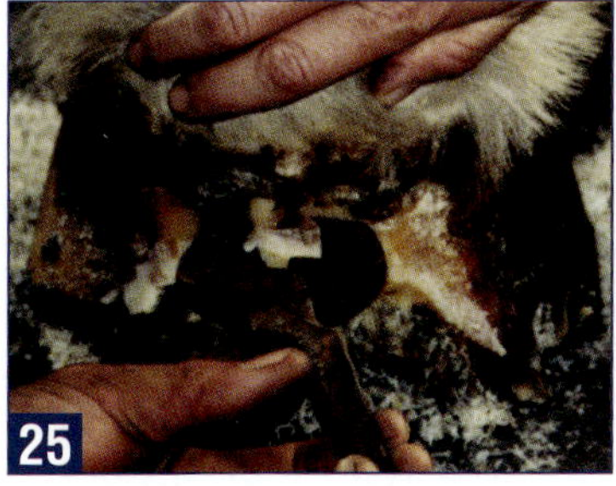

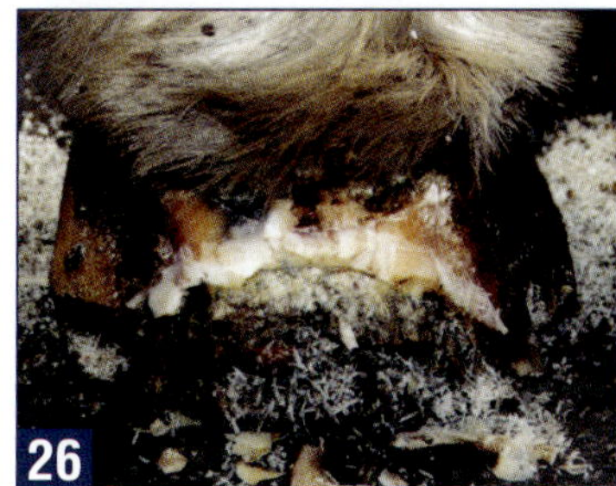

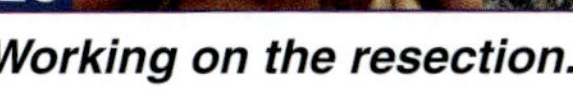

Working on the resection.

This next horse is a Clydesdale mare named

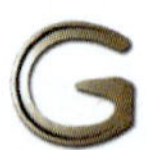

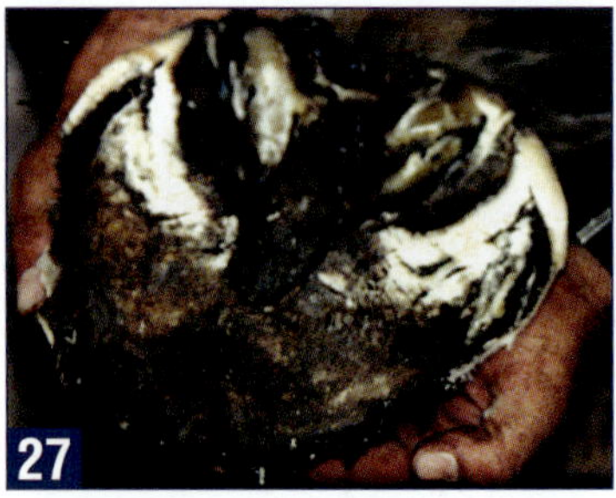

Trimmed and resected foot.

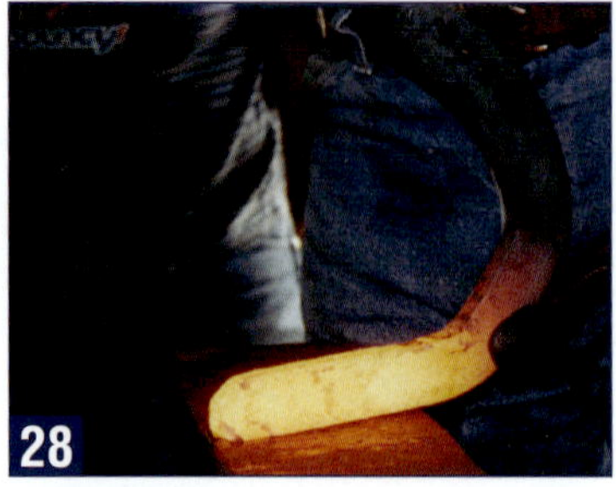

Making a draft W-shoe.

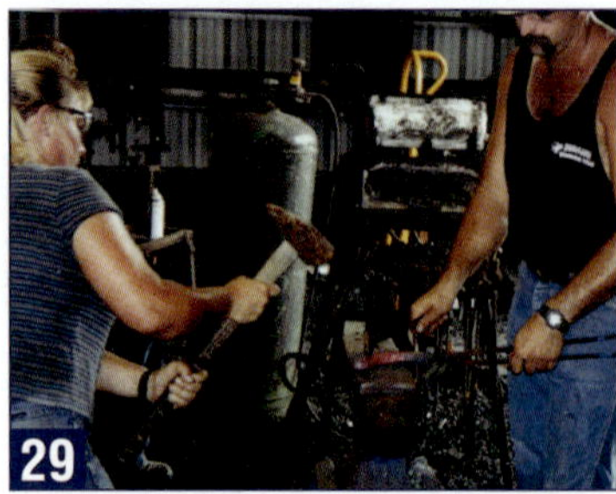

Kelly striking.

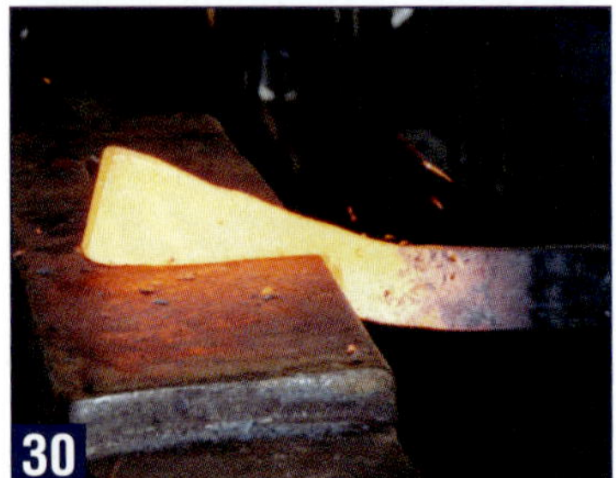

Making the frog plate.

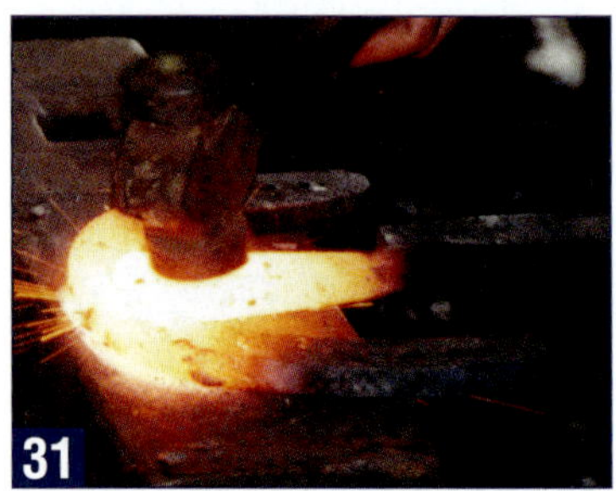

Jump welding the frog plate to the shoe.

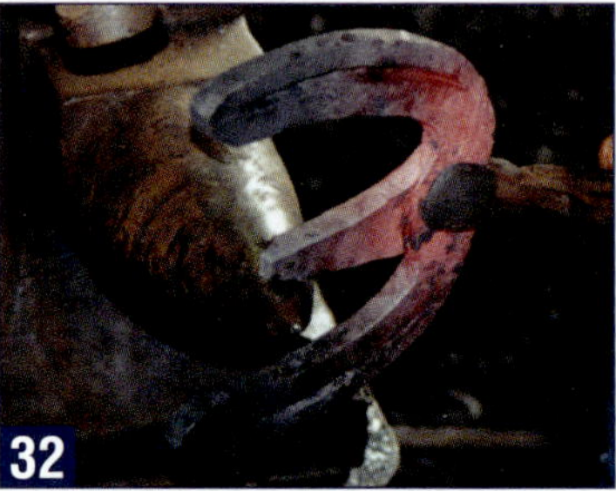

Shaping.

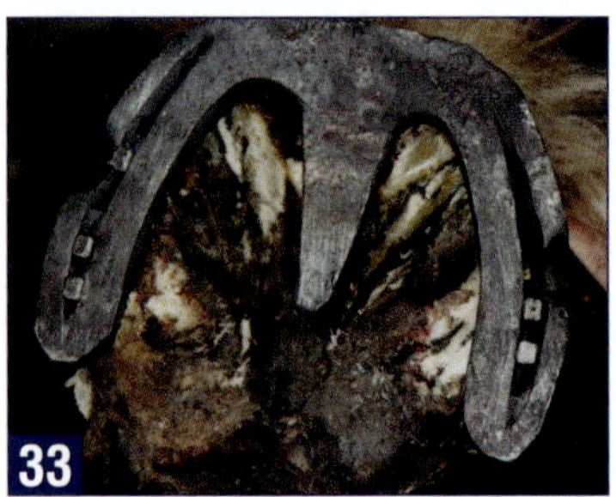

Finished job.

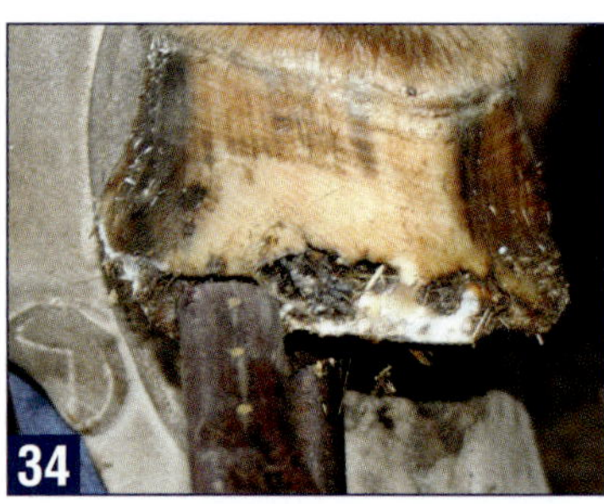

Foot with WLD, notice the knife sticking out of the separation.

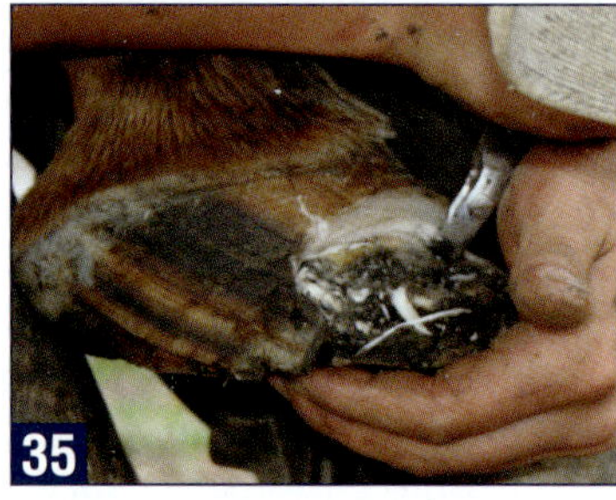

Cody doing a resection.

Sarah. A local vet had been treating Sarah for thrush for 11 months, but the foot continued to deteriorate. **Figure 21** shows the foot when we first saw her. In **Figure 22**, I have the blade of my hoof knife inserted into the white line area as far as the hilt will allow it to go. I began with the resection, **(Figures 23-26)** and ended up with the foot you see in **Figure 27**. Since so much of the toe is gone, I made a W-shoe for the foot. It is handy to have a striker anytime when making draft shoes, so Kelly has been recruited for the job in **Figure 29**. Most of the heart bars and W-shoes that I use have the frog plate jump-welded to the back of the shoe. That is what is taking place in **Figure 30**. The finished product is nailed on the foot in **Figure 31**. Sarah was shod with that shoe for about four resets and made a complete recovery. She was a difficult horse to treat due to her disposition, so her recovery was mainly due to the resection and not the application of a topical solution.

Cody is doing a similar job on a horse in the next series. In **Figure 34**, the WLD has destroyed a lot of the connection between the wall and coffin bone. Cody did a resection, **(Figure 35)**, and the

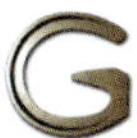

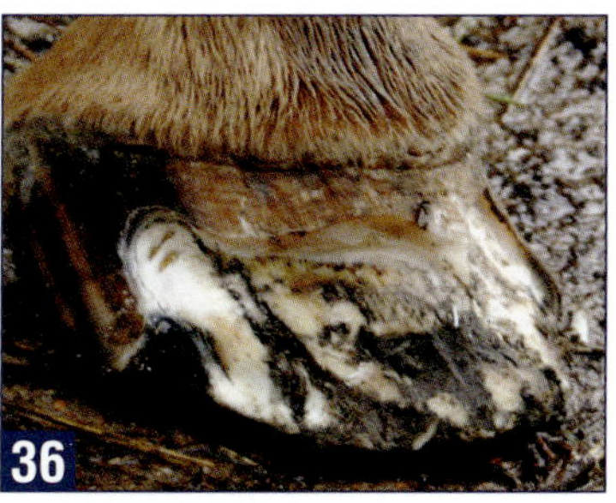

Resected foot.

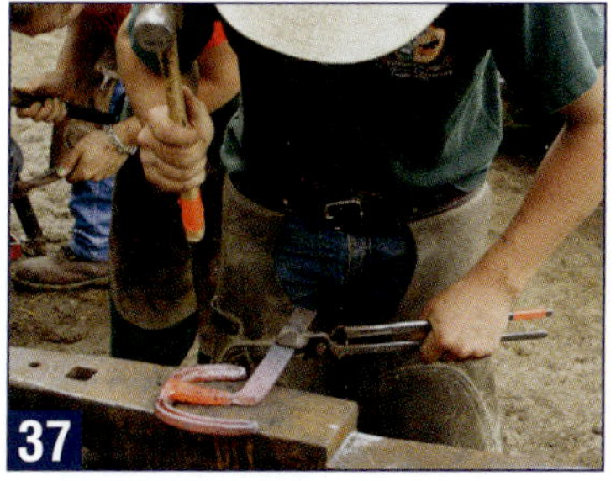

Cody making the W-shoe.

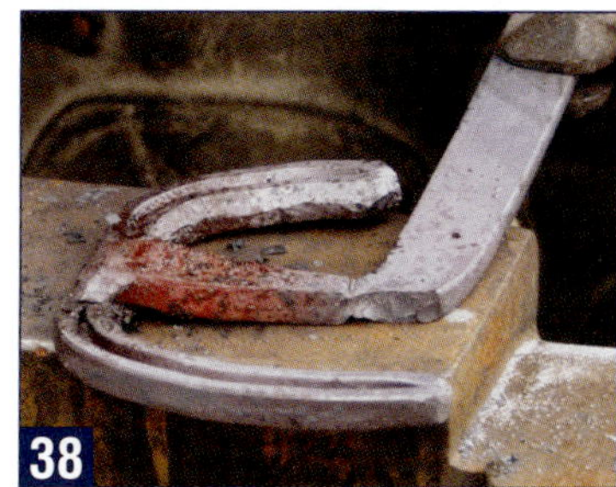

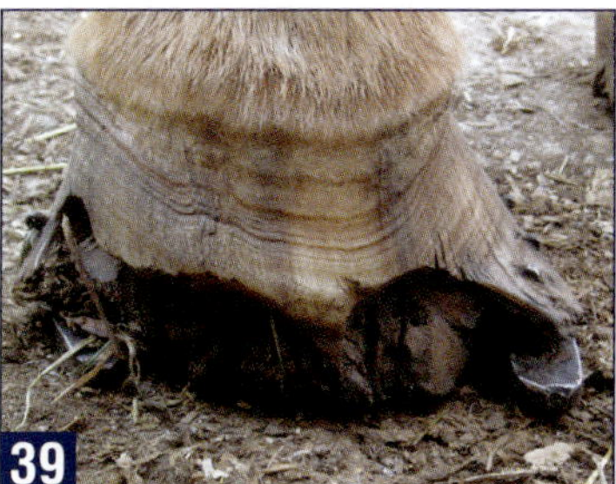

9-weeks later.

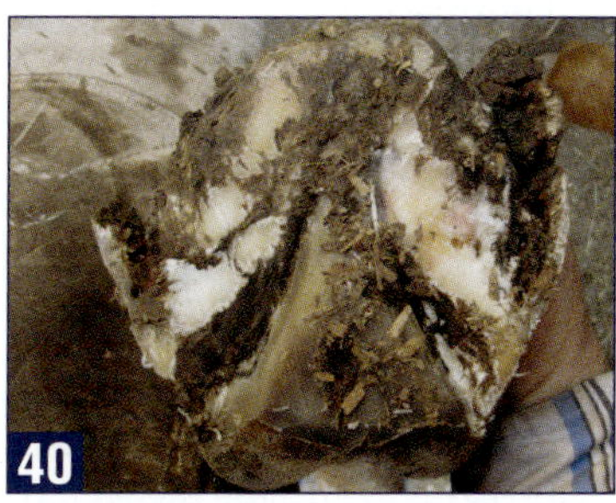

Trimmed foot ready to reset W-shoe.

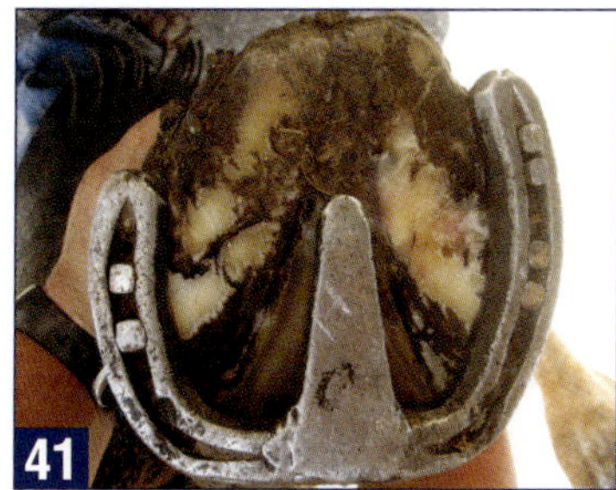

Views of foot with W-shoe.

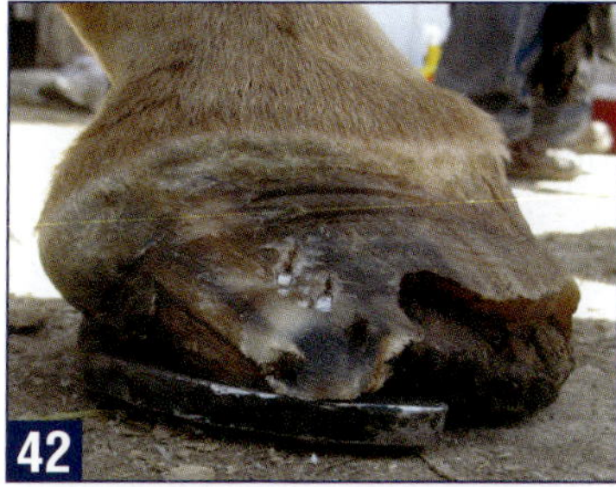
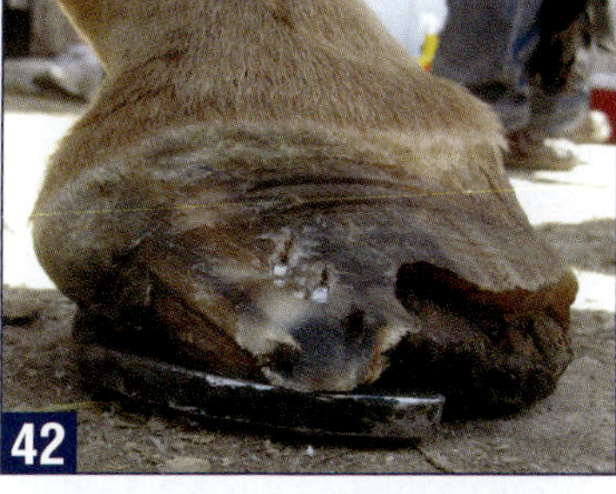

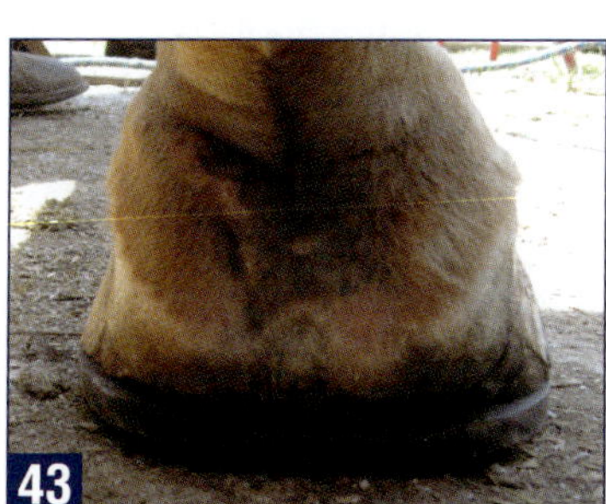

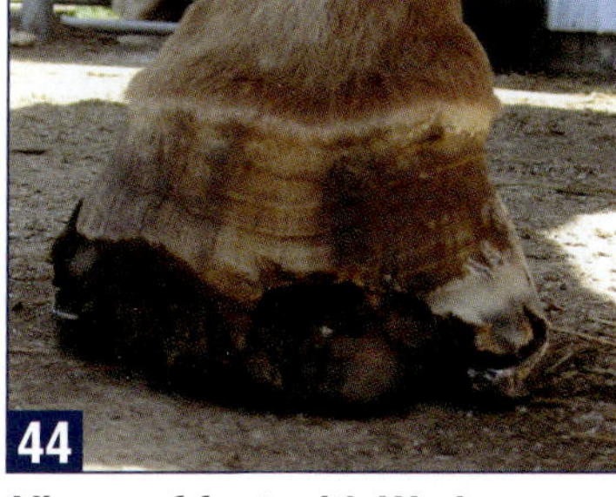

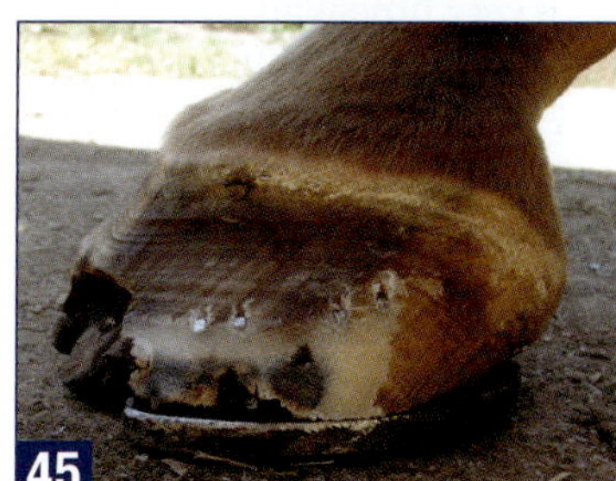

Views of foot with W-shoe.

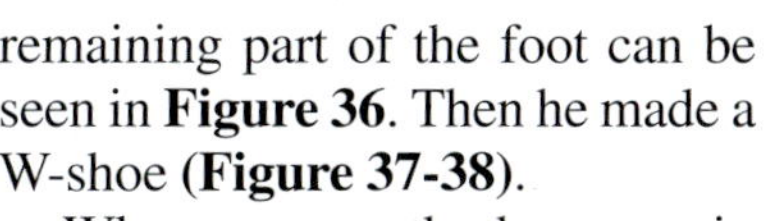

remaining part of the foot can be seen in **Figure 36**. Then he made a W-shoe **(Figure 37-38)**.

When we saw the horse again in about 9 weeks, the shoe was still on, and the foot had grown down **(Figure 39)**. **Figure 40** shows the shoe off and the foot trimmed. The W-shoe was nailed back on **(Figures 41-45)**, and the horse was more comfortable. At this writing, we were still waiting to see if it

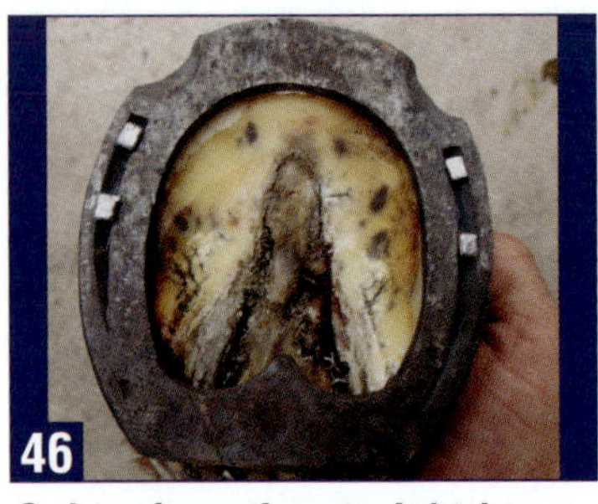

Solar view of a straight bar on a foot with some of the toe resected for WLD.

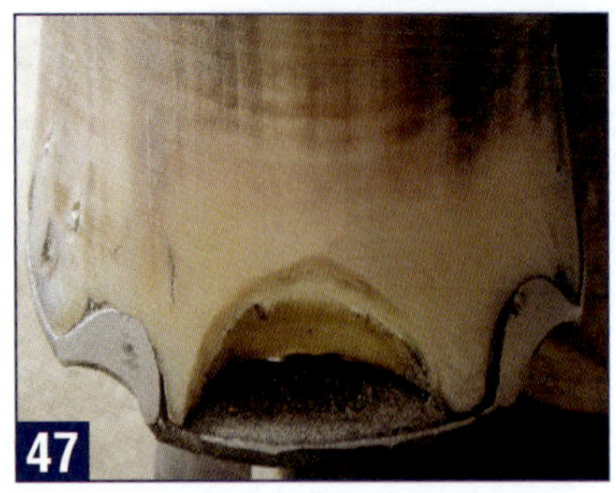

Dorsal view of the foot with the bar shoe from figure 46.

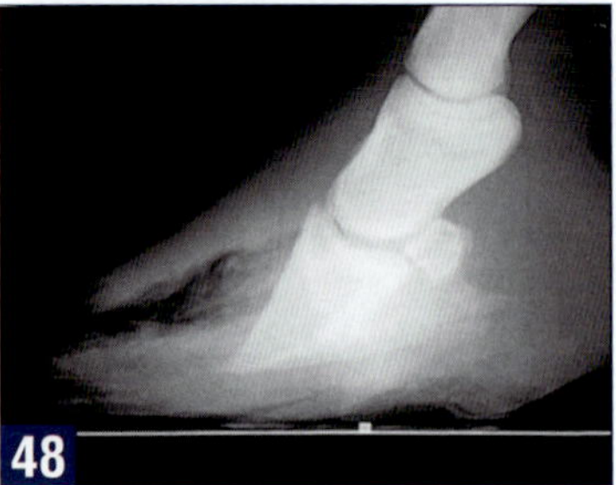

Radiograph of WLD.

would grow out all the way and return to normal.

Depending on how much material I have to remove and where it is, I prefer a bar shoe on any weakened foot. The foot in **Figures 46 and 47** was fairly weak to start with, so I decided that there was enough foot removed from a weakened foot to warrant the straight bar. This is a simple thing to do and is likely to keep the horse more comfortable.

Figure 48 is a radiograph of what WLD has done to a foot. This was taken by Dr. Scott Morrison.

On the feet that I am not requiring the customer to treat, I like to mix copper sulfate crystals with Keratex, then place it in the cavity where I have removed some hoof tissue. Copper sulfate is used as a root killer in septic systems as well as in ponds. You can buy it at most farm supply and hardware stores. The Keratex will keep the copper sulfate against the area where the white line disease is eating the foot, and this seems to help quite a bit as well. I only use this method on the smaller areas of white line disease, not the large ones.

Another thing I should mention is that we hot fit virtually every foot that we shoe. We also deal with very little white line disease, and I believe that the hot fitting is a big part of that. By hot fitting, we kill any fauna and flora on the bottom of the foot at least once every 5 to 7 weeks. The only proof I have that this works is the fact that we deal with so little WLD compared with a lot of shoers I know who only cold shoe.

Support the damaged foot until it grows sufficiently to be used as a normal foot again. This means that you have to be very direct with your customer since the horse is not lame. Using the horse too hard before the foot is strong enough can be devastating. The foot can be ripped apart, and dealing with that may make dealing with the white line disease seem small.

The vet can play a vital role in diagnosing WLD as well as recommending chemical remedies. For the owner's part, they need to follow the instructions for care from the vet and farrier to the letter. It may be labor intensive, but if the horse is worth it, the work involved won't be a problem.

ANTICIPATED OUTCOME

Some horses seem to really suffer with white line disease, so with these, you want to always be on the lookout for problems. Properly treating white line disease will generally allow the foot to return to normal once it grows out.

IN SHORT

D: Consumption of the white line and stratum internum by a bacteria and fungus combination.

T: Resection to allow exposure to oxygen followed by a shoeing strategy that supports whatever portion of the foot is left. Heart bar and W-shoe are commonly employed. Commercial remedies may be used as well.

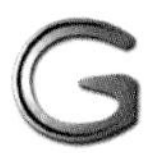

Chapter

46-1 BOWED TENDONS

DEFINITION

One of the flexor tendons has become injured from being strained. The fibers of the tendon have been stressed, and in almost all cases there is some degree of injury to the tendon itself.

REASON

A horse can bow a tendon for a variety of reasons, but the most common ones are: Overworking an under conditioned horse, poor conformation, taking a misstep, bad trimming and shoeing, and material fatigue. This injury is more common during hot and humid conditions, although it can happen in any climate.

ANATOMY

The majority of bowed tendons involve the superficial flexor tendon on the front leg, although the deep flexor can also be bowed. It is rare to see on the hind leg. Due to the mechanics, the palmar/plantar aspect of the tendon will have the most stress on it, thus it is the part of the tendon that generally has the most damage.

SYMPTOMS

A bowed tendon will present itself as a swelling on the back of the leg, and the horse will be quite lame. The more drastic the bow, the sorer the horse will be. This is a physical injury, which leads to inflammation of the tendon and the covering or sheath, so there will be pain, heat, and swelling. The bow can happen anywhere on the tendon, but it is most common in the middle in front leg injuries **(Figure 1)** and lower down in the rare hind leg bow **(Figure 2)**.

If the owner was using the horse when the tendon was injured, then you may have a story that goes with it to aid in diagnosis. You may also be able to determine the cause by looking at the shoeing or trimming on the foot as well as the conformation of the animal.

The horse will react to palpation of the inflamed

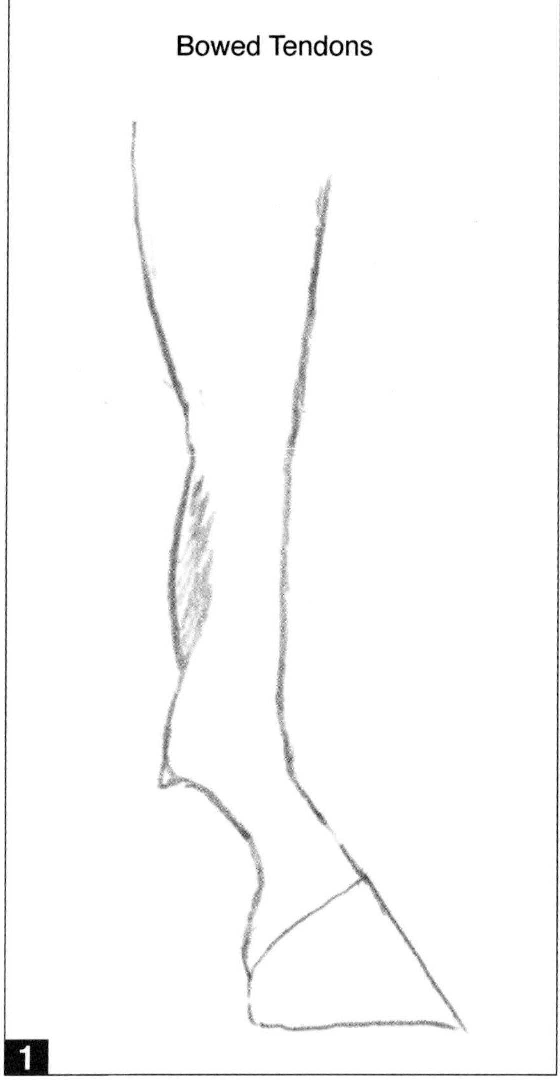

Drawing of a bowed tendon.

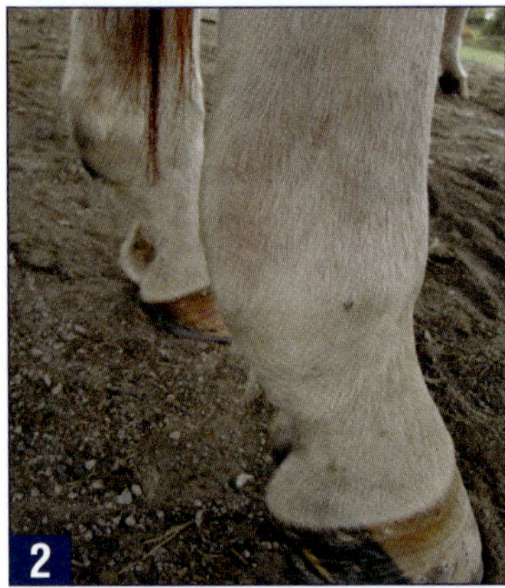

Swollen area from a sprained suspensory ligament where a bowed tendon on a hind leg will occur, close to the fetlock.

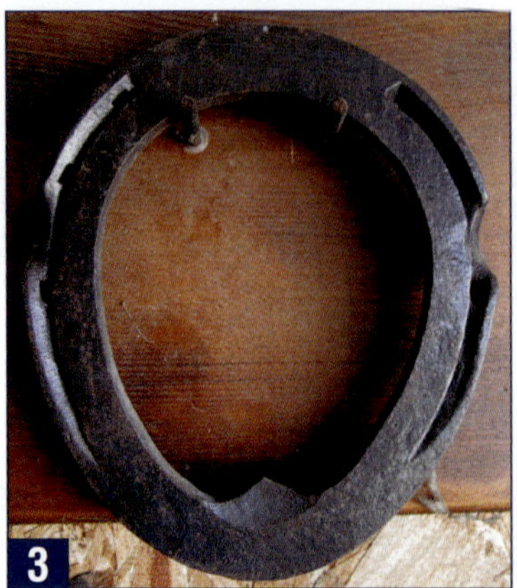

Egg bar shoe, although this one is missing the rocker toe.

tendon, and a vet can do an ultrasound to get a good picture of the damage.

TREATMENT

The first part of treating this horse is to determine which tendon is involved. You need to know with certainty so that you can trim to help the right anatomical structure. Trimming to help one tendon will end up placing stress on the other, so that makes knowing which one so important. If you cannot find out without a doubt, trim to the natural angle and follow the shoeing strategy outlined below.

If the deep flexor tendon is damaged, it can be relieved by increasing (long heel, short toe) the angle of the foot. The opposite is true if the injury occurred to the superficial flexor tendon. In that instance, you should decrease (low heel, long toe) the angle of the foot. Refer to the section on angles in **Chapter 12 Biomechanics** of this textbook if needed.

Regardless of which tendon is involved, you can shoe the horse with an egg bar shoe **(Figure 3)** and rocker toe. Putting a shoe that extends behind the heels will give support to the flexor tendons, and the rocker toe will keep them from having to work as hard when the horse is moving.

The leg should also be wrapped to help support the damaged tendon. Both legs should be wrapped since both legs went through the same thing. Even though just one got injured, that does not mean the other one was not stressed. The good leg should be trimmed to natural angle, but still should be shod with the egg bar and rocker toe.

This horse needs stall rest for the first 30 days, and then stall rest with a small run for the next 5 to 9 months. Hand-walk the horse for 10 minutes a day after 30 days and increase that slowly over time. Reset the shoes at shorter than normal intervals. Doing so will keep the injured tendon from becoming stressed from improper hoof angles or excessive leverage from too long a toe.

Veterinarians may use anti-inflammatory medicines, prescribe ice or cold water therapy, suggest astringents if they desire, and can assist in the diagnosis. Pressure from tendon swelling under a tight annular ligament can complicate treatment. Annular ligaments are not elastic, so if there is swelling within them, they may need to be surgically released by the veterinarian. The owner's role is to stable the horse, change the wraps, and apply the therapy prescribed.

There is such a thing as a "bandage bow." This happens when a leg wrap has been left on too long and is too tight. The tendon itself is not necessarily damaged, just the connective tissue around it. Rest for up to a week will generally allow this to heal with no long-term problems.

ANTICIPATED OUTCOME

Once the tendon heals, it will generally have a thickened and woody feel to it. The collagen fibers that have healed the tendon will not be as strong as the original tendon, and they tend to be more elastic. The horse may become sound, but it will be prone to having tendon issues again. Be certain to shoe this horse forevermore with the injury in mind. This means trimming to accommodate the tendon that was bowed and applying as much extension as safely possible behind the heel.

IN SHORT

D: Inflamed tendon, mainly the superficial flexor tendon.

T: Trim to relax injured tendon and shoe with an egg bar and rocker toe. Horse needs to be on stall rest for several months, and both legs need wrapped.

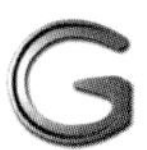

Chapter

46-2 BROKEN BONES

DEFINITION

With a broken leg, any of the bones in the limb may be fractured. When any of the long bones are broken, it is usually a devastating and fatal

REASON

Direct trauma is the usual reason, and the variables are numerous; from getting kicked by another horse to running into an object at speed.

ANATOMY

Any long bone in the limb may be involved. Fractures of the coffin bone and cuboidal bones are not being addressed in this section.

SYMPTOMS

In this section, I am going to cover a couple kinds of breaks. One is called a saucer fracture, and the other is a complete break.

With a saucer fracture, there will be a small portion of the bone that has been splintered away from the main bone. This can be seen in **Figure 1**. The saucer fracture will often be the result of a direct trauma, and if the skin is broken, there will be a sore and possibly proud flesh that will not heal. With an X-ray, the portion of the bone that has been splintered will be readily apparent **(Figure 1)**.

With a complete break, there will be a bone in the leg that has been broken into two or more pieces. This has happened to the horse in **Figures 2-5**. The horse is unable to bear weight on the injured limb and there is quite a bit of swelling. As you can see in **Figure 5**, the leg can be bent at unnatural angles and from unusual locations.

The broken bone in **Figures 6-7** is the radius of a brood mare that was kicked by another horse. The amount of change that occurred as the body tried to deal with the break over a long time is evident from the broken ends of the bone. I destroyed this horse for the owner and was appalled that the horse was allowed to suffer for so long. With an injury of this magnitude, euthanasia or heroic effort at fixing are called for.

TREATMENT

The saucer fracture falls under the vet realm, and the splinter of bone is surgically removed. A farrier may end up putting a rest shoe like the patten bar on the horse if the wound is in a place that has a lot of movement, and the owner will have to doctor the horse through the healing process. Depending on the location, the horse may or may not be lame.

With the catastrophic complete break, it is often in the best interest of the horse to destroy it. The horses that I have been involved with do not seem to be in extreme pain in the first few hours after the break. This is probably a result of shock. Plates, screws, surgery, prosthetics, and other options can

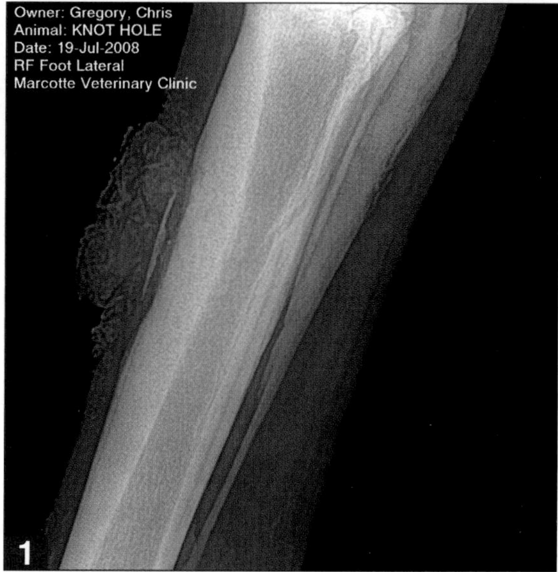

Radiograph of a saucer fracture on the cannon bone.

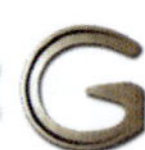

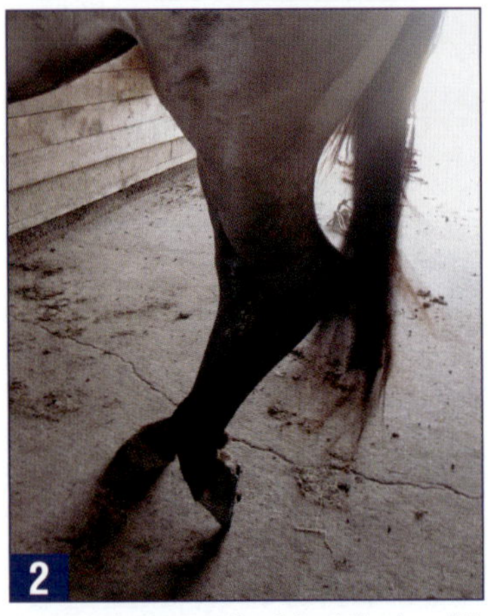

Lateral view of a hind limb with a broken tibia.

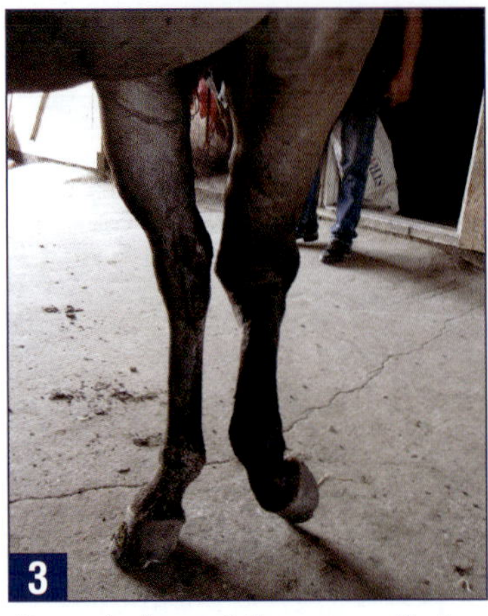

Dorsal view of the same limb.

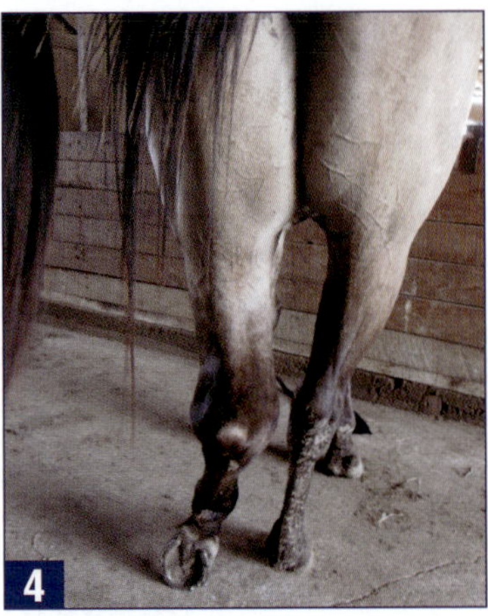

Caudal view of the broken tibia.

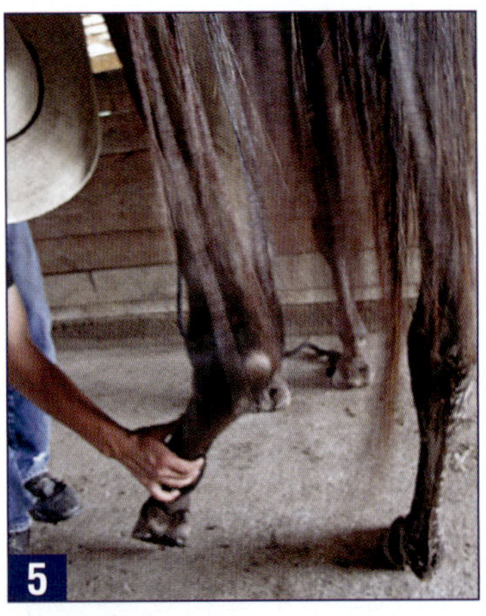

The leg is being pulled out to show where the break occurred. Compare to Figure 4.

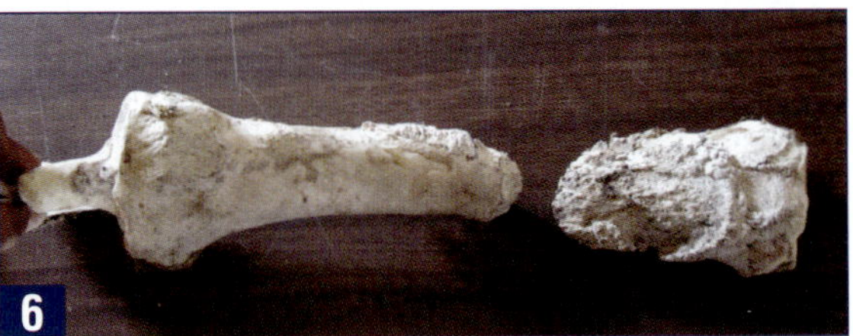

Cranial view of a broken humerus.

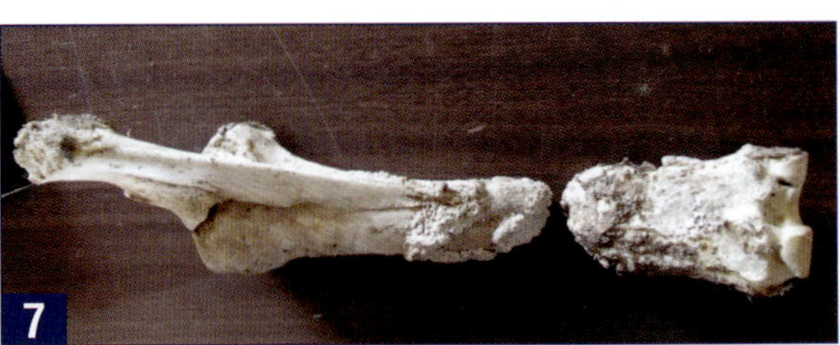

Caudal view of a broken humerus.

be tried, but the limitations of the animal should be carefully considered.

ANTICIPATED OUTCOME

With the saucer fracture, horses tend to heal with a scar but no lameness. With the complete break, euthanasia is often the outcome. In the event that the horse is salvaged, return to work is not likely.

IN SHORT

D: A bone has been fractured.

T: Surgery, possible rest shoe, (patten bar), cast, and stall rest; or euthanasia.

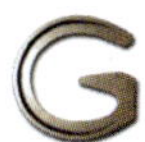

Chapter 46-3 BUCKED SHINS

DEFINITION

The cannon bone has become bowed toward the dorsal aspect.

REASON

This happens most often in young racehorses. As they race, the cannon bones will flex and bend from the forces put on them, and this can cause small cortical fractures on the dorsal part of the cannon bone. The body responds by laying down more bone cells, and this causes the cortex to thicken and the bone to bow.

ANATOMY

Primarily the cannon bone.

SYMPTOMS

When it is first occurring, there may be mild lameness, but inflammation on the front of the cannon bones will be present. Once it has become a complete bucked shin, there will not be inflammation, but the cannon bone will appear bowed from a lateral view.

TREATMENT

The horse should be examined every time it is worked out for pain or swelling over the front of the cannon bones. If either is present, then the workload should be decreased. This doesn't mean stopped, rather, just less and slower. As the inflammation disappears, the horse can be pushed again. This usually takes about 30 days. This is a bone modeling process.

It used to be common to pinfire horses with bucked shins, but as far as I know, this does not speed the recovery. Once a horse has been pinfired, there will often be scars that identify the spots of trauma (**Figures 1-3**).

If the shoes have excessive toe grabs or traction, then backing off may be preventive. Ice and water therapy may help.

ANTICIPATED OUTCOME

This is generally not too bad a problem unless owners or trainers who don't know what they are doing push the horse beyond reason. It will result in a blemish, but not a permanent lameness.

IN SHORT

D: The cannon bone has become bowed.

T: Careful training to prevent irreparable damage.

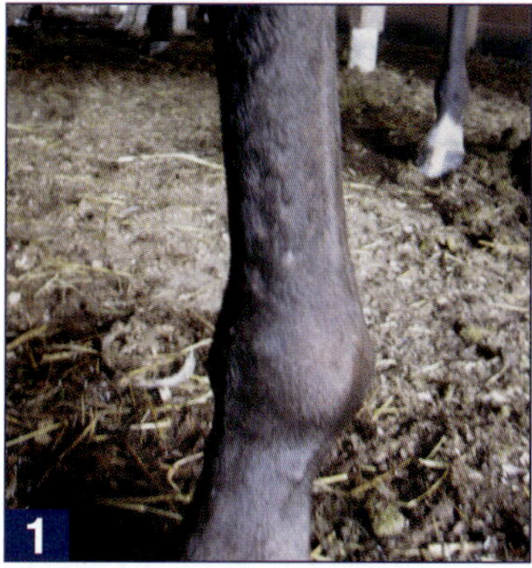

Photo of a horse that was pin-fired for bucked shins.

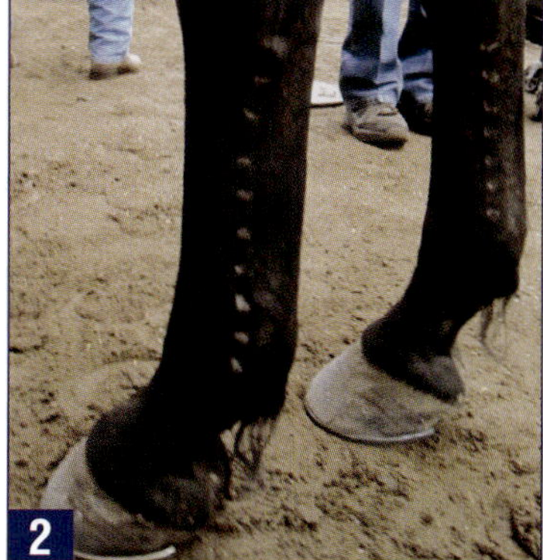

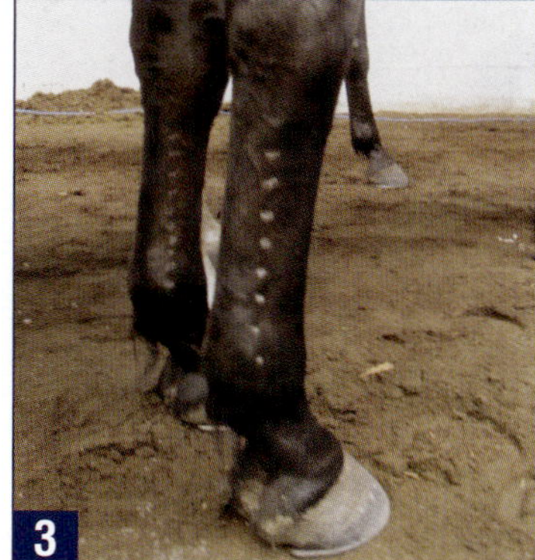

A horse that was pin-fired, but I don't know what they were pin-firing it for.

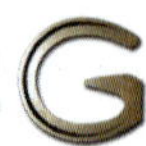

Chapter

46-4 CAPPED HOCKS AND ELBOWS

DEFINITION

Capped hocks and capped elbows are large soft swellings at the point of the hock and the point of the elbow, respectively. This is a swelling of the subcutaneous bursae (acquired bursitis) over the tuber calcaneus (hock) or olecranon process (elbow). A capped elbow is also known as a shoe boil, especially when long extended heels on a foot with a lot of action have caused the capped elbow.

REASON

These swellings happen from direct and repeated trauma to these locations. In the case of the capped hock, the horse is often a stall kicker. Poorly made roping boxes can also put repeated and direct trauma on this area. Capped elbows often result from horses laying down on hard ground, long-term injuries that cause a lot of lying down, or a shoe hitting the elbow from extreme action in that limb. The shoes on opposite feet have been implicated, with people claiming that these feet hit the elbow, but I have not seen this. Some blame the hind foot on the same side, some the hind foot on the opposite side, and many think it is caused by the inside of the opposite front foot. In any of these instances, I think it is more likely that the ground the horse was rolling around on is the culprit.

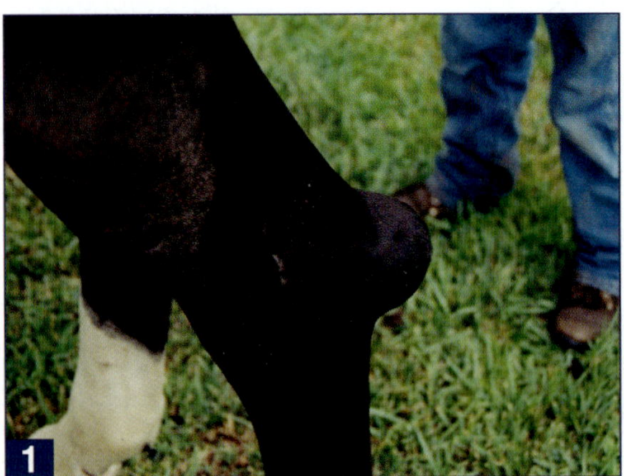

Old capped hock.

ANATOMY

The bursae of the point of hock and the point of elbow.

SYMPTOMS

In the early stages, the swelling can be as large as a grapefruit. Lameness is not associated with capped hocks and elbows, and the swelling will be soft at first. Within weeks, a firm fibrous capsule forms. It will end up being a tough pad of scar tissue.

TREATMENT

In the early stages of a capped hock or elbow, cold water or ice can be helpful. Capped hocks and elbows can also be drained. Draining is especially important if the swelling becomes infected. Older injuries can be surgically removed by a veterinarian. If these are left untreated, the body will absorb the fluid, and the horse will end up with a pad of scar tissue as a blemish. This is what has happened to the horses in **Figures 1-4**. **Figure 1** shows an old capped hock, and **Figures 2-4** show old capped elbows.

To prevent these, direct trauma to this area has to be removed. This can be done by preventing stall kicking and using better-made roping boxes for the capped hocks. For capped elbows that occur from laying on hard surfaces, deep bedding is an obvious

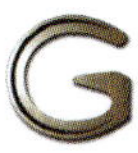

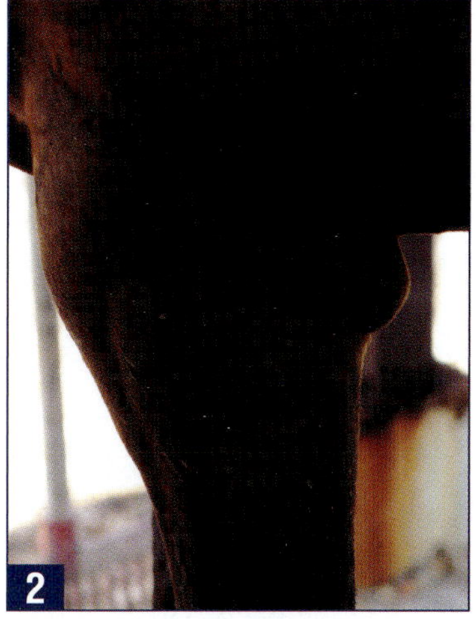

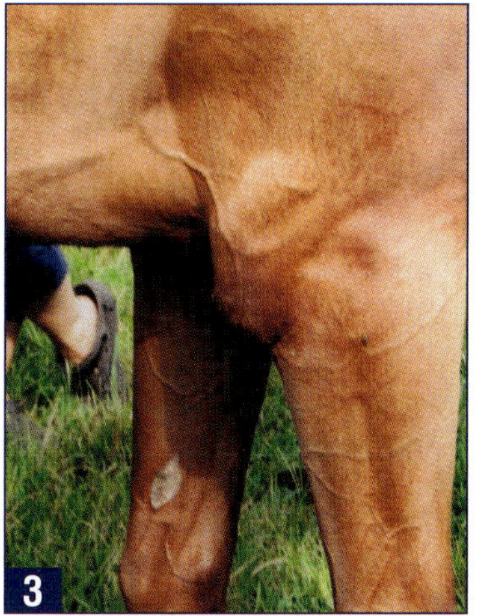

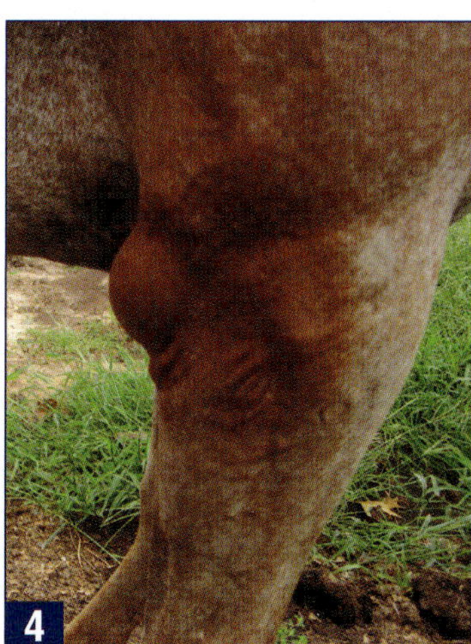

Old capped elbows.

answer. I don't think that horses hit themselves in the elbow that often with other feet while lying down, so shoeing to prevent that is not likely to help. Horses that hit themselves in movement can be shod with lighter or shorter shoes to prevent the collision between the shoe and the elbow. A device known as a sausage pad, shoe boil roll, or donut can also be placed on the pastern to prevent the hit. **Figure 5** is a drawing of a shoe boil roll. It is a padded protective apparatus that is attached to the leg with buckles or Velcro.

Vets may inject corticosteroids or do surgery to drain or remove the scar tissue. They may also advise on the use of ice or liniments. The owner can provide an environment that eliminates the trauma, such as the roping boxes and bedded stalls. They can also provide protection as seen in **Figure 5**.

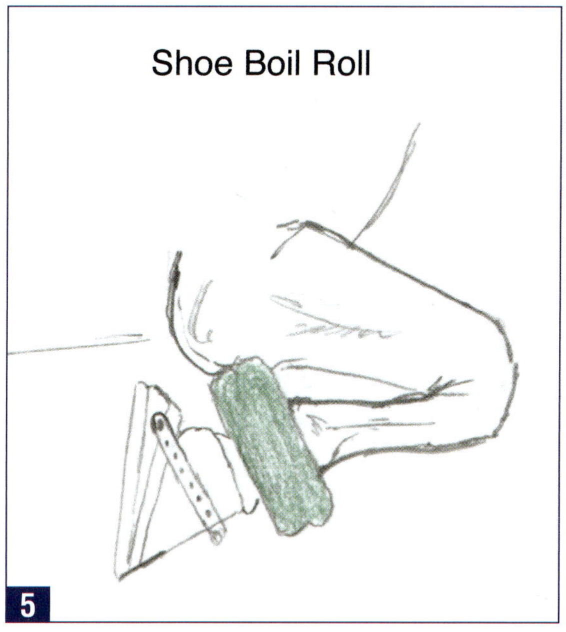

ANTICIPATED OUTCOME

Since the horse is not lame, I would expect the horse to continue to be sound.

IN SHORT:

D: Soft swelling at the point of hock or elbow.

T: Ice or cold water early, possible drainage, or nothing.

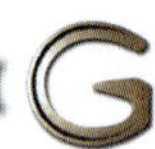

Chapter

46-5 CARPITIS

DEFINITION

If you break the word down, this term would mean inflammation in the knee. However, most of the time it is used, it is referring to actual osteoarthritis (degenerative joint disease) of the knee.

REASON

The most common reason for this condition is conformation and use of the horse. Heredity plays a big role in conformation, and horses that suffer from carpus varus seem to be the most prone to carpitis. This condition is also common in horses that have been used with heavy loads or on hard terrain.

ANATOMY

Any of the carpal bones can be affected, but the resulting bone growths are generally dorsal medial. As such, the intermediate carpal bone is almost always involved.

SYPTOMS

Carpitis can be articular or nonarticular. If it is nonarticular, there will be a hard swelling on the dorsal medial aspect of the carpus, but the horse will not be lame. If a flexion test is performed on the knee, it may elicit a response. All three of the horses in **Figures 1-3** would be considered sound if judged solely on how they moved, even though their knees are obviously abnormal.

If the bone growth is articular, the horse will be lame and reluctant to bend the knee. This can be a real challenge working on the foot. **Figure 4** is of a relatively small bone growth, yet this horse was quite lame. This indicates that articular carpitis may not always look that bad, but it can be devastating nonetheless. The horses in **Figures 5-17** are all suffering from the disease and all are lame, varying from Grade 2 to Grade 4.

If the knee finally fuses completely, the horse will become comfortable again because the damaged knee is not being moved. At this point, it is all but impossible to work on the feet without being inventive. When a horse with a fused knee moves, the limb is moved forward as a whole without flexing at the knee. It is very obvious when you see a horse moving like that, especially if they are moving at anything faster than a walk.

TREATMENT

There is not much that can be done for a horse with carpitis. From a farrier's perspective, all that can be done is to trim, level, and balance the foot (TLB). We will sometimes put shoes on to protect from uneven and unusual wear. When working on these horses, try to bend the knee as little as

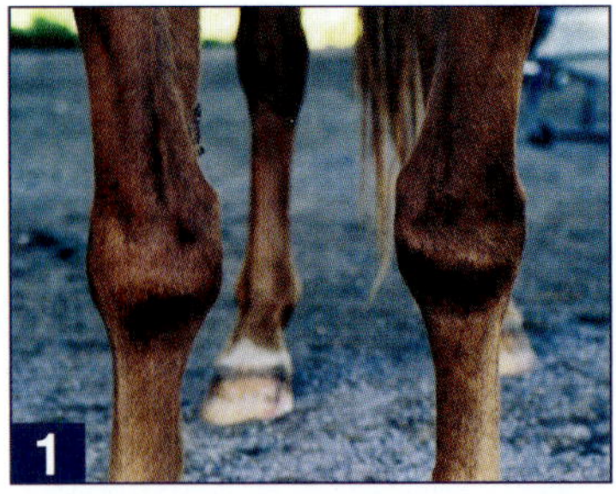

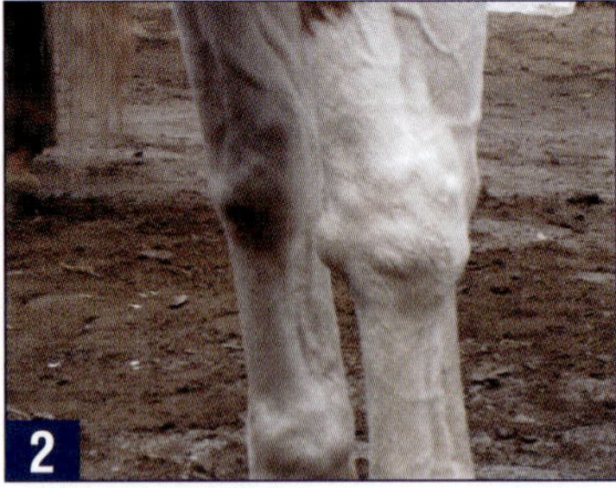

3

Pictures of some horses with nonarticular carpitis.

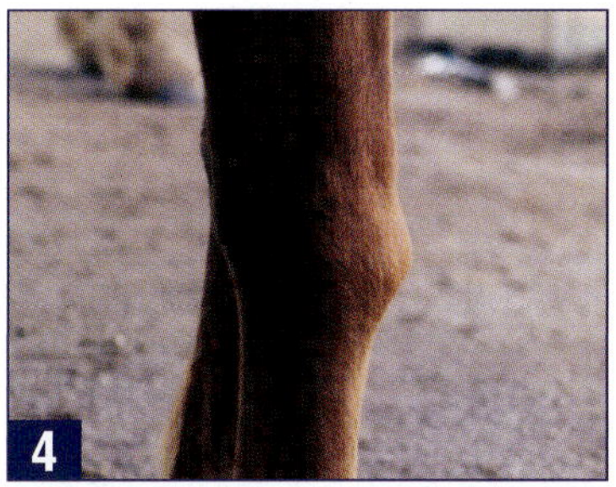
Lateral view of a small bone growth in the knee, yet the horse is still lame.

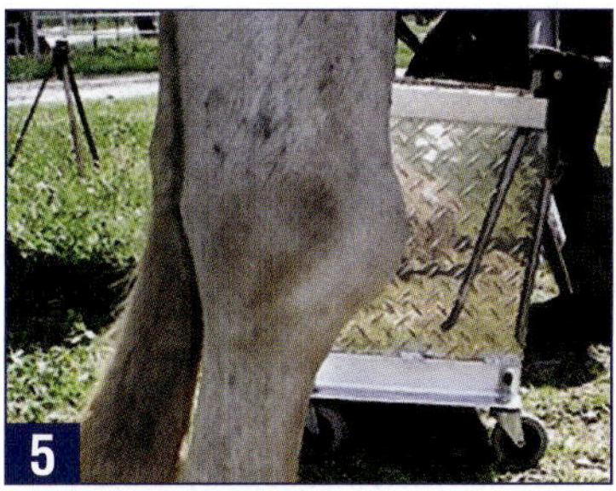
Lateral view of a big bone growth in the knee.

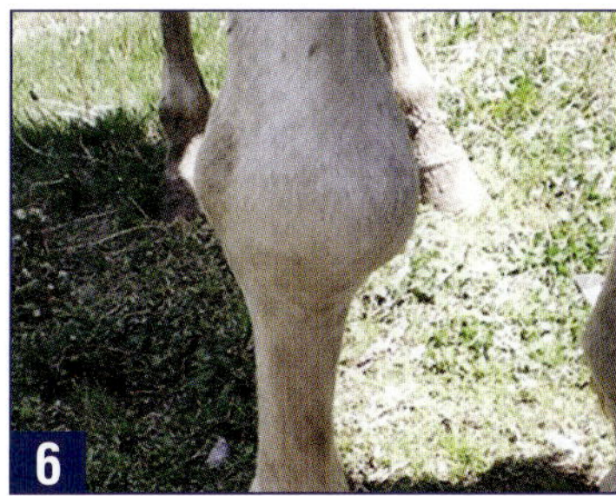
Dorsal view of the knee in Figure 5.

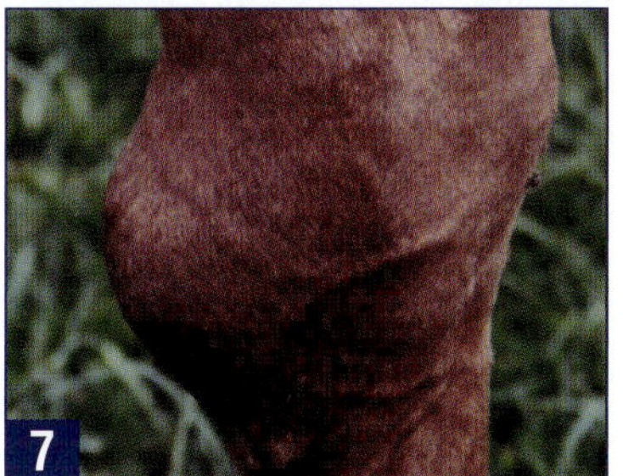
Lateral view of big growth.

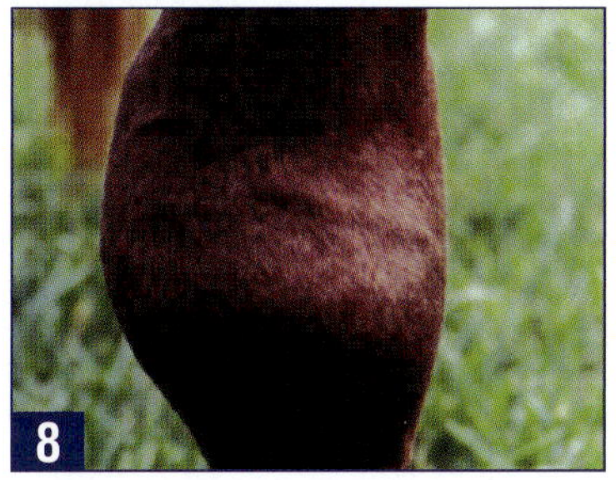
Dorsal view of the knee in Figure 7.

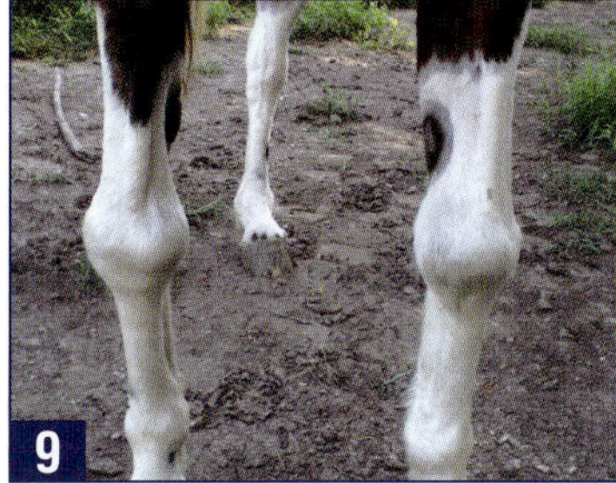
Dorsal view of carpus varus with carpitis.

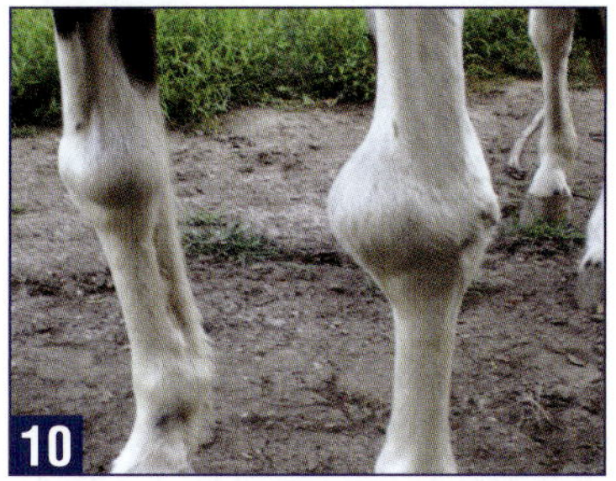
Dorsal lateral view of the horse in Figure 9.

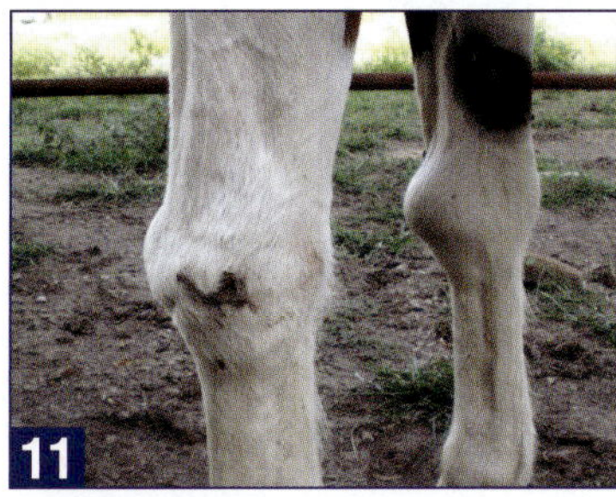
Lateral view of the horse in Figures 9 and 10.

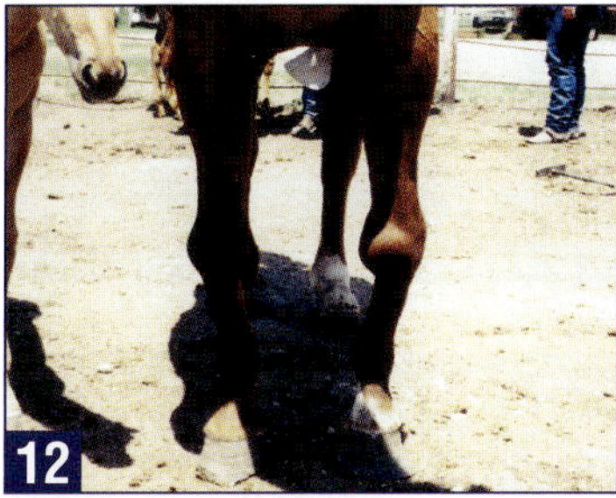
Brood mare with bad carpitis.

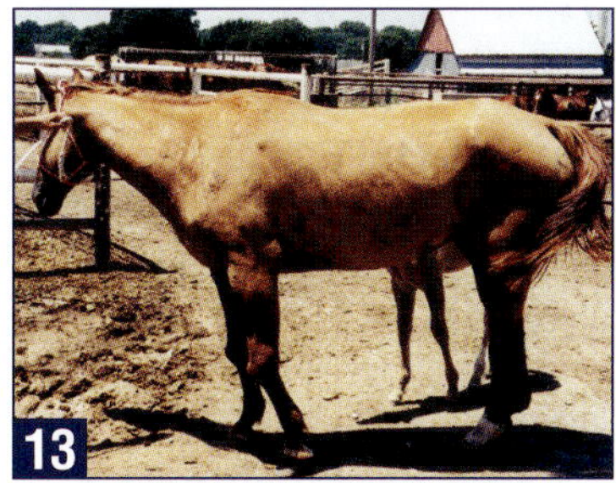
Lateral view of the horse in Figure 12.

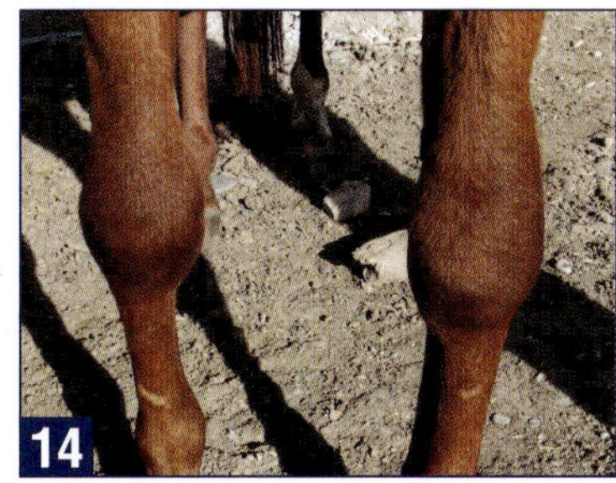
Dorsal view of carpitis.

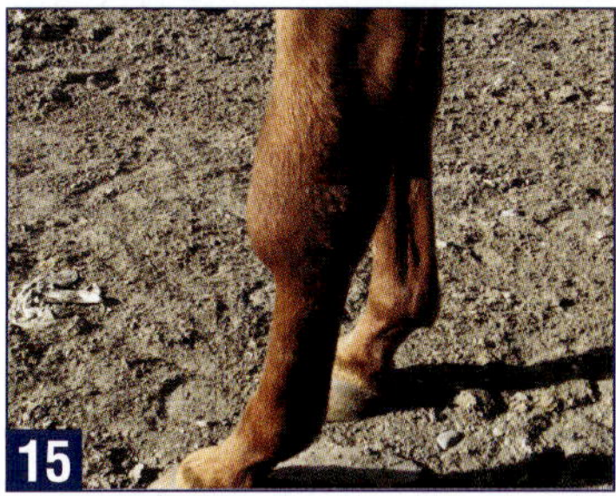
Lateral view of the horse in Figure 14.

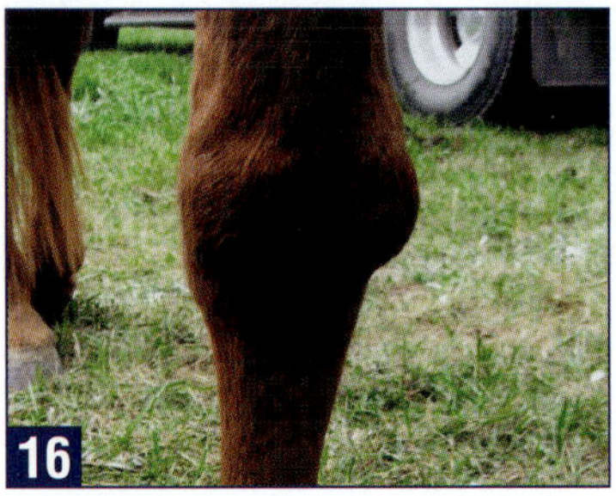

16

17

Carpitis.

18

19

20

21

22

23

24

25

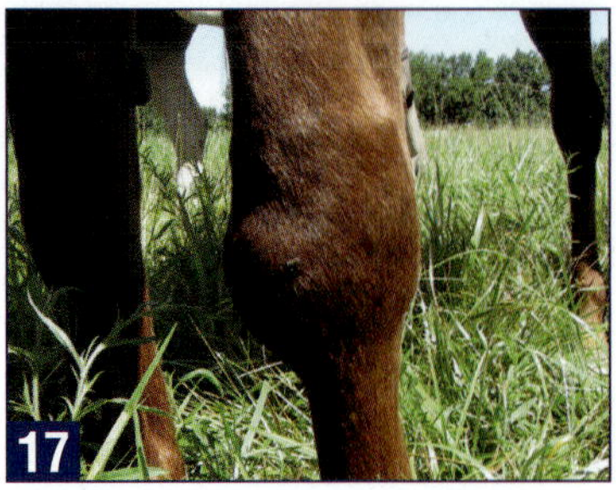

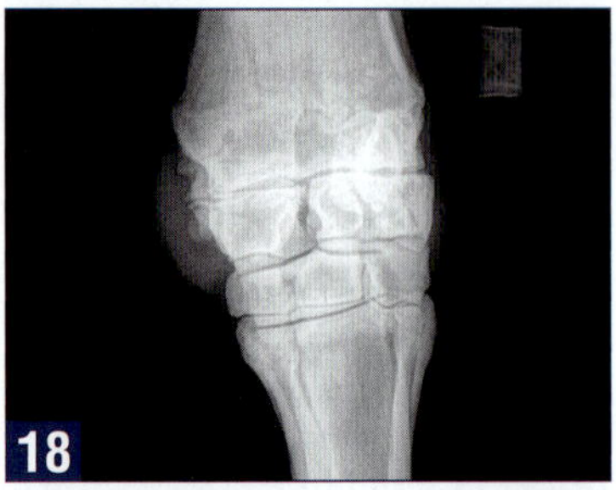

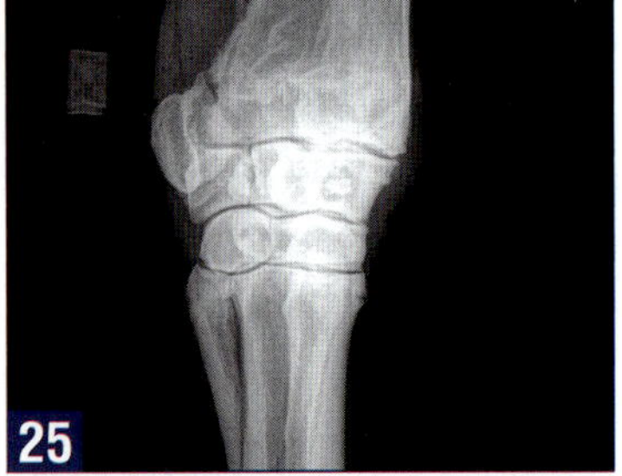

Figures 18 - 24 are various bad knees, courtesy of Dr. Marcotte.

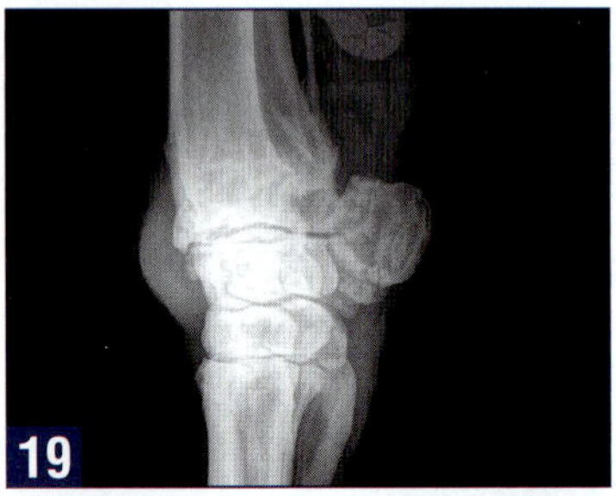

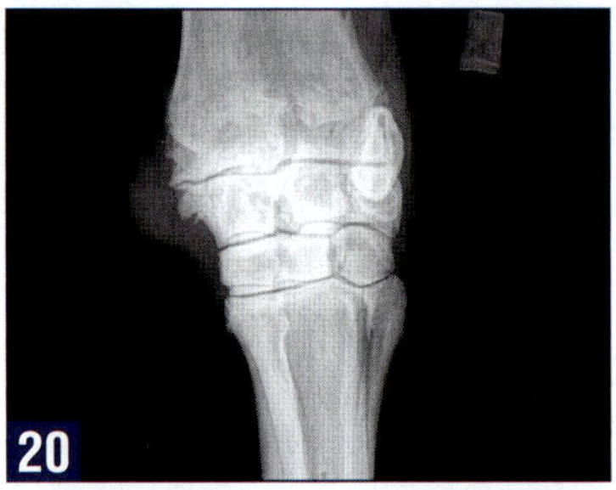

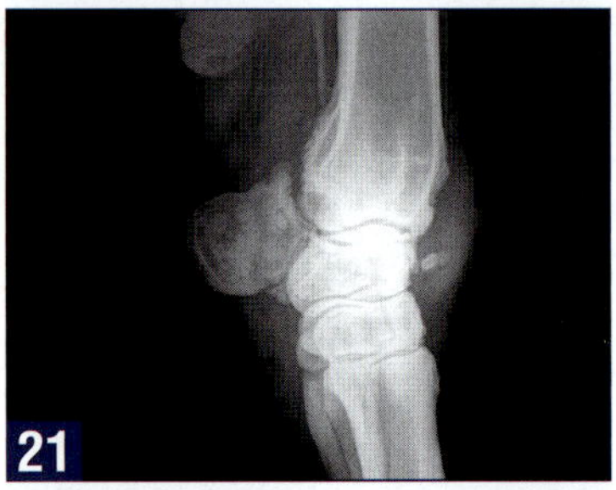

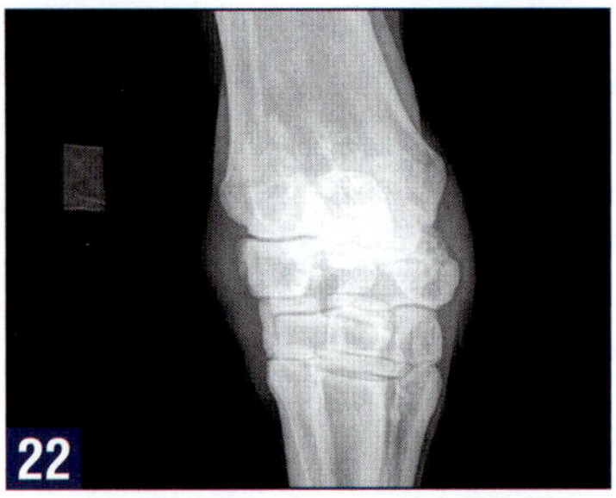

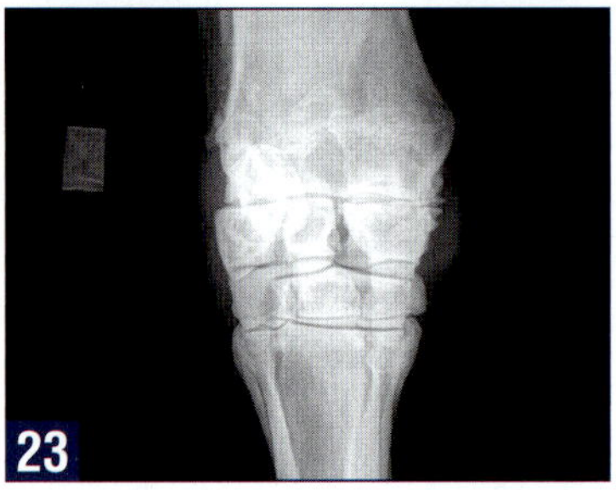

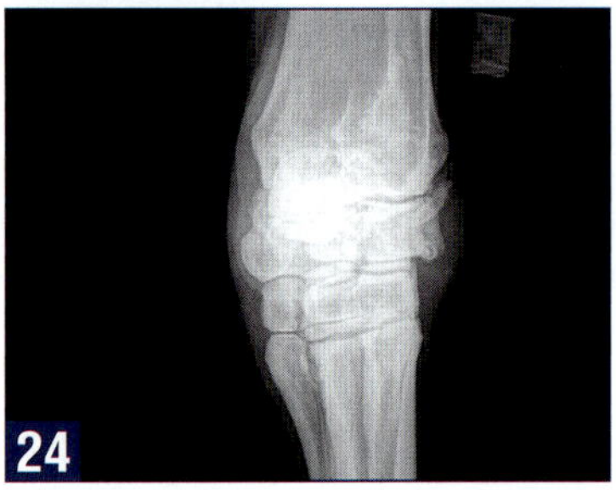

possible, working close to the ground. If you are only trimming, try to catch the horse lying down so that you can work on the foot without bending the knee at all.

Veterinarians can take radiographs to determine the extent of the problem. They can also inject the joint in the early stages to make the horse a little more comfortable. **Figures 18-25** are of some really bad knees that Dr. Marcotte has X-rayed. If you study them, you will see that there are a lot of bone changes and even some fractures in these radiographs.

The owner should stop using the horse once any lameness is present.

ANTICIPATED OUTCOME

Once bone growth begins, there is not much to stop it. If the growth becomes articular, the usefulness of the horse is over.

IN SHORT

D: Bone growth in and around the carpus.

T: TLB the foot and protect from uneven wear if needed.

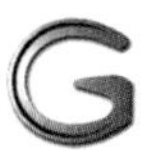

Chapter

46-6 CURB

DEFINITION

Inflammation of the plantar ligament, with swelling occurring about four inches below the point of the hock.

REASON

This area is generally stressed by poor conformation. Horses that are sickle-hocked and cow-hocked tend to put more strain on the soft tissue in the plantar region of the hock. Even horses with normal conformation can acquire curb if they stress this area by stopping hard, jumping, or taking a bad step.

ANATOMY

The superficial flexor tendon can be involved with curb, but the plantar ligament is most often the primary anatomic structures involved.

SYMPTOMS

When a horse has curb, there will be inflammation below the point of the hock. There will be swelling in this area as well as heat. The horse may be reluctant to put its heels on the ground and may travel on its toes. Lameness associated with curb is generally Grade 2 or less, and the swelling may remain as a permanent blemish after the pain is over. I have seen very few curbs with the type of horses that I shoe. **Figure 1** is a drawing of a sickle-hocked hind leg with curb. In **Figure 2**, the horse has a curb that has healed, resulting in a blemish.

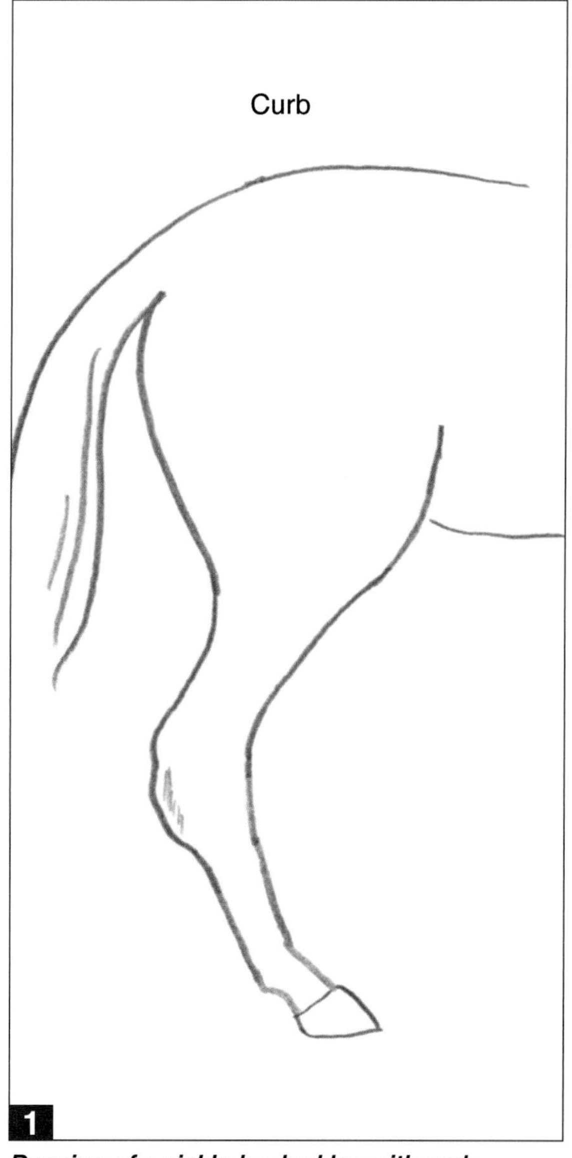

Drawing of a sickle-hocked leg with curb.

TREATMENT

The primary treatment for curb is rest and ice. Shoeing with wedged heels may give the horse some relief when they are reluctant to put their heels on the ground. In severe cases, a patten bar can allow the limb to rest and heal.

Given enough time, the horse should make a full recovery, even if the swelling below the point of the hock remains. A veterinarian may wish to prescribe anti-inflammatories as well as inject the curb on a case-by-case basis.

ANTICIPATED OUTCOME

Once the acute phase is over, the horse should make a full recovery. A large hard swelling may remain as a permanent blemish.

IN SHORT

D: Inflammation about four inches distal to the point of the hock.

T: Rest, ice, possible wedged heels or patten bar.

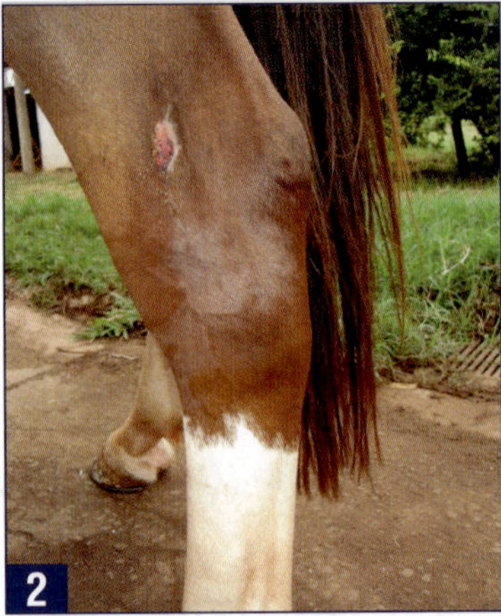

Lateral view of a hind leg with curb.

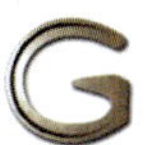

Chapter

46-7 OSSELETS

DEFINITION

Osselets is the term used to describe arthritic bone growth at the dorsal aspect of the fetlock joint. In fact, the term osselets means "little pieces of bone," although it is directed at the dorsal fetlock joint when talking about the lameness problem of osselets.

REASON

Osselets are caused by the fetlock sinking so far that the dorsal aspect of the joint becomes damaged. This is referred to as dorsiflexion, which means that the angle of the joint is being decreased in a dorsal aspect, the opposite of palmar flexion.

Bone growth can occur around the fetlock and not be articular or classified as osselets (**Figures 1-2**). This horse is actually not lame. Osselets refers to the dorsal aspect, specifically.

ANATOMY

The anatomy involved will be the dorsal distal cannon bone and the dorsal proximal P1. Of course, the main extensor tendon will be affected as well.

SYMPTOMS

When a horse has osselets, it may not be severely lame when not worked. However, these horses almost always get sore when asked to do anything strenuous. When osselets are in the beginning stages of formation, the affected horse will be sore and have some soft swelling at the dorsal aspect of the fetlock joint. As the condition progresses into a full-blown bone growth, the horse will avoid trotting or running on its own and will become sore when it does.

The radiograph in **Figure 3** from Dr. Scott Morrison shows how osselets affect the fetlock joint. The horse in **Figure 4** has an advanced case of osselets on the off front, and **Figure 5** is a medial palmar view of the off front fetlock. This horse cannot be used.

Figures 6-7 are from Dr. Marcotte. In both of these radiographs, there is evident bone fragments and changes in the dorsal fetlock joint, and this horse is beyond help from shoeing.

TREATMENT

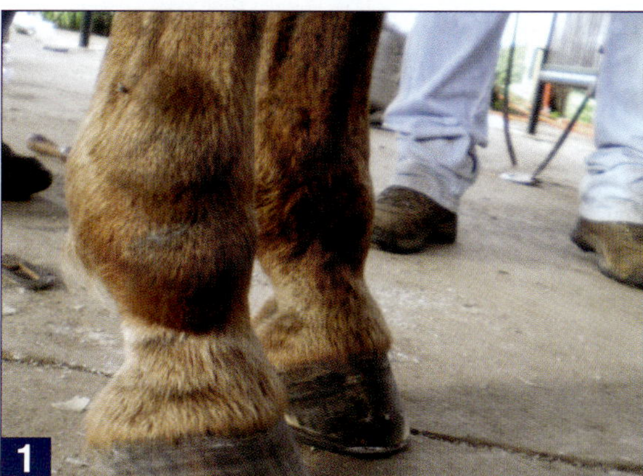

A horse in Brazil with bone growths around the fetlock.

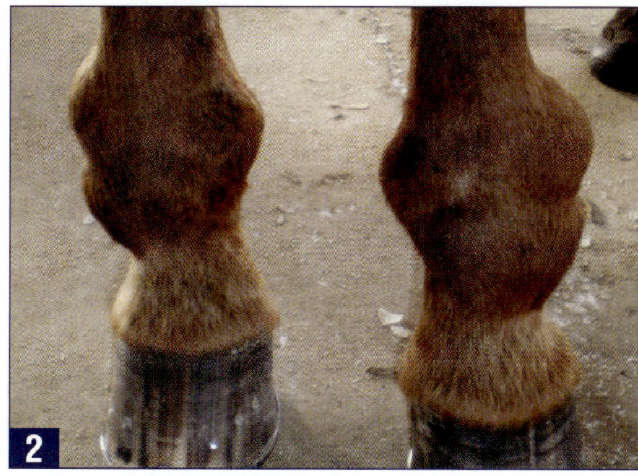

Surprisingly, this horse is not lame.

Unfortunately, there isn't any real good solution for osselets. For shoeing, a severe rocker toe or square toe is recommended, but this is only a measure of comfort for the horse, and not a remedy.

Veterinarians have traditionally pin-fired horses with the beginning stages of osselets, although I don't have any experience with that. One of the benefits of pin-firing may be the rest that the horse will receive after the treatment. Allowing a horse six months of stall rest at the very first stage of dorsal fetlock joint inflammation can be helpful in the prevention of a full blown case of osselets. Injection of the joint and rest may be of help in the early going, but there is little that can be done once articular bone growth has occurred.

Owners of a horse with osselets should be advised that using the horse only hurts it, and the horse should be retired or euthanized if it cannot stay pasture sound.

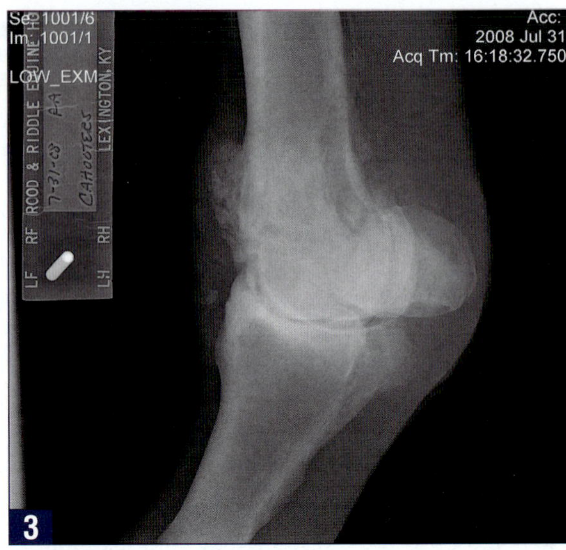

Radiograph of osselets.

ANTICIPATED OUTCOME

This is a career-ending problem for the horse.

IN SHORT

D: Arthritic bone growth at the dorsal aspect of the fetlock joint.

T: Severe rocker toe or square toe shoe may give the horse some comfort.

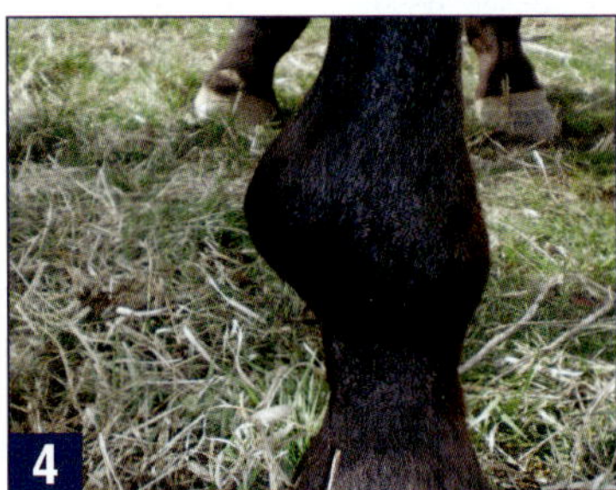

Dorsal view of a horse with osselets.

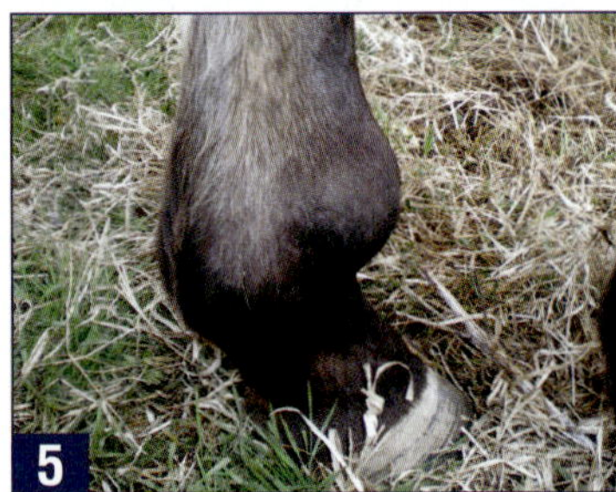

Medial palmar view of the horse in Figure 4.

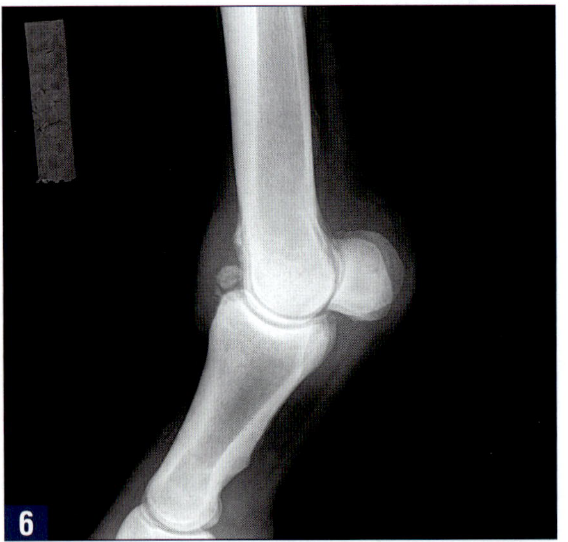

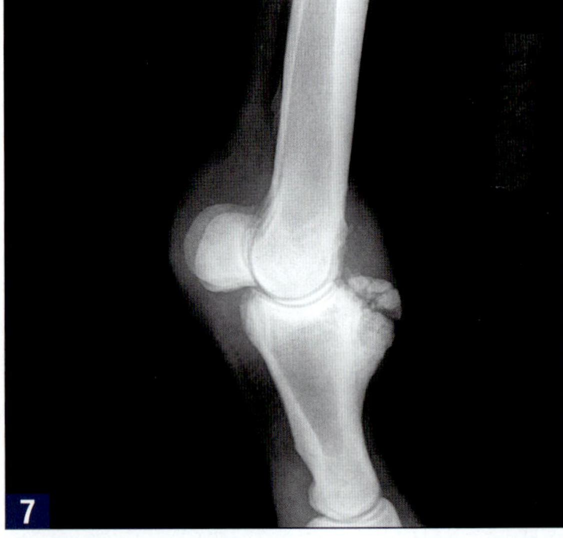

Radiographs of fetlock joints severely damaged by osselets.

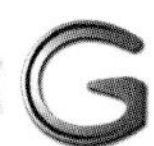

Chapter

46-8 RADIAL NERVE PARALYSIS

DEFINITION

The radial nerve has become damaged, resulting in the horse being unable to bring the forelimb forward as well as experiencing difficulty bearing weight on the affected limb.

REASON

The radial nerve may be damaged from blunt-force trauma, such as hitting a fence or being kicked. In the case of humerus fractures, the radial nerve may be severed. Horses that are put under general anesthesia may have the radial nerve damaged from being placed on one side for an extended period of time.

ANATOMY

The radial nerve passes over the humerus and supplies the extensor muscles.

SYMPTOMS

A horse with radial nerve paralysis will be unable to bring the forelimb forward. The toe will drag, and the horse may have difficulty getting the foot forward far enough to bear weight. **Figure 1** is a drawing of how most horses with radial nerve paralysis will stand, with the toe of the affected leg on the ground.

TREATMENT

There are few treatments for this condition, and if the nerve is severed, the horse should be euthanized. From the farrier's realm, all that can be done is to shoe the foot normally to reduce the wear at the toe from being drug on the ground. The opposite foot may benefit from a heart bar as a preventive measure against founder, but if the horse has not recovered pretty quickly, it will probably not recover at all. A veterinarian may want to inject DMSO and/or anti-inflammatory medication. The owner can only provide a safe stall.

ANTICIPATED OUTCOME

If the horse does not have significant recovery in the first few weeks of treatment, the chance of recovery is not good. Horses that do not recover will not be usable nor have any quality of life.

IN SHORT

D: Damage to the radial nerve.

T: Protect the toe of the foot from excessive wear, vet involvement, possibly euthanize of the horse.

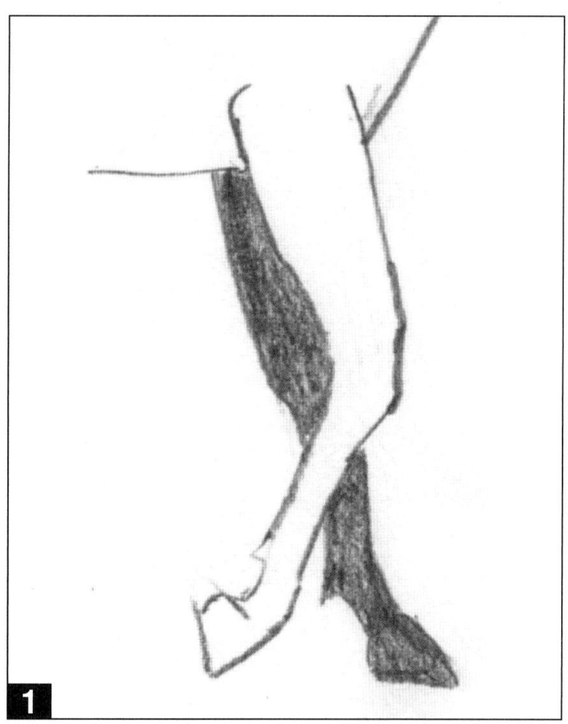

Drawing of how a horse with radial nerve paralysis will generally stand.

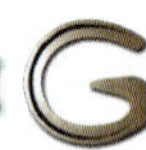

Chapter

46-9 RINGBONE

DEFINITION

Ringbone is the term given to bone growth in the pastern or coffin joint areas. False (nonarticular) ringbone if it does not include the joint surface, and true (articular) ringbone if it does involve the joing surface. High ringbone is the bone growth that is in the pastern joint region, and low ringbone is bone growth in the coffin joint region.

REASONS

Poor conformation is a leading cause of ringbone, and horses that are naturally steep are more susceptible to develop ringbone from constant concussion. With crooked conformation, there will be uneven joint spaces that may lead to articular ringbone, and excessive pull on collateral ligaments or tendons can lead to nonarticular ringbone.

Direct trauma such as a cut that involves the periosteum of the pastern bones can also lead to the development of ringbone.

ANATOMY

Ringbone will involve the long pastern, short pastern, and coffin bone. The pastern joint and coffin joint will be involved with articular ringbone.

SYMPTOMS

With nonarticular ringbone, the main symptom is that there is hard growth in the pastern or coffin area, but the horse is not lame. It may develop a buttress foot, and there may be large lumps all around the pastern joint, but the horse is still not sore. Radiographs will show this new bone

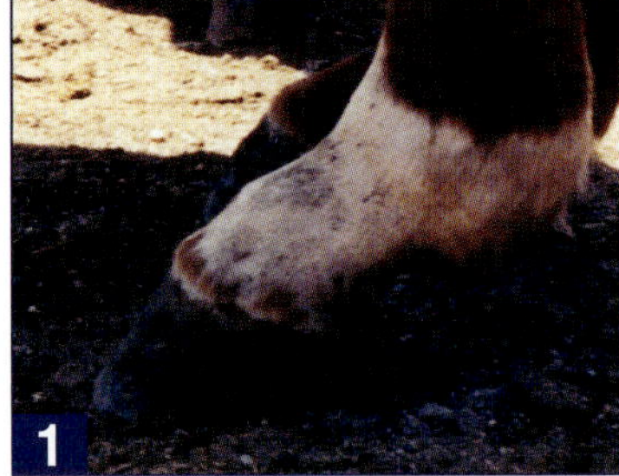

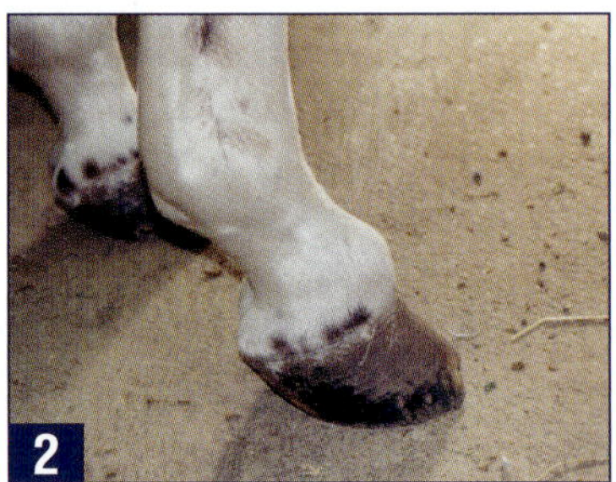

High nonarticular ringbone.

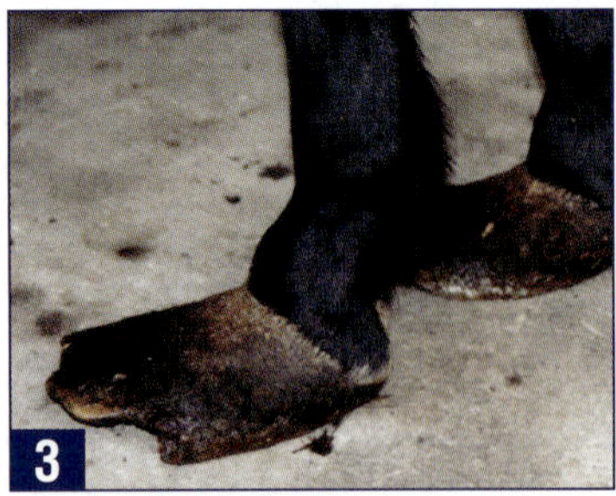

High ringbone, whether articular or not is unknown.

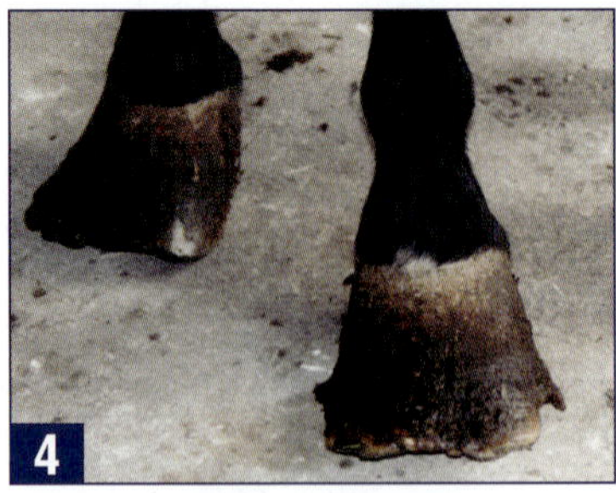

Dorsal view of the horse in Figure 3.

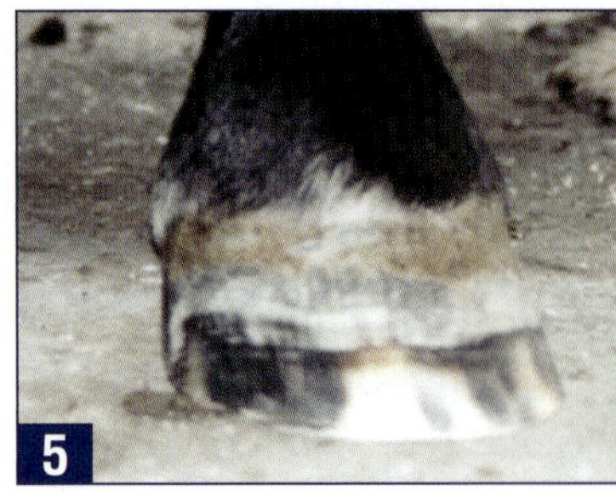

The foot in Figure 3 is now trimmed.

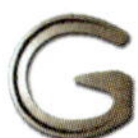

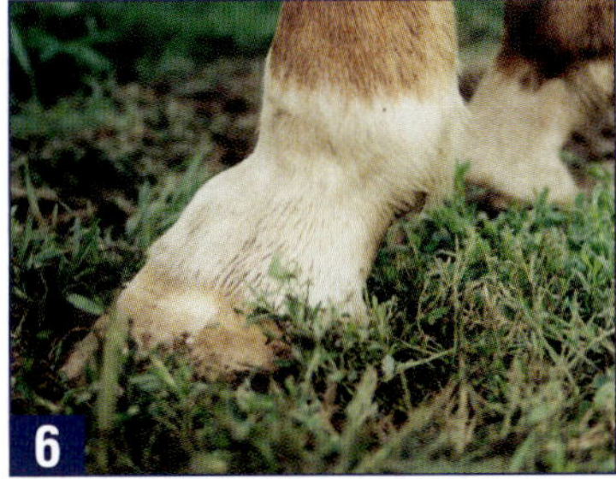

High ringbone leading to the look of a buttress foot.

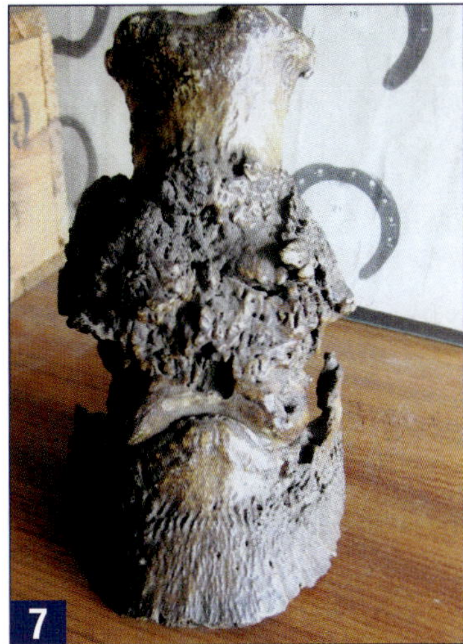

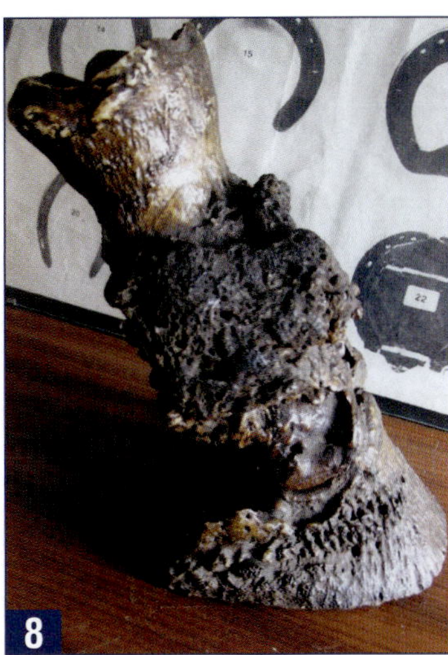

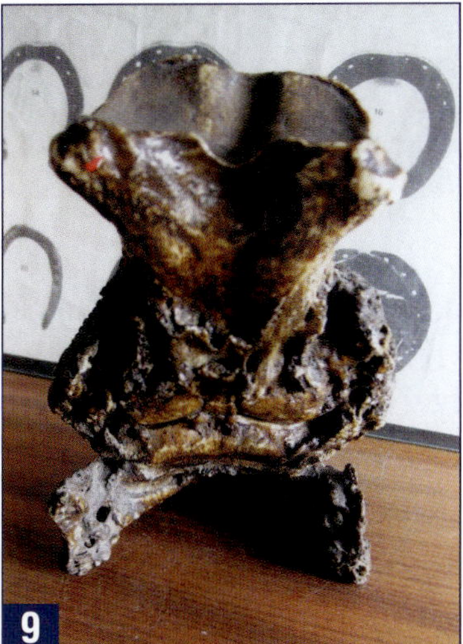

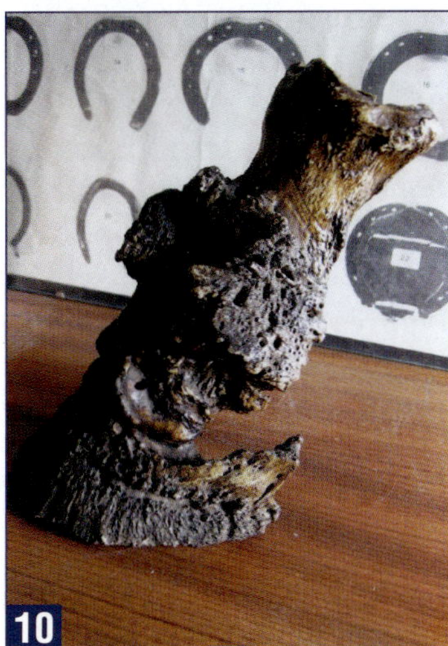

Bone model of a horse with severe ringbone.

growth. **Figures 1-2** are pretty classic-looking nonarticular high ringbone. The horse in **Figures 3-4** was quite lame, but you can see the neglect that the horse suffered by looking at the toe length. Once the foot was trimmed **(Figure 5)**, the horse was more comfortable, but I never saw him again to find out if he had returned to soundness. **Figure 6** shows a foot that looks like a buttress foot from the ringbone, as you would see with an extensor process of P3 fracture.

The bones in **Figures 7-10** are the digit of a horse that suffered with massive high ringbone. This model is at the Army School of Farriery for the British Army in Melton Mowbray, United Kingdom. One of the things that did happen for this horse is that the pastern joint completely fused, which could have made the horse sound.

With articular ringbone, the horse will be lame. You will need a radiograph to see the extent and location of the bone growth. **Figures 11-12** are X-rays taken by Dr. Morrison of ringbone. Dr. Marcotte took the X-rays in

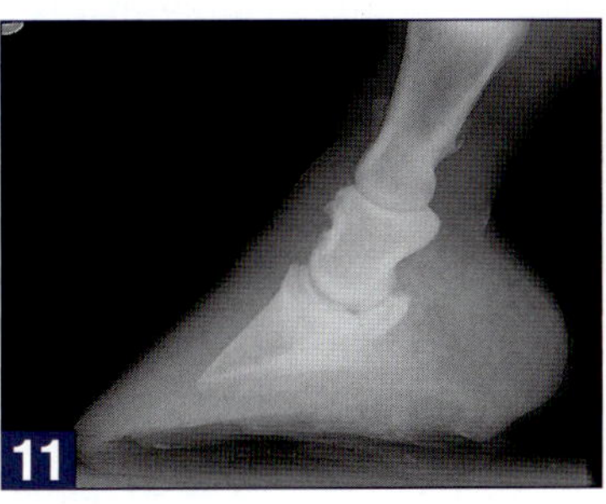

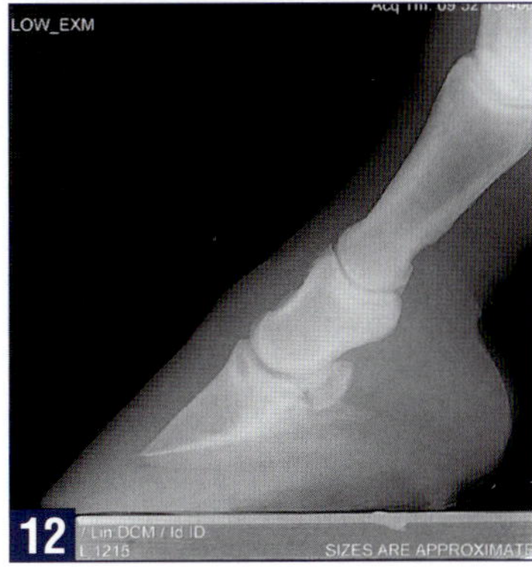

Radiograph of ringbone.

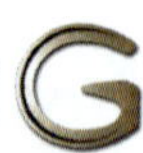

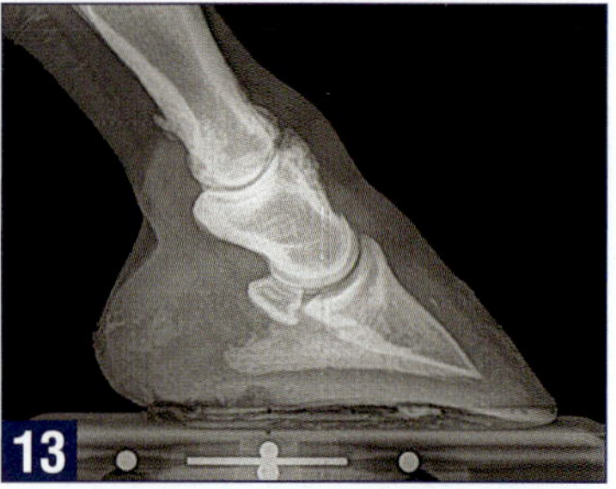

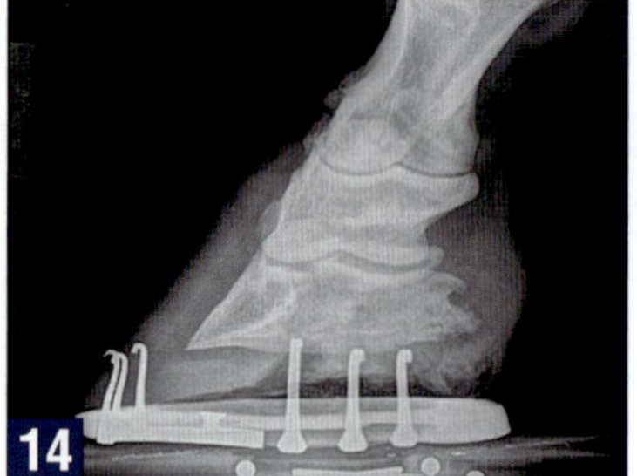

Radiograph of ringbone.

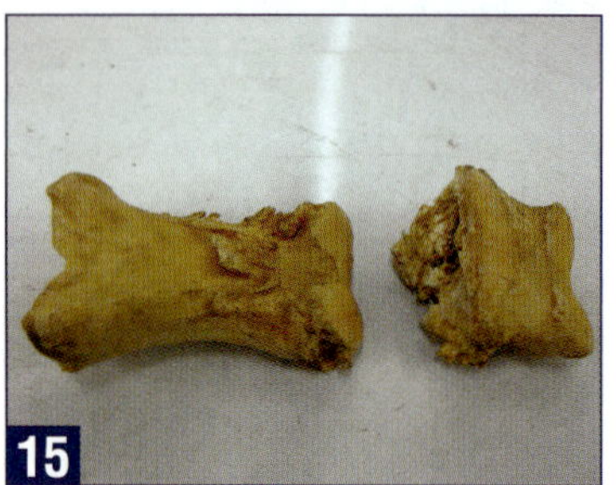

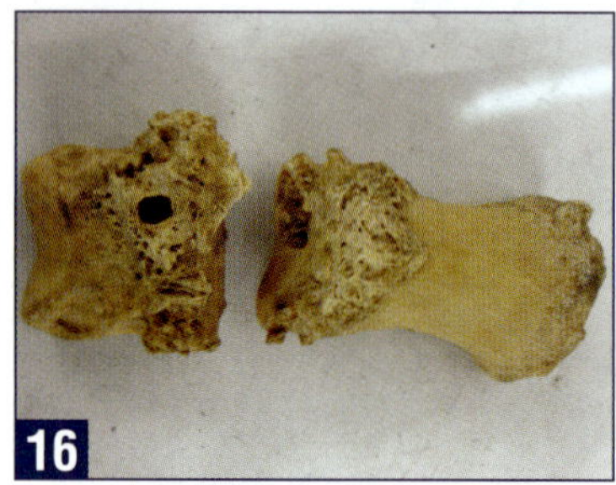

Bones of a horse that had articular high ringbone

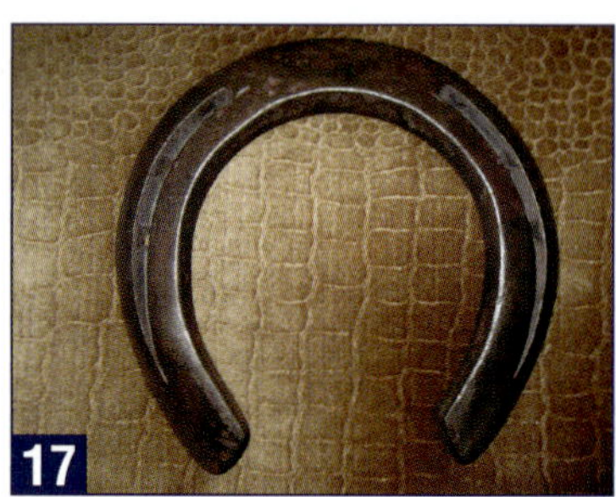

Cupped breakover shoe.

Figures 13-14. Notice the dorsal aspect of the pastern joints and the margin of the bones. Chris Pardoe, AWCF, had the bones in **Figures 15-16**. Look carefully at the joint surface to see the major damage and erosions that this horse endured.

Although shoeing alone will not fix a horse with ringbone, you may make the horse more comfortable by using a half-round or beveled shoe. The Equilibrium shoe from Delta Mustad Hoofcare Center or the Grand Circuit Open Roller shoe could be used, or you can make it yourself, like the shoe in **Figure 17** that Cody made. I call it a cupped breakover shoe. There have been several horses that were much more comfortable in this shoe.

For high articular ringbone, fusing of the pastern joint by the veterinarian may allow the horse to return to useful service. This can be done in several ways, from laser surgery to bone grafts to screws across the joint. If it is low articular ringbone, the prognosis is not good, and the owner should be advised that there is very little chance of this horse becoming sound again. Even if the coffin joint fuses, the horse will be lame if used over rough terrain.

The horse in the next series is one that has the worst case of low ringbone that I have ever encountered. There was an injury to the pastern joint at some point, and the resulting bone growth has made the coffin bone, navicular bone, and P2 basically one whole structure. When this horse walked, it would place the injured near foot in front of the good off front, and roll from the broken lateral heel through the medial toe. The horse is extremely lame. **Figures 18-20** are of the foot before trimming, and **Figures 21-22** are after being trimmed. **Figures 23-24** are the really important ones; these are the radiographs of this unbelievable leg.

When I shod this horse, I tried to make the foot as level on the long axis as I could. It is important in these instances to be aware that this is not something that is going to be fixed, just something that you are doing to make the horse more comfortable. This means that I am not going to make great big changes in an attempt to put this horse back in the arena, just small ones to make it move and bear weight in a better position.

The shoe I chose was a cupped bar shoe. Details of this shoe can be seen in **Figures 25-28**. There are a lot of nails around this shoe. Because the foot was so damaged, I wanted to have a lot of nailing options. I nailed this shoe on, and the horse immediately felt better. It gave many of the signs that you

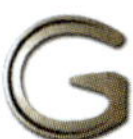

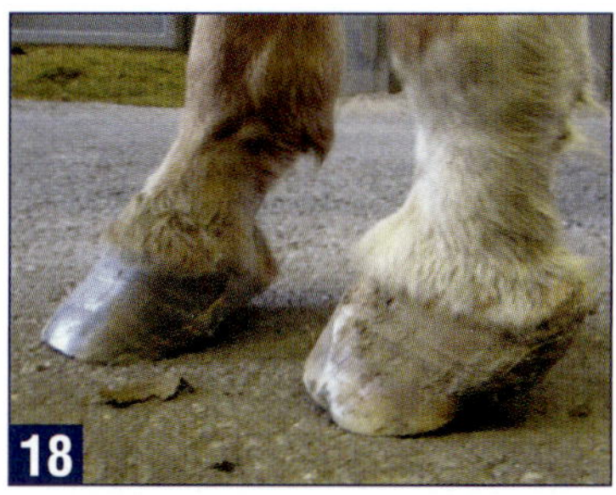

Lateral view of the near front foot of a horse that has severe ringbone.

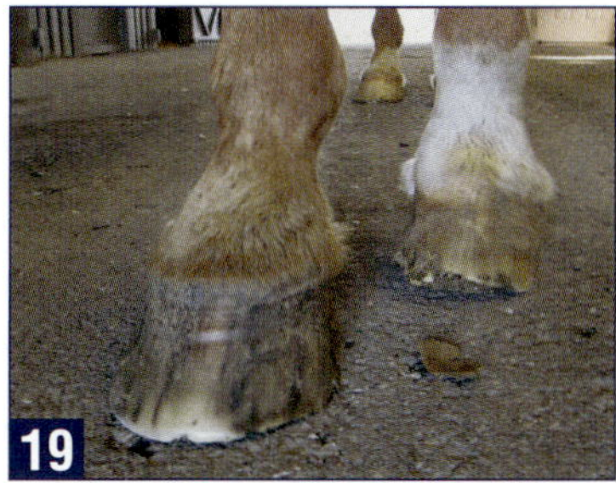

Dorsal view of the same foot.

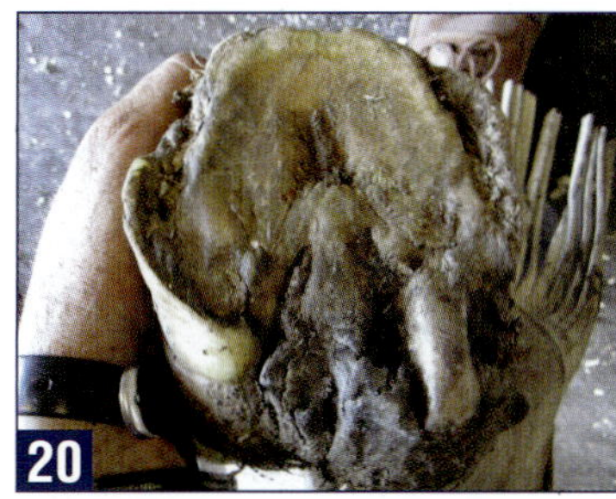

Solar view of the foot in the injured horse, pre-trim.

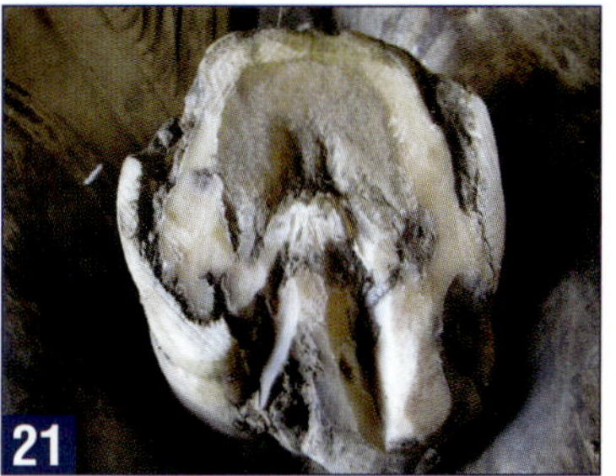

Solar view of the foot after trim.

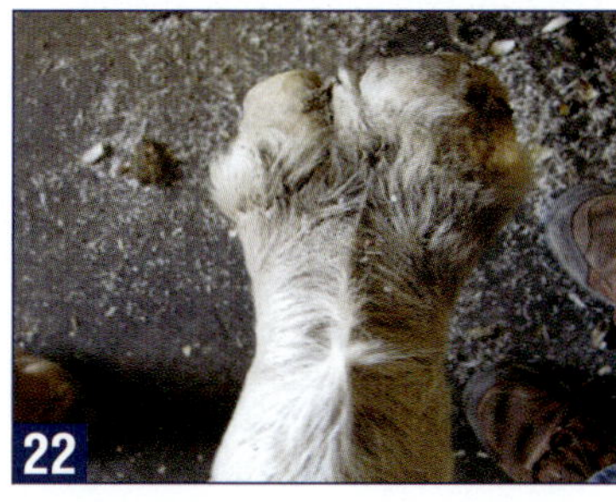

View of the bad mediolateral balance of this leg.

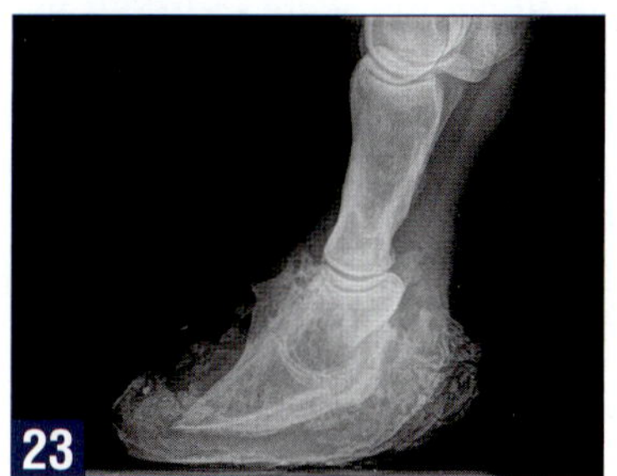

Lateral radiograph of the damaged leg. Notice that there is no real definition between the coffin bone, navicular bone, and the short pastern.

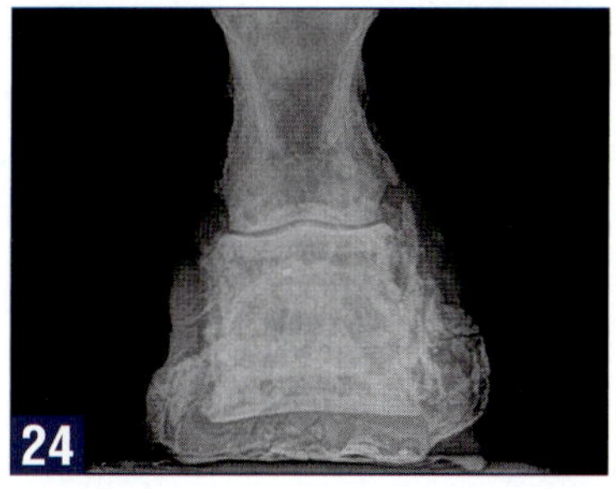

Dorsal view of the injured digit.

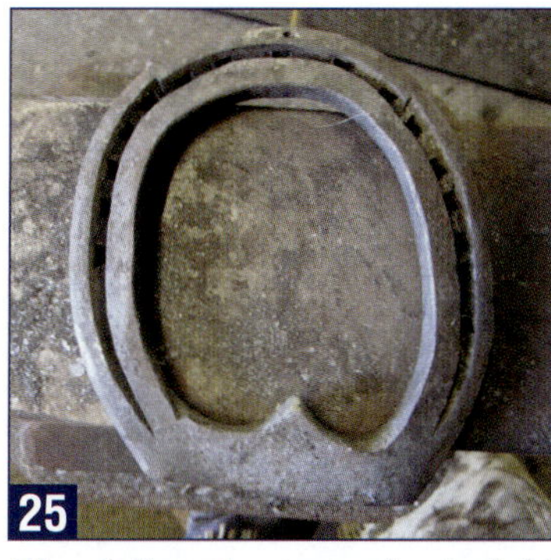

The fullered, cupped, straight bar that I am putting on this foot.

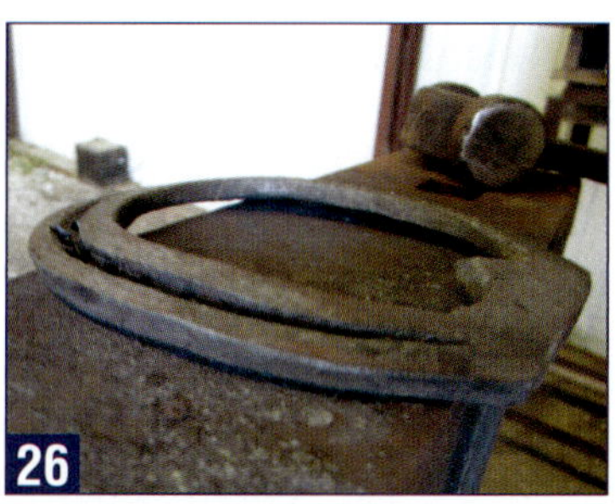

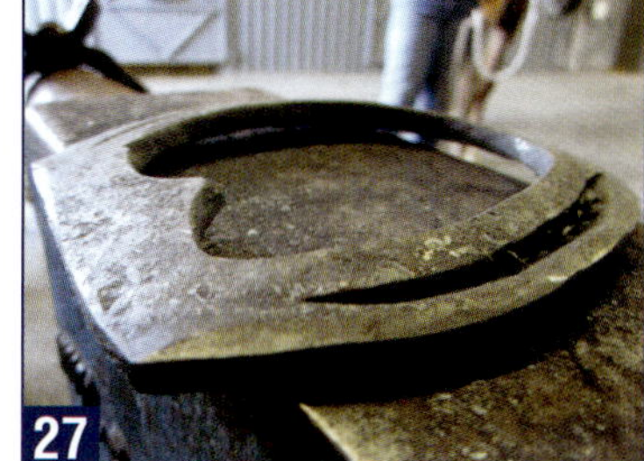

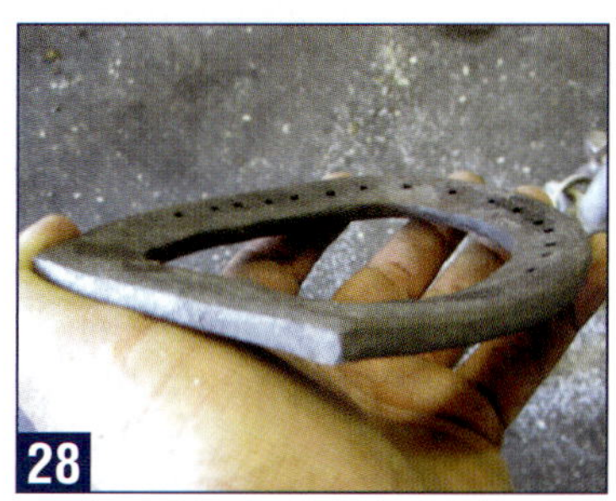

Pictures showing the amount of cup in the bar shoe.

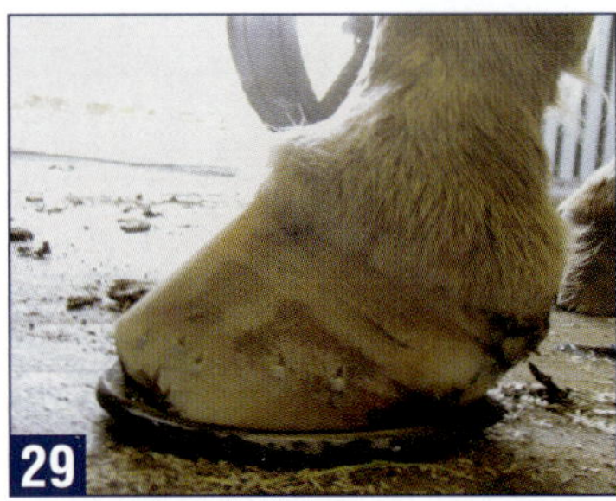

Lateral view of the shod foot.

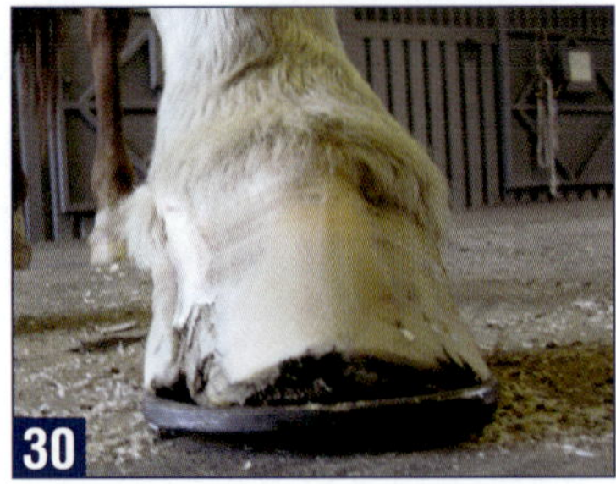

Dorsal view of the shod foot.

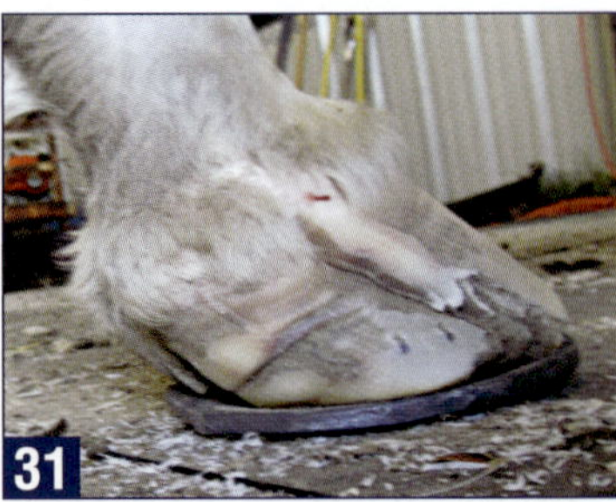

Medial view of the shod foot.

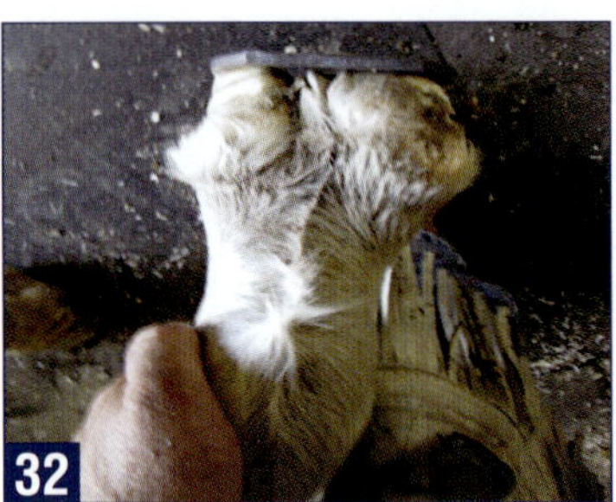

Balance of the leg after being shod.

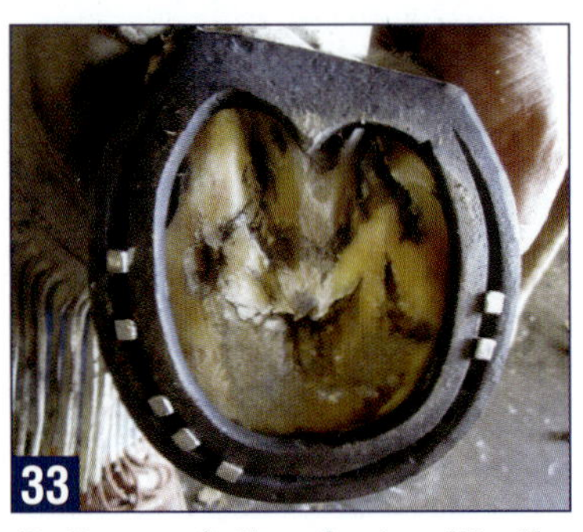

Bottom of the foot with the shoe on.

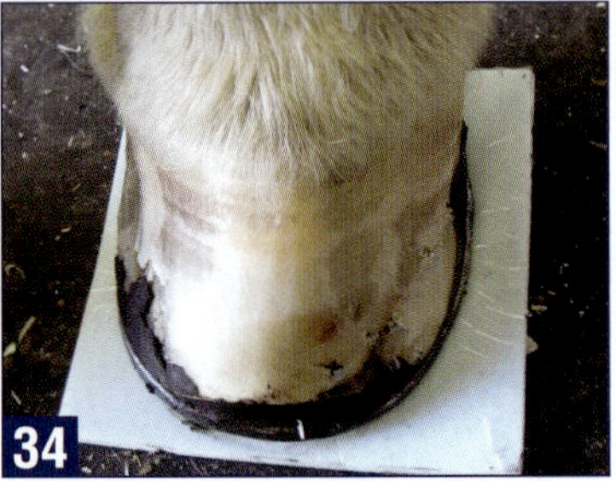

Putting the Styrofoam pad on the foot for pour-in pad. The black substance around the edges of the foot is Sole Pack to block the gaps between the shoe and the foot from letting the Equi-Pak out.

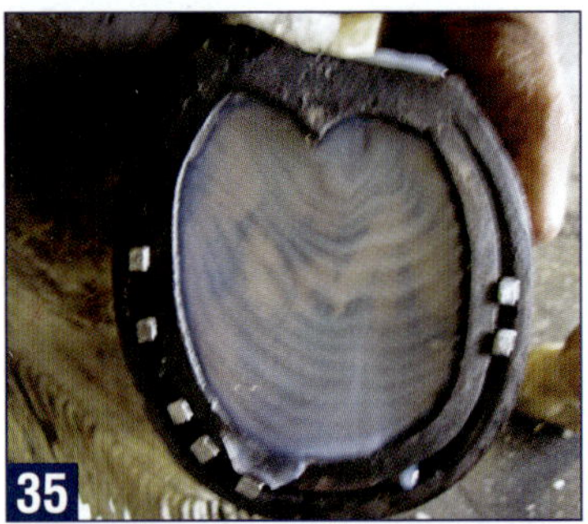

Finished foot with pour-in pad.

look for in a horse that has been relieved of pain; placing weight on the foot, better head carriage, the look in the eyes, as well as the posture of the back and hind legs. It is a satisfying thing to see in a horse that you are working on getting relief from pain. **Figures 29-33** show the shoe on the foot. To finish the job, I decided to use a pour-in pad. **Figure 34** is the shod foot with the styrofoam pad on it, and **Figure 35** is the finished job with the pour in complete.

ANTICIPATED OUTCOME

Nonarticular ringbone, high or low, can be considered a blemish. The horse is not lame, so it can be used normally. Be aware though, that nonarticular ringbone can become articular ringbone, or the bone growths may become fractured, causing lameness. With high articular ringbone, there is surgical potential for relief, but if it is low articular ringbone, the horse is probably not going to be useable again.

IN SHORT

D: New bone growth in the pastern and coffin joint areas.

T: Rocker toes, beveled shoes, half-rounds, and potential surgery to fuse the pastern joint.

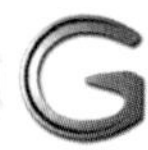

Chapter

46-10 SEVERED TENDONS

DEFINITION

Severed tendons refer to a tendon being lacerated. The tendon can be completely cut through or partially torn.

REASON

A severed tendon can result from a cut from a physical item such as a piece of tin or wire. If the tendon tears without physical trauma from a sharp object, it is referred to as a ruptured tendon (spontaneous tendon rupture), which is a result of degeneration or a previous infection.

ANATOMY

Any tendon can be involved, but in this instance we are specifically referring to the flexor and extensor tendons below the knee and hock. With the spontaneous tendon rupture from degeneration or infection, the peroneus tertius, superficial flexor on the hind limb and the gastrocnemius are most commonly involved.

SYMPTOMS

There should be physical evidence of the lesion in the form of a traumatic wound; blood, cut skin and so forth. In the case of a cut flexor tendon, the horse will be unable to bear weight normally, and the toe of the foot may actually point up in the air. **Figures 1 and 2** are radiographs from Dr. Marcotte that show a horse with severed flexor tendons. Notice the misalignment of the bones in **Figure 1** and the extreme damage in **Figure 2** when the leg is bearing weight. With the extensor tendons, the horse may knuckle over and stumble when walking, yet be able to bear weight normally.

TREATMENT

The shoe of choice when dealing with severed flexor tendons is a patten bar. This shoe is often overlooked by hoof-care providers for a couple of reasons. First, it is considered hard to make by a lot of farriers, so they don't learn how to put one together. Many veterinarians don't work with farriers who can make the shoe, so they don't prescribe it. Also, a lot of people do not understand how the shoe works. The angle change is not the portion of the shoe that is important; rather its main purpose is to let the horse use the foot and leg less, as well as provide a lot of palmar/plantar support.

The patten bar can be considered a rest shoe. Because it works by elevating the foot, the horse is less likely to use that limb. Consider when you are standing with one foot up on a step and the other

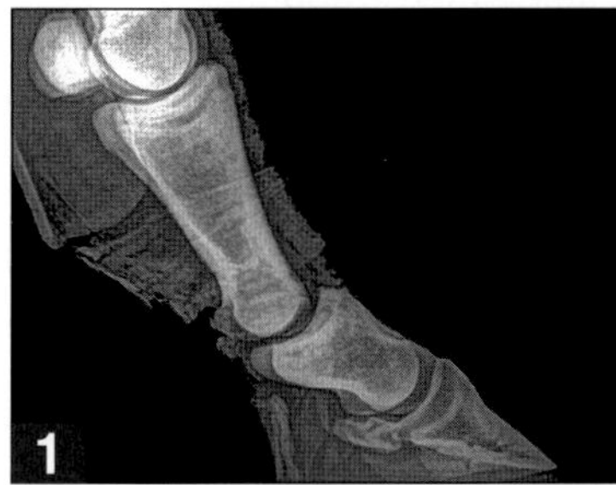

Radiograph of a leg with a cut tendon.

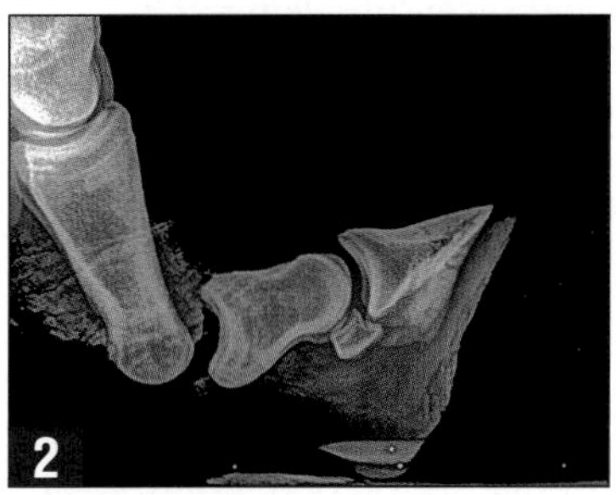

Same leg as Figure 1 with weight applied.

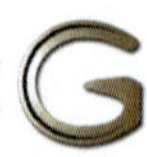

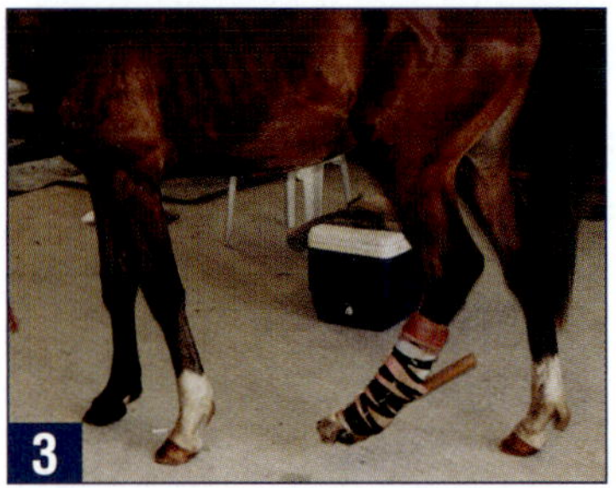
3
Horse with a cut tendon on a hind leg.

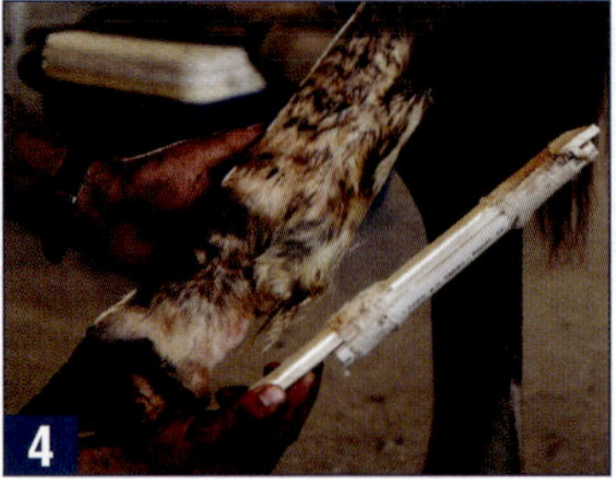
4
The brace that the vet made and applied.

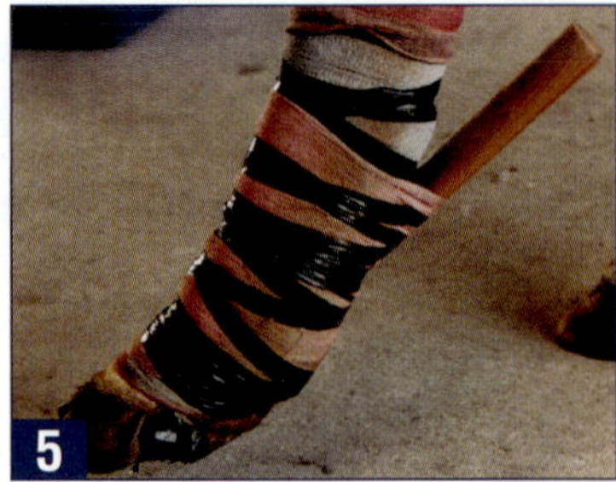
5
The owner tried to supplement the brace with a hammer handle.

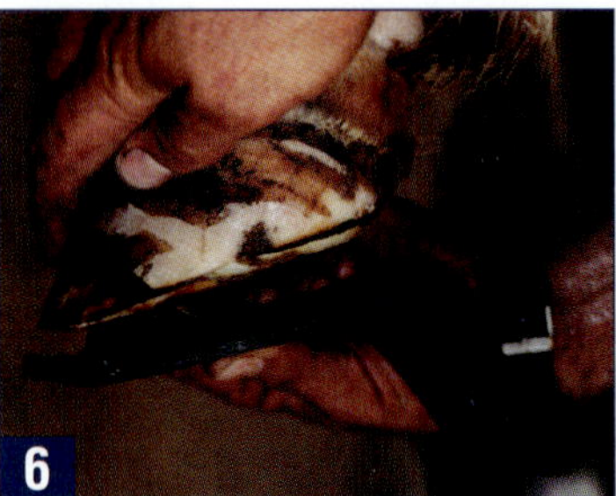
6
Patten bar ready to be applied.

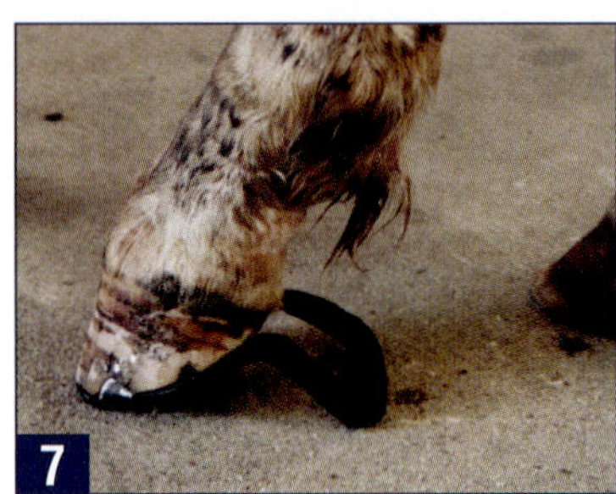
7
Patten bar on the foot.

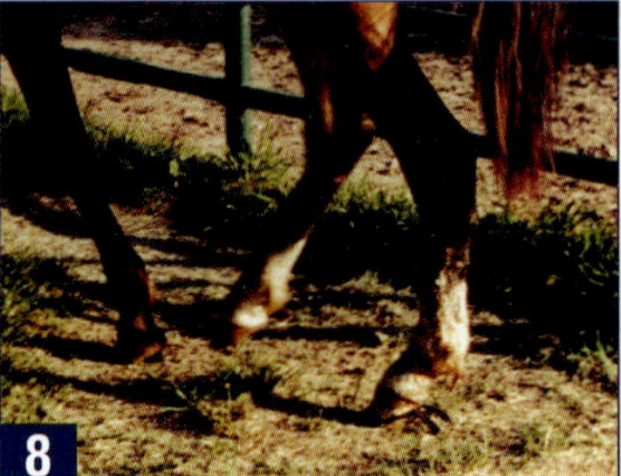
8
The horse bearing weight on that foot without the toe popping up in the air for the first time in many days.

foot on the ground. The foot on the step (elevated) will be bearing very little of your weight, while the one on the ground (not elevated) will be bearing the brunt of the weight. You can test this by attaching a short piece of two-by-four lumber to your foot. After a while you will find that the foot and leg with the board on it has done a lot less work than the other. This fact, instead of the angle change, is the real reason that the patten bar works in these cases.

The shoe should be reset every four to six weeks, and the height of the bar reduced at each reset. Generally, I will make the patten bar with a bar height of 1.5 inches for the first shoeing. It will then be lowered half an inch on the first reset, and then another half inch on the second reset. Of course this depends on how well the wound is healing, and there are instances where it is not lowered at all with some cases. I would like the horse to be in a wedge-heel bar shoe by the fourth reset if everything is going well, then a normal shoe after that.

The patten bar is effective on both the front and hinds, but more so on the hinds. Since the front limbs do not have a reciprocal apparatus, there is a chance that the bar can become a fulcrum for even more stress on the tendon. If a horse places the leg in front of itself far enough, then leans back, it can end up actually causing more damage to the tendons. To prevent this from happening, make certain that the bar is extended as far behind the foot as possible. In the hind leg, this is not a problem.

While this should go without saying, the patten bar is not a turn-out shoe or the type of shoe that a horse can be used to work or ride. It should only be used until there is enough healing that the horse can be shod without it, and the horse should be kept confined to a stall or small paddock while wearing it.

The horse in **Figure 3** cut its leg on the bucket of tractor. When it first came to the shop, the vet had sewn the tendon back together and made a brace **(Figure 4)**. Because the brace was ineffective and the toe of the foot popped up in the air every time the foot bore weight, the owner had taped a hammer handle to the leg **(Figure 5)**. Just my advice, but anytime you have a horse brought to you with a hammer handle taped to its leg, get your camera out.

The patten bar was made and applied **(Figures**

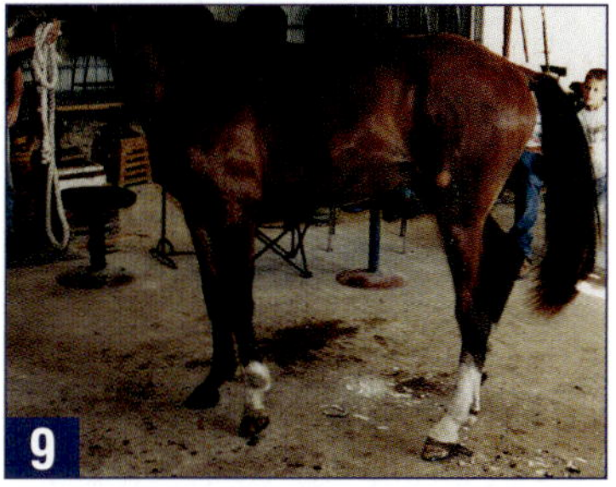

The horse at the first reset.

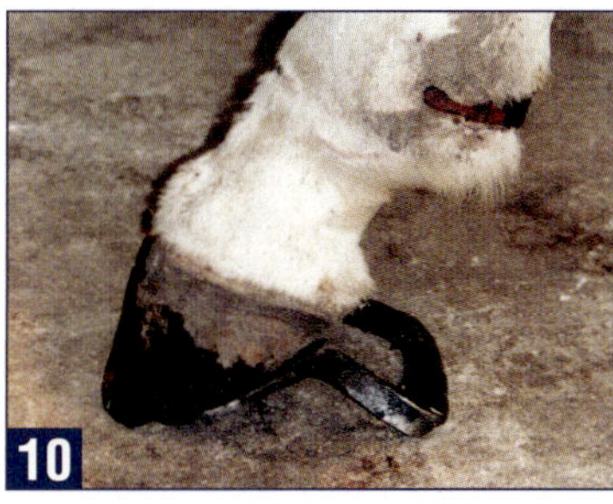

Foot and shoe at first reset before.

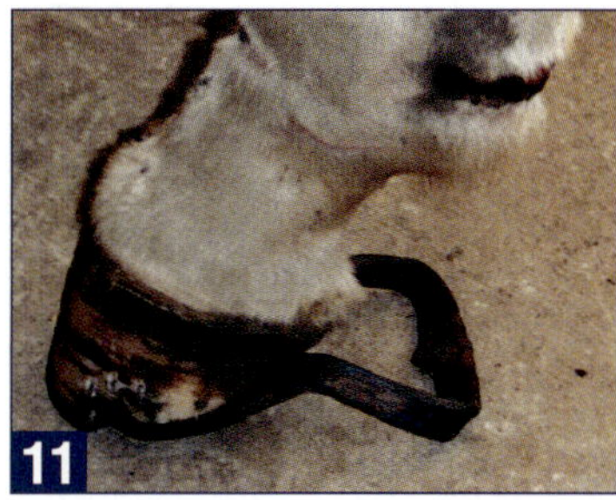

Foot and shoe at first reset after.

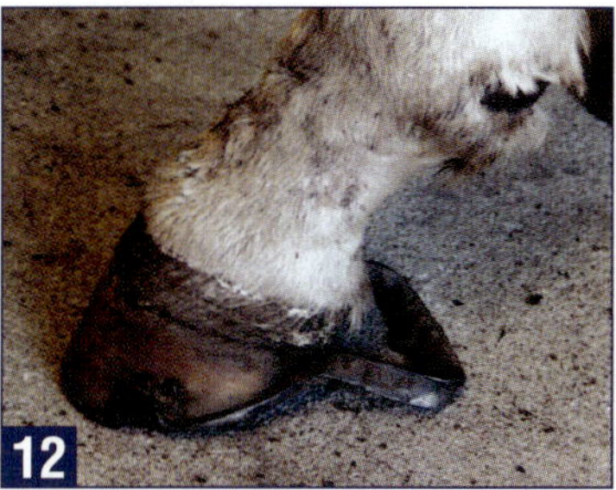

Foot and shoe returning for second reset.

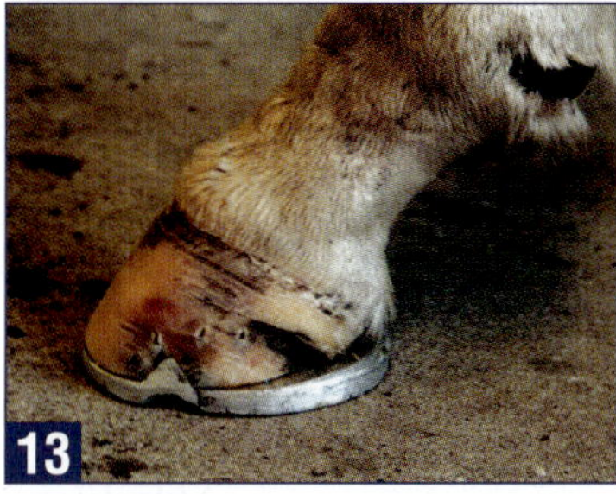

Foot shod with an aluminum wedged-heel bar shoe.

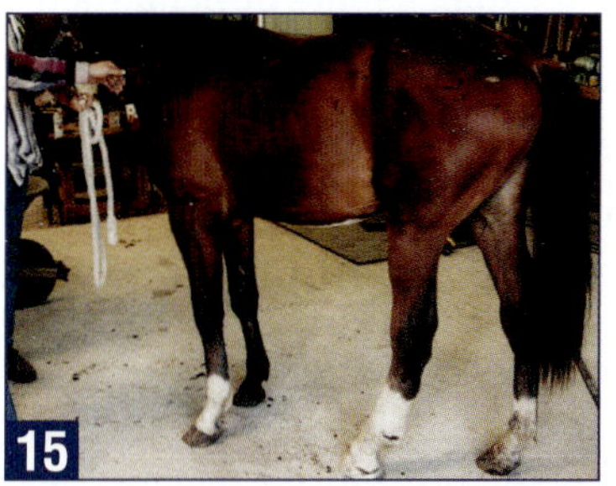

The horse at the last shoeing. Notice how well the rest of the horse looks.

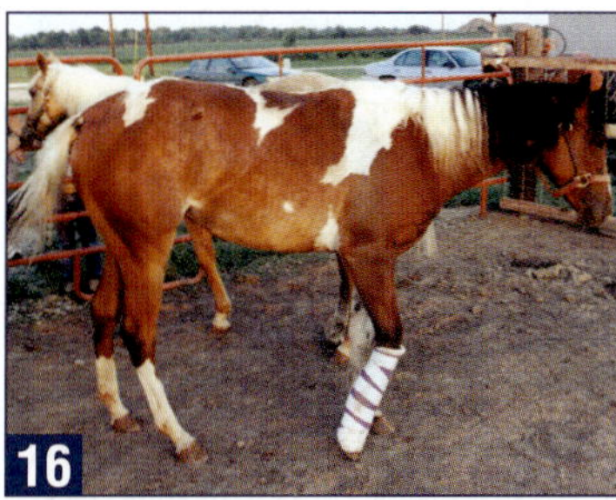

Horse with a cut tendon on a front leg.

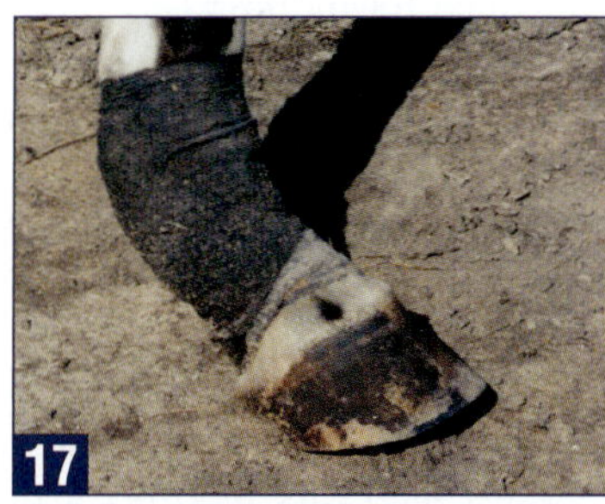

The foot bearing a little weight, but the toe coming up off the ground.

6-7), and the horse was able to bear weight on the foot without the toe coming up for the first time in several days **(Figure 8)**. **Figure 9** shows the horse when it came back for the first reset at about six weeks. The foot before the reset is shown in **Figure 10**. You can see how much I dropped the bar at that time in **Figure 11**. This horse recovered so fast that when he returned **(Figure 12)**, I decided it was time to go with the wedge-heel shoe **(Figures 13-14)**. The whole horse at this time is shown in **Figure 15**. If you compare his body score to what can be seen in **Figure 3**, it is amazing how much the whole horse recovered once the leg was feeling better. After that, the horse was shod normally and was sound. The only remnant was some thickening and scarring at the area of the cut.

Figure 16 shows a horse that was treated by the same vet for a severed tendon in the front leg. After several days of misery from the cast and inability to bear weight on the leg whatsoever **(Figure 17)**, the owner called for some relief. A patten bar was made and applied **(Figure 18)**, and the horse was able to

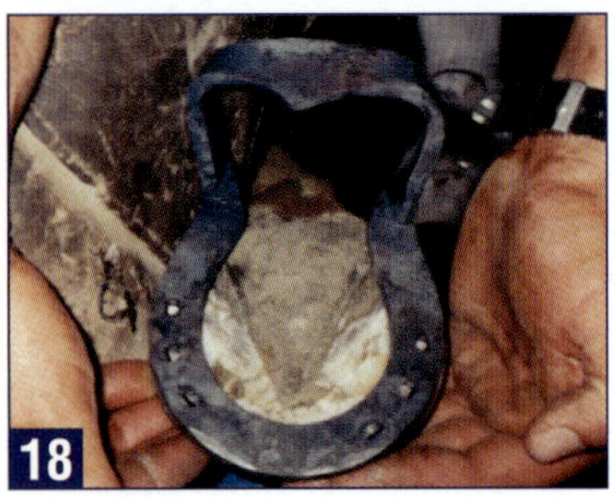

18

Patten bar on the front foot of this horse.

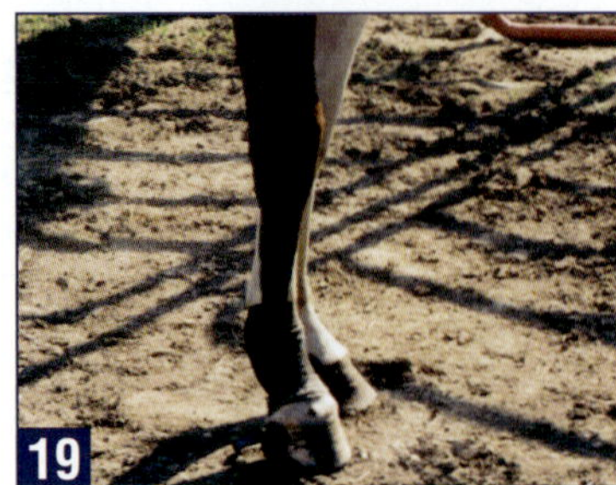

19

The horse able to bear weight on the injured leg without the toe coming off the ground.

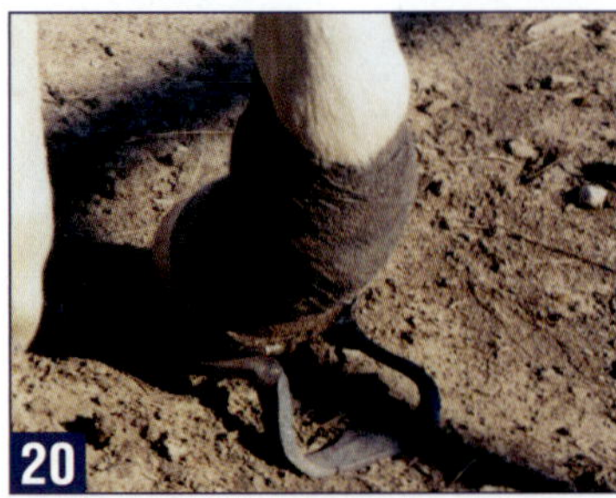

20

Patten bar extending quite a way back from the foot on a front leg.

bear weight on that leg **(Figure 19)**. Notice how far the bar extends behind the foot in **Figure 20**. This horse also returned to soundness.

The first thing that should be done in the event of a complete cut through the tendon is for the vet to suture the tendons back together. If this can be done within the first six hours or so, and the horse is then shod with a patten bar, there is a good chance of repair.

In the instance of extensor tendons being severed, the tendons should be sutured and the leg placed in a cast so that it cannot knuckle over. A patten bar is not called for in these cases; rather, a normal trim, level, and balance is all that a farrier can do. It may be appropriate in some cases to put a toe extension on the foot, but I would only do that if the vet was adamant about it and the horse had a big problem with knuckling over. The problem with the toe extension is that it can possibly lead to a stumble, which could have very bad results on the recently injured tendon. Casting is often done with severed tendons, and this requires a good vet and some careful care from the owner. I have seen several bad casts that were not applied correctly, which caused more damage than good.

The owner needs to provide the horse with stall rest as advised. There is often hydrotherapy (spray the wound with water) and medication application prescribed as part of the recovery. This will require some time and attention from the owner on a daily basis.

ANTICIPATED OUTCOME

One of the biggest factors in recovery is the amount of time between injury and treatment. If more than six hours pass between injury and suture, there is a good chance of bacterial contamination, and successful repair is much more difficult. In the cases of extensor tendon tears, the prognosis is good to excellent. In the cases of flexor tendon tears, the prognosis is always guarded due to the amount of weight these tendons support.

IN SHORT

D: Tendon has been cut through.

T: Suture by vet, patten bar for flexor tendons, normal shoeing, if any, for extensor tendons, and careful aftercare by owner.

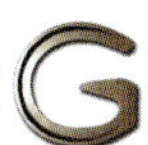

Chapter

46-11 SPAVIN

DEFINITION

The term spavin is used to specifically identify a bone growth in the hock of a horse. It is sometimes used to denote a bone growth in the knee, and referred to as a knee spavin; however, this would be a misuse of the word. The term "spavined" refers to old and decrepit.

There are a couple of soft swelling issues in the hocks that are also called spavin. One is blood spavin, which is simply the equivalent of varicose veins in humans. These enlarged veins run across the medial side of the hock (Figures 1-2). Blood spavin is not a concern.

Another is called a bog spavin, and it is a distension of the joint capsule of the distal intertarsal and tarsometatarsal joint. A bog spavin may look exactly like a bone spavin, but it is soft compared to the bone spavin. This is a sign of stress and damage in the hock and should be checked to determine if preventive measures can be taken.

REASON

Spavin occurs for many of the same reasons that bone growths happen in other areas, specifically, conformation, use of the animal, and age. Horses that are straighter through the hock are prone to spavin, and any horses that are required to work hard on the hindquarters are at risk. In my practice, I primarily see it in cutting horses, calf horses, and drafts.

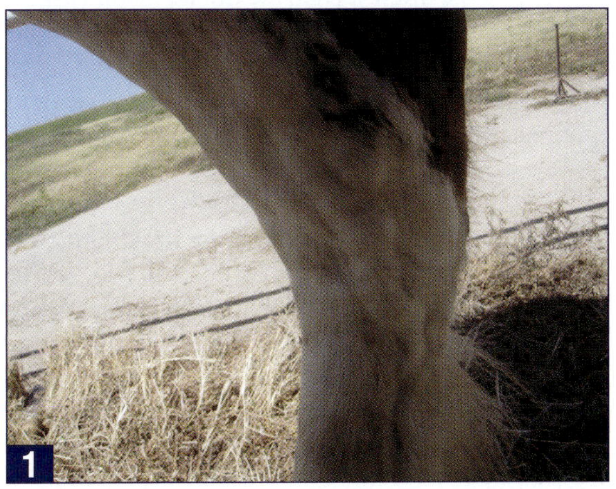

1

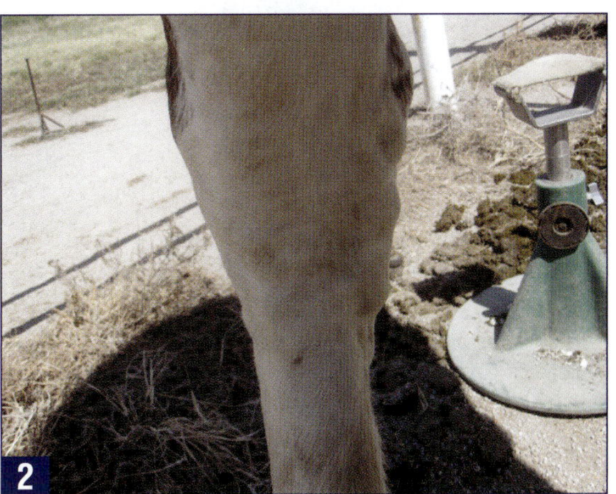

2

Blood spavin on the inside hock of a Clydesdale.

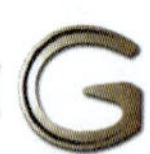

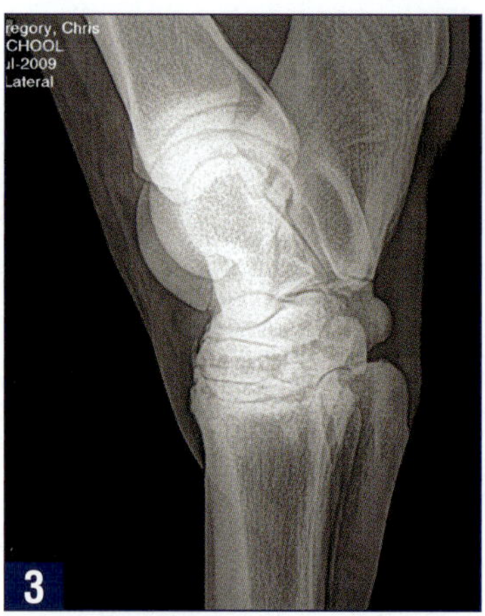

Lateral radiographic view of a hock with spavin.

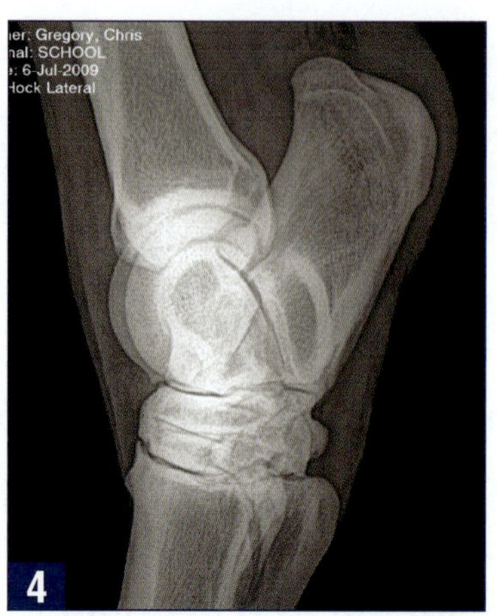

Lateral radiographic view of a bone spur on the cannon bone.

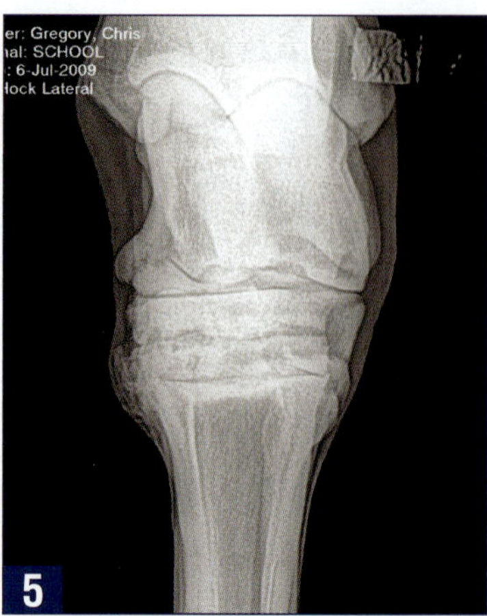

Dorsal radiographic view of a hock with spavin.

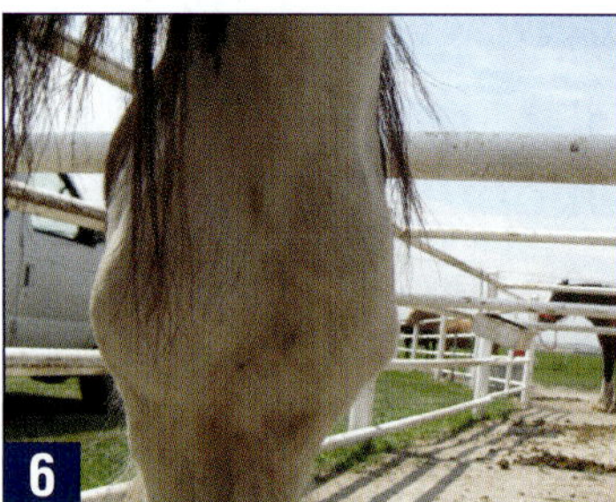

Dorsal picture of large bone spavins in a hock.

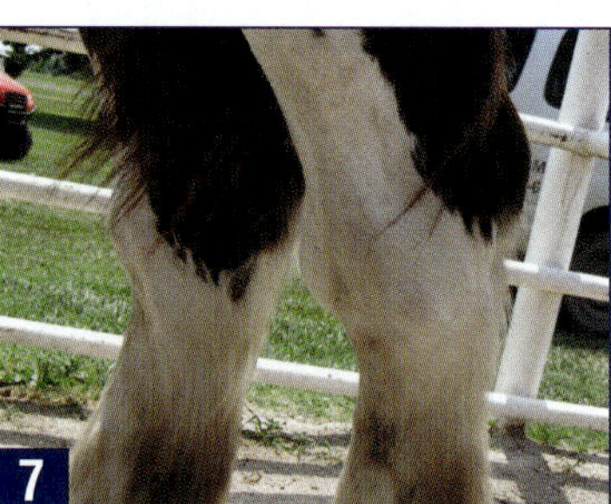

Lateral view of the hocks on the horse in Figure 6. Notice the large dorsal bone growth in the hock.

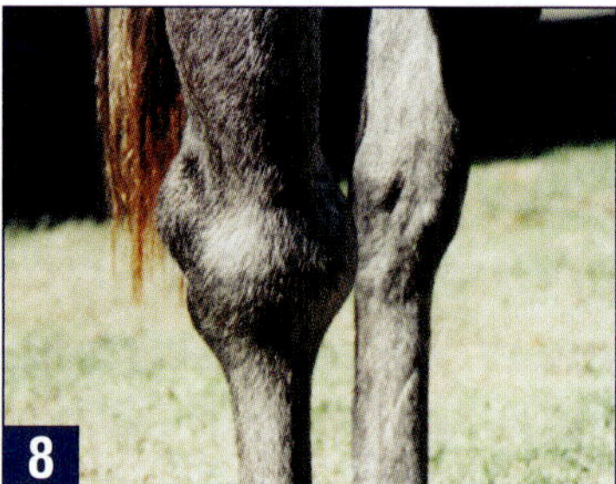

Dorsal view of the right hock with spavin.

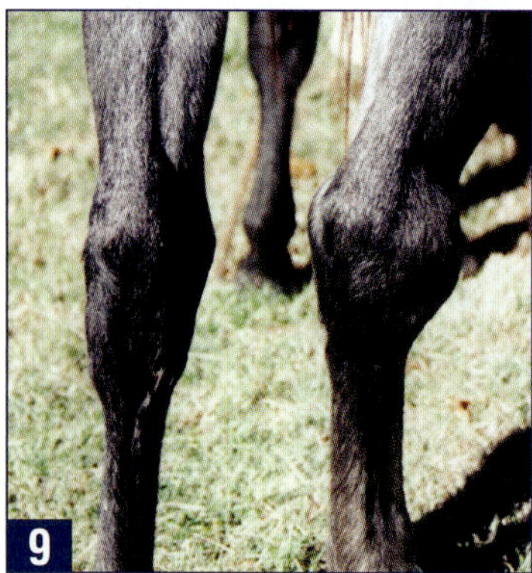

Plantar lateral view of the same hock as Figure 8.

ANATOMY

Any of the tarsal bones can be affected, but spavin is most often seen in the dorsal medial aspect of the hock. This means that the central tarsal bone is generally involved. Most of the time, the distal intertarsal and tarsometatarsal joint are the ones affected.

SYMPTOMS

Spavin will start as osteoarthritis and lameness is often the first sign that an owner will see. As the problem progresses, the bone growth can involve a large area of the joint and cause severe lameness and bring an end to a horse's competitive career.

There will be a bone growth on the tarsus if the spavin is external. It is possible that the growth is internal, and these are called blind spavins. Some of these spavins are really large, and some are not.

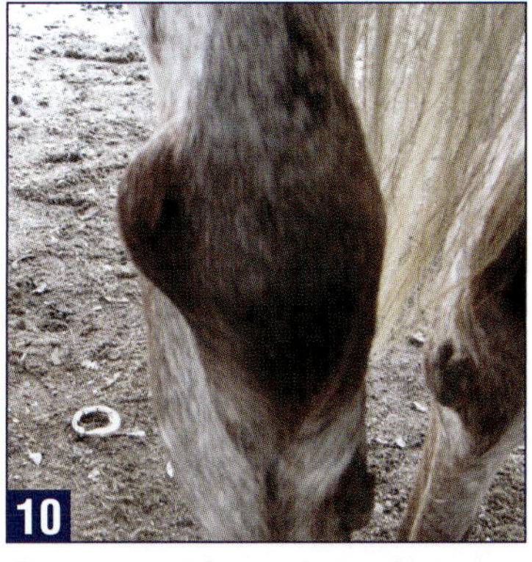

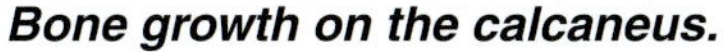
Bone growth on the calcaneus.

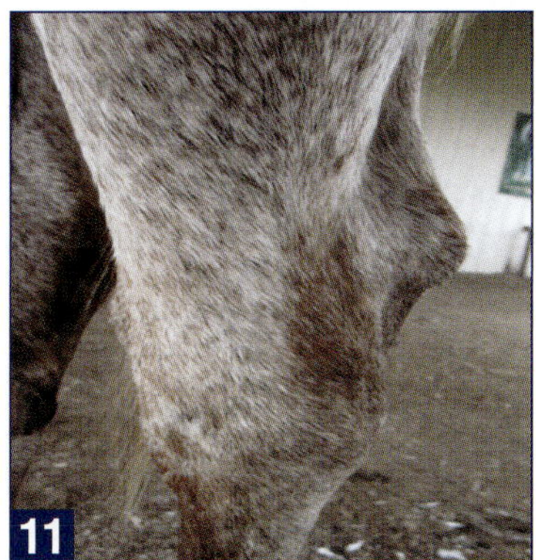

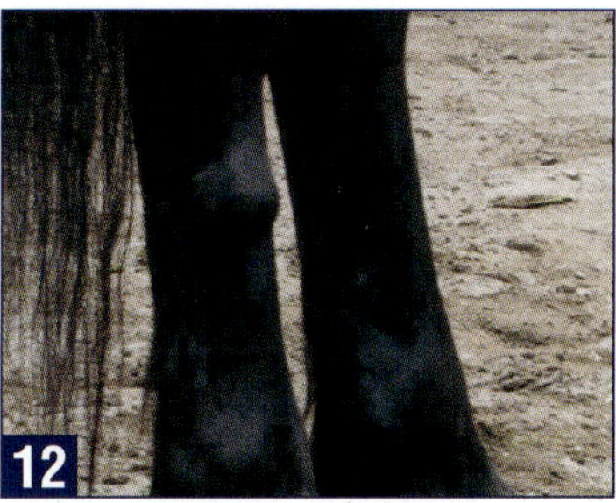

Bone growth on the cannon bone that is not a spavin.

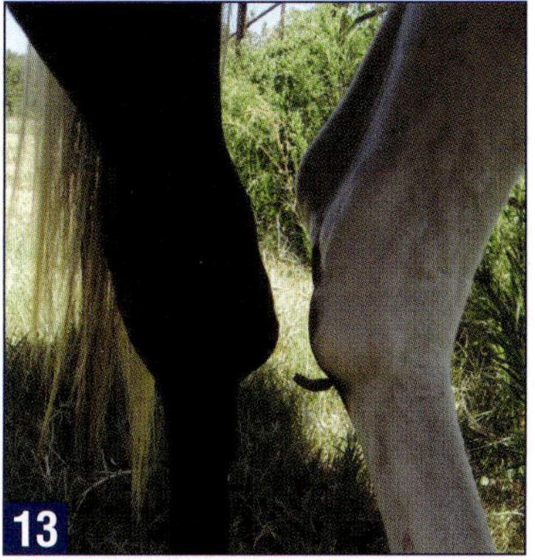

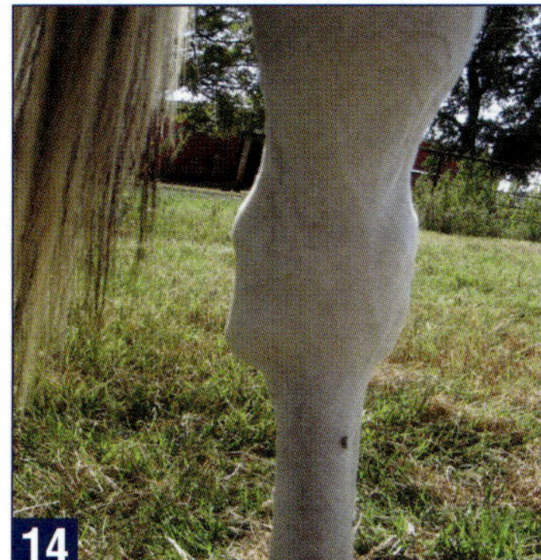

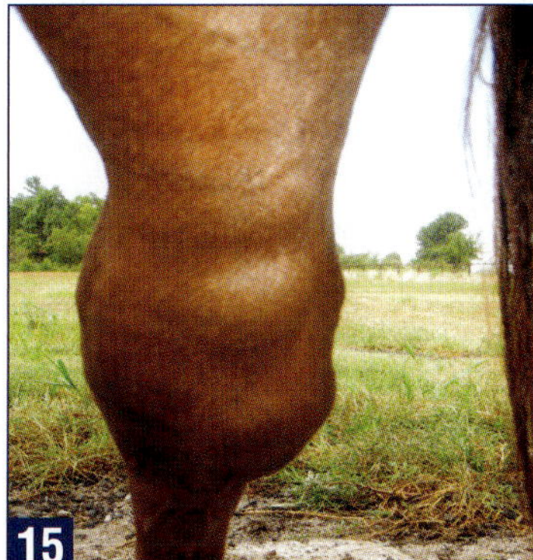

Bad spavins.

Radiographs will show the changes in the hock.

Figure 3 is a lateral radiograph with a pretty bad bone growth occurring in the distal intertarsal and tarsometatarsal joints. In **Figure 4**, there is a large bone spur on the proximal dorsal cannon bone, and **Figure 5** is a dorsal view of a hock with spavin.

The horse in **Figure 6** is a young Clydesdale that had such bad hocks that he couldn't be used on the Budweiser Hitch. Notice the large size of his tarsus, both medial and lateral. In **Figure 7**, the hocks on this horse can be seen from the side. Both hocks have bone growth that extends dorsally.

Figures 8-9 are of the right hock of a horse with large bone spavins that is not actually lame. Since there aren't radiographs, it can only be assumed that the joints are completely fused. It is not that common to have it only on one leg unless the horse has suffered a traumatic injury to that leg. By definition, (bone growth in the hock), the growth shown on the horse in **Figures 10-11** would be called spavin. However, these growths on the outside of the calcaneus do not bother this horse in the least and can be considered a blemish. The bone growth on the cannon bone in **Figure 12** is also just a blemish and not considered a spavin because the hock is not involved.

The spavins in **Figures 13–15** are common of the type of bone spavin that I see with the typical rodeo horse. All three of these horses are sore, and working on their feet causes them to become more so from the movement in the hock.

A flexion test can be performed on the tarsus, and the horse will respond with some lame steps (See **Chapter 43, Lameness**). Horses with spavin also tend to stab the hind foot into the ground when they land, and the shoes may be worn extremely fast from this action.

TREATMENT

Shoeing for spavin traditionally involves making a shoe that will withstand a lot of wear. A spavin shoe has a thick heel with a shoulder just behind

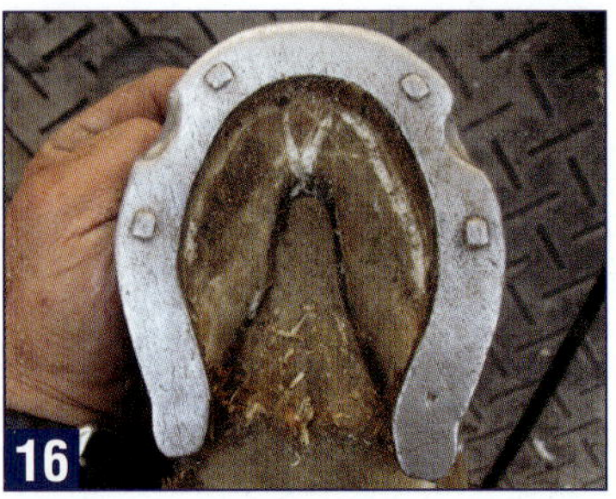

Normal shoe for the hind feet of a lot of rodeo and cutting horses that I shoe.

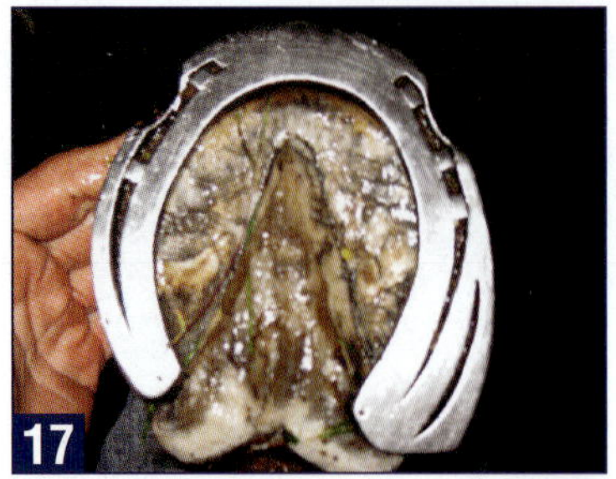

Hind shoe with a lateral heel extension. May make the horse more comfortable while the joints are fusing.

the last nail hole. It also has a rocker toe. This type of shoe will allow for a lot of grinding that occurs when the foot lands with the stabbing gait. The rocker toe will help keep the toe of the shoe off the ground, limiting wear and making the shoe last longer. There is not really anything that can be put on the foot that will fix this problem, but shoes are essential to prevent uneven and excessive wear.

A lot of our customers' rodeo and cutting horses are shod behind with plain stamped handmade shoes in an effort to reduce the stress on the hocks. Since these shoes have a little less traction than traditional shoes, they allow these horses to work in soft ground on their hindquarters without as much stress as other shoes would create. The foot in **Figure 16** is shod with my most commonly used type of hind shoe. **Figure 17** shows a foot that Cody shod with a lateral heel extension. This is used a lot when the horse is sore from the developing spavin,as well as in horses that are cow-hocked.

Most of the treatment for this type of problem will come from the veterinary side. The horse can have everything done to it from injecting the joint capsules to having surgery to fuse the joints. The distal intertarsal joint and the tarsometatarsal joint can be fused, and the horse will become comfortable and usable again.

For the owner, the horse can be carefully monitored to determine when the joints need injecting again. They can also try to reduce the demands on the horse until the joints are fused or whatever other treatment is judged best has been completed.

ANTICIPATED OUTCOME

This is determined on a horse-by-horse basis. Some horses that develop spavin are done for good, while there are others who will end up feeling and moving fine. Regardless, a spavin is a sign of stress, and a horse with spavin should be considered damaged.

IN SHORT

D: Bone growth in the hock.

T: Shoe to prevent wear.

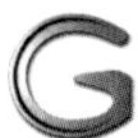

Chapter

46-12 SPLINTS

DEFINITION

The splint bones are attached to the cannon bone by interosseous ligaments. When these become damaged, the splint bone tears away. It is also possible for the splint bone to break. The resulting inflammation and eventual bone growth in this area is referred to as a splint.

REASON

A splint can be the result of a direct trauma to the splint bone. This is most likely when the splint bone has become broken. The splint bone can also have an area torn away from the cannon bone from mediolateral imbalance or severe twisting of the cannon bone. In the case of a cannon bone twisting, the horse has enough traction on its shoe that the body twisted without the shoe moving. This can cause the splint bone to separate from the cannon bone.

ANATOMY

Cannon bone, splint bones, interosseus ligaments. Most commonly the medial splint bone on the front leg (2nd metacarpal).

SYMPTOMS

When a splint first occurs, the horse may be a little bit off. There will be swelling on the leg in the area where the splint bone was damaged. At this point, it is known as a green splint.

In the event of a broken splint bone, the horse

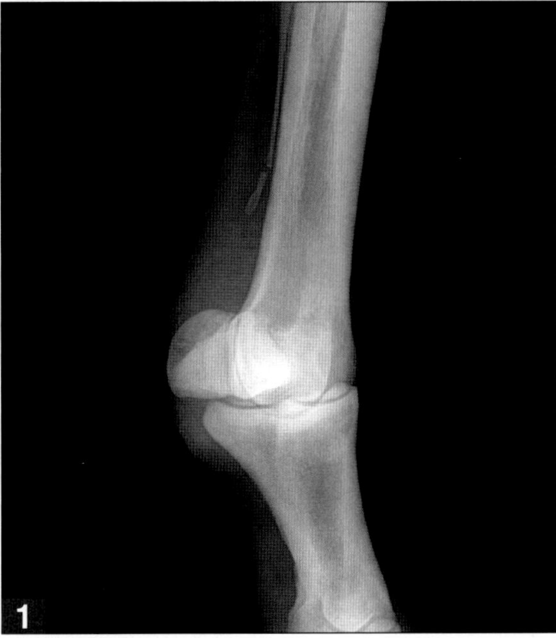

Radiograph from Dr. Marcotte showing a broken distal splint bone.

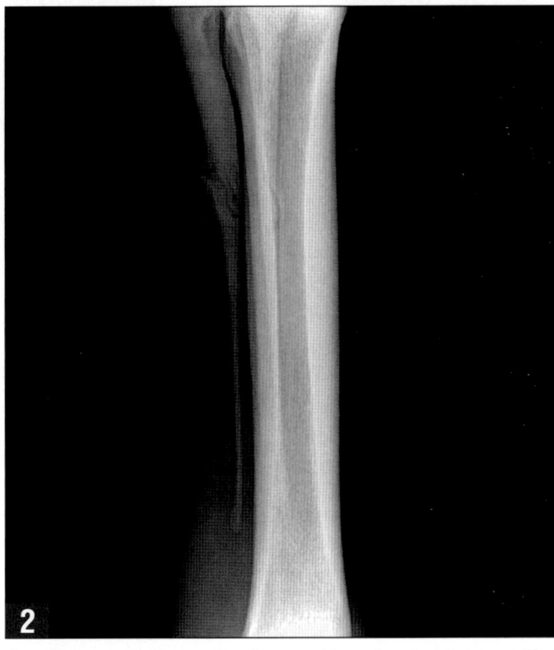

Radiograph from Dr. Marcotte of a broken splint bone.

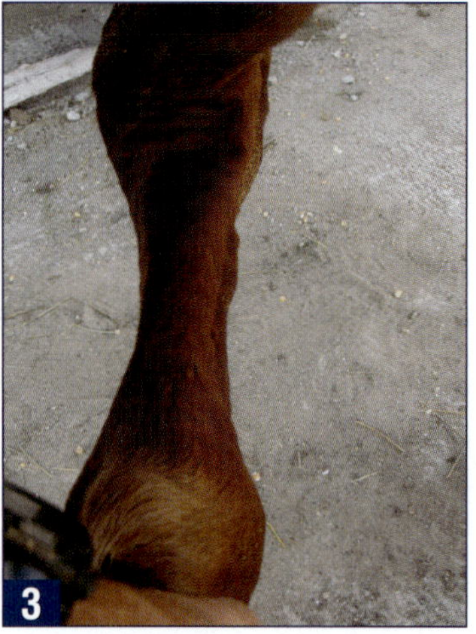

3

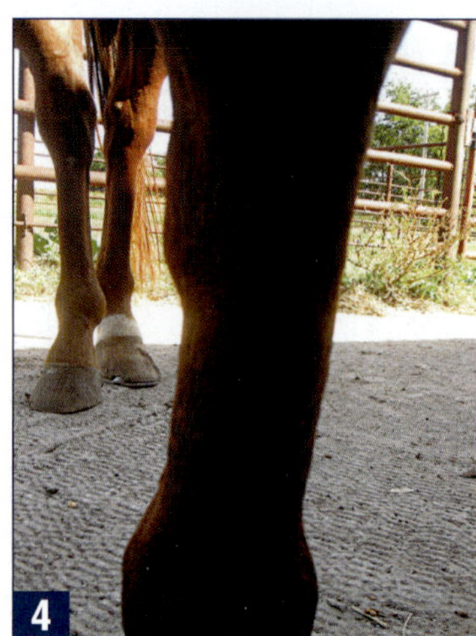

4

Medial splint on a front leg.

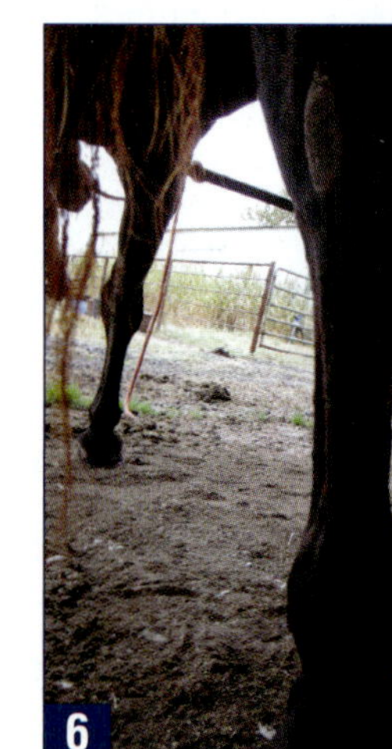

5

6

Lateral splint on a hind leg.

may be very lame. The area of the break, as well as the amount of interosseus ligament and cannon bone involvement, will play a big part in determining just how sore the horse will be. If an X-ray is taken, the damaged or broken splint bone will be evident. In **Figure 1**, the distal nodule of the splint bone has been broken off, and in **Figure 2**, the splint bone has been broken through the body of the bone. **Figure 2** is likely to be Grade 3 or 4 lame, while **Figure 1** may be anywhere from Grade 1 through Grade 4, depending on several factors.

TREATMENT

A normal splint that does not have a break in it will generally resolve itself within a few weeks. Stall rest is recommended if the horse is lame, but shoeing will consist of simply a balanced job. If the cause was from too much traction, then you will want to change the style of shoe on the horse. Once it heals, there will be a hard swelling where the injury occurred. This blemish is called a splint. In **Figures 3-4**, there is a splint on the 2nd metacarpal. This is where they most generally occur. In **Figures 5-6**, there is a splint on the 4th metatarsal. This is unusual, and the one in the pictures is quite large.

In the case of a broken splint bone, a veterinarian must be part of the equation. Whether to surgically remove the piece or not will be determined by the amount of pain the animal is in, and the potential to heal without surgery.

Owners must stay off the horses until they have healed. Getting the feet shod on a good schedule will also help to prevent splints from happening, by preventing foot imbalance from uneven growth. Using quality splint boots will help prevent splints.

ANTICIPATED OUTCOME

When a horse suffers with a splint, I expect the horse to be sore for about 21 days, but continually improving. A permanent bone growth will result, but no long term lameness.

IN SHORT

D: The splint bone has become separated from the cannon bone or broken.

T: Rest and time, possible surgery for broken splint bone.

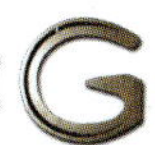

Chapter

46-13 SPRAINED SUSPENSORY LIGAMENT

DEFINITION

The suspensory ligament has become injured and over stressed.

REASON

The primary reasons are the same as those that cause a bowed tendon. However, instead of the superficial flexor tendon failing, in this case the suspensory ligament fails. The primary reasons are: overworking an unconditioned horse; a bad step; poor conformation; and bpoor quality shoeing or trimming.

ANATOMY

The primary anatomy is the suspensory ligament, but the sesamoids are also involved.

SYMPTOMS

In the early stages, the horse will be lame, and there will be inflammation in the suspensory ligament. Most of the time, this will occur close to the fetlock. If left untreated, the fetlock may descend and the foot may change from the unusual weight bearing. Once the injury heals, there will often be a swelling that can be considered a blemish.

Figure 1 shows a hind leg on a horse that had suffered a sprained suspensory ligament. It has healed, but the result is a large and somewhat hard area above the fetlock. **Figure 2** is a fishtail shoe. This shoe will give the maximum amount of support to the back of the leg, but I mainly recommend them on the hind feet. **Figures 3-5** show a horse that had a sprained suspensory ligament, but was left to heal on its own. Over time, the sesamoids may descend from their normal position, as is evident on the radiograph in **Figure 6**.

This horse in **Figures 7-9** was shod with a reverse shoe to really pull the toe back and extend the heels. While this did not make the horse sound, it definitely made it more comfortable. If left long enough, the horse may develop a condition called sesamoiditis. This comes from the sprained suspen-

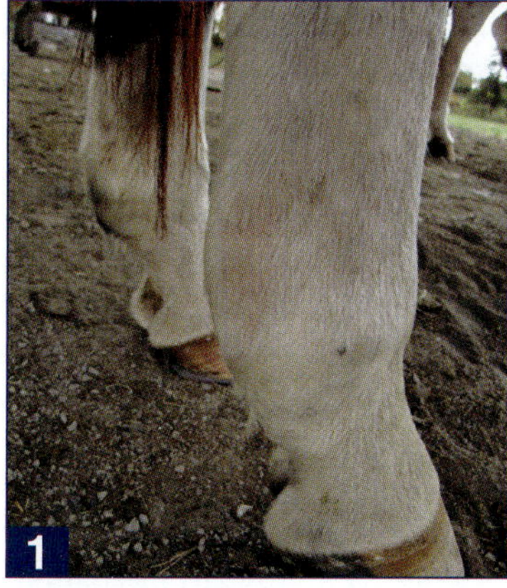

1

Healed sprained suspensory ligament.

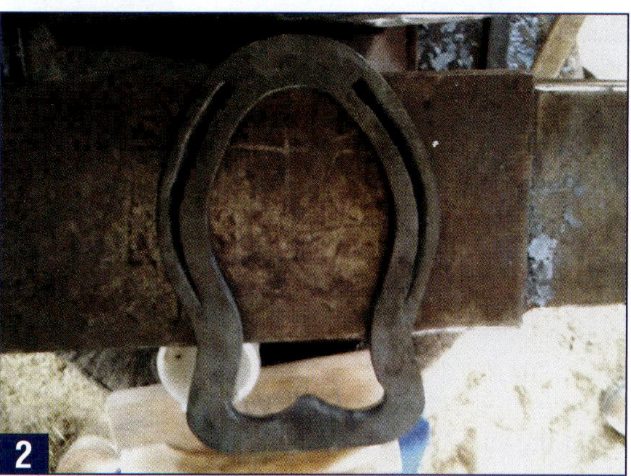

2

Fishtail shoe used to support the back of the leg.

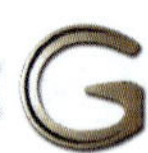

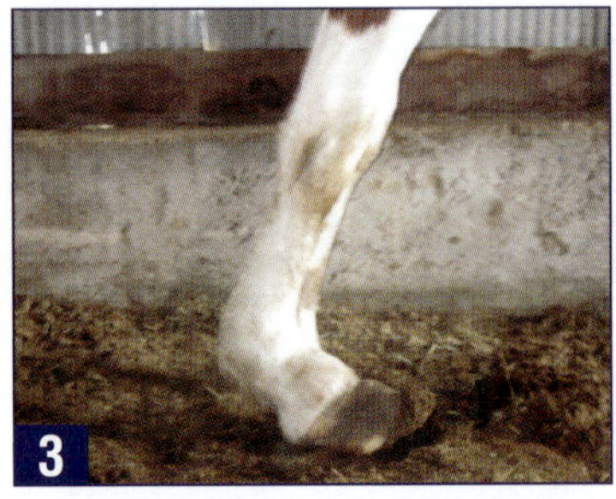

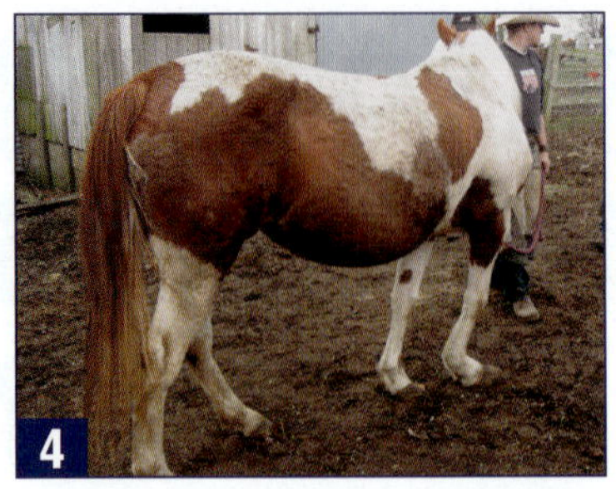

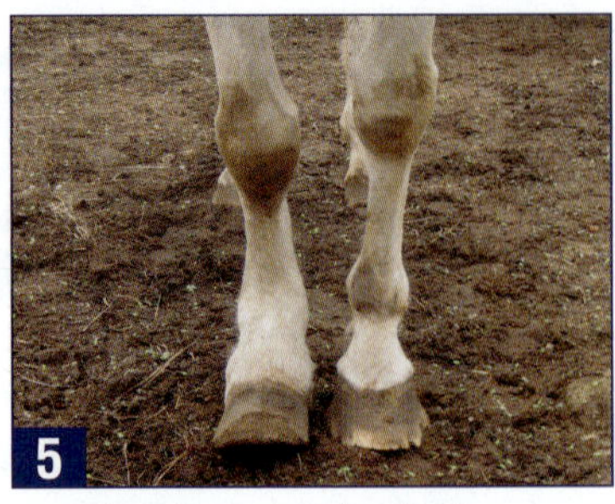

Badly crippled horse from a long-standing sprained suspensory ligament that has not healed.

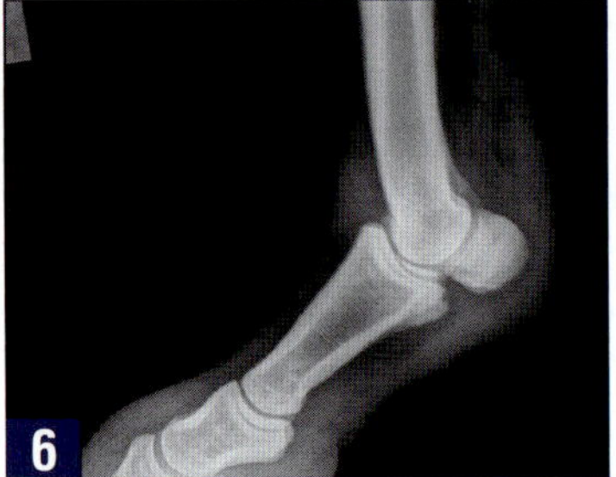

Radiograph of a horse that had suffered with a sprained suspensory ligament long enough that the sesamoids had descended.

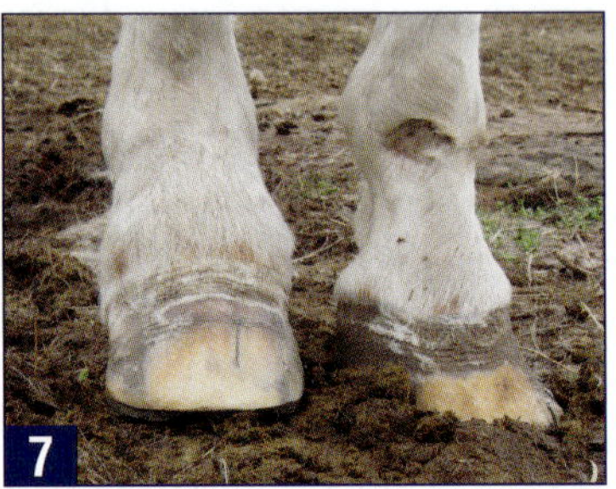

Dorsal view of the crippled horse with the reverse shoe on the foot.

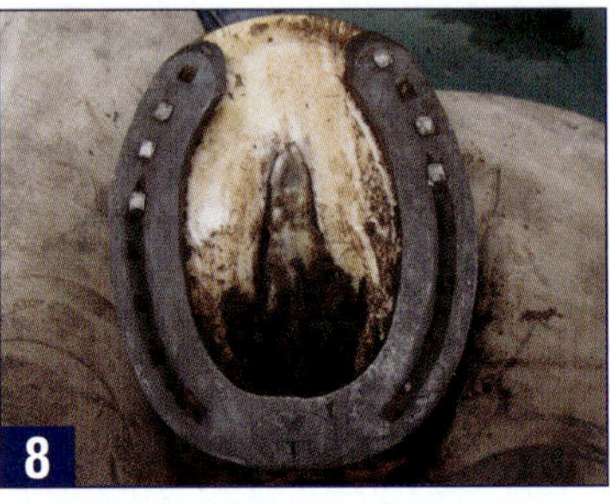

Solar view of the reverse shoe.

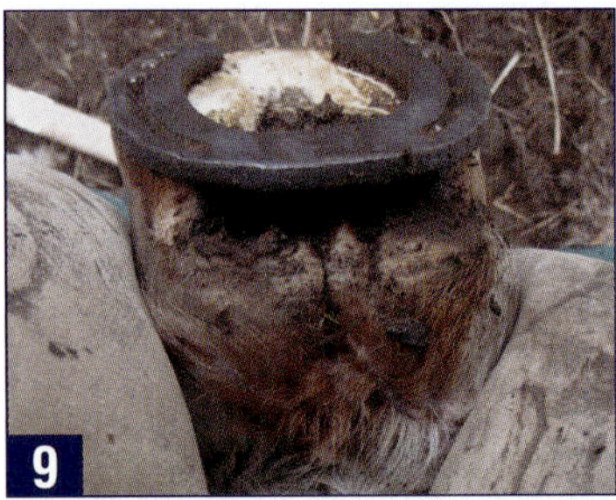

View showing the amount of heel extension from the reverse shoe.

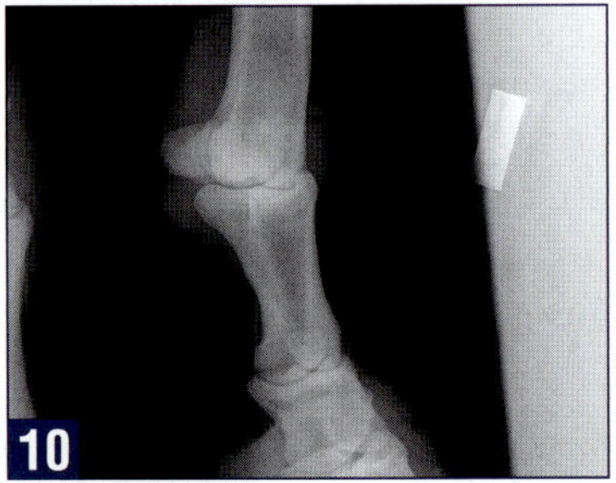

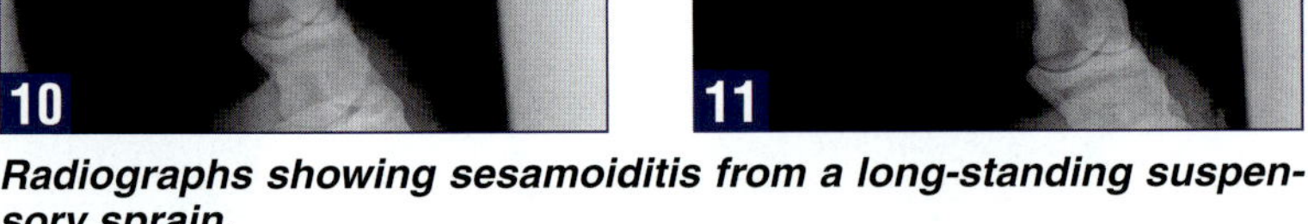

Radiographs showing sesamoiditis from a long-standing suspensory sprain.

sory ligament. The results can be seen in **Figures 10-11**. In these X-rays, the borders of the sesamoids appear to have a lot of striations in them as a result of demineralization.

TREATMENT

In the early stages, stall rest, wrapping the legs, shoeing with a heel extension, and trimming to take stress off of the suspensory ligament should all be done. The trim strategy will generally involve lowering the heels. This will recruit the deep flexor tendon to do more work while letting the superficial flexor tendon and suspensory ligament have a little bit of a break. The extended heels will support the back of the leg.

Depending on the cause, a patten bar in the early stages may be very helpful. If the horse just took a bad step, I would lean toward the patten bar. If the horse was ridden to the point of material fatigue, then a patten bar may make the opposite leg do too much work. Just because one leg was injured, bear in mind that the other leg was on the same ride.

For the veterinarian, there are drugs that can be injected into the leg, shock wave therapy, and the possibility of casting or other devices that may be used. The vet also has the potential to use and interpret an ultrasound machine. This is a great diagnostic tool when looking at a sprained tendon or ligament **(Figure 12)**.

The owner needs to be committed to the time and care it will take for this horse to heal. Even though the horse may appear sound earlier than expected, please don't use them ahead of schedule.

ANTICIPATED OUTCOME

There are several factors that come into play with the potential outcome of a horse with a sprained suspensory ligament. First is the extent of the damage. The worse it is hurt, the more difficult the recovery. Next is the conformation of the animal. The time from injury to treatment is a factor, as is the willingness of the owner to follow all of the instructions for fixing the problem.

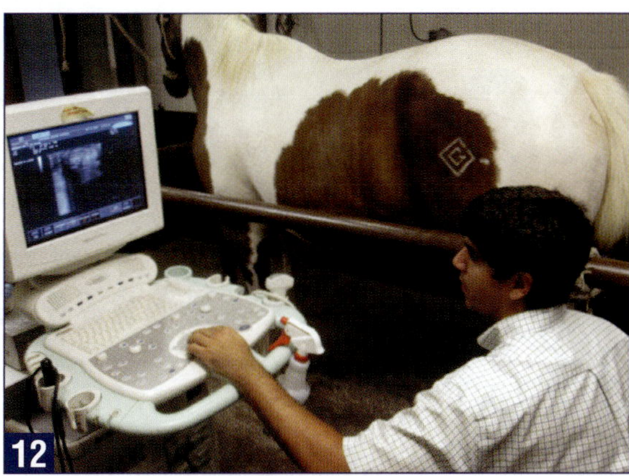

Dr. Lamb at Oakridge Equine Hospital using an ultrasound machine.

IN SHORT

D: Injured suspensory ligament.

T: Stall rest, wrap legs, shoe to alleviate stress, extended heels, and vet attention.

Chapter

46-14 STIFLED AND STIFLE LAMENESS

DEFINITION

Stifled refers to the upward locking of the patella on the distal end of the femur, causing the limb to be locked in extension. Stifle lameness, on the other hand, is lameness that results from damage in the stifle joint.

REASON

A horse's patella becomes locked because it has become hooked on the bulbous medial ridge of the femoral trochlea. The quadriceps normally contracts to raise the patella, and the biceps femoris contracts to pull the patella off the medial ridge. When these muscles are not toned or the patella is loose, the potential to lock in place on the medial ridge of the femoral trochlea is present. This is more common in horses with a straighter conformation.

With stifle lameness, the horse has become injured for a variety of reasons, including osteochondrosis, arthritis, fracture, ligament avulsion, and falling.

ANATOMY

The stifle joint comprises the distal femur, the patella, and the proximal tibia. Since there is a reciprocal apparatus on the hind limb, a problem in the stifle area will affect the entire limb.

SYMPTOMS

When a horse has a tendency to being stifled, it will be going along at a walk, trot, or pace, and the hind limb will become fixed in an extended position. This may be frequent or rare, depending on the conformation of the horse. It can happen from a misstep or working a horse that is not in shape for the job being demanded of it.

With stifle lameness, there will generally be changes in the joint as can be seen in these x-rays

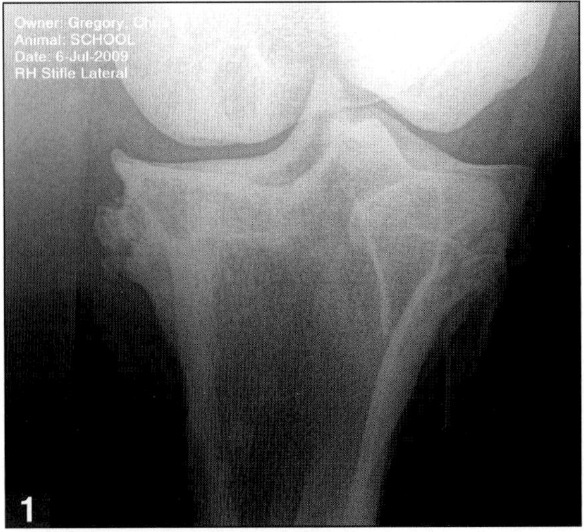

Bone spur on the proximal tibia.

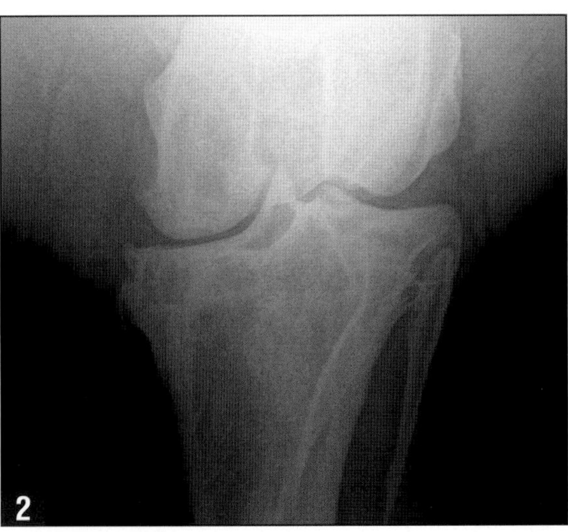

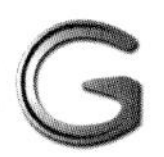

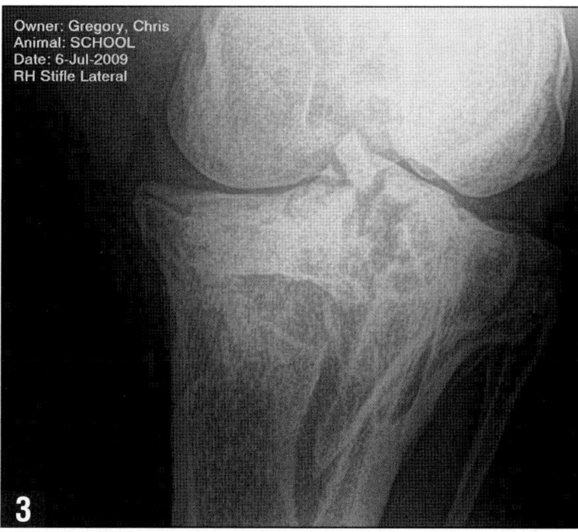

Arthritis in the stifle joint.

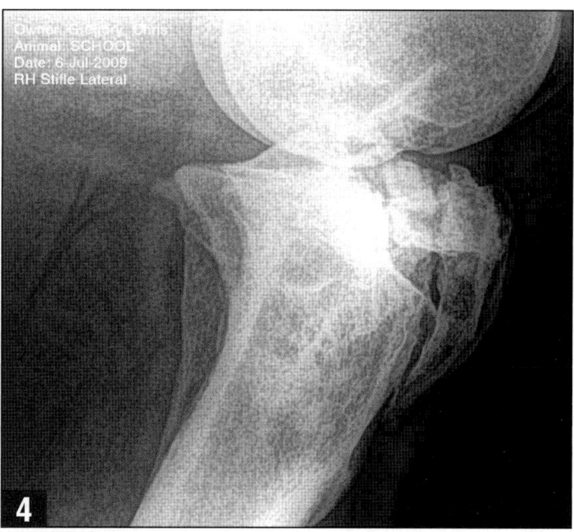

Major damage to the proximal tibia.

by Dr. Marcotte. These will be seen as osteophyte and enthesiophyte growths, arthritis, and bone spurs. **Figures 1-5** are several stifle joints that have suffered from injury and damage.

TREATMENT

If a horse has a problem becoming stifled, working the horse on hills to strengthen the quadriceps and biceps femoris will be quite beneficial. The veterinarian may blister the media patellar ligament or may do surgery to shorten the ligament. At one time, the vet might have done a desmotomy (to cut a ligament) of the medial patellar ligament, but that is uncommon now. Completely cutting the ligament will prevent the upward fixation, but it also destroys the passive stay apparatus. If you are with a horse when the patella gets locked, you may be able to unlock it by scaring the horse backwards. A locked patella can also be manually manipulated by straightening the leg even more, and then pushing the patella out.

With stifle lameness, there is often little to be done. Joint injections and therapy such as swimming may provide some relief, but a lot will depend on the extent of the injury.

From the farrier's perspective, the only thing we can do with shoeing to affect the stifle is to protect the foot from uneven wear with a good shoe on a well-balanced foot.

The vet may have a whole range of suggestions, and the owner should take the advice that is given and do what can be done for the horse.

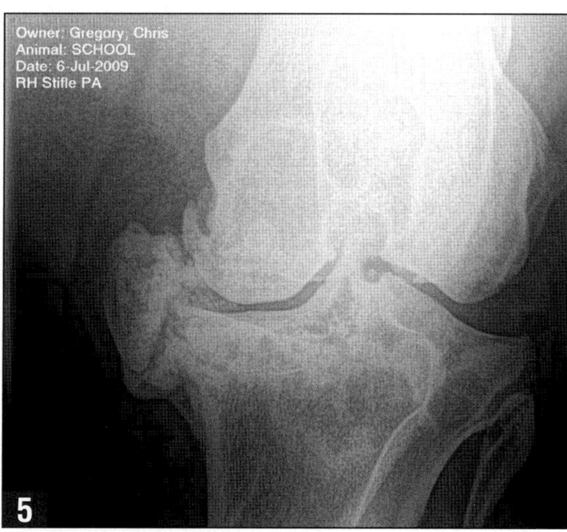

Large bone growth.

ANTICIPATED OUTCOME

There have been a lot of stifled horses that have returned to work without problem once they have gained muscle tone or had surgery or injections. For the horse with stifle lameness, the outcome is based entirely on the extent of the injury, the stage the injury is detected, and the ability of the horse to heal.

IN SHORT

D: Stifled is upward fixation of the patella. Stifle lameness is seen in a horse that moves with pain from injury to the stifle joint.

T: Trim, level, and balance, protecting the foot from uneven wear. Use a good vet.

Chapter

46-15 STRINGHALT

DEFINITION

The term stringhalt is used to describe the unintentional, jerky, sudden, and spastic lifting of the hind foot as a horse is walking.

REASON

There has been a lot of speculation about the exact cause of stringhalt. As of now, the best suggestion is that it is a nervous condition caused by a brain injury, spine injury, or if unilateral, an injury to the nerve that controls the lateral extensor muscle.

ANATOMY

The nervous system is implicated, as well as the lateral extensor muscle and tendon.

SYMPTOMS

When the horse is being worked, it will have a sudden lifting of the hind foot in flight in an unusual manner. In severe cases, the horse may actually hit itself in the belly with the leg. The condition can be unilateral (one leg) or bilateral (both legs).

TREATMENT

Treatment for stringhalt is completely out of the farrier realm. The farrier may have to be careful to avoid injury when working on these horses, since the leg can come up violently.

There has been success with preventing the movement from being so spastic by doing a tenotomy of the lateral extensor tendon. This may not fix the problem, but it can make the symptoms less severe.

Some horses do better with rest but generally have symptoms return once they are worked.

ANTICIPATED OUTCOME

I have only dealt with a couple of horses with this problem, both Missouri Foxtrotters. They were unusable, but that may depend on the severity of the problem.

IN SHORT

D: Sudden and jerky movement of the hind legs.

T: Tenotomy of the lateral extensor tendon of the hind legs involved.

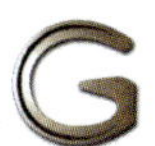

Chapter

46-16 THOROUGHPIN

DEFINITION

Thoroughpin refers to the distension of the deep flexor tendon sheath where it passes in front of the calcaneus in the hock. This condition is also called hollows.

REASON

This is a sign of stress. The horse is being worked hard enough that there is an inflammation of the tendon and sheath in this area.

ANATOMY

Deep flexor tendon and its sheath in the hock.

SYMPTOMS

The horse will not be lame from this, but there will be a soft swelling in hock, just dorsal to the calcaneus, primarily on the lateral side. One of the interesting features is that if the swelling is pushed on, it will often disappear temporarily or sometimes cause distension on the medial side.

The picture of the hock in **Figures 1-2** is of a thoroughpin. Notice that this one is big enough that there is swelling on both sides of the hock in front of the calcaneus. **Figure 3** shows a hock that has swelling in the area where thoroughpin occurs, but this happens to be a bone growth, not a thoroughpin. Palpation of the area will tell you if the swelling is hard or soft.

TREATMENT

Since the horse is not sore, there isn't a shoeing-related treatment. The veterinarian and owner may treat the condition as you would a windpuff; with cold water, liniment, and backing off of the training. The shrunken thoroughpin often returns once training is resumed.

ANTICIPATED OUTCOME

The horse isn't sore and generally doesn't become sore.

IN SHORT

D: Soft swelling in the deep flexor tendon sheath where it passes through the hock.

T: Nothing that is farrier related.

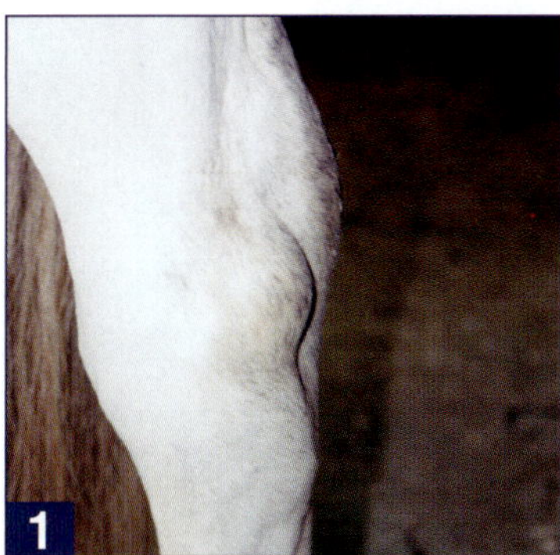

1

Lateral view of a hock with a large thoroughpin.

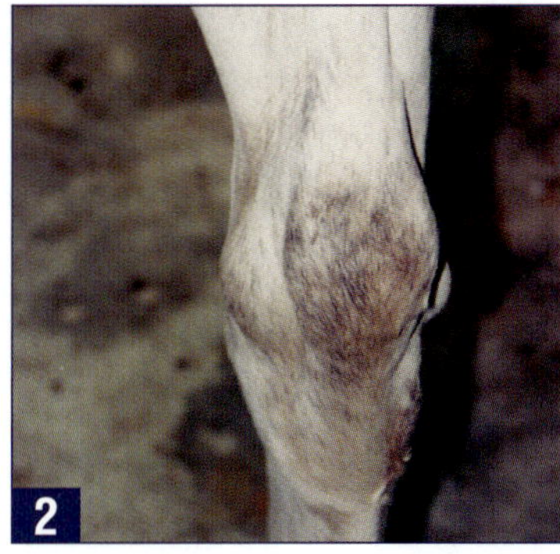

2

Plantar view of the same hock in Figure 1.

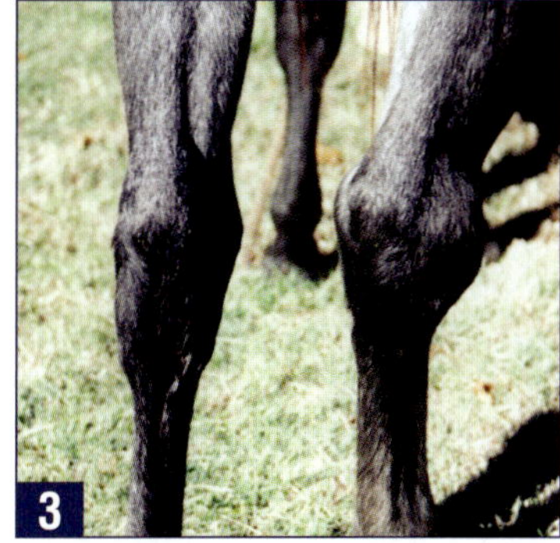

3

A hock with a large bone growth.

Chapter

46-17 WINDPUFFS

DEFINITION

This is a chronic soft puffy swelling that occurs in the fetlock region. It is also known as road puffs and hygromata. There are two types of windpuffs. Articular windpuffs are a distension of the fetlock joint capsule, and tendinous windpuffs are distension of the deep flexor tendon sheath at the level of the pastern.

REASON

The actual cause of windpuffs is not known. The swellings are not associated with any lameness, heat, tenderness, inflammation or changes in the synovial fluid. They are thought to be sign of stress from overwork, poor conformation, or poor shoeing and trimming.

ANATOMY

Tendinous windpuffs involve the deep flexor tendon sheath, and articular windpuffs involve the joint capsule of the fetlock. Front and hind legs can be affected.

SYMPTOMS

The only symptom is the swelling behind the fetlock. There is no lameness or pain associated with this condition. **Figure 1** is a drawing that represents the areas where windpuffs will occur. **Figures 2-5** are different angles of a hind leg with both articular and tendinous windpuffs.

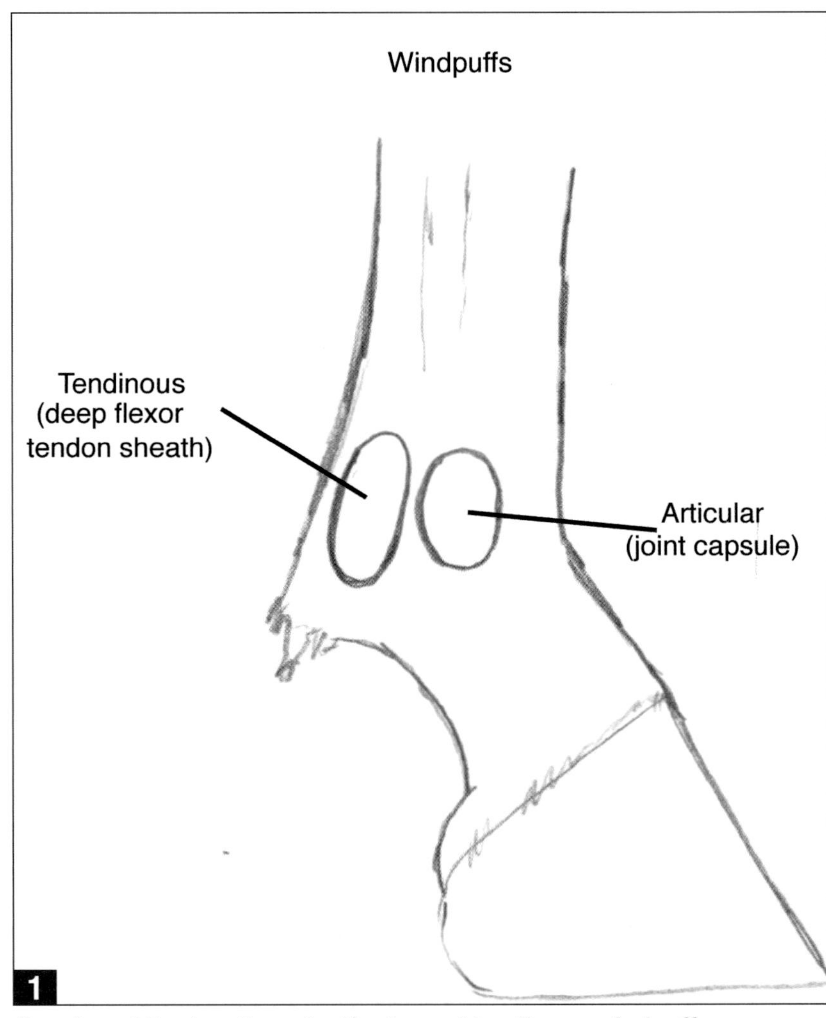

Drawing of the location of articular and tendinous windpuffs.

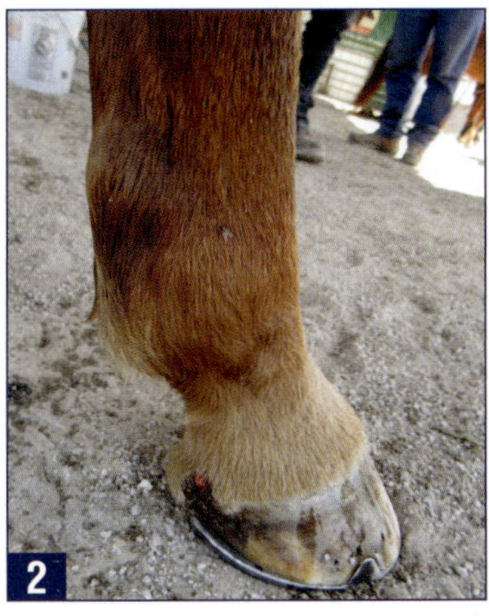

Lateral view of a leg with windpuffs.

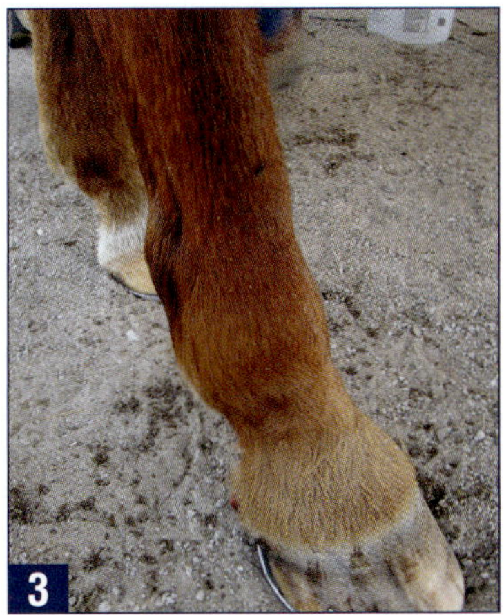

Dorsolateral oblique view.

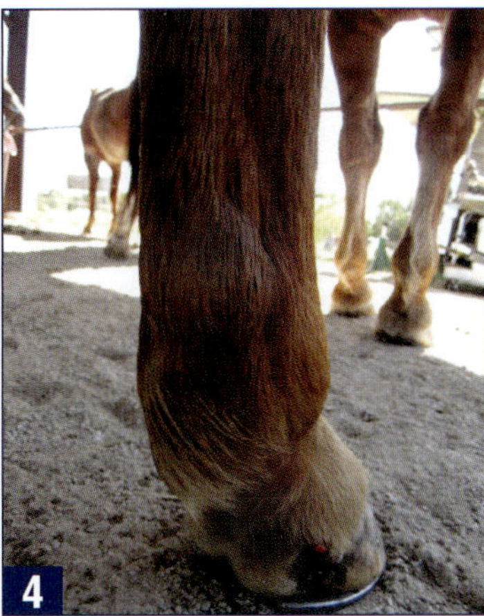

Plantarlateral view.

TREATMENT

Pressure bandages and/or the application of a liniment are really all that can be done, and some horses will still continue to have windpuffs. Be careful that a strong liniment is not covered with a bandage since that can cause some serious skin irritation. Ice and water therapy may also have some beneficial effect.

A vet can drain them if the owner is concerned with aesthetics, and the owner can bandage or apply liniment if desired.

ANTICIPATED OUTCOME

Since the horse is not lame, I rarely worry about windpuffs. They may go away if treated, but there is no difference in how the horse feels.

IN SHORT

D: Soft puffy swelling behind the fetlock joint.
T: Liniment, bandaging, or ignore.

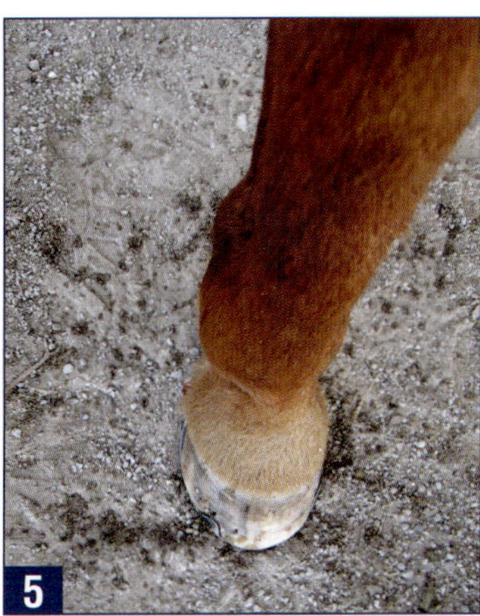

View from the hip.

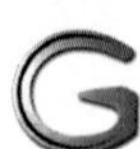

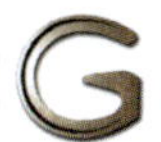

Section

11

Shoe Arsenal

Chapter 47: Farrier's Arsenal 532

Chapter 48: Straight Bar Shoe 536

Chapter 49: Egg Bar Shoe 551

Chapter 50: Heart Bar, W-Shoe and G-Bar 561

Chapter 51: Patton Bar 569

Chapter 52: Z-Bar 573

Chapter 53: Aluminum Fundamentals For Farriers 578

Chapter 54: Hospital Plate 590

Chapter 55: Extensions 594

"[7] And the staff of his spear was like a weaver's beam; and his spear's head weighed six hundred shekels of iron: and one bearing a shield went before him."

—Samuel 17:7

—New King James Version

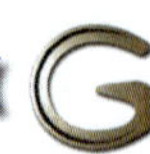

Chapter

47 FARRIER'S ARSENAL

INTRODUCTION

This section will cover making and fitting the main pathological shoes that every farrier should learn to make and use.

Throughout your career, you will find the need to shoe horses that present a challenge to the average farrier. From lameness to conformation abnormalities, you will have to be equipped to cope with some interesting feet. To be a great farrier requires that one is great in every aspect of farriery. You cannot be considered a great all-around farrier if you don't know anatomy, can't handle horses, or are unable to make and apply certain shoes.

I have known some that said they were great farriers based on their ability to trim feet. They claimed that the trim is the bulk of the job, and the shoe does not matter as much as the trim. When it comes to pathological shoeing, they are wrong.

There are a handful of shoes that you should learn to make and fit well. Doing so will mean you can decrease your inventory of factory-made shoes yet still provide a service that is above and beyond that of the normal horseshoer. The savings in inventory alone will make it worth it, however, the fact that you can charge a much higher price for these shoes and save money by making them yourself means you are going to get paid for your skills.

The earlier you learn to make these shoes, the more money you will make throughout your career. It works like this. As of 2010, a pair of heart bar shoes will run around $25 from a local supplier. There is about $2 worth of steel in them. Once they are applied to a horse, most farriers will charge around $50 extra for the heart bars. If you made the shoes, you made $48, not to mention the pride in craftsmanship. Beyond that, you weren't hauling

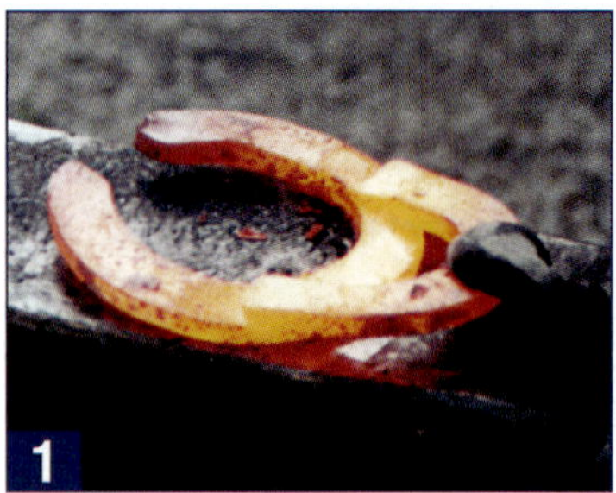

1 *Jump welding a toe extension.*

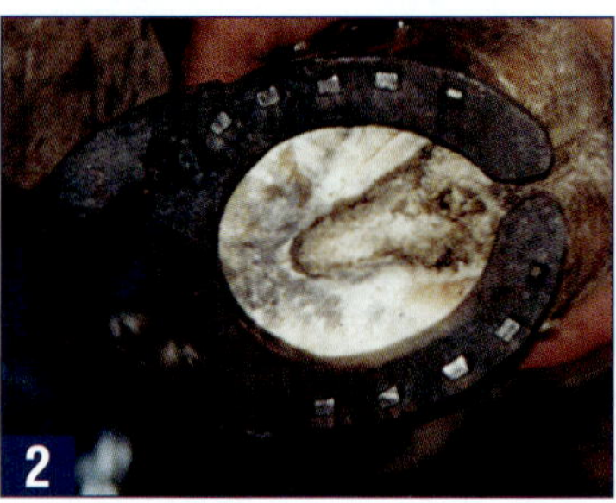

2 *Toe extension on the crippled mare.*

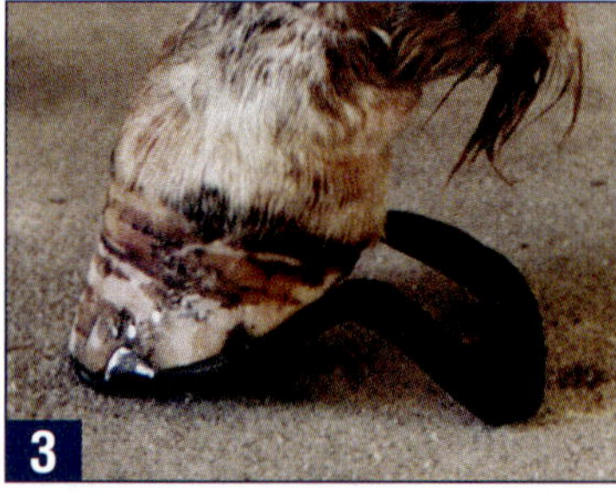

3 *Patton bar on horse with torn tendon.*

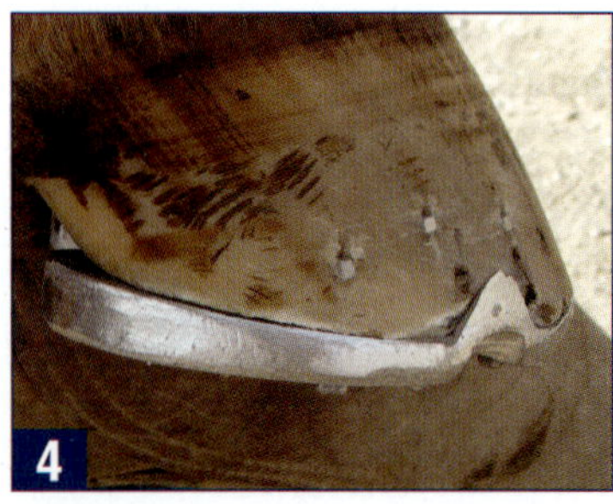

4 *Wedge-heel handmade aluminum shoe*

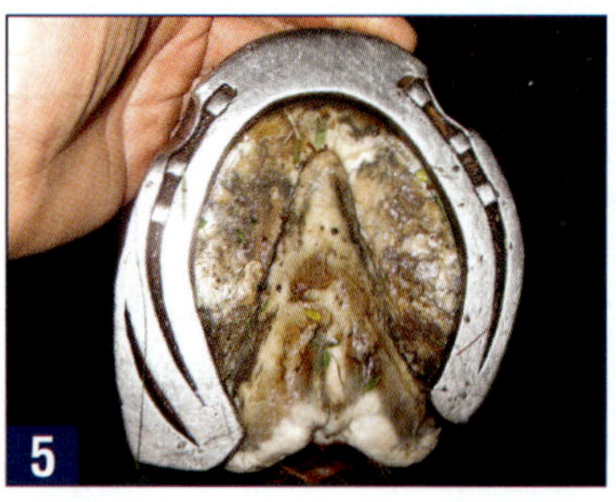

5 *Lateral heel extension hind.*

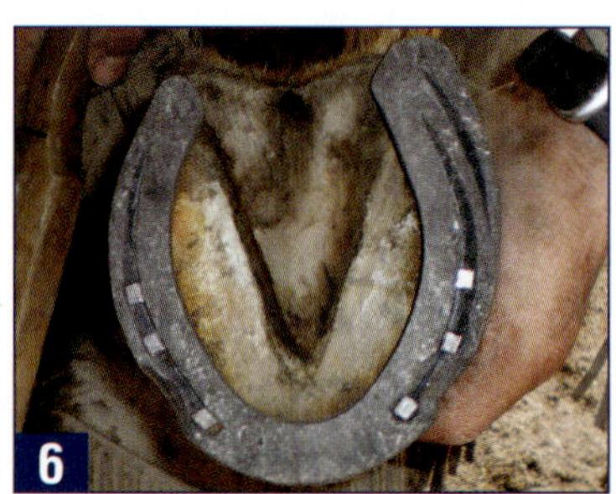

6

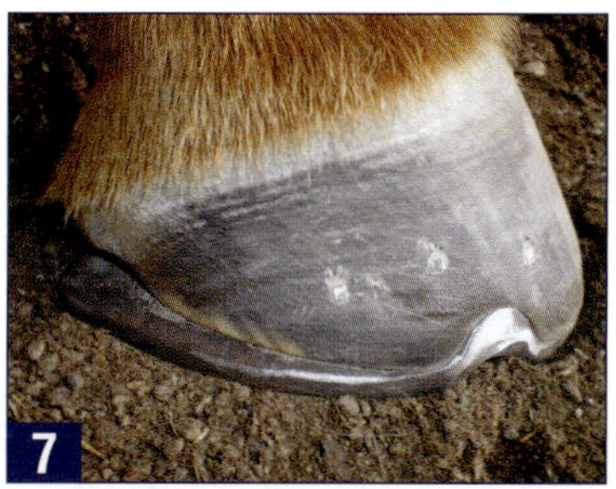

Lateral heel extension from a lateral view.

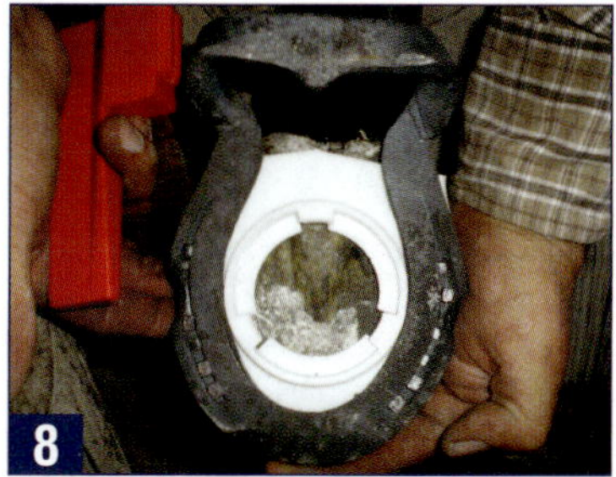

Patten bar with a hospital plate pad.

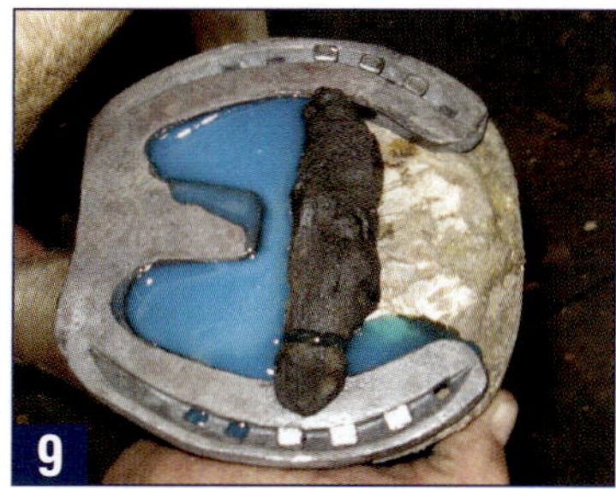

W-shoe with an Equi-Pak pour in.

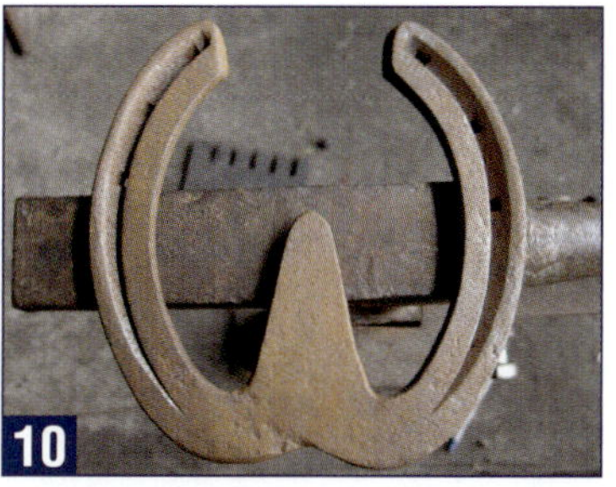

W-shoe made by the late Steve Casey, AWCF.

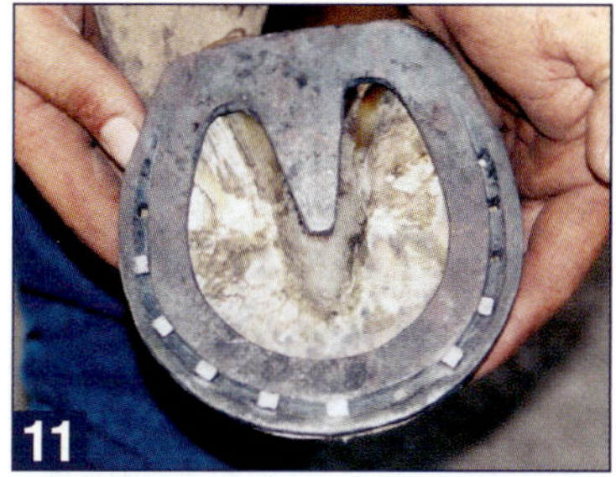

Heart bar on foot.

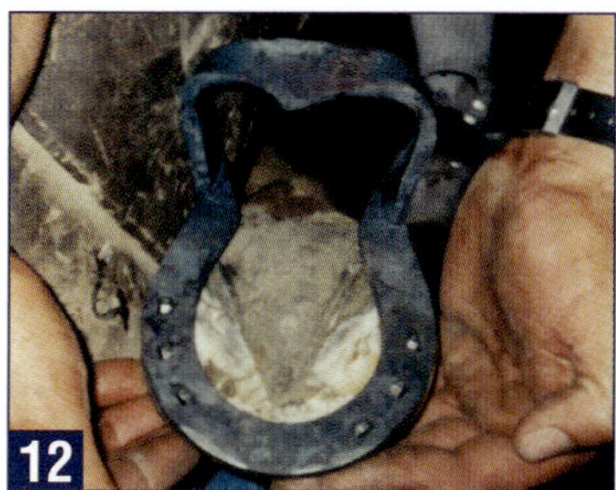

Front patten bar.

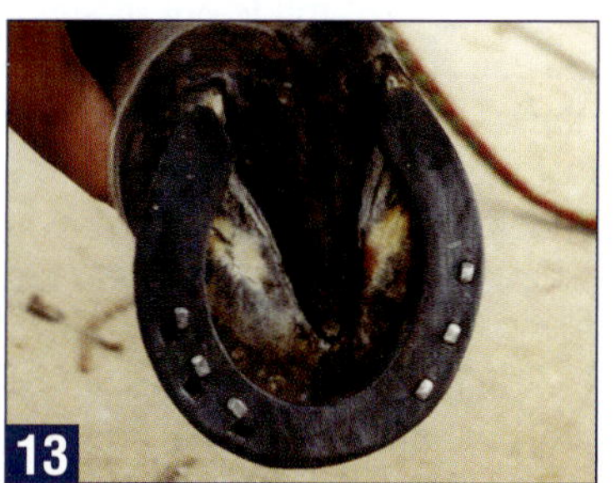

Lateral extension front.

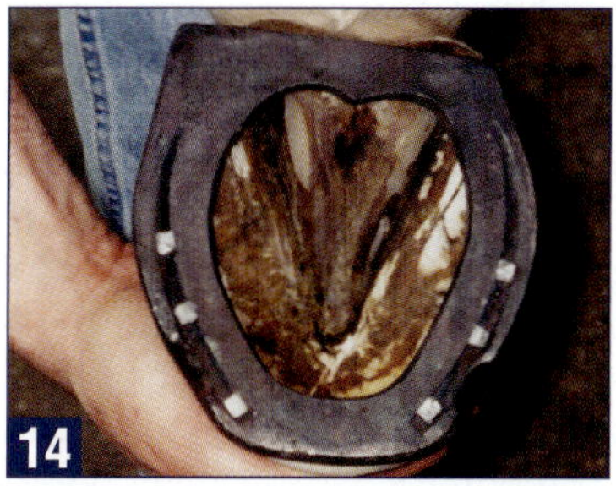

Lateral heel extension hind bar shoe.

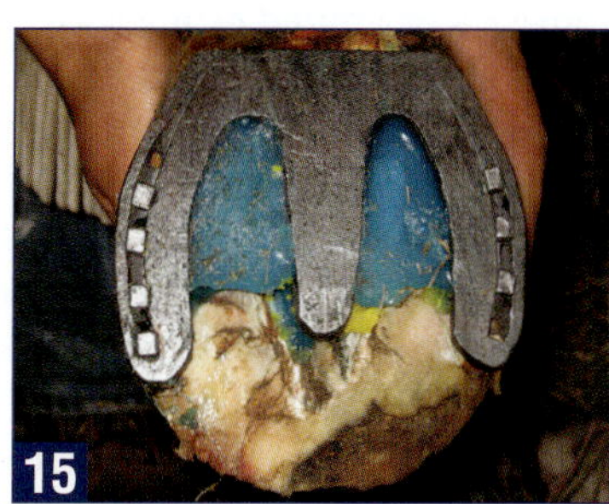

W-shoe made by Cody.

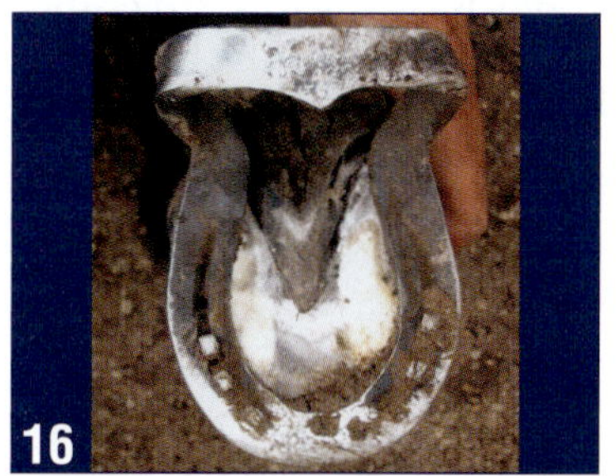

Patton bar on a mule with a broken humerus.

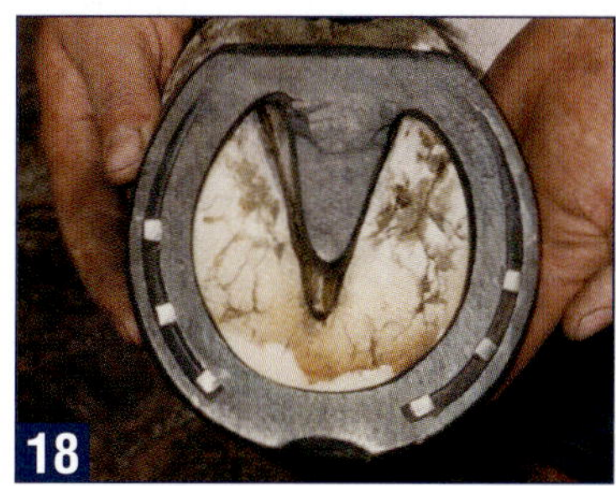

Heart bar.

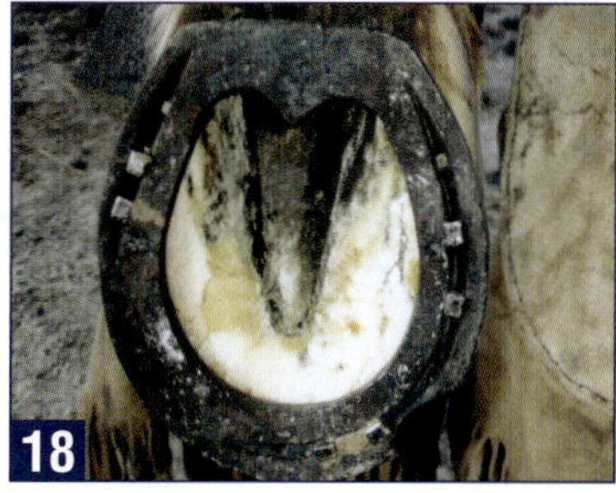

Straight bar.

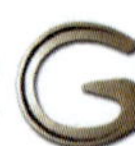

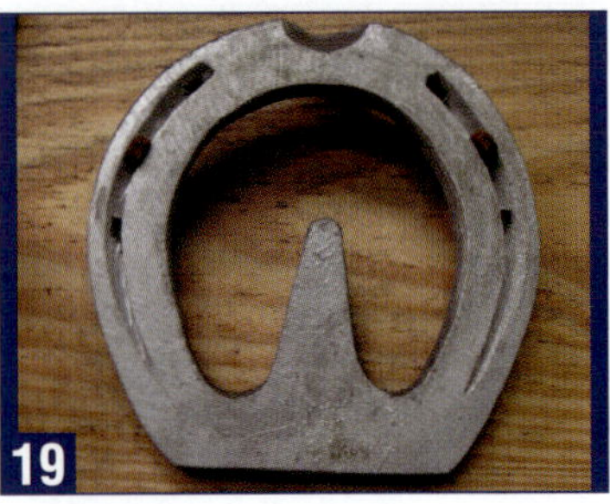
Aluminum heart bar.

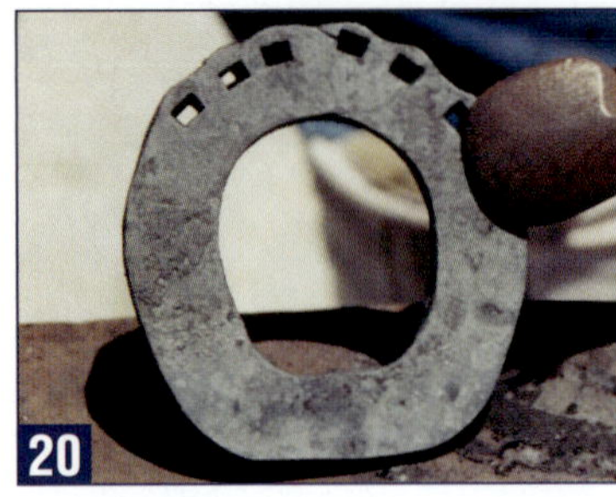
Foal straight bar.

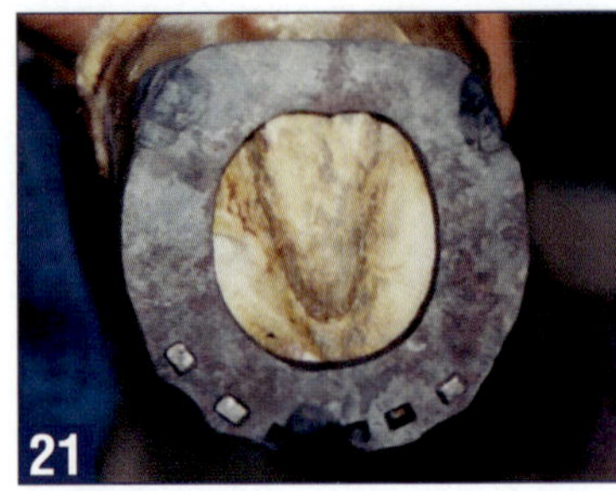
Foal straight bar, broken coffin bone.

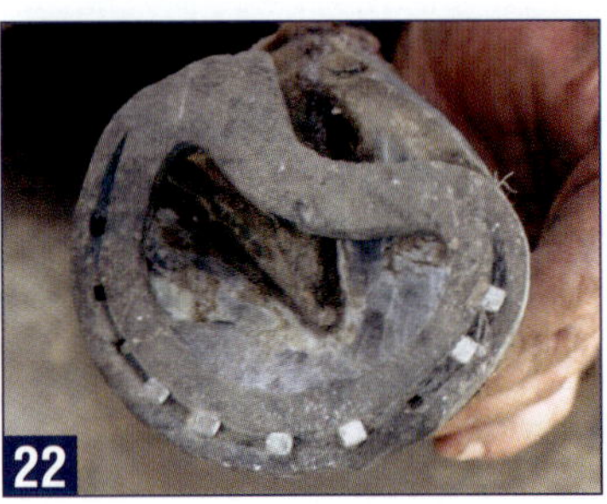
Z-bar.

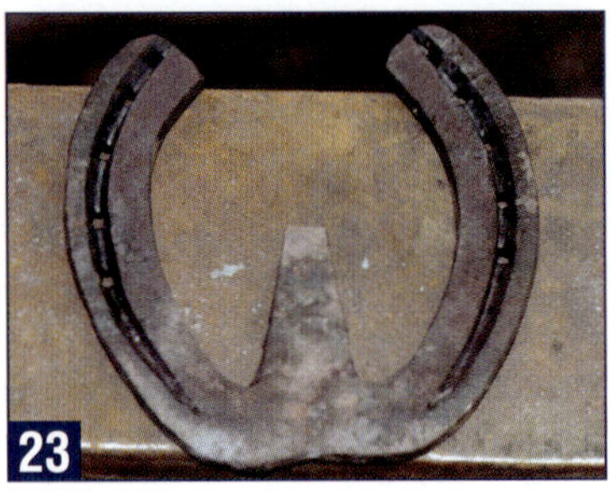
W-shoe.

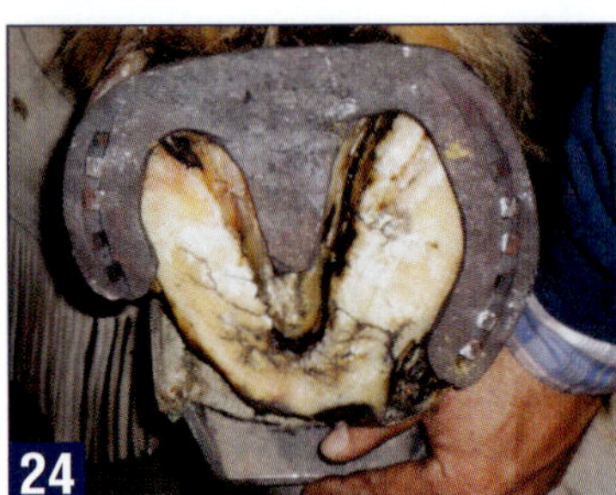
Modified W-shoe on draft horse.

those shoes around as inventory for months. Every time I make and nail on a pair of specialty shoes, I think about how much that client is paying for the practice that I put in learning to make those shoes.

There is the argument about time being money, so I recommend you become competent enough at making these shoes that it does not take very long. Then your time really is money. However, you will find that when you are self-employed, your time has a different value than if you were working for someone else and a wage.

The main shoes I think that you need to know how to make at a minimum are:

- Straight bar
- Egg bar
- Heart bar/W-shoe/G-bar
- Patten bar
- Z-bar
- Lateral extension
- Wedges

Some of these shoes are best made out of steel, some aluminum. You can add hospital plates, pads, pour-ins, and other things to the shoes above, but the basis is the making of the shoe itself.

None of these shoes are worth making if you do not also learn to fit them correctly. They should generally be fullered or creased, since they are often used on an injured foot. It is sometimes necessary to remove individual nails to put less stress on the foot. A plain stamped shoe does not allow this. Although I will give you suggestions for measurements, you will have to make some of these shoes yourself to determine what your formula is.

Turn the page, and let's start making some shoes.

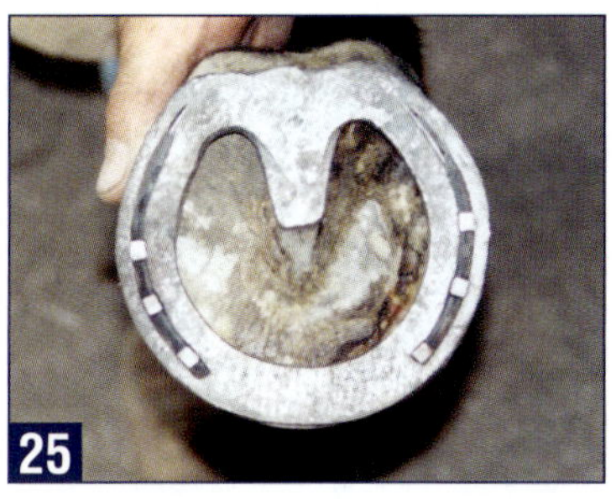
Heart bar.

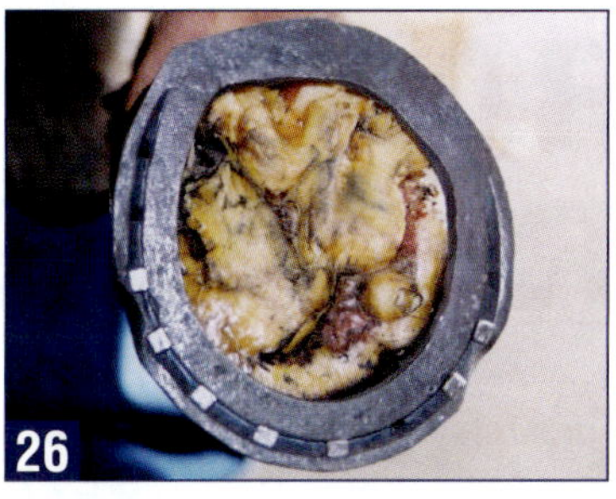
Modified straight bar.

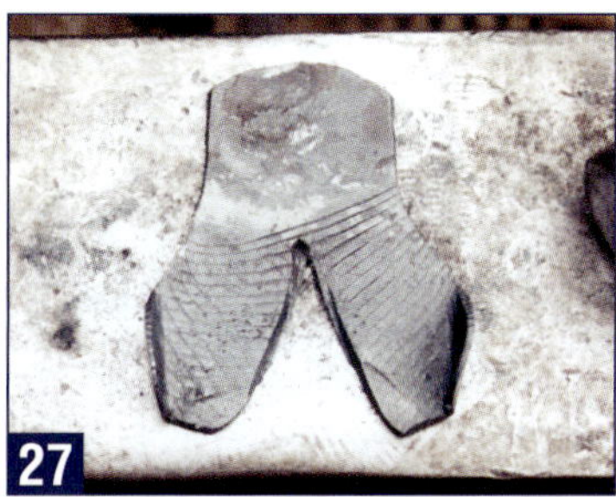
Foal toe extension made from rasp.

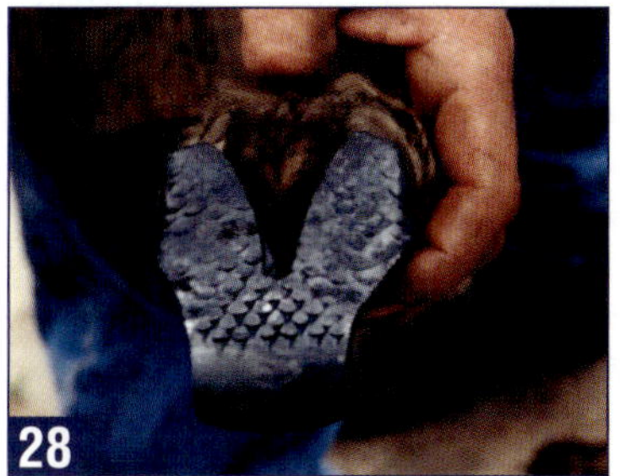
Toe extension applied to foot, ready to be glued.

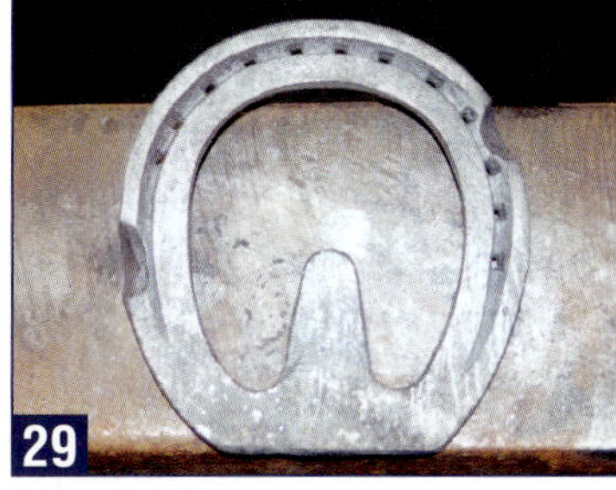
Heart bar.

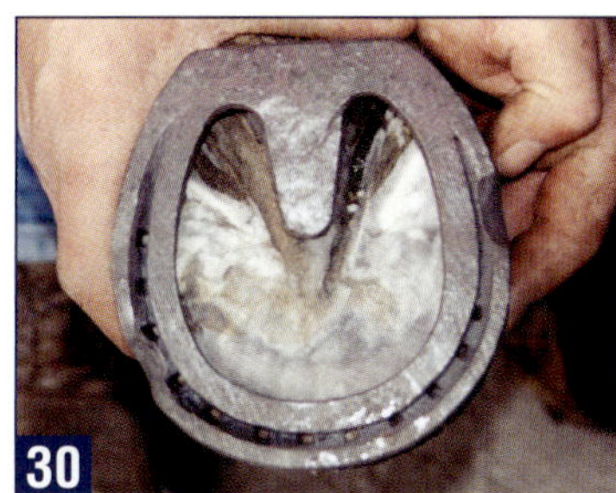
Heart bar on foot.

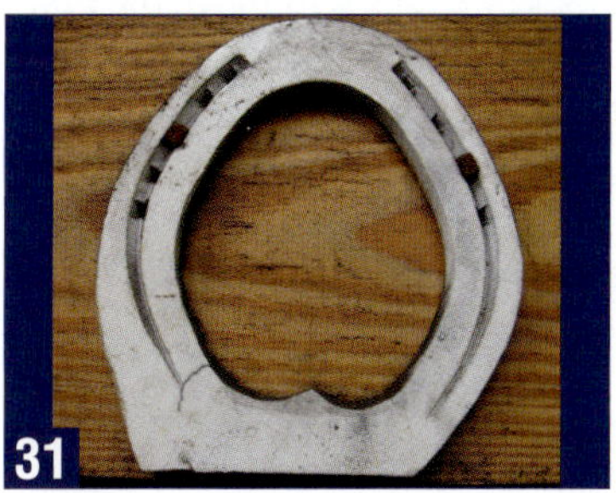
Lateral heel extension bar shoe.

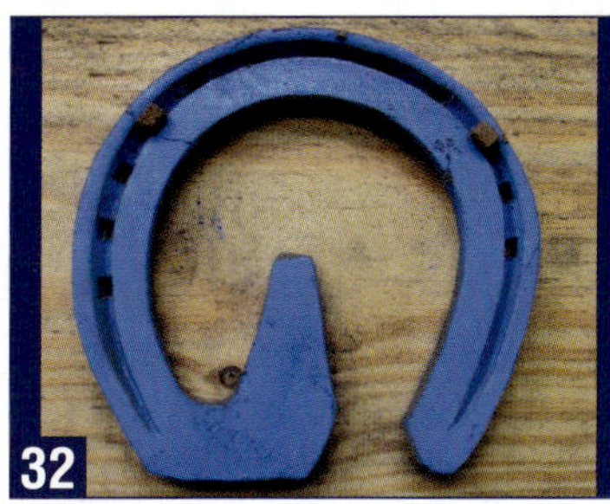
G-bar.

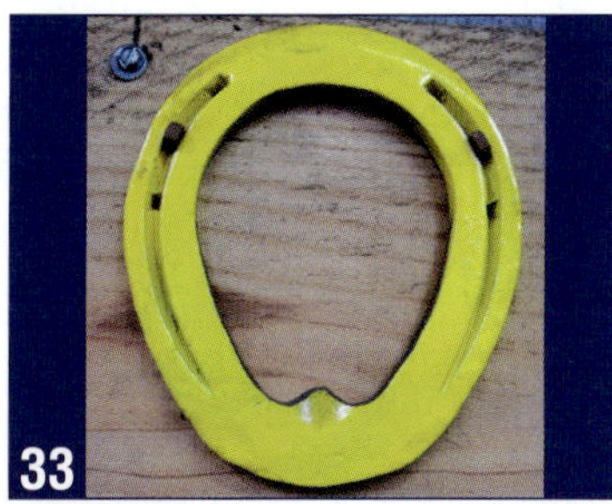
Egg bar.

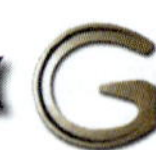

Chapter 48 STRAIGHT BAR SHOE

This is the foundation for pathological shoeing. In essence, the straight bar's main function is to stabilize the hoof capsule. There is also some advantage from web width across the heel that will reduce ground penetration in softer footing and give the foot protection from more shoe, but the main factor is to make a foot more rigid.

To measure for a straight bar, I am going to give you the formula Cody used when he was working on passing his AFA Certified Journeyman Exam. Using bar stock that was 3/4-inch wide, he would measure the circumference of the foot from heel to heel. Then he would measure the width of the bar at the heels. If the bar width was 2 1/2 inches or less, he would cut the steel the same length as the foot measured from heel to heel. Whatever distance the heels measured beyond 2 1/2 inches, he would add that amount to the measurement. For instance: A foot measures 14 inches from heel to heel, and the bar width has to be 3 1/4 inches. For this shoe, it would require 14 3/4 inches of steel. 14 + (3 1/4 - 2 1/2) = 14 3/4. If you use wider bar stock, you will need less steel. An average of 1/4 inch less length of bar stock for every 1/8 inch wider the stock is.

STRAIGHT BAR SHOE SEVEN HEATS TO A BLANK

SETUP

If you are just learning to make a bar shoe, and it is not for a given foot, begin by cutting two pieces of 5/16-by-3/4-by14 inch stock.

It is just as easy and quick to make two shoes at the same time if you are using a propane forge. This fact makes using propane an advantage for people who are taking the bar shoe portion of the AFA Certified Journeyman exam. With coal or coke, begin by making one shoe at a time unless you are already proficient in working more than one piece in a coke fire.

I recommend that beginners don't mark the stock in the straight since it can be difficult to keep the center mark in the center of the toe. Any small discrepancy in the hockey sticks will move the mark in the toe. If you have your nails marked as well, then the whole pattern will be racked.

HEAT 1

Heat the middle of the stock and make a toe bend

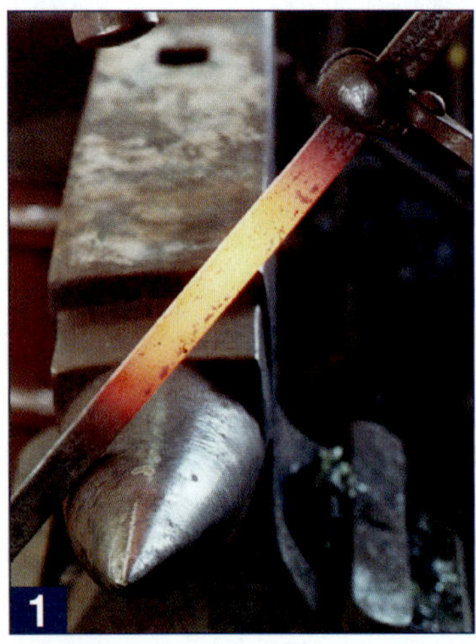

Choking up on the stock to make the toe bend in the middle of the stock.

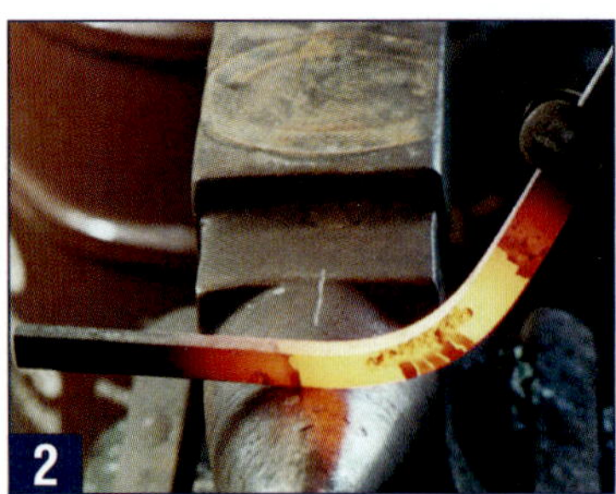

Beginning of the toe bend.

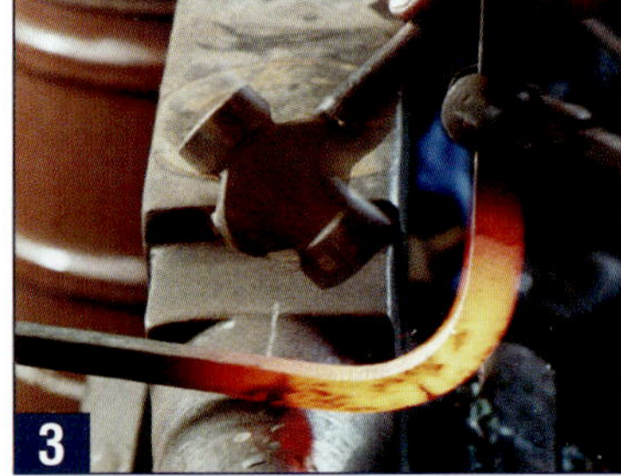

Bend past 90 degrees, and keep your hammer, tongs and steel in as close to the same plane as possible.

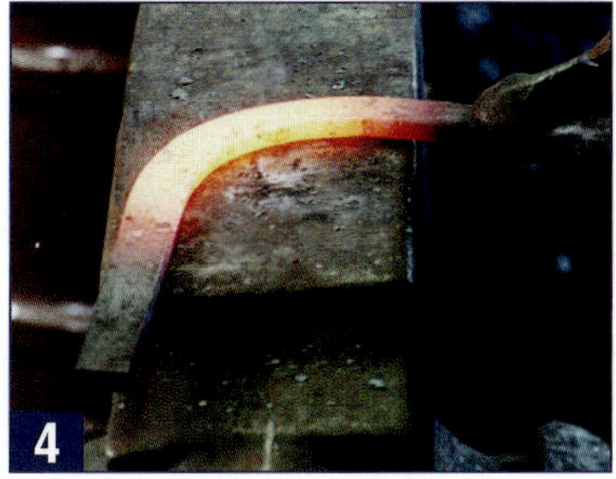

Position for seating out the toe.

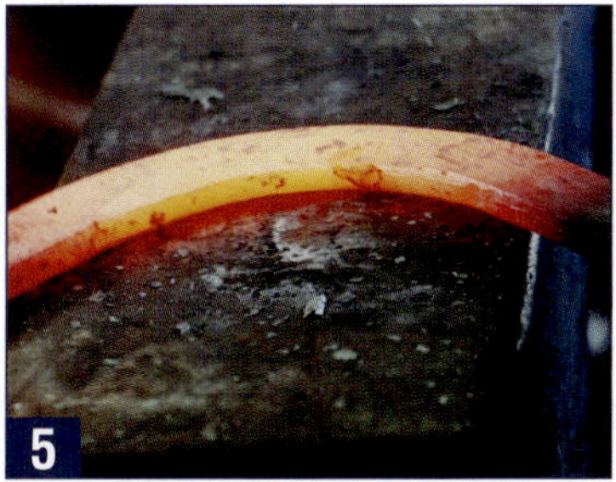

The inside of the toe bend once it is seated out.

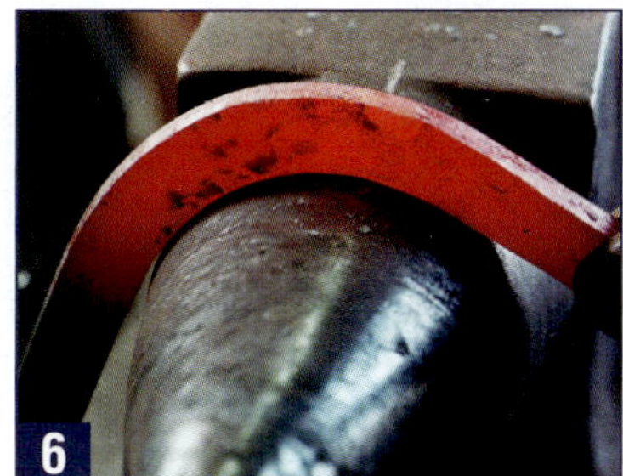

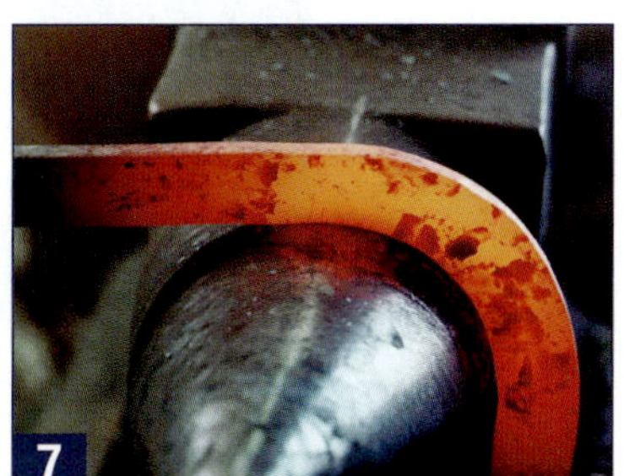

Making the toe radius

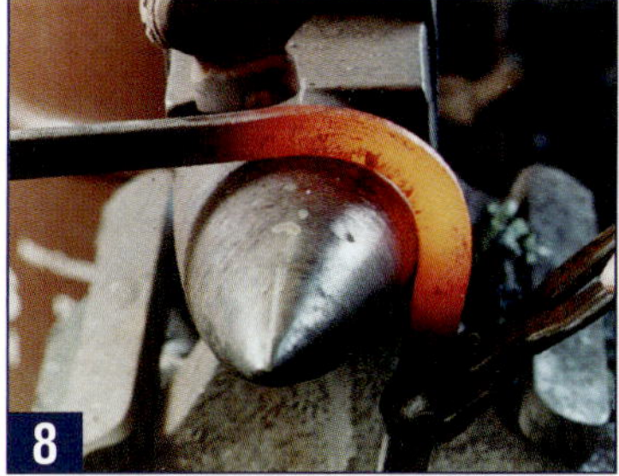

Set the toe by hitting just past the point of contact on the horn.

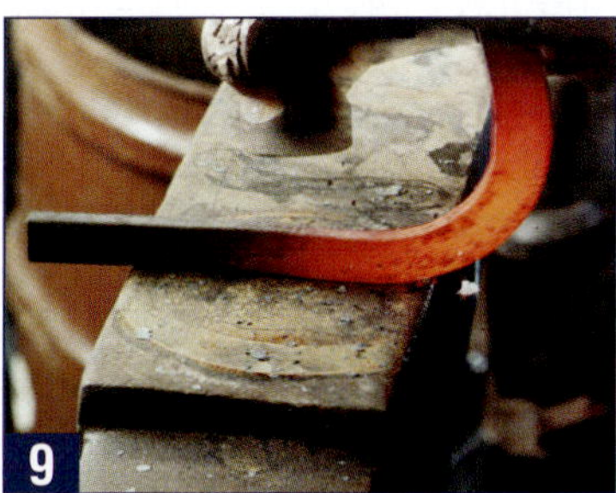

Straighten the branch where inertia caused it to bend.

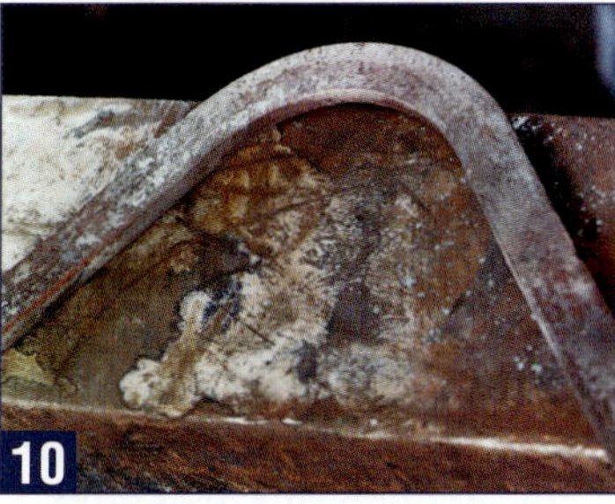

The finished toe bend.

for either a front or hind shoe. If you are in propane, I recommend cooling one end of the stock so that your heat is in the middle of the stock **(Figures 1-3)**. Since there are no marks on the stock, you will have to estimate where the middle of the stock is. Notice that there is as much material past the tongs as there is past the horn. On a regular open-heeled shoe, the amount beyond the tongs would be close to the width of the stock.

Seat out the toe **(Figures 4-5)**, then set your toe on the horn **(Figures 6-8)** the same way you would if making a normal shoe. Straighten the bend that was created by inertia **(Figure 9)** and you have a toe bend for a straight bar **(Figure 10)**.

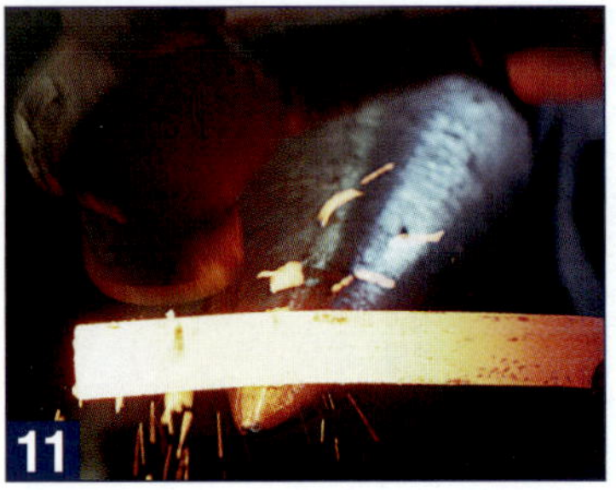

Placement of the steel to start the hockey stick bend.

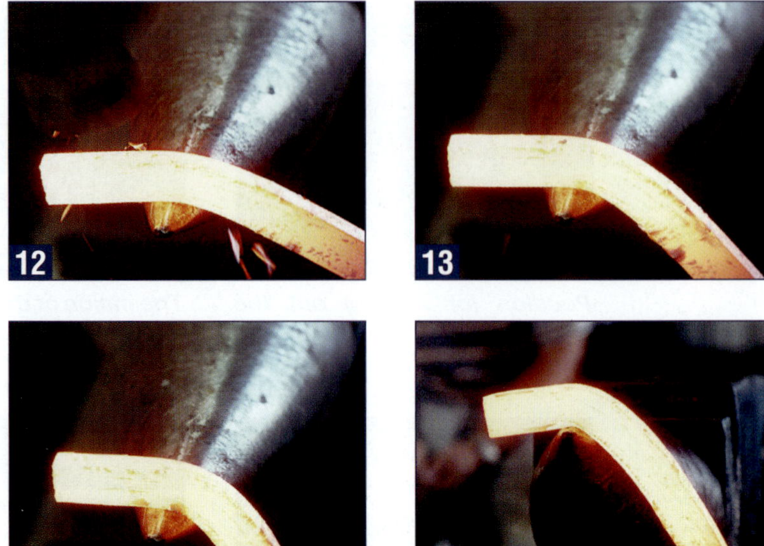

Notice that the area beyond the horn is in the same place, but the stock in the tongs is at a different angle.

HEAT 2

The first part of making the heel and bar is called a hockey stick. It is a real sticking point for some, so we will spend a little extra time on trying to completely understand everything that is happening during this phase of the straight bar.

Heat one branch and bend about 2 inches of the end of the stock on the tip of the horn. **(Figures11-14)**. The area to be bent can be marked if you have trouble determining 2 inches without a mark. Bend the stock by moving your tong hand, not by changing the angle of your hammer swing. Because I am dropping my hand, the stock past the horn seems to stay in the same place. Imagine that the horn and hammer are the jaws of a vise, and you have placed the hot stock in the vise and are bending it by pushing down on your tongs.

Once it is bent, it should be just shy of 90 degrees **(Figure 15)**. The stock will bend tighter if you hit it closer to where the stock contacts the horn. If you hit too far toward the end of the stock (away from that contact point with the horn), you will cause it to bow in a long radius instead of a tight bend.

One thing that the bar shoe is judged by is the dimensions of the bar. It must maintain the width of the parent stock, 3/4-inch in this case. By bending the stock at such a tight angle, the dimensions across the corner of the heel are automatically diminished. Since this happens, it is necessary to upset material into the corner to increase the mass. Doing this is what is referred to as making a hockey stick.

Try to put more steel than needed into the corner so that it can be forged out later in the bar and still maintain the original width in the corner. The stock will actually be wider directly across the corner of the heel. The added width here makes the corner of the shoe sharp and crisp but still allows you to maintain a minimum width of 3/4 inch in all other areas of the bar shoe.

Turn the stock over, and place it on the face of the anvil so that the end of the stock is up and the branch of the shoe is as close to flat on the anvil face as possible **(Figure 16)**. You will notice that there will be a long bend in the branch between the toe and the heel that formed when the end of the stock was bent over the tip of the horn. It will straighten during the first few upsetting blows on the end of the stock.

Swing the hammer so that the force of the blow is coming at a slight angle toward your feet **(Figure 17)**. Press downward with your tong hand and continue to hammer at an angle **(Figure 18)**. After the first few blows, you can feel the branch straighten as the corner becomes solid on the anvil face. There will be a different, more solid feeling blow as you upset the steel for the side of the bar.

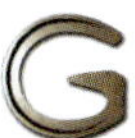

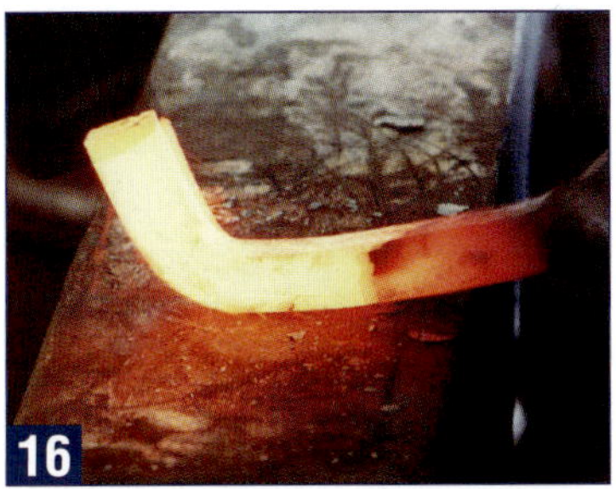
Turn the hockey stick portion up to begin upsetting it into the corner.

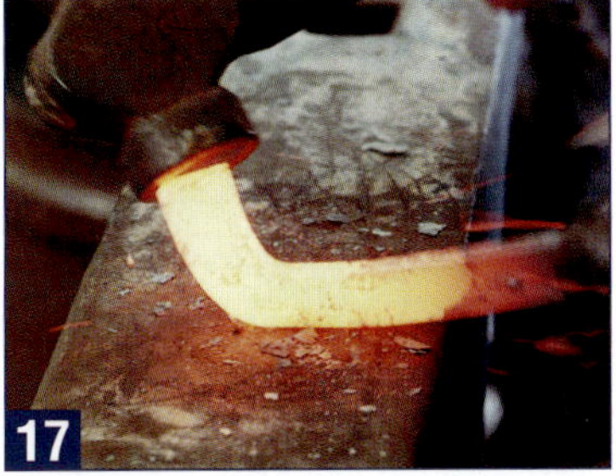
Notice the angle of the hammer coming in to start the hockey stick.

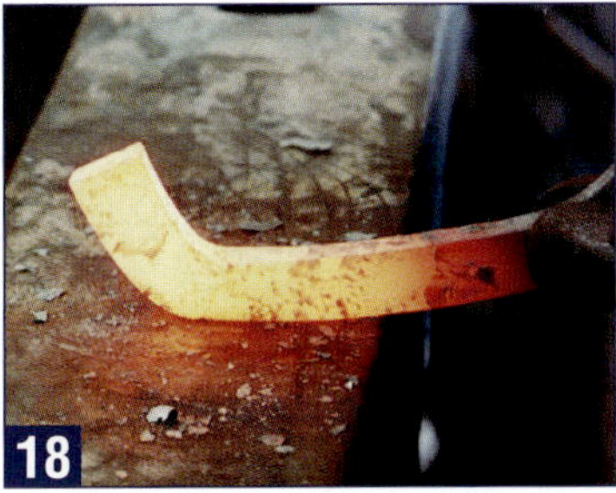
Hockey stick being upset.

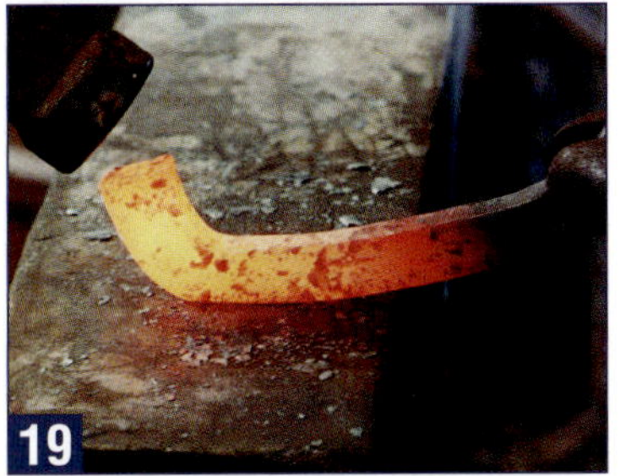
Change the angle of the hammer to close the bend on the inside of the hockey stick.

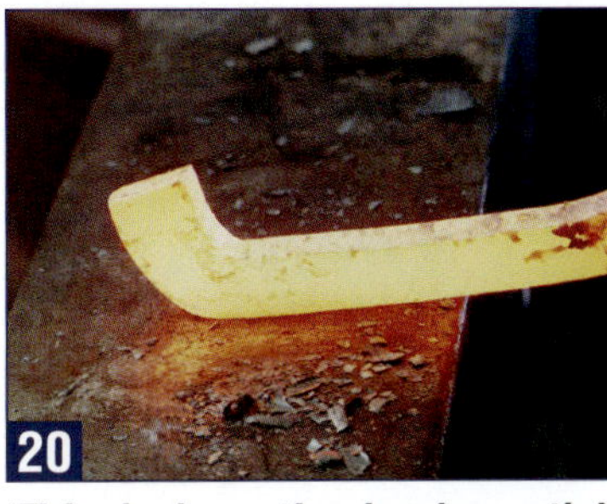
This is how the hockey stick should look when you are done upsetting it.

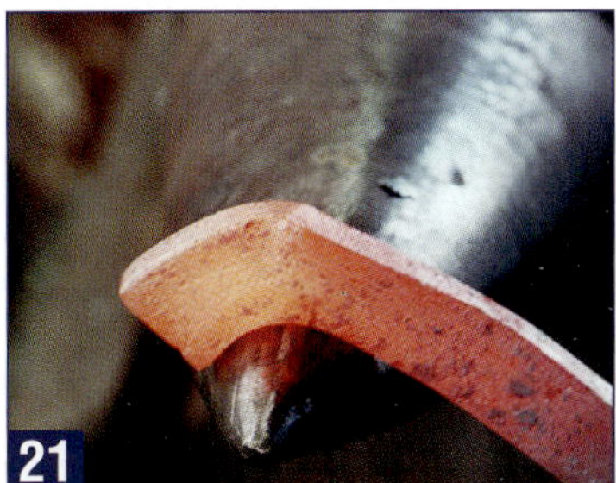
Place on the end of the horn to forge the inside of the bar and crisp the outside corner.

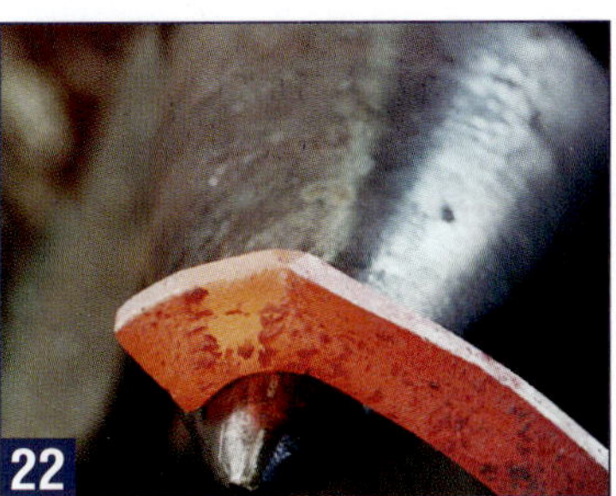
Stay in the same place while you forge the hockey stick.

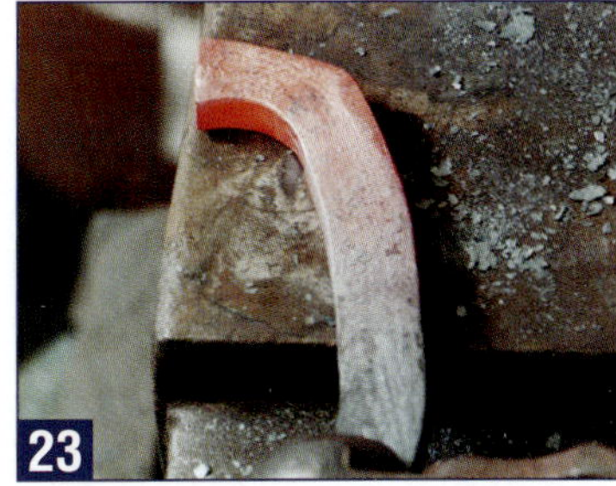
Position to scarf the end of the hockey stick.

A common problem when building a hockey stick is for the angle to open up. Most of the time, the problem is in your tong hand and you are letting the branch come off the face of the anvil. By pressing down with your tong hand and changing the arc of the hammer, you can easily control the direction of the piece you are upsetting. Eventually you will learn to control whether it opens or closes with ease.

If you want the angle to close, change the arc of the hammer swing. Aim the swing so that the hammer would hit higher up your shin if there were not an anvil in the way **(Figure 19)**. If you want it to open away from the shoe, lift on the tongs and allow the hammer to come down in a more perpendicular arc. Continually level the piece being upset as you forge it.

When you are done upsetting the one half of the bar, it should look like the piece in **Figure 20**.Turn the shoe over, move to the tip of the horn, and hold the shoe at an angle so that the branch of the shoe is pointing to just above your knee on your tong side **(Figure 21)**. Hammer directly down on the outside of the hockey stick, thinning the width to approximately 7/8 inch. This move makes the appropriate angle for the junction of the branch and the bar, while also sharpening the heel **(Figure 22)**. Be careful to keep your tong hand still for forging the back of the hockey stick. I have seen people either hammer around the horn, or drop their tong hand while they are at this point in the process. When that happens, they end up making the back of their bar round instead of straight.

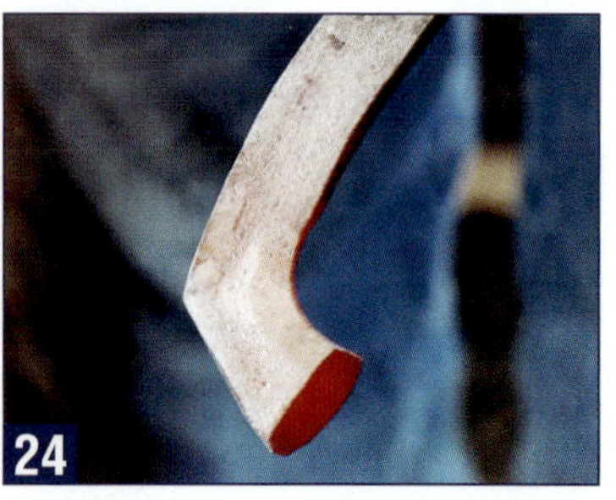

Your piece should look like this when the hockey stick is done.

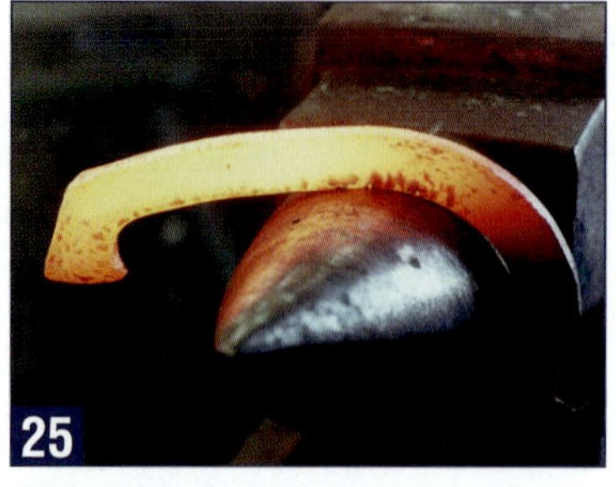

Third heat, bend around horn. Notice tong position.

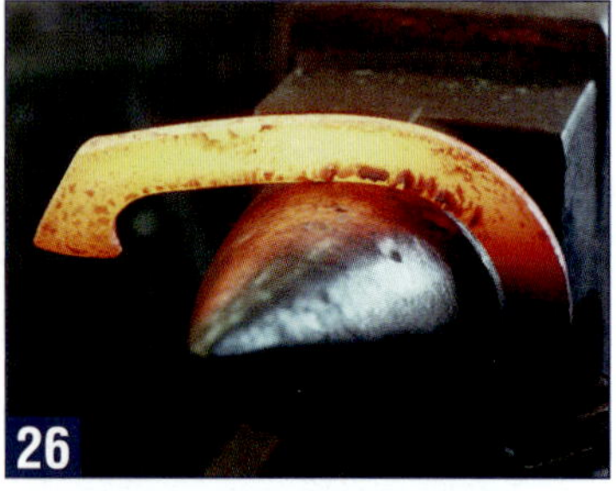

Continue around the horn.

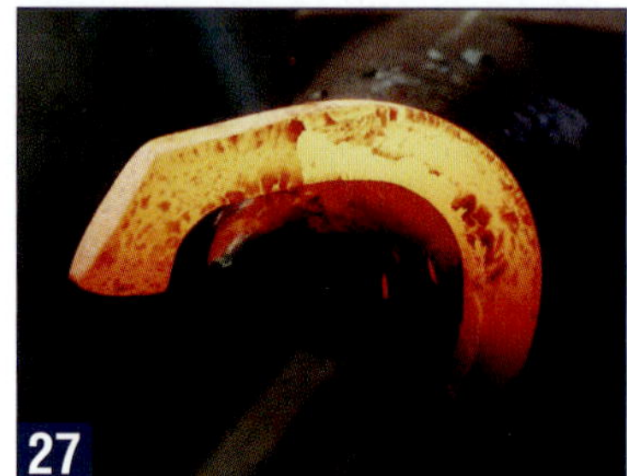

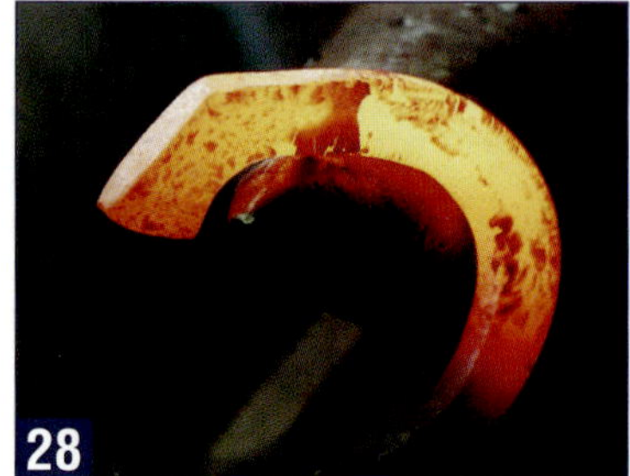

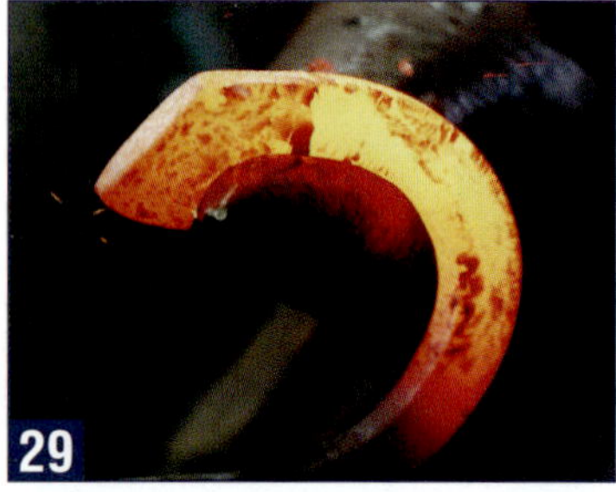

When you get to the end of the branch, move your hammer over the shoe instead of the shoe under the hammer.

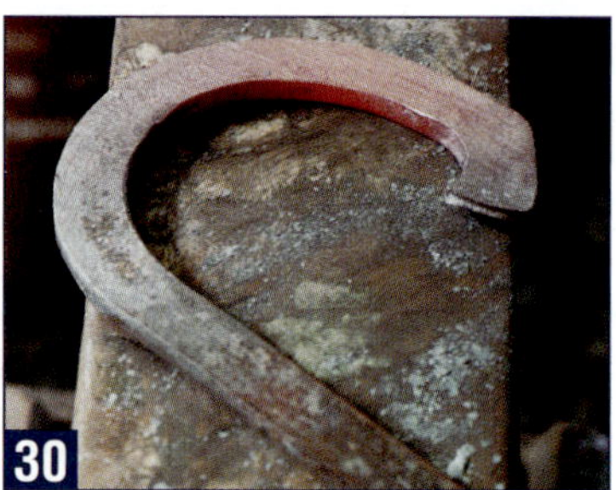

Your shoe should look like this.

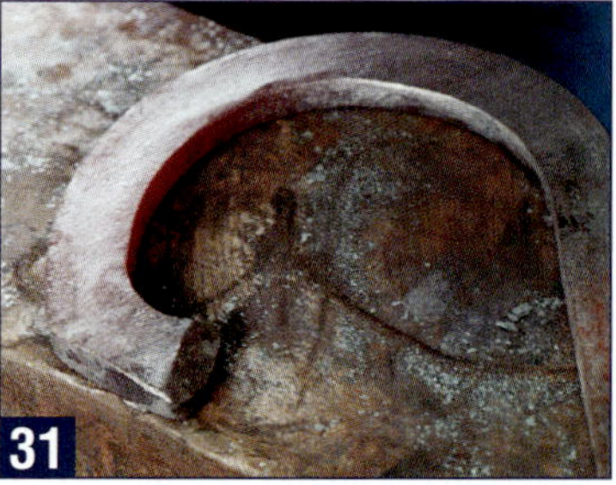

Place the end of the bar directly at the edge of the anvil to scarf it **(Figure 23)**. Scarf by turning the hammer in your hand and swing with a straight hammer blow to thin the end of the stock that will be welded. Once this heat is finished, it should look like **Figure 24**.

HEAT 3

Heat the branch and turn it on the horn to the desired shape. It will not be possible to do this exactly as you would with a normal shoe, because the hockey stick is in the way. Bend the branch around the horn until the hockey stick portion of the bar contacts the horn. Move to the end of the horn and place the shoe so that the appropriate radius can be achieved from the widest point of the shoe back. We generally move the stock under the hammer, but for this particular shoe, we hold the shoe in one place and move the hammer over the stock **(Figures 25-29)**.

Place the shoe on the anvil so that the bar is parallel to the near edge of the anvil face **(Figure**

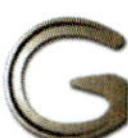

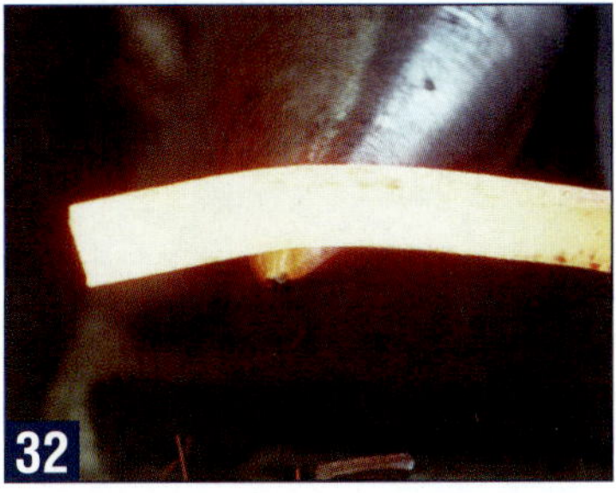

Begin the second hockey stick.

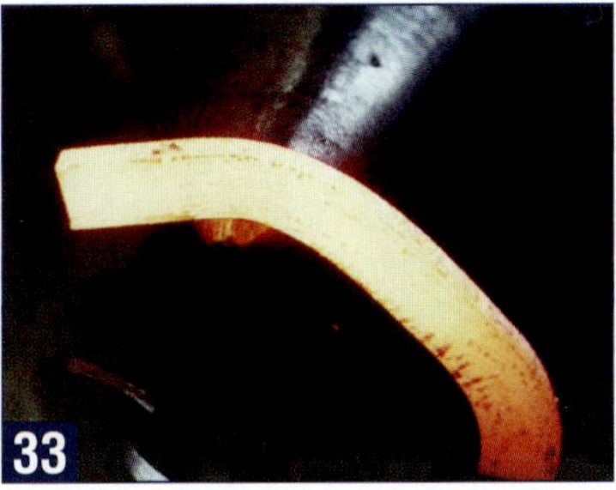

Move your tongs, not the hammer.

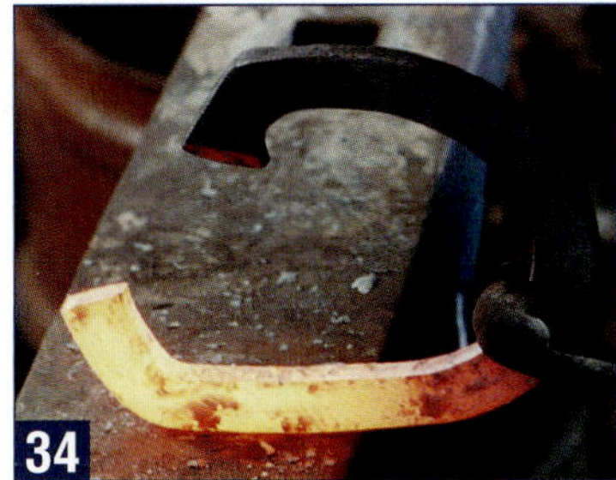

Forge the hockey stick.

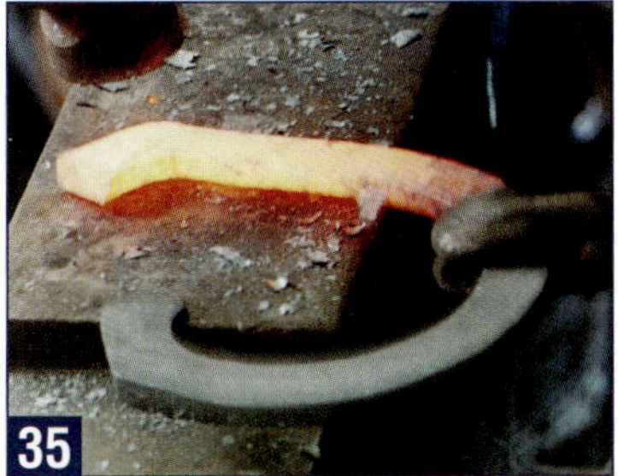

Keep the hockey stick level.

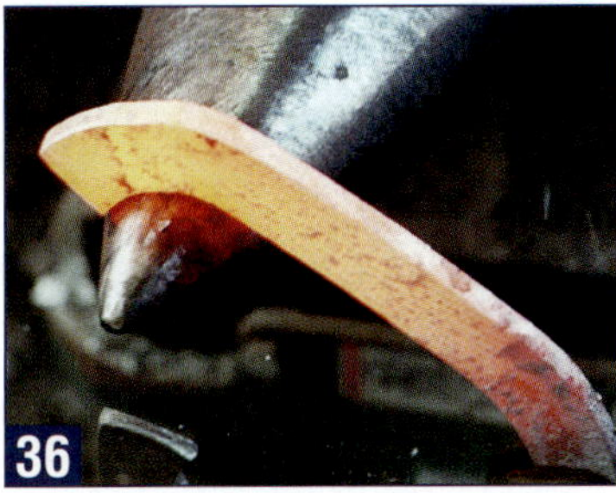

Forge the back of the hockey stick to forge the corner of the bar.

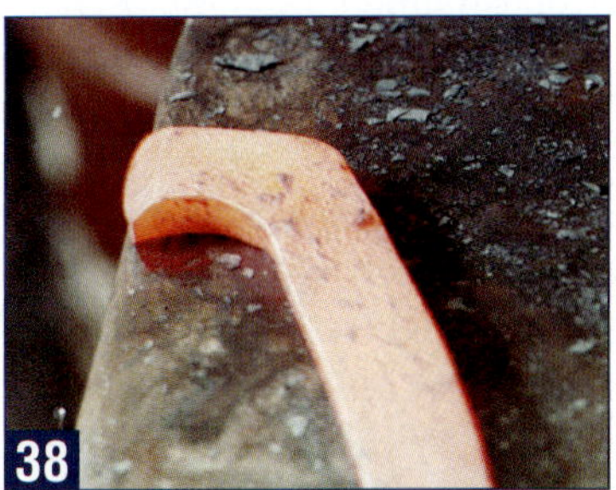

Scarf the hockey stick.

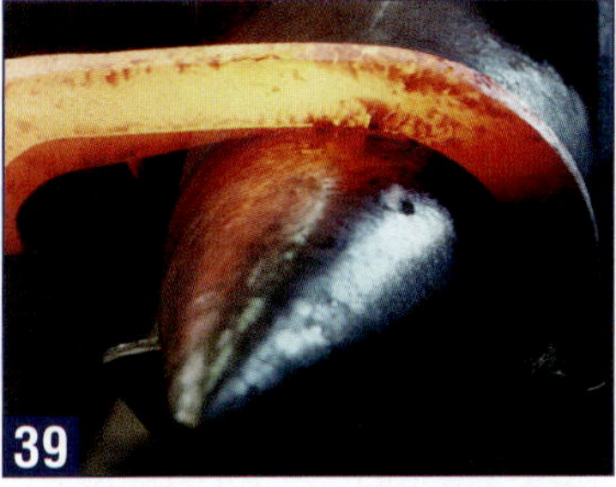

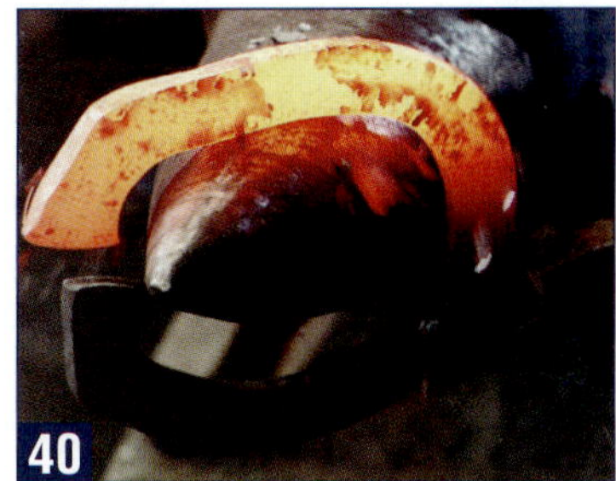

Bend the branch around the horn.

30-31). It can be helpful to place a finished shoe over the top of the half finished bar shoe to help evaluate the shape. Train your eye to see the shoe in halves. The scarffed edge of the bar should be in line with the center of the toe bend. If you marked center of the stock in the straight, the mark should line up with center of the bar.

HEATS 4 And 5

Both of these heats are the same as the previous ones. Sometimes the shoe will be too tight in the toe bend, which can make it difficult to upset the second hockey stick. In these cases, simply take the toe bend back to the horn and find a larger radius to move the ends of the shoe apart. Study **Figures 32-40** carefully, and try to get your shoe to the exact same point at each step. **Figures 32-38** are Heat four, and **Figures 39-40** are Heat five.

How the bar is set up for welding at the end of the fifth heat is important. Some people like to weld with the heel of the hammer, and some like to use the toe. I personally use the toe of the hammer for the first welding heat, because there is less chance of thinning the bar at the weld and digging a hole.

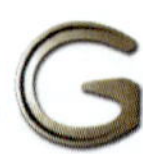

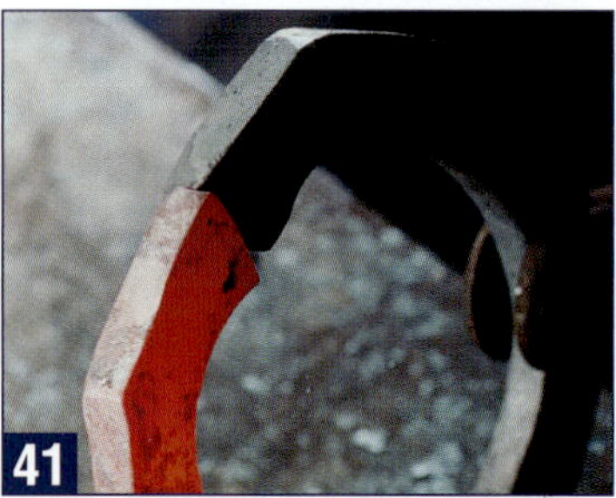
Bring the scarves together.

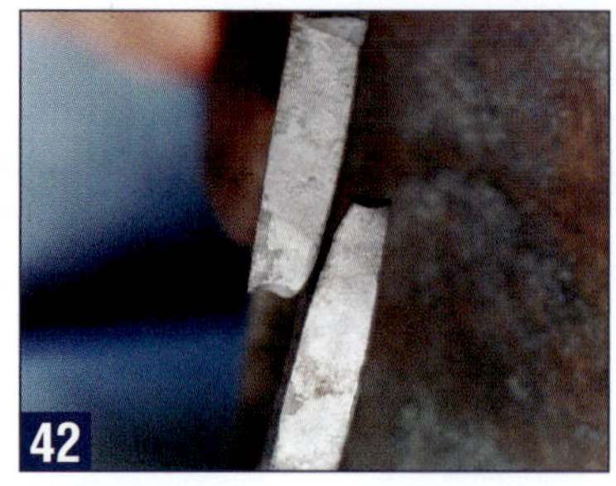
In this picture, you can see how much the scarves overlap.

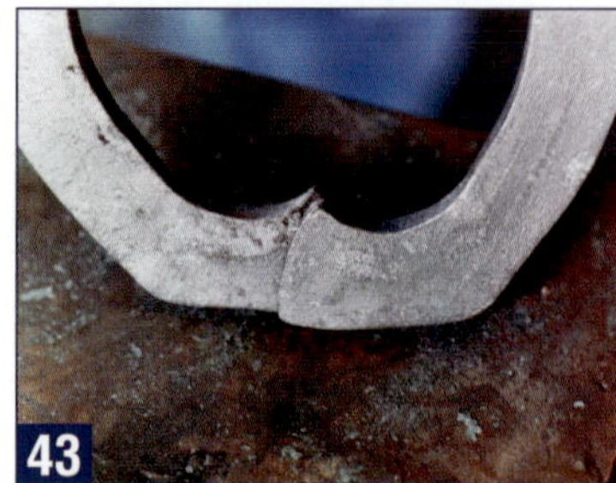
Line up the sharp points on the hockey sticks.

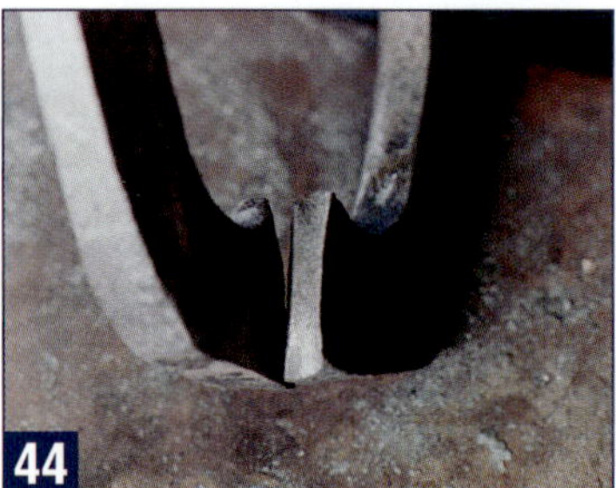
Here is the overlap.

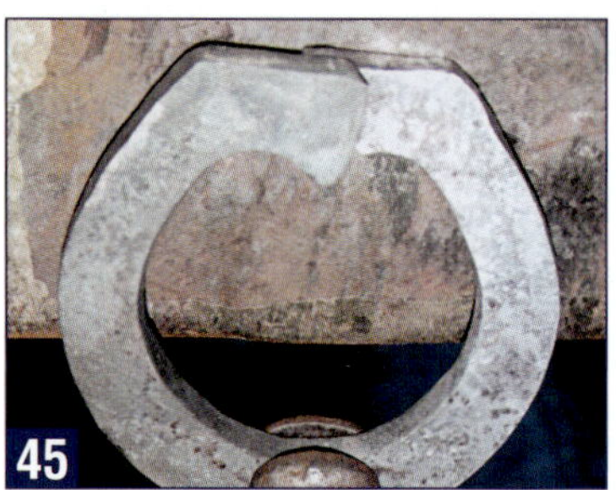
The left branch is on top of the right branch because I am hammering right handed.

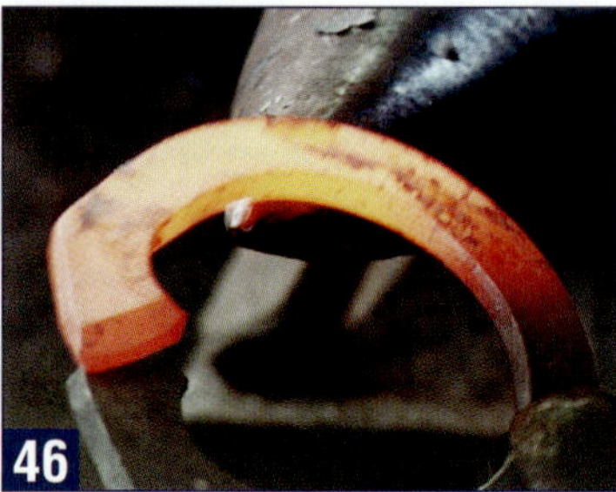
This is overlapped the wrong way for me, but it would be right for a left handed person.

If you are going to use the toe of the hammer, set up the bar so that when you are holding the toe of the shoe, the half of the bar on top is on your tong-hand side **(Figures 41-45)**. The opposite is desired if you are going to weld with the heel of the hammer **(Figure 46)**. It is possible to use a cross peen to do the initial welding, in which case, it doesn't matter which side is on top.

Line up the points on the inside of the upset halves of the bar and try to get the scarves as close together as possible. While holding the shoe flat on the face of the anvil, hit the bottom branch of the shoe to bring the scarves together. This hit will cause the branch to bow, pushing it into the scarf above.

If the shoe has lost all iridescent heat, heat lightly before fluxing (we are not counting that as one of the heats). Flux the weld, then place the shoe in the fire. If you are working in coke, any flux (or none at all, if you are able) will work. In **Figure 47**, you can see that I am using Borax. For welding in propane, you have to use flux. Russell Colvin, CJF, and Mike Miller, CJF, FWCF, from Alabama have created a flux called Iron Mountain Flux. It is sold through Blackwater Forge, and it has the longest welding window of any commercial flux that I have ever used. I am putting Iron Mountain Flux on the shoe in **Figure 48**.

HEAT 6

The next two heats are the welding heats. Place the area to be welded in the hottest part of the fire. With propane, you will know that it is ready to weld when the shoe disappears in the fire. This means that when you glance in the forge, it takes just a second or two for you to focus on the shoe. At this point, the shoe is as hot as the liner of the forge and as hot as it will get. The flux can be burned away and turn into scale, so get to welding as soon as it is ready.

With coke, place the shoe in the center of the fire and wait until the steel sweats. This means that the steel has a wet look. Molten flux will make it look wet at a lower temperature, but I am referring to how the steel will look right before it starts to spark. You cannot wait until the shoe disappears in the fire with coke forges, since doing so will make the shoe really disappear — as it burns away. The coke is so much hotter than propane that the shoe will still be colder than the fire when it is ready to weld. **Figure 49** is a picture taken at Calgary by Bob Garner, the owner of G.E. Forge & Tools. If you look closely at the detail

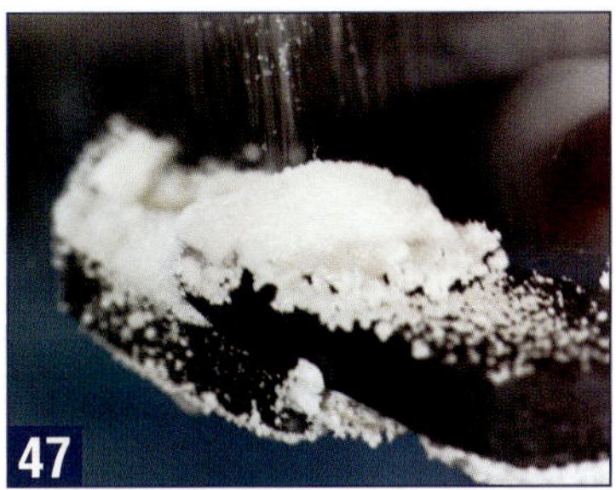

Fluxing with Borax.

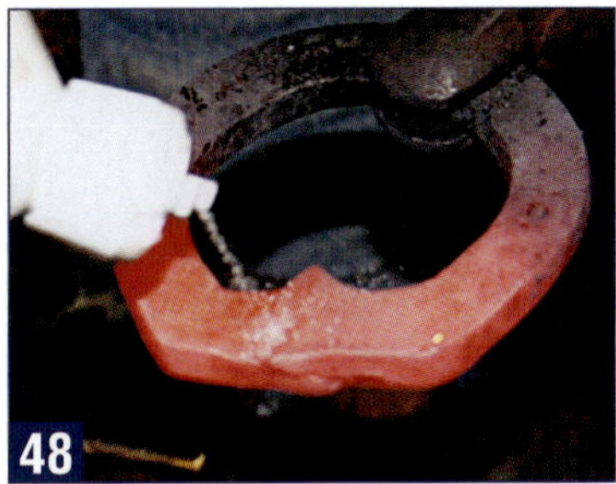

Fluxing with Iron Mountain Flux.

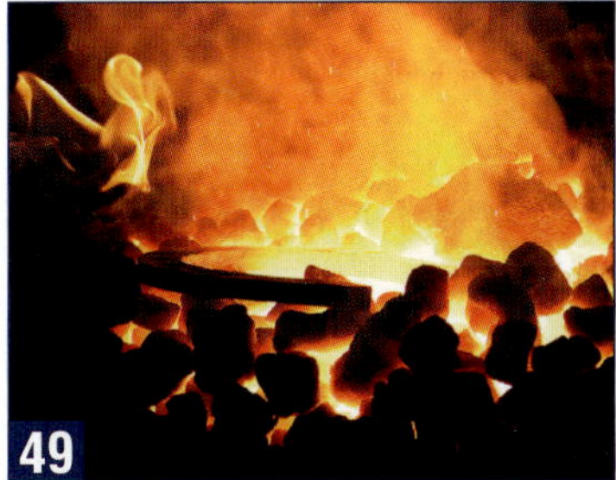

A great photo by Bob Garner from G.E. Tools showing the colors in a coke fire.

in the fire, you can see just how hot it is toward the center of the fire. A light spark is acceptable, however, this is an indication that the steel is burning. A heavy spark, and the shoe is going to be ruined.

Achieving the correct heat is critical, regardless of the type of forge used. Remove the shoe from the fire, holding the toe. Place the area to be welded on the anvil, and hit with one or two light, quick, flat hammer blows **(Figures 50-51)**. The first few blows will lightly weld the inside while also squeezing out any flux, scale, or graudu (a word for forge crap from Frank Turley) from between the two halves of the bar. Be certain that any spectators are warned about the possibility of sparks flying off the anvil — especially children since their eyes are at about anvil level.

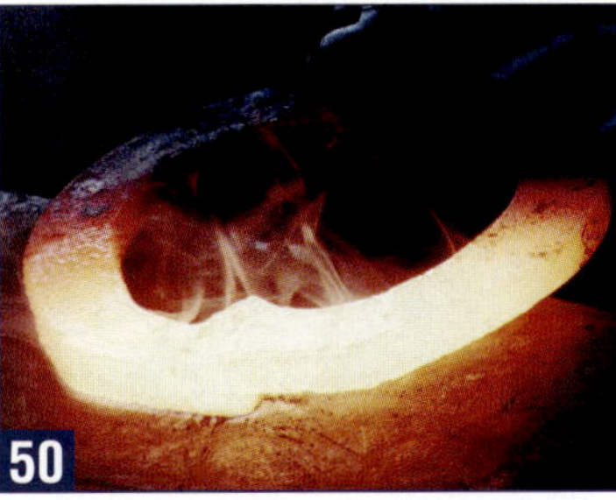

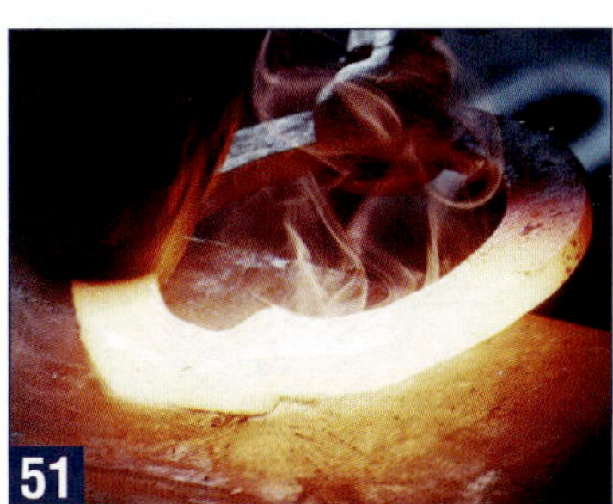

Beginning of first welding heat

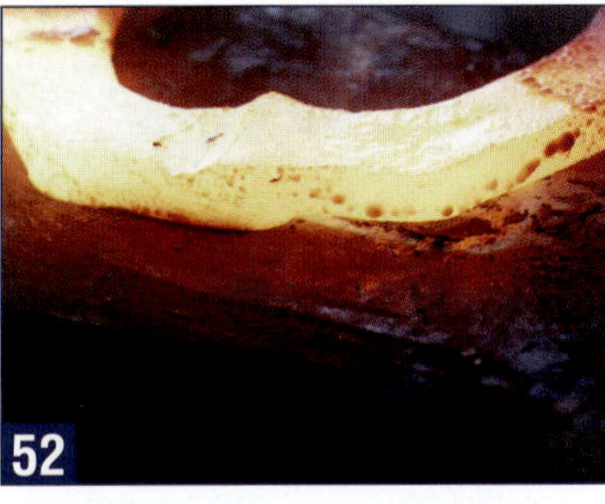

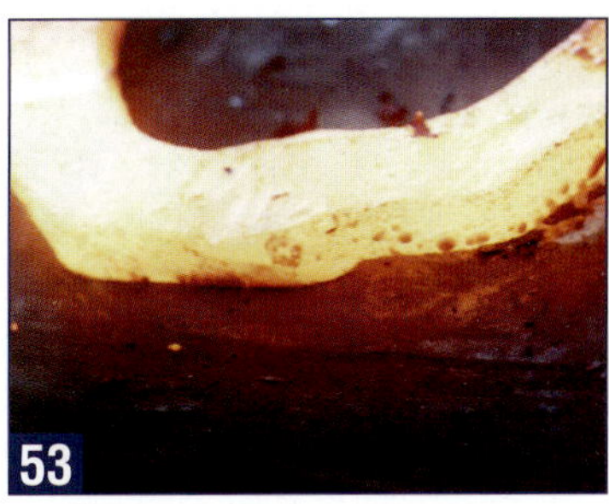

Blending away the seams.

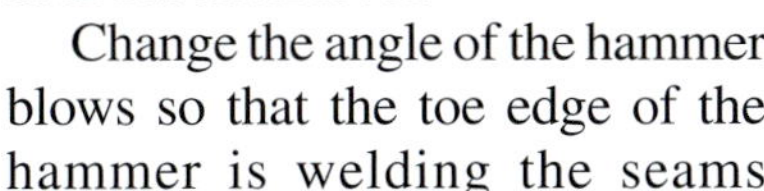

Change the angle of the hammer blows so that the toe edge of the hammer is welding the seams between the two pieces **(Figures 52-53)**. I use the toe of the hammer face, so I simply have to lift on the hammer handle slightly to make the seam disappear with an angled blow. It should only take about 10 hammer blows to make the seam disappear. Quickly turn the shoe over and repeat exactly the same sequence of blows on the other side. When the seams disappear, quit hitting the shoe. You have accomplished what you needed to on the first welding heat, and continuing to hit the shoe only increases the potential of the weld breaking.

Try to weld the ground surface first and flip to the hoof surface for the second part of the heat. There is a better chance that the first seam welded will look better than the second seam, and shoes are looked at from the ground surface when they are on the hoof.

The first welding heat should be a very quick heat. Brush the bar **(Figure 54)**, flux again, and get the shoe back in the fire as soon as you can **(Figure 55)**. If everything went correctly, the shoe will still be hot when you go back into the fire for the second welding heat.

HEAT 7

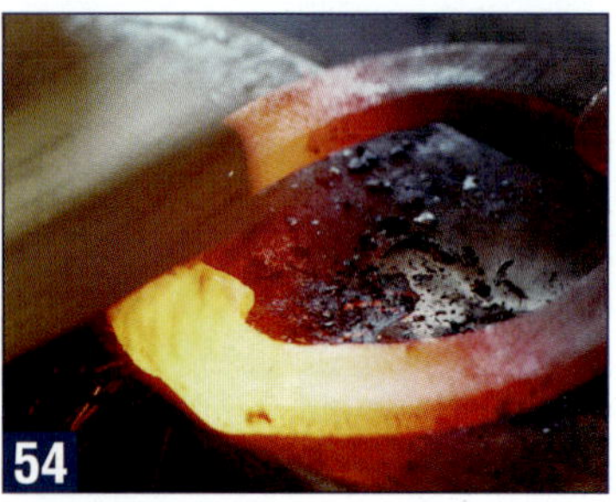

Brush to remove scale.

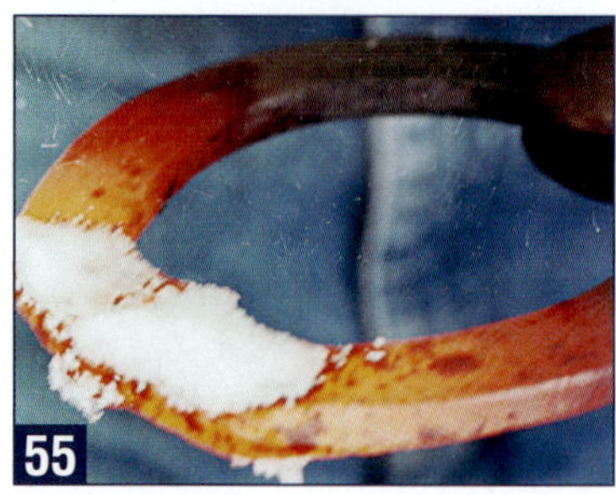

Flux again and head back to the fire. Notice how hot the shoe still is.

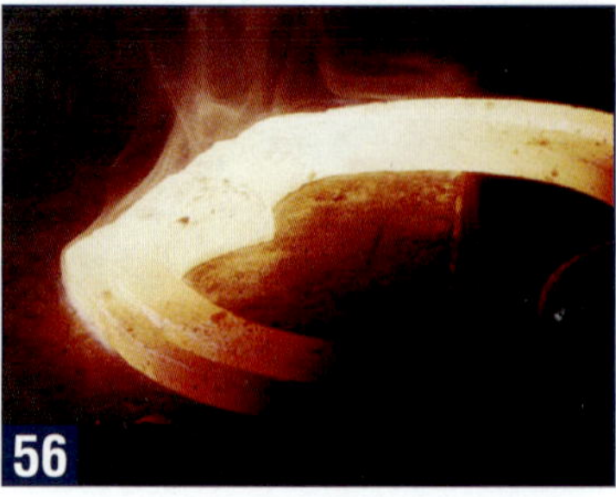

Hit flat on the weld for the second welding heat.

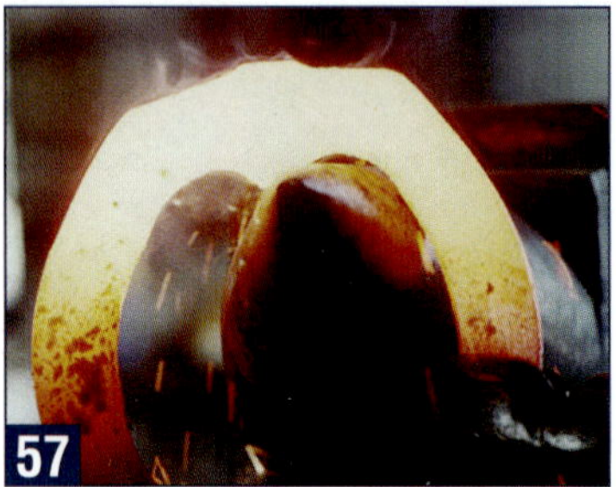

On the horn, hit the weld.

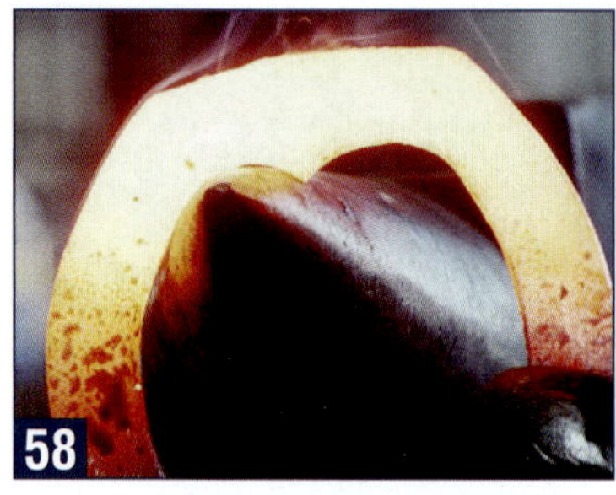

Move the bar to the other side of the sex appeal and hit the weld.

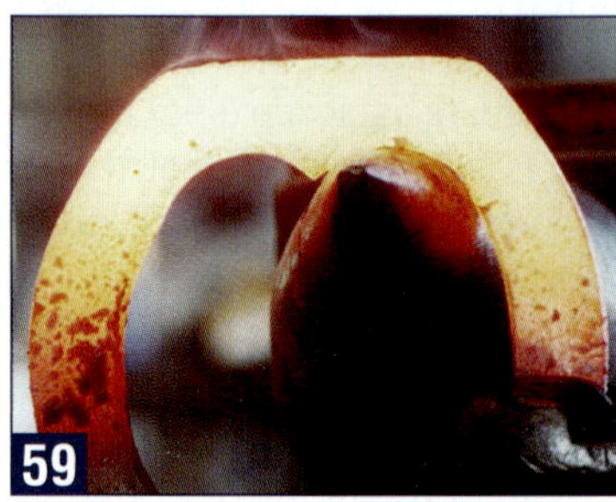

Go back to the position as in figure 57, and hit the weld.

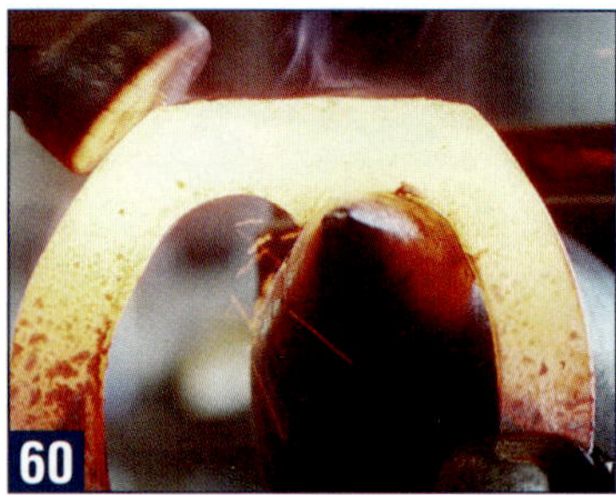

Stay in this position, and hit the outside of the heel to crisp it up as you forge the sex appeal as well.

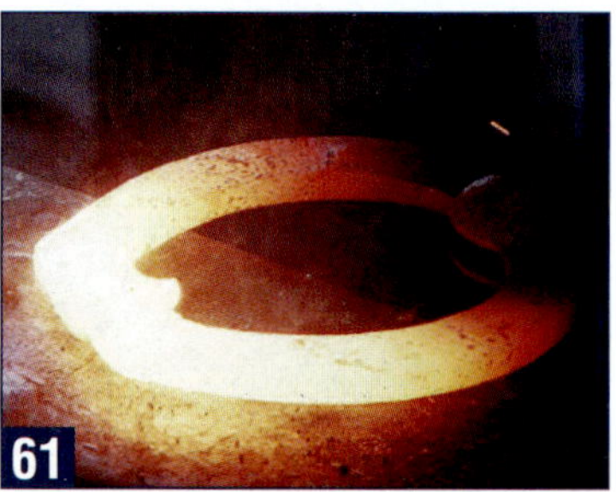

Forge the bar back to original thickness.

Since the shoe returned to the fire while it was still rather hot, it should not take long to get to a good welding heat for the second weld. Get the shoe to the correct temperature, remove it from the fire holding the toe, and hit with light, quick, flat hammer blows directly over the weld, as you did making the rings earlier **(Figure 56)**. Move to the end of the horn and place one side of the bar over the desired radius of the horn **(Figure 57)**. Notice that the welded area is really wide from being forged on the thickness. Hammer on the weld, not directly over the horn.

You want to hit the weld so that you don't thin the bar on either side of the sex appeal. Move the shoe once more so that the other side of the bar is at the same place on the horn as the first side was **(Figure 58)**. Again, hammer on the weld. The area of the weld will thicken, and the back of the bar will straighten while you are forging the back of the weld. Move once again to the first position **(Figure 59),** and after you hit on top of the weld, change the hammer so that it is coming in at an angle. This will crisp up the outside of the heel with the hammer and

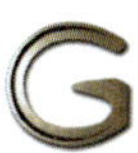

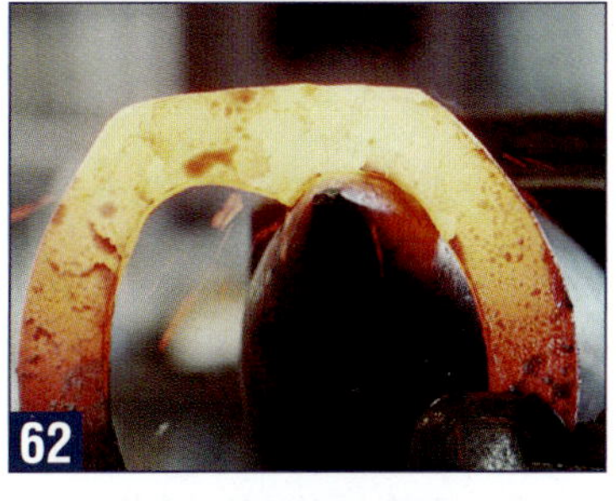

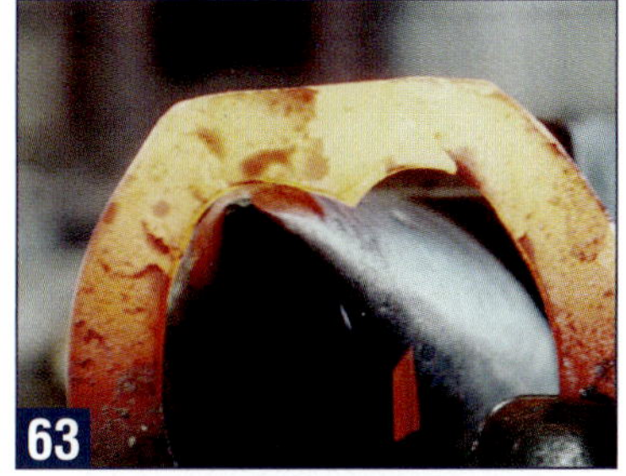

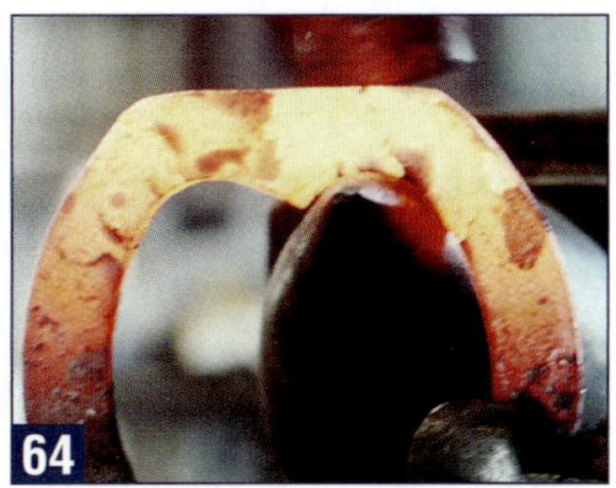

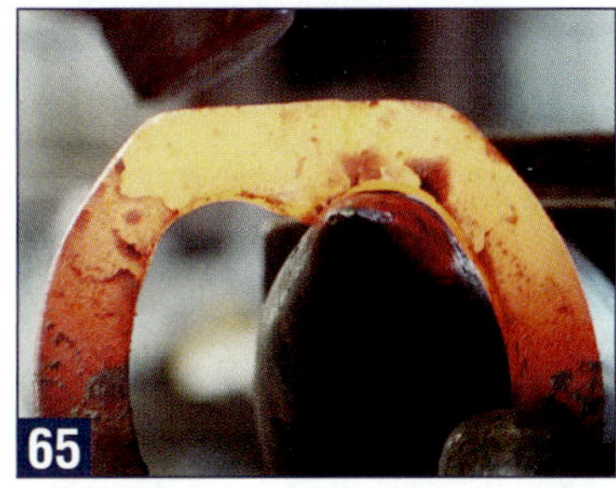

Same moves as Figures 57 through 60.

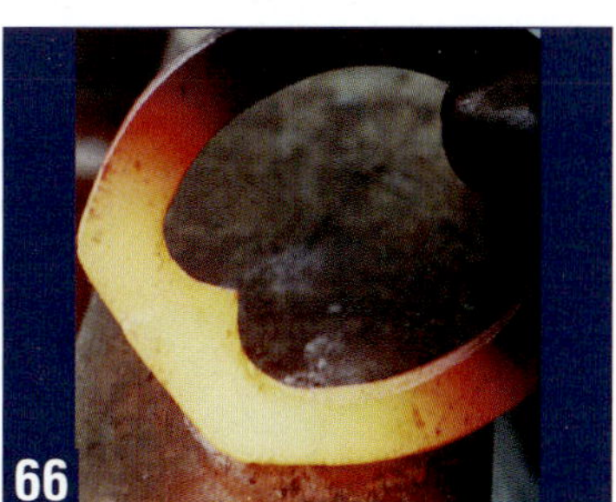

Position to crisp both corners on the outside of the heels.

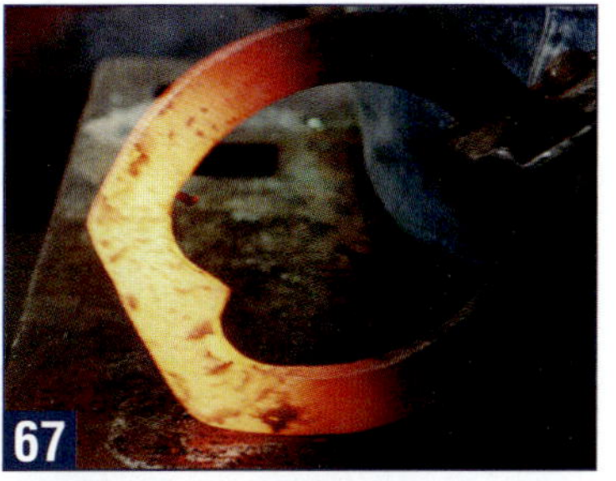

Forging the outside of the heels.

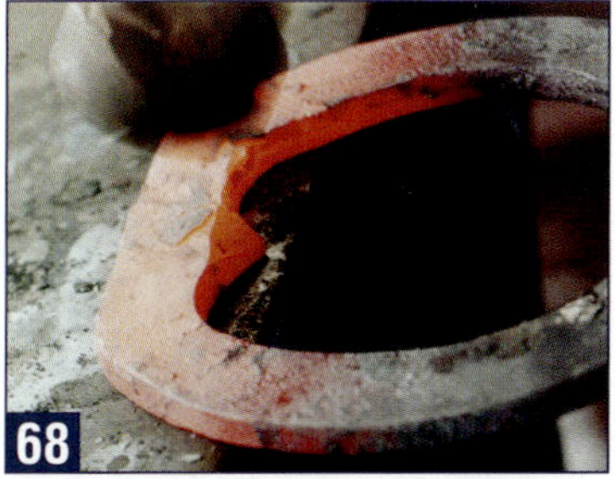

Forging the bevel on the sex appeal. This position allows the hammer to clear anvil face.

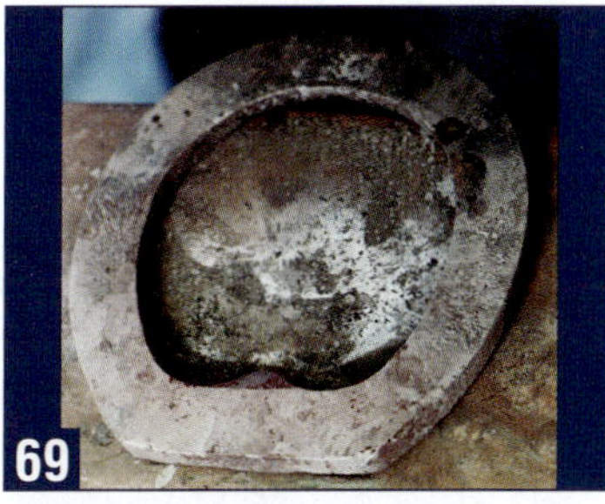

Finished blank in 7 heats.

the inside of the sex appeal on the horn **(Figure 60)**.

Since the bar thickened, you need to forge it back to the original thickness on the face of the anvil **(Figure 61)**. Move back to the horn and repeat the previous steps until the back of the bar is straight and the thickness matches the parent stock **(Figures 62-65)**.

Another move that can be used to crisp up the heels is to hold the shoe at an angle to the face of the anvil, and hammer at an angle on the opposite heel **(Figures 66-67)**. Quenching the toe can prevent the shoe from distorting during this move. This move can also be used to narrow the shoe.

To finish, you can bevel the inside of the sex appeal. Do this by placing the inside of the bar at the near edge of the anvil, and forge with an angled hammer blow **(Figure 68)**. The finished product should look like **Figure 69**, or the shoe that Cody made, shown in **Figure 70**.

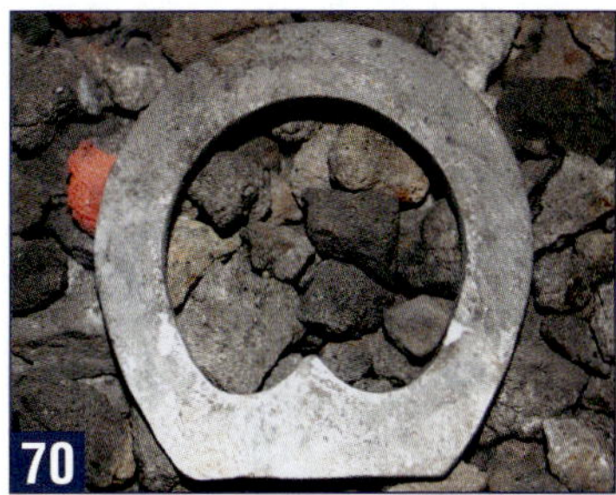

Here is one that Cody made.

FULLERED STRAIGHT BAR

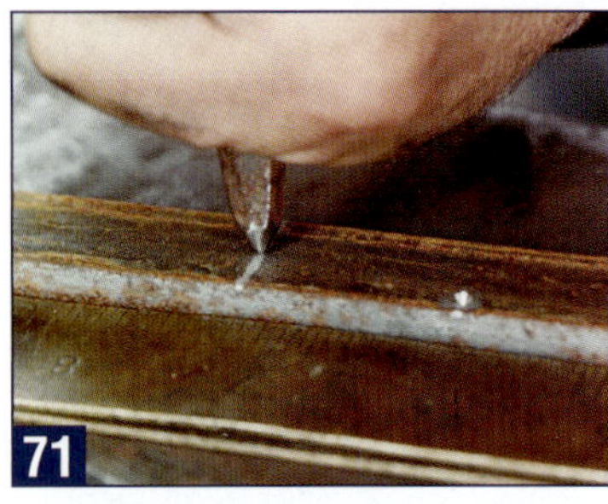

Marking the shoe for the beginning of the fullering.

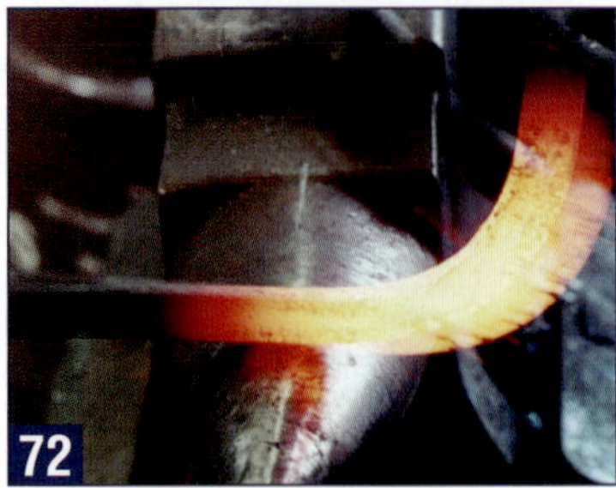

Making the toe bend.

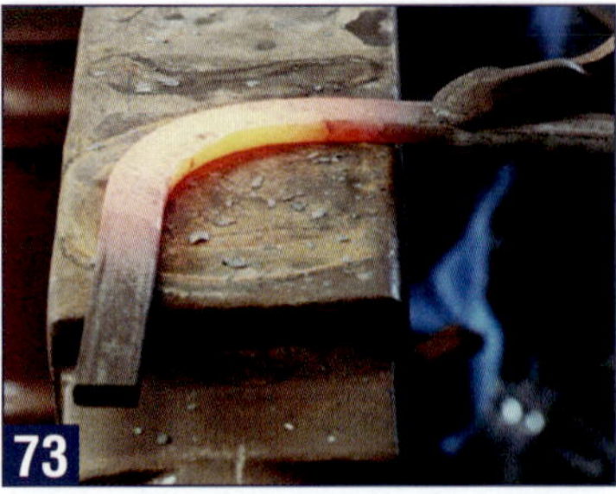

Seat out the inside of the toe bend.

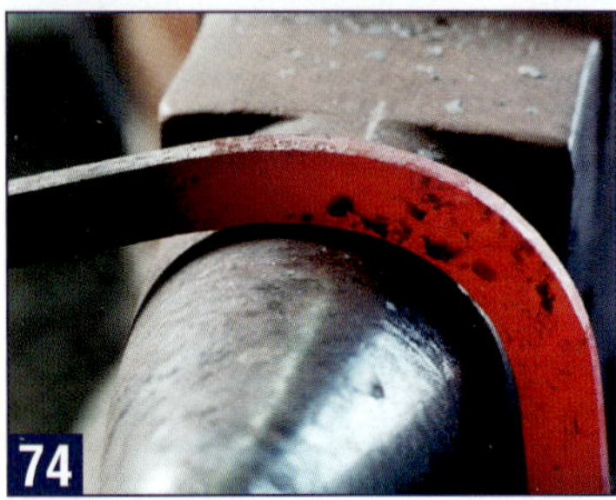

Setting the toe.

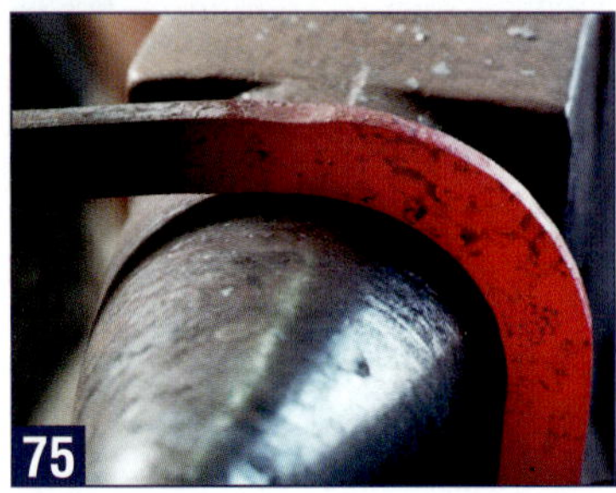

Hemming the shoe where the fullering is going to start.

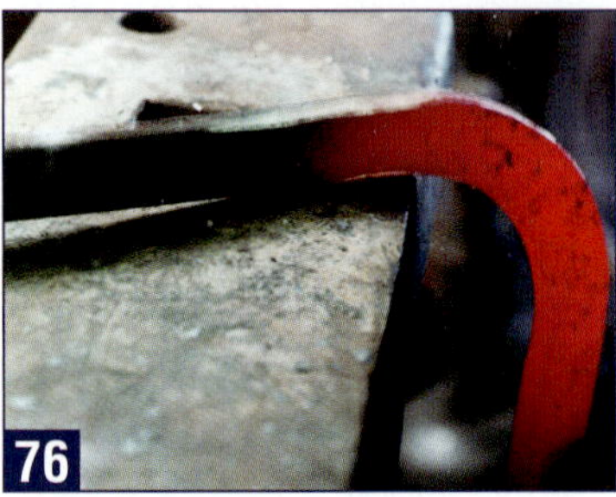

Continue the hemming on the face of the anvil.

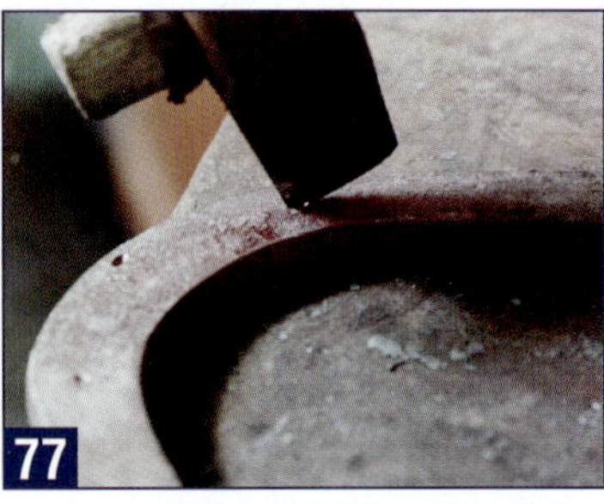

Marking the start of the crease. The creaser is held up at an angle to get a crisp corner.

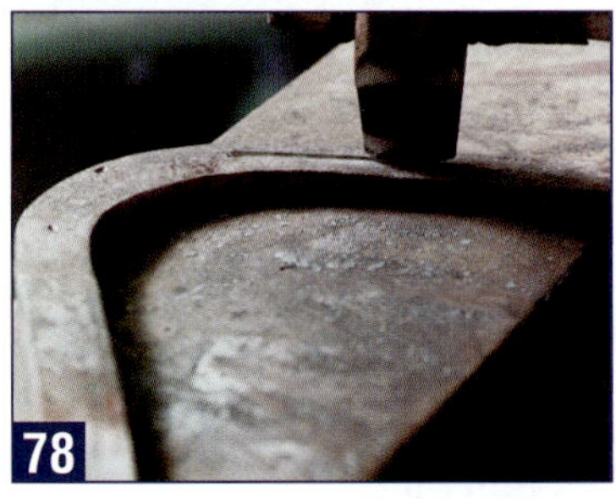

Continue marking the crease.

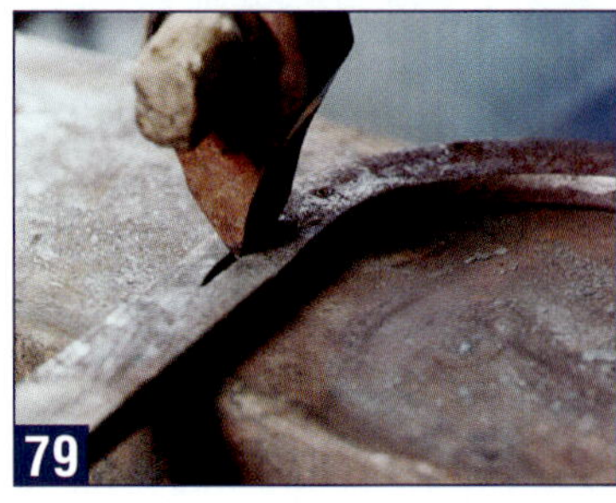

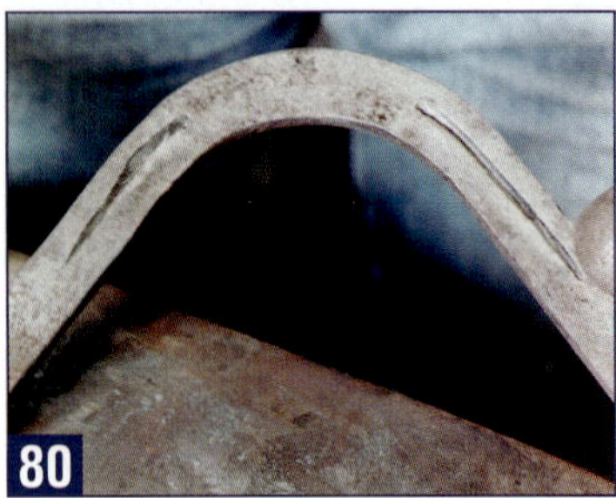

This is what the toe bend and the marked fullering should look like at the end of the first heat.

IN FIVE HEATS

To make this shoe, you will want to mark the stock in the straight. Begin with 14 inches of 5/16-by-3/4 inch stock. Mark center and 1 5/16 inches from center for the beginning of the crease, just as you did for your fullered front shoe **(Figure 71)**.

HEAT 1

Heat the center of the stock and make a toe bend as you would for a front shoe **(Figure 72)**. Seat it out heavily **(Figure 73),** set the toe, and hem both branches **(Figures 74-76)**. Mark the fullering as deep as the heat will allow **(Figures 77-80)**.

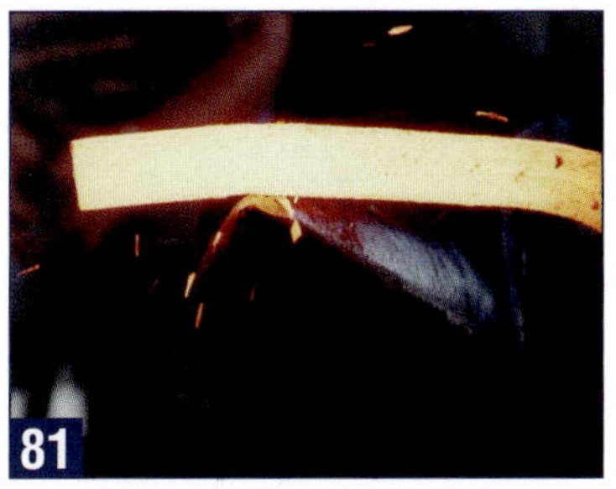

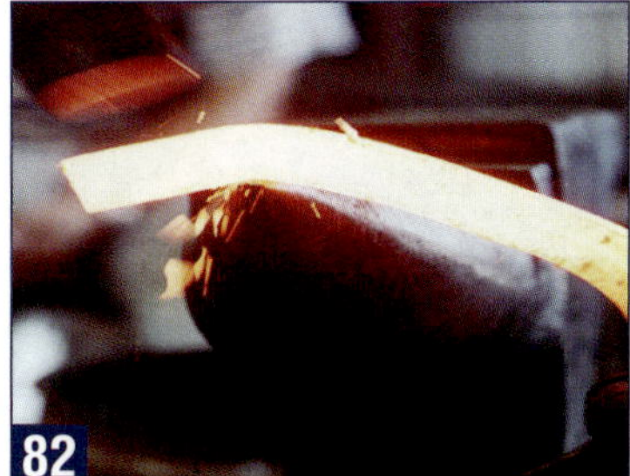

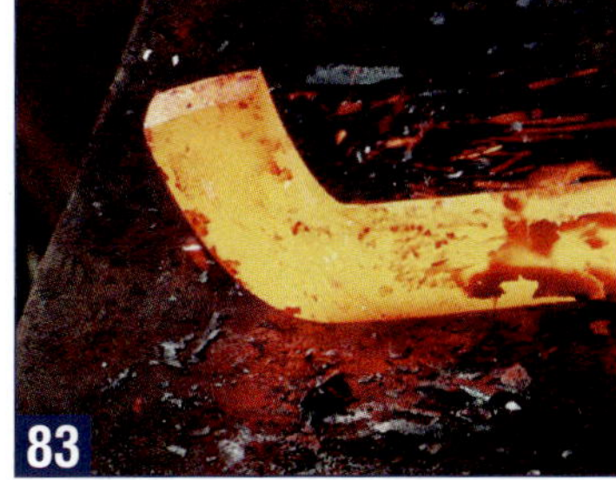

Make the hockey stick.

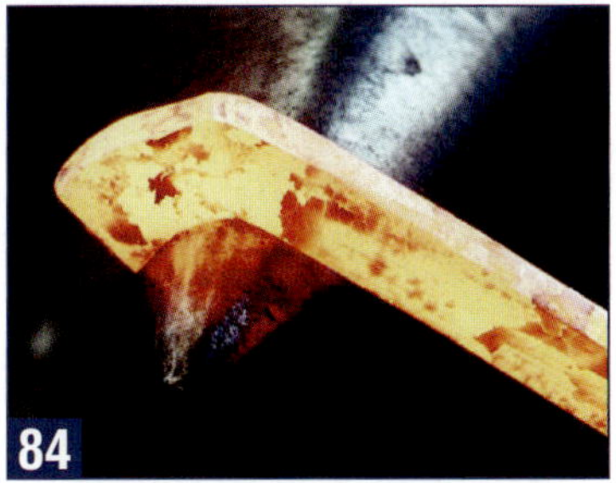

Forge the back of the bar.

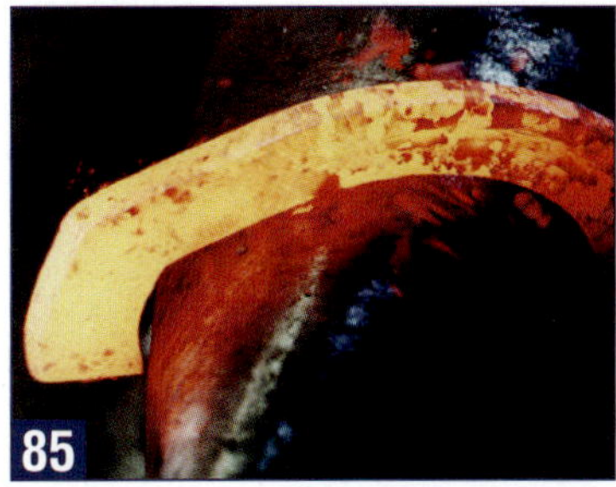

Bend the branch around the horn.

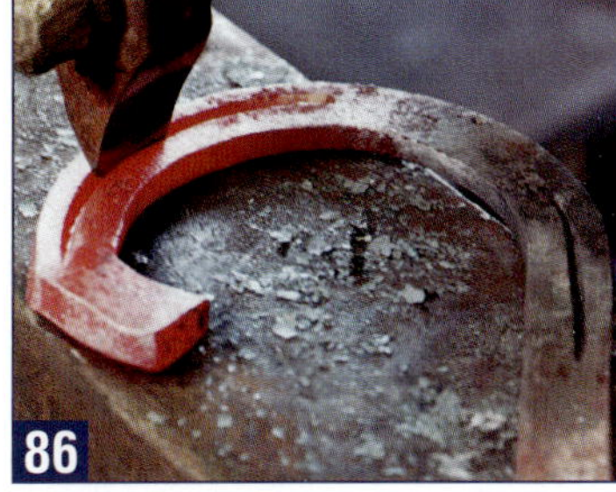

Finish the crease.

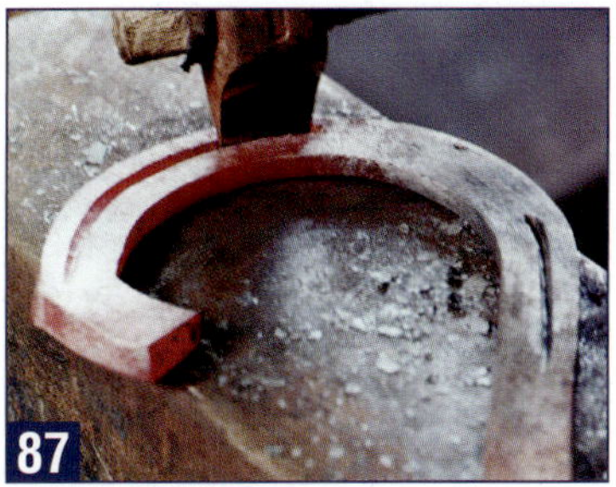

Finish the crease.

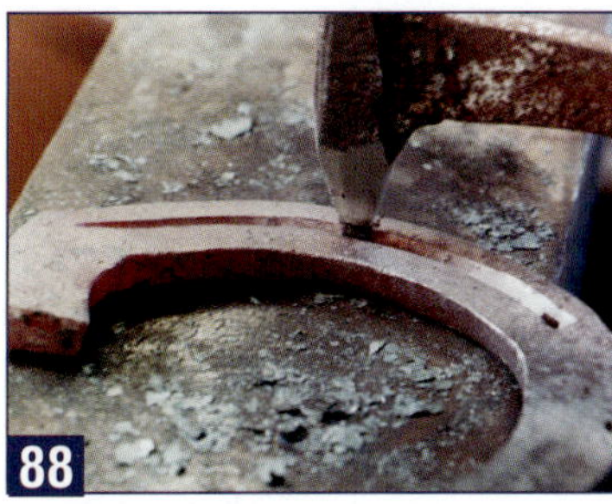

Drift the holes.

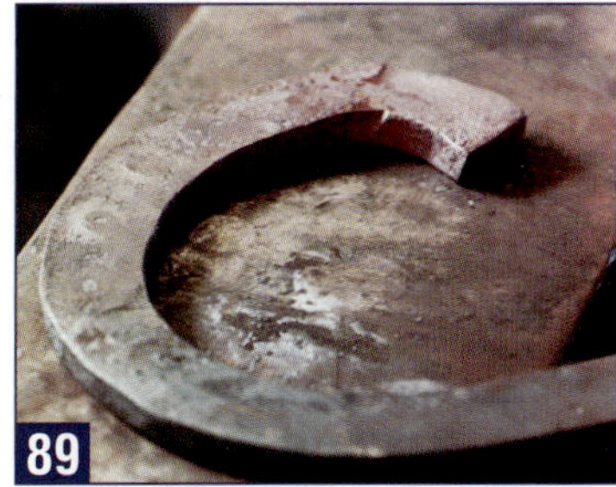

Hammer on the hoof surface of the shoe after the nails have been drifted.

HEAT 2

Heat one branch, bend the end of the stock and upset the hockey stick to make half the bar **(Figures 81-83)**. Forge the appropriate angle over the end of the horn **(Figure 84)**. Bend the branch around the horn **(Figure 85)**. There should still be enough heat in the branch to finish the crease **(Figures 86-87)** and drift the nail holes **(Figure 88)**. Hammer the hoof surface **(Figure 89)**, forge out the frog eyes **(Figure 90),** and pritchel **(Figure 91)**.

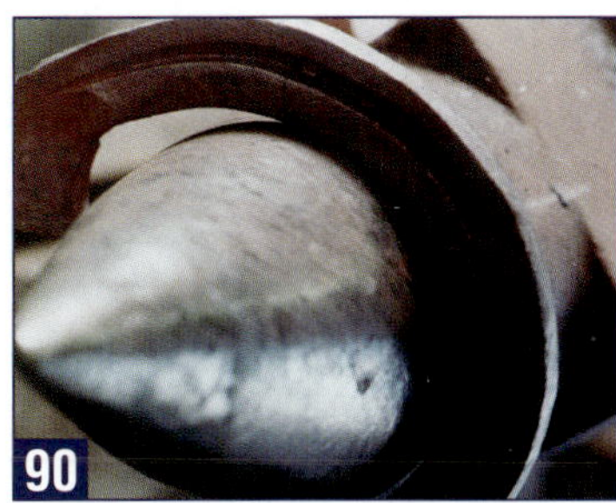

Clean up frog eyes on the horn.

HEAT 3

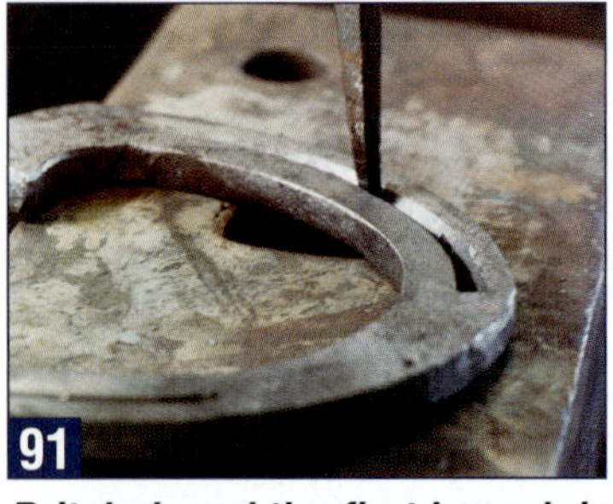

Pritchel, and the first branch is complete.

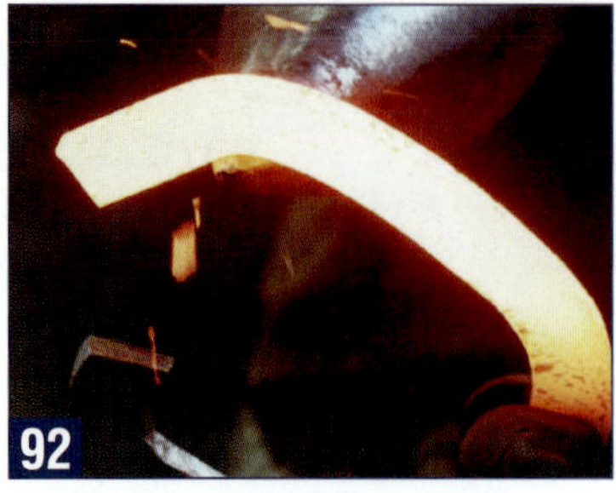

Make second hockey stick.

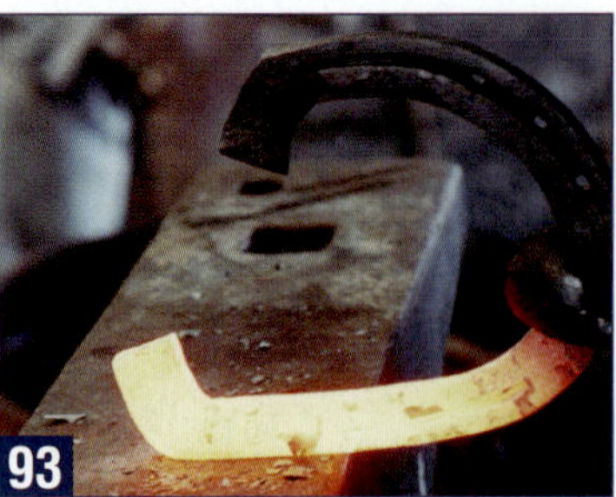

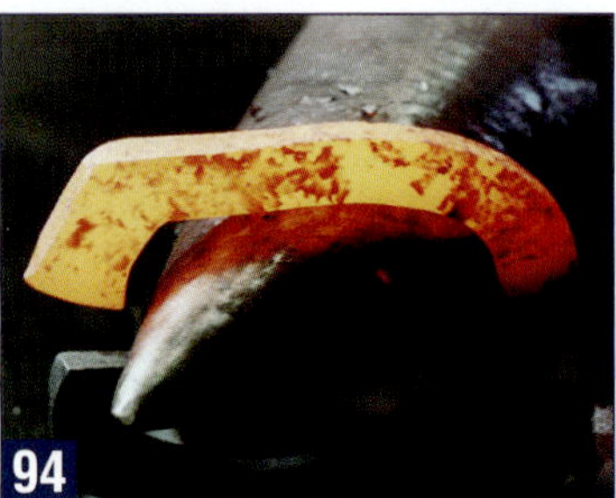

Bend branch around the horn.

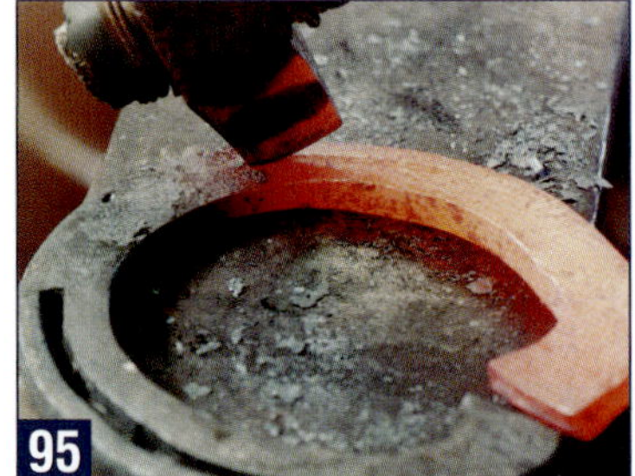

96

Fuller second branch. Do not let the scarves cross each other before creasing the second branch.

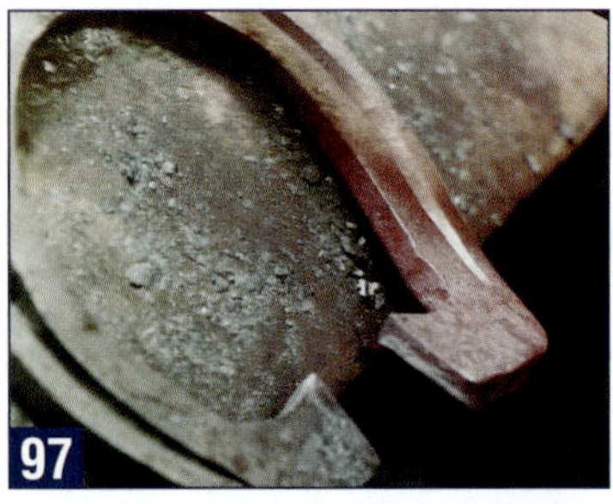

The branch will bend upward when you fuller it, especially when you have the excess mass on the end of the branch.

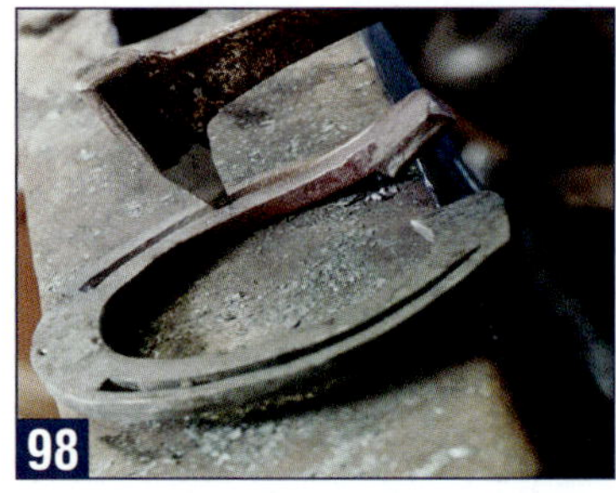

Level enough to work, and drift the holes.

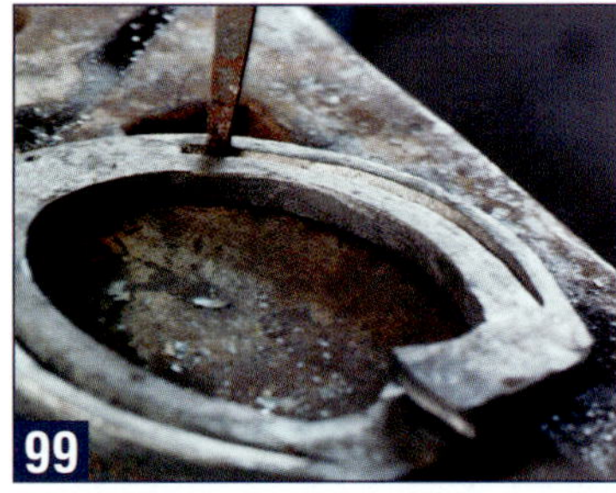

Put the scarves together and pritchel.

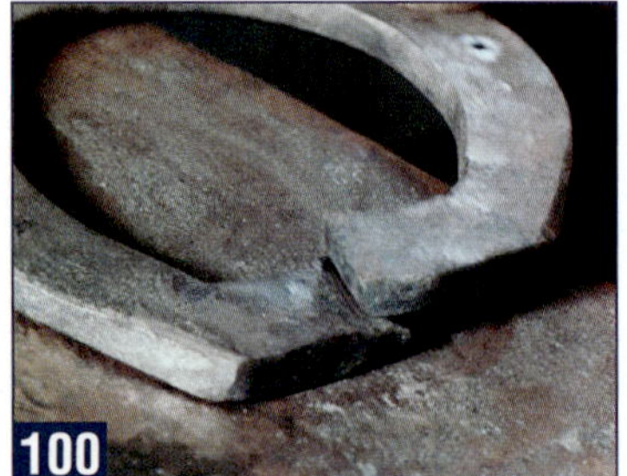

Hammer on the hoof surface to force the scarves together.

Repeat all the same steps as in Heat 2 on the second branch **(Figure 92-100)**. During the fullering process, the end of the stock will bend upward as in **Figure 97**. Don't lose efficiency by getting too concerned about this. A lot of people lose too much time leveling the shoe four or five times while it is being built. The only level that matters at all is the final one, so just keep the shoe flat enough to work safely and keep the shoe on the anvil.

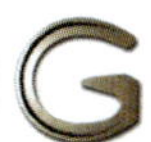

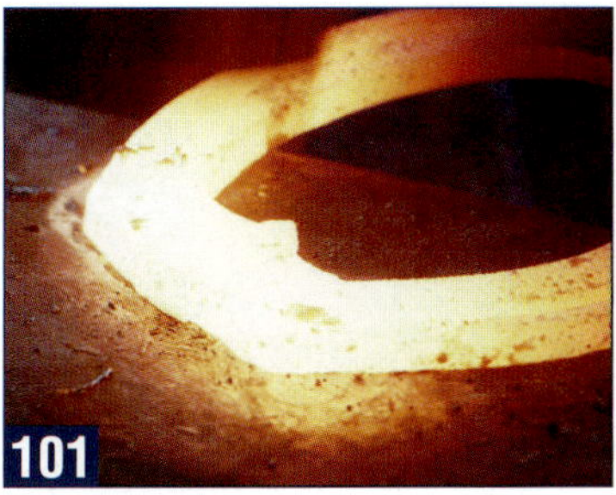

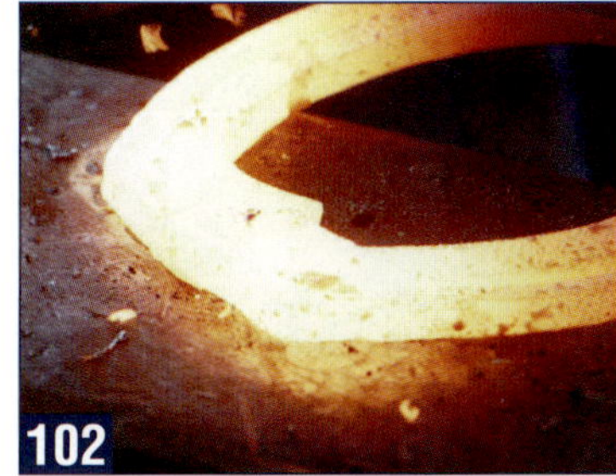

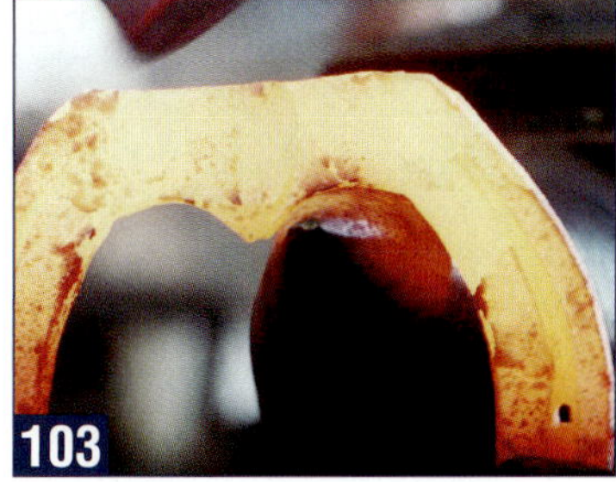

Weld the bar.

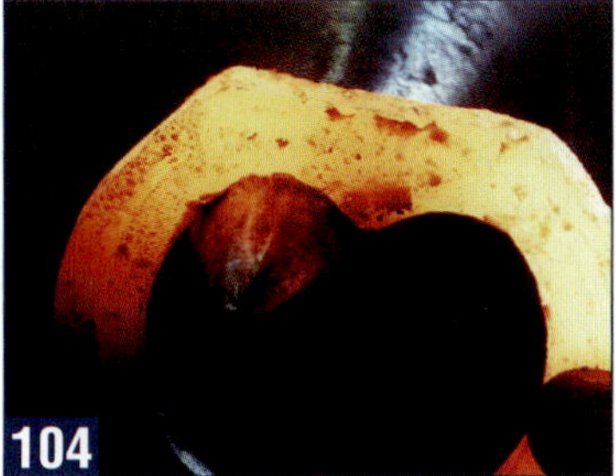

Weld the bar.

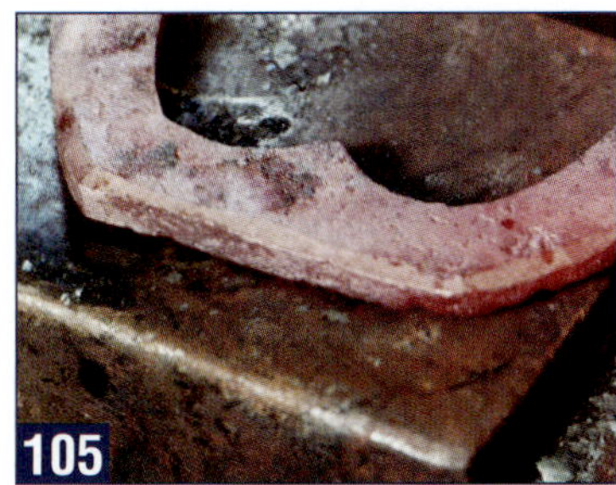

Hammer box the bar and the back of the heels.

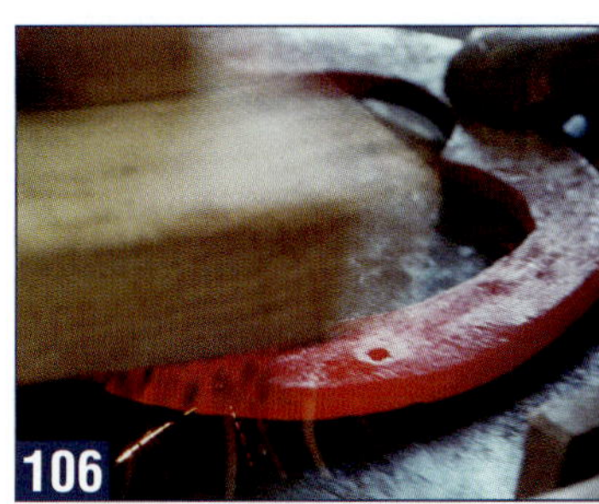

Vigorously brush the hot shoe.

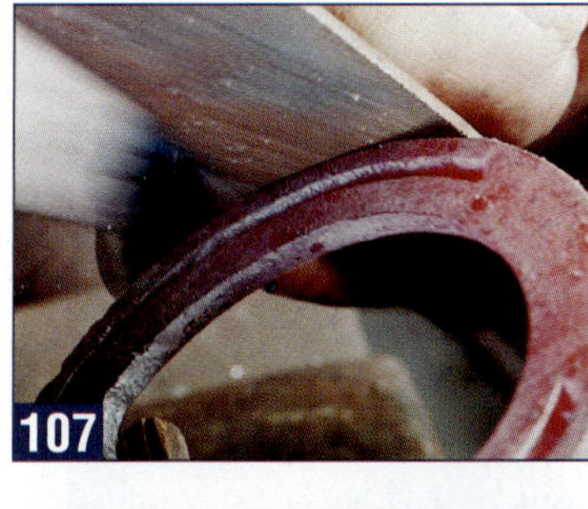

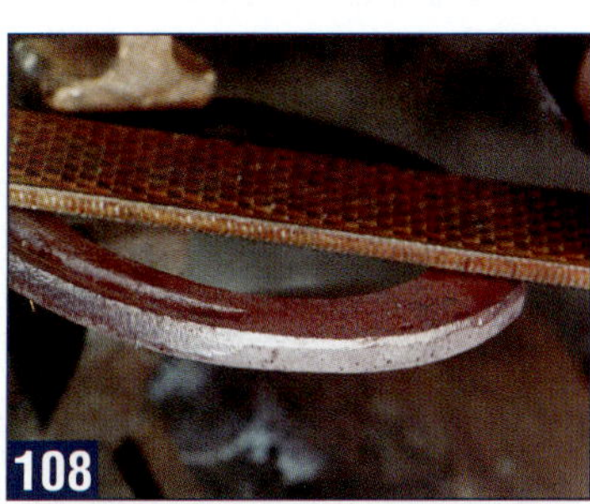

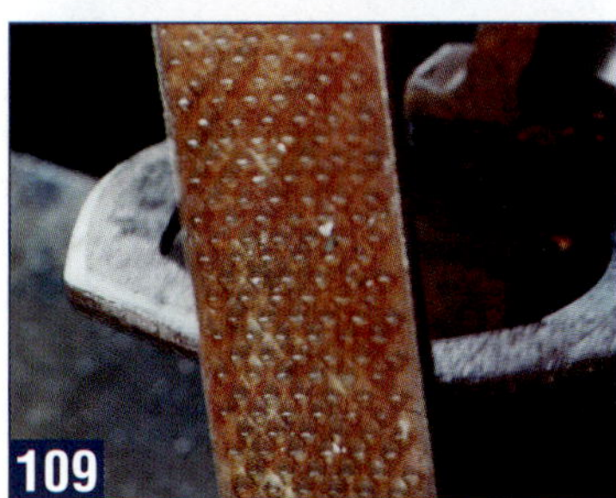

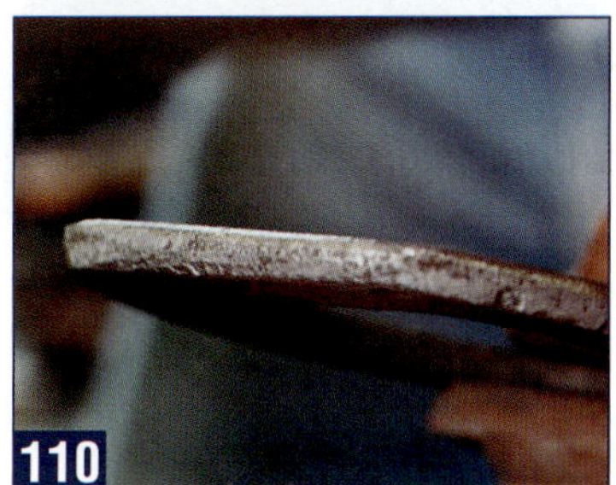

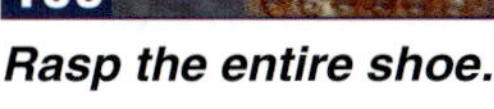

Rasp the entire shoe.

HEATS 4 And 5

These are the welding heats. Both of these should be done as the welding heats described for making the blank. Here it is pictured as **Figures 101-104**. The second welding heat is not always needed, but it will give you a little insurance for a strong weld.

Box both heels and the back of the bar with your hammer **(Figure 105)**. Brush and rasp to make a nice looking specimen **(Figures 106-110)**. The inside of the bar can be cleaned up with a half-round

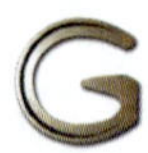

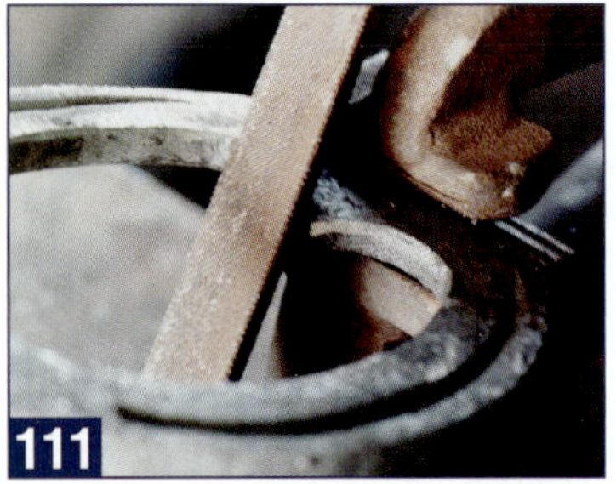

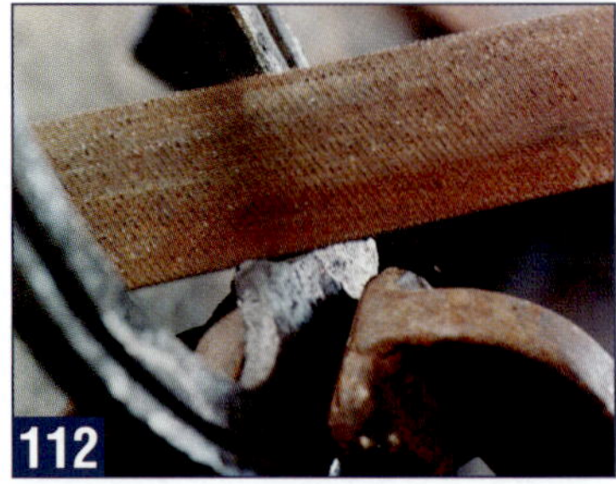

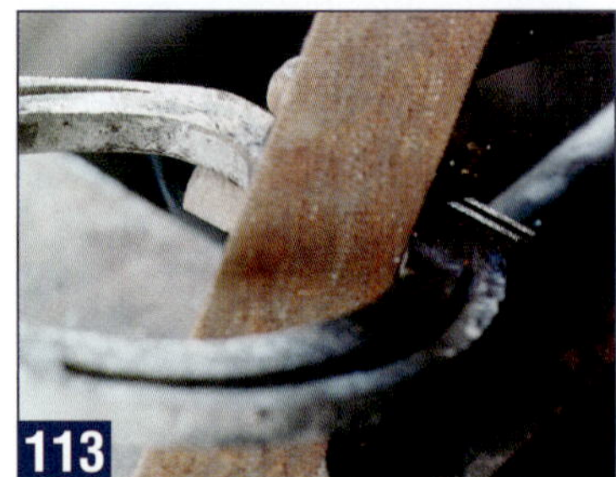

Use a half-round file on the inside of the bar and shoe.

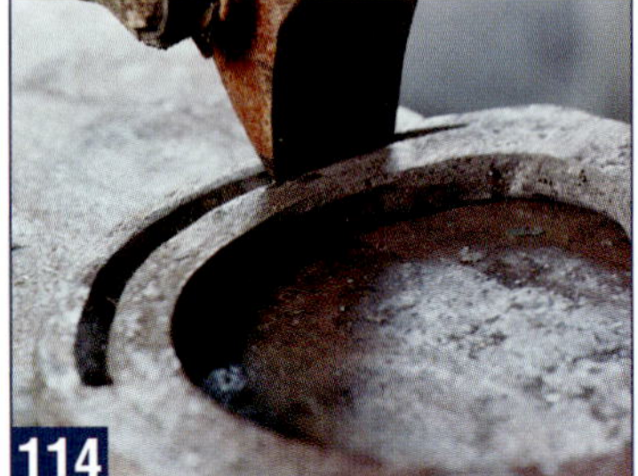

Make another pass through the fullering to clean up the crease.

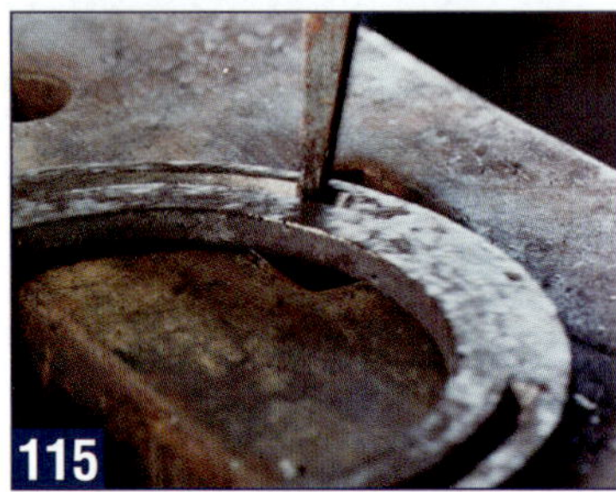

Check and clean out the nail holes.

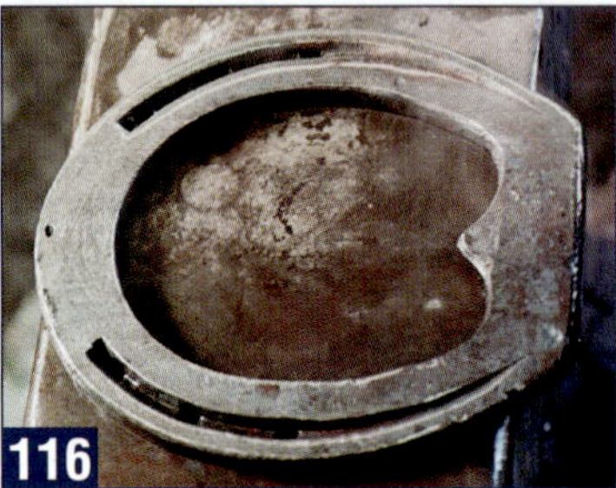

The finished fullered straight bar in 5 heats.

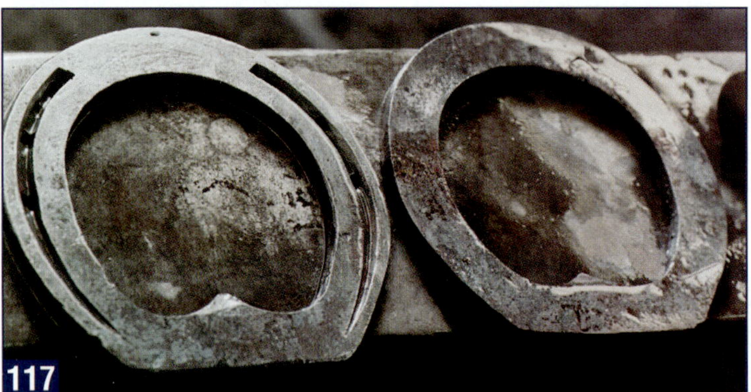

The 2 straight bars sitting next to each other.

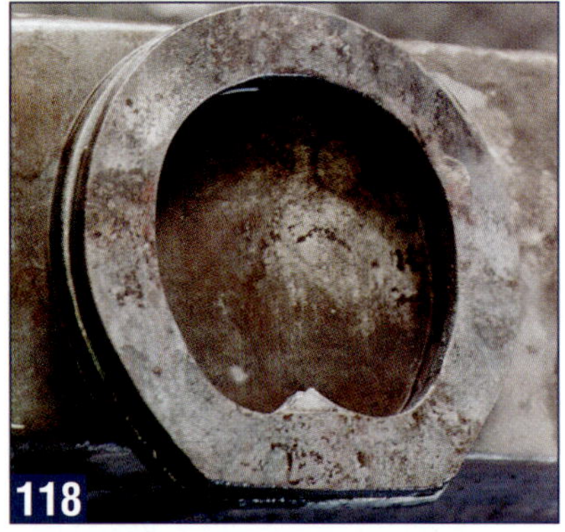

When you place the blank on top of the fullered straight bar, you can see the difference in sizes.

file **(Figures 111-113)**.

One of the problems with welding after the nails are punched is that the crease and nail holes suffer from the extreme heat, flux, and scale. It may be necessary to run the fuller through at a black heat, and reshape the nail holes with the pritchel **(Figures 114-115)**. You should end up with a nicely made straight bar **(Figure 116),** and it will be slightly larger than the blank from the fullering **(Figures 117-118)**.

Making this shoe in four or five heats will take many hours of practice. You may find that someday you can win bets at clinics by making this shoe in two heats and adding a toe clip if it goes well. (If you ever have me do a clinic for you, we will have to get a bet going.) Don't get discouraged; rather focus on what is going well and how your goal is getting closer with every shoe.

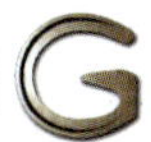

Chapter

49 EGG BAR SHOE

In Five Heats to a Blank

The egg bar is a popular and very usable shoe. It differs from a straight bar shoe in that it provides for palmar or plantar support. Like most specialty shoes, these shoes are expensive to buy but easy to make. As I go back over the pictures from throughout my career, I am surprised to find that I have not utilized this shoe very much. I would estimate that I have put on only three egg bars for every 20 straight bars, although you can make an egg bar a little easier and a little faster.

Some downsides to this shoe are the pressure that can be placed on the heels as well as the potential for losing this shoe with the excess material extending beyond the foot.

The method I recommend for measuring a foot for a fullered egg bar is to measure around and behind the foot where you want the shoe to go, then subtract three inches from that total measurement. Different forging styles will cause different measurements, so, as with most shoes, make a few from a known length, measure those, and develop a formula that works for you.

SETUP

Begin by cutting a 14-inch piece of 5/16-by-3/4-inch steel. Don't mark anything if you are a beginner, since it can be difficult to match the sex appeal on the bar to the center punch mark at the toe of the shoe. You will mark later when you are fullering this shoe before welding. For now, just concentrate on making a nice blank.

HEAT 1

Heat the middle of the stock and make a front

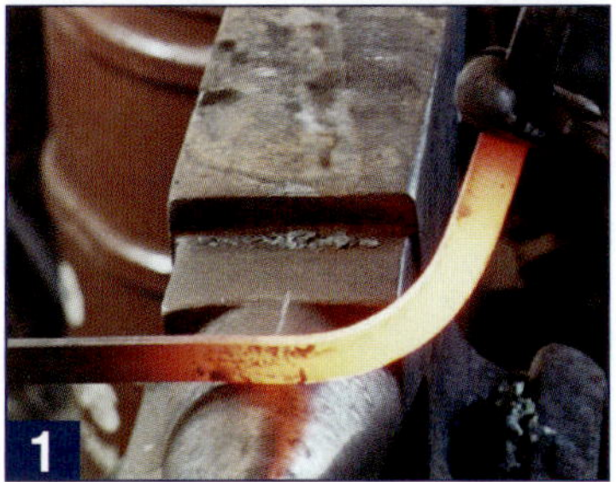

Making the toe bend.

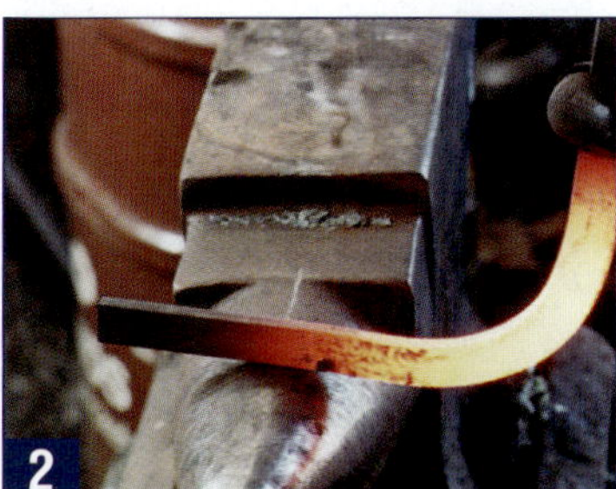

Making the toe bend.

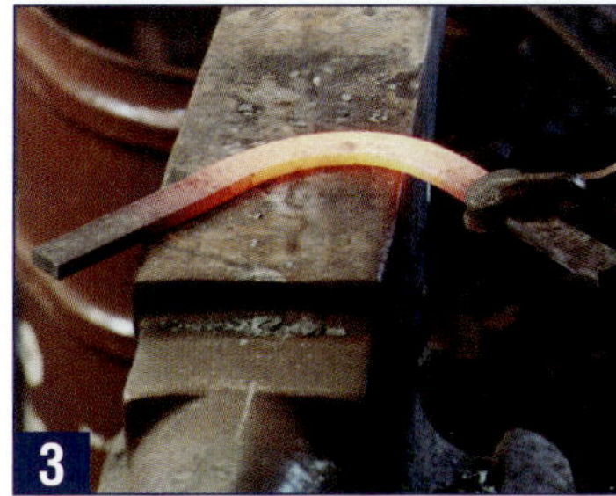

Seat out the bend.

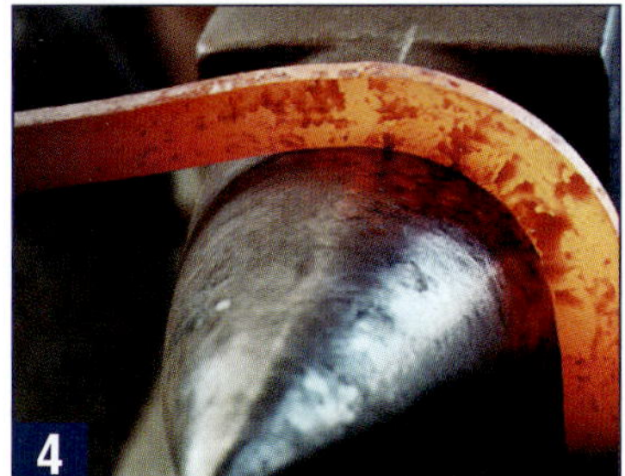

Set the toe.

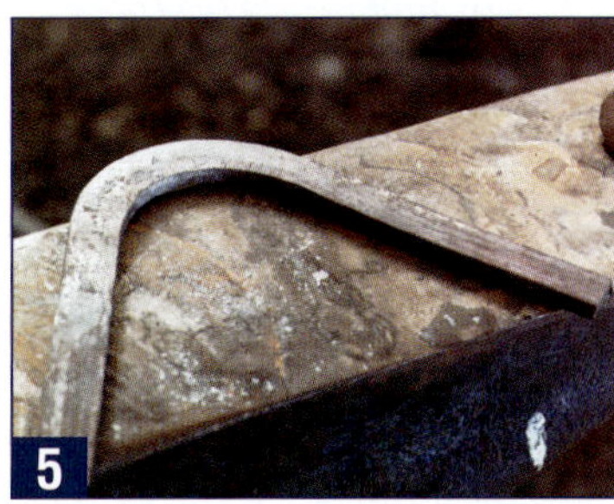

Finished toe bend for the egg bar.

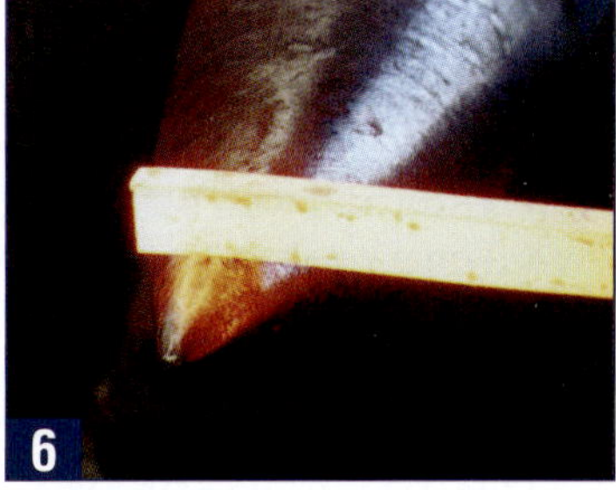

Place the heated end of the bar on the horn.

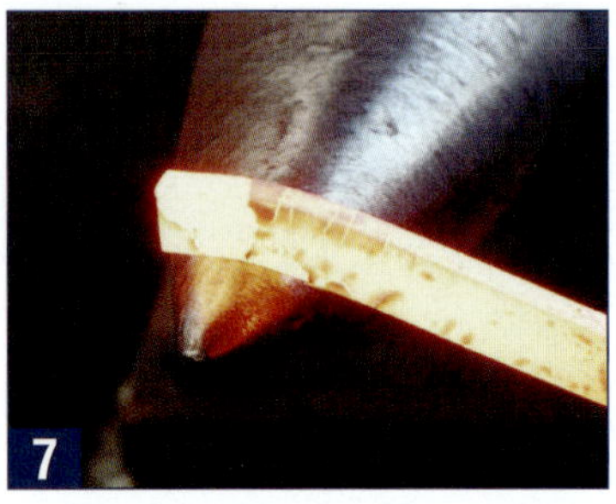

Lower your tongs as you bend it.

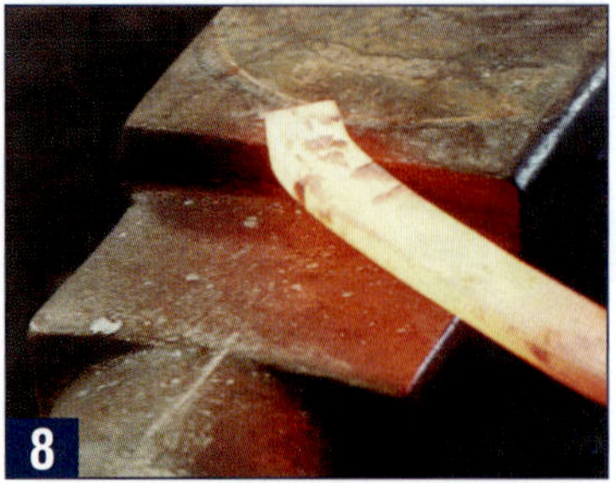

Move to the step of the anvil, and hammer with half-faced blows.

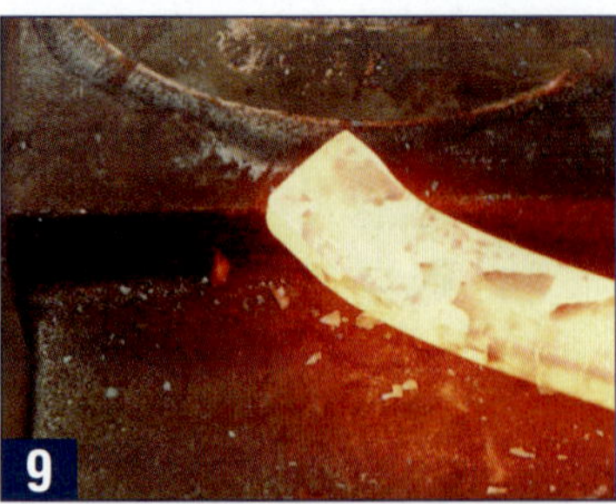

Pivot on the inside corner of contact with the step.

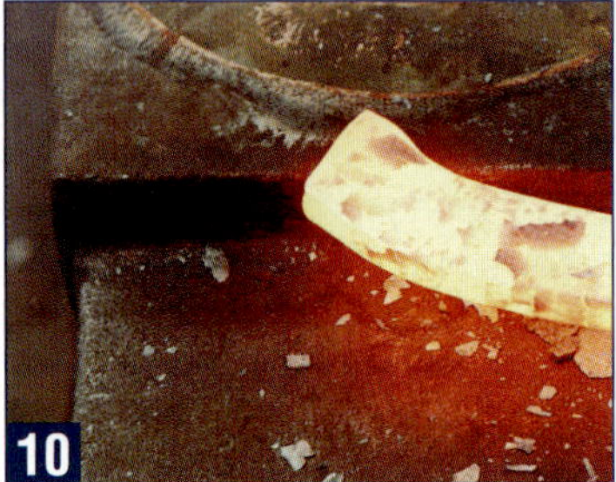

Move every blow.

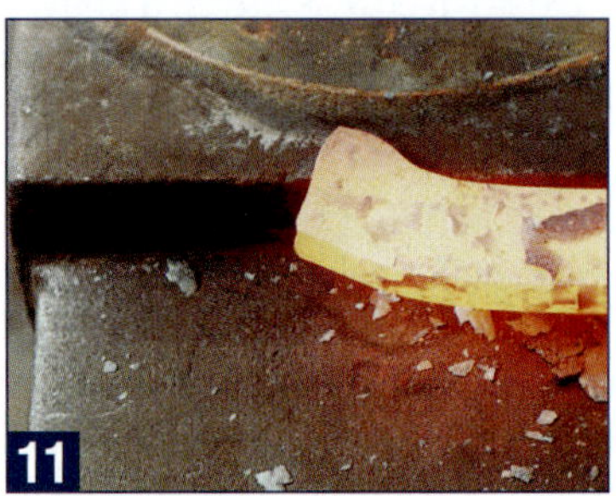

That's right, every blow.

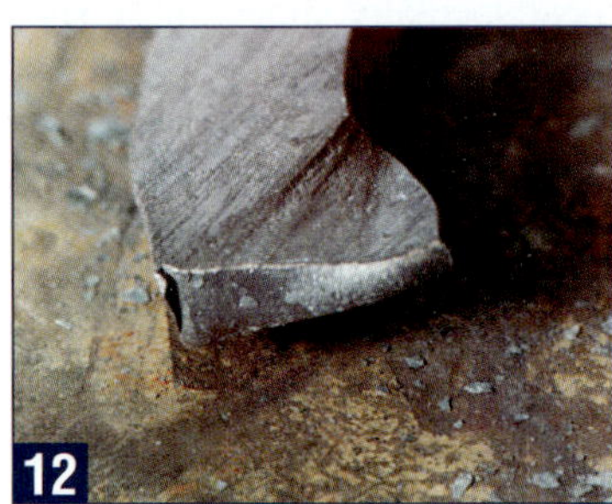

Your chain link scarf should look like this.

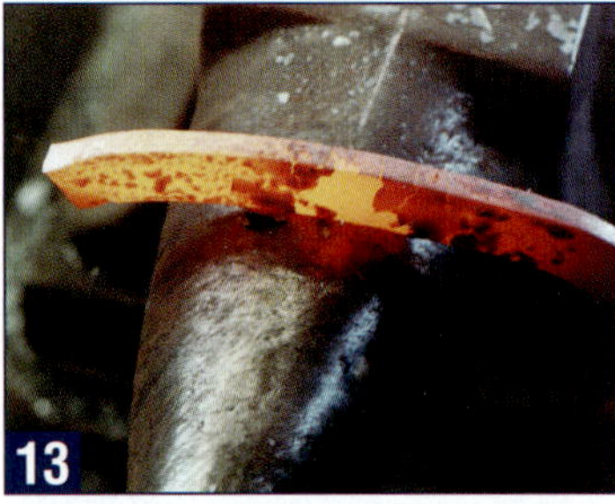

Bend the branch on the horn.

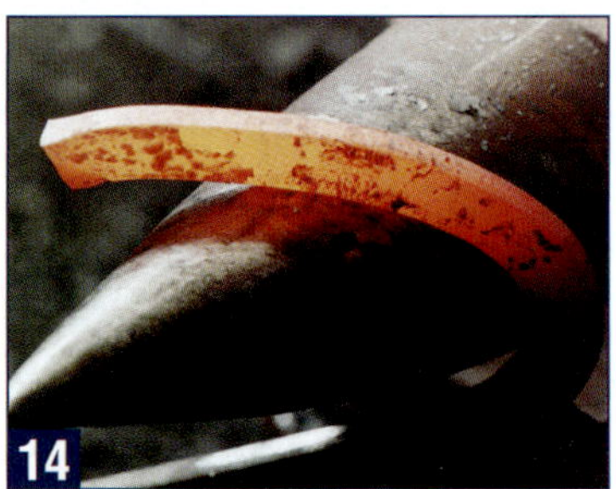

More bending.

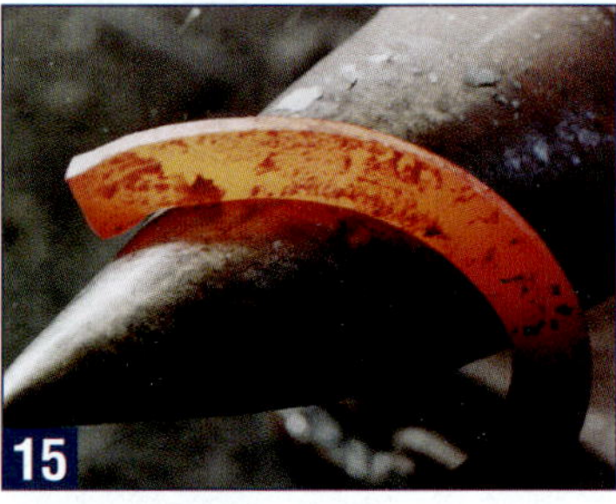

Still more bending.

toe bend **(Figures 1-4)**. At this point, it will look just like the toe bend on your plain front shoe with some added length. Place more stock past the tongs and past the horn when forging on a longer piece of steel, as you did with the straight bar.

Anytime you have a shoe with excess material in it, you can isolate the toe bend by the placement of your tongs. The closer your tongs are to what you are hitting, the more you work on just the part of the steel that is being hit. The finished toe bend should look like **Figure 5**.

HEAT 2

Heat one branch and bend approximately 3/4 inch over a tight radius at the tip of the horn **(Figure 6-7)**. I weld my egg bars using a chain-link scarf. To make a chain-link scarf, hold the end of the stock over the step at a 45-degree angle **(Figure 8)** and hammer with a half-faced blow **(Figure 9)**. Move the shoe toward the body of the anvil as you continue to hit with a half-faced blow **(Figures 10-11)**. The steel is pivoting at the point where the inside of the steel meets the corner of the anvil at the step.

Once you reach the edge of the stock, turn it over

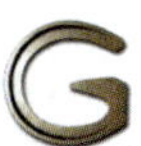

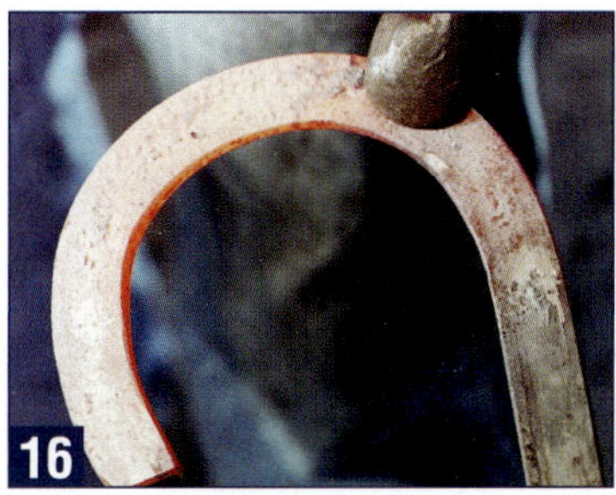

You should have it bent like this, even though this is a picture for the ring excercises.

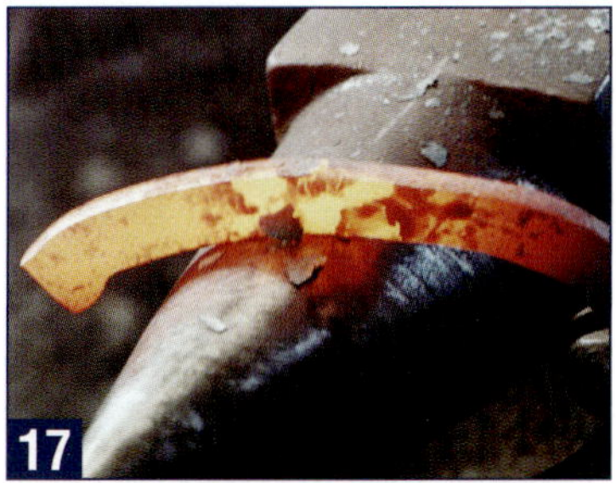

Repeat all the same steps on the second branch.

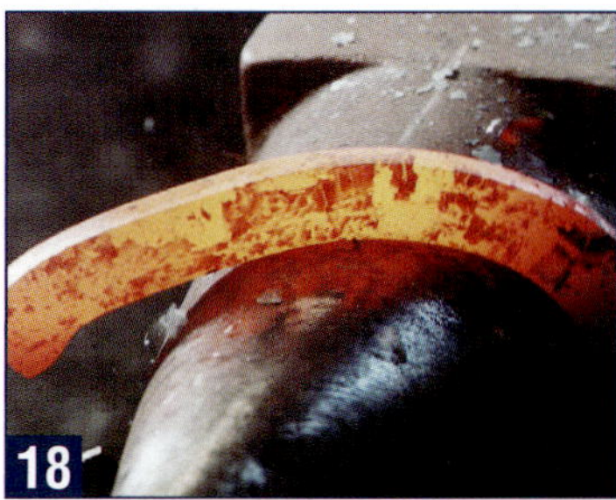

That's right, all the steps.

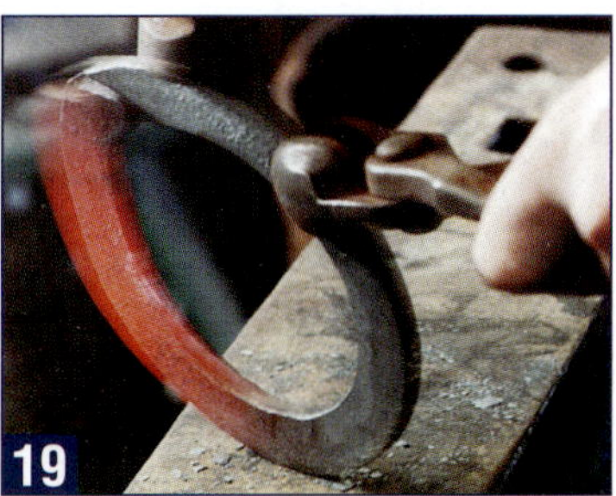

Close the shoe to overlap the scarves.

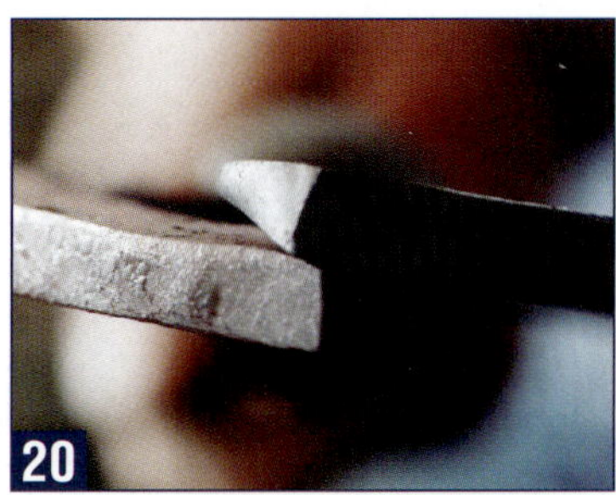

Both corners at the end of the shoe should overlap like this.

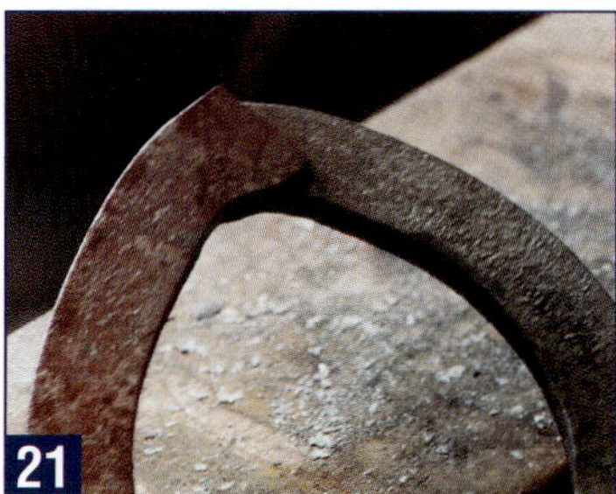

The left is over the right as I hold the toe.

and look at the scarf. It should look like a series of lines that are wide at one edge and converge at the inside corner **(Figure 12)**. There is still some thickness toward the outside edge of the stock, but it should be quite thin on the inside edge.

Bend the branch around the horn **(Figures 13-15)**. Lay the shoe on the anvil and evaluate the toe bend through the branch to the scarf. The end of the steel should line up with the center of the toe bend. It will look similar to **Figure 16**. (I lost the actual picture of this stage of this exact shoe, so **Figure 16** is a stand-in from the ring exercise.) Laying an open-heeled shoe on top of the half-finished egg bar can help to train your eye so that you can compare the bends that you made to the bends in the open-heeled shoe.

HEAT 3

Do the exact same things to the second branch **(Figures 17-18)** and close the shoe so that the scarves overlap **(Figure 19)**. The portions of the scarves with the lines from the step of the anvil should be against each other. Make certain that the corners on the outside of the weld overlap each other **(Figure 20)**.

If the shoe is not closed up enough, there will not be enough steel in the weld. As you hold the toe of the shoe, the scarf from your tong-hand side should be over the scarf from your hammer-hand side. I am right-handed, so you can see in **Figure 21** how the shoe looks in my tongs.

Brush and flux the steel, then return to the fire to get the first welding heat.

HEAT 4

Come from the fire and hit with a few light, quick, flat hammer blows directly on top of the weld **(Figures 22-23)**. Use the toe of the hammer to blend out the seam. Flip the shoe over and repeat on the opposite side. If you look closely at **Figures 24-26**, you can see what the bar should look like after the first weld. In **Figure 24**, there is still quite a bit of thickness in the material, and you can see the lines made by the toe of the hammer in **Figures 25-26**. Brush and flux before returning to the fire.

HEAT 5

Come from the fire and quickly hit the weld with fast, flat blows **(Figures 27-28)**. Once the metal has returned to the original thickness, move to the tip of

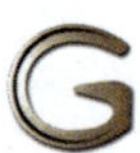

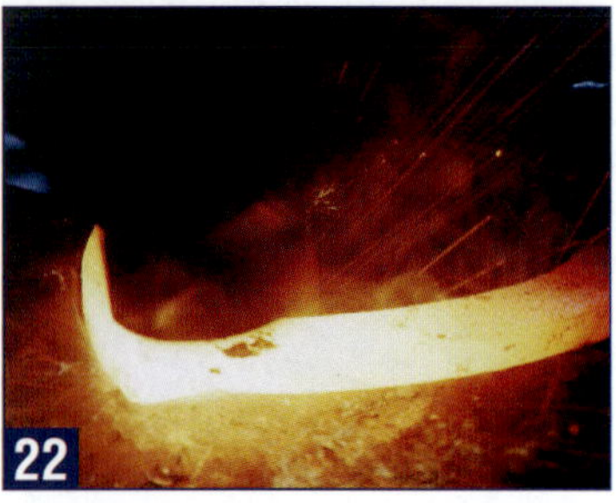
First part of the weld is flat, quick and light.

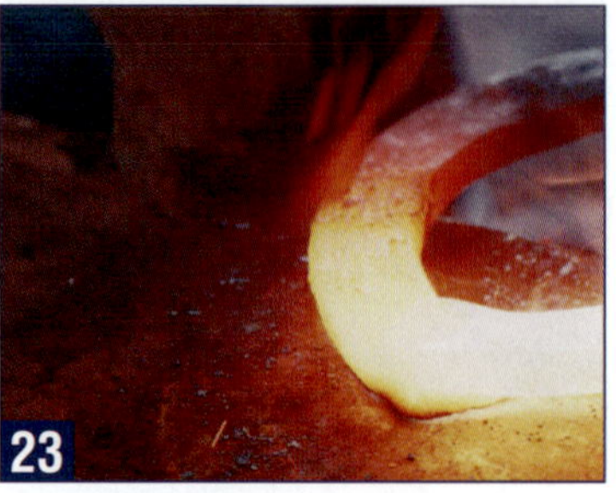
Blend seams with the toe of your hammer.

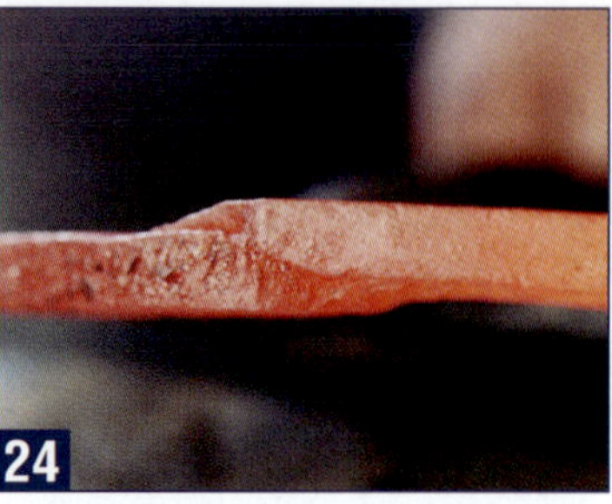
It should look like this after the first weld.

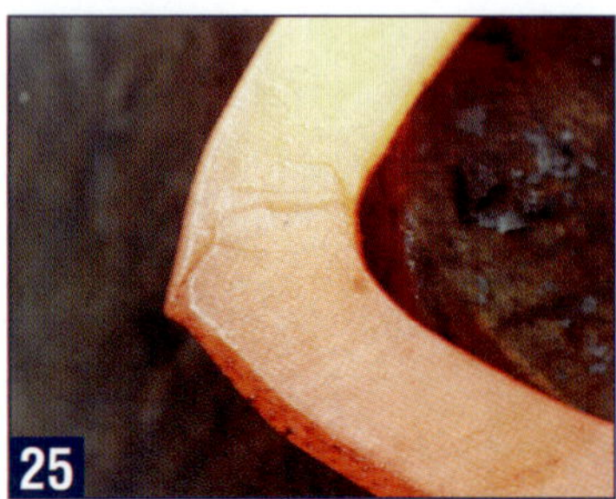
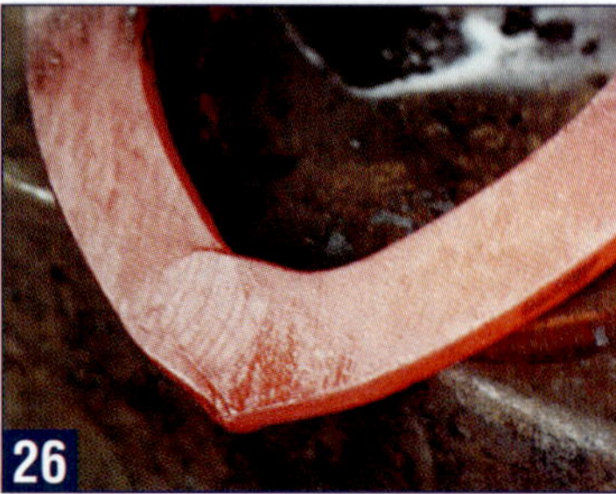
It should look like this after the first weld.

On the second welding heat, start by hitting flat on the face of the anvil.

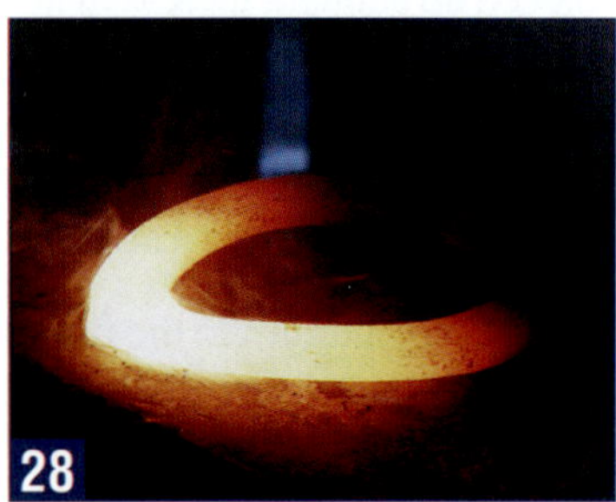
Continue to hit flat on the weld until the stock is back to its original thickness.

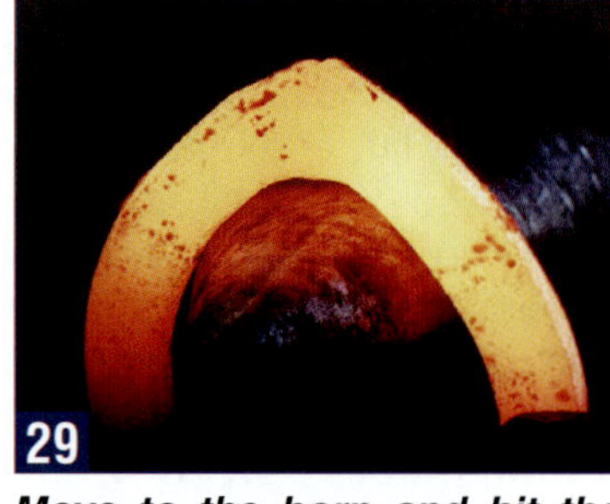
Move to the horn and hit the center of the weld lightly on a fairly large radius.

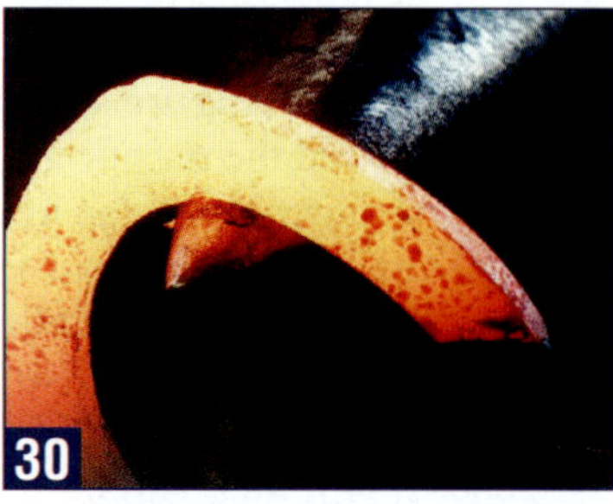
Move the shoe so that the weld is past the top of the horn. Hit the weld.

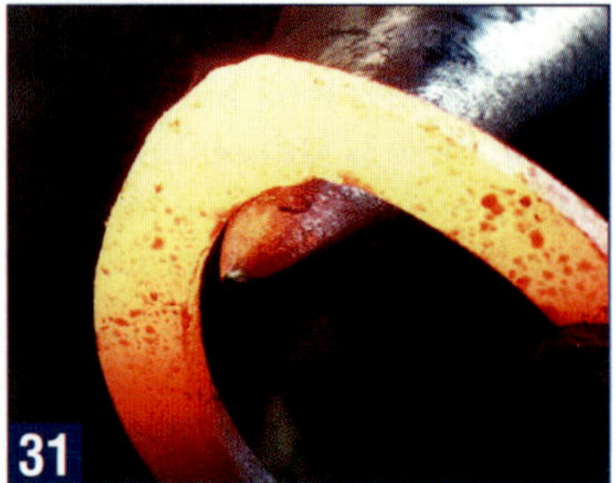
Pull the shoe toward you, and hit the weld.

the horn. Since there is so much metal in the weld, it is easy to forge a nice sex appeal into the weld.

The sex appeal, or the "tallinga," as it is called in Iowa, is the sharp point in the middle of the weld pointing toward the toe of the shoe. Having this on a handmade shoe makes no difference at all to the job that the shoe will do on the foot. However, it is an indication that the person who made the shoe has a higher degree of skill than those who makesshoes without one. Even though this is only style and fashion, shoes without it don't look as nice.

Start by slightly flattening the area of the weld with some light hammer blows on top of the horn **(Figure 29)**. Place the center of the weld just beyond the anvil ridge — much like the move for a square toe

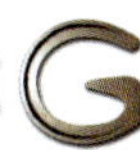

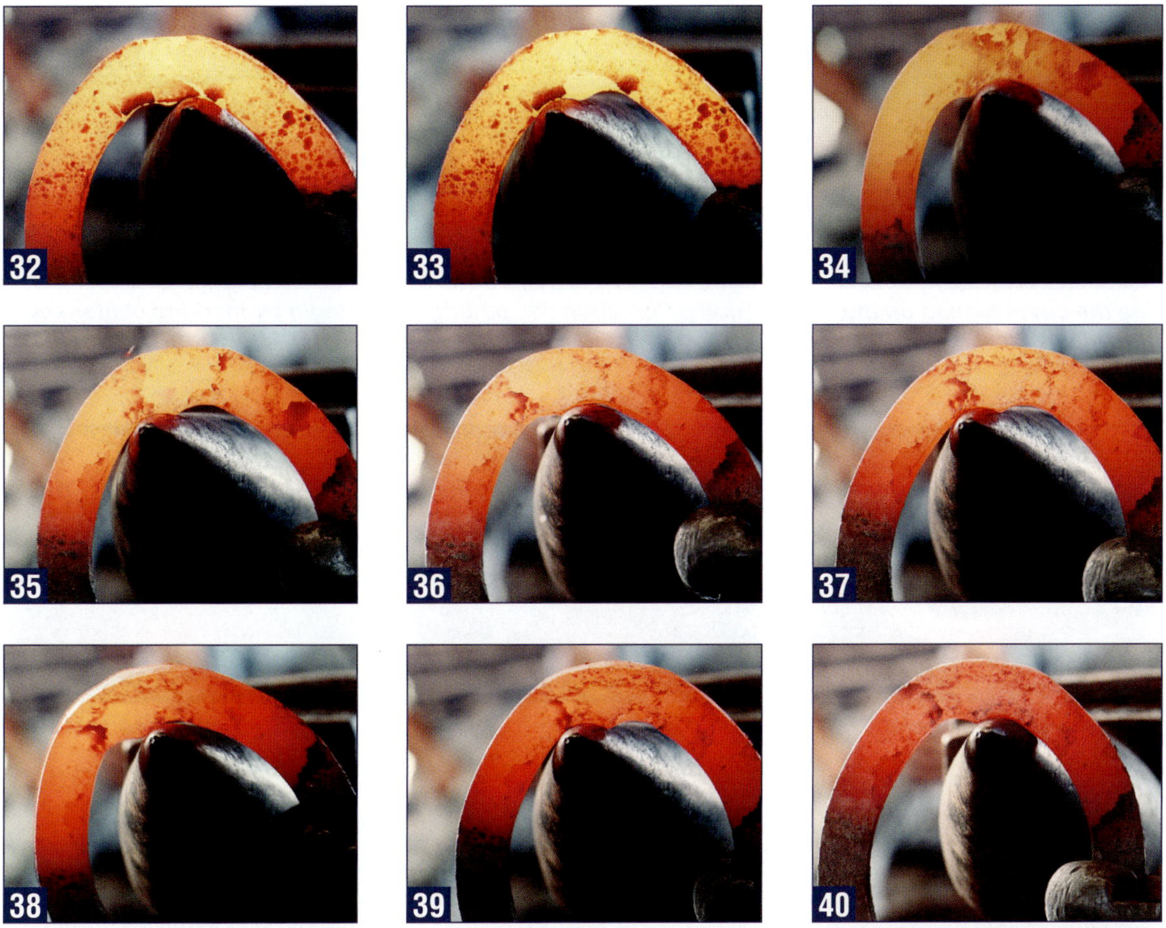

Figures 32-40. Move back and forth on top of the horn to make your sex appeal. Protect the center of the weld, but forge either side of it.

— **(Figure 30)** and hammer directly into the weld. You want to have the force of the hammer directed just past the top center of the anvil to avoid simply smashing the steel.

After a couple of hammer blows, move the weld to the near side of the horn at the same point on the tip of the horn **(Figure 31)**. Hammer so that the force of the hammer comes down just near the side of the point of contact. A small point will begin to appear on the inside of the weld. This is the sex appeal for a bar shoe. Continue the forging sequence until the bar has returned to the original width. The next nine pictures are a step-by-step method for making the sex appeal on an egg bar **(Figures 32-40)**. Be careful with your placement of the shoe on the tip of the horn so that you maintain the sex appeal, not destroy it.

Place the shoe on the face of the anvil and bring the thickness back to 5/16 inch at the weld and clean up the sex appeal on the tip of the horn. If you want to have a bevel on the inside of the sex appeal, you can do this by placing the shoe on the top of the horn with the ground surface down and hammering into the weld **(Figure 41)**.

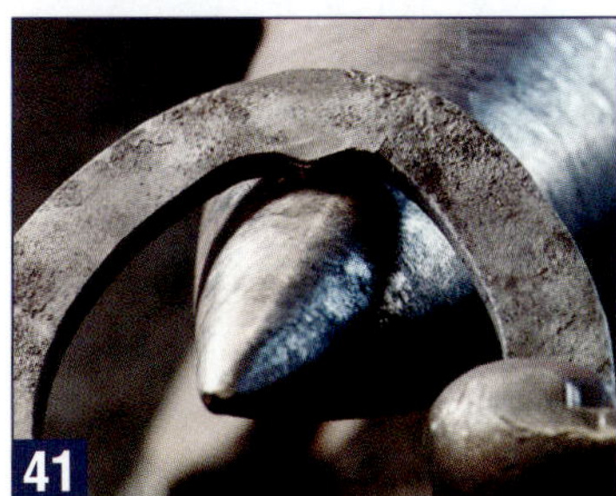

You can enhance the sex appeal a little bit on the top of the horn in this position.

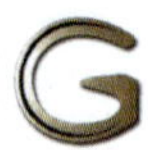

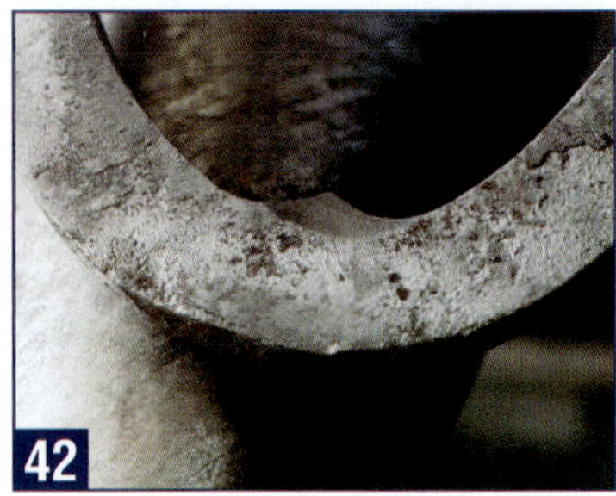

See the bevel formed on the horn.

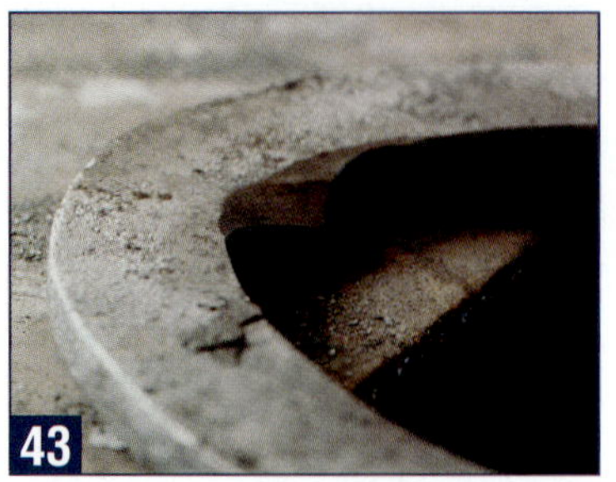

Another position for putting a bevel on the sex appeal.

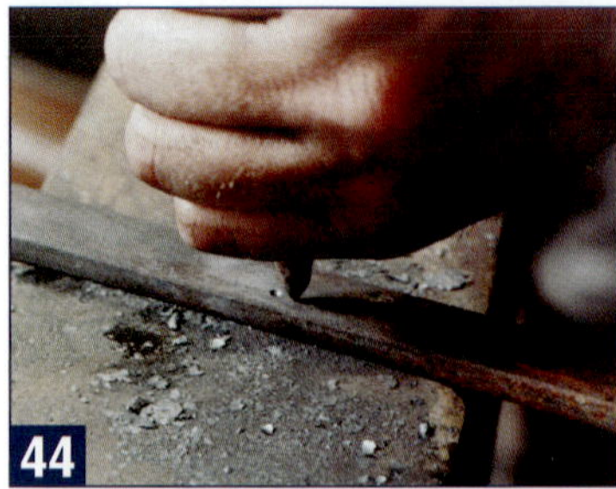

Begin by marking center and start of fullering.

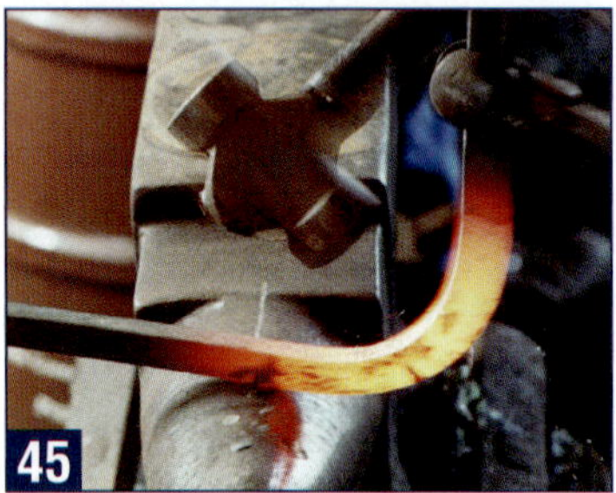

Make the same toe bend.

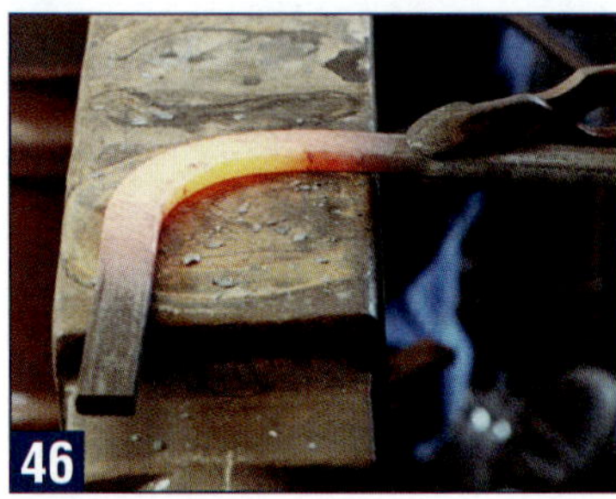

Seat it out.

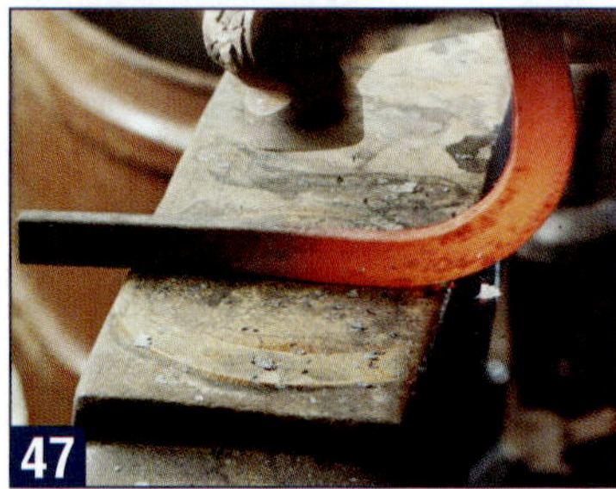

Straighten branches that were bent by inertia.

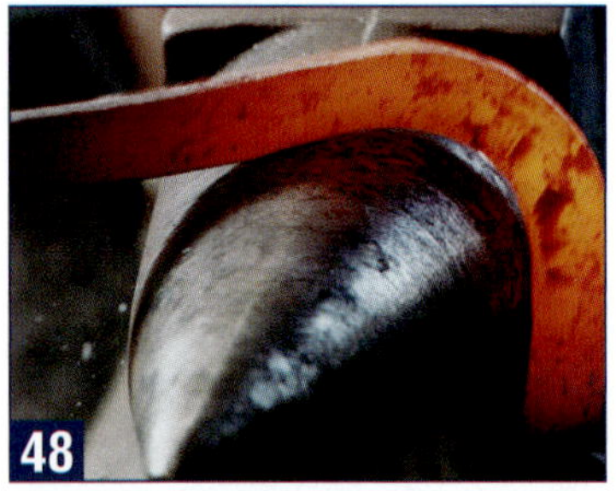

Set the toe and hem the start of the fullering.

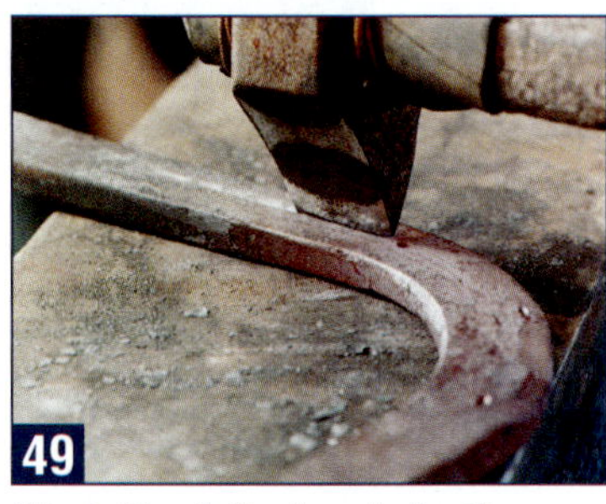

Mark the fullering in both branches.

Figure 42 shows how the beginning of this method looks on the ground surface. You can see that it is a little off center. Just turn the shoe over and move it so that the bevel is centered up. It is a good idea to do this for the first time on someone else's anvil, because it is hard to make the bevel without denting the horn with the corner of your hammer.

Another method is similar to the way you would make the bevel on a straight bar. Place the shoe so that the foot surface is on the face of the anvil and hammer the inside of the weld with the round side of your hammer **(Figure 43)**.

All that is left is to level the shoe, and you will have an egg bar blank.

FULLERED EGG BAR IN FIVE HEATS

Anytime that you are nailing on a bar shoe, there is a good chance you are shoeing a damaged foot. With this in mind, I crease all of my bar shoes. This allows for removal of one nail at a time, which is easier on damaged feet. (You may have heard this before.)

Now that we will be placing nail holes in the shoe, it will be helpful to mark the steel in the straight. Cut 14 inches of 5/16-by-3/4 inch stock and mark center. Mark the beginning of the fullering at 1 5/16 inches from center, just as you did for your plain front shoes **(Figure 44)**. I know that the heading is allowing for five heats, but you will find that four heats is often plenty for making this shoe when you have had a little practice.

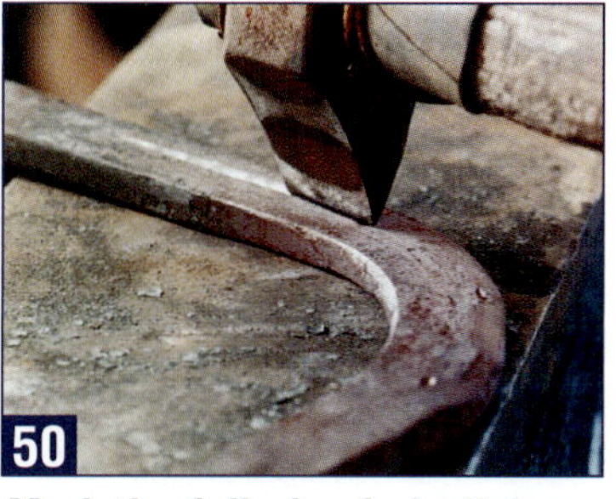

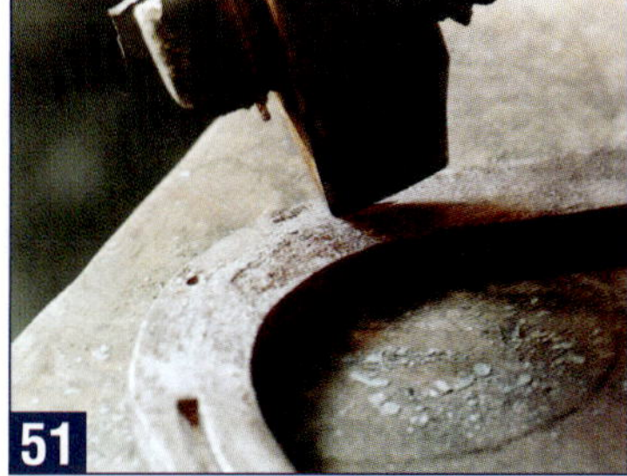

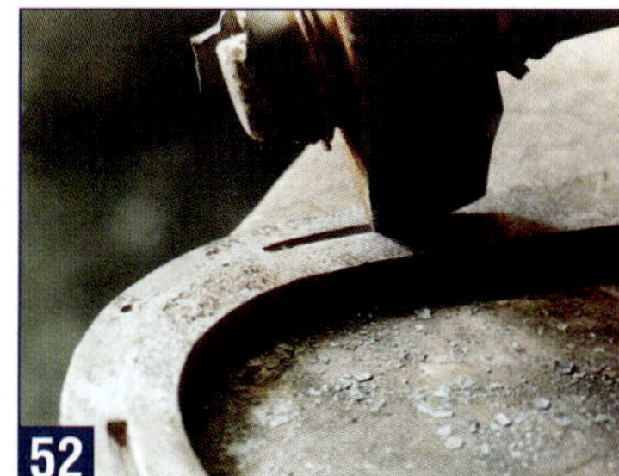

Mark the fullering in both branches.

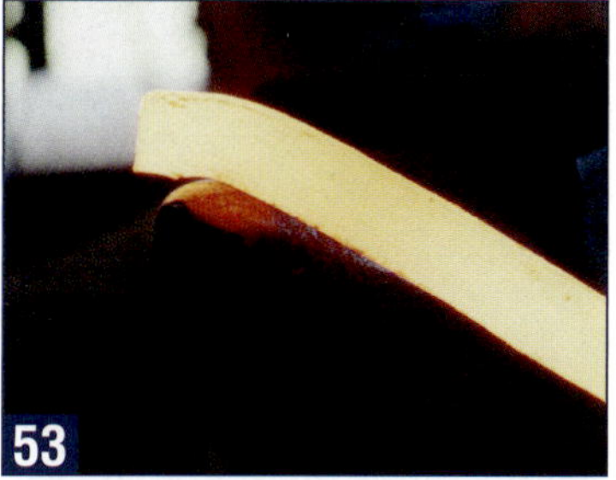

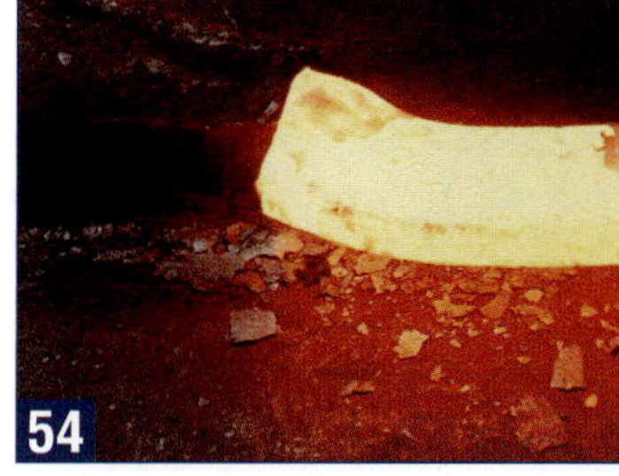

Make the scarf on the first branch.

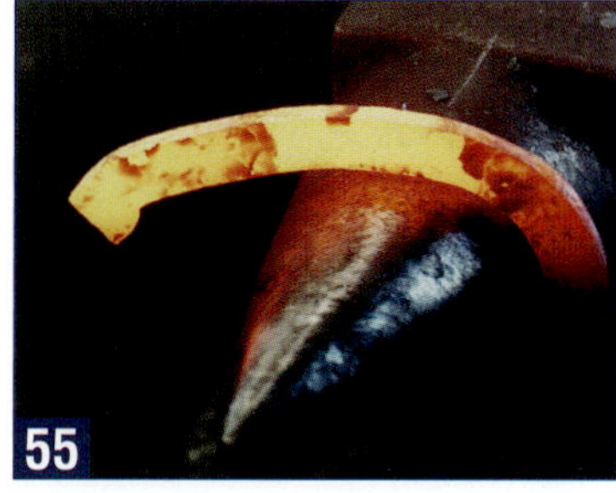

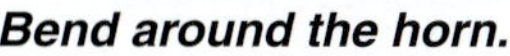

Bend around the horn.

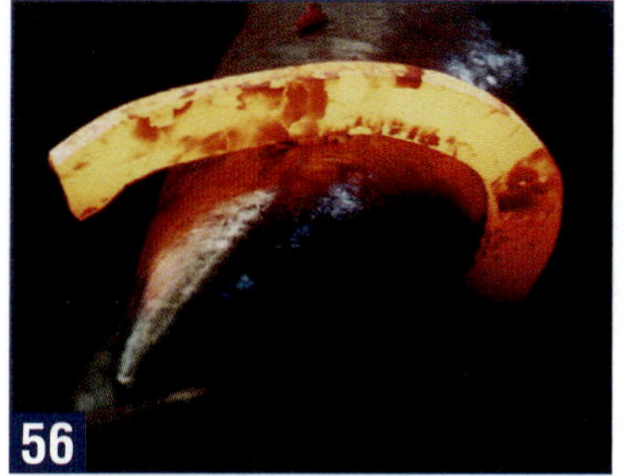

Bend around the horn.

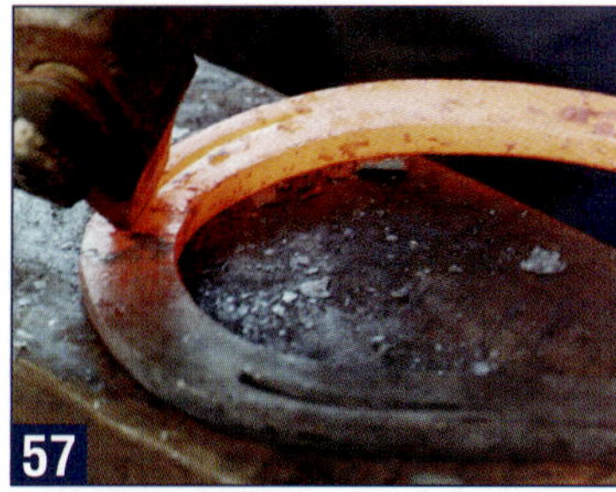

Finish fullering.

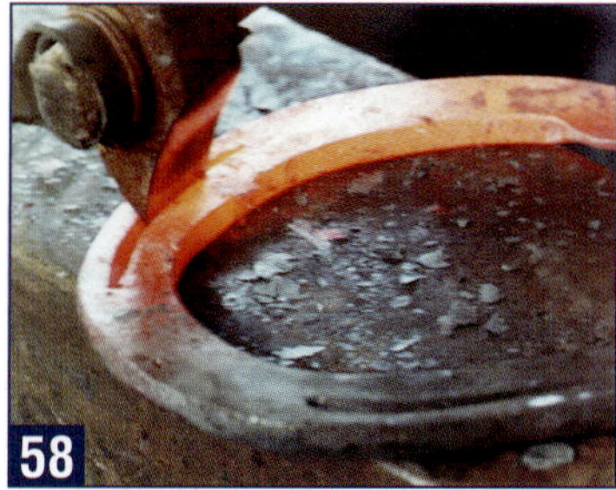

HEAT 1

Heat the center of the stock and make a proper front toe bend **(Figure 45)**. Seat out heavily to widen the web at the toe **(Figures 46)**. Set the toe and clean up the inertia bends **(Figure 47)**. Hem from the mark for the start of the fullering **(Figure 48)** and mark the fullering on both branches as deep as the remaining heat will allow **(Figures 49-52)**.

HEAT 2

Heat one branch, bend around the tip of the horn **(Figure 53)**, scarf **(Figure 54)**, and bend around the horn **(Figures 55-56)**. There should still be enough

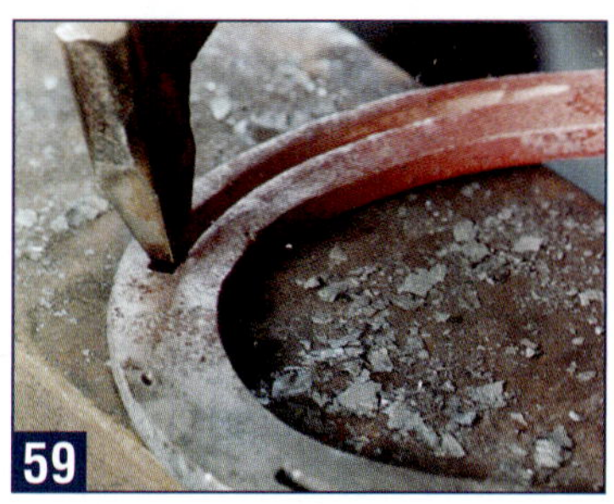

Drift the nail holes.

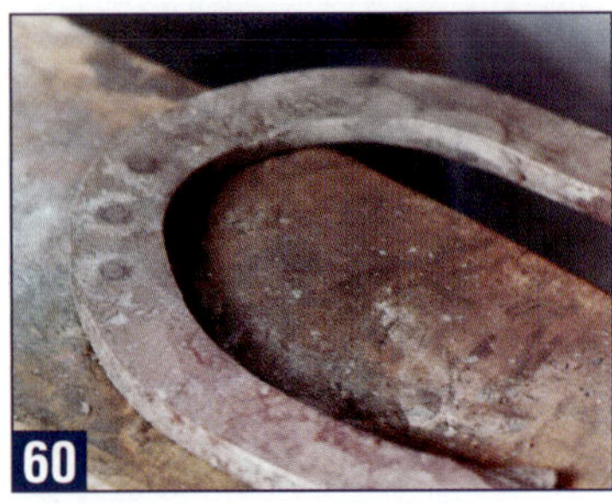

60 Hammer across the hoof surface.

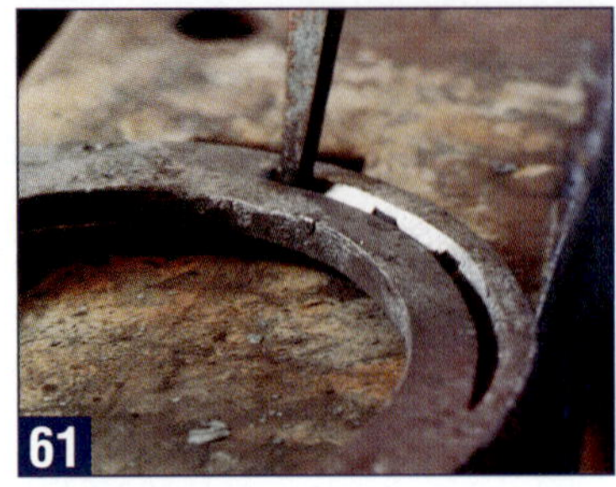

61 Pritchel.

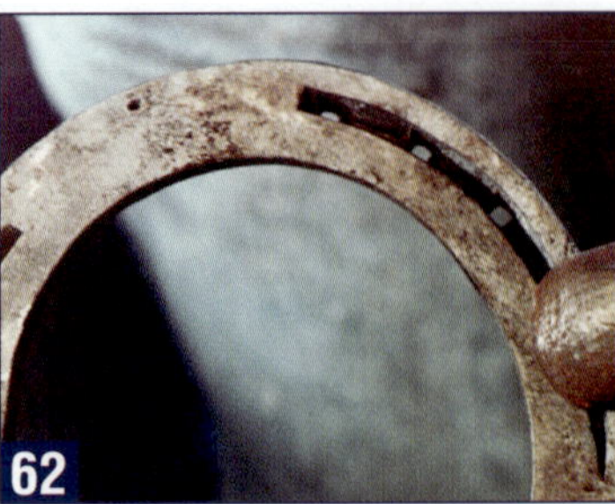

62 The shoe should look like this after the second heat.

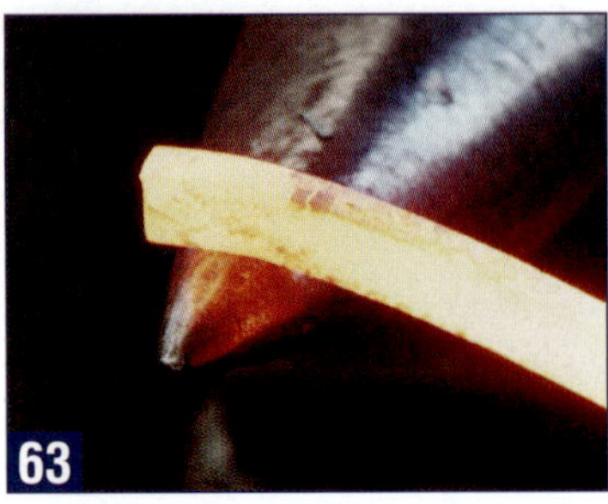

63 Bending the end of the stock on the horn.

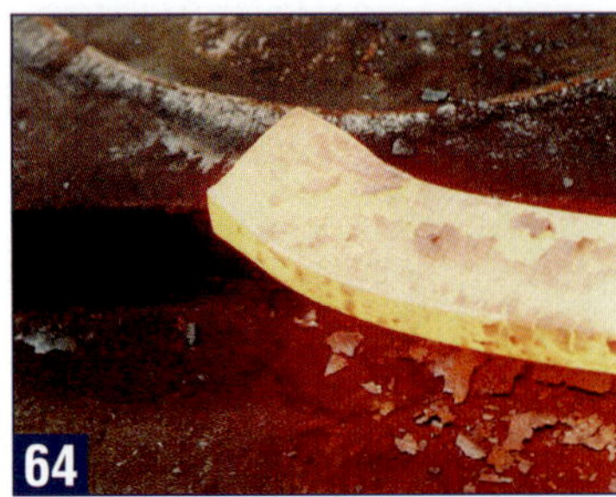

64 Scarfing second branch.

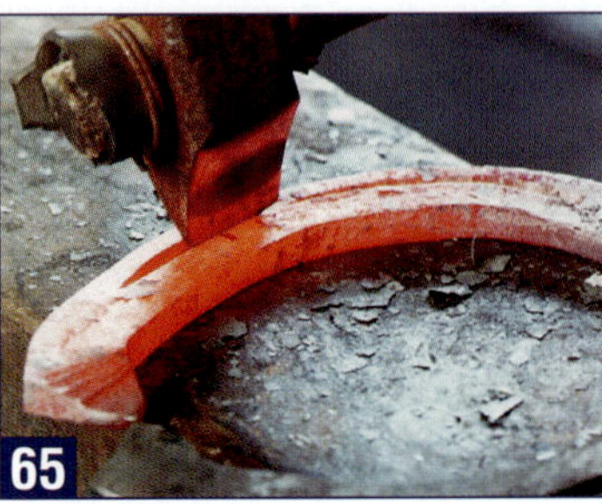

65 Fullering second branch. Don't let the scarves cross yet.

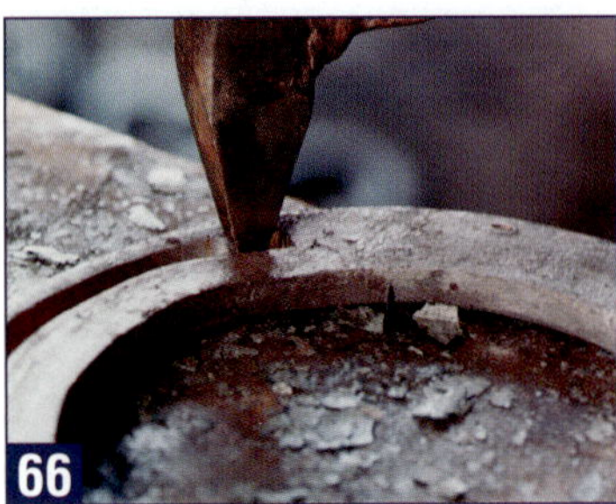

66 Drifting the nail holes.

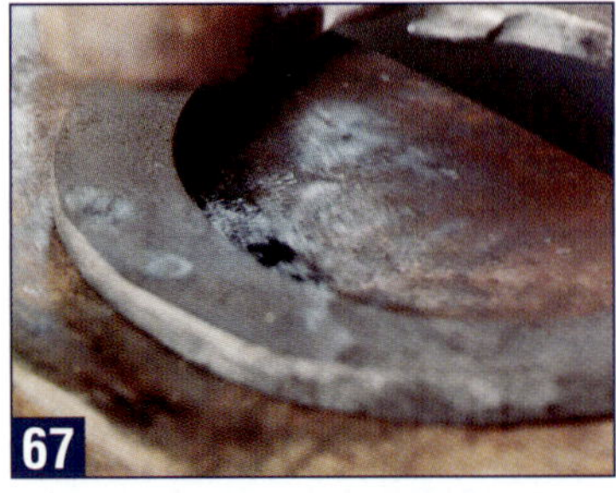

67 Hammer on the hoof surface across shiny spots where you drifted the nail holes.

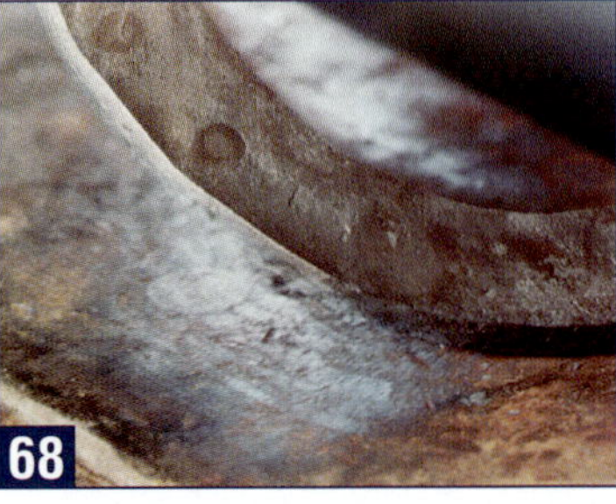

68 Hammer on the hoof surface across shiny spots where you drifted the nail holes.

heat to run the fuller (**Figures 57-58**).

Now you can drift the nail holes (**Figure 59**), hammer along the hoof surface (**Figure 60**), forge out any frog eyes, and pritchel (**Figure 61**).

You should have half the shoe built (**Figure 62**). Try to line up the scarf with the center of the toe.

HEAT 3

Repeat the steps from Heat 2 (**Figures 63-69**). You will notice that while I am fullering the second branch, I don't have the scarves over each other. Because of the way that the metal will bow when it is fullered, if you overlap the scarves you will have trouble keeping the shoe on the anvil as it warps. The shoe will be a little cold when I place the scarves together (**Figures 70-71**) Now you just brush and apply flux prior to returning the shoe to the fire.

HEAT 4

Weld the bar like you did when making the blank (**Figure 72**). This is a very fast heat, and you will be going back to the fire while the shoe is still quite hot. It is tempting to continue hammering the shoe

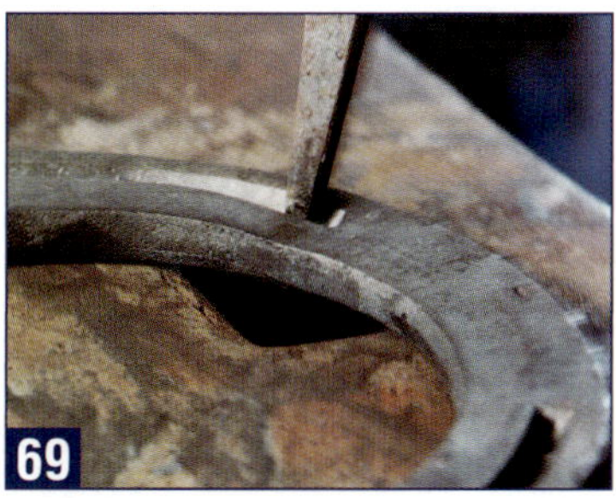

Pritchel.

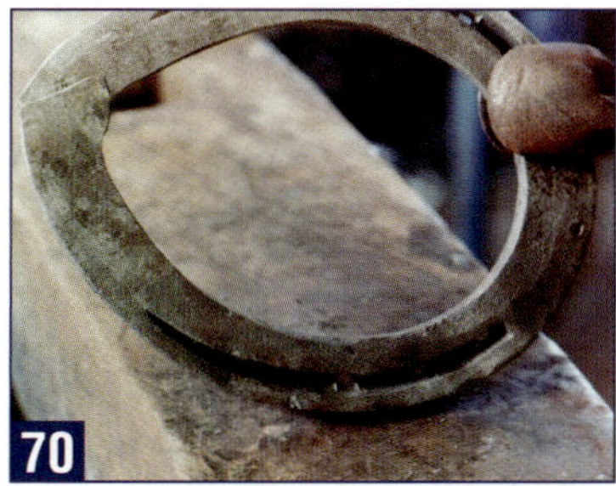

It should look like this after heat number 3.

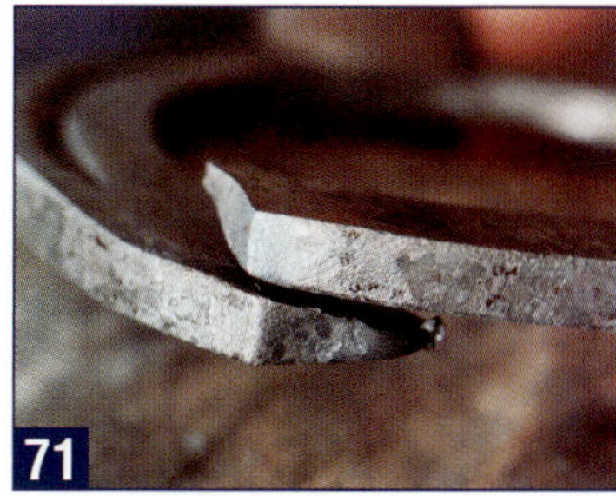

Be certain that the scarves cross each other far enough.

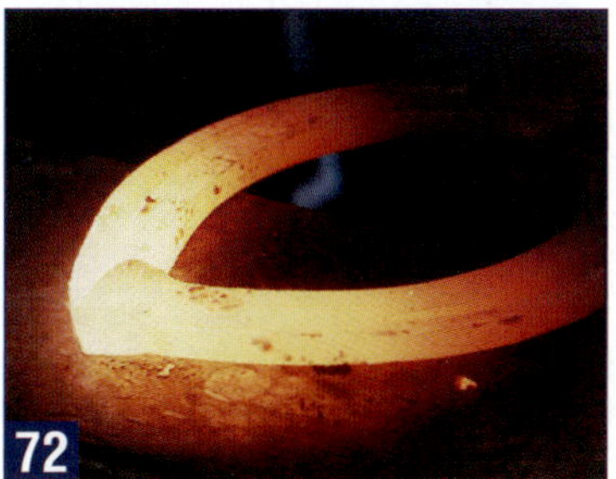

First welding heat.

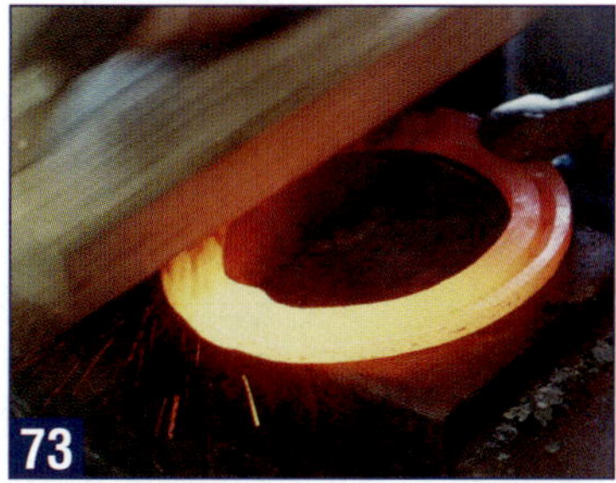

Brush before fluxing and going back for second welding heat.

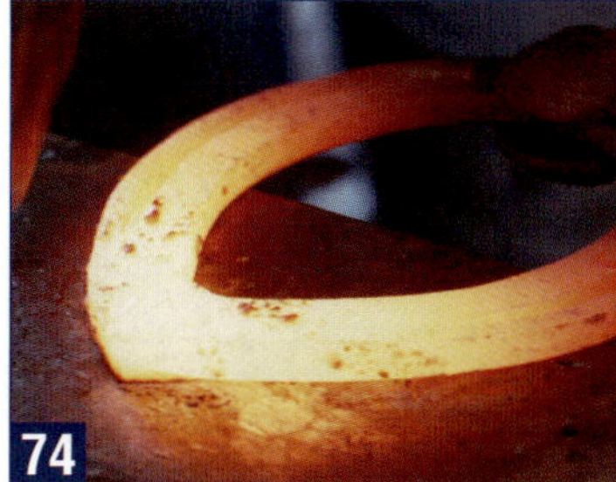

Second welding heat.

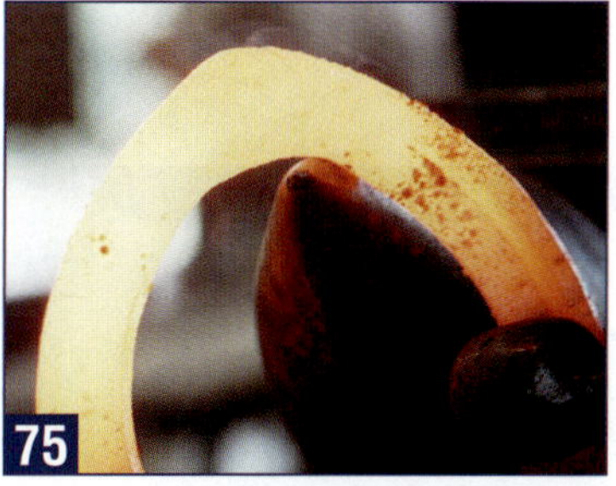

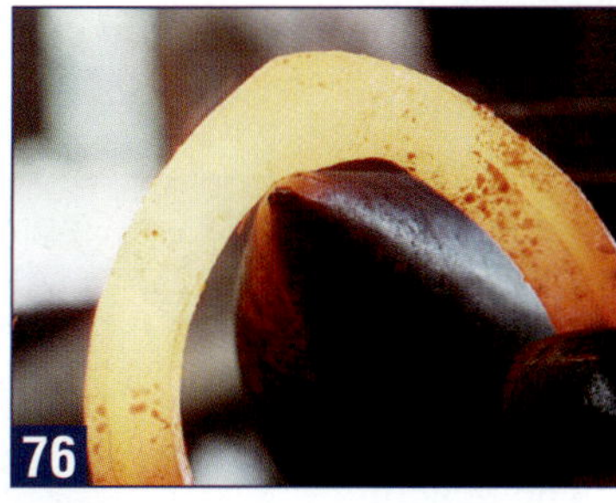

Forge on the horn to make the sex appeal.

77

Forge on the horn to make the sex appeal.

since it is at a forging heat. With experience you will find that you can finish this weld in one heat, but I would suggest that you exercise patience and take a fast first welding heat, brush, flux, and get back to the fire as soon as the seams of the weld have disappeared **(Figure 73)**.

HEAT 5

Forge the area of the weld back to the original thickness as you finish welding the bar. Move to the horn and create the sex appeal as you did with the blank **(Figures 74-77)**, Here are some better pictures of the additional move you can do to bevel the sex appeal on the top of the horn. Lay the welded area of the bar on the horn and hammer on the inside of the web **(Figures 78-80)**. This move will really clean up the bar if done correctly **(Figure 81)**.

The finished shoe should be attractive and nailable **(Figure 82)**. If you place the blank on top of the fullered shoe, you will once again find that there has been extra growth in the fullered shoe **(Figure 83)**. As a general rule, fullering will make an average shoe around 1/4inch longer on each branch, but your forging style will greatly influence that. The

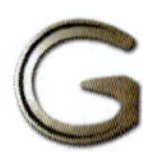

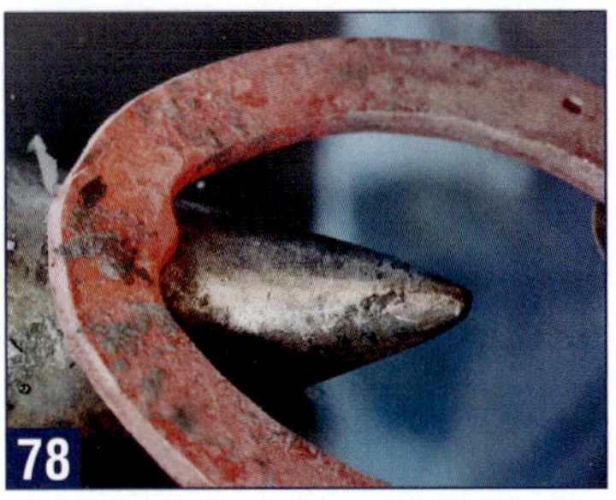

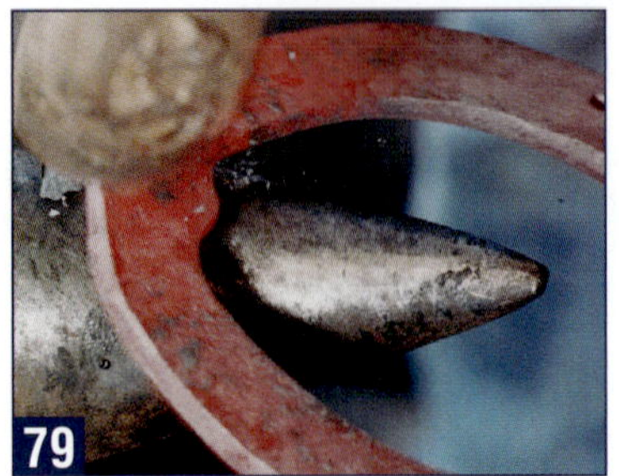

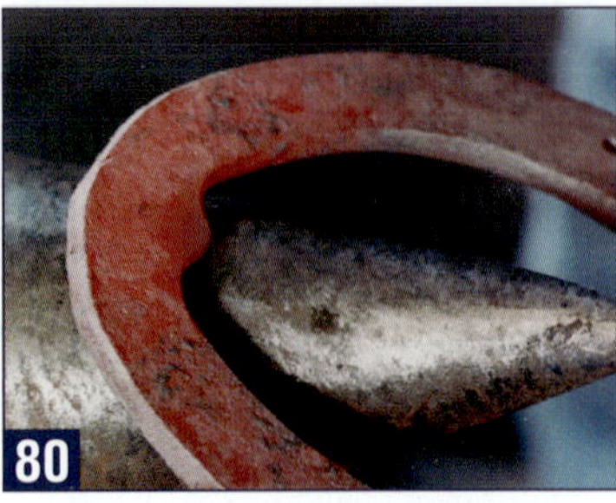

For this shoe, I am going to make the bevel on the inside of the sex appeal on the top of the horn.

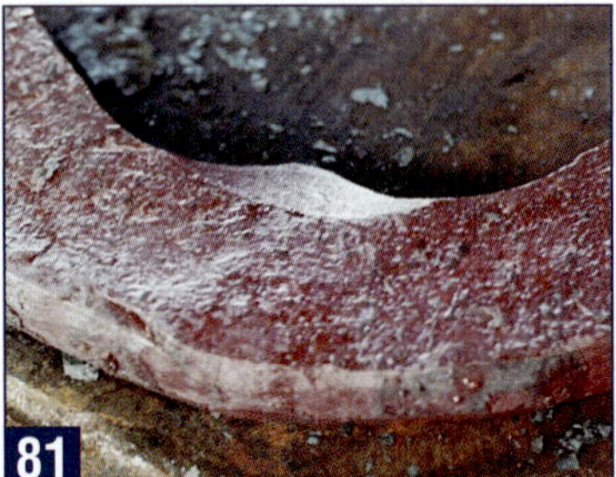

Detail of the bevel.

dimensions of the stock used will also have a lot to do with how much growth you get from fullering.

Since this shoe has an area that extends past the heels of the foot, people often punch the nail holes too far back. Our eyes are trained to compare distances and unless you make a lot of these shoes, you may naturally try to place the heel nail closer to the back of the shoe than is appropriate. Try balancing the shoe on the edge of the anvil so that you can see daylight through both heel nails. In **Figure 82**, all of the nails are past the edge of the anvil, and the shoe is not falling off. The general rule is that if the nail holes can extend past the edge of the anvil without the shoe falling off, you are not punched too far back. Of course making an extremely heavy bar could affect that rule.

The egg bar is an easy shoe to make, and in some farrier practices, it is used quite extensively. Once you have made a few of these, you will get a lot of enjoyment out of nailing them on feet. There is something about nailing on your own handmades that you just can't get from a keg shoe, and that seems to be doubled when you are nailing on a handmade that helps a horse.

Photos in this chapter were taken by Jonathan Brisbin.

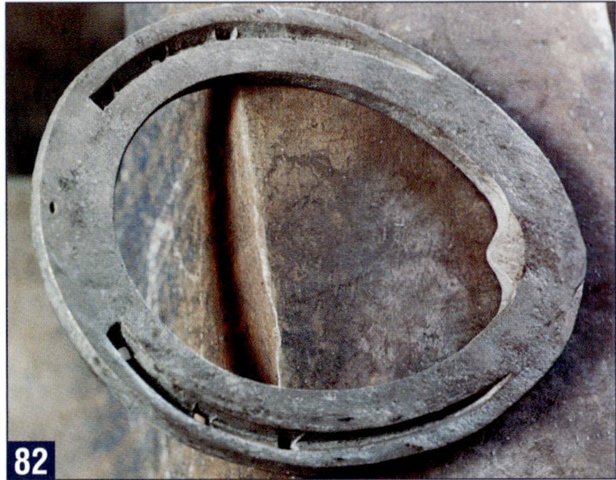

Finished shoe.

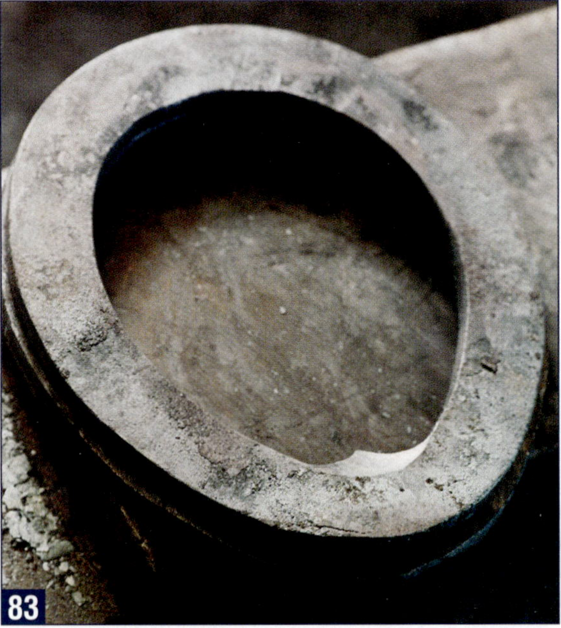

The blank sitting on top of the fullered shoe. You can see a size difference.

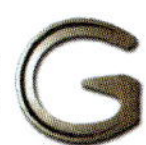

Chapter

50 HEART BAR, W-SHOE, AND G-BAR

These shoes are part of a group of very usable shoes. They are all designed to take weight off of the hoof wall and place it on the frog. By recruiting the frog as a weight-bearing structure, you are able to give a horse relief from pain that comes from bearing weight on the hoof wall. This principle of transferring weight is the advantage that this shoe offers as a weapon in your arsenal. One disadvantage shared by all three is that they trap a lot of stuff in the commissures if you do not use a pour-in pad material such as Equi-Pak. Beyond that, each one has its advantages and disadvantages. To begin this section, let's look at those individually.

W-Shoe (Figure 1): A modified heart bar, often called an open-toed heart bar, this is my favorite shoe for foundered horses. It can be easier to shape and fit, because if you come too long, it is only a matter of cutting some off the open ends. It does not offer the ground contact or the hoof stabilization that you can get from a heart bar, but it does eliminate any pressure from the toe of a foundered hoof that can be hurt worse with that pressure.

Heart Bar (Figure 2): Perhaps the most widely used of the three, the biggest advantage that it offers over the others is that it stabilizes the hoof like a bar shoe. The disadvantage is that it can be a little harder to shape and fit, but that is a skill level problem that can be fixed with practice.

G-Bar (Figure 3): This is also known as a half bar. The G-bar has an advantage in that it can be made without welding, and fitting is a matter of simply trimming off a little of the open heel. The disadvantage of this shoe is that it is difficult to shape, and it does not offer as much stability as the heart bar. It can also put pressure on the toe if you are using it on foundered horses. Surprisingly enough, I have only nailed on two of these shoes that I can remember.

MAKING THE W-SHOE

First let's make the W-shoe. For measurements, I would measure as you would for a square toe, only the heel of the foot will be where the square toe goes, and the typical heels of the shoe will go toward the toe of the foot. You will see what I mean here in a picture or two.

Begin by making a pretty normal, square-toed type of shoe (**Figures 4-6**). I don't punch the nail holes until after I weld, unless I am in a real hurry, such as in a contest. Next, I forge the frog plate. To do this, take a piece of stock that is the appropriate width for the base of the frog. Heat the end of the piece, and place it on the face of the anvil, hammering with a half-faced blow to forge a triangle **(Figures 7-8)**. Lay the end of the frog plate past the far edge of the anvil and forge a little grab **(Figure 9)** like the one on the

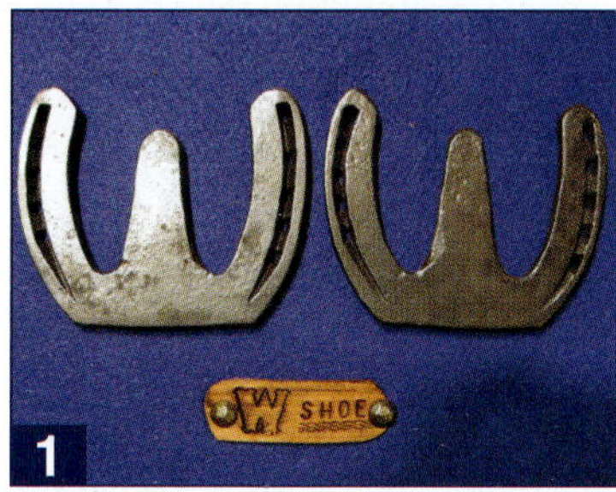

1

W-shoe on Cody's AWCF Shoe Display

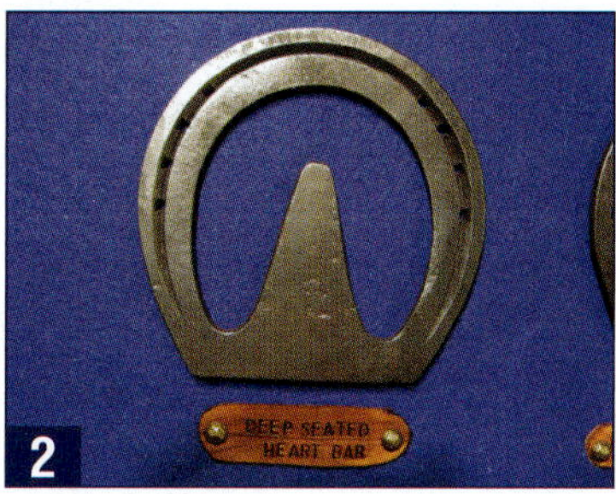

2

Heart bar on Cody's AWCF Shoe Display.

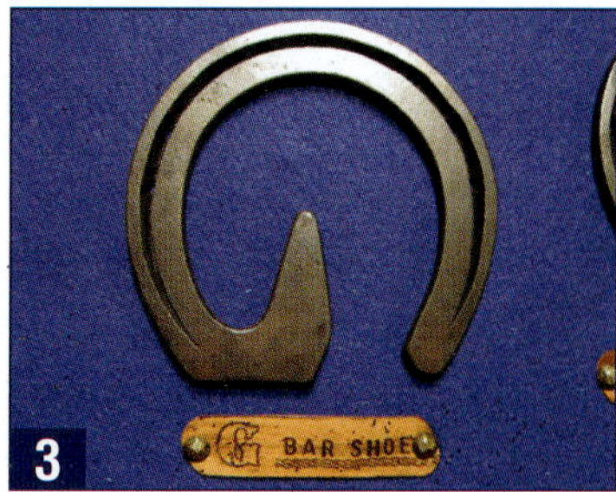

3

G-bar on Cody's AWCF Shoe Display.

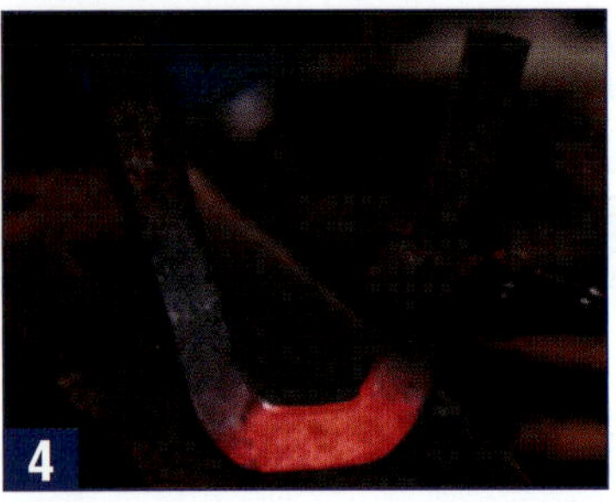

Bend in the bar to make a W-shoe

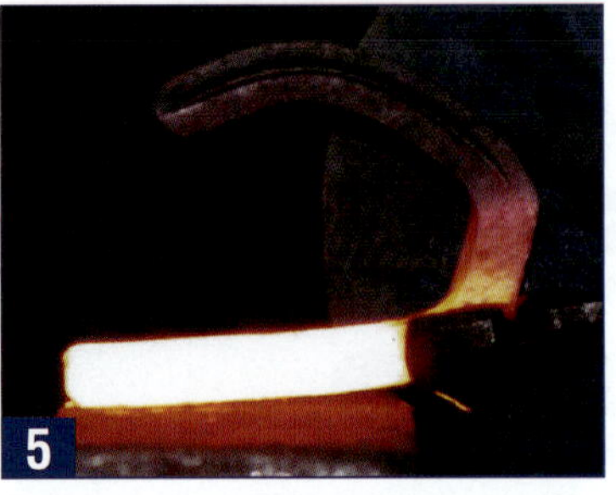

Making the ends of the toe like you would forge a heel.

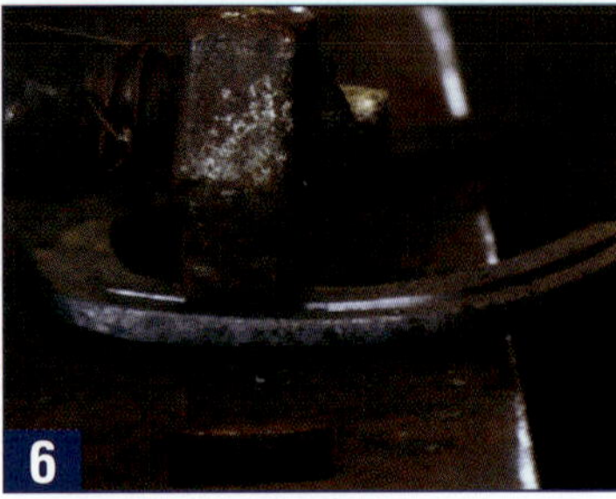

Fullering the shoe.

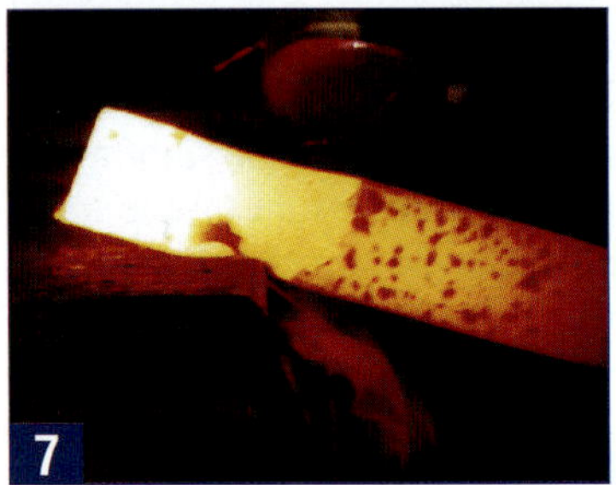

Forging the frog plate.

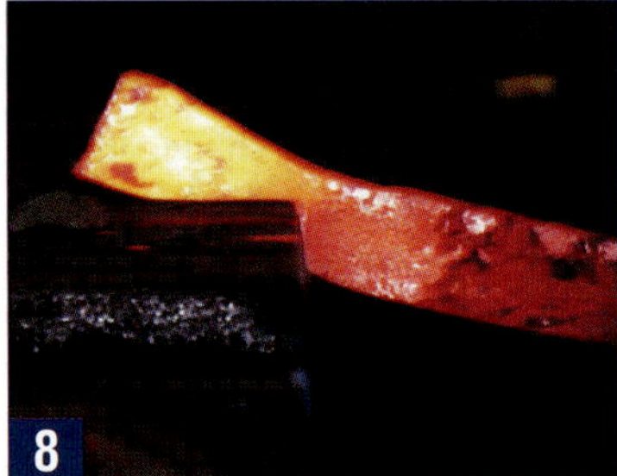

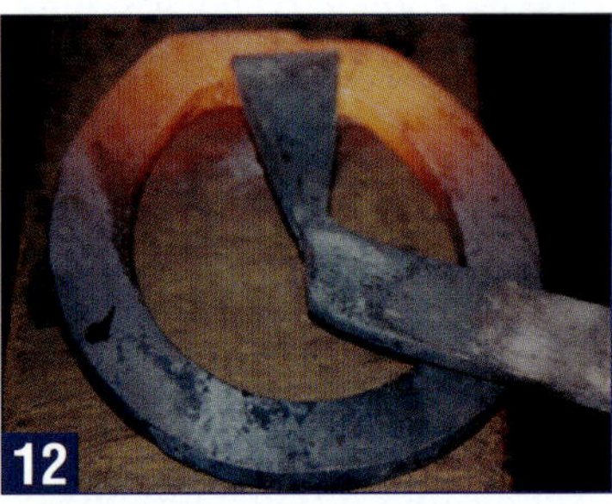

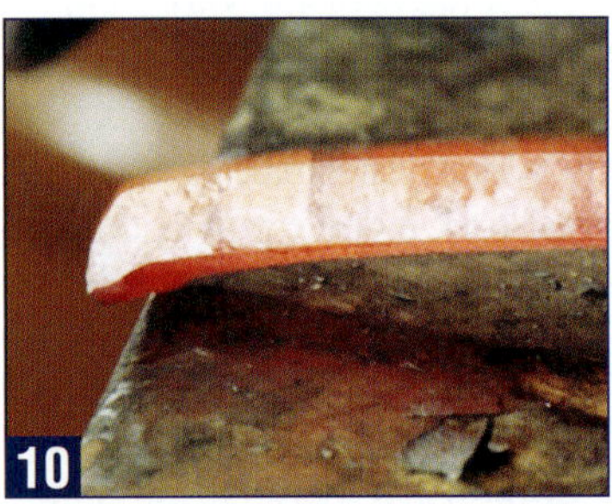

You can see the grab that was forged to catch when jump welding.

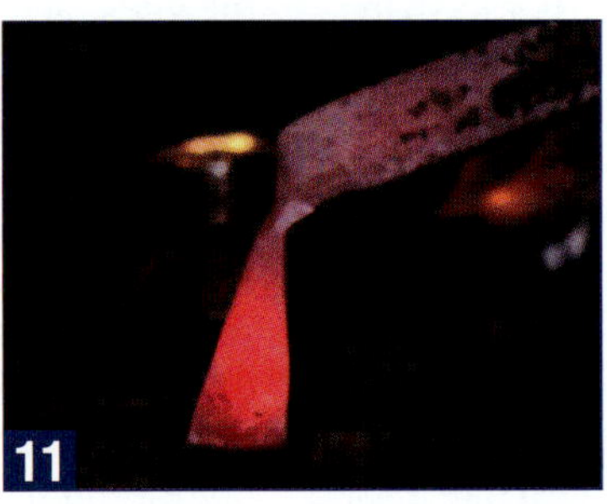

Bend the frog plate at an angle to the bar.

Choreograph the moves needed for jump welding the frog plate.

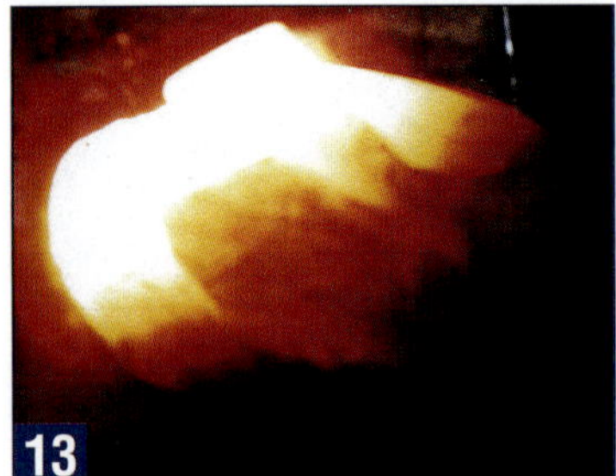

Place the pieces together at a welding heat.

piece in **Figure 10**. Bend the shouldered area so that it is easier to jump weld when you come out of the fire at a welding heat **(Figure 11)**.

The next step is to jump weld the frog plate to the shoe. You may want to choreograph the moves a couple of times before getting the pieces hot **(Figure 12)**. This is a good idea so that you have a plan when the steel is hot. Heat both pieces to the same welding temperature, come out of the fire with the shoe in your tong hands, place the shoe on the anvil, then place the plate on the shoe and weld it **(Figure 13-14)**. Take a second welding heat **(Figure**

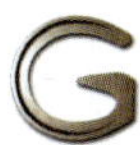

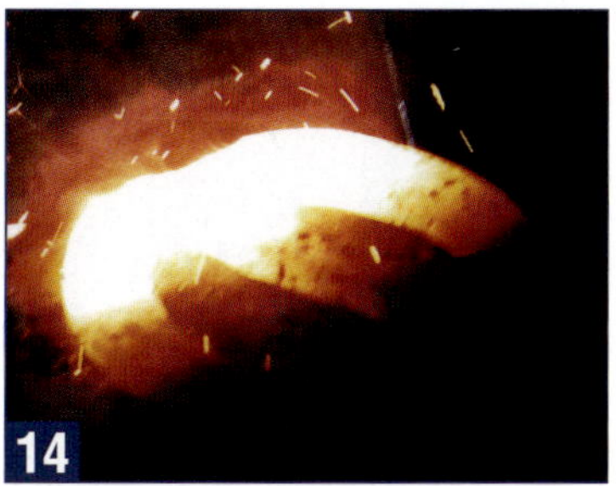
14
Hit lightly and fast.

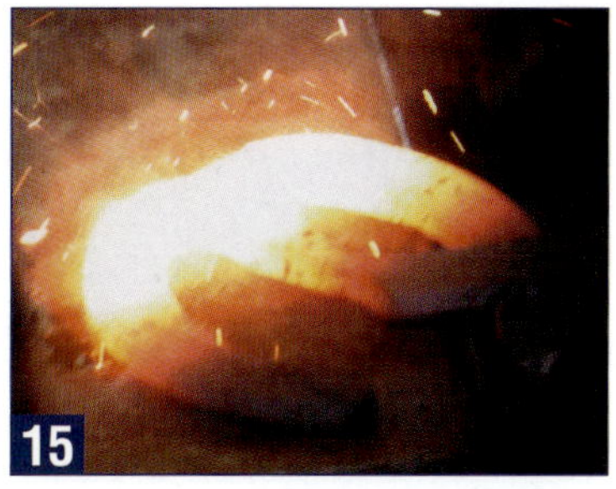
15
Continue to weld as long as there is a welding temperature.

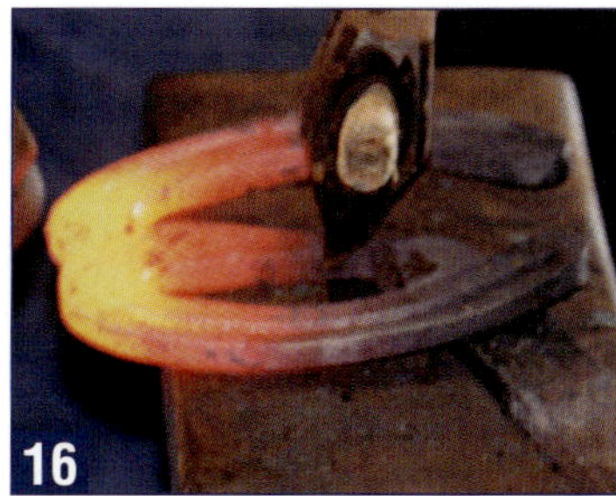
16
Cut off the bar.

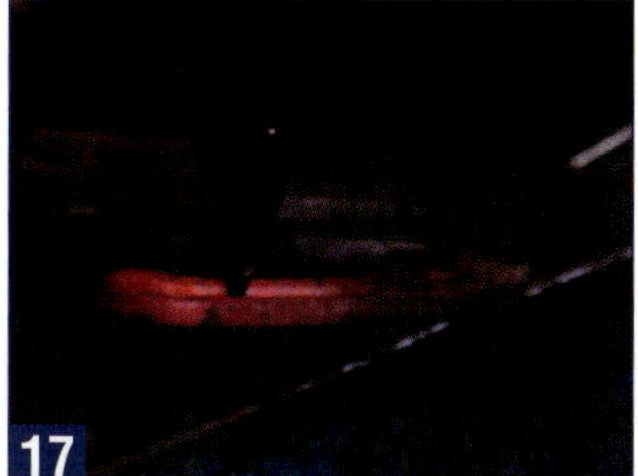
17
Finish the shoe.

18
Pritchel.

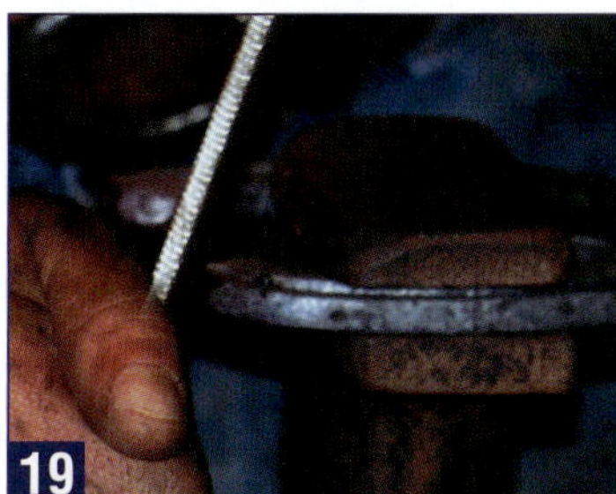
19
Rasp.

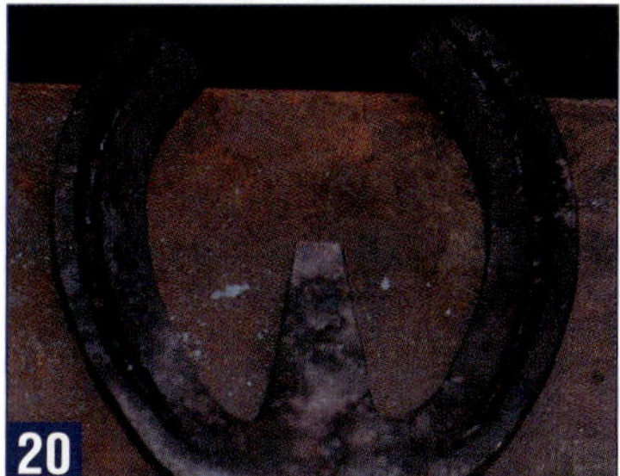
20
Finished shoe, ready to nail.

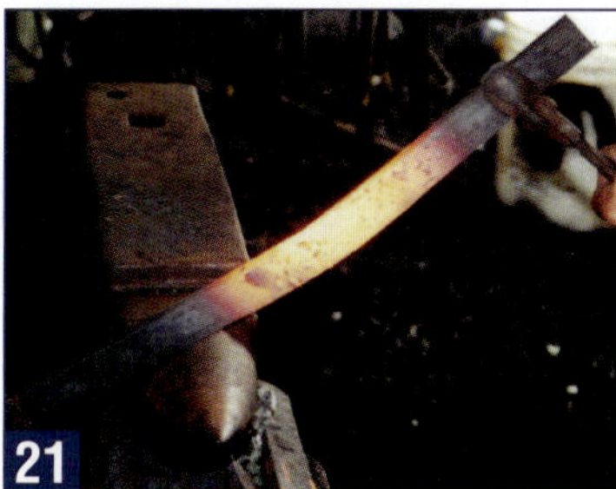
21
Toe bend for a draft bar shoe.

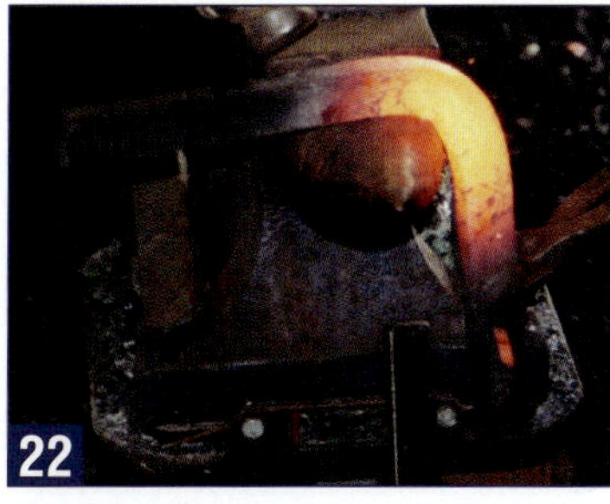
22
Setting the toe.

15) and cut off the long piece that is still attached to the frog plate **(Figure 16)**. Finish the shoe by drifting **(Figure 17)**, pritchelling **(Figure 18)** and rasping **(Figure 19)**. The finished shoe is shown in **Figure 20**.

MAKING THE HEART BAR

Making a heart bar is a very similar process with the exception that we are welding into the bar. For this demo, I am making a heart bar for a draft horse hind foot. Begin by making the straight bar **(Figure 21-24)**. I like to weld my frog plate on right after the first weld of the bar, so put the bar shoe aside for now and make the frog plate.

Since this one has to be so big, I am going to upset the end of the bar to get the thickness that I need. **Figures 25 and 26** show the piece being upset on the end. I am using the horn to get an even larger spread in **Figure 26**. It is good to have a strong wife when building draft bar shoes, so here I am having Kelly strike for me to make the shoulder for the frog plate **(Figures 27-29)**. It is the exact same process that we did on the W-shoe frog plate, just bigger.

Bring the shoe and the frog plate to a welding

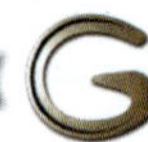

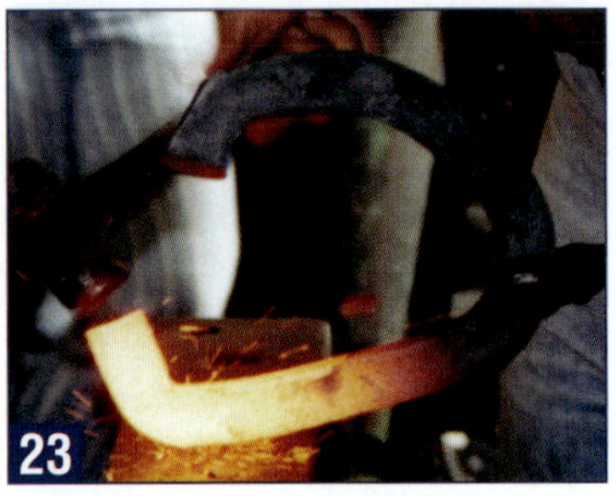
Making a hockey stick.

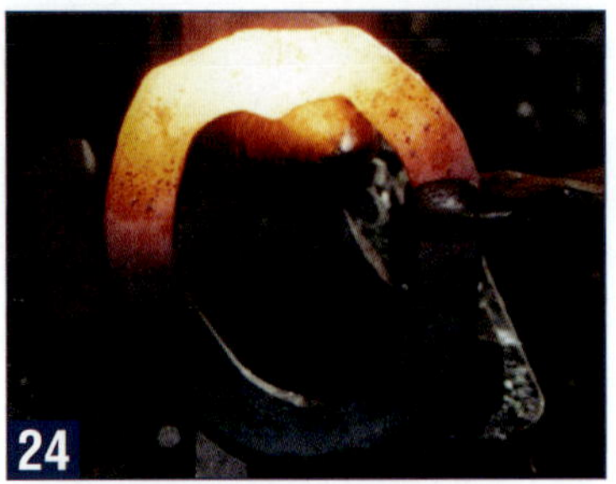
Cleaning up the weld.

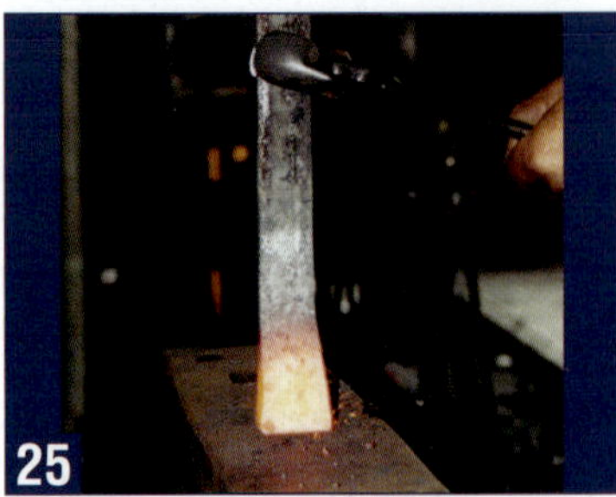
Upsetting the end of the stock to make a wider frog plate.

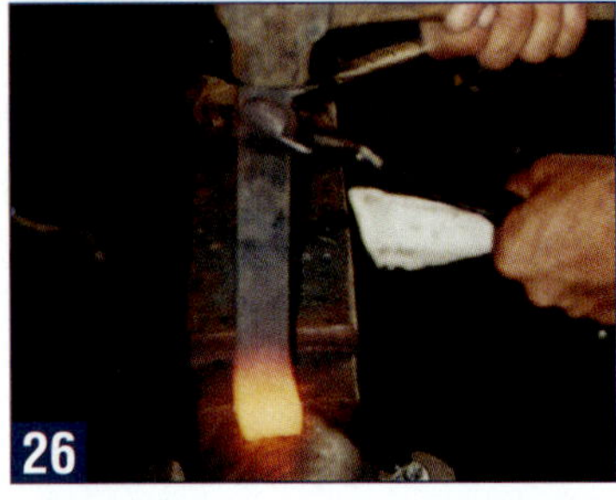
Using the horn to spread the end of the stock even more.

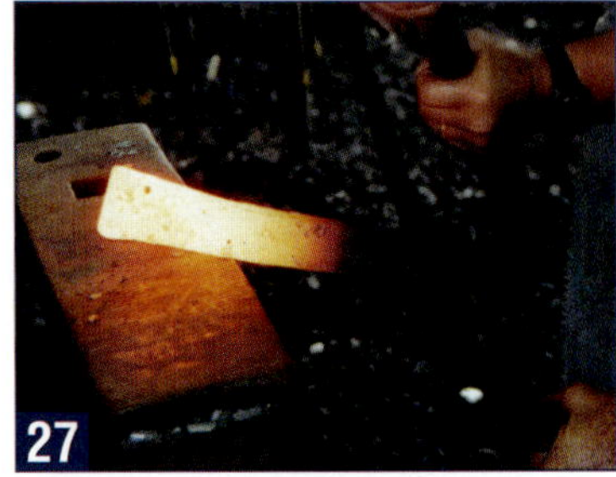
Making the frog plate.

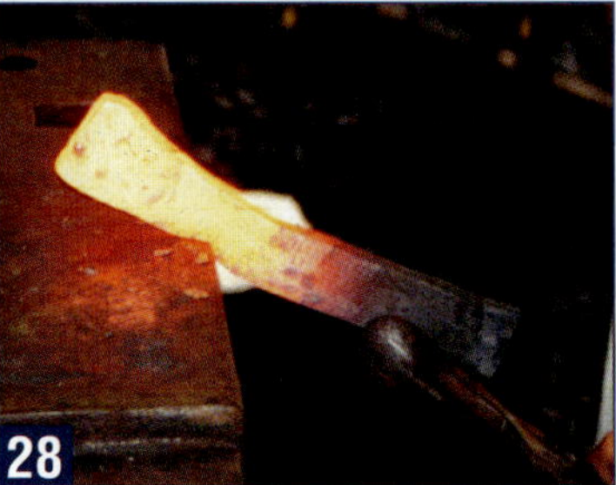
Kelly striking for me to make the frog plate.

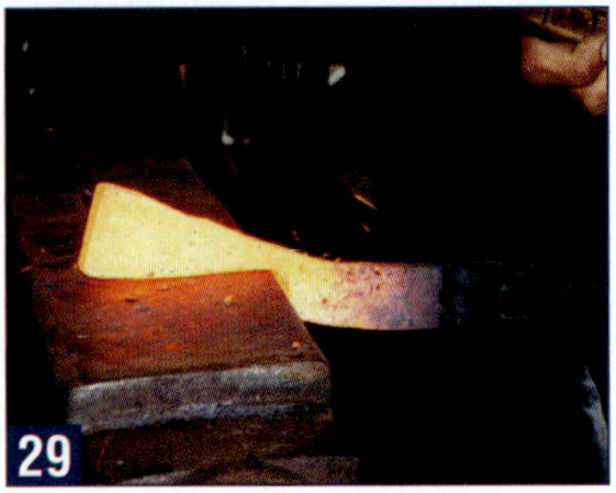
Finishing the frog plate.

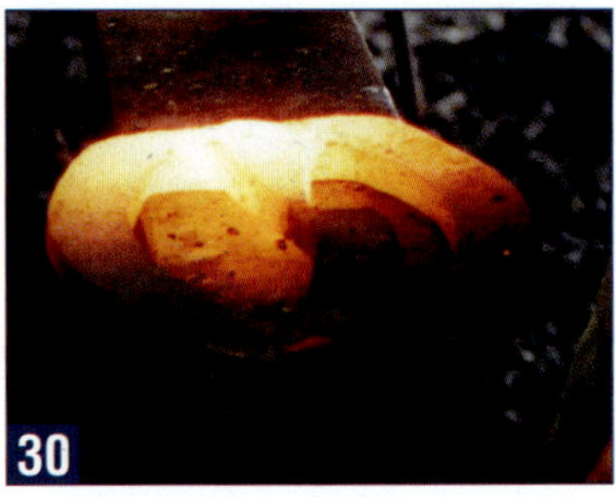
Finishing the weld.

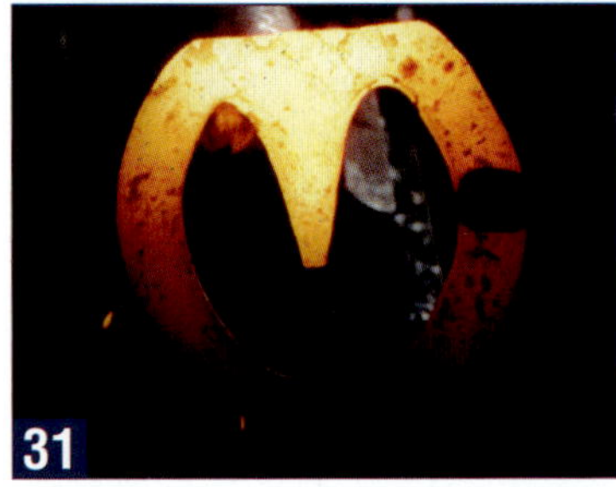
Cleaning up the bar on the horn.

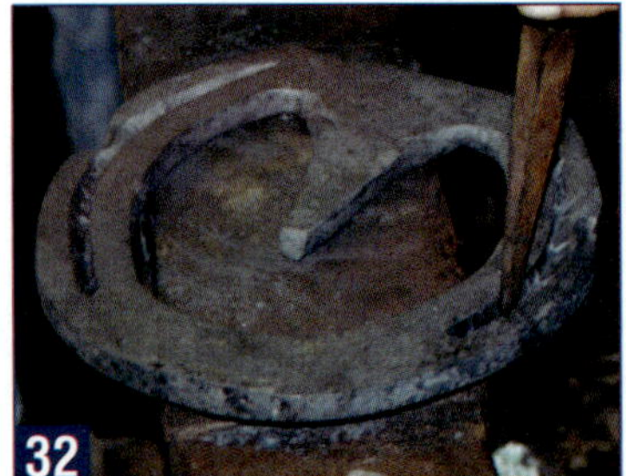
Pritchelling the shoe.

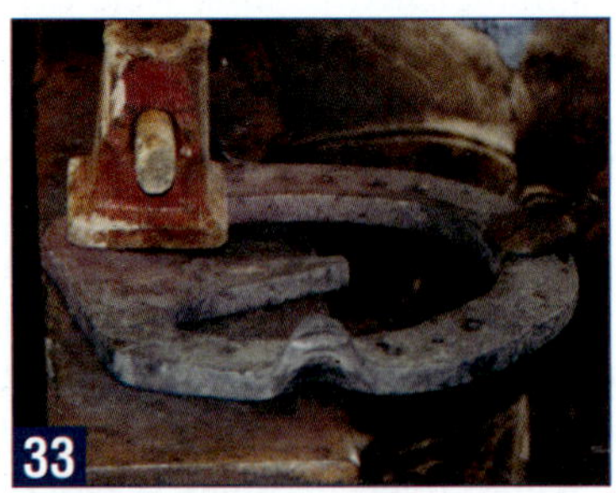
Using a fatter to finish.

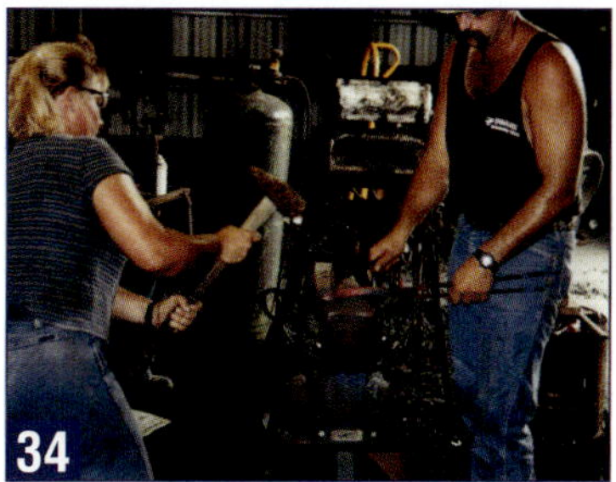
Make sure your striker puts their back into it.

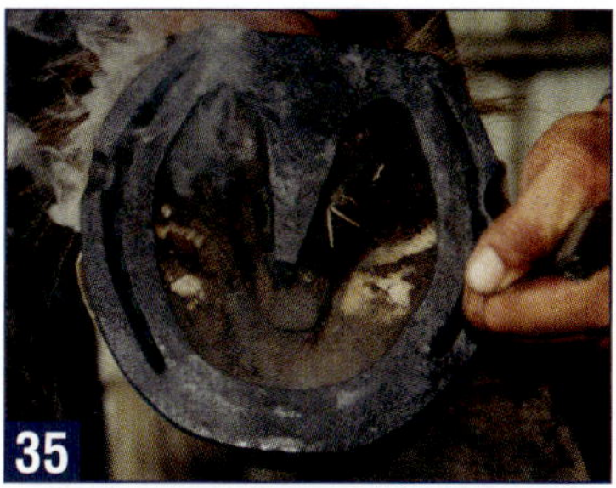
Hot fit any shoe with frog coverage at a colder heat and don't burn long.

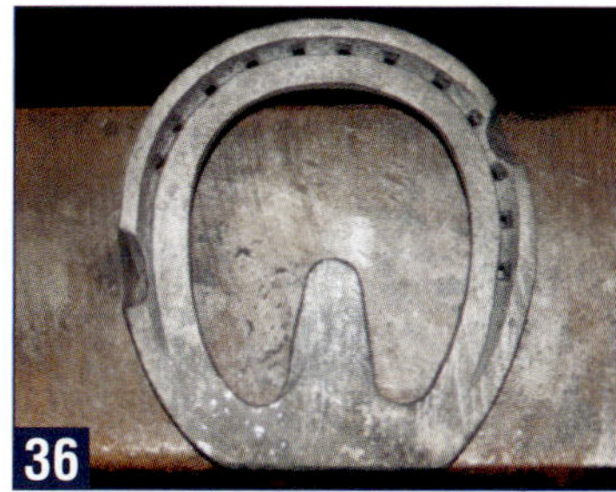
Heart bar shoe with a lot of nailing opportunities.

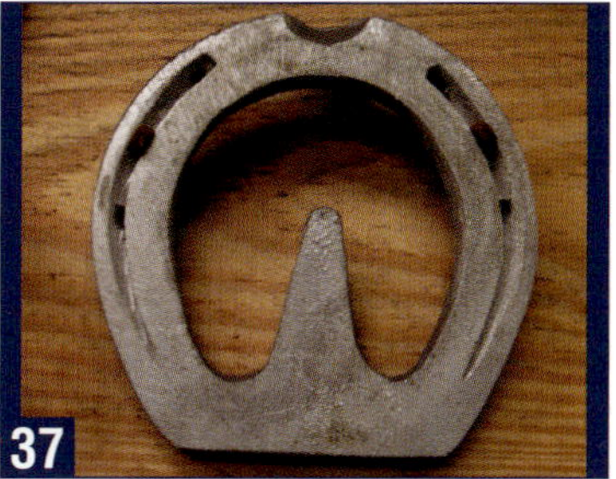
Aluminum heart bar shoe.

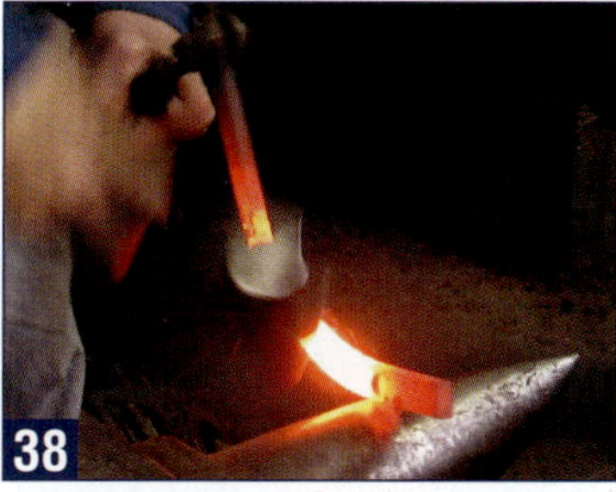
Making a bend in the stock.

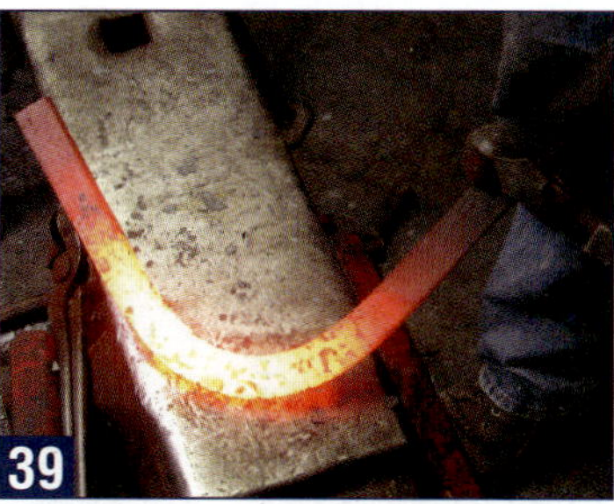
Toe bend that is not committed to.

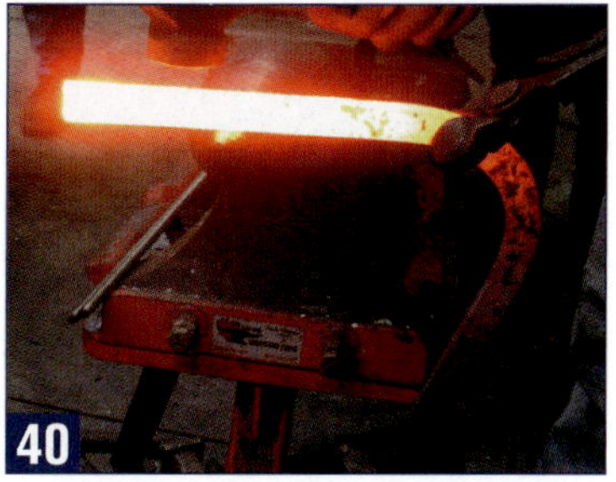
Starting a large hockey stick.

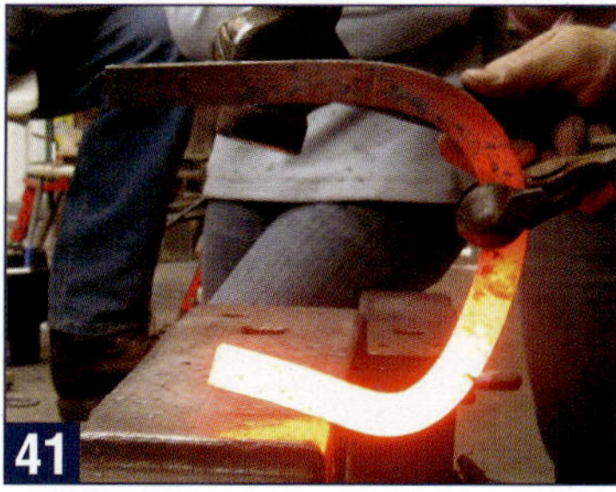
Making the S curve.

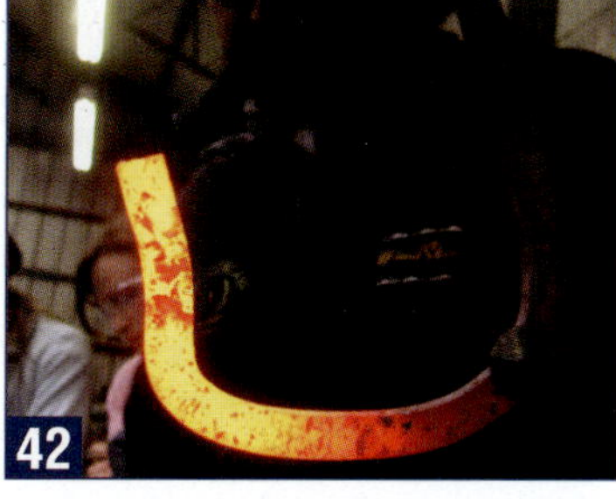
Close up of the S curve in the hockey stick for the frog plate.

heat and weld the plate into the bar. **Figure 30** is the final weld. Crisp and shape everything on the tip of the horn **(Figure 31)** and finish the shoe **(Figure 32)**. In **Figures 33-34**, I am using a flatter on the shoe while Kelly strikes. Hot fit the shoe at a cool heat **(Figure 35)** and nail it on.

Figure 36 is a heart bar with fullering and nails all around the shoe to allow nailing it on a badly damaged foot, and **Figure 37** is heart bar made from aluminum to give a lot of coverage without the added weight of steel.

MAKING THE G-BAR

To make a G-bar shoe, begin by making a general bend off center in the stock **(Figures 38-39)**. This is going to be close to your regular toe bend, but not something that you want to become committed to at this time. Heat the long end of the stock and make a large hockey stick. You will be bending over about twice what you would for a normal hockey stick **(Figure 40)**. Put an S-curve in the material to make it stick in the corner **(Figure 41)**. You can see this move on this shoe **(Figure 42)** and read more about it in the section on lateral extensions where I talk

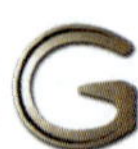

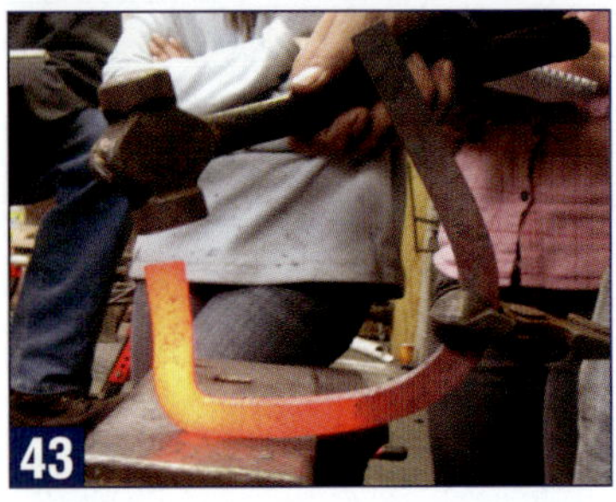

Starting to upset the hockey stick.

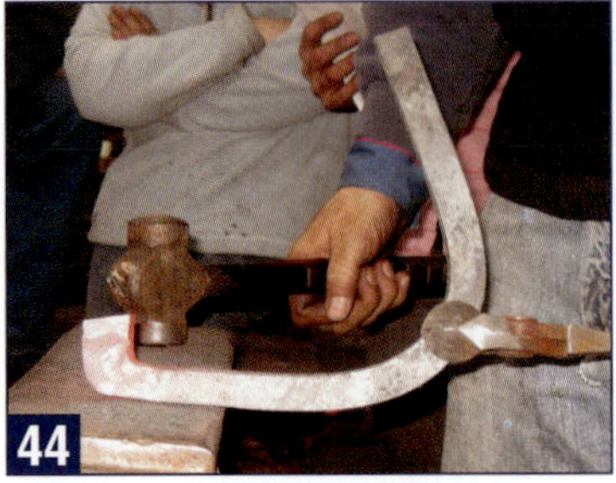

Finishing the hockey stick.

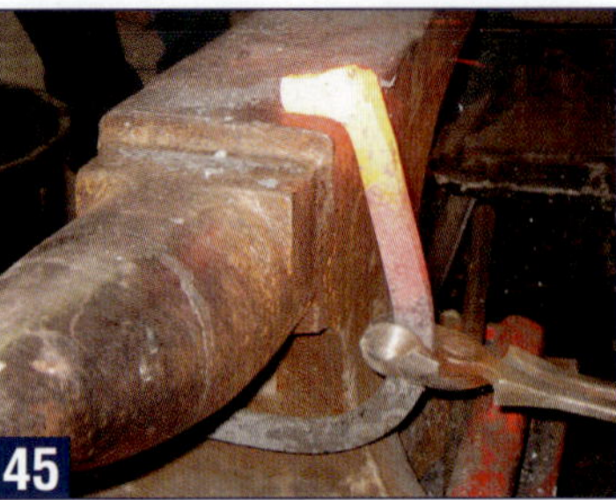

Forging the hockey stick into a frog plate.

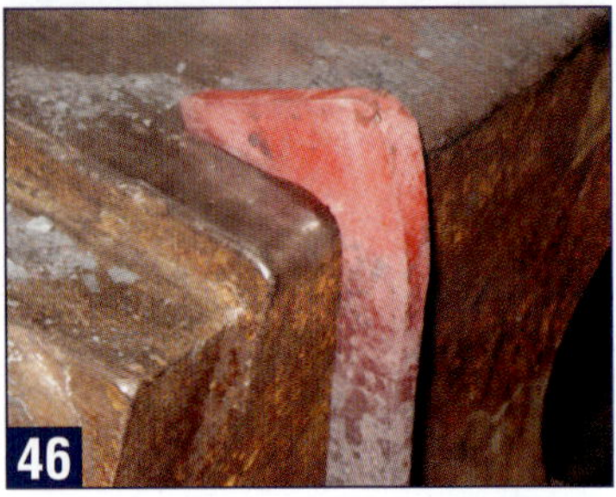

Sharpen the end of the plate to match the frog you are fitting.

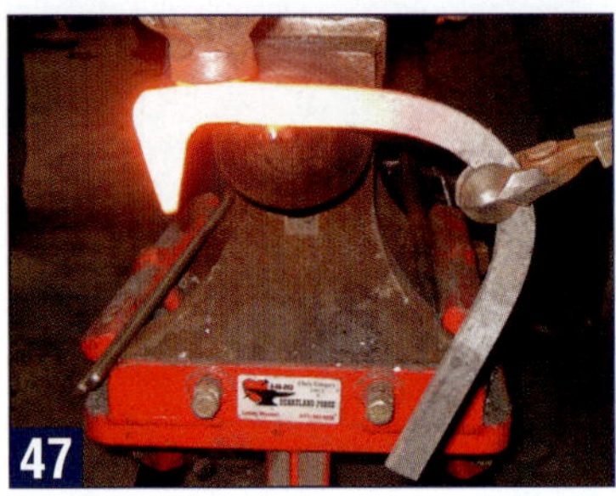

Bend over a lot of steel for the back of the bar.

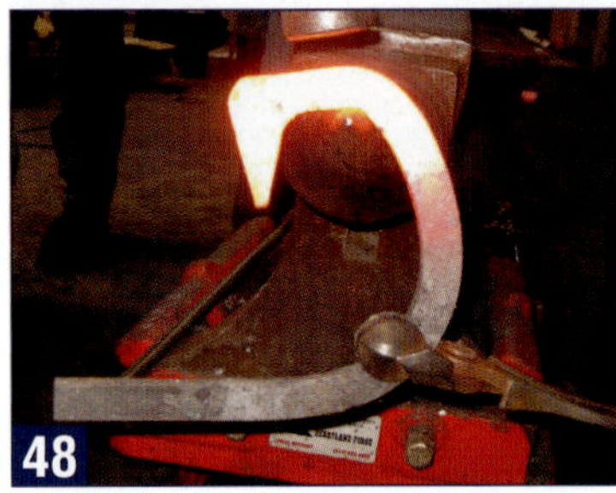

Bend the piece on the tip of the horn by dropping your tong hand.

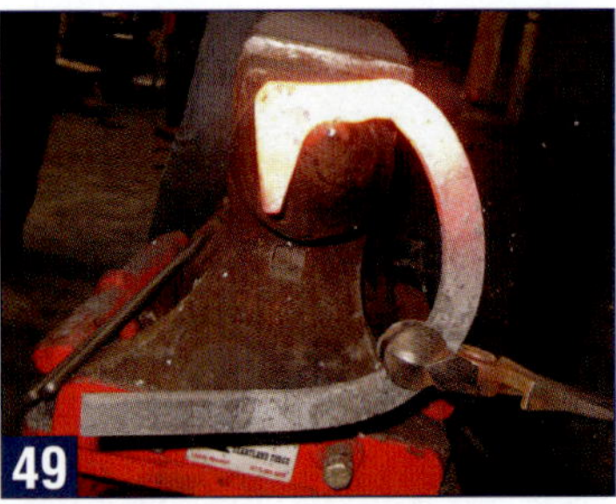

Make a small bend in the piece that will become the bar.

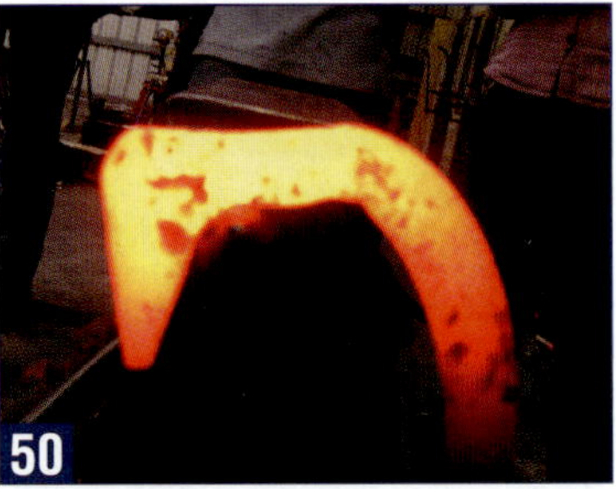

Detail of that bend.

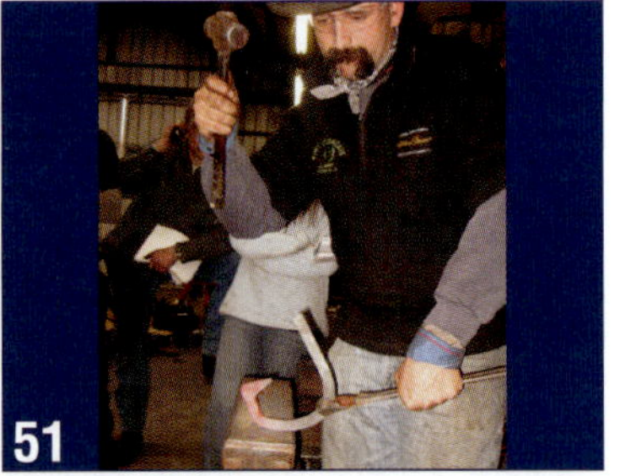

Position of the tongs, shoe, hammer, and body to make the back of the bar crisp.

about whip across bar shoes. Forge the hockey stick until it is a large rectangular shape **(Figures 43-44)**.

Sharpen the upset hockey stick into a frog plate **(Figures 45-46)**. This next move is one that took quite some time to figure out, but here is the secret for getting a nice corner on the outside heel of the bar that has the frog plate on it. Typically, when you try and make a good hockey stick on the piece with the frog plate, it will bend over on itself, and the back of the bar gets round.

Start by bending over a bit more than you would think you need for a good hockey stick **(Figures 47-48)**. Now you are going to forge a small bow in the material toward the inside of the shoe **(Figures 49-50)**. Hold the shoe in your tong hand so that your hammer handle is at 90 degrees to the plane of the shoe. Position the shoe carefully to place the branch as flat on the face of the anvil as possible. Turn your hammer in your hand so that the face is turned approximately 45 degrees to the face of the anvil and come down hard with a straight hammer swing. You are hammering straight, but the hammer is hitting at an angle from being turned in your hand. Study **Figures 51-53** to see how this works.

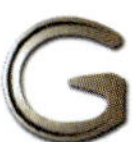

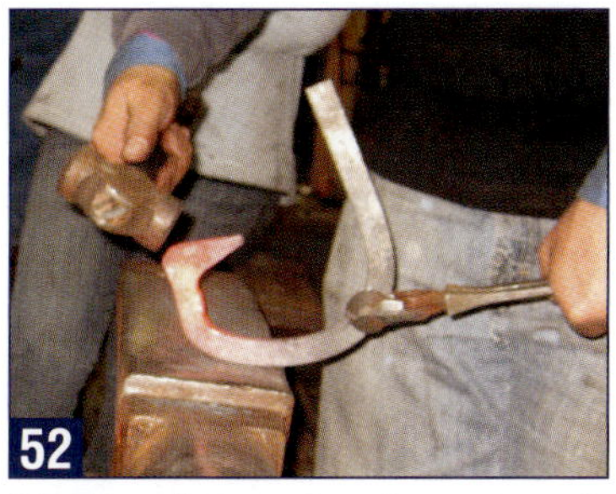

Notice how the hammer is swung straight, but the face hits at an angle.

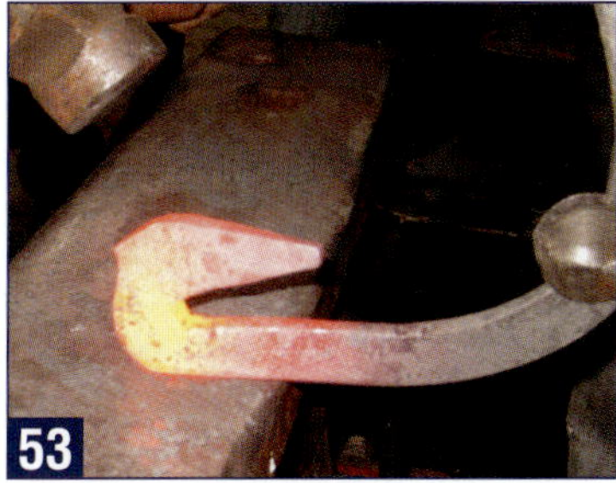

Forge to make the bar.

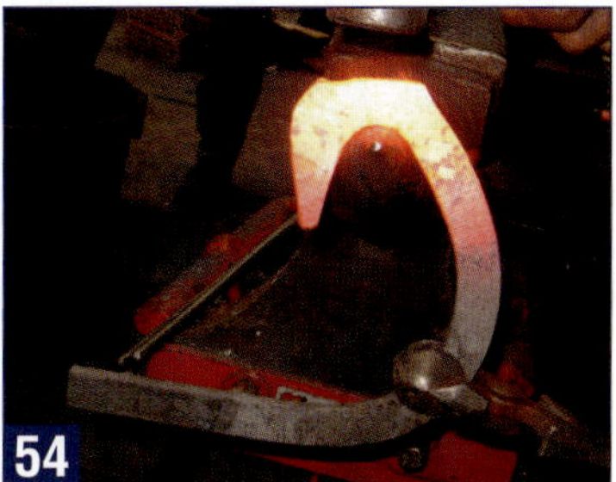

Shape the bar on the horn.

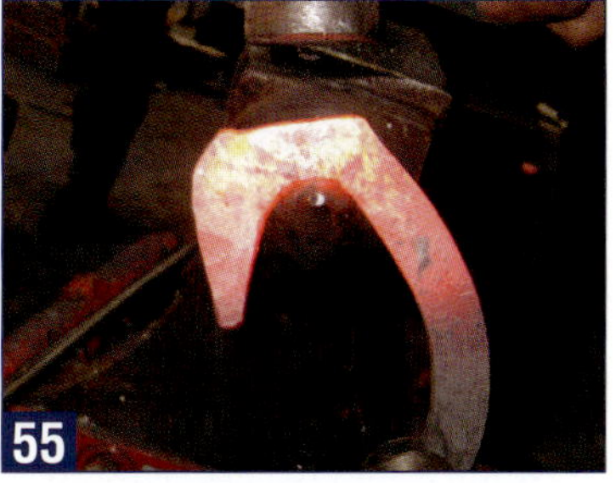

Shape the bar on the horn.

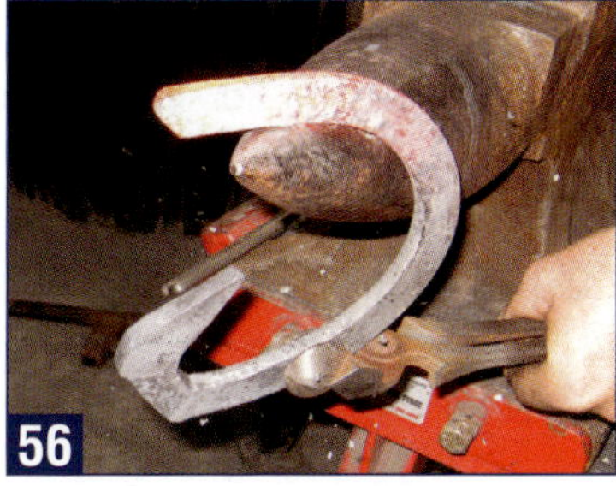

Bend the other branch.

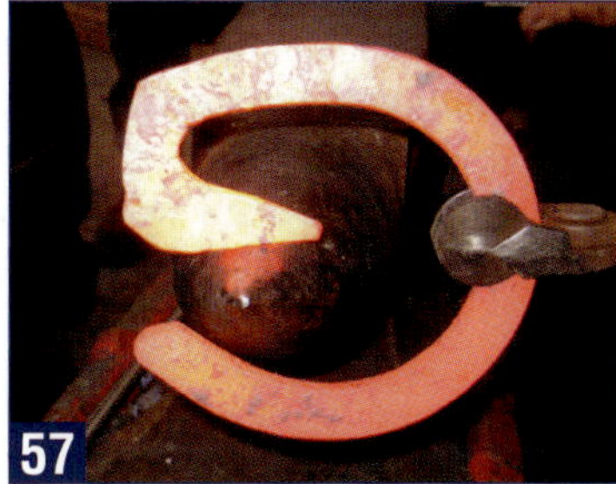

Shape the shoe.

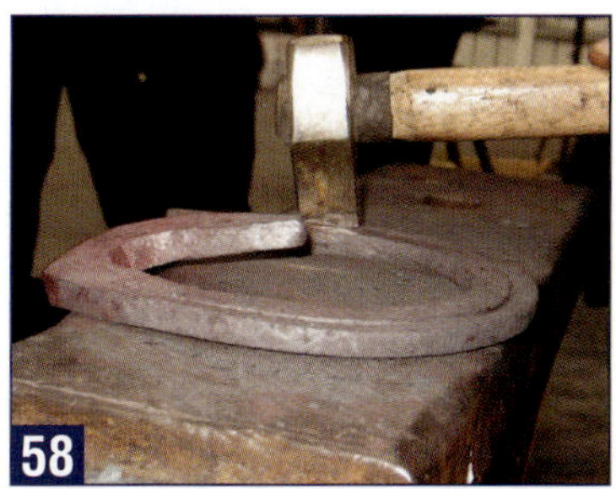

Fuller the shoe. Notice that I have bent the frog plate up so that it is not causing problems with the level of the shoe while I fuller.

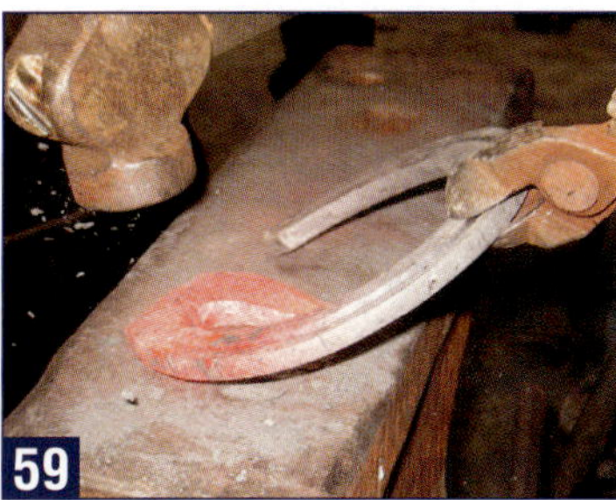

Hammer on the frog plate while you lift the shoe.

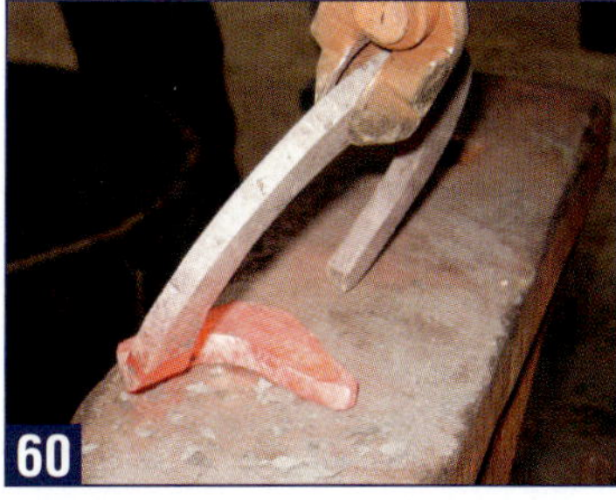

Lift until the frog plate is bent out far enough to forge on.

You will have to play with this till you feel the steel upset. It will feel like building a hockey stick when the steel "sticks" to the face of the anvil. It feels, sounds, and looks solid.

Upset so that you have enough mass to make a good outside corner and maintain the width of your bar. Move to the tip of the horn and position the shoe like you would if you were building a normal hockey stick. Hammer into the piece to form a nice heel **(Figures 54-55)**. This is an outstanding move to use if you are making a one-piece heart bar as well.

Build the rest of the shoe, forging, fullering, drifting, pritchelling, and shaping **(Figure 56-58)**. There is one more move that I want to include on this shoe to allow forging on the frog plate. This move can be used on heart bars that are welded solidly as well. Heat the heel of the shoe, place it on the anvil and hammer on the frog plate while you lift on the shoe **(Figures 59-60)**. The frog plate is now bent out from the shoe, and you can forge

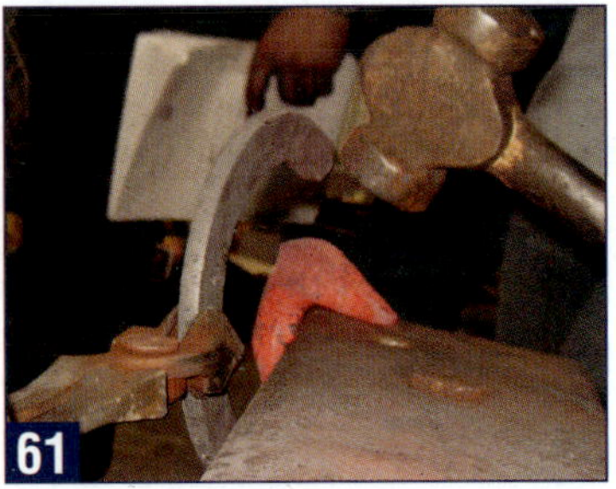

Shape the frog plate on the anvil.

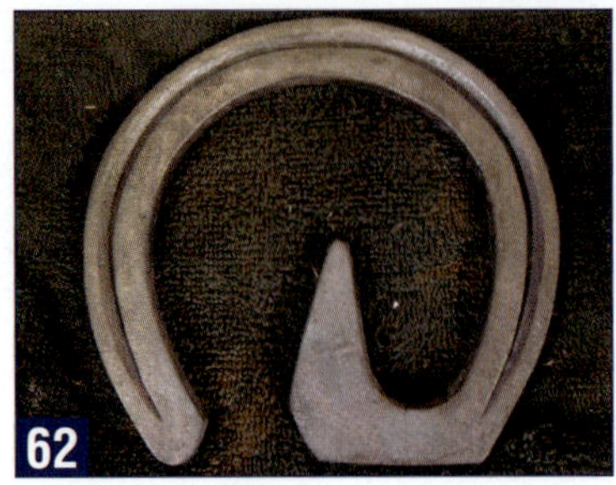

Shoe in the demo without the nails punched.

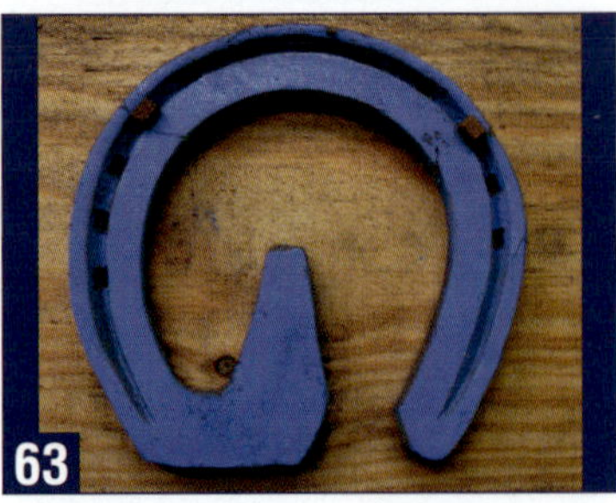

Another G-bar with the bar coming from the opposite side of the shoe.

on it as I am doing in **Figure 61**. **Figure 62** is the shoe without the nails punched. You can see another G-bar built with the frog plate attached to the opposite heel in **Figure 63**.

Now you have a few ways of building a nice frog-support shoe. You will find one that you like better than the other, and you will also find that each has a place. Make a few of these before you get to the horse, and you can look like a hero in front of the customer or vet or both. The horse will think you are a hero for sure.

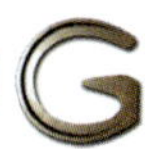

Chapter

51 PATTEN BAR

Here is one of my favorite weapons in the battle against lame horses. This shoe is not well understood and is not used nearly as much as it could be. The patten bar has a few disadvantages that have hampered its popularity, but they pale in contrast to the advantages.

First among the disadvantages is the difficulty in making one. Like other difficult shoes, it will become easy when you get good at making them. (I know, that sounds so easy.) So that disadvantage is taken care of. The next disadvantage is the fact that the shoe is thought of by most farriers and vets alike for the angle change instead of the real purpose — creating a rest period for the injured limb. The angle change is part of what a patten bar does, but the main function is rest. Finally, it is not a shoe that you can use on a horse that is to be turned out or used. With several bar shoes, the horse can be stabled however the owner wants. They can also be ridden in many situations. However, if a horse is injured badly enough that it needs a patten bar, it should not be ridden anyway, and the stall rest will be good for the horse as well.

To measure for this shoe, determine how much steel you would need to cover the foot alone. In this case, let's assume that a normal, fullered handmade would need to be 12 inches. Next, determine how much lift you are going to need for that foot. As a jumping- off place, for me, it takes six inches of additional steel to make a 1-inch lift on an average foot. The bar should be as wide as the widest part of the foot, so if your foot is abnormally wide, you may need more than the 6 inches. If we needed 12 inches for the shoe and six inches for the bar, we are looking at 18 inches to make a patten bar with a 1-inch lift for this foot. For more lift, double the amount of additional lift you want, and add that to the stock. 1 1/2 inches of lift would then require seven inches of steel.

THE SHOE

Begin by marking the center of the toe and the start of the fullering, as well as the area where the bar begins. For this shoe, that mark would be at about three inches from the end of the stock. There are six inches in the bar, so three inches on each side. Get a heat in the middle of the stock, and if you are in a gas forge, you may want to quench the ends to isolate the heat in the center. It was important to choke up on a normal bar shoe, and it is even more important to choke up on a shoe that is this long **(Figure 1)**. If you don't, you will find that it is hard to control where the toe bend is going to end up. Seat out the toe, hem the area to be fullered, set the toe, and mark the fullering **(Figure 2)**.

On the next heat, you are going to start making the bends for half the bar. Heat one end of the shoe and place the amount you want to bend on the face of the anvil. Hammer close to the edge of the anvil and lower your tong hand as you hammer into that corner **(Figures 3-4)**. As you bend this piece away from the toe, the branch will bow the opposite way. You will want to take care of that now, as you would on a normal shoe, to counteract inertia. Put the piece

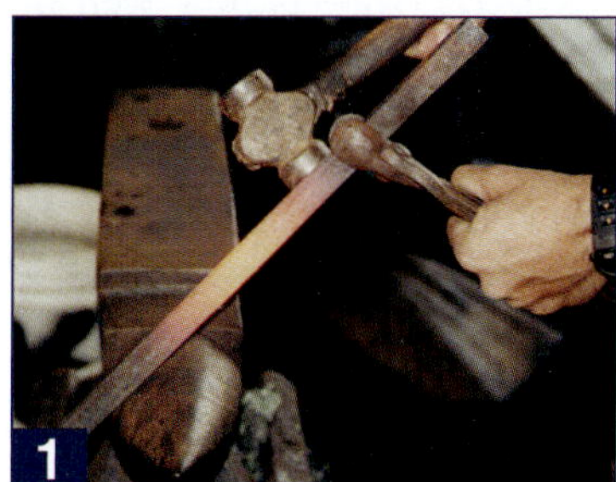

1

Toe bend. Notice tong position and the amount of steel past the horn.

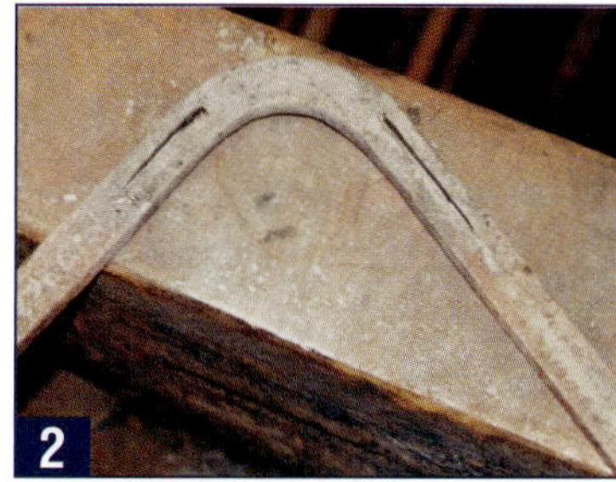

2

The fullering is marked and the toe bend is done.

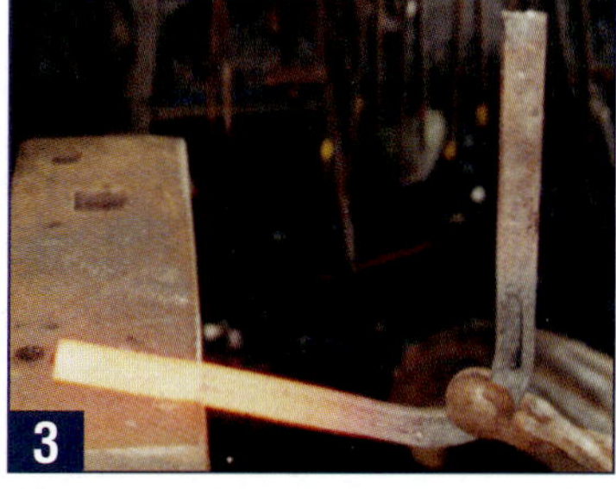

3

First bend to make one half of the bar.

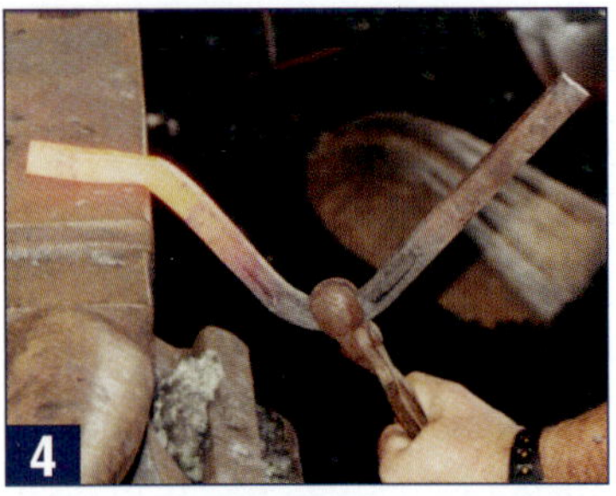

Continue the bend by dropping your tong hand.

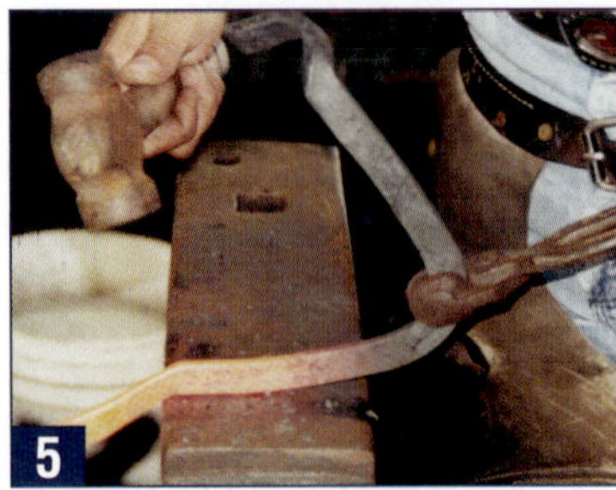

Taking care of inertia.

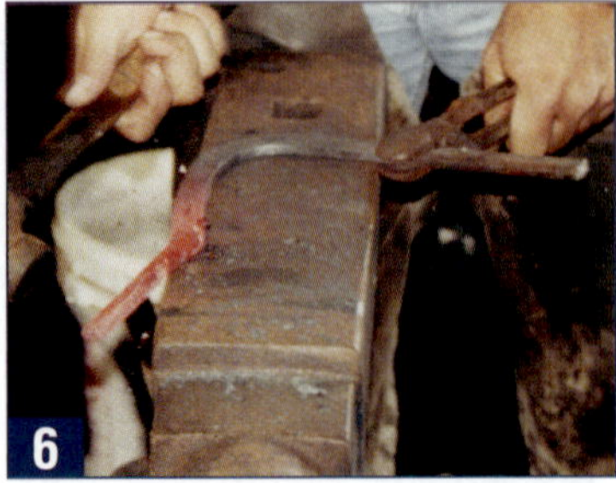

Position to bend the piece for the bar down the side of the anvil.

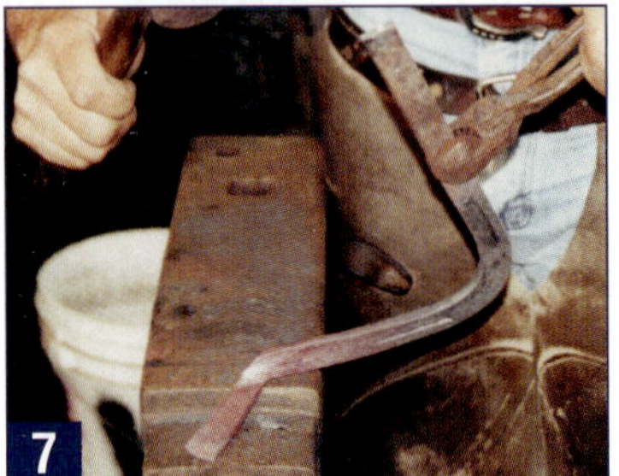

Start the bends in the bar on the step of the anvil.

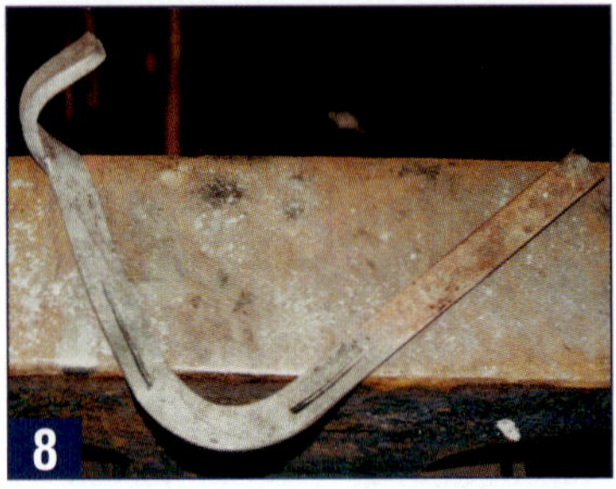

You should have a piece that looks like this after the second heat.

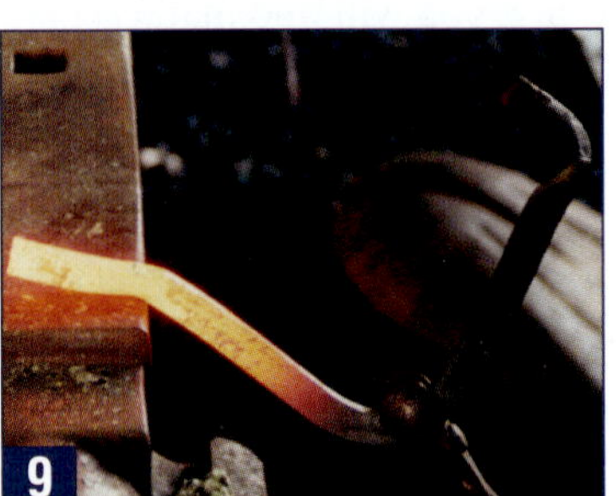

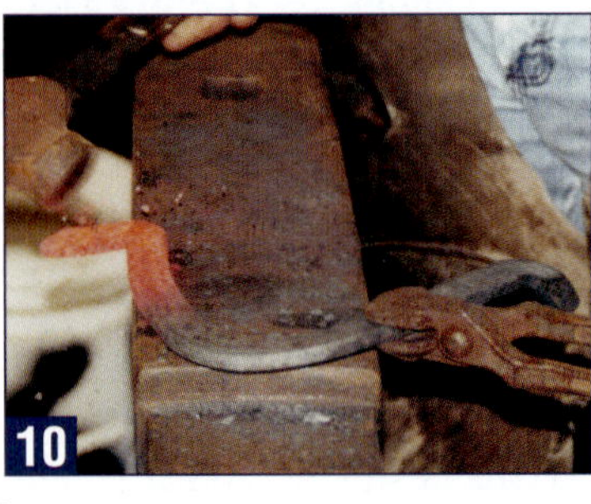

Repeat the steps from the first side.

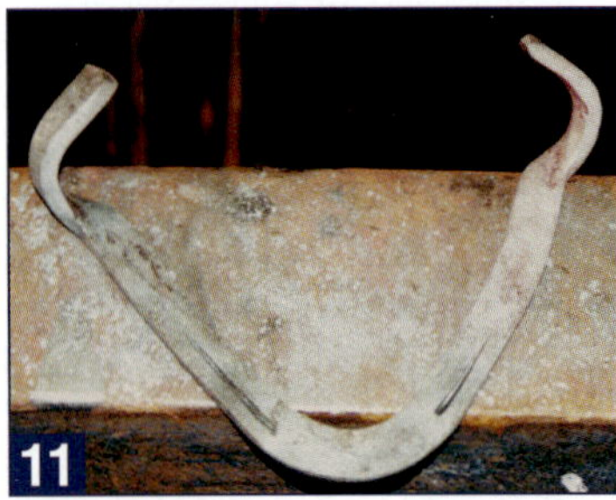

The shoe is ready to be put together.

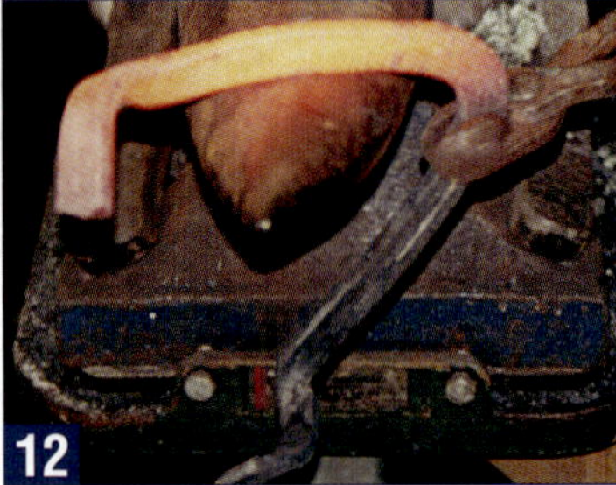

Bend the branch around the horn.

for the bar past the far edge, and hammer on the inside where the quarter is going to be **(Figure 5)**.

Now, lay the shoe on the face of the anvil, ground surface down, and with the bent piece beyond the far edge of the anvil. Bend the piece for the bar down the far side of the anvil. You can see this position in **Figure 6**.

The next position is to bend the piece to make the area of the bar that will bear weight. Move to the step of the anvil and start that bend as in **Figure 7**. You can move to the tip of the horn if you need to, but continue to bend the piece until it looks like the one in **Figure 8**.

The next heat is on the opposite side of the shoe, and you are going to repeat what you just did to the first branch. **Figures 9 and 10** are the sequence on the opposite branch. Be certain that you are bending the piece for the bar in the right direction, toward the ground surface. The shoe is now well on the way to being a good patten bar, and it should look like **Figure 11**.

Bend one branch around the horn **(Figure 12)**. If you only have one fuller, I would recommend that you go ahead and finish creasing and punching now. When you crease, there is a chance for the bar to get in your way on one side, since you fuller toward the toe on one side and toward the heel on the

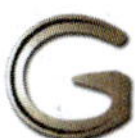

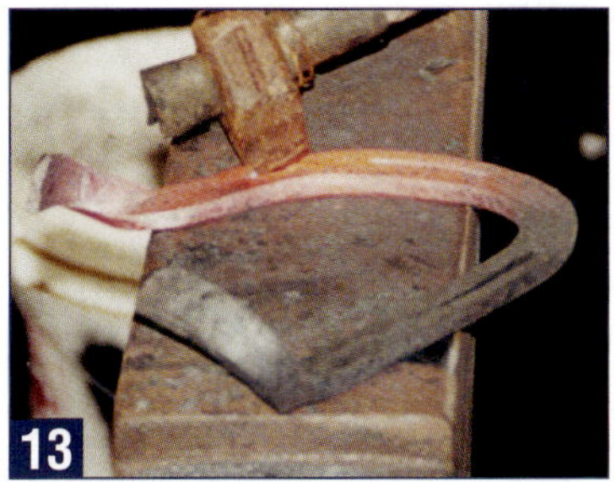

Fuller the branch.

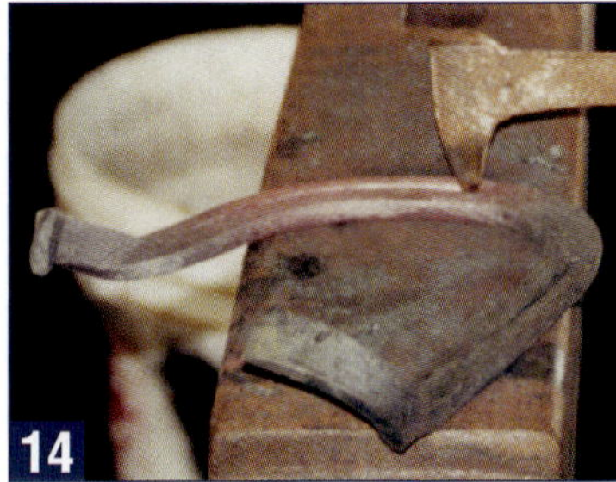

Drift a lot of nail holes.

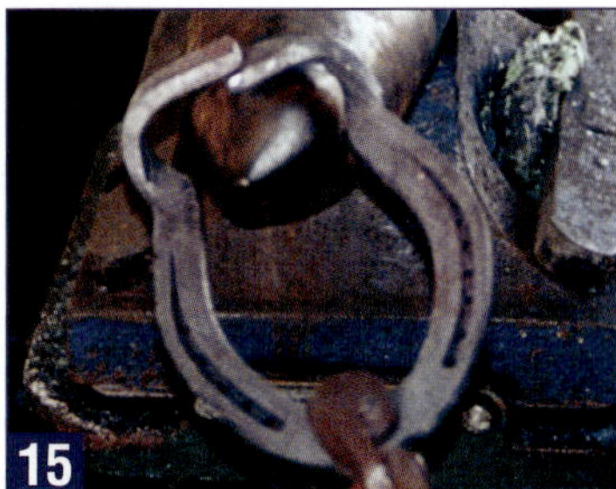

Put the bar together and prepare it to weld.

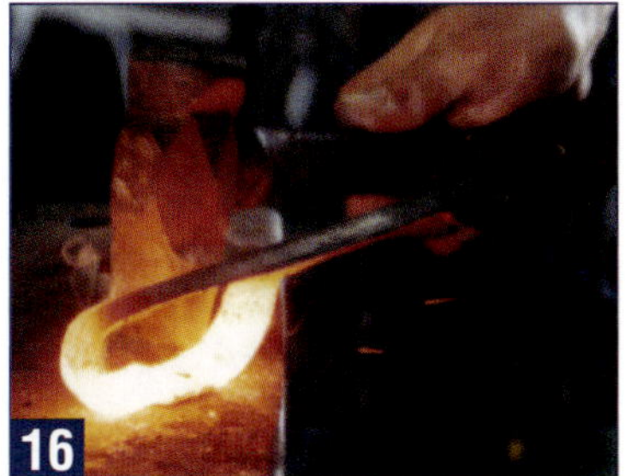

Using a cross peen to weld the hoof surface of the bar.

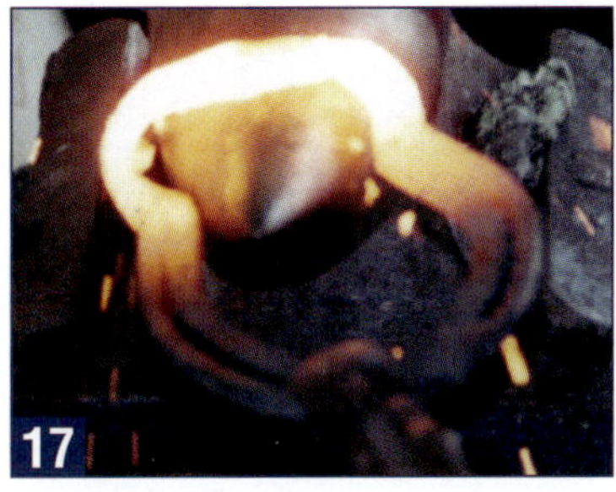

Position the shoe on the horn to weld the ground surface of the bar.

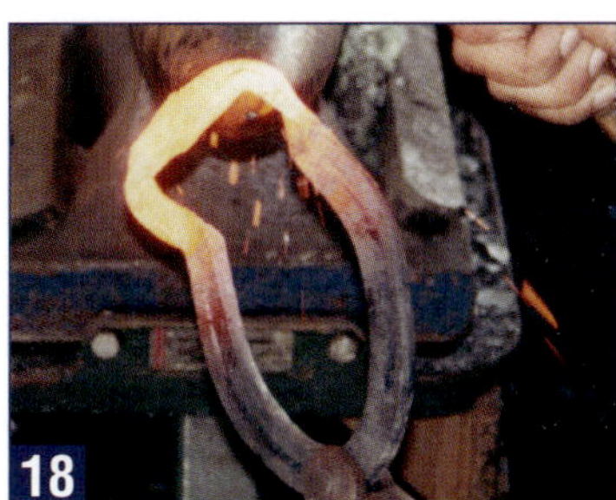

Position on the horn to shape the bar.

other. Before the bar is welded, you can easily bend it out of the way to crease so that there is no interference. **Figures 13-14** show fullering and drifting the nails. Put a lot of nail holes in a shoe like this so you have several options when you get to the foot. If you have two fullers, you can fuller towards the toe on both sides by setting one fuller up as a left handed fuller and one as a right handed fuller.

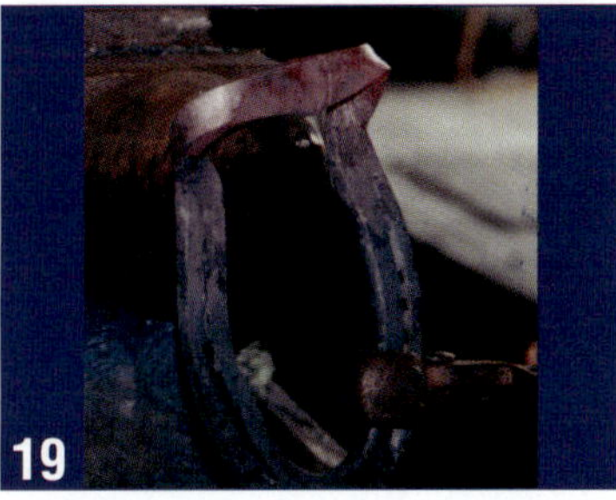

Cleaning up the bar.

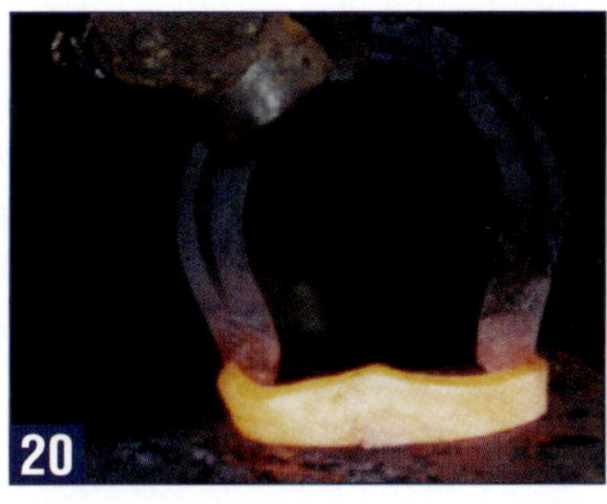

Forging the leading edge of the bar.

Now we are ready to put the shoe together and weld the bar. Get a heat to shape the shoe and place the ends of the bar over each other. Just as with the other bar shoes, I like to have the left side on top of the right side as I hold the toe of the shoe **(Figure 15)**. The weld on the bar of a patten bar shoe is a very hard weld to get. This is primarily because you cannot get the toe of your hammer into the seams, but also because you cannot just turn it over and place it flat on the anvil to weld the opposite side. You have to move from the face of the anvil to the horn to weld both sides. You may want to choreograph these moves prior to getting the welding heat.

Bring the bar to a welding heat, place the bar down on the anvil face, and weld the inside of the bar. In **Figure 16**, I am using a cross peen hammer. This allows me to weld the seam between the heels of the shoe. As soon as the seam disappears, move to the horn to weld the opposite side **(Figure 17)**. Take a second welding heat and use some of that heat to shape the corners of the bar. In **Figures 18-19**, you can see a couple of positions on the horn. In **Figure 20**, I am forging the leading edge of the bar while the rear edge is being straightened on the anvil face. To get the bar in this position, hold the shoe with the

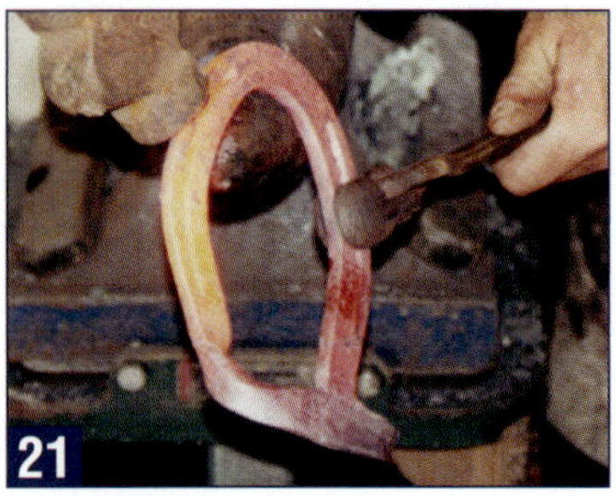

Shaping the shoe.

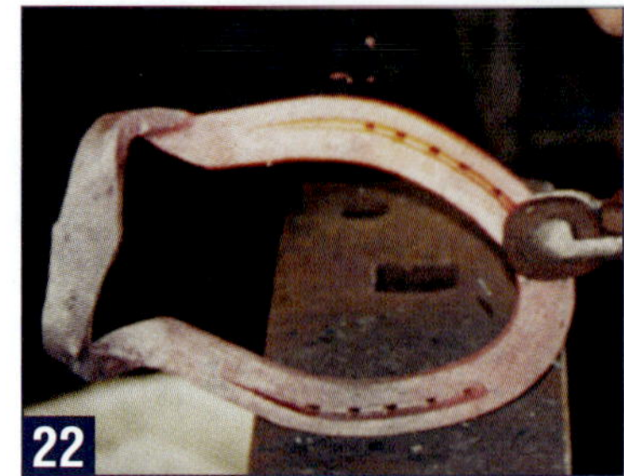

Using a flatter to clean up the hoof surface of the bar.

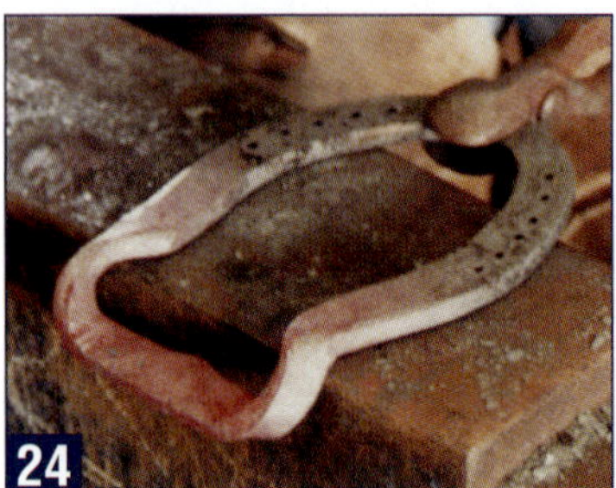

Changing the angle of the bar.

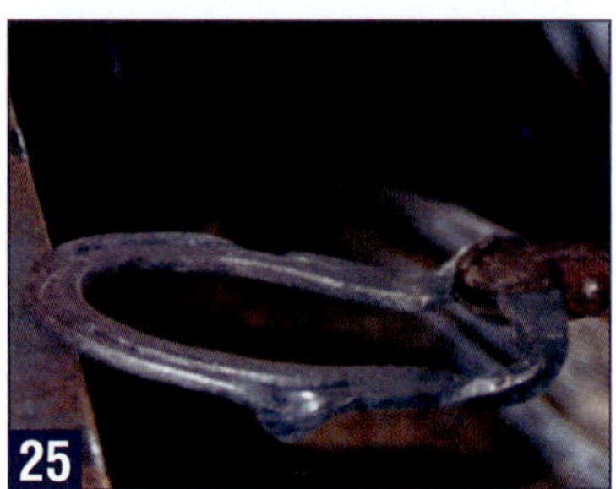

Forging the rocker toe.

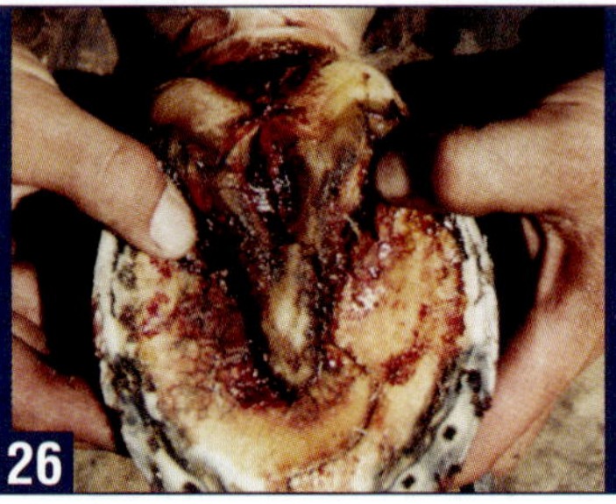

Badly injured foot.

hoof surface up, hammer on the bar lightly as you lift the shoe. This will turn the bar out so that it can be forged as in **Figure 20**.

Put the finishing touches on the shape (**Figures 21-22**). I like to shape the bar by itself in one heat,and the shoe in another. If both are hot at the same time, it is hard to do something to one part without changing the other. The bar can be shaped on the horn, flattened with a flatter (**Figure 23**), and aligned with the rest of the shoe by hitting it over the edge of the anvil (**Figure 24**).

With a patten bar, there are two levels to consider. There is the level of the foot on the shoe, and there is the level of the shoe on the ground. You need to have a rocker toe on a patten bar that is at the same level as the bar so the shoe will sit flat on the ground. To make this rocker toe, place a portion of the toe on the face of the anvil and lower the shoe as you hit the toe until the bar is at the same level as the toe (**Figure 25**). It is important that this shoe is as stable on the ground as possible.

Figure 26 is a foot that was sliced through the middle by a galvanized culvert. The patten bar in this series was made for this foot, and you can see it being nailed on in **Figure 27**.

Your patten bar is now complete. I have found numerous uses for this shoe, and you will as well, once you see the results that can be achieved. Introduce this shoe to your favorite vet if it is not already being used, and you will be well on the way to helping a lot more horses.

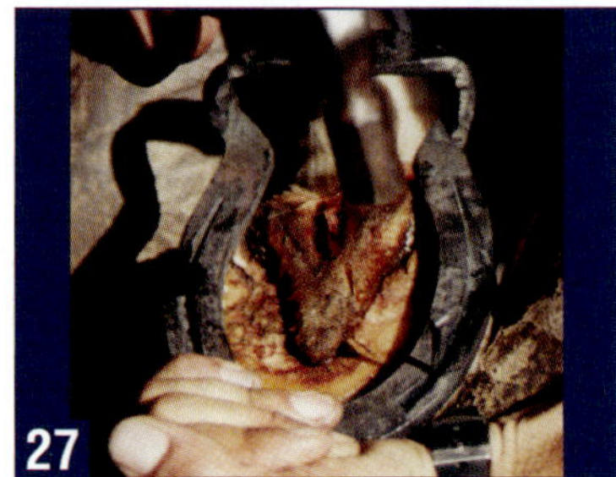

Patten bar being nailed on the injured foot.

It is possible to fabricate this shoe by taking an oversized keg shoe, fitting it with long extended heels, and then welding a piece of light pipe or tubing to the back of it. To change the height of the bar, you simply heat the pipe and smash it to make it taller or shorter. I haven't used one like that, but I have seen them. As long as the horse is helped, that is what is important.

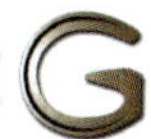

Chapter

52 Z-BAR SHOE

Here are a few ways to make this useful shoe. The first and second shoes are made from one piece, and the other is a two-piece method. When making this shoe out of two pieces, the bar portion of the shoe is jump-welded for the first weld. After making these shoes for these photos, I think I prefer the one-piece method. It seemed to flow off the anvil easier, but you will have to try making this shoe each way to see if you like one more than the other. The main point though, is to have a shoe that will help a wounded horse feel better and improve.

For the one-piece method, begin with a normal toe bend. Then bend one branch towards the inside of the shoe with a sharp bend **(Figures 1-3)**. Next, bend this piece the opposite direction, somewhere in the middle **(Figure 4)**. Move to the heel region of the other branch and make a short hockey stick. Bring the ends of the shoe together **(Figure 5)** and line them up so that they overlap at around 90 degrees to each other **(Figures 6-7)**. Weld at this corner **(Figure 8)** and move to the tip of the horn to shape and forge the weld **(Figure 9)**.

The next five pictures **(Figures 10-14)** are the same sort of shoe being made for a foot. The difference is that I made the branch without the Z-bar bend in it first. The great thing about doing it this way is that it allows you to see the foot in the shoe a little easier **(Figures 11-12)**. I still make a perfect fit by cutting the excess off **(Figure 13)**. The shoe will look like **Figure 14** when it is ready to be fullered and punched.

When nailing shoes on injured feet, I like to have multiple nailing options as well as a crease to allow

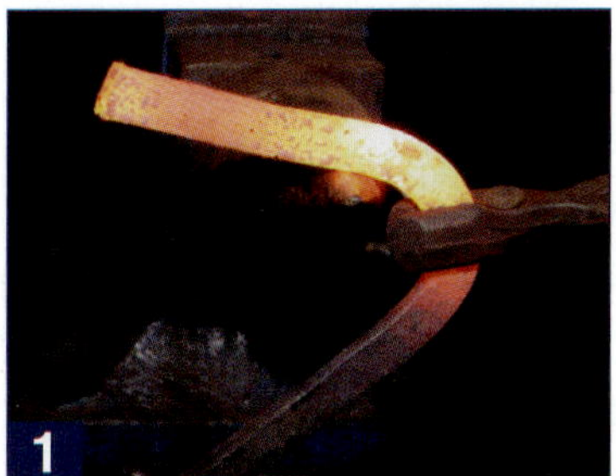

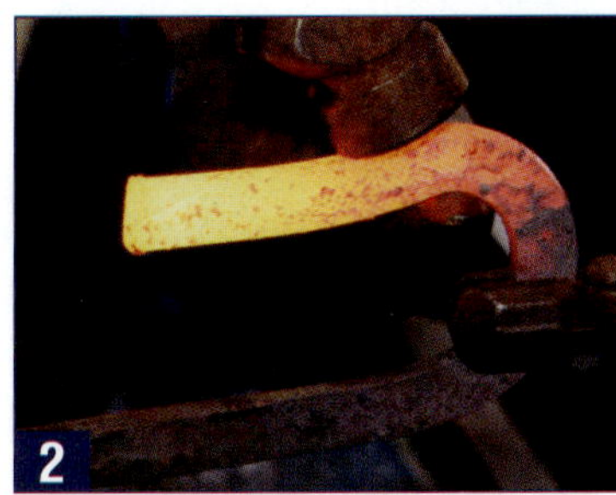

After making the toe, bend one branch sharply toward the inside.

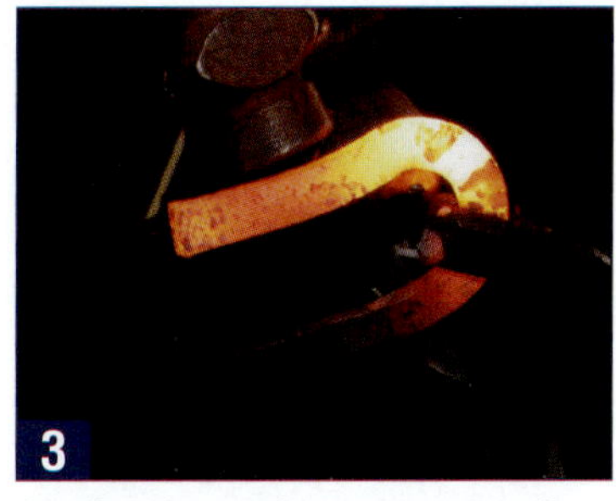

Notice how the tongs are in a position to have a lot of power.

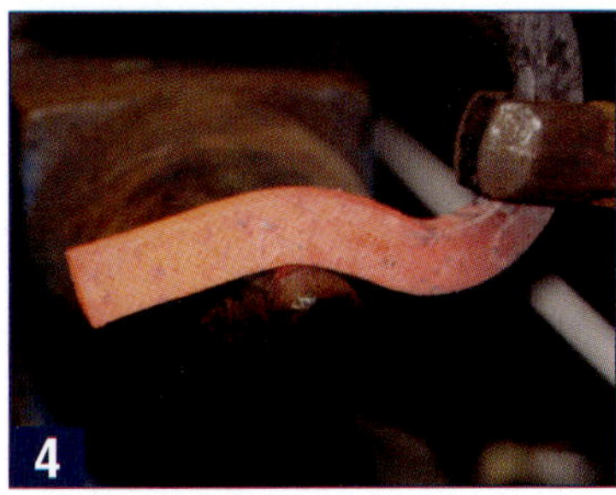

Bend that piece away from the middle now.

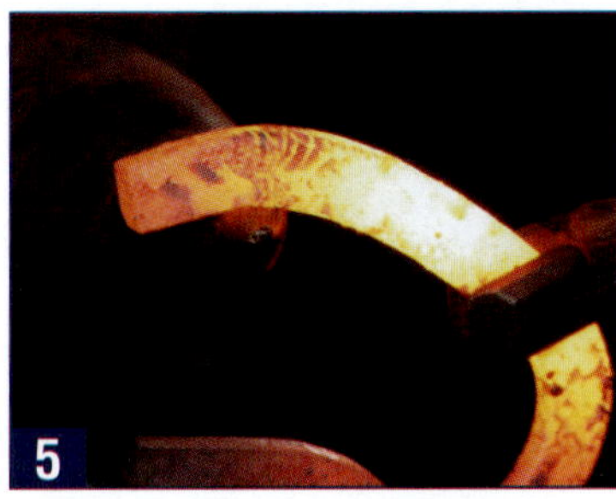

Bend a small amount toward the middle on the opposite branch.

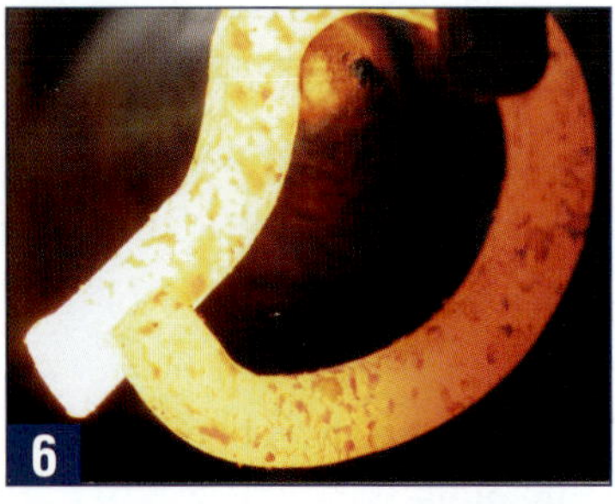

Bring the two ends together.

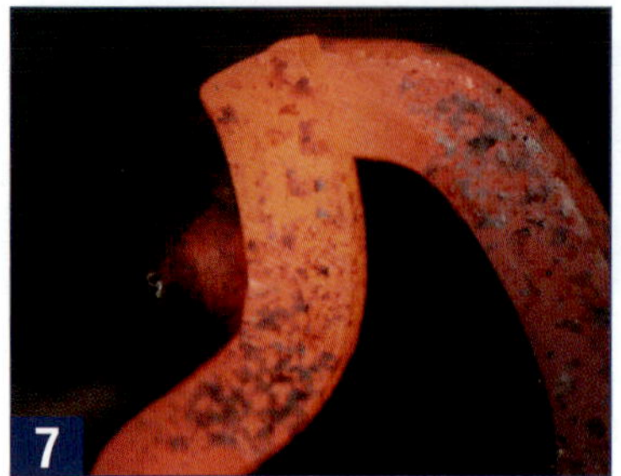

8

Weld in the corner where the two pieces meet.

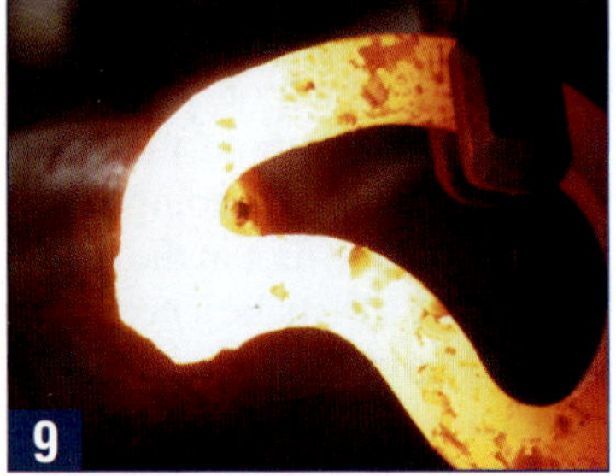

Shape the weld on the tip of the horn.

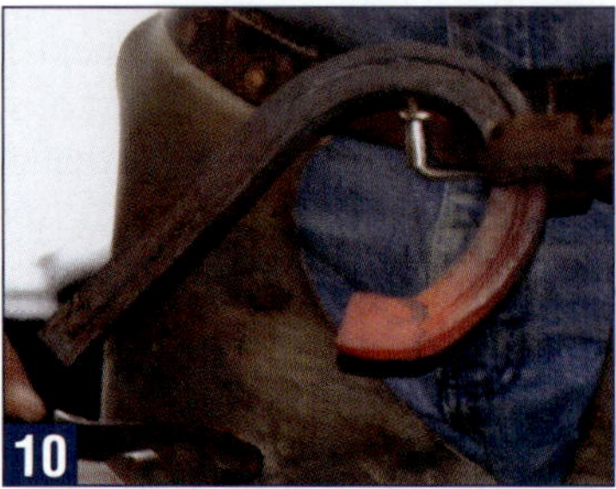

Another method is to start with the other branch.

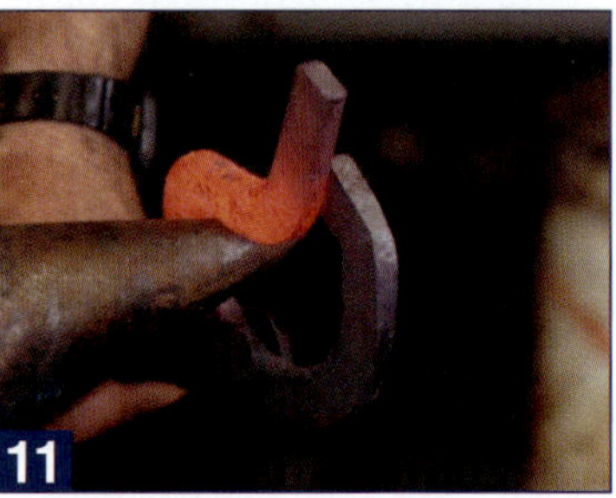

Shape the Z-bar branch.

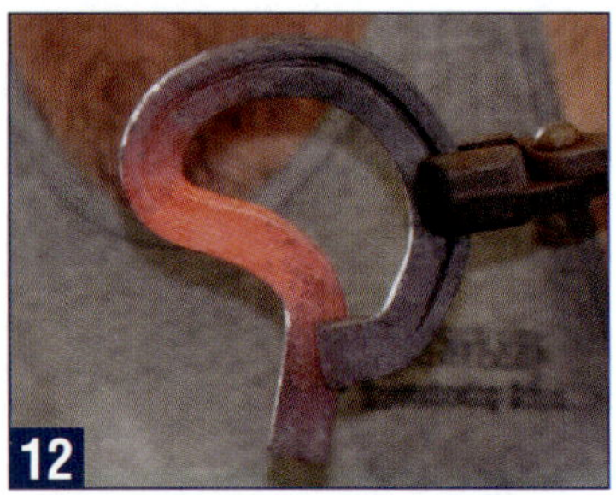

Bring the pieces together.

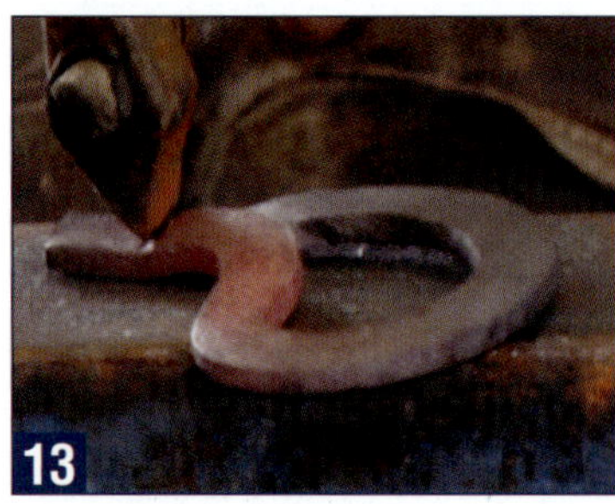

Cut off the excess.

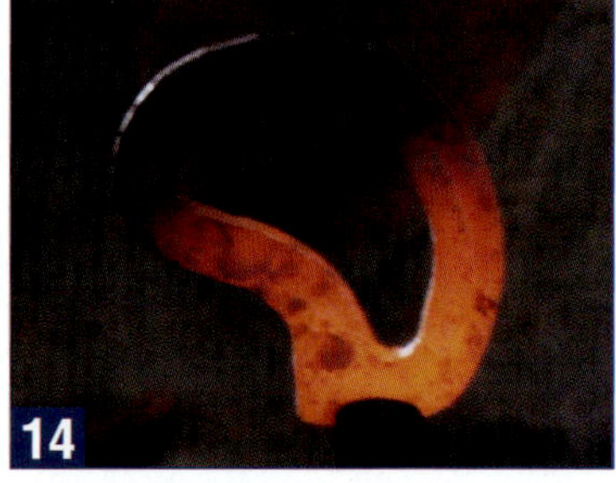

Weld the back of the bar.

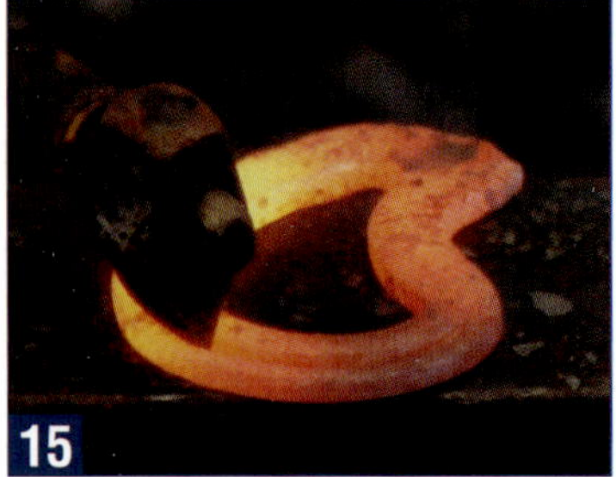

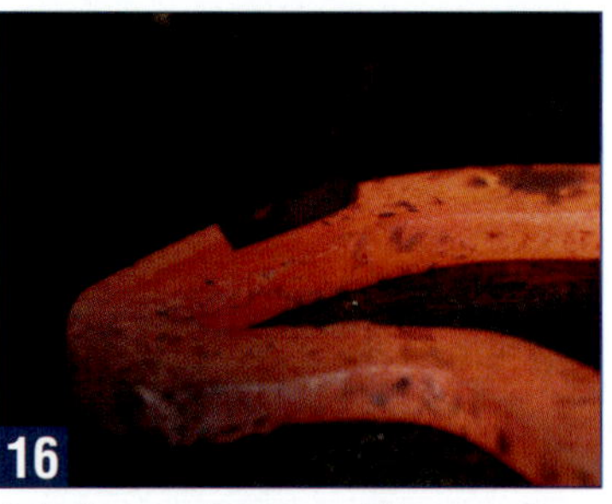

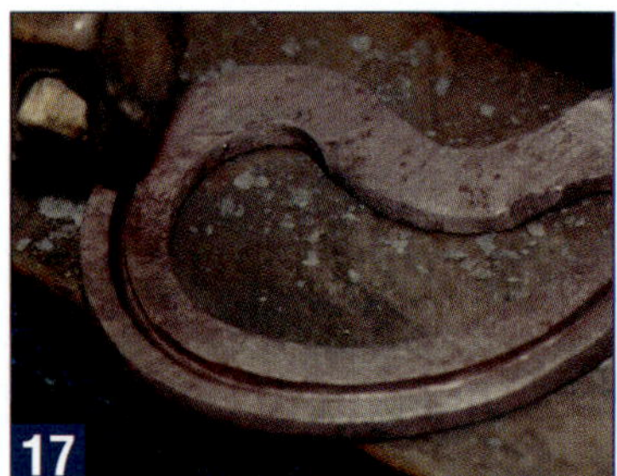

Fuller as much of the shoe as possible for multiple nailing options.

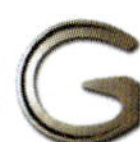

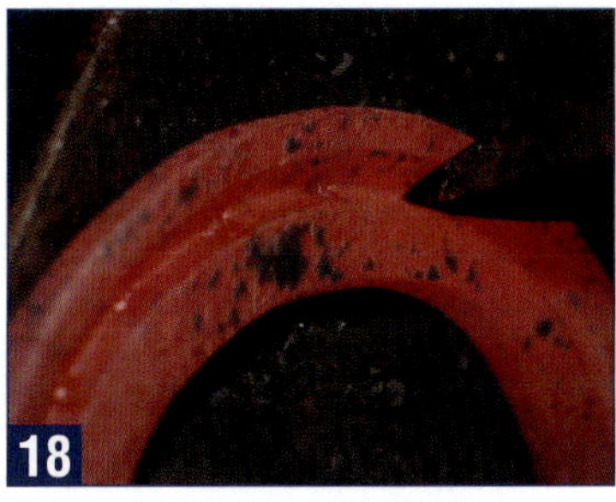

Drift a bunch of nail holes.

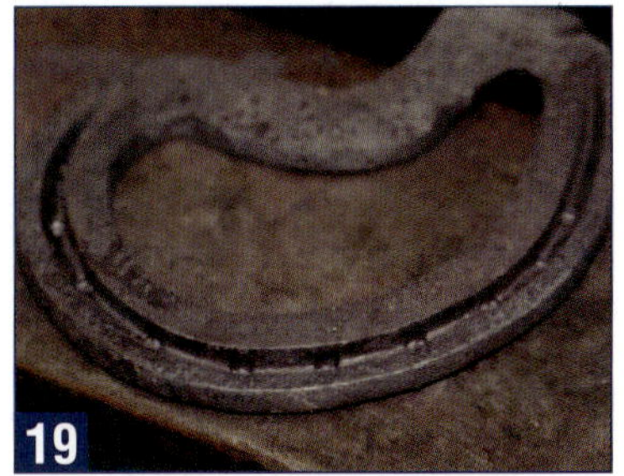

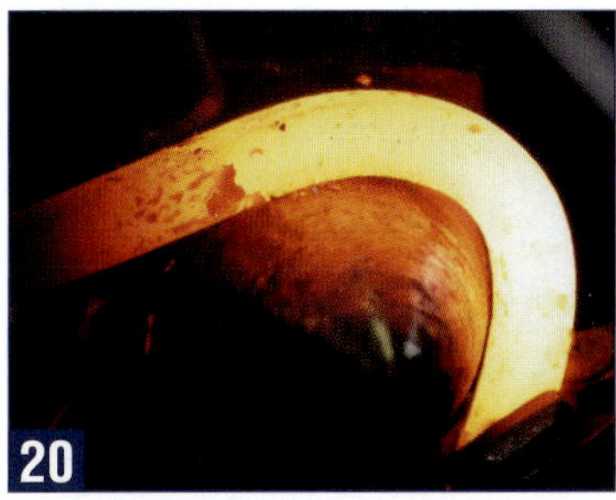

For the two-piece method, begin with the toe bend.

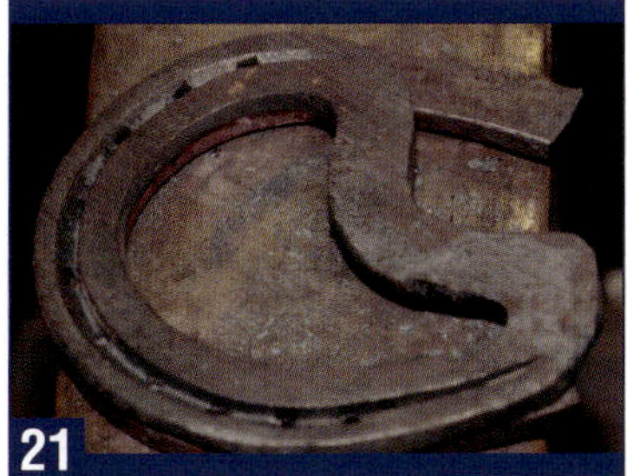

Make the toe bend appropriate for the foot you are shoeing.

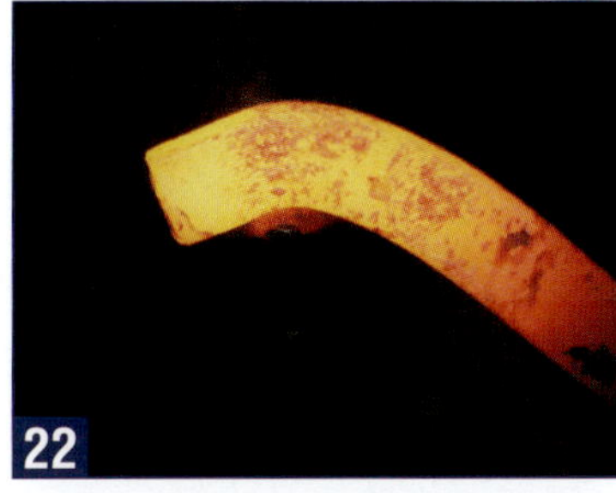

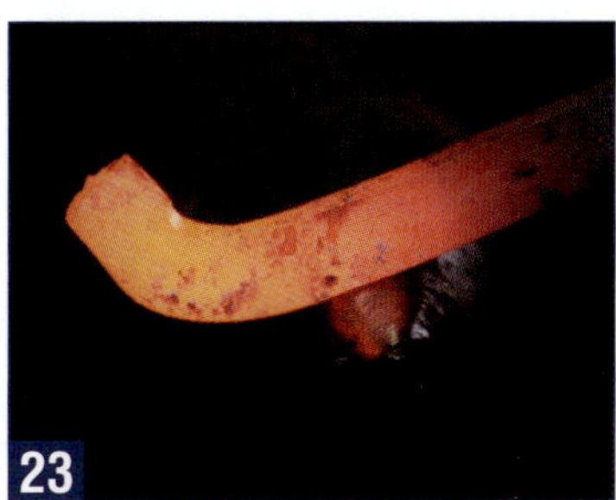

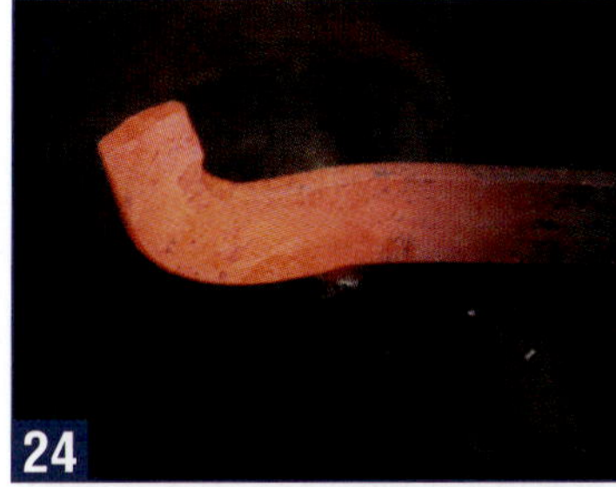

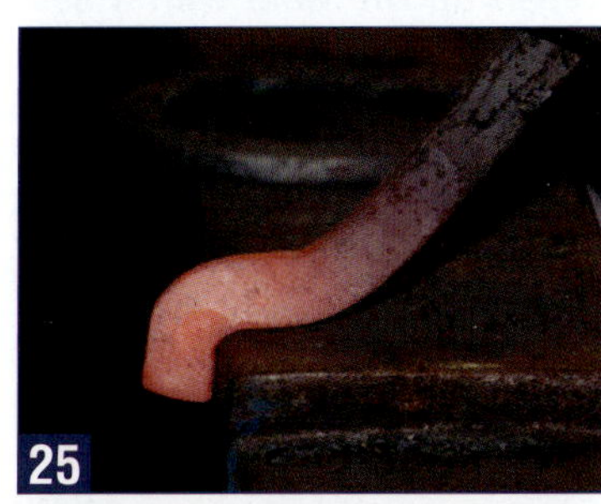

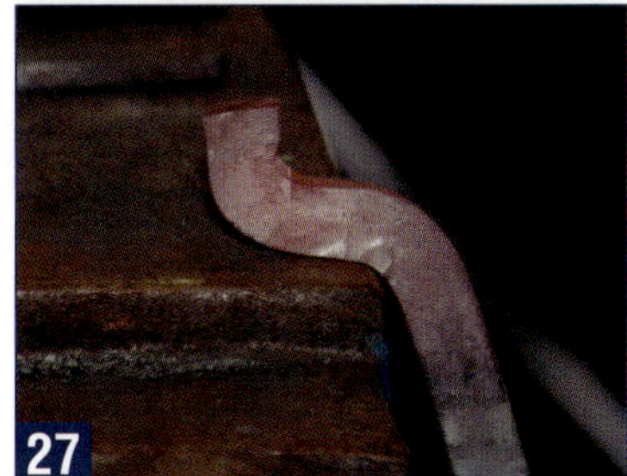

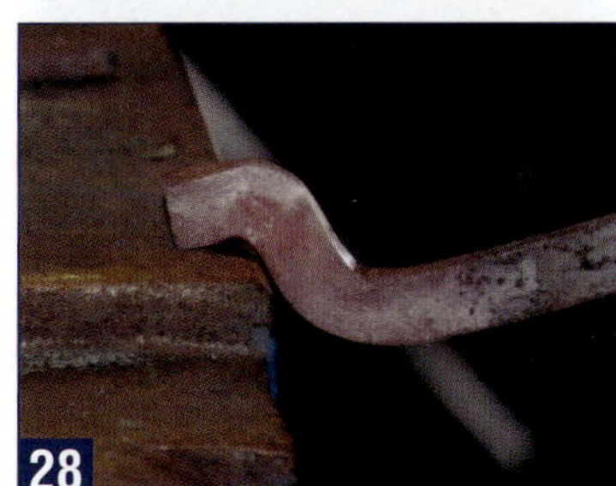

Shape the bar portion on another piece of stock.

individual nail pulling. With this in mind, fuller the shoe from the heel to opposite branch **(Figures 15-17)**, drift and pritchel several extra nail holes around the shoe **(Figures 18-19)**.

This next shoe is made using the two-piece method. Begin with a toe bend **(Figure 20)**. You can see that it matches the first shoe **(Figure 21)**, so you could take this blank to the foot to determine where to cut the shoe and come across to the frog with the bar portion of the shoe if you wanted to insure you were on the right path.

Take another piece of stock and shape it to fit

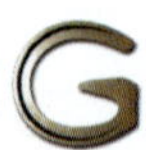

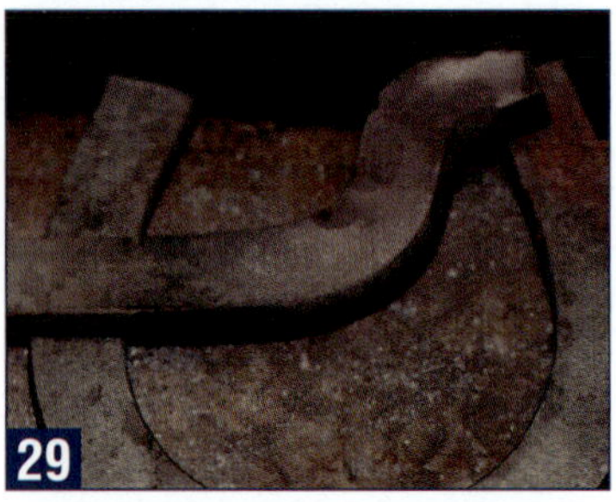

29

Place the piece in position to determine if it is correct.

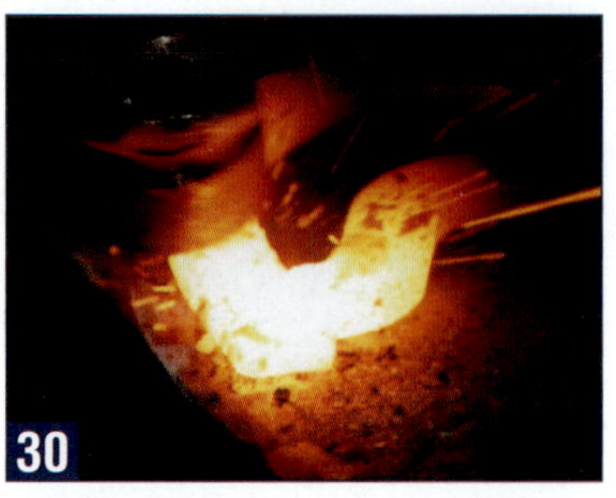

30

Jump-weld the bar portion to the heel of the shoe.

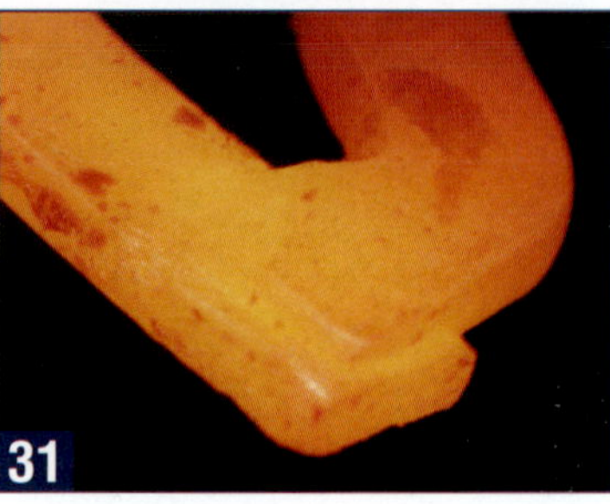

31

You can see the detail of the first welding heat.

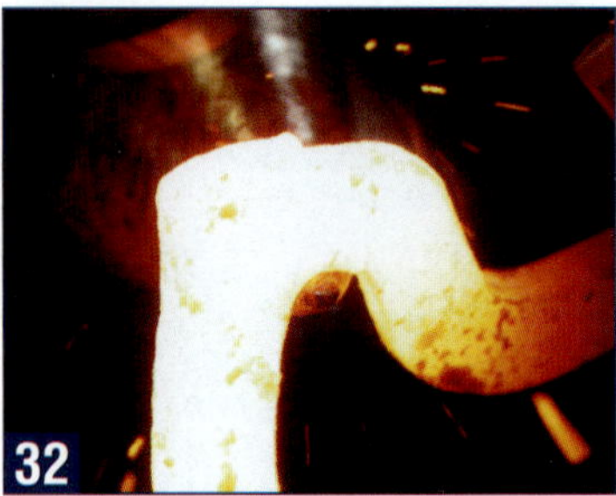

32

Clean up the weld with a second welding heat.

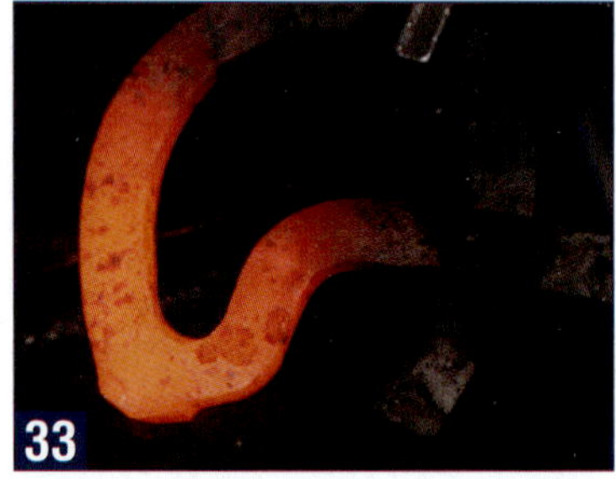

33

At this point, you can move the bar or shape the shoe so that it is exactly what you are after.

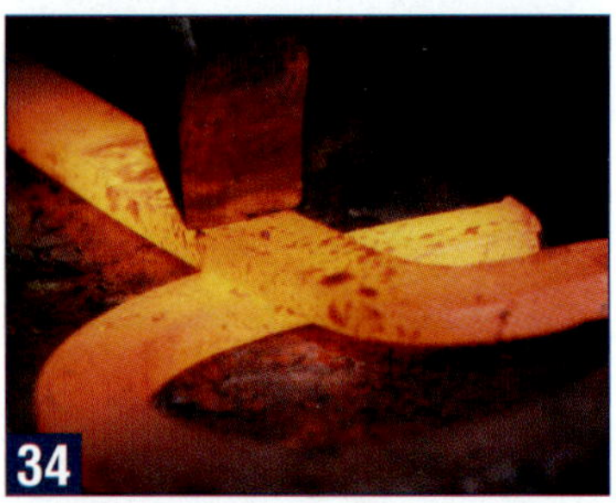

34

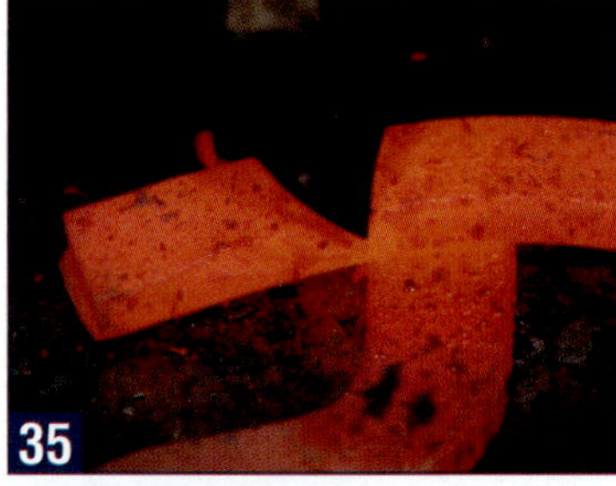

35

Cut both pieces so that you can weld the second area.

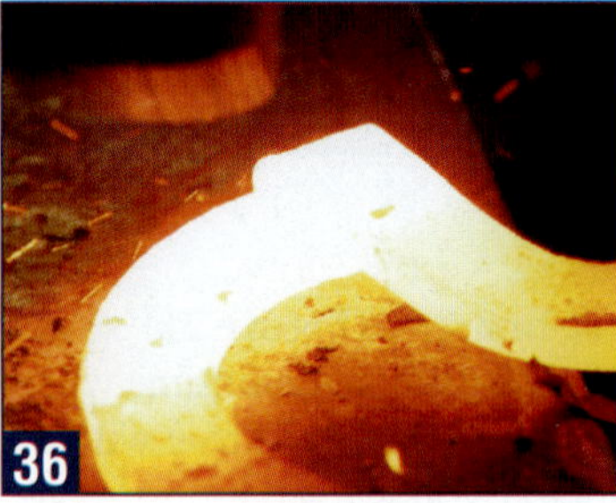

36

Weld the second place where they come together.

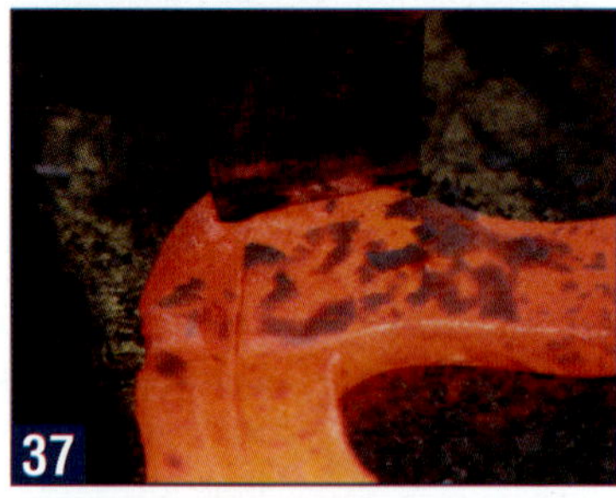

37

Cut off any excess from welding such a large area.

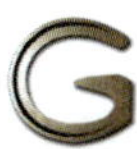

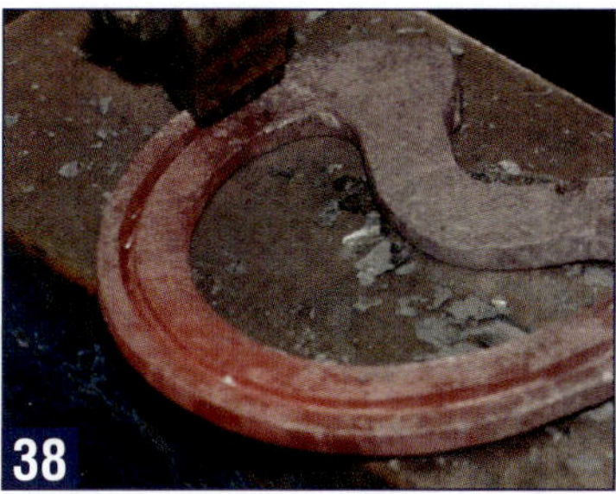
38

Fuller around the shoe.

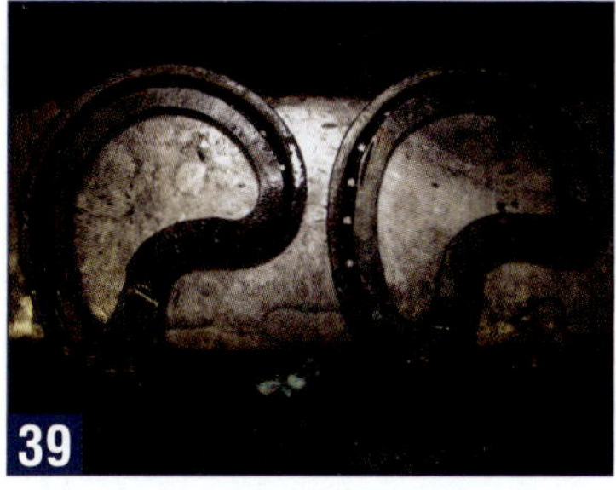
39

Here are the two shoes, each made differently, but each able to do the exact same job.

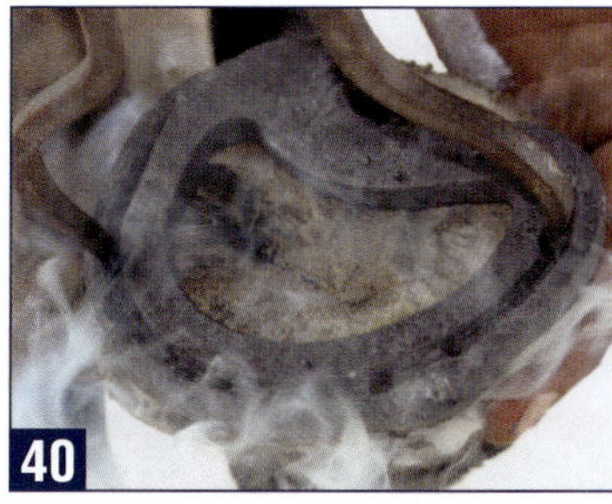
40

Hot fitting a Z-bar to a foot.

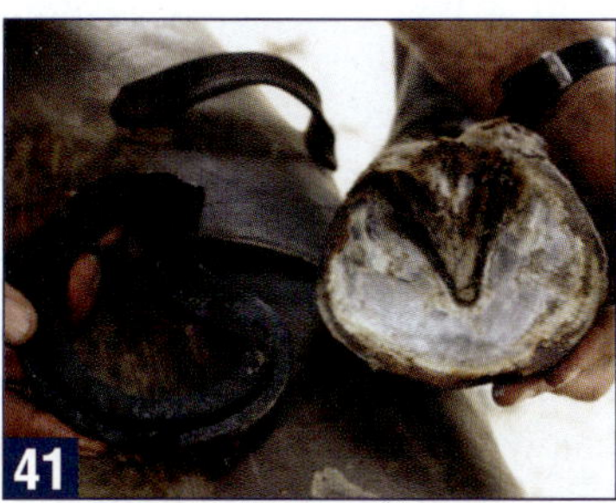
41

You can see how it matches part of the foot.

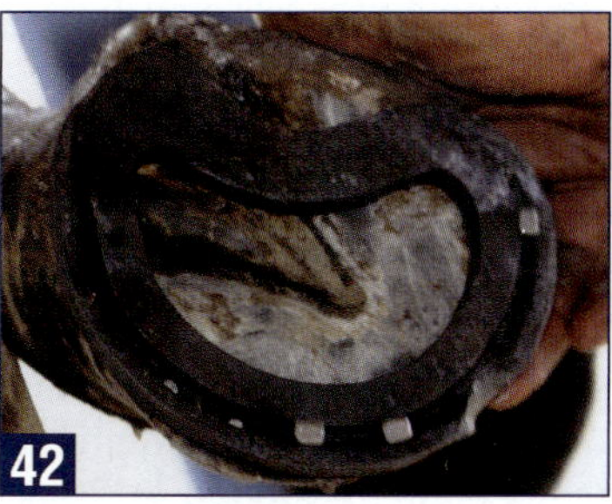
42

Z-bar nailed on.

inside the shoe from the area you want to cut to the area of the heel. An advantage of this method is that you can jump weld in a bar that has a different dimension than the shoe if the foot called for it. I begin on the tip of the horn and make the first bend to get to the heel of the shoe **(Figure 22)** The next bend will be the opposite direction at an appropriate distance to cover the frog **(Figures 23-24)**. Once the initial bends are made, you can move to soft corners of the anvil to clean up and define your bends **(Figures 25-28)**. Place this piece on the blank to check your bends **(Figure 29)**.

Jump-weld the heel of the blank to the end of the piece with the bend **(Figures 30-31)**. Take another welding heat and clean up the first weld **(Figures 32-33)**. Now heat the opposite branch and cut off the pieces with your fuller so that they are square **(Figures 34-35)**. Flux, reheat, and weld **(Figure 36)**. The corner at the second weld may need a little cleaning up, so I am doing this with my fuller in **Figure 37**. Fuller around the shoe as in **Figure 38**. **Figure 39** Shows the finished shoes.

From this point, you can handle this shoe like any other. One thing to bear in mind, like the heart bar, this may not be the best shoe to hot fit too hot over the frog **(Figure 40)**. When you try to pick up a hot plate with a wet rag, the heat can transfer through the wet rag rapidly. For this reason, I don't like to hot fit over a frog at a very hot temperature. **Figure 41** is the shoe beside the foot and **Figure 42** is in the process of being nailed on.

This is another one of the shoes that is not commercially available. Because you can't buy it, being the farrier that can build it is another way of putting you in a whole new category as a farrier. Learn to make this shoe well, and you have another weapon in your arsenal to fight against lameness' in horses.

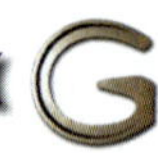

Chapter

53 ALUMINUM FUNDAMENTALS FOR FARRIERS

In our own farrier practice, there is little demand for aluminum shoes. I use them primarily for therapeutic cases where I am after a lot of coverage but very little weight. The big advantage to aluminum is how little it weighs. The disadvantage is how fast it wears away.

FORGING ALUMINUM IS DIFFERENT

First, you need to know how to tell when the stock is ready to forge. Unlike steel, aluminum does not change color. Aluminum has a low melting temperature of around 1,220 degrees Farenheit, or 660 degrees Celsius. This temperature is easily reached in a forge; thus aluminum is commonly turned into a puddle when you are first giving it a try. For this reason, you should find some old aluminum shoes to play with in the forge before using bar stock or new shoes. Old aluminum shoes make outstanding practice for pulling clips.

Place your stock in the fire and start a mental count. At 30, take the stock from the fire and check it. With experience, you will develop a feel for the right heat with your brush **(Figure 1)**. However, the best way to check is with a piece of wood. Your hammer handle should be perfect for this. Run your handle over the stock, and it should feel slightly slippery and leave a black line **(Figure 2)**. If there is a lot of smoke, or the line burns away **(Figure 3)**, the stock is too hot. Hitting it this hot will cause it to crumble **(Figure 4)**. It will feel like hitting an ice cube with your hammer when it is crushed.

Once you have brought the stock to the correct

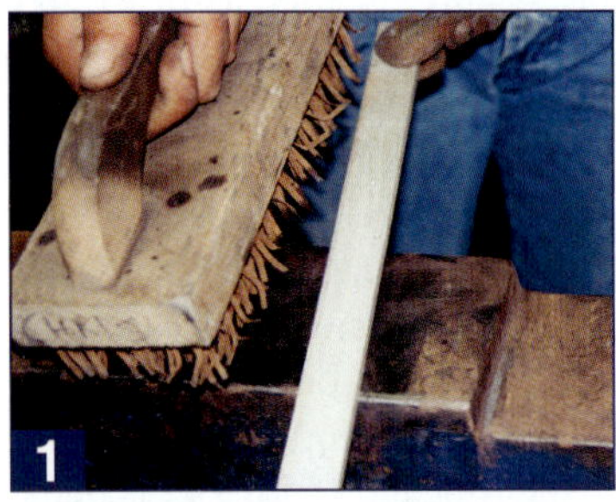

1 *Feeling the stock with a brush to see if it is the right temperature.*

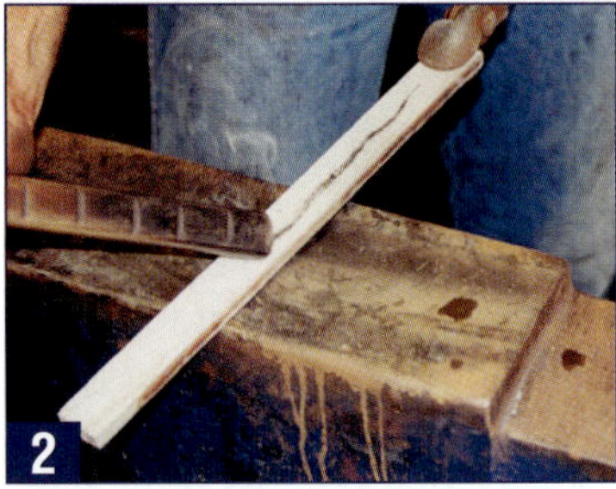

2 *Using a hammer handle to test the heat on a piece of aluminum.*

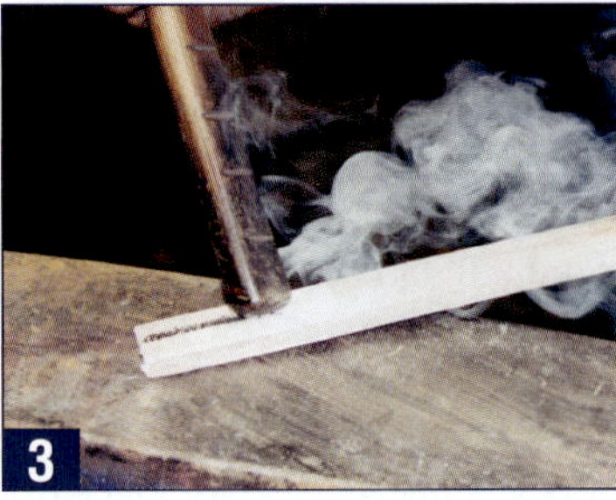

3 *The stock is too hot to hit. Notice the large amount of smoke.*

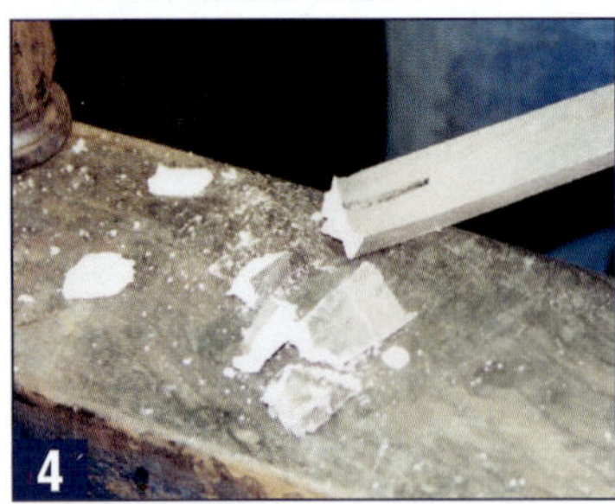

4 *If it is hit while too hot, it will crumble like an ice cube.*

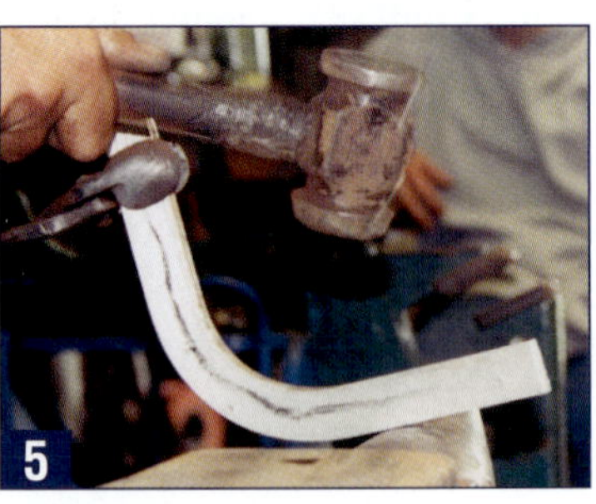

5 *Make your toe bend.*

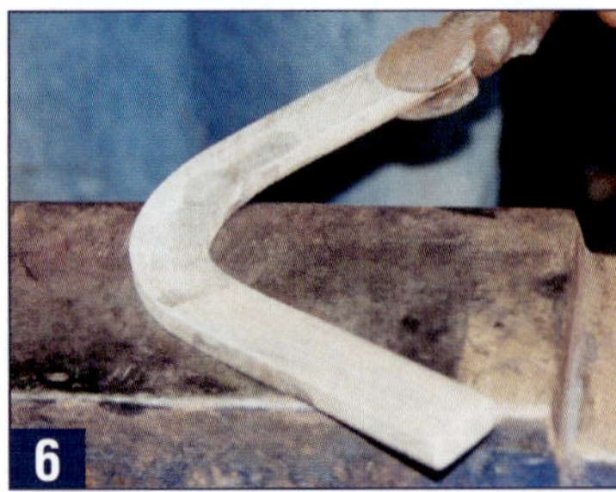

6 *Seat out the toe bend.*

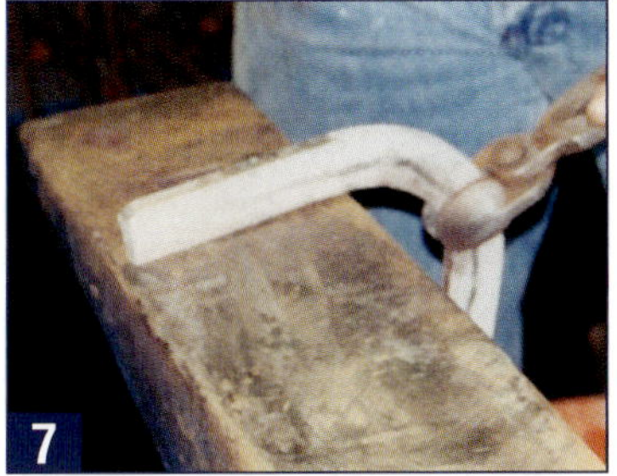

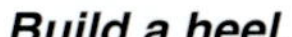

Build a heel.

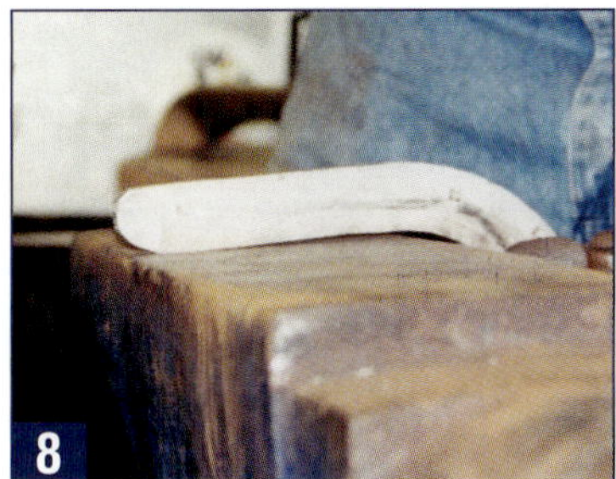

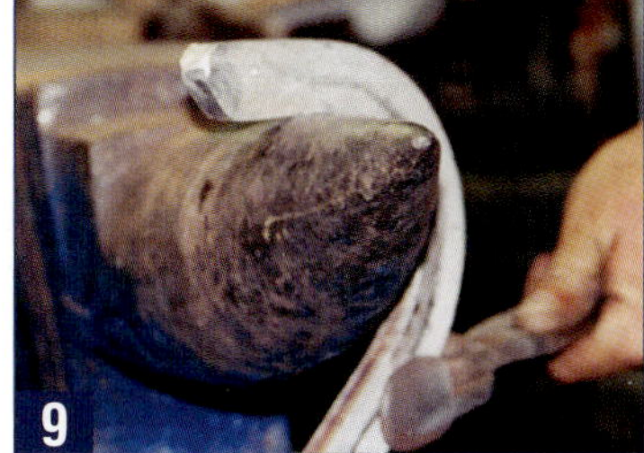

Turn the branch on the horn.

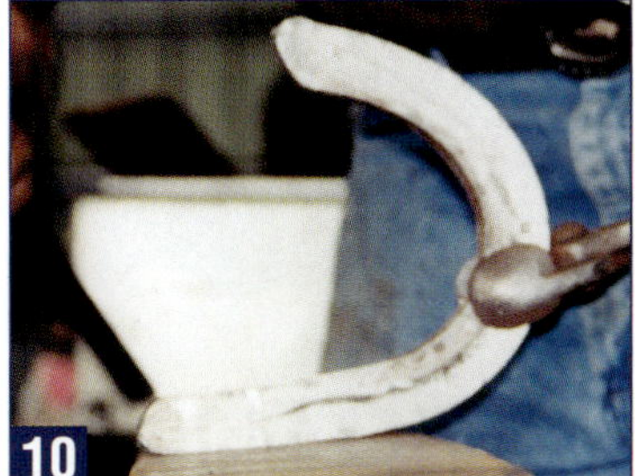

Build the other heel.

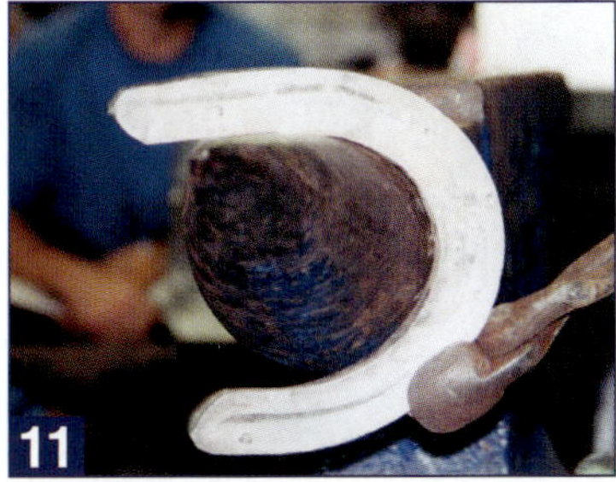

Turn the second branch.

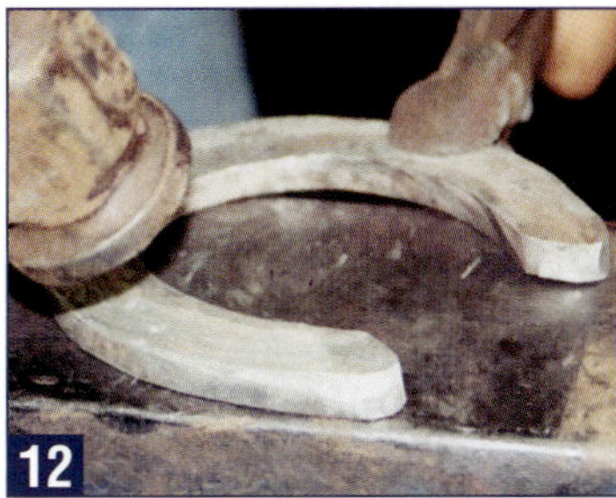

Hammer box the heels from the widest point of the shoe back.

forging temperature, the rest of it is just shoe-making basics. Do a toe bend **(Figure 5)** seat it out **(Figure 6)**, make a heel **(Figures 7-8)**, and turn it on the horn **(Figure 9)**. **Figures 10-11** are the second branch. You can do most of the boxing with your hammer at this stage, as in **Figure 12**. All of this has been done in one heat, and it is not a struggle. The aluminum stays malleable for a long time, so this is a good shoe to make at a clinic of horse owners. You look like you can really get a lot finished in one heat.

Aluminum will not lie to you. Every hammer blow makes a mark, and you may learn that you hammer differently than you thought. Also, aluminum does not move like steel. With steel, you displace metal and it stays displaced. With aluminum, it feels as if you are continually pushing it around. This is especially true for areas like hemming, fullering, and building heels. Aluminum is also a dead material to hit. With steel, the hammer rebounds upwards, making it easier to lift for the next blow. Aluminum absorbs the entire blow, and you must do all the work of lifting the hammer. The first time you forge aluminum, you may wonder why your arm is getting tired so quickly. It is mainly due to this absorbing quality, and partially due to the fact that it allows you to work so long. The long working heats don't allow the break in tempo that forging steel does.

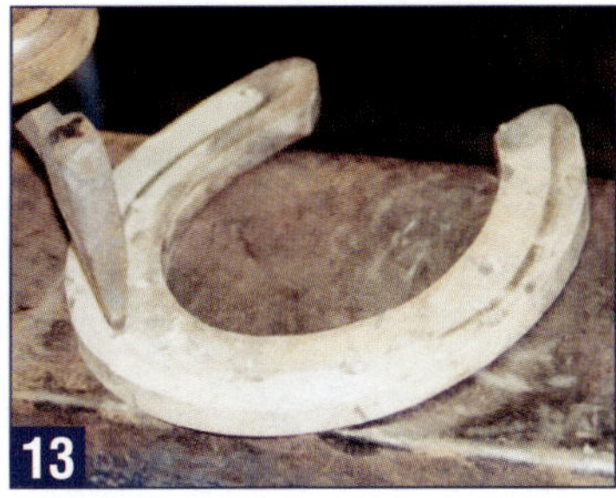

Use the fore punch, but be careful to not go too deep.

Still on the same heat, punch your nail holes **(Figure 13)**. If you reheat to punch your nail holes, you will find that the extra heat is actually a detriment with aluminum. At a forging heat, the aluminum displaces more than when it is a little colder. When you punch the hole, a lot of material is pushed out for the frog eye, and when you forge it back, your nail hole collapses. With it colder, the material does not move as much, making it easier

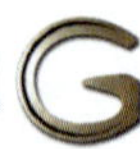

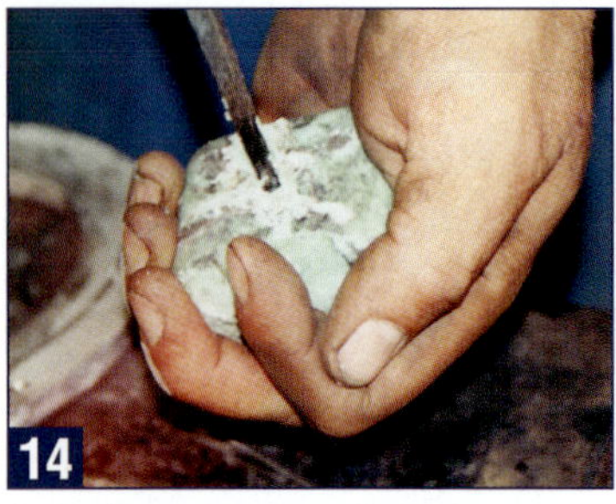
Lubricate your pritchel.

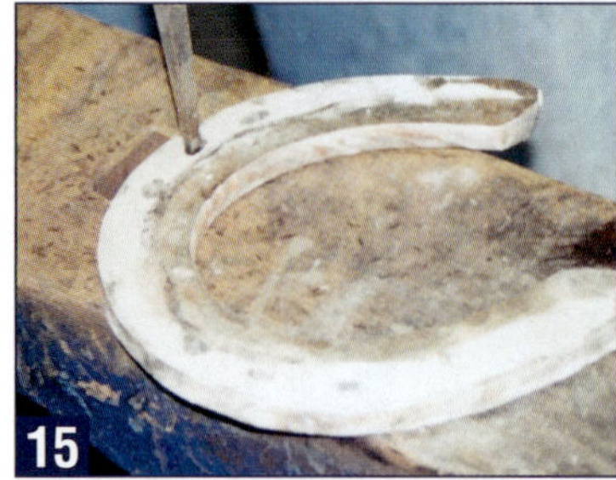
Pritchel out the nail holes.

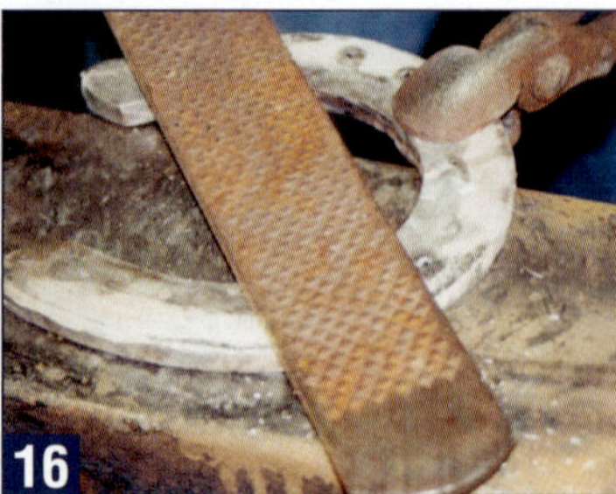
Rasp off the flashing that comes through the holes.

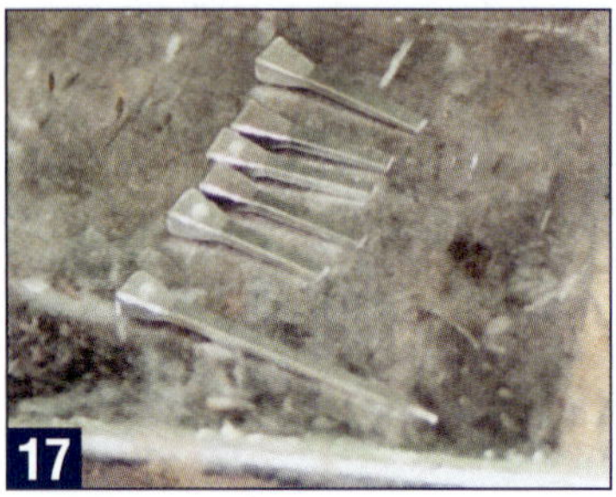
Cut off several nails to use as fore punches to make the perfect shaped hole.

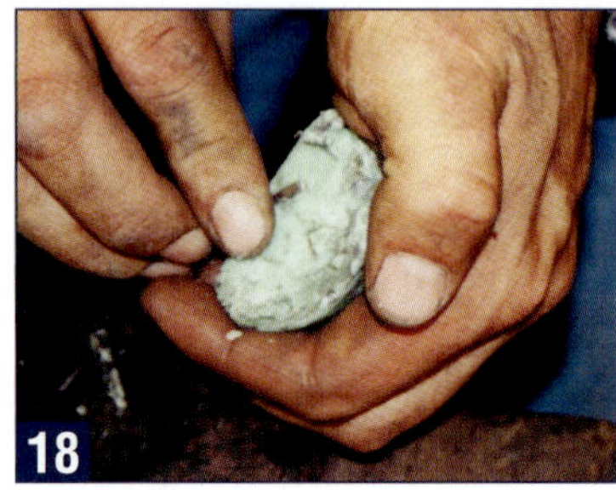
Lubricate the nails.

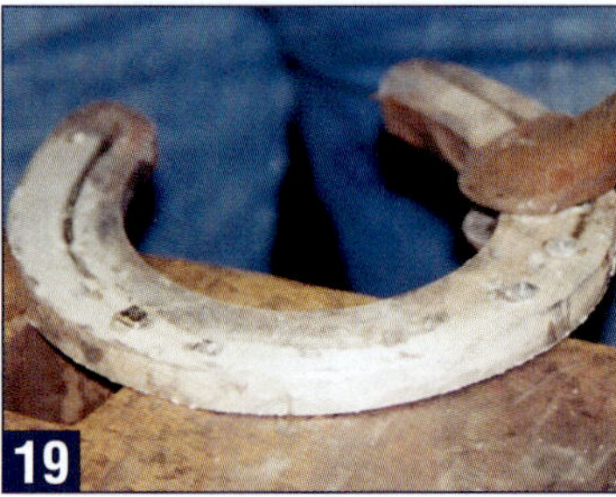
Drive the nails into the holes.

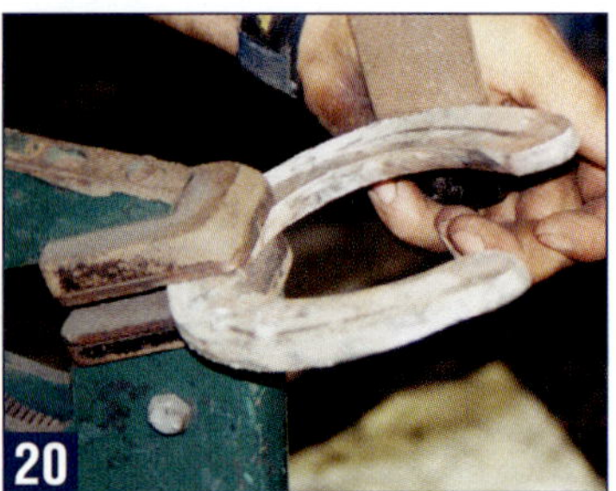
Rasp the shoe to clean it up.

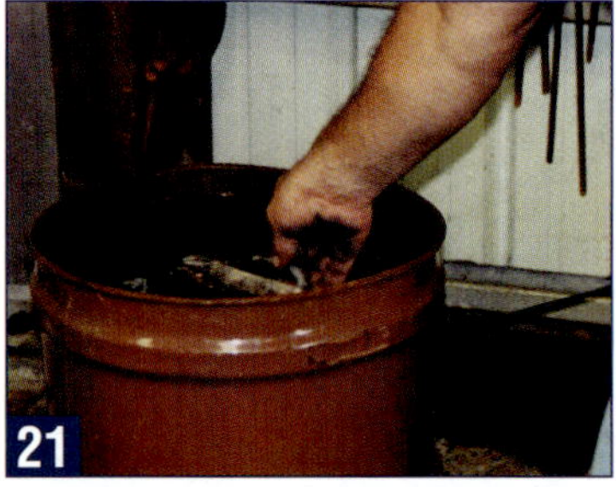
Dip a fine wire brush in the quench tub.

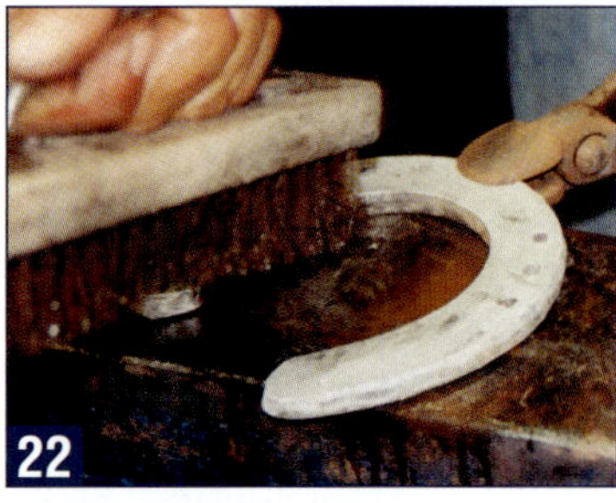
Wet brush the shoe.

to pritchel and forge out frog eyes.

To pritchel, it is essential that you have lubricant of some sort on the tool. You can see that I am using soap in **Figure 14**, but you can use beeswax or whatever else you like to cool your punches. Before driving the pritchel through the shoe, I bottom it out lightly on the face of the anvil. The light tap on the face chills the little piece of aluminum you are trying to shear out, and this makes it a cleaner hole. When it is hot, you just end up dragging the material through the hole and make it difficult to clean up. Hit the pritchel with a sharp blow **(Figure 15)**.

After pritchelling, before you hit the shoe flat on the anvil face, take a rasp and clean up the flashing that has been pushed through the hole **(Figure 16)**. You don't have to put the shoe in a vise for this. Aluminum is soft enough that rasping on it is easy. To size the hole exactly for the nail that you are using, cut half the shank off several nails **(Figure 17)**. In **Figure 18**, I am soaping the nails up just as I did with the pritchel. Then I drive the nail into the nail hole to shape it exactly to that particular nail **(Figure 19)**. I put the shank of the nail into the hole, and move the shank so that it is in the corner of the

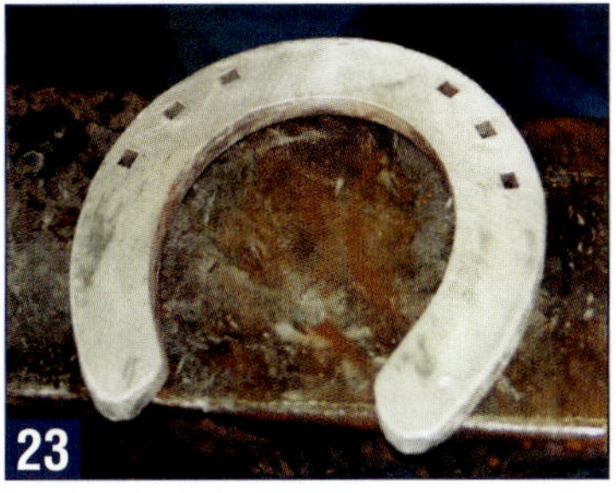
Here is your finished aluminum shoe.

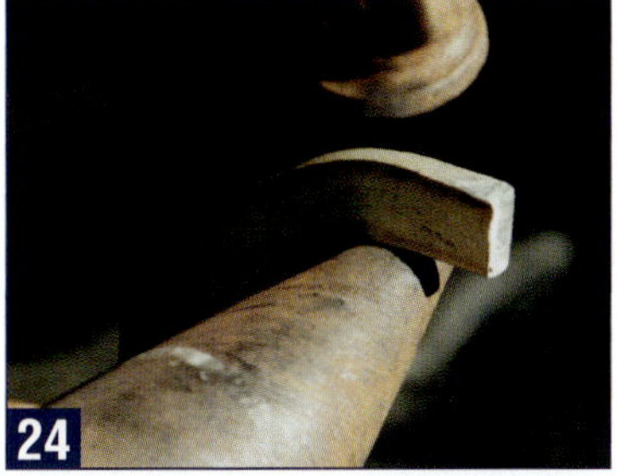

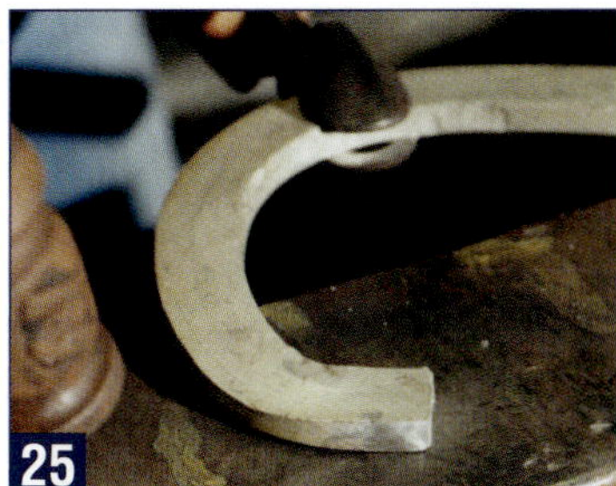

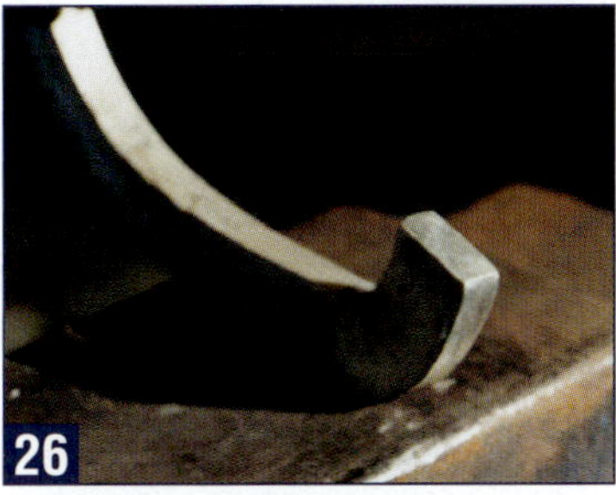

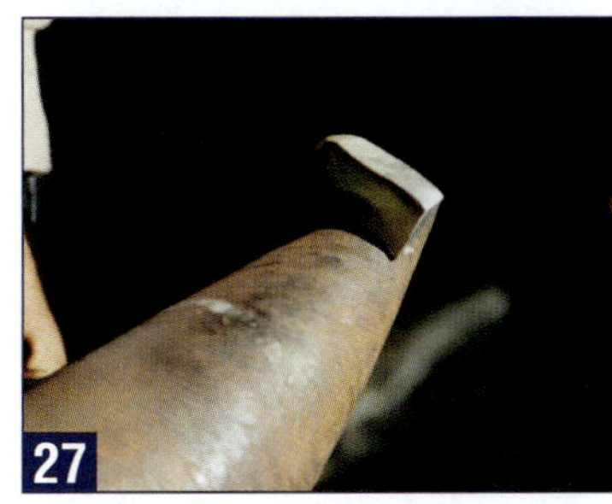

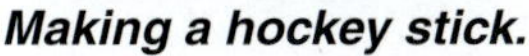
Making a hockey stick.

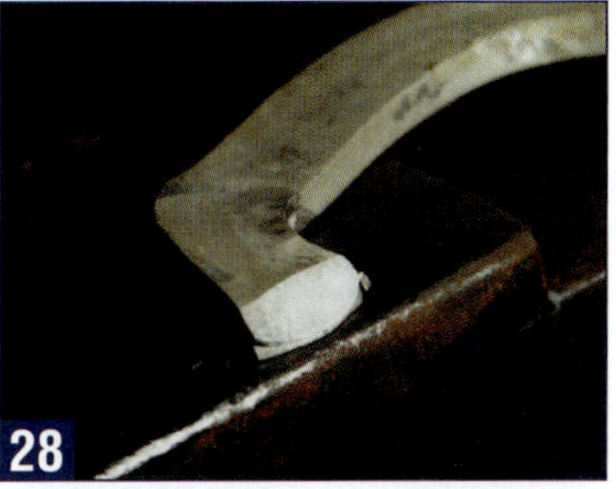
Scarf the hockey stick like you did on the steel straight bar.

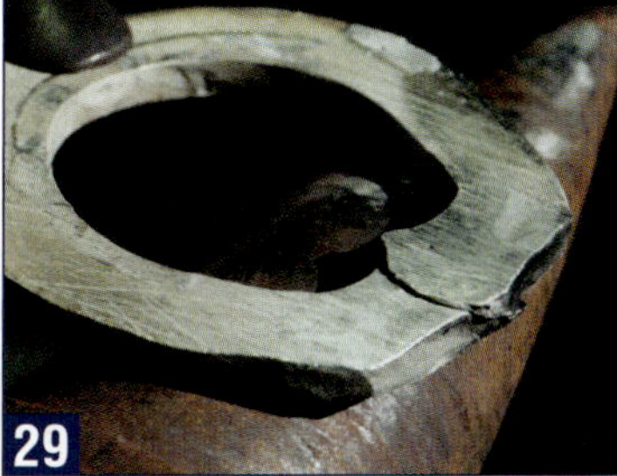
Do the exact same moves to the other branch.

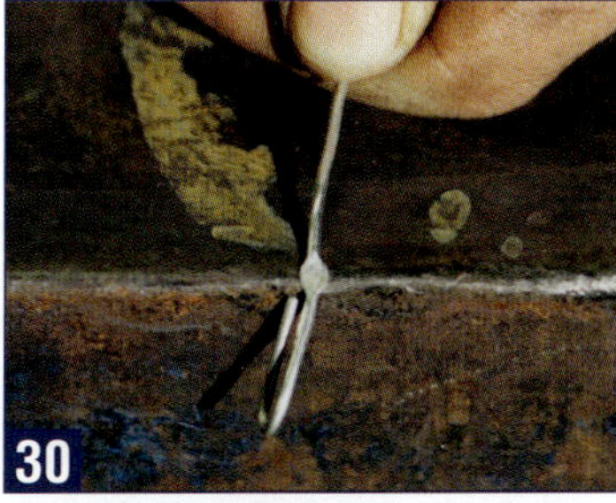
Cut the brazing rod.

hardy hole when I tap it.

It does not require heat to rasp an aluminum shoe, but it will rasp faster if it is hot. I recommend putting it in the fire for a count of 10, and then rasping it up **(Figure 20)**. To shine the shoe, use a fine-bristle wire brush that has been wet down. This is what I am doing in **Figures 21-22**. **Figure 23** is the finished shoe.

ALUMINUM STRAIGHT BAR SHOES

Next we are going to build a straight bar out of aluminum in a gas fire. (We will forego pictures of steps that occur elsewhere.) Begin by heating and testing the heat of the stock. Make a toe bend, then bend a piece at the end of the stock to make your first hockey stick **(Figure 24)**. It should look like **Figure 25** before you start making the hockey stick as in **Figure 26**. Move to the end of the horn and forge the outside corner of the heel like you would with steel **(Figure 27)**. Place the hockey stick at the edge of the anvil face and make your scarf **(Figure 28)**. Repeat the same process on the other branch, and bring the pieces together so that you have a shoe that looks like the one in **Figure 29**. The scarves need to be clean, so you should brush them before you put them together. Another important aspect is to get the scarves as tight as possible. A steep scarf makes aluminum easier to weld in the fire.

"Welding" aluminum in a forge is really a bit of a misnomer. You do weld steel in a forge, because nothing is added to bond the two pieces. When you attach two pieces of aluminum in a forge, it requires

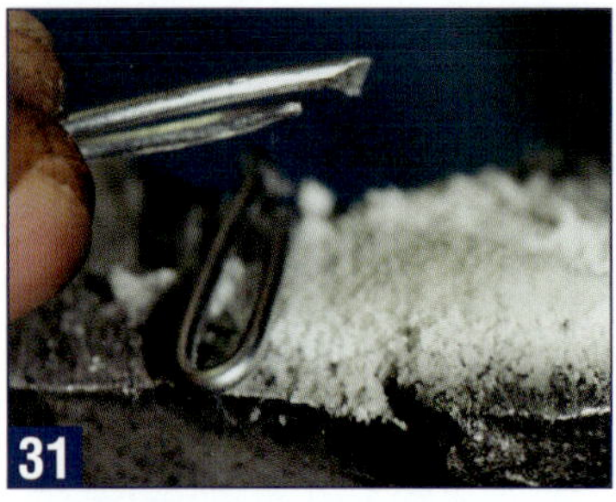

Place the rod and flux on the bar of the aluminum shoe.

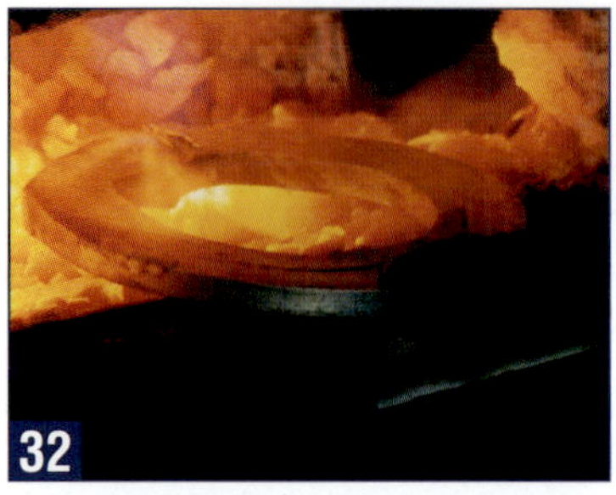

Steadily place under the flame in a propane fire.

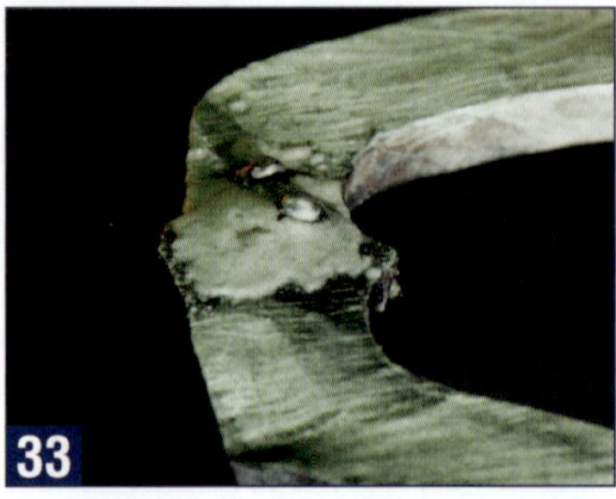

I pulled it out of the fire early to show you what it looks like when the rod puddles up.

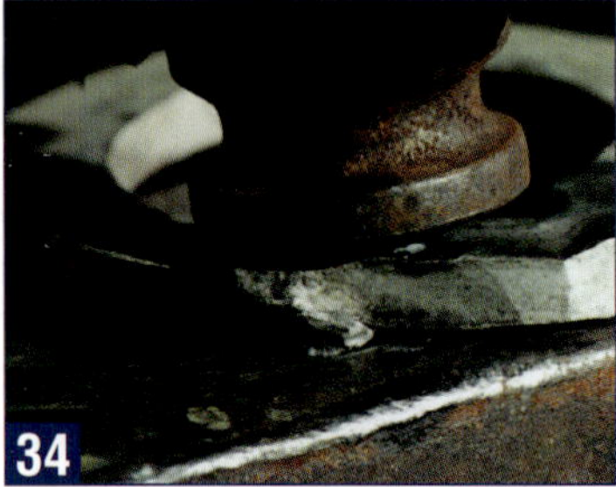

When it melts, bring the shoe out of the fire and press on the weld.

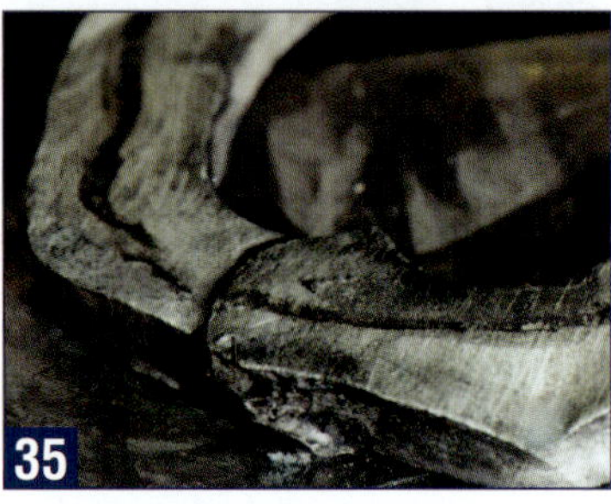

Check that it has cooled down before working it.

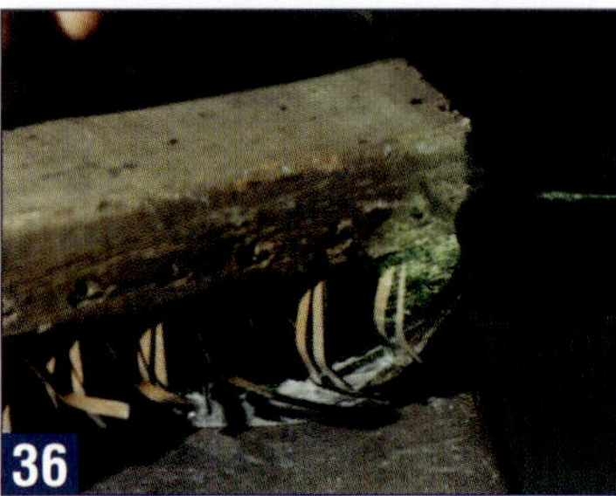

Brush the weld.

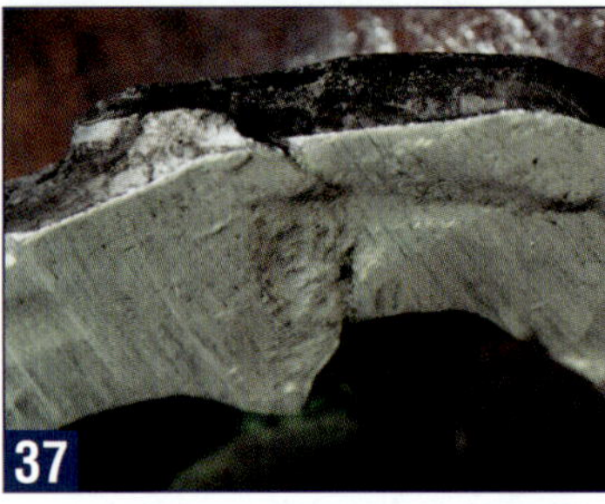

Here is the first weld. Notice the little crack on the right side from getting too hot. I will weld the crack on the next heat.

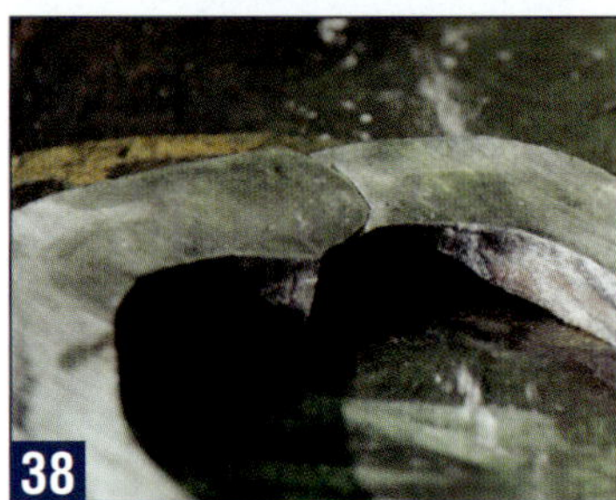

Forge it flat.

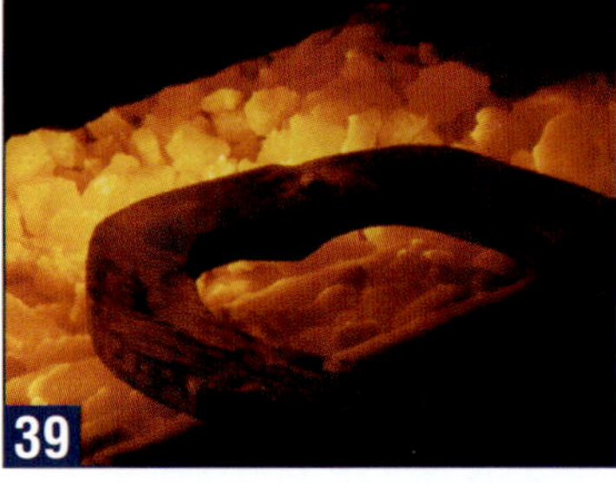

Flux, place rod on the bar, and go back to the fire for second weld.

adding material in the form of an aluminum brazing wire, so we are really brazing instead of welding.

Take some brazing wire and cut it on the end of the anvil face **(Figure 30)**. Bend the pieces of wire so they won't roll around on the shoe. In **Figure 31**, I have placed the aluminum welding flux on the area of the shoe to be welded, then placed the pieces of brazing rod on top of the flux. Flux needs to go all around the area to be brazed, because when it gets molten, it has to coat the entire surface of the scarves to provide a capillary action and draw in the molten brazing rod. (It may help to hammer the brazing rod flat. This increases the surface area, allowing the rod to heat and run more quickly, and avoids overheating the shoe.)

With a very steady hand, place the bar with the flux and wire under the flame in the forge, as in **Figure 32**. I brought it out of the fire for **Figure 33** so that you can see how the brazing rod has balled up into little puddles of molten aluminum. The reason you need to be so steady is that the molten aluminum can fall off of the shoe if you happen

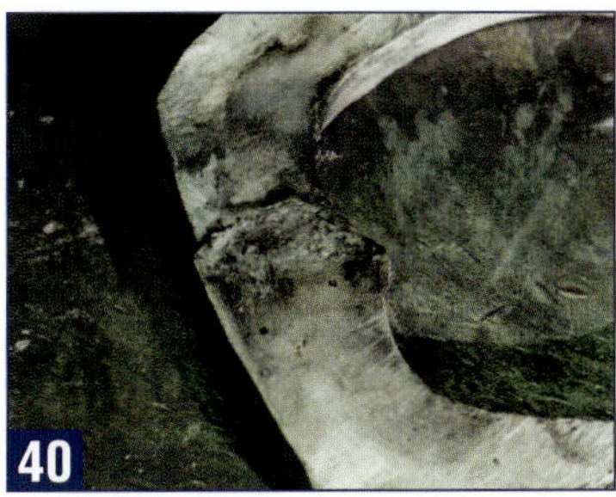
40
Second weld is done.

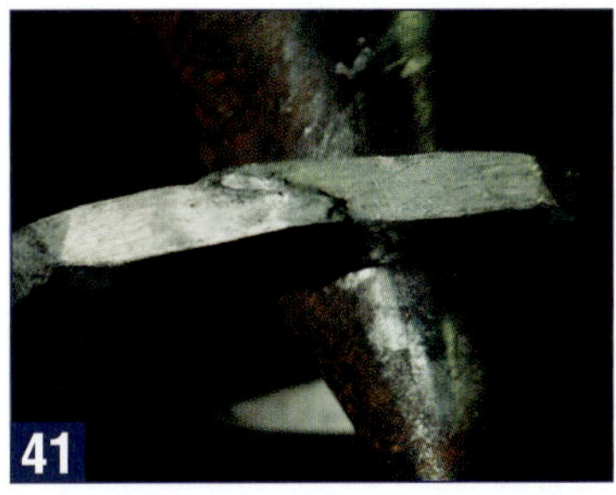
41
You can see the outside of the bar. It may not look like it, but it is welded.

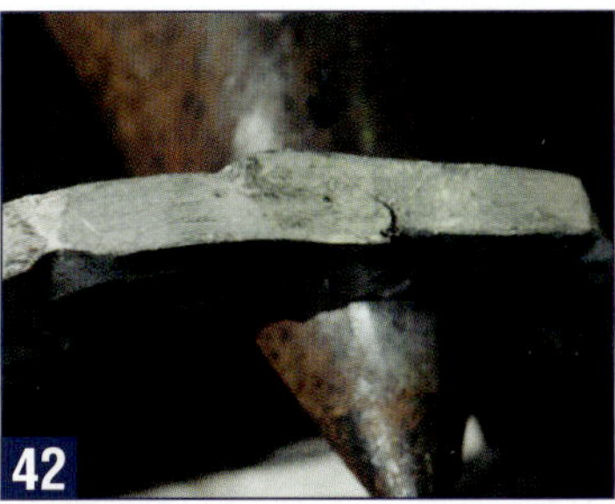
42
Forge the outside of the bar on the horn.

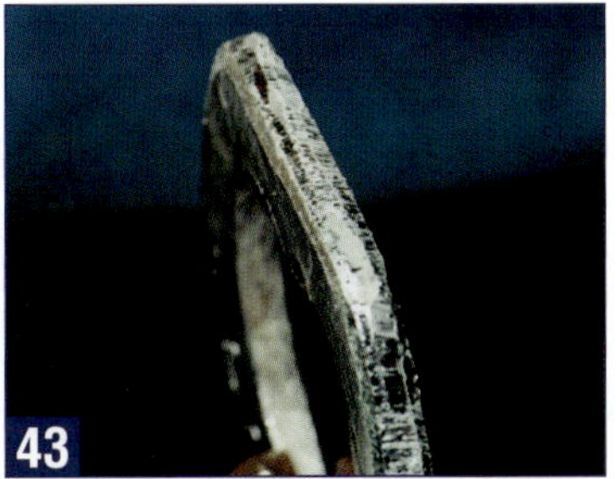
43
Here is the bar after welding, forging and rasping.

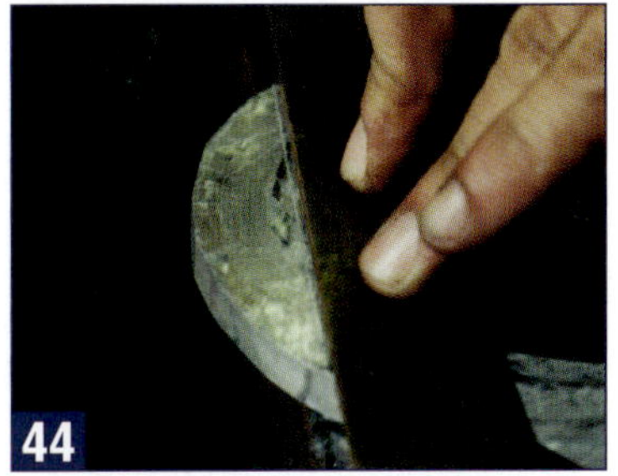
44
Layout start of fullering.

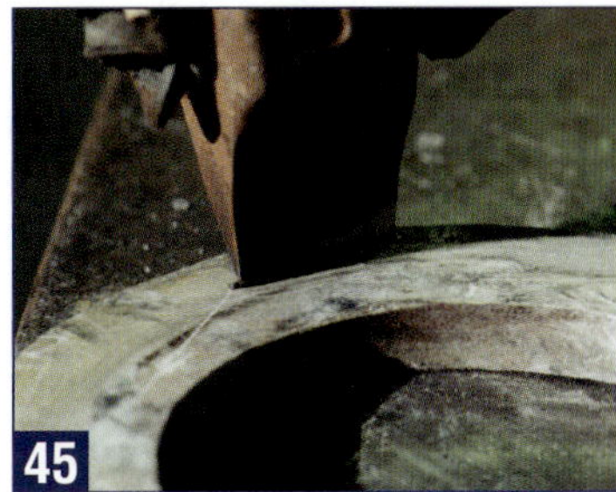
45
Mark fullering.

to tilt it. Go back to the fire and let the shoe get hot enough that the molten brazing rod is sucked between the scarves by the capillary action.

Once the little puddles of brazing rod are sucked into the weld, come out slowly without tilting the shoe, place it on the anvil, and push down on the weld with your hammer **(Figure 34)**. Notice I said to press with your hammer, but don't actually hammer, just press. The rod is still molten, so if you tilt the shoe or hammer on it, the molten material will be squeezed out. Besides, the aluminum in the bar shoe itself is too hot to hit.

Be patient. If you are at a contest, you may want to place this shoe off to the side. When it is cool enough to work, you can see the black mark stays on the stock **(Figure 35)**. Brush the shoe up well before hammering on it so that you don't drive any of the flux into the stock **(Figure 36)**. Look carefully at the right side of the bar in **Figure 37** and you will see a crack where I actually got this shoe a little too hot. Surprisingly, this is not a problem. As long as I let it cool down far enough, I can braze that crack together when I finish up the brazing.

Figure 38 is the opposite side of the bar. I am brazing from the other side in **Figure 39**, and

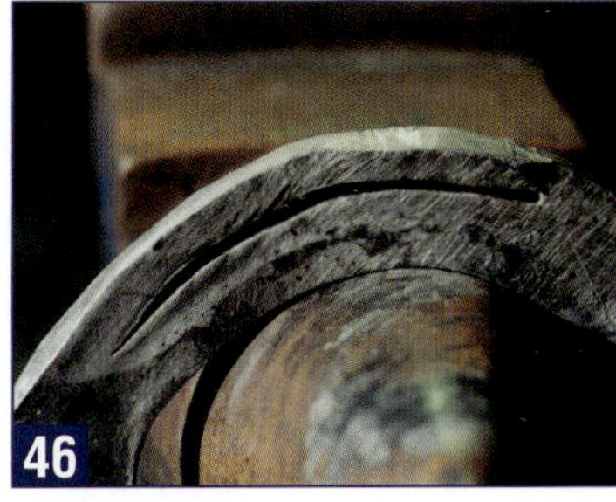
46
Hem the shoe.

Figure 40 is how the shoe will look when it is brazed but is not yet cleaned up. There are some small cracks where the pieces come together, but these will forge and rasp out, so you will not even see where the shoe came together.

Figure 41 shows the outside of the bar before I hit it, and **Figure 42** is after a couple of hammer blows. **Figure 43** shows the shoe after it is rasped.

Now I am going to fuller this shoe. I wait until it is cool enough to crease, and then I mark the beginning of my fullering **(Figure 44)**. Make one light pass with the fuller to mark the crease **(Figure**

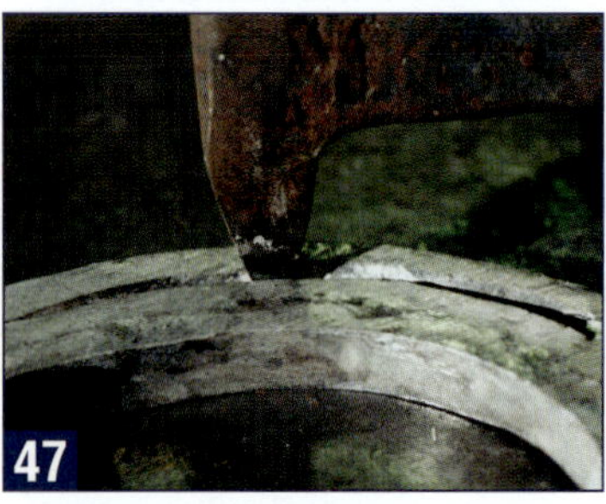

Fuller, drift, pritchel, and use nails to finish holes.

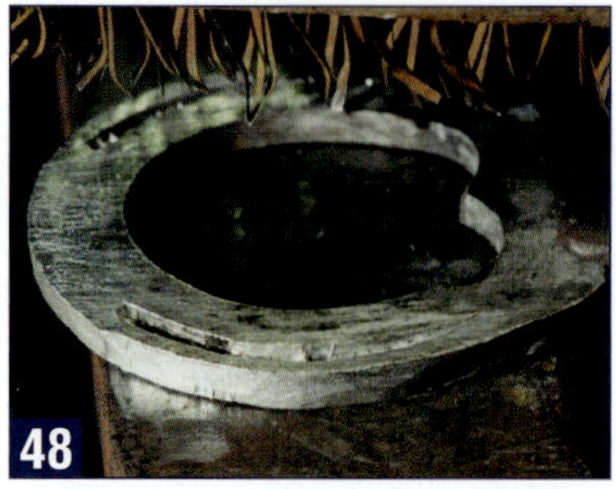

Clean up the shoe with a butcher block brush.

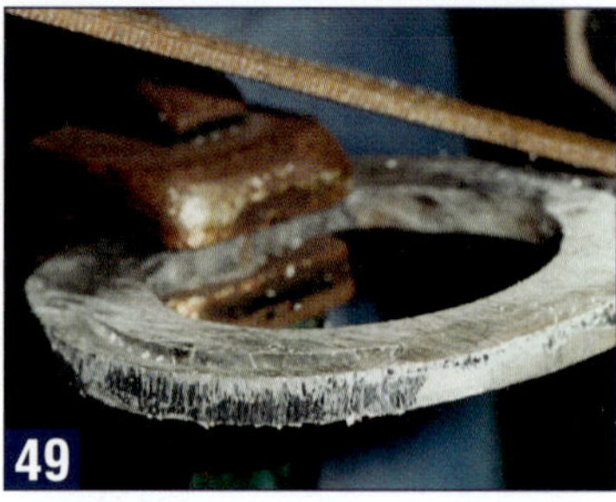

Rasp it.

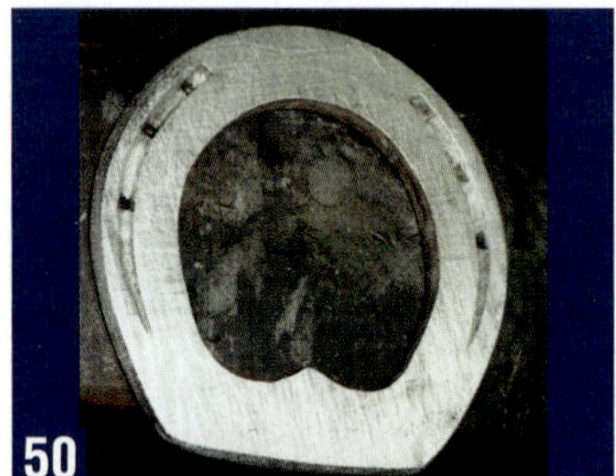

The finished product.

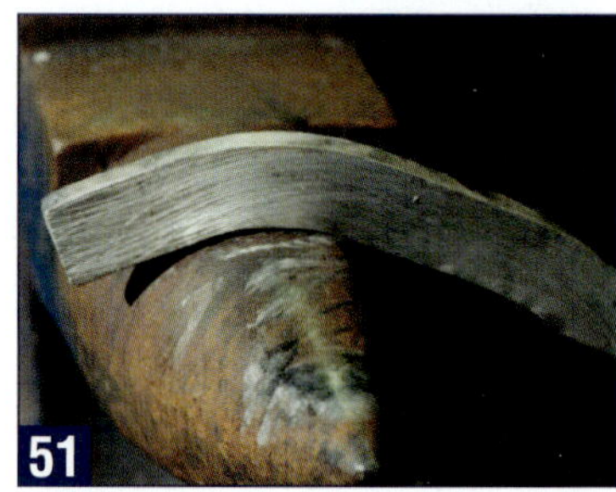

Bend the end of the branch around the horn.

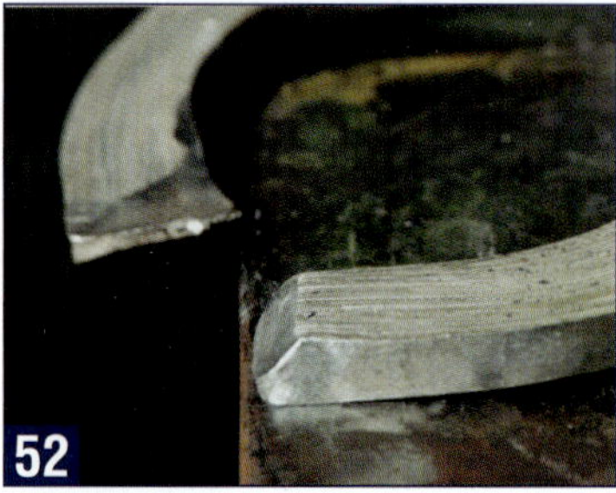

Scarf both ends of the stock for welding.

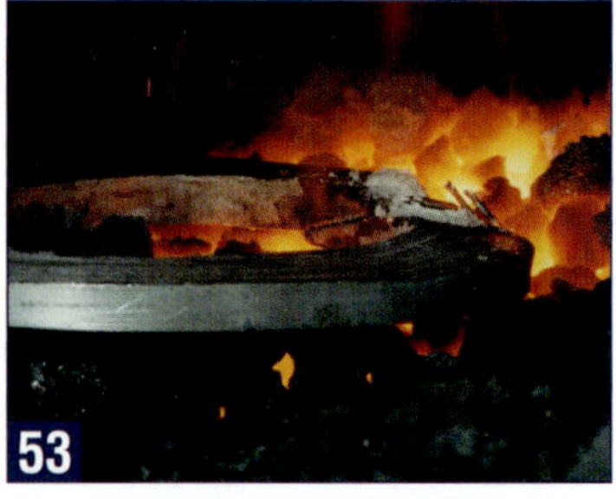

Put together, apply flux and rod, and place in the coke fire.

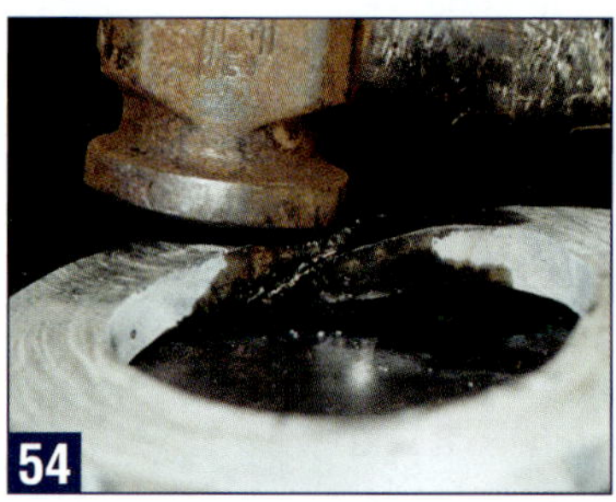

When it runs, bring it out of the fire and press with hammerhead.

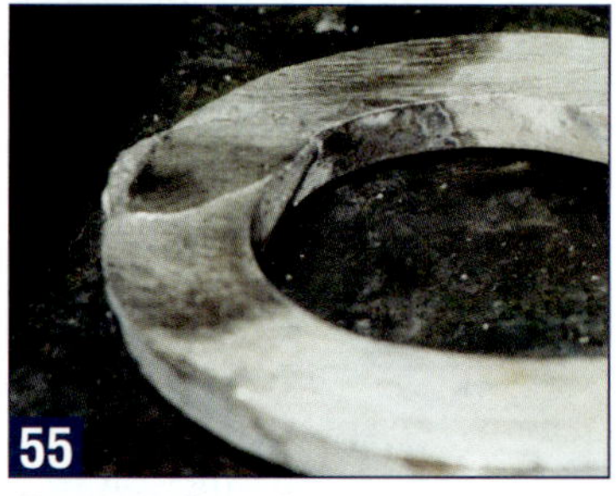

Forge it flat after the first weld, once it is cool enough to hit.

45), then hem the shoe on the horn **(Figure 46)**. Aluminum does not act like steel, and you will find that a lot of the finish in this shoe is going to come from the rasp, not the hammer. Finish fullering and drift the holes **(Figure 47)**. Pritchel and size the holes as described on the previous aluminum shoe with nail heads, then clean it up. Brush the shoe with a butcher block **(Figure 48)** move to the vise to rasp and file the shoe **(Figure 49)**. Use the fine brush to finish, and you will end up with a shoe that looks like the one in **Figure 50**.

ALUMINUM EGG BAR SHOES

Our next aluminum project is to weld an egg bar. We are going to make this one in the coke forge. A coke fire is so much hotter than propane fires that working aluminum in coke is risky. Just be aware of that, and you should have no problems. Begin with the toe bend, then bring the end of the stock around as in **Figure 51**. Do the same to the opposite branch, then make short beveled scarves as in **Figure 52**. Build your fire up so that you have a lot of hot coals in the top of the fire. Scarf and place the brazing rod on the area to be brazed. Place the shoe

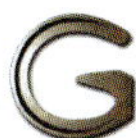

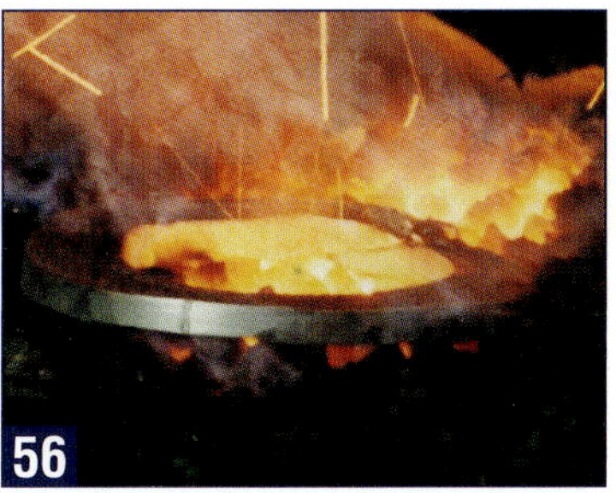

56

Take second welding heat.

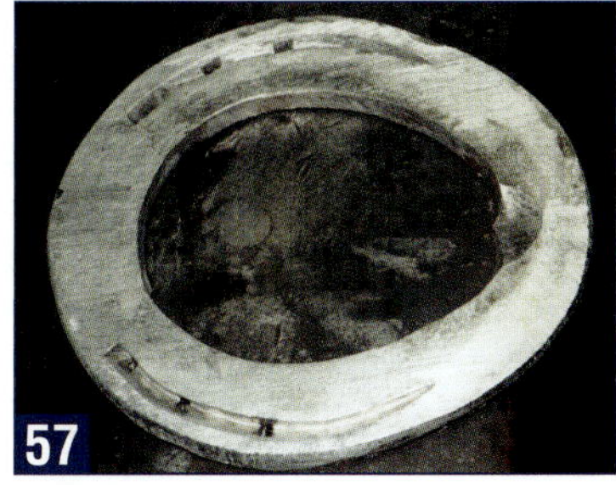

57

Finished egg bar.

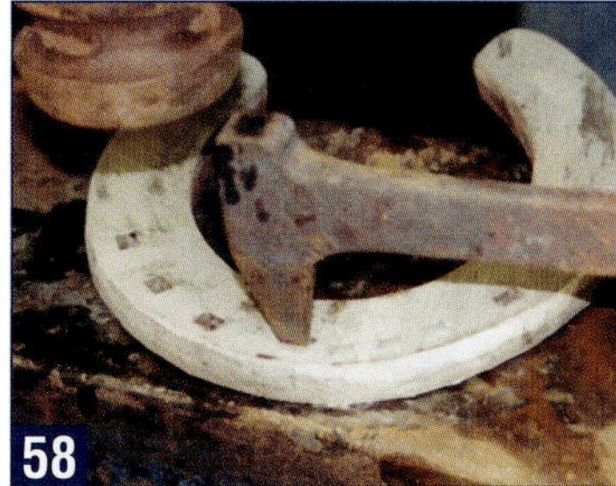

58

Drift a series of nail holes across the toe.

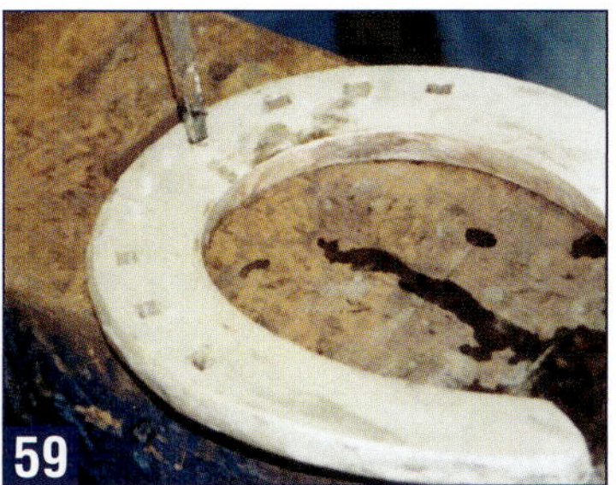

59

Pritchel.

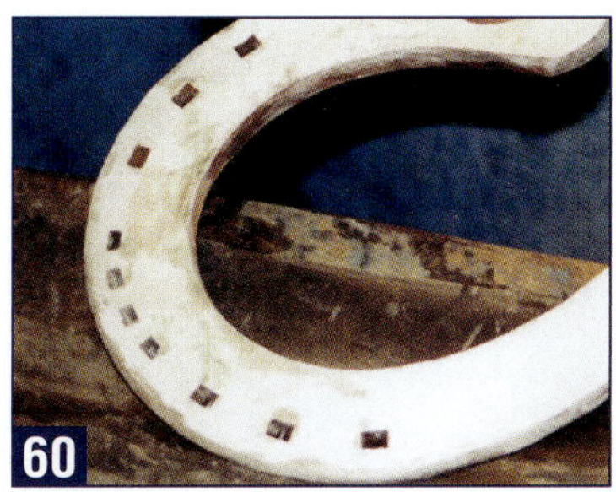

60

Place one nail at a time into a hole.

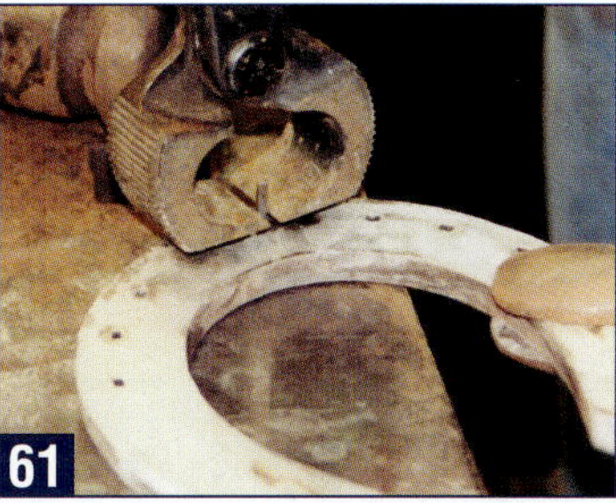

61

Cut off short on the hoof surface.

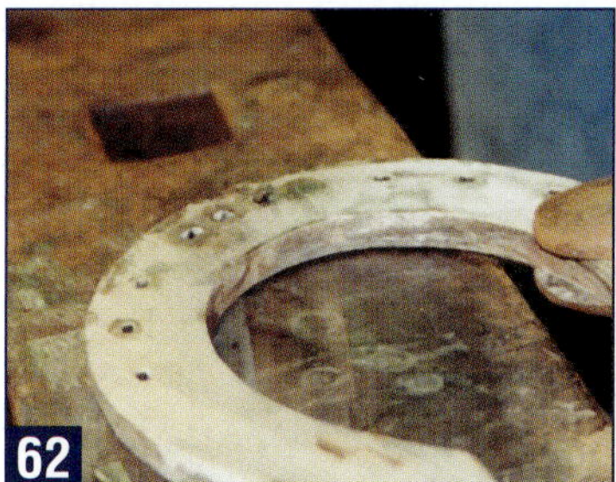

62

Brad up the end that was cut.

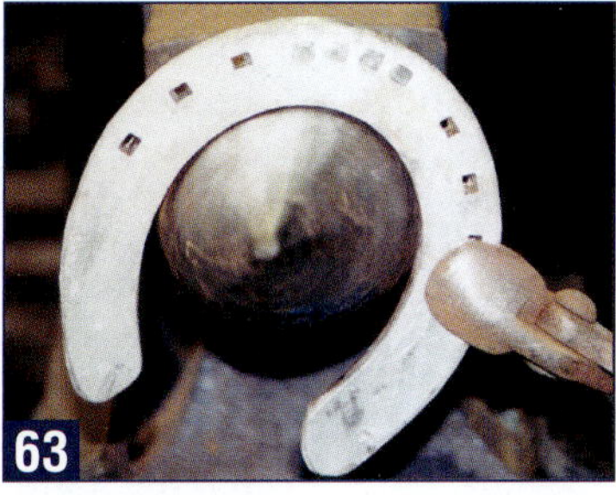

63

Forge back to original dimensions.

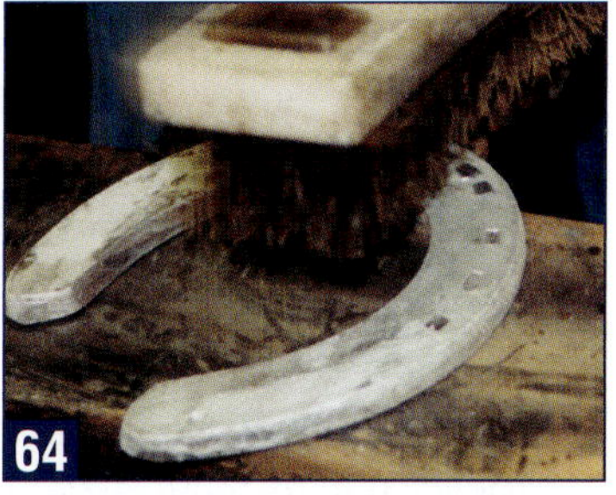

64

Brush to clean up the shoe.

on the top of the fire and watch for the rod to melt and run into the joint **(Figure 53)**. Bring the shoe out of the fire and press on it with your hammer as I am doing in **Figure 54**. Let the shoe cool to at least forging temperature, brush it up, turn it over to flux again and apply brazing rod, then return to the fire **(Figures 55-56)**. Fuller, punch, and finish the shoe. It should look like **Figure 57**.

WEAR PLATE OPTIONS

As stated earlier, one of the downsides with aluminum is that it wears too quickly. Most commercial aluminum shoes will have a small steel plate in the toe of the shoe to increase the wearability. With a handmade aluminum shoe, you can add your own wear plate. Here are a couple of common methods that work pretty well.

If you want to use nails for the wear plate, punch a series of holes with your fore punch across the toe **(Figure 58)**. Pritchel **(Figure 59)**, and the shoe will look like the shoe in **Figure 60**. Drive one nail in at a time and cut it off on the hoof surface with about 1/8-inch inch showing **(Figure 61)**. Brad up the piece of nail that is sticking out of the shoe like I

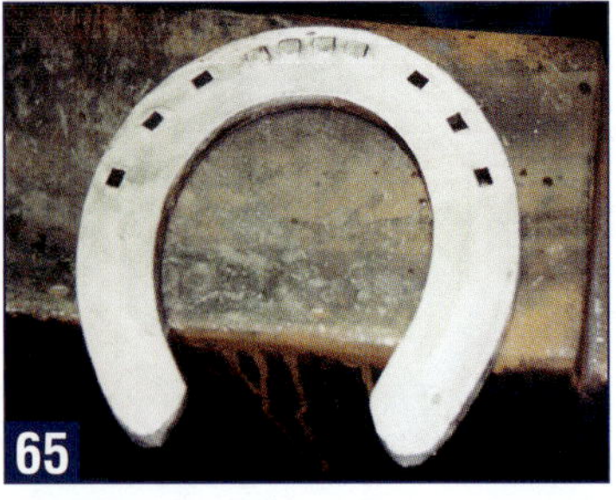
Finished shoe with nails for wear plate.

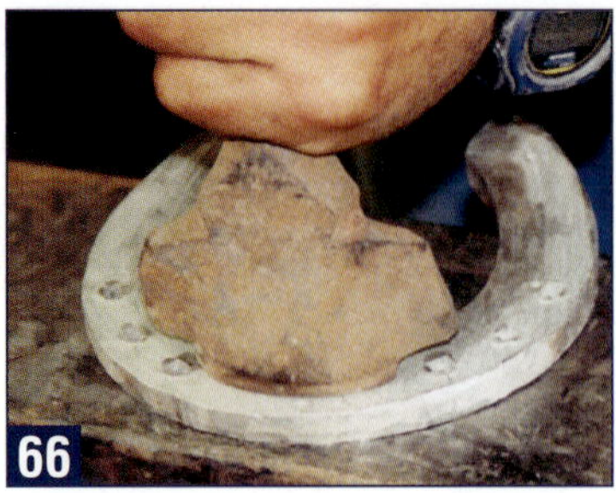
Jim Keith wear plate tool.

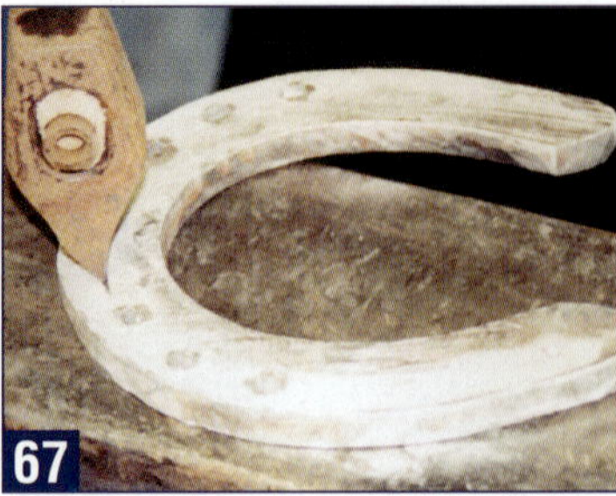
Fullering the wear plate area in the toe.

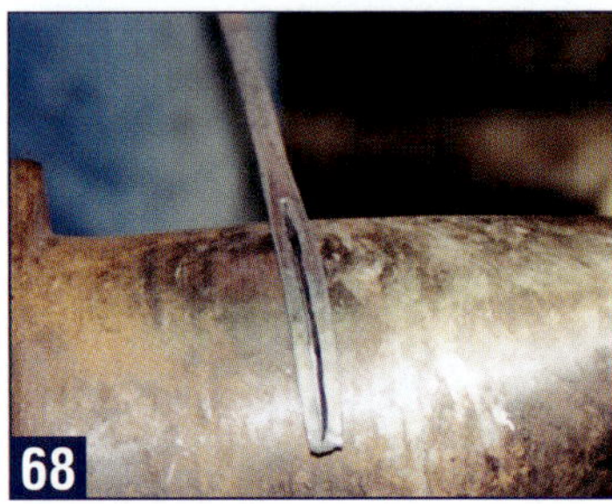
The piece that is going to be the wear plate. Forged, creased, and bent around the horn.

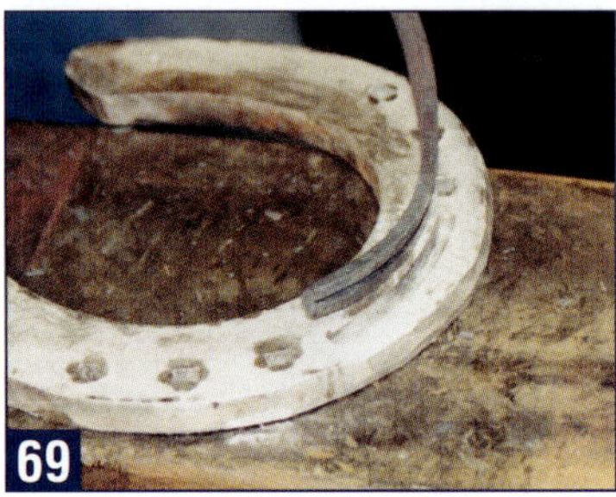
Measure over the cut area.

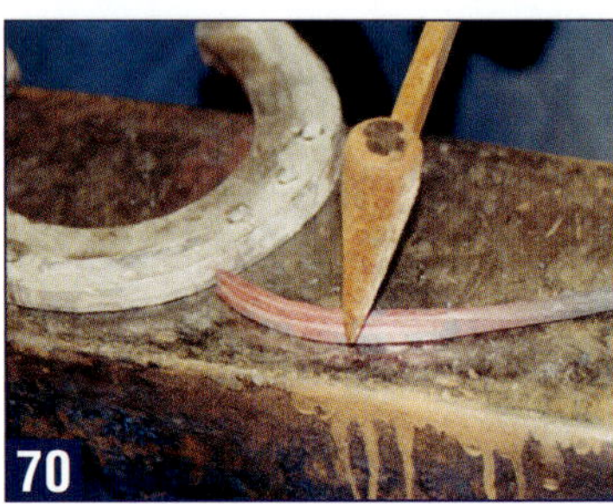
Cut off the wear plate.

am doing in **Figure 62**, and then do the next nail. Do only one at a time so that one won't interfere with the next. When they are all in and bradded up, move to the horn to forge the frog eyes from punching the holes back into the shoe **(Figure 63)**. Finish as before **(Figure 64)**, and your shoe will look like the finished shoe in **Figure 65**. If you are going to clip this shoe, I recommend that you put the wear plate nails into the toe prior to making the toe clip. That's experience talking there.

Another type of wear plate can be made by placing a piece of metal into the toe. This is similar to the type of wear plate you will see on a keg shoe. In **Figure 66**, I am using a tool that Jim Keith made for me that he designed to make the cut for a wear plate. He made it in his trip hammer by smashing the upset end on a piece of sucker rod and then putting a slight radius in it. This tool is like a curved cold chisel.

Since a tool like that is not easily found, I am going to show you how to place this wear plate while using tools that you already have. Determine where you want the wear plate, and then run your fuller through that area **(Figure 67)**.

Forge a piece of 1/4-inch round into a piece that is rectangular, roughly 1/8-by-1/4 inch. Whatever you do, be certain that the piece is not wider than the stock that the shoe is made from is thick. In other words, if you have a shoe made out of 3/8-by-1 inch, your wear plate should be about 1/8 inch less than 3/8 inch. When you are done forging the piece, cut a small groove in it and bend it to the radius that matches the toe of the shoe **(Figure 68)**. Some people call this a blood groove from the tradition of making a groove in a knife blade. We put a groove on the wear plate so that there is an area to drive the aluminum into to hold the wear plate in place. The groove should be on the outside of the wear plate.

Conversely, you can forge the wear plate so that it is a slightly wedge-shaped cross section. By doing this, you can put the large part into the bottom of the crease, and when you close up the material in the shoe, the wear plate is dovetailed into the shoe. I like the blood groove better, but you can try both.

Match and measure the radius of the plate and shoe **(Figure 69)**. Cut it off with a sharp hot cut **(Figure 70)**. Cool the plate and heat the shoe. Drive the cold plate into the hot shoe **(Figure 71)**, and it will look like the shoe in **Figure 72**. Move to the horn and forge the material into the groove

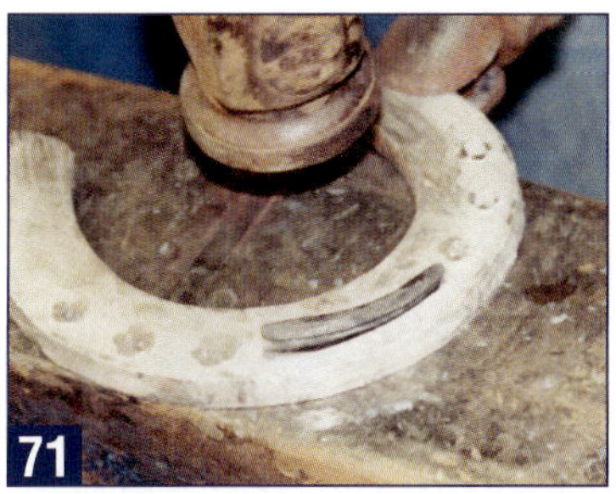

Warm the shoe, cool the wear plate, and drive it into the area creased through the toe.

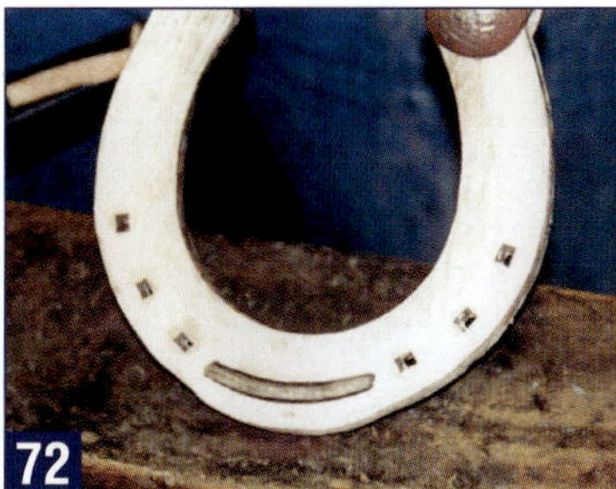

Piece in the shoe.

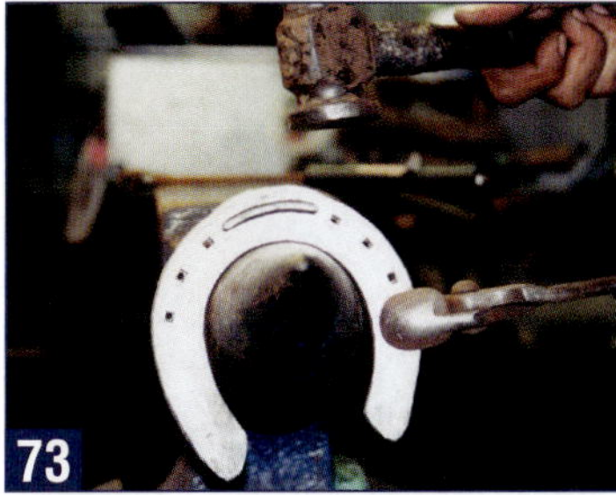

Forge back to original dimensions.

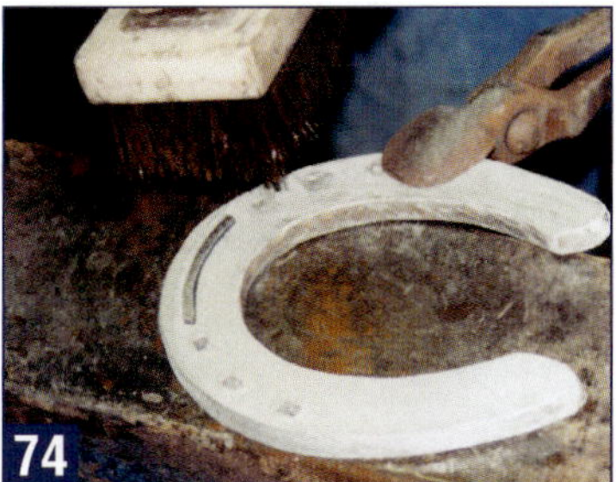

Brush to clean up.

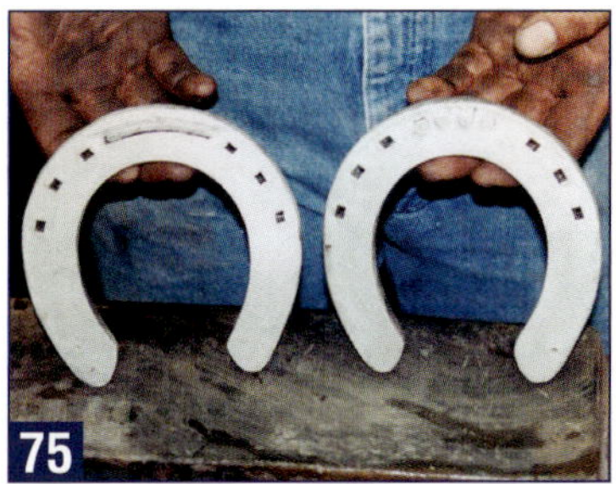

Both shoes with different types of wear devices in the toe.

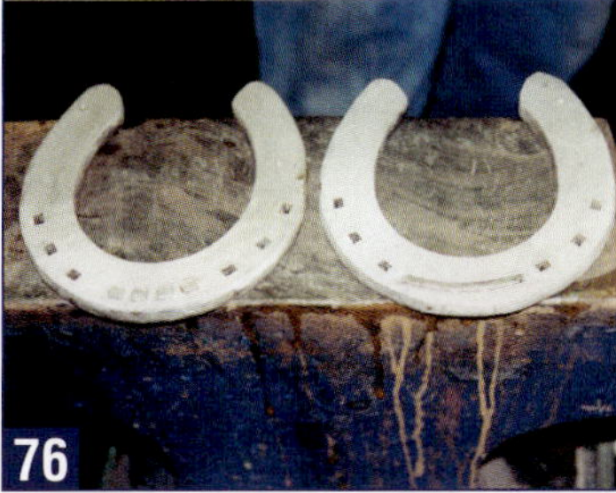

Another view of the wear devices.

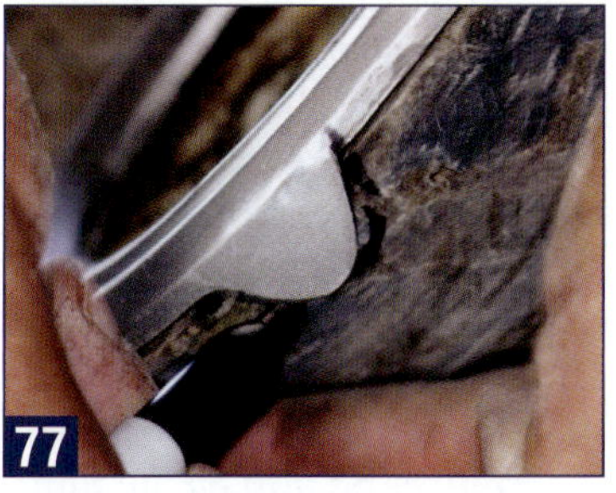

Draw around clip with a marker.

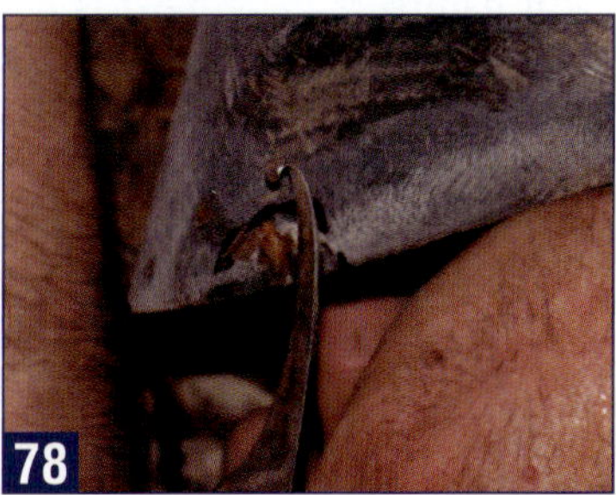

Cut out the area with a hoof knife.

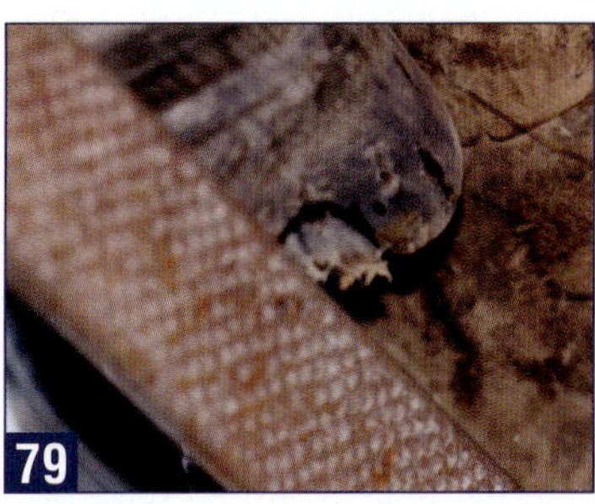

You can also rasp out the clip area.

on the wear plate **(Figure 73)**. Clean it up as before **(Figure 74)**, and you should have a pair of aluminum shoes with increased wearability **(Figure 75)**. **Figure 76** is another look at the wear plates.

USING CLIPPED ALUMINUM SHOES

When you are nailing aluminum shoes on feet with clips, you can't get the shoe hot enough to hot fit, so fitting clips is a little more difficult. Begin by shaping the shoe to the foot. In **Figure 77**, I am marking the area of the clip with a marker. This tells me where the clip will be so that I can cut it into its fit. To cut out the area for the clip, you can use your knife **(Figure 78)** or you can use your rasp **(Figure 79)**. Nail the shoe on the foot and hammer the clip into the foot **(Figure 80)**. If you look closely at **Figure 80**, you will see that I am holding the opposite foot in the air while I tap on the clip. I like the foot to be loaded if I am going to hammer on a clip.

Generally, I am opposed to hammering on clips for several reasons. First, there is the positive pressure that is left on the foot by the metal being bent into the foot. Next, there is the pressure from either

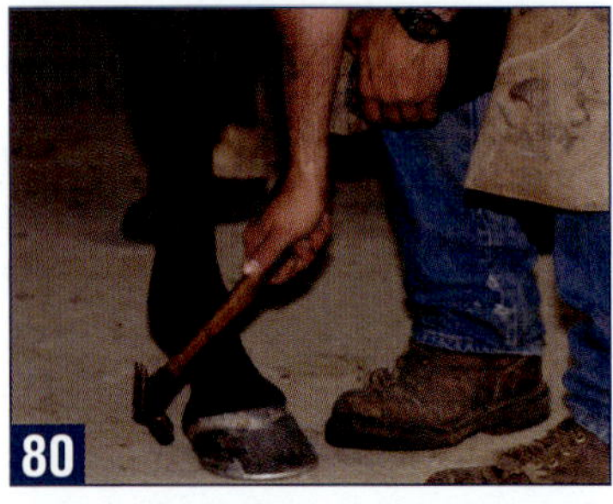

When the shoe is on, you may have to hammer on the aluminum clip. Notice that I am holding the other foot up.

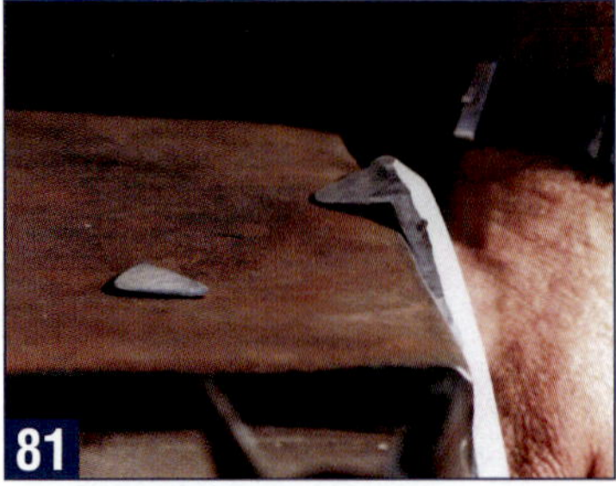

Breaking clips off of an aluminum keg shoe on the edge of the anvil.

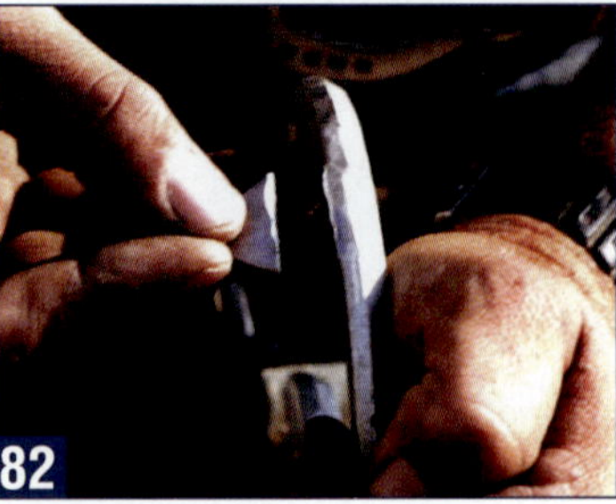

The shoe with the clip broken off.

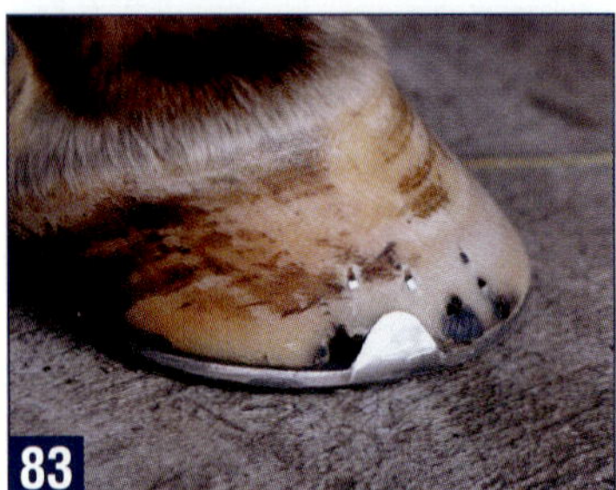

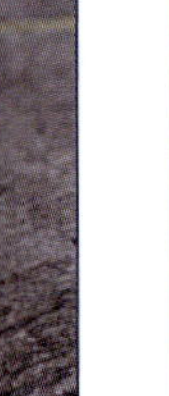

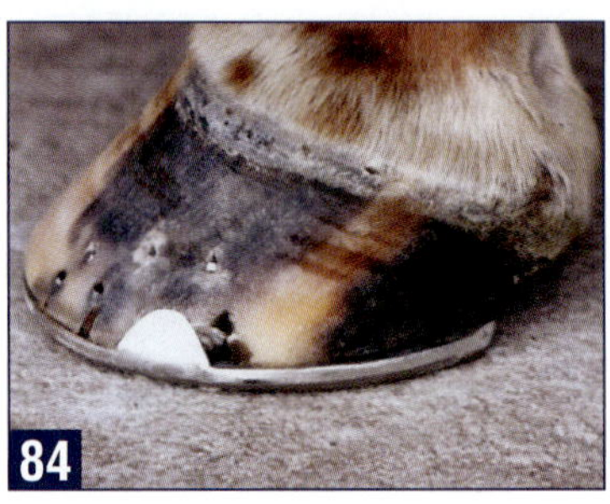

Finished foot with cold fit aluminum clips.

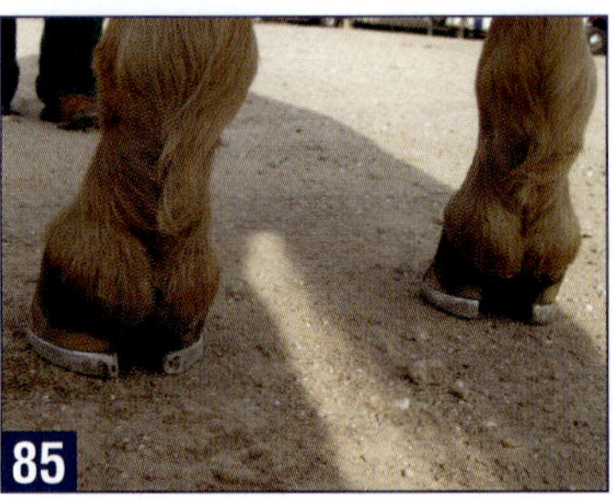

Palmar view of Cody's customer's horse with navicular syndrome.

side clamping across the foot when you hammer on quarter or side clips. Finally, having to hammer steel clips is a sign that you lack skill in fitting clips. Clips should be cut and burned into position when shoeing hot, but you may have to hammer with aluminum. At least aluminum is not as strong as steel and should not leave so great a positive pressure.

When you do hammer in a clip, be certain that you hammer from the base of the clip and stop as soon as the clip is tight against the foot.

If you don't like clips on your aluminum keg shoes, they are very easy to break off on the edge of the anvil as shown in **Figure 81**. **Figure 82** shows how clean the clip breaks off, but you will still have to rasp off the sharp area where the clip was attached. **Figures 83 and 84** are a couple of finished feet with aluminum clips.

Next is a series from one of Cody's customers who had a horse with navicular syndrome. I was helping Cody shoe that day, and he was going to make handmade shoes for this horse. Cody was 17 years old, so he wanted to play the old-bull, young-bull game. So, here is the result of a horse that Cody and I shod together. **Figure 85** gives the palmar view where you can see the heel fit and elevation in the wedged aluminum shoes. **Figures 86 and 87** are Cody's work, and **Figures 88 and 89** are mine. You can pick your bull. He has a better clip fit, but my rocker toe is a little cleaner.

I want to end this chapter with a picture of a shoe that you won't see too often: This is a tooled and fullered aluminum shoe that Cody made out of 1/2-by-1 inch aluminum bar stock for his AWCF shoe display. I was honored to be his striker.

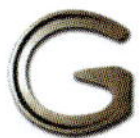

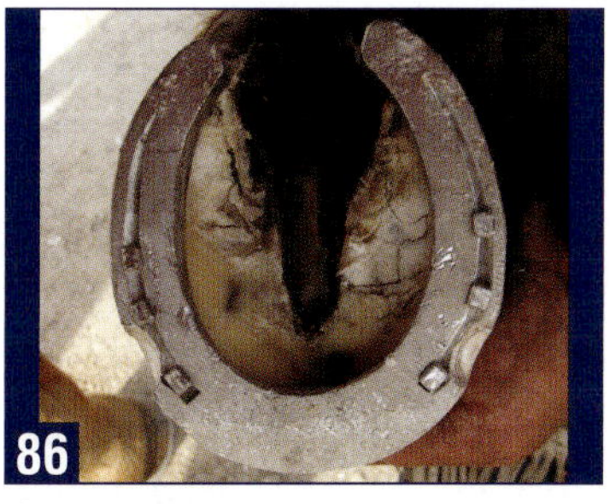

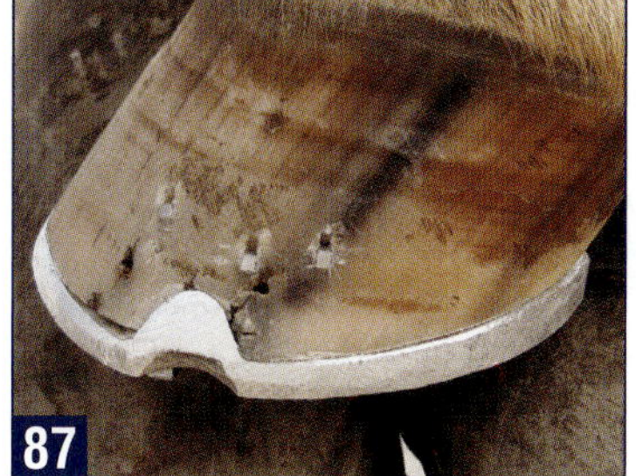

Cody's job.

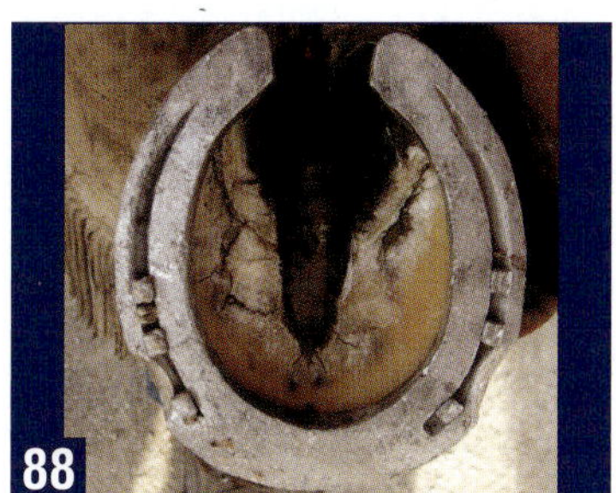

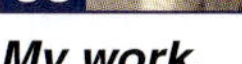

My work.

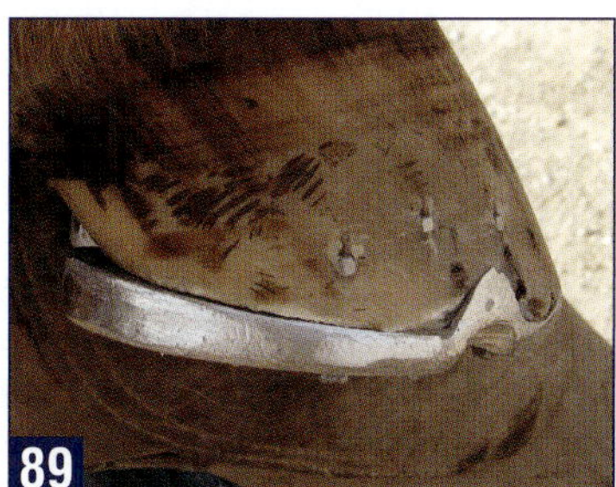

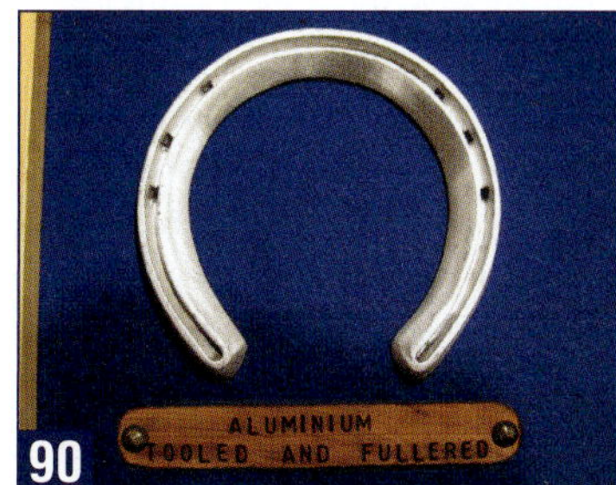

Aluminum tooled and fullered shoe from Cody's AWCF shoe display.

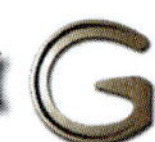

Chapter

54 HOSPITAL PLATE

A hospital plate is the ultimate in protection for an injured foot. There are several ways to protect the foot, from boots, to bandages to pour-ins, to pads. **Figure 1 and 2** are a boot and a bandaged foot. Regardless of the type of horses they shoe, almost every farrier will encounter a time when the hospital plate is the ideal method.

Traditionally, the hospital plate is bolted to the horseshoe with four bolts. **Figures 3 and 4** show a W-shoe with a four-bolt hospital plate. With a W-shoe, the four-bolt method is preferred. This is a secure way to attach the plate, but if I can attach the plate with one bolt, it makes changing the dressing less complicated for the customer. The easier I can make their job, the more likely it will be done. That turns into success not only for the horse, but for the customer and the farrier as well.

The hospital plate explained in this chapter is not a new idea. Several years ago I attended a Dave Farley, CF, clinic in Arkansas. He had a collection of shoes with him, and this hospital plate was among them. Since that time, I have had it on countless horses.

There is also another method that was on a shoe display that was made by Rodney King, CJF, AWCF, of New Zealand. Rodney worked at Rood & Riddle Equine Hospital in Kentucky, and he came to the school to take his AWCF. I took a picture of his hospital plate and included it here. It is a pretty neat way to make one as well **(Figures 5-7)**.

For the horse in this series, we had been dealing with a chronic infection that was a result of founder. You can see that it is in the later stages **(Figure 8)**, but there had been the appearance of a slice in the sole. The founder was a result of having to bear weight on this foot while the opposite foot was healing from severe damage incurred from kicking a barn.

The one-bolt hospital plate requires a straight-bar shoe. Begin with a normal straight bar. Once it is built, forge the sex appeal out of the bar and make

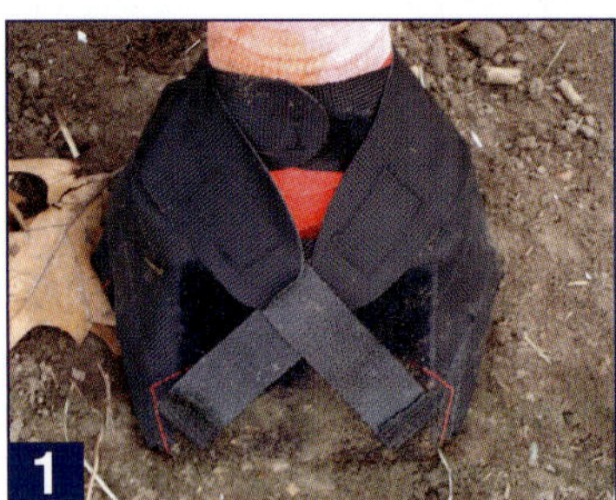

Temporary abscess boot from Kaeco.

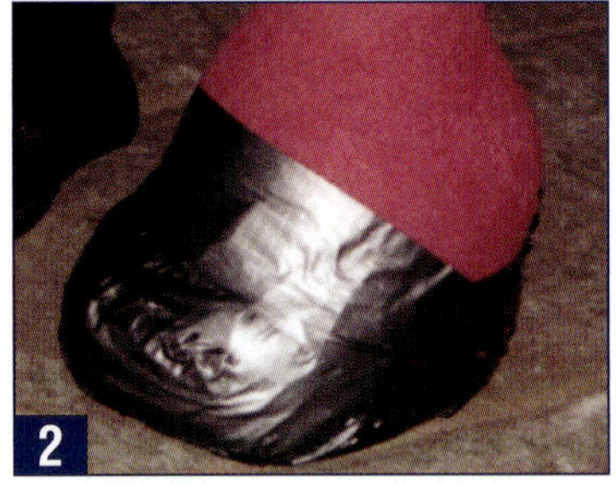

Bandaged foot with elastic bandage and duct tape.

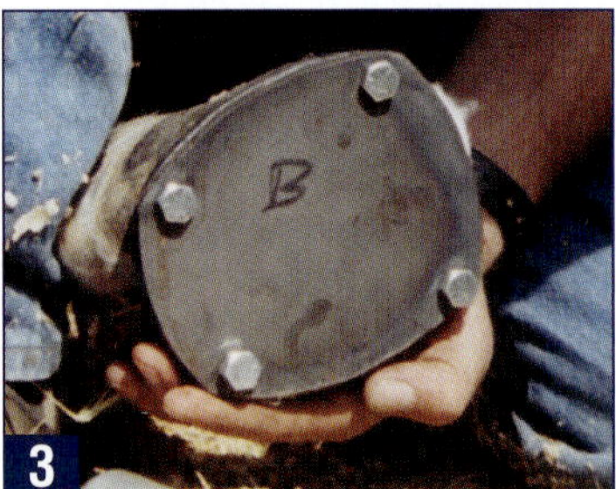

four-bolt hospital plate.

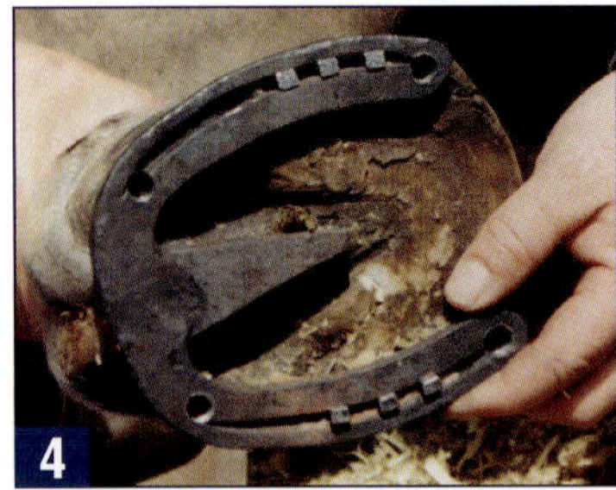

W-shoe that had the four-bolt plate on it.

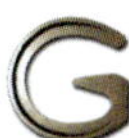

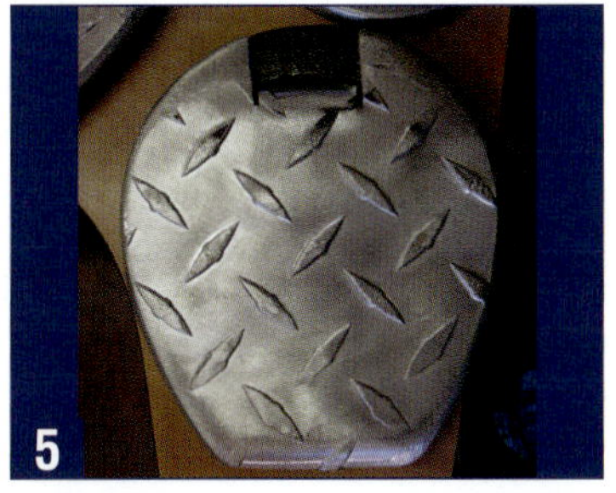

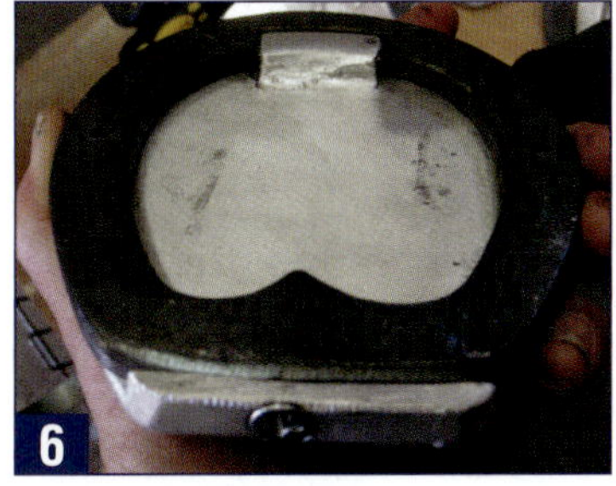

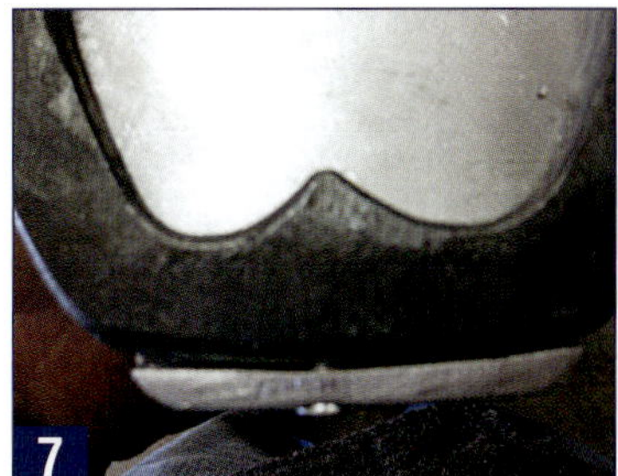

Another method of making the one-bolt hospital plate.

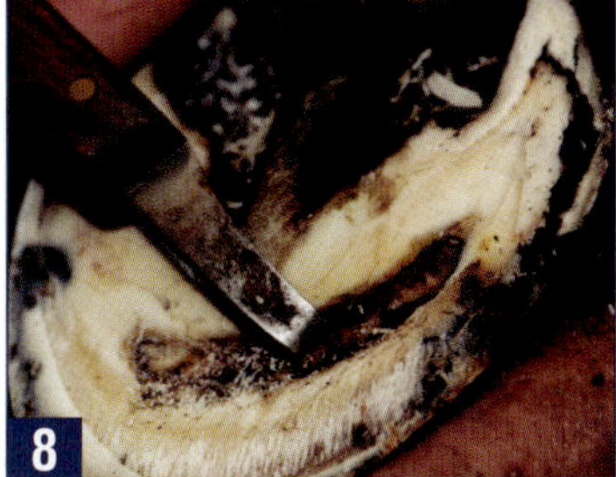

Foundered foot with chronic abscess.

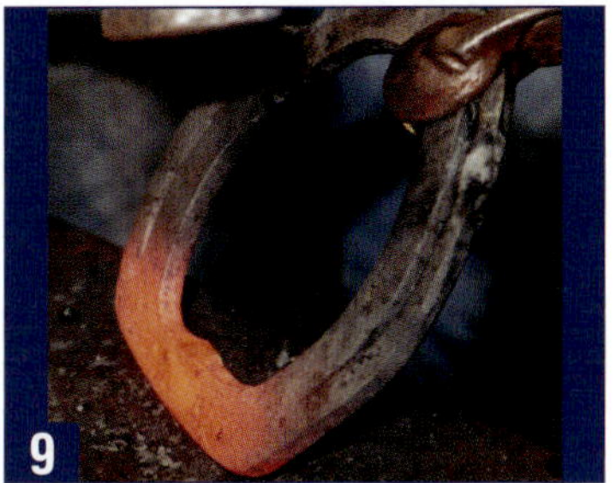

Forging on the bar of the straight bar shoe.

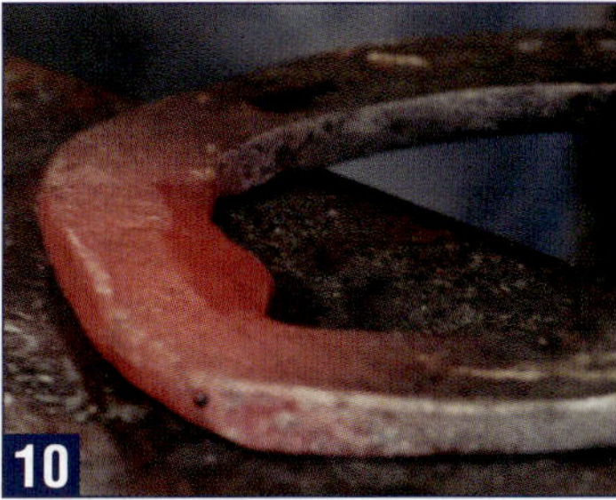

Making the bevel for the hospital plate to fit in.

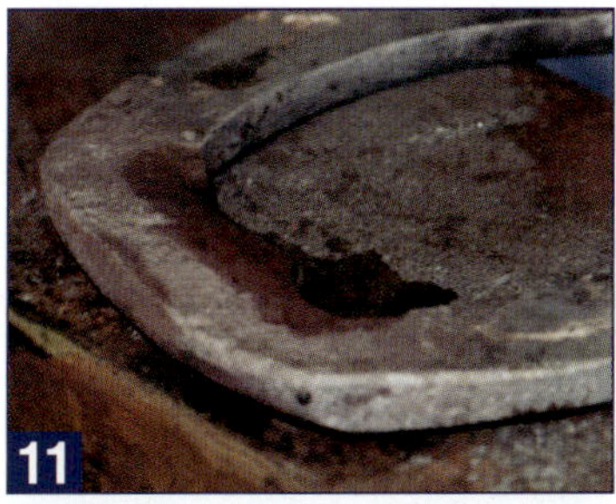

The shoe with the bevel finished.

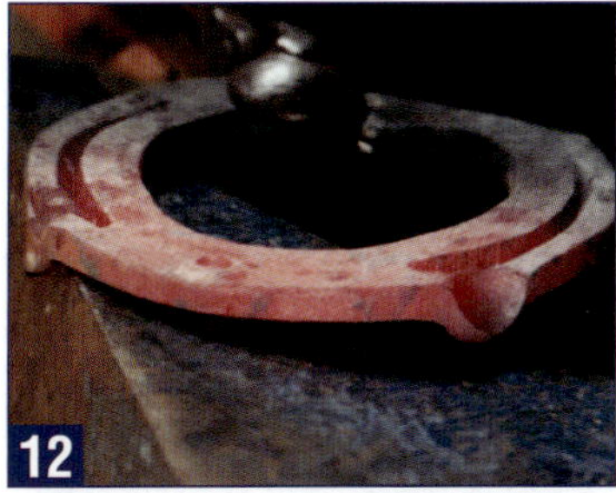

Making the clips with a good source.

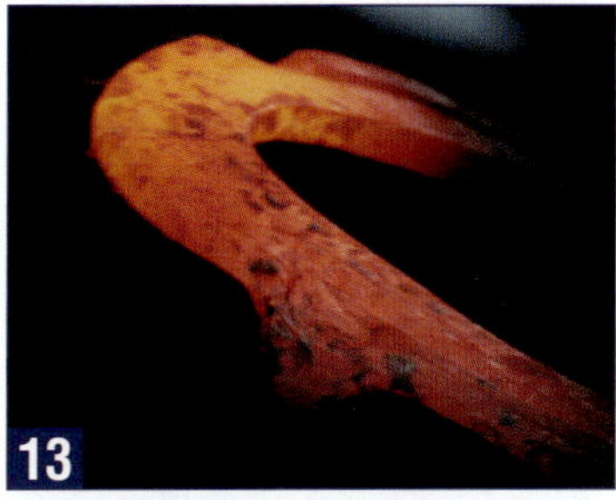

Bending the rocker toe.

a good bevel on the hoof surface of the bar **(Figures 9-11)**. Draw a pair of clips with a ball peen, and make a well- defined source hole and a rocker toe **(Figures 12-13)**.

Once the shoe is complete, draw around the shoe on the material you are going to use to make the plate **(Figure 14)**. Mark it cold with your hot-cut **(Figure 15)**. Heat the plate and cut it out. After the plate is cut out, you need to cut the flange on the bottom of the plate to fit into the bevel you forged on the bar. Reheat the plate and bend the flange so that it will fit into the bar **(Figures 16-17)**. Place the hot plate on the bar shoe, and bend it to match the rocker toe and

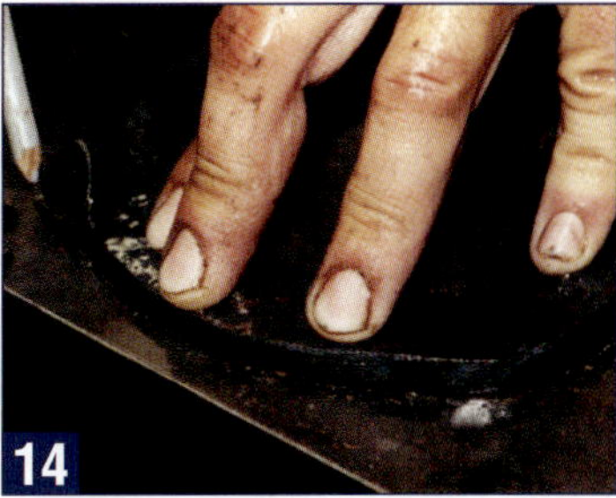

Mark the plate with a piece of soapstone, silver sharpie, or a silver pencil.

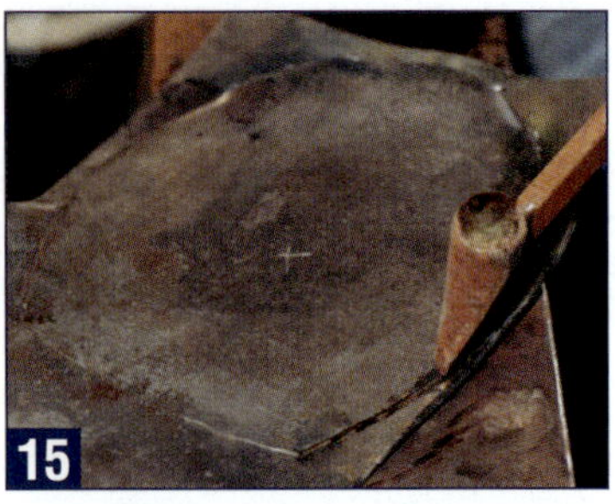

15 *Use a hot-cut to mark and cut the plate.*

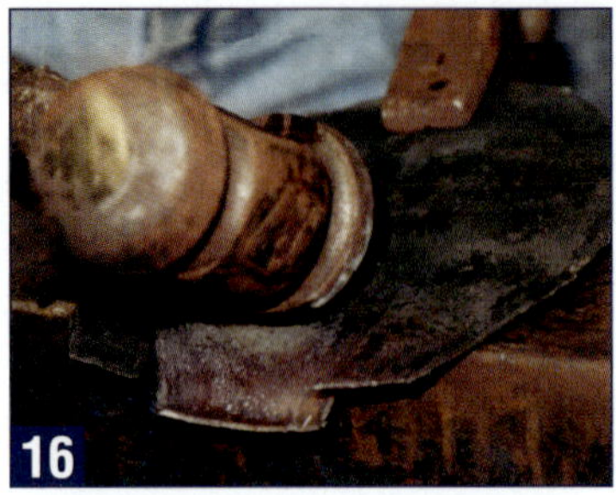

16 *Begin bending the flange.*

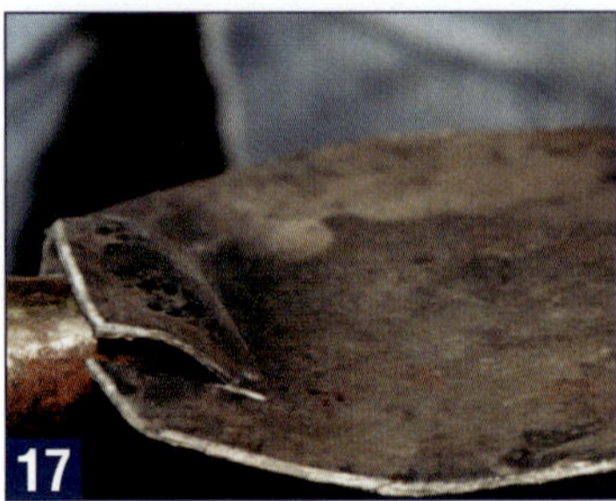

17 *You can use the horn to work on the angle of the flange.*

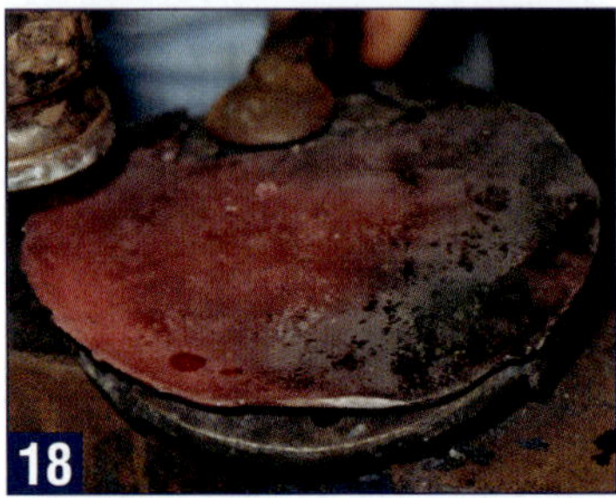

18

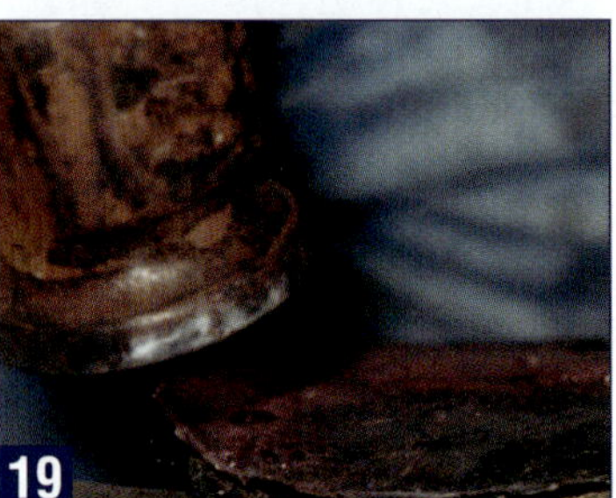

19

Heated plate being formed to the shoe.

20 *Forge the plate into the clip source.*

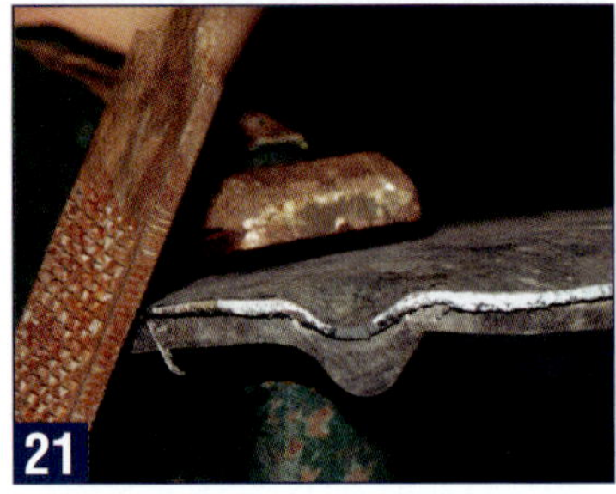

21 *Rasp the plate to fit with the shoe and plate in a vise.*

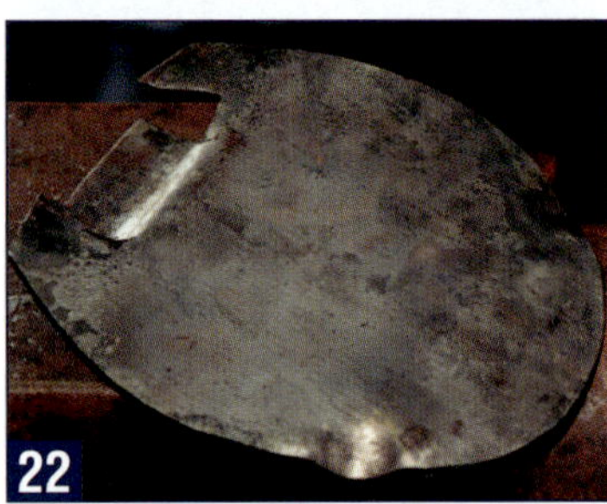

22 *Finished plate.*

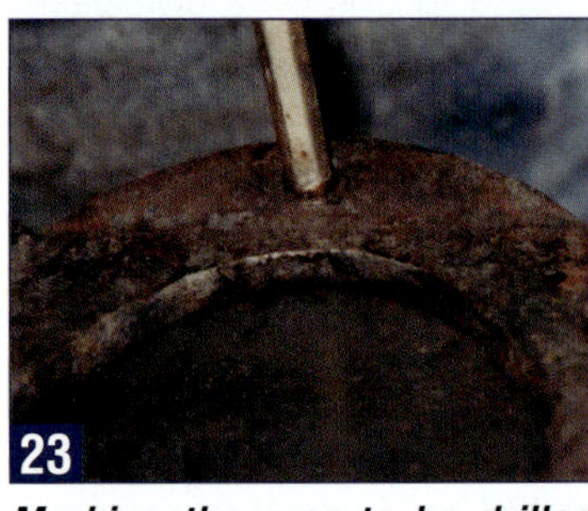

23 *Marking the area to be drilled on the plate.*

clip areas of the shoe **(Figures 18-20)**. Place the shoe and plate in a vise and rasp the plate to exactly match the shoe **(Figure 21)**. Once the plate is finished, it should look like **Figure 22**.

All that is left to finish the shoe is to tap the hole. We generally punch the shoe with a 5/16-inch punch and tap with a 3/8-inch tap. Use a narrow center punch to mark the plate **(Figure 23)** and drill a hole for the bolt in the plate. Next, use a tap to thread the hole for the bolt that will hold the plate in place **(Figure 24)**. The plate should now slide into position easily, and once you thread the bolt into the hole, your hospital plate is finished **(Figure 25)**.

To use the hospital plate, trim and hot fit the foot **(Figure 26)** and nail it up **(Figure 27)**. Clinch the foot **(Figure 28)** and rasp the nail heads off from the ground side **(Figure 29)**. Be certain to clinch prior to rasping off the nail heads. If you get the order reversed, you may push the nails out of the holes during the clinching process.

Apply whatever medication is needed for the foot **(Figure 30)**. **Figure 31** shows the hands of my customer placing gauze into the shoe. When you have hands like that, you appreciate a one-bolt

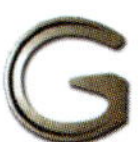

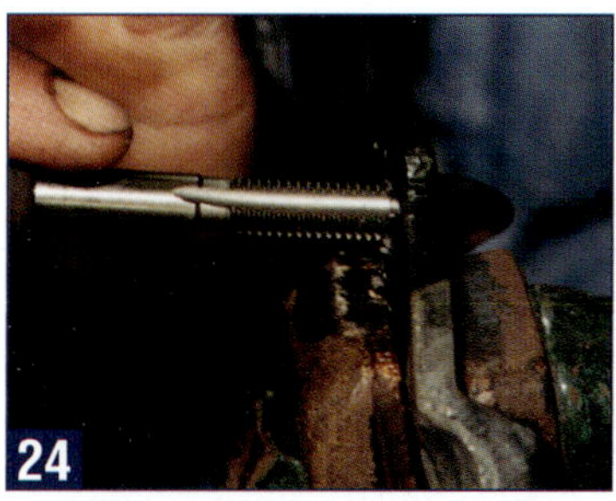
24
Tapping the hole for the bolt.

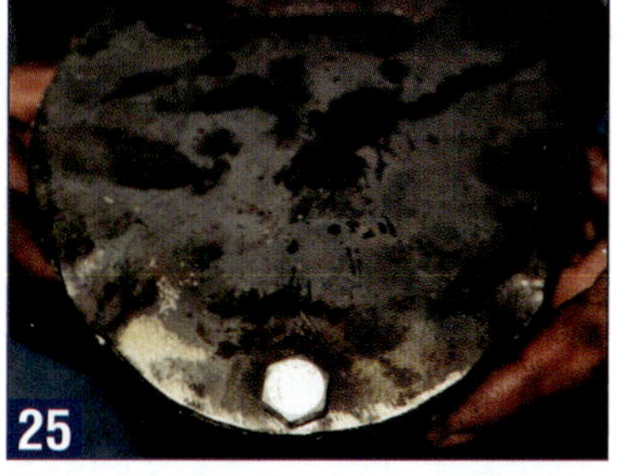
25
The finished shoe with the plate attached.

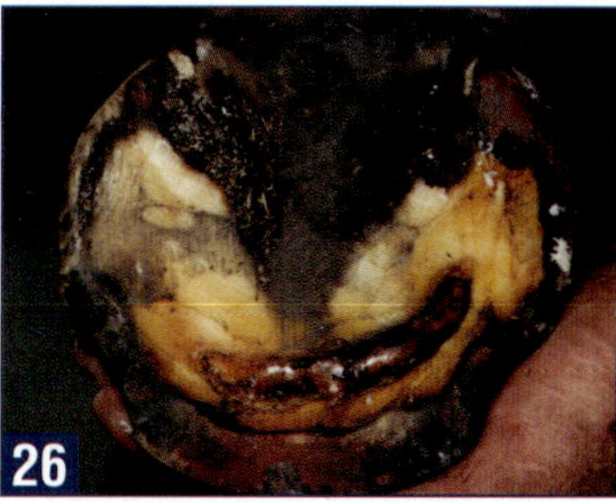
26
Hot fit the trimmed foot.

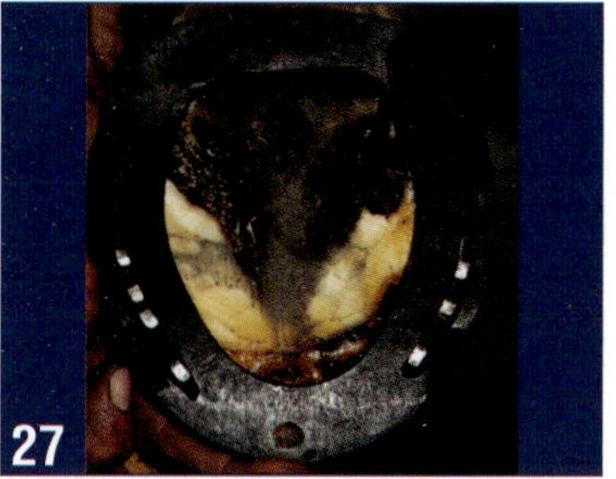
27
Nailed bar shoe.

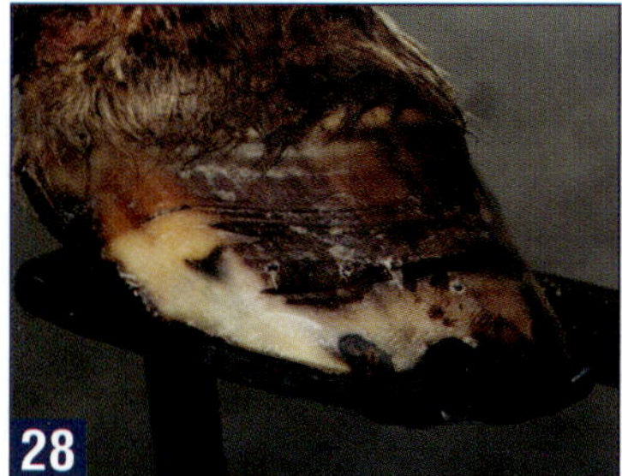
28
Clinching.

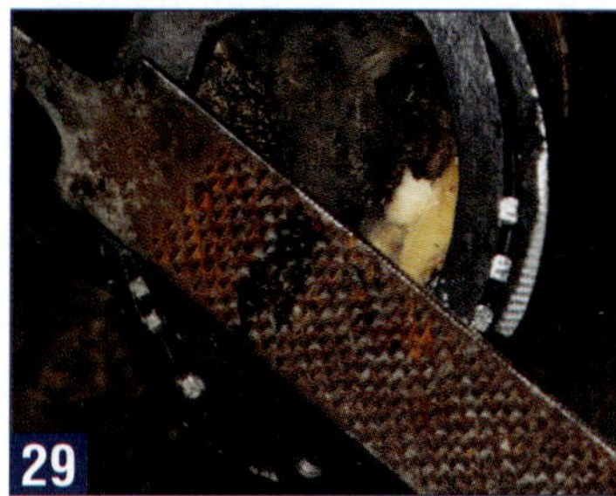
29
Rasping off the nail heads.

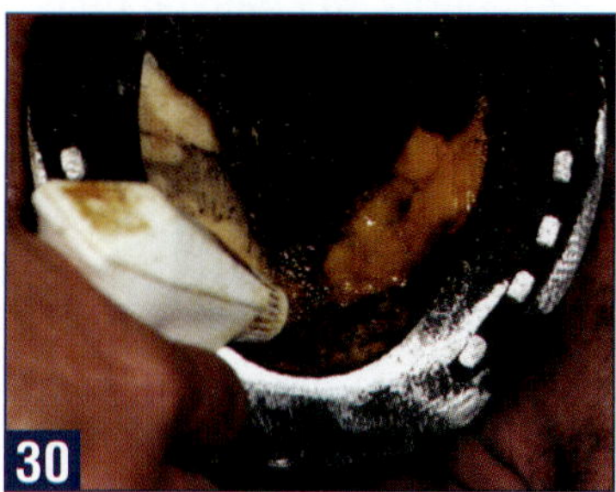
30
Applying medication.

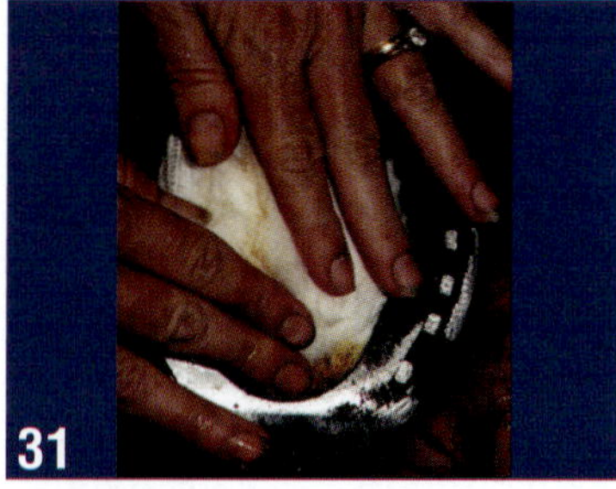
31
My customer's hands.

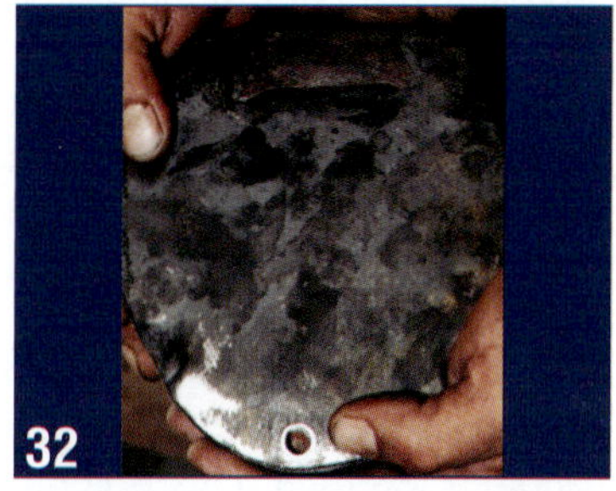
32
Sliding the plate into position.

hospital plate. Slide the plate into position **(Figure 32)** and put the bolt in the hole at the toe. The rocker toe should be angled enough that the foot is still flat on the ground even though there is a bolt head sticking past the shoe at the toe **(Figure 33)**.

I have used this type of hospital plate with great success on numerous horses. The customers who have experience with both this type of hospital plate and the traditional kind really appreciate the user-friendly nature of the one-bolt system. Make a couple in the shop for practice before doing the first one at the horse.

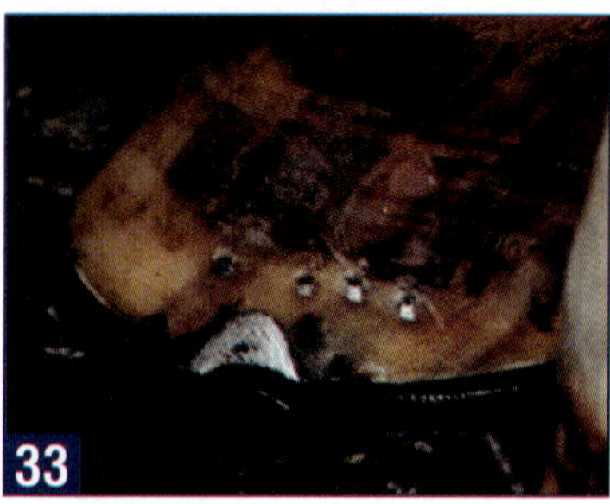
33
The finished foot with the bar shoe and hospital plate on the ground.

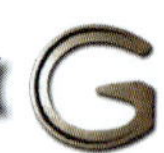

Chapter 55

EXTENSIONS

Extending a shoe beyond the perimeter of the foot is a common way to change the way that the foot supports the limb above it. Extensions are used to change the actual base of support that is under the bony column. If the extension is placed behind the heel, it can also change the way a foot lands. The larger the extension, the greater the pressure and leverage it can place on the foot.

Anytime you have shoe extending beyond the foot, the last point of contact with the foot will be the place that has the most weight on it. To understand this concept, consider a foot with an egg bar on it. When the foot is unshod, the solar surface of the hoof wall contacts the ground, and the weight is appropriate for each aspect of the foot. Once the egg bar is applied, there is the same amount of weight on that leg, but the shoe is now what is reacting with the ground instead of just the foot. Since there is more shoe behind the heels of the foot, the weight that is being born by the back of the shoe is being applied to the heels. While an egg bar may be a great shoe for a horse with a damaged suspensory apparatus, it may have a detrimental effect on the heels of some horses.

An extension should be as small as is needed to get the job done. There is a fine line where support becomes leverage. This is certainly not the sort of situation where if a little is good, a lot is better.

A lateral extension is pretty much any apparatus that extends medially or laterally beyond the perimeter of the foot. This can be a little confusing to people who are new to the industry and see a picture of an extension on the medial side of a foot, and it is being called a lateral extension. I know that it was confusing for me at one time.

There are several ways to make extensions. Some are made of traditional materials such as steel or aluminum. A lot of them are made from acrylic or polyurethanes, especially on young stock that have thin-walled and weaker feet that will not accept nails. Extensions made out of acrylic or urethane are covered in **Chapter 32, Modern Materials and Methods**, so in this section, I am going to cover those that are forged.

The most common extension that I use in my practice is the lateral heel extension **(Figures 1-3)**. With a horse that is cow-hocked or has any weakness in the hock or stifle, a lateral heel extension can really increase its comfort. My daughter has a barrel horse that has suffered some hock and stifle troubles, and he goes lame without the extensions, and sound with them. The difference is dramatic.

To make an open heeled lateral extension, add at least 1/2-inch more material to the shoe than you would need to cover the foot. The more you add, the more you need to upset into the heel. You can add as much as you need; just bump until you are at the right length.

Begin with a short heat on the lateral heel. This heat is about two inches, and I will put the additional 1/2-inch that I cut into that 2-inch area **(Figure 4)**.

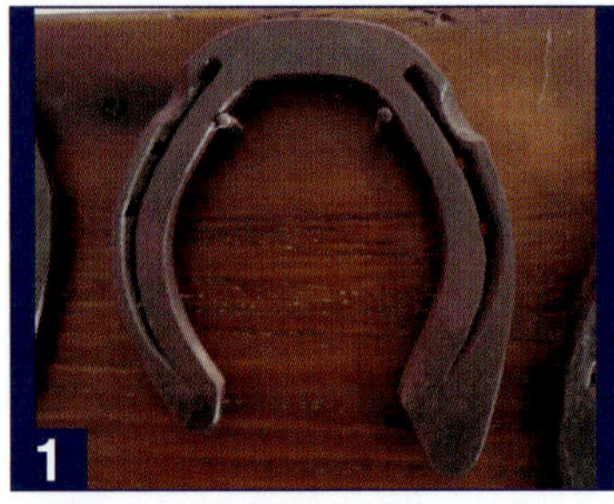

Lateral heel extension from my AWCF shoe display.

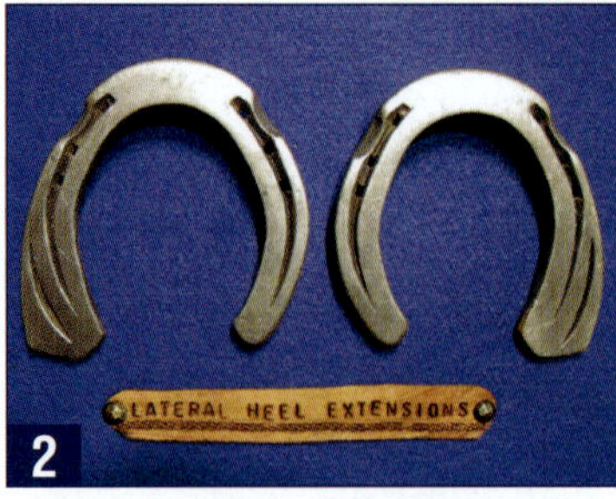

Lateral heel extension from Cody's AWCF shoe display.

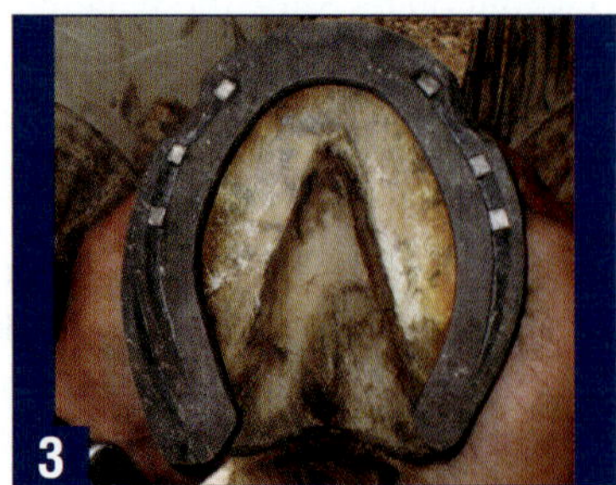

Lateral heel extension on a foot.

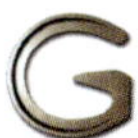

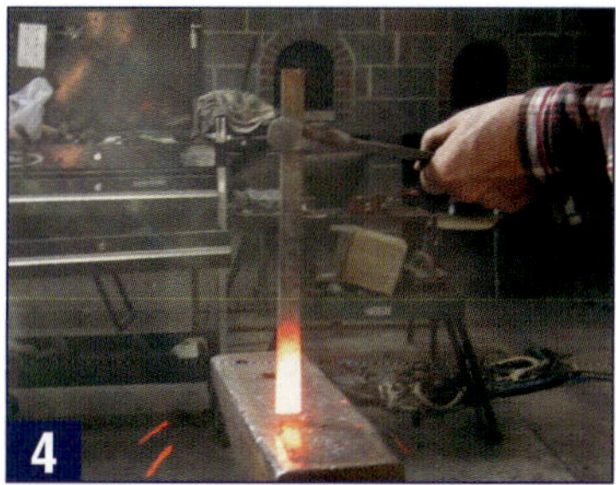

Bumping the heel.

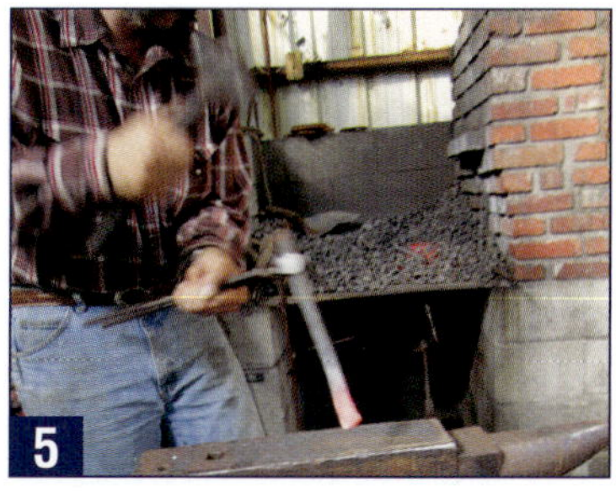

Making an angle on the end of the stock.

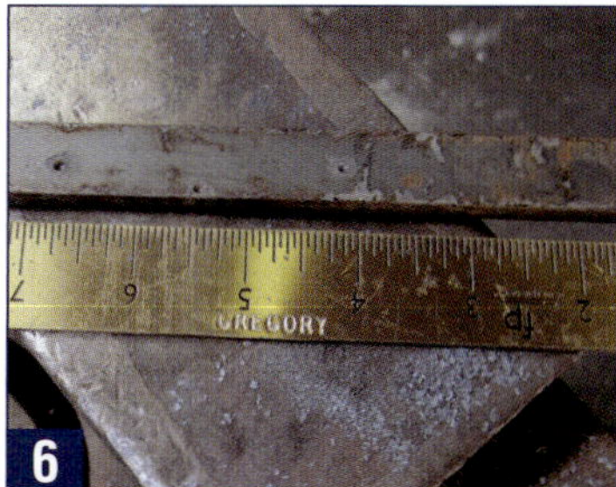

Marking the stock for center and start of fullering.

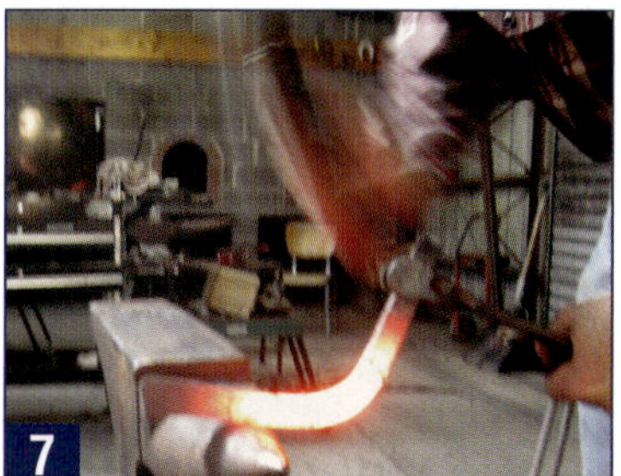

Making the toe bend.

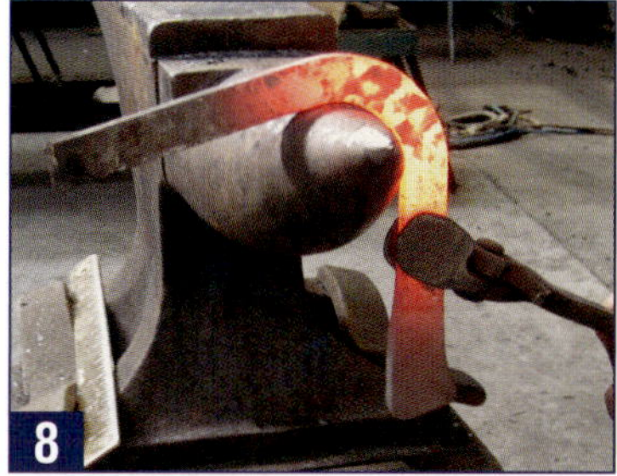

Setting the toe.

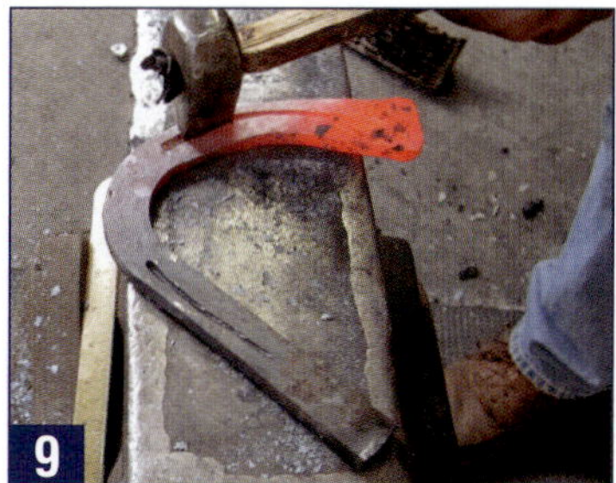

Fullering the lateral branch.

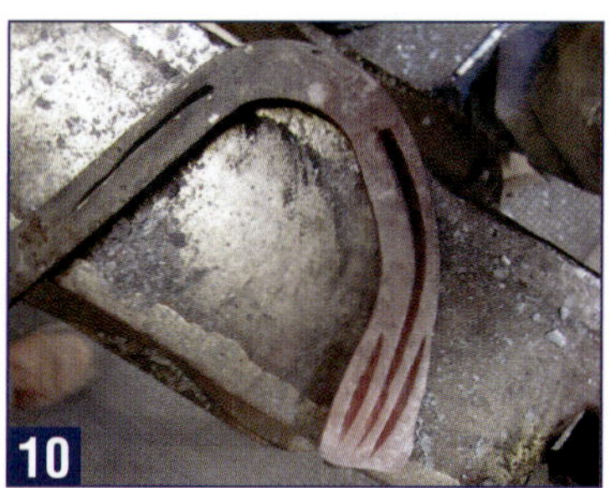

Lateral branch fullered.

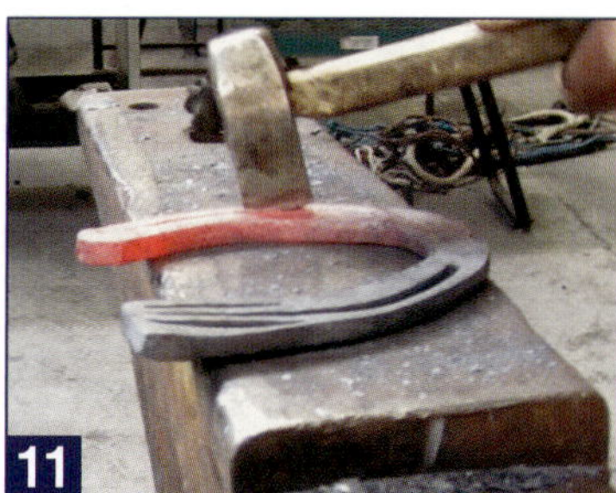

Making the medial branch.

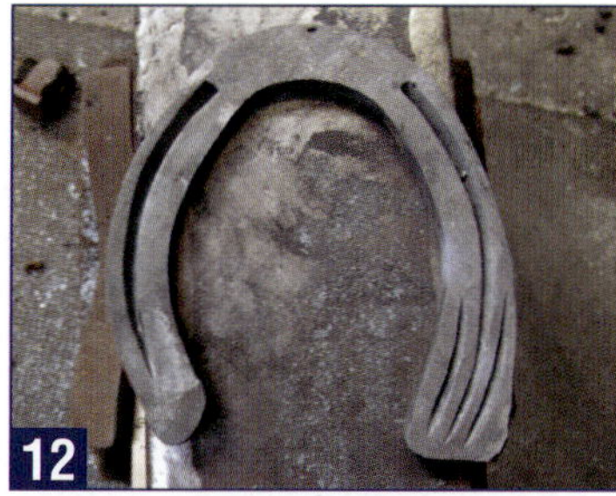

Lateral heel extension shoe.

As you bump, try to gain width, but maintain your original thickness. At the end of the bumping heat, you can angle the steel to pull the corner back and make building a heel easier **(Figure 5)**. Mark center after finishing the bump **(Figure 6)**. From here it is normal shoe building.

Make a toe bend as in **Figures 7-8**. Mark the fullering, hem the stock, and go back for the next heat. Heat the lateral branch and make a heel on the end. The lateral heel style you choose can range in style from a blocky one (like I am making here), to the ones on the shoes at the beginning of this series. You can do some heavy boxing on the hoof surface to gain width if you want more than just the bumping provided. Turn the branch, fuller, and finish **(Figures 9-10)**. On the medial branch, you do everything as you would on a normal shoe **(Figure 11)**. You should have a shoe that looks like **Figure 12**.

Figures 13-14 show the amount of extension that is commonly put on a lateral extension hind shoe. In **Figures 15-16**, the changes of the foot on the ground in relation to the leg are easily apparent with the addition of a lateral extension.

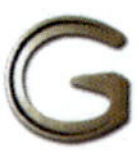

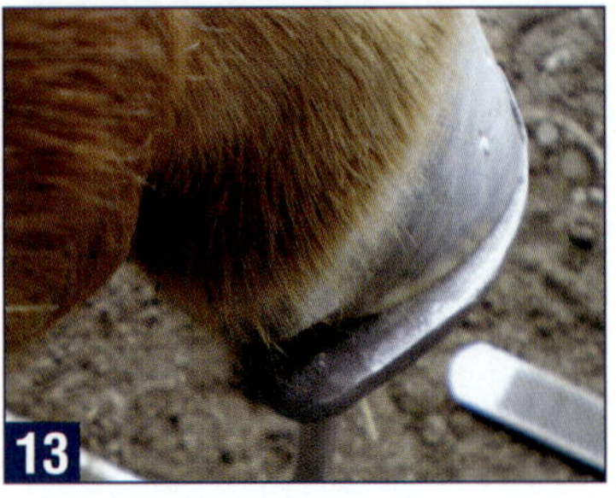

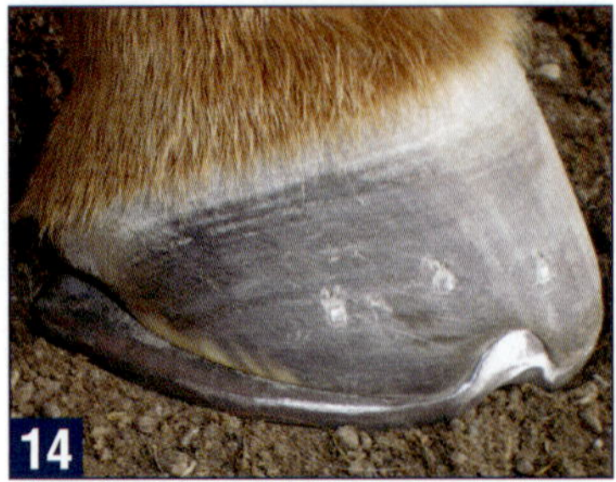

13, 14 Lateral heel extension on a foot showing the amount of extension.

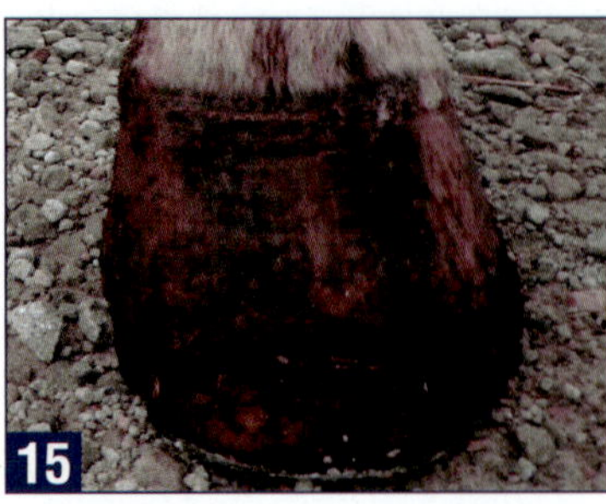

15 Foot that is not under the bony column.

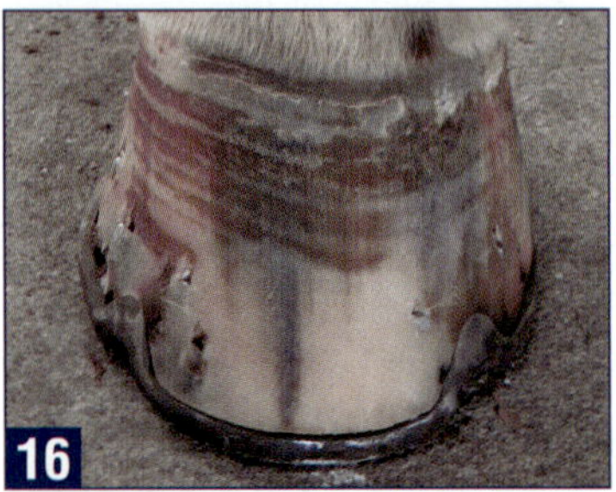

16 Same foot after being shod with the lateral heel extension shoe.

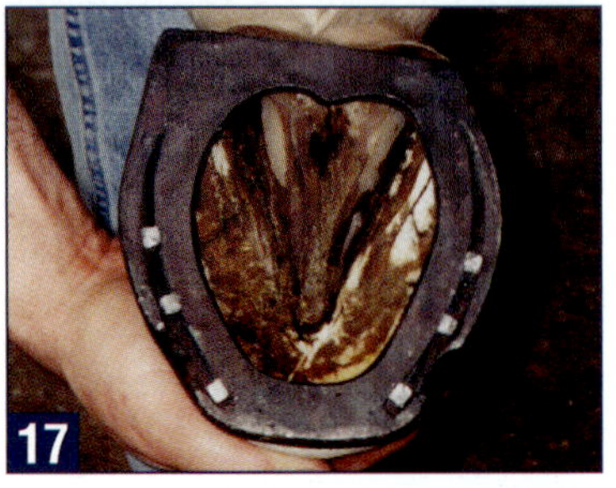

17 Lateral heel extension bar shoe on a cow hocked horse.

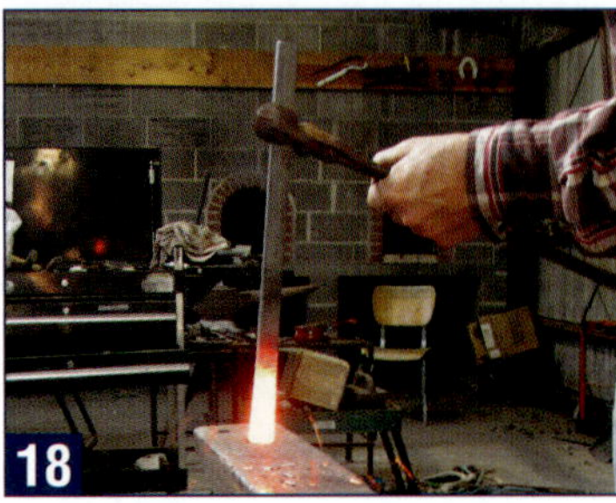

18 Bumping the lateral heel.

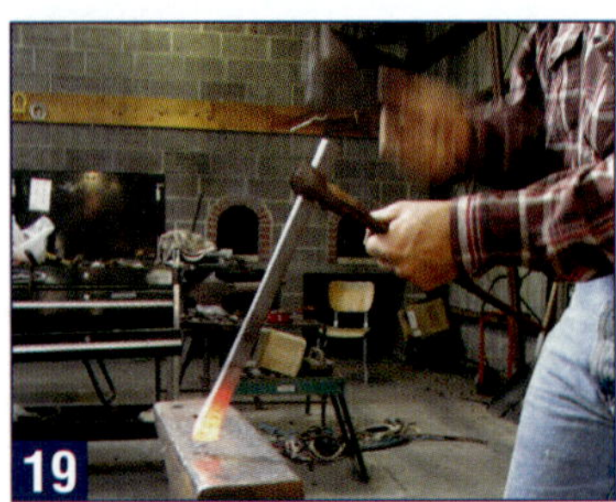

19 Making an angle by the way that I am bumping.

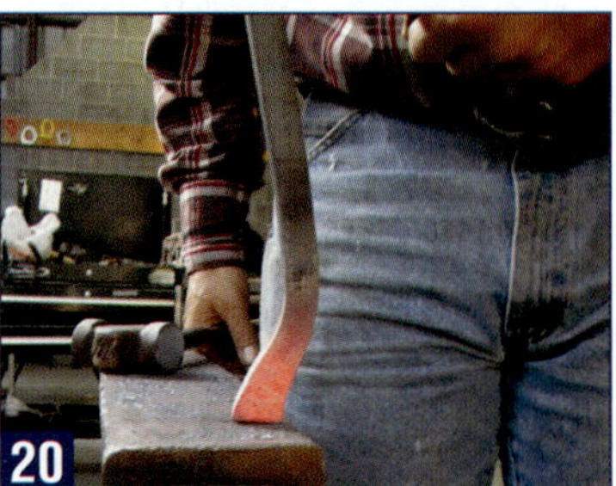

20 Bending the quarter to show how the angle on the stock makes the outside heel.

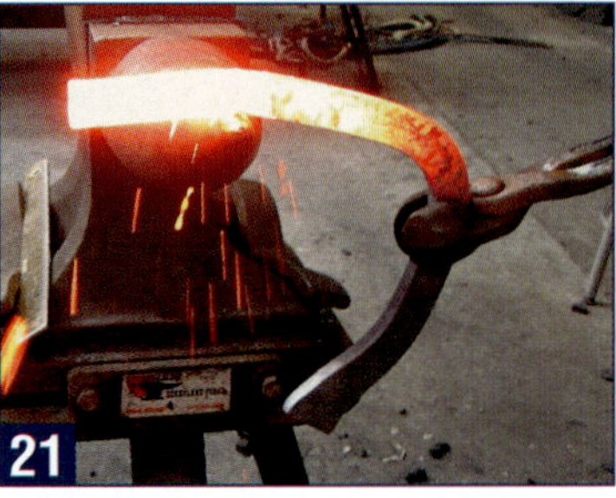

21 Bending for a long hockey stick.

Another way to make these types of shoes is to weld with a whip-across method. The shoe in **Figure 17** is one that I put on a horse in Melton Mowbry, United Kingdom, in 1997 when I was getting ready for my AWCF exam. This horse was cow-hocked, and the effect of this shoe was quite dramatic.

Cut more stock than you would need to make a normal fullered bar shoe for the foot you are working on. Put a light bump into the area that is going to have the extension **(Figure 18)**. As I bump, I can change the angle that I am bumping at **(Figure 19)** so that the end of the stock will have an angle to it. This will end up being the outside corner of the bar, which is readily apparent when I bend the quarter into the branch **(Figure 20)**.

After making a toe bend, bend up about twice the amount that you need for a normal hockey stick on the side of the shoe that was not bumped **(Figure 21)**. After the hockey stick is forged, the material has good thickness to make a nice bar **(Figure 22)**. Move to the same position that you would when making a normal hockey stick on a regular bar shoe. Forge the stock to form a good corner as you would

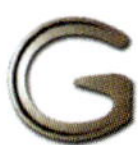

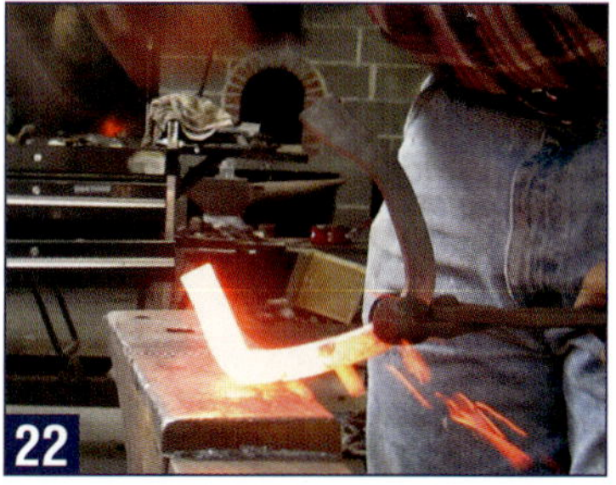

Bumping into the corner for the inside heel.

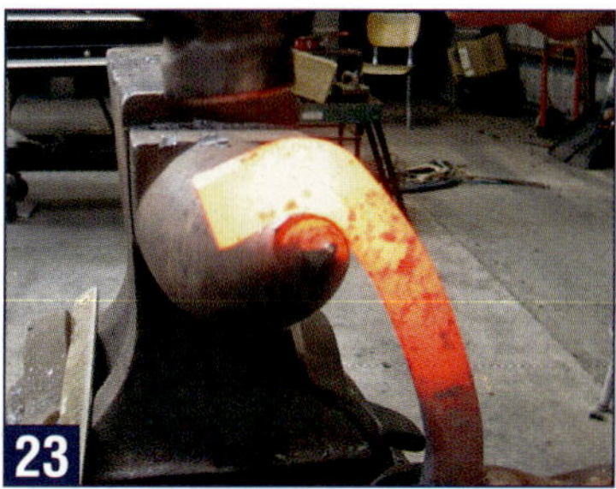

Making the bar.

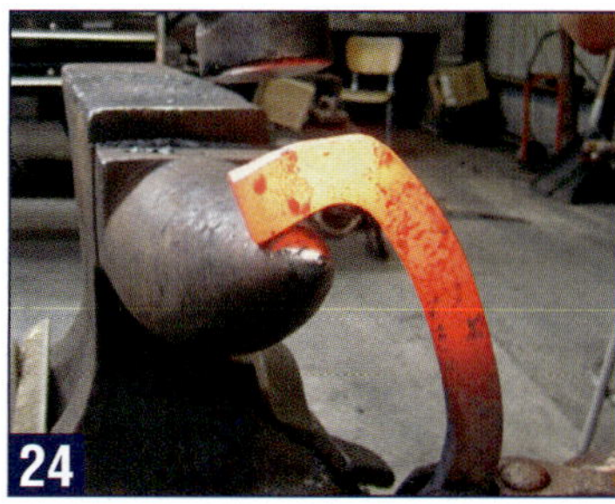

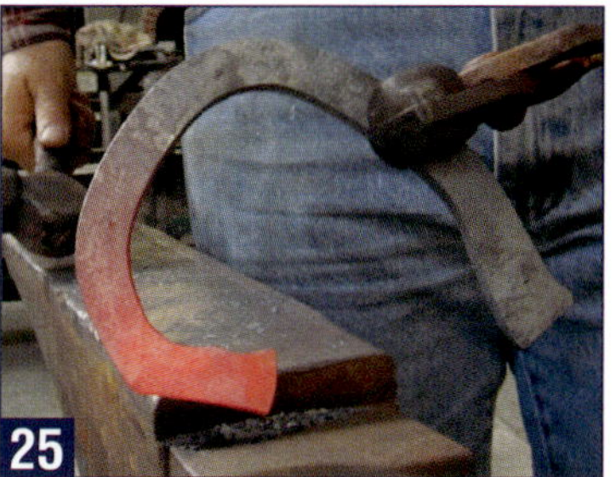

Bar ready to be welded.

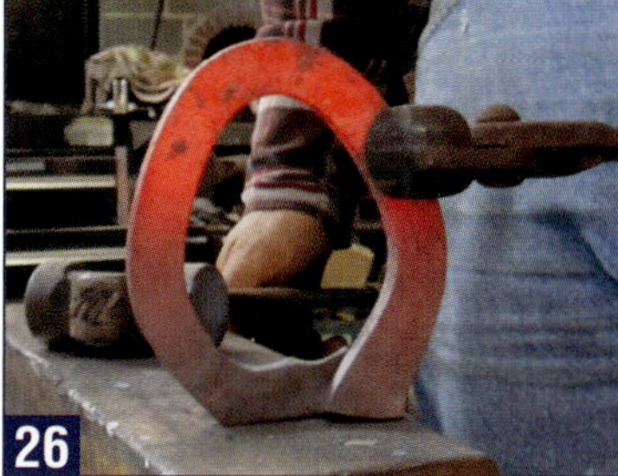

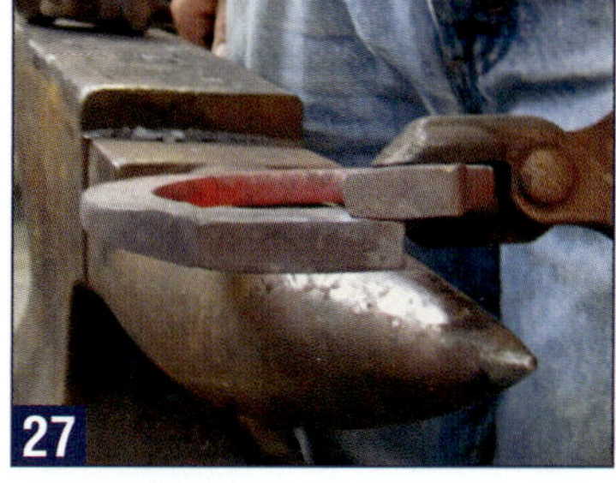

The shoe put together and ready to be welded.

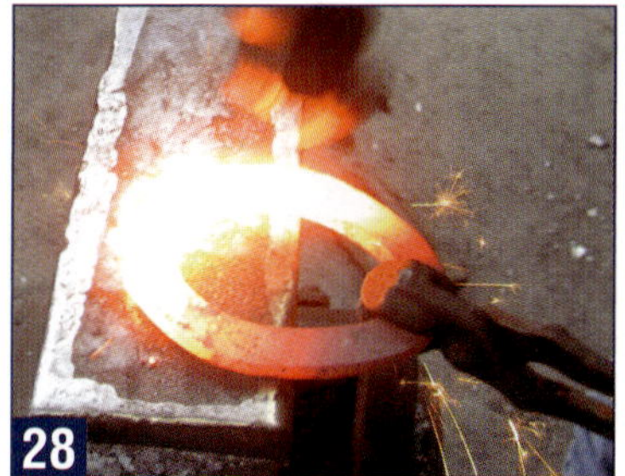

Welding.

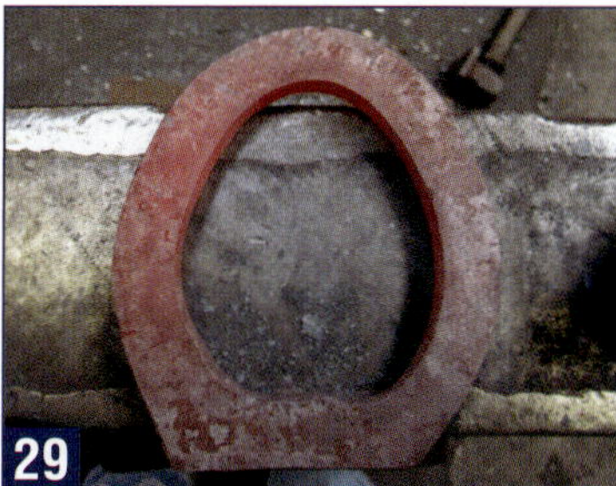

Finished blank.

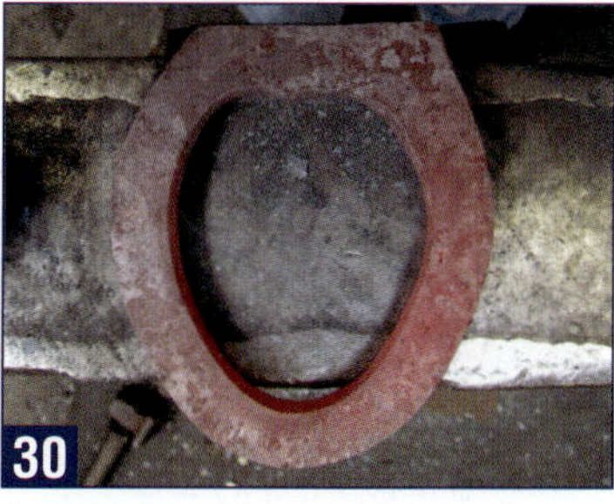

Looking at the blank from another angle to see how it could be used for a toe extension.

on a bar shoe. Pull the stock back slightly and begin making the sex appeal **(Figures 23-24)**. It should look like **Figure 25** when it is done.

There was only a light bump on the extension side, so the rest of the extension will be formed by where we make the weld. Put the shoe together as seen in **Figures 26 and 27**. When you weld the bar to the heel of the shoe, you will end up with plenty of material to make the extension. Weld the corner of the shoe **(Figure 28)**, and you should end up with something that resembles **Figure 29**. If you want a larger extension, bump more into the branch before welding. Looking at this shoe from another angle, it is possible to imagine a nice toe extension. **Figure 30** is just **Figure 29** turned 180 degrees. I use the same method for a toe extension shoe, and if I don't want it to be a square toe too, I just weld at the corner without making the hockey stick **(Figure 31)**.

For extensions that are going to engage the entire side of a foot, you can use wider than normal bar stock, punch one side fine, and the punch other side coarse **(Figure 32)**. Place the nails in the white line, and the whole shoe is moved over and you end up

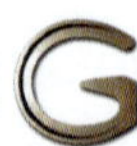

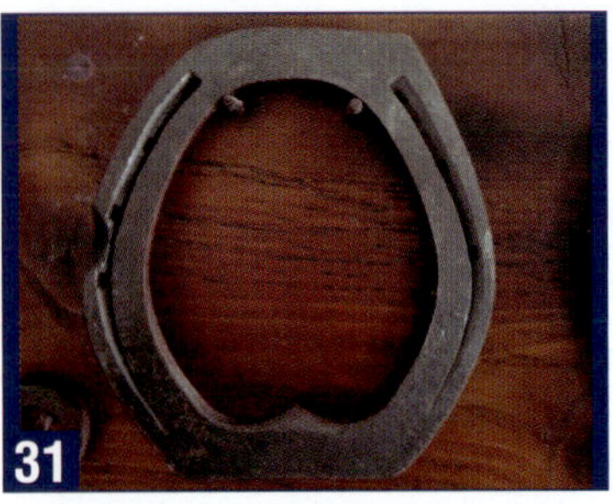

Lateral toe extension from my AWCF shoe display.

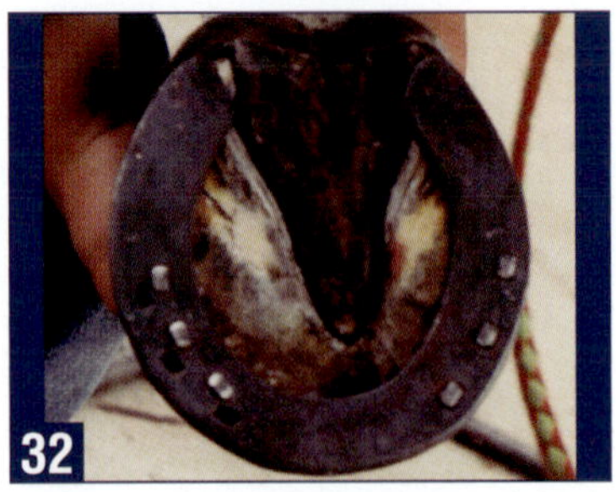

Lateral extension shoe with nails punched coarse on one side.

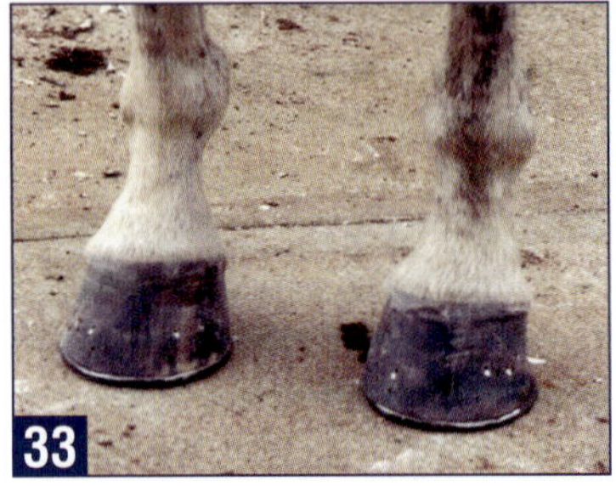

The shoe under the bony column.

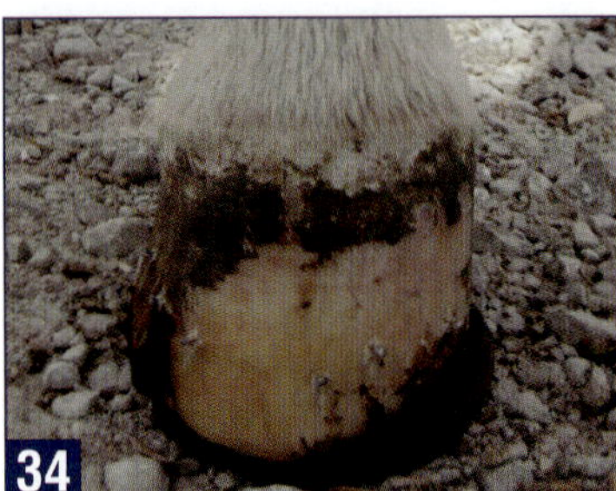

Toe extension bar shoe from Cody's AWCF shoe display.

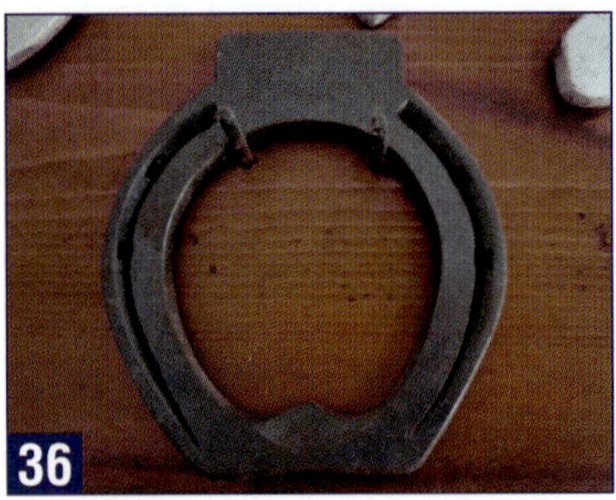

Toe Extension bar shoe from my AWCF shoe display.

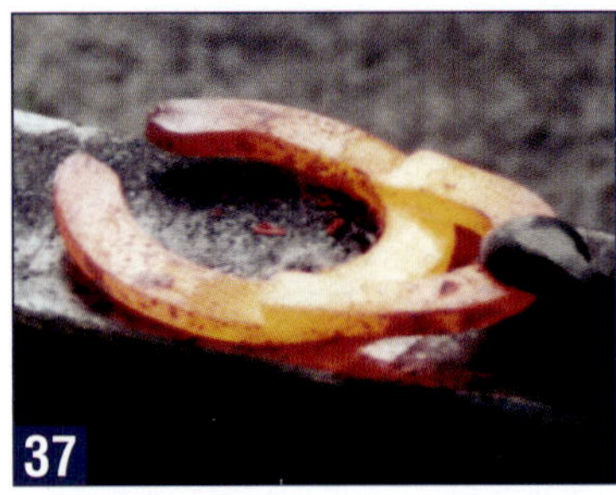

Jump welding a toe extension on a shoe.

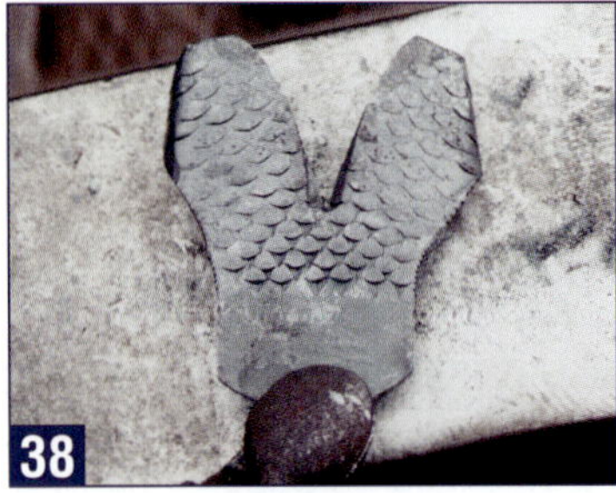

Toe extension for a baby made from a rasp.

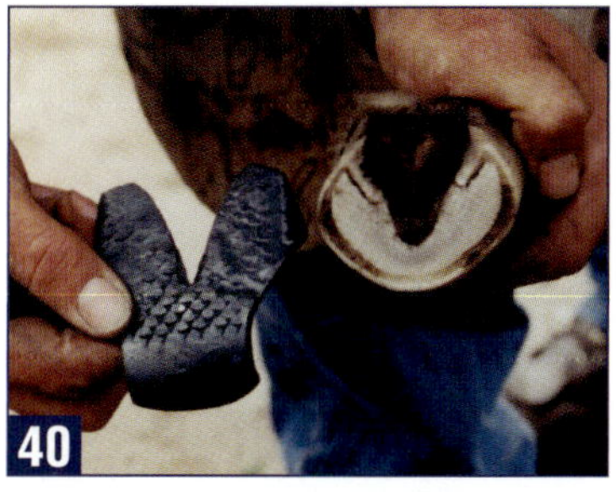

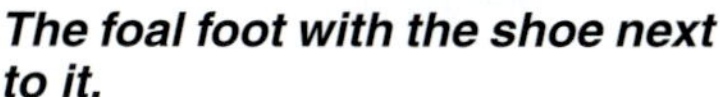

The foal foot with the shoe next to it.

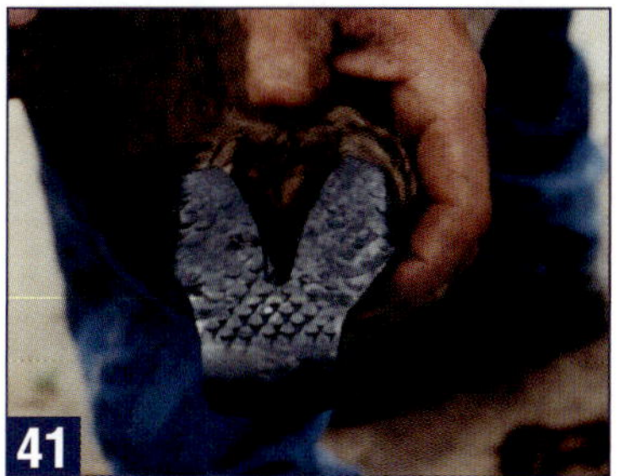

The shoe on the foot.

with shoe sticking out one side. You can also forge half the stock down on one side to make the shoe a bit more of a custom fit. The main thing to get right is to have the shoe under the bony column **(Figures 33-34)**.

Toe extensions, **(Figures 35-36)** are commonly used in conjunction with a deep flexor tendon tenotomy or a check ligament desmotomy. This shoe allows the foot to be held in the correct position after the deep flexor tendon or check ligament has been cut. **Figures 35-36** were made by forging hockey sticks on the end of the stock, turning the toe away from the bend of the hockey sticks, and welding the hockey sticks to make the toe extension. This shoe can also be made by welding an additional piece of steel to the toe, as seen in **Figure 37**.

On young stock that has not fully formed, the extensions will be applied without the surgery that would accompany this shoe on an older horse. You can make this shoe out of aluminum or thin steel like the one for a foal made out of a rasp, **(Figure 38)**. I made some small clips to help hold it on at the heels **(Figure 39)**, and it fit the foot pretty well. **(Figures 40-41)**. We glued it on and helped the limb develop with a more ideal conformation.

Extensions come with a cost. There is a greater chance of losing a shoe, and they also put a lot of stress on the foot, leg, and limb. Use them with care, caution, and a healthy dose of anatomical understanding, and they can do a lot to make a horse grow, move, and feel better.

G

Section

12

Practical Application of Sound Basics

This section is several short descriptions of some of the horses I have worked on that had problems, and the shoes used to help them. You will see that the shoes recommended in *Section 11: The Shoe Arsenal*, are applicable, and I hope that you will see the need for learning to make them.

Chapter 56: Treating Lame and Abnormal Feet

-1 Patten Bar Cases..602

-2 Z-Bar Cases...611

-3 Straight Bars...615

-4 Drastic Changes 622

-5 Heart Bar and W-Shoe 630

" 7 For unclean spirits, crying with loud voice, came out of many that were possessed with them: and many taken with palsies, and that were lame, were healed. "

—Acts 8:7

—King James Version

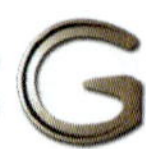

Chapter

56-1 PATTEN BAR SHOE

CASE STUDY

The patten bar is a horseshoe that is not well understood and is not used nearly as often as it could be. This shoe is a rest shoe, and the principle behind it is not the angle change created, but rather the elevation that is achieved, which allows that limb to work less. In effect, the patten bar is a rest shoe.

Imagine if you were to tape a piece of 2-by-4 to the bottom of your shoe for a day. In fact, you can do this and you won't have to imagine. As you went about your day, you would find that when you were not moving, the foot and leg without the 2-by-4 would be doing the bulk of the labor. When you stood, the woodless leg would take the most weight. When you walked, you would find that you would come down heavier on the woodless leg. This is how a patten bar helps a horse.

This first case hits pretty close to home. Cody owns an amazing stud horse that he calls Spiderman. I have always thought that a good stud would make a great gelding, but this horse is special. He's the type of animal that should be passing on his genetics. Anyway, Spiderman tried to get over a pipe fence. When he did, he ended up catching the second bar with his back foot, and his hock was over the top of the fence. We don't know how long he was trapped like this, but when we found him, he had lost a lot of blood and was quite weak.

Figures 1-5 show how he looked that first day. Notice in **Figure 4** where the proximal end of his cannon bone is exposed. **Figure 5** is a plain, stamped handmade with extended heels, which probably had a hand in trapping that foot. Kelly bedded Spiderman down **(Figure 6)**, and we called

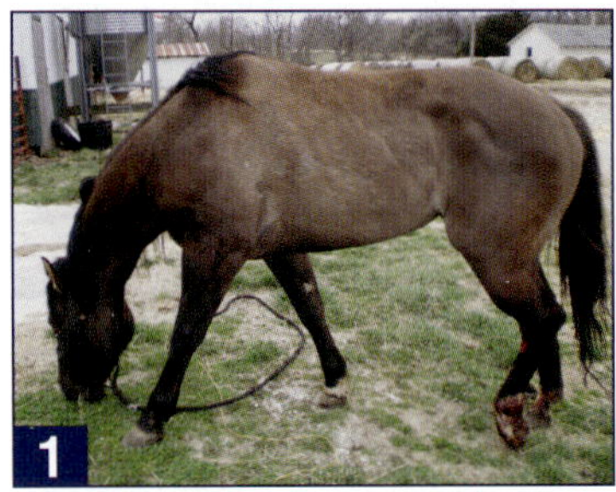

1

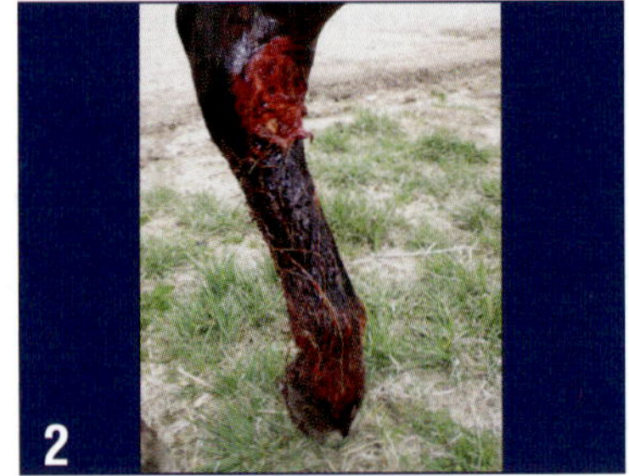

2

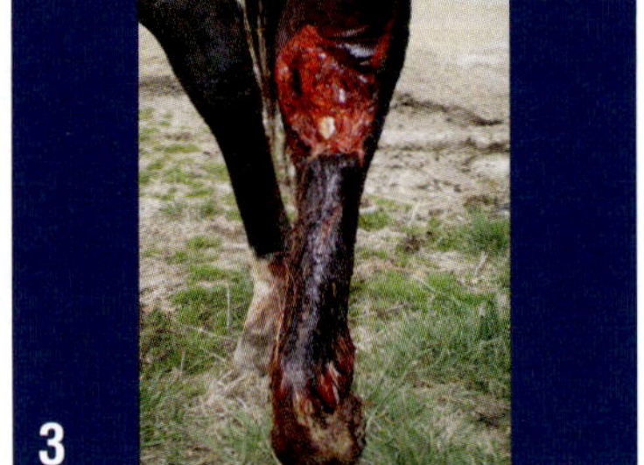

3

Spiderman following his injury.

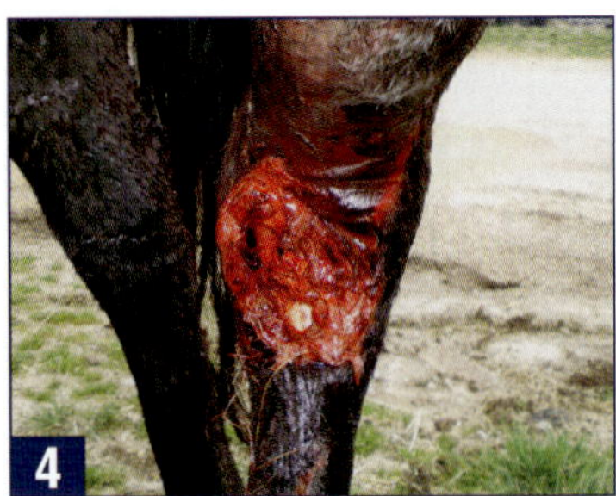

4

Notice the end of the cannon bone.

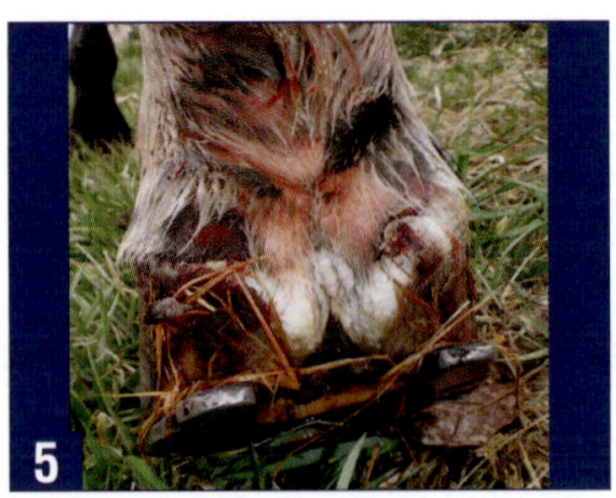

5

This shoe may have helped trap the foot.

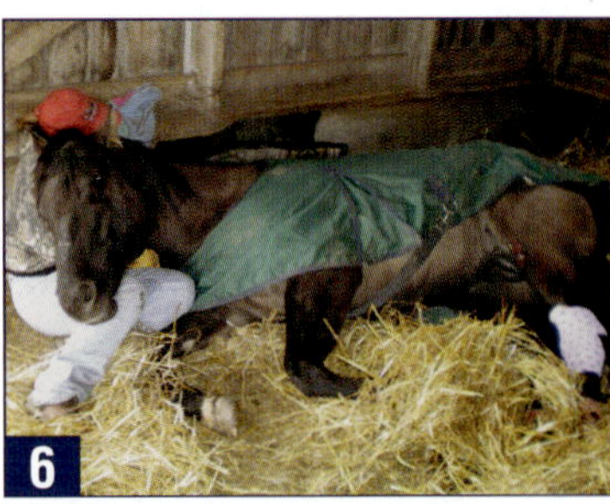

6

Bedding the patient down.

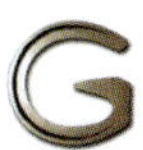

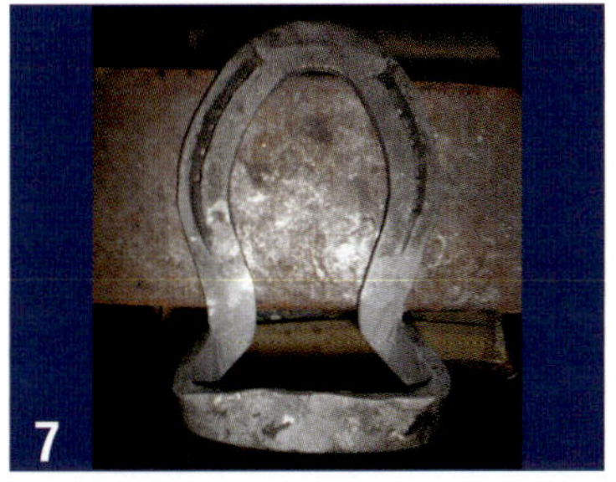

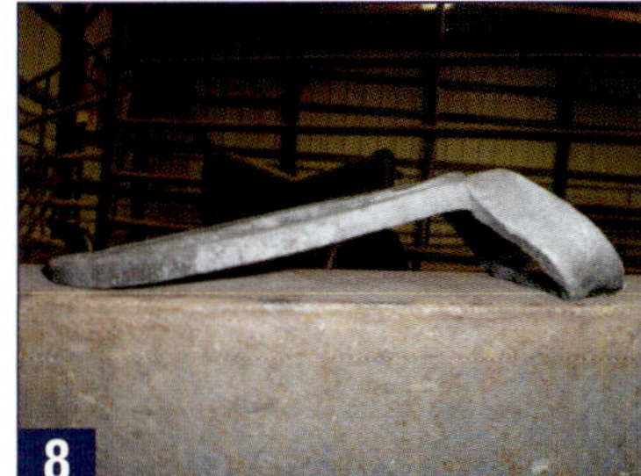

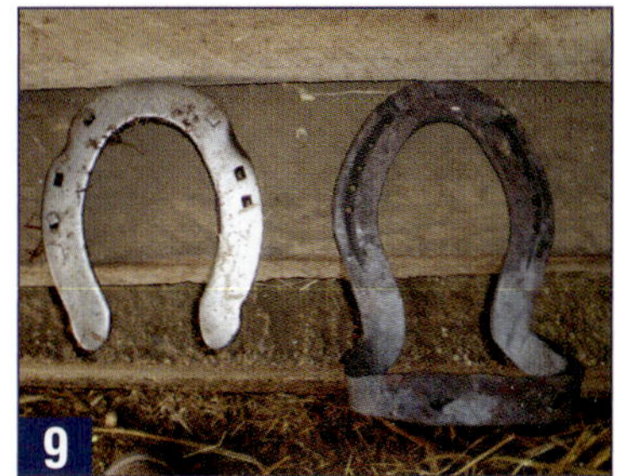

The patten bar shoe.

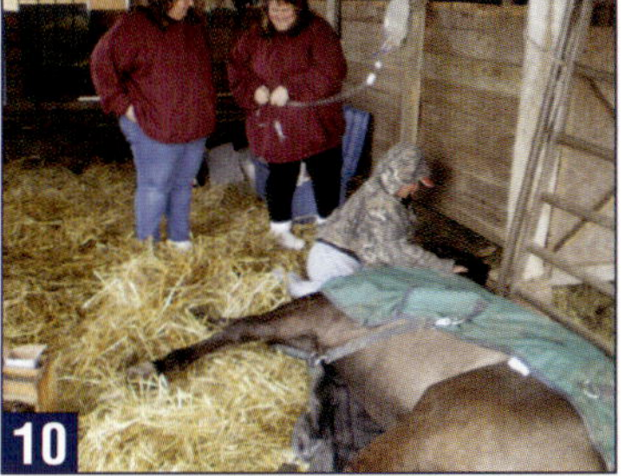

Badly needed fluids from the veterinarians.

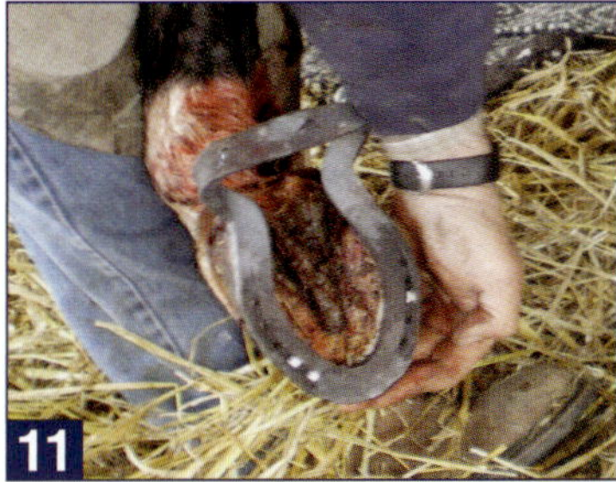

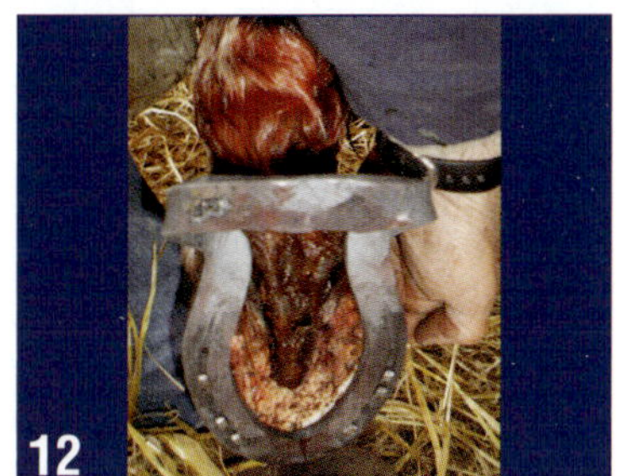

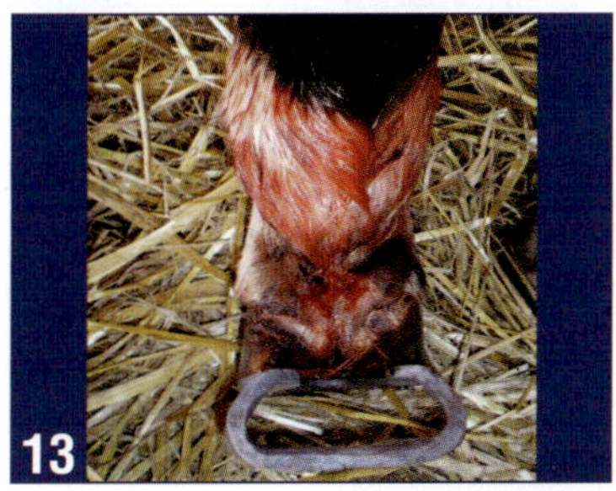

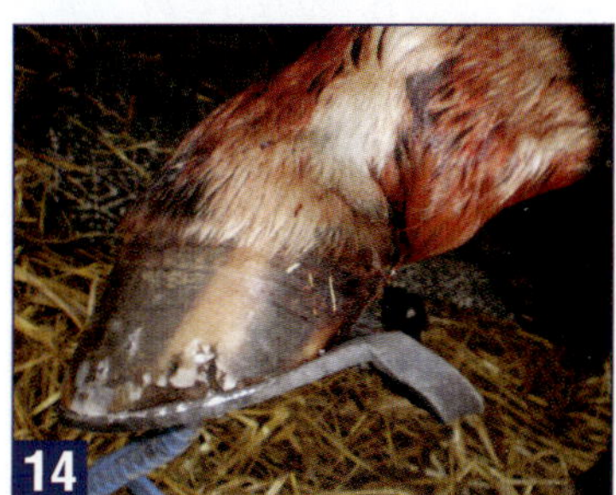

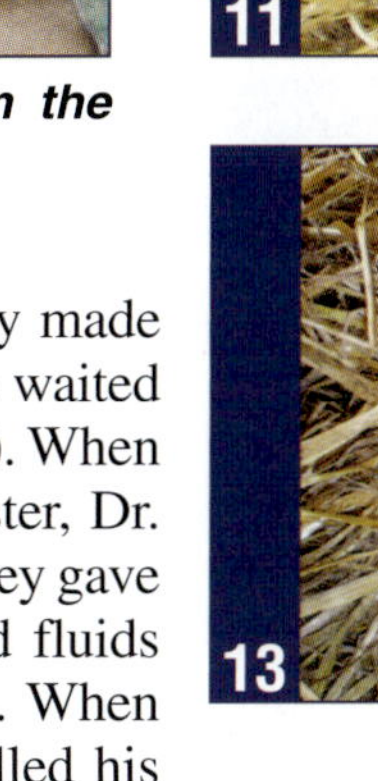

the local vet. I immediately made him a patten bar while we waited for her arrival **(Figures 7-9)**. When Marilyn Nance and her sister, Dr. Christine Martin arrived, they gave Spidey some badly needed fluids for blood loss **(Figure 10)**. When he was able to stand, I pulled his old shoe, trimmed the foot, and nailed on the patten bar as quickly and easily as possible **(Figures 11-15)**.

When shoeing in this manner, you are trying to get the shoe on as fast as possible so that the animal does not have to suffer longer than needed. Get the shoe on and the nails bent over. Finish is not an important part of shoeing a horse that is in this sort of pain. The next day, there was a major bleed from a ruptured blood vessel **(Figure 16)**, but it quit when we wrapped the wound fairly tightly **(Figure 17)**. Over the next week or two,

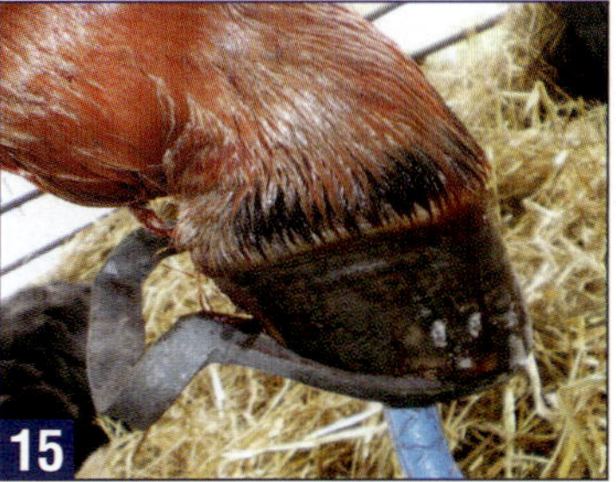

Nailing on the patten bar.

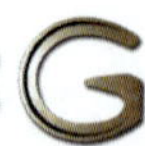

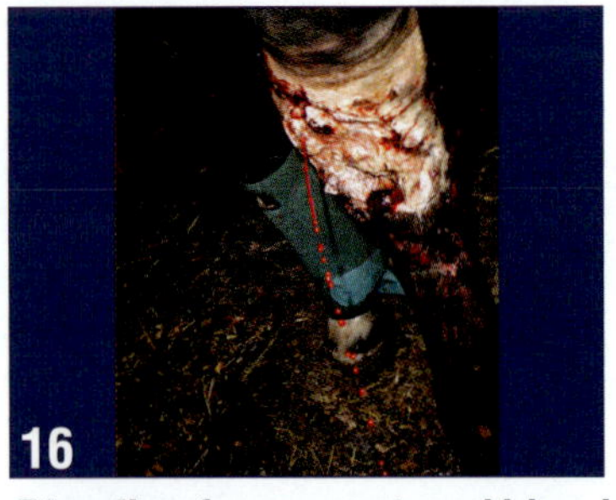

Bleeding from a ruptured blood vessel.

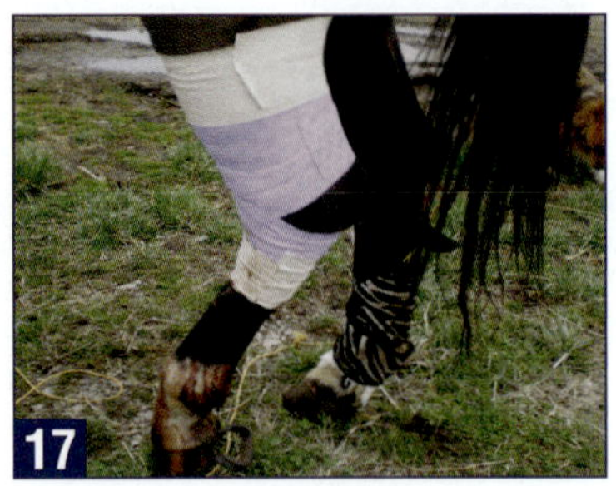

Wrapping the wound.

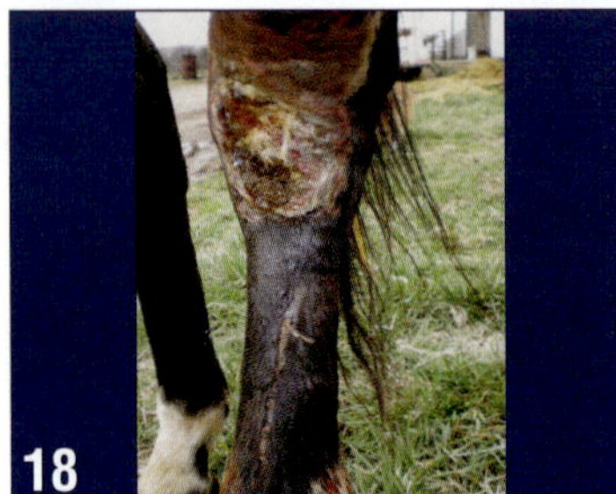

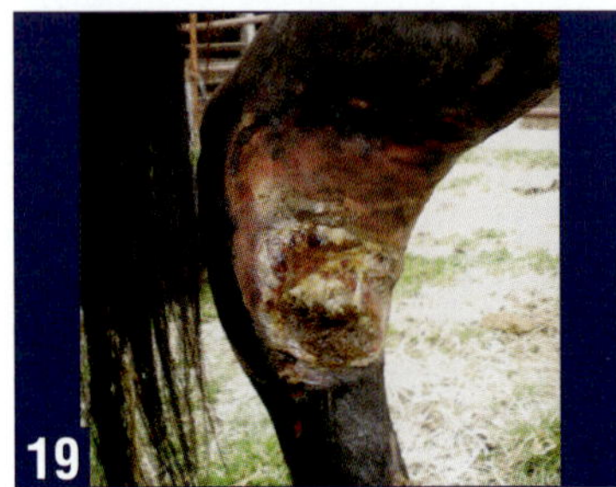

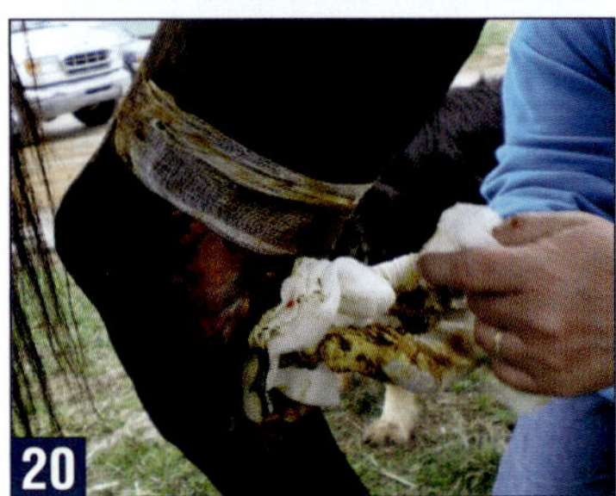

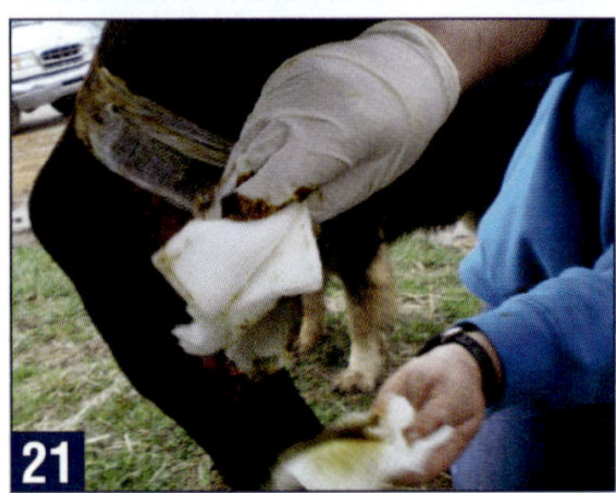

Doctoring the patient: Herbal remedies and water treatment.

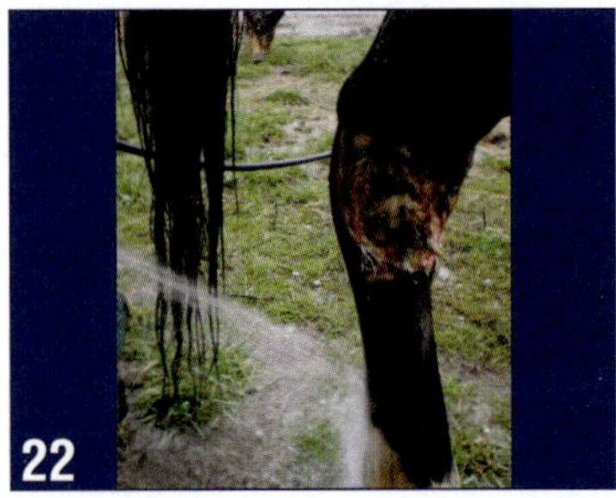

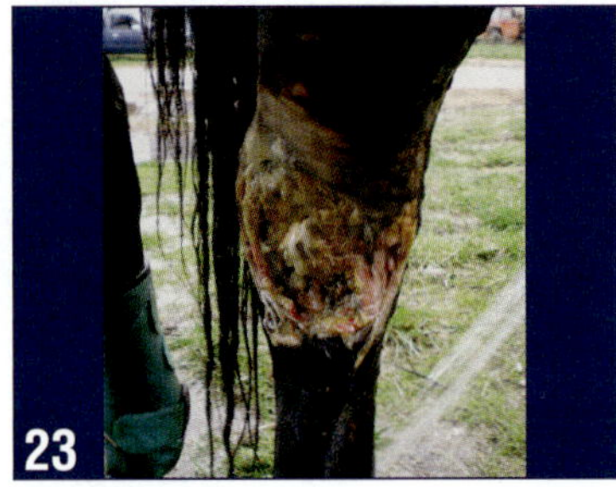

The healing process continues. Water treatment two weeks after the injury.

Kelly doctored the leg with an herbal remedy, did water therapy, and wrapped the leg **(Figures 18-21)**. You can see how the tissue looked as it was filling in and healing. In **Figures 22 and 23**, the wound is about two weeks old, and Kelly is doing water therapy on it.

The leg continued to heal, forming scabs and draining as is the norm with a wound of this magni-

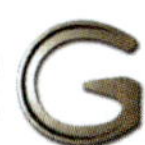

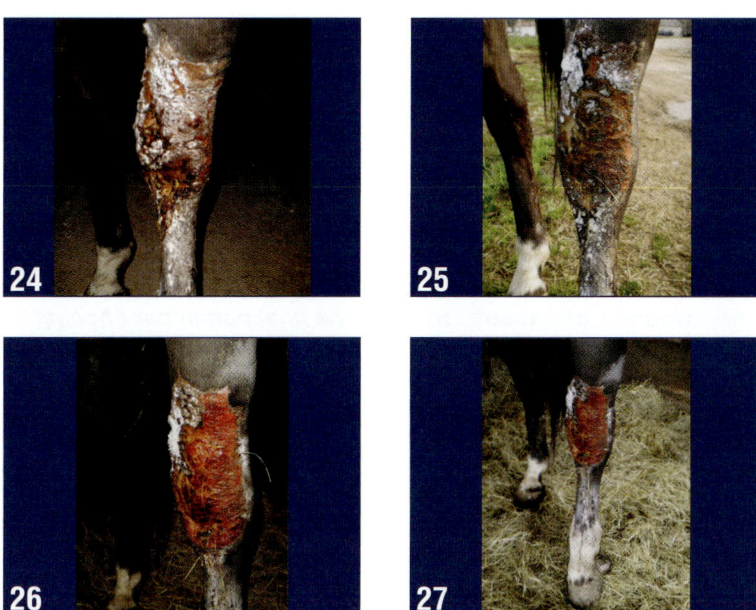

The wound continues scabbing up and draining.

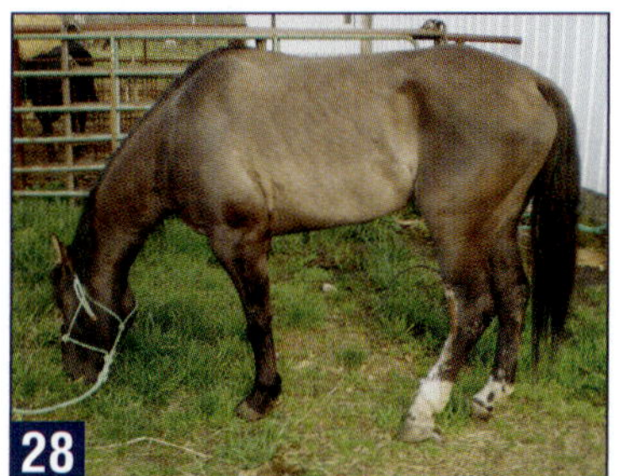

Spiderman was using the leg at about 80% at this stage.

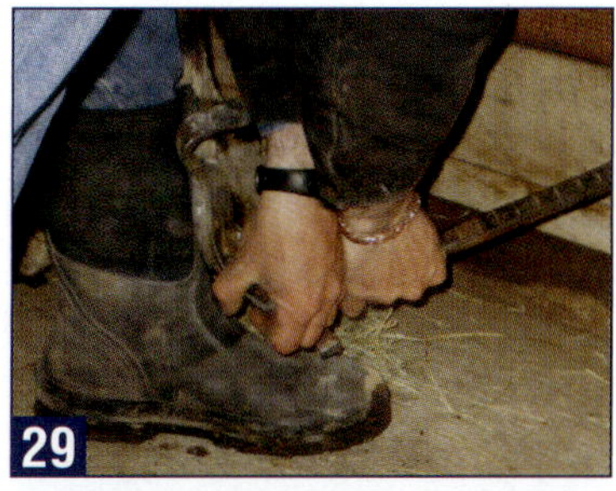

Replacing the patten bar and staying low.

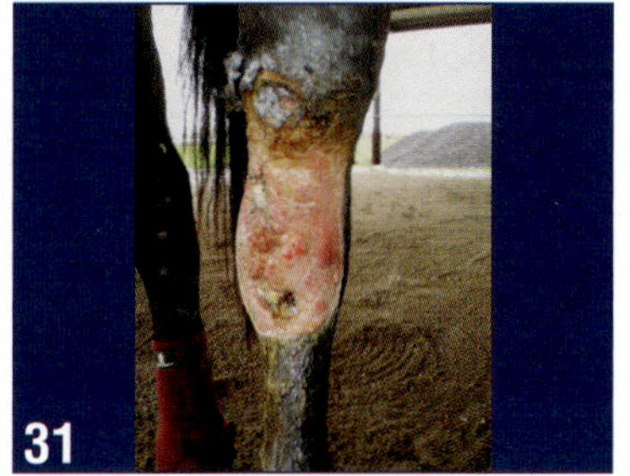

Wound treatment continues.

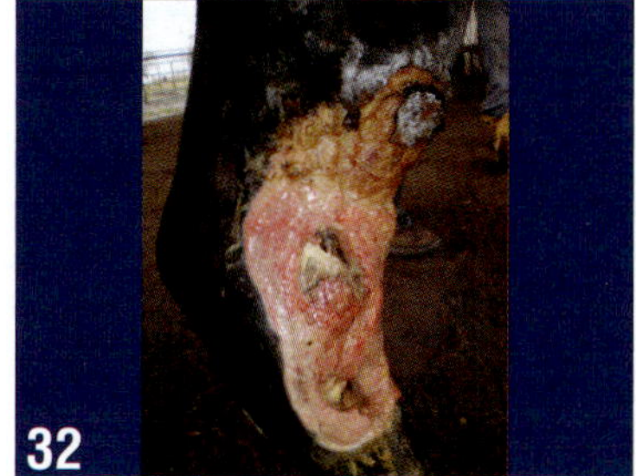

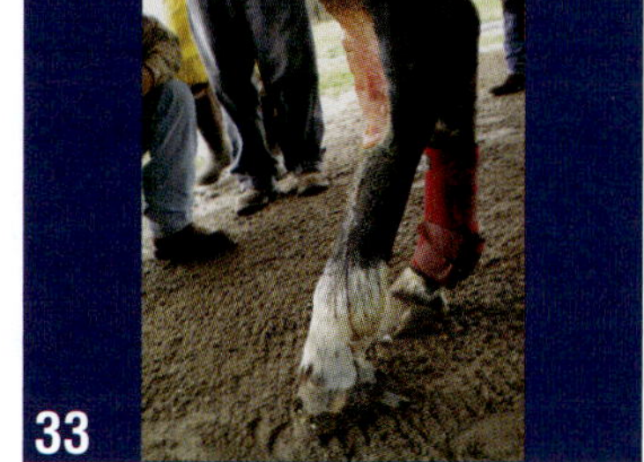

tude. **Figures 24-28** show this process.

In about six weeks, the wound was healing nicely, and it was time to reset the patten bar. Spiderman was using the leg at about 80% by this stage of the healing process. You can see in **Figures 29 and 30** how low to the ground I am working while nailing the shoe back on. In **Figures 31-33**, Kelly has been treating the wound with gauze and saline. This has

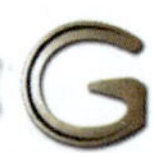

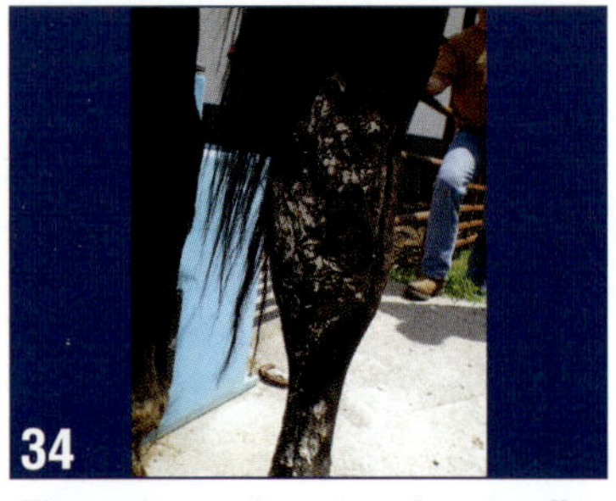

34

The wound at about five months.

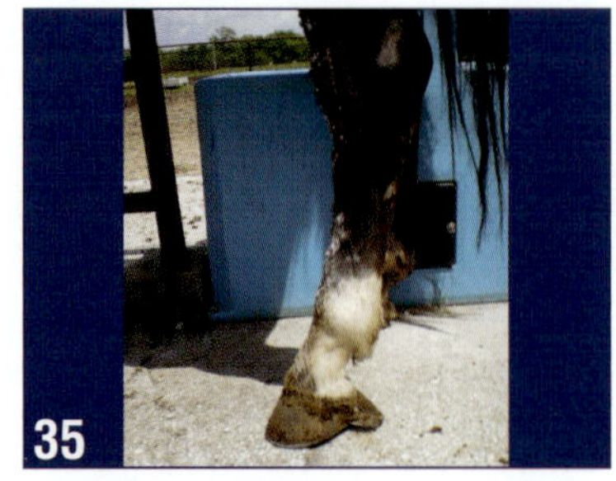

35

The final patten bar shoeing.

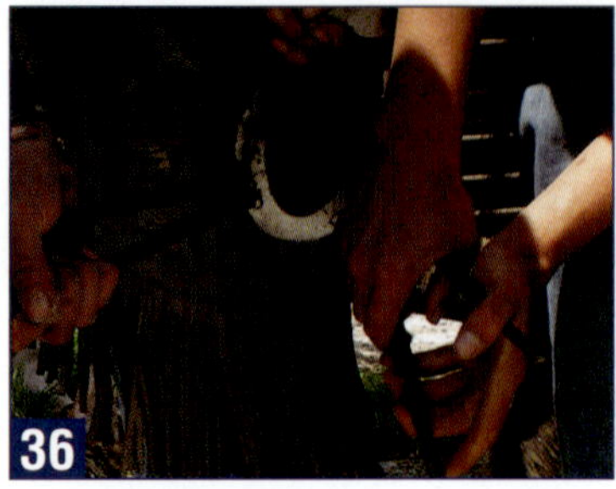

36

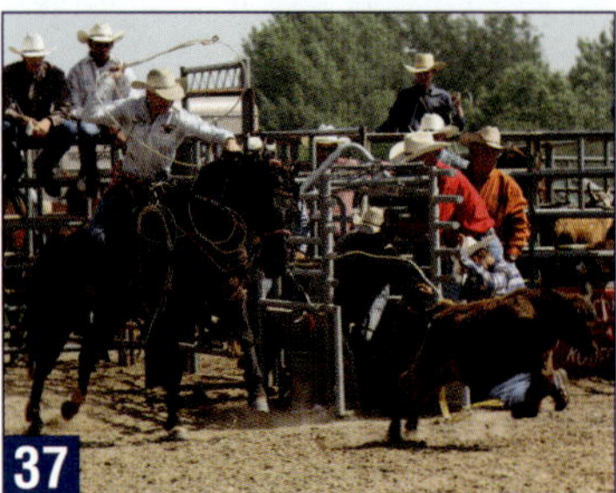

37

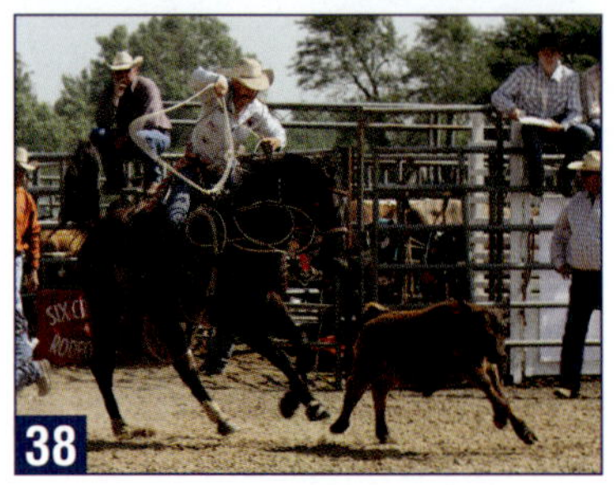

38

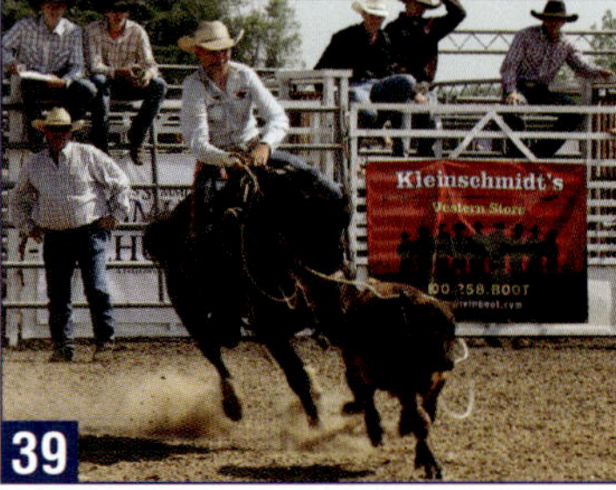

39

Cody back in the saddle on Spiderman in August, following the Feburary injury.

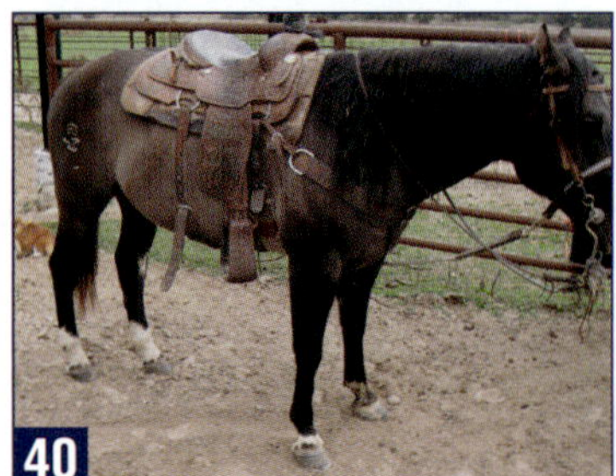

40

Just a white scar remains.

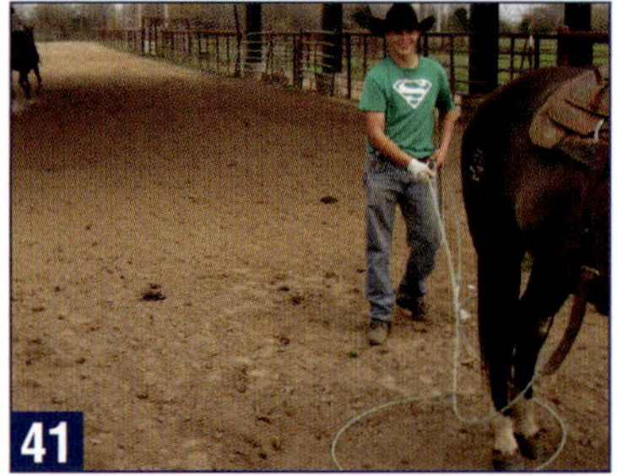

41

Cody is able to do anything he wants with Spiderman (within reason).

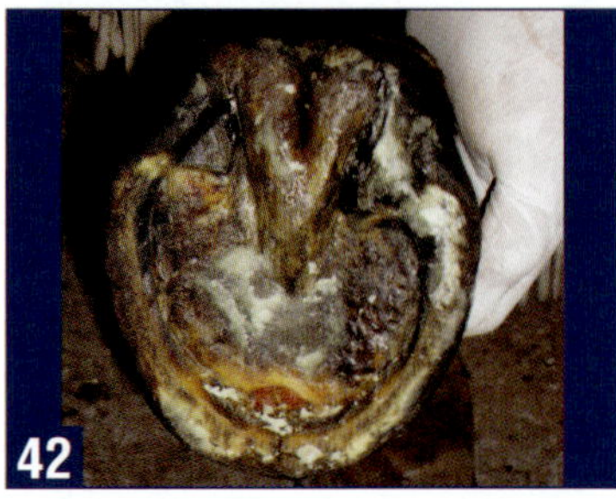

42

Sole damage from a bad abscess caused by sole pressure and a hot nail.

really made the wound look better, but the exposed bone was a pretty big concern. Throughout, the opposite leg was wrapped daily to support it while it supported Spidey.

The last shoeing was done in July, and the injury was about five months into the treatment **(Figures 34-36)**. Spiderman is able to bear weight and use his leg about as much as he wants to at this stage.

This injury happened in February, and Cody was able to rope on Spiderman by August **(Figures 37-39)**. Today the scar is just a white area that says little about how dramatic the original injury was **(Figures 40-41)**. There were several factors involved in this remarkable recovery. First, the patten bar was applied within hours of the injury. Second, Kelly did every bit of doctoring needed to make this horse feel better, and third, we had a vet involved from the beginning. Remember that combination when dealing with any traumatic injury.

Next is a horse that suffered a major abscess. When Dr. Marcotte called, he said we were about to have an avulsion, and he didn't care what I did. When I suggested the patten bar, he thought it would be fine, but with the problems this horse was having, he did not hold out much hope.

This horse had been shod badly, and the farrier had left major sole pressure and a hot nail in this

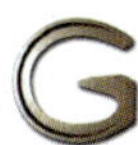

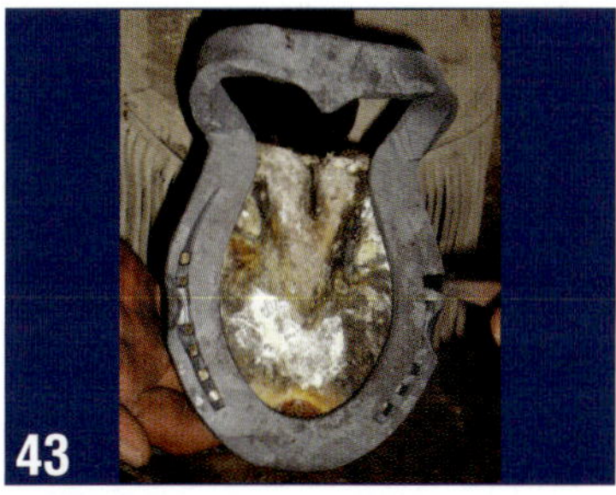

Fitting the patten bar.

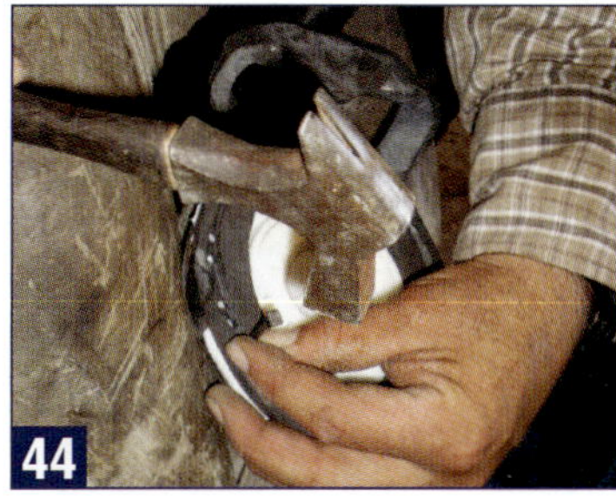

Securing the foot.

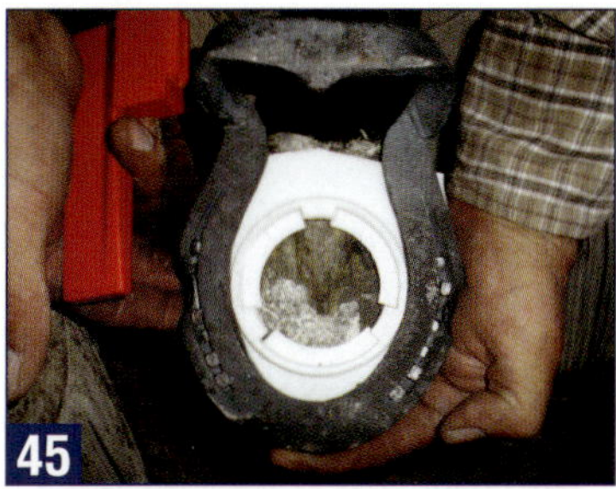

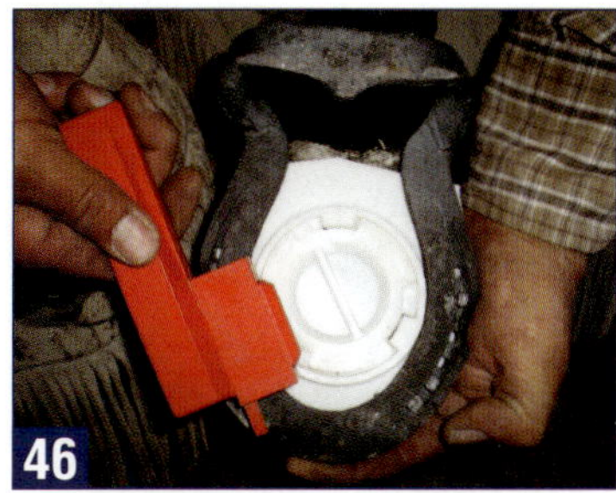

A Mustad hospital pad, equipped with a removable center.

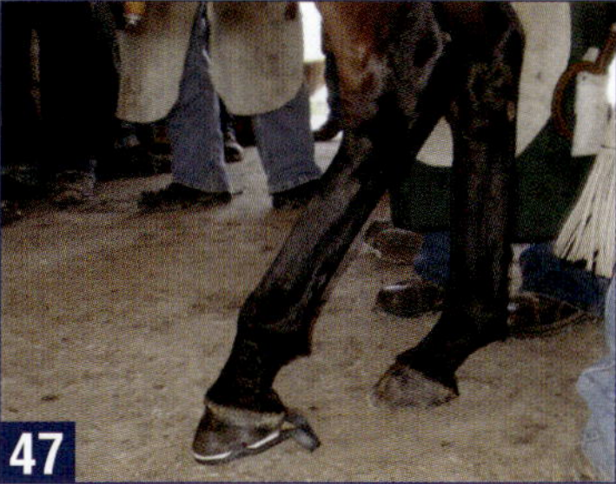

The horse was still leery of putting too much weight on the foot.

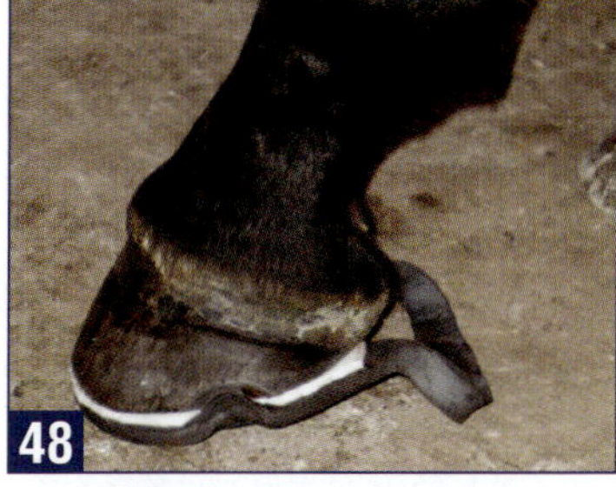

The clips are far back because of the thickness of the pad.

foot. The resulting infection was so bad that there was very little attachment between the hoof and the sensitive structures. The foot was easily spread and manipulated from the major infection, and it felt like one bad step would wrench it off the coffin bone.

In **Figure 42**, the damage to the sole is apparent. Drainage has been achieved, and we want to protect this area but still be able to treat it with medication. The perfect answer would be a hospital plate, but not with the patten bar. I decided to use a Mustad hospital pad. This is a hard plastic pad with a removable center for the application of medication. It was a great solution.

I made the shoe and fit it **(Figure 43)**. The pad was attached, and I nailed the shoe on. I was careful with how I held the foot while nailing, so that the concussion of nailing wouldn't hurt the horse, or even worse, hammer the hoof capsule off of the coffin bone. With feet that are this injured, it is good to secure and stabilize the hoof capsule as much as possible when nailing **(Figure 44)**. It is easier to do on a front foot than a hind, and I will use my tong hand to hold the foot tightly against my leg while nailing.

In **Figures 45-46**, the removable portion of the hospital pad is evident. Even with the patten bar on, this horse does not want to put much weight on that foot **(Figure 47)**. That is great with me. Notice

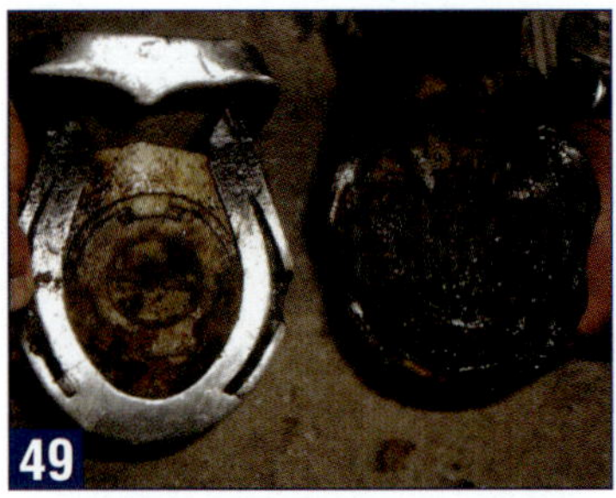

The sole, right, after six weeks. The shoe and pad are at left.

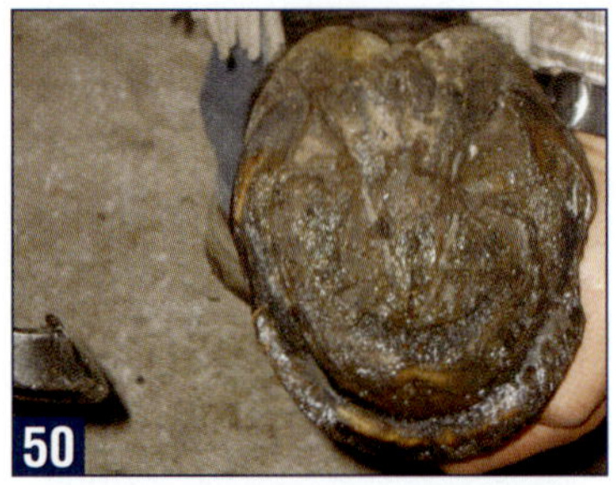

Some growth had occurred and the horse went back to normal shoes.

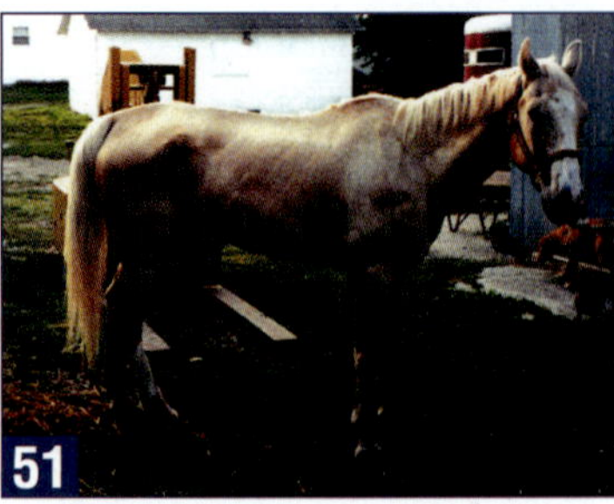

A severe tendon cut had caused this horse to lose weight.

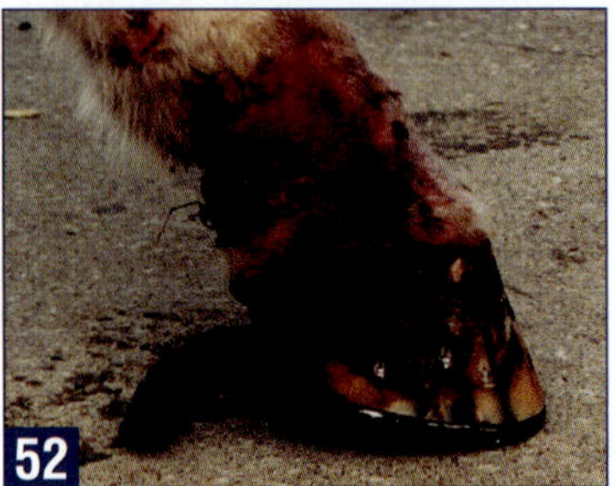

First shoeing cycle.

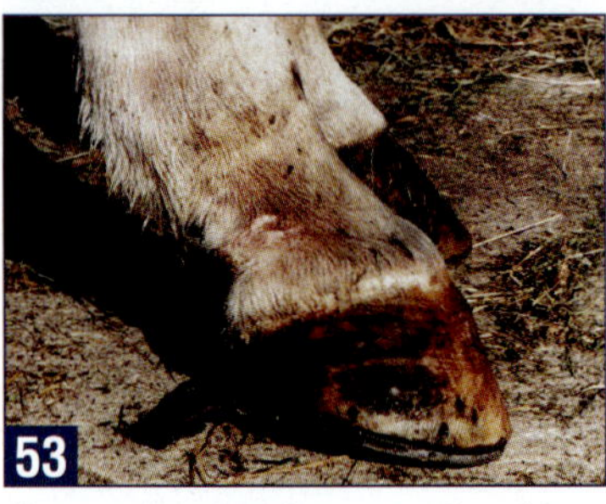

Second shoeing cycle. Note the improvement.

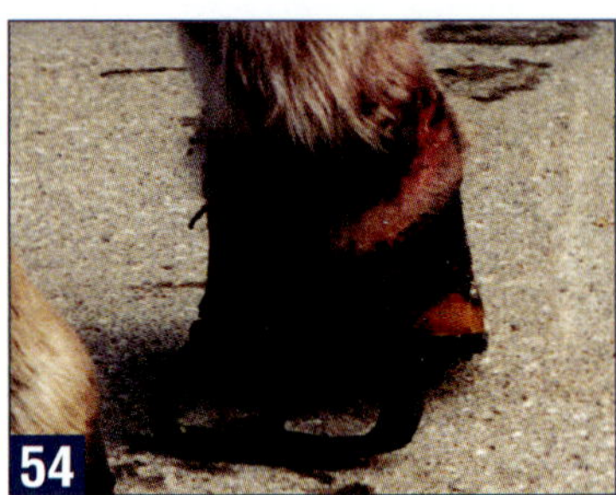

First shoeing cycle.

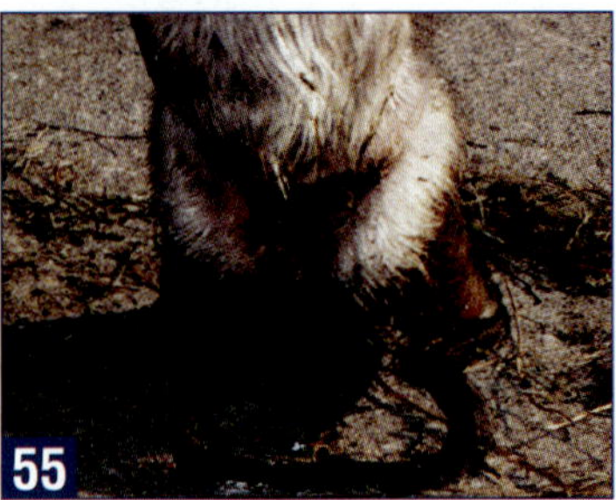

Second shoeing cycle. Again, note the improvement.

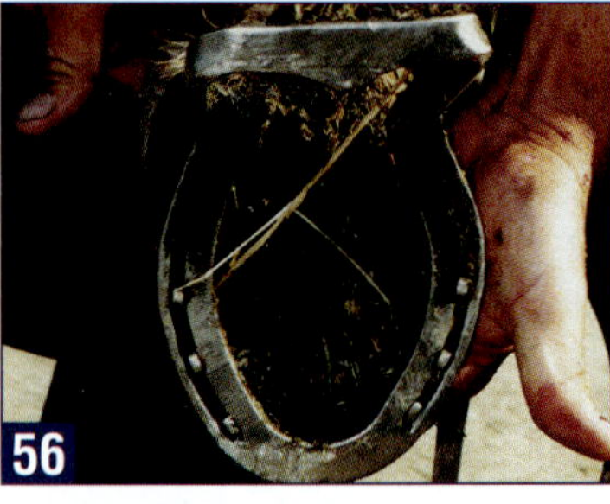

Patten bar shoe on the foot from the bottom.

in **Figure 48** that I have clips pretty far back in an effort to help hold this foot together. When clips are fit to a foot and then a pad is added, it can be really hard to get a clean and solid clip fit. This clip fit has been fouled by the use of a pad and my lack of attention to that detail when I was fitting. When using a pad, especially a thick one, it is difficult getting a good burned-in clip.

When the owner brought the horse back six weeks later, the foot felt significantly better. There has been some growth, and the shoe and pad had done their job **(Figures 49-50)**. I nailed a set of shoes on this horse, and he continued his recovery. He was back barrel racing after the next set of shoes. Dr. Marcotte was as surprised and happy as I was.

The next horse is one that had a severe cut in the back of his pastern. It was in an area that would not heal because of movement, and this horse was sick as a result of the injury. He had lost a lot of weight **(Figure 51)** and had had a lot of trouble dealing with the injury. If you compare **Figure 52** to **Figure 53** and **Figure 54** to **Figure 55**, you can see the difference that one shoeing cycle with the patten bar made in his progress of healing. **Figure 56** is the patten bar on the foot from the bottom. That is what a patten bar is supposed to do: Allow the horse to

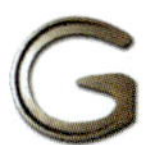

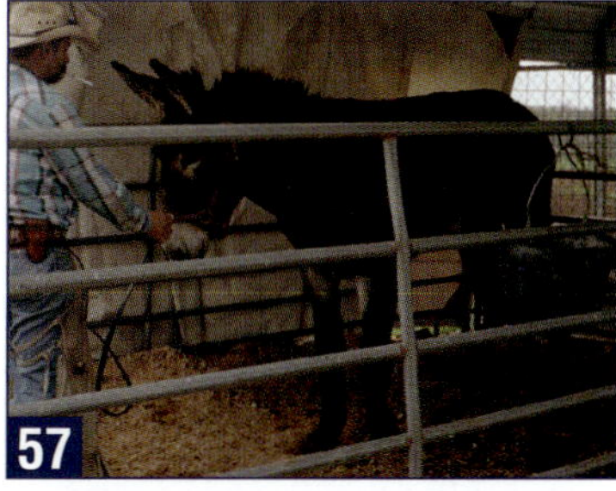

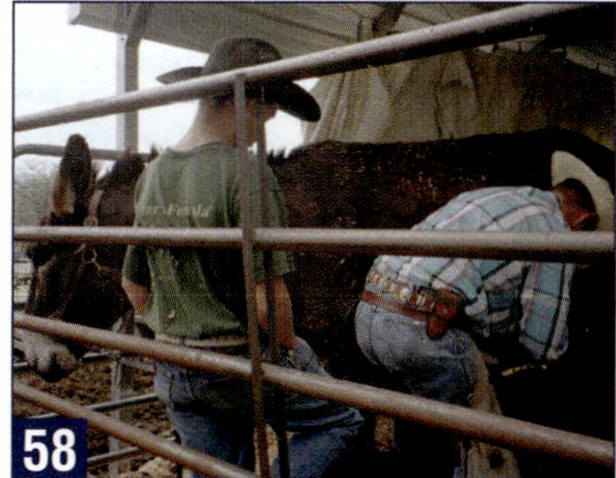

Treating the injured jack.

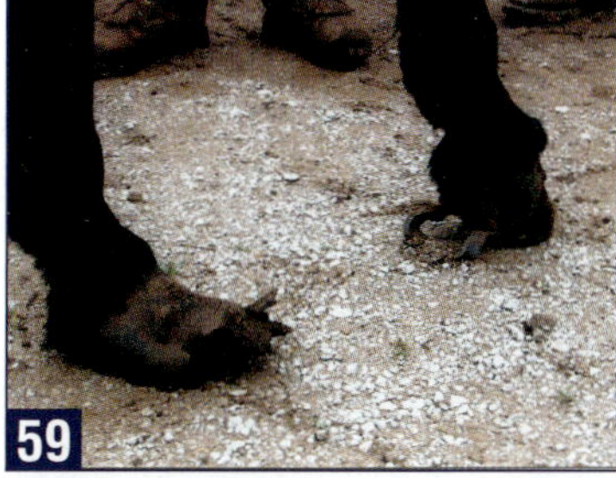

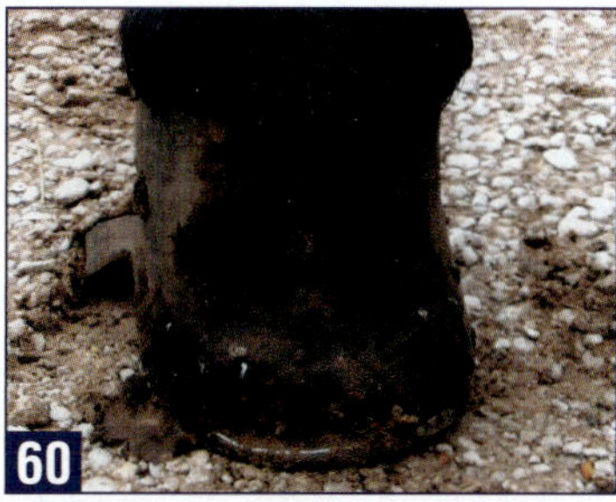

Much improved at the second shoeing.

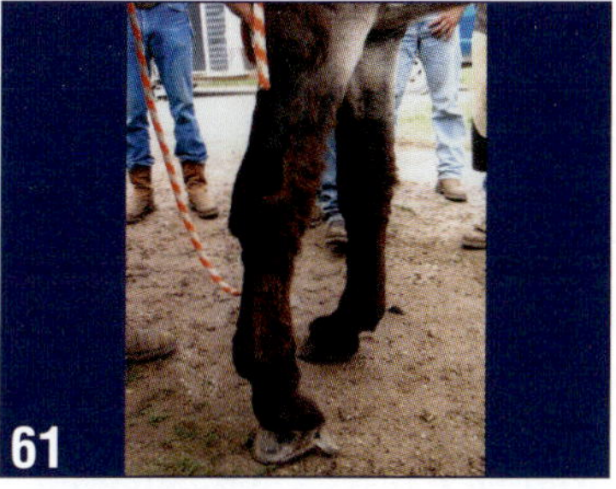

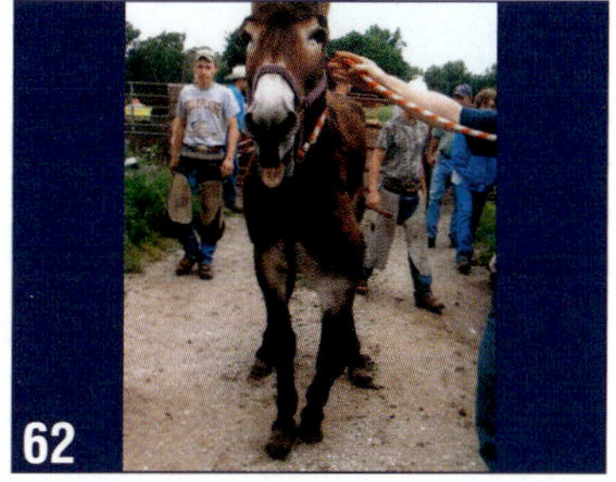

Continued improvement.

survive and heal whatever wound needs healing.

So far, we have had a lot of patten bars on hind feet. It can be effective on the front feet as well, but you need to take some things into consideration. First, it is a little more dangerous, since a horse is likely to step on one in the front end with the hind feet. Second, if you don't have the bar far enough back, it can actually become a pivot point for the leg with a damaged tendon to rock back on. I have used it on several front feet with good results. Here is one of the more interesting ones.

A customer called with a mammoth jack that had been kicked while trying to breed a Belgian mare. This jack had never been handled, and was quite an ornery type of animal. When the mare kicked him, she broke his humerus. Remember from the anatomy chapters that this is a huge bone.

When I got the call, the customer was going to put the jack down. We went out to see him, and I gave him a shot of Torbejesic and Domosedan **(Figures 57-58)**. It was pretty gruesome, but when you pulled his leg forward, you could feel and hear the grating of the two pieces of bone against each other. I don't have pictures of the first shoeing, but when we came back six weeks later, he had been using that leg a little bit. He stood on his toe, pulled that foot forward with his shoulder, and placed weight lightly on the patten bar. The owner couldn't believe it **(Figures 59-60)**. **Figures 61-62** show what he was looking like when we returned. Notice the condition of his other foot, as well as the way the foot with the patten bar is quite deformed.

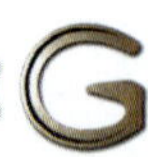

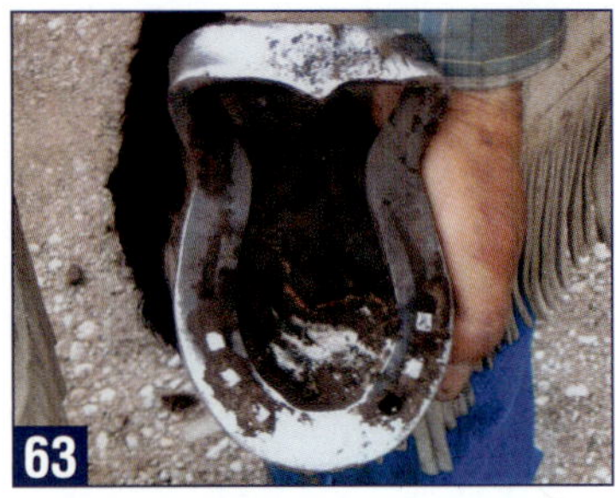

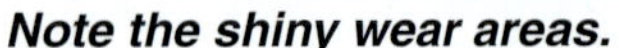

Note the shiny wear areas.

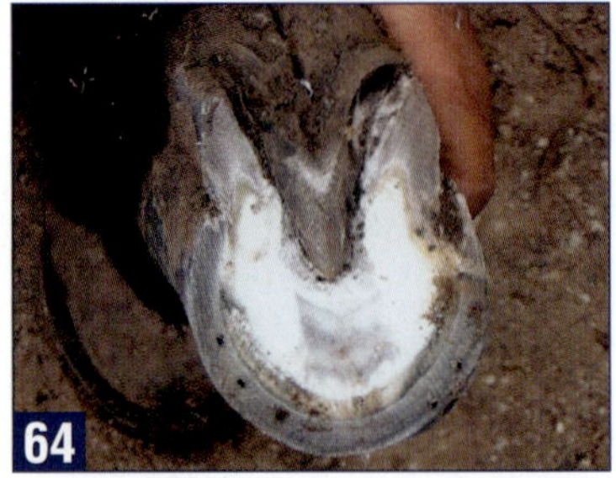

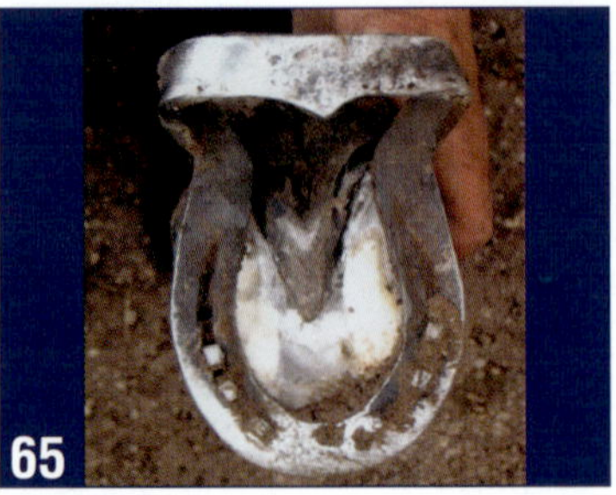

Resetting the shoe at the same height.

66

The jack today.

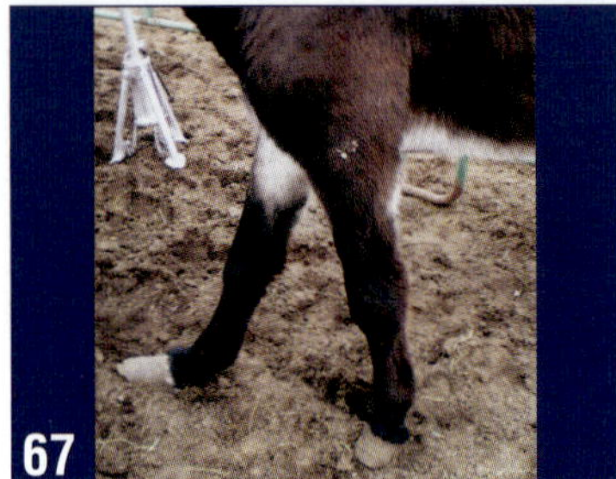

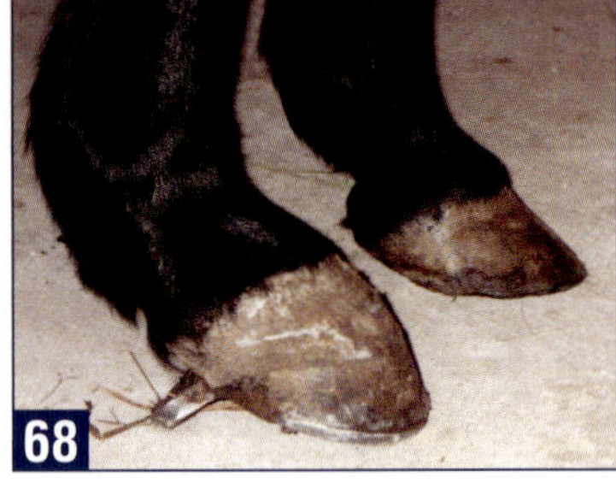

A patten bar that has been left on an injured foot for too long a period. Note the hoof distortion.

Since he had not been handled, the feet were in a very neglected state when we first worked on him.

When looking at the bottom of the foot with the patten bar, it is easy to see where the shoe was being used because those areas are shiny **(Figure 63)**. I trimmed him up and reset the shoe **(Figures 64-65)** without lowering the height of the bar. We let him go for another couple of months while he continued to heal. **Figures 66-67** show what he looks like today. There is a large amount of bone where the two pieces of the humerus came together, but he is breeding mares like his owner wanted him to.

The last picture, **Figure 68**, is of a horse that has had a patten bar on too long. This is neglect on the owner's part, and you can see what a change it made in the hoof capsule. One of the things to take from this photo is just how much a foot can change in a short time. Remember that when you trim a foot out of balance or nail something a little crazy on a foot.

The patten bar is a great weapon in your arsenal, but like all weapons, it must be used carefully and with understanding of what it can do.

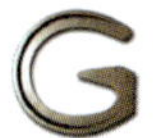

Chapter

56-2 Z-BAR SHOE

CASE STUDY

The principle behind the use of this shoe is to take weight off an area of the foot that has been injured. This shoe is not hard to make, and it can give the horse some real relief.

As you can see from **Figure 1**, dealing with a cut hoof can be quite bloody. You may want to wear an old apron as well as take precautions if you are shoeing in clothes that you don't want stained.

The first horse pictured here injured its foot by kicking a fence. It broke a large part of the lateral foot away from the coffin bone as well as cut through the coronary band. This was a young horse, and it was Grade 3 lame when we arrived to work on it. In **Figure 2**, the damaged horn is being pulled back to reveal the top of the lateral cartilage. When this was removed from the cavity, there was a small piece of coffin bone attached. In **Figure 3**, the extent of the damage to the coronary band and the skin above it is apparent. The first visit, I made and applied a Z-bar shoe to the foot that was still solid **(Figure 4)**. The horse was more comfortable immediately and remained so for the rest of the treatment.

In **Figure 5**, the outside of the foot is healing, and I put the same Z-bar back on. At the 12-week mark, we came back to shoe for the third time. At this point, the area that had been injured was being held in place only by the frog, so I removed it **(Figures 6-9)**. Once it was removed, the foot

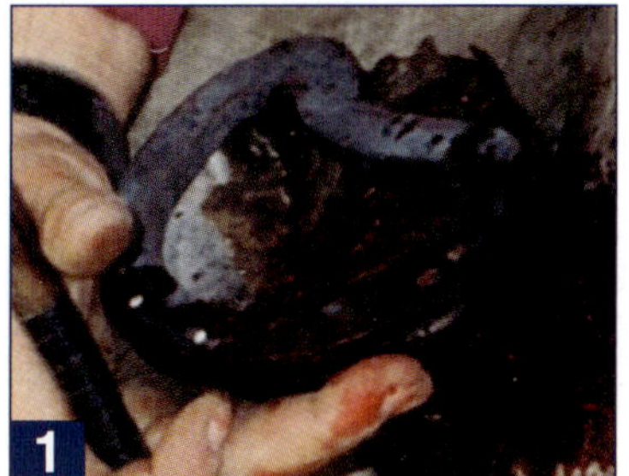

1

Bloody injured foot with a Z-bar on it.

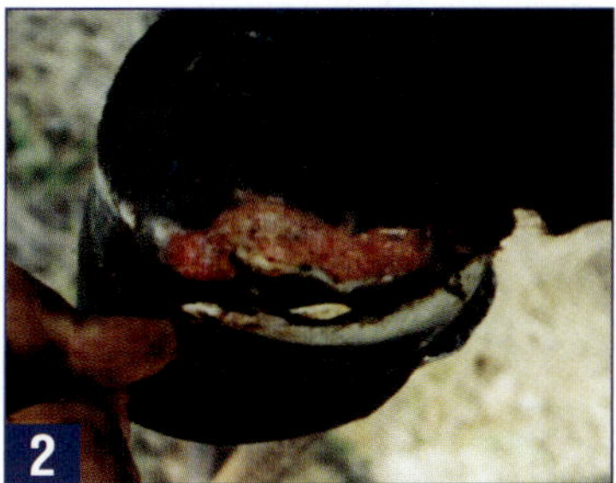

2

Pulling the wall back to expose the injury on a different foot.

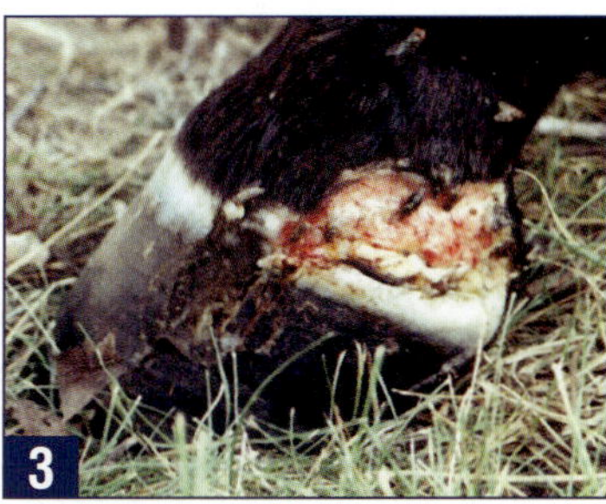

3

Lateral view of injury.

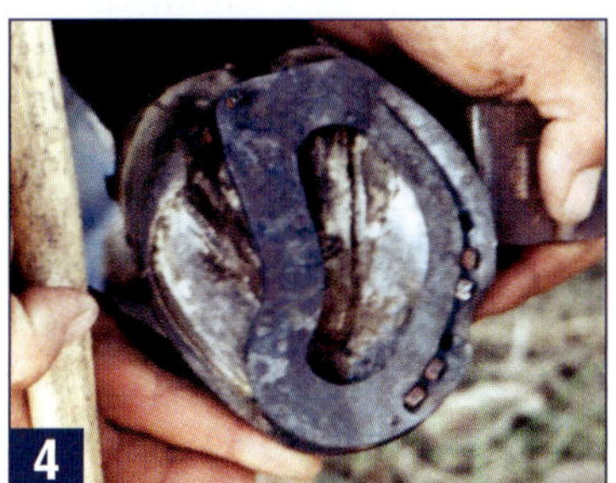

4

Z-bar on the foot.

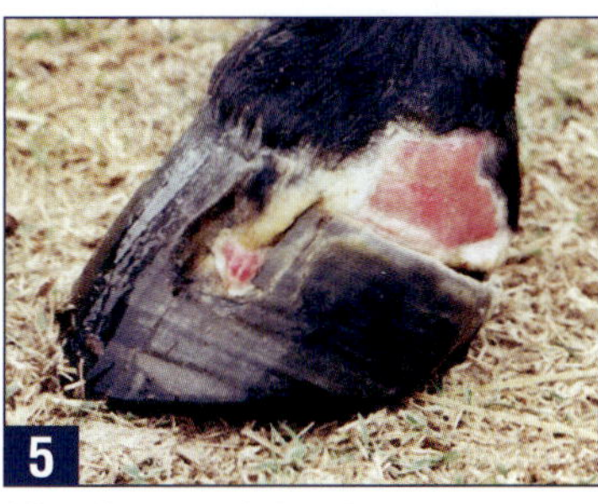

5

The foot as it heals.

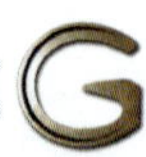

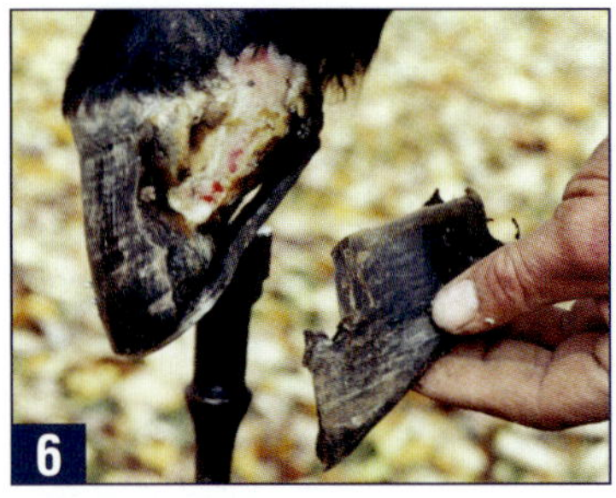

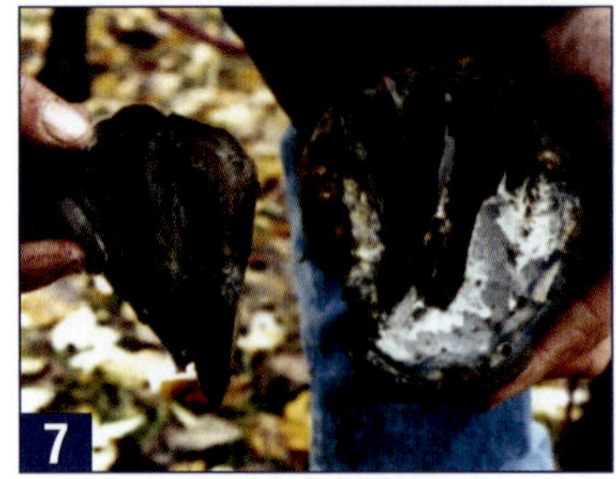

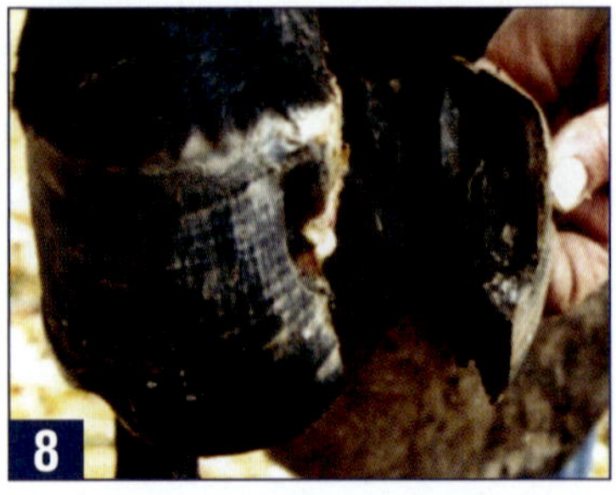

Removing the detached and dead portion of the foot. This was the area that was unsupported by the Z-bar.

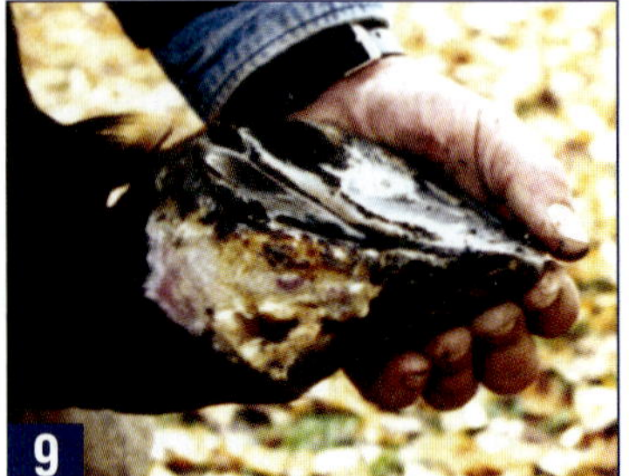

Trim and reset.

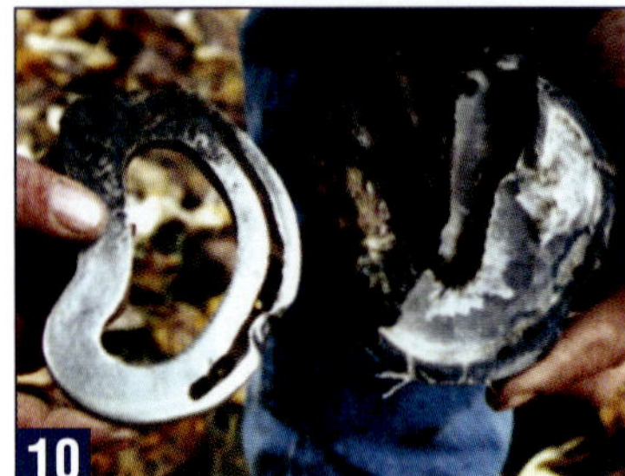

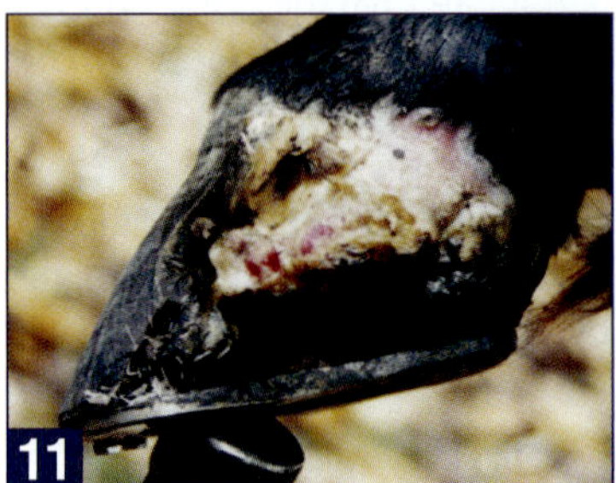

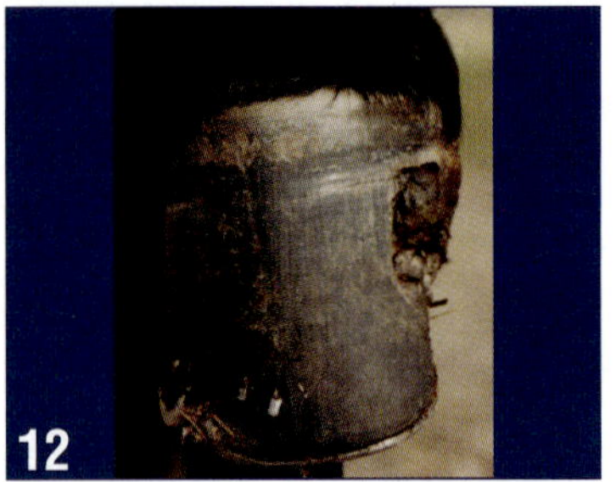

Next trip back.

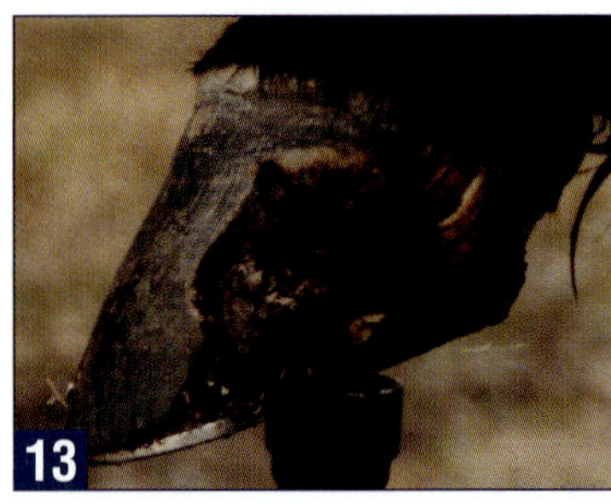

Lots of growth.

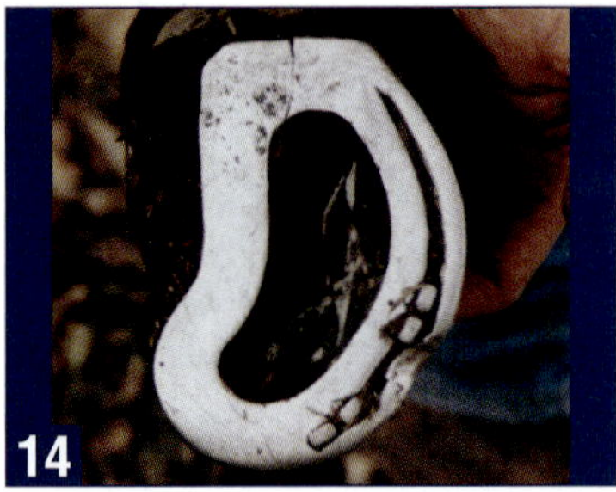

Z-bar doing the job intended.

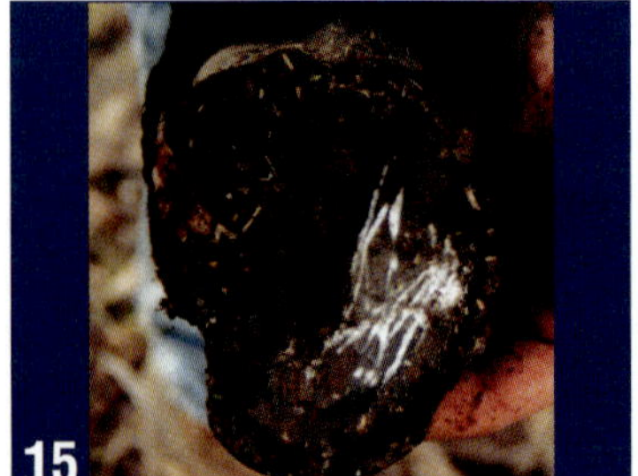

Foot without shoe.

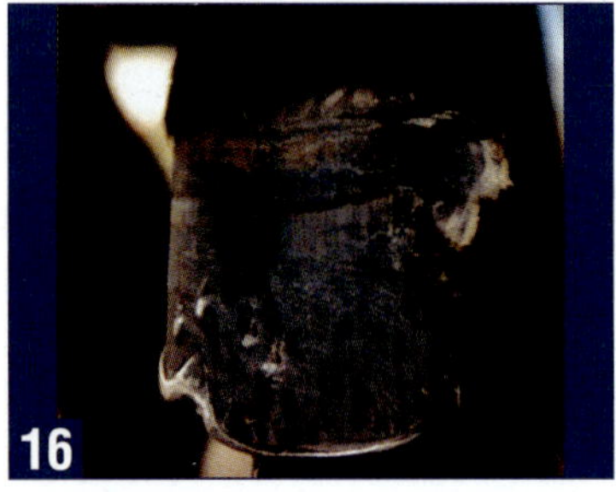

Final shoeing.

that remained was trimmed, and the same Z-bar was nailed back on **(Figures 10-11)**. The last time I saw the horse was when I came back about two months later. The horse was still sound, and there was an amazing amount of new growth at the coronary band where the injury had occurred. I was surprised that foot was growing in an area where I thought the coronary band had been completely destroyed **(Figures 12-13)**. The

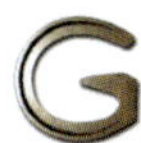

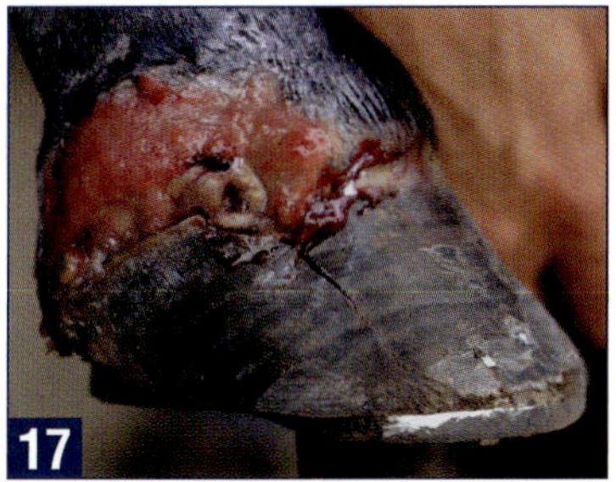

Injured foot with Z-bar on it.

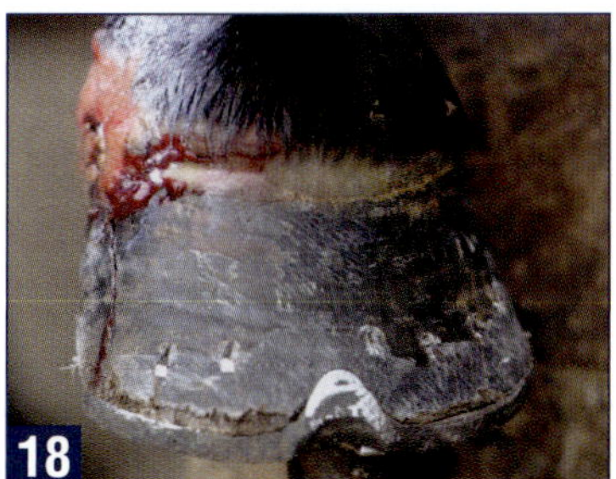

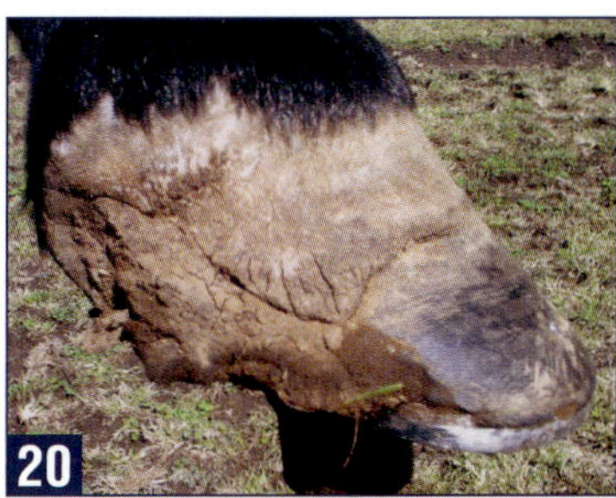

Return trip as foot heals.

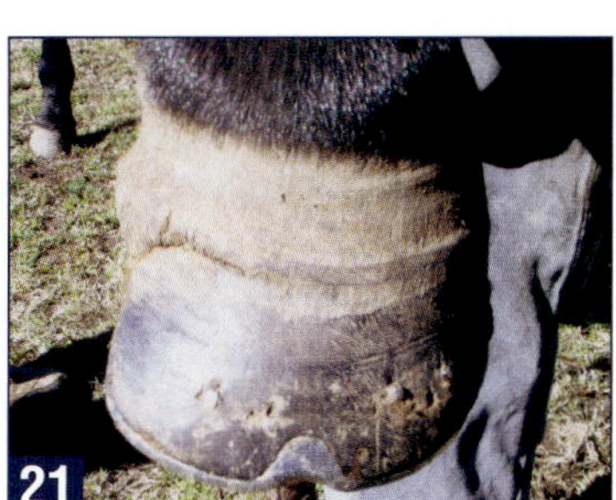

Bottom of foot. Equi-Pak pour-in.

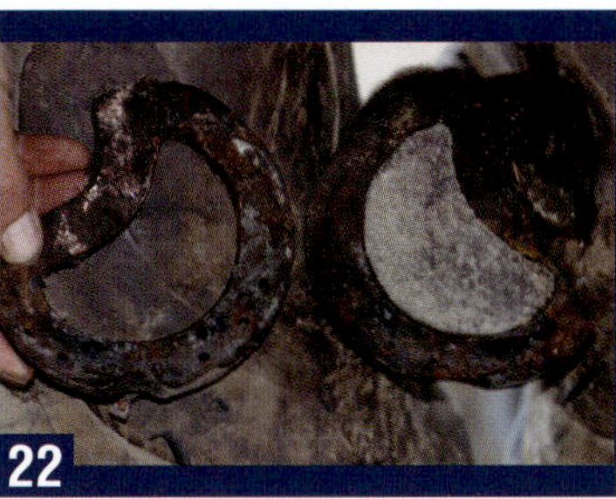

The pour-in has stayed stuck to the foot.

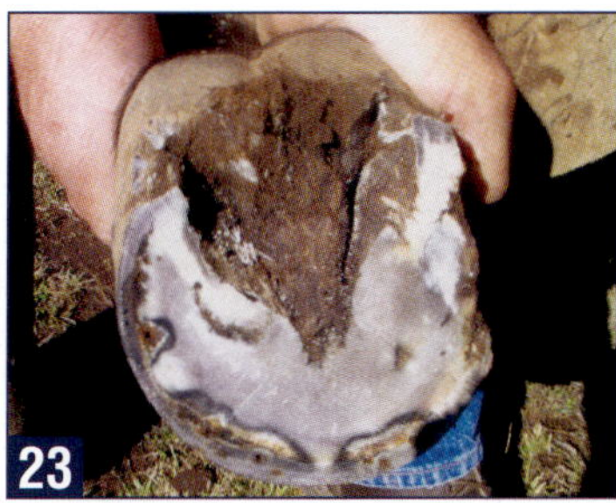

Trimmed for reset.

Z-bar is allowing this horse to heal **(Figures 14-15)**. I reset him for the last time **(Figure 16)**, and from what I have heard since, this horse ended up a success.

On another occasion, a horse had a traumatic hoof injury of unknown origin. The woman brought this horse to the shop, and I used a Z-bar with Equi-Pak. This animal was Grade 4 lame when it came to the shop, as can be seen in **Figures 17 and 18**. Once the shoe was on and clinched, we applied the Equi-Pak (**Figure 19**). The horse improved to Grade 3 lame, and the owner called a week later to tell me that she did not think the horse was limping at all.

The horse was Grade 1 lame on the next visit, but this was a remarkable recovery. When the horse came back, the cut area was much healed **(Figures 20-21)** and you can see that the Equi-Pak has held in well **(Figure 22)**. To remove a shoe on a foot like this, pull the nails individually, which is one of the main reasons for fullering this shoe. At this point, the foot was in much better shape **(Figure 23)**, and I reset it. This horse was shod about three times with a Z-bar, and is now simply trimmed and left without shoes. The foot is pretty strong and doing well **(Figure 24-26)**. There is permanent scarring,

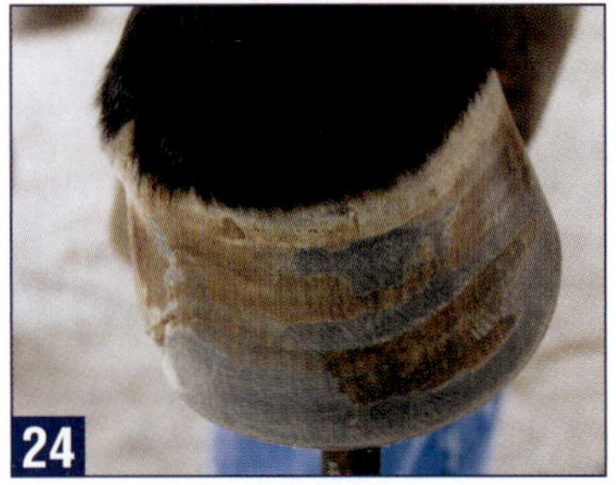

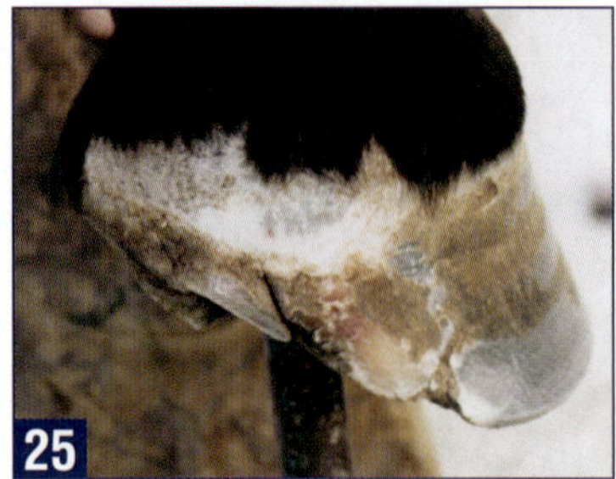

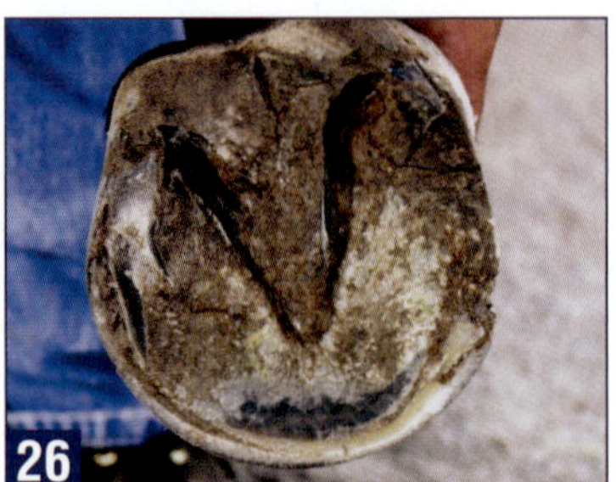

The foot as it is now.

but that is a minimal problem when you consider how badly injured that foot was.

One of the main things to consider when dealing with badly injured feet is that shoes can be created to place weight on good tissue and relieve stress from the injured area. This principle of shifting weight is easily accomplished with a shoe such as the Z-bar, since the injured portions are completely unsupported. Unsupported also means not having to support any weight, which is exactly what makes this shoe work and makes it a good thing for you to be able to make and fit.

I have found the Z-bar easy to use and make, and I am sure that most farriers will find a use for this shoe on an injured horse someday.

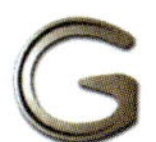

Chapter

56-3 STRAIGHT BARS

CASE STUDY

Section 11, Chapter 48, Straight Bars, which tells you how to build straight bars is one of the longest chapters of this book. The reason is that the straight bar is useful in so many pathological shoeing scenarios and is the basis for a lot of other pathological shoes. Since it is used pretty often and fits very similarly to a regular horseshoe, I will not waste too much time here with a lot of straight bars, just a few interesting ones.

It can be made in more than one way, and being able to make and fit a straight bar is paramount if you are to be a great farrier. This chapter contains a few examples of practical application of this shoe.

This horse was severely lame. He had suffered a massive abscess, and his entire sole had been damaged. **Figure 1** is what the foot looked like when the horse came in. What was left of the frog was an odd yellow color, the sole was disconnected, and someone had done a little bit of nipping on the wall. That is about as helpful to a farrier as disassembling your motor at home before you take your car in to the mechanic. Notice the frog in **Figure 2** and the piece of wall that pulled free in **Figures 3 and 4**. The whole horny sole covering came off to expose a sore and damaged sole **(Figure 5)**.

Feet like this can be really challenging, since there is no way to recruit frog, sole, or bars for part of the weight bearing. A heart bar or Z-bar would have been a fantastic choice if the frog wasn't as damaged as the sole. As such, you have to figure out how to shape a shoe to maximize the hoof wall that you do have available. To make this bar shoe, I made a modified whip-across, ending up with a bar that covered that damaged medial heel without putting

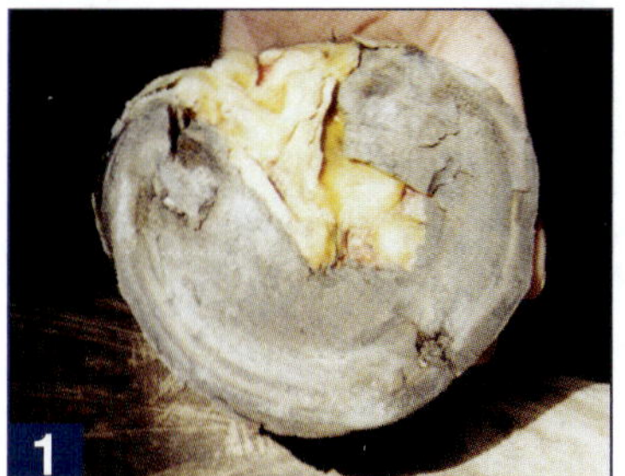

Badly abscessed foot.

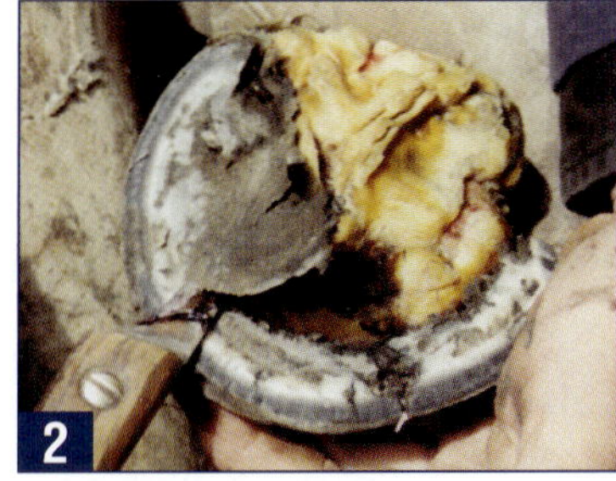

Pulling off the sole.

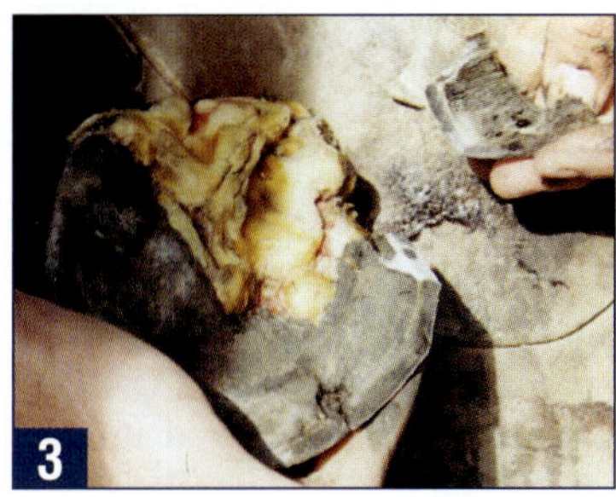

Large chunk of heel broke free.

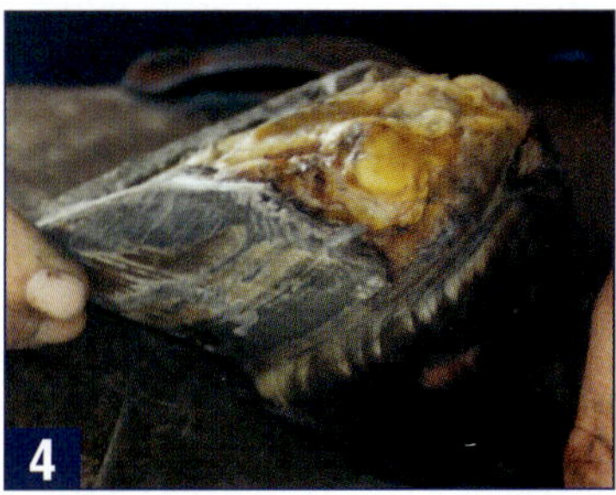

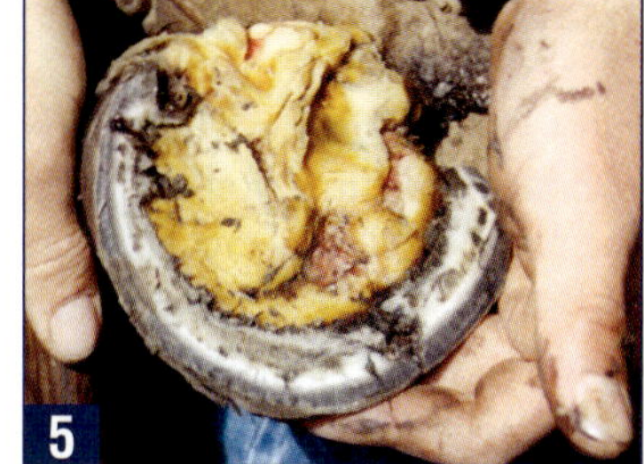

Foot ready to be shod.

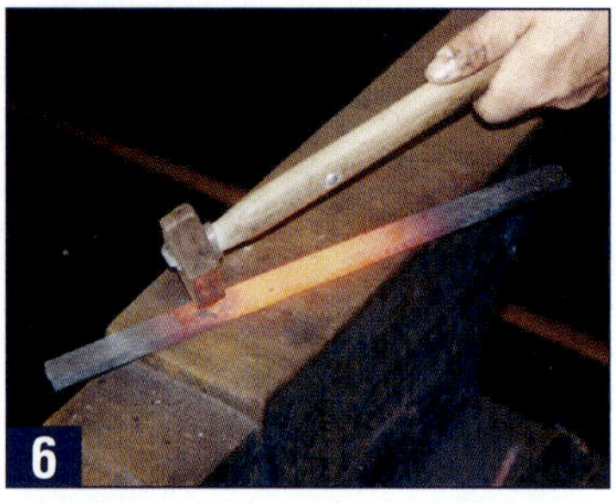

6 *Fullering through the toe in the straight.*

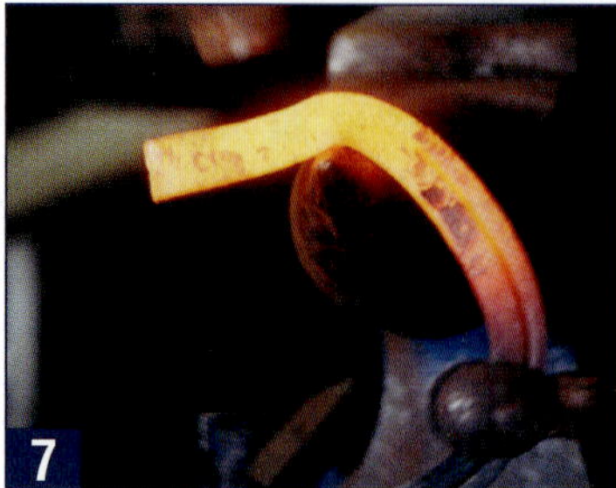

7 *Long side.*

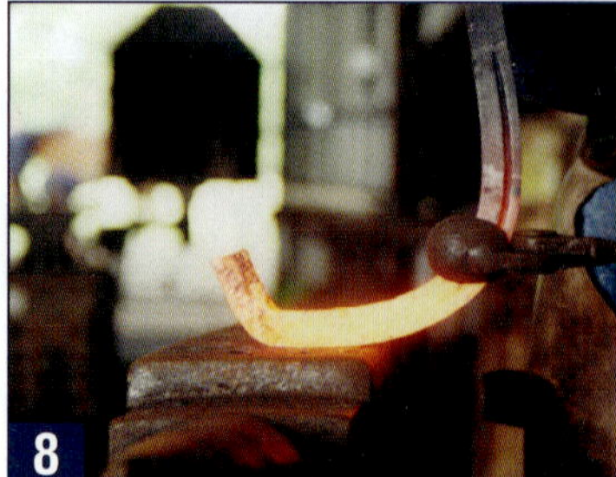

8 *Short side.*

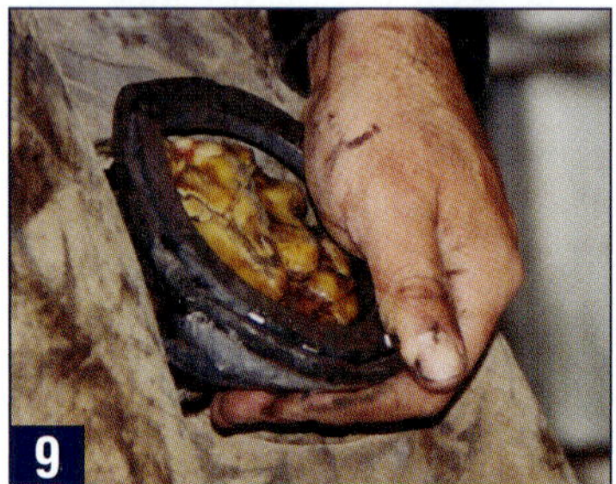

9 *Nailing up, holding the hoof capsule itself securely.*

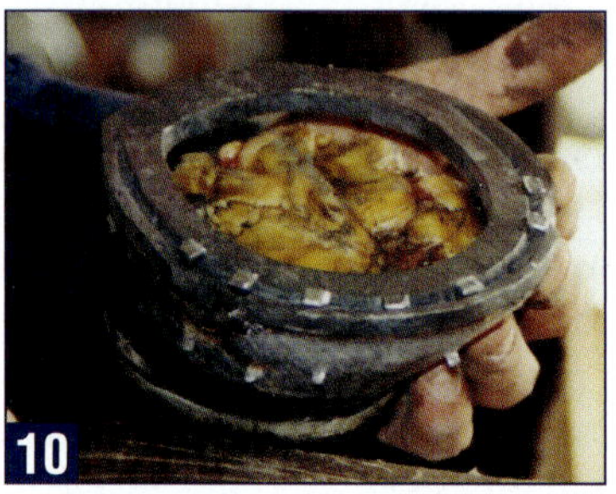

10 *Lots of nails around the shoe.*

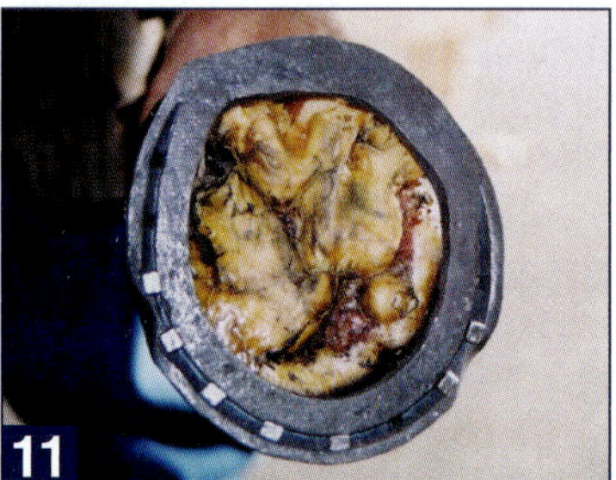

11 *Shoe nailed up.*

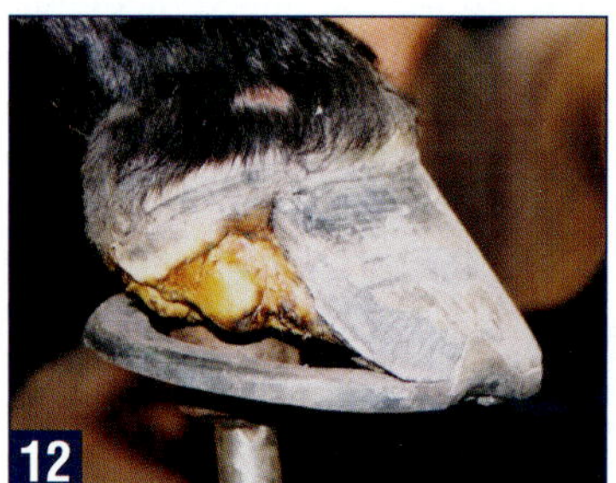

12 *Lateral view of broken heel with bar shoe on the foot.*

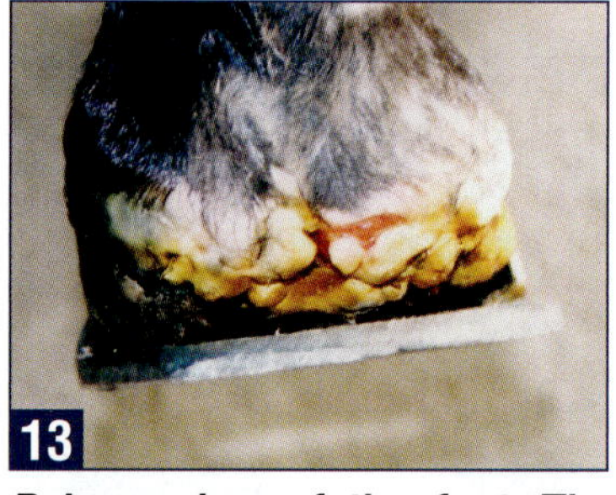

13 *Palmar view of the foot. The tissue of the frog is badly damaged.*

too much pressure on the foot around it.

I always want to have a lot of nailing options with feet that are in this sort of shape. Fullering through the toe allowed me to place nails all around the shoe. Anytime you are going to crease through the toe, you should crease about 70% of the depth of the fullering in the straight **(Figure 6)**. By doing this, when you bend the toe, the fullering will collapse instead of the outside edge being thinned out. Creasing in the toe after the bend is hard to do without messing up the stock dimension. When the crease collapses, you can simply open it back up with the fuller after you bend the toe.

I bent less from one side of the shoe for my hockey stick **(Figure 7)** and more on the other side **(Figure 8)**. That gave me a good, strong lateral heel and a weak corner on the medial side where I wanted coverage without too much expansion.

When I nailed on this shoe, I was intent on holding just the foot with my knees and not the pastern **(Figure 9)**. This is a good technique to use when you have a hoof that is as sore as this horse's

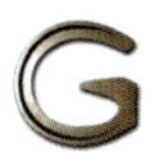

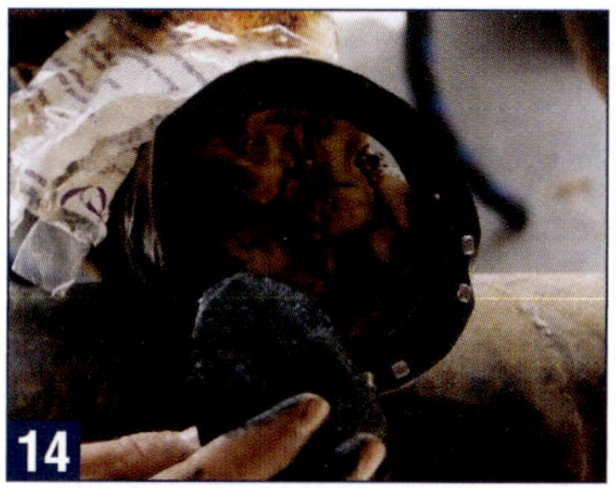

Packing the foot with Hawthorne's Sole Pack.

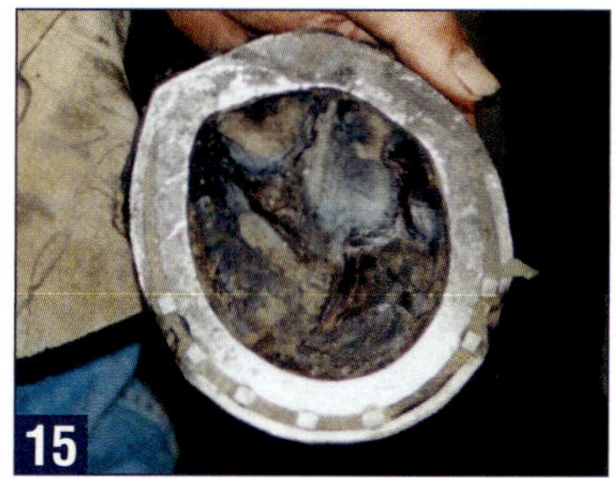

Look of the foot when it returned.

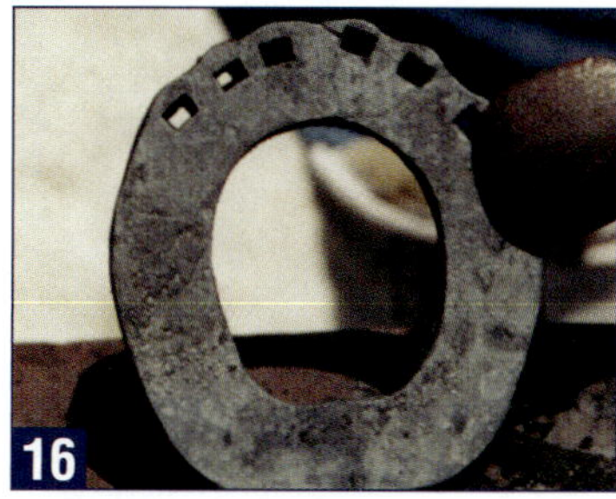

Tiny bar shoe for foal with a broken coffin bone.

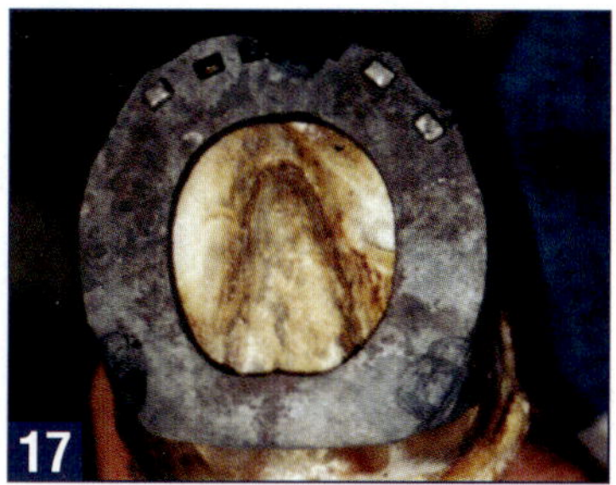

Shoe on the foot.

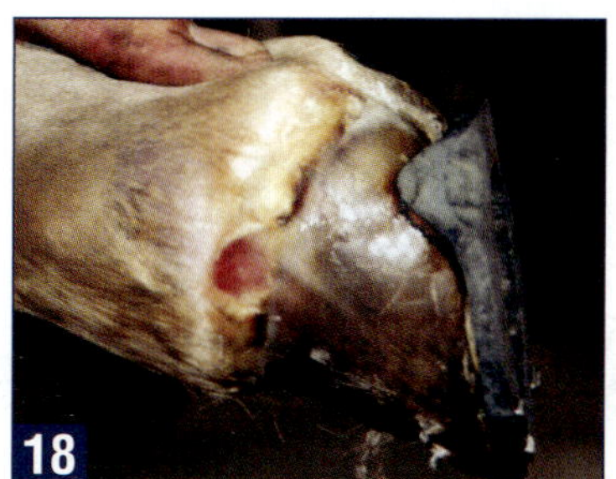

was. The reason is that you can dampen some of the blow from the hammer by securing the foot tightly. Another thing you can do is to hammer with an intermittent cadence on an injured foot.

Figures 10-13 show how this foot nailed up. The horse was instantly better, as long as he did not land on any rocks. I sent the horse home with a supply of Hawthorne's Sole Pack and had the owner pack the foot and bandage it daily **(Figure 14)**.

Unfortunately, I only got to see this horse one more time, and this was for a reset a couple months later. The sole was looking better at that time **(Figure 15)**, but I would have liked to have had more that just the one reset. That is the nature of doing pathological work. My goal is to get the horse good enough that it can go back to the care of its previous farrier. However, some owners jump the gun.

One day, a lady asked me to trim her 4-month-old foal. It had been running out, and its feet did not need trimmed in the least. I told her that it would be a waste of her money and that I wouldn't trim it if it were mine. She agreed, and I went on to trim her mares.

About a week later, Dr. Martin calls to tell me that there is a foal in the clinic with a fractured coffin bone. When I went to the clinic, I found out it was this foal. I was very thankful of my policy of not doing horses that don't need it, because had I trimmed that foal, I would have been the first person blamed, even though I would not have been the cause of the problem. That's something to think about. There are so many horses to be shod and trimmed, taking money and doing horses that don't need to be done is not a good business decision.

Anyway, getting to the foot. **Figure 16** shows the bar shoe I made for the little foot. The tongs are holding the shoe, giving you a size comparison. In **Figure 17**, the shoe is on the foot. I have two clips back in the heels to stabilize the foot and a toe clip to help hold the shoe on. When clips are opposing each other in angle, it may be necessary to stand them up slightly for the hot fit. Otherwise, their angles will not allow the shoe to get to the foot. The shoe has

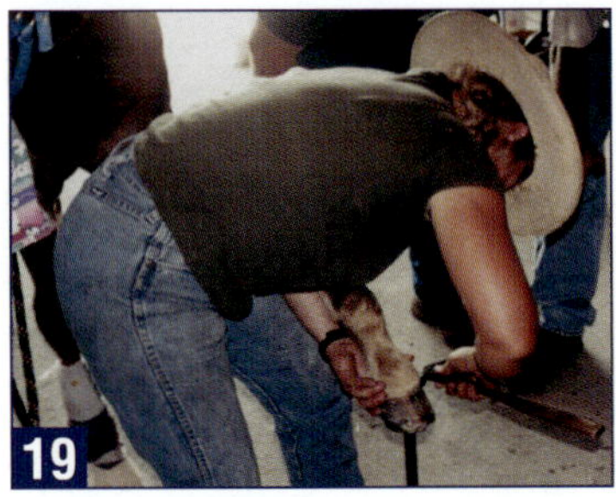
19 Kelly clinching.

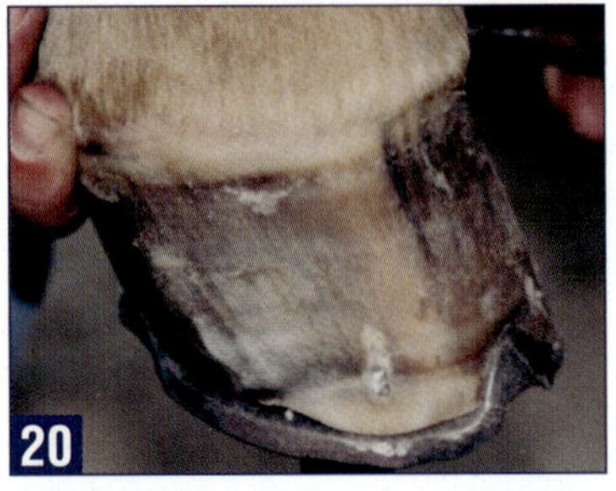
20 Medial view of the foot with the shoe on it.

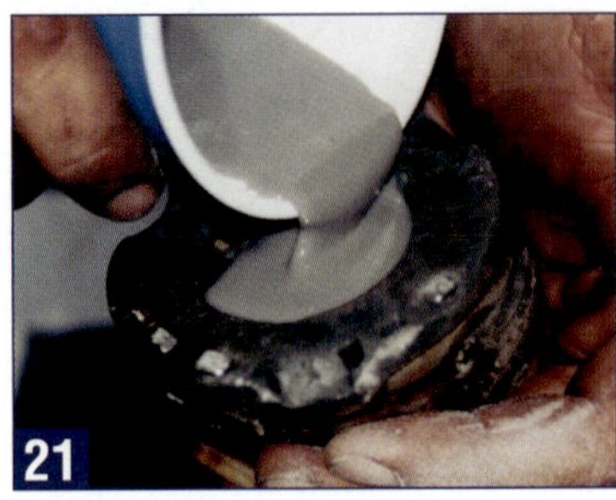
21 Old type of pour-in.

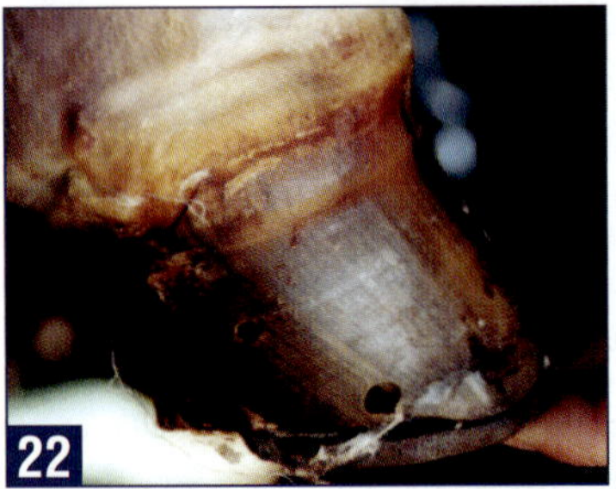
22 Drill holes in the wall where antibiotics had been injected into the bone.

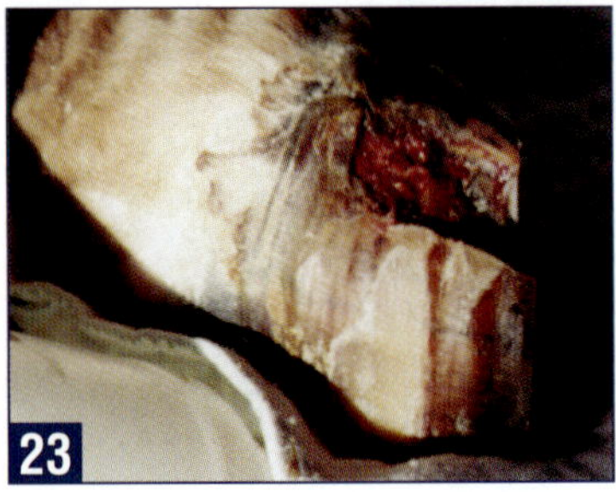
23 Large area of heel resected.

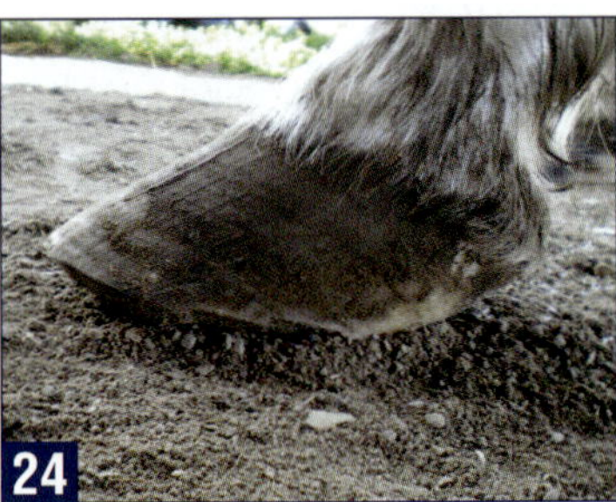
24 Foot needing a square toe and egg bar shoe.

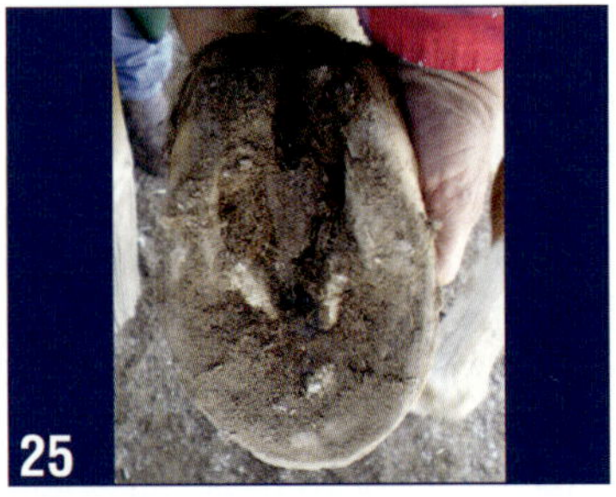
25 Solar view pre-trim.

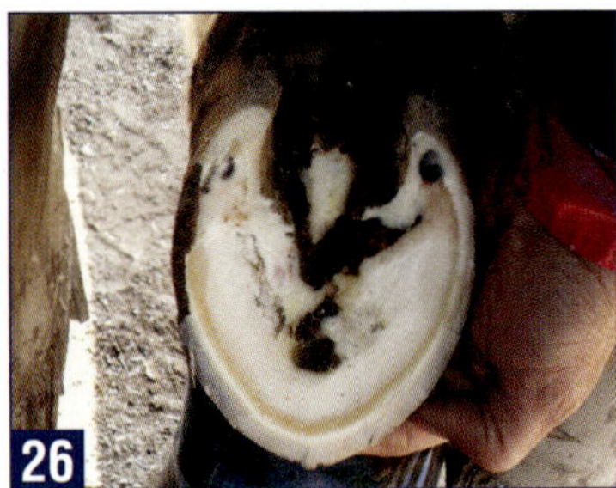
26 Post trim.

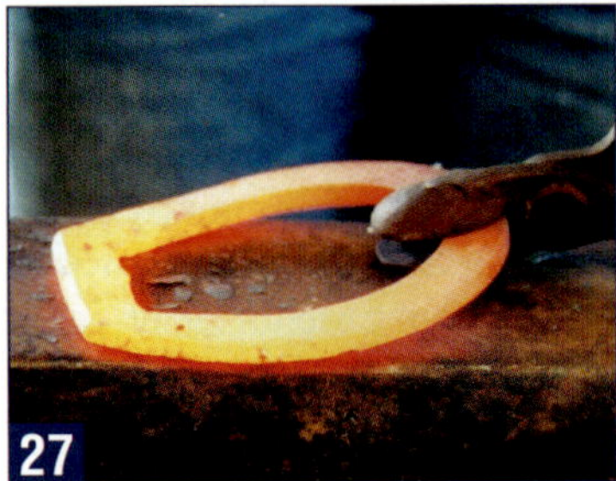
27 Making the square toe out of the bar.

been nailed with a few nails **(Figure 18)** and Kelly clinched it up **(Figures 19-20)**. This was before Equi-Pak was common, so Dr. Martin used to use a powder that mixed with a liquid and smelled like a dental clinic **(Figure 21)**. A portion of the coffin bone became infected, and it was injected with antibiotics. The holes in the hoof wall in **Figure 22** show the injection sites. Eventually, we ended up removing a fairly large portion of hoof wall at the heel due to the infection **(Figure 23)**. Although the coffin bone finally healed, the foal had developed with a crooked and unsound conformation on the other limb from the incredible stress of doing all the work for so long on one leg. It was finally destroyed as a 2-year-old because of the trauma suffered by the good leg while the broken coffin bone healed.

In **Figure 24**, we have the lateral view of a horse that ended up with an egg bar. (Notice that the customer had put a trim on it before bringing it in. I wonder if they do this to their mechanic as well?

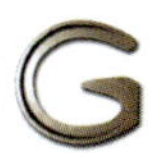

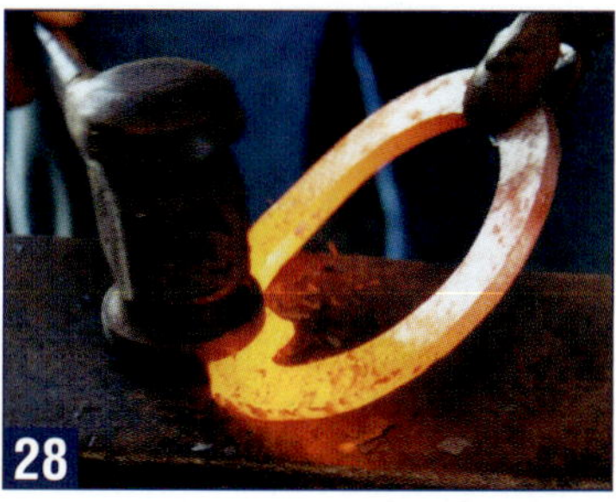

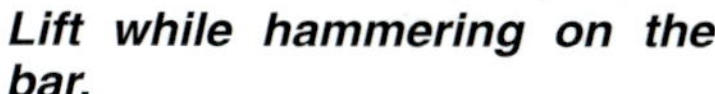
Lift while hammering on the bar.

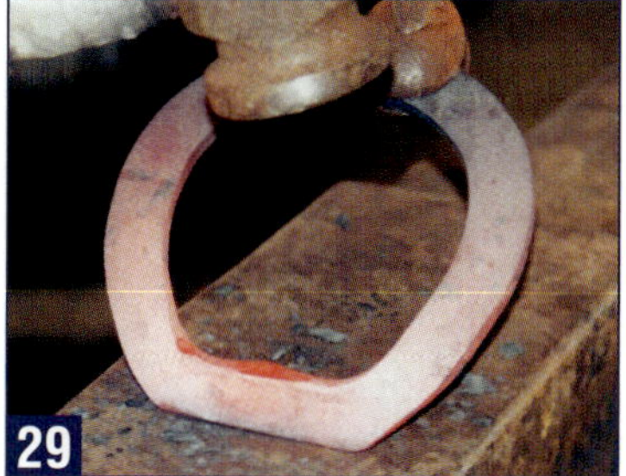

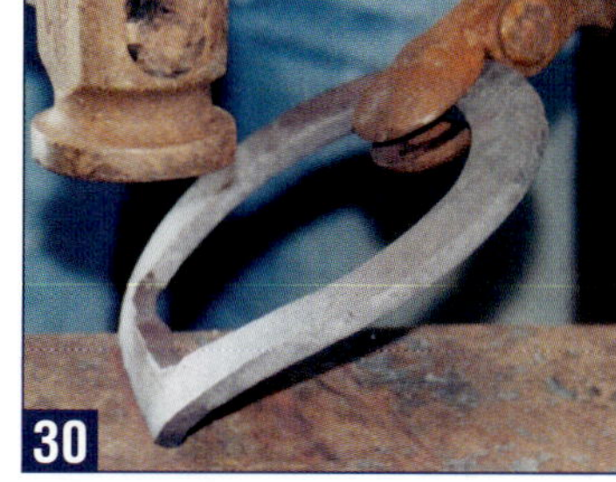

Access with a hammer to the inside of the bar.

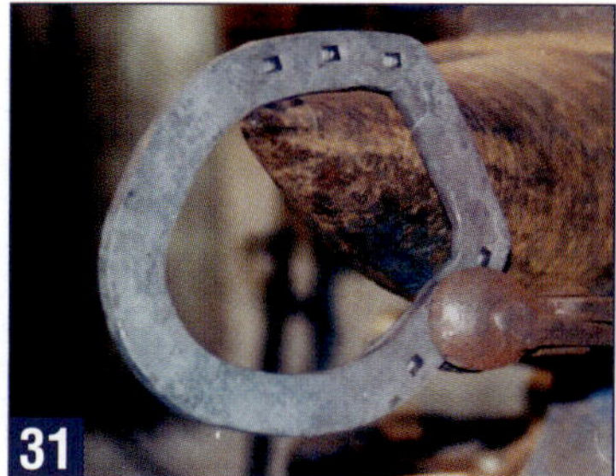

Shape as a square toed shoe.

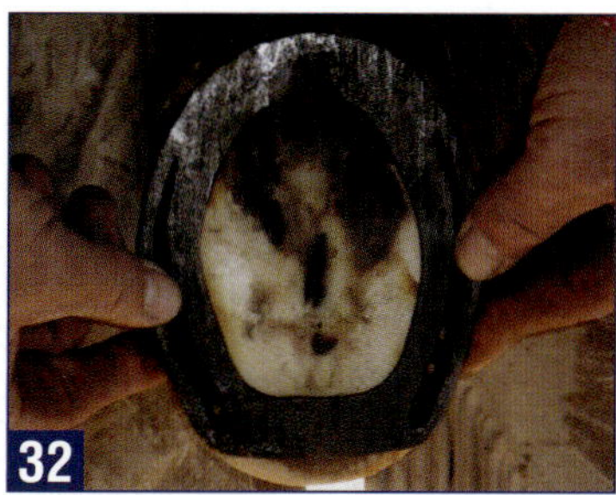

Fitting the shoe.

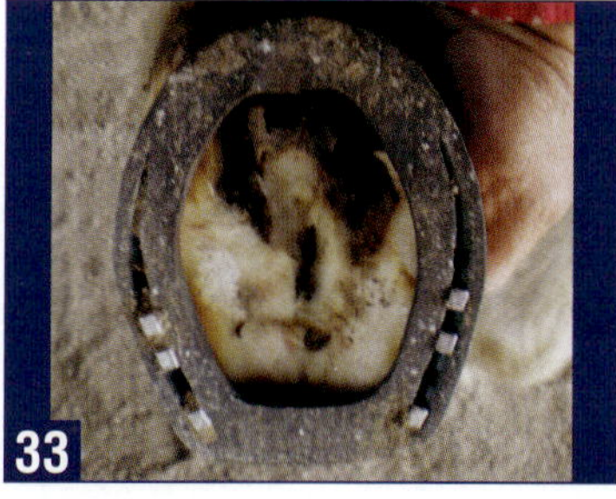

Nailed up.

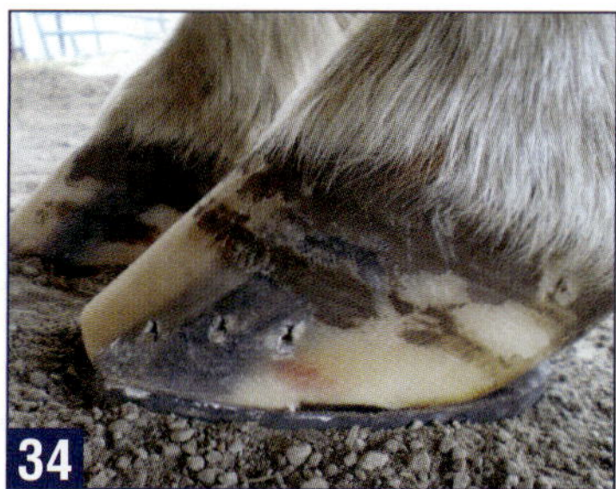

I am certain they must.) However, it was a square-toed egg bar, which is just like a straight bar that has been nailed on backwards. The method of doing this deserves mention, so here it is. **Figure 25** is the bottom pre-trim and **Figure 26** is post trim.

The straight bar is made in the normal way. Heat the shoe and hold the toe of the shoe with the tongs while hammering on the bar and lifting the toe of the shoe **(Figures 27-28)**. This allows access for the hammer to work the sex appeal out of the bar, making it flat and straight **(Figures 29-30)**. From there, it can be shaped like and punched like a square-toed shoe **(Figure 31)**. (Yes, dear reader. I know that the shoe in **Figure 31** is different than the shoe in **Figure 32**. I just needed the photo of shaping a square-toed egg bar.) The shoe is fit and nailed up in **Figures 32 and 34**.

Anytime I come across weak feet, I like to use a straight bar. The draft horse in **Figure 35** is a good example. This foot was in bad shape, so I trimmed

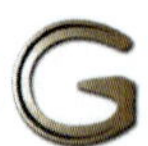

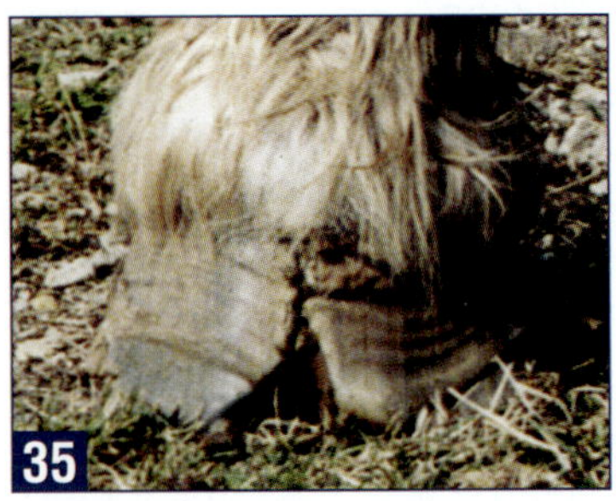
Damaged foot.

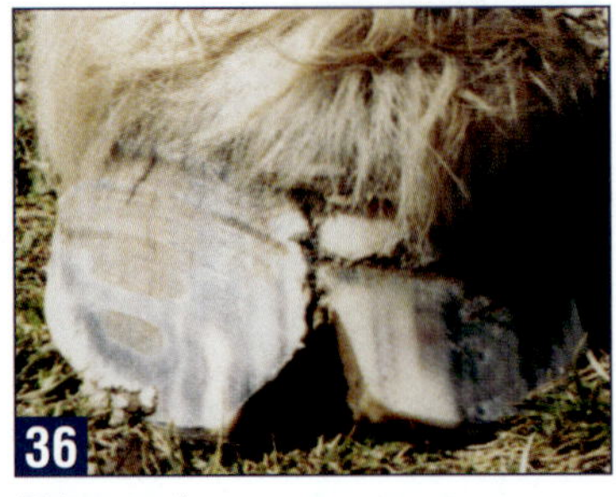
Trimmed.

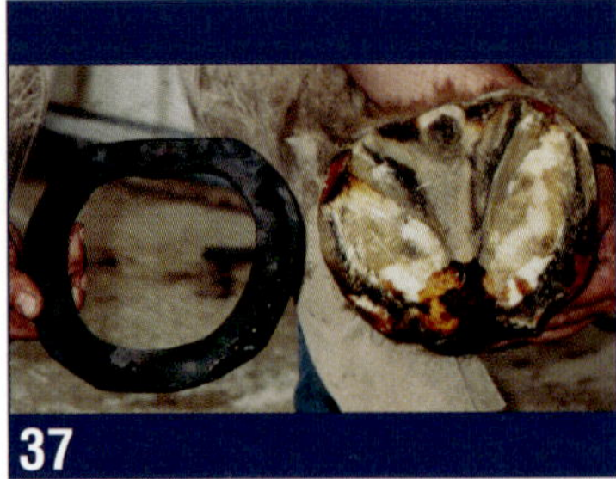
Fit with bar shoe.

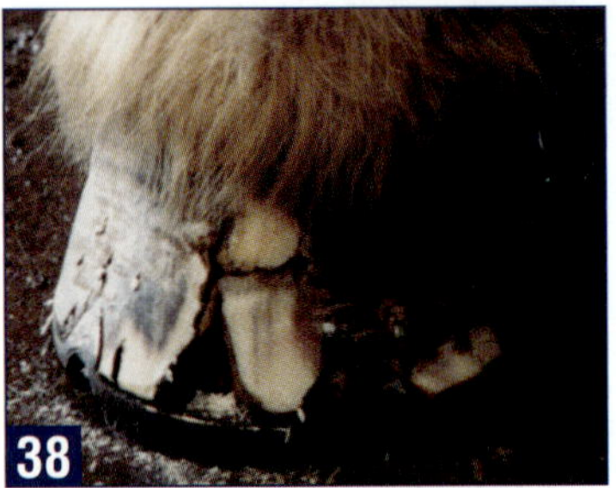
Nailed up.

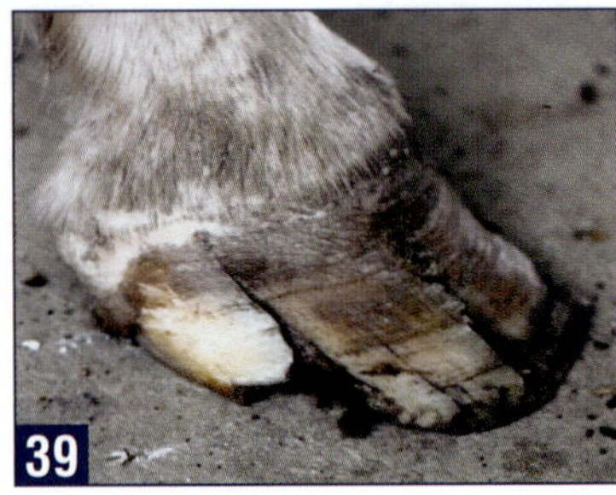
Damaged foot.

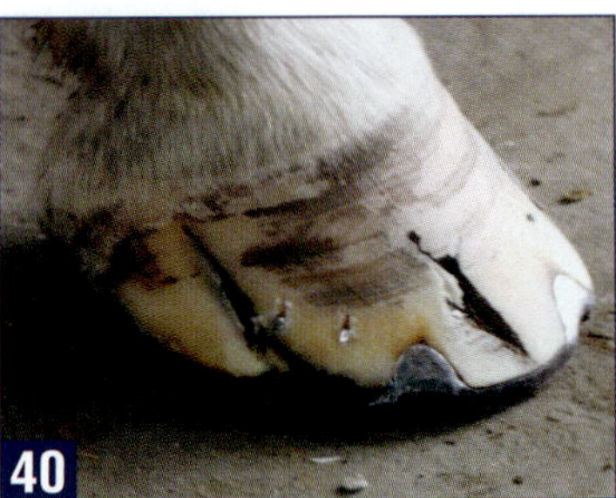
Nailed up.

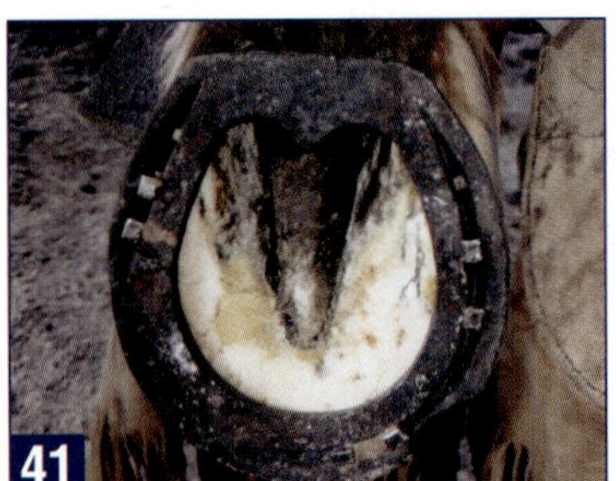
Unusual nail scheme.

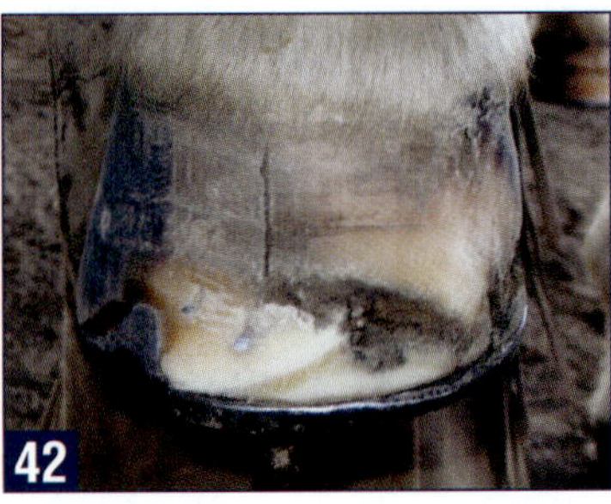
Dorsal view of the foot from Figure 41.

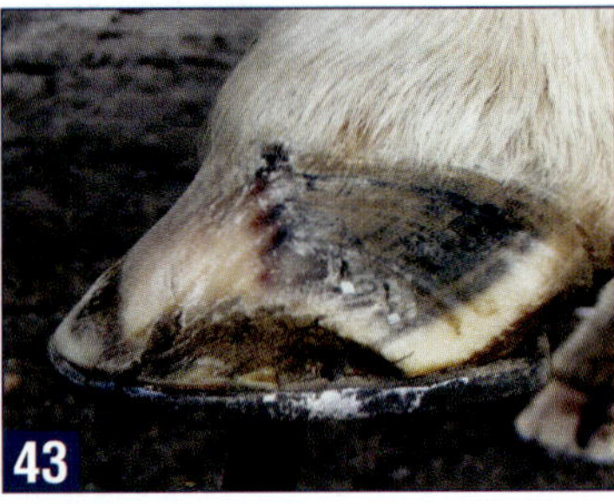
Medial view of the foot from Figure 41

it **(Figure 36)**, and fit and nailed a bar shoe on it **(Figures 37-38)**.

Figures 39-40 are the lateral views of a foot before and after shoeing with a straight bar. Nothing too special here, just another example of the kind of foot that benefits from a straight bar.

In **Figure 41**, notice the unusual nail pattern to accommodate a broken, weak, and abnormal foot. This foot is nailed up in **Figures 42-43**.

Figure 44 is the hind foot of a reining horse with a slider plate on it that cut a piece out of its foot on some tin on a barn. In **Figure 45**, it is sound now that there is a straight bar on it.

Figure 46 is a horse that has a bad near front foot that had been shod with a W-shoe. The straight bar on the off front foot **(Figure 47)** was good support. I like to use a straight bar with a rocker toe and a toe clip for a lot of horses **(Figure 48)**. They fit nicely and last for a long time. In **Figure 49**, there is a whip-across straight bar with a heel extension that is on the back of a cow-hocked horse. Another one of these handy straight bars can be seen in **Figure 50**.

I have found the straight bar **(Figure 51)** to be an extremely useful shoe throughout my career. It

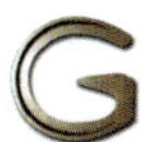

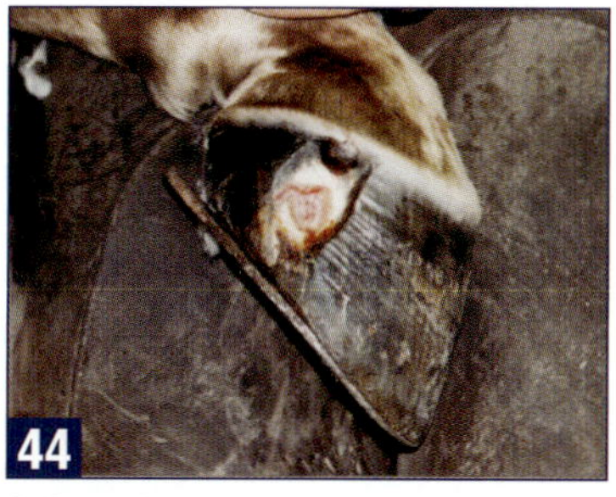

Injured hind foot with a slider plate on it.

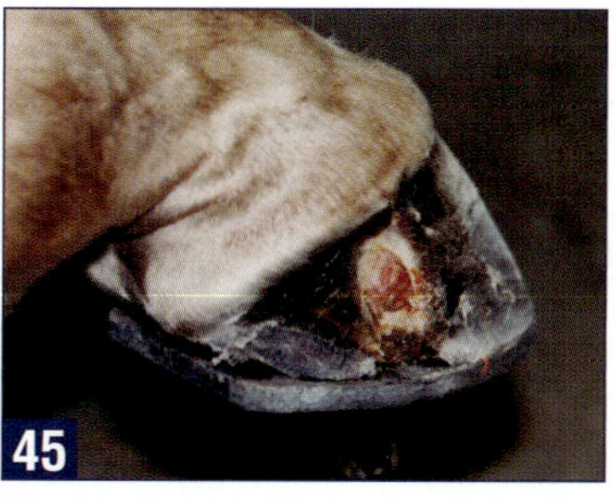

Same foot with a straight bar on it.

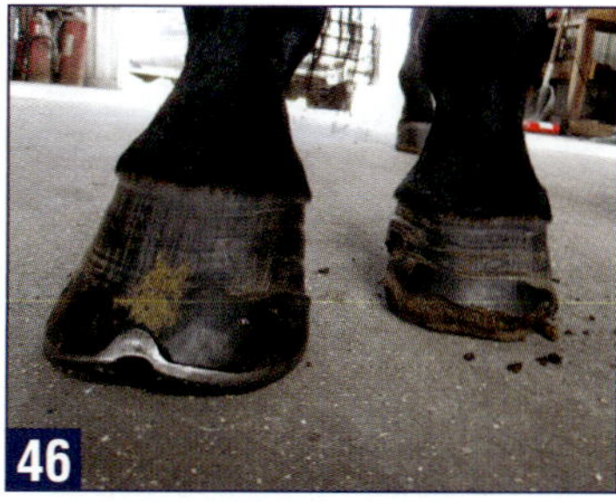

Good foot on a lame horse wearing a straight bar.

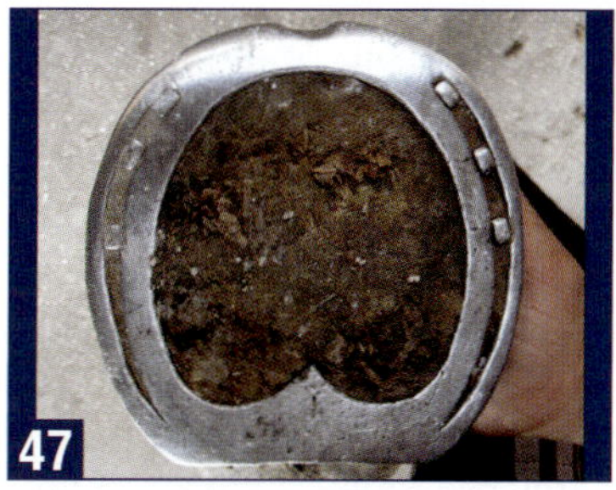

Same horse as Figure 46, solar view.

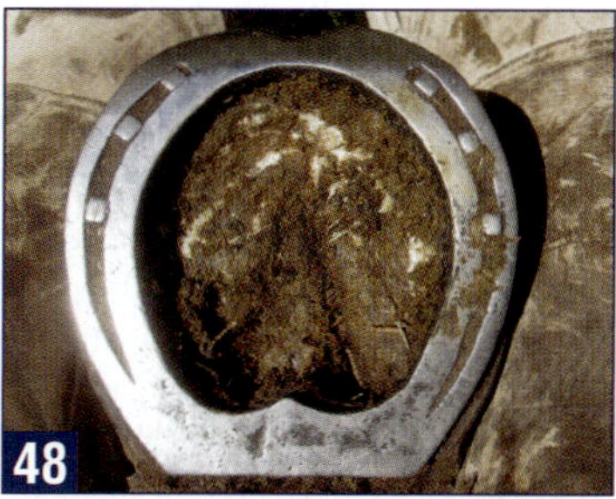

Straight bar with a rocker toe and toe clip.

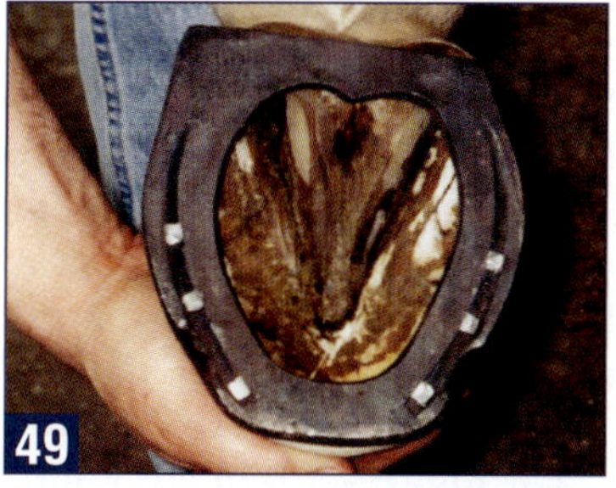

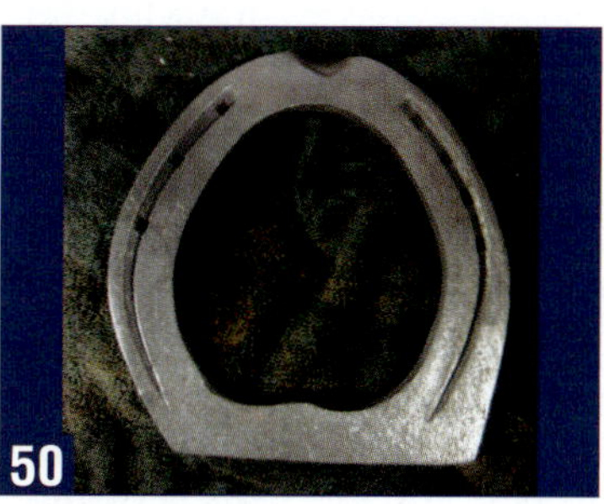

Whip-across lateral extension hind straight bar.

Straight bar shoes.

is easy to make, easy to fit, and gives the foot a lot of stability and strength. Take the time you need to learn how to use this shoe, and you will find that there are a lot of horses that you can help.

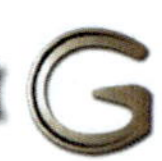

Chapter

56-4 DRASTIC CHANGES

CASE STUDY

In **Chapter 22, Trimming Feet,** we discussed the concept of the Wooden Indian. It is basically the idea that in order to carve a Wooden Indian, you take a chunk of wood and remove everything that does not look like a Wooden Indian. This can be applied to trimming feet. A simple and straightforward example can be seen in the before and after photos of **Figures 1-2**.

With a normal foot that has not grown out of control, trimming becomes an easy part of the job of farriery. However, with some feet that have become wildly overgrown or misshapen, the farrier must have enough vision to see what a finished foot (wooden Indian) can and should look like. With that in mind, this chapter has examples of feet that were outliers and shows what was done to bring them closer to normal.

It is common for cattle ranchers in the Midwest to have a donkey that runs with the cows. This donkey will help ward off predators, and provides security to the herd. One problem faced by donkeys in that line of work is that their hoof care is often handled as if they were cows. If they don't travel enough, they don't wear their feet enough. Founder is also a big problem for these animals. The donkey in **Figure 3** was part of a cow herd, but he had injured a flexor tendon as a youngster and it had caused his foot to be pulled around in such a steep position that he ended up walking on the dorsal aspect of the wall. Once a year, the foot would grow so long that it would interfere with the fetlock above it **(Figures 4-5)** signaling the rancher that another trim was needed. **Figure 6** shows the two hind feet of the donkey together, and **Figure 7** is looking at the dorsal wall of the foot from a plantar position.

When trimming feet that are this deformed, the position of the coffin bone and sensitive structures will not be where expected. I don't like to use a saw on feet that are severely deformed because at times I have hit bone and blood where I didn't think it would be. I prefer to trim with conventional tools, nippers, knife and rasp, until I have the foot where I want it, or I hit the first bit of blood. **Figure 8** shows the foot partially trimmed, and close inspection of **Figure 9** will show that I hit just a speck of blood in the white line area on the left side of the foot. That made it a good spot to stop, and a lateral view of the finished foot can be seen in **Figure 10**.

While a problem like this one is often created during development of the animal, bad injuries that do not heal properly can also create some unusual feet. **Figures 11-13** show the back leg of a horse that was caught in wire. When it healed, the foot was pulled back and rolled around as well. **Figure 14** is of the horse, and **Figures 15-16** are a little closer photos of the foot. Since we knew how this happened and how long the horse had been hurt, the position of the coffin bone was not hard to deter-

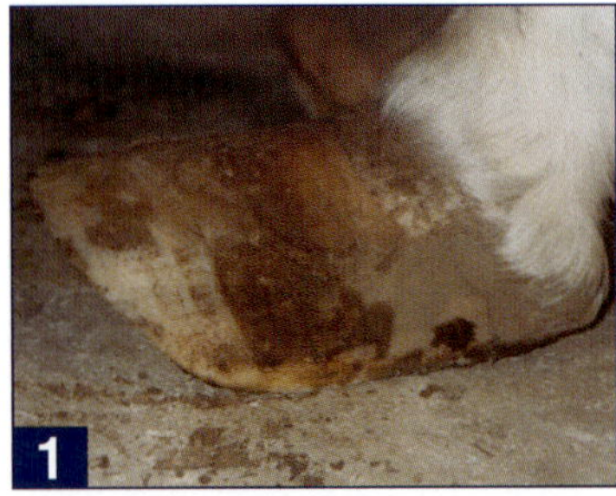

1 ***Lateral view of an untrimmed and neglected foot.***

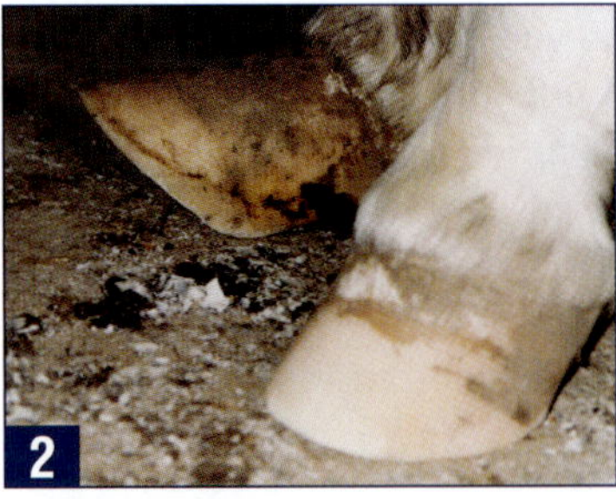

2 ***Lateral view of the foot after being trimmed.***

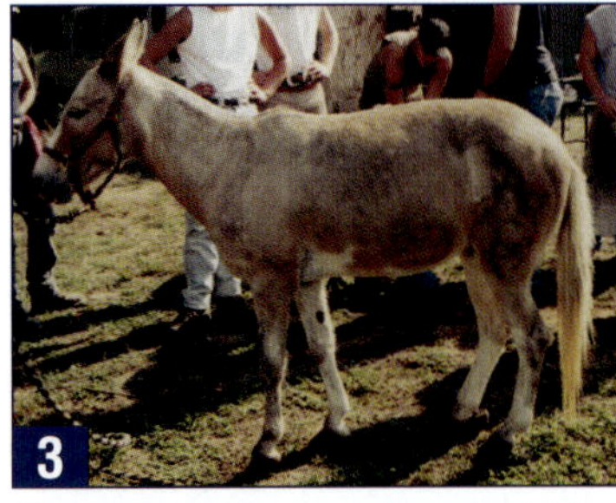

3 ***Donkey with a deformed hind foot.***

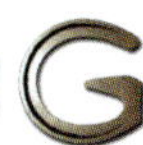

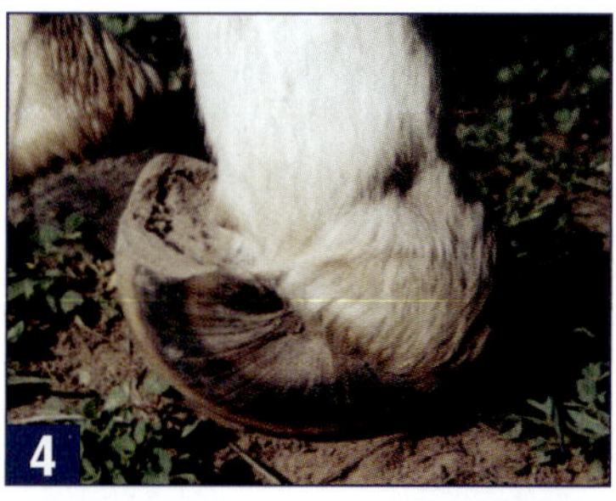

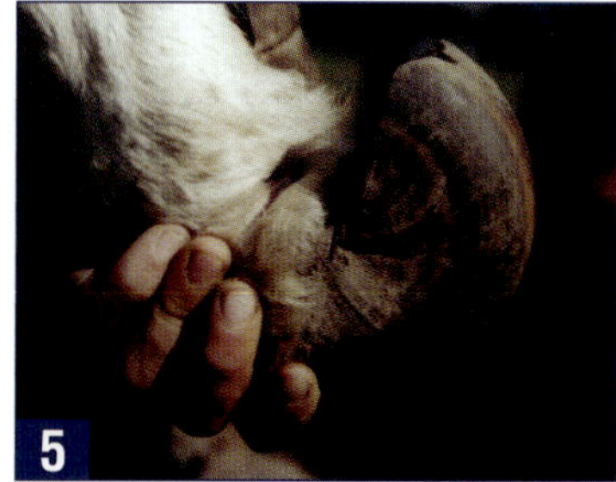

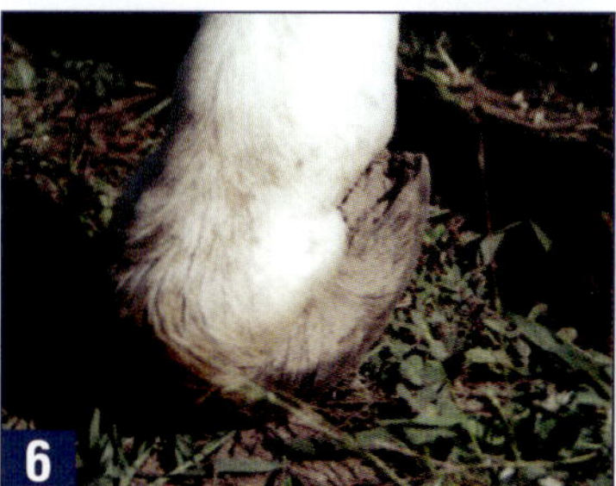

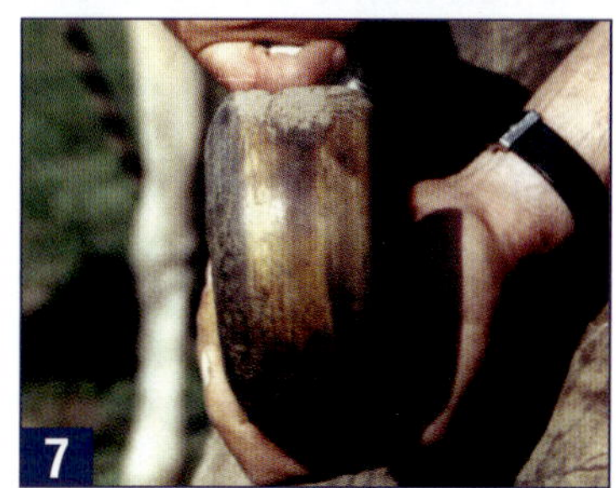

Detail of the foot.

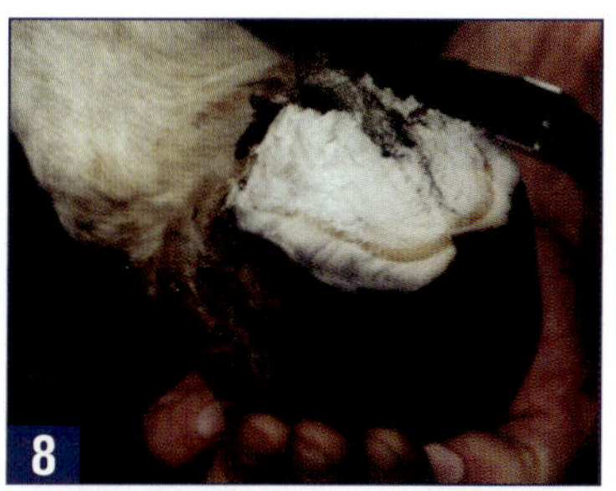

The foot partially trimmed.

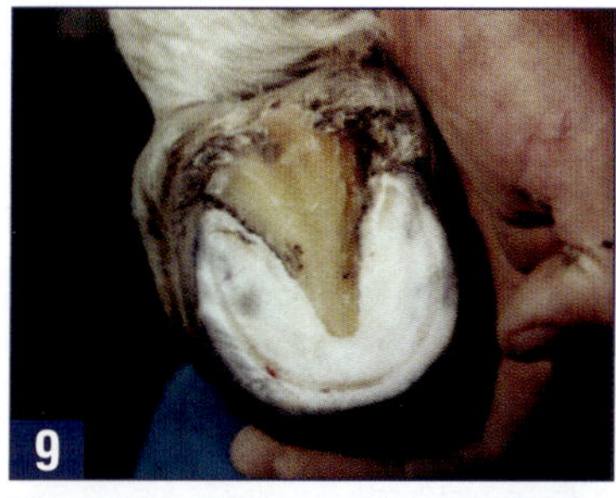

The foot trimmed. There is a speck of blood on the left side of the white line area, an indication that the foot is trimmed short enough.

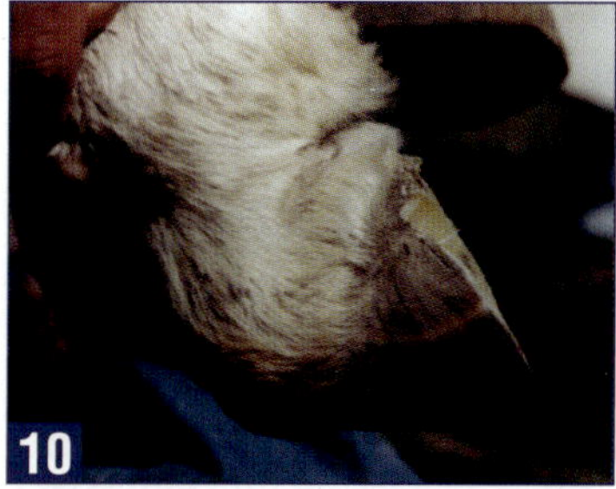

Lateral view of trimmed foot.

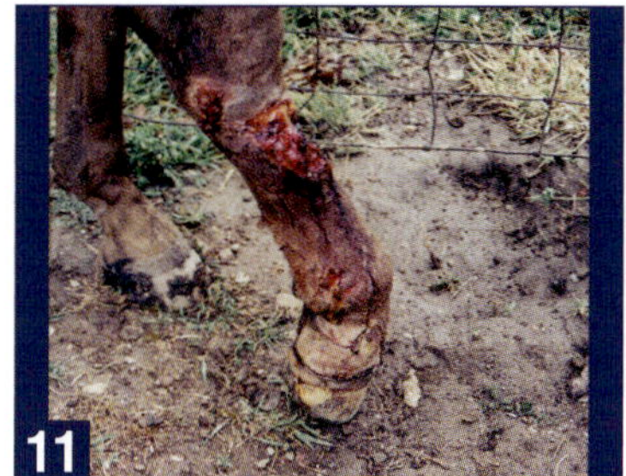

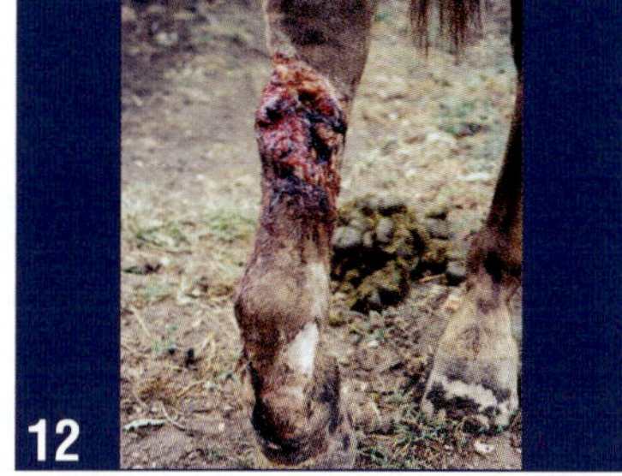

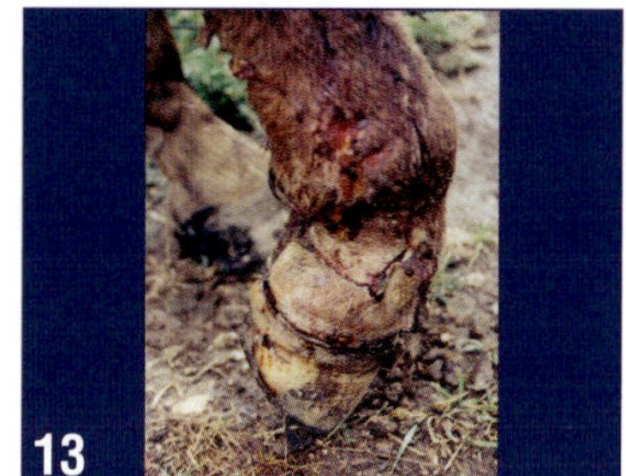

Hind leg of a horse that was badly cut in wire.

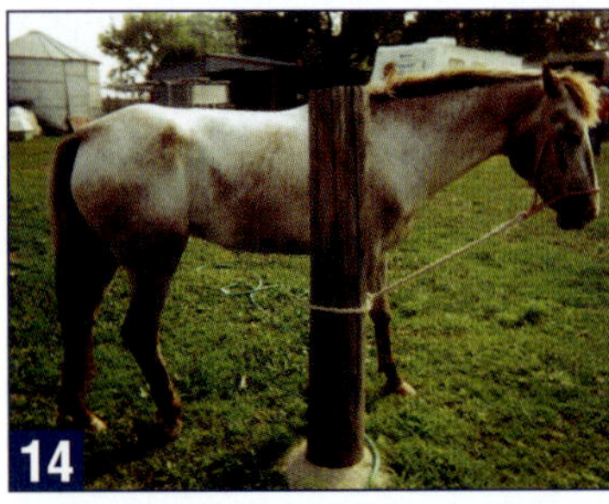

14 *The horse once the leg wound had healed.*

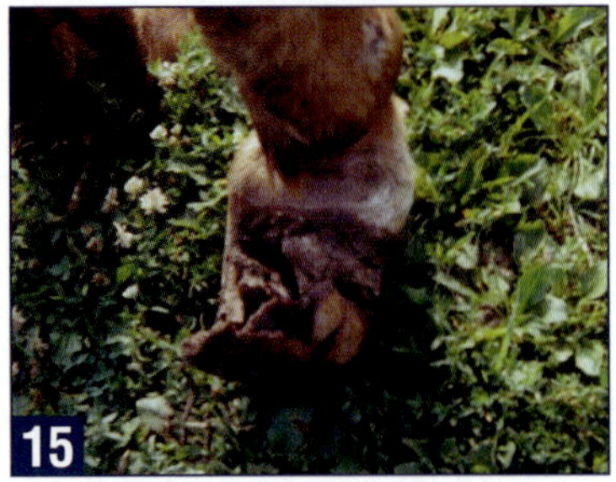

15

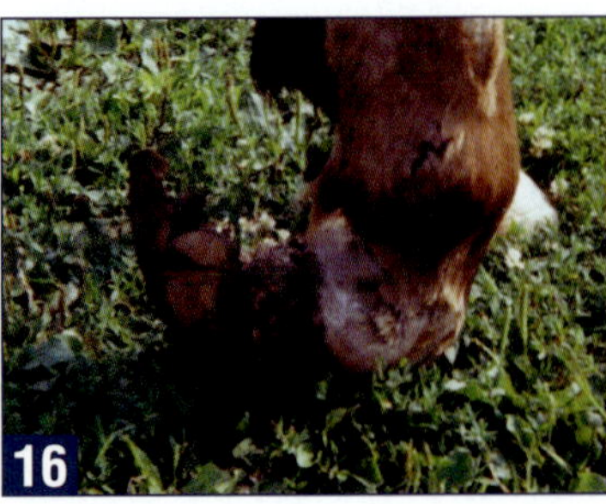

16

The abnormal foot after the leg healed.

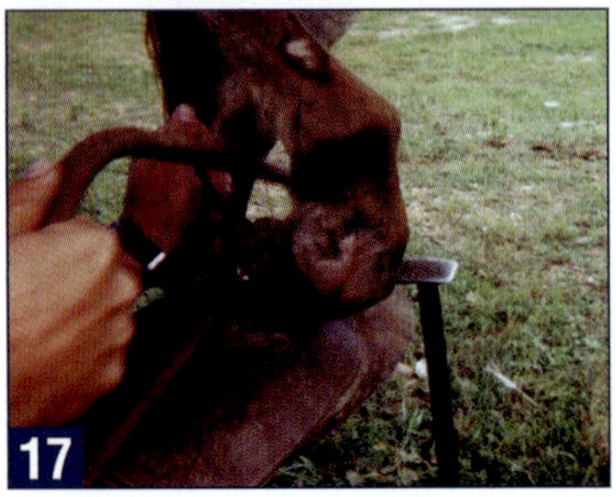

17 *Cutting off hoof growth with a saw.*

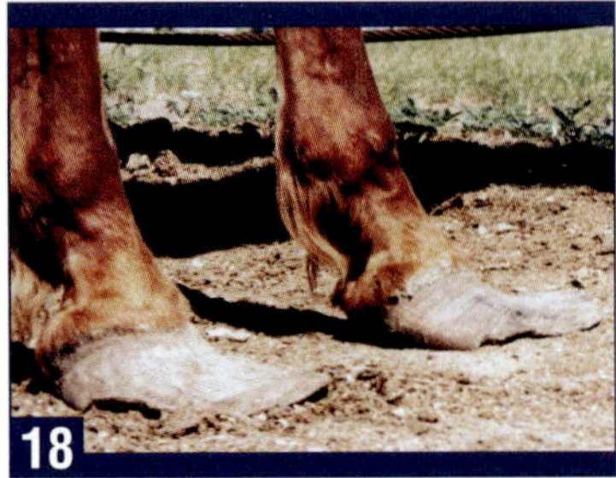

18 *A long foot without a lot of vertical depth.*

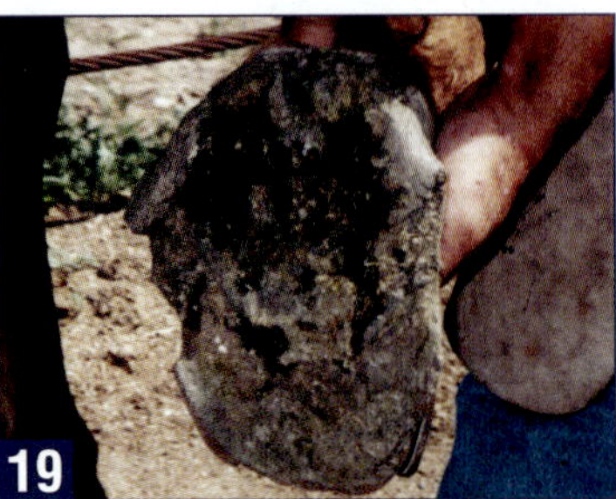

19 *Bottom of this foot.*

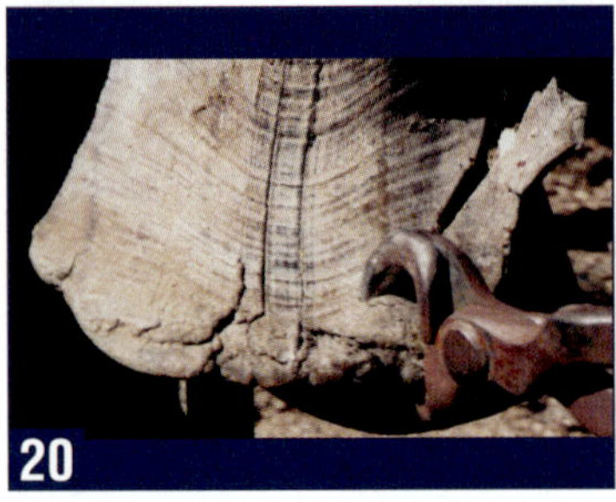

20 *Trimming the foot back on the stand.*

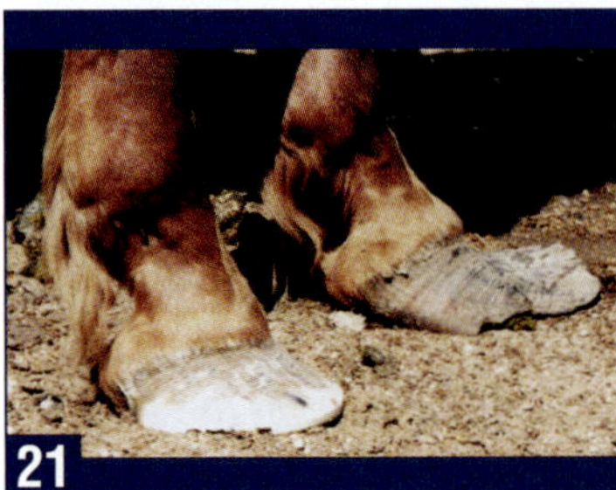

21 *Post-trim.*

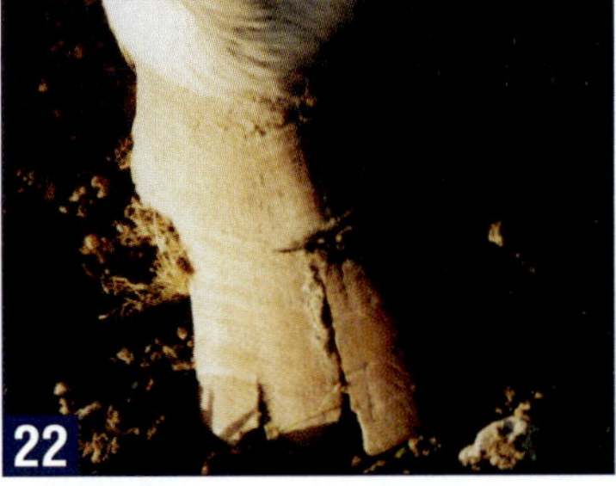

22 *Foot that broke off around the center of the toe.*

mine, and a saw could be used to remove the large amount of hoof **(Figure 17)**. On a side note, if we had this horse to deal with again, a patten bar shoe would have probably saved him and resulted in a normal foot when the wound healed.

Figure 18 is a foot worth mentioning and knowing about. Feet like this can be deceiving because it looks like there is a lot of length. There is length but not vertical depth. This means that the coronet is pretty close to a normal distance from the ground, but the excess growth of wall has spread laterally and dorsally **(Figure 19)**. When you encounter feet like these, be careful to not remove too much sole, just the excess wall. This is most easily done from the outside of the foot instead of the bottom **(Figure 20)**. **Figure 21** shows a lateral view of the finished trim.

The foot in **Figure 22** is one that had grown a lot of length, then broke off at the sides, leaving a long and skinny piece of wall at the toe. These feet are very satisfying to work on since they easily are returned to normal. **Figure 23** is the bottom pre-trim, and **Figures 24-25** show the normal, healthy looking, regular foot that was hiding under all the

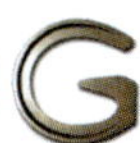

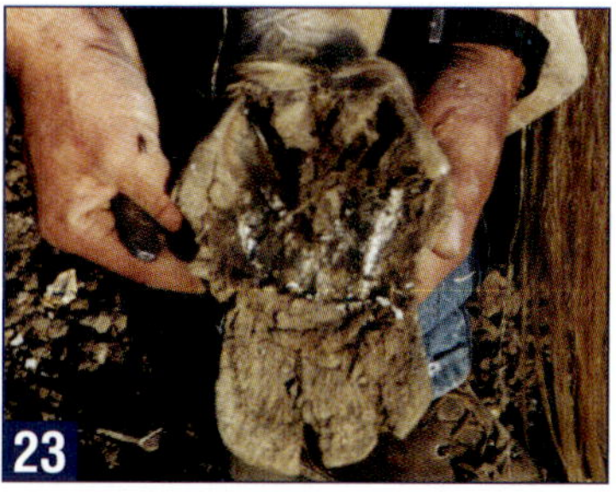

Bottom of the foot.

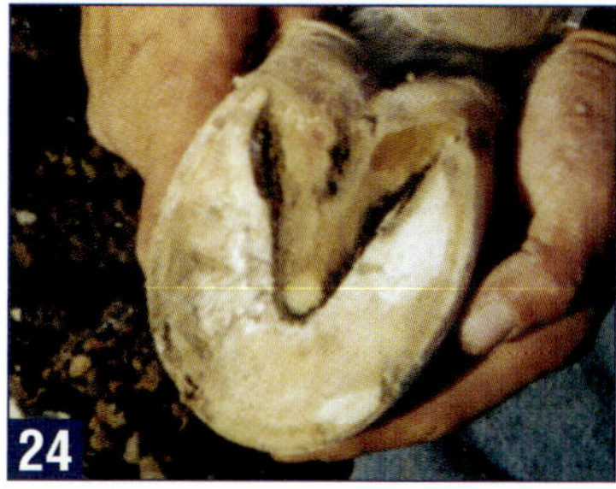

Post-trim.

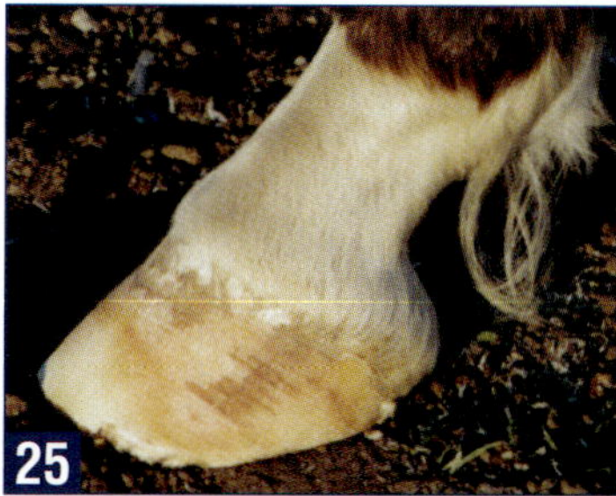

Trimmed foot on the ground.

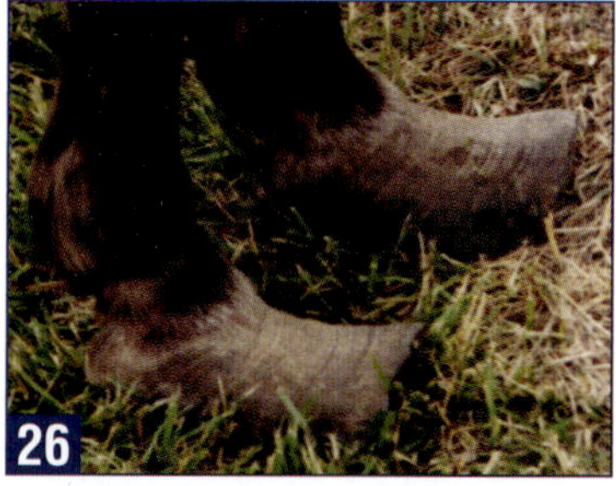

Chronic founder on the hind feet.

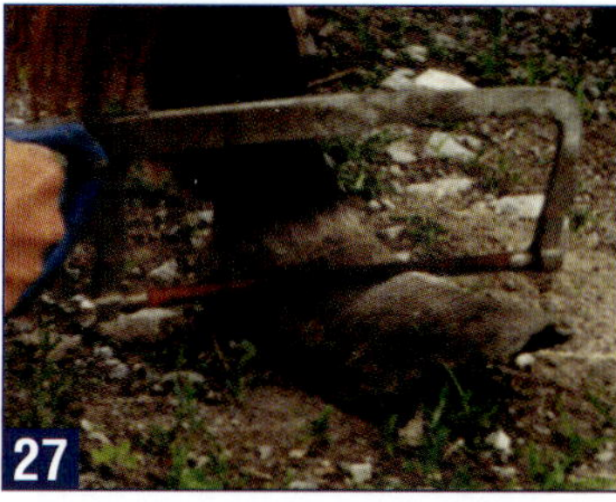

Sawing off the excess toe.

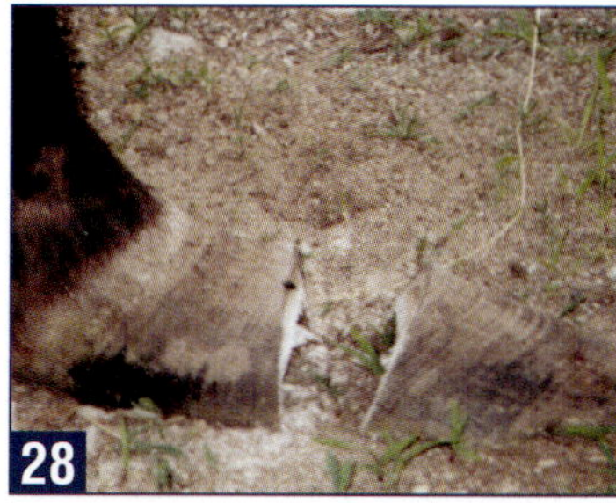

The piece of sawed-off toe sitting in front of the foot on the ground.

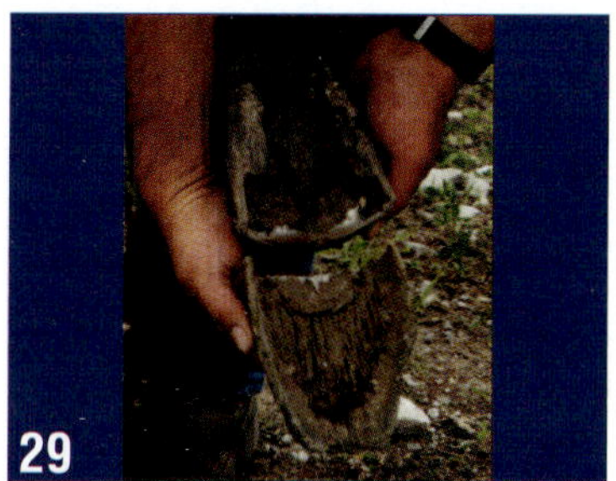

Holding the piece of toe in front of the foot in the air.

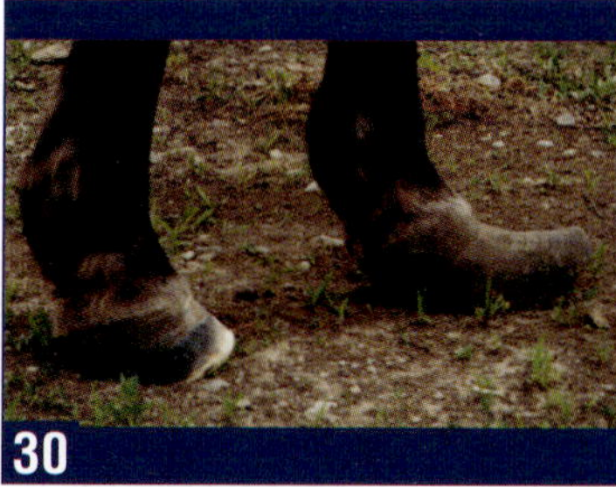

The foot post-trim.

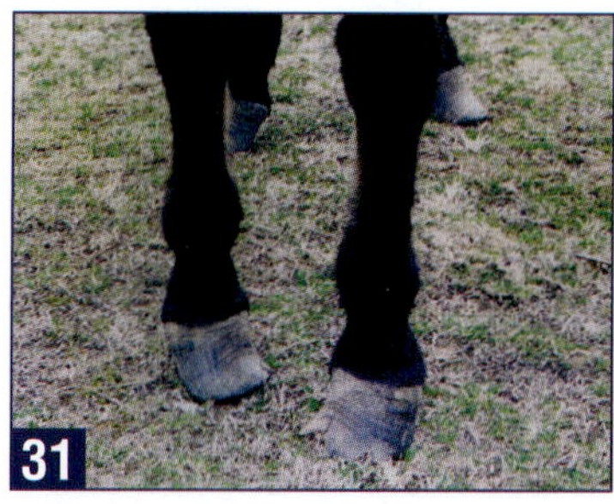

Broken-out front feet on a mule

mess.

Figure 26 shows the hind feet of a horse that has chronic founder. Shoeing in the Midwest makes you good at feet like these. I began by sawing off a pretty good length of wall **(Figures 27-29)**, and **Figure 30** shows the resulting, normal looking foot post-trim.

The next series of photos shows the feet of a mule that had collapsed laterally. With mules and donkeys, the wall is thick enough in the quarters that they will sometimes end up severely broken-in or broken-out when there is a mediolateral imbal-

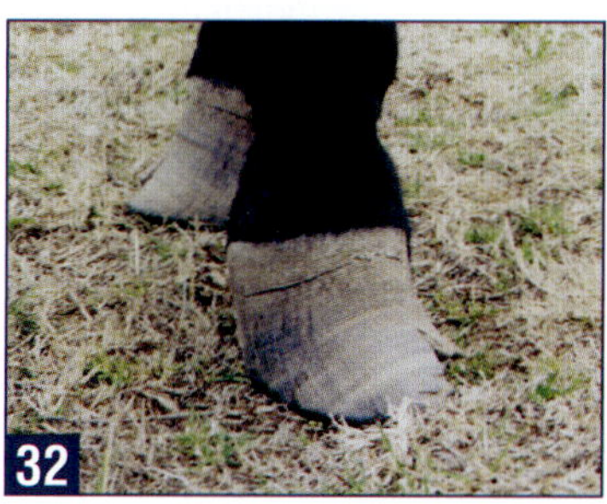

Broken-in hind feet on a mule.

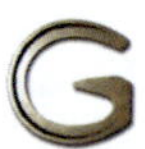

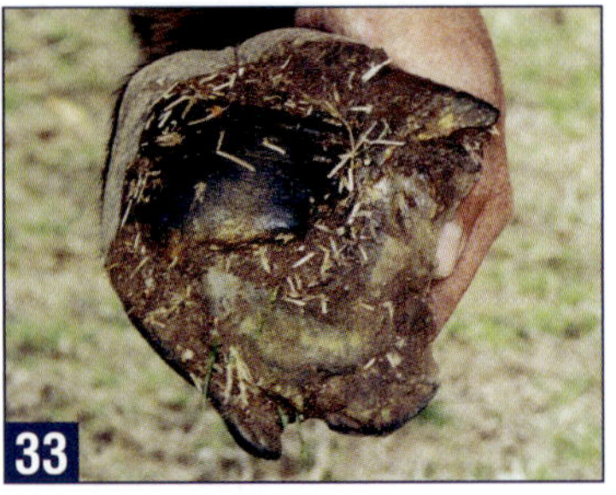
Near front before.

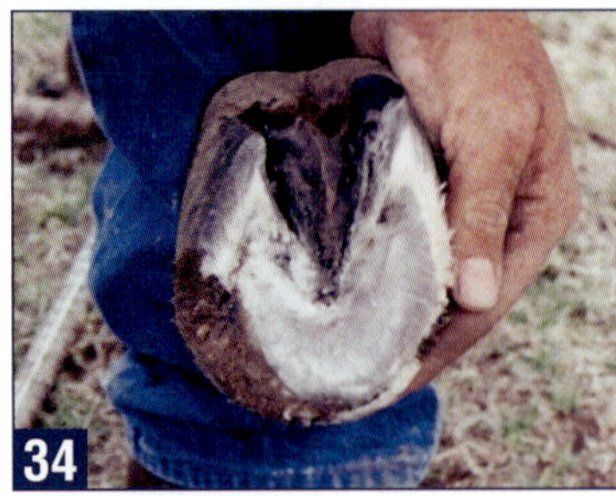
Near front after.

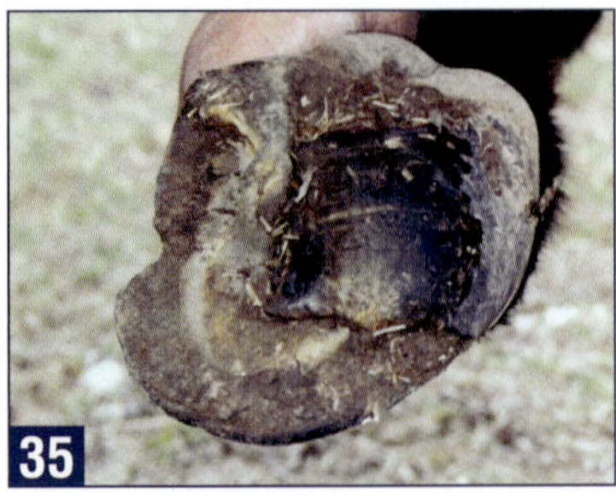
Off front before.

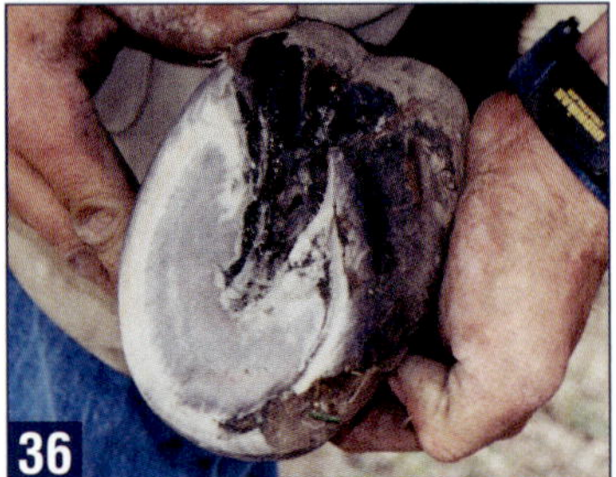
Off front after.

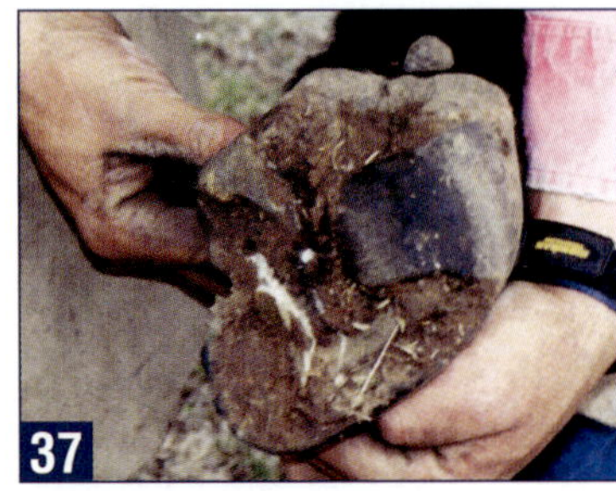
Near hind before.

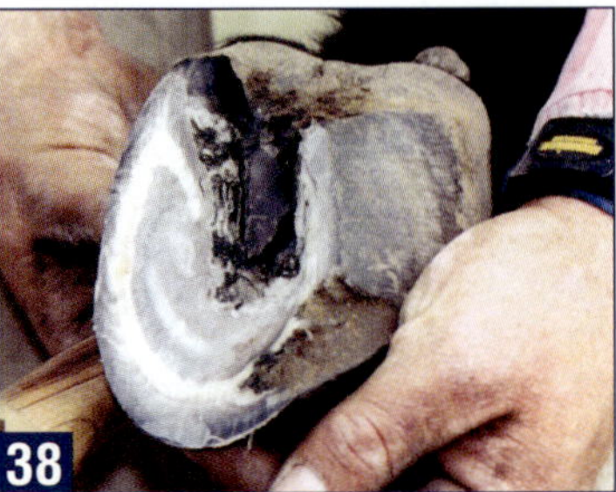
Near hind after.

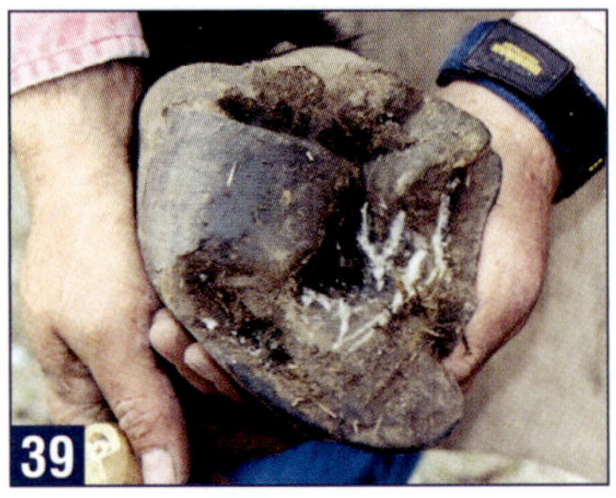
Off hind before.

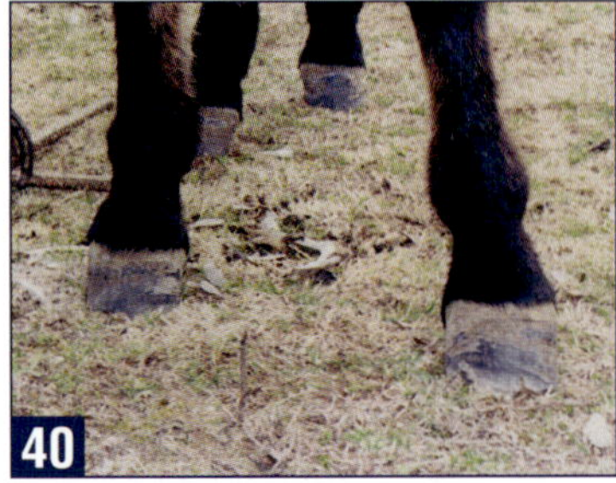
Dorsal view of the feet on the ground after trimming.

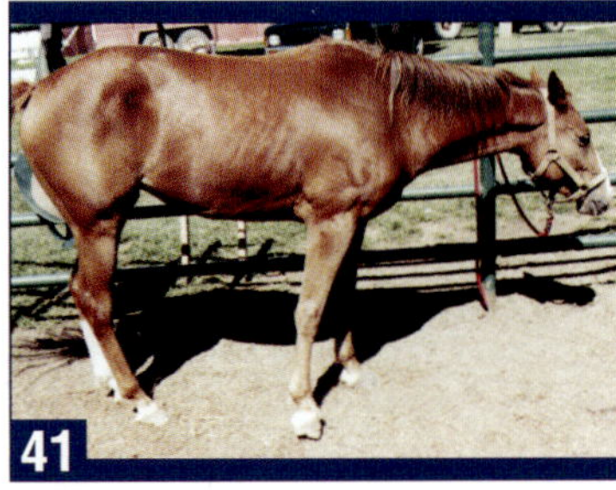
Mare in obvious distress from pain.

ance. With the normal horse foot, the wall in the heels and quarters will generally wear on one side while it flares on the opposite. When this does not happen with a donkey or mule, the results are what you see in **Figures 31 and 32**. **Figures 33-39** show the bottom of the feet, either pre-trim or post-trim, which is easy to see. Notice how much of the wall has collapsed and covered the frog and sole on these feet. **Figure 40** is the feet on the ground when the trim is finished.

The horse in **Figure 41** had caught its foot in a panel as a foal. This had caused it to grow up with some abnormal foot. The horse generally got around pretty well until the good foot (near front) developed an abscess. This required the bad foot (off front), to go into more service than it was used to and caused the horse major discomfort. Notice how the horse looks in **Figure 41**, and its discomfort is evident.

To relieve some of this horse's pain, the bad foot needed some support in the way of shoeing. **Figures 42-44** are the pre-trim, and **Figure 45** is trimmed and hot-fit. What I imagined here is what the foot would look like if it were normal, then I created that platform

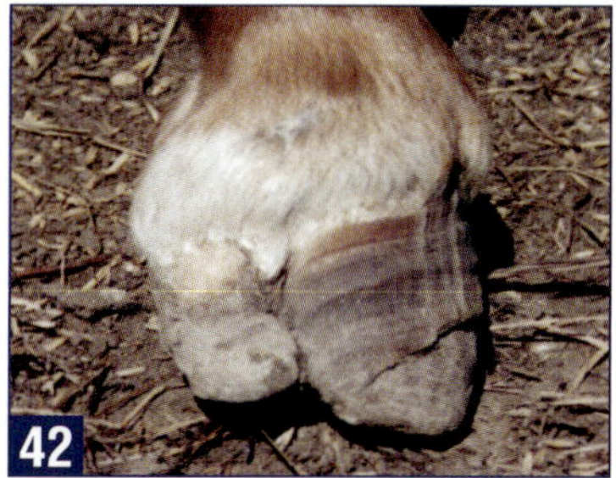

Damaged front foot, lateral view.

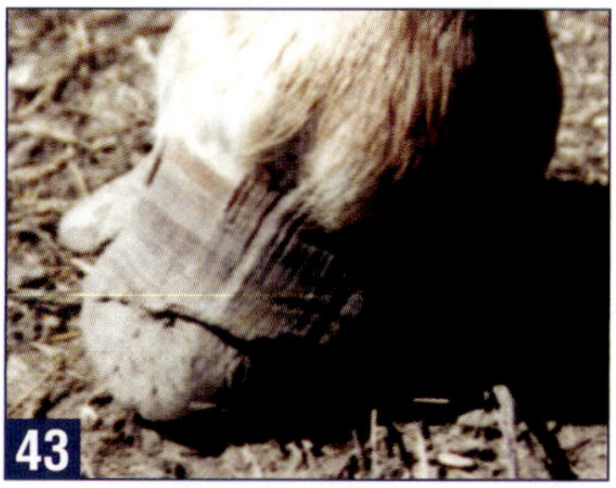

Dorsal view.

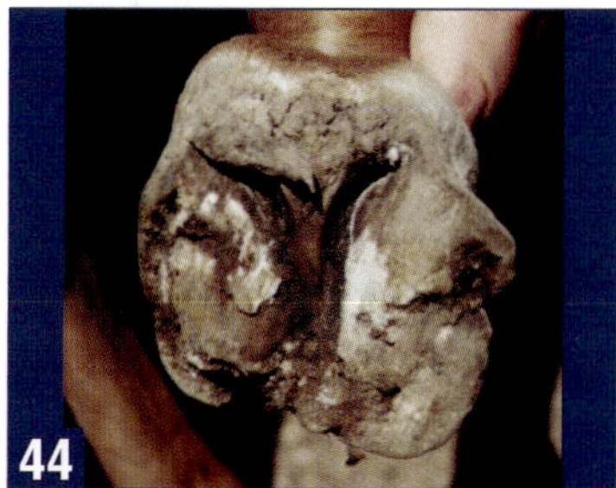

Solar view.

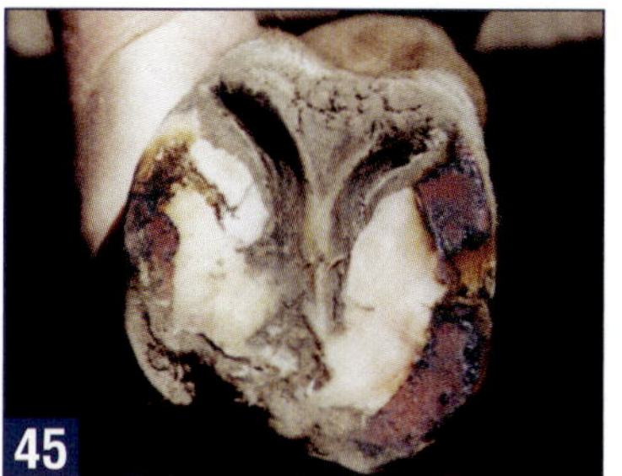

Trimmed and hot fit.

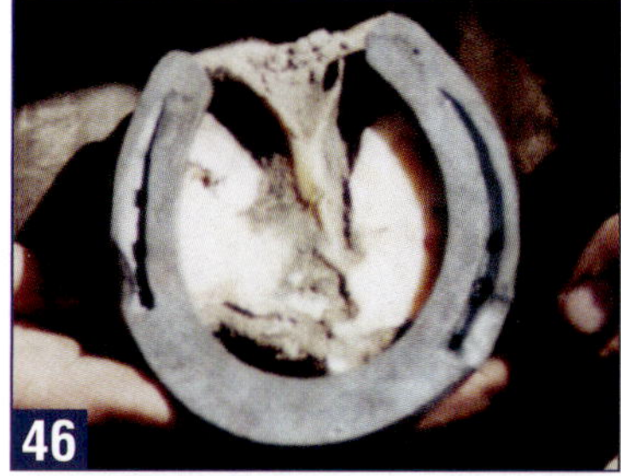

Shoe on the foot.

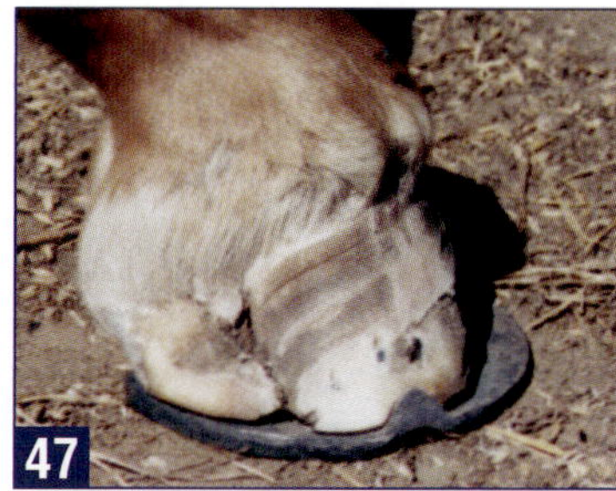

Lateral view of the shod foot on the ground.

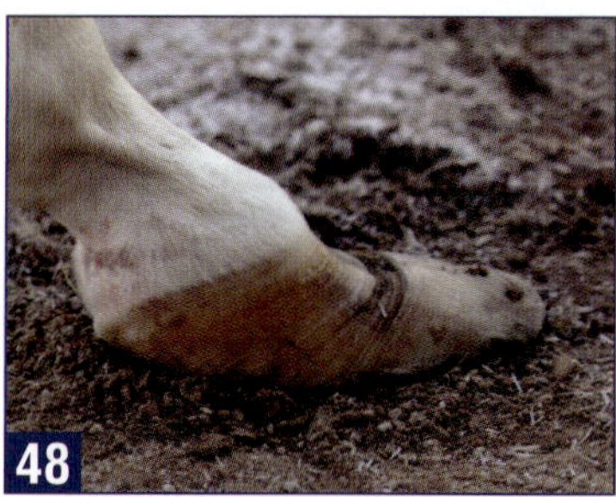

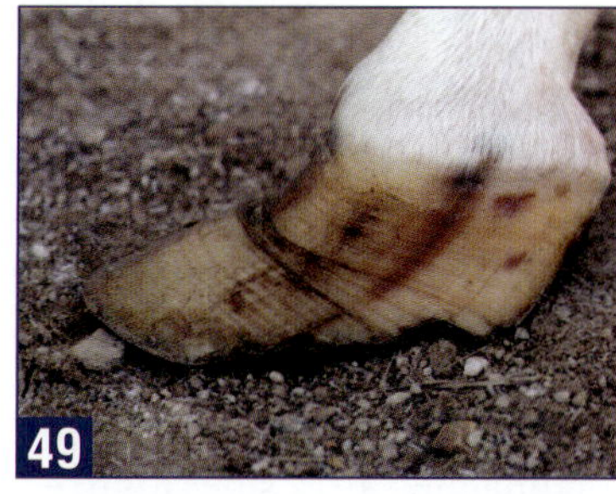

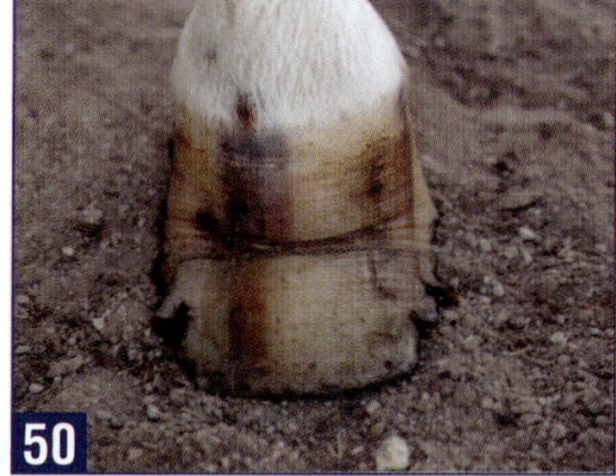

A foot with a large fever line showing that there had been a problem fro the horse at some point.

for the foot with a shoe. **Figures 46 and 47** are the foot with the shoe on it, and the horse was much more comfortable.

The foot in **Figures 48-50** had a big growth ring in it that suggested there had been a systemic problem for the horse many months previous. Depending on the rate of hoof growth, the horse had suffered the problem between six and ten months before. The excess wall

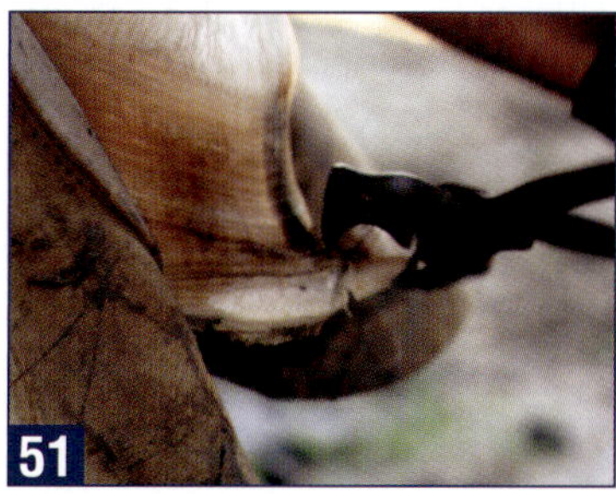

Trimming the foot.

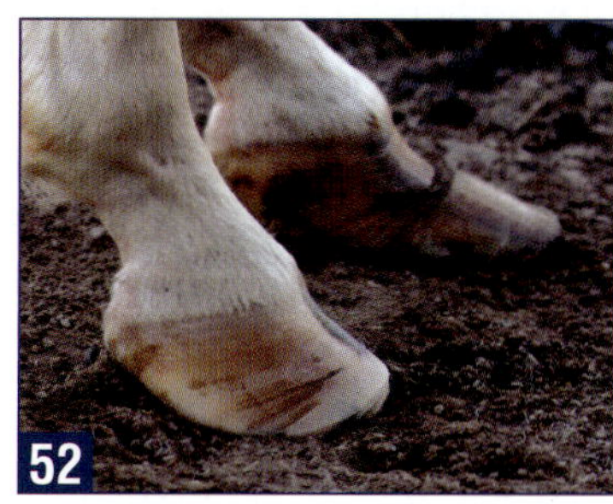

Post-trim.

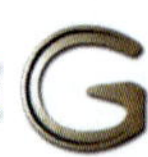

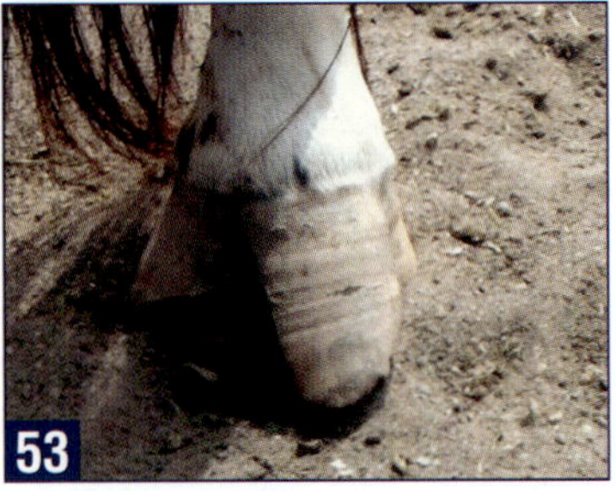

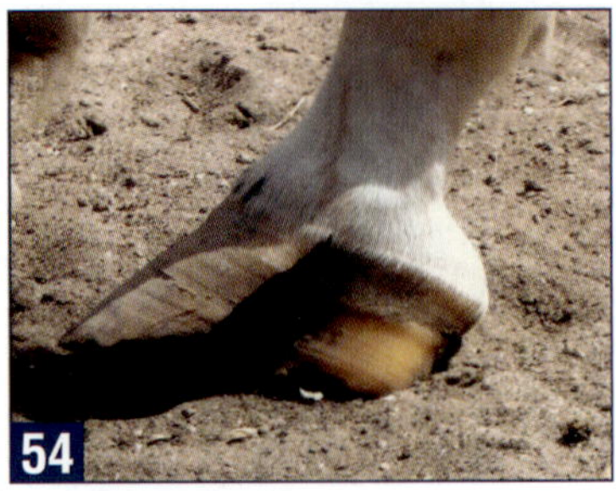

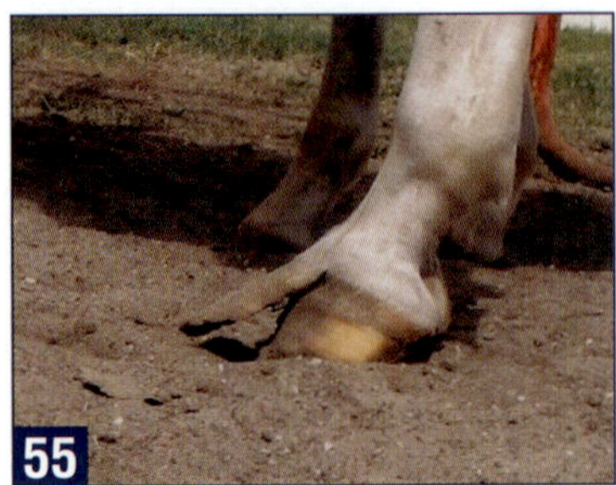

Cracked foot on a mare with a violent disposition.

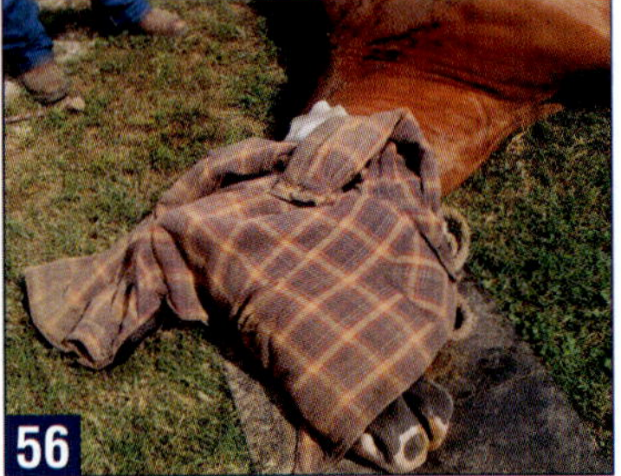

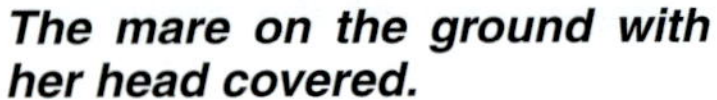

The mare on the ground with her head covered.

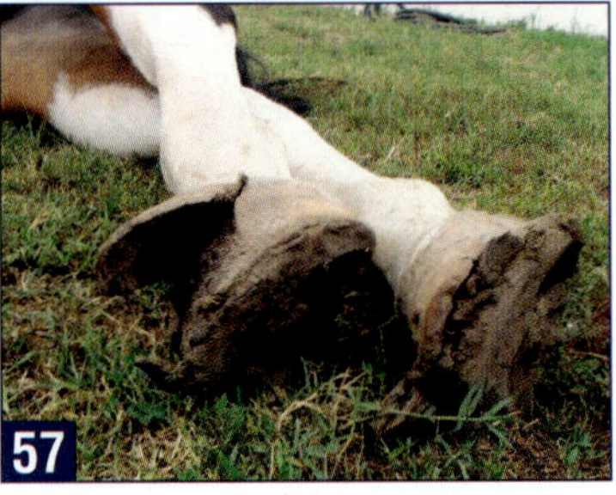

Detail of the damaged foot.

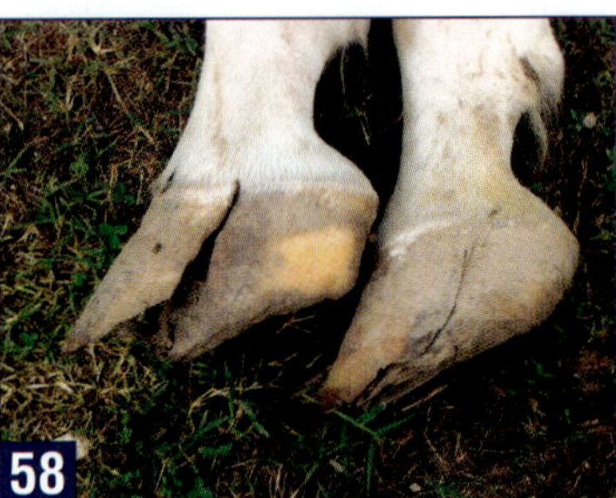

was trimmed (**Figure 51**), and **Figure 52** was the result.

The hind foot on this next horse is hard to do justice to in pictures. She was a recipient mare. That is a mare that is implanted with the fertilized embryo of another mare so that the genetics of a well-bred horse could be developed and raised by another horse. This is a common practice among many breeders and is a good way to prevent the wear and trauma of pregnancy from damaging a good horse. This particular mare was extremely mean. The only way to catch her was to rope her, and she put up a fight that was beyond the abilities of most horses once she was caught. Because of her disposition, her feet were left alone. Her near hind foot developed a crack that became a big problem, and finally had to be dealt with. Had she been a nicer mare, regular trimming would have prevented the problem from becoming such a big one.

Figures 53-55 show the foot on the ground before she was drugged. The vet drugged and dropped her. **Figure 56** shows her head wrapped to protect her eyes. When a horse is tranquilized with certain drugs, their eyes remain open and can be injured by debris on the ground. Once she was on her side, I took a couple pictures of the damaged foot (**Figures 57-58**). We trimmed this horse on her side (**Figure 59**). I removed horn on the injured foot all the way to blood at the coronary band (**Figures 60-62**). The vet doctored the foot while we finished the other feet (**Figure 63**).

I hope you were able to get some good out of these examples. I would also encourage you to get a camera and keep it with you. There are hundreds of horses I did in the first ten years of my career that I wish I had taken pictures of. Create a portfolio of

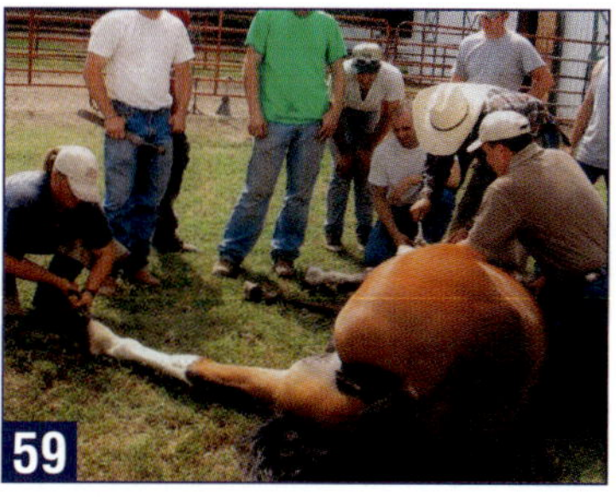

Trimming the feet.

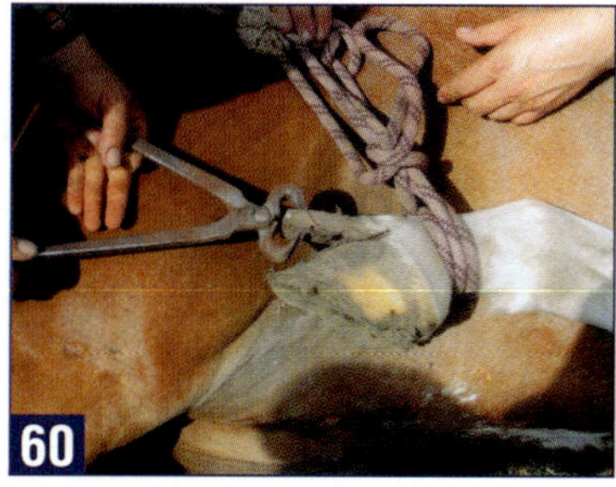

Trimming the bad foot.

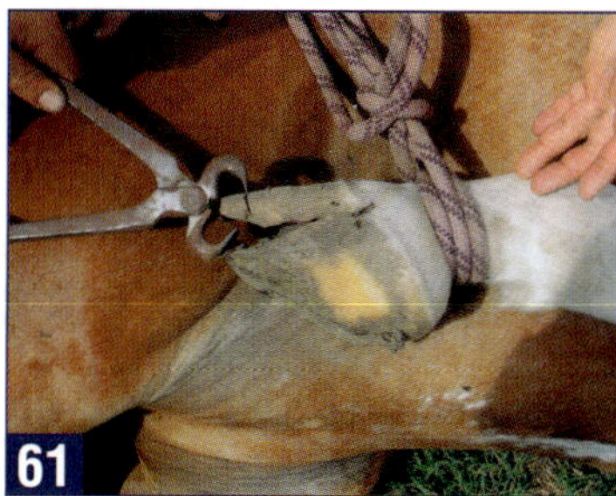

before-and-after photos. They'll make the stories about these feet so much better.

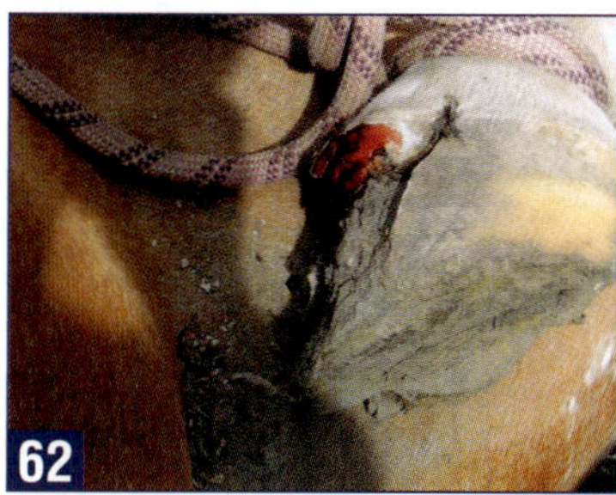

The wall was removed all the way to the coronet.

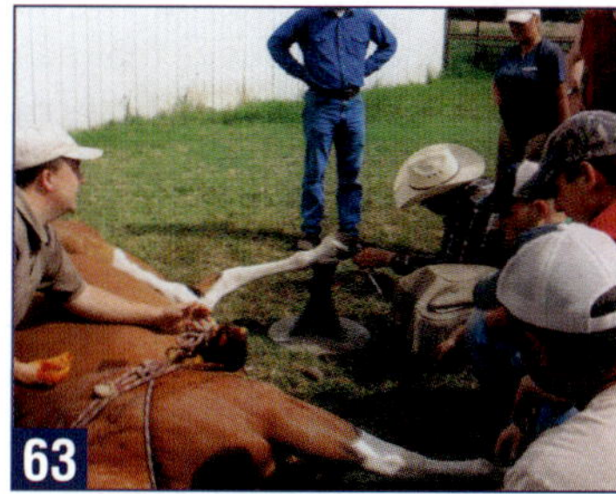

Finishing off the other feet while the vet doctors the bad foot already trimmed.

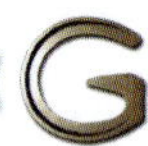

Chapter

56-5 HEART BAR AND W-SHOE

CASE STUDY

The heart bar, W-shoe and G-bar shoes have been implicated as bad shoes by many vets and farriers. Each of these shoes itself is a great tool for helping horses. Rather, it is the application of the shoes that has been the problem. When a shoe is applied that causes an area of the foot to bear more weight than it was meant to, there is always danger of causing problems. When that shoe is applied without a high degree of knowledge and skill, the chance of problems is multiplied. In this chapter, I will show the use of the heart bar and W-shoe on several horses. I have used these shoes for many years with results that are sometimes unbelievable. Before using this shoe, be certain that you have a good understanding of the principles and anatomy involved.

Remember that a shoe with a frog plate design is intended to take some of the weight off of the wall and apply that weight to the frog. It is a simple as that. Anytime I have a foot with an injury to the wall, I know that the heart bar, G-bar or W-shoe may be a way for the horse to have some comfort and healing. I generally jump weld the frog plate onto the shoe **(Figure 1)**, and this is detailed in **Chapter 50, Heart Bar, W-Shoe and G-Bar**. **Figures 2 and 3** show a foot that had a bad cut at the coronet. **Figure 4** is the heart bar that allowed this foot to heal. This is an example of a straight forward and common sense approach to using a heart bar shoe.

Figures 5-8 show a foot that was shod by a shoer who was trying very hard to do the right thing but found himself in over his head. This horse was

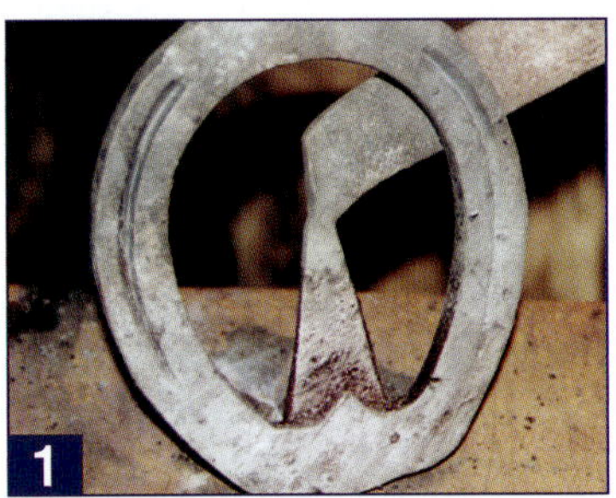

1 *Frog plate on the first jump weld.*

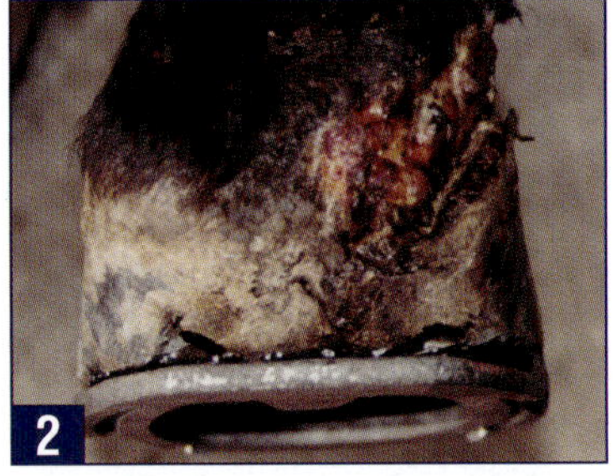

2 *Injured foot with a heart bar on it.*

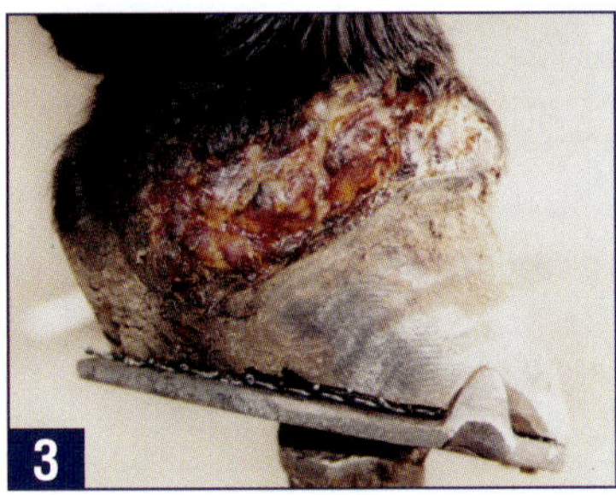

3 *Lateral view of the same foot.*

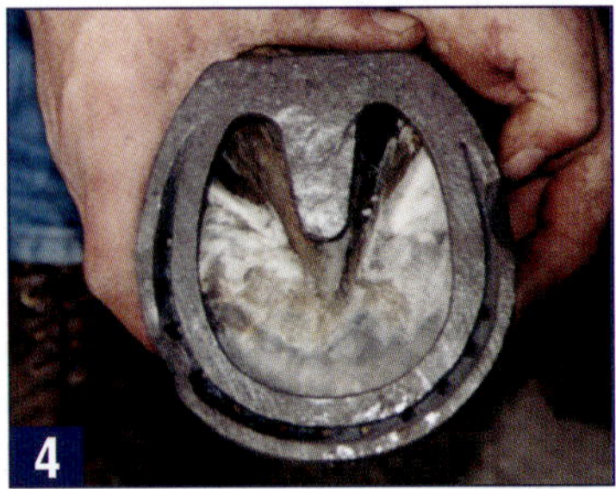

4 *Bottom of the foot with the heart bar on it.*

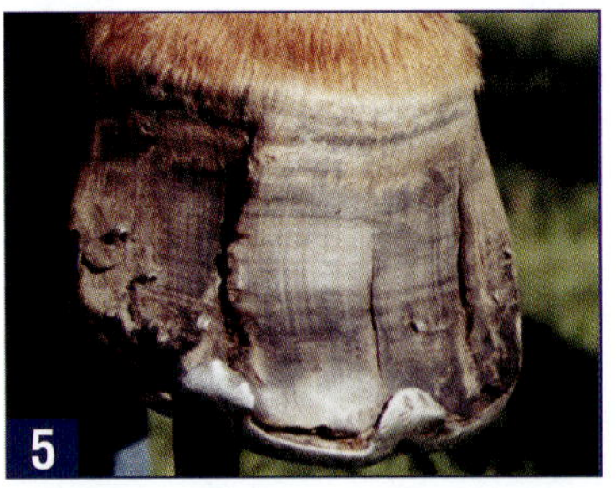

5 *Before: Dorsal view of a cracked, dished, and misshapen foot.*

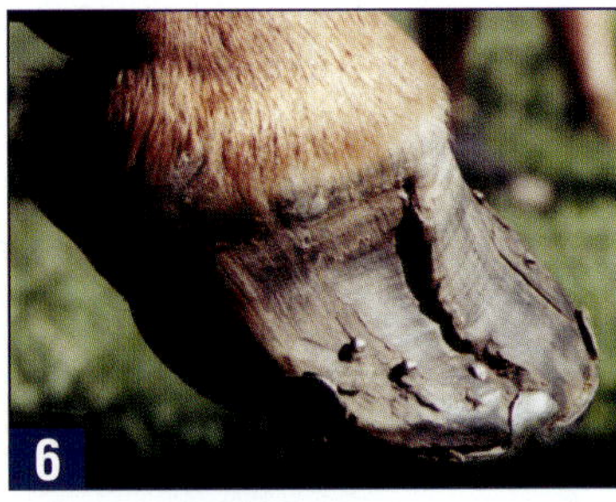

6 *Before: Medial view.*

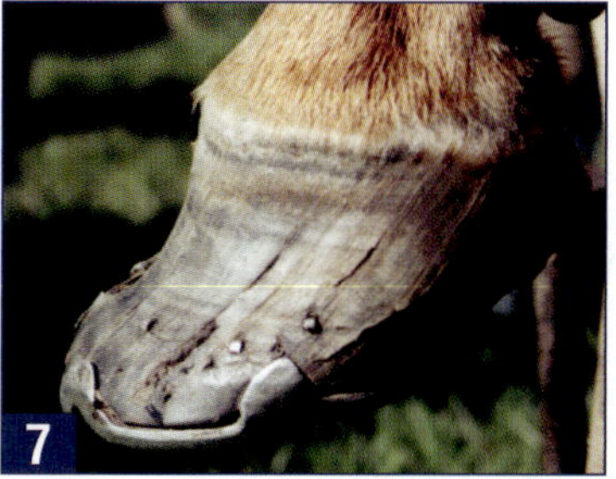

Before: Lateral view.

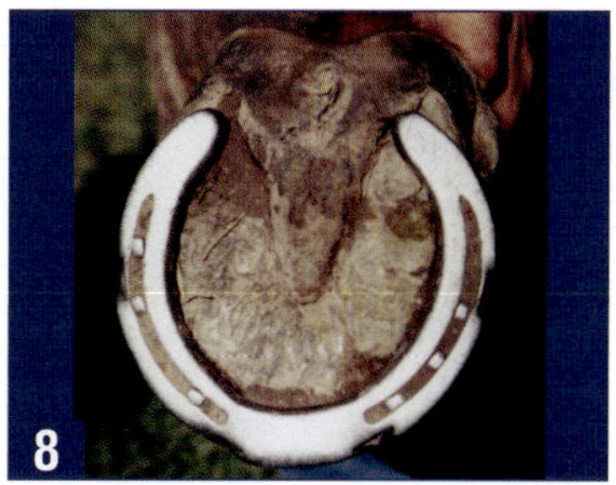

Before: Solar view.

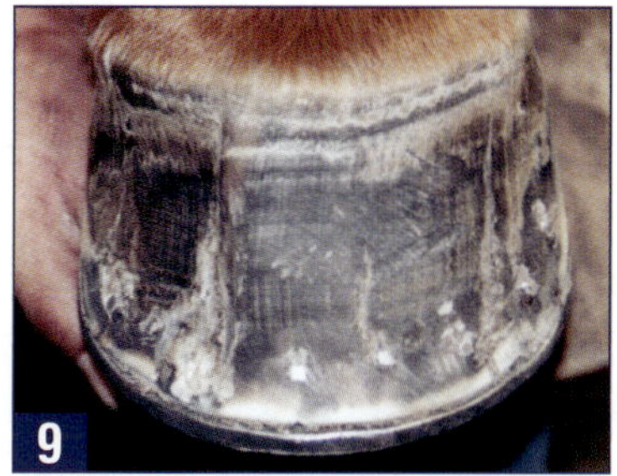

After: Dorsal view.

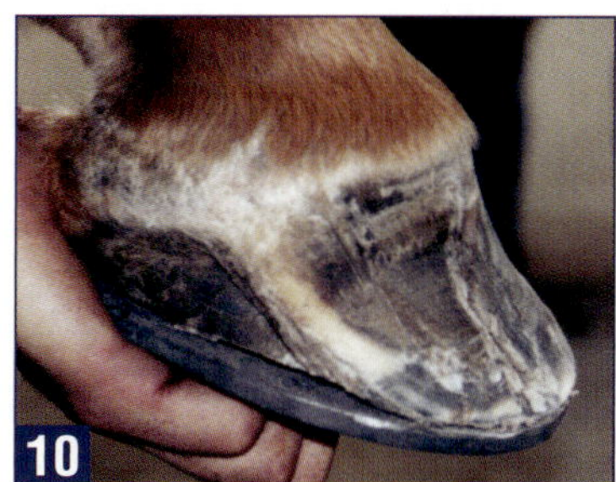

After: Medial view.

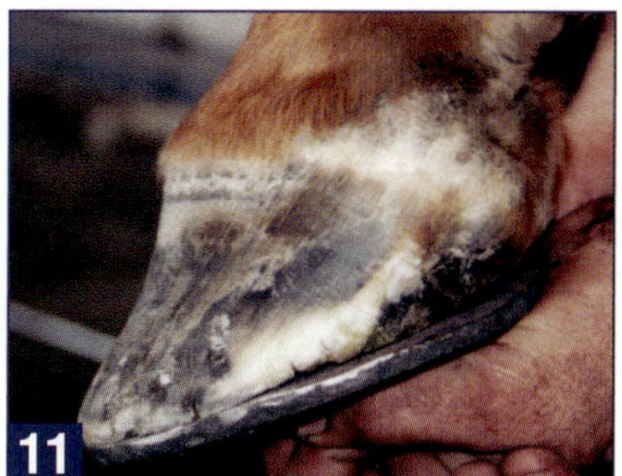

After: Lateral view.

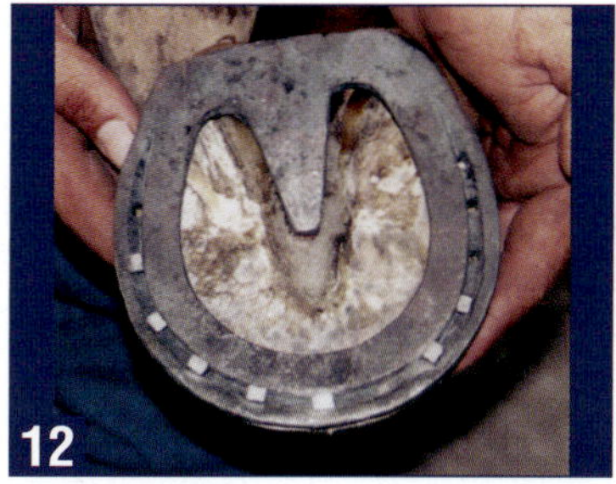

After: Solar view with a heart bar in place.

brought to the school as a vet referral, and I invited the shoer to come as well. When the horse showed up, I was disappointed to find out that the shoer could not come because he had an appointment at the hair salon. Anyway, in **Figures 5-7**, the outside of the foot can be seen from several views. There are cracks and dishes in this very weak hoof. The shoe on the foot is shown in **Figure 8**. There are four clips on the shoe to help hold it in place.

Figures 9-11 show the same foot after I trimmed it and applied a heart bar. Nothing special was done to this foot. I just applied solid, basic principles of farriery to the trimming, and then made a heart bar that could take some of the load off of a very weak hoof wall. **Figure 12** shows the heart bar on the bottom of the foot. Notice all of the nails in the toe of the foot. The toe is actually the best place for nailing. There is very little movement in the wall compared to the heels, the wall is quite thick here, and it is solidly attached to the coffin bone. The reason that the toe is not nailed very often is due to the fact that this is the area of highest wear. Nail heads would wear off here faster than on the sides of the foot. However, anytime I have an unusual foot

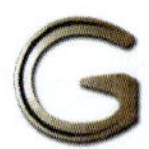

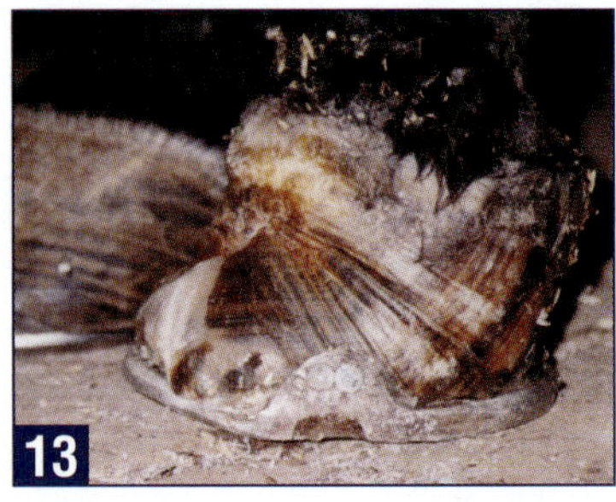

Near front foot, badly foundered.

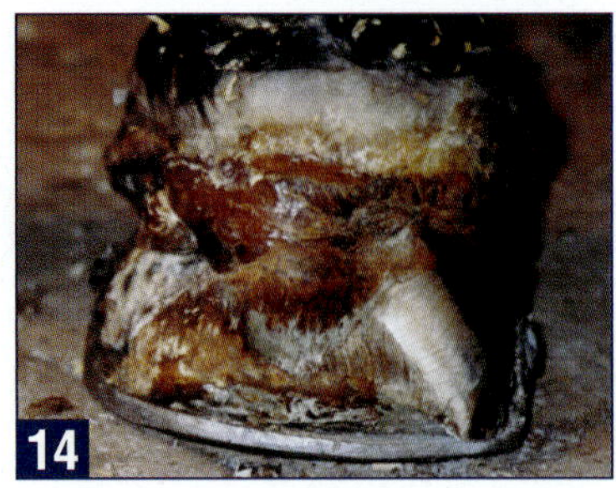

Dorsal view of the foot.

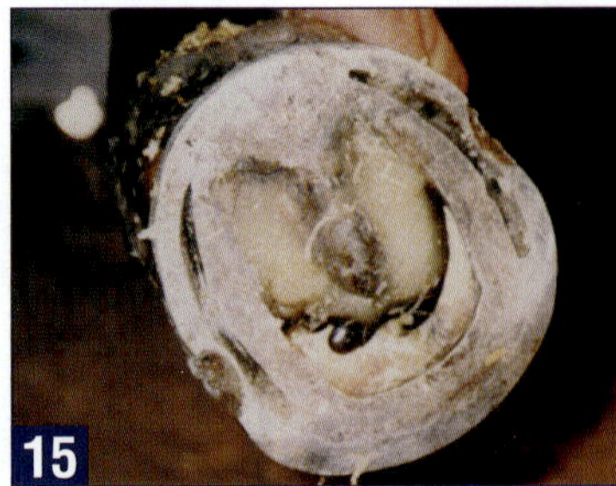

Solar view of the foot.

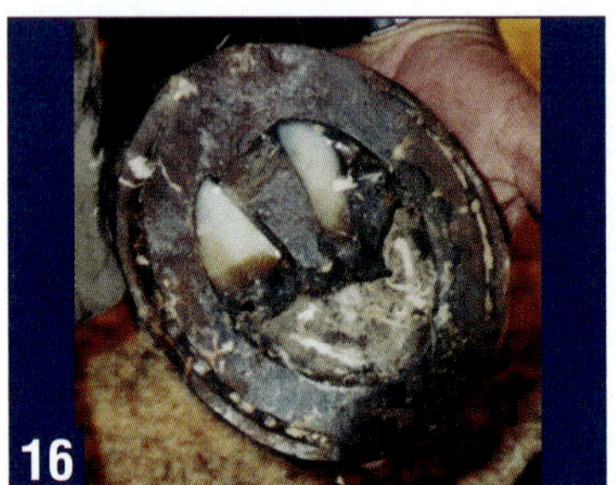

Egg bar/heart bar shoe on the foot.

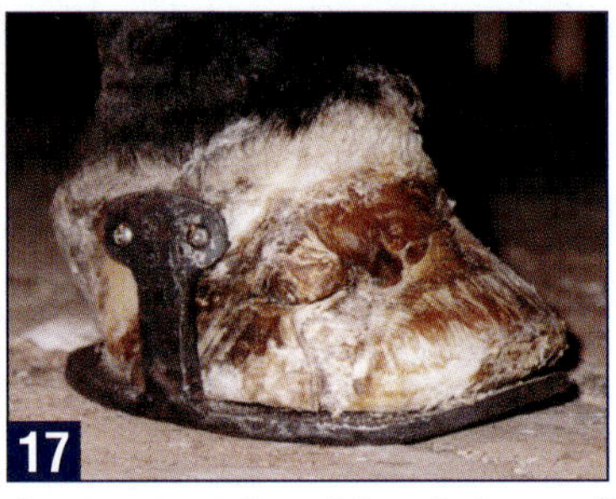

A strut up the side of the wall was screwed into the good horn available near the top of the foot.

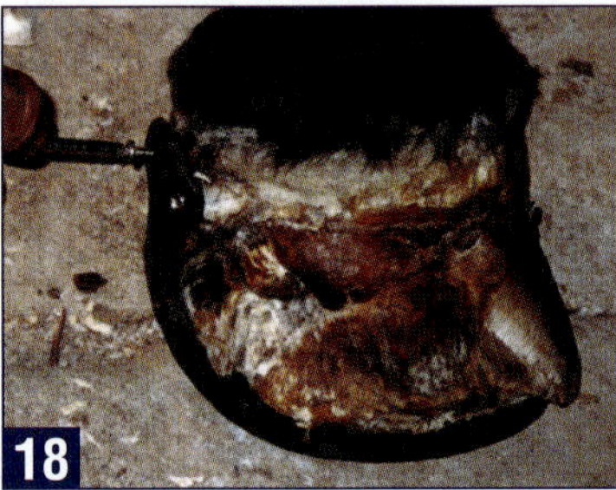

Screwing in the strut.

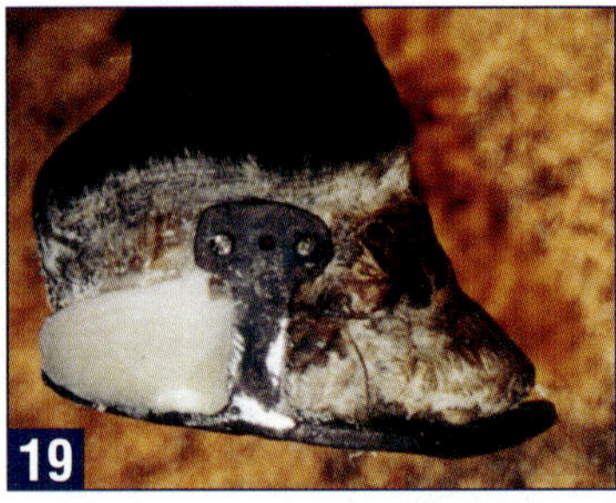

Super Fast around the back of the shoe to help hold it on. Notice the rocker toe and the gap between the toe and the shoe.

that I am putting a shoe on, I consider the toe a great place to put nails.

In 1996, I used a W-shoe for the first time on a foot that I had originally used a heart bar for. This horse introduced me to the W-shoe out of necessity, and I thought at the time that I might be doing something wrong because I had never seen a W-shoe or anything like it before. Once I used it and began to see results and understand the principles behind the application, I found that the W-shoe was one of the best options for founder there is. Here is the horse that taught me this.

Figures 13-15 show the foundered and injured front foot of a horse that was reportedly hit by lightning, with the lightning grounding out at that foot. I made and applied a heart bar/egg bar with a strut up the side that could be screwed to the wall that was available **(Figures 16-18)**. Vettec Super Fast was put around the heel of the shoe and foot to help hold it on **(Figures 19)**, and there is a rocker toe on the shoe. The rocker toe was not added so much for breakover as it was for simply trying to decrease the

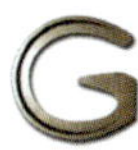

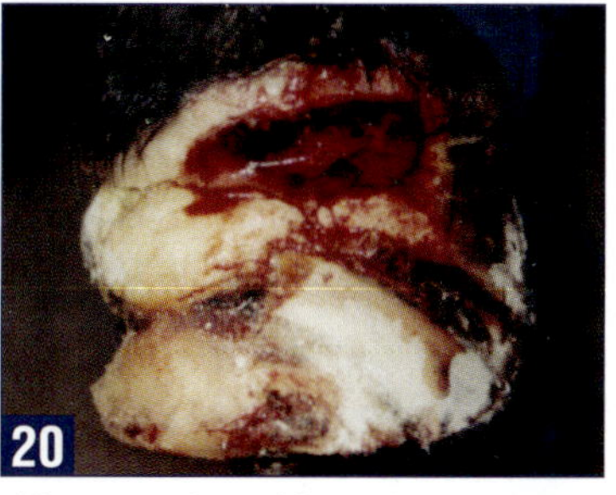

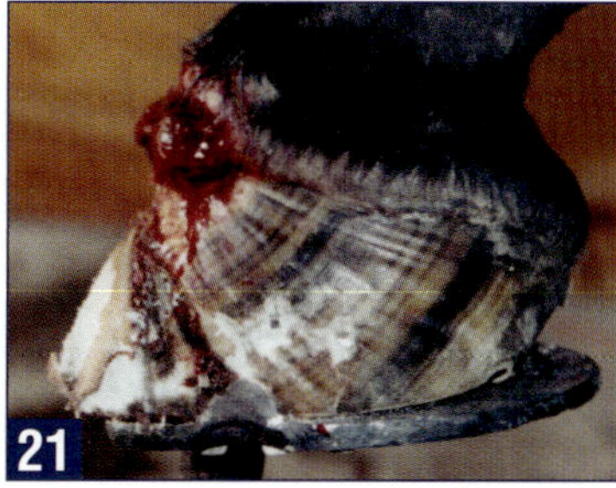

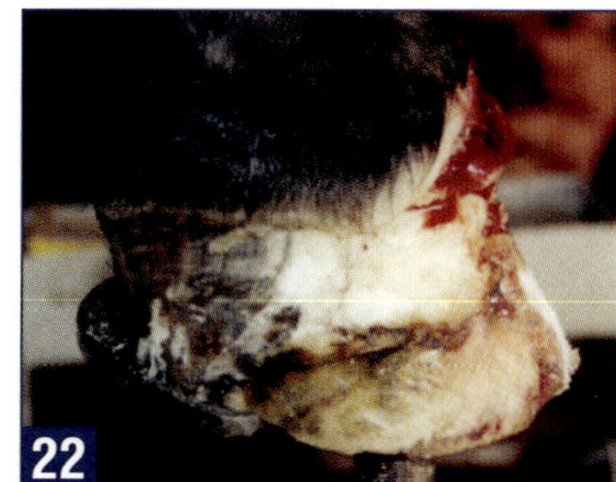

Abscess breaking out at the coronet.

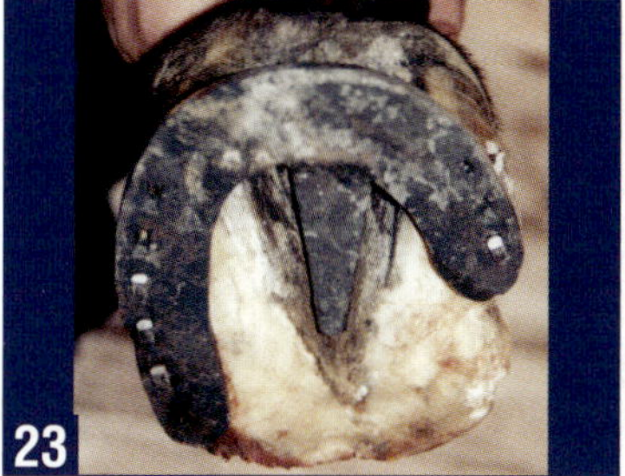

My first kind of W-shoe.

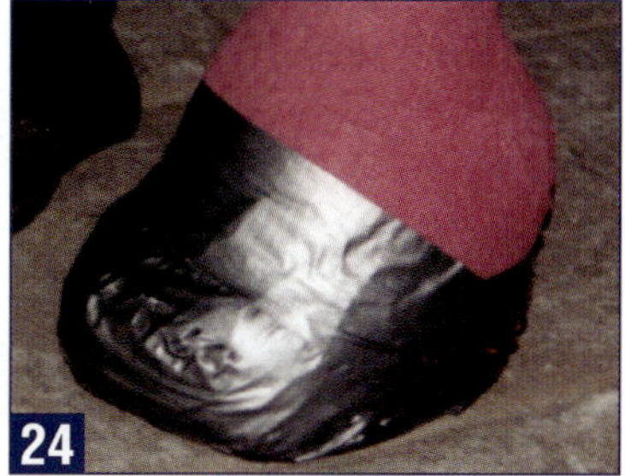

The foot, bandaged.

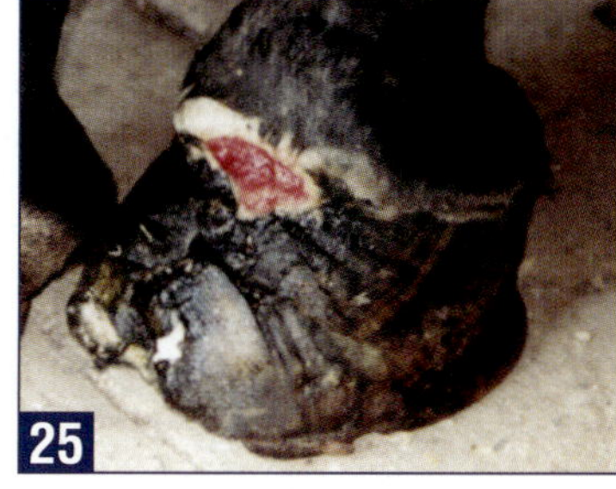

As it healed.

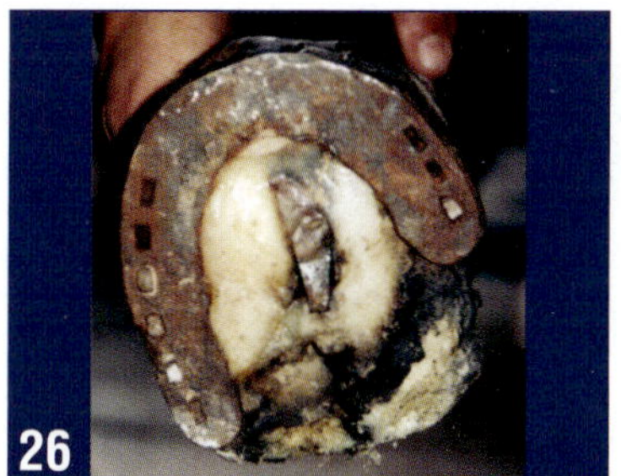

Time for reset

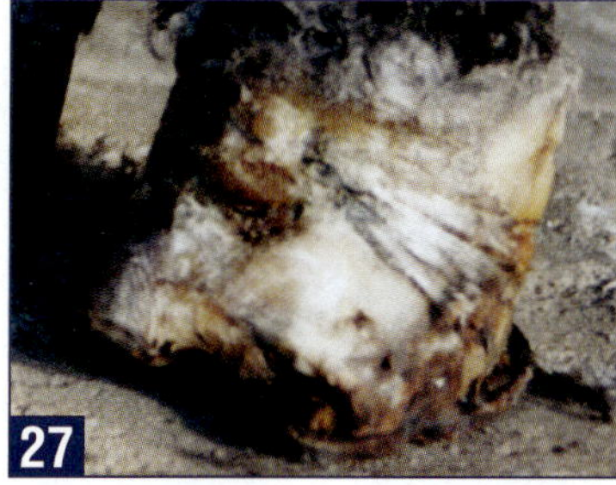

gap between the toe and the shoe where the toe of the foot was destroyed.

In those days, I didn't know what else to do with the area of the shoe that was against such damaged horn. The idea of completely cutting it out never occurred to me. I had enough sense not to put pressure on the wall at the toe with a shoe, but not enough sense to cut it out — at least not yet. But this horse was about to school me.

The gap at the toe ended up getting some debris in it, and this caused the horse to develop an abscess — and not just a normal abscess, but a dramatic infection **(Figures 20-22)**.

Using a heart bar was no longer an option, so I made my first W-shoe **(Figure 23)**, which resembled a J more than a W at the time. The owner did a lot of work doctoring and caring for the foot, and the abscess finally healed **(Figures 24-25)**. Over the course of 11 months, the foot grew and improved, while my skill at making and using the W-shoe grew with it. **Figures 26-31** show some of this evolution. By the end of that year, the foot would look like **Figures 32-33** at the end of a shoeing cycle, and **Figures 34 and 35** once it was reset. This horse

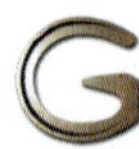

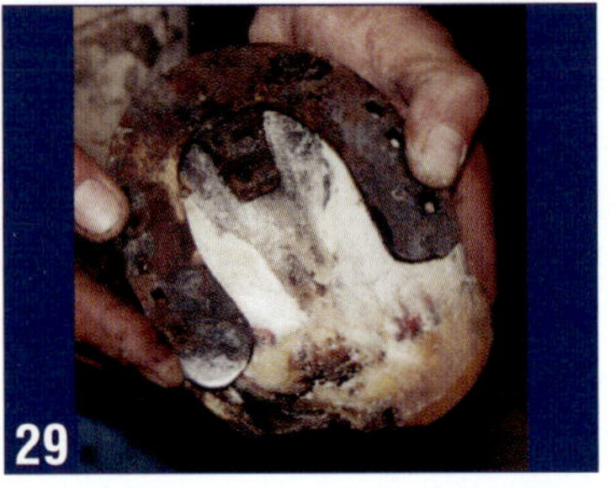
29

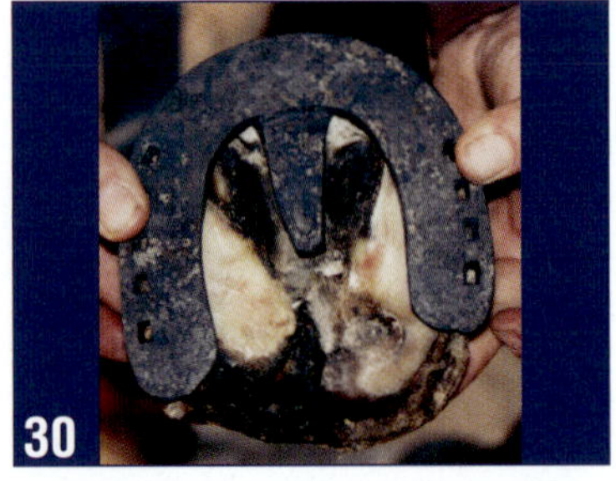
30

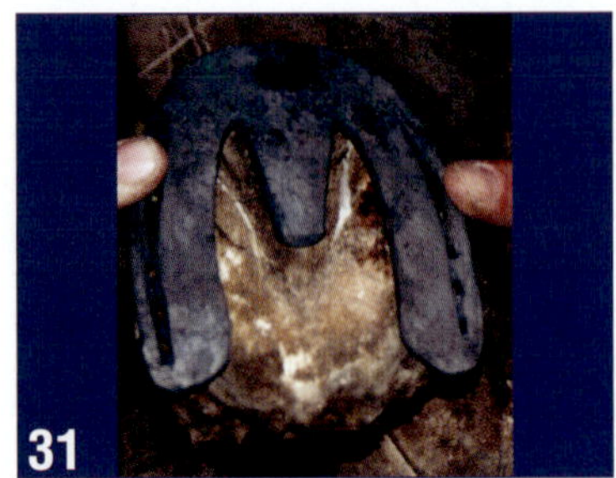
31

Evolution of my W-shoes as the foot allowed for different lengths.

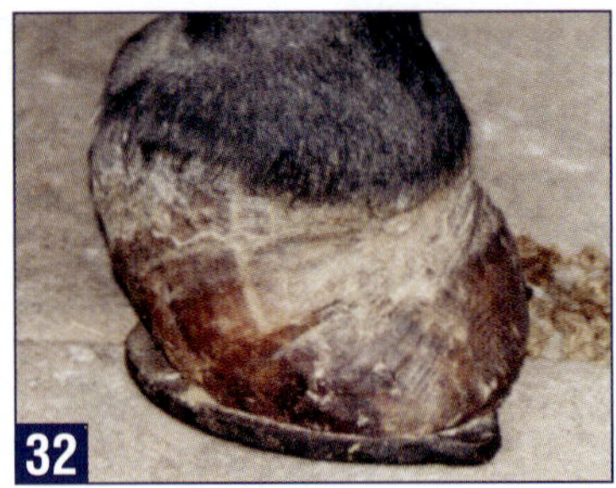
32

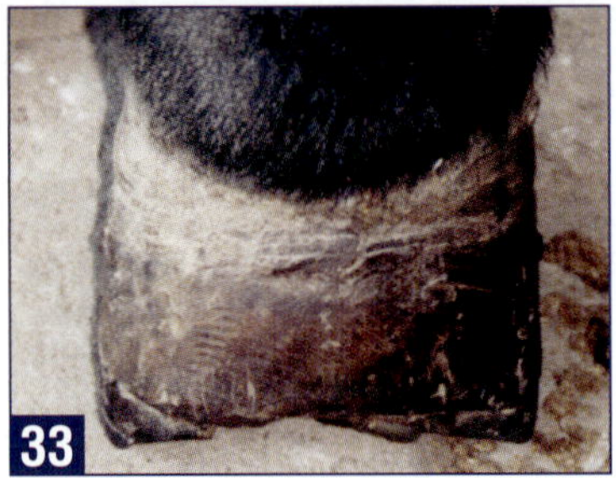
33

Still growing lots of heel, but getting to be a better foot.

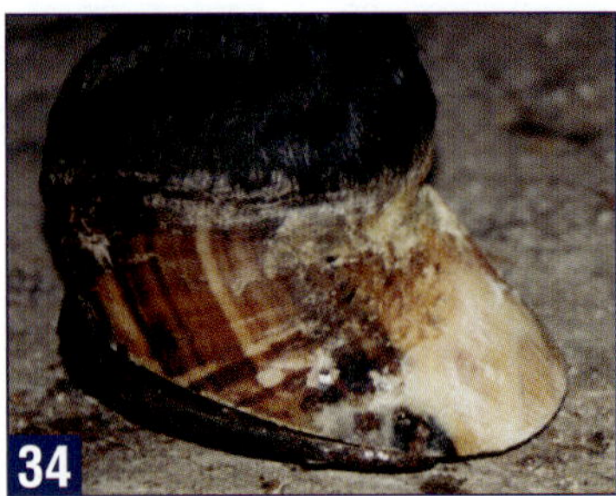
34

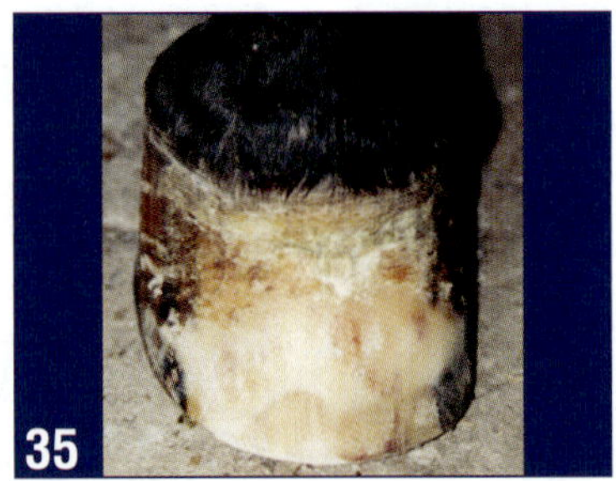
35

Where the foot ended up.

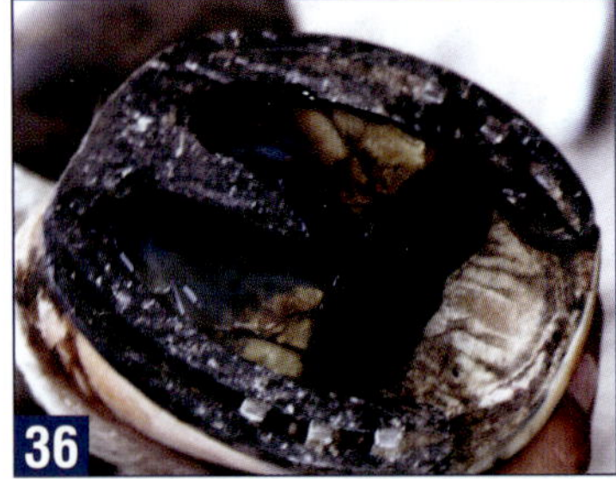
36

W-shoe with pour-in pad.

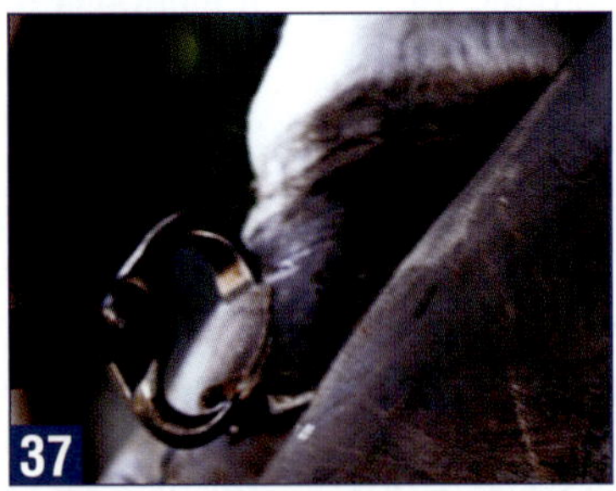
37

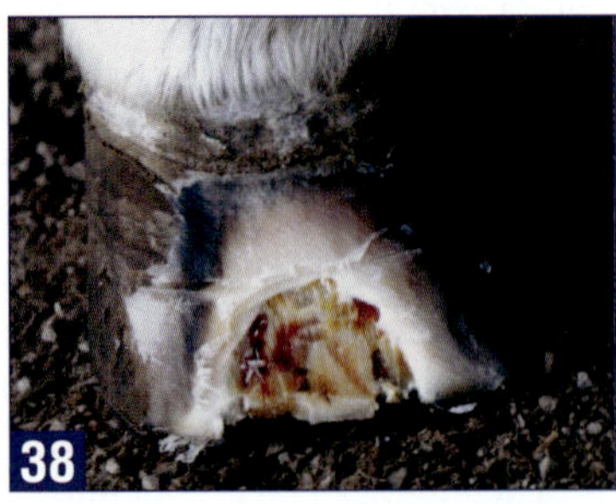
38

Doing a resection.

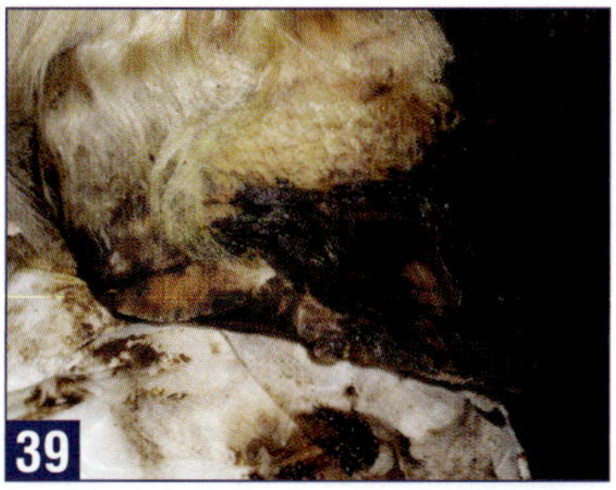

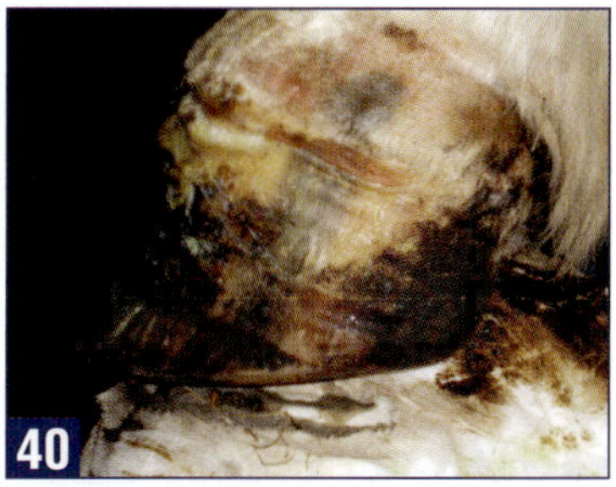

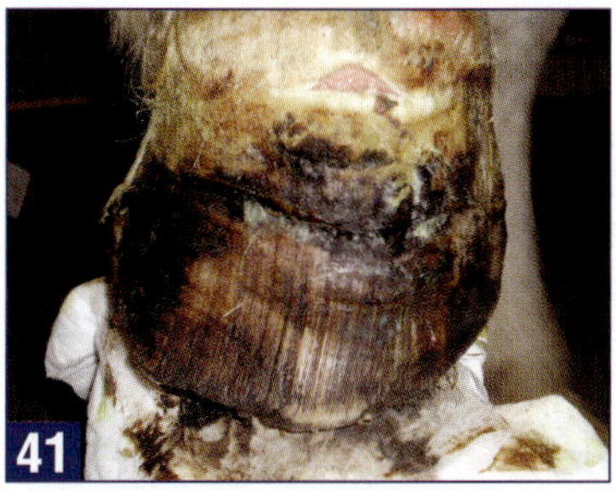

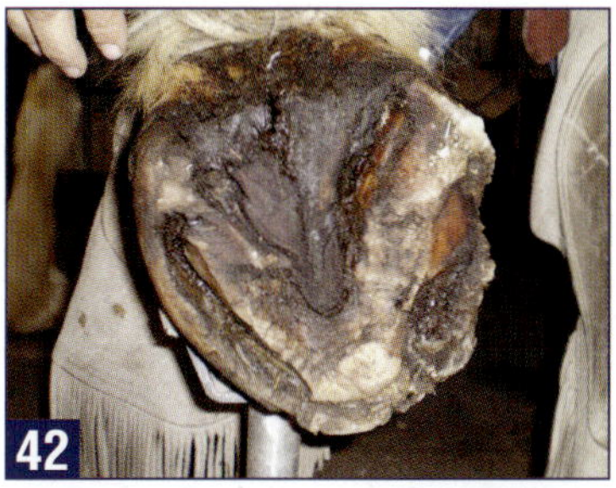

Dallas's foot, first visit.

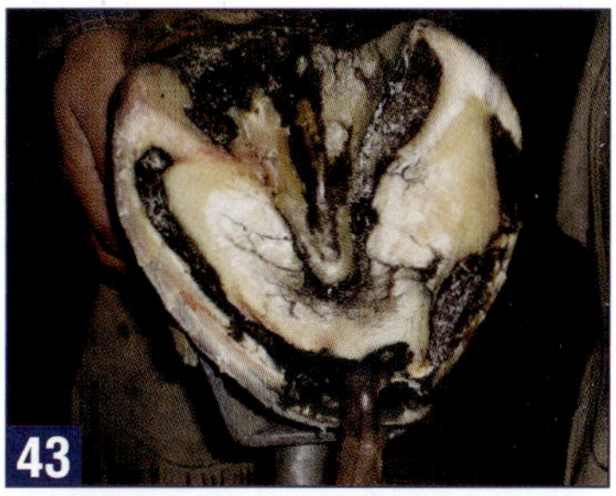

First trim in progress.

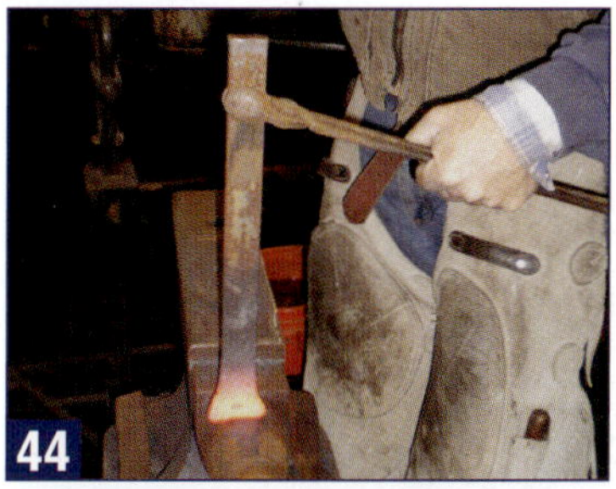

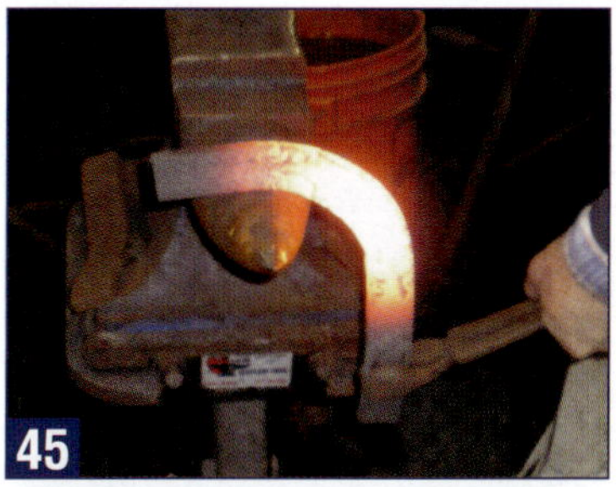

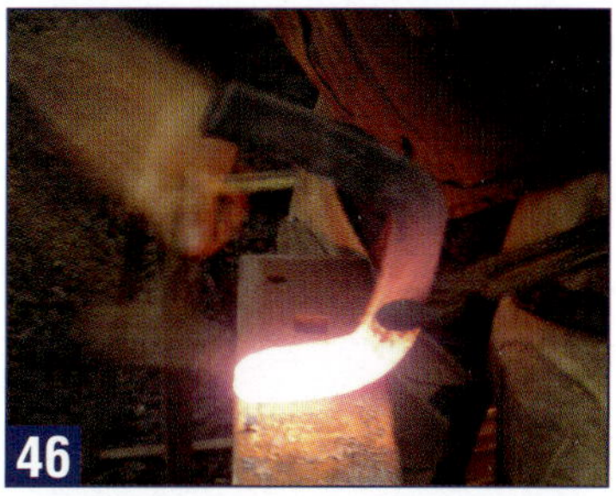

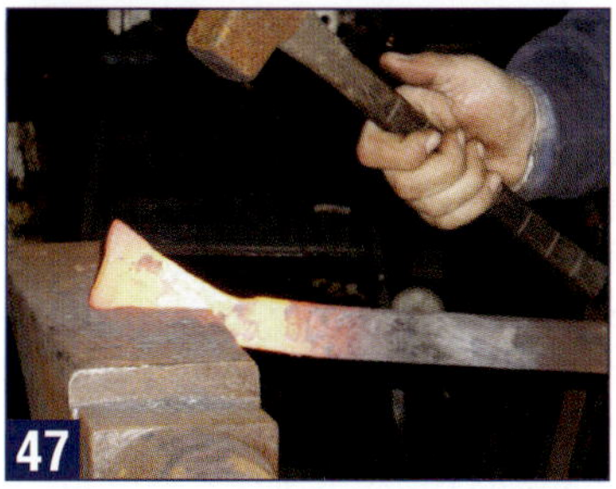

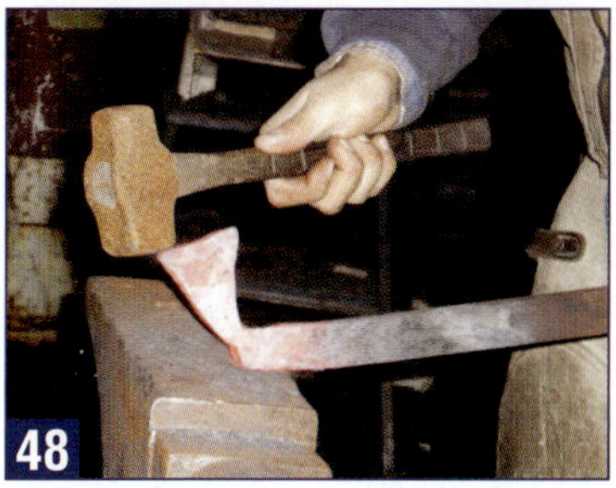

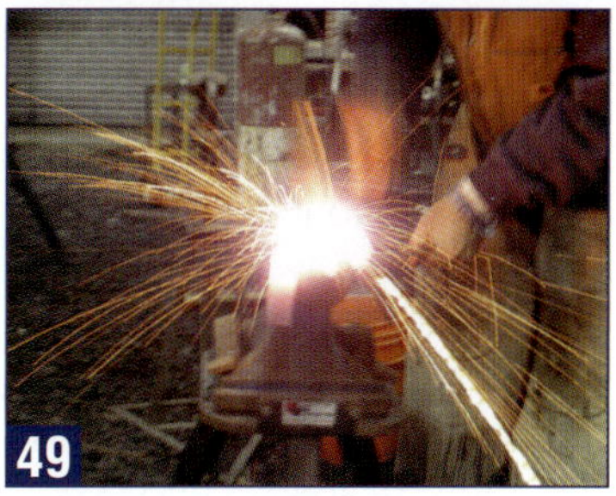

Figures 44-52, making a W-shoe for Dallas, a draft horse. *continued next page*

went on to have several babies and ended up having a pretty nice life.

The W-shoe became a common part of my practice. I especially like using it when doing resections **(Figures 36-38)**. Consider what happens when the foot has had a resection, and then the steel toe of the shoe is allowed to extend beyond the foot in the newly resected toe. The pressure put on both sides of the toe is multiplied, made worse because it is in an area that is already in potential crisis from the founder.

Next we have Dallas, a retired Budweiser Clydesdale. Dallas had been diagnosed with white line disease, and the vet sent him to see us so that we could put a shoe on to support what foot Dallas had. **Figures 39-42** show the foot the first time we

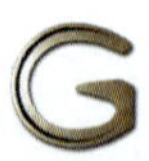

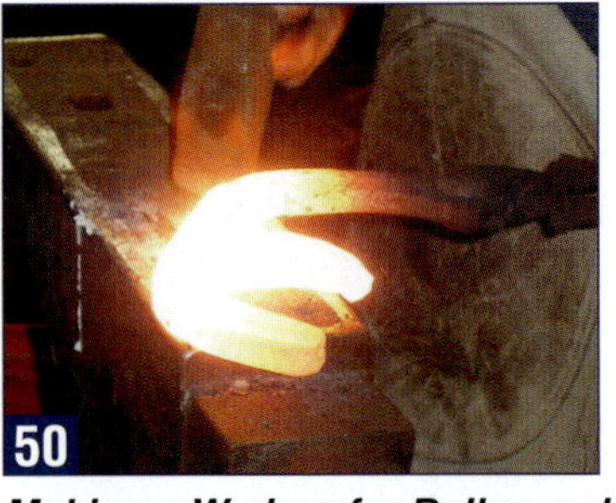

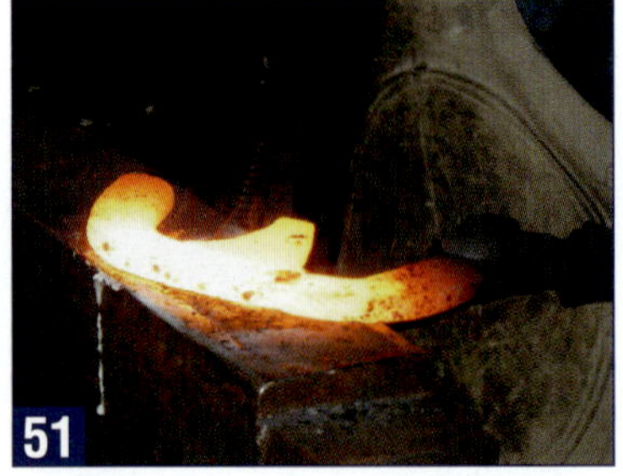

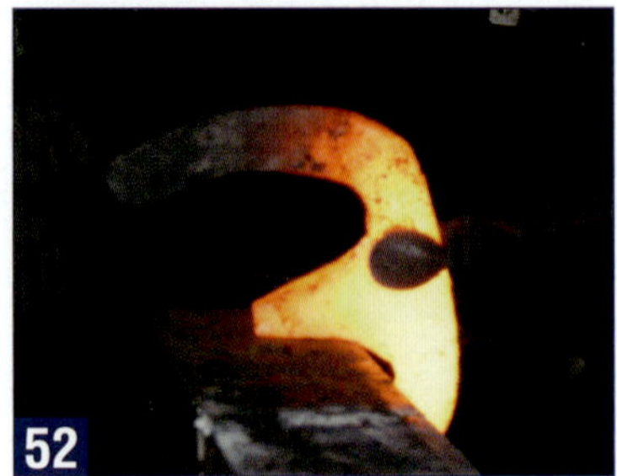

Making a W-shoe for Dallas, a draft horse.

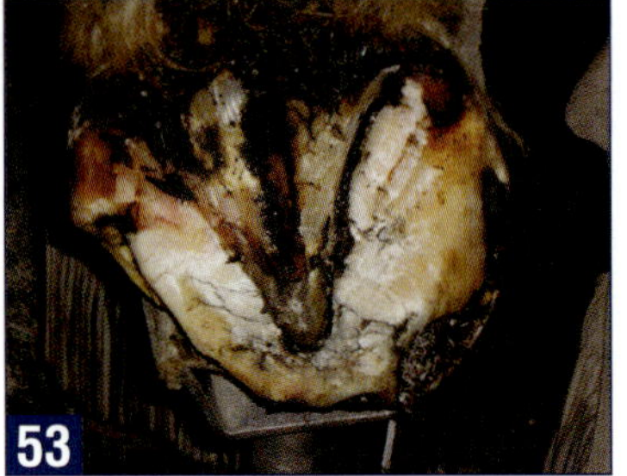

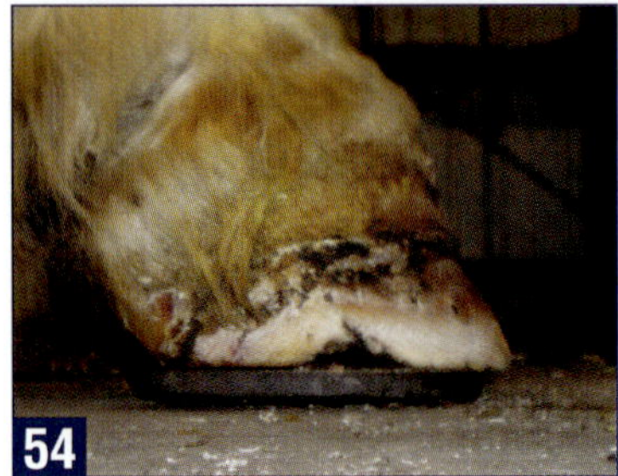

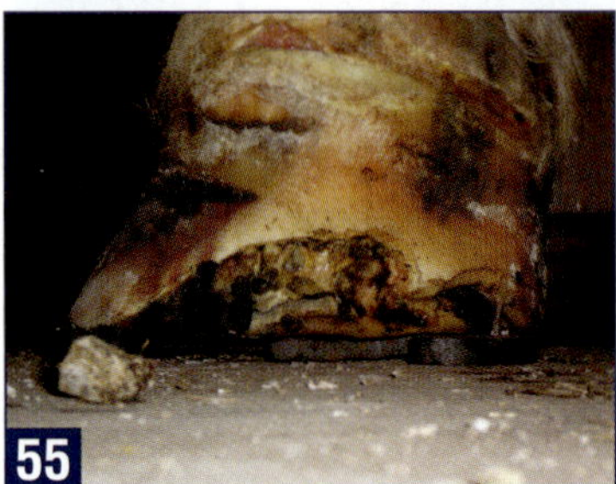

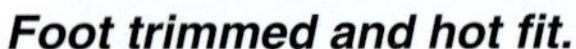

Foot trimmed and hot fit.

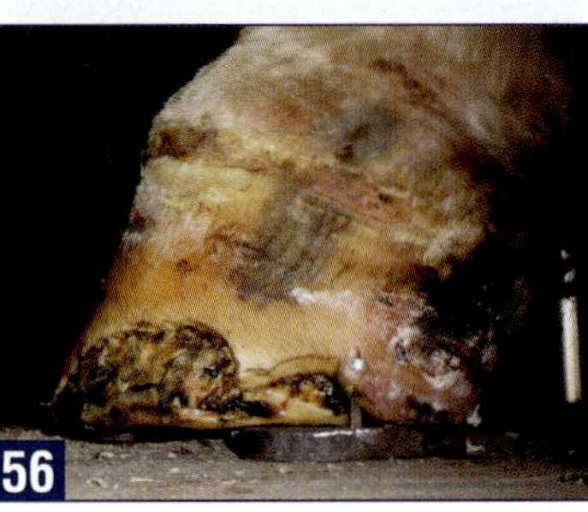

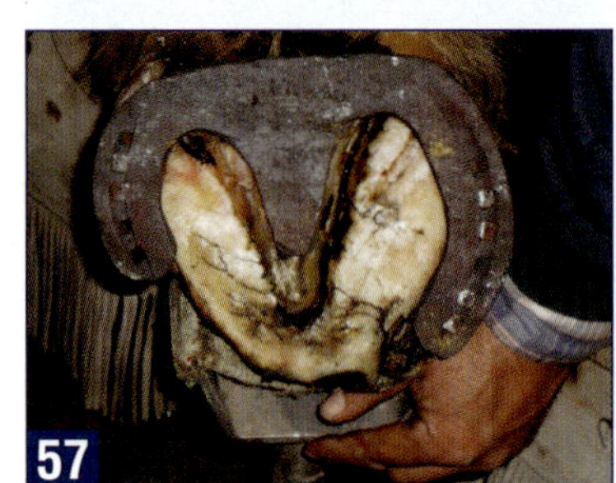

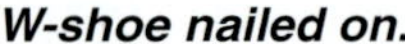

W-shoe nailed on.

saw it. **Figure 43** is his foot on a cradle after the initial trim. Notice the nippers going into the toe of the foot to cut away some of the wall that was not attached to the coffin bone.

One of the principles that I have tried to get across in this book is to put shoe where you have foot in these sorts of cases. This becomes even more important when dealing with a horse the size of a draft. The best option here in my opinion was a W-shoe. **Figures 44-52** are a recap of making this shoe. Notice that it is longer on one branch than the other, due to having more foot on one side than the other. **Figure 53** is a view of the bottom of the foot after the hot fit, showing most of the affected wall removed.

I nailed the shoe on. If you look carefully, you will see that I only got two nails on the left side as you view the photo **(Figures 54)**. **Figures 55-57** show the foot on the shoe on the ground from a few angles. Now comes the hard part. Putting Equi-Pak in an area of foot on a horse that size that does not want to bend his fetlock. Gravity is against you here, so get ready to get messy. In **Figure 58**, you can see where the Hawthorne's Sole Pack is making a dam in front of the frog plate as Kelly heats the bottom of the foot with a heat gun. **Figure 59** is the application of the material itself. Put it in slowly enough that you can kind of shape it.

Dallas came back to the shop in about six weeks, and the foot was looking better **(Figures 60-62)**, but there was a sore area at the top of the coronary band. In hindsight, that should have thrown up a big red flag. But at the time, I thought it was the result of infection and inflammation from the white line disease. We trimmed the foot, hot fit it, reset

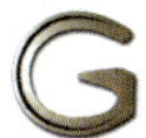

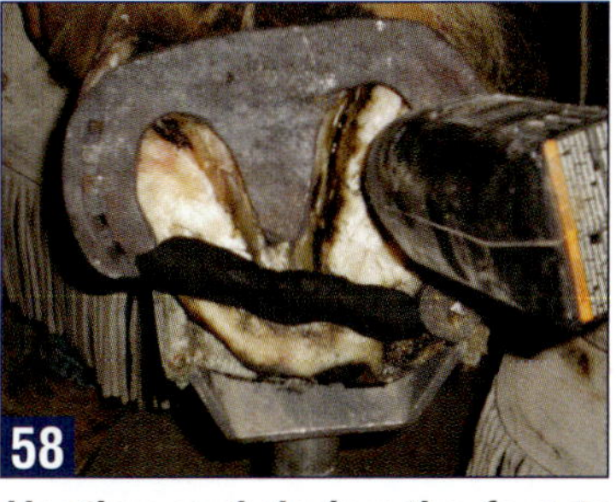

58 *Heating and drying the foot to apply Equi-Pak.*

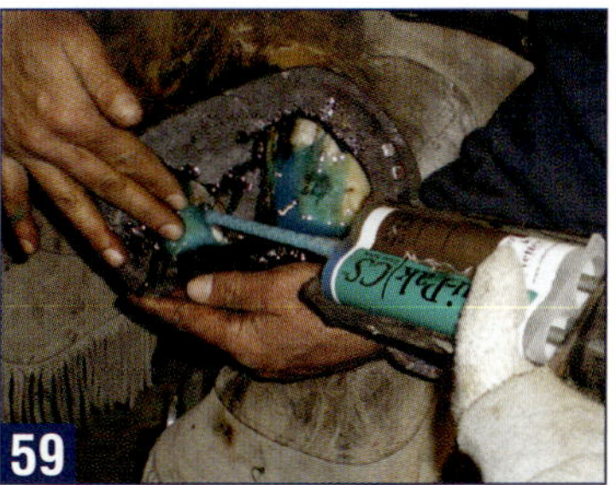

59 *Doing the pour-in.*

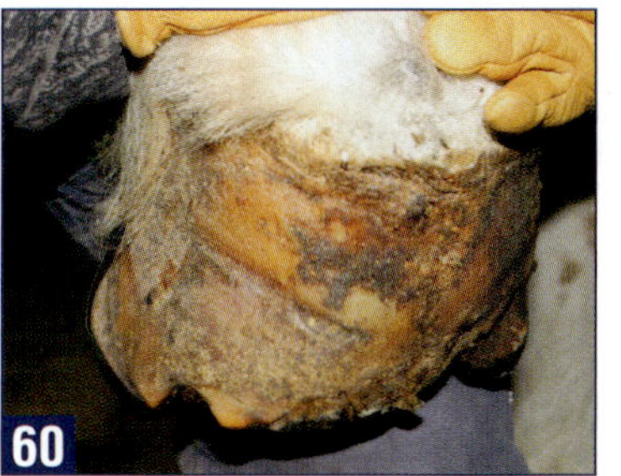

60

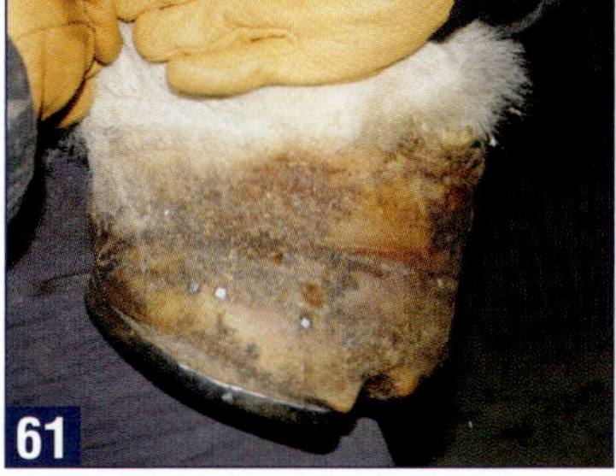

61

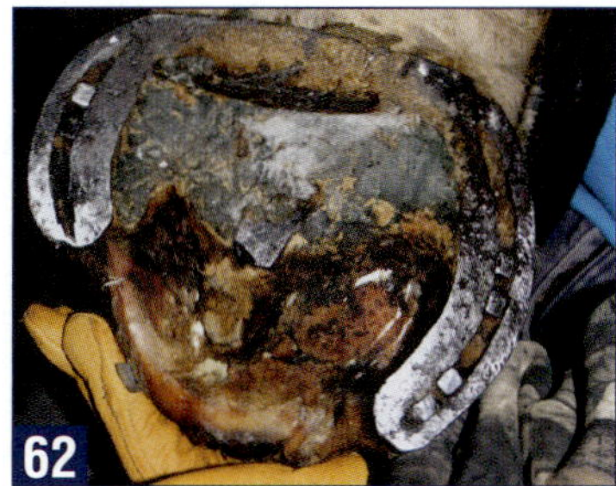

62

First reset, before picture when Dallas came in at six weeks.

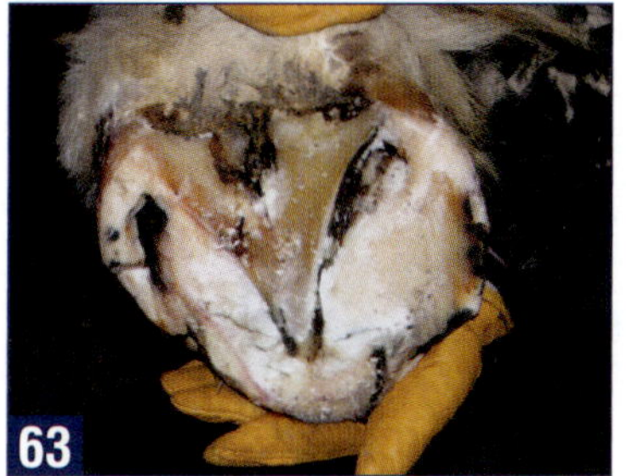

63 *Foot trimmed.*

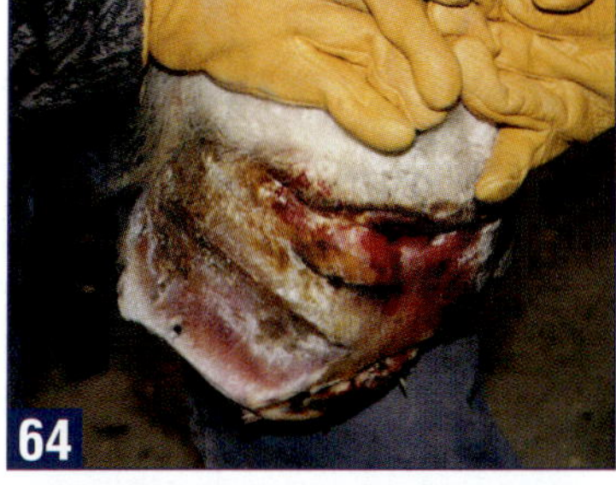

64 *Bleeding sore at the coronet.*

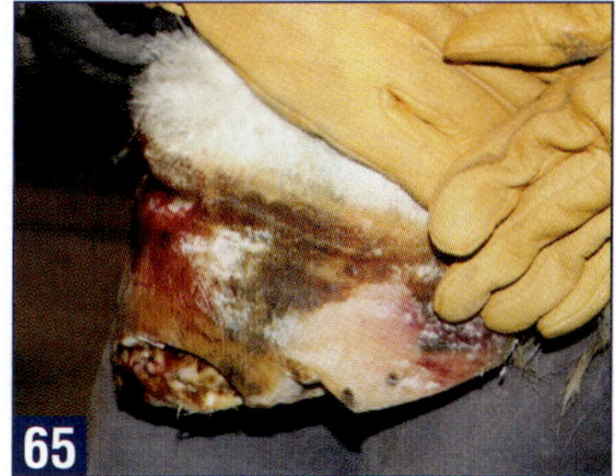

65

66

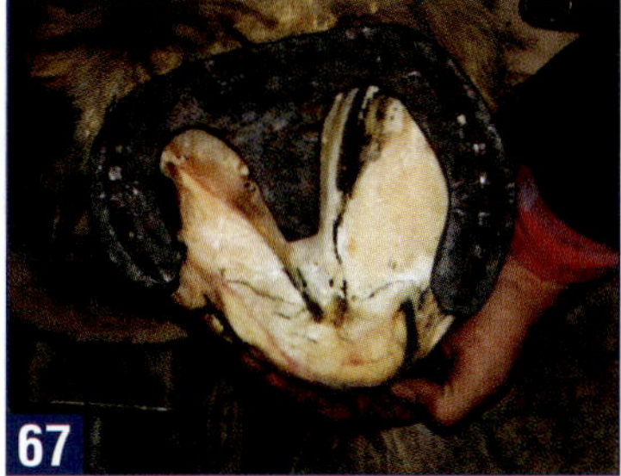

67 *Nailed up.*

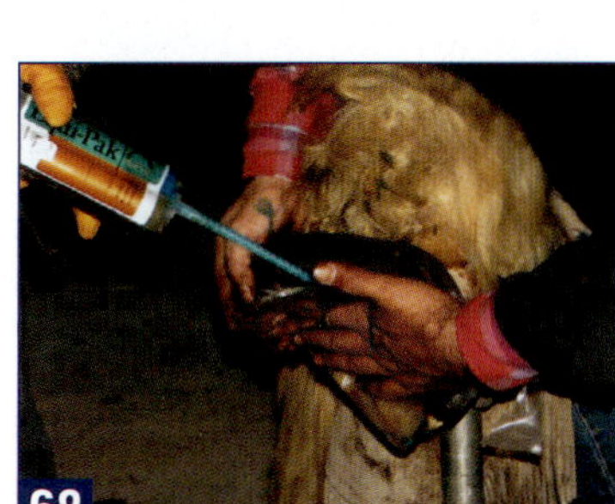

68 *Doing the pour-in.*

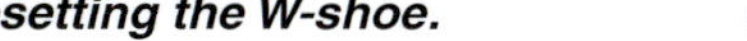

Resetting the W-shoe.

the W-shoe, and filled it with Equi-Pak (**Figures 63-68**). Dallas was a little sore, but less than he had been before the first shoeing. We all thought that we were making pretty good headway.

Dallas continued to do pretty well and we were happy to see how he had grown down when we saw him a couple months later. The place that had been bleeding at the dorsal coronary band had grown down, as seen in

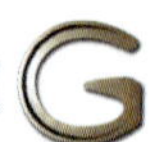

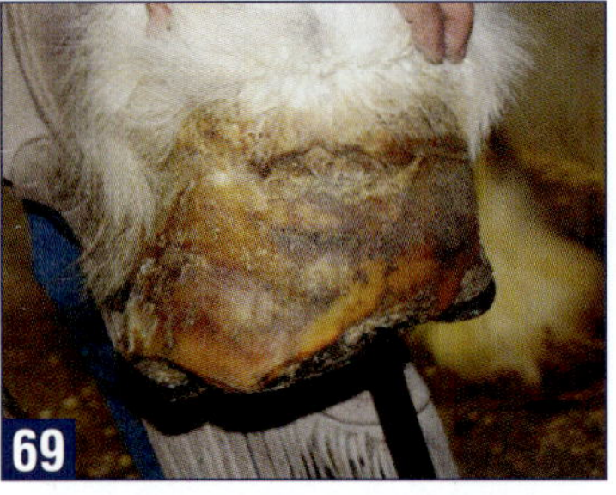

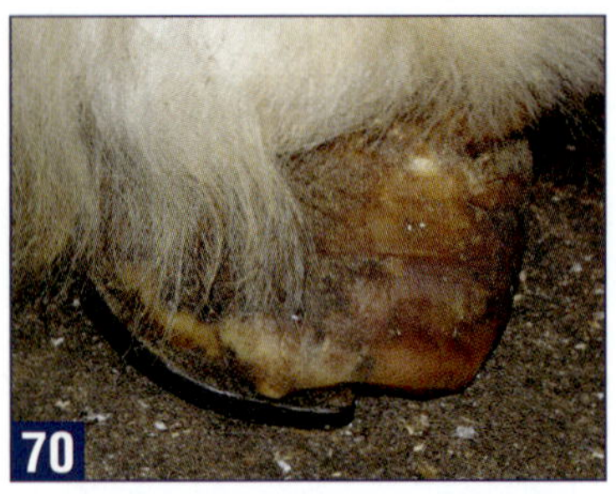

Next visit, major progress.

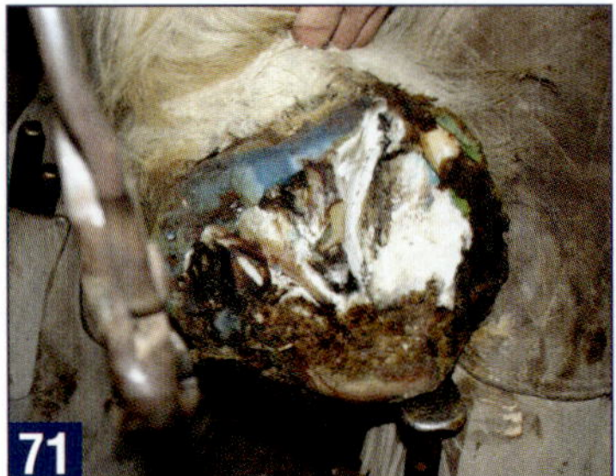

The shoe pulled.

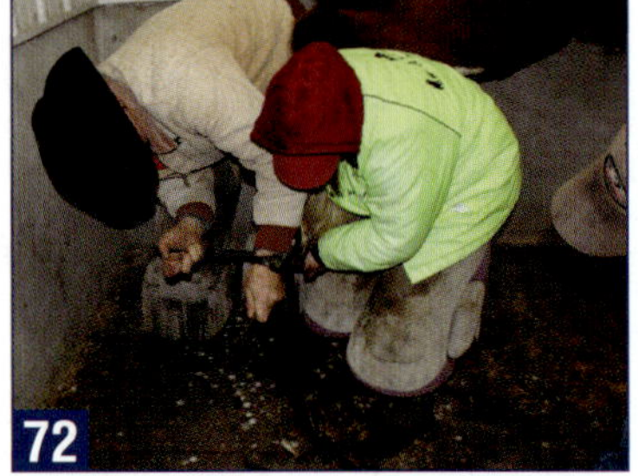

Kelly and I trimming together.

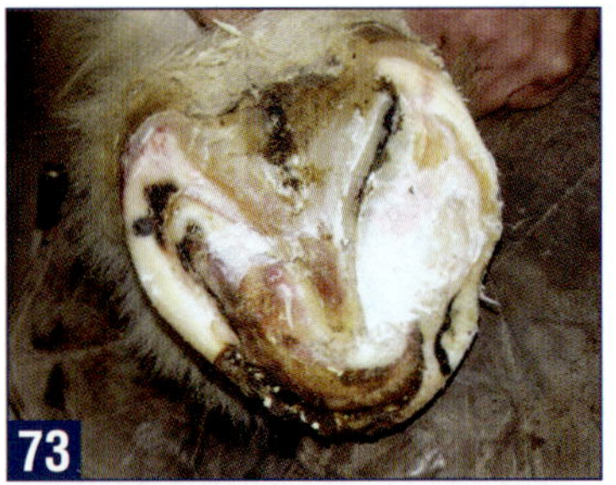

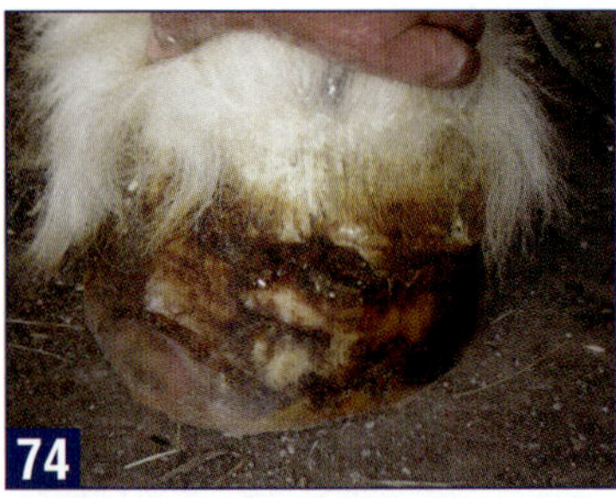

Trimmed, and it appeared to be healing.

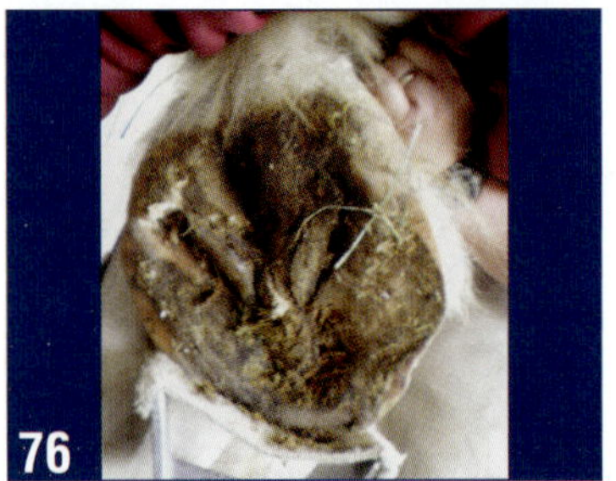

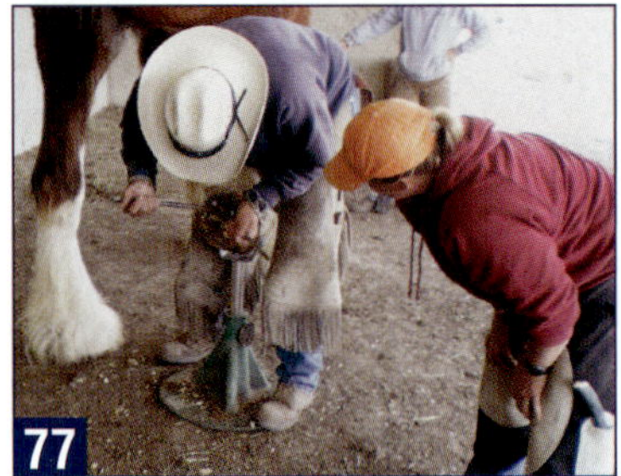

Last trim we did before Dallas went to Oakridge Equine Hospital for keratoma surgery.

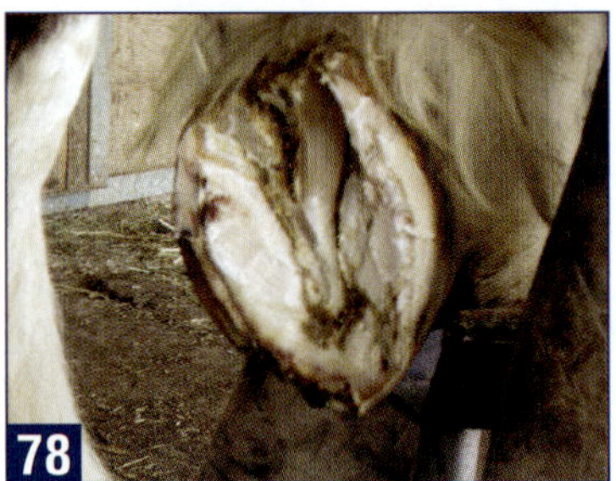

The foot was looking good at this point, but the continued lameness caused the owner to look deeper, which turned out to be a good thing.

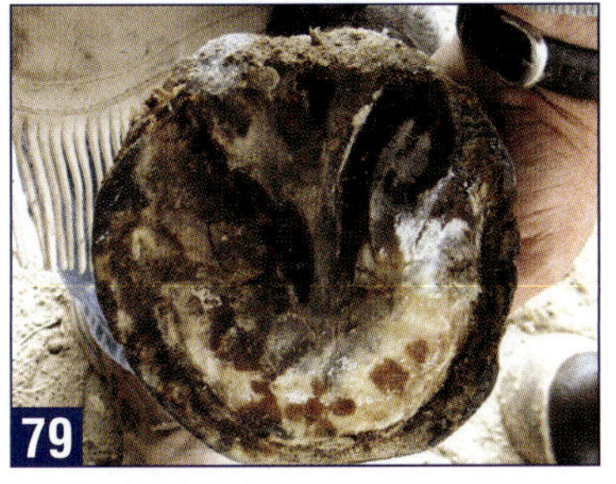

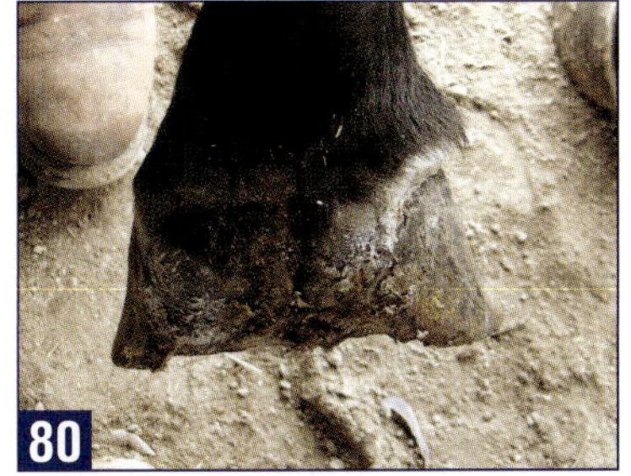

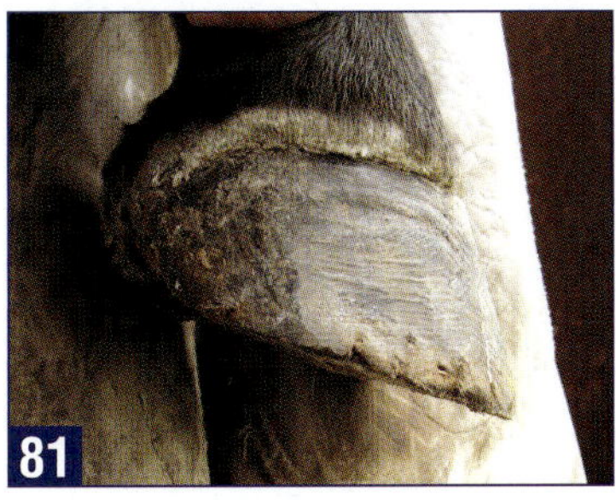

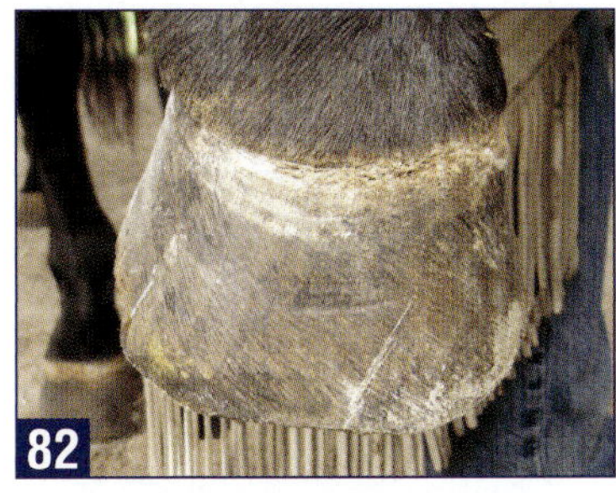

First look at a sore, misshapen, and badly growing foot.

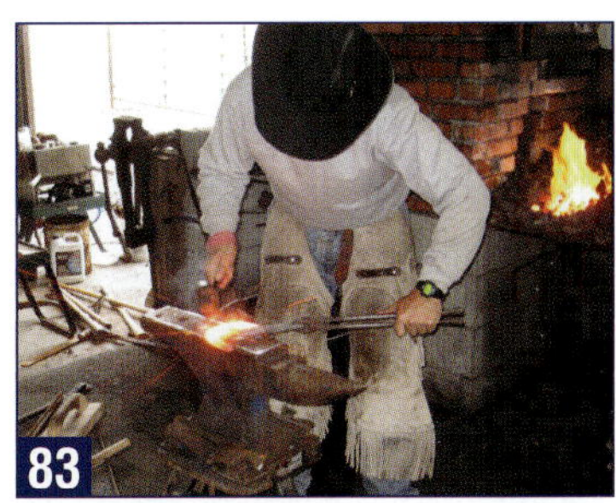

Making a W-shoe for the foot.

Figures 69 and 70. I pulled the shoe, and you can see by the white on the sole in **Figure 71** just how much that Equi-Pak CS had stuck to the sole. Kelly and I are working on the foot together in **Figure 72**, which is not uncommon when doing drafts that stand well. His foot ended up looking pretty good at this point in the treatment **(Figure 73)**.

The last time we trimmed Dallas, he was still a bit lame, but the foot was looking outstanding **(Figures 74-78)**. However, with Dallas still having some trouble, the vet started digging a little deeper. It turned out that Dallas actually had something like 18 keratomas in the laminae. The amazing thing is that he was not limping worse than he was, and I was really impressed by how well the W-shoe performed. Had it been white line disease from the outset, this would have been an easy happy ending. Once Oakridge Equine took over the case, Dallas received farrier treatment at their clinic by farrier John Muldoon. Dallas is making a good recovery from the keratoma surgery as this book is going to print.

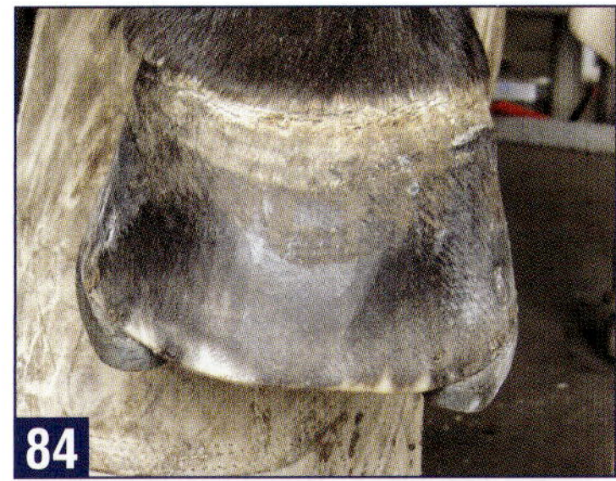

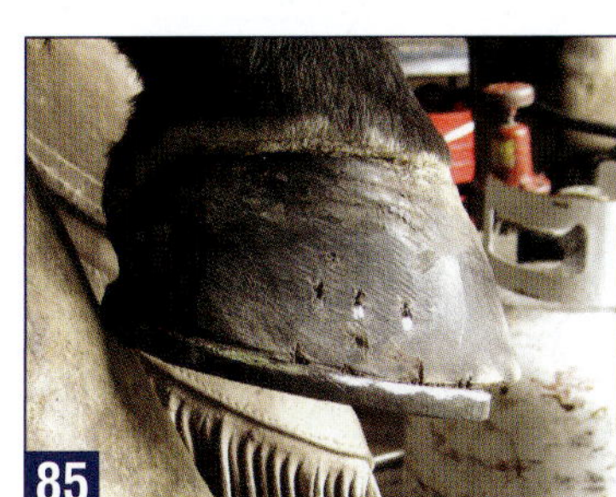

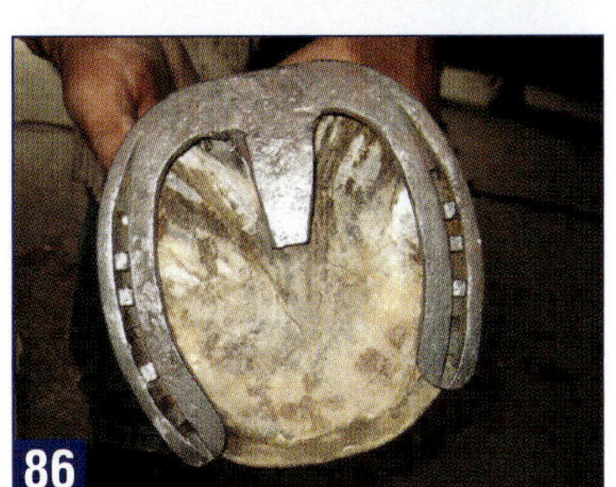

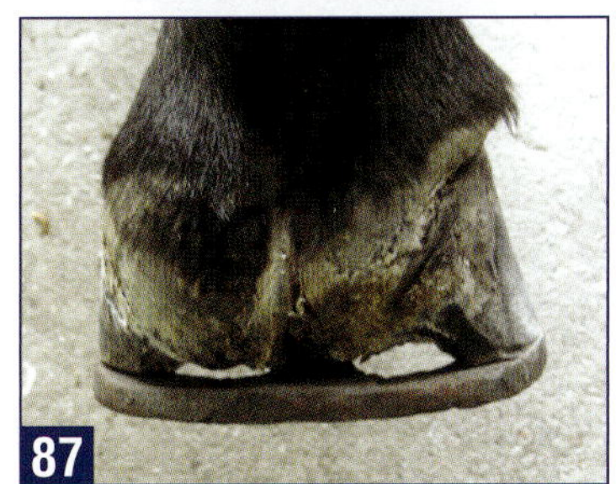

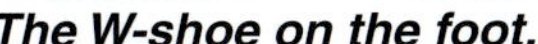

The W-shoe on the foot.

The foot shown in **Figures 79-81** belongs to a halter horse that was Grade 4 lame. On the medial side, there was a large ledge just below the coronet **(Figure 82)**, and the foot was growing pretty much all laterally. The previous farrier had done a lot of heavy dressing on the foot, but it had not been done well.

I trimmed the foot and made a W-shoe for it **(Figure 83)**. Once the shoe was nailed on **(Figures 84-87)**,

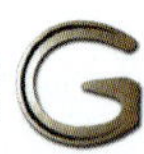

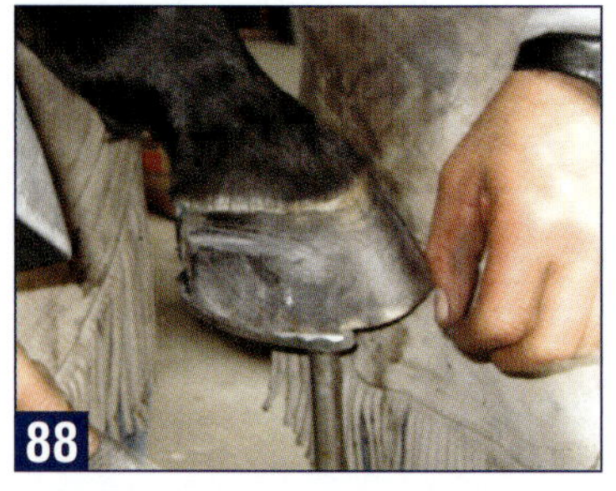

Making a horizontal groove with my rasp.

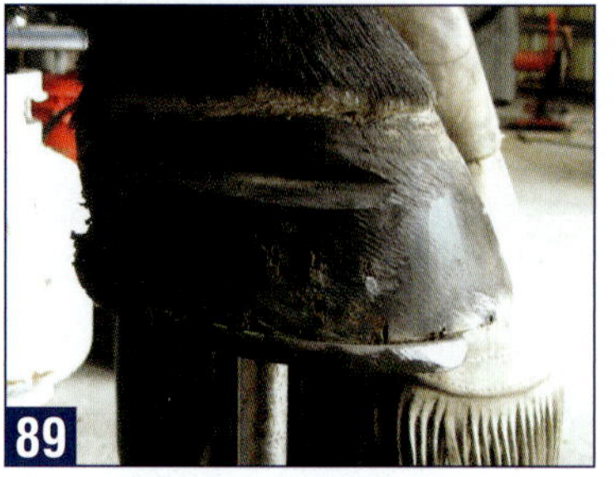

The foot after shoeing a grooved.

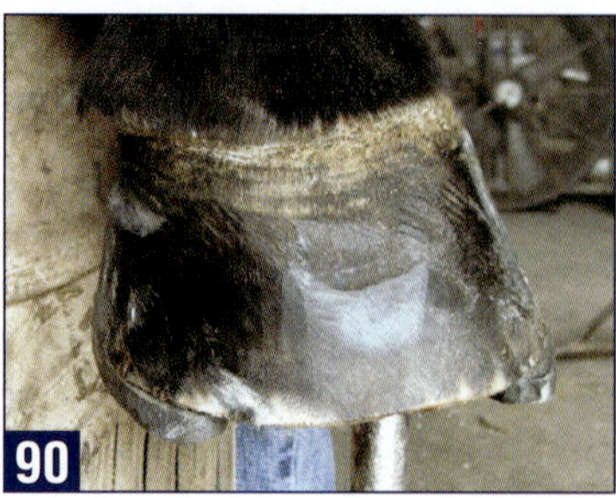

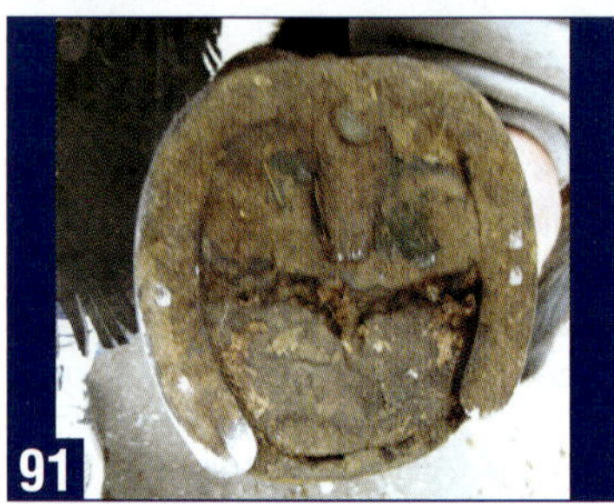

First return.

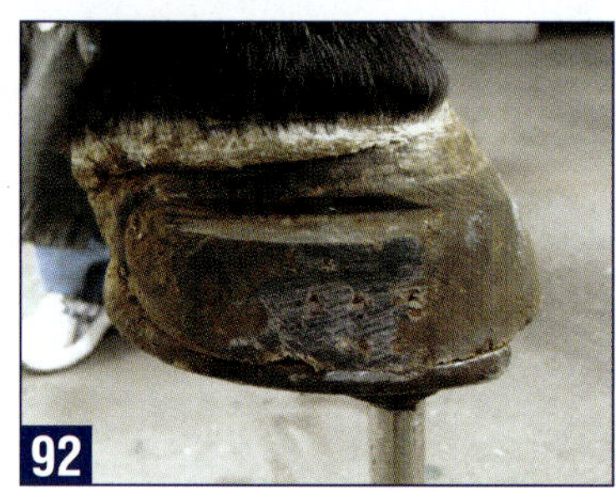

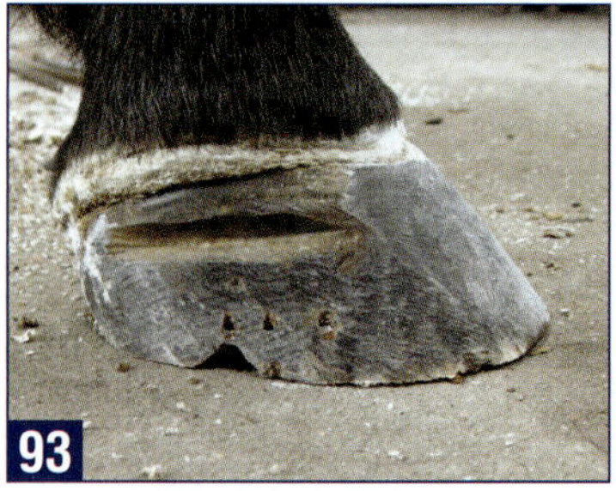

Kelly's trim.

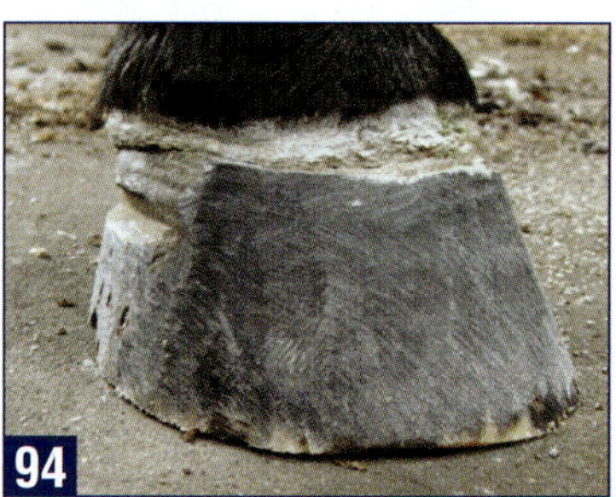

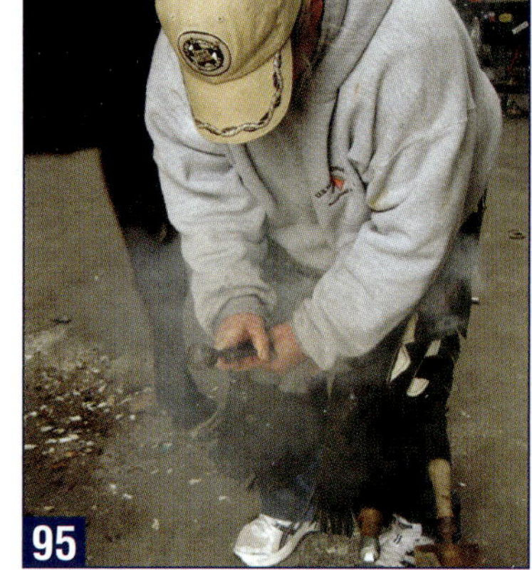

Hot fitting.

I grooved the medial side horizontally with a rasp **(Figures 88-90)**. Look carefully at **Figure 87** to see the ledge on the medial side. This side of the foot was badly jammed and not growing. The horse left at about Grade 2 lame.

When the horse returned in six weeks, the foot had improved immensely. The shoe and Equi-Pak were still in place **(Figure 91)**. I was amazed at how the medial side had grown down from the coronet **(Figure 92)**. Since I had just had shoulder surgery, Kelly trimmed and reset the horse this time. **Figures 93-94** are the trimmed foot, **Figure 95** is the hot fit, and **Figures 96-100** are the foot, freshly shod. Notice the sheared heel and jammed up medial side of the foot in **Figure 100**. After the Equi-Pak pour, the horse was ready to go again **(Figure 101)**. He was getting sounder by the day.

On the next visit, the foot had improved even more. **Figures 102-103** show the pre-trim, and **Figures 104-105** are the post-trim. In **Figure 105**, the coronet is still suffering from proximal displacement, but the groove in the wall is growing down nicely. I decided

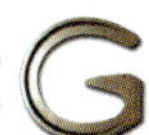

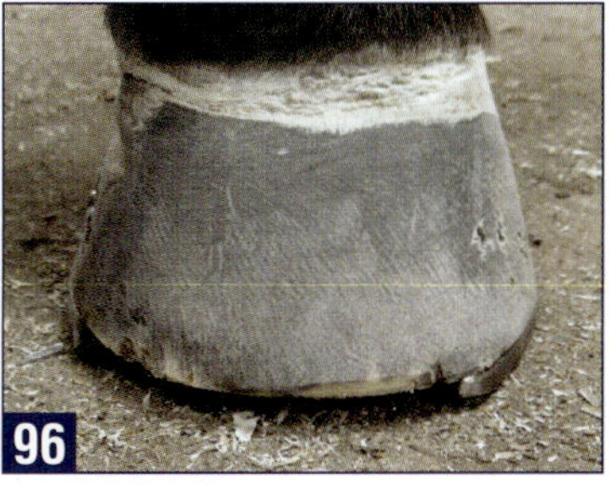

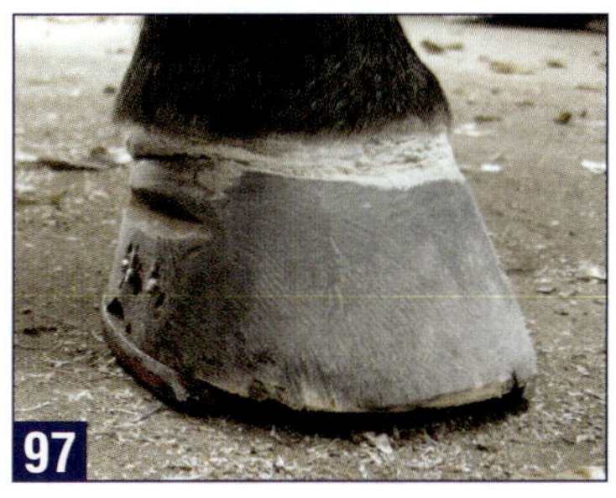

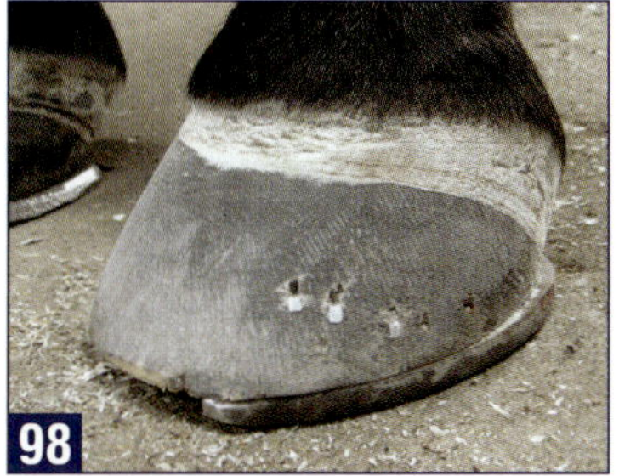

Foot reset and finished.

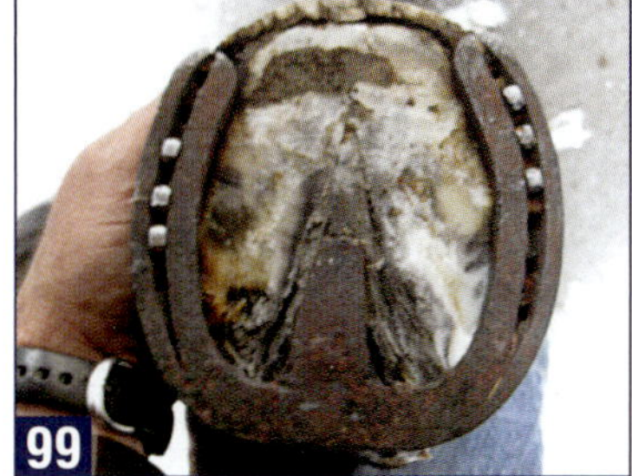

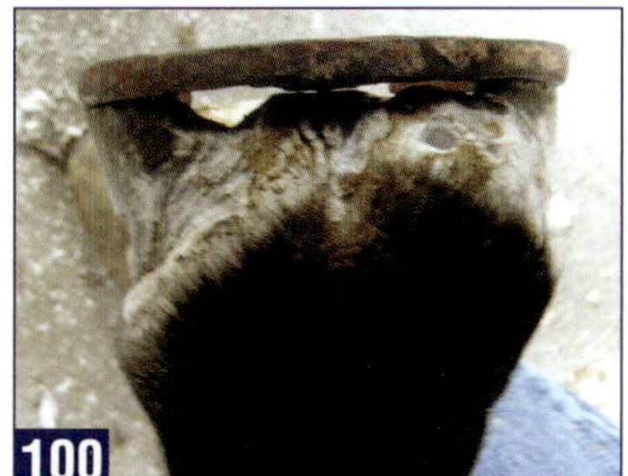

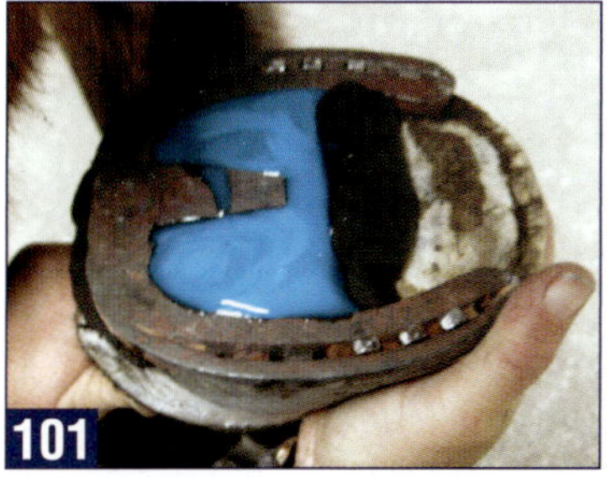

Pour-in pad.

102

Second return.

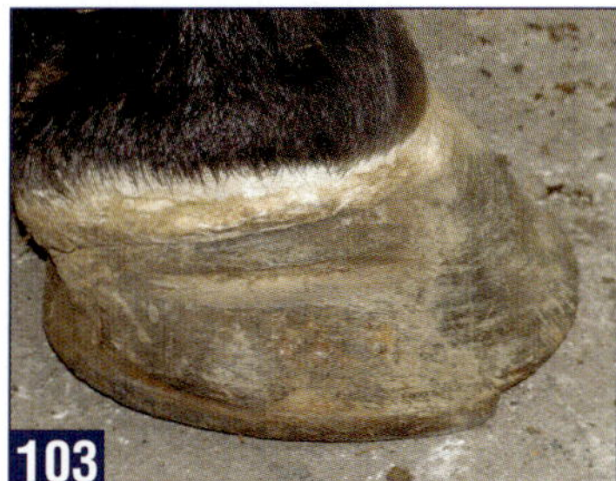

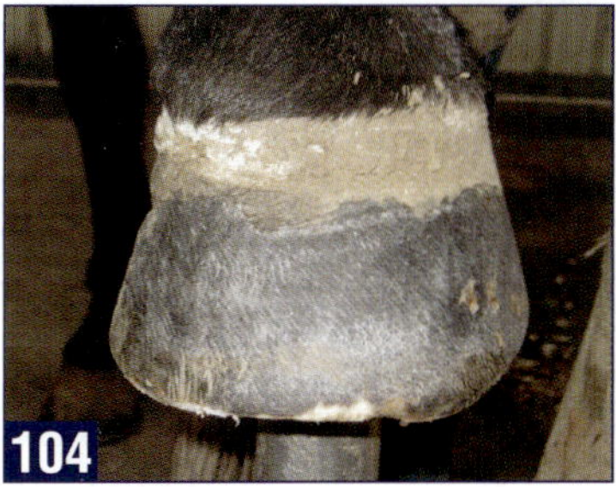

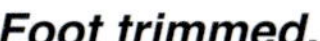

Foot trimmed.

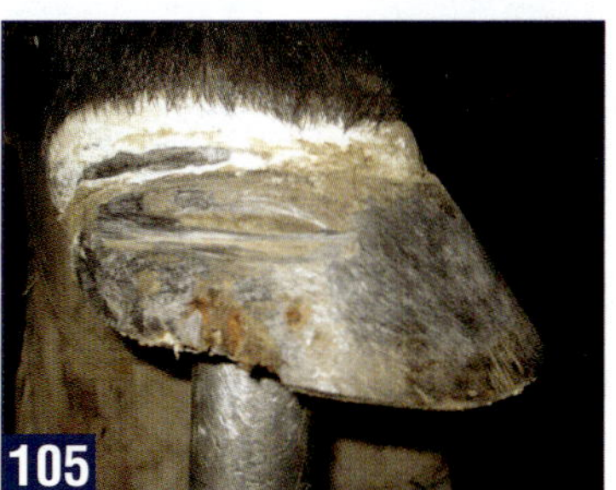

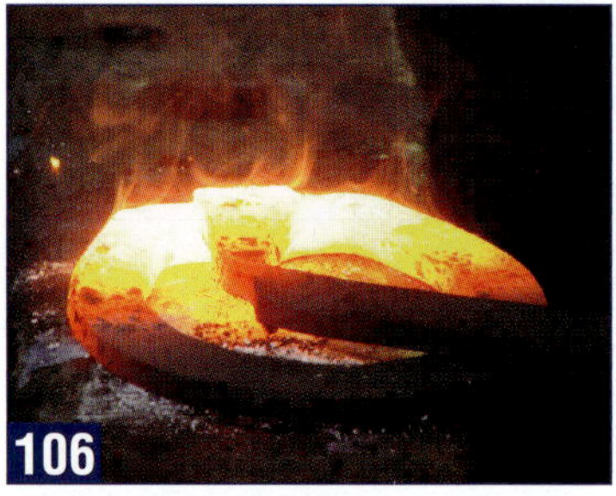

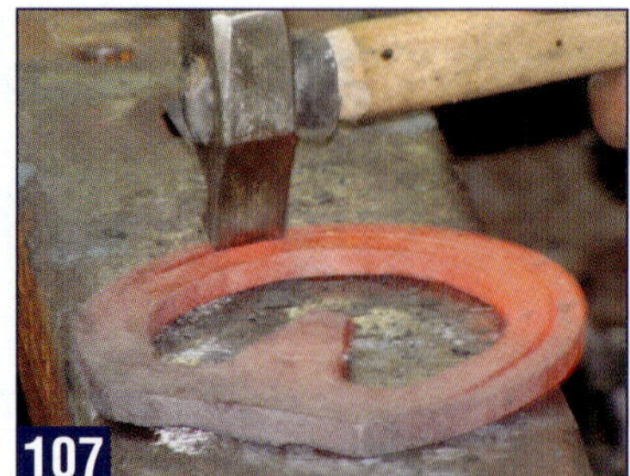

Making a heart bar.

108

Heart bar nailed on.

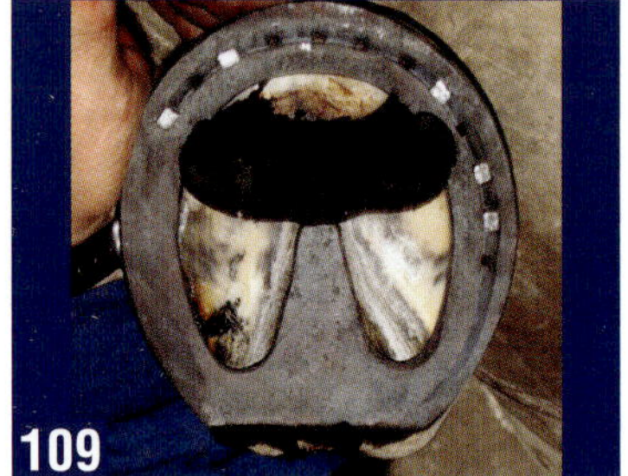

Sole Pack in the toe to make a dam.

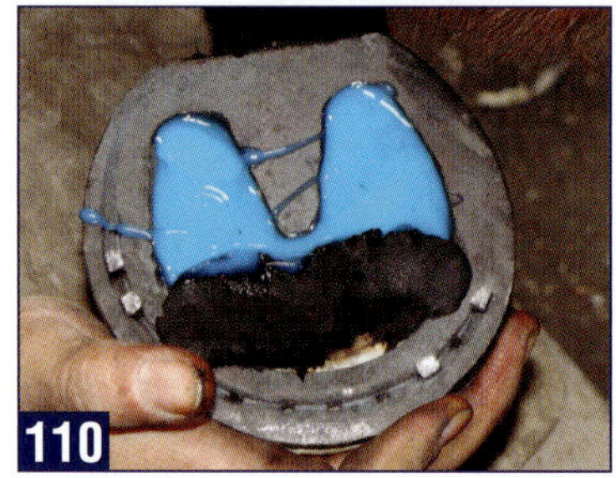

Pour-in pad.

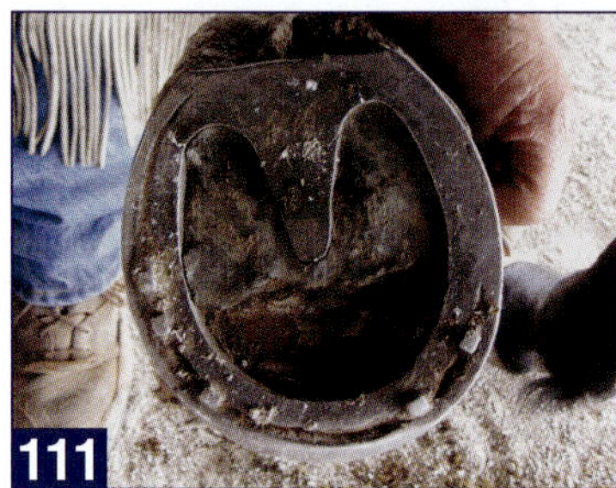

Third return.

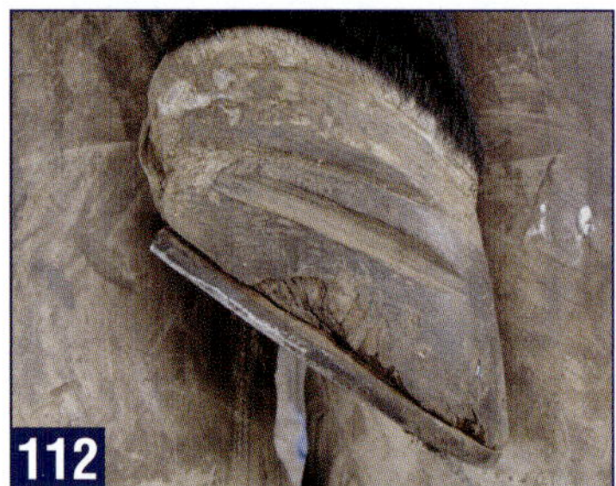

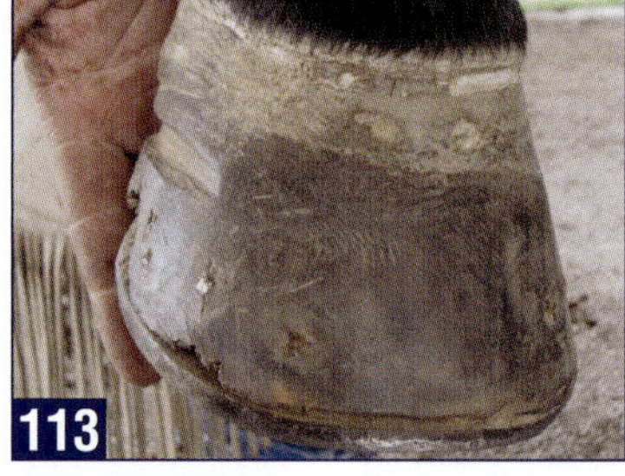

Major progress was made with the heart bar.

that it was time to put this horse into a heart bar **(Figures 106-108)**. Since the sole in front of the frog was still not growing that well, I did the Equi-Pak pour-in without getting into the soft area of the sole in front of the frog **(Figures 109-110)**.

The heart bar had a great impact on the foot. **Figures 111-113** show the foot when it returned. There was more growth than at any other time, and the ledge on the medial side was making good progress growing downward. I reset the heart bar **(Figures 114-116)**, and did a complete pour-in **(Figures 117-118)**. I also decided to do an additional groove at this time **(Figures 119-122)**. The horse was as sound as it had been in years, and the foot was improving with every visit.

As you deal with damaged, diseased, and injured feet in your career as a farrier, you can draw on some of the principles that are presented in this chapter to help you decide how to deal with those feet. I have had great success with a straightforward and traditional approach. I hope that you will decide to replace inventory with skill, and find the enjoyment from helping horses that I have. This is a fun way to spend a life.

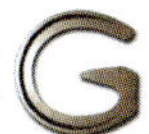

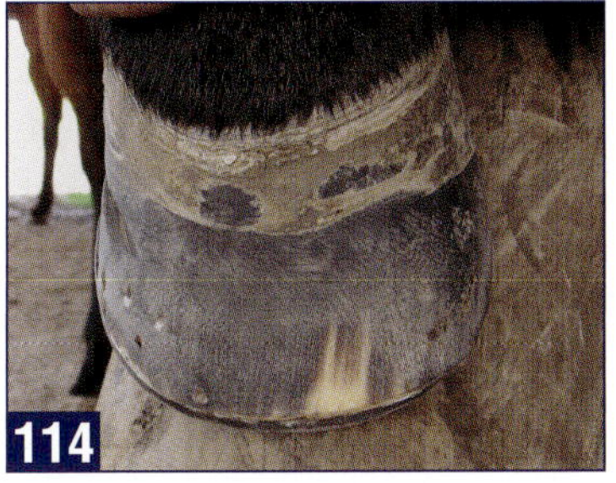

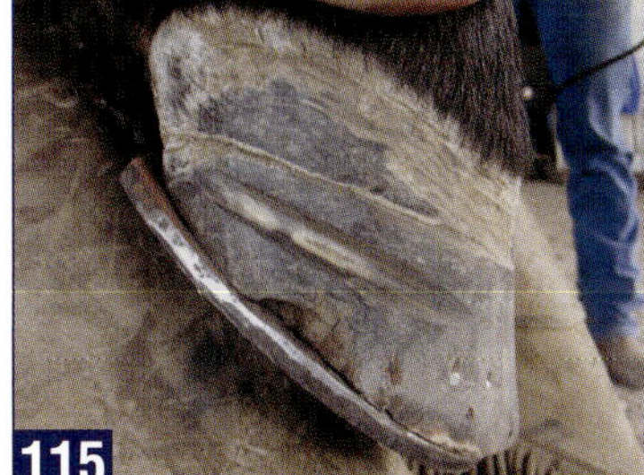

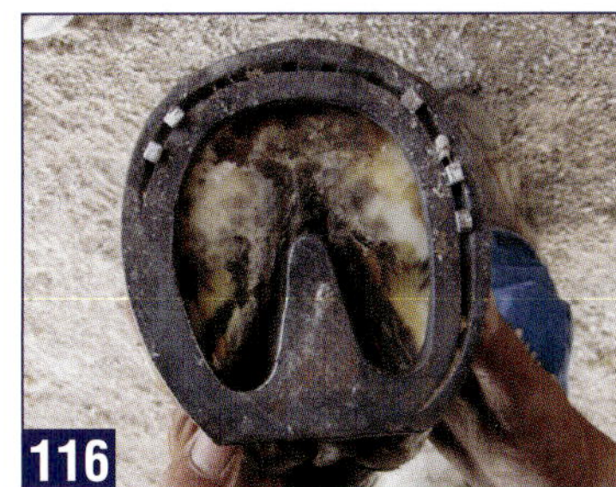

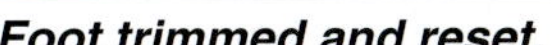
Foot trimmed and reset.

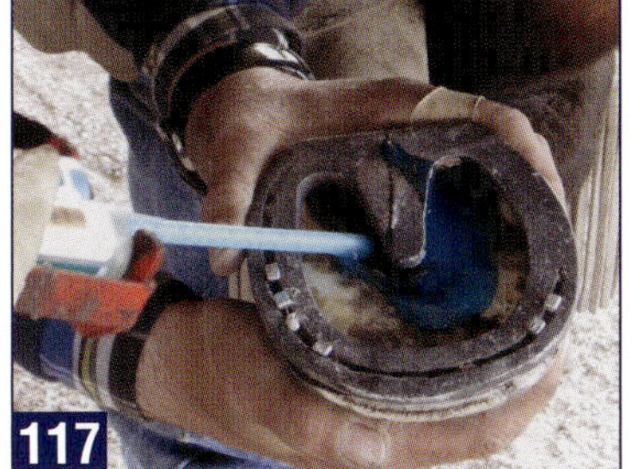

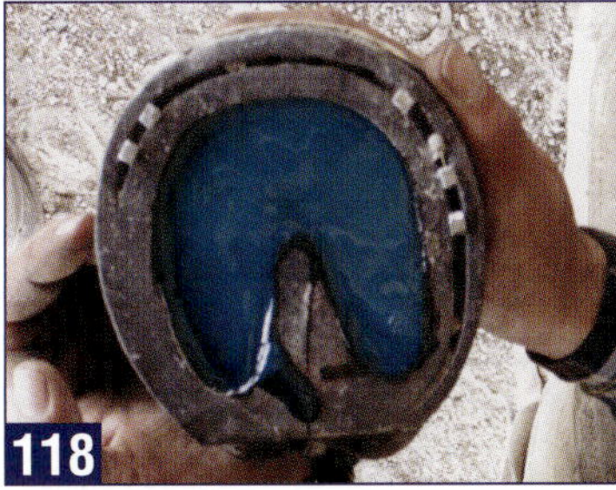

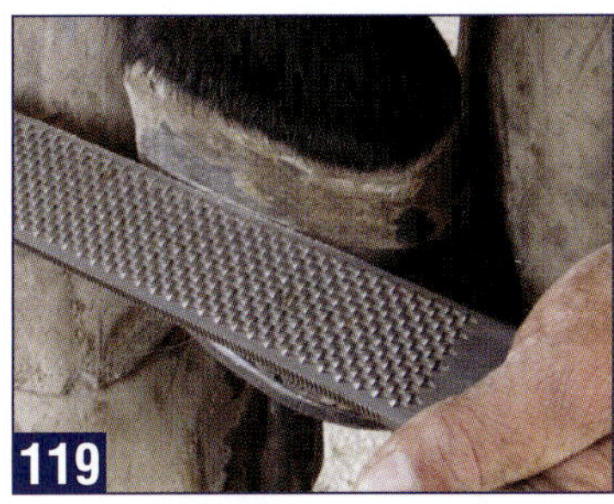

Doing a full pour-in pad this time.

Making a second groove.

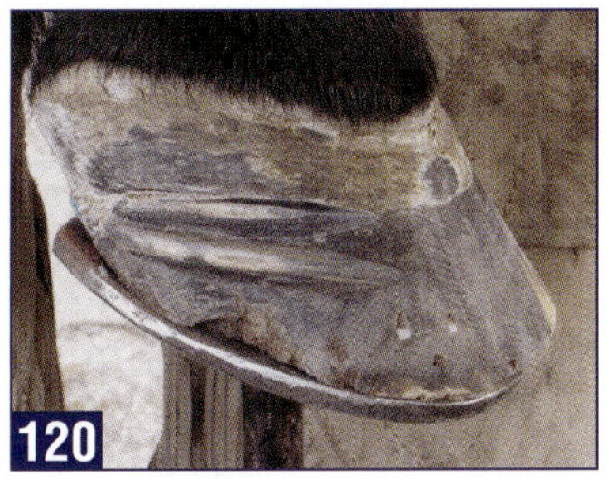

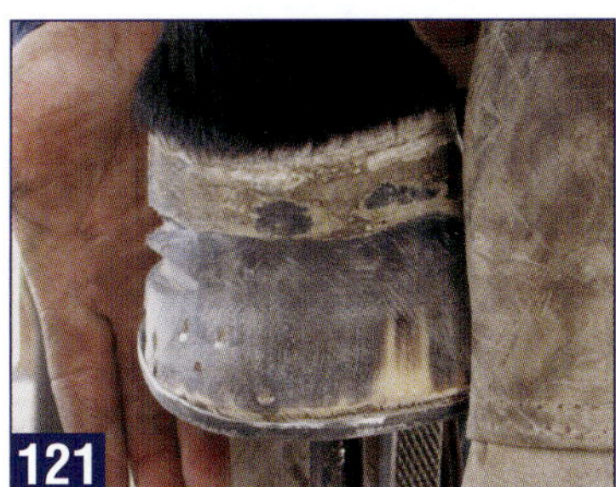

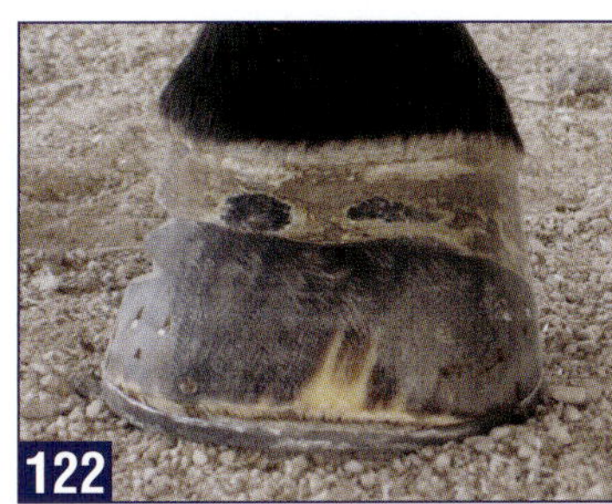

Foot finished.

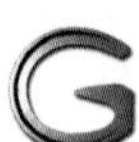

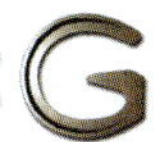

Section

13

Business

Chapter 57: General Thoughts On Farriery and Standards 646

Chapter 58: Starting Your Business 649

Chapter 59: Farrier Economics................................ 656

Chapter 60: Business Plan.................................... 662

" [7] Howbeit there was no reckoning made with them of the money that was delivered into their hand, because they dealt faithfully. "

—2 Kings 22:7

—King James Version

Chapter

57 GENERAL THOUGHTS ON FARRIERY AND STANDARDS

You obviously have some interest in this incredible trade or you would not be reading this book. I congratulate you on your choice of industries, and if it becomes to you half of what it has been to me, you are in for a great life. There are few jobs and no industries that I know of that will give back like this one. I hope you enjoy the ride.

Paul Harvey once quoted someone on his radio show who said, "Find something you love to do. Do that thing for a living. You will never work a day in your life." As I look back on my career, I feel that there were never truer words spoken. As with all jobs, there are the down sides: bad weather, bad horses, bad customers, and just plain old bad days. For me, however, those have been few and far between when compared with the good side. Sometimes the bad horses and the bad customers even became the game of the day and helped to break up the monotony.

Shoeing horses is a day of breaks. While you are working at the anvil, you have a break from the horse. When you are under the horse, you have a break from the anvil. You will sometimes look around you with a smile as you realize that someone is actually paying you for all the fun you are having. If my customers had any idea how much I was enjoying myself, they might have charged me!

Do not be fooled by this. Horseshoeing is not for everyone. It takes a special person to make it in this industry. You must be a self-starter to be self-employed. Making decisions in the short term that will make you prosperous in the long term takes discipline and foresight.

You must have a desire to help horses above all else. Shoeing for the money will end up leaving you without any joy in the job, while shoeing horses for the horse will make you crave it even more.

No matter how efficient and competent a farrier you become, you will never reach the summit of knowing it all. If you someday feel that you have reached that point, you'll know it is time to find something else to do.

I have known a lot of great farriers, and they all shared some common traits. Foremost among these was the fact that they never quit learning. I am amazed how often a horse, a student, my wife, my son, a clinician, or an article teaches me something new about this thing that has been my obsession for as long as I can remember.

Another thing shared by these greats was their love of the horse. There are those that become competent mechanics who don't like horses, but I don't know of any great farriers that don't like horses. If you do not like horses, you might think about looking elsewhere right now. You can't shoe horses for the money and remain happy. You have to shoe horses for the horse. Do that, and it will be a good trade for you. And if you do it for the horse, the money will follow.

SAFETY

You are going to be sore. You will get burned. Your hoof knife is going to cut the thumb on your off hand. New rasps will remove your skin easier than they will hoof. A horse will kick you. Someday one will bite you. You will be able to brag about the large number of broken toes you have suffered — or you will wear boots to protect them. All of this and more awaits you. If this is enough to make you turn away, then perhaps this is not the trade for you. However, if you are aware of this and more prior to starting, you won't be surprised the first time a horse paws you into next week.

Horses are bigger and stronger than we are.

However, they lack opposable thumbs. They also fall under the category of prey, while we are predators. That fact alone causes some problems for the horse, right at the beginning. Getting around untrained and mean horses is something of a wrestling match. There are moves you can learn to keep yourself safe, as well as moves a horse can and will do to try and prevent you from accomplishing your task. Handling some bad horses to learn safe areas and safe moves is a good idea, if you can arrange it.

The hind feet are much safer than the fronts. You can often win the battle of shoeing the hind feet on a bad horse. They are safer because the horse cannot see you as easily when you are working on the hind feet, and getting kicked is only kind of like being punched really hard. Couple that with the fact that the horse's reciprocal apparatus allows us to lock the joints in a flexed position so that we only have to battle the weaker extensor muscles, and you have a safer working area.

On the front feet, a horse can see you, bite you, and paw you. Pawing can be like someone jumping off a building and landing on you. It's much worse than being punched. The extensor muscles of the front limbs are quite strong, and there is no reciprocal apparatus to give us a mechanical advantage when we are in a fight.

This makes it difficult to do a good job.

There are several restraint methods that are common and useful. In this book, you will find a few that I have used and like, so I will limit this text to those. Like most things with shoeing horses, there is more than one approach to getting the job done. As long as the final result is a sound horse, a sound holder, a sound farrier, and a barn that does not look like a biker bar after a brawl, you can't argue with it too much.

A lot of potential farriers tell me that their back is keeping them from the trade. Do not worry. Once you start using your back, God will make it stronger and build you a back brace out of muscle. Once you start using your hands, God will make the skin thicker and stronger to make using your hands in tough situations easier. You just have to get through the initial painful part, and you are good to go.

QUALITY AND STANDARD

I have made the bulk of my living by teaching people to shoe horses for a living. My school has always been small, and the advertising budget was spent almost entirely on rodeo. My truck and trailer were a travelling billboard, and the majority of students that have passed through my shop have done so because other farriers guided them here. That has made my job easier, because I feel that I have had the cream of the crop when it comes to students.

My school was not designed for just anybody. It was based on the principle of having the highest standard of teaching, attracting the highest standard of students, and turning out graduates that were able to stand above the rest.

These are the principles that you need to apply to your own shoeing business. Each horse needs to be approached as if it were your own. Each shoe needs to be shaped and leveled as if it were going to be inspected at a contest. Your standard needs to be almost like religion to you. If you are too tired to do that next horse at a high standard, you are too tired to do that horse.

There will be times where you do as good a job as the horse will allow you to. When dealing with raucous and untrained animals, you will sometimes end up having to take what you can get. Those situations aren't the ones I'm referring to. I am talking about your everyday horse and your everyday standard. Make it high, strive to keep it high, and bring your shoeing to the next level with every horse.

When you do a good horse to a bad standard, you lower your standard. Consider it this way. Your standard will be an average of the work you normally do. When you do one horse at the bottom of the curve, it brings your standard down. Try to always be pushing that average up, not letting it come down.

RESPONSIBILITY

Put yourself in the horse's shoes for a minute. You are caught and taken out of your stall, pasture, arena, etc. A maybe good, maybe bad halter that has had the sweat, dirt, and manure from who-knows-where is placed over your nose and buckled onto your face.

Next, you are tied to something, somewhere. Hopefully it is safe, because you might not be. If it is your lucky day, a competent, caring, conscientious, skilled, able, experienced (should I go on?) person is on hand to work on your feet. Why does it matter? It matters because you are going to have to deal with what this person does to your feet. Trimmed flat? Hope so. Level? That would be nice.

Shoe fits? Another nice touch. Friendly and polite? Respects and admires your attributes as a horse that is a product of its environment? All of these become important if you put yourself in the horse's shoes.

Now, put your daughter (or son, mom, wife, dad, significant other), in the horse's shoes. What the incoming farrier is, or is not, has now really started to matter.

Now, I could take a little bit, so long as I was saving money, didn't hurt too bad, or whatever else was the case. But if you ask me to have my wife, Kelly, suffer? No way. Now I need the best that I can find.

For the horses that you are going to shoe, you need to be the best that can be found. You need to be the person who gets his or her name inserted every time someone mentions the best farrier in the area. Keep working hard and presenting the highest standard until your name comes up every time someone mentions the best farrier in the state. Then try for the United States; then the hemisphere. Eventually, you will have a group of customers that are certain, with no reservations, that you are the best farrier in the world — all because you take the responsibility of shoeing the horse seriously; because you know what you are doing every day matters. If not to the owner, then at least it matters to the horse.

All of this has to come from within. If you have it in you, it will show up on the feet. I hope you do. Most of my graduates have it in them. Going to my school is extremely hard for those who do not have it. This is important. Take it to heart and do what you have to do to become the best farrier that ever swung a hammer.

It is my hope that this book will help you reach your goals, and if that includes making life a little better for some horses, my goal has been achieved.

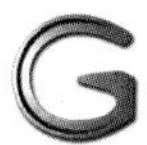

Chapter

58 STARTING YOUR BUSINESS

If you want good, clean, high-quality oats, you will have to pay a good and honest price for them. If you want oats that have already been through the horse, those come cheaper, and you will have to get them somewhere else.

Everyone wants a high-quality product that is done cheaply and fast. The customer can pick two of those: If it is cheap and fast, it won't be high quality. If it is fast and high quality, it won't be cheap, and if it is high quality and cheap, it won't be fast. You can decide which two you are going to provide.

There are a few basic rules in running any self-employed business venture. Foremost among these is: treat your customers the way you would like to be treated if you were them, and they were you.

A lot of the farriers that I have known entered this trade because they were frustrated customers. Unable to get a horseshoer, or worse, getting an incompetent horseshoer, has lead a lot of people to this industry. If you are a farrier that was once a customer, you realize just what it takes to make a horseshoeing customer happy. Doing that which makes a customer satisfied will make your customers happy, which will lead to your prosperity.

Shoeing horses takes many skills in a lot of different areas. Due to demand, being a good mechanical farrier may not be the most important requirement for having a successful business. (I hate saying this, but it is a fact I have seen around the world.) I have known several farriers with average abilities who had businesses that were well above average in volume and profit. By and large, these individuals were exceptional businessmen. They offered timely service, listened to their customers, were prompt, called when they were running behind, scheduled around their customers' needs and ultimately were better at running a business than doing the actual hoof-care work.

On the other hand, I have also known some farriers with superior shoeing skills whose businesses were barely surviving, or they had to find other employment altogether. Some of these people simply lacked some of those skills that a successful entrepreneur in a service industry needs, even though they are unrelated to horseshoeing.

That being said, the most important things you can do is to become proficient and competent. Do that and then add some people and business skills, and you will have the world at your fingertips.

I once had a student that came to my Farrier Blacksmith Course in February, took the six-month Journeyman Farrier Course from March to August, and became an AFA Certified Journeyman Farrier by the end of September. He was as talented a farrier as you could ever find. I would show this person how to build a shoe, and he would make one better than the demo on his first try. I would correct a portion of his trimming, and I would never have to do it again because he would not make the same mistake twice. However, he was probably here for three months before he said 20 words altogether to me. He never made eye contact, regardless of the situation. He shook hands without a grip and with his head lowered.

As a result of these personality traits, this young, gifted farrier was unable to keep a shoeing business going. His customers didn't really like or dislike him — rather they felt pretty neutral about him. He did not call or follow up with customers about problems with their horses. He failed to push scheduling or products, or even visit with his customers about their needs. As a result, he soon found that he did not have repeat business, despite a higher level of competence than the majority of people who are shoeing for a living.

In contrast, I had a student when I ran the school in Colorado who was as charismatic as they come. You wanted to spend time with this kid because he made you feel good about yourself. There was something about the way he shook your hand and looked you in the eye that made you want to make him happy. I would not have let him shoe a horse I borrowed from my mother-in-law — but I would have enjoyed his company while the horse was being shod.

During the last week of a 20-week course, this young man made $1,600. This was in the early 1990s, and $1,600 for a beginning farrier was quite a substantial sum. He built a big, profitable practice that was based on his personality, not his mechanical skills - those were barely adequate. But he was a natural businessman that made people believe in him.

I once had a customer call to schedule us to shoe one of several horses the family owned. They only wanted us to work on one, because it was the one that was the lamest. A few of the others were also lame, but this one was extremely so. When we went to their farm, the lady explained that the horses were always lame for at least a week after being shod. They would always have a couple more shod than they wanted to make up for the lameness downtime and to improve the odds of having at least a couple of sound horses at a time.

The shoeing was horrible — and that's sugar-coating the description. None of the shoes were shaped properly. They were nailed on twisted and off-center. The fact that there was not more lameness was actually a big surprise in light of the shoeing.

It is not appropriate to bad-mouth another farrier for any reason, so we did our best to keep from it. We said things like: "Well, that is not exactly how we would have done it," or "There is no way to tell what the guy had to start with." (These are good statements to store in your memory for when you come across equally awful shoeing and can't think of anything nice, but have to say something.)

We pulled the shoe off the front foot of the crippled horse and dealt with the obvious abscess. While working, I asked the lady about her farrier. She said, "He is a pretty terrible horseshoer, but he is one of the nicest guys you could ever want to meet." When she said that, a light went on that shone on some of the intricacies of this industry. Basically this man had a good profitable business because he was "one of the nicest guys you would ever want to meet."

Keep that in mind as you run your business.

STARTING OUT

The average beginning farrier does not walk into a six-figure business when they first get out of horseshoeing school. For most, the first year is tough, very tough; the kind of year you call your cell phone from another phone, just to make sure it is still working.

Don't let it bother you. It is part of paying your dues. Most of us have been down this road and some of the best learning of your career can happen during this time if you allow it to.

You have a lot more time in this first year than you will ever have again. Use it wisely. Hone your forging skills by building your shoe inventory for the time when you are going to be busy. Study your textbooks. Do some reading about the business of starting and running a business. This can be a good year.

Historically, most beginners will double their income in the second year, then double that amount again in the third. By the fourth year, most of the beginners that I have trained have been able to make whatever they wanted, so long as they have stayed in the same area.

Keeping that in mind can help you get through that first lean year. It can also provide you with benchmarks to check your progress in those first years.

To build your business initially, here are a few things that I have seen work for a lot of beginners.

First, have some nice business cards and fliers made. Your business card is your travelling bill-board. Even though the first year is a hard time to spend money on something like a business card, it is important that you don't skimp. I also suggest that you put a line on your business card that reads "Next Appointment." This gives you a reason to schedule, which allows you to control your income a little better. It also gives you a reason to hand the customer another of your travelling billboards every time you shoe their horse. Pretty soon, they have a few of these in their wallet, and when someone asks about shoeing, that little billboard can go to work.

When you are done with a horse, get your

appointment book out and suggest to the owner when you think this horse should be worked on again. In the Midwest, we don't mind going 8 weeks in the dead of winter, but insist on 6 weeks from March through September. There are horses that are able to go longer and some that need to go less, but you will quickly identify these and can adjust the schedule appropriately.

Before you leave customers, shake hands, thank them for the work, and hand them a couple extra cards. Tell them you are trying to build a business and their help would be appreciated. That little act can do a lot for getting you more work. By stating the obvious, "I am building a business," you are planting the seed that you hope will grow into a forest.

Put your fliers up in every feed store, farm store, vet clinic, sale barn, tack shop, gas station, western store, and anywhere else you think a horse person might see it. Having your name seen over and over is a good thing. Pretty soon, the local horsemen and horsewomen are associating your name with horseshoeing. It is then a very small step for them to think of you every time the subject of horseshoes or horseshoers comes up.

The next suggestion for the young farrier is to get into every horseshoer's truck that will have you. Donate a day to other shoers; more if you find one that is easy to get along with as well as competent.

Remember when you go with someone else that there are some unwritten laws and ethics in the world of farriery that you must be aware of. First and foremost, you cannot take a customer that you meet as a result of riding with another guy.

Consider this scenario. You get out of school and call John the farrier to see if you can ride with him. He accepts, you meet one morning, and head to the barn. When you get there, low and behold, the customer is from the same state where you used to live. You find out that you know a lot of the same people. He once dated your cousin. You and his brother played football together.

That guy is probably going to be calling you the next time that horse needs to be shod. You have a responsibility to handle this correctly. Not doing so can cause complications in the local farrier community that you may come to regret for years to come.

Your first duty is to John the farrier. When the customer calls, you need to let him know that you cannot shoe his horses without John being there. This makes for a delicate situation, but I recommend honesty. Tell the customer that in this magnificent trade, there is a code of honor that does not allow you to do those horses.

Next, you need to call John and tell him that his customer called you. There is a good chance that John will suggest that you take the customer anyway, but you must not assume that. John can do what he wants here. He may fire the customer, he may give the customer to you, or he may continue to shoe for the customer. It doesn't matter. What does matter is that you did the right thing.

There is always the possibility that you meet the customer through means that don't involve John. In that case there is no problem with doing the horses. You have to get horses from somewhere, and if you are getting horses to shoe, some farrier in the area is losing those horses. Just remember: any horse owner you meet as a direct result of spending the day with John cannot be your customer unless John is okay with it.

Break this unwritten rule and the local farrier community will not accept you. When this happens, the community gets just a little bit more cutthroat, and individual farriers get a little bit more isolated from each other instead of banding together.

In a tight-knit community, farriers help each other, tacking on lost shoes, covering an injured farrier's shoeing book, and taking care of each other's businesses so that at least someone can get a vacation. You want to be on the inside of this, not the outside. Think of this in the same way as I suggested you do about customer-relations issues. Put yourself in John's shoes and you will know what to do.

You will gain several things from riding with other shoers. First, you will make new friends who share the same interest that you do. Next, most established farriers have all that they can do and more, so when they are looking for a place to send customers, the first person they will think of will often be the last one who helped them. Finally, you get to see up close and personal how other horseshoers shoe their horses and deal with their businesses.

When you go to help, don't expect to get paid. If you are lucky, you will get lunch (although I do advise packing one if you are in the habit of eating one). If you happen to get paid, that is a tremendous bonus. Unlike some trades, in farriery, the occasional day help is often more hindrance than help. If you prove your worth and capability, you may get offered a more regular position and a paycheck, but don't go with expectations.

The next suggestion is to find local horse groups that are willing to let you do a clinic. Bear in mind that horseshoeing as a spectator sport is primarily enjoyable only to other farriers. Most horse owners will not appreciate a two-hour lecture followed by a three-hour shoeing job. With that in mind, I would suggest that you do one foot or perhaps half of a horse. Bring a cooler full of soda pop and water, be on your best behavior, and make a professional impression on the local horsemen and horsewomen.

When you do these clinics, be very particular about the horse you get. If they bring you an outlaw, you may end up doing a horse-fighting clinic instead of a horseshoeing one. If you are great with bad horses, then this may be a perfect example to show off that skill, but there is always a strong chance of a disaster with a bad horse.

Since these clinics are done locally, I often take my own horse. There are some really good reasons for this. You will know the horse as well as the feet. This gives you an advantage in shaping and fitting the shoe in the first attempt. Besides, once you are a farrier, your horse will always need trimming and shoeing.

I have done clinics for saddle clubs, FFA classes, 4-H clubs, historical societies, home school groups, rodeo clubs, and at county fairs. You never know where someone who just happens to be tapped into the local horse community will see you. Get them on your side, and the business might just take off faster than you can imagine.

Another good way to get some advertising is by doing a shoeing day with a local farm store or veterinarian clinic. Go to a feed store and ask the owner if he would like to sell more horse feed. You know the answer before you ask, but it will plant the right seed in his mind, and get him to say "yes." (That's a sales trick all on its own.) Once he's answered yes, suggest that he host a horse-appreciation day. This includes having you there to shoe at a slight discount while the store offers discounts on feed, tack, wormer, or whatever.

The plan could include a local veterinarian being on hand for Coggins papers, shots, or even worming. You could invite an equine chiropractor or even a horse masseuse. The idea is to give a horse owner a reason to come to the feed store on that weekend.

One thing to insist on is that your name appears in all ads for the event. I've often seen my name put on the sign out front for a couple weeks ahead of time.

This gives you a lot of advertising for the effort, and again, people will associate your name with horseshoeing.

There are a couple things to consider when you use this tactic. First, make sure that the business you are going in with is reputable. Doing this with an incompetent vet or at a feed store that most horse owners don't like or use can hurt you more than help. You want your business to benefit by being associated with another good business — not have your reputation sullied.

Next, make sure that the horses coming in are scheduled, so having too many show up doesn't snow you under. That can make you look bad. A couple of options are to have a contact number so that you can schedule appointments throughout the day. Once you hit the number you want, you can extend the discount offer for another time. The other option — which is more fun — is to have several farrier friends come to visit on that weekend. If tons of horses show up, you have it covered. If none do, you can visit and have a forge day.

For those of you in a shoeing school, this could be a class reunion. You could have these little get-togethers amongst friends all around the country.

We have done these shoeing days on numerous occasions. Some have been hits and some haven't. One cold Saturday a few years ago, we only had seven students stay behind for the shoeing day and they were only three weeks in to the course. We had over 30 horses signed up when we got there, and a line of trailers out the driveway. Needless to say, Kelly, Cody and I shod a lot of horses that day.

When I started shoeing horses, it was a common thing to see a horse at a farm, and drive on in. While I was in college, Kelly and I would set out after she was done with track practice, and I was done with rodeo practice, and hit the local back roads to find horses. Some nights I would get two or three to trim, sometimes two or three to shoe, sometimes I'd get skunked. Sometimes there would be a week's worth of work lined up. It was a great time for us. I was getting $23 to shoe a horse with new shoes, $18 for resets and $12 a trim. My rent was only $125 per month, so it was not as bad as it sounds. I could make half the rent in a couple hours, so we thought we were cutting a fat hog.

Compared to my fellow college students in 1987, we were wealthy. In fact, we graduated from college in 1991 with $12,000 in the bank and no debt.

That year of starting a shoeing practice was irreplaceable. I made a lot of mistakes, but since we moved, I didn't have to live with those mistakes.

Like a lot of young rodeo cowboys that start shoeing without any real guidance, I made a lot of mistakes I wish I hadn't on feet. But my biggest mistakes were business ones. By reading about these mistakes, I hope that you are able to avoid them.

First, don't get in the habit of letting customers negotiate the price with you based on volume. This is not the sort of job in which you are trying to build huge volume. You want to do a few horses for a lot of money, not a lot of horses for a little bit of money. As Wayne Allen, CJF, of Georgia is fond of saying, "They's only so many bend-over and getups in ya." He is right.

You may feel like you are doing a great thing for a customer by shoeing for less, but you are only hurting yourself as well as the local farrier community. It is not part of our job as farriers to make horses affordable.

A case in point: I knew a shoer that literally did 60 horses a week for over 20 years. He began in 1976 for around $20 per horse. When I met this individual he was making $30 a horse in 1992. I was talking to him about raising his rates, and he explained that he just couldn't do that to his customers. He would lose his business and make all these people mad.

I did not see him again until 1997. I was in a McDonald's and I recognized the guy emptying the trash. We visited for a couple of minutes and he asked me if I would buy his anvil for $50 because he could no longer physically shoe horses and was in the process of selling his house and moving to a trailer park.

I've never forgotten this, and thinking about it scares me to death. If he had set some standards for his customers to meet, he might have had something to fall back on. Don't be this guy!

When you accept lesser payments for shoeing based on the fact that the individual had 10 horses, you have taken the time out of your schedule for 10 horses. Those 10 horses will be shod for less money in the same time you could have shod 10 other horses at regular price. In the very beginning, you might go ahead and shoe these horses because you didn't have anything to do at that time anyway. But, I would explain to the customer that it was a one-time thing so that they could have a sample of your outstanding craftsmanship.

The next thing is to establish very early in the relationship with your customers how things are going to be handled. (That goes for getting married as well.) If a customer calls at 3 p.m. on Friday, and you go out and shoe that horse that night in the glow of your headlights, there will not be any incentive for that customer to call early to schedule next time. This can be handled by adding an emergency charge. When you agree to shoe that horse that night by headlights, you can let them know that there is an additional 25% added to the bill. You'll either earn more for the night or they'll decide that the horse can wait until you can get it in your schedule.

I have had customers who would not send a check until the horses were due again. Every time the check arrived in the mail, Kelly would say, "Gail's about to call." That is a bad thing to let get established, but it is even worse to shoe a horse when you're still owed for the last shoeing. Do that and you can really get burned. One of the problems with shoeing is that the value of the service is lost as time goes on. The horse needs to be reshod because the old shoeing has run its course. This makes it hard to get paid for old work.

Think about how you're going to deal with lost shoes before they come up. Lost shoes are a fact of life for a farrier. The wonder is that we don't have more lost shoes. When you consider that a metal shoe is nailed between a massive animal and the hard ground, the animal wears that shoe all the time, and only a few rectangular nails hold it in place, lost shoes are no surprise.

Many customers will judge the quality of your shoeing based solely on whether a shoe stays on or not. This is not an appropriate criterion to base the ability of a shoer on, but you will find that it is a common one. Some shoers end up shoeing improperly to prevent lost shoes. The long-term problems that can occur for the horse are not worth the short-term benefits of keeping the shoe on.

When a horse I have shod loses a shoe, I generally replace it for free, even when the horse or owner is at fault. The little that I could charge to compensate me for replacing a lost shoe is not enough to make up for a lost customer who gets cross about having to pay for it. Each case is individual, so you can decide this for yourself. Just have a policy in place before it comes up so that you don't have to make a permanent policy in haste.

If I were to map out the ideal way for a new farrier to go about building a good trade, it would be as follows.

Find somewhere with a large horse population where you do not wish to live for the rest of your career. Move there for at least two years and start a shoeing business while you concentrate on attaining your AFA Certified Journeyman status. This would also be an excellent time to attend a few college classes.

Shoe horses in this area as well as humanly possible and put everything you can into building your skills. Once you achieve the CJF, you can move to the area where you wish to live the rest of your career. The mistakes you make early on will haunt you if you stay in the first area (and you will make mistakes), but moving will give you a fresh start. You will be moving into the area as an already proven expert by having CJF behind your name. People remember the bad much longer than the good, so it is nice to come into the new area with a clean slate and a high degree of competence.

When you arrive in your new home, advertise like you don't need the work. The ad can say something like:

Cody Gregory, American Farriers Association
Certified Journeyman Farrier.
Experienced shoer, handling all
types of shoeing. Handmades a specialty.
Accepting limited number of appointments.
Call 417-262-3060.

This reads a lot more like someone who knows how to shoe than the ads you normally see; such as;

Hot, Cold, Corrective.
Have anvil, will travel.
Please call so I don't starve.

This leads to a discussion about print ads in local shoppers and newspapers. When you begin shoeing in an area, you need to let the local horse owners know that you are here and available. One method is to use print ads. The customers who find farriers from print ads know that you paid for that ad, and they also know that you need business or you would not have an ad in the paper.

Since there is such a demand for competent farriers, most of the good ones get so busy that they don't ever advertise, don't have business cards, nothing on their truck indicates what they do, and many don't take new customers. The downside is, you have to get through the first few years to get to that point.

I recommend putting a tasteful ad in the papers that indicates you are available, but do not let it sound desperate. Run the same ad for no more than three months, then pull it, regardless of how many horses you have to shoe. If you don't have enough business yet, try an alternative way of advertising.

Get a product or other service that you can advertise. A lot of my graduates sell Farriers' Formula. The new ad will read something like:

Farriers' Formula available
from Cody Gregory's Farrier Service.
Available in regular or double strength.
Call Cody Gregory's Farrier Service
at 417-262-3060.

That is a great way to get the word out that Cody Gregory is a farrier, yet it doesn't seem like Cody needs any horses. You want the customer to feel like you are doing them a favor by showing up to shoe their horses, not the other way around. When you are new and desperate, the customer may pick up on that and take advantage of you.

CUSTOMER APPRECIATION

Horses are great to work for, but the owner is the one who pays the bill. Realizing that early in your career is important.

Once you have been going for a few years you will find that the demand for farriers far outstrips the availability in most of the world. This means that most of us can have far more work than we can deal with. At the end of a long day, the last thing most busy farriers want to do is deal with 20 messages. Even if each message only takes three minutes (Please, take only three minutes!) then you have an

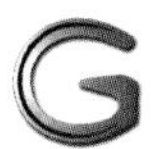

additional hour of phone time to add to the end of a long day of shoeing.

The temptation is great to ignore those messages and disregard the needs of those customers. Once you do that the first time, it gets a little easier the next. And again the next, until finally, blowing off customers is more the norm than not.

Now imagine that you are shoeing 10% more horses than you want to. This means you are working 10% harder than you intended to, dealing with 10% more horses, 10% more customers, and 10% more needs.

You decide that you can become a little arrogant and disrespectful (not consciously, it just happens). After all, you are also making 10% more money than you expected. You come home to a list of messages from 2% of your customers at the end of a long Monday. You decide to disregard them. Tuesday, another 2% of your customers call, as well as half the ones from Monday. You disregard them again. After all, you are a shoeing god. Your long list of horses and customers confirms this.

This disregarding of calls goes on for some time; let's say for 20 days in a month. You have now ignored 40% of your business. Even your most loyal customers will take this for only so long. You are getting more difficult to deal with and be around because of the stress of all these customers. Pretty soon you are doing 25% less horses than you wanted as well as 25% less of everything, including money.

If you think you were stressed earlier when you had too much to take care of, try having not enough.

This has happened to quite a few farriers I have known over the years. Simply running your business in a way that would make you want to be your own customer will help you avoid this potential pitfall.

All in all, this is an incredible trade that you are associated with. The way it makes me feel to help a horse is hard to replace with anything else I have ever done. Learn a high standard and work to it everyday. Treat fellow farriers, horse owners, and horses well, yet demand the respect and pay to which you are entitled. Make this business about the horse first, and get up every morning happy to be a farrier. If you enjoy it half as much as I have, you are in for a blessed life.

Chapter 59 FARRIER ECONOMICS

When you shoe horses full-time for a living, there is a lot more you need to be aware of than just the mechanical act of shoeing. Doing a good job for the equine customer is important, but to survive as a businessman, you must have a grasp of the economic side of this business.

A lot of people who don't shoe horses think that farriers are making an easy living. For the most part, farriers are very well paid for the time invested, but there is more to it than meets the eye. Those folks don't see the thousands that try every year but don't make it to become a full-time shoer. They don't see the difficulty in learning how to shoe horses at a high standard, and they also do not understand the economic reality of shoeing horses.

To be fair, there are several businesses that look better from the outside than they do once you know where all the corners are. Running a horseshoeing school is a great example. Until I actually ran my own school, I had no idea what kind of overhead went into it.

I knew a guy that washed cars at dealerships for a living. He had all his equipment on a trailer, made washing the cars look simple, and pretty much looked like he was printing money. We got to visiting one day, and there was more to it than I ever imagined. There was dealing with car dealers to start with, and that cost him some profit. Those guys are natural negotiators that are good at getting the deal they want. Then there was the cost of fuel for the power washer, insurance for working on new cars, insurance for working at dealerships, taxes for washing cars in other states, cost of soap, extra clothes, brass nozzles and new hoses for the washer, on and on and on. Here I thought all he did was show up, wave a wash-wand around for a couple of hours, and take his sack of money to the bank.

TAXES AND INSURANCE

These two items are some of the costs of doing business that will drive you over the edge. Even so, you cannot become a successful businessman without considering and understanding a few things about insurance and taxes.

In the United States today, there is a litigious atmosphere. You will be working on some valuable horses, and if something goes wrong, you can find yourself in a huge fight. And it's not only if something goes bad. You don't have to be wrong to be sued. There are many examples of people or companies who lost a legal battle that should have never happened. Refer to McDonalds and the temperature of their coffee.

Anyhow, you need to be aware of the fact that you live in a time where differences are more likely to be settled in court than behind the barn. If you decide to have or reject insurance coverage, you should only do so after careful deliberation and much discussion. I will not tell you what you should do, but I will let you know that I have never had liability coverage. Remember, I was lucky enough to start this career in the 1980s, and liability coverage for farriers in those days was pretty rare. I will also tell you that if I ever had a situation where I felt even remotely uncomfortable with a customer or circumstance, I would load my rig and get out of there. The quickest way to get rid of me as your farrier is to tell me about how you sued the last farrier or vet, or anyone for that matter.

One of my best friends is an orthopedic surgeon who paid his way through medical school as a farrier. This man is the ultimate overachiever. He has been shoeing since 1969, has an MBA, MD, CJF, and is one of only 35 currently living Fellows of the Worshipful Company of Farriers. His name is Mike Miller, and if you are really interested in liability insurance, I suggest that you look him up. As a medical doctor, he has a lot more information and experience with liability insurance than I ever hope to.

Now, on to taxes. My dad, Mike Gregory, is an incredibly brilliant man. When I was a kid, he was a lawyer who owned a ranch. Nowadays, he is a rancher who has to go to his law office every once in a while. He understands taxes extremely well, and has given me advice throughout my career. One of the earliest pieces was, "The small businessman who does not consider taxes at the beginning of his venture, is the one that fails the fastest."

So often, we get caught up in the doing the physical part of our job, and all the other little things of running a business, that we don't take the tax part into account. I think this is in large part because taxes are harder to understand than anatomy, and we assume that they will take care of themselves.

Every state has different laws that govern taxes on services rendered and products sold. You need to spend the money to get a good CPA who understands the intricacies of what you are doing for a living. A good CPA will save you more than they cost every year. Discuss becoming incorporated, the value of hiring people, home offices, leasing vs. buying your truck, etc. Once you become self-employed, your tax situation becomes increasingly complicated. There are more words in the US Tax Code than there are in the King James Bible. I don't have specific advice on taxes because what I print today is apt to change tomorrow, just make sure that you don't forget they are a part of having a business in the United States.

Kelly used to do our taxes when we lived in Colorado and she was home with the kids instead of shoeing with me. When she had a question, she would call the IRS until she got the same answer at least twice. This might mean only two calls on a good day, but there were times when it would take four. This means we have a tax system where the people who are in charge of implementing it don't even know how it is supposed to be done. Hire a good CPA. Scratch that. Hire a GREAT CPA.

INITIAL FARRIER BUSINESS BUDGET

There are a few things that you are going to have to have to shoe horses for a living. Like all small businesses, there are start-up costs that cannot be avoided. Sacrificing some aspect, or even doing without a tool that is not absolutely necessary, can diminish some of these, but there are some tools that you just have to have.

As this book is being written in 2010, the average cost for the recommended tool list that I send my students is going to come to about $1,700 for the Advanced and Journeyman Farrier students. The students in my long classes have a few additional tools in the way of tongs, punches, pritchels, and more rasps than the shorter course students.

Add an anvil at $600, an anvil stand at $500, and a forge at $500. We have just made it over $3,000, and that is only part of the budget. As we continue from here, you will learn how to apply some basic business principles. Understand that you have to spend a little money so that you can make some money. Kelly struggles with that one. She is so tight that when she opens her purse, George Washington squints. However, having a frugal wife has absolutely kept me out of the poor house.

These initial costs are quite insignificant when you compare starting a shoeing business to almost any other start-up business that I know of (at least to have the earning potential that you will have with these small costs). In farriery, the majority of your income is based on your skills, not the actual physical product itself.

Shoeing horses is much more than the cost of four shoes and a handful of nails. Although these are the costs that your customer sees and understands, it is not the end of the story by a long way.

Part-time shoers can shoe horses without seeing this. There are some who have a regular job, but shoe a couple horses for a little money every night. These part-time farriers don't understand what they have to charge for shoeing a horse because they have not broken down exactly what they are making in the way of profit. Many of them get paid in cash, so they consider the money they make shoeing as extra income, and it does not really get put into the financial equation for that family at the end of the month. With all this cash, these shoers feel flush with money in their pockets.

A lot of them buy their supplies with their checkbook, not the money they made shoeing. This gives them a false sense of what they are making from the shoeing. Now, don't get me wrong, there is perhaps no better part-time job in the world than shoeing. But if you are going to be a part-timer, you need to understand the business side of what you are doing as well.

I give my students a handout that breaks down what it costs to shoe horses during their first year. When you fill it out, the results may surprise you. It is included here *(next page)*, and everyone will have to fill it in to fit his or her individual situation.

I know that how this is written is ignoring the fact that things can be paid for in payments and you can also depreciate a lot of items. For now, let

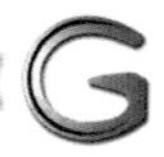

Heartland Horseshoeing School

Truck ______________________

Fuel ______________________

Maintenance______________________

Insurance ______________________

Education:

Tuition ______________________

Cont. Ed. ______________________

Library______________________

Associations______________________

Equipment:

Initial Tools ______________________

Anvil ______________________

Forge ______________________

Supplies:

Nails______________________

Shoes ______________________

Rasps/tools______________________

Misc. ______________________

Business Expenses:

Accounting______________________

Printing ______________________

Phone______________________

Signage ______________________

Personal:

Health ins. ______________________

Retirement ______________________

Entertaining ______________________

Advertising:

Free horses______________________

Print adds______________________

Donations______________________

us just consider this as the first year of expenses for becoming a farrier. Having this hypothetical situation gives us a foundation to start talking about farrier economics. (Imagine if there were no such thing as a hypothetical situation.)

Most people are surprised when they fill this form out that the figures come to between $25,000 and $40,000. I know that it can be substantially increased or diminished based on several items — truck expenses especially. However, let us use the figure of $26,000 for the purpose of this discussion.

Contemplate this fact. If your expense sheet came out to $26,000, this means you have to make $500 per week with no weeks off just so that you can make these first year expenses. Pretty sobering if you think about it that way. You have to shoe $26,000 worth of horses just to make your expenses. Wow! How can that be possible?

Every horse on your books will have a weekly dollar value to you. Let us do some simple math. Let us say that you are able to charge $80 to shoe a horse. If you put your horses on an 8-week schedule, each horse will be worth $10 per week to you. You only get paid once, but if they paid you weekly for that shoeing, it would be in the amount of $10 each week.

That was easy. Now, we know that we have to make $500 per week to break even. In order to make that $500 in a week, we need to have 50 horses on the books. Fifty horses X $10 per week = $500 per week. What this means is: you need to shoe 50 horses over an 8-week period in order to make $26,000 per year.

That doesn't sound too bad; only a little more that 6 horses per week. Even if you are really slow, you can get that done.

Most people will end up where they average an hour for normal flat shoes on a short-footed horse. If you are doing horses at that speed, you can work for 6.5 hours, one day a week, and still make your basic first year expenses. Pretty cool, huh?

Let us consider that you want to make more

than just your expenses. Well, what do you want to make? Do you want to gross $1,200 per week? Okay, with the math we have established, you need 120 horses on your books. That will require you to work 120 hours over an eight-week period. That is only 15 horses per week, and that is still fewer hours than the average part-time job.

If you take a vacation and spread out the schedule, you have lost income. Of course, you could bunch up the horses before and after, but if you don't, you lost some revenue. So if you had 100 horses on the books, making you $1,000 per week, and all of a sudden they went from and eight-week to a ten-week schedule, that $80 per horse is now going to be spread further. Each horse will be worth only $8 per week. That is a 20% hit for taking a couple of weeks off. And, once you shoe the horse again at the end of those ten weeks, they are back to normal, and the two-week extension in the last shoeing cycle can never be made up again.

It is hard to take time off as a shoer for that reason. You will find that there is so much work before and after leaving for a vacation that doing so is almost not worth it. Sorry, but that is how it is. Most farriers will only take one week off at the most, and they will work until the minute they leave, then do a horse on the way home from the beach. Oh well, being that busy is certainly preferable to not being that busy.

You may find that your business will ebb and flow through the shoeing cycle. I don't know why, but it has always seemed to happen to me with every shoeing business that I have ever started, and I have started five personal shoeing practices, not including the school customers at two different schools.

You will end up with a really busy four weeks, and a slower two weeks over the course of six. I finally got to where I didn't fight it, and I tried to exploit the situation by giving myself some time off during the downturn portion of the cycle.

Jeff Houston takes it one further, and he will decide he wants a week off in early March to come to the school and meet the next shoeing stars of our industry. Jeff is such a kindhearted soul that he comes here every year at his own expense just to be a part of the next generation. Because he is going to be gone that week in March, he counts backwards from that week, and manipulates his calendar in October and November the year before to accommodate the week he wants free in March.

All of that will come with experience, but for now, I want you to think of each horse as having a weekly dollar value. Trims also have a weekly value; you just have to do the math. If you get $35 to trim a horse and you do those horses every 6 weeks, each trim has a value of roughly $5.83 (35 divided by 6 = 5.833333). If you want to make $583 per week, just get 100 horses to trim on your books.

For the supplies and equipment portion, I have another handout. It is hard to estimate what will be needed in a year for a new farrier, but this list will come pretty close. If you are shoeing quarter horses, the shoe sizes and quantities should work fine. For those who are doing warmbloods or other larger breeds, just move everything up one or two sizes.

I also recommend for people who are going to be cold shoers that they get shoes like the St. Croix Euro or Eventer instead of generic-shaped compromise patterns. These shoes have a great front and hind pattern that nails up quite easily on most breeds.

A quick note on skill that will also be addressed in other parts of this book: If you have the skill to shape and clip your own shoes, you don't have to buy shoes that have those features. Consider two farriers that are both shoeing for $100 per horse, yet one uses shoes that he modifies himself while the other buys all modifications for twice the price of the first farrier. To give it a number, let us imagine that the one doing the modifications is paying $2 per shoe, and the other farrier is paying $4 per shoe; this is a difference of $8 per horse. If each farrier does 30 horses in a week, the one who does his own modification is making an extra $240 per week just for his skill in the fire. Look at that over a career, and you start to understand the necessity of becoming good at that aspect of the job. Back to the subject at hand.

RECOMMENDED INVENTORY FOR INITIAL BUSINESS START-UP

✔ 1 case MX50
✔ 3 cases .... 5 CH Mustad Slim

✔ St. Croix shoes:

	Plain	Rim
000	1 box	½ box
00	3 boxes	1 box
0	5 boxes	2 boxes
1	3 boxes	1 box

2................................1 box ....½ box
✔ 100 feet...........................3/8" X 3/4" barstock
✔ 300 feet ....5/16" X 3/4" barstock
✔ 1 dozen rasps
✔ Kaeco Epson Salts Poultice and Abscess Kits
✔ Miscellaneous pads
✔ Vettec Equi-Pak and Super-Fast

This is by no means a complete list. You will find that you may need things that are not on it, and you will also end up with some things that you haul around for five years and never use.

Okay, now that we understand this, let's talk about what you need to charge for shoeing a horse. I have seen it recommended charging a multiple of the average haircut in the area, but I don't really like that method. Haircuts seemed to be unrelated to the cost of living in an area, and like shoeing, there can also be a huge range from the top of the scale to the bottom. In fact, until 2007 you could get a haircut from old Claude Higgins on the Lamar square for $2 (It was only $1.75 if you were an old customer). He cut hair in the trenches during World War II and was quite an American hero. Anyway, if you multiplied his $2 by 50 times, you would still be less than what I charge to shoe a horse in the same area.

What I have found to be a pretty good guide is to take the average mortgage payment in an area and charge 10% of that. If you are able to do that, then you are living in an area where you can make a good living. This means you have to shoe 10 horses to pay for housing every month. That is not too bad.

There are some places that are hard to do that. Take Hawaii for instance. I have a graduate there by the name of Tom Richmond. He is an excellent hand and pretty much took the Big Island by storm when he started shoeing there. Very quickly, Tom was doing as many horses as he could at $100 per horse. However, the average mortgage payment in Hawaii is way beyond $1,000. This meant that Tom was working in an area where he was not able to make his housing payment with ten horses. That means you have to work a little harder, and sacrifice some of the things you want to afford the things you have to have. But then again, he does get to live in Hawaii.

Best-case scenario is to live in an area where you can charge $150 to shoe a horse and the average mortgage payment is only $1,000. Now you are way ahead of the game. You are able to make your housing payments with less than seven horses. That puts you in a powerful position.

After you have been shoeing for a while, you will find like most that you could be making a little more. In the self-employed, single farrier shoeing business, there are two good ways I know of to make more money. You can charge more or shoe more. Either one works, but the first is the preferable.

Grant Moon, AWCF, a good friend of mine and a person who knows a tremendous amount about money, gave me this advice when we judged a contest together one time. "Never say no to a new customer. Raise your prices when your diary is full, and keep the new business coming in at a higher rate." That is superb advice. If you say no to new business because you are full up, pretty soon the word gets out that you are not taking any new customers, and before you know it, you won't have the option. You will be stuck with the clientele that you have. Also, no one likes to be rejected, for any reason. Hearing the word "no" is as direct a rejection as you can give, regardless of why.

If, on the other hand, you go up a substantial amount when the new customer calls, one of two things will happen. Either you will shoe some more horses for more money, or the prospective new customer will be the one to say no. At least you were not the one to say it. Later, if that person has a change of fortune or needs your expertise, at least they will still call because they were not rejected.

Throughout my career, I have used prices to keep me from doing things that I did not want to do. If you put your prices way up, you will often not have to do what you did not want to do, or in the event that you do, you are really well paid.

Here is what happens, you are shoeing away, doing six horses a day for six days a week. You are working too hard but are making a great living at $100 per horse. The phone rings, and a horse owner has heard of your incredible skill. They need you to do their horses. You quote this new customer a price of $125, and amazingly, they say, "Okay, when can you shoe my five horses?" Man, you didn't see that coming. But hey, you just got one heck of a raise. It does come with a little more work, but just wait till you see how easy it is to shoe those horses when you are making an additional $25 each. On the down side, it does make it hard to then shoe your normal horses at $100.

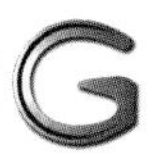

So, you will fit in this new client. And later, you will realize that you are worth that extra money, so you tell all of your current customers that you are going up to $125. Will they balk? Some will. Will you lose 25% of them? Very doubtful. But, for the sake of arguments, let's say that you do lose 25%.

Well, you went up 25% and lost 25% of your business. But here is what the reality is. You will still make the same amount of money yet do 25% less work. Not only that, but you actually are doing a little better than that, because you won't have the expenses involved with those 25% of the horses that you lost.

I know that these figures are not exact, and if an accountant put a pen to it, there would be discrepancies that would only confuse the point I am trying to make. If you try this experiment on your own business, what you may find is that you don't lose any horses, and now all of a sudden you are needing to figure out how to do all of these extra horses for all that extra money. Often, the fact that you are now so much more expensive will put you in even greater demand as the horse-owning public decides you must be a farrier god based on what you charge to shoe a horse, and everyone owns a horse that deserves a shoeing god.

This has led some enterprising business-minded farriers to start up multi-farrier practices. In concept, this is an outstanding idea. Think about the local plumbing shop. They have a central location, several trucks that have supplies on them, and a journeyman plumber with an apprentice in each one. The shop has an inventory, and there is probably a secretary to order supplies and schedule the workdays for each truck. It is a fantastic system that works very well for plumbers.

There are a couple of problems when you apply that model to the farrier industry. The first is: most farriers become farriers because they want to be self-employed. Not everyone has what it takes to be self-employed, and there are times when I wish my day had a start time and an end time as well. When it is hot and heavy around here, I think I might enjoy going home at five, and not have to worry about the stresses of running a business. If you would rather not have to schedule customers, order supplies, deal with all the calls, and generally do the things that you have to do when you own a business, then finding a multi-farrier practice to work for may be perfect for you.

I have a friend in California named Mike Deleonardo, CJF. Mike is famous in this industry for his outstanding multi-farrier practice. I did a clinic for him one time, and I was truly impressed to see how their business was put together and run. Mike is made to take that stress, and he thrives under it. If you are considering starting a multi-farrier practice, talk to Mike about it.

Another famous Hall of Fame Farrier is Red Renchin, CJF, out of Wisconsin. Red has had one of the most successful multi-farrier practices in the United States for many years, and he would also be a great resource if you were wanting advice in this area.

Another problem with the multi-farrier practice is that customers will generally see their farrier more than the plumber, they form a relationship with an individual farrier, and most owners want a particular farrier. With a multi-farrier practice, the clients may get whatever farrier the secretary schedules. This can lead to dissatisfaction amongst clients.

From the multi-farrier practice owner's perspective, you have to worry about employees moonlighting and taking your business. You have to pay well enough that you get empoyees with enough talent to do the job. Turnover can be a problem, and you have to deal with way more customers than you would if you were a one-person operation. I think that there is a real chance that you will stop being a farrier and become a mentor, secretary, coach, counselor, HR professional, PR man, marketer or head mechanic – when in fact what you wanted to be was a farrier.

We all have different wants and needs, and this is just another piece of this dynamic trade that may fit you.

At the end of the day, the economics of running a successful shoeing business are not much different than running any small business. There are numerous courses, books, and resources for the small businessman, and you can gather this data and apply it to the farrier industry.

Chapter 60 THE BUSINESS PLAN

A Farrier Plan For Success

If you were hoping for a get-rich-quick scheme, let me redirect you to the back of the comic books. Farriery is not that. It is, on the other hand, a very lucrative trade for those who are willing to invest the time and effort to become good at it.

There is such a broad range of skills needed to be a great farrier that most of us are lucky to master a few of them. For our part, both Kelly and I are not good at bookkeeping. We don't like it, it is not natural to us, and our business has suffered as a result of that failing. On the bright side, we have been fortunate enough that the other skills have been enough that we were able to survive.

I highly recommend that you do your best to find out what your weaknesses are, and then do what you can to improve them. For us, that meant we pay more for accounting services. If your weakness had to do with mechanical skills, you can't hire a CPA for that, so get in the forge and fix it.

I used to hate clips. I loved to forge. Bump, weld, draw, crease, punch, make caulks, all of it but the clips. We would go to a contest and I would make a nice shoe at the beginning of a multi-shoe class, and place it on top of the forge without a clip. The next shoe would be the same, and the next. Kelly would be looking at me, look at the clock, and say, "You need to get those clips on." I would nod, knowingly.

With only a few minutes left, I would throw the shoes in the fire, and then go about destroying them with my clips. Now bear in mind that I would practice for hours on those shoes before coming to the contest, but I was not practicing on the clips.

In everyday shoeing, I would not use clips (in those days, you couldn't buy clipped shoes). If a horse needed clips, well, that was unfortunate for that horse. Finally, Bob Marshall taught me how to pull a proper clip. Wow. That was a big event in my life. He also said, "You need to practice your weaknesses." When I write that now, it seems so evident. I don't know how I couldn't see it before, but it has become a mantra to me. Once I finally figured out that I could get good at pieces and parts that I didn't like, the forge work really started coming around.

The first step is to identify the weakness. The second step is to determine a plan to change that weakness, and the final step is to turn your weakness into your strength.

One of the best illustrations of this concept is from an old friend of mind named Dave Showen. Dave was a farrier in Colorado, and we used to get together and compete and practice when we lived there. Dave is well known for his hammers, and I own the hammer with serial number 02 stamped in it from his first production line. If Lee Liles, CJF, is reading this, he will probably call me to see if he can put it in his Horseshoeing Museum in Sulphur, Oklahoma.

Dave hated to work aluminum. Back then, there were not a lot of clinicians who would do anything with aluminum. This was the early 1990s, and the American forging skills as a whole were not what they are today. Dave had tried aluminum, but it ended up in a puddle in his forge or wound up shattering.

Dave got frustrated — and determined. The first thing he did was to bolt a pair of hinges from the front of his forge to the front of his forge stand. This allowed him to dump the molten aluminum out of the bottom of the hot forge liner when a shoe melted. He would shut off the forge, grab the top of it, and swing it forward when it was full of liquid aluminum. Next, he bought a pile of aluminum bar stock and began to make everything out of aluminum. He had aluminum Scotch-bottom draft shoes, aluminum roadsters, and aluminum toe weights. You name it, he made it out of aluminum.

Pretty soon, he was welding all sorts of bar shoes out of aluminum. He figured out what wire he needed, what flux (not available at farrier supplies like it is now), and what method worked best.

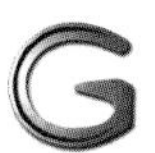

Remember, this was the early 90s, so Dave was pretty far ahead of his time.

Before long, Dave became known for his skill in working aluminum. He did several clinics for farriers wanting to see this man work aluminum, and I still have some of those shoes he made back then. What a fantastic story about determination, and turning weakness into a strength. It can be applied to most aspects of farriery, and I would encourage you to look carefully at where you want to be and make a plan to get there.

With that in mind, here is an adaptation of a business plan that Jim Keith, CJF, used to give to his beginning students when he taught at Tucumcari Area Trade School in the 1980s and early 90s. I still hand it out to my students today.

THE BUSINESS PLAN

Personal Evaluation:

A. Identify Strengths and Weaknesses
   1. Technical skills
   2. Management skills
   3. Personal characteristics
   4. How can weaknesses be compensated for?

B. Goal Setting
   1. Define your lifetime goals
   2. Define 1-year goals
   3. Define 5-year goals
   4. Define 10-year goals

(Repeat this process for your personal goals and your business goals)

Purpose of this Business:

A. Define the purpose of this business
   1. What is your personal reason to run this business?
   2. What is the business reason to run this business?
   3. Are these purposes compatible?

B. Identify specific, measurable goals:
   1. Sales volume
   2. Sales volume growth
   3. Profit
   4. Personal compensation
   5. Time commitments
   6. Personal growth and education

Management:

A. Form of business
   1. Self proprietorship
   2. Partnership
   3. Corporation
   4. Identify owners

B. Identify outside consultants
   1. Accountants
   2. Financial management
   3. Marketing

Products and Services:

A. Identify any products this business will sell
   1. What products can you sell?
   2. Who will be your suppliers?
   3. Who will buy these products?
   4. Why will they buy them from you?

B. Economics of product sales
   1. What will you charge for these products?
   2. What is your cost for these products?
   3. What level of inventory is required?
   4. Warehousing issues

C. Identify services offered
   1. What services do you offer?
   2. What problems do these services fix?
   3. What makes these services unique?
   4. What sets you apart in this industry?

D. Economics of services offered
   1. What will you charge for your services?
   2. What will it cost you to provide these services?
   3. Will it be profitable?
   4. Will you be competitive?

Customers:

A. What distance will you have to travel?

B. Will customers be coming to you?

C. How many customers live in your geographic area?

D. How many of these will chose your business?

E. What will the average customer spend per year?

Geographic Location:

A. Business address

B. Why is this a good location?

C. What nearby business will help attract customers?

D. What are the features of your facility or rig?

E. What renovations or repairs are needed, and what will they cost?
F. What are the prospects for growth in this area?
G. What are the fixed annual costs in this area?

Competitive Analysis:

A. Identify four major competitors:
B. Compare your business to theirs on a scale of 1-5; 1-worst. 5-best
    1. Image – What is the customer perception of your business?
    2. Location – Compare travel for customers and suppliers
    3. Products – Completeness of your line of goods
    4. Services – Consider quality
    5. Services – Consider quantity
    6. Pricing – Who offers the most for the money?
    7. Advertising – Does the target market know about you?
    8. Sales methods – What is done for repeat business?
C. Identify changes needed to improve your competitive position

Marketing Strategy:

A. Pricing Strategy
    1. How do you calculate pricing?
    2. What factors influence price?
    3. What are your discount policies?
B. Customer Service
    1. What special customer services to you offer?
    2. What, if any, payment options do you offer?
    3. How are customer complaints handled?

This plan can be applied to almost any aspect of your life. You can use it for skill improvement, marriage, spiritual life, or, as intended, to build your business. It is personal to you, but there is a power to be gained by sitting down and writing out what you are trying to achieve. Experts say that you are many times more likely to achieve any goal that you are trying to reach by simply putting it to paper. The business plan puts all of that in place, you just need to fill in the blanks.

Section

14

Educators Manual

Chapter 61: Tips on Teaching 666

Chapter 62: Practical Testing Strategies............. 669

Chapter 63: Test Questions 676

Chapter 64: Judging 685

> **" [11] Who teacheth us more than the beasts of the earth, and maketh us wiser than the fowls of heaven? "**
>
> **—Job 35:11**
>
> **—King James Version**

Chapter 61

TIPS ON TEACHING

Almost every farrier will become involved in teaching at some point in his or her career. It may be as simple as teaching members of a 4-H pony club how to pick up and clean the feet, showing a customer how to pull a shoe, doing farrier clinics, or taking on apprentices. For a few, there is a career in the field of farrier education. They will have the responsibility of teaching a lot about the basics of shoeing to people who may know nothing about the trade. Whatever situation you find yourself in, there are some principles of vocational training that you may find helpful.

There are several ways that a thing can be taught. It can be written about, demonstrated, talked about, and the student can actually do it. These all involve different styles of learning. There are several different categories for types of learning. Visual, auditory and read-write learners are the basic ones. As an educator, you have to use all of these types of teaching, then identify which has the most benefit for which students so that you can concentrate on each individually with his or her preferred method.

I have found that farriery is a difficult trade for students to become great at. A lot of people get good enough to put metal on a foot, but to be truly great at shoeing horses takes a lot of dedication and work ethic. Often, students who have always excelled with ease at other endeavors will suffer frustration as they try to learn the fine points of shoeing a horse. Their mentor has to identify these times and coach them through the tough spots so who they can enjoy the good spots.

There are a lot of skills that must be mastered to be a great farrier. Some of these are horsemanship, business skills, people skills, and mechanical skills with a hammer, tongs, knife, nippers, rasp, punches, creasers, pritchels, and anvil. There is also the skill set that involves the academic side of shoeing, and this includes anatomy, conformation, pathology, gaits, shoeing strategies and theories, as well as exposure to new techniques and materials. It is a tremendous body of knowledge that one must master, and the job of teaching it can be daunting. With that in mind, I thought having a chapter about teaching would be a good addition to this book. Following, not in any particular order, are some random things I have learned over my career as a farrier educator.

Begin by breaking down each aspect of the job into tasks. For instance, the way that I teach basic shoe building is to break down the whole into several tasks. For a basic shoe, these tasks are: Toe bend, heel, branch, nail holes, heel, branch, nail holes, clips. Each task should be able to be practiced on its own. Hypothetically, a person could practice each task hundreds of times, and never yet have made a complete shoe. Once all of the tasks are mastered, putting them all together will make a fantastic shoe.

People learn best by doing a task in a repetitive nature. I want my students to do each task at least six times in a row before moving to the next task, and that is why I break down the shoe building into the areas that I do. If two students were made to make six shoes, the first one making one shoe after another, and the second making each task of the shoe over and over till the six shoes were complete, the second student would have a better technique and grasp of shoe building than the first. This method can be used for most forging projects, and I also like to assign projects that require repetitive hammering for the first several. The first projects that my students do are a hoof pick, horseshoe sandwiches, simple punches, and clinch block. These require less bending and more forging than building shoes, so students get to do a lot of direct forging and hitting.

It is hard to teach in this way when it comes to shoeing live horses, since a student who does repetitive knife work on the sole will soon run out of sole. What I will do is put students together to do horses when there are a couple of students with different needs. Perhaps I have one student who needs to work on rasping the bottom of the foot and dressing work with another who needs to work on nipping and nailing. I will have them do horses together for a couple of days, with each one being assigned the tasks that are their weak spots.

Most people like to practice what they are good at. That's just human nature. This can cause a student to become really great at some aspect, while another suffers. For me, in my early career it was clips. With no one to guide my education, I ended up sabotaging my early farrier competitions by refusing to practice clips that I didn't like or make well. This caused me to have some nice shoes with terrible clips, and more often than not, the clips ruined the shoe. In your own case, as well as those you may teach, try to identify any weak areas and concentrate on making them into strengths.

"Quality comes not from tools, but from the hands that use them." This was the featured saying on an old poster I used to have in the shop, and it had a picture of some old rough hands setting a nail on a shoe. The shoe had been on for some time, was already clinched and full of dirt, and anyone could see that it was a posed sort of photo, but I still liked it. While the saying is true, it is only true up to a point. It is all but impossible to do a great job when you don't have good equipment. A highly skilled farrier can shape on a flat horned anvil, using a pair of pulloffs for a hammer and clinchers for tongs, but that is true only once the skills have been developed. Whether you are a teacher or a student, having the right equipment is a necessity. Make the investment to provide the right equipment to create the best learning environment you can.

Horseshoeing can be dangerous, especially for those who are so focused on the job at hand that they have blinders on to what else is happening around them. A young farrier may be concentrating so hard on something like trimming or fitting that he or she is oblivious to the horse, which may be an outlaw. As the experienced farrier on scene, you have to be aware of everything that is happening in the situation, and try to keep the young farrier safe.

Learning to shape is one of the hardest parts of learning to shoe horses. My personal method of shaping requires some vision. I like to look at a foot, and imagine that foot already wearing the shoe that I am about to make or fit for it. In this way, I have already seen the foot with the ideal shoe fitted in the ideal way. When I go to the anvil, I simply recreate what I already imagined. If students can comprehend this, and have the ability to imagine the shoe on the foot, they are going to get the shape easier than those that can't. What happens a lot of the time in the early going is that a student will get to the anvil without a plan on how to shape the shoe. They didn't take the time to pay close attention to the foot so that they could see the shape of the shoe they are about to burn on. This can cause them to ruin shoes and end up frustrated.

I don't have any shortcuts for learning to shape, but I do have my students spend six hours shaping old keg shoes. I suggest that they shape a shoe from front to hind to front to hind, until the shoe is ruined. Once one shoe is used up, another takes its place. These six hours should be in a straight marathon of forge time, and once it is over, the student will have a better grasp of how shoes move on the horn when hot, and they are now ready to learn how to shape. Throughout my career as an educator, those who have done this shaping marathon end up leaps and bounds ahead of those who refuse to.

Being in the position of running a school creates an unusual social dynamic. The teacher is actually an employee of the student yet must also be in charge of that student. Be aware of this if you become an educator. Try to make the interactions positive. Never ask a student to do something that you would be unwilling to do. Show the students how to do the difficult stuff instead of just talking about it, particularly when it comes to mean horses. Those students who can't do a bad horse are going to have a much harder time surviving their first few years than those who know how to get around that horse with confidence.

Try to limit the number of horses that you put a student under in the first few weeks of training. If I could create the perfect system, I would have students only trimming for the first three weeks of a class, doing no more than two horses in a day. Mixed with those trims would be a lot of forging and shaping practice based on the feet they were working on. In the fourth week, the student would shoe two feet per day, and move to shoeing one horse a day from the fifth week to the seventh. From the eighth week on, the students would do as many horses as they could handle. Since customer needs don't allow this, we have to do the horses as they are presented. Make the most out of each horse when they are scarce, and watch out for your students when they are overly abundant.

There is a fine line between knowing enough to be nervous about shoeing and knowing so little that you are full of confidence that is born of ignorance. Students coming from short courses tend to be confident because they know so little that they think they can actually shoe with the best of them. That is a strategy used by some schools to make money, however, it is at the expense of the horse and student and should not be tolerated.

I think that a student should spend a couple days studying anatomy, shoe a dead foot, and dissect it before they are able to work on a live horse. By doing this, they know a lot more about what they are working on, and they will have a healthy respect for it. Putting a student under horses to do anything beyond pulling a shoe or cleaning a foot on the first day they get to school gives them the impression that there is so little to know about it that anyone can just get going. I personally find that to be a bad idea, but that is my thought on the subject, and I have been wrong before.

When teaching anatomy, use the correct terminology. If students do not learn the proper terms for the anatomical structures, they are at a decided disadvantage when it comes to shoeing for the public and working with vets. Even reading articles and textbooks will become a stumbling block if students do not understand what they are reading.

My last thought on teaching is this; many of the students a farrier school attracts do not like theory and have not excelled in the academic side of school. They are for the most part good, hard-working, hands-on, solid people. However, for some, their teachers gave up on them and did not expect them to succeed, so they didn't. Make your expectations of your students so high that they are almost unattainable and believe they are going to achieve those standards. When I believe in my students, it is transferred to them and they believe in themselves. Pretty soon, they are doing work and expressing knowledge in a time frame that no one else had ever thought possible of them. I have seen some changes in people through farrier education that you have to witness to believe, and it has led to some great careers.

The horse is a noble beast that deserves our respect and the very best craftsmanship that we can deliver. Making decisions about shoeing that are based on laziness or cost does not benefit the horse as much as it could be when the decisions are based on what is best for the horse. Read the chapter on hot fitting to gain a perspective on this ideal, where the reason for doing something in shoeing is about the end result being the best for the horse, even if it is not the easiest for the farrier. Put the horse first when making decisions about what to do, both in shoeing and teaching, and you won't go wrong.

I have had a great life working as a farrier educator and have always felt blessed being in this great trade. If you were made to shoe, teach, or both, I hope that you have as wonderful a life as I have.

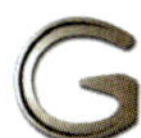

Chapter 62 PRACTICAL TESTING STRATEGIES

As your skills develop, you may find that you want to test those skills against standards that are established by farrier associations and companies around the world. This is a great goal for any young farrier, and the preparation required to take any of the exams will cause you to learn a lot about the trade that you may not already know.

There are some things to know about failing before you start your quest. First, every time you fail, it is actually a gift that will only make you better if you view it in the right way. Getting mad and walking away from the process will not hurt anyone but you, so turn the failures into launch pads to make yourself a better farrier.

Second, if you fail, that does not say anything about you as a person. It only means that another farrier's opinion on one day was not in line with your opinion. Sometimes the examiner is wrong, but more often, the candidate is wrong. Candidates will be looking at the job with more bias, and it may be years before they can look back on that failure and acknowledge to themselves that it was not up to standard. Again, avoid anger.

Next, there is no way to take the subjective nature out of grading farrier work. In some things, there is an exact right answer or method. In farriery, the nature of the craft creates situations where farriers can disagree with a method, yet both can be right. This makes judging and being judged that much harder. From a candidate's point of view, the more you know about the shoeing style of the examiner or tester, the better. Testers, on the other hand, should always ask themselves if what the candidate did is harmful, and if there was any chance that the judge could live with the job had he done it himself. This is especially important when judging shoe displays. The shoe display is a chance to fail almost any shoe, since there is no such thing as a perfect shoe. I have seen some fantastic shoe displays failed for the silliest reasons, and it has become quite a problem with some judges.

Finally, some of the best farriers I know have had major problems passing exams that I thought they would sail through. Not everyone is good at taking exams, which in itself is a skill. If you are one of those people, then I suggest that you practice taking exams. While that may require failure, you can also set up some situations with prep courses where you are examined over and over as you get better at the exam-taking skill set.

EXAMS

American Farrier's Association:

There are several different farrier bodies that offer exams. In the United States, we currently have the American Farrier's Association, which offers a

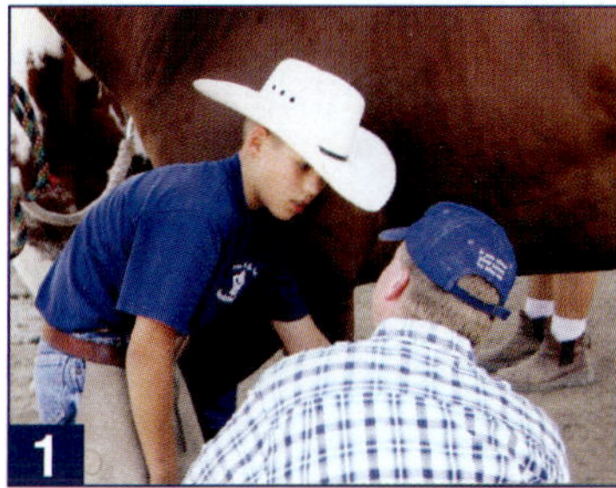

1 *Cody taking his first AFA Certified Farrier exam, 12 years old.*

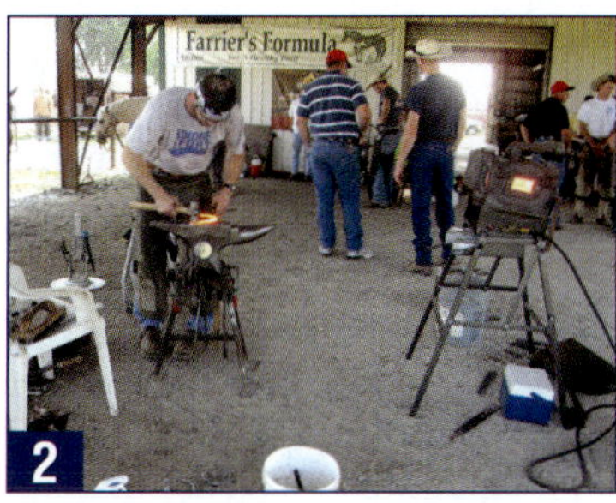

2 *AFA Certification at HHS*

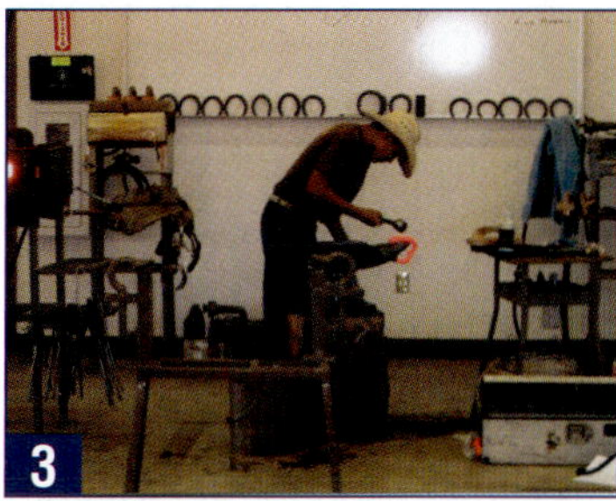

3 *CJF Bar Shoe exam in Walla Walla, Washington.*

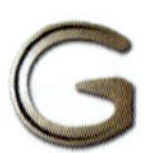

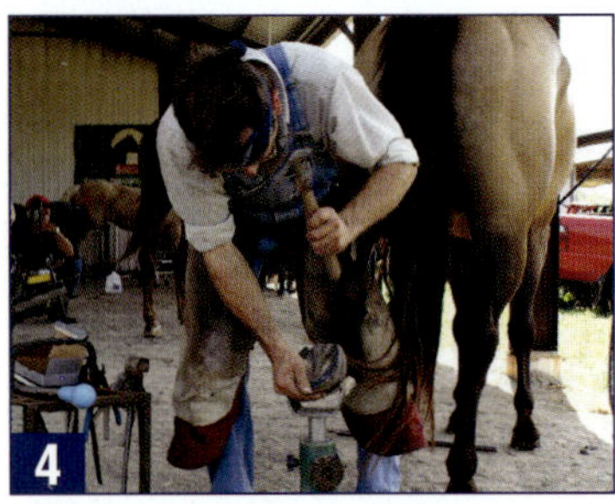

AFA candidate, Jason Kropf, CF

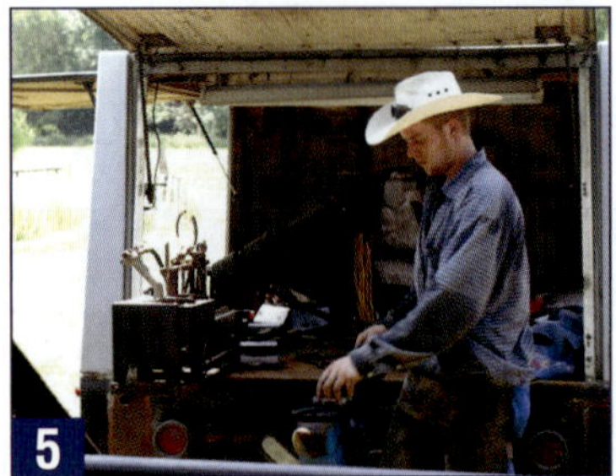

AFA Candidate, Tyler Brefles

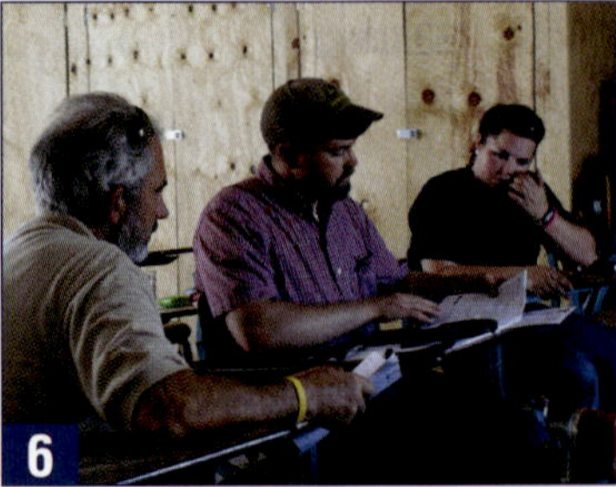

Marking the written exams, Ed Reardon, CJF, on left.

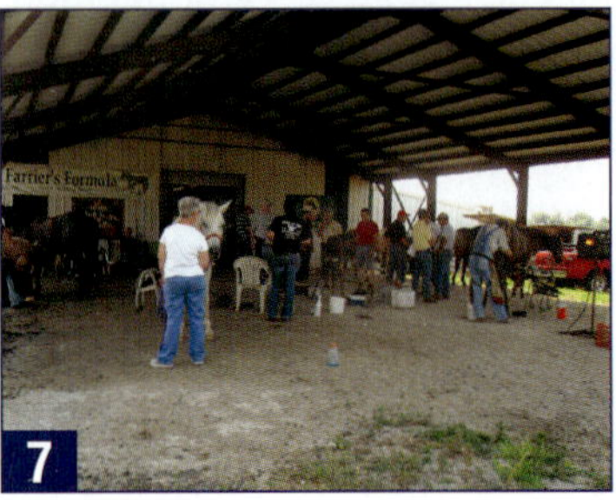

AFA Exam.

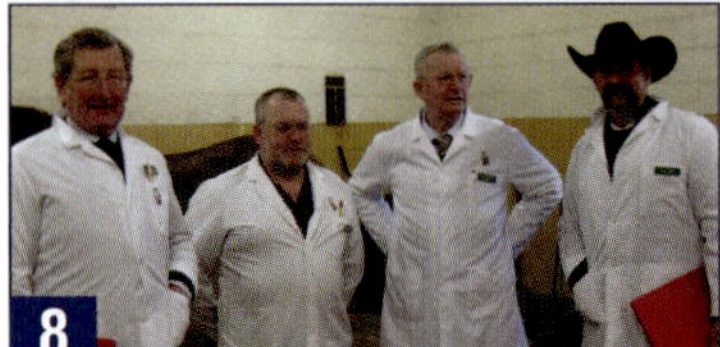

Diploma of the Worshipful Company of Farrier Exam in Hereford, England. Examiners are, Dr. Killingbeck, Veterinary Examiner, Chris Pardoe, Farrier Examiner, Bob Rush, Senior Farrier Examiner, and Chris Gregory, Provisional Examiner. January, 2010.

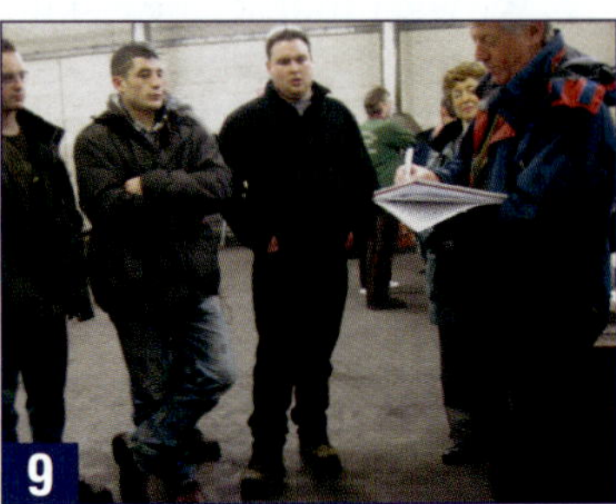

Captain David Goodall on right, Registrar of the WCF, giving the candidates the shoeing assignment.

few exams at different levels. The Certified Farrier (CF) level requires a candidate to shoe two feet with keg shoes in an hour, present a shoe display with 13 modifications, and take a multiple-choice test. The candidates must also recreate a shoe or modification from their shoe display in 30 minutes at the exam so that the examiners can see the candidate's abilities.

The next level is the Certified Tradesman Farrier (CTF). This test requires the candidate to shoe a horse with keg shoes that they clip in an hour and a half, make a fullered shoe to a pattern, and take a multiple-choice test.

The top level is the Certified Journeyman Farrier (CJF). This requires a candidate to shoe a horse with clipped, plain-stamped handmades in two hours, make a fullered straight bar to a pattern in 35 minutes, and take a multiple-choice test.

Beyond that, there are some endorsements that can be given above CJF, such as a Therapeutic Endorsement.

It is a good system and has done an incredible amount of good for the American farrier. Having a good standard has elevated the trade in this country faster than perhaps any other one thing. However, there are some flaws in the fact that the written tests have some ambiguity in the wording that have caused controversy, and there are some people involved in the judging that should not be. Like most systems, it is not perfect, but it is the best we have in the United States.

Worshipful Company of Farriers

In the United Kingdom, there is the Worshipful Company of Farriers (WCF). This is an ancient craft company with roots that date back to 1356. The WCF has literally set the standard for farriery for the world, and even their easiest test has aspects that are more difficult than the AFA Certified Journeyman Farrier examination.

The lowest level of exam in the WCF is the DipWCF, (Diploma of the Worshipful Company of Farriers). This is the entry-level exam that a farriers must pass to be allowed to shoe horses on their own in the United Kingdom The shoeing for this exam is easier than the AFA CJF, but the rest is harder. The candidate must shoe two feet with specified hand-

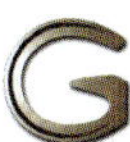

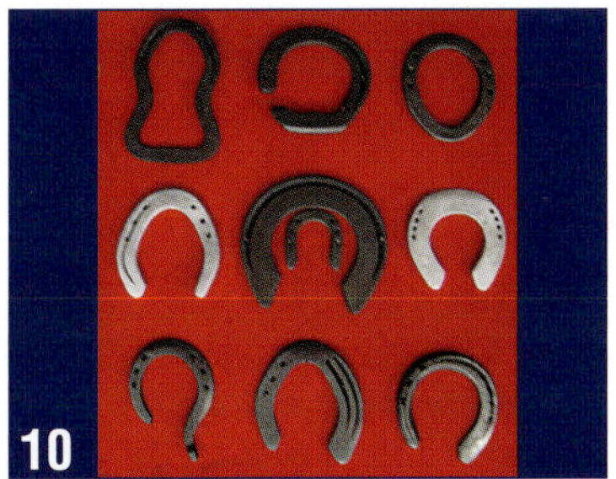
DipWCF shoe display

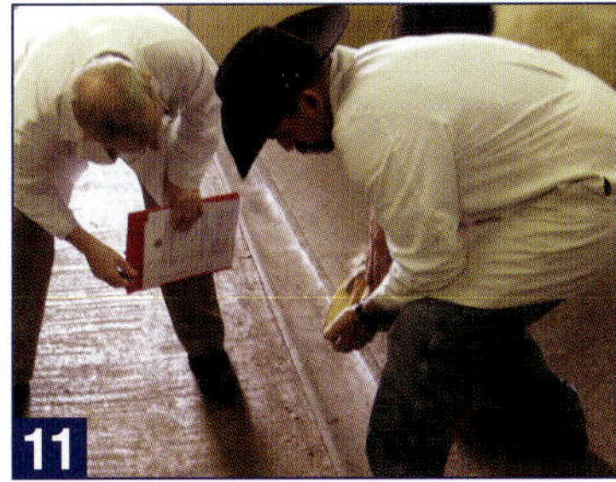
Bob Rush, FWCF, examining me examining a horse.

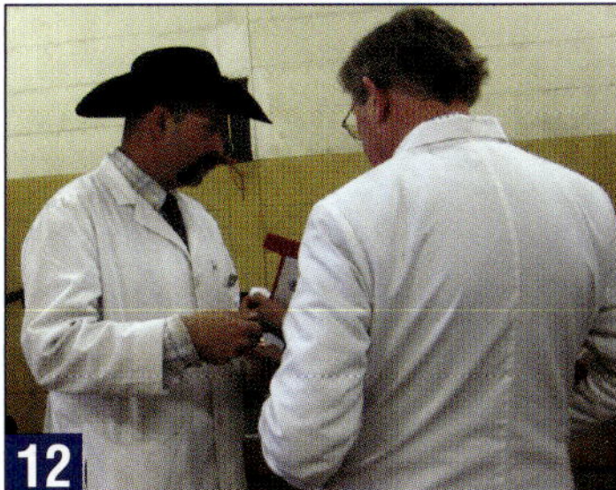
Dr. Killingbeck and I discussing a horse.

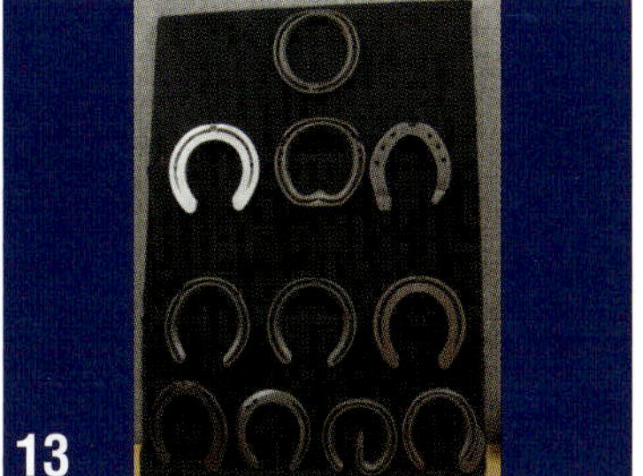
DipWCF shoe display.

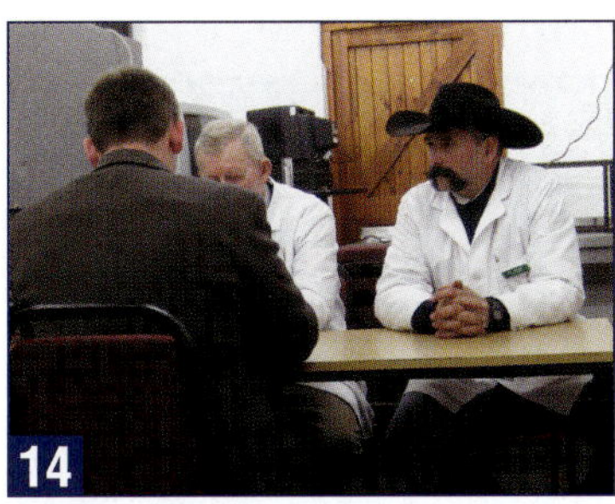
Oral exams.

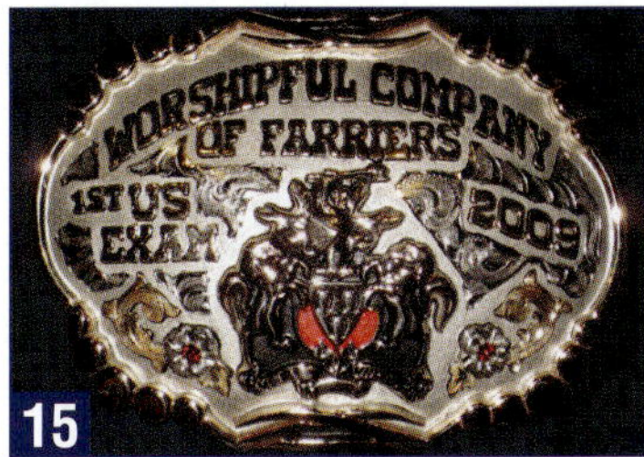

Buckle presented to everyone involved with the first AWCF exam on foreign soil, held at Heartland Horseshoeing School in 2009.

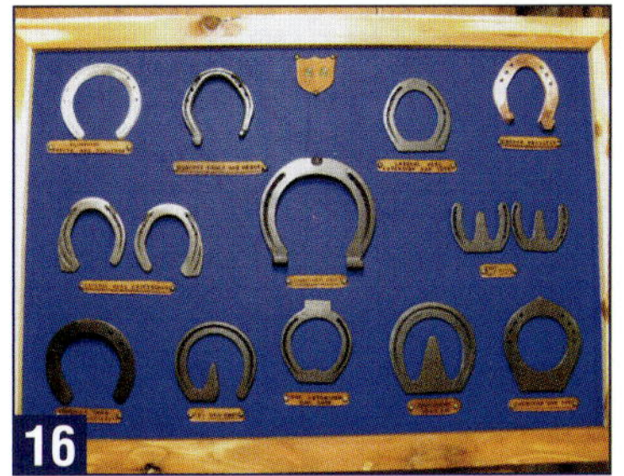
Cody's AWCF shoe display.

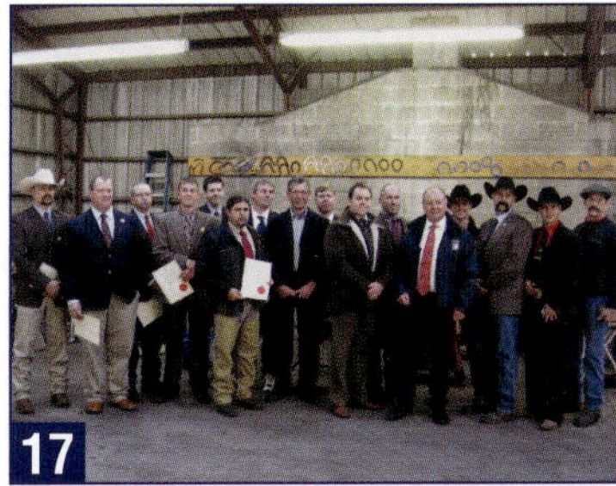
Candidates, examiners, horse holders, and others involved in the first AWCF in the U.S.

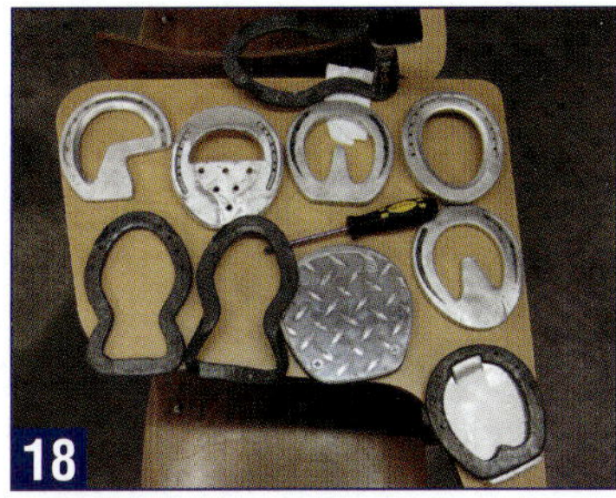
Rodney King, CJF, AWCF, from New Zealand, AWCF shoe display.

mades in two hours. Generally, this involves a front and hind, and the shoeing may require fullering, clipping, stud holes, plain-stamped, rocker or rolled toe, and perhaps concave bar stock. The easier part is that it is only two feet in the two hours. The harder part of the shoeing is the variety of shoes that might be called for, requiring the candidate to be competent in more than just plain-stamped, clipped handmades.

The theory (written) portion of this exam is much harder than the American multiple-choice test and does a better job of determining what a candidate knows, and not just whether or not the candidate is a good guesser at multiple-choice questions. The WCF uses essay tests, which have the disadvantage of being much harder to grade, but the advantage of no ambiguity in the questions causing confusion. The WCF also requires a shoe display of six shoes and has an oral portion on the exam that can be the deciding factor to help a candidate prove his or her knowledge.

The next level is the Associateship of the Worshipful Company of Farriers (AWCF), and this

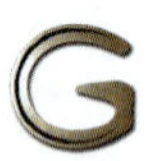

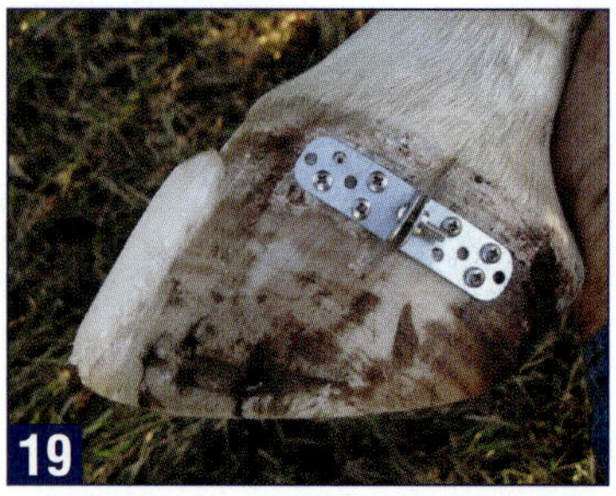

Foot that was used for the modern farriery portion of the exam.

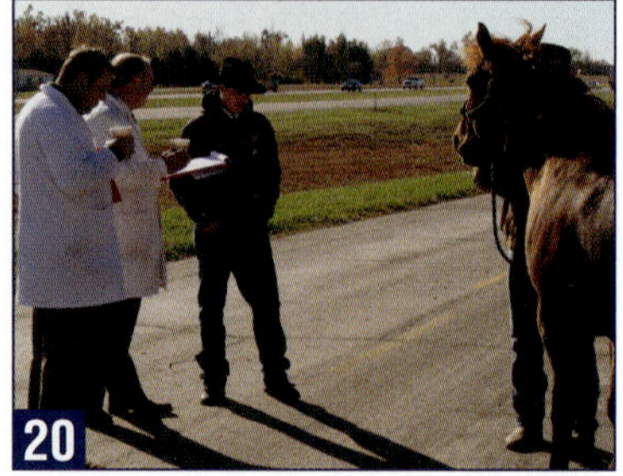

Horse assessment during the AWCF.

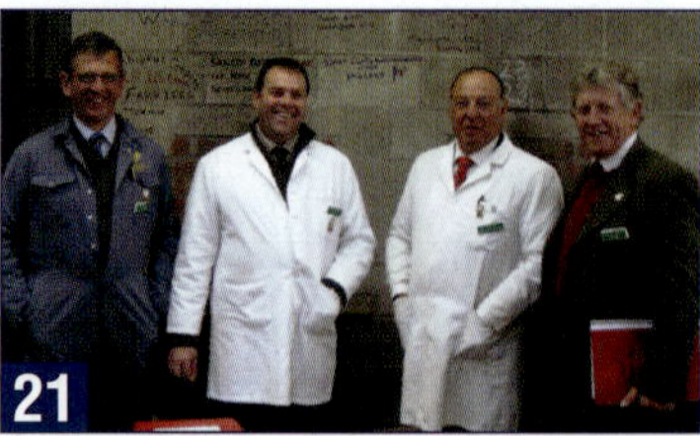

Examiners and registrar for the exam in the U.S. Left to right, Dr. James Sutton, Sandy Beveridge, Simon Curtis, and David Goodall.

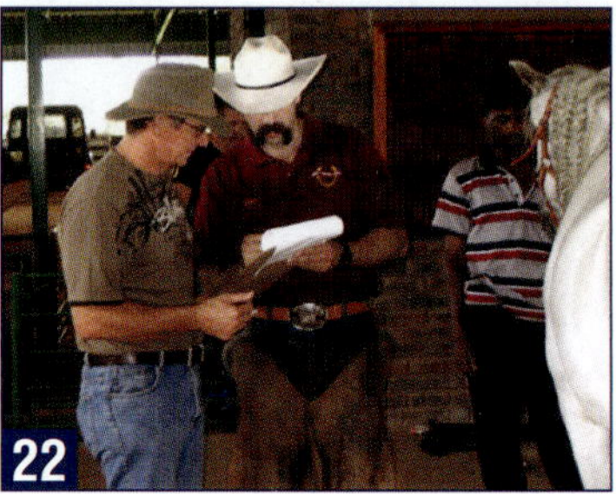

First exam in South Africa, 2005.

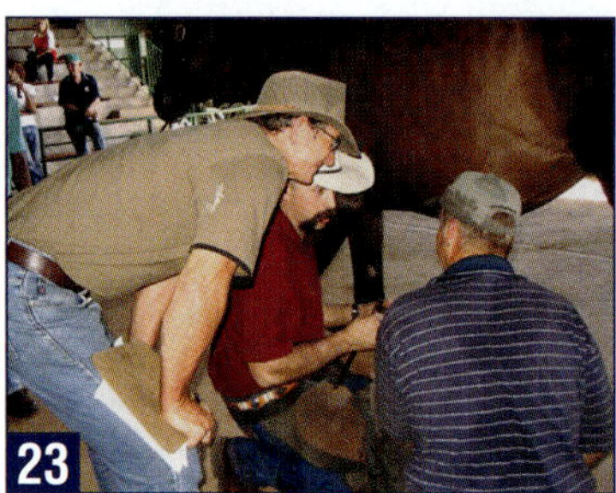

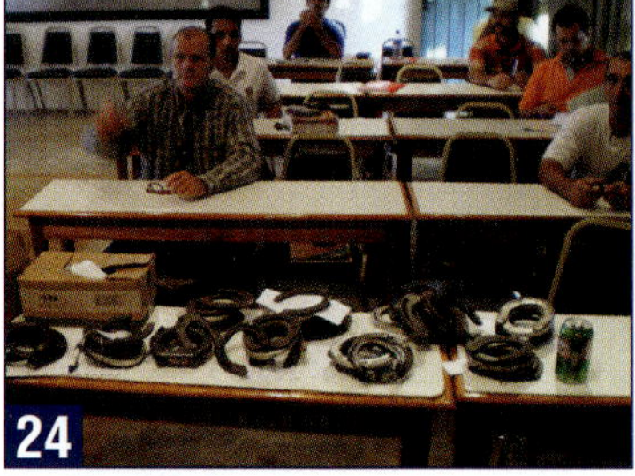

First AFB exam.

is the hardest test of practical farriery in the world. There are several aspects to this exam. They include a horse assessment, radiograph assessment, modern materials, ten shoes in the shoe display, an oral exam, and shoeing two feet with a huge potential assortment of shoes. Candidates have to be able to make and fit such a large variety of shoes that there is very little chance of someone just having a good day and getting by. The preparation required for this exam will vault you to the next level and make you a much better farrier.

The top level is the Fellowship of the Worshipful Company of Farriers (FWCF). As of the writing of this book, there are 35 FWCF farriers in the world, with four Americans having achieved this level. This test is primarily academic, with the practical only being the making of a complex shoe to a dead foot and a shoe display of remedial shoes. The theory portion is very demanding, requiring a thesis or dissertation to be handed in prior to the exam, presentation of a lecture on a farrier-related topic given to the candidate with only an hour to prepare, and an intense oral exam.

Association of Brazilian Farriers (Associacao Dos Ferradores Do Brasil)

The AFB is a newer group of farriers in Brazil that has an exam that I put together for them. It is an exam that has a combination of both the AFA and WCF exam styles, yet still something that is different. There are two levels. First is the Certified level and the second called the Graduate Farrier level. Graduate Farrier is the same level as the Advanced Skills Farrier in the Farrier International Testing System, (FITS) exam. The term Journeyman does not translate into anything for Brazil.

The Certified level requires successful completions of a shoe display, multiple-choice test, an oral exam, and shoeing a pair of feet with keg shoes, toe-clipped by the candidate in one hour. For the Graduate level, there is a written test with 20 essay questions, from which the candidate must choose 10 to answer. There is a shoe display, an oral exam, and a shoe-making demonstration where the candidate is assigned a remedial shoe from a list of 35. The candidate must shoe a horse with three-quarter-fullered and clipped handmade hinds, and the fronts can be straight bars, egg bars, heart bars or W shoes, as drawn from a hat. It is quite an intense test, and

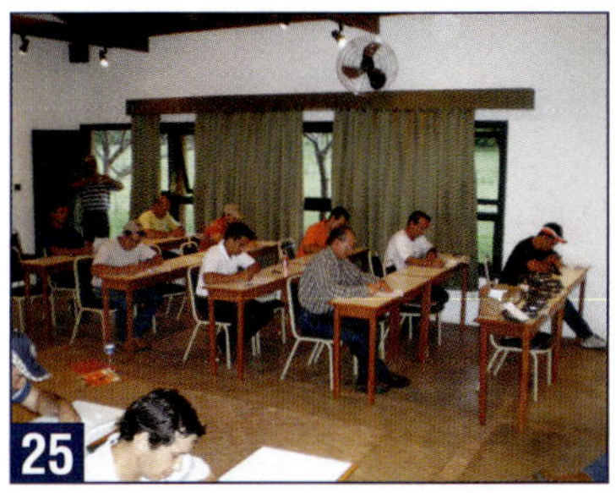

AFB candidates taking the written test.

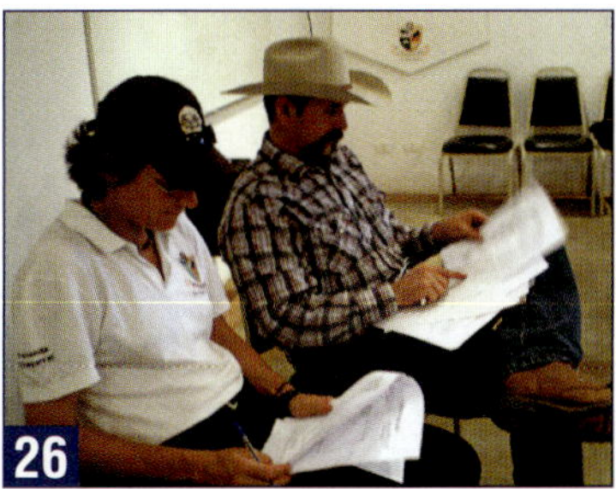

Marking the written exam with outstanding interpreter, Dr. Claudia Leschonski.

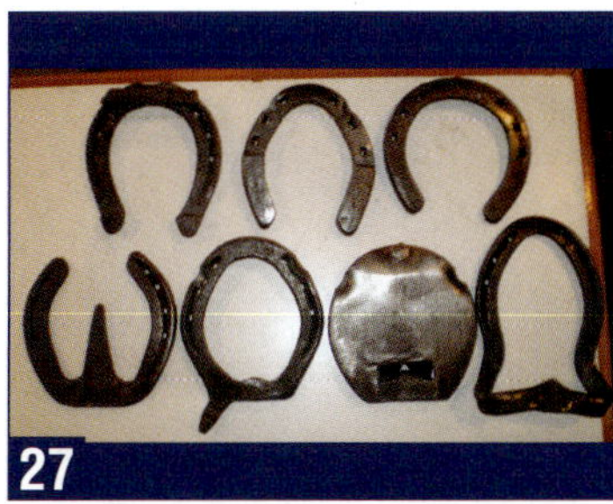

AFB Graduate Farrier shoe display.

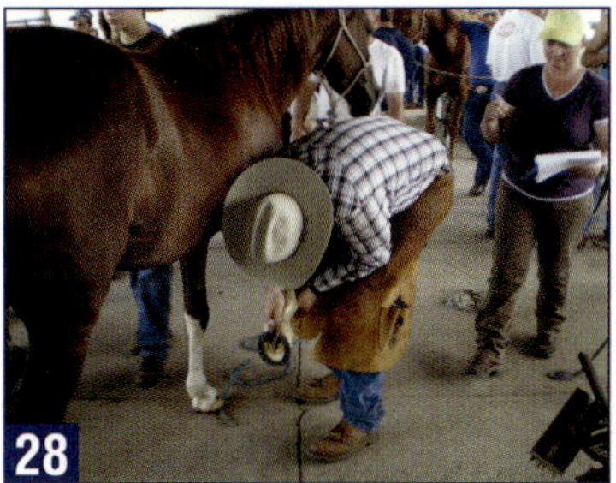

Judging the shoeing.

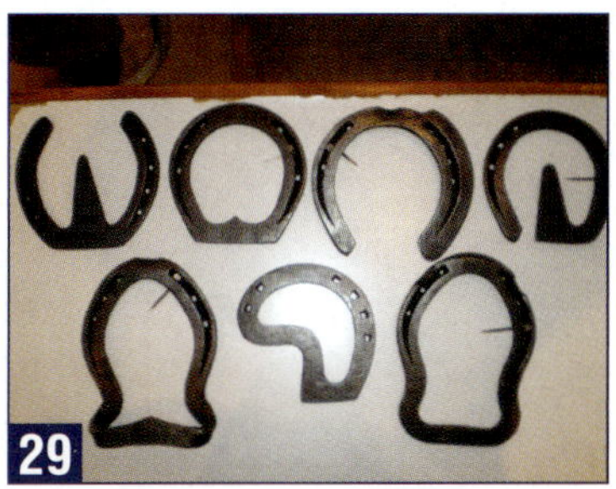

AFB Graduate Farrier shoe display.

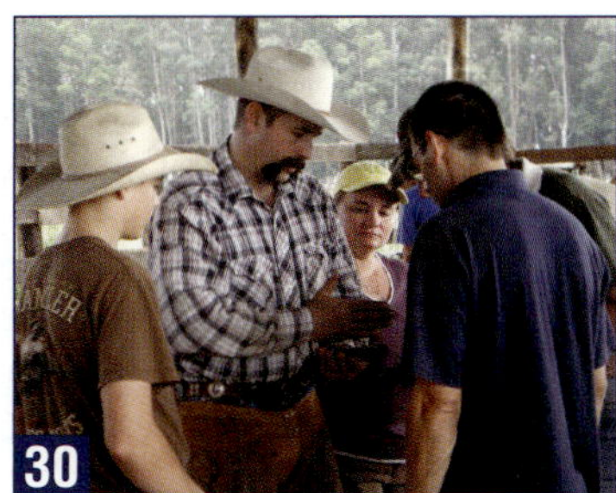

Explaining to an AFB candidate what we are looking for on a shoe.

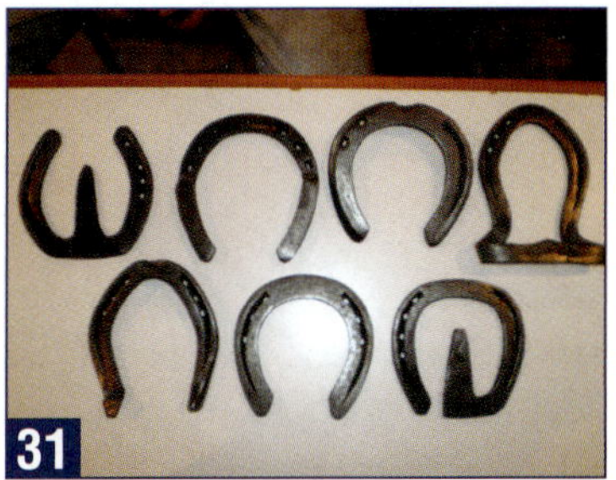

AFB Graduate Farrier shoe display.

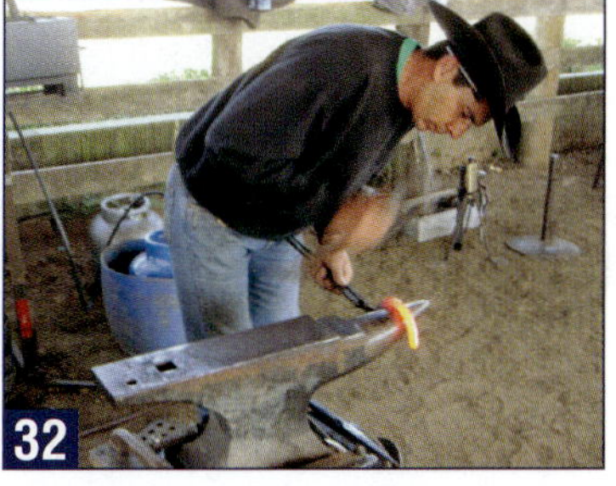

President of the AFB, and one of the first two men to pass the Graduate Farrier exam, Flavio Souza.

those who have attempted the exam have learned a lot from the process.

Farrier International Testing System (FITS)

Beyond those mentioned, I have put together something I call FITS for use by other countries that want to have an exam. This test is offered at two levels and is very close to the exams that I wrote for the AFB. The main difference is that FITS has a photographic element as part of the candidate's record, which I feel will make the exam fairer. Any examiners will be putting their name to the job, and if there is a photo of a great job that fails, or a lousy job that passes, it will be on record. The trial run for this system was held for the South African Farrier's Association in November of 2010, and it was a resounding success. The top level is referred to as the Advanced Skills Farrier, or ASF.

Another cool thing that has happened with the advent of the FITS exam is that the farriers who

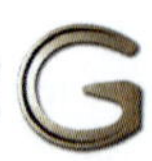

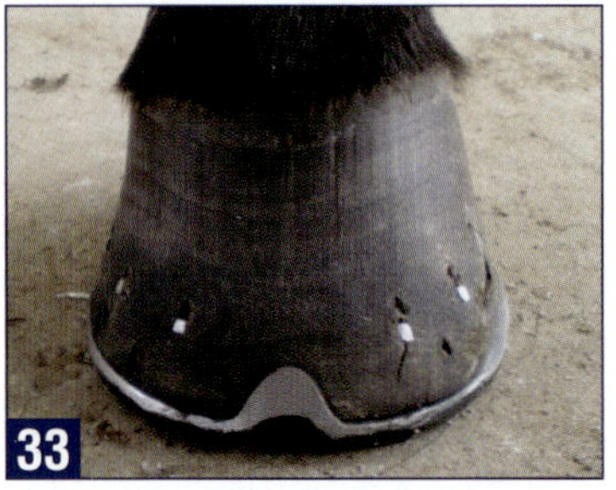

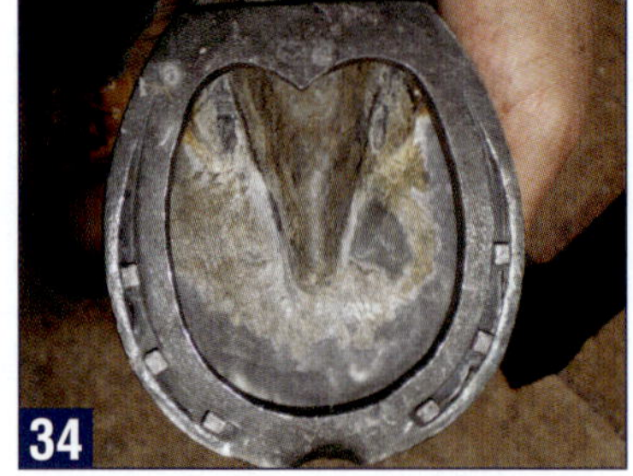

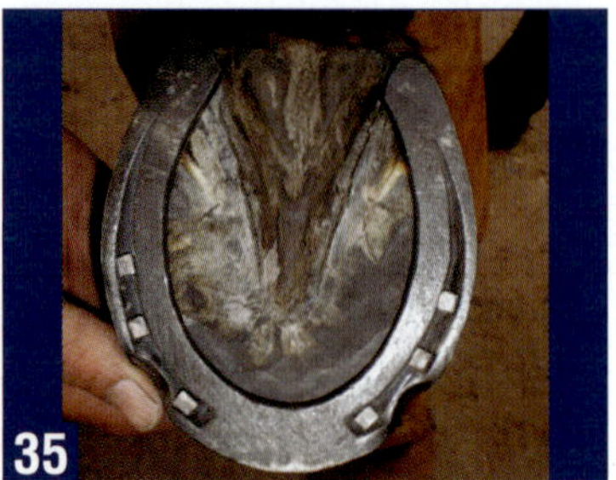

Pictures of Flavio's passing shoeing

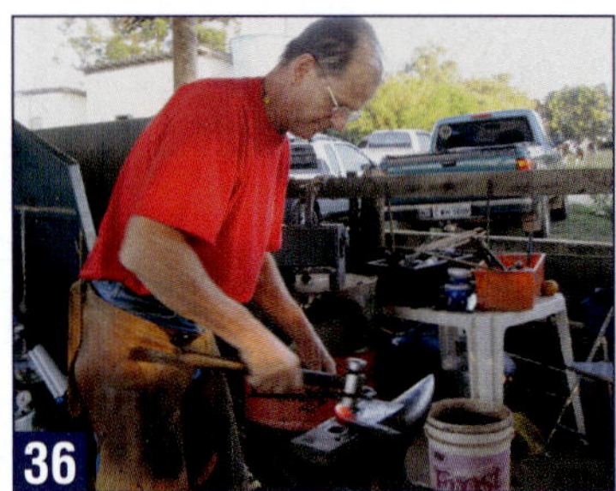

Vice President of the AFB, and one of the first two men to pass the Graduate Farrier Exam, Fabio Furquim.

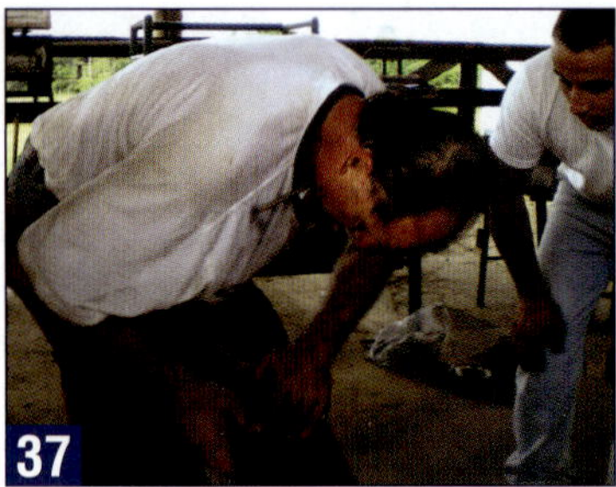

Fabio working.

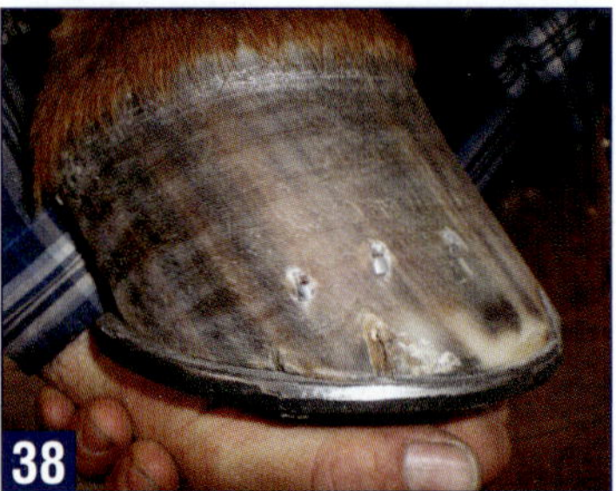

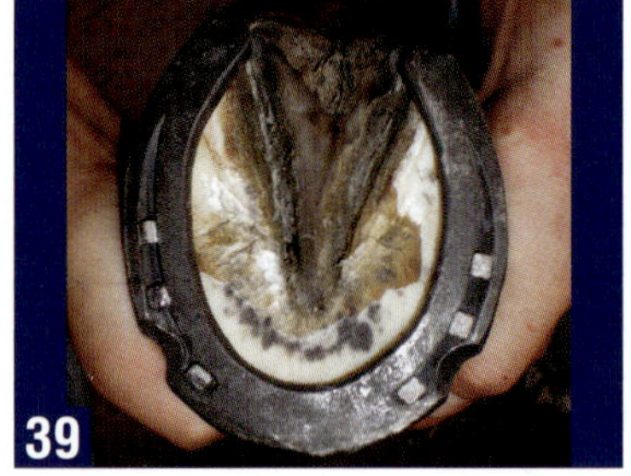

Pictures of Fabio's passing job.

pass a level in one country are accepted at that level in the other participating countries. Also, a member of the AFB could travel to South Africa to take the exam, and vice versa. It is a pretty neat thing to see happening in the international farrier community.

STRATEGIES FOR TAKING A PRACTICAL FARRIER EXAM

The first thing that any candidate should do is to read and understand the rules governing an exam. There should not be any doubt about what is being tested, what is considered a good job, and what the candidate can be failed for. With this knowledge, let's take the AFB Graduate Farrier exam as an example, and go about devising a strategy for taking the test.

This exam requires a candidate to shoe two hind feet with fullered, quarter clipped, handmade shoes. Those are a given and can be practiced at length. The front feet can be a pair of several different bar shoes, so the candidate has to prepare for at least four scenarios. Preparation should find the candidate making several pairs of each type of bar shoe to different patterns and keeping track of the time it takes to make the shoes. The candidate should also come to the exam with bar stock cut and marked at different lengths. I like to have bar stock in lengths from 10 inches to 12.5 inches in half-inch increments for the hinds, and from 13 to 16 inches in half-inch increments for the bar shoes. I will also have a few long bars in the event that my horse has a foot beyond the norm.

For our example, let's say that the candidate drew the straight bars from the hat, and there is a 2.5-hour time limit for shoeing the horse with the straight bars in front and the fullered shoes behind. I would begin by trimming three feet completely, as well as the bottom of the fourth foot. With only the dressing of the fourth foot remaining, I would put the stock for the front bar shoes in the fire, return to the horse to dress the foot, and finish the trim. The stock is heating while I am dressing, and my holder can call for the judge while I begin making the shoes. There will always be one foot that you will like better than the others. I always let my holder know which foot that is, so he can present the horse in such a manner that the judge sees my best foot first. This sets up a better score due to human nature.

No time was lost waiting on a heat. I allow myself six minutes per foot or a total of 24 minutes for the trim.

I should be able to make and fit the straight bars in 40 minutes, so I work on the bar shoes until they are done, then place the stock for the hind shoes in the fire as I am finishing the bar shoes. I want to insure that I get a look at the shoes cold before the examiner, so I take the minute needed to have a cold look, check nail holes, and have my holder call for the examiner. Again, handing the best shoe for the best foot to the judge first creates that good impression.

While the examiner is judging the fit, I am working on the hinds. Again, no time was lost, and I should be right around an hour and five minutes into the job. It will take about 30 minutes to make and fit the hinds, so I work on them until they are ready. I give the hinds a cold look, check nail holes, and have my holder call for the judge while I am nailing up the fronts.

Nailing will require only about a minute per shoe, and I love to have three minutes to clinch. This means that 16 minutes is plenty for finishing the entire horse, so we should be on a good pace here. When the examiner gets to the horse, I stop, have a short break while the hinds are checked, and this is a good time to wipe away the sweat, take a drink, and have a breather. By the time the examiner is done with the hinds, I should have plenty time to nail and finish the horse.

As you can see from this timeline, there is a lot of time to do the job if everything falls into place. I suggest that you do some horses as if you were being examined, keep close track of your times, and try to get them to fall into the schedule I just laid out. If you are working on the AFA CJF, the same schedule can easily work. Just shorten the time for making the fronts.

The key to any of these exams is in the fit. More time is lost on fitting shoes than any other portion of the exam. Never take a shoe to the horse without a clip if a clip is called for. I have seen so many people take a lot of time to make the perfect fit without clips, waste time checking it, and then ruin their shape when they went back to the anvil to pull a clip. Go ahead and trust yourself to clip the shoe and take it to the horse with the clips ready to burn.

As with everything in life worth having, there is work involved. If it were easy, it would not have any value, and everyone would have the title. Anyone can achieve it if they are willing to work. Find a mentor that can and will help you, take some prep courses, and surround yourself with great farriers to become a great farrier. Diligent, correct, and constant practice will help you achieve your dreams.

Chapter

63 TEST QUESTIONS

One of the best ways to learn anything is to study the questions and standards of that thing so that you can make certain that you are learning the right subject matter. With that in mind, I have included numerous questions here that I have used on tests for years, as well as several that I have included as part of the AWCF Prep Courses. Mike Miller, CJF, FWCF, added about 20 of these questions when he helped me with one of the prep courses.

Mark Watson, AWCF, the Sargeant Major of Farriery at the Defence Animal Centre in Melton Mowbray, United Kingdom, put together a prep course for AWCF candidates that had some very good information in it about the definition of exact words when taking an exam. I am including it here with his permission. Understanding what exactly is being asked is the first step to having a successful answer. Here is the basic outline of test preparation that Mark created. I have added and changed some of it to suit me, but the basics are all from Mark.

THE PAPER

- Read the test twice
- Make notes
- Answer an easy question first
- Be aware of the time
- Leave at least half a page between answers. By doing this, you can add more to the answer if it occurs to you, or if time allows.
- Write legibly
- Allow time for checking answers
- Make certain that you answer all required questions
- If time is short, get something down.

TYPES OF ANSWERS

- **Essay:** Write the answer as if you were doing a report.
- **List:** This is a fast and simple way to answer, but you can embellish on each item if you have the time.
- **Illustration:** Practice drawing diagrams and make them appropriate to the question. A diagram of an anatomical structure should be fairly accurate, while a diagram of a conformational defect may be as simple as a stick figure.

UNDERSTANDING THE WORDS IN THE QUESTION

- **Define –** State or show precisely the meaning of.
- **List –** Catalog or inventory the items of a class in a logical format.
- **Describe –** Give characteristics in words.
- **Explain –** Give the full details in an understandable, logical format that is written as if you were explaining to someone with no prior knowledge of the subject.
- **Discuss –** Consider the subject from several points of view, giving supporting evidence from each stance.
- **Illustrate –** Use a drawing or diagram.
- **Compare –** Evaluate similarities and differences between different subjects.
- **Contrast –** Reveal differences, similarities, and opposing qualities. Similar to compare, but with more detail.
- **Note –** A short record or statement about the subjects.

Beyond this, it is common for an exam to ask you to fully describe, or contrast in detail, or explain completely, etc., to give emphasis to the question and the desired answer. By knowing the exact definition of what the test is asking, you are better able to give an appropriate answer. This allows you to spend the time where you should.

If you are a student, learn this information cold and there won't be much that the teacher can ask you that you won't be able to answer. If you are an educator, you can pluck your test from these pages. I hope that you are able to get some good from the experience of taking these test questions and giving a complete answer. Be aware that this is only a sampling, and it would be easy to simply ask many of the same questions about other anatomical structures, conformations, or pathologies.

1. Describe the tendons of the pelvic limb.
2. Describe in detail the tendons of the thoracic limb.
3. Explain the concussion-reducing structures in the foot.
4. What are the effects of uneven weight bearing in the forelimb?
5. Describe in detail the functions and parts of the foot.
6. Explain the reciprocal apparatus and stay apparatus.
7. From where does the hoof wall grow? Fully describe this process.
8. What are the sesamoidian ligaments, and how do they function?
9. Discuss the horny hoof and the coriums that produce it.
10. What are the types of synovial joints in the limb, how do they work, and give examples.
11. What is meant by the term "natural angle," and how can it be achieved?
12. Describe the state and function of the 3rd phalanx.
13. What is the position and function of the digital cushion?
14. Defend the position of leaving horses barefoot at all times.
15. Compare the use of a leather pad to pour-in pad material such as Equi-Pak.
16. Fully describe the anatomy of the carpus.
17. Define pedal osteitis, and explain how a farrier can help a horse with this condition.
18. Describe the differences and similarities between the front and hind legs.
19. What is the approach that a farrier should take when trimming a neglected horse suffering from chronic laminitis?
20. What are splints, how do they occur, and how can they be dealt with?
21. Describe in detail the anatomy of the navicular bursa. Include the radiographic anatomy in your answer.
22. Describe any differences between the foot of a donkey and the foot of a horse. When a donkey's foot has been neglected, how do you trim that foot?
23. What is meant by the term:
    A.) Breakover
    B.) Point of breakover
    C.) Time of breakover

    Include at least two diagrams. How can farriery speed up breakover, or can it? Suggest four reasons for doing so if it can be done.
24. Define and describe the following conditions that may affect the hind limb of a horse: Stringhalt, shivering, locking patella, bone spavin.
25. List the various angular limb deformities that may affect a young foal. Discuss fully how you would manage a 3 week old foal with unilateral carpal valgus, including your reasoning.
26. Discuss how vertical hoof cracks develop. Describe in detail how you would treat a quarter crack that involved the full thickness of the wall, including the coronary band and the sole.
27. Discuss how you would shoe the following:
    A.) Fractured P3 in the hind limb.
    B.) Horse that has had surgery for a penetrating wound to the navicular bursa.
    C.) Badly sheared heels.
    D.) Early onset degenerative joint disease of the proximal interphalangeal joint.
28. Discuss indications for using the heart bar, describe how to fit a heart bar, and list possible alternative shoes or shoeing systems that would perform a similar function.
29. Describe what a keratoma is, where it occurs, how it affects a foot, and how a vet-farrier team could deal with it.
30. Fully describe the pedal bone.
31. Discuss shoeing strategies for a foot with bad corns in both heels.
32. How is bone formed? Explain the anatomy of a long bone in the horses' leg. Compare the third metacarpal to the distal phalanx. Include diagrams.
33. Describe in detail the epidermal hoof wall, growth, structure and function.
34. Describe each of the following and how a farrier could help a horse with these conditions:
    A. Seedy toe
    B. Quittor
    C. Canker

D. Side bone

35. Write an essay on how a farrier can cause foot lameness.
36. Explain how a farrier can help a horse with rotation of the pedal bone using modern materials.
37. Describe in detail the circulation of the blood in the horse's forelimb from the knee downward. How can uneven weight bearing affect the circulation?
38. What causes a hoof to flare? How can it be corrected?
39. Describe the articulation of the metacarpophalangeal joint and name all the tendons and ligaments involved.
40. Describe the articulation of the distal interphalangeal joint and the function of the ligaments and tendons involved.
41. Describe in detail the circulation of the blood and lymph in the lower limb.
42. Describe the function and all elements of the stay apparatus.
43. What do you understand by "a broken back hoof pastern axis?" Why might a horse have differing hoof/pastern angles and axis in its front feet?
44. A horse fore foot is described as being "toed-in and base narrow". How would you expect it to move? How would you expect the hoof to be shaped?
45. What is the function of (a) the Bars (b) the White Line (c) the Periople
46. What effects does laminitis have on the structures and functions of the foot?
47. A horse has asymmetrical front feet. What may be the causes?
48. Describe the structure of the frog, its relationship to other parts of the foot, and its functions.
49. Radiography shows that a horse has a sagittal fracture of the pedal bone of a hind foot. What are the principles of treatment? Describe how a farrier can assist the healing process.
50. What would make you suspect that a horse was suffering from a developing infection under the sole? How can a farrier help?
51. Give the uses for mediolateral extensions. Describe the different methods of making them.
52. What do you understand by the expression "collapsed heels?" What may be the causes? How would you shoe for it?
53. How would a horse that turns out the toes of its forelimb move? What effect would it have on the limb if not corrected? How could it be corrected?
54. For what purposes are studs used? What problems may result from their use over a long period of time?
55. Describe five different types of pathological shoes and their intended use. What are the advantages and disadvantages of each?

As an added bonus, the Worshipful Company of Farriers (WCF) has allowed me to print an

Associateship of the Worshipful Company of Farriers (AWCF) and a Diploma of the Worshipful Company of Farriers (DipWCF) exams in their entirety. This should serve as a warning that you don't want to come to one of their exams unprepared. I think that you will be impressed when you get a look at just what kind of standards these folks represent. Both of these exams are in the exact format that a candidate will receive when they sit the exams, from the color of the paper to the exact wording. The WCF exams change from exam to exam, so these exams are examples of some that have already been given to candidates. It is great to have a testing body that holds such high standards of knowledge, as you can see from these examples on the following pages.

THE WORSHIPFUL COMPANY OF FARRIERS

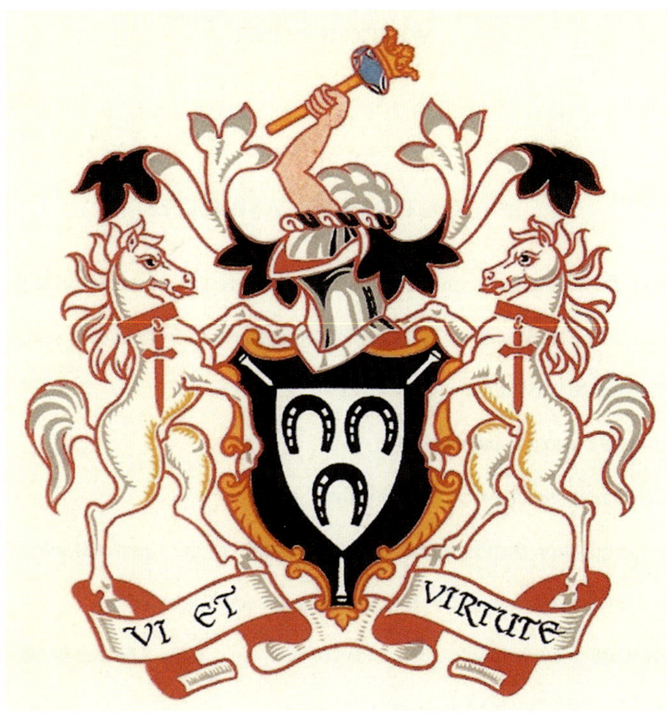

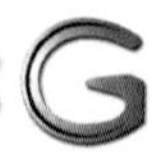

THE WORSHIPFUL COMPANY OF FARRIERS

8

First established as a Fellowship by the Court of Mayor & Aldermen 1356
Incorporated by Charter of King Charles II 1674
Supplemental Charter granted by H.M. Queen Elizabeth II 1983

ASSOCIATESHIP EXAMINATION (THEORY)

WRITTEN PAPER

INSTRUCTIONS TO CANDIDATES

1. Do NOT state your name on the Answer Book or on any of the additional papers.
2. The Candidate must answer AT LEAST ONE question from EACH section.
3. The Candidate is required to answer FIVE questions.
4. All questions carry equal marks.
5. Questions may be answered in any order.
6. Insert the question number in the left-hand margin of the Answer Book.
7. Draw a line across the page before answering a new question.
8. Answers are to be written on both sides of the pages in the Answer Book.
9. TIME ALLOWED – 2 hours and 30 minutes.

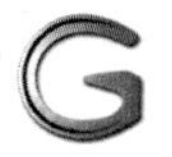

THE WORSHIPFUL COMPANY OF FARRIERS

First established as a Fellowship by the Court of Mayor & Aldermen 1356
Incorporated by Charter of King Charles II 1674
Supplemental Charter granted by H.M. Queen Elizabeth II 1983

2

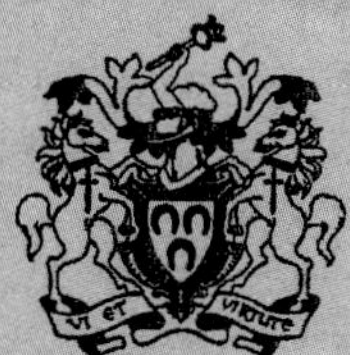

ASSOCIATESHIP EXAMINATION (THEORY)
15th October 2007

Questions

<u>SECTION A</u>. Anatomy.

1. Describe in detail the anatomy of the navicular bursa and its associated structures. Include the radiographic anatomy in your answer. *(20 marks)*

2. Draw and label cross sections (transverse) of the gross anatomy of the limb at the following locations:-
    a) Just distal to (below) the carpus. *(6 marks)*
    b) Just proximal to (above) the proximal (abaxial) sesamoids. *(6 marks)*
    c) Just distal to (below) the fetlock joint. *(8 marks)*

<u>SECTION B</u>. Physiology and Function.

3. You have been asked to speak to a meeting of the British Horse Society on the subject, 'All horses should go bare foot'. Outline the arguments that you would give for and against this statement. *(20 marks)*

4. Describe the gross changes that occur in a horse's foot affected by chronic laminitis – describe how these changes are thought to occur. *(20 marks)*

5. For each of the following state how the condition can be identified and its cause. Briefly suggest ONE shoeing plan to help each problem.
    a) Contraction of the deep digital flexor tendon. *(5 Marks)*
    b) A medial suppurative corn. *(5 Marks)*
    c) A shoe boil (capped elbow). *(5 Marks)*
    d) A seedy toe. *(5 Marks)*

<u>SECTION C</u>. Farriery Theory.

6. How would you assist a veterinary surgeon in treating a horse with:-
    a) A completely severed superficial digital flexor tendon in a hind leg. *(10 marks)*
    b) A horse that has had a deep flexor tendon tenotomy (surgical transection) for chronic laminitis in a fore leg. *(10 marks)*

7. A veterinary surgeon asks for your advice on appropriate shoeing for a 7 year old hunter that has recently been diagnosed with bilateral degenerative joint disease of the distal intertarsal joint (spavin). How would you expect the horse to move? What would your preferred shoeing plan be and why? What other methods of shoeing could be used? *(20 marks)*

8. Describe with the aid of diagrams the various types of PEDAL bone fracture that can occur. *(7 marks)* From your own experience discuss how a farrier may help in the treatment of one of these fractures. *(13 marks)*

THE WORSHIPFUL COMPANY OF FARRIERS

First established as a Fellowship by the Court of Mayor & Aldermen 1356
Incorporated by Charter of King Charles II 1674
Supplemental Charter granted by H.M. Queen Elizabeth II 1983

66

FARRIERY DIPLOMA EXAMINATION

WRITTEN PAPER

10:00 – 12:30 on Friday 16 January 2009

INSTRUCTIONS TO CANDIDATES

1. *Do NOT state your name on the Answer Book or on any additional paper.*
2. *Answers are to be written in the Answer Book on both sides of the pages.*
3. *Insert the question number in the left-hand margin of the Answer Book and on any additional papers.*
4. *Answer ALL questions.*
5. *Questions may be answered in any order.*
6. *Note the different marks carried by different parts of the questions.*
7. *Draw a line across the page before starting a new question.*
8. *TIME ALLOWED is two-and-a-half hours.*

QUESTIONS

(Marks)

1. Describe both of the following conditions and suggest how a farrier and veterinary surgeon might work together to treat them.
   a) Navicular disease / syndrome. (10 Marks)
   b) A septic pipe corn of the medial heel. (10 Marks)

2. Describe, using diagrams to help, how a horse moves in each of the following gaits: The walk, trot, canter, and gallop. Explain which of these gaits is the most useful in determining if a horse is sound, giving your reasons. (20 Marks)

3. Describe, in detail, the blood supply to, and venous drainage from, the lower limb and foot from the CARPUS downwards. You may use diagrams D & E supplied to assist your answer and / or draw your own. (20 Marks)

4. Describe in detail, remembering to mention foot preparation, style of shoe, and material used, how you would shoe both in front and behind:-
   a) Working hunter. (10 Marks)
   b) A hackney driving horse for road work. (10 Marks)

5. Answer all of the following:-
   a) What is a splint, and what causes them? (5 Marks)
   b) What is bone spavin? Briefly describe how an affected horse moves. (5 Marks)
   c) What is a sand crack? Suggest possible causes. (5 Marks)
   d) What is epiphysitis? How can it be recognised? (5 Marks)

I am also including an exam from the Association of Brazilian Farriers (Associacao Dos Ferradores Do Brasil), which had their first exam in 2008. I was extremely lucky to be selected to write and administer their certification, so this exam is exactly as it appeared for them, although it was translated into Portuguese by Dr. Claudia Leschonski. I was amazed at the level of knowledge the Brazilian farrier was able to express through this test, and there was a very high success rate. These exams serve as an example of the international tests that I administer as part of the FITS exams. These are discussed in **Chapter 63, Practical Testing Strategies.**

BRAZILIAN
FARRIERS ASSOCIATION

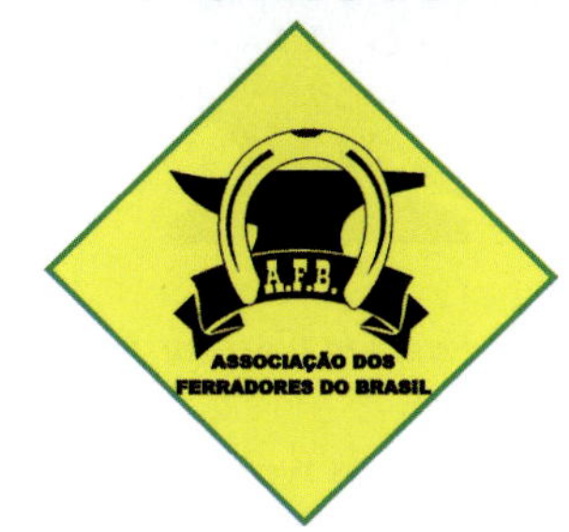

Graduate Farrier Written Test 2

Answer 5 questions from each section, 10 questions total.

Section A. Anatomy:

1. List at least 20 ligaments below the knee or hock.
2. Draw the sesamoidian ligaments.
3. Draw and label the parts of a bone.
4. Describe in detail the relationship of the palmar tendons to changes in hoof pastern axis.
5. Draw and label the pelvic limb, including the dorsal tendons.
6. Describe the vascular system as it pertains to the hoof.
7. Draw and describe the navicular ligaments.
8. Explain the coriums and the insensitive structures of the foot.
9. Draw and label the bones and joints in the carpus from at least 2 views.
10. Describe in detail the concussion reducing structures in the pelvic limb.

Section B. Horseshoeing:

1. Describe spavin in the hock, and strategies for shoeing a spavined horse.
2. How would you treat a horse that has a bowed deep flexor tendon?
3. Give the treatment and shoeing options for a horse with quittor.
4. What is happening when a horse has sesamoiditis, and how can a farrier help?
5. Explain the shoeing and treatment options for a horse with a sprained suspensory ligament on the pelvic limb.
6. Describe in detail the uses and applications of patten bar shoes.
7. What shoeing strategies can be used for shoeing a horse with sloping heels.
8. What can cause navicular syndrome, and what can a farrier do for a horse diagnosed with navicular?
9. What has happened to a horse that is stifled, and what are the treatment options.
10. How can a farrier help a horse with a new, bleeding, quarter crack.

This final test is one of the tests that I give to my 24-week students in the Journeyman Farrier Course. I have multiple versions, and if you are a Journeyman Farrier Course student who is right now reading this, I would not count on getting one of these exact exams.

HEARTLAND
HORSESHOEING SCHOOL

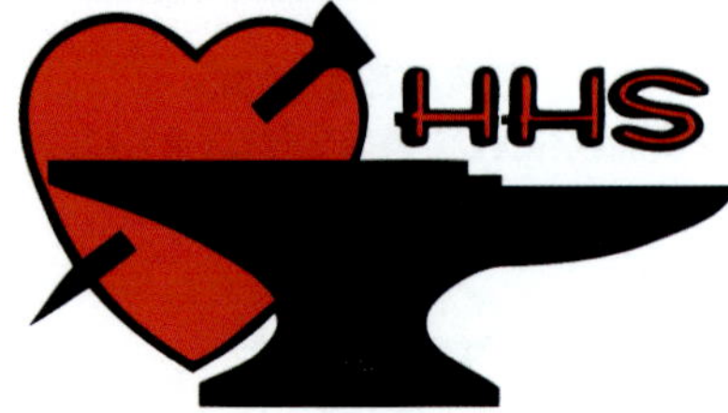

Journeyman Farrier Course Final Exam II

Answer 5 questions, one from each section, as well as 2 additional questions of your choice.

QUESTIONS:

Section A:

1. Discuss the position, composition and function of the horny sole, white line and horny frog.
2. Name the tendons that flex the limbs, describing their origin, insertion and function for both front and hind. Explain the properties of these tendons as well.

Section B:

1. Describe and discuss the anti-concussion mechanism of the horses fore limb.
2. Explain the nerve and blood supply of the hoof, as well as the effect on hoof growth.
3. Discuss the anatomical effects of uneven weight bearing on the forelimb.

Section C:

1. State the difference between unilateral and bilateral sidebone, as well as the type of shoeing demanded for these maladies.
2. In what instances would you use a heart bar? Discuss advantages and disadvantages.
3. Give the what, when, where, why and how for the use of a hospital plate.

There is a lot more to being a good farrier than just the physical and practical aspect. I hope these questions inspire you to study hard to improve your knowledge of the craft and encourage you to pursue some testing that will make and keep you sharp.

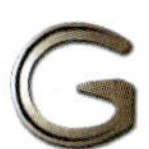

Chapter 64

JUDGING

As you progress in this profession, there will come a time when your skills and abilities are recognized to the point that you will be called upon to judge other farriers. When this happens to you, take it as the honor it is and do your best to avoid being condescending and arrogant about it.

I will always remember with disdain some of the people in this industry who tried to belittle me when I was a beginner and felt small enough already. But, I will also remember with great respect and admiration those who were accepting and welcoming. Everyone is reading these words fits into the picture somewhere. For the beginner, you have as much right to be a farrier as anyone else (courtesy Danny Ward), and for the veteran, help that beginner become a leader in this trade by being a good example. You never know when you just might be teaching a future world champion to pull a clip or make a heel.

The first contest I legitimately judged was in Hutchison, Kansas, in 1994. Man, did I learn a lot. Unfortunately, it was at the expense of the competitors. First, I learned that you have to go with your gut instinct and make sure that you can live with how you place the shoes and feet. Second, it is a lot more fun to compete than it is to judge. And finally, the people who compete have willingly made themselves vulnerable to your judgment, and that is a great responsibility. When I was done with that contest, I was absolutely spent.

Everything went well except for the draft class. I had been advised to judge based on what would be the easiest to fix. With that approach, a shoe that was out of level would be easier to fix than a shoe that had a bad shape. Bad shape would be easier to fix than bad nails, etc. This is a good method, but it should be only one part of how you judge. Just as in trimming feet, if you tried to apply the old advice to always take the heels to the widest, highest part of the frog, there would be some horses that you would cripple in the attempt. When judging others, use several criteria to make certain that the best work wins, or passes the exam, as the case may be.

I placed that draft class in Hutchinson, and later, didn't like the way they looked as I had placed them. That one bad class has haunted me ever since, but I think it was good for me. (Sorry to those that were in it, though.)

With shoeing, I don't want to leave a horse with something that will keep me up at night. With judging, I also want to get my sleep. If you can't arrive at that place, you don't want to be a judge. The insomnia alone will kill you.

I recommend that every judge should evaluate at least one class in front of the competitors, preferably before the contest, so that everyone will know what you are looking for. When you do that, it helps to level the playing field (**Figure 1**).

When that is impossible, try your best to keep the shoes in order so that you can talk to the competitors after the contest. Leaving a contest without

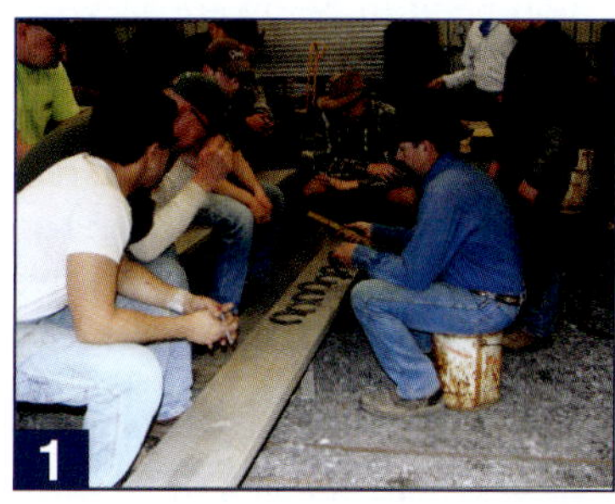

Judging the shoes in front of the competitors.

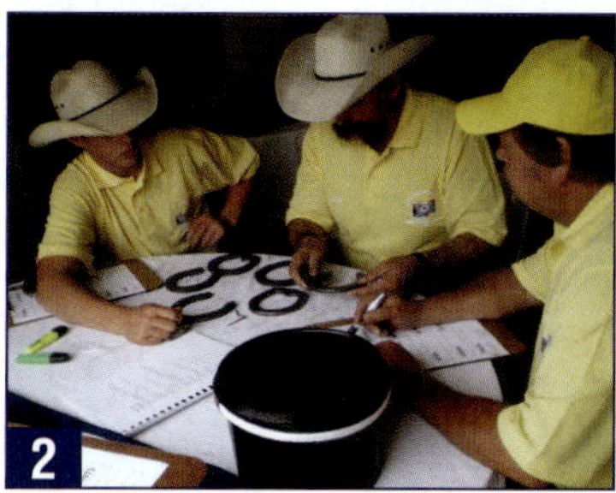

Laying out the shoes.

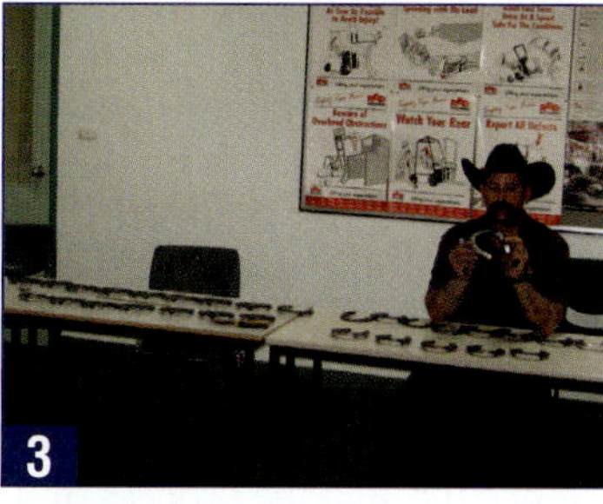

Judging the forging at a contest in Australia.

a ribbon can be hard for a lot of competitors, but if they leave with some insight, they will be more content **(Figure 2)**.

Every time you judge farriery, you are having an impact on the future of this industry. If it is done negatively, the impact is negative. On the bright side, the opposite is true. There have been a lot of potentially great farriers decide to stay out of contests and certifications over one small incident they suffered at the hands of a judge with a weekend badge. Imagine if someone would have chased Bob Marshall away when he was a beginner. The craft would have missed the opportunity to have his insight and contributions.

JUDGING SHOES

Here is the process I now use to judge shoes. I lay out all of the similar shoes in the class **(Figure 3)**. They are ground surface up to start, and I go through quickly to see if there are any that can be tossed off the table — for instance, a shoe with a toe clip when the class called for quarter clips. I get rid of all the shoes that are missing elements, then I place the shoes with a quick glance from first to last.

All of the shoes are then turned over, and I quickly put the badly punched shoes at the bottom. If I have a heel nail inside center of the stock or too far back, that shoe will move right down the line.

Once all of that is done, I judge my last placed shoe against the shoe just ahead of it. I look at level, nail fit, nail placement, shape, finish, forging, and overall quality. All of these are part of the equation, and when one item is to be weighted more than another, that should be explained ahead of time. If I find that this shoe is a better shoe than the one that was placed ahead of it, I will change their places.

From that point, I judge the second to last against the third to last, and so on, right up the line. Grant Moon told me he plays a game when he does this of trying to get the last shoe into first place. That is a good thing to think about as you do this. Once you are done, pick up two random shoes, let's say third and seventh. Judge those two against each other to make sure that there is a good distance between them and you feel good with the results.

If time is not important, I leave everything on the table and take a little break. Then I come back and go through the process of judging again. I do it quickly on my second pass. I am just making sure that I will be sleeping when I go to bed.

KNOW THE JUDGE

When I am going to a contest, I try to know as much about that judge as possible. If you have a good idea of what a particular judge finds important, you can try and mimic the style that judge likes. For instance, Dallas Morgan, CJF, a great friend of mine from New York by way of Australia, really likes flat. He judged me in a contest one time, and I saw just how much emphasis he put on level. It was much more than I do when I judge, but that is fine. It is his particular style, and I respect his judging immensely. Anyway, I placed a distant second in the first class, based primarily on level. For the rest of the day, every shoe I turned in was as flat as I could possibly make it. I have a buckle to show just how flat those shoes were.

I am also picky about who I allow to judge my work. If you go to a contest that is being judged by someone you do not respect, the results of the contest are meaningless. For Convention or Calgary, you may have to go even if you don't really respect the judges just because of the venue, but I won't waste the time at a local contest with an incompetent judge. The winner may as well have his or her name pulled out of a hat. Since I feel that way, it is a huge honor for me to judge someone else. When a competitor is willing to put their work in front of me, I really appreciate it.

JUDGING HORSES

Judging horses can be trickier than judging shoes because everyone does not get to start with the same thing. With a shoe, everyone gets a certain type and size of stock. This allows you to judge the craftsmanship that each competitor could apply to that piece of steel. With horses, there can be a huge difference, not only with the feet, but with the attitude of the horses as well **(Figures 4-6)**.

Because of this, you need to be aware of what each person started with. It is not an exact science, but they did invite you for your opinion, so that is what you have to give them. I like to look at the feet with the competitor prior to the exam or contest so that I know what they started with. Also, I always pencil in the scores of the first two or three horses that I judge. I then go back and re-evaluate the feet after I have looked at a few more. It is amazing how badly the first few people will be scored in most contests. It comes down to human nature, and going back to the feet will prevent my human nature from

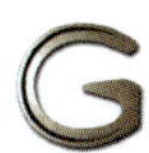

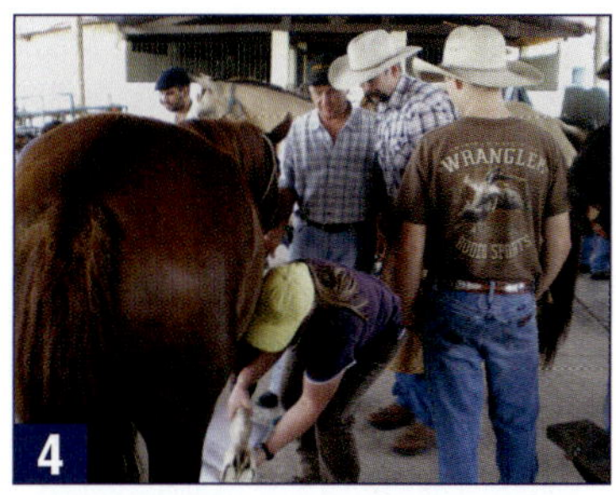

Kelly judging the feet during an Association of Brazilian Farriers certification in Brazil.

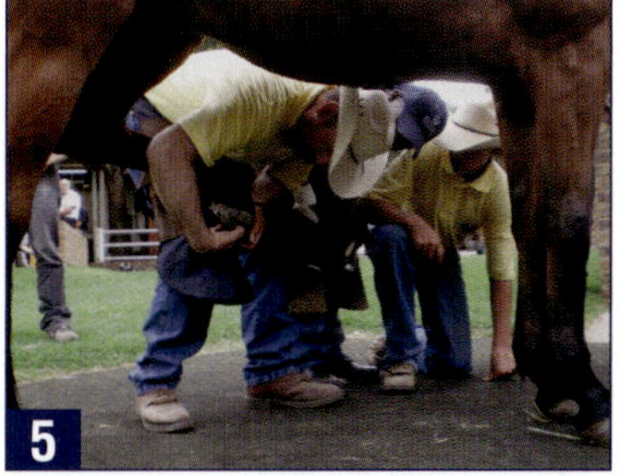

Judging the shoeing at a contest in South Africa.

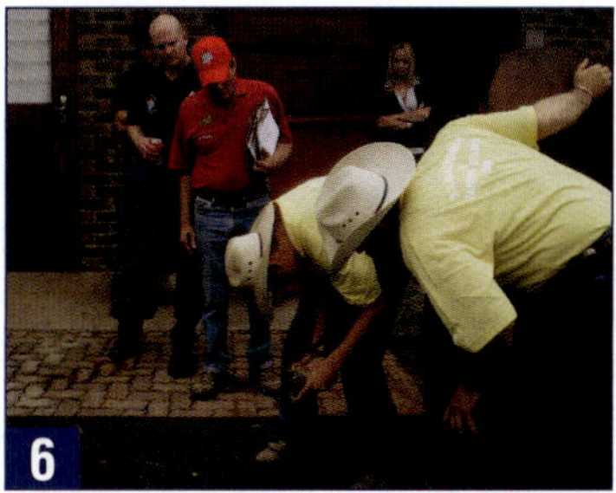

Cody judging the horses in South Africa.

making a bad call just because it is the first horse I am looking at.

Anytime it is possible, I like to at least trim a foot for the competitors so that they can be comfortable knowing what I see as just good, basic work. Farriery is not rocket surgery, so try to do good clean work when you do clinics, and hopefully you will get to judge good clean work in the contest **(Figure 7)**.

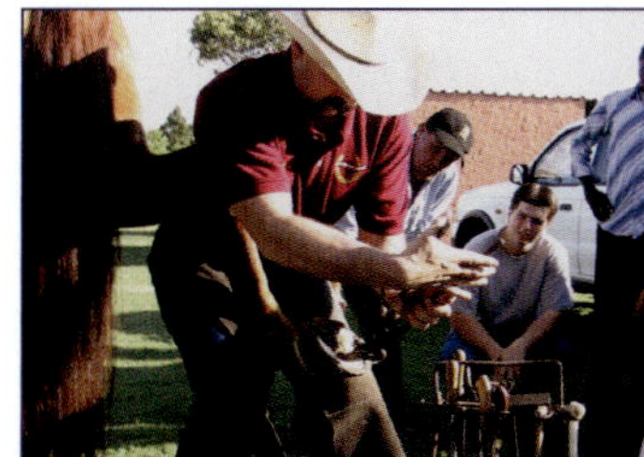

Trimming a foot at a clinic.

When you are getting judged on a horse, you can use a few tricks to help you out. First, make sure that you have a good holder, someone that can handle horses and guide the judge to see your best work first. My holder should know which foot is best, and then call the judge when they are standing on that side of the horse. If there is a mediolateral balance problem on a front foot, the holder can help me by turning the horse's head. The holder can also hurt me by turning the head if everything is perfect.

When you are competing on a bad horse, warn the judge or steward before they pick up the feet. This is common courtesy, but not doing it will cause the judge to be thinking other things when he gets under your horse. Also, don't call for a judge if you are not ready to be judged. The person judging the contest is going to get to do enough walking around, and having them come to your horse when you are not ready is not a good idea.

JUDGING YOUR OWN WORK

You can gain a lot becoming a critical and accurate judge of your own work. For many in the farrier industry, isolation hampers growth. There is a saying about some of the old time farriers with a low level of skill. It is said that they shod horses for one year, 25 years in a row. This basically means that they stopped learning and improving, and never achieved the level they could have. Their skill level never improves because the industry does not require it. There is such a large demand for farriers, that a person who is willing to do this job can make a living, even if their skills are substandard. It can be very hard for isolated farriers to judge the quality of their own work since they may be unaware of what work done to a high standard looks like. It is imperative for these farriers to expose themselves to farrier associations, periodicals, and textbooks, as well as other competent tradesmen.

For the beginner, the exposure is even more important, as the horse-owning public continues to become better educated about the differences that exist between the skill levels of various farriers. Regardless of how well a book is written or how clear the pictures are, there is no way to replace one-on-one instruction from a skilled craftsman. Finding those skilled individuals and spending some time in their shops is the best advice I can give when it comes to learning how to judge your own work.

There are a few things that can be expressed in text to help you learn how to critique your skills in the forge. To judge symmetry of a shoe, try placing the shoe on a piece of paper and tracing around the outside edge with a colored pen or pencil **(Figure 8)**. Turn the shoe over and trace around it again with

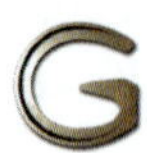

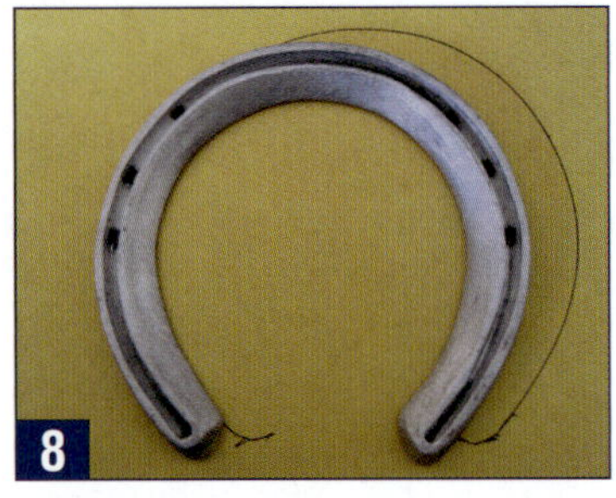

Shoe that has been traced around with a pen.

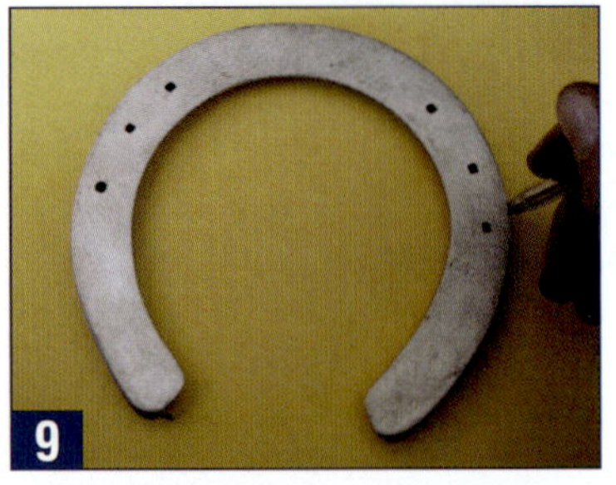

Turning the shoe over to trace with a different colored pen.

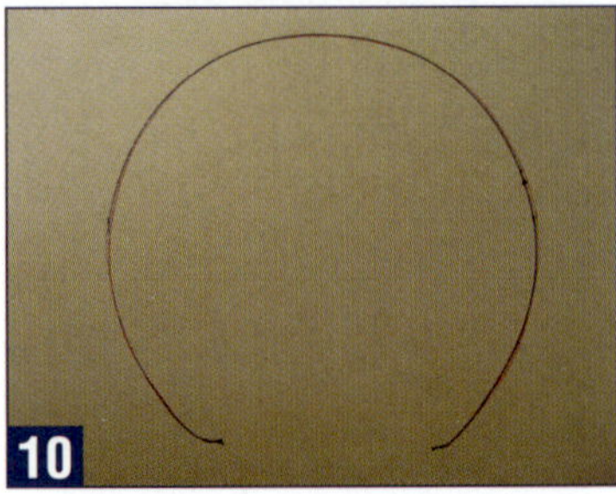

The results that show very little asymmetry.

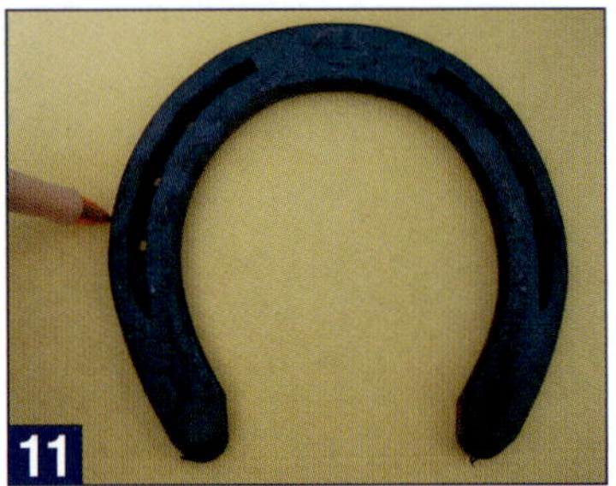

Mustad Basic front.

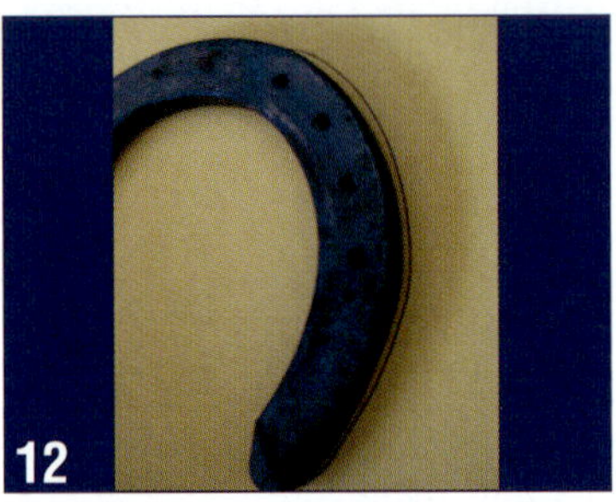

Traced the other way.

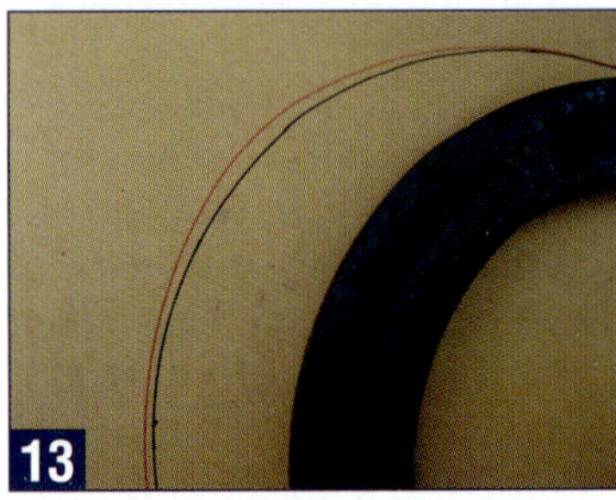

The difference in symmetry that is part of the shoe designed for a right front foot.

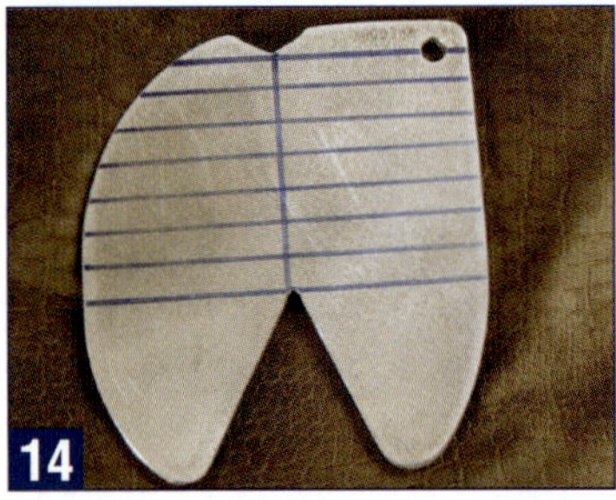

The plate that Kent Misner, CJF, gave me.

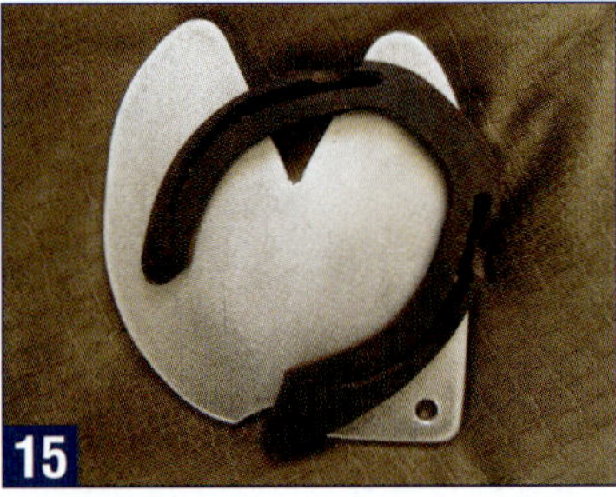

Placing a shoe with quarter clips on the plate.

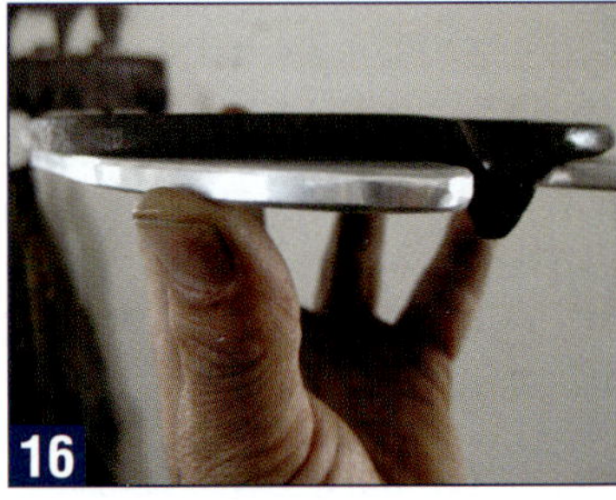

Shoe out of level.

a different color **(Figure 9)**. Any discrepancies in the shape of the shoe will then show up by the gap between the two lines **(Figure 10)**. Whatever the distance is between the lines is actually twice the amount of error in the shoe. Ideally, one line will be exactly superimposed over the other. The aluminum shoe pictured is quite symmetrical, and there is little variation. The second shoe is a Mustad pre-shaped keg shoe that is made for a right foot. The dimple in the crease behind the last nail indicates the lateral side **(Figure 11)**. Since this shoe is designed to be for a side, it is intentionally asymmetrical. You can see how much by the differences in the two lines **(Figures 12-13)**. This shoe is out of symmetry exactly half the distance between the red and black lines in **Figure 13**.

To judge level, cut out a plate of aluminum or steel approximately seven inches by seven inches. It may be helpful to cut out an area on one edge to accommodate shoes with clips, as well as large frogs **(Figure 14-15)**. Lay the finished shoe on the plate and hold it so that you can see whether the shoe matches the level of the plate. The shoe in **Figure 16** is not level, while the one in **Figure**

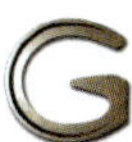

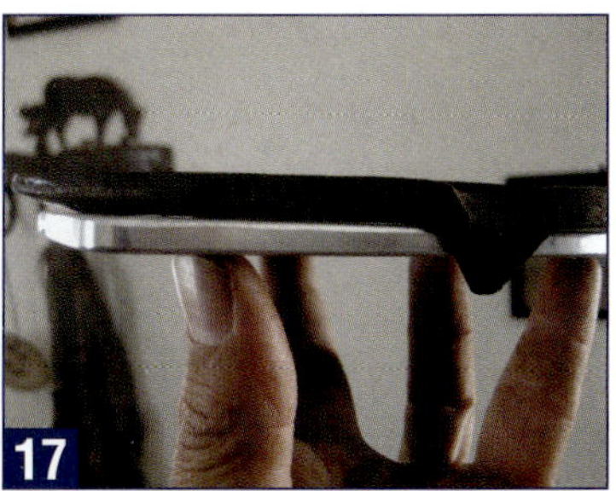

Shoe that is level.

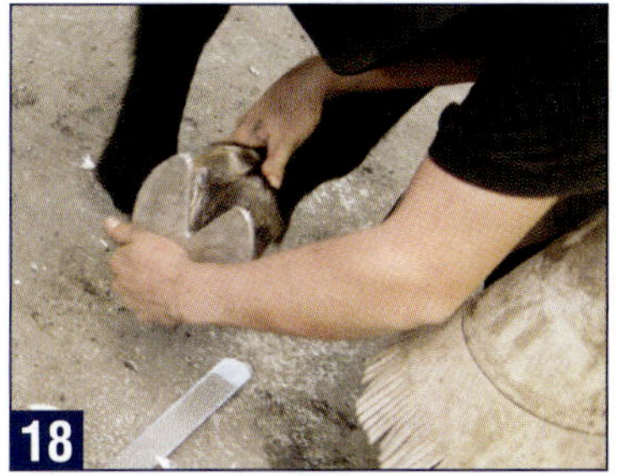

Cody using the plate to check the level of a trimmed foot.

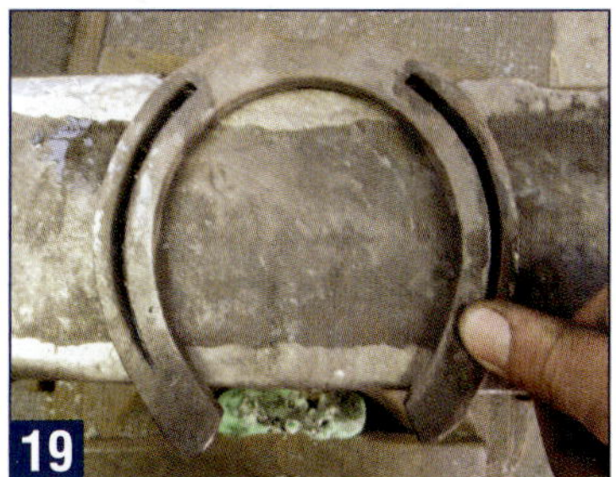

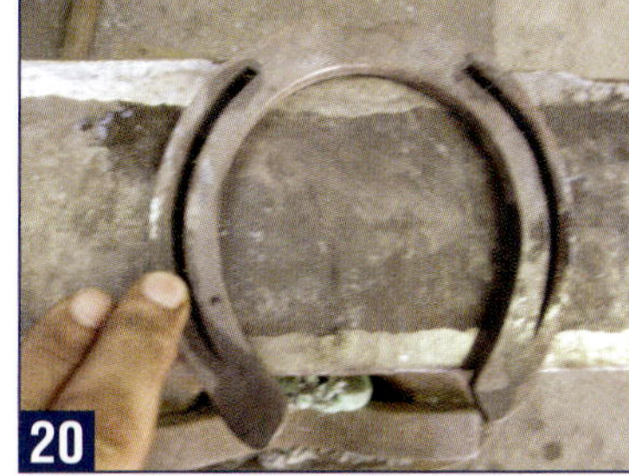

Checking level by pushing on the shoe sitting on the anvil.

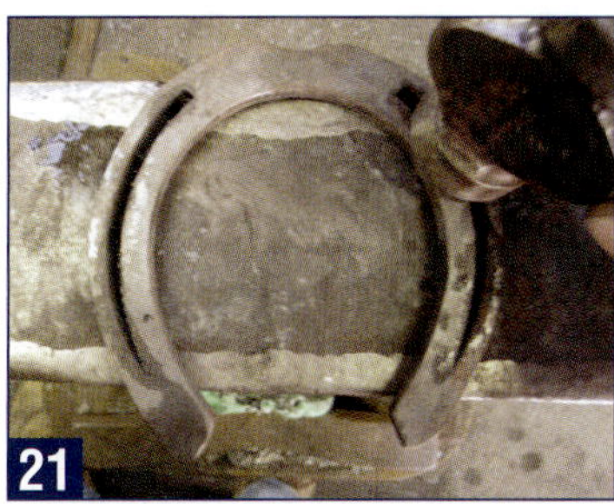

Using a hammer to check level on a hot shoe.

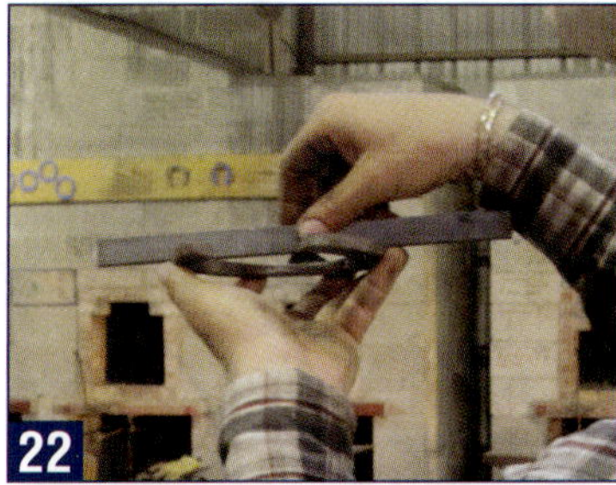

Looking at the area of the shoe that is in contact with the bar stock.

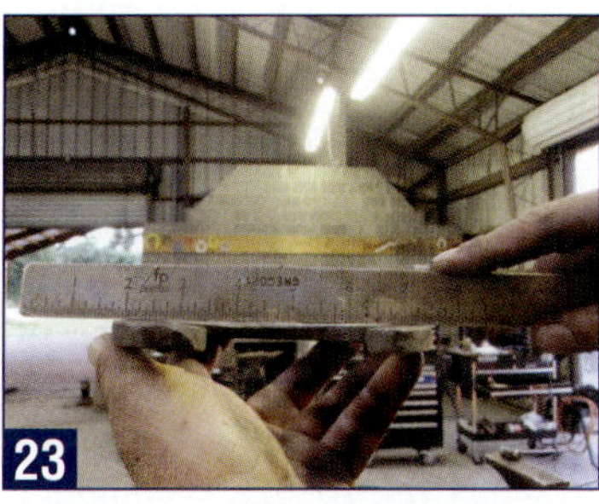

Using a ruler the same as I was using the bar stock in Figure 22.

17 is. This level judging plate can also be used on feet, as recommended by Professor Russell in the last century **(Figure 18)**. The plate pictured was made for me by a farrier friend of mine named Kent Misner, CJF. He helps judge AFA Certifications at the school, and when I complimented a plate he was using, he made me a couple. How many industries have stuff like that happen? Probably not even a fraction compared to the farrier industry. Kent sent those plates to me, and I called to ask what I owed, and he wouldn't even take anything for postage.

Another helpful method to judge level is by placing the shoe on the face of a flat anvil and either getting down to eye level with the shoe or pressing around the outside of the shoe to see if there are any gaps. If it is cold, you can use your hands **(Figures 19-20)**, but use a hammer or tongs if it is still hot **(Figure 21)**.

When a shoe is ready to nail, you want to insure that there is contact with the outside of the hoof wall and not with the sole on the inside of the web. To determine this, hold the shoe at eye level and draw a piece of bar stock or a ruler across the shoe to see where there is contact **(Figures 22-23)**. If there is

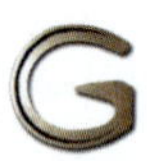

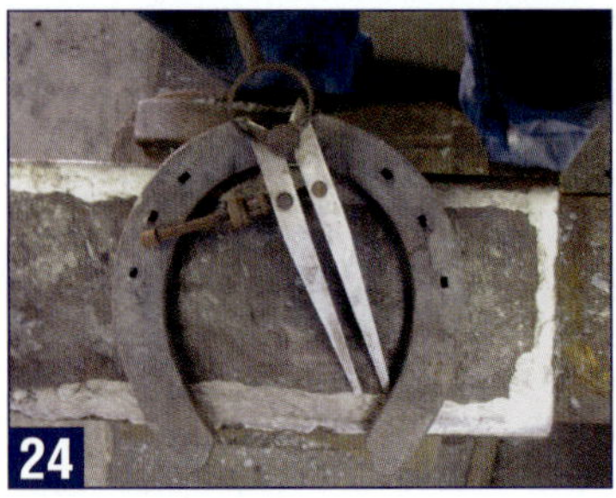

Pair of dividers.

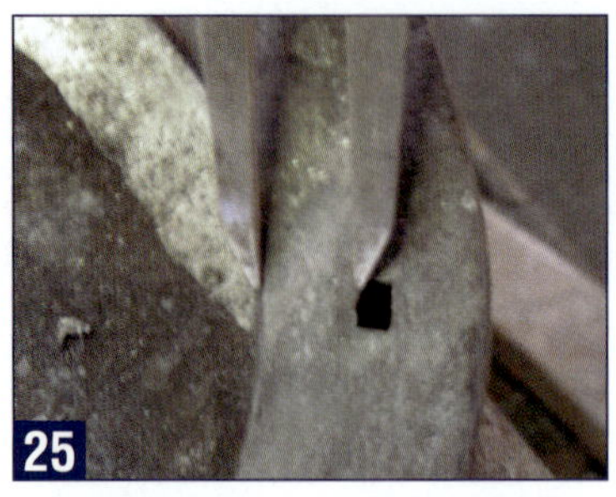

Checking the nail exit depth of the toe nail.

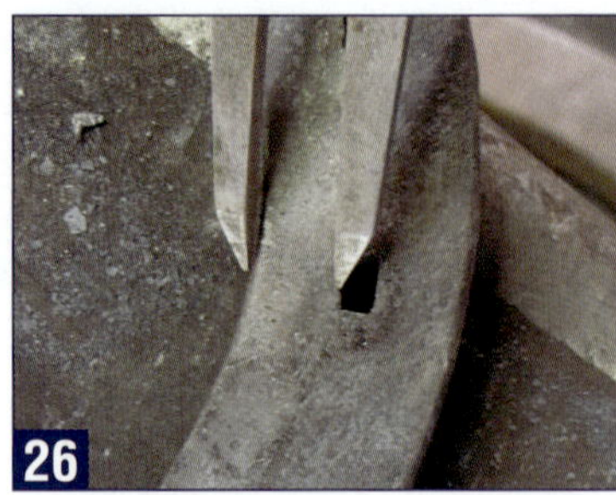

Comparing the nail exit depth of the second nail.

contact with the inside edge of the shoe, the shoe has not been properly leveled. Hammer around the inside hoof surface of the shoe to make certain that there is contact with the outside of the hoof wall. Flat bar stock naturally upsets on the inside of a bend and draws on the outside edge, which leads to this problem.

Beginners will often diminish the width of the stock from overforging on the horn. Take a pair of dividers and set them to the measurement of the stock. Move them around the finished shoe to find any areas where the shoe has been overforged. Dividers **(Figure 24)** are also helpful to determine the nail hole exit depth and compare the toenails to the heel nails. **Figures 25-27** show dividers that are set at the exit depth of the inside of the toe nail **(Figure 25)**. You can see how the second nail **(Figure 26)** and heel nail **(Figure 27)** are at different exit depths.

Ask other tradesmen to help you and judge your work. When you are at a clinic, if the clinician asks for a volunteer to clinch, nail, pull shoes, or whatever, be that volunteer. Doing so may be a little intimidating, but you are certain to get some feedback.

One final thought in this chapter. Throughout this industry, we have people who have not been proven competent, but may be quite charismatic and vocal. If you want to be great at anything, mimic those that have shown their competence, and not just those that talk of it. Why did I begin hot fitting when I did? Because the best in the world were all hot fitting. There are only 35 FWCF farriers alive right now and guess what? Almost all of them who still shoe, shoe hot. There is only a fraction of farriers who are able to achieve the status of AFA Certified Journeyman Farrier. Well, guess what? Those that have are mostly hot shoeing.

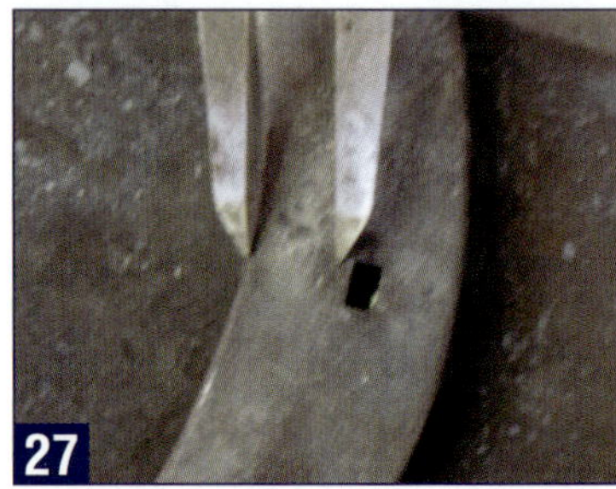

Comparing the nail exit depth of the heel nail.

I never set out to be an adequate or average anything, and most of the people I know are the same. Do you know anyone that gets up in the morning and says to themselves, "I hope that I just barely do good enough today." No, you don't. I don't either.

Surround yourself with people who have proven their ability to reach a measurable high standard. It is hard to soar like an eagle if you are surrounded by turkeys. By competing, measuring yourself against the best, and striving to be like the best, you will find that one day, you are that farrier whom the beginner looks at, hoping to someday achieve what you have achieved. It is easy to get sidetracked with slick salesmanship and fancy product. Inventory has replaced a lot of skills in this trade. I hope you decide to keep the standards of good craftsmanship alive. Not just for your own benefit, but for that wonderful animal that this is really all about — the horse.

REFERENCES

The content of this book has come from the experiences I have enjoyed in a career as a farrier and farrier educator. Part of that has meant the creation of a library, and a zest for reading about farriery. Although I do not think that there are any direct quotes out of any one book, these are the ones that have influenced this work the most as well as provided a world of knowledge as I came across issues in my own work that needed answers. Any omission of influence is completely accidental.

Budras K-D., Sack W.O., Rock S. (2003) *Anatomy of the Horse, An Illustrated Text, Fourth Edition*. Schlutersche GmbH & Co. Hanover, Germany.

Clayton H.M., Flood P.F., Rosenstein D.S., Mandeville, D. (2005) *Clinical Anatomy of the Horse*. Mosby Elsevier.

Curtis S.J. (Ed). (2002) *Corrective Farriery, A Textbook of Remedial Horseshoeing, Volume I*. Newmarket Farriery Consultancy, England.

Curtis S.J. (1999) Farriery - *Foal to Racehorse*. Newmarket Farriery Consultancy, England.

Denoix J-M. (2000) *The Equine Distal Limb*. Iowa Sate University Press/Ames, Iowa.

Dollar J.A.W., Wheatley A. (1897) (1993) *A Handbook of Horseshoeing*. Centaur Forge Ltd.

Floyd A.E., Mansmann R.A., (2007) *Equine Podiatry*. Saunders, Elsevier.

Grossman D.G., (1938) *The Anatomy of the Domestic Animals*. W.B. Saunders Company.

Harris S.E., (1993) *Horse Gaits, Balance and Movement*. Simon & Schuster Macmillan Company.

Harrison J.C., (1968) *Care and Training of the Trotter and Pacer*. The United States Trotting Association.

Hedge J. (Ed) (2003) *Photos and Drawings for Conformation and Anatomy*. Equine Research Inc.

Hickman J., Humphrey, M., (1988) *Hickman's Farriery. A Complete Illustrated Guide. Second Edition*. J.A. Allen & Co.

Holmes C.M., (1949) *The Principles and Practice of Horse-Shoeing*. The Farriers' Journal Publishing Co. Ltd.

Lungwitz A., Adams, J.W., (1884) (1904) *Horseshoeing*. J.B. Lippincott Company, (originally) Oregon State University Press. (facsimile edition).

Miller M.E., (2010) *The Mirage of the Natural Foot*. Michael E. Miller.

Pollitt C.C. (1996) *Color Atlas of the Horse's Foot*. Mosby – Wolfe.

Price H., Fisher R., (1989) *Shoeing For Performance*. The Crowood Press.

Richardson M.T. (Ed) (1890) (1991) *The Practical Horseshoer*.

Rooney J.R. (1998) *The Lame Horse*. The Russell Meerdink Company, Ltd. USA.

Russell W. (1903) (1987) *Scientific Horseshoeing*. Loose Change Publications.

Simpson S.J. (2005) *The Contemporary Horseshoer*. J. Scott Simpson, USA.

Stashak T.S. (Ed) (1987) *Adams' Lameness in Horses, 4th Edition*. Lea and Febiger.

Smythe, R.H. (1993) *Horse Structure and Movement*. J.A. Allen & Co. Ltd.

In addition to these books, I have been a voracious reader of our trade magazines, and have had the joy of reading many years of these great magazines, some of them now no longer being published. Those that are no longer in print are:

Anvil Magazine. Editor, Rob Edwards.

Loose Shoe. Editor, Craig Trnka.

The ones that are still in print that I read are:

American Farriers Journal. Editor, Frank Lessiter.

Forge Magazine. Editor, Gill Harris.

Professional Farrier

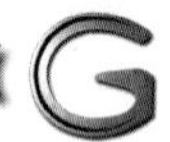

INDEX

A

Abscess 403-412
Acrylics 288
Adams, Bill 215
Allen, Wayne, CJF 655
Aluminum 578-589
  Welding 581-585
American Farriers Association 4, 671
Anatomy terminology 45-49
Angles 145-150, 159
Angular Limb Deformities, (ALD) 159
Anesthesia, (regional) 395-396
Annular ligaments 99, 114
Anvils:
  General information 31
  Round-horned 17
  Stand 17
Apprenticeship 3
Apron 13
Army School of Farriery 24, 25
Arteries 49, 126-127
Associateship of the Worshipful Company of Farriers 4
Association of Brazilian Farriers 672-673
  Exam 683
Avolio, Ed 30

B

Back (gait) 184
Bailey, Mike, CJF 32
Bandage bow 492
Bars, (hoof) 56-57
Bar shoes:
  Aluminum 581-585
  Egg Bars 551-560
  G-bar 561-568
  Heart Bars 561-568, 634-643
  Patten Bar 569-572, 602-610
  Shaping 255-257
  Straight Bars 536-550, 615-621
  Z-bar 573-577, 611-614
Bar Stock 312
Base Narrow 164, 174
Base Wide 164, 174
Bell, Ivon, FWCF (hons) 3, 237
Beveridge, Sandy, FWCF 672
Bench-kneed 164
Blood supply, see Vascular system 126-130
Blood spavin 515
Bog spavin 515
Bone spavin 515-518
Bones 47
  Development 65
  Parts of bones 66-67
  Types of bones 65
Boots:
  Overreach 191
  Scalpers 192
  Speedy cutting boot 194
  Splint 187-188
Bowed Tendons 491-492
Bowlegged, see carpus varus 163, 170, 174
Bradley, Dan, CJF 273
Brazing 320-321
Broken back 160
Broken bones 493-494
Broken forward 160
Broken in 165
Broken out 165
Brushing 186-188
Buck kneed 161-162
Bucked shins 495
Bulbs 61

C

Calcaneus 79-81, 95
Calf kneed 161-162
Caulks 347-349
Camped behind 165-166
Camped in front 161, 166
Canker 413-414
Cannon bone 83
Canter 183
Capped elbow 496-497
Capped hock 496-497
Capsular ligament 100, 120
Carpal joints 94
Carpitis 170, 498-500
Carpus 75
  Diagrams 75-78
Carpus valgus, knock-kneed 163, 170, 174
Carpus varus, bowlegged 163, 170, 174
Cartilage 56-66, 84-86, 90
Casey, Steve, AWCF 533
Cattle 292-293
Caudal 46
Central sulcus 61
Certified Farrier, AFA 3
Certified Journeyman Farrier, AFA 3
Certified Tradesman Farrier, AFA 3
Check ligaments:
  Radial – superior 98, 104
  Subcarpal – inferior 98, 105
  Subtarsal 98, 105
Chondrocompedal ligament 98, 106
Chondrocoronal ligament 99, 106
Chondrotendinous ligament 99, 106
Chondroungular ligament 99, 106
Circumflex artery 126-129
Cleft 408-409
Clark, Tom 26, 33
Clinch block 14, 343-345
Clinch cutter 13
Clinch gouge 14
Clinching 271-277
Clinchers 14
Clinkers 29
Clipping hammer 19
Clips:
  Cold fitting 259-261, 587-588
  Fitting 258-261
  Forging 327-331, 340-341
Clinchers 273-275
Clinching 271-277
Club foot 415-417
Coal 28
Cobrasox 431-432
Coffin bone, see P3, pedal bone, third phalanx, distal phalanx 88-90, 97
Coffin bone fractures 418-421
Coffin joint 96
Coke 30
Collateral cartilages 90
Collateral ligaments 100, 121
Collateral sesamoidian ligament 99, 112
Colvin, Russell, CJF 542
Commissures 50, 61
Common extensor tendon, see Main extensor tendon 122-125
Concussion 141-144
Conformation:
  Pelvic limb 165-166
  Thoracic limb 160-165
Corium 46, 51
Cornification 62
Corns 422-424

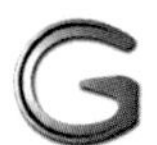

Coronary band 53-59, 62
Coronary bone, see P2, short pastern,
 second phalanx, middle phalanx........ 86-87, 96-97
Coronary cushion........ 53
Coronary venous plexus 129
Corrective shoeing........ 389
Cow hocked 165-166
Cracks:
 Between the bulbs 477-478
 Hoof........ 425-433
 Lacing........ 428-430
 Quarter........ 463-467
 Repair 290-291, 427-433, 464-465
 Vertical, see sand cracks 425-433
Cranial........ 46
Crease nail puller........ 14
Creaser 20
Creasing, see fullering........ 331-333
Crossfiring 192-192
Cupped bar shoe 508-510
Cupped break-over shoe........ 466-467, 475
Cupped shoe 436-437
Cresty neck 444
Curb 501-502
Curtis, Simon, FWCF........ 33, 283-284, 674
Cut-out under the knees........ 161-162

D

Daniels, Bruce, CJF........ 236
Deep sesamoidian ligament, (X or cruciate)........ 99, 110
Deep flexor tendon 122-125, 152
Deleonardo, Mike, CJF 661
Developmental orthopedic disorders, (DOD)........ 159
Digit 45, 85
Digital cushion, (plantar cushion)........ 61, 126, 132
Diploma of the Worshipful Company of Farriers 4
Distal........ 46
Distal digital annular ligament 99, 114
Distal navicular ligament, see Impar........ 100, 115-116
Distal interphalangeal joint 91-92, 96
Distal phalanx, see P3, pedal bone, coffin bone, third phalanx 88-90, 97
Distal sesamoid, see Navicular........ 86
Dorsal........ 45
DRASTA........ 399
Draw steel 313
Dropped sole........ 435-437

E

Egg Bar Shoe 551-560
Elbow Hitting........ 194
Epiphyseal plate, see physis, (growth plate) 65-67
Epson Salt Poultice........ 410, 437
Equi-Pak 280-282, 420
Equilibrium shoe 508
Equilox........ 284-289
Extend 46
Extended Heels........ 253-255
Extensions........ 594-599
 Acrylic and Urethane 282-287
 Lateral........ 597-598
 Lateral heel........ 594-597
 Toe........ 417, 597-599

F

Farley, Dave, CF 590
Farrier International Testing System, (FITS)........ 673-674
Fascia 48
Fellowship of the Worshipful Company of Farriers 4
Ferrie, Jim, FWCF........ 470
Fetlock 84-86, 91-93, 96-97
Figure-eight 352-353
Final common pathway 438-439
Finishing feet........ 276-277
Finishing shoes 379-380
Firepots 25-26
Fires 25-30
First phalanx, see P1, long pastern, proximal phalanx. 86-87, 96-97
Fisher, Phil, CJF........ 400
Flares........ 624-627
Flex 46
Flexural deformities........ 171-172
Flux:
 Iron Mountain welding 542
 Red Mountain brazing 320
Foot 50-64
Foot stand........ 22-23
Fore punch 21
Forge
 Coal 26, 2
 Coke 25, 29
 Gas........ 17, 30
 Lighting 28
Forging........ 188-191
Founder........ 438-449
Four-point trim........ 304-306
Frog........ 61
Frog eyes........ 323-324
Front limb 68-70
Fuller, see creaser 20
Fullering, see creasing 331-333
Furquim, Fabio, GF 674

G

G-bar shoe........ 561-568
G.E. Forge and Tool........ 274
Gait:
 2-beat........ 180
 3-beat........ 180
 4-beat........ 180
 Definition 178
 Diagonal 180
 Faults 185
 Lateral........ 180
Gallop 184
Garner, Bob........ 542-543
Gillis, Matt, CJF 215
Glue-ons........ 287-293
Goodall, David, Capt. RN. 672
Gravel........ 308-309
Greenburg, Stuart........ 333
Gregory, Mike........ 656

H

Hague, Brent, DVM........ 453
Hammers:
 Clipping........ 19
 Driving 15
 Rounding........ 19
Handmade shoes:
 Concave........ 381-386
 Finishing........ 379-380
 Fronts........ 371-378
 Hinds 359-370
 Measuring feet for........ 236-238
Hawthorne's Products........ 411
 Hot Nail........ 411
Hayes, Steve, CJF........ 321
Heart bar shoe........ 561-568, 634-643
Heartland Horseshoeing School exam 684
Heel caulks........ 347-349
Heels 325-327, 338
Hereford School, (England):
 Blacksmithing 25
 Farriery 25
Hershfield, Abner 26
Hind limb........ 71-75
Hock, see tarsus 79-81
Hockey stick 538-541
Hoof........ 50
 Angles 145-150
 Avulsion 450-451
 Circulation........ 144-145

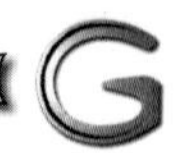

Cradle 22
Drawing 50
Gouge 274-275
Grooving 640-643
Growth 62
Knife 16
Moisture 63
Nippers 14
Regions 50-52
Shape 63
Stands 22
Testers 16, 392-394
Wall 54
Trimming 218-228

Horn:
Intertubular 55-56
Tubular 55-56

Horse:
Anatomy 43-156
Handling 198-206
Psychology 207-208

Hospital plate 590-593
Hot fitters 20
Hot fitting 245, 262-265
Houston, Jeff 39, 263
Humerus 68-70
Hygroma 528-529

I

Impar ligament, see distal navicular 100, 115-116
Intertubular horn 55-56
Interference 186-187
Interosseus 100, 118
Intersesamoidian ligament 99, 112
Iron Mountain flux 542-543

J

Jar caulks 243, 320-321
Jim Keith Tools 273
Joints 47, 90, 93
Digit 96
Front limb 91
Hind limb 92

K

Kaeco Abscess Kits 412, 459
Keg shoes 239, 242
Shaping 245-248
Keith, Jim, CJF 322, 663
Keratoma 452-454
Kicking horse 202-204
Killingbeck, DVM 671
King, Rodney, CJF, AWCF 590
Kirkpatrick, Bill 289
Knee hitting 186-187

Knees:
Back at 161-162
Bench 161-162
Calf 161-162
Cut out under 161-162
Offset 161-164, 167-168

Knife
Hoof 16
Loop 16, 221-222

Knock-kneed 163, 170, 174
Knuckling over 415-417
Kohler, Jack, CJF 236

L

Lameness:
Cause 401-402
Definition 389
Examination 390-398
Grades 398-399
Treatments 399-400

Laminae 62, 164
Laminitis 438-449
Lateral 46
Lateral extensor tendon 122-125
Lechonowski, Claudia, DVM 673, 683
Leg 45, 75
Definition 45, 75
Ligaments 48, 98-121
Annular 98, 114
Capsular 100, 120
Check 98, 104-105
Collateral 100, 121
Interosseus 100, 118
Navicular 100, 115-116
Of the ergot 98, 103
Of the collateral cartilages 98-99, 106
Pastern 100, 117
Plantar 100, 119
Sesamoidian 99, 108-113
Suspensory 98, 101
T – ligament (see Tranverse lamina) 99, 107

Limb 45
Front – thoracic 69
Hind – pelvic 71

Limb deformities 159-172
Long pastern bone, see P1, first phalanx, proximal phalanx. 86-87, 96-97
Long extensor tendon, see Main extensor tendon 122-125
Lost shoes 653-654
Lymphatic system 132-133

M

Magic Cushion 411
Magnetic resonance imaging, MRI 398
Main extensor tendon 122-125
Marcotte, John, DVM ....406, 448, 456, 457, 474, 500, 503, ...507, 511, 519, 524-525, 606
Marshall, Bob 315, 327, 371, 662
Martin, Christine, DVM 603, 617
Martin, Edward, FWCF 299
Medial 46
Medial lift bar shoe 475-476
Merocrine gland 406
Middle phalanx, see P2, short pastern, second phalanx, coronary bone 86-87, 96-97
Miller, Michael, MD, CJF, FWCF 25, 216, 303, 352, 411, 438, 542, 656, 676
Miller, Robbie, CF, (FITS) 284-287
Middle sesamoidian ligament, (V or oblique) 99, 109
Mirage of the Natural Foot 216, 303
Misner, Kent, CJF 688-689
Moon, Grant, AWCF 660, 686
Morgan, Dallas, CJF, DWCF 32
Morrison, Scott, DVM 406, 442, 454, 457, 461, 468, 490, 503, 507
Muldoon, John 639
Muscles 48
Mustad Delta Hoofcare Center 274
Mustad hospital pad 607

N

Nail holes 322-325, 338-340
Nailing 266-270
Nails 266-267
Nance, Marilyn 603
Narrow in front 163-164

Navicular
Bar shoe 458
Bone, see distal sesamoid. 86
Bursa, (podotrochlear bursa) 107
Ligaments 100, 115-116
Syndrome 455-460

Near 46
Neurovascular bundle 126, 128, 131
Nerves 49, 131-132
Noavel Headstall 204-206, 208
Northern Melbourne Institute of TAFE 24
Nuclear scintigraphy 397-398
Nutrient foramen 66-67

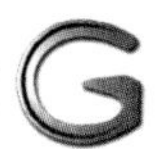

O

O'Dwyer 32
Obel lameness grades 398-399
Off 46
Offset knees 164, 167
Onion heel shoe 459
Open roller shoe....508
Osselets 503-504
Ossification 65, 67
Overreach....188-191, 306
Ozark School of Blacksmithing 26

P

P1, see long pastern, first phalanx, proximal phalanx. 86-87, 96-97
P2, see short pastern, second phalanx,
  middle phalanx, coronary bone....86-87, 96-97
P3, see pedal bone, coffin bone, third phalanx, distal phalanx 88-90, 97
Pace....184
Packing 411
Pads....411-412
Palmar....45
Palmar annular ligament....99, 114
Palmar digital nerves 131-133
Paracuneal sulci, see commisures 61
Pardoe, Chris, AWCF 507-508
Pastern:
  Angles and axis 145-150, 160
  Bones....85-87
  Joint 96
  Ligaments....100, 117
Patella....68, 73
Pathological shoeing....389
Patten bar shoe....512-514, 569-572, 602-610
Pedal bone, see P3, coffin bone, distal phalanx, 3rd phalanx 88-90, 97
Pedal osteitis 461-462
Pelvic limb....68, 71-74, 92
Periople....53
Periosteum 65-66
Peroneus tertius.... 139-140
Physis, epiphyseal plate, growth plate....65-67
Pinfire....495
Plantar....45
Plantar cushion, see also, digital cushion....61, 126, 132
Plantar ligament....100, 119
Plexuses:
  Coronary....129
  Dorsal....129
  Solar 129
Podotrochlear bursa, see navicular....107
Poor, Jim, CJF....25
Post-legged 165-166, 171
Pritchel....21
Pritchelling.... 324-325
Propane 17
Proximal....46
Proximal digital annular ligament 99, 114
Proximal phalanx, see P1, long pastern, first phalanx. 86-87, 96-97
Pulloffs....13
Punches....21

Q

Quarter cracks....463-467
Quittor.... 468-469

R

Radial check ligament, (superior) 98, 104
Radial nerve paralysis....505
Radius 68-70
Radiography....397
Rasp:
  Finish....16
  Handles....16
  Regular 15
Rasping a foot.... 223-225
Rasping a shoe 379-380, 584-585
Reciprocal apparatus 139-140
Red Mountain flux....320
Reddin, Ric, DVM....303
Renchin, Red, CJF....661
Resection.... 447-448
Resets....234
Richardson, M.T. 264
Richmond, Tom, CF 660
Rikard, Mark, CF....352
Ring exercise 336-337
Ringbone....506-510
Rocker toe....248-250
Rolled toe....250-251
Rotational deformities 159
Ruler, Brass....22

S

Safety 7-8
Sand cracks 425-433
Saucer fracture....493
Scalping 191-192
Scapula.... 68-70
  Angle 158
Schwartz, Marvin 281
Scotch hobble 200
Second phalanx, see P2, see short pastern,
  middle phalanx, coronary bone....86-87, 96-97
Sensitive structures, see coriums....46, 51
Sesamoid bones 84
Sesamoidean ligaments 99, 108-113, 153-154
Sesamoiditis....521-522
Setting shoes 267-269
Severed tendons 511-514
Shaping 245-248
Sheared heels 470-472
Shin buck 495
Shoe boil 496-497
Shoe spreaders 16
Shoeing apron....13
Shoeing box 13
Shoeing rig:
  Trailer....35
  Truck 35
Shoes:
  Aluminum 578-589
  Aluminum egg bar 584-585
  Aluminum straight bar....581-584
  Concave....381-386
  Cupped 436-437
  Egg bar 551-560
  Eventers....240-241
  G-bar....561-568
  Glue on 287-293
  Heart bar....561-568, 634-643
  Keg 239-242
  Lateral extension 594-596
  Onion heel 459
  Navicular bar....458
  Open roller 508
  Patten bar....569-572, 602-610
  Rim....239-241
  Shaping....350-351
  Sigafoos....287-289
  Square toed....251-253
  St. Croix 239-240, 242, 244
  Straight bar....536-550, 615-621
  Toe extension....597-599
  W-shoe....561-568, 634-643
  Wedged aluminum 459-460
  Z-bar....573-577, 611-614
Short pastern bone, see P2, second phalanx,
  middle phalanx, coronary bone....86-87, 96-97
Short sesamoidian ligaments....99, 111
Showen, Dave, CJF....662
Sickle hocks....165-166, 175
Sidebone 473-476
Sigafoos shoes 287-289

Soft heel cracks....477-478
Solar....46
Solar corium....59-60
Sole....59, 154
Sole bruises....479-481
Sound Horse Technologies....287-289, 431
Souza, Flavio, GF, CF....673
Spavin....515-518
Speedy-cutting....193
Splint bones....82
Splints....519-520
Sprained suspensory ligament....521-523
Square-toe
- Egg bar....618-619
- Hind shoe....251-253

St. Croix Forge....239, 242, 274
Standing under....161
Stay apparatus....134-140
Step....178-180
Stifled and stifle lameness....524-525
Stone Well Bodies....39
Straight bar shoes....536-550, 615-621
Straight behind, see also post-legged....165-166, 171, 175
Stratum externum, see stratum tectorium....54-59
Stratum internum....54-59
Stratum medium....54-59
Stratum tectorium, see stratum externum....54-59
Street nails....404-405
Stride....178-179
Stringhalt....527
Studs....243-244
Stumbling....185
Subcarpal check ligament (inferior)....98, 105, 152
Subtarsal check ligament....98, 105
Sulcus....61
Super Fast....282-285, 290-292
Superficial flexor tendon....122-125, 152
Superficial sesamoidian ligament, (Y or straight)....99, 108
Surgical shoeing....389
Suspensory ligament....98, 101, 152-153
Suspensory navicular ligament....99, 115
Suspensory sprain....521-523
Sutton, James, MRCVS....672
Sway backed, (lordosis)....172
Synovial fluid....96
Synovial joints....90-97

T

T-Square....229-230, 346-347
Tarsal joints....95
Tarsus....79
- Diagrams....79-81

Tendons....48, 122-125
- Deep flexor....122-125
- Lateral extensor....122-125
- Main extensor....122-125
- Superficial flexor....122-125

The Practical Horseshoer....264
Therapeutic shoeing....389
Thermography....398
Third phalanx, see P3, pedal bone, coffin bone, distal phalanx....88-90, 97
Thoroughpin....527
Thrush....482-483
Tibia....68, 74
Toe bend....337-338
Toe-dragging....195
Toed-in....164
Toed-out....164
Tongs:
- Farrier....18
- Making....354-358
- Position....317-318

Tools....12-23
Trailers....253-255
Traction....239-240
Transverse lamina, see T- ligament....99, 107
Trimming....218-228
Trot....182
Turley, Frank....26,32, 218, 333
Twitch....202

U

Ultrasound....396, 523
Upsetting steel....313-314

V

Valgus....163
Varus....163
Vascular system....126-130
Veins....49, 129-130
Venogram....130
Venous plexuses....129
Vettec....280
Vibram hoof pads....411
Vise....18

W

W-shoe....416-417, 561-568, 634-643
Walk....181
Wall (hoof)....53-59
Ward, Danny, CJF....685
Water content of hoof....63
Watson, Mark, AWCF....676
Wear plates....585-587
Wedged aluminum....458-459
Welding....314, 333-335, 341-343
- Egg bar....553-555
- Frog plate (W-shoe and heart bar)....562-564
- Jump or "drop-tong"....345-346
- Patten bar....571
- Straight bar....542-545
- Z-bar shoe....574-576

Wheat, Rick....204
White line....57
White line disease....484-490
Windpuff, (articular, tendinous)....528-529
Wire brushes....21, 22
Worshipful Company of Farriers....4, 670-672
- Crest....679
- Written exams....681-683

X

X-rays
- Abscess....406, 412
- Angle....147
- Carpitis....500
- Diagnostic....397
- Founder....441-443, 449
- Fractured coffin bone....419
- Fractured navicular bone....457
- Keratoma....453
- Navicular....457
- Osselets....504
- Pedal osteitis....461
- Quittor....469
- Ringbone....507-509
- Saucer fracture....493
- Sesamoiditis....522
- Severed tendons....511
- Sidebone....474
- Spavin....516
- Splints....519
- Stifle....524-525
- Venogram....130
- White line disease....490

Z

Z-bar shoe....573-577, 611-614